Pediatric Kidney Disease

Franz Schaefer · Larry A. Greenbaum
Editors

Pediatric Kidney Disease

Third Edition

Volume II

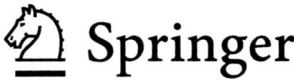 Springer

Editors
Franz Schaefer
Division of Pediatric Nephrology
Heidelberg University
Heidelberg, Germany

Larry A. Greenbaum
Emory School of Medicine
Emory University
Atlanta, GA, USA

Previously published as COMPREHENSIVE PEDIATRIC NEPHROLOGY with Elsevier, The Netherlands, 2008

Springer-Verlag Berlin Heidelberg 2016
ISBN 978-3-031-11664-3   ISBN 978-3-031-11665-0   (eBook)
https://doi.org/10.1007/978-3-031-11665-0

This Springer imprint is published by the registered company Springer Nature Switzerland AG
The registered company address is: Gewerbestrasse 11, 6330 Cham, Switzerland

Preface

We are delighted to welcome you to the new edition of Pediatric Kidney Disease. As in the previous versions of this textbook, our goal has been to bridge the gap between multivolume "library-level" books and numerous pocket handbooks available in our specialty. We hope that Pediatric Kidney Disease will continue to be the standard textbook for reference to busy clinicians, who need to obtain an up-to-date, easy-to-read, review of virtually all kidney disorders that occur in children.

Following a critical review of the previous edition and the downloadable figures of each chapter, the table of contents was revised to optimally reflect the needs and expectations of our readers. One-third of the chapters were written by new authors. For chapters with unchanged authorship, each author was asked to thoroughly update the materials, which has resulted in extensive revisions of most chapters. A number of new topics have been included, such as metabolic disorders affecting the kidney, pediatric kidney tumors, sickle cell nephropathy, diabetic kidney disease, and strategic choices in kidney replacement therapy.

For all chapters, we have requested the authors to ensure the relevance and clinical usefulness of their chapter for busy pediatric and pediatric nephrology clinicians as well as the multidisciplinary team members. We hope that the included material and its presentation are of value and will contribute to the expansion of knowledge in the field of pediatric nephrology.

Heidelberg, Germany Franz Schaefer
Atlanta, GA, USA Larry A. Greenbaum

Contents

Part VII

Renal Tubular Disorders

Differential Diagnosis and Management of Fluid, Electrolyte and Acid-Base Disorders

34

Giacomo D. Simonetti, Sebastiano A. G. Lava, Gregorio P. Milani, and Mario G. Bianchetti

Introduction

In this chapter, the disturbances of fluid, electrolyte and acid-base balance will be addressed in different subchapters that deal with water, salt, K^+, acid-base, Ca^{++}, Mg^{++}, and phosphate. This traditional presentation is didactically relevant. It is worth mentioning, however, that more than one disturbance in fluid, electrolyte and acid-base

G. D. Simonetti (✉)
Pediatric Institute of Southern Switzerland, EOC, Bellinzona, Switzerland

Università della Svizzera Italiana, Lugano, Switzerland
e-mail: giacomo.simonetti@eoc.ch

S. A. G. Lava
Pediatric Cardiology Unit, Department of Pediatrics, Centre Hospitalier Universitaire Vaudois (CHUV) and University of Lausanne, Lausanne, Switzerland
e-mail: webmaster@sebastianolava.ch

G. P. Milani
Pediatric Unit, Fondazione IRCCS Ca'Granda Ospedale Maggiore Policlinico, Milan, Italy

Department of Clinical Sciences and Community Health, Università degli Studi di Milano, Milan, Italy

Pediatric Insitute of Southern Switzerland and Universtity of Southern Switzerland, Bellinzona, Switzerland

M. G. Bianchetti
University of Southern Switzerland, Lugano, Switzerland
e-mail: mario.bianchetti@usi.ch

homeostasis often concurrently occurs in the same subject.

Overall, the etiology of fluid, electrolyte and acid-base disorders is straightforward, since the most commonly occurring causes are easily recognized on clinical grounds. In some cases, however, the cause is not readily apparent, and a comprehensive systematic approach is recommended. The diagnostic approach to initially unexplained "isolated" disturbances involving the fluid, electrolyte and the acid-base balance should include both very careful history and clinical examination as well as the concurrent assessment of an extended "electrolyte spectrum". In the setting of initially unclassified and apparently "isolated" disturbances involving the fluid, electrolyte and acid-base balance, the concomitant measurement in blood of pH, pCO_2, HCO_3^-, Na^+, K^+, Cl^-, Ca^{++} (either total or ionized), Mg^{++}, inorganic phosphate, alkaline phosphatase, total protein level (or albumin), uric acid, urea and creatinine is advised.

Water and Salt

Introduction

Body Fluid Compartments

Water accounts for $\approx$50–75% of the body mass. The most significant determinants of the wide range in water content are age and gender: (a) the

© The Author(s), under exclusive license to Springer Nature Switzerland AG 2023
F. Schaefer, L. A. Greenbaum (eds.), *Pediatric Kidney Disease*,
https://doi.org/10.1007/978-3-031-11665-0_34

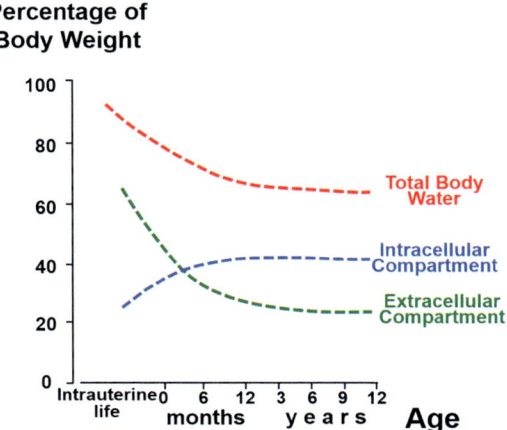

Fig. 34.1 Influence of age on the subdivision of total body water, intracellular fluid and extracellular fluid. For clinical purposes, "the rule of 3" is suggested: (1) total body water makes up 2/3 of the body mass; (2) the intracellular compartment contains 2/3 of the total body water; (3) the extracellular compartment is further subdivided into the interstitial and the intravascular compartments (blood volume), which contain 2/3 and 1/3 of the extracellular fluid, respectively

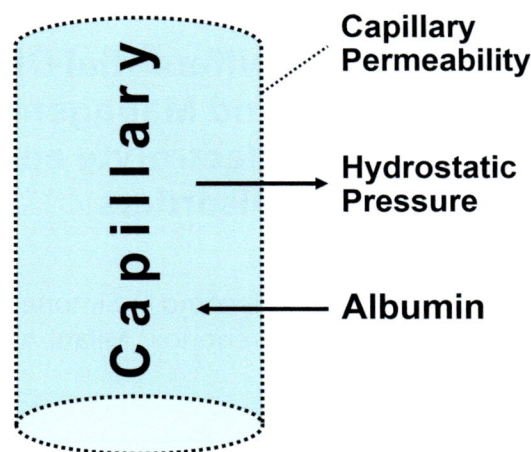

Fig. 34.2 Distribution of ultrafiltrate across the capillary membrane. The barrel-shaped structure represents a capillary. A high hydrostatic pressure or increased capillary permeability causes fluid to leave the vascular space. By contrast, an increased intravascular albumin concentration (and, therefore, an increased oncotic pressure) causes fluid to enter the vascular space

water content of a newborn, an adolescent and an elderly man are ≈75, ≈60 and ≈50%; (b) after puberty males generally have 2–10% higher water content than females (Fig. 34.1). The intracellular compartment contains about two-third of the total body water and the remaining is held in the extracellular compartment. The solute composition of the intracellular and extracellular fluid differs considerably because the sodium pump (=Na^+-K^+-ATPase) maintains K^+ in a primarily intracellular and Na^+ in a primarily extracellular location. Consequently, K^+ largely determines the intracellular and Na^+ the extracellular compartment [1–4]. The extracellular compartment is further subdivided into the interstitial and the total intravascular compartments (total blood volume), which contain ≈2/3 and ≈1/3 of the extracellular fluid [1–4], respectively (the transcellular fluid compartment, which comprises the digestive, cerebrospinal, intraocular, pleural, peritoneal and synovial fluids, will not be further addressed in this review).

The size of the total intravascular compartment is determined by the overall size of the extracellular fluid compartment and by the

Starling forces. Three major forces control the distribution of fluids across the capillary membrane (Fig. 34.2): (a) the hydrostatic pressure, which causes fluids to leave the vascular space, and; (b) the higher concentration of proteins in the intravascular compartment as compared with that in interstitial fluid, which causes fluids to enter the vascular space. This force, which is called oncotic pressure, is due both to the concentration gradient of albumin (blood proteins other than albumin account for 50% of the weight of proteins in blood but only for 25% of the oncotic pressure) as well to the fact that albumin is anionic and therefore attracts cations (largely Na^+) into the vascular compartment (Gibbs-Donnan effect). (c) Capillary permeability, which is a further modulator of the distribution of fluids across the capillary membrane (and can be increased, for example, during inflammatory states like infection, post-operatively or in the context of an idiopathic capillary leak syndrome).

Recent data suggest that an extrarenal system might also contribute to sodium homeostasis. Sodium might be stored on negatively charged glycosaminoglycans in the skin interstitium,

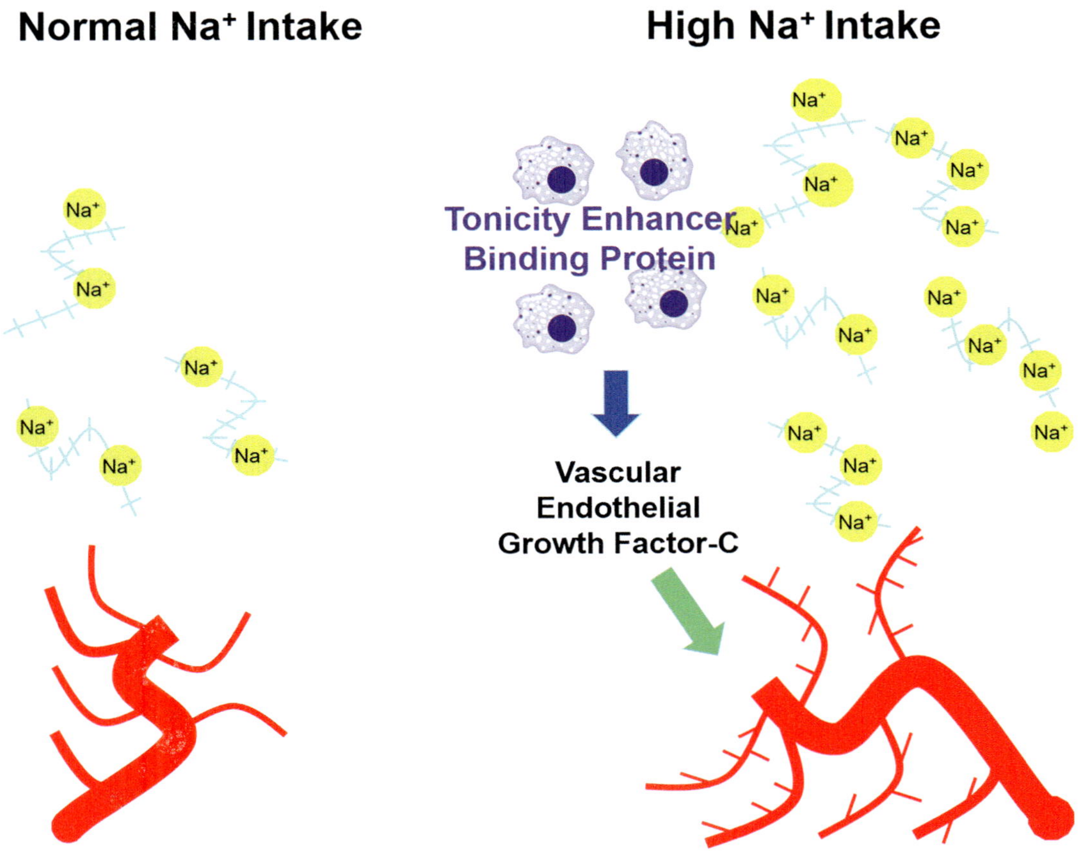

Normal Na⁺ Intake

High Na⁺ Intake

Fig. 34.3 Sodium is stored on negatively charged glycosaminoglycans in the skin interstitium. Excess sodium modulates lymphangiogenesis, and osmotically inactive sodium accumulates in the skin interstitium, binding proteoglycans. Excess sodium recruits macrophages, and subsequently activates within subcutaneous macrophages (cells with blue nucleus) a transcription factor, tonicity-enhanced binding protein, which in turn induces the production of the angiogenic protein vascular endothelial growth factor-C. Vascular endothelial growth factor-C stimulates lymphatic vessel (red) growth and creates a new fluid compartment, which buffers the increased body sodium (yellow) and ameliorates the tendency to excess body fluid linked with excess salt intake [5–7]

becoming osmotically inactive [5]. The skin interstitium might therefore represent a sort of fluid-buffering system, able to store sodium without commensurate water retention and potentially limiting accumulation of excess body fluid following high salt intake (Fig. 34.3) [6, 7].

Effective Circulating Volume

The total intravascular compartment is subdivided into the effective (≈ arterial) and the ineffective (≈ venous) compartment. Effective circulating volume denotes the part of the total intravascular compartment that is in the arterial system and is effectively perfusing the tissues.

The effective circulating volume is biologically more relevant than the total intravascular (respectively the ineffective) compartment and usually varies directly with the extracellular fluid volume. As a result, the regulation of extracellular fluid balance (by alterations in urinary Na⁺ excretion) and the maintenance of the effective circulating volume are intimately related. Na⁺ loading will tend to produce volume expansion, whereas Na⁺-loss (e.g., due to vomiting, diarrhea, or diuretic therapy) to volume depletion. The body responds to changes in effective circulating volume in two steps: (a) the change is sensed by the volume receptors that are located in the cardiopulmonary circulation, in the carotid sinuses and aortic arch, and in the kidney; (b) these receptors activate effectors that restore normovolemia by varying vascular resistance, cardiac output, and renal water and salt excretion. In brief, the non-renal receptors primarily govern the activity of the sympathetic nervous system and natriuretic peptides, whereas the renal receptors affect volume balance by modulating the renin-angiotensin II-aldosterone system [1–4].

In some settings the effective circulating volume is independent of the extracellular fluid volume. For example, among patients with heart failure the extracellular fluid volume is increased but these patients are effectively volume depleted due to the low volume of blood pumped by the heart [1–4].

Blood Osmolality: Measurement of Sodium

Osmolality is the concentration of all solutes in a given weight of water (the similar concept of osmolarity denotes the concentration of all of the solutes in a given volume of water). The total (or true) blood osmolality is equal to the sum of the osmolalities of the individual solutes in blood. Most osmoles in blood are Na^+ salts, with lesser contributions from other ions, glucose, and urea. However, under normal circumstances, the osmotic effect of the ions in blood can usually be estimated as two times the Na^+ concentration. *Blood osmolality* (in mosm/kg H_2O) can be measured directly (via determination of freezing point depression) or estimated from circulating Na^+, glucose and urea (in mmol/L[1]) as follows [3, 4, 8–12]:

$$\left(Na^+ \times 2\right) + glucose + urea$$

The *effective blood osmolality*, known colloquially as blood tonicity, is a further clinically significant entity, which denotes the concentration of solutes impermeable to cell membranes (Na^+, glucose, mannitol) and are therefore restricted to the extracellular compartment (osmoreceptors

sense effective blood osmolality rather than the total blood osmolality). These solutes are effective because they create osmotic pressure gradients across cell membranes leading to movement of water from the intracellular to the extracellular compartment. Solutes that are permeable to cell membranes (urea, ethanol, methanol) are ineffective solutes because they do not generate osmotic pressure gradients across cell membranes and therefore are not associated with such water shifts. Glucose is a unique solute because, at normal concentrations in blood, it is actively taken up by cells and therefore acts as an ineffective solute, but under conditions of impaired cellular uptake (like diabetes mellitus) it becomes an effective extracellular solute.

Since no direct measurement of effective blood osmolality (which is biologically more important than the total or true blood osmolality) is possible, the following equations are used to calculate this entity [3, 4, 8–12]:

$$\left(Na^+ \times 2\right) + glucose$$

measured total blood osmolality – urea

Plasma normally consists of about 93% water and 7% solids (proteins and lipids). Electrolytes are dissolved exclusively in the water portion of plasma. Blood Na^+ (normal range between 135 and 145 mmol/L) can be determined either by indirect or direct potentiometry. The two techniques show good agreement as long as protein and lipid concentrations are normal. However, while assessed by indirect potentiometry in diluted samples, increased protein or lipid concentrations result in spuriously low Na^+ (pseudo-hyponatraemia) whereas decreased protein or lipid concentrations result in spuriously high Na^+ (pseudo-hypernatraemia). A spuriously normal Na^+ value (pseudonormonatraemia) might also occur [13]. Direct potentiometry measures Na^+ in undlituted samples and avoids this problem. Therefore, it is the currently recommended technique [14].

Flame photometry, the traditional assay for circulating Na^+, measures the concentration of Na^+ per unit volume of solution, with a normal

---

[1]To obtain glucose in mmol/L divide glucose in mg/dL by 18. To obtain urea in mmol/L divide urea nitrogen in mg/dL by 2.8 or urea in mg/dL by 6.0.

range between 135 and 145 mmol/L. In fact, Na^+ is dissolved in plasma water, which accounts for 93% of the total volume of plasma. Ion selective electrodes, that have replaced flame photometry in most laboratories, determine the activity of Na^+ in plasma water, which ranges between 145 and 155 mmol/L (that, multiplied by 0.93, gives the traditional range of 135–145 mmol/L). For convenience, laboratories routinely apply a correction factor so that the reported values still correspond to the traditional normal range of 135–145 mmol/L. A kind of "pseudohyponatremia" caused by expansion of the non-aqueous phase of plasma—for example, due to hyperlipidemia or paraproteinemia—is no longer seen because determination by selective electrodes in undiluted samples is not affected by this (the recommended name for this quantity is ionized sodium). Although, strictly speaking, a Na^+ concentration outside the range of 135–145 mmol/L denotes dysnatremia, clinically relevant hypo- or hypernatremia is mostly defined as a concentration outside the range of 130–150 mmol/L [3, 4].

Dehydration and Extracellular Fluid Volume Depletion

Although dehydration[2] semantically and in general usage means loss of water, in physiology and medicine the term denotes both a loss of water and salt. Depending on the type of pathophysiologic process, water and salts (primarily Na^+Cl^-) may be lost in physiologic proportion or lost disparately, with each type producing a somewhat different clinical picture, designated as normo-

tonic (mostly isonatremic), hypertonic (mostly hypernatremic), or hypotonic (always hyponatremic) dehydration. Dehydration develops when fluids are lost from the extracellular space at a rate exceeding intake. The most common sites for extracellular fluid loss are (1) the intestinal tract (diarrhea, vomiting, or bleeding), (2) the skin (fever, excessive sweating or burns), and (3) the urine (osmotic diuresis, diuretic therapy, diabetes insipidus, or salt losing renal tubular disorders). More rarely, dehydration results from prolonged inadequate intake without excessive losses [3, 4, 8–12].

The risk for dehydration is high in children and especially infants for the following causes: (a) infants and children are more susceptible to infectious diarrhea and vomiting than adults; (b) there is a higher proportional turnover of body fluids in infants compared to adults (it is estimated that the daily fluid intake and outgo, as a proportion of extracellular fluid, is in infancy more than three times that of an adult, Fig. 34.4); (c) young children do not communicate their need for fluids or do not independently access fluids to replenish volume losses.

Dehydration reduces the effective circulating volume, therefore impairing tissue perfusion. If not rapidly corrected, ischemic end-organ damage occurs.

Three groups of symptoms and signs occur in dehydration: (a) those related to the manner in which fluids loss occurs (including diarrhea, vomiting or polyuria); (b) those related to the electrolyte and acid-base imbalances that sometimes accompany dehydration; and (c) those directly due to dehydration. The following discussion will focus on the third group.

When assessing a child with a tendency towards dehydration, the clinician needs to address the degree of extracellular fluid volume depletion. More rarely the clinician will address the laboratory testing and the type of fluid lost (extracellular or intracellular fluid).

Degree of Dehydration
It is crucial to correctly assess the degree of dehydration since severe extracellular fluid volume depletion calls for rapid isotonic fluid resuscita-

---

[2]The terms dehydration and extracellular fluid volume depletion are mostly used interchangeably. However, these terms denote conditions resulting from different types of fluid losses. Volume depletion refers to any condition in which the effective circulating volume is reduced. It is produced by salt and water losses (as with vomiting, diarrhea, diuretics, bleeding, or third space sequestration). Strict sense dehydration refers to water loss alone. The clinical manifestation of dehydration is often hypernatremia. The elevation in serum Na^+ concentration, and therefore effective blood osmolality, pulls water out of the cells into the extracellular fluid. However, much of the literature does not distinguish between the two terms.

Fig. 34.4 Fluid turnover in infancy and adulthood. There is a proportionally greater turnover of fluids and solutes in infants and children as compared with adults. The figure depicts fluid intake, extracellular fluid volume and fluid outgo (diuresis and perspiratio insensibilis) in a healthy 6-month-old infant weighing 7.0 kg (input represents ≈50% of extracellular fluid volume) and in a healthy adult weighing 70 kg (input represents ≈15% of extracellular fluid volume)

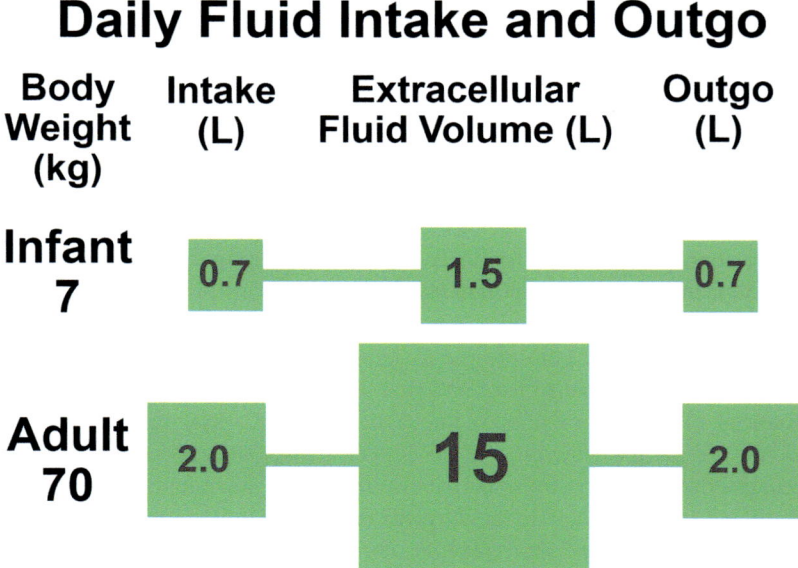

tion. Dehydration is most objectively measured as an acute change in weight from baseline (acute loss of body weight reflects the loss of fluid, not lean body mass; thus, a 1.3 kg weight loss reflects the loss of 1.3 liters of fluid). In most cases, however, an accurate recent weight is unavailable.

As a result, a pertinent history and a number of findings on physical examination are used to help assess dehydration. The signs and symptoms of dehydration include static (reduced general appearance, dry mucous membranes, reduced skin turgor, sunken eyes and fontanelle, colder extremities) and dynamic signs (delayed capillary refill, deep respiration with or without increased respiratory rate, tachycardia, weak peripheral pulses, reduced blood pressure, reduced urine output, reduced or absent tears' production). Skin turgor, sometimes referred to as skin elasticity, is a sign commonly used to assess the degree of hydration (the skin on the back of the hand, lower arm, or abdomen is grasped between two fingers, held for a few seconds and then released: skin with normal turgor snaps rapidly back to its normal position but skin with decreased turgor remains elevated and returns slowly to its normal position). However, decreased skin turgor is a late sign in dehydration that is associated with moderate or, more fre-

quently, severe dehydration. Like decreased skin turgor, arterial hypotension is a late sign in hypovolemia (in children with minimal to mild dehydration blood pressure is often slightly increased).

Several attempts have been made to determine a measure of dehydration by using combinations of clinical findings. In children ≤4 years of age with a diagnosis of acute diarrhea or vomiting, four clinical items ((a) general appearance, (b) eyes, (c) mucous membranes, (d) tears), which may be summed up to a total score ranging from 0 to 8, accurately estimate dehydration (Table 34.1) [15].

Laboratory Testing and the Type of Fluid Lost

Laboratory testing can confirm the presence of dehydration. The *fractional clearance of Na⁺* (which measures the amount of filtered Na⁺ that is excreted in the urine)

$$\frac{\text{Urinary Na}^+ \times \text{Circulating creatinine}}{\text{Circulating Na}^+ \times \text{Urinary creatinine}}$$

is $<0.5 \times 10^{-2}$ (or $<0.5\%$) and the *urine spot Na⁺ concentration* <30 mmol/L (unless the disease underlying dehydration is renal).

Furthermore, in dehydration, the urine is concentrated with an *osmolality* >450 mosm/kg

Table 34.1 "4-item 8-point rating scale" clinical dehydration scale. The score consists of 4 clinical items, which may be summed for a total score ranging from 0 to 8. The final 3 categories are no or minimal dehydration (<3%; score of 0), mild dehydration ($\geq$3% to <6% dehydration; score of 1–4), and moderate to severe dehydration ($\geq$6% dehydration; score of 5–8)

Characteristic	Score		
	0	1	2
General appearance	Normal	Thirsty, restless or lethargic but irritable when touched	Drowsy, limp, cold, or sweathy; comatose or not
Eyes	Normal	Slightly sunken	Very sunken
Mucous membranes (tongue)	Moist	Sticky	Dry
Tears	Tears	Decreased tears	Absent tears

H_2O. The urinary concentration is measured with an osmometer or fairly estimated, in the absence of proteinuria and glucosuria, from the specific gravity, as determined by refractometry (dipstick assessment of specific gravity is unreliable), as follows:

$$(\text{specific gravity} - 1000) \times 40$$

Furthermore, laboratory testing can detect associated electrolyte and acid-base abnormalities but determination of circulating electrolytes and acid-base balance is typically limited to children requiring intravenous fluids. These children are more severely volume depleted and are therefore at greater risk for dyselectrolytemias. Laboratory testing is less useful for assessing the degree of volume depletion.

- *Bicarbonatemia* $\leq$17.0 mmol/L is considered by some a useful laboratory test to assess dehydration.
- The *blood urea* level might be a further good biochemical marker of dehydration because it reflects both the decreased glomerular filtration rate and the enhanced Na^+ and water reab-

sorption in the proximal tubule. Unfortunately, this test is of limited usefulness since it can be increased by other factors such as bleeding or tissue breakdown (on the other side the rise can be minimized by a concomitant decrease in protein intake).

- The *serum Na^+* concentration varies with the relative loss of solute to water. Changes in Na^+ concentration play a pivotal role in determining the type of fluid depletion (Fig. 34.5):
  - Hyponatremic (and hypotonic) dehydration: Here, hyponatremia reflects net solute loss in excess of water loss. This does not occur directly, as fluid losses such as diarrhea are not hypertonic. Usually solute and water are lost in proportion, but water is taken in and retained in the context of hypovolemia-induced secretion of antidiuretic hormone. Since body water shifts from extracellular fluid to cells under these circumstances, and since signs of dehydration mostly depend on effective intravascular volume and tissue perfusion, signs of dehydration easily become profound.
  - Normonatremic (and isotonic) dehydration: in this setting, solute is lost in proportion to water loss.
  - Hypernatremic (and hypertonic) dehydration: this setting reflects water loss in excess of solute loss. Since body water shifts from intracellular to extracellular fluid under these circumstances, these children have less signs of dehydration for any given amount of fluid loss than do children with normonatremic (or normotonic) dehydration and especially those with hyponatremic dehydration. Clinical assessment can therefore underestimate the degree of dehydration in these children.
- *Bioimpedance devices* can also be helpful in determing hydration status in children as they measure fluid deficit in relation to extracellular water content or body weight, or consider absolute resistance [16].

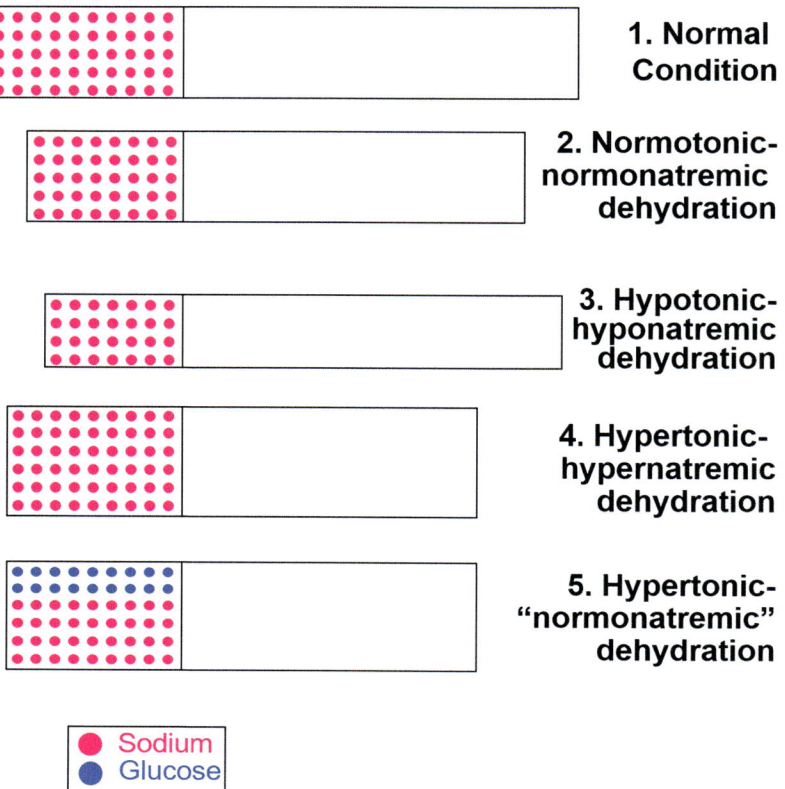

Fig. 34.5 Extracellular and intracellular compartments in children with dehydration. Normally, the extracellular compartment makes up approximately 20% and the intracellular 40% of the body weight (panel 1 of the figure). The second, third and fourth panels depict the relationship between extracellular and intracellular compartment in three children with dehydration in the context of an acute diarrheal disease: dehydration is normotonic-normonatremic in the first (panel 2), hypotonic-hyponatremic (mainly extracellular fluid losses) in the second (panel 3), and hypernatremic (mainly intracellular fluid losses) in the third child (panel 4). The lower panel depicts the relationship between extracellular and intracellular compartment (mainly intracellular fluid losses) in a child with dehydration in the context of diabetic ketoacidosis (hypertonic-"normonatremic" dehydration; the brackets indicate that in the context of diabetic ketoacidosis the concentration of circulating sodium is normal or even reduced). In each panel the red circles denote sodium and blue circles impermeable solutes that do not move freely across cell membranes (in the present example glucose). For reasons of simplicity, no symbols are given for potassium, the main intracellular cation

Dysnatremia

Consequences, Symptoms and Diagnostic Work Up

Under normal conditions, blood Na^+ concentration is maintained within the narrow range of 135–145 mmol/L despite great variations in water and salt intake. Na^+ and its accompanying anions Cl^- and HCO_3^- account for 90% of the extracellular effective osmolality. The main determinant of the Na^+ concentration is the plasma water content, itself determined by water intake (thirst or habit), "insensible" losses (such as metabolic water, sweat and respiration), and urinary dilution. The last of these is under most circumstances crucial and predominantly determined by anti-diuretic hormone. In response to this hormone, concentrated urine is produced.

Dysnatremias produce central nervous system dysfunction. While hyponatremia may induce brain swelling, hypernatremia may induce brain shrinkage, yet the clinical features elicited by opposite changes in tonicity are remarkably similar [3, 4, 8–12].

Hyponatremia

Introduction

Hyoponatremia is classified (Fig. 34.6) according to the extracellular fluid volume status, as either "hypovolemic" (= depletional) or "normo-hypervolemic" (= dilutional). Vasopressin is released both in children with low effective circulating volume, the most common cause of hyponatremia in everyday clinical practice, as well as

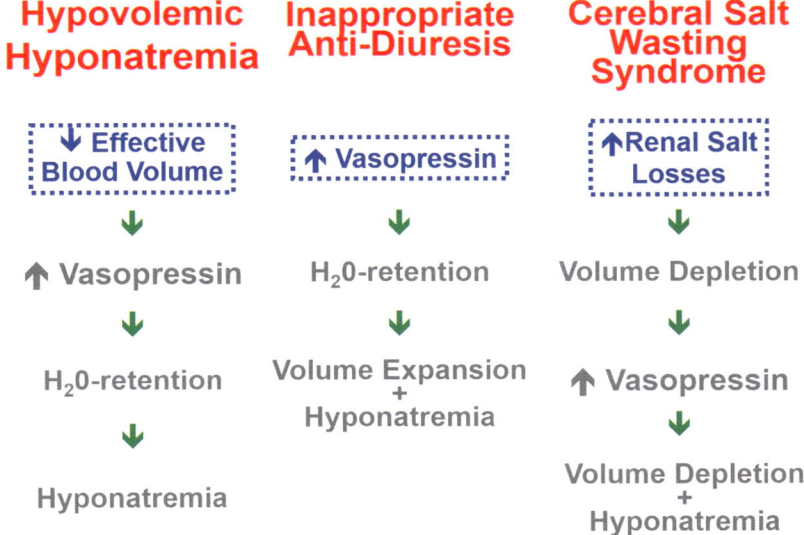

Fig. 34.6 Extracellular fluid volume status in children with hyponatremia. Hyoponatremia is classified according to the extracellular fluid volume status, as either hypovolemic (= depletional) or normo-hypervolemic (= dilutional). In most cases (left panel) hyponatremia results from a low effective arterial blood volume and is termed hypovolemic hyponatremia (the term appropriate anti-diuresis is sometimes used in this circumstance). The true syndrome of inappropriate anti-diuresis results from persistently high levels of vasopressin or, more rarely, activation of its renal receptor (middle panel). Cerebral salt-wasting syndrome is a further form of hyponatremia that sometimes develops in patients with intracranial disorders (right panel). In this condition, renal salt-wasting is the primary defect, which is followed by volume depletion leading to a secondary rise in vasopressin

in those with normo-hypervolemic hyponatremia. In hypovolemic hyponatremia, vasopressin release is triggered by the low effective arterial blood volume (this condition is also referred to as 'syndrome of appropriate anti-diuresis'). In dilutional hyponatremia, the primary defect is a euvolemic, inappropriate increase in circulating vasopressin levels (this condition is also termed 'syndrome of inappropriate anti-diuresis').

Assessing the cause of hyponatremia may be straightforward if an obvious cause is present (for example in the setting of vomiting or diarrhea) or in the presence of a clinically evident extracellular fluid volume depletion [3, 4, 8, 11, 12]. Sometimes, however, assessing the volume status and distinguishing hypovolemic from normo-hypervolemic hyponatremia may not be straightforward. In such cases, the urine spot Na^+ and the fractional Na^+ clearance are helpful, as patients with dilutional hyponatremia have a urinary Na^+ >30 mmol/L (and fractional Na^+ clearance >0.5%), whereas those with extracellular fluid volume depletion (unless the source is renal) will have a urinary Na^+ <30 mmol/L (and fractional Na^+ clearance <0.5%). Since effective blood osmolality is mostly low in hyponatremia, and urine is less than maximally dilute (inappropriately concentrated), blood and urine osmolalities, although usually measured, are rarely discriminant.

A decrease in Na^+ concentration and effective blood osmolality causes movement of water into brain cells and results in cellular swelling and raised intracranial pressure. Nausea and malaise are typically seen when the Na^+ level acutely falls <125–130 mmol/L. Headache, lethargy, restlessness, and disorientation follow, as its concentration falls <115–120 mmol/L. With severe and rapidly evolving hyponatremia, seizures, coma, permanent brain damage, respiratory arrest, brain stem herniation, and death may occur. In more gradually evolving hyponatremia, the brain self regulates to prevent swelling over hours to days by transport of, firstly, Na^+, Cl^-, and K^+ and, later, solutes like glutamate, taurine, myoinositol, and glutamine from intracellular to extracellular compartments. This induces water loss and ameliorates brain swelling, and hence leads to few symptoms in subacute and chronic hyponatremia.

Evaluating the Cause

In normovolemic subjects, the primary defense against developing hyponatremia is the ability to dilute urine and excrete free-water [3, 4, 8, 11, 12]. Rarely is excess ingestion of free-water alone the cause of hyponatremia. It is also rare to develop hyponatremia from excess urinary Na^+ losses in the absence of free-water ingestion. In order for hyponatremia to develop, both a relative excess of free-water as well as an underlying condition that impairs the ability to excrete free-water are typically required. Renal water handling is primarily under the control of vasopressin, which is released from the posterior pituitary and impairs water diuresis (hence the synonymous name "anti-diuretic hormone") by increasing the permeability to water in the collecting tubule.

There are osmotic, hemodynamic and non-hemodynamic stimuli for release of vasopressin. In most cases, hyponatremia develops when the body attempts to preserve the extracellular fluid volume at the expense of circulating Na^+ (therefore, a hemodynamic stimulus for vasopressin production overrides an inhibitory effect of hyponatremia). However, there are further stimuli for production of vasopressin in hospitalized children that make virtually any hospitalized patient at risk for hyponatremia (Table 34.2).

Some specific causes of hypotonic hyponatremia deserve further discussion.

– **Hospital-acquired hyponatremia** is most often seen in the postoperative period or in association with a reduced effective circulating volume.
– Postoperative hyponatremia is a serious problem in children, which sometimes is caused by a combination of nonosmotic stimuli for release of anti-diuretic hormone, such as pain, nausea, stress, narcotics, and edema-forming conditions. Subclinical depletion of the effec-

Table 34.2 Causes of hypotonic hyponatremia in childhood

Hypovolemic	Normovolemic (or hypervolemic)
Intestinal salt loss	*Increased body water*
– Diarrheal dehydration	– Parenteral hypotonic
– Vomiting, gastric	solutions
suction	– Exercise-associated
– Fistulae	hyponatremia
– Laxative abuse	– Habitual (and
	psychogenic)
	polydipsia
Transcutaneous salt loss	*Non osmolar release of*
– Cystic fibrosis	*antidiuretic hormones*[a]
– Endurance sport	– Cardiac failure
	– Sever liver disease
	(mostly cirrhosis)
	– Nephrotic syndrome
	– Glucocorticoid
	deficiency
	– Drugs causing renal
	water retention
	– [Hypothyroidism][b]
Renal sodium loss	*Syndrome of inappropriate*
– Mineralocorticoid	*anti-diuresis*
deficiency (or	– Classic syndrome of
resistance)	inappropriate
– Diuretics	secretion of
– Salt wasting renal	antidiuretic
failure	hormone
– Salt wasting	– Hereditary
tubulopathies	nephrogenic
(including Bartter	inappropriate
syndromes)	antidiuresis
– Gitelman syndrome,	
and De Toni-Debré–	
Fanconi syndrome)	
– Cerebral salt wasting	
Perioperative (e.g.:	*Reduced renal water loss*
preoperative fasting,	– Chronic renal failure
vomiting, third space	– Oliguric acute renal
losses)	failure

[a] Effective arterial blood volume mostly reduced
[b] Evidence supporting this association is rather poor

tive blood volume and administration of hypotonic fluids are currently considered the most important causes of postoperative hyponatremia.

– More rarely, hospital-acquired hyponatremia is seen in association with the syndrome of inappropriate anti-diuresis, which is caused either by elevated activity of vasopressin or, less commonly, by hyperfunction of its renal (= V2) receptor, independently of increased effective blood osmolality and hemodynamic stimulus (i.e.: reduced effective circulating volume). It is currently assumed that this condition results not only from dilution of the blood by free-water but also from inappropriate natriuresis. The syndrome of inappropriate anti-diuresis (Fig. 34.6) should be suspected in any child with hyponatremic hypotonia, a urine osmolality >100 mosmol/kg H_2O, a normal fractional Na^+ clearance (>0.5%), low normal or reduced uric acid level, low blood urea level and normal acid-base and K^+ balance.

– The longstanding assumption that hypontremia associated with meningitis or respiratory infections is caused by inappropriate anti-diuresis is not substantiated by reports that adequately assessed the volume status. On the other hand, dysnatremia is frequently observed in many other community-acquired infections. Hyponatremia develops in approximately 50% of acute moderate gastroenteritis cases, often associated with metabolic acidosis and potassium disturbances. Up to 60% of infants with bronchiolitis tend to develop an isolated hyponatremia, while 70% of infants with pyelonephritis might develop hyponatremia. In these patients, metabolic acidosis and hyperkalemia are also often present, suggesting silent renal resistance to aldosterone [17].

– **Desmopressin**, a synthetic analogue of the natural anti-diuretic hormone, is used in central diabetes insipidus, in some bleeding disorders, in diagnostic urine concentration testing and especially in primary nocturnal enuresis with nocturnal polyuria. Desmopressin is generally regarded as a safe drug and adverse effects are uncommon. Nonetheless, hyponatremic water intoxication leading to convulsions has been reported as a rare side effect of desmopressin therapy in enuretic children. This complication mostly develops in subjects managed with the intranasal formulation ≤14 days after starting the medication, following excess fluid intake and during intercurrent illnesses (Table 34.3) [18].

Table 34.3 Drug-induced hyponatremia

Diuretics (thiazides more commonly than loop diuretics)

Drugs blocking the renin-angiotensin-aldosterone system (converting enzyme inhibitors, sartans or renin inhibitors)

Antidiuretic drugs

- ↑ **water permeability of the renal collecting tubule:** arginine-vasopressin, vasopressin analogues like desmopressin and oxytocin
- ↑ **antidiuretic hormone release, ↑ antidiuretic hormone action:** carbamazepine, lamotrigine, valproate, barbiturates, antidiabetic drugs (chlorpropamide, tolbutamide), clofibrate, colchicine, nicotine, vincristine, cyclophosphamide
- ↓ **synthesis of prostaglandins:** nonsteroidal anti-inflammatory drugs including salicylates, paracetamol
- **Mechanism unknown:** haloperidol, tricyclic antidepressants, selective serotonin-reuptake inhibitors, monoamine oxidase inhibitors, narcotics like morphine

- Male infants have been described with hyponatremia and laboratory features consistent with release of vasopressin but who had no measurable circulating levels of this hormone. This rare condition results from gain-of-function mutations of the X-linked receptor gene that mediates the renal response to vasopressin, resulting in persistent activation of the receptor. The condition, which has been termed **hereditary nephrogenic syndrome of inappropriate anti-diuresis**, represents a kind of mirror image of the X-linked nephrogenic diabetes insipidus, the result of loss-of-function genetic defects in the aforementioned renal receptor.
- **Cerebral salt wasting syndrome** is a peculiar form of depletional hyponatremia that sometimes occurs in patients with cerebral disease (Fig. 34.6). It mimics the syndrome of inappropriate anti-diuresis, except that salt-wasting is the primary defect with the ensuing volume depletion leading to a secondary release of vasopressin. Salt wasting of central origin might result from increased secretion of a natriuretic peptide with subsequent suppression of aldosterone synthesis. The distinction between cerebral salt wasting and inappropriate activity of vasopressin is not always sim-

ple since the true volume status is sometimes difficult to ascertain.

- **Endurance athletes** sometimes replace their diluted but Na^+-containing sweat losses with excessive amounts of severely hypotonic solutions: the net effect is a reduction in the circulating Na^+ level. The effect is likely compounded by a reduced renal function during exercise (such individuals may also be taking non-steroidal anti-inflammatory drugs, which can impair the excretion of free water).
- A tendency towards low normal blood Na^+ level is sometimes seen in children who drink excessively and present with polyuria and polydipsia. Usually the problem is simply one of habit, particularly in infants who are attached to a bottle (= **habitual polydipsia**). In childhood, polydipsia is rarely a symptom of significant psychopathology (= **psychogenic polydipsia**).
- Diuretics (thiazides more frequently than loop diuretics) and **drugs** that block the renin-angiotensin-aldosterone system (converting enzyme inhibitors, sartans or direct renin inhibitors) make up a common cause of hyponatremia (Table 34.3). More rarely, other drugs sometimes cause renal retention of fluids and therefore dilutional hyponatremia.

Hypernatremia

Introduction

Hypernatremia (Na^+ >145 mmol/L) reflects a net water loss or a hypertonic Na^+ gain, with inevitable hypertonicity [3, 4, 8–10]. Severe symptoms are usually evident only with acute and large increases in Na^+ concentration ≥160 mmol/L. Importantly, the sensation of thirst protecting against the tendency towards hypernatemia is absent or reduced in patients with altered mental status or with hypothalamic lesions and in infancy.

The cause of hypernatremia is almost always evident from the history. Determination of urine osmolality in relation to the effective blood osmolality and the urine Na^+ concentration helps if the cause is unclear. Patients with diabetes insipidus present with polyuria and polydipsia (and not hypernatremia unless thirst sensation is impaired). Central diabetes insipidus and nephrogenic diabetes insipidus may be differentiated by the response to water deprivation (failure to concentrate urine) followed by desmopressin, causing concentration of urine uniquely in patients with central diabetes insipidus.

Non-specific symptoms such as anorexia, muscle weakness, restlessness, nausea, and vomiting tend to occur early. More serious signs follow, with altered mental status, lethargy, irritability, stupor, or coma. Acute brain shrinkage can induce vascular rupture, with cerebral bleeding and subarachnoid hemorrhage.

Evaluating the Cause

Two mechanisms protect against developing hypernatremia or increased effective blood osmolality: the ability to release vasopressin (and therefore to concentrate urine) and a powerful thirst mechanism. Release of vasopressin occurs when the effective blood osmolality exceeds 275–280 mosmol/kg H_2O and results in maximally concentrated urine when the effective blood osmolality exceeds 290–295 mosmol/kg H_2O. Thirst, the second line of defense, provides a further protection against hypernatremia and increased effective osmolality. If the thirst mechanism is intact and there is unrestricted access to free-water, it is rare to develop sustained hypernatremia from either excess Na^+ ingestion or a renal concentrating defect (Table 34.4).

Hypernatremia is primarily a hospital-acquired condition occurring in children who have restricted access to fluids. Most children with hypernatremia are debilitated by an acute or chronic disease, have neurological impairment, are critically ill or are born premature. Hypernatremia in the intensive care setting is common as these children are typically either intubated or moribund, and often are fluid restricted, receive large amounts of Na^+ as blood products or have renal concentrating defects from diuretics or renal dysfunction. The majority of hypernatremia results from the failure to administer sufficient free-water to children who are unable to care for themselves and have restricted access to fluids.

Two special causes of hypernatremia deserve some further discussion.

– A frequent cause of hypernatremia in the outpatient setting is currently **breastfeeding-associated hypernatremia**, which should more properly be labeled "not-enough-breastfeeding-associated hypernatremia" [19]. This condition occurs between days 7 and 15 in otherwise healthy term or near-term newborns of first-time mothers who are exclusively breast-fed. In all cases feeding had been

Table 34.4 Causes of hypernatremia in childhood

Hypovolemic	Normovolemic	Hypervolemic
Inadequate intake	**Hypodypsia** (essential hypernatremia)	**Inappropriate intravenous fluids** (e.g.: hypertonic saline, $NaHCO_3$)
– Breast feeding hypernatremia	**Hyperventilation**	**Salt poisoning** (accidental, deliberate)
– Poor access to water	**Fever**	**Primary aldosteronism** (and other conditions that cause low-renin hypertension)
– Altered thirst perception (uncosciousness, mental impairment)		
Intestinal salt loss (diarrheal dehydration)		
Renal water and salt loss		
– Postobstructive polyuria		
– Diuretics		
– Diabetes insipidus (either primary or, more rarely, secondary[a])		
– Medullary renal damage		

[a] Secondary nephrogenic diabetes insipidus may develop as a complication of inherited renal diseases such as nephropathic cystinosis, Bartter and Gitelman syndromes and nephronophthisis

difficult to establish and the volume of milk ingested was likely to have been low. The underlying problem is water deficiency: Na$^+$ concentration raises predominantly as a result of low volume intake and a loss of water, demonstrating that inadequate feeding is the cause of hypernatremic dehydration. Monitoring postnatal weight loss provides an objective assessment of the adequacy of nutritional intake allowing targeted support to those infants who fail to thrive or demonstrate excessive weight loss ($\geq$10% of birth weight).

– Diarrhea or vomiting are a further reason of hypernatremia in the outpatient setting, but are much less common than in the past, presumably due to the advent of low solute infant formulas and the increased use and availability of oral rehydration solutions.

Management

The discussion will exclusively focus on some features of parenteral hydration, and the management of hyponatremia with V2 anti-diuretic hormone receptor antagonists [3, 4, 8–12].

Maintenance and Perioperative Fluids

Intravenous maintenance fluids are designed to provide water and electrolyte requirements in a fasting patient. The prescription for intravenous maintenance fluids was originally described by Holliday (Table 34.5), who rationalized a daily H$_2$O requirement of 1700–1800 mL/m^2 body surface area and the addition of 3 and 2 mmol/kg body weight of Na$^+$ and K$^+$ respectively (approximating the electrolyte requirements and urinary excretion in healthy infants). This is the basis for the traditional recommendation that hypotonic intravenous maintenance solutions are ideal for children. This approach has subsequently been questioned because of the potential for these hypotonic solutions to cause hyponatremia. Surgical patients appear as the subgroup of children with the highest risk to develop severe hypo-

Table 34.5 Intravenous maintenance fluids designed to provide water and electrolyte requirements in a fasting patient. Both the recommendation originally described by Holliday and the most recent recommendation are given. The addition of KCl 2 mmol/kg body weight is also recommended

	Holliday's recommendation	Current suggestion
Solution	5% dextrose in water supplemented with NaCl 3 mmol/kg body weight daily	Isotonic saline in 5% dextrose in water
Amount (mL/m^2 body surface area^a daily)	1700–1800	1400–1500
Clinical practice	100 mL/kg body weight for a child weighing less than 10 kg^b + 50 mL/kg for each additional kg up to 20 kg + 20–[25] mL/kg for each kg in excess of 20 kg	80 mL/kg body weight for a child weighing less than 10 kg^b + 40 mL/kg for each additional kg up to 20 kg + 15–[20] mL/kg for each kg in excess of 20 kg

^{a} The Mosteller's formula may be used to calculated the body surface area (in m^2): $\sqrt{\dfrac{height\,(cm) \times body\,weight\,(kg)}{3600}}$

^{b} In children weighing $\leq$5.0 kg the daily parenteral water requirement is 120 mL/kg body weight

natremia with the use of hypotonic intravenous solutions, likely because they tend to be hypovolemic. Furthermore, traditional maintenance fluid recommendations may be much greater than actual water needs in children at risk of hyponatremia.

Most authors currently suggest (Table 34.5) that hyponatremia should be prevented by (a) using isotonic (usually normal saline, which contains NaCl 9 g/L) or near isotonic (usually Ringer's lactate) solutions and (b) reducing by $\approx$20% the daily volume of maintenance fluid to 1400–1500 mL/m^2 body surface area. Considering the potential for hypoglycemia in infancy, ringer's lactate or normal saline in 5% glucose in water (which contains glucose 50 g/L) is considered the safest fluid composition for most children.

Dehydration

Oral rehydration therapy is currently the treatment of choice for children with minimal, mild or moderate dehydration due to diarrheal diseases. However, in the practice of pediatric emergency medicine, mainly because of rapidity, intravenous rehydration is a commonly used intervention for these children.

Treatment approaches to parenteral rehydration in the hospitalized child vary. There are numerous ways to estimate the degree of dehydration (the "4-item 8-point rating scale" is currently widely recommended; Table 34.1), to calculate fluid and electrolyte deficits, and to deliver the deficits to the patient. For many years, the recommendation was to accomplish 100% (or even less) replacement of the volume deficit during the first 24 h of treatment. More recently, the aim of treatment has generally been to accomplish a more rapid full repletion within ≤ 6 h. In many children with mild to moderate dehydration, especially those resistant to initial oral rehydration therapy, and in children with severe dehydration, we currently administer intravenous isotonic (or near isotonic) crystalloid solutions such as normal saline or lactate Ringer's as repeated boluses of 10–20 mL/kg body weight (administered over 20–60 min).

In children with diarrhea or vomiting, reduced carbohydrate intake leads to free fatty acid breakdown, excess ketones, and an increased likelihood of continued nausea and vomiting. Consequently, some authorities have suggested the use of a glucose containing normal solution (mostly the lactate Ringer's in 5% glucose in water), which will stimulate insulin release, reduce free fatty acid breakdown, and therefore reduce treatment failure due to persisting nausea and vomiting (owing to hyperketonemia) [20].

The child with hypovolemic circulatory shock presents with (a) increased heart rate and weak peripheral pulses, (b) cold, pale and diaphoretic skin, and (c) delayed capillary refill. The initial management recommended by the American Academy of Pediatrics includes the administration of a high concentration of O_2 (ensuring that 100% of the available arterial hemoglobin is oxygenated). Common errors in the child with hypovolemic circulatory shock secondary to a diarrheal disease are delayed or inadequate (i.e. with hypotonic crystalloid solution) fluid resuscitation.

Children with hypernatremic dehydration are also hydrated parenterally with isotonic crystalloid solutions until diagnosis of the dyselectrolytemia, followed by slightly hypotonic solutions (e.g.: half-saline) in order to slowly correct the circulating Na^+ concentration (abruptly correcting hypernatremia using a Na^+ free glucose solution creates an increased risk of brain edema; Fig. 34.7). In acute dysnatremic dehydration, Na^+ should be corrected slowly at a rate not exceeding 0.5 mmol/L per hour (or more than by 12 mmol/L per day). Subacute or chronic hypernatremia should be corrected even more slowly.

Hydration in Infectious Diseases Associated with a Tendency Towards Hyponatremia

Fluid restriction has been widely advocated in the initial management of infectious diseases such as meningitis, pneumonia or bronchiolitis, which are often associated with a low Na^+ level. However, there is no evidence that fluid restriction is useful. Furthermore, hyponatremia results from appropriate, volume-dependent antidiuresis in these disease conditions. In clinical practice, initial restoration of the intravascular space with an isotonic crystalloid followed by isotonic maintenance fluids 1400–1500 mL/m^2 body surface area per day (Table 34.5, right panel) are currently advised. In cases presenting with overt hyponatremia, frequent monitoring of electrolytes is also required with adjustments to be made according to laboratory findings.

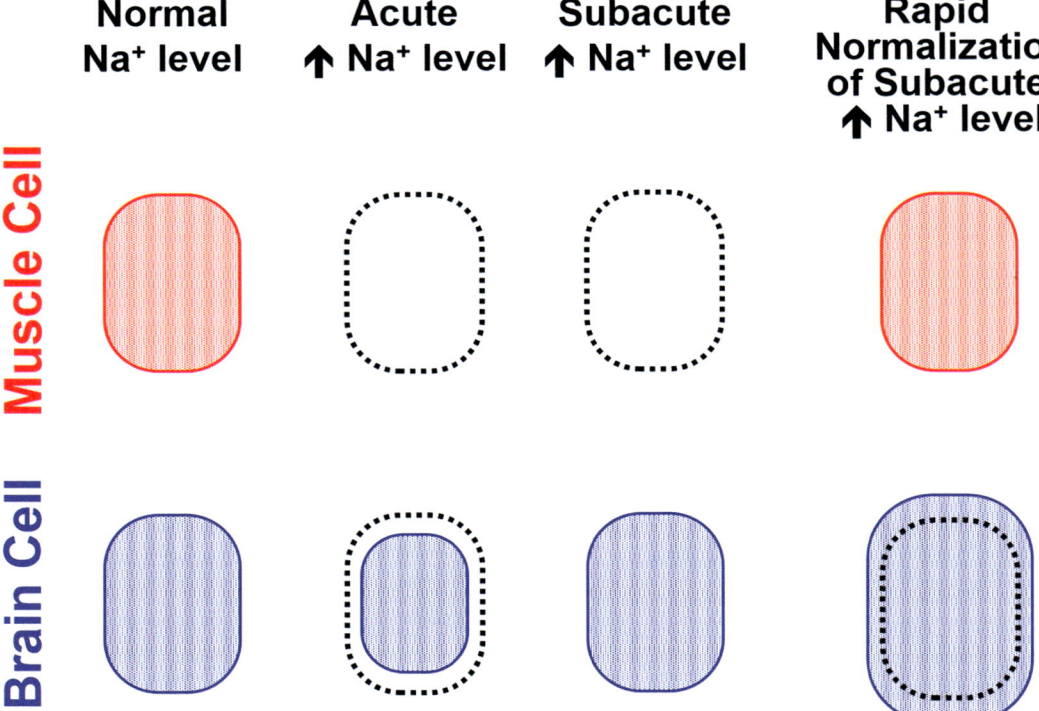

Fig. 34.7 Cell volume in acute or subacute hypernatremia and after rapid correction of hypernatremia. When hypernatemia develops acutely, all cells are reduced in size (the degree of cell volume reduction reflects the degree of hypernatremia). When hypernatremia is present for 36–48 h or more (= subacute hypernatremia), cell volume reduction persists in most cells, including muscle cells (upper panel). However, brain cells and red blood cells tend to restore their normal cell volume (lower panel). A rapid normalization of sodium level in children affected with subacute or chronic hypernatremia pathologically increases the volume of brain cells (and red blood cells). Swelling of cells, which does not have serious consequences when it occurs in most organs, may have damaging consequences when it occurs in the brain (lower panel, right)

Hyponatremia

Chronic normovolemic (or hypervolemic) hyponatremia is usually managed either by restricting water intake or by giving salt. An alternative may be the use of nonpeptide vasopressin receptor antagonists. There are three receptors for vasopressin: the $V1_a$ receptors that mediate vasoconstriction, the $V1_b$ receptors that mediate adrenocorticotropin release, and the V2 receptors that mediate the anti-diuretic response. Vaptans, oral V2 receptor antagonists, have been approved for the management of normovolemic and hypervolemic hyponatremia: these agents produce a selective water diuresis (without affecting Na^+ and K^+ excretion) that raises the circulating Na^+ level. Only limited information is currently available with these agents in childhood.

Vaptans do not correct hyponatremia in patients affected by nephrogenic syndrome of inappropriate childhood anti-diuresis. In these patients, a way to enhance water excretion is the oral administration of urea (dosage in adults: 30 g per day). This regimen, which may be effective because it causes simultaneously water diuresis and renal Na^+ retention, is well tolerated, and has been used chronically in pediatric outpatients.

Potassium

Balance

Most (98%) of the K^+ in the body (40–50 mmol/kg) is within cells. The maintenance of distribution of K^+ across cells is largely dependent on the activity of the sodium pump (= Na^+-K^+-ATPase). In healthy humans, the extracellular K^+ concentration is maintained between 3.5 and 5.0 mmol/L. K^+ balance, like that of other ions, is a function of intake and urinary excretion. In adults, the daily K^+ intake averages 0.5–2 mmol/kg body weight (Fig. 34.8). The homeostasis goal of the adult is to remain in zero K^+ balance. Thus, ≈90–95% of the typical daily intake of 1 mmol/kg is ultimately eliminated from the body in the urine (the residual 5–10% is lost through the stool). Infants maintain a positive K^+ balance (the estimated requirement for growth is 1.2 mmol/day during the first 3 months of life, 0.8 mmol/day up to 1 year and 0.4 mmol/day thereafter). The net accretion of K^+ ensures the availability of adequate substrate for incorporation into cells newly formed during periods of somatic growth. Postnatal growth is associated with an increase in total body K^+ from ≈8 mmol/cm body height at birth to >14 mmol/cm body height by 18 years of age. The rate of accretion of body K^+ per kg body weight in the infant is more rapid than in the older child, reflecting both an increase in cell number and K^+ concentration, at least in skeletal muscle, with advancing age [21–23].

Regulation of Circulating Potassium

Circulating K^+ concentration is regulated by the total body K^+ content, which depends upon (a) the external balance, i.e. the difference between intake and excretion in the urine, feces and sweat, and (b) the internal balance, which represents the relative distribution of K^+ between the intracellular and the extracellular spaces [21–23].

External (≈ Renal) Potassium Homeostasis

Virtually all regulation of urinary K^+ excretion and therefore of external K^+ homeostasis occurs in the **renal cortical collecting tubule**. Indeed, almost all of the filtered K^+ is reabsorbed in the proximal tubule and the loop of Henle, so that <10% of the filtered load is delivered to the cortical collecting tubule. This tubular segment adjusts the external homeostasis of K^+ by modulating its secretion.

- The major physiologic regulators of K^+ secretion within the cortical collecting tubule are "hyperkalemia" and aldosterone, which act in concert to promote the tubular secretion and therefore the urinary excretion of this ion.
- Increasing the flow rate traversing the cortical collecting tubule is a further factor that may increase the K^+ excretion. This response is most prominent in the presence of hyperkale-

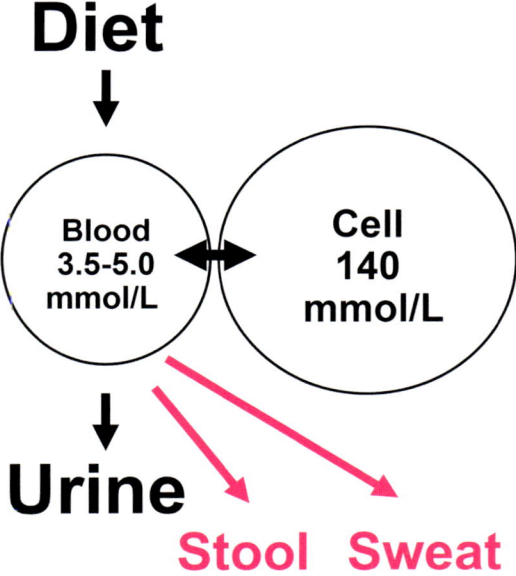

Fig. 34.8 Major factors governing the homeostasis of potassium. Most of the potassium in the body resides within cells. The maintenance of distribution of potassium across cells is largely dependent on the activity of the sodium pump. Potassium balance, like that of other ions, is a function of intake and urinary excretion. Since only small amounts of potassium are normally lost in the sweat and in the stool, they are depicted in a different color. However, substantial intestinal potassium and therefore potassium depletion can be seen with vomiting, diarrhea or other intestinal disease conditions or when sweat production is chronically increased

mia, since the concurrent elevations in aldosterone and circulating K^+ concentration produce a high level of K^+ secretion within the cortical collecting tubule.

Internal Potassium Homeostasis

The main modulators of the distribution of K^+ between the intracellular and the extracellular spaces are insulin, the sympathetic nervous system (via β_2-adrenergic receptors) and the acid-base balance.

Prenatal and Neonatal Potassium Balance

During fetal life K^+ is actively transported across the placenta from the mother to the fetus (indeed, the fetal K^+ concentration is maintained at levels ≥ 5.0 mmol/L even in the face of maternal K^+ deficiency). The tendency to retain K^+ early in postnatal life is reflected by the observation that infants, especially premature newborns, tend to have higher circulating K^+ levels than children. Furthermore, in infancy the ability to increase urinary K^+ excretion is blunted (see: non-oliguric hyperkalaemia of the premature infant).

Symptoms, Signs, and Consequences of Hypokalemia and Hyperkalemia

Excess or deficient K^+ in the extracellular space impairs cardiovascular, neuromuscular, renal and endocrine-metabolic body functions [21, 22]. The most dangerous clinical consequence of these dyselectrolytemias is the predisposition to life-threatening cardiac arrhythmias. The manifestations of hypokalemia are outlined in Table 34.6, those of hyperkalemia in Table 34.7.

The severity of hypokalemic manifestations is proportionate to the degree and duration of hypokalemia and symptoms generally do not become manifest until the K^+ concentration is below 2.5–3.0 mmol/L. Hypokalemia causes characteristic

Table 34.6 Body functions impaired by hypokalemia

- Cardiovascular abnormalities
Cardiac arrhythmias (premature atrial and ventricular beats, sinus bradycardia, paroxysmal atrial or junctional tachycardia, atrioventricular block, and ventricular tachycardia or fibrillation)
    Increased systemic vascular resistance
- Neuromuscular disturbances
Skeletal muscle weakness (usually beginning with the lower extremities and progressing to the trunk and upper extremities; sometimes involvement of the respiratory muscles)
    Muscle cramps, rhabdomyolysis
    Smooth muscle dysfunction (intestinal and urinary system)
- Renal effects
Decreased urinary concentrating ability (decreased expression of the antidiuretic hormone-sensitive water channel aquaporin-2)
    Increased renal ammonium production (and therefore $\uparrow$ generation of HCO_3)
Hypokalemic nephropathy[a] (interstitial fibrosis, tubular atrophy, cyst formation in the renal medulla)
- Endocrine and metabolic effects
    Negative nitrogen balance (causing growth retardation)
    Glucose intolerance (with tendency towards diabetes mellitus)
Decreased aldosterone release (direct adrenal action), increased renin secretion
    Hepatic encephalopathy (in susceptible individuals)

[a] Following prolonged hypokalemia

Table 34.7 Body functions impaired by hyperkalemia

- Cardiovascular abnormalities
Cardiac arrhythmias (ventricular fibrillation or standstill are the most severe consequences)
    Reduced systemic vascular resistance
- Neuromuscular disturbances
Skeletal muscle weakness (usually beginning with the lower extremities and progressing to the trunk and upper extremities; rarely involvement of the respiratory muscles)
    Smooth muscle dysfunction (intestinal and urinary system)
- Renal effects
Reduced renal ammonium production (and therefore reduced generation of HCO_3)
- Endocrine and metabolic effects
    Increased aldosterone release (direct adrenal action), reduced renin secretion

K⁺   **Ca⁺⁺**

High

Normal

Low

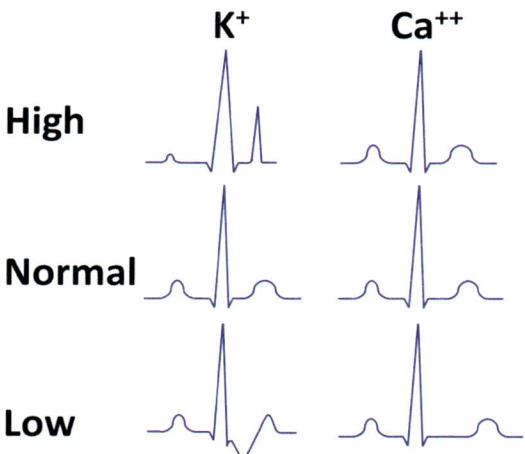

Fig. 34.9 Diagram illustrating some electrocardiographic consequences of hyperkalemia, hypokalemia, hypercalcemia and hypocalcemia. The electrocardiographic changes of hyperkalemia include tall and "peaked" T waves, PR prolongation, QRS widening and, at very high K⁺ concentrations, ventricular arrhythmias (not shown). Hypokalemia produces a decreased amplitude of the T wave, a depression of the ST segment and an increased amplitude of U waves, which occur at the end of the T wave. Hypercalcemia manifests with a shortened, hypocalcemia with a prolonged QTc interval

electrocardiographic changes (Fig. 34.9): depression of the ST segment, a decreased amplitude of the T wave, and an increased amplitude of U waves which occur at the end of the T wave.

There are very few symptoms or signs of hyperkalemia, and these tend to occur only with very high levels. Symptoms generally do not become manifest until the K⁺ concentration exceeds 7.0 mmol/L, unless the rise in concentration has been very rapid. Hyperkalemia produces the following elecrocardiographic changes: peaked T wave with shortened QT interval is the first change, followed by progressive lengthening of the PR interval and QRS duration. The severity of hyperkalemia is classified as follows: (a) mild: K⁻ between 5.1 and 6.0 mmol/L and absent or equivocal electrocardiographic changes; (b) moderate: K⁺ between 6.1 and 7.0 mmol/L and definite eletrocardiographic changes in reploarization ("peaked" T waves); (c) severe: K⁺ ≥7.1 mmol/L and severe definite eletrocardiographic changes including atrial standstill, advanced atrio-ventricular heart block, QRS wid-

ening or ventricular arrhythmia (usually associated with weakness of skeletal muscles). The electrocardiographic signs of hyperkalemia are given in Fig. 34.9.

Evaluating the Causes of Hypokalemia and Hyperkalemia ("Diagnostic Tests")

The following tests have been developed to evaluate and distinguish the various causes of hypo- or hyperkalemia in childhood [21–23].

(a) The **t**rans**t**ubular **K+** concentration **g**radient, colloquially referred to as TTKG, measures the K⁺ secretion within the cortical collecting tubule and represents an estimate of the aldosterone activity. This parameter can be easily calculated assuming (a) that the urine osmolality at the end of the cortical collecting tubule is similar to that of blood, and (b) that no K⁺ secretion or reabsorption takes place in the medullary collecting tubule. If these assumptions are accurate, then the K⁺ concentration in the final urine will rise above that in the cortical collecting tubule due to reabsorption of water in the medullary collecting duct. This effect can be accounted for by dividing the urine K⁺ concentration by the ratio of the urine to blood osmolality. If, for example, this ratio is 2, then 50% of the water leaving the cortical collecting tubule has been reabsorbed in the medulla, thereby doubling the luminal K⁺ concentration. This parameter is calculated as follows:

$$\frac{\text{Urinary K}^+ \big/ \text{Urinary Osmolality}}{\text{Blood Osmolality} \big/ \text{Circulating K}^+}$$

Blood osmolality (in mosm/kg) can be measured with an osmometer or very reasonably estimated from circulating Na⁺, glucose, and urea (in mmol/L) as follows: (Na⁺ × 2) + glucose + urea. On the other hand, urinary osmolality (in mmol/kg H₂O) can be measured with an osmometer or estimated, in the absence of proteinuria and glucosuria, from the specific gravity, as determined by refractometry, as follows: (specific gravity − 1000) × 40.

(b) The fractional clearance of K^+ (which measures the amount of filtered K^+ that is excreted in the urine)

$$\frac{\text{Urinary}\,K^+ \times \text{Circulating Creatinine}}{\text{Circulatory}\,K^+ \times \text{Urinary Creatinine}}$$

and the molar urinary potassium/creatinine ratio (mol/mol)

$$\frac{\text{Urinary}\,K^+}{\text{Urinary Creatinine}}$$

are two further frequently used tests, which are strongly correlated.

(c) The fractional clearance of Cl^- (which measures the amount of filtered Cl^- that is excreted in the urine)

$$\frac{\text{Urinary}\,Cl^- \times \text{Circulating Creatinine}}{\text{Circulating}\,Cl^- \times \text{Urinary Creatinine}}$$

and especially the molar urinary chloride/creatinine ratio (mol/mol; see above)

$$\frac{\text{Urinary}\,Cl^-}{\text{Urinary Creatinine}}$$

are two further, closely correlated tests that have been suggested.

The molar urinary potassium/creatinine and the urinary chloride/creatinine indices are based on a near-constant creatinine excretion rate and consequently have a limited significance in patients with a very low body mass index.

(d) The 24-h K^+-excretion is a further useful diagnostic test. The use of this traditional diagnostic test is not generally advised considering that 24-h urine collections are troublesome and difficult to obtain (and often imprecise) in children who are not hospitalized, are not practical in a medical emergency, and almost impossible without invasive techniques such as bladder catheterization in infants.

In our experience, the following three "urinary tests" are useful to distinguish the various causes of hypokalemia and hyperkalemia:

• In normotensive children with hypokalemia the transtubular K^+ gradient and the urinary potassium/creatinine ratio (and perhaps the fractional clearance of K^+) easily help distinguish hypokalemia due to a short-term shift of the ion into cells (transtubular K^+ gradient <2.5; urinary potassium/creatinine <2.5 mol/mol) from hypokalemia resulting from a deficit of this ion, including renal K^+ losing conditions and hypokalemia complicating intestinal diseases (in patients experiencing diarrhea, secondary hyperaldosteronism caused by circulating volume depletion leads to an increased urine K^+ excretion).

• In normotensive children with hypokalemia and metabolic alkalosis the urinary excretion of Cl^- helps distinguish renal (urinary chloride/creatinine ratio >10 mol/mol) from non-renal causes (urinary chloride/creatinine ratio <10 mol/mol), as explained in the subchapter metabolic alkalosis.

• It has sometimes been incorrectly assumed that, when hypokalemia occurs in the context of non-renal conditions, the fractional clearance of K^+, the molar urinary potassium/creatinine ratio and the 24 h K^+-excretion are very low, allowing discrimination of non-renal and renal conditions. However, in most children with non-renal hypokalemia extracellular volume depletion is present also, leading to secondary activation of the renin-angiotensin II-aldosterone system, and therefore to an increased urinary K^+ excretion. As a consequence, the urinary K^+ excretion sometimes does not discriminate between non-renal and renal conditions associated with hypokalemia.

- In hyperkalemia the molar urinary potassium/creatinine ratio and the transtubular K^+ gradient help distinguish impaired from unimpaired urinary K^+ excretion. In subjects with unimpaired urinary K^+ excretion the molar urinary potassium/creatinine ratio is expected to be >20 mol/mol, the transtubular K^+ gradient >7.

Hypokalemia

The clinician evaluating a child with hypokalemia (<3.5 mmol/L) should consider five groups of causes [21–26]: (a) spurious hypokalemia; (b) redistribution; (c) true K^+ depletion due to non-renal (mostly intestinal) conditions; (d) true K^+ depletion due to renal conditions; and (e) hypokalemia associated with an expanded "effective" circulating volume and therefore with systemic hypertension due to enhanced mineralocorticoid activity (Table 34.8).

The total K^+ stores are reduced only in subjects with hypokalemia due to non-renal or renal conditions. On the other side, the body K^+ content is normal in children with spurious hypokalemia, in those with an increased shift of K^+ into cells and in those with hypokalemia associated with an expanded "effective" circulating volume.

Table 34.8 Causes of hypokalemia

- **Spurious hypokalemia** (cells take up potassium after blood has been drawn)
- **Hypokalemia associated with normal or low blood pressure**
  - **Increased shift of potassium into cells (total body K^+ content normal)**
    - Activation of β_2-adrenergic receptors
      - Endogenous: stress, hypothermia
      - Exogenous: β_2-adrenergic agonists (e.g.: albuterol), xanthines
    - Hormones
      - Insulin
        - Endogenous: anabolism (e.g.: refeeding syndrome)
        - Exogenous: treatment of diabetic ketoacidosis
      - Aldosterone (possibly)
    - Alkalosis (metabolic)
    - Rare causes
      - Hypokalemic periodic paralysis
        - Congenital (autosomal dominant inheritance)
        - Complicating thyrotoxicosis (particularly in Chinese males)
      - Barium-induced hypokalemia, acute chloroquine intoxication
      - Maturation of red cell precursors after treatment of megaloblastic anemia with vitamin B_{12} or folic acid
      - Paraneoplastic hypokalemia secondary to increased cell synthesis in acute myeloid leukemia[a]
  - **True potassium depletion (= total K^+ body content reduced)**
    - **Extrarenal "conditions"**
      - Prolonged poor potassium intake, protein-energy malnutrition
      - Gastrointestinal conditions
        - Gastric (associated with alkalosis): Vomiting, nasogastric suction
        - Small bowel
          - Associated with acidosis: biliary drainage, intestinal fistula, malabsorption, diarrhea (including diarrhea associated with AIDS), radiation enteropathy
          - Associated with alkalosis: Congenital chloride diarrhea
        - Large bowel
          - Associated with acidosis: uretero-sigmoidoscopy
          - Acid-base balance unpredictable: bowel cleansing agents, laxatives, clay ingestion, potassium binding resin ingestion
      - Sweating, full thickness burns

(continued)

Table 34.8 (continued)

    Cystic fibrosis

    Dialysis

  Renal "conditions"

    Interstitial nephritis, post-obstructive diuresis, recovery from acute renal failure

    With metabolic acidosis: renal tubular acidosis (type I or II), carbonic anhydrase inhibitors (e.g.: acetazolamide and topiramate), amphotericin B, outdated tetracyclines

    With metabolic alkalosis

      Inherited conditions: Bartter syndromes, Gitelman syndrome and related syndromes

      Acquired conditions: normotensive primary aldosteronism, loop and thiazide diuretics, high dose antibiotics (penicillin, naficillin, ampicillin, carbenicillin, ticarcillin), magnesium depletion

    Acid-base balance unpredictable: cetuximab

• **Hypokalemia associated with high blood pressure (often linked with metabolic alkalosis; total K^+ body content normal)**

    Low renin: primary aldosteronism (either hyperplasia or adenoma), apparent mineralocorticoid excess (= defect in 11-β-hydroxysteroid-dehydrogenase), Liddle syndrome (congenitally increased function of the collecting tubule sodium channels), dexamethasone-responsive aldosteronism (synthesis of aldosterone promoted not only by renin but also by adrenocorticotropin), congenital adrenal hyperplasia (11-β-hydroxylase or 17-α-hydroxylase deficiency), Cushing disease, exogenous mineralocorticoids, licorice-ingestion (= 11-β-hydroxysteroid-dehydrogenase blockade)

    Normal or high renin: renal artery stenosis, malignant hypertension, renin producing tumor

[a] The pathogenic mechanism includes also hyperkaluresis due to activation of the renin-angiotensin II system

Occasionally, metabolically active cells (in the blood sample) take up K^+ after blood has been drawn and before it has been tested in the laboratory. This condition, which has been called **spurious hypokalemia**, has been noted in patients with acute myeloid leukemia associated with a very high white blood cell count and in hot weather. The problem of spurious hypokalemia, which is much less common than spurious hyperkalaemia, can be avoided if plasma (or serum) is rapidly separated from the cells or if the blood is stored at 4 °C.

Normal total body K^+ content with hypokalemia results from an **increased shift of this ion into cells**. Metabolic alkalosis, increased endogenous secretion or exogenous administration of insulin, sympathetic activation and exogenous administration of β_2-adrenergic receptors are the main causes of hypokalemia caused by cellular uptake of K^+. Hypokalemic periodic paralysis is an uncommon form of hypokalemia resulting from an increased shift of K^+ into cells, which is characterized by recurrent episodes of hypokalemia (associated with hypophosphatemia and mild hypomagnesemia) and muscular weakness or paralysis that occurs primarily in males of Asian descent. The hypokalemic episodes are precipitated by rest after exercise, a carbohydrate meal or the administration of insulin or β-adrenergic agonists.

The K^+ stores may be depleted when **dietary K^+ is very low** and therefore fails to counterbalance the obligatory K^+ losses and, in infancy and childhood, the required K^+ accretion. Since the kidney is able to lower K^+ excretion to very low figures in the presence of K^+ depletion, decreased intake alone will cause hypokalemia only in rare cases. However, it contributes to the severity of K^+ depletion when another problem is superimposed. Under normal circumstances the net fluid loss from the skin and the gastrointestinal tract is small, therefore preventing the development of K^+ depletion. Sometimes, however, in cases such as prolonged exertion in hot, dry environment, in cystic fibrosis (in these patients sweat contains large amounts of Na^+, K^+ and Cl^-), and especially in the context of various gastrointestinal conditions (Table 34.8) K^+ loss occurs. In most of these cases extracellular volume depletion is present also, leading to secondary activation of the renin-angiotensin II-aldosterone system, and further worsening the K^+ deficiency. It has even been noted that in some patients with diarrheal states, an increased urinary K^+ excretion plays a more important role than intestinal losses in the development of K^+ deficiency. Hypokalemia is mostly associated with metabolic alkalosis after poor dietary K+ intake, in the context of "upper" gastrointestinal conditions or in conditions associated with increased sweating and with acidosis in "lower" gastrointestinal conditions. Finally, **renal K+ losses** occur either associated with acidosis or, more frequently, with alkalosis.

Excessive mineralocorticoid activity is the main cause of hypokalemia associated with metabolic alkalosis and arterial hypertension. The underlying mechanism will be discussed elsewhere.

Clinical Work Up

The clue to the diagnosis of spurious hypokalemia is a normal electrocardiogram without the characteristic changes (Fig. 34.9). Considering that the great majority of children with true hypokalemia have either a gastrointestinal condition or take drugs associated with renal K+ wasting, the causes of hypokalemia can almost always be discerned clinically. When the data obtained from the clinical history fail to establish a presumptive diagnosis, the following simple steps are suggested:

- Repeated measurement of blood pressure;
- Concurrent determination of the acid-base balance, Na+, Cl−, Ca++, Mg++, inorganic phosphate, alkaline phosphatase, uric acid, and especially urea and creatinine;
- In normotensive subjects the molar urinary potassium/creatinine ratio distinguishes hypokalemia due to a short-term shift of K+ into cells (ratio <2.5 mol/mol) from hypokalemia resulting from a deficit of the ion;
- In normotensive subjects with hypokalemia and metabolic alkalosis the urinary chloride/creatinine ratio discriminates renal (ratio >10 mol/mol) from non-renal causes (ratio <10 mol/mol).

Management

Considering the numerous origins of hypokalemia, this section will focus exclusively on the urgency and the mode of substitution in patients with normotensive hypokalemia [24–26].

- The urgency for substitution is dictated by following factors: (a) Conditions that increase the likelihood of dangerous cardiac arrhythmias (and/or concurrent cardiac pathologies reducing the hemodynamic tolerance of arrhythmias); (b) The possibility that K+ will shift into cells (e.g.: during recovery from diabetic ketoacidosis); (c) Severe muscle weakness in a child who must intensively hyperventilate because of metabolic acidosis, (d) Magnitude of the ongoing K+ losses (e.g.: during severe diarrhea); and (e) Degree of hypokalemia.
- Potassium preparations
  - Potassium chloride: preferred in metabolic alkalosis due to diuretic therapy or vomiting;
  - Potassium citrate or potassium bicarbonate: prescribed in hypokalemia and metabolic acidosis (typically renal tubular acidosis);
  - Potassium phosphate: administered in the recovery from diabetic ketoacidosis, in subjects at risk of refeeding syndrome and during total parenteral nutrition.
- The concurrent intravenous administration of K+Cl− with glucose or bicarbonate is not advised in patients with severe hypokalemia, because glucose and bicarbonate cause a shift of K+ into cells and transiently reduce circulating K+ concentration.
- Route of administration. The safest way to administer K+ is by mouth. Intestinal conditions that limit intake or absorption of K+, severe hypokalemia (<2.5 mmol/L), characteristic electrocardiogram abnormalities (with or without cardiac arrhythmias) or respiratory muscle weakness and an anticipated shift of K+ into cells mandate intravenous substitution.
- Intravenous K+Cl−
  - Bolus of K+Cl− is recommended exclusively in very severe degree of hypokalemia and abnormal electrocardiogram. The aim will be to raise K+ to 3.0 mmol/L in

1–2 min.[3] The amount of intravenous K^+Cl^- (in mmol) will be chosen from measured K^+ (in mmol/L) and body weight (in kg) using the formula: $(3.0 - $ measured $K^+) \times$ body weight $\times 0.04$. Following this bolus, the rate of infusion of K^+ should be reduced to 0.015 mmol/kg body weight per minute, and measurement of K^+ concentration should be repeated each 5–10 min.

> N.B.: The K^+Cl^- supplementation should be minimal if hypokalemia is due exclusively to an abnormal distribution of the K^+ stores (e.g.: exogenous administration of β_2-adrenergic receptors or hypokalemic periodic paralysis).

- In conditions demanding intravenous K^+ but without any acute emergency the rate of infused K^+ should not exceed 0.5–1.0 mmol/kg body weight hourly. Furthermore the K^+ concentration in intravenous solutions should be less than 40 mmol/L for use in peripheral veins because higher concentrations lead to local discomfort, venous spasm and sclerosis.

- Parenteral supplemental K^+ administration is the most common cause of severe hyperkalemia. Consequently, the safest route to give K^+ is by mouth. A traditional approach to minimizing hypokalemia is to ensure adequate dietary K^+ intake (unfortunately the K^+ contained in foods that have a high K^+ content is almost entirely coupled with phosphate rather than with Cl^- and therefore is not effective in repairing K^+-loss associated with Cl^--depletion, including use of diuretics, vomiting or nasogastric drainage). In most circumstances, oral replacement with K^+Cl^- (1–3 mmol/kg body weight daily in divided doses) is effective in correcting hypokalemia.

Hyperkalemia

The clinician evaluating a child with hyperkalemia (>5.5 mmol/L) will initially consider the possible diagnosis of **spurious hyperkalemia** (Table 34.9) [21–23, 27–29]. The term refers to those conditions in which the elevation in the measured K^+ is due to K^+ movement out of the cells during or after the blood specimen has been drawn. The major cause of this common problem is mechanical trauma during venipuncture, resulting in the release of K^+ from red cells and a characteristic reddish tint of the serum (or plasma) due to the release of hemoglobin. A normal electrocardiogram without the characteristic signs (Fig. 34.9) is the initial clue to this diagnosis.

In very rare instances, however, red serum (or red plasma) represents severe intravascular hemolysis rather than a hemolyzed specimen.

Furthermore, spurious hyperkalemia can also occur in hereditary spherocytosis and in familial pseudohyperkalemia, a rare autosomal dominant disorder recognized as a laboratory artifact. In the circulation, the Na^+ and K^+ content of red cells is normal. However, the measured plasma or serum K^+ concentration is elevated because of an abnormally high rate of efflux of K^+ from the red cells when the temperature is lowered below 22 °C. The in vitro K^+ efflux can be reversed by incubation at 37 °C.

K^+ also moves out of white cells and platelets after clotting has occurred. Thus, the serum K^+ concentration normally exceeds the true value in the plasma by 0.1–0.5 mmol/L. Although in normal individuals this difference is clinically insignificant, the measured serum K^+ concentration may be as high as 9 mmol/L in patients with marked leukocytosis or thrombocytosis. Spurious hyperkalemia is suspected whenever there is no apparent cause for the elevation in the serum K^+ concentration in an asymptomatic patient.

True hyperkalemia (Table 34.9) occurs rarely in healthy subjects, because cellular and urinary adaptations prevent substantial extracel-

---

[3]The basis for this decision is as follows: the total blood volume approximates 7% of body weight (this volume circulates each minute, cardiac output being at least 70 mL/min/kg body weight) and plasma volume 60% of blood volume, i.e. approximately 4% of body weight. Consequently a 50.0-kg adolescent with a very severe hypokalemia of 1.5 mmol/L will be given $(3.0 - 1.5) \times 50 \times 0.04 = 3.0$ mmol of K^+Cl^- in 1–2 min. Considering that infused K^+ will mix with interstitial fluid (approximately 3–4 times the plasma volume) before reaching cell membrane, there will be a much smaller increase in K^+ concentration near cell membranes.

Table 34.9 Causes of hyperkalemia (drugs associated with hyperkalemia appear in Table 34.10)

- **Spurious hyperkalemia** (potassium movement out of the cells during or after blood has been drawn)
  - Mechanical trauma during venipuncture
  - Hereditary spherocytosis
  - Familial pseudohyperkalemia
- **True hyperkalemia**
  - **Increased potassium load**[a]
  - **Increased shift of potassium out of cells**
      Normal anion gap metabolic acidosis
      Insulin deficiency
      Extracellular hypertonicity
      Increased tissue catabolism (severe hemolysis, rhabdomyolysis, tumor lysis syndrome, immediately after
  cardiac surgery)
      Severe exercise
      Familial hyperkalemic periodic paralysis (= Gamstorp disease)
      Hyperkalaemia of the premature infant
  - **Impaired renal potassium excretion**
      Global renal failure: acute or chronic
      Hyperreninemic hypoaldosteronism: adrenal insufficiency (= Addison disease), salt-losing congenital
      adrenal hyperplasia (21-hydroxylase deficiency)
      Hyporeninemic hypoaldosteronism: idiopathic, complicating acute glomerulonephritis or mild-to-
      moderate renal failure)
      Pseudohypoaldosteronism
          Type 1 (cortical collecting tubule)
          Primary
              Autosomal recessive[b]: reduced sodium channel activity
              Autosomal dominant: mutations in the gene for the mineralocorticoid receptor, phenotype mild and
              transient
          Secondary: complicating obstructive uropathy (with or without urinary tract infection), systemic lupus
          erythematosus, sickle cell disease, renal transplantation, renal amyloidosis
          Type 2 (= Familial hyperkalemic hypertension or Gordon syndrome[c])

[a] Not a cause of hyperkalemia, unless very acute (and important) or occurring in subjects with impaired potassium excretion (due, for example, to underlying kidney disease)
[b] Autosomal recessive pseudohypoaldosteronism type 1 is opposite to Liddle syndrome
[c] The clinical phenotype of Gordon syndrome is opposite to Gitelman syndrome

lular K$^+$ accumulation. Furthermore, the efficiency of K$^+$ handling is increased if K$^+$ intake is enhanced, thereby tolerating what might be a fatal K$^+$ load. These observations lead to the following conclusions concerning the development of hyperkalemia:

(a) **Increasing K$^+$ load** is not a cause of hyperkalemia, unless very acute or occurring in a patient with impaired urinary K$^+$ excretion. In special conditions, acute hyperkalemia can be induced (primarily in infants because of their small size) by the intravenous administration of unusual large doses of K$^+$ or the use of stored blood for transfusions.

(b) The net **release of K$^+$ from the cells** can cause a transient elevation in the circulating K$^+$ concentration (in the presence of normal or even low total body K$^+$ stores). Four causes of hyperkalemia resulting from release of the ion from cells will be discussed: (a) extracellular hypertonicity; (b) tumor lysis syndrome; (c) hyperkalemic familial periodic paralysis; and d. non-oliguric hyperkalaemia of the premature infant.

An *elevated extracellular tonicity* results in water movement from the cells into the extracellular fluid. This is linked with K$^+$ movement out of the cells by two mechanisms. First, the loss of water raises the intracellular K$^+$ level, creating a gradient for passive K$^+$ exit. Second, the friction forces between water and solute result in K$^+$ being carried along with water. Hypertonicity-induced hyperkalemia occurs in hyperglycemia, in hypernatremia, and following administration of mannitol.

The phenotype of acute *tumor lysis syndrome* is opposite to refeeding syndrome. The term denotes the metabolic abnormalities that occur either spontaneously or immediately after initiation of cytotoxic therapy in neoplastic disorders. The findings include hyperuricemia, hyperkalemia, hyperphosphatemia, hypocalcemia (due to precipitation of calcium phosphate), and acute renal failure. The syndrome has been noted in children with a tumor characterized by rapid cell turnover such as lymphomas (particularly non-Hodgkin lymphoma) and some leukemias.

Hyperkalemic familial periodic paralysis, or Gamstorp disease, is a rare inherited autosomal dominant disease that causes patients to experience episodes of flaccid weakness[4] associated with increased K^+ levels. In this syndrome, hyperkalemia occurs with increased K^+ intake, cold weather, exercise or at rest. The attacks of paralysis, however, are not always linked with hyperkalemia.

Non-oliguric hyperkalemia (>6.5 mmol/L) of the premature infant is a common and serious condition. The features are a rapid rise of K^+ concentration to excessively high values at 24 h after birth, a tendency towards cardiac arrhythmia, and occurrence only within 72 h after birth exclusively in premature infants. This peculiar condition mainly results from a K^+ loss from the intra- into the extracellular space. Moreover, renal K^+ excretion that is dependent on both glomerular filtration rate and urinary output is slightly decreased in this setting. Finally, aldosterone unresponsiveness, rather than a decreased concentration of aldosterone, also contributes to the degree of hyperkalemia. However, since there is no significant K^+ intake during the first days of life of premature infants, even total absence of renal K^+ excretion cannot increase

K^+ concentration, if there is no intra- to extracellular K^+ shift.

(c) Persistent hyperkalemia requires an **impaired urinary K^+ excretion** (the total body K^+ stores are increased in this condition). Two factors modulate renal K^+ homeostasis in the cortical collecting tubule: "hyperkalemia" and aldosterone, which act in concert to promote the tubular secretion and therefore the excretion of K^+, and the flow rate traversing the cortical collecting tubule. Consequently, a decreased aldosterone release or effect or a decreased renal tubular flow rate are the major conditions impairing urinary K^+ excretion.

– *Reduced aldosterone secretion or effect*: Any cause of decreased aldosterone release or effect can diminish the efficiency of K^+ secretion and lead to hyperkalemia. The ensuing tendency towards hyperkalemia directly stimulates K^+ secretion, partially overcoming the relative absence of aldosterone. The net effect is that the rise in the K^+ concentration is generally small in patients with normal renal function, but can be clinically important in the presence of underlying renal insufficiency or with multiple insults.

– *Decreased renal tubular flow rate*: The ability to maintain K^+ excretion at near normal levels is habitually preserved in advanced renal disease as long as both aldosterone secretion and distal flow are maintained. Thus, hyperkalemia generally develops in oliguria or in the presence of an additional problem including high K^+ diet, increased tissue breakdown or reduced aldosterone bioactivity. Impaired cell uptake of K^+ also contributes to the development of hyperkalemia in advanced renal failure. Decreased distal tubular flow rate due to marked effective volume depletion, as in heart failure or "salt-losing" nephropathy, can also induce hyperkalemia.

– Acute and chronic renal failure, the most recognized causes of impaired urinary K^+ excretion, will be discussed elsewhere (See Chaps. 51 and 58). Hyperkalemia

---

[4]Please note that hyperkalemic skeletal muscle paralysis results from hyperkalemia of any cause, rather than this rare inherited disorder.

and a tendency towards hyponatremia and metabolic acidosis characteristically occur in children with hyperreninemic hypoaldosteronism (including classic congenital adrenal hyperplasia), hyporeninemic hypoaldosteronism, and end-organ resistance to aldosterone, mostly referred to as pseudohypoaldosteronism. In North-America, Japan, and most European countries neonatal screening (measurement of 17-hydroxy-hydroxyprogesterone in filter paper blood) identifies children affected by classic congenital adrenal hyperplasia due to 21-hydroxylase deficiency before salt-losing crises with hyperkalemia develop. Consequently, in these countries classic congenital adrenal hyperplasia is nowadays an uncommon cause of hyperkalemia. In our experience, secondary type 1 pseudohypoaldosteronism is, together with advanced renal failure, a common cause of true hyperkalemia, at least in infancy. Secondary type 1 pseudohypoaldosteronism develops in infants with urinary tract infections, in infants (but not older children) with urinary tract anomalies (either obstructive or vesicoureteral reflux), and especially in infants with both urinary tract infections and urinary tract anomalies [30].

– Finally, the syndrome of (acquired) *hyporeninemic hypoaldosteronism*, which is characterized by mild hyperkalemia and metabolic acidosis, is due to diminished renin release and, subsequently, decreased angiotensin II and aldosterone production. The syndrome, which mostly occurs in subjects with mild renal failure, has been first reported in subjects with overt diabetic kidney disease and has been occasionally noted in children with acute glomerulonephritis or mild-to-moderate chronic renal failure.

– Prescribed medications, over-the-counter drugs, and nutritional supplements may disrupt K⁺ balance and promote the development of hyperkalemia, as shown in Table 34.10. Although most of these prod-

Table 34.10 Drugs that have been associated with hyperkalemia

Medication	Mechanism of action
Increased K⁺ input	K⁺ ingestion or infusion
K⁺ supplements (and salt substitutes)	
Nutritional and herbal supplements	
Stored packed red blood cells	
Potassium containing penicillins	
Transcellular K⁺ shifts	
β-adrenergic receptor antagonists	↓ β₂-driven K⁺ uptake
Intravenous amino acids (Lysine, Arginine, Aminocaproic acid)	↑ K⁺ release from cells
Succinylcholine	Depolarized cell membranes
Digoxin intoxication	↓ Na⁺-pump
Impaired renal excretion	
Potassium sparing diuretics	
Spironolactone, eplerenone	Aldosterone antagonists
Triamterene, amiloride	Na⁺ channels blocked (collecting tubule)
Trimethoprimᵃ, pentamidine	Na⁺ channels blocked (collecting tubule)
Nonsteroidal anti-inflammatory drugs	↓ Aldosterone synthesis, ↓ glomerular filtration rate, ↓ renal blood flow
Blockers of the renin-angiotensin II-aldosterone system (converting enzyme inhibitors, angiotensin II-antagonists, renin inhibitors)	↓ Aldosterone synthesis
Heparins (both unfractionated and low molecular weight heparins)	↓ Aldosterone synthesis
Calcineurin inhibitors (e.g.: cyclosporineand tacrolimus)	↓ Aldosterone synthesis, ↓ Na⁺-pump, ↓ K⁺-channels

ᵃ Including cotrimoxazole, the fixed combination of trimethoprim with sulfomethoxazole

ucts are well tolerated, drug-induced hyperkalemia may develop in subjects with underlying renal impairment or other abnormalities in K^+ handling or with concurrent, combined use of multiple drugs potentially inducing hyperkalemia. Their hyperkalemic action is less evident in children than in elderly subjects.

Clinical Work Up

The clue to the diagnosis of spurious hyperkalemia, the most common cause of elevated K^+ levels in clinically asymptomatic infants and children, is a normal electrocardiogram without the characteristic changes.

Considering that the great majority of children with true hyperkalemia have renal failure (either acute or chronic), secondary type 1 pseudohypoaldosteronism or take drugs that can cause hyperkalemia, the cause of hyperkaemia can mostly be discerned clinically. When the data obtained from the clinical history fail to establish a presumptive diagnosis, the following simple steps are suggested [21–23, 27–29]:

- Repeated measurement of blood pressure;
- Concurrent determination of the acid-base balance, Na^+, Cl^-, Ca^{++}, Mg^{++}, inorganic phosphate, alkaline phosphatase, uric acid, and especially urea and creatinine;
- In subjects with true hyperkalemia unrelated to an impaired urinary K^+ excretion, the expected molar urinary potassium/creatinine ratio is >20 mol/mol and the transtubular potassium gradient >10.

Management

Because many conditions account for true hyperkalemia, there is no universal therapy for this dyselectrolytemia. The following measures deserve consideration upon recognition of hyperkalemia with increased total body K^+ stores: (a) Interruption of excessive dietary K^+ intake; (b) Discontinuation of drugs that may cause hyperka-

lemia; (c) Increasing renal K^+ excretion (for this purpose children without end-stage renal failure or physical signs of fluid overload must have substantial salt intake[5] via oral or parenteral routes; the use of a loop diuretic, less frequently a thiazide diuretic, also increases renal K^+ excretion); (d) Increasing gastrointestinal K^+ excretion using cation exchange resins; and (e) Institution of dialysis in children with end-stage renal failure.

Emergencies: Because of the serious deleterious cardiac effects, severe hyperkalemia (≥ 7.1 mmol/L) with electrocardiographic abnormalities requires emergency intervention. The following measures, which are listed according to their rapidity of action, have been recommended:

(a) Intravenous Ca^{++}, which directly antagonizes the membrane actions of hyperkalemia;
(b) Intravenous insulin (and glucose), which lowers extracellular K^+ level by driving K^+ into cells;
(c) Intravenous or nebulised ß$_2$-adrenergic agonists, which, like insulin, drive K^+ into cells; and
(d) Intravenous $NaHCO_3$, which results in H^+ ion release from cells (as part of the buffering reaction), a change that is accompanied by K^+ movement into cells to preserve electroneutrality.

Available data indicate (1) that nebulized (or inhaled) albuterol, a ß$_2$-adrenergic agonist, or intravenous insulin (and glucose) are the best supported recommendations; (2) that their combination may be more effective than either alone; (3) that although there are no properly conducted studies assessing the efficacy of Ca^{++}, there remains little doubt of its effectiveness in treating or preventing arrhythmias; and (4) that evidence for the use of intravenous $NaHCO_3$ is equivocal. For practical purposes, the emergency interventions given in Table 34.11 are advised.

---

[5]A low salt intake and extracellular fluid volume depletion are the most commonly observed contributing factors in the development of hyperkalemia in children with renal failure. In patients with a salt-retaining disease, proper management is achieved by avoiding severe restriction of dietary salt while concurrently administering diuretics.

Table 34.11 Currently recommended emergency intervention for severe hyperkalemia (≥ 7.1 mmol/L) with electrocardiogram abnormalities. Albuterol and intravenous glucose (with insulin) lowers extracellular potassium level by driving potassium into cells, while calcium directly antagonizes the membrane actions of hyperkalemia but does not modify extracellular potassium concentration. None of the recommended emergency interventions modifies the total body potassium content

Medication	Dosage	Onset (min)	Length of effect (h)	Comments—Cautions
Nebulized albuterol	10–20 mg (diluted in 4 mL of saline) over 10 min	15–30	4–6	May increase heart rate
Intravenous albuterol	10 µg/kg body weight over 15 min	15–30	4–6	May increase heart rate
Glucose and insulin	Glucose 0.5–1.0 g/kg body weight and insulin 0.1 U/kg body weight intravenously over 15 min	15–30	4–6	Tendency towards hypoglycemia (monitor blood glucose level)
Intravenous calcium	20–50 mg/kg body weight over 1–3 min	Immediate	½–1	Does not lower potassium level

Acid-Base Balance

Introduction

Maintenance of acid-base balance within narrow limits (i.e. pH 7.00–7.30 within the cell depending on the cell type and tissue of origin and pH 7.35–7.45 in extracellular fluids) is a crucial function of the living organism, largely because of its effects on body proteins. The "pCO2-HCO$_3^-$-pH"-based approach, popularized by Relman and Schwartz in the 1960s, relies upon the definition of pH in blood as a function of the ratio between the partial pressure of carbon dioxide (pCO$_2$; mmHg or kPa) and the bicarbonate (HCO$_3^-$; mmol/L or meq/L) concentration, as indicated by the (simplified) Henderson-Hasselbalch equation [31, 32]:

$$pH = pK + \frac{HCO_3^-}{pCO_2}$$

Arterial blood is the standard sample for the determination of acid-base balance but arterial blood sampling, which can be painful, is often unavailable in childhood. In this age group, acid-base balance is mostly assessed in arterialized capillary blood samples (from the finger pulp following hand warming during ≥ 10 min or the earlobe following spreading the lobe with a vasodilating cream during ≥ 10 min) or in venous blood samples. Normal values for peripheral venous blood differ from those of arterial blood due to the uptake and buffering of metabolically produced CO$_2$ in the capillary circulation. If a tourniquet is used to facilitate phlebotomy, it should be released about one minute before blood is drawn to avoid changes induced by ischemia. The peripheral venous pH range is ≈ 0.02–0.04 pH units lower than in arterial blood, the pCO$_2$ ≈ 3–8 mmHg higher and the HCO$_3^-$ concentration ≈ 1–2 mmol/L lower. Automated blood gas analyzers measure pH and pCO$_2$, while the HCO$_3^-$ concentration is calculated from the Henderson-Hasselbalch equation. Most currently available blood gas analyzers determine circulating L-lactate as well (the assay does not detect D-lactate). Abnormalities of blood pH result from a deviation in circulating bicarbonate (HCO$_3^-$; mmol/L) or in partial pressure of carbon dioxide (pCO$_2$; mmHg[6]). There are four primary disturbances of acid-base balance (Fig. 34.10). Since alveolar ventilation regulates pCO$_2$, any disturbance in pH that results from a primary change in pCO$_2$ is called respiratory acid-base disorder: retention of CO$_2$ leads to a reduction in pH (<7.35) called respiratory acidosis, a fall in pCO$_2$ leads to a rise in pH (>7.45) called respiratory alkalosis. On the other side, primary changes in the concentration of HCO$_3^-$ are called metabolic acid-base disorders: a primary reduction in

---

[6]To obtain SI units (kPa) divide by 7.5.

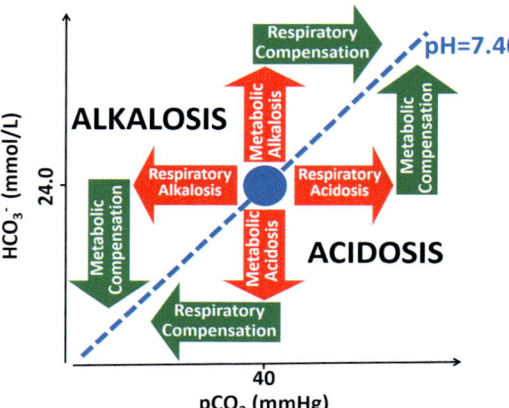

Fig. 34.10 Common sense diagram depicting the four primary disturbances of acid-base balance with the expected compensation. There are four primary disturbances (red arrows) of acid-base balance. Since ventilation modulates pCO_2, any disturbance in pH that results from a primary change in pCO_2 is called respiratory acid-base disorder: retention of CO_2 leads to a reduction in pH (<7.35) called respiratory acidosis, while a fall in pCO_2 leads to a rise in pH (>7.45) called respiratory alkalosis. On the other side, primary changes in the HCO_3^- concentration are called metabolic acid-base disorders: a primary reduction in HCO_3^- is termed metabolic acidosis and a primary increase in HCO_3^- is called metabolic alkalosis. Since blood pH is determined by the ratio between HCO_3^- and pCO_2, and not either one alone, primary respiratory (primary changes in pCO_2) disturbances invoke compensatory metabolic (secondary changes in HCO_3^-) responses (green arrows), and primary metabolic (primary changes in HCO_3^-) disturbances elicit compensatory respiratory (secondary changes in pCO_2) responses (green arrows)

HCO_3^- is termed metabolic acidosis and a primary increase in HCO_3^- is called metabolic alkalosis.

Blood pH is determined by the ratio between HCO_3^- and pCO_2, not either one alone. Thus, primary respiratory disturbances (primary changes in pCO_2) invoke compensatory metabolic responses (secondary changes in HCO_3^-), and primary metabolic disturbances (primary changes in HCO_3^-) elicit compensatory respiratory responses (secondary changes in pCO_2). For instance, metabolic acidosis due to an increase in endogenous acids (e.g., ketoacidosis) lowers extracellular fluid HCO_3^- and decreases extracellular pH. This stimulates the medullary chemoreceptors to increase the ventilation in an attempt to return the ratio of HCO_3^- to pCO_2, and thus pH,

towards normal. The physiologic metabolic and respiratory compensations to simple primary acid-base disturbances can be guessed from the relationships displayed in Table 34.12.

"Base excess" and "standard HCO_3^-" are *in vitro* generated parameters of the acid-base balance that are of little value and often even misleading [31, 32].

Systemic Effects of Metabolic Acid-Base Abnormalities

The systemic effects of acid-base abnormalities will be briefly addressed below [31, 32].

Respiratory System

Primary metabolic acid-base balance disturbances (primary changes in HCO_3^-) elicit compensatory respiratory responses (secondary changes in pCO_2). Metabolic acidosis (=primary reduction in HCO_3^-) stimulates the ventilation to correct the ratio of HCO_3^- to pCO_2, and thus pH, towards normal (Fig. 34.10). The rise in ventilation occurs within minutes but may take several hours to reach its fullest expression. The increase is more the result of increased tidal volume than respiratory rate. This degree of hyperventilation, called Kussmaul respiration, may cause some dyspnea and be appreciated on physical examination. In a child with simple metabolic acidosis, the pCO_2 is expected to decrease by 1.3 mmHg for each mmol per liter decrease in HCO_3^- (Table 34.12), reaching a minimum of 10–15 mmHg. Thus, a patient with metabolic acidosis and HCO_3^- of 16.0 mmol/L would be expected to have a pCO_2 of ≈30 mmHg, i.e. between 27 and 33 mmHg. Values for pCO_2 <27 or >33 mmHg define a mixed disturbance (metabolic acidosis and respiratory alkalosis or metabolic acidosis and respiratory acidosis, respectively).

Primary metabolic alkalosis (= primary increase in HCO_3^-) may lead to compensatory hypoventilation and consequent CO_2 retention. Uncomplicated metabolic alkalosis is usually not associated with profound alveolar hypoventilation. Metabolic alkalosis should be repaired

Table 34.12 Predicted compensations to simple primary acid-base disturbances

Disorder	Primary change	Compensatory response
Metabolic acidosis	↓ HCO_3^-	↓ pCO_2 by 1.3[a] mmHg for ↓ 1.0 mmol/L[b] in HCO_3^-
Metabolic Alkalosis	↑ HCO_3^-	↑ pCO_2 by 0.6[a] mmHg for ↑ 1.0 mmol/L[b] in HCO_3^-
Respiratory Acidosis	↑ pCO_2	
Acute		↑ 1.0 mmol/L[c] in HCO_3^- for ↑ 10 mmHg[d] in pCO_2
Chronic		↑ 3.5 mmol/L[c] in HCO_3^- for ↑ 10 mmHg[d] in pCO_2
Respiratory Alkalosis	↓ pCO_2	
Acute		↓ 2.0 mmol/L[c] in HCO_3^- for ↓ 10 mmHg[d] in pCO_2
Chronic		↓ 5.0 mmol/L[c] in HCO_3^- for ↓ 10 mmHg[d] in pCO_2

[a] Range approximately ±3 mmHg
[b] From 25 mmol/L
[c] Range approximately ±2.0 mmol/L
[d] From 40 mmHg

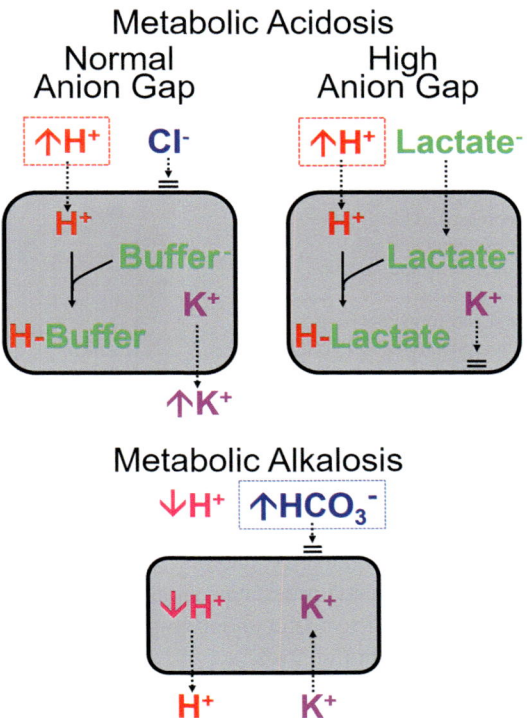

Fig. 34.11 Effect of metabolic acidosis or alkalosis on circulating potassium level. Both in normal (= hyperchloremic) and high (= normochloremic) anion gap metabolic acidosis some extracellular H^+ shifts into the intracellular fluid volume (the squares denote the cell membrane). In normal anion gap (left upper panel) metabolic acidosis, Cl^- remains largely in the extracellular fluid volume. On the contrary, in high anion gap (right upper panel) metabolic acidosis (e.g.: L-lactate acidosis) some organic anions enter the intracellular fluid. Hence, a tendency towards hyperkalemia, the consequence of a shift of K^+ from the intracellular to the extracellular fluid volume, occurs almost exclusively in normal anion gap metabolic acidosis only. Please note that hyperkalemia is followed by a stimulated aldosterone release and results in the urinary excretion of the extra K^+. No tendency towards hyperkalemia occurs in respiratory acidosis. In metabolic alkalosis (lower panel) some intracellular H^+ shifts into the extracellular fluid volume. Hence, a tendency towards hypokalemia, the consequence of a shift of K^+ from the extracellular to the intracellular fluid volume, occurs. No tendency towards hypokalemia occurs in respiratory alkalosis

before surgery (e.g.: before pyloromyotomy in infantile hypertrophic pyloric stenosis) because this acid-base abnormality predisposes to respiratory depression in the immediate postoperative course.

Potassium Balance

There are major interactions between the internal K^+ balance and acute metabolic acid-base changes. In patients with normal anion gap metabolic acidosis the excess hydrogen ions are buffered in the cell and electroneutrality is maintained by movements of intracellular K^+ into the extracellular fluid. Interestingly, metabolic acidosis is much less likely to raise the extracellular K^+ concentration in patients with high anion gap acidosis like L-lactate acidosis or ketoacidosis. The underlying mechanisms are briefly explained in Fig. 34.11 (upper panel). For similar reasons, some tendency towards hypokalemia is noted in metabolic alkalosis (Fig. 34.11, lower panel). Respiratory acidosis and alkalosis do not significantly modulate K^+ balance.

Ca^{++} (and Mg^{++}) Balance

Acid-base disorders affect circulating Ca^{++}, Mg^{++}, inorganic phosphate, and K^+. Acidemia increases calcium phosphate dissociation, increasing free (ionized) Ca^{++}. Acidemia also allows greater dis-

Fig. 34.12 Effect of Alkalemia on the concentration of ionized calcium and magnesium in blood. In the context of alkalemia (e.g.: hyperventilation) blood H⁺ concentration decreases. As a consequence, freely ionized calcium and magnesium concentrations decrease. The opposite is observed in the context of acidemia

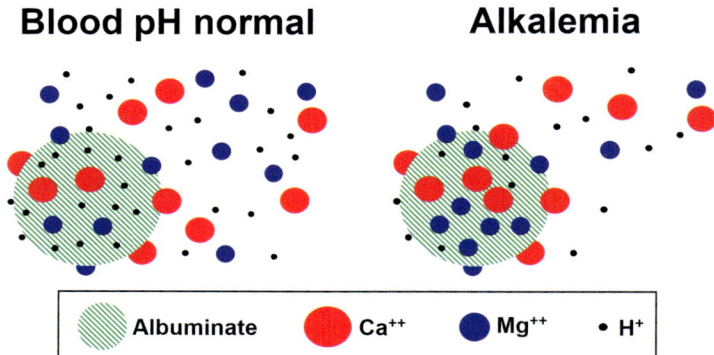

sociation of Ca^{++} and Mg++ from plasma protein. The effect of acidosis on Ca^{++} salt dissociation extends to the bone. Alkalemia might increase calcium phosphate precipitation and lowers ionized Ca^{++} and Mg^{++} (the underlying mechanisms are explained in Fig. 34.12).

Hemoglobin Oxygen Affinity

Blood pH alters hemoglobin oxygen binding and tissue oxygen delivery. Acidemia decreases hemoglobin oxygen affinity, shifts the oxygen dissociation curve "to the right" and increases tissue delivery of oxygen (Bohr effect). On the contrary, alkalemia shifts the curve to the left, increasing the oxygen binding to hemoglobin and tending to decrease tissue delivery.

Cardiovascular System

Acidemia impairs cardiovascular function in four ways: (a) it depresses vascular tone; (b) it alters the release of, and the response to, catecholamines; (c) it depresses myocardial contractility inducing diastolic dysfunction; and (d) it induces arrhythmias (in mild to moderate acidemia, increased catecholamines produce sinus tachycardia; when acidemia is severe, vagal activity increases and bradycardia ensues; there is also an increased risk of ventricular fibrillation). Alkalemia exerts fewer effects on the cardiovascular system. The predominant clinical problem is an increase in myocardial irritability. Alkalemia reduces the free Ca^{++} and Mg^{++} inside the cell and out, and most alkale-

mic patients are also hypokalemic. Changes in both ions contribute to the increased potential for arrhythmias.

Alkalemia has significant effects on vascular tone in the cerebral circulation: hypocarbia constricts the cerebral vasculature as indicated by the fact that subjects with respiratory alkalosis develop lightheadedness and lack of mental acuity, but coma does not occur.

Central Nervous System

Acidosis and alkalosis impair central and peripheral nervous system function. Alkalemia increases seizure activity. If pH is ≥7.60, seizures may occur in the absence of an underlying epileptic diathesis. Acidosis depresses the central nervous system (this most frequently occurs in respiratory acidosis). Early signs of impairment include tremors, myoclonic jerks, and clonic movement disorders. At pH ≤7.10, there is generalized depression of neuronal excitability. Central effects of severe hypercarbia include lethargy and stupor at pCO_2 60 mmHg or more, coma occurs at pCO_2 ≥90 mmHg. Metabolic acidosis causes central nervous system depression less commonly. Fewer than 10% of diabetics with ketoacidosis develop coma (hyperosmolarity and the presence of acetoacetate may be more important than acidosis per se).

Metabolism

A final aspect of acid-base pathophysiology is the effect of pH on metabolism. The most often

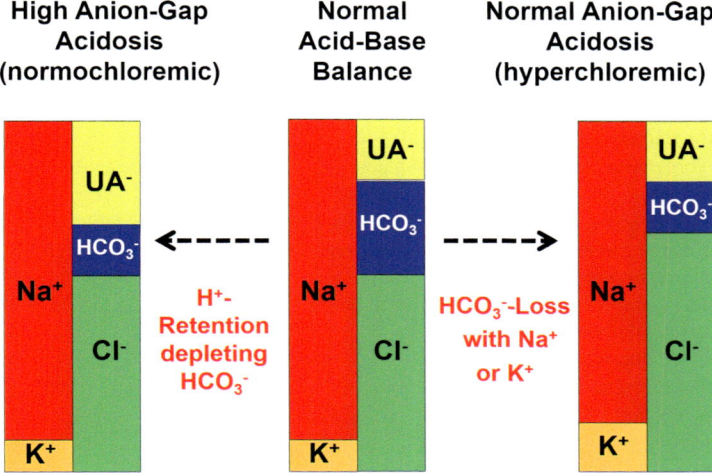

High Anion-Gap Acidosis (normochloremic) | **Normal Acid-Base Balance** | **Normal Anion-Gap Acidosis (hyperchloremic)**

H^+-Retention depleting HCO_3^-

HCO_3^--Loss with Na^+ or K^+

UA^- = unmeasured anions = $(Na^+ + K^+) - (Cl^- + HCO_3^-)$

Fig. 34.13 High anion gap (= normochloremic) and normal anion gap (= hyperchloremic) metabolic acidosis. Calculation of the blood anion gap, the difference between the major measured cations (Na^+ and K^+; mmol/L) and the major measured anions (HCO_3^- and Cl^-; mmol/L), is a crucial laboratory diagnostic tool in patients with metabolic acidosis. The blood anion gap separates two major types of metabolic acidosis. High anion gap (= normochloremic) metabolic acidosis results from retention of fixed acids, which deplete HCO_3^- stores by releasing their protons (most cases develop following excessive endogenous or exogenous acid load). Most cases of normal anion gap (= hyperchloremic) metabolic acidosis result from an intestinal or a renal loss of HCO_3^- (accompanied either by Na^+ or K^+). The figure also emphasizes the tendency towards hyperkalemia (the result of a K^+-shift from the intracellular to the extracellular fluid volume) in normal anion gap (hyperchloremic) metabolic acidosis (as explained in Fig. 34.11)

cited example of pH control of enzyme activity is the pH regulation of phosphofructokinase, which catalyzes a rate-controlling step in carbohydrate metabolism. Glycolysis terminates in lactic and pyruvic acid; and accumulation of these acids reduces pH. This is but one example of pH feedback. Most enzymes operate most effectively at a specific optimum pH. As pH varies from the optimum, enzyme activity changes. The integrated response of the individual enzyme alterations may serve to maintain or restore normal pH.

Metabolic Acidosis

Primary hypobicarbonatemia and, therefore, metabolic acidosis mostly occurs when endogenous acids are produced faster than they can be excreted, when HCO_3^- is lost from the body, or when exogenous acids are administered [31–35].

The main laboratory tool in metabolic acidosis is the calculation of the blood anion gap

(Fig. 34.13), the difference between the major measured cations (Na^+ and K^+; mmol/L) and the major measured anions (bicarbonate and Cl^-; mmol/L) by means of the equation:

$$AG = (Na^+ + K^+) - (Cl^- + HCO_3^-)$$

Because electroneutrality must be maintained, the anion gap results from the difference between the unmeasured anions (primarily albumin, which is largely responsible for the normal anion gap, but also phosphate, sulfate, and organic anions such as lactate) and the remaining cations (Ca^{++} and Mg^{++}).

The calculation of blood anion gap (reference: ≤ 18 mmol/L[7]) allows separation of the two major types of metabolic acidosis: one type has an increased anion gap (>18 mmol/L; high anion

---

[7]The blood anion gap sometimes does not include the blood concentration of K^+: $Na^+ - (HCO_3^- + Cl^-)$. The approximate upper value of this anion gap is lower by 4 mmol/L: 14 mmol/L.

Table 34.13 Causes of metabolic acidosis

- **Metabolic acidosis with increased anion gap**
  - Excessive acid load
    - Endogenous sources of acid (due to abnormal metabolism of substrates)
      - Ketoacidosis (largely β-hydroxybutyric acid)
      - Congenital organic acidemias (e.g.: methylmalonic acidemia and propionic acidemia)
      - L-lactate acidosis
        - Type A (impaired tissue oxygenation; e.g.: sepsis, hypovolemia, cardiac failure)
        - Type B (altered metabolism of L-lactate with normal tissue oxygenation in the context of a mitochondrial impairment)
          - Inherited metabolic diseases: either altered production of glucose from lactate or altered degradation of pyruvate derived from pyruvate
          - Thiamine deficiency
          - Drugs (e.g.: biguanides, antiretroviral agents)
          - Toxins (e.g.: ethanol)
          - Chronic diseases (mostly hepatic)
      - Overproduction of organic acids in the gastrointestinal tract (D-lactate)
      - Conversion of alcohols (methanol, ethylene glycol) to acids and poisonous aldehydes
  - Defective renal excretion of acids due to generalized renal failure ("uremic acidosis")
- **Metabolic acidosis with normal anion gap**
  - Losses of bicarbonate (HCO_3^-)
    - Intestinal: diarrhea, surgical drainage of the intestinal tract, gastrointestinal fistulas resulting in losses of fluid rich in HCO_3^-, patients whose ureters have been attached to the intestinal tract (the alkali of intestinal secretion is lost by titration with acid urine)
    - Urinary: carbonic anhydrase inhibitors (e.g.: acetazolamide), proximal renal tubular acidosis (= type 2)
  - Failure to replenish HCO_3^- stores depleted by the daily production of fixed acids
    - Distal renal tubular acidosis (either classic, also called type 1, or type 4)
    - Diminished mineralocorticoid (or glucocorticoid) activity (adrenal insufficiency, selective hypoaldosteronism, aldosterone resistance)
    - Administration of potassium sparing diuretics (spironolactone, eplerenone, amiloride, triamterene)
  - Exogenous infusions
    - Amino acids like L-arginine and L-lysine (during parenteral nutrition)
    - HCl or NH_4Cl
  - Rapid administration of normal saline solution (= "dilutional" metabolic acidosis)

gap metabolic acidosis) and the other does not (normal anion gap metabolic acidosis or hyperchloremic metabolic acidosis), as shown in Fig. 34.13 and Table 34.13.

High Anion Gap Metabolic Acidosis

The HCO_3^- deficit observed in high anion gap metabolic acidosis results from retention of fixed acids, which deplete HCO_3^- stores by releasing their protons. Two mechanisms lead to this form of metabolic acidosis (Fig. 34.13 and Table 34.13): (a) excessive acid load (endogenous or exogenous) overwhelming the normal capacity to decompose or excrete the acid; and (b) diminished capacity to excrete the normal load of fixed acids in the context of renal failure.

In health, the blood anion gap is predominantly due to the net negative charge of albumin. Abnormally low serum albumin levels influence acid-base interpretation as calculated by the anion gap. For example, in a patient with increased production of endogenous acids, elevation of the anion gap may be masked by concurrent hypoalbuminemia. In this condition the anion gap corrected for albumin may be calculated by means of the following formula (albumin in g/L):

$$\left(Na^+ + K^+ \right) - \left(Cl^- + HCO_3^- \right) + \frac{1}{4}\left(40 - \text{Albumin} \right)$$

Considering that many currently available blood gas analyzers determine circulating L-lactate, the determination of the albumin and lactate corrected anion gap has been recently suggested (upper reference: 15 mmol/L):

$$\left(Na^+ + K^+\right) - \left(Cl^- + HCO_3^- + Lactate\right) + \frac{1}{4}\left(40 - Albumin\right)$$

Normal Anion Gap Metabolic Acidosis (= "Hyperchloremic")

This form of metabolic acidosis develops (Fig. 34.13 and Table 34.13): (a) from a primary loss of HCO_3^-, (b) from the failure to replenish HCO_3^- stores depleted by the daily production of fixed acids (H^+: 1–3 mmol/kg body weight) in subjects with normal glomerular filtration rate, or (c) from the administration of exogenous acids (including the rapid administration of large volumes of normal saline solution and other Cl^- rich fluids).

The following factors account for the metabolic acidosis that is observed after administration of normal saline solution, which is called "dilutional" (or "chloride overload") acidosis: (a) Volume expansion, which results from infusion of normal saline, reduces the renal threshold for HCO_3^- leading to bicarbonaturia; (b) The infusion of normal saline with a Na^+ level almost identical to that of blood results in a relatively stable Na^+ level in blood. By contrast, the concentration of Cl^- in the infused solution, which is much higher than that of normal blood, leads to progressive hyperchloremia and hypobicarbonatemia.

Urine Net Charge

The kidney prevents the development of metabolic acidosis by modulating the HCO_3^- concentration in blood. This is done by (a) preventing loss of large amounts of filtered HCO_3^- (primarily a task of the proximal tubule, which may reclaim the filtered HCO_3^-) and (b) generating HCO_3^- (primarily a task of the distal tubule). The main mechanism by which the distal tubule generates HCO_3^- is the conversion of glutamine to NH_4^+, which is excreted in the urine, plus HCO_3^-,

which is added to the blood. As a consequence, the urinary NH_4^+ excretion reflects the renal HCO_3^- generation, and the renal NH_4^+ excretion can be equated with HCO_3^- regeneration on a 1:1 basis. In a child with normal anion gap metabolic acidosis and normal renal mechanisms of acidification a very low urinary concentration of HCO_3^- and, more importantly, a large concentration of NH_4^+ will result. The measurement of these parameters, which is complicated by the need to avoid significant changes in urine composition after voiding,[8] is usually unavailable in clinical practice. In the context of metabolic acidosis, a urinary pH significantly <6.2 indicates a very low urinary concentration of HCO_3^- and argues against an altered renal mechanism of urinary acidification. Furthermore, and more importantly, the crucial concept of urinary net charge or urine anion gap[9] (which results from urinary Na^+, K^+ and Cl^-) was developed as an indirect assessment of urinary NH_4^+ concentration. Usually, because ammonium (an unmeasured cation) accompanies Cl^- in the context of metabolic acidosis, the concentration of Cl^- should be greater than the sum of Na^+ and K^+, and the net charge negative ($Na^+ + K^+ < Cl^-$). A positive net charge ($Na^+ + K^+ > Cl^-$) indicates impaired ammonium secretion and, therefore, impaired distal acidification of renal tubule. For instance, in the aforementioned context of metabolic acidosis with normal renal mechanisms of acidification (e.g. a child with normal anion gap metabolic acidosis

---

[8]The changes are due to bacterial overgrowth, especially at room temperature, as well as to open exposure to the atmosphere, which produces gas loss.

[9]The term urine anion gap is a misnomer for what should have been named urine cation gap.

Table 34.14 Indirect assessment of urinary excretion of NH_4^+ by means of the urinary net charge in subjects with normal anion gap metabolic acidosis

Distal acidification of the renal tubule	Urinary NH_4^+	Urinary net charge
Normal	↑ NH_4^+	$Na^+ + K^+ < Cl^-$
Impaired	↓ NH_4^+	$Na^+ + K^+ > Cl^{-a}$

[a] The urine osmolal charge is a more precise estimate of the urinary NH_4^+ concentration in this setting:

$$\frac{\text{Measured Osmolality} - \left[2 \times (Na + K) + Urea + Glucose\right]}{2}$$

due to mild diarrhea) the enhanced urinary NH_4^+ excretion will result in a large urinary level of urinary NH_4Cl and consequently the measured urinary cations (= $Na^+ + K^+$) will have a concentration lower than that of the measured anion Cl^-: $Na^+ + K^+ < Cl^-$. On the contrary, in a child with an impaired renal acidification, the urine net charge will be as follows: $Na^+ + K^+ > Cl^-$ (Table 34.14).

When the urine net charge is positive ($Na^+ + K^+ > Cl^-$) and it is unclear whether increased excretion of unmeasured anions is responsible, the urinary NH_4^+ concentration can be estimated from calculation of the urine osmolal gap (Table 34.14). This calculation requires measurement of the urine osmolality (in mosm/kg) and the urine Na^+, K^+, urea, and, if the dipstick is positive, glucose concentrations[10] (in mmol/L). In the context of metabolic acidosis, an estimated urinary NH_4^+ concentration of <20 mmol/L indicates an impaired NH_4^+ excretion.

Metabolic Acidosis During the First Months of Life

During the first months of life bicarbonatemia is lower by 2–4 mmol/L than in older children, and it is even lower in preterm infants. This is the consequence of a lower renal threshold for bicarbonate. In addition, in preterm infants and in growing children the daily production of H^+ is higher by

50–100% than that noted in adults (this is mainly explained by the fact that the growing skeleton releases 20 mmol of H^+ for each 1 g of Ca^{++} that is incorporated). The clinical implications of these data are that, as compared with older children, newborns and infants have a relatively limited capacity to compensate for hypobicarbonatemia. In this age, the tendency towards metabolic acidosis is compensated for by the large intake of milk, whose alkali content is high. Infants are therefore more prone to develop metabolic acidosis in conditions associated with a decreased milk intake.

Symptoms, Signs, Consequences

The signs and symptoms of acute metabolic acidosis include (1) high respiratory rate (in young children and infants, the increase in depth of respiration, as observed in classic Kussmaul type deep breathing, may not be as apparent as in adults and the response to metabolic acidosis may be tachypnea alone); (2) abdominal pain and vomiting; (3) irritability and lethargy.

The gastrointestinal absorption and excretion of dietary base plays a major role in acid-base homeostasis in infants in whom the predominantly milk-based diet supplies a considerable amount of alkali. Infants are therefore more vulnerable to developing metabolic acidosis in illnesses associated with decreased milk intake.

Since an excessive chronic acid burden interferes with Ca^{++} deposition in the bone and Ca^{++} intestinal absorption, metabolic acidosis of any form can impair growth in children. Other signs and symptoms are abdominal pain, vomiting, irritability, lethargy, seizures and coma. However, the latter manifestations are primarily due to the underlying disease (e.g.: organic acidemias or hyperosmolality in diabetic ketoacidosis) and not primarily to the acidosis itself.

Clinical Work Up

The causes of metabolic acidosis, which appear in Table 34.13, can almost always be discerned clinically. A careful history and physical exami-

---

[10]The obtain urea and glucose in mmol/L divide blood urea nitrogen (in mg/dL) by 2.8 and glucose (in mg/dL) by 18.

nation and the determination of the blood anion gap direct an accurate evaluation. For the initial diagnostic approach to metabolic acidosis of unknown origin, the following initial steps are taken [31–35]:

– Confirm the diagnosis of metabolic acidosis
– Confirm that the respiratory response is appropriate
– Distinguish high from normal anion gap metabolic acidosis:

> Normal anion gap: consider intestinal loss of HCO_3^-
> High anion gap: assess urinary ketones, blood glucose and blood L-lactate

The major causes of high anion gap acidosis are L-lactate acidosis, which results from impaired tissue oxygenation (type A acidosis) or from an altered metabolism of L-lactate with normal tissue oxygenation in the context of a mitochondrial impairment (type B acidosis), diabetic ketoacidosis, which mainly results from the accumulation of ß-hydroxybutyrate, and "uremic" metabolic acidosis, which is characterized by the accumulation of phosphate, sulfate, and organic anions.

In children, normal anion gap metabolic acidosis mostly results from intestinal bicarbonate losses due to diarrhea. Renal bicarbonate wasting is much less common. In children with normal anion gap acidosis but without history of diarrhea, the concurrent determination of urinary Na^+, K^+, Cl^- will provide information on the renal mechanisms of acidification.

Sometimes there is overlap between the causes of a normal and high anion gap metabolic acidosis. Diarrhea, for example, is most often associated with a normal anion gap. However, severe diarrhea and hypovolemia can result in an increase in the anion gap due to hypoperfusion-induced lactic acidosis and starvation ketosis.

Management

The management of metabolic acidosis includes the following four points:

- Emergency measures:
  – Avoidance of further production of H^+ including measures to ensure a proper airway, adequate peripheral perfusion and O_2 delivery. For instance, in a child with type A L-lactate acidosis in the context of severe dehydration, delivery of O_2 and the rapid administration of normal saline will regenerate adenosine triphosphate. On the other hand, in a child with accidental methanol intoxication the administration of ethanol might stop the production of toxins leading to acidosis.
  – Increasing pH level by lowering the pCO_2, ensuring an adequate degree of hyperventilation, if necessary by mechanical ventilation.
- Correction of the underlying condition. For example, the administration of insulin, in addition to normal saline, in diabetic ketoacidosis.
- Administration of $NaHCO_3$. The use of $NaHCO_3$ is controversial, considering the possible benefits ((a) metabolic advantage of faster glycolysis with better availability of adenosine triphopsphate in vital organs; (b) improved cardiac action) and the risks ((a) extracellular fluid volume expansion; (b) tendency towards hypernatremia; (c) development of hypokalemia and hypocalcemia; (d) worsening of intracellular acidosis). The following guidelines have been suggested for administration of $NaHCO_3$:
  – Diabetic ketoacidosis: $NaHCO_3$ should be considered when hyperkalemia persists despite insulin therapy, when acidemia worsens despite insulin therapy (suggesting insulin resistance as a result of acidemia) and perhaps when HCO_3^- is <5.0 mmol/L. We are very reluctant to use bicarbonate in diabetic ketoacidosis because the administration of $NaHCO_3$ is a risk factor for cerebral edema.
  – Type A L-lactate metabolic acidosis: In this form of acidosis the primary effort should be directed at improving delivery of O_2. $NaHCO_3$ should be given when HCO_3^- is <5.0 mmol/L.

– Since the "HCO_3^- space" is ≈ 0.5 L/kg body weight the dose of $NaHCO_3$ in severe metabolic acidosis may be calculated from

body weight (in kg), current blood HCO_3^-, and desired blood HCO_3^- (both in mmol/L), using the equation:

$$Body\ weight \times 0.5 \left(desired\ HCO_3^- - current\ HCO_3^- \right)$$

– Hence, a child weighing 20.0 kg with a severe hypobicarbonatemia of 3.5 mmol/L will be given 40 mmol of $NaHCO_3$ over several minutes (i.e. 2.0 mmol/kg body weight) if the "desired" blood HCO_3^- level is 7.5 mmol/L. In most cases, however, the initial dosage of $NaHCO_3$ is 1.0 mmol/kg body weight, a dosage that is expected to increase blood HCO_3^- by 2.0 mmol/L.

• Correction of metabolic acidosis tends to decrease circulating K^+ level. Hence, one must avoid a severe degree of hypokalemia when $NaHCO_3$ is given. K^+ depletion and metabolic acidosis are associated in three settings: classic distal renal tubular acidosis, acute diarrheal disease and diabetic ketoacidosis, as shown in Table 34.15. The management of renal tubular acidosis will be discussed in the chapter "Renal tubular acidosis", that of uremic acidosis in the sections discussing renal replacement therapy.

Table 34.15 Conditions associating metabolic acidosis and potassium depletion

Condition	Basis of potassium depletion
Classic distal renal tubular acidosis	Renal loss
Diarrhea	Intestinal and renal (secondary hyperaldosteronism due to circulating volume depletion) loss
Diabetic ketoacidosis	Renal loss (osmotic diuresis)[a], cellular shift following insulin therapy

[a] Circulating potassium is often initially normal in diabetic ketoacidosis

Metabolic Alkalosis

Primary hyperbicarbonatemia and, therefore, alkalemia, are the hallmarks of metabolic alkalosis [31, 32, 36, 37]. In this peculiar acid-base disorder (Table 34.16) hyperbicarbonatemia, alkalemia and the compensatory hypoventilation (resulting in a rise of the pCO_2) are almost always associated with hypokalemia (see: systemic effects of acid-base abnormalities).

With the constraints of electroneutrality, the ways to add HCO_3^- to extracellular space are loss of the anion Cl^- or retention of Na^+. Hence circulating HCO_3^- may be raised either (1) associated with a normal or contracted "effective" circulating volume (blood pressure normal or low) or with (2) an expanded "effective" circulating volume (blood pressure increased).

• **Metabolic alkalosis associated with normal or contracted "effective" circulating volume (= "unaccompanied" Cl^- deficiency syndrome or normotensive hypokalemic metabolic alkalosis) = chloride depletion metabolic alkalosis**
• In this clinical-laboratory entity Cl^- is lost from the extracellular space "not accompanied" by the major cations Na^+ and K^+ but "accompanied" by H^+ or NH_4^+. Since a loss of H^+ or NH_4^+ is equivalent to a gain of HCO_3^-, the final effect is loss of Cl^- and gain of HCO_3^-.
• Two further steps complete the development of metabolic alkalosis:
  – "Extra" HCO_3^-, which is filtered by the kidney, is mostly reabsorbed and only a little HCO_3^- is excreted.

Table 34.16 Causes of metabolic alkalosis (linked with hypokalemia)

- Associated with normal (or contracted) "effective" circulating volume (and therefore with normal or even low blood pressure)
  - (a) Nonrenal causes (low urine chloride excretion: chloride/creatinine <10 mol/mol)
    Intestinal causes
    Low dietary chloride intake (e.g.: soybean formula with a low chloride content in infancy, "tea and toast diet")
    Loss of gastric secretions (vomiting, nasogastric suction)
    Posthypercapnia
    Congenital chloridodiarrhea (uncommon), villous adenoma (uncommon)
    Cutaneous cause
    Cystic fibrosis
    Excessive sweating (uncommon, associated with low dietary chloride intake)
    "Posthypercapnia" (= posthypercapnic alkalosis)
    Refeeding syndrome
    Transient neonatal metabolic alkalosis in infants of mothers affected by chloride deficiency (eating disorders associated with chloride deficiency, Bartter syndromes, Gitelman syndrome)
  - (b) Renal causes (high urine chloride excretion: chloride/creatinine >10 mol/mol)
    Primary chloride losing tubulopathies (Bartter syndromes, Gitelman syndrome)
    Secondary chloride losing tubulopathies (some cases of chronic cisplatin tubulopathy)
    Current diuretic use (including surreptitious use)[a]
- Associated with an expanded "effective" circulating volume (and therefore with high blood pressure)
    Enhanced mineralocorticoid activity
    Primary aldosteronism (either hyperplasia or adenoma)
    Apparent mineralocorticoid excess (= defect in 11-β-hydroxysteroid-dehydrogenase), Liddle syndrome (congenitally increased function of the collecting tubule sodium channels), dexamethasone-responsive aldosteronism (synthesis of aldosterone promoted not only by renin but also by adrenocorticotropin), congenital adrenal hyperplasia (11-β-hydroxylase or 17-α-hydroxylase deficiency), Cushing disease
    Secondary hyperaldosteronism (including renal artery stenosis, malignant hypertension, and renin producing tumor)
    Exogenous mineralocorticoids, licorice-ingestion (= 11-β-hydroxysteroid-dehydrogenase blockade)
    Reduced renal function plus a source of HCO_3^-: alkali ingestion, ingestion of ion-exchange resin plus nonreabsorbable alkali

[a] The urinary chloride excretion is low in subjects with remote use of diuretics

- Contraction of the circulating volume activates the renin-angiotensin II-aldosterone system resulting in urinary K^+ excretion, which further aggravates hyperbicarbonatemia.
- Secondary hyperaldosteronism resulting in urinary K^+ excretion is the main cause of hypokalemia that accompanies this form of metabolic alkalosis.
- This clinical-laboratory entity, termed in the past volume contraction hypokalemic alkalosis, is currently termed Cl^- depletion hypokalemic alkalosis because balance and clearance studies indicate that Cl^- repletion in the face of persisting alkali loading, volume contraction, and K^+ and Na^+ depletion repairs alkalosis. During the first months of life metabolic alkalosis is often not associated with hypokalemia (alternatively it is associated with mild hypokalemia) because the ability of the kidney to excrete K^+ is reduced early in life.
- Maternal Cl^- depletion, deficient Cl^- intake, gastrointestinal Cl^- losses, cutaneous Cl^- losses in the setting of cystic fibrosis, diuretics and renal tubular disturbances are the most important causes of normotensive hypokalemic metabolic alkalosis (Table 34.16). The urinary excretion of chloride is low in patients with non-renal and normal or high in subjects with renal causes of this peculiar form of metabolic alkalosis. In our experience the determination of the molar urinary chloride/

creatinine ratio in spot urine samples from patients with normotensive metabolic alkalosis distinguishes between renal (urinary chloride/creatinine ratio largely >10 mol/mol) and non-renal causes (urinary chloride/creatinine ratio <10 mol/mol). In clinical practice this simple parameter is useful in patients in whom the etiology of metabolic alkalosis with normal or low normal blood pressure is not obtainable from the history. Please note that the urinary chloride/creatinine ratio is also usually >10 mol/mol in patients with metabolic alkalosis associated with expanded effective circulating volume (see below).

- **Posthypercapnic alkalosis (= "posthypercapnia").** Chronic respiratory acidosis is associated with a compensatory hyperbicarbonatemia. In those patients with a tendency towards a contracted circulating volume when pCO_2 falls to normal, there will be a stimulus for persistently increased HCO_3^- levels and hypokalemia. In addition, a rapid correction of chronic respiratory acidosis (e.g.: mechanical ventilation) results in an acute rise in cerebral pH that can produce serious neurologic sequelae or even death. Consequently, pCO_2 should be lowered slowly and carefully in chronic hypercapnia.
- **Metabolic alkalosis associated with an expanded "effective" circulating volume (= hypertensive metabolic alkalosis)**
- The second way to add HCO_3^- to the circulating volume and preserving electroneutrality is to retain HCO_3^- along with Na^+, therefore expanding the extracellular fluid volume and increasing blood pressure. Obviously, to retain extra Na^+ (along with HCO_3^-), "permission" of the kidney is required.
- The mechanisms for renal retention of Na^+ and HCO_3^- include either (1) an enhanced reabsorption of filtered HCO_3^- or (2) a reduced glomerular filtration rate plus a source of HCO_3^- (e.g.: the ingestion of large amounts of milk and the absorbable antacid $CaCO_3$).
- Excessive mineralocorticoid activity is the main cause of metabolic alkalosis associated with hypokalemia and expanded circulating volume. The corresponding causes appear in Table 34.16.

Symptoms, Signs, Consequences

There are no specific diagnostic symptoms or signs of metabolic alkalosis [23, 31, 32, 36, 37]. Physical examination may reveal neuromuscolar irritability, such as tetany or hyperactive reflexes. These signs will be more pronounced if hypocalcemia is an accompanying feature, since the ionized Ca^{++} concentration decreases as pH rises. The symptoms and signs of accompanying hypokalemia have been discussed above.

It is recognized that in children with both normal (or contracted) and expanded circulating volume and metabolic alkalosis the assessment of the fluid volume status by physical examination and history may be quite inaccurate. This assumption is supported by the experience in infantile hypertrophic pyloric stenosis where the clinical assessment of the fluid volume status may be quite inaccurate, and the severity of metabolic alkalosis helps to define the amount of fluid replacement required.

Management

The most frequent causes of hypokalemic metabolic alkalosis associated with a normal or contracted "effective" circulating volume include intestinal (mostly gastric) or cutaneous fluid losses, and excessive diuretic therapy. These forms of metabolic alkalosis are termed "chloride responsive", because they are reversed by the oral or intravenous administration of Na^+Cl^-, K^+Cl^- and water. Many institutions hydrate infants with hypertrophic pyloric stenosis with a "near isotonic" parenteral solution containing glucose 5% (= 50 g/L), Na^+Cl^- 80–90 mmol/L and K^+Cl^- 20–30 mmol/L until correction of the acid-base and K^+ balance. The initial parenteral repair consists of a normal saline solution at least in children with both hypokalemic alkalosis and rather severe hyponatremia (≤ 120 mmol/L).

Occasionally, severe metabolic alkalosis is additionally treated with (1) a carbonic anhydrase inhibitor like acetazolamide, which induces bicarbonaturia accompanied by Na^+- and K^+- losses, (2) with NH_4Cl, or (3) with HCl (through a central venous line). Finally, hemodialysis (or hemofiltration) with a low dialysate HCO_3^- in association with saline infusion has been advised for the treatment of severe metabolic alkalosis in advanced kidney disease.

In "chloride responsive" metabolic alkalosis the oral administration of K+ with any anion other than Cl^- (e.g.: citrate) prevents the correction of alkalosis.

Respiratory Acid-Base Disturbances

These acid-base disorders will not be discussed in this textbook of clinical nephrology with the exception of Table 34.17, which depicts the main causes.

Table 34.17 Causes of respiratory acidosis (hypoventilation) and alkalosis (hyperventilation)

- Respiratory acidosis (hypoventilation)
  - Central nervous system (patient will not breathe!)
    - Cerebral
      - Posthypoxic brain damage
      - Cerebral trauma
      - Intracranial disease
      - Psychotropic drugs
    - Brain stem
      - Brain stem herniation
      - Encephalitis
      - Central sleep apnea
      - Severe metabolic alkalosis
      - Sedative or narcotic drugs
    - Upper airway reflexes
      - Bulbar palsy
      - Anterior horn cell lesion (including Guillan-Barré and poliomyelitis)
      - Disruption of airway
  - Peripheral disorders (patient cannot breathe)
    - Respiratory muscle disease
      - Myasthenia, Guillain-Barré syndrome, myopathy, muscular dystrophy
      - Muscle fatigue or paralysis (including hypokalemic paralysis)
    - Airway and pulmonary disease
      - Interstitial lung disease (including lung fibrosis)
      - Obstructive disease (including upper airway obstruction, asthma, bronchiolitis, cystic fibrosis)
    - Obstructive sleep apnea
    - Obesity, kyphoscoliosis
- Respiratory alkalosis (hyperventilation)
  - Hypoxia: intrinsic pulmonary disease, high altitude, congestive heart failure, cyanotic congenital heart disease
  - Pulmonary receptor stimulation: pneumonia, asthma, interstitial lung disease, pulmonary edema, pulmonary thromboembolism
  - Drugs: salicylates, nikethamide, catecholamines, theophylline, progesterone
  - Central nervous disorders: subarachnoid hemorrhage, Cheyne-Stokes respiration, primary hyperventilation syndrome
  - Miscellaneous: panic attacks with hyperventilation (rare before puberty), fever, sepsis, recovery from metabolic acidosis

Calcium

Balance

A 70 kg man contains one kg of Ca^{++} (= 25 mol), 99% of which resides in the skeleton in the form of hydroxyapatite and 1% of which is found in soft tissues and the extracellular space. Since Ca^{++} plays a crucial role in neuromuscular function, blood coagulation, and intracellular signaling, circulating Ca^{++} concentrations are maintained within a tight physiologic range. The Ca^{++} (and phosphate) homeostasis involves intestinal, bone, and renal function. Regulation of intestinal function is important because, in contrast to the complete absorption of dietary Na^{+}, K^{+} and Cl^{-}, that of Ca^{++} (like Mg^{++} and phosphate) is incomplete. This limitation is due both to the requirement for vitamin D and to the formation of insoluble salts in the intestinal lumen, such as calcium phosphate, calcium oxalate, and magnesium phosphate.

A normal adult ingests $\approx$1000 mg (= 25 mmol) of Ca^{++} per day, of which $\approx$40–50% may be absorbed. However, 300 mg (approximately 8 mmol) of Ca^{++} from digestive secretions is lost in the stool, resulting in the net absorption of no more than 10 to 20%. In the steady state, this amount of Ca^{++} is excreted in the urine. Within the blood Ca^{++}, $\approx$40% is bound to albumin, 15% is complexed with citrate, sulfate, or phosphate, and 45% exists as the physiologically important ionized form [38–40].

Considering that a large proportion of circulating Ca^{++} is bound to albumin, the determination of albumin (or the direct measurement of ionized Ca^{++}) is essential to the diagnosis of true hypocalcemia or hypercalcemia. The so-called Payne's formula [38–41] may be used for correction of total calcium to account for albumin binding:

$$\text{Adjusted}\,Ca^{2+}\left[\text{mmol}\,/\,L\right] = \text{measured}\,Ca^{2+}\left[\text{mmol}\,/\,L\right] + \frac{40 - \text{albumin}\left[g\,/\,L\right]}{40}$$

Although only a small fraction of the total body Ca^{++} is located in the plasma, it is the blood level of ionized Ca^{++} that is under control of calciotropic hormones:

(a) **vitamin D**,
(b) **parathyroid hormone** and
(c) the **Ca^{++}-sensing receptor**. This receptor, which is found on the cell surface of tissues such as the parathyroid gland, kidney, and bone, detects hypocalcemia and leads to enhanced secretion of parathyroid hormone. Summarizing the process briefly, a fall in circulating Ca^{++} in normal subjects leads to a compensatory increase in parathyroid hormone secretion, which returns the Ca^{++} level to normal by two major actions: increased Ca^{++} release from bone and stimulated production of 1,25-dihydroxyvitamin D, the active metabolite of vitamin D, resulting in an increase in intestinal Ca^{++} absorption [38–40].

(d) **Parathyroid hormone related peptide** is a further calciotropic hormone with the following identified actions: (1) During pregnancy, Ca^{++} is transferred from the maternal circulation to the fetus by a pump regulated by this hormone; (2) Parathyroid hormone related peptide levels are elevated during lactation and contribute substantially to the movement of Ca^{++} from the maternal skeleton to the mammary glands; (3) Finally, this peptide is involved in the pathogenesis of hypercalcemia of malignancies [38–40].

Hypocalcemia

Non-neonatal Hypocalcemia

Symptoms and Signs
Symptoms and signs of hypocalcemia, which is often asymptomatic, result from neuromuscular, ocular, ectodermal, dental, gastrointestinal, car-

diovascular, skeletal or endocrine dysfunctions, and are related to the severity and chronicity of the hypocalcemia (Table 34.18). Hypocalcemia manifests with a prolonged QT interval on standard electrocardiogram (Fig. 34.9). However, some signs and symptoms are unique to chronic

Table 34.18 Clinical signs and symptoms of hypocalcemia

- **Neuromuscular**
  - **Tetany**
    - sensory dysfunction: circumoral and acral paresthesias
    - muscular dysfunction
      - Stiffness, myalgia, muscle spasms and cramps
      - Forced adduction of the thumb, flexion of the metacarpophalangeal joints and wrists, and extension of the fingers
      - Laryngismus stridulus (spasm of respiratory muscles and of glottis causing dyspnea)
    - Autonomic dysfunction: diaphoresis, bronchospasm, biliary colic
    - Trousseau sign: inflation of a sphygmomanometer above systolic blood pressure for 3–4 min induces a carpal spasm
    - Chvostek sign: ipsilateral tapping of the facial nerve just anterior to the ear followed by contraction of the facial muscles (the complete sign is contraction of corner of the mouth, the nose and the eye; contraction of the corner of the mouth alone often occurs in normal subjects)
  - **Myopathy:** generalized muscle weakness and wasting with normal creatine kinase (myopathy represents more a feature of vitamin D deficiency than hypocalcemia per se; elevated parathyroid hormone level or hypophosphatemia may contribute to the myopathy)
  - **Extrapyramidal disorders:** Bradykinetic movement disorders, sometimes dystonia, hemiballismus, choreoathetosis, oculogyric crises
  - **Convulsions** (generalized or partial)
  - **Mental retardation, psychosis**
- **Ocular**
  - Cataract (rarely keratoconjunctivitis)
  - Papilledema (often associated with benign intracranial hypertension; rarely optic neuritis is present)
- **Ectodermal** (especially in the context of severe, chronic hypocalcemia)
  - Dry scaly skin
  - Hyperpigmentation, dermatitis, eczema, and psoriasis
  - Course, brittle, and sparse hair with patchy alopecia
  - Brittle nails, with characteristic transverse grooves
  - Candidiasis: usually as a component of **A**utoimmune **P**oly**E**ndocrinopathy-**C**andidiasis-**E**ctodermal **D**ystrophy (= APECED-association)
- **Dental** (dental hypoplasia, failure of tooth eruption, defective enamel and root formation, and abraded carious teeth)
- **Gastrointestinal**
  - Loose stools (steatorrhea due to impaired pancreatic secretion)
  - Gastric achlorhydria
- **Cardiovascular**
  - Systemic hypotension, decreased myocardial function, congestive heart failure
  - Prolonged QTc interval on standard electrocardiogram with tendency towards cardiac arrhythmias (clinically relevant if hypocalcemia is associated with hypokalemia and hypomagnesemia)
- **Skeletal**
  - Rachitic findings
    - Delayed closure of the fontanelles
    - Parietal and frontal bossing
    - Craniotabes
    - Rachitic rosary: enlargement of the costochondral junction visible as beeding along the anterolateral aspects of the chest
    - Harrison sulcus caused by the muscular pull of the diaphragmatic attachments to the lower ribs

(continued)

Table 34.18 (continued)

> Enlargement and bowing of the distal radius, ulna, tibia and fibula
>
> Progressive lateral bowing of the femur and tibia

- Children with hypoparathyroidism: increased bone mineral density, osteosclerosis and thickening of the calvarium
- Children with pseudohypoparathyroidism: Albright's hereditary osteodystrophy, osteitis fibrosa cystica (due to normal skeletal responsiveness to parathyroid hormone)

• **Endocrine manifestations**
  - Impaired insulin release
  - Hypothyroidism, prolactin deficiency, and ovarian failure associated with polyglandular autoimmune syndromes

hypoparathyroidism and not hypocalcemia: these include candidiasis and dysmorphic changes in **A**utoimmune **P**oly **E**ndocrinopathy-**C**andidiasis-**E**ctodermal **D**ystrophy (= APECED-association). Among the symptoms of hypocalcemia, tetany, papilledema and seizures may occur in patients who develop hypocalcemia acutely. By comparison, ectodermal and dental changes, cataracts, basal ganglia calcification, and extrapyramidal disorders are features of chronic hypocalcemia and are common in hypoparathyroidism [38–40, 42].

Causes

Deficiency or impaired function of (a) parathyroid hormone, (b) vitamin D or (c) Ca^{++}-sensing receptor are major causes of reduced blood level of ionized Ca^{++}. Because bone Ca^{++} stores are so large, the major reason for hypocalcemia is decreased bone resorption. Sometimes acute events such as hyperphosphatemia, can produce hypocalcemia even though the regulatory systems are intact. The main causes of hypocalcaemia include vitamin D deficiency, Ca^{++} deficiency, impaired vitamin D metabolism, impaired parathyroid hormone action (secondary to end organ resistance), reduced production of parathyroid hormone, and abnormal Ca^{++}-sensing receptor or impaired renal function (Table 34.19).

Diagnostic Work Up

Hypocalcemia is a rather common clinical problem, the cause of which can very often be determined from the history (as with a breast-fed infant not receiving any supplementation of vitamin D presenting with non-febrile generalized convulsions, enlargement of the costochondral junction along the anterolateral aspects of the chest and enlargement of the wrist). In some cases, however, the underlying condition is not readily apparent. A detailed history documenting diet, lifestyle, family, and drug history, as well as development and hearing is important. The examination should include an assessment of skin, nails, teeth, and the skeleton, as well as the cardiovascular system. A comprehensive range of investigations should be performed at baseline, which have been divided into first and second line (Table 34.20). The objective of assessing urine Ca^{++} excretion is to establish whether the molar urine calcium/creatinine is inappropriately high in the presence of hypocalcemia. Reference values for urine calcium/creatinine ratio in young children are not well defined and will vary according to factors such as diet. The upper limits of normal urine Ca^{++} excretion in healthy children appear in the footnote of Table 34.20. Renal phosphate handling may be abnormal despite a blood phosphate within the quoted laboratory normal range, and should be assessed in more detail by determining the tubular maximum reabsorption threshold of phosphate (see phosphate).

Checking biochemistry of the parents and possibly siblings is crucial when inherited diseases such as hypocalcaemic hypercalciuria and hypophosphataemic rickets are suspected. It is also important to measure maternal Ca^{++} and vitamin D levels in the case of hypocalcaemia in infancy because of the link with maternal vitamin D deficiency and hyperparathyroidism. Maternal hyperparathyroidism is linked with adverse preg-

Table 34.19 Causes of hypocalcemia in infants and children

Parathyroid hormone level low
- **Abnormal production of parathyroid hormone**
  - Magnesium deficiency[a]
  - Following neck surgery
  - Hypoparathyroidism (autosomal recessive, autosomal dominant, or X-linked)
  - Di George anomaly (= 22q11 deletions), 10p13 deletion, Hall-Hittner or CHARGE-association (=Coloboma, Heart anomaly, Choanal Atresia, mental Retardation, Genital hypoplasia, and Ear anomalies), HDR-association (= Hypoparathyroidism, Deafness, Renal dysplasia)
  - Autoimmune PolyEndocrinopathy-Candidiasis-Ectodermal Dystrophy (= APECED-association)
  - Infiltrative lesions such as Wilson's disease and thalassemia
  - Mitochondrial diseases (e.g. Kearns Sayre syndrome)
- **Altered "set point"** (calcium sensing receptor activating mutations)

Intact parathyroid hormone level high
- **Hypovitaminosis D, calcium deficiency, impaired vitamin D metabolism**
  - **Hypovitaminosis D**
    Reduced vitamin D intake or production in the skin
    Decreased intestinal absorption (e.g. celiac disease and cystic fibrosis)
  - **Calcium deficiency**
  - **Impaired vitamin D "metabolism"**
    Severe liver disease
    Drugs that "inactivate" vitamin D: anticonvulsants (phenobarbital, phenytoin, carbamazepine, oxcarbazepine), antimicrobials (isoniazid and rifampicin), antiretroviral drugs
    Enzyme deficiency: defects of the 1-α-hydroxylase gene (= vitamin D dependent rickets type I)
    End organ resistance to vitamin D (= vitamin D dependent rickets type II)
- **Signaling defects: pseudohypoparathyroidisms**
- **Renal failure, osteopetrosis, excessive fluoride intake**

[a] Severe chronic magnesium deficiency ($\leq$0.45 mmol/L) causes hypocalcaemia by impairing parathyroid hormone secretion as well as parathyroid hormone action

Table 34.20 First and second line investigations in childhood hypocalcemia when the cause cannot be determined from the history and clinical examination

First line investigations	Second line investigations
• **Blood values**	
Phosphate[a], Magnesium	Autoantibody screen
Alkaline Phosphatase	Parental (and siblings)
Sodium, Potassium, Bicarbonate, Creatinine	Maternal Vitamin D₃-status
Intact Parathyroid Hormone	1,25-hydroxy vitamin D3
25-Hydroxyvitamin D₃ (= calcidiol)	Genetic studies (e.g. 22q11 deletion)
• **Urinary values**	
Urinalysis (for glucose, protein and pH)	
Calcium[a], Phosphate[b], Creatinine	
• **Imaging**	
Hand and wrist radiograph	Renal ultrasound Skull radiograph

[a] The upper limit of normal for urine calcium/creatinine in healthy children is 2.20 mol/mol (or 0.81 mg/mg) in infants aged 6–12 months, 1.50 mol/mol (or 0.56 mg/mg) in infants aged 13–24 months, 1.40 mol/mol (or 0.50 mg/mg) in infants aged 25–36 months, 1.10 mol/mol (or 0.41 mg/mg) in children aged 3–5 years, 0.80 mol/mol (or 0.30 mg/mg) in children aged 5–7 years and 0.70 mol/mol (or 0.25 mg/mg) in older children
[b] Calculate the maximal tubular reabsorption of phosphate as indicated in the section on phosphate

nancy outcome and causes transient hypocalcemia in the newborn because the fetal parathyroids are suppressed following exposure to high Ca⁺⁺ levels in utero. An autoantibody screen including adrenal, parathyroid, smooth muscle and microsomal antibodies is useful in cases of isolated hypoparathyroidism and where APECED-association is suspected. Renal ultrasound scan looking for evidence of nephrocalcinosis or renal dysplasia is also often advised.

The biochemical picture of hypocalcemia can be categorized according to the presence of undetectable, normal or high levels of circulating parathyroid hormone, an approach that reflects the underlying pathophysiology [42].

- Undetectable or low levels of this hormone in the hypocalcemic child suggest hypoparathyroidism (Table 34.19). Aplasia or hypoplasia of the parathyroids is most commonly due to the DiGeorge syndrome associated with deletion of chromosome 22q11. In this syndrome, the characteristic clinical signs of the so called "CATCH-22" might be noticed: Cardiac malformations (especially conotruncal anomalies like tetralogy of Fallot, truncus arteriosus communis or interrupted aortic arch), Abnormal facies, Thymic aplasia, Cleft palate and Hypocalcemia/Hypoparathyroidism). A similar phenotype including hypoparathyroidism has also been associated with deletions of chromosome 10p, while the HDR-association (**H**ypoparathyroidism, **D**eafness, and **R**enal dysplasia) is due to defects in the GATA3 gene. Defects in the parathyroid hormone gene are rare. Diseases such as APECED can present with hypoparathyroidism in the absence of the two other major manifestations, which are candidiasis and adrenal failure. There should be a high index of suspicion for this disease in all cases of hypoparathyroidism presenting in children older than 4 years. Children with APECED may have other "minor" features such as malabsorption, gallstones, hepatitis, dysplastic nails and teeth. Screening should be considered in the siblings of affected individuals. Mitochondrial disease is a rare cause of hypoparathyroidism but is not usually an isolated finding.

- Detectable parathyroid hormone values (low-normal or normal) in an asymptomatic individual raise the possibility of hypocalcemic hypercalciuria, an abnormality of the Ca^{++}-sensing receptor which can be assessed in more detail by determining urinary Ca^{++} excretion. This parameter is typically low in longstanding hypoparathyroidism, and a relatively high urine Ca^{++} excretion (molar urinary calcium/creatinine ratio ≥ 0.30) suggests hypocalcemic hypercalciuria. This abnormality is due to activating mutations of the Ca^{++}-sensing receptor with downshift of the setpoint for Ca^{++} responsive parathyroid hormone release. Mg^{++} levels are low in this disorder because the Ca^{++}-sensing receptor also detects this cation. Interestingly, the biochemical picture of hypocalcemic hypercalciuria sometimes resembles Bartter syndromes and includes hypokalemia and hyperbicarbonatemia.

- If blood creatinine is normal, thereby excluding renal insufficiency, then increased parathyroid hormone levels point towards a diagnosis of rickets[11] or pseudohypoparathyroidism. Vitamin D deficiency is still prevalent in the Western world. High-risk groups include families, where the maternal and child diet may be low in Ca^{++} and vitamin D and where exposure to sunlight can be limited. The diagnosis of Fanconi-De Toni-Debré syndrome should be considered in any hypocalcemic child with persistent glycosuria, phosphaturia, and acidosis. Pseudohypoparathyroidism is a heterogeneous disorder that results from signaling defects of the cell surface receptors. Patients may become hypocalcemic despite a compensatory increase in parathyroid hormone concentration, and may have other endocrine problems, such as primary hypothyroidism and hypogonadism that are also manifestations of an abnormal signaling mechanism. Some patients are overweight and mentally retarded.

Neonatal Hypocalcemia

Hypocalcemia is a common metabolic problem in newborns. During pregnancy, Ca^{++} is transferred from the maternal circulation to the fetus by a pump regulated by parathyroid hormone-related peptide. This process results in higher blood Ca^{++} in the fetus than in the mother and leads to fetal hypercalcemia, with total Ca^{++} level of $\approx 2.50–2.75$ mmol/L in umbilical cord blood [38–40, 42].

The cessation of placental transfer of Ca^{++} at birth is followed by a fall in total blood Ca^{++} concentration to $\approx 2.00–2.25$ mmol/L and ionized Ca^{++} to $\approx 1.10–1.35$ mmol/L at 24 h. Ca^{++} subsequently rises, reaching levels seen in older children and adults by 2 weeks of age.

The definition of hypocalcemia depends upon birth weight: (a) in term infants or premature infants >1.50 kg birth weight, hypocalcemia is defined as a total Ca^{++} concentration <2.00 mmol/L or a ionized fraction <1.10 mmol/L; (b) premature infants with birth weight <1.50 kg are hypocalcemic if they have a total Ca^{++} concentration <1.75 mmol/L or a ionized fraction of <1.00 mmol/L [38–40, 42].

---

[11] In hypophosphataemic rickets, circulating parathyroid hormone and calcium are usually normal.

Symptoms and Signs

Neonatal hypocalcemia is usually asymptomatic. Among those who become symptomatic, the characteristic sign is increased neuromuscular irritability. Such infants are jittery and often have muscle jerking. Generalized or partial clonic seizures can occur. Rare presentations include inspiratory stridor caused by laryngospasm, wheezing caused by bronchospasm or vomiting possibly resulting from pylorospasm [38–40, 42].

Causes

The causes of neonatal hypocalcemia are classified by the timing of onset. Hypocalcemia is considered to be early when it occurs in the first 2–3 days after birth.

Early Neonatal Hypocalcemia

Early hypocalcemia is an exaggeration of the normal decline in Ca^{++} concentration after birth. It occurs commonly in premature infants, in infants of diabetic mothers, and after perinatal asphyxia or intrauterine growth restriction.

- Prematurity: One-third of premature infants and the majority of very-low-birth-weight infants develop hypocalcemia during the first 2 days after birth. Multiple factors contribute to the fall. They include hypoalbuminemia and factors that lower both total and ionized Ca^{++}, such as reduced intake of Ca^{++} because of low intake of milk, possible impaired response to parathyroid hormone, increased calcitonin and increased urinary Ca^{++} losses.
- Infants of diabetic mothers: Hypocalcemia occurs in 10–20% of infants of diabetic mothers. The lowest concentration typically occurs between 24 and 72 h after birth and often is associated with hyperphosphatemia. Hypocalcemia is caused by lower parathyroid hormone concentrations after birth in this condition compared to normal infants. Hypoparathyroidism is likely related to intrauterine hypercalcemia suppressing the fetal parathyroid glands. Concurrent hypomagnesemia is a further contributing factor.

- Birth asphyxia: Infants with birth asphyxia frequently have hypocalcemia and hyperphosphatemia. Possible mechanisms include increased phosphate load caused by tissue catabolism, decreased intake due to delayed initiation of feedings, renal insufficiency, acidosis, and increased serum calcitonin concentration.
- Intrauterine growth restriction: Hypocalcemia occurs with increased frequency in infants with intrauterine growth restriction. The mechanism is thought to involve decreased transfer of Ca^{++} across the placenta.

Late Neonatal Hypocalcemia

Late hypocalcemia develops after the second or third day after birth. It typically occurs at the end of the first week.

- Hypoparathyroidism: Hypoparathyroidism associated with excess phosphorus intake is the most common cause of late neonatal hypocalcemia. Hypoparathyroidism often occurs as part of a syndrome, including DiGeorge syndrome or, more rarely, mitochondrial cytopathies.
- Maternal hyperparathyroidism: Infants born to mothers with hyperparathyroidism frequently have hypocalcemia. The mechanism is related to increased transplacental Ca^{++} transport caused by maternal hypercalcemia, which results in excessive fetal hypercalcemia that inhibits fetal and neonatal parathyroid secretion. Affected infants typically develop increased neuromuscular irritability in the first 3 weeks after birth, but they can present later.
- Hypomagnesemia: Hypomagnesemia causes resistance to parathyroid hormone and impairs its secretion, both of which can result in hypocalcemia. The most common etiology in newborns is transient hypomagnesemia, although rare disorders of intestinal or renal tubular Mg^{++} transport can occur.
- Other causes: Critically ill or premature infants are exposed to many therapeutic interventions that may cause transient hypocalcemia including bicarbonate infusion resulting

in metabolic alkalosis, transfusion with citrated blood or infusion of lipids leading to formation of Ca^{++} complexes and decreased ionized Ca^{++}. Finally, mild hypocalcemia has been associated with phototherapy. Other rare causes include acute renal failure of any cause, usually associated with hyperphosphatemia, any disorder of vitamin D metabolism and rotavirus infections.

- High phosphate intake: Intake of excess phosphate is an historically important cause of late hypocalcemia that was seen in term infants fed bovine milk or a formula with a high phosphorus concentration. It has been postulated that the high phosphorus levels antagonize parathyroid hormone or may produce increased Ca^{++} and phosphorus deposition in bones. Symptomatic infants typically present with tetany or seizures at 5–10 days of age. Severe hyperphosphatemia and hypocalcemia also can be caused by phosphate enemas.

Hypercalcemia

Signs and Symptoms

Hypercalcemia is more difficult to diagnose than hypocalcemia because of the nonspecific nature of symptoms and signs (Table 34.21). Hypercalcemia manifests with a shortened QT interval on electrocardiogram (Fig. 34.9). Major symptoms include sekeletal pain, fatigue, anorexia, nausea and vomiting, and particularly important are polyuria and polydipsia. Changes in behavior and frank psychiatric disorders may also be a result of hypercalcemia. The extent of symptoms and signs is a function of both the degree of hypercalcemia and the rate of onset of the elevation in the blood concentration. Thus, a rather severe hypercalcemia of 3.50 mmol/L is asymptomatic when it develops chronically, while an acute rise to these values may cause marked changes in sensorium. It is worthy of mention, however, that symptoms and signs associated with hypercalcemia may be due to the elevation in the Ca^{++} concentration but also to the underlying disease [38–40, 43, 44].

Table 34.21 Symptoms and signs of hypercalcemia

- **General**
  - Weakness
  - Depression
  - Anorexia
- **Central nervous system**
  - Impaired concentration
  - Increased sleep requirement
  - Altered state of consciousness
  - Mental retardation
  - Polydipsia (and polyuria)
- **Muscular:** weakness
- **Ocular**
  - Palpebral calcification
  - Band keratopathy
  - Conjunctival calcification
- **Dermal:** Pruritus and skin calcifications
- **Gastrointestinal**
  - Constipation
  - Anorexia, nausea, vomiting
  - Pancreatitis
  - Peptic ulcer
- **Cardiovascular**
  - Shortened QTc interval on standard electrocardiogram[a]
  - Arterial hypertension
- **Skeletal: joint pains (pseudogout)**
- **Renal dysfunction**
  - Altered urinary concentration ability with polyuria and polydypsia
  - Nephrolithiasis, nephrocalcinosis, renal failure
  - Distal renal tubular acidosis

[a] without any major tendency towards cardiac arrhythmias

Causes

Hypercalcemia results when the entry of Ca^{++} into the circulation exceeds the excretion of Ca^{++} into the urine or deposition in bone. Since the major sources of Ca^{++} are the bone and the intestinal tract, hypercalcemia mostly results from increased bone resorption or from increased intestinal absorption. In some cases, however, multiple sites are involved in the development of hypercalcemia. The great majority of adult patients with elevated Ca^{++} level will be found to have either **primary hyperparathyroidism** or **malignancy** (this form of hypercalcemia is thought in many instances to be caused by secretion of parathyroid hormone related peptide), although the differential diagnosis is much longer. For these other causes of hypercalcemia, which include **vitamin D (or A) intoxication**, **sarcoidosis**, **tuberculosis**, some **fungal infections**, **thyreotoxicosis**, **Addison's disease**, milk-alkali syndrome (= **calcium-alkali syndrome**) related to the prescription of Ca^{++}, absorbable alkali and vitamin D supplements, treatment with **thiazides** or **lithium** carbonate, **familial hypocalciuric hypercalcemia**, **prolonged immobilization** in subjects with high skeletal turnover (including adolescents) and the recovery phase of **rhabdomyolysis**, the use of the mnemonic VITAMINS TRAPS (Table 34.22) has been suggested. Children present with hypercalcemia less frequently than adults, but the

Table 34.22 Causes of hypercalcemia (please note that some causes of hypercalcemia are given twice)

- **Classical causes (Mnemonic VITAMINS TRAP)**
  - **V**itamin D and vitamin A
  - **I**mmobilization
  - **T**hyrotoxicosis
  - **A**ddison's disease
  - **M**ilk-alkali syndrome (= calcium-alkali syndrome)
  - **I**nflammatory disorders (granulomatous diseases with excessive production of calcitriol)
  - **N**eoplastic-related disease[a]
  - **S**arcoidosis
  - **T**hiazides[b] and other drugs
  - **R**habdomyolysis (recovery phase)
  - **A**IDS
  - **P**arathyroid disease[a] (including familial hypocalciuric hypercalcemia), **p**arenteral nutrition
- **Hypercalcemia associated with elevated calcitriol (1,25-dihydroxyvitamin D₃)**
  - Sarcoidosis
  - Acute granulomatous pneumonia, lipoid pneumonia
  - Tuberculosis (and other mycobacterial infections)
  - Wegener's granulomatosis
  - Crohn's disease
  - Hepatic granulomatosis
  - Talc and silicone granulomatosis
  - Cat scratch disease
  - Neonatal subcutaneous fat necrosis
- **Hypercalcemia associated with elevated parathyroid hormone related peptide**
  - Hypercalcemia of malignancy
  - Some benign tumors (ovary, kidney, pheochromcytoma)
  - Systemic lupus erythematosus
  - HIV-associated lymphadenopathy
  - Massive mammary hyperplasia
  - During late pregnancy and lactation in hypoparathyroidism
- **Drugs associated with the development of hypercalcemia**
  - **Common:** calcium, vitamin D, vitamin A, lithium, thiazides[b] (e.g.: hydrochlorothiazide, chlortalidone)
  - **Less common:** omeprazole, theophyllin (toxic doses), recombinant growth hormone, foscarnet, hepatitis B vaccination, manganese toxicity
- **Rare causes of hypercalcemia with an unknown underlying mechanism**
  - Infections: nocardiosis, brucellosis, cytomegaloviric infection (in AIDS), berylliosis
  - Juvenile idiopathic arthritis
  - Advanced chronic liver disease
- **Rare causes of hypercalcemia in infancy and young children**
  - Reduced function of the calcium-sensing receptor
    - Deactivating mutations
      - Heterozygous: Familial hypocalciuric hypercalcemia

(continued)

Table 34.22 (continued)

> Homozygous: Severe neonatal hyperparathyroidism
> Autoantibodies directed at the calcium-sensing receptor

- Congenital hypoparathyroidism
- Idiopathic infantile hypercalcemia
- Jansens metaphyseal chondrodysplasia[c]
- Williams-Beuren syndrome
- Down syndrome
- Hypophosphatasia
- Congenital lactase deficiency
- Phosphate depletion in severe prematurity
- Renal tubular acidosis
- Primary hyperoxaluria
- Neonatal subcutaneous fat necrosis

[a] Malignancy and primary hyperparathyroidism account for 80–90% of cases of hypercalcemia in adulthood
[b] Although thiazides are frequently cited as a cause of hypercalcemia, it is more usual that they bring mild pre-existing hypercalcemia to light
[c] Consequence of a constitutive activation of the parathyroid hormone receptor

causes that are common in adults are also common in children. Young children and infants, however, present with hypercalcemia in association with some rather rare conditions seen almost exclusively in that population. **Idiopathic infantile hypercalcemia** is characterized by an increased sensitivity to vitamin D. It is the consequence of loss of function mutations in the gene that encodes the enzymatic system responsible for the inactivation of 25-hydroxyvitamin D, resulting in its decreased conversion into inactive metabolites [38–40, 43, 44]. Hypothermia treatment for neonatal asphyxia can sometimes lead to neonatal subcutaneous fat necrosis and consequently hypercalcemia by elevated calcitriol (Table 34.22).

Diagnostic Work Up

The causes of hypercalcemia are often discerned clinically. Clinical history (calcium-alkali syndrome, which replaces the traditional term of milk-alkali syndrome, is currently a cause of hypercalcemia that results from the widespread use of over-the-counter Ca^{++} and vitamin D supplements), physical examination and rather simple laboratory data (circulating phosphate and creatinine; urinary Ca^{++}, phosphate and creatinine) and chest x-ray (looking for sarcoidosis) provide the correct diagnosis in many cases.

- **Step 1: Assess clinical and simple laboratory data**
- Clinical history and physical examination are useful in establishing the diagnosis of hypercalcemia induced by immobilization, medication or thyreotoxicosis, and the diagnosis of "syndromic" hypercalcemia, including Williams-Beuren syndrome, Down syndrome and Jansens metaphyseal chondrodysplasia. Measurement of the serum phosphate concentration and urinary Ca^{++} excretion also may be helpful in selected cases: hyperparathyroidism and the humoral hypercalcemia of malignancy induced by secretion of parathyroid hormone related peptide often present with hypophosphatemia resulting from inhibition of renal proximal tubular phosphate reabsorption. In comparison, the serum phosphate concentration is normal or elevated in granulomatous diseases, vitamin D intoxication, immobilization, thyrotoxicosis and metastatic bone disease. Calciuria is usually raised or high-normal in hyperparathyroidism and hypercalcemia of malignancy. Two conditions lead to relative hypocalciuria: thiazides, which directly enhance active reabsorption of Ca^{++} in the distal tubule, and familial hypocalciuric hypercalcemia, in which the fractional excretion of Ca^{++} is often <1.0% (further clues to

the possible presence of this disorder are a family history of hypercalcemia and few if any hypercalcemic symptoms).

- **Step 2: analyze parathyroid hormone level**
- An elevated parathyroid hormone concentration indicates the presence of primary hyperparathyroidism or a patient taking lithium. 10–20% of patients with primary hyperparathyroidism have a parathyroid hormone concentration in the upper end of the normal range: such a "normal" level, which indicates that the secretion is not suppressed, is virtually diagnostic of primary hyperparathyroidism, since it is still inappropriately high considering the presence of hypercalcemia. A low or low-normal parathyroid hormone level is consistent with all other non-parathyroid hormone-induced causes of hypercalcemia.
- **Step 3: Analyze vitamin D metabolites**
- The levels of vitamin D metabolites 25-hydroxyvitamin D and 1,25-dihydroxyvitamin D are assessed if there is no obvious malignancy and parathyroid hormone levels are not elevated. An elevated 25-hydroxyvitamin D is indicative of either vitamin D intoxication or idiopathic infantile hypercalcemia. On the other hand, increased 1,25-dihydroxyvitamin D may be induced by direct intake of this metabolite or non-renal production in granulomatous diseases or lymphoma.

Management

The degree of hypercalcemia and the rate of rise of Ca^{++} level habitually determine symptoms and urgency of treatment [42, 43]:

- asymptomatic or mildly symptomatic hypercalcemia (total Ca^{++} <3.00 mmol/L) does not require immediate treatment. Similarly, Ca^{++} of 3.00–3.50 mmol/L is often well-tolerated chronically, and may not require urgent treatment (however, an acute rise to these concentrations may cause marked sensorium changes, which require more urgent measures).
- Total Ca^{++} concentration >3.50 mmol/L requires immediate treatment, regardless of symptoms.

The nonsurgical management of childhood hypercalcemia includes following points:

(a) Avoidance of the cause. For example, removal of exogenous vitamin D and Ca^{++} in children with vitamin D intoxication, calcium-alkali syndrome or idiopathic infantile hypercalcemia.

(b) Specific management. Steroids inhibit the effects of vitamin D and are particularly effective in hypercalcemia secondary to granulomatous diseases. The bisphosphonates, which inhibit skeletal Ca^{++} release, are effective in hypercalcemia that results from excessive bone resorption of any cause (including among others hypercalcemia of malignancy, hypercalcemia associated with neonatal subcutaneous fat necrosis and vitamin D intoxication). Pharmacologic doses of calcitonin reduce the Ca^{++} levels by decreasing bone resorption. The effect of calcitonin, which is limited to the first 48 h, is most beneficial in subjects with total Ca^{++} >3.50 mmol/L when combined with a bisphosphonate and administration of saline.

(c) Normal saline, administered at a rapid rate (initially 2800–3000 mL/m² body surface area daily), corrects possible volume depletion due to hypercalcemia-induced renal salt wasting and promotes renal Ca^{++} excretion. The loop diuretic furosemide is no longer recommended with the exception of cases with volume overload.

Magnesium

Balance

A 70 kg man contains ≈1 mole of Mg^{++}. About half of it is present in bone tissue, the other half in soft tissue, whereas no more than 1–2% of the total body Mg^{++} is present in extracellular fluids. Intracellular Mg^{++} serves as cofactor for many enzymes that produce and store energy via hydrolysis of adenosine triphosphate [40, 45, 46].

In healthy humans the total circulating Mg^{++} concentration is maintained within narrow limits and ranges between 0.75 and 1.00 mmol/L.[12] Approximately 1/4 of circulating Mg^{++} is bound to albumin. For the remaining 3/4 of circulating Mg^{++} ≈10% is complexed to inorganic phosphate, citrate and other compounds, while 90% (≈2/3 of total circulating Mg^{++}) is in the form of free ion.

Mg^{++} balance, like that of other ions, is a function of intake and urinary excretion. In adults the daily Mg^{++} intake averages 0.23–0.28 mmol/kg (5.6–6.8 mg/kg) body weight. About 1/3 of this Mg^{++} is absorbed. In healthy adults there is no net gain or loss of Mg^{++} from bone so that balance is achieved by the urinary excretion of the absorbed 0.06–0.08 mmol/kg (1.5–1.9 mg/kg) body weight.

Only 15–25% of filtered Mg^{++} is reabsorbed in the proximal tubule and 5–10% in the distal tubule. The major site of Mg^{++} transport is the thick ascending limb of the loop of Henle where 60–70% of the filtered load is reabsorbed [40, 45, 46].

With negative Mg^{++} balance, the initial loss comes primarily from the extracellular fluid (equilibration with bone stores begins after several weeks). Thus, circulating Mg^{++} falls rapidly with negative Mg^{++} balance, leading to a conspicuous decrease in Mg^{++} excretion unless urinary Mg^{++} wasting is present. The fractional clearance of Mg^{++}, which is 3–5% in healthy subjects ingesting a normal diet, can fall to <0.5% with Mg^{++} depletion due to non-renal losses. This parameter is calculated from the following equation:

$$\frac{Urinary\,Mg^{++} \times Circulating\,Creatinine}{Circulating\,Mg^{++} \times Urinary\,Creatinine}$$

There is no protection against hypermagnesemia with loss of renal function. In this setting, high intake leads to extracellular Mg^{++} retention.

Hypomagnesemia

Hypomagnesemia, which is not rare, results either from intestinal (including dietary insufficiency) or renal losses (Table 34.23). In the presence of hypomagnesemia, the healthy kidney lowers Mg^{++} excretion to very low values. Hence, the diagnosis of hypomagnesemia caused by intestinal Mg^{++} losses (or low dietary Mg^{++} intake) is established by the demonstration of low urinary excretion of Mg^{++}. Conversely the diagnosis of hypomagnesemia caused by renal losses is established by the demonstration of inappropriately high (= "normal") urinary Mg^{++} excretion [40, 45, 46].

Table 34.23 Causes of hypomagnesemia

Decreased magnesium intake and intestinal losses
– Dietary deprivation
– Small bowel disorders, including acute or chronic diarrhea, malabsorption and steatorrhea, and small bowel bypass surgery
– Acute pancreatitis
– Paunier disease[a] (= hypomagnesemia with secondary hypocalcemia)
– Chronic management with proton-pump inhibitors

Renal losses
– Primary renal magnesium wasting diseases
– Drugs
  Loop and thiazide-type diuretics
  Drugs other than diuretics (aminoglycoside antibiotics, amphotericin B, cisplatin, pentamidine, cyclosporine, tacrolimus, foscarnet, cetuximab[b])
– Volume expansion
– Hypercalcemia
– Miscellaneous: recovery from acute tubular necrosis, following renal transplantation and during a postobstructive diuresis

Further causes
– Alcohol
– Refeeding syndrome
– Diabetes mellitus
– Following surgery
– "Hungry bone syndrome" following parathyroidectomy for hyperparathyroidism

Neonatal hypomagnesemia
– Maternal hypomagnesemia (including maternal diabetes mellitus)
– Intrauterine growth retardation

[a] Often combined with impaired renal magnesium conservation
[b] A monoclonal antibody against the epithelial growth factor receptor

---

[12]Circulating magnesium levels can be reported in mmol/L, meq/L, mg/dL or mg/L. The valence of magnesium is 2 and its molecular mass 24.3 g/mol; therefore 0.50 mmol/L is equivalent to 1.00 meq/L, 1.22 mg/dL and 12.2 mg/L.

Decreased Intake, Poor Intestinal Absorption or Intestinal Loss

Intestinal secretory losses, which contain some Mg^{++}, are continuous and not regulated. Although the obligatory losses are not large, marked dietary deprivation can lead to progressive Mg^{++} depletion. Mg^{++} loss will also occur when the intestinal secretions are incompletely reabsorbed as with most disorders of the small bowel, including acute or chronic diarrhea, malabsorption and steatorrhea, and small bowel bypass surgery. Prolonged use of proton pump inhibitors is an increasingly recognized cause of hypomagnesemia (these drugs interfere with the transport of this ion across the intestinal wall) [47]. Hypomagnesemia can also be seen in acute pancreatitis (saponification of Mg^{++} and Ca^{++} in necrotic fat is the underlying mechanism). Paunier disease or hypomagnesemia with secondary hypocalcemia is a very rare defect of intestinal Mg^{++} resorption (usually combined with impaired renal Mg^{++} conservation), which presents early in infancy with hypocalcemia responsive to Mg^{++} administration. The disease is caused by a loss of function mutation in an ion channel of the transient receptor potential gene family called TRPM6 [45, 46].

Renal Losses

Urinary Mg^{++} losses can be induced by different mechanisms.

Primary renal Mg^{++} wasting: these disorders are discussed in Chap. 37.

Drugs: Both loop and thiazide diuretics can inhibit net Mg^{++} reabsorption, while the K^+-sparing diuretics may lower excretion of Mg^{++}. The degree of hypomagnesemia induced by the loop and thiazide diuretics is generally mild, in part because the associated volume contraction will tend to increase proximal Na^+, water, and Mg^{++} reabsorption. Many further drugs can also produce urinary Mg^{++} wasting, as depicted in Table 34.23.

Volume expansion: Expansion of the extracellular fluid volume can decrease passive Mg^{++} transport. Mild hypomagnesemia may ensue if this is sustained.

Hypercalcemia: Ca^{++} and Mg^{++} seem to compete for transport in the thick ascending limb of the loop of Henle. The increased filtered Ca^{++} load in hypercalcemic states will deliver more Ca^{++} to the loop; the ensuing rise in Ca^{++} reabsorption will diminish that of Mg^{++}.

Miscellaneous: Mg^{++} wasting can be seen as part of the tubular dysfunction seen with recovery from acute tubular necrosis, following renal transplantation and during a postobstructive diuresis.

Alcohol: Excessive urinary excretion of Mg^{++} is common in alcoholic patients. Dietary deficiency, acute pancreatitis, diarrhea and refeeding also contribute to hypomagnesemia in these patients.

Further Causes

- Hypomagnesemia, together with hypophosphatemia, hypokalemia and increasing extracellular fluid volume, occurs in the context of refeeding syndrome (See: hypophosphatemia).
- Hypomagnesemia sometimes occurs in diabetes mellitus and is related in part to the degree of hyperglycemia.
- Hypomagnesemia can be seen following surgery, at least in part due to chelation by circulating free fatty acids.
- Hypomagnesemia can occur as part of the "hungry bone" syndrome in which there is increased Mg^{++} uptake by renewing bone following parathyroidectomy (for hyperparathyroidism).
- Hypomagnesemia is often encountered in cystic fibrosis patients with advanced disease, although sweat Mg^{++} concentration is normal in these patients. The causes are multiple, including aminoglycoside toxicity inducing renal magnesium-wasting and impaired intestinal magnesium balance. Interestingly, magnesium supplementation may lead to an improvement in respiratory muscle strength and mucolytic activity [48].

Neonatal Hypomagnesemia

Like in older children, in newborns hypomagnesemia may result from decreased Mg^{++} intake, intestinal losses or renal losses. However, two peculiar causes of neonatal hypomagnesemia deserve consideration: (1) maternal hypomagnesemia and (2) intrauterine growth retardation.

- **Maternal hypomagnesemia:** Neonatal hypomagnesemia secondary to maternal hypomagnesemia is a recognized feature of maternal diabetes mellitus. However, maternal hypomagnesemia from any cause has been associated with neonatal hypomagnesemia.
- **Intrauterine growth retardation:** Hypomagnesemia sometimes occurs in infants whose birth weight is small in relation to their gestational age.

Symptoms, Signs, Consequences

Mg^{++} depletion is often associated with two biochemical abnormalities: (1) hypokalemia and (2) hypocalcemia. As a result, it is often difficult to ascribe specific manifestations solely to hypomagnesemia. The typical signs and symptoms of Mg^{++} depletion include tetany, positive Chvostek, Trousseau and Lust signs (the Lust sign, also called peroneal sign, is the dorsal extension and abduction of the foot, which is elicited by tapping the peroneal nerve on the lateral aspect of the fibula), or generalized convulsions. Generalized weakness and anorexia sometimes also occur. In addition, Mg^{++} depletion can induce ventricular arrhythmias, particularly during myocardial ischemia or cardiopulmonary bypass [40, 45, 46].

Hypokalemia

Hypokalemia, mostly accompanied by metabolic alkalosis, is common in hypomagnesemia. This association is in part due to underlying disorders that cause both Mg^{++} and K^+ loss, such as diuretic therapy and diarrhea. There is also evidence that concomitant Mg^{++} depletion aggravates hypokalemia and renders it refractory to treatment by potassium because Mg^{++} depletion increases distal K^+ secretion, as depicted in Fig. 34.14 [45, 46].

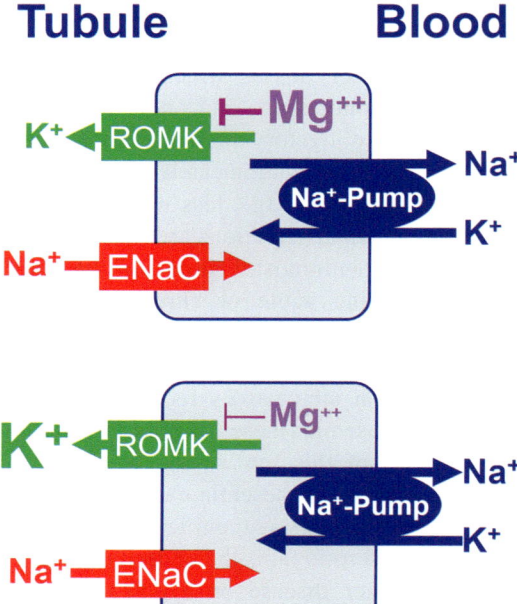

Fig. 34.14 Renal mechanism underlying hypokalemia in Mg^{++} depletion. In the distal nephron K^+ is taken up into cells across the basolateral membrane via Na^+ pump (blue oval) and secreted into luminal fluid via the apical ROMK K^+ channels (green rectangle). Na^+ is reabsorbed via epithelial Na^+ channels (ENaC, red rectangle). Intracellular Mg^{++} inhibits the ROMK K^+ channels and decreases K^+-secretion (upper panel). A decrease in intracellular Mg^{++} releases the Mg^{++}-mediated inhibition of ROMK K^+ channels, increases K^+-secretion (lower panel) and results in hypokalemia that is refractory to treatment by K^+. ROMK denotes renal outer medullary K^+ channel

Hypocalcemia

Hypocalcemia is the classical consequence of severe hypomagnesemia (≤ 0.50 mmol/L). The following factors account for this tendency [40, 45, 46]:

- Inappropriately low circulating **parathyroid hormone** secretion.
- Inappropriately low **1,25-dihydroxyvitamin D**, the active metabolite of vitamin D.
- Bone resistance to **parathyroid hormone** (hypomagnesemia interferes with G protein activation in response to parathyroid hormone, thereby minimizing the stimulation of adenylate cyclase).

Repletion

Repletion of Mg^{++} is controversial in asymptomatic (mostly mild) hypomagnesemia. Oral repletion using lactate, oxide, pidolate or chloride salts is usually preferred. Because of the laxative effect of oral Mg^{++}, the amounts administered must be tailored to the individual patients (0.30 mmol/kg body weight of Mg^{++} per day in divided doses results in diarrhea in ≈10% of patients). The parenteral route is preferred in critically ill patients but the exact dosage is poorly understood. For true emergencies (e.g. generalized convulsions or ventricular arrhythmias) Mg^{++} is administered (either as sulphate or as chloride) intravenously over 1–2 min in a dosage of 0.15–0.20 mmol/kg body weight[13] (repeated if no response 5–10 min later). In subjects with moderate to severe but rather oligosymptomatic Mg^{++} deficiency, the mentioned dose is given over 4–6 h until circulating Mg^{++} returns to normal.

Inorganic Phosphate

Balance

In a 70 kg man, the body phosphate content amounts to ≈1% of the body weight, or 700 g, of which 85% is contained in the bone tissue and teeth, 14% in the soft tissues, and the remaining 1% in extracellular fluids [49].

In the blood, phosphate is found both as organic as well as inorganic salt but clinical laboratories measure the inorganic form. Of the circulating inorganic phosphate, ≈10% is bound to proteins, 5% is complexed with Ca^{++}, Mg^{++} or Na^+ and 85% exists as ionized phosphate. The normal blood concentration of inorganic phosphate is highest during the neonatal period and early childhood and declines thereafter (Table 34.24) because infants and children retain phosphate avidly. There is a mean diurnal variation in concentration of phosphate of ≈0.20 mmol/L (≈0.6 mg/dL) with a nadir at

---

13 Approximately 3.5–4.5 mg/kg body weight of elemental magnesium.

Table 34.24 Fasting values for circulating inorganic phosphate, fractional phosphate excretion and maximal tubular phosphate reabsorption in infancy and childhood

Age	Blood inorganic phosphate, mmol/L[a]	Fractional phosphate excretion, 10^{-2}	Maximal tubular reabsorption of phosphate, mmol/L[a]
0–3 months	1.62–2.40	11.9–38.7	1.02–2.00
4–6 months	1.78–2.21	3.50–34.9	1.27–1.88
6–12 months	1.38–2.15	10.3–20.0	1.13–1.86
1–2 years	1.32–1.93	5.50–23.3	1.05–1.74
3–4 years	1.02–1.92	≤18.4	0.90–1.78
5–6 years	1.13–1.73	0.60–15.0	1.02–1.62
7–8 years	1.06–1.80	≤16.8	0.98–1.64
9–10 years	1.13–1.70	1.80–14.1	1.00–1.58
11–12 years	1.04–1.79	1.80–12.1	0.97–1.65
13–15 years	0.97–1.80	≤12.6	0.91–1.68

[a] To obtain traditional units (mg/dL) multiply by 3.1

11.00 h, subsequently rising to a plateau at 16.00 h and peaking in the early night.

The average diet of a 70 kg man provides 800–1500 mg phosphate daily. As much as 2/3 of the dietary phosphate is absorbed in the gut but intestinal secretion, mainly in saliva and bile acids, adds 200 mg of phosphate into the intestinal lumen daily. Under steady-state conditions, the kidney is the most important modulator of the blood phosphate level, ensuring that urinary phosphate output is equivalent to the net phosphate absorption from the intestine. Phosphate is freely filtered across the glomerulus, and 80–90% of the phosphate is reabsorbed by the renal tubules (mostly in the proximal tubule) in subjects aged 6 months or more (Table 34.24). The renal tubular handling of phosphate is best expressed as fractional excretion of phosphate or, more precisely, as maximal tubular reabsorption of phosphate, which clarifies the relationship between circulating phosphate and urinary phosphate excretion. The fractional clearance of phosphate, the tubular phosphate reabsorption and the maximal tubular phosphate reabsorption are easily calculated, following an overnight fast, from plasma (P_{Ph}) and urinary (U_{Ph}) phosphate, and plasma (P_{Cr}) and urinary (U_{Cr}) creatinine, as follows [50]:

$$\text{Fractional excretion} = \frac{U_{Ph} \times P_{Cr}}{P_{Ph} \times U_{Cr}}$$

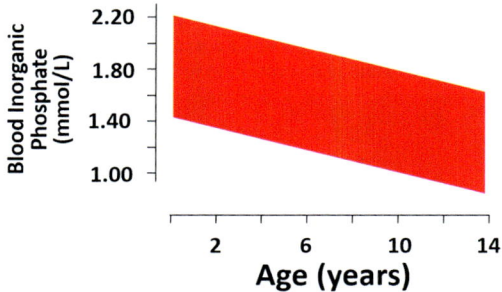

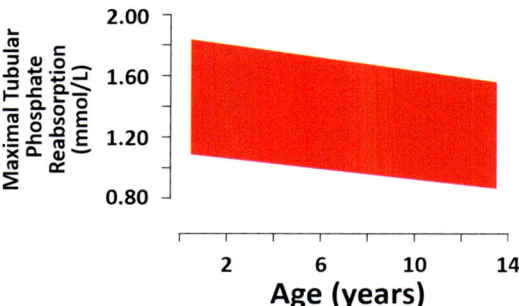

Fig. 34.15 Influence of age on fasting blood inorganic phosphate and maximal tubular reabsorption of phosphate. Blood inorganic phosphate and maximal tubular reabsorption of phosphate measured in infants, children and adolescents [50]

$$\text{Tubular phosphate reabsoption} = 1 - \frac{U_{Ph} \times P_{Cr}}{P_{Ph} \times U_{Cr}}$$

$$\text{Maximal reabsoption} = P_{Ph} - \left(\frac{U_{Ph} \times P_{Cr}}{U_{Cr}} \right)$$

The reference values [50] for the fractional excretion of phosphate and the maximal tubular reabsorption of phosphate are age dependent and appear in Table 34.24 and Fig. 34.15.

Three groups of hormonal factors regulate phosphate homeostasis [49]:

(a) **1,25-dihydroxyvitamin D** stimulates the intestinal phosphate absorption;
(b) **Parathyroid hormone** decreases the renal tubular reabsorption and causes phosphaturia;
(c) **"Phosphatonins"** are phosphaturic factors other than parathyroid hormone. **Fibroblast growth factor 23** (FGF-23) is currently considered the most important phosphatonin.

FGF-23 is secreted by osteocytes and osteoblasts in response to phosphate loading or increased serum $1,25(OH)_2D_3$ levels and mainly targets the kidney in order to regulate the reabsorption of phosphate, the production and catabolism of 1,25-dihydroxyvitamin D and the expression of α-Klotho, an FGF-23 co-receptor and anti-ageing hormone.

Hypophosphatemia

Hypophosphatemia does not necessarily mean phosphate depletion since it can occur in the presence of a low, normal, or high total body phosphate. On the other hand, phosphate depletion may exist with normal, low, or elevated levels of blood phosphate [51, 52].

The normal phosphate level in adolescents and adults ranges between 0.97 and 1.80 mmol/L (2.9–5.4 mg/dL). In this age group, hypophosphatemia is arbitrarily divided into moderate cases (phosphate 0.32–0.65 mmol/L or 0.96–1.95 mg/dL) and severe cases (phosphate <0.32 mmol/L or <0.96 mg/dL). There are three major mechanisms by which hypophosphatemia can occur: (1) low dietary intake or poor intestinal absorption, (2) internal redistribution, and (3) increased urinary loss. In patients with hypophosphatemia caused by decreased intestinal absorption or internal redistribution the fractional excretion of phosphate and the maximal tubular reabsorption of phosphate are normal (Table 34.25). On the contrary, these parameters are low or inappropriately normal in patients with increased urinary losses [51–53].

Low Dietary Intake or Poor Intestinal Absorption

Given the fact that phosphate is ubiquitous in foods, the development of deficiency would be anticipated only in severe cases of malnutrition or in very-low-birth weight infants at the time of rapid postnatal growth. If phosphate restriction is severe and prolonged, or if intestinal absorption is reduced by the chronic use of phosphate binders, then the constantly reduced intestinal delivery may induce phosphate depletion.

Table 34.25 Causes of hypophosphatemia

- **With normal maximal tubular phosphate reabsorption and fractional excretion of phosphate**
  - Low dietary intake or poor intestinal absorption
    Low dietary intake: severe malnutrition, very-low-birthweight infants
    Poor absorption: steatorrhea, chronic diarrhea, use of phosphate binders
  - Internal redistribution
    Refeeding syndrome in malnutrition (including diabetic ketoacidosis treated with insulin)
    Respiratory alkalosis
    Hungry bone syndrome after parathyroidectomy
- **With increased fractional excretion of phosphate**
  - Hyperparathyroidism
  - De Toni-Debré–Fanconi syndrome (= general impairment of the proximal tubule)[a]
  - Gitelman syndrome and Bartter syndromes[b]
  - Hypophosphatemic rickets[c]
  - After kidney transplant (= posttransplant hypophosphatemia)

[a] Various drugs may cause an incomplete or, more rarely, a complete form of De Toni-Debré–Fanconi syndrome with hypophosphatemia including paracetamol poisoning, and treatment with ifosfamide, valproic acid, the iron chelator deferasirox or ß$_2$-adrenoreceptors (e.g.: albuterol)
[b] Hypophosphatemia is rather mild in these post-proximal tubular disorders
[c] At least in part explained by increased activity of fibroblast growth factor 23

Internal Redistribution

In the majority of cases, an acute shift in phosphate from the extracellular to the intracellular compartment is primarily responsible for lowering phosphatemia. The most frequent cause is refeeding syndrome, a recognized and potentially fatal condition that occurs when previously malnourished patients are fed. The fluid and electrolyte abnormalities noted in the refeeding syndrome and those noted in severe diabetic ketoacidosis following the administration of insulin therapy are similar.

Patients who are malnourished develop a total body depletion of phosphate, Mg^{++} and K^+. Nonetheless, their blood levels are maintained by redistribution from the intracellular space. The delivery of glucose as part of a feeding strategy causes a huge increase in the circulating insulin level that induces a rapid uptake of glucose, K^+, phosphate and Mg^{++} into cells. The blood concentration of these metabolites falls dramatically. In addition, the body begins to retain fluid, and the extracellular space expands. Although hypophosphatemia is the predominant feature of the syndrome, rapid falls in K^+ and Mg^{++} levels, together with some tendency towards metabolic alkalosis, predispose to cardiac arrhythmias, while extracellular space expansion can precipitate acute heart failure in patients with cardiovascular disease. The most effective way to treat refeeding syndrome is to be aware of it. One should start feeding slowly and aggressively supplement and monitor phosphate, K^+ and Mg^{++} for 4 days after feeding is started.

Another cause of hypophosphatemia in hospitalized patients is respiratory alkalosis. Severe hyperventilation can be seen in patients with anxiety, pain, sepsis, and in patients during mechanical ventilation. The fall in carbon dioxide will result in a similar change in the cells because carbon dioxide readily diffuses across cell membranes. The elevated pH stimulates the glycolysis, leading to an accelerated production of phosphorylated metabolites and a rapid shift of phosphate into the cells.

The hungry bone syndrome, characterized by massive deposition of Ca^{++} and phosphate in the bone, can occur after parathyroidectomy for long-standing hyperparathyroidism (both primary and secondary).

Urinary Loss

1. In hyperparathyroidism, both primary and secondary, there is an increased urinary loss of phosphate.
2. Fanconi-De Toni-Debré syndrome is characterized by a general impairment of the proximal tubule leading to urinary loss of compounds normally reabsorbed by the proximal tubule. It results in hypophosphatemia, glucosuria, hyperaminoaciduria, uricosuria, and hyperbicarbonaturia (causing renal tubular acidosis).
3. The urinary phosphate excretion is also increased in patients with hereditary hypophosphatemic rickets and tumor-induced osteomalacia and rickets, as discussed in Chap. 55.

4. Recent data demonstrate a mild tendency towards urinary loss of phosphate in Gitelman and Bartter syndromes [54].

5. Following kidney transplant, hypophosphatemia has been described in the absence of both hyperparathyroidism and other signs of proximal tubule dysfunction.

Symptoms, Signs, Consequences

Phosphate depletion can cause a variety of symptoms and signs [49, 51–53]. Two major mechanisms are responsible for these symptoms: (a) decrease in intracellular adenosine triphosphate, and (b) in diphosphoglycerate. In adults, hypophosphatemia is symptomatic when the phosphate level is <0.35 mmol/L. Hypophosphatemia may be asymptomatic under certain clinical situations: patients recovering from diabetic ketoacidosis and patients with prolonged hyperventilation are usually asymptomatic because often there is not real phosphate depletion. The clinical features of phosphate depletion appear in Table 34.26.

Management

Hypophosphatemia does not automatically mean that phosphate replacement is indicated. To determine whether treatment is indicated, it is necessary to establish the cause of the hypophosphatemia, in which the history and the clinical setting are important. The identification and

Table 34.26 Symptoms, signs and consequences of phosphate depletion

- Skeletal muscle and bone: proximal myopathy, rhabdomyolysis[a]
- Cardiovascular system: impaired myocardial contractility
- Respiratory system: respiratory failure (and failed weaning)
- Neurological system: paresthesias, tremors, seizures, features resembling Guillain-Barré syndrome or Wernicke encephalopathy
- Hematological system: hemolysis, impaired granulocyte chemotaxis and phagocytosis causing Gram-negative sepsis, altered platelet function and thrombocytopenia

[a] In patients with rhabdomyolysis, hypophosphatemia can be masked by the release of phosphate from the injured muscle

treatment of the primary cause usually leads to normalization of the circulating phosphate level. As an example, the hypophosphatemia found in patients with diabetic ketoacidosis will usually correct spontaneously with normal dietary intake. However, replacement therapy is needed in patients with hypophosphatemia in combination with evidence of renal or gastrointestinal phosphate loss, the presence of underlying risk factors, and particularly if there are the clinical manifestations described above [53].

The safest mode of therapy is oral. Cow's milk is a good phosphate source: it contains 1 g (32 mmol) elemental phosphate per liter. Alternatively, oral preparations in the form of sodium phosphate or potassium phosphate can be used. The average adult patient requires 1–2 g (32–64 mmol) phosphate per day for 7–10 days to replenish body stores. An important side effect of oral supplementation is diarrhea.

Intravenous phosphate, usually 2.5–5.0 mg/kg (0.08–0.16 mmol/kg) over 6 h is given in symptomatic patients, who cannot take milk or tablets. More aggressive repletion with phosphate has been advocated but the magnitude of the response is unpredictable (close monitoring of phosphate level is crucial). Side effects of intravenous phosphate repletion are hypocalcemia, metastatic calcification, hyperkalemia associated with K+-containing supplements, volume excess, hypernatremia, metabolic acidosis, and hyperphosphatemia.

Burosumab, a fully human monoclonal antibody against FGF-23, is used for the treatment of hereditary hypophosphatemic rickets. The drug has demonstrated superior efficacy in correcting hypophosphatemia and clinical symptoms compared to conventional therapy consisting of oral phosphate and active vitamin D (Chap. 55).

Hyperphosphatemia

Spurious or artefactual hyperphosphatemia has been observed if hemolysis occurs during the collection or processing of blood samples. Spurious hyperphosphatemia due to interference with analytical methods occurs in patients with hyperglobulinemia, hyperlipidemia or hyperbilirubinemia and following contamination with heparinized saline from indwelling catheters or in subjects receiving liposomal amphotericin [55]. True hyperphosphatemia indicates either an increased phosphate load or a decreased renal phosphate excretion, as shown in Table 34.27. High dietary ingestion of phosphate alone rarely causes hyperphosphatemia with the exception of newborns and infants fed cow's milk, whose phosphate content is six times greater than human milk [49].

Table 34.27 Causes of hyperphosphatemia

- **Artifactual or spurious**
- **Increased phosphate load (with normal fractional excretion of phosphate and normal maximal tubular phosphate reabsorption)**
  - High dietary intake or increased intestinal absorption
    Newborns and infants fed cow's milk (rather than breast milk or adapted formula milk)
    Parenteral administration of phosphate salts
    Large amounts of phosphate-containing laxatives, phosphate enemas[a]
    Vitamin D intoxication
  - Internal redistribution
    Tumor lysis syndrome (before treatment and after initiation of cytotoxic therapy)
    Rhabdomyolysis
    Lactic and ketoacidosis (or severe hyperglycemia alone)[b], including severe dehydration in the context of acute diarrhea
- **Decreased renal phosphate excretion**
  - Reduced renal function (either acute or chronic)
  - Increased renal tubular phosphate reabsorption (= decreased fractional phosphate excretion and increased maximal tubular phosphate reabsorption)
    Hypoparathyroidism (and pseudohypoparathyroidism)
    Acromegaly
    Drugs: growth hormone, bisphosphonates, dipyridamole
    Idiopathic childhood nephrotic syndrome
    Familial hyperphosphatemic tumoral calcinosis

[a] The danger of hyperphosphatemia secondary to phosphate enema is especially high in children less than 2 years of age
[b] Metabolic acidosis blunts glycolysis and therefore cellular phosphate utilization. In addition, tissue hypoxia or insulin deficiency also play a crucial role

Acutely or chronically impaired renal function plays at least a partial role in most instances of hyperphosphatemia, including physiologically low glomerular filtration rate to explain the inability of the neonate to eliminate excess phosphate, mild renal insufficiency (due to volume contraction secondary to diarrhea) in subjects ingesting large amounts of phosphate-containing laxatives or mild to moderate tubulointerstitial injury secondary to intrarenal accumulation of uric acid in tumor lysis syndrome (see "hyperkalemia").

Familial hyperphosphatemic tumoral calcinosis is a recessive disorder characterized by hyperphosphatemia due to an increased maximal tubular phosphate reabsorption. Affected subjects present with extra-articular soft tissue deposition of calcium phosphate. This very rare disease (a kind of mirror image of some forms of hypophosphatemic rickets) results from inactivating mutations that lead to deficiency of circulating fibrolast growth factor 23 [49].

References

1. Moritz ML, Ayus JC. Disorders of water metabolism in children: hyponatremia and hypernatremia. Pediatr Rev. 2002;23:371–80.
2. Moritz ML, Ayus JC. Preventing neurological complications from dysnatremias in children. Pediatr Nephrol. 2005;20:1687–700.
3. Bianchetti MG, Simonetti GD, Bettinelli A. Body fluids and salt metabolism—part I. Ital J Pediatr. 2009;35:36.
4. Peruzzo M, Milani GP, Garzoni L, Longoni L, Simonetti GD, Bettinelli A, Fossali EF, Bianchetti MG. Body fluids and salt metabolism—part II. Ital J Pediatr. 2010;36:78.
5. Lava SA, Bianchetti MG, Simonetti GD. Salt intake in children and its consequences on blood pressure. Pediatr Nephrol. 2015;30:1389–96.
6. Titze J. Sodium balance is not just a renal affair. Curr Opin Nephrol Hypertens. 2014;23:101–5.
7. Marvar PJ, Gordon FJ, Harrison DG. Blood pressure control: salt gets under your skin. Nat Med. 2009;15:487–8.
8. Reynolds RM, Padfield PL, Seckl JR. Disorders of sodium balance. BMJ. 2006;332:702–5.
9. Sam R, Feizi I. Understanding hypernatremia. Am J Nephrol. 2012;36:97–104.

10. Haycock GB. Hypernatraemia: diagnosis and management. Arch Dis Child Educ Pract Ed. 2006;91:8–13.
11. Haycock GB. Hyponatraemia: diagnosis and management. Arch Dis Child Educ Pract Ed. 2006;91:37–41.
12. Ball SG. How I approach hyponatraemia. Clin Med. 2013;13:291–5.
13. Lava SA, Bianchetti MG, Milani GP. Testing Na+ in blood. Clin Kidney J. 2017;10:147–8.
14. Spasovski G, Vanholder R, Allolio B, et al. Clinical practice guideline on diagnosis and treatment of hyponatraemia. Nephrol Dial Transplant. 2014;29(Suppl 2):i1–i39.
15. Bailey B, Gravel J, Goldman RD, Friedman JN, Parkin PC. External validation of the clinical dehydration scale for children with acute gastroenteritis. Acad Emerg Med. 2010;17:583–8.
16. Dunkelmann L, Bucher BS, Tschumi S, Duppenthaler A, Simonetti GD. Estimation of dehydration using bioelectric impedance in children with gastroenteritis. Acta Paediatr. 2012;101:e479–81.
17. Mazzoni MB, Milani GP, Bernardi S, Odone L, Rocchi A, D'Angelo EA, Alberzoni M, Agostoni C, Bianchetti MG, Fossali EF. Hyponatremia in infants with community-acquired infections on hospital admission. PLoS One. 2019;14(7):e0219299.
18. Lucchini B, Simonetti GD, Ceschi A, Lava SA, Bianchetti MG. Severe signs of hyponatremia secondary to desmopressin treatment for enuresis: a systematic review. J Pediatr Urol. 2013;9:1049–53.
19. Lavagno C, Camozzi P, Renzi S, Lava SA, Simonetti GD, Bianchetti MG, Milani GP. Breastfeeding-associated hypernatremia: a systematic review of the literature. J Hum Lact. 2016;32:67–74.
20. Canziani BC, Uestuener P, Fossali EF, Lava SA, Bianchetti MG, Agostoni C, Milani GP. Nausea and vomiting in acute gastroenteritis: physiopathology and management. Eur J Pediatr. 2018;177:1–5.
21. Daly K, Farrington E. Hypokalemia and hyperkalemia in infants and children: pathophysiology and treatment. J Pediatr Health Care. 2013;27:486–96.
22. Dussol B. Equilibre potassique, hypokaliémie et hyperkaliémie. Nephrol Ther. 2010;6:180–99.
23. Jain G, Ong S, Warnock DG. Genetic disorders of potassium homeostasis. Semin Nephrol. 2013;33:300–9.
24. Greenlee M, Wingo CS, McDonough AA, Youn JH, Kone BC. Narrative review: evolving concepts in potassium homeostasis and hypokalemia. Ann Intern Med. 2009;150:619–25. (Erratum in: Ann Intern Med 2009; 151: 143–4).
25. Palmer BF. A physiologic-based approach to the evaluation of a patient with hypokalemia. Am J Kidney Dis. 2010;56:1184–90.
26. Unwin RJ, Luft FC, Shirley DG. Pathophysiology and management of hypokalemia: a clinical perspective. Nat Rev Nephrol. 2011;7:75–84.
27. Nyirenda MJ, Tang JI, Padfield PL, Seckl JR. Hyperkalaemia. BMJ. 2009;339:1019–24.
28. Lehnhardt A, Kemper MJ. Pathogenesis, diagnosis and management of hyperkalemia. Pediatr Nephrol. 2011;26:377–84.
29. Masilamani K, van der Voort J. The management of acute hyperkalaemia in neonates and children. Arch Dis Child. 2012;97:376–80.
30. Bertini A, Milani GP, Simonetti GD, Fossali EF, Faré PB, Bianchetti MG, Lava SA. Na+, K+, Cl−, acid–base or H2O homeostasis in children with urinary tract infections: a narrative review. Pediatr Nephrol. 2016;31:1403–9.
31. Adrogué HJ, Gennari FJ, Galla JH, Madias NE. Assessing acid-base disorders. Kidney Int. 2009;76:1239–47.
32. Carmody JB, Norwood VF. A clinical approach to paediatric acid-base disorders. Postgrad Med J. 2012;88:143–51.
33. Kraut JA, Madias NE. Metabolic acidosis: pathophysiology, diagnosis and management. Nat Rev Nephrol. 2010;6:274–85.
34. Morris CG, Low J. Metabolic acidosis in the critically ill: part 1. Classification and pathophysiology. Anaesthesia. 2008;63:294–301.
35. Morris CG, Low J. Metabolic acidosis in the critically ill: part 2. Causes and treatment. Anaesthesia. 2008;63:396–411.
36. Gennari FJ. Pathophysiology of metabolic alkalosis: a new classification based on the centrality of stimulated collecting duct ion transport. Am J Kidney Dis. 2011;58:626–36.
37. Luke RG, Galla JH. It is chloride depletion alkalosis, not contraction alkalosis. J Am Soc Nephrol. 2012;23:204–7.
38. Allgrove J. Disorders of calcium metabolism. Curr Paediatr. 2003;13:529–35.
39. Carmeliet G, Van Cromphaut S, Daci E, Maes C, Bouillon R. Disorders of calcium homeostasis. Best Pract Res Clin Endocrinol Metab. 2003;17:529–46.
40. Hoorn EJ, Zietse R. Disorders of calcium and magnesium balance: a physiology-based approach. Pediatr Nephrol. 2013;28:1195–206.
41. Payne RB, Little AJ, Williams RB, Milner JR. Interpretation of serum calcium in patients with abnormal serum proteins. Br Med J. 1973;4(5893):643–6.
42. Singh J, Moghal N, Pearce SH, Cheetham T. The investigation of hypocalcaemia and rickets. Arch Dis Child. 2003;88:403–7.
43. Inzucchi SE. Understanding hypercalcemia—its metabolic basis, signs, and symptoms. Postgrad Med. 2004;115:69–70, 73–6.
44. Jacobs TP, Bilezikian JP. Clinical review: rare causes of hypercalcemia. J Clin Endocrinol Metab. 2005;90:6316–22.
45. Alexander RT, Hoenderop JG, Bindels RJ. Molecular determinants of magnesium homeostasis: insights from human disease. J Am Soc Nephrol. 2008;19:1451–8.

46. Dimke H, Monnens L, Hoenderop JG, Bindels RJ. Evaluation of hypomagnesemia: lessons from disorders of tubular transport. Am J Kidney Dis. 2013;62:377–83.

47. Janett S, Camozzi P, Peeters GG, Lava SA, Simonetti GD, Goeggel Simonetti B, Bianchetti MG, Milani GP. Hypomagnesemia induced by long-term treatment with proton-pump inhibitors. Gastroenterol Res Pract. 2015;2015:951768.

48. Santi M, Milani GP, Simonetti GD, Fossali E, Bianchetti MG, Lava SA. Magnesium in cystic fibrosis—systematic review of the literature. Pediatr Pulmonol. 2016;51:196–202.

49. Goretti M, Penido MG, Alon US. Phosphate homeostasis and its role in bone health. Pediatr Nephrol. 2012;27:2039–48.

50. Brodehl J. Assessment and interpretation of the tubular threshold for phosphate in infants and children. Pediatr Nephrol. 1994;8:645.

51. Gaasbeek A, Meinders AE. Hypophosphatemia: an update on its etiology and treatment. Am J Med. 2005;118:1094–101.

52. Amanzadeh J, Reilly RF Jr. Hypophosphatemia: an evidence-based approach to its clinical consequences and management. Nat Clin Pract Nephrol. 2006;2:136–48.

53. Ritz E, Haxsen V, Zeier M. Disorders of phosphate metabolism—pathomechanisms and management of hypophosphataemic disorders. Best Pract Res Clin Endocrinol Metab. 2003;17:547–58.

54. Viganò C, Amoruso C, Barretta F, Minnici G, Albisetti W, Syrèn ML, Bianchetti MG, Bettinelli A. Renal phosphate handling in Gitelman syndrome—the results of a case-control study. Pediatr Nephrol. 2013;28(1):65–70. https://doi.org/10.1007/s00467-012-2297-3.

55. Molinaris V, Bianchetti MG, Milani GP, Lava SAG, Della Bruna R, Simonetti GD, Farè PB. Interferences in the measurement of circulating phosphate: a literature review. Clin Chem Lab Med. 2020;58(12):1971–7. https://doi.org/10.1515/cclm-2020-0281. Epub ahead of print.

Renal Fanconi Syndromes and Other Proximal Tubular Disorders

35

Detlef Bockenhauer and Robert Kleta

Introduction

Fanconi first described the concept that defective renal proximal tubule reabsorption of solutes might contribute to "non-nephrotic glycosuric dwarfing with hypophosphataemic rickets in early childhood" [1]. Rickets and albuminuria secondary to kidney disease was described some 50 years previously but attributed to a disorder of adolescence [2]. Fanconi's first case presented at 3 months with rickets and recurrent fevers. She had glycosuria and albuminuria and progressed to terminal renal failure by 5 years of age. At autopsy the renal tubule cells appeared filled with crystals, which were thought to be cystine. In subsequent reports, Debré, de Toni and Fanconi all described series of children with rickets, glycosuria and albuminuria [3–5]. In acknowledgment of this pioneering work, we now refer to this symptom constellation as Fanconi-Debre-de Toni syndrome, or just short as "renal Fanconi syndrome" (RFS). The presentation, course and outcome of the described children, however, varied markedly. This reflects that RFS is not a uniform entity, but a diagnosis of proximal tubular dysfunction, which can be due to a variety of different causes (see Tables 35.1 and 35.2). RFS can be isolated or in the context of multiorgan disorders, congenital or acquired, transient or permanent, associated with progression to end-stage kidney disease (ESKD) or with stable kidney function throughout. Moreover, it can differ in the extent and severity of tubular dysfunction. Severe and generalized proximal tubular dysfunction is seen in cystinosis whilst many children with e.g. Dent disease or Lowe syndrome may have no clinically significant disturbance of phosphate and bicarbonate transport [39]. Indeed, there is some debate at what point proximal tubular dysfunction can be called RFS [40].

Here, we use the term RFS to include disorders with dysfunction of multiple proximal tubular pathways, but recognize that not every transport system need be affected. This clinical and biochemical heterogeneity is likely to arise from the multiple mechanisms involved in proximal tubular transport, reflecting not only the bulk of solute and water reabsorption but also the re-uptake of proteins, amino acids, vitamins, cytokines and many other substances. RFS do not therefore have a common and single pathogenetic basis but reflect the interplay of a number of different biochemical processes. Identification of the underlying etiology is therefore of utmost importance, as it informs management and prognosis.

D. Bockenhauer (✉) · R. Kleta
Department of Nephrology,
Great Ormond Street Hospital, London, UK

Department of Renal Medicine,
University College London, London, UK
e-mail: d.bockenhauer@ucl.ac.uk; r.kleta@ucl.ac.uk

© The Author(s), under exclusive license to Springer Nature Switzerland AG 2023
F. Schaefer, L. A. Greenbaum (eds.), *Pediatric Kidney Disease*,
https://doi.org/10.1007/978-3-031-11665-0_35

Table 35.1 Congenital causes of renal Fanconi Syndrome (RFS) by age of onset. (Adapted from [6])

Onset	Disorder	Associated features	Diagnostic test
Neonatal	Galactosemia	Liver dysfunction, jaundice, encephalopathy, sepsis	Red cell galactose 1-phosphate uridyl transferase
	Mitochondrial disorders	Usually multisystem dysfunction (brain, muscle, liver, heart)	Lactate/pyruvate (plasma lactate may be normal due to urinary losses), muscle enzymology
	Tyrosinemia	Poor growth, hepatic enlargement and dysfunction	Plasma amino acids, urine organic acids (succinylacetone)
Infancy	Fructosemia	Rapid onset after fructose ingestion, vomiting, hypoglycemia, hepatomegaly	Hepatic fructose-1-phosphate aldolase B
	Cystinosis	Poor growth, vomiting, rickets ± corneal cystine crystals	Leukocyte cystine concentration, molecular diagnosis (*CTNS*)
	Fanconi Bickel syndrome	Failure to thrive, hepatomegaly, hypoglycemia rickets, severe glycosuria, galactosuria	molecular diagnosis (*GLUT2*)
	Lowe's syndrome	Males (X-linked), cataracts, hypotonia, developmental delay	Clinical and molecular diagnosis (*OCRL*)
	RFS—GATM	Autosomal dominant, RFS recognisable in infancy, usually "mild" RFS, advanced CKD in adulthood	molecular diagnosis (*GATM*)
	RFS—EHHADH	Autosomal dominant, RFS recognisable in infancy, no progressive CKD	molecular diagnosis (*EHHADH*)
Childhood	Cystinosis	see above	
	Dent disease	Males (X-linked), hypercalciuria, nephrocalcinosis	Molecular diagnosis (*CLCN5, OCRL*)
	Wilson's disease	Hepatic & neurological disease, Kayser-Fleischer rings	Copper, coeruloplasmin, molecular diagnosis (*ATP7B*)

Table 35.2 Acquired causes of the renal Fanconi syndrome

Drugs and toxins
  Anti-cancer drugs
    Ifosfamide (see text)
    Streptozocin [7, 8]
  Antibiotics
    Aminoglycoside (see text)
    Expired tetracyclines [9, 10]
Anti-retrovirals
  Adefovir/Cidofovir/Tenofovir [11–15]
  ddI [16, 17]
Heavy metals
  Lead poisoning [18]
  Cadmium [19]
Sodium valproate [20]
Aristolochic acid (Chinese herb nephropathy) [21–23]
Toluene/Glue sniffing [24]
Fumaric acid [25]
Suramin [26]
Paraquat [27]
L-Lysine [28]
Renal disorders
  Tubulointerstitial nephritis [29]
  Membranous nephropathy with anti-tubular basement antibodies [30–38]

Clinical Features

The presenting clinical features of RFS in childhood are usually failure-to-thrive and rickets, although patients with RFS in the context of a systemic disorder may first be identified via the extra-renal manifestations, such as the cataracts in Lowe syndrome, or myopathy in mitochondrial cytopathies.

The failure-to-thrive is presumably due to the high-volume losses, with patients preoccupied with drinking, rather than caloric intake. Some patients exhibit features of a secondary nephrogenic diabetes insipidus, further compounding the water losses from impaired proximal reabsorption [41, 42].

Rickets is the consequence of renal phosphate losses (see below), as well as impaired proximal hydroxylation of vitamin D. The critical step in the formation of active Vitamin D (i.e. 1,25 OH-cholecalciferol) is mitochondrial 1α-hydroxylation in the proximal tubule. For this to occur, cholecalciferol, bound to its carrier vitamin D-binding protein (a low-molecular weight protein) needs to be reabsorbed from the tubular lumen, a process impaired in RFS [43].

Biochemical Abnormalities

Excessive urinary levels of a wide range of solutes and substances normally reabsorbed in the proximal tubule are the biochemical hallmarks of RFS.

Proteinuria

Proteinuria **in RFS** is made up of albumin, low molecular weight proteins and tubular enzymes, such as retinol binding protein (RBP), α-1 microglobulin, β-2 microglobulin, N-acetylglucoseaminidase, alanine aminopeptidase. The urinary level of these very sensitive markers of proximal tubular dysfunction is markedly elevated, especially if RBP is assayed [44, 45]. Albuminuria can be highly variable in RFS, but is typically below nephrotic range proteinuria [46]. In a family with autosomal dominant isolated RFS without apparent glomerular dysfunction the total amount was roughly 1g per day in affected adults [47]. This is consistent with some estimates of the amount of filtered albumin, which would usually undergo tubular reabsorption, at 0.4–1 g albumin per 1.73 m^2 per day [48, 49]. However, more recent estimates suggest that the amount of filtered albumin may actually be much higher, reaching several grams per day [50]. Indeed, there are multiple reports of patients with genetically defined defects in proximal tubular protein reabsorption, such as pathogenic variants in *OCRL*, *CLCN5* or *CUBN*, excreting several grams of protein in the urine per day [51–53]. Whether this amount of albuminuria is solely tubular or does reflect secondary glomerular damage remains controversial [54]. Interestingly, patients with proximal tubular disorders, even when they have nephrotic range proteinuria, typically have normal levels of plasma albumin and do not exhibit oedema [53]. Thus, the total amount of protein loss in RFS can be variable, reflecting the degree of impairment of reabsorption and potential concomitant glomerular dysfunction.

It is important to remember that urine dipsticks primarily detect larger proteins including albumin and thus can miss the mostly low-molecular weight proteinuria of RFS. Tubular proteinuria may be seen in some forms of nephrotic syndrome, likely reflecting associated tubulointerstitial damage [55, 56].

Aminoaciduria

The aminoaciduria seen in RFS is generalized and its pattern is influenced by plasma values, so that in rare situations of severe protein malnutrition, aminoaciduria as analyzed on thin-layer chromatography, may be recorded as "normal" or "mild" [44]. Quantitative analysis in urine and plasma by ion-exchange chromatography should be used to determine the degree and specific nature of aminoaciduria.

Organic Aciduria

Organic acids, including citrate and uric acid, are also exclusively reabsorbed in the proximal tubule and excretion is thus increased in RFS [57]. Consequently, patients with RFS typically have hyperuricosuria with hypouricemia, as well as hypercitraturia [58]. Moreover, transport of drugs, such as probenecid, furosemide or penicillin, can be affected, potentially altering pharmacokinetics [59]. The increased excretion of lactate can lead to normalization of plasma lactate levels in mitochondrial cytopathies, resulting in another potential diagnostic pitfall [60].

Glycosuria

Renal glycosuria in RFS reflects the impaired proximal tubular ability for glucose reabsorption, so that glycosuria occurs with normal blood glucose levels. As RFS is typically associated with marked polyuria, the urinary glucose concentration may be less than the 5 mmol/L and thus missed by dipstick measurement [39]. Formal laboratory measurement, ideally of a 24-h urine collection, should thus be used to detect and quantify glycosuria. Normally, less than 1.5 mmol (300 mg)/day/1.73 m^2 are excreted [61], but this can increase to several grams daily with defects in proximal tubular reabsorption [62].

Renal Tubular Acidosis

Since the proximal tubule is the key site for bicarbonate reabsorption, bicarbonaturia is a typical feature of RFS with consequent metabolic acidosis (see also Chap. 35). The degree to which the threshold for reabsorption is reduced is variable, according to the underlying cause of RFS. In severe acidosis, filtered bicarbonate is reduced to a level below the threshold for proximal reabsorption and urine pH falls below 5.3 if distal acidification is intact. The hyperchloremic metabolic acidosis contributes to loss of skeletal calcium and consequent hypercalciuria. Unfortunately, treatment with alkali supplementation is complicated by the ongoing proximal losses, as soon as the plasma bicarbonate level rises above the threshold capacity for reabsorption. Frequent daily dosing of alkali supplementation can help to sustain bicarbonate levels in the normal range, or at least closer to it.

Phosphaturia

Renal phosphate wasting with secondary hypophosphatemia is another hallmark of proximal tubular dysfunction, leading to rickets or bone disease. Urine phosphate handling is usually assessed as the tubular reabsorption (TRP), the complement to the fractional excretion of phosphate (FEP). Thus, it is calculated as: TRP [%] = 100 − FEP [%]. Usually, a TRP >70% is considered normal, however this can be misleading. If the plasma phosphate level is decreased, the filtered load of phosphate may be close to or below the threshold of tubular phosphate reabsorption and TRP can therefore be misleadingly "normal". To account for the filtered load, uri-

Table 35.3 Normal age-specific values for TmP/GFR (derived from [64–66])

Age	mmol/L
<1 month	1.48–3.43
1–3 months	1.48–3.30
4–6 months	1.15–2.60
7 months–2 years	1.10–2.70
2–4 years	1.04–2.79
4–6 years	1.05–2.60
6–8 years	1.26–2.35
8–10 years	1.10–2.31
10–12 years	1.15–2.58
12–15 years	1.18–2.09
>15 years	0.80–1.35

nary phosphate excretion can be assessed using the tubular threshold concentration for phosphate excretion, corrected for glomerular filtration rate (TmP/GFR) [63]. It is calculated as follows: TmP/GFR = (Phosphate plasma − Phosphate urine/Creatinine urine × Creatinine plasma). Normal values are age-dependent and listed in Table 35.3.

Hypercalciuria

Approximately 70% of filtered calcium is reabsorbed in the proximal tubule and, consequently hypercalciuria is another characteristic of RFS. It is further compounded by the acidosis-mediated calcium release from bone (see above). Nephrocalcinosis and stone formation can ensue, but interestingly is rather uncommon. Presumably, the polyuria inherent in RFS is protective against these complications, as may be the increased luminal concentration of citrate (see organic aciduria, above) [67].

Hypokalemia

Potassium, like almost all other electrolytes, is predominantly reabsorbed in the proximal tubule, making hypokalemia another typical feature. It can further be compounded by hyperaldosteronism if electrolyte and fluid losses result in volume contraction [68–70].

Other Substances

Carnitine is reabsorbed in the proximal tubule and is therefore lost in excess in RFS. Low plasma carnitine concentrations have been reported in children with cystinosis and tyrosinemia [71, 72] leading to plasma and muscle deficiencies of carnitine, which could contribute to the myopathy in these disorders. Moreover, losses of vitamins, carrier proteins and chemokines have all been described in RFS [46, 73].

Pathogenesis

The variation in etiology, manifestations and severity of RFS make it unlikely that there is a single common pathogenetic mechanism. Most studies of the pathogenesis have, of necessity, focused on one biochemical pathway. However, *in vivo*, it is more likely that a number of interlinked biochemical processes are disrupted in a variable manner.

Disruption of Energy Production

The high transport activity of the proximal tubule requires a large amount of energy. Thus, disruption of the energy supply is an obvious etiology of RFS. Consequently, it is not surprising that RFS is a frequent complication of mitochondrial cytopathies [60]. In fact, most inherited primary forms of RFS that have been genetically solved to date appear to be associated with mitochondrial dysfunction [74–76] (see below: Primary renal Fanconi syndromes).

Mitochondrial dysfunction has also been implicated in the development of RFS in cystinosis (see Chap. 30). Similar studies have been undertaken in models of tyrosinemia, which is associated with excessive accumulation of succinylacetone (SA). SA reduced sodium-dependent uptake of sugar and amino acids across rat brush border membranes [77] and intra-peritoneal injection of SA to rats led to development of RFS [78]. SA inhibits sodium-dependent phosphate transport by brush border membrane vesicles, decreases ATP production and inhibits mitochondrial respiration [79]. Administration of maleic acid, used to create an animal model of RFS, causes a reduction in ATP and phosphate concentrations, NaK ATPase activity and coenzyme A [80].

Glutathione Depletion

Historically, another line of investigation has looked into the role of glutathione (GSH) in the pathogenesis of RFS. GSH has a number of key cellular roles including post-translational protein modification, xenobiotic detoxification and it acts as a major antioxidant. Some such studies have mainly focused on cystinosis (Chap. 30), yet deficiency of GSH has also been implicated in other forms of the RFS. Ifosfamide toxicity, which leads to RFS, may be mediated by its interaction with γ-glutamyl transpeptidase, a precursor of GSH synthesis, and by hepatic metabolism to chloroacetaldehyde [81]. Incubation of chloroacetaldehyde with isolated human renal proximal tubules was associated with depletion of GSH, coenzyme A, acetyl-coenzyme A and ATP [82]. Wistar rats injected with ifosfamide develop RFS, associated with GSH depletion which is attenuated by treatment with melatonin [82]. Addition of ochratoxin A, the presumed toxin causing RFS in Balkan Endemic Nephropathy, to rat proximal tubular cells causes an elevation of reactive oxygen species and depletion of cellular GSH [83]. However, other data suggest that specific renal proximal tubular uptake and metabolism of ifosfamide is causative for the side effect of RFS [84].

Reduced Activity of Cotransporters

Increased solute excretion in RFS could result from reduced expression or activity of sodium-coupled cotransporters, which mediate proximal tubular reabsorption. In the animal model of maleic acid induced RFS, decreased *Slc34a1* mRNA expression and consequent reduced NaPi2a protein were observed [85].

Mice lacking hepatocyte nuclear factor 1 alpha (HNF1α), a transcription factor expressed in liver, pancreas, kidney and intestine, develop RFS, abnormal bile metabolism and diabetes [86]. HNF1α −/− mice had reduced expression of sodium-coupled transporters for glucose (SGLT2) and phosphate (NaPi1 and NaPi4) but normal levels of NaPi2a, the major phosphate transporter [87]. In addition, one primary form of proximal tubular dysfunction (see below: Primary renal Fanconi syndromes) is associated with a homozygous mutation in *SLC34A1* [88].

Disruption of the Endocytic Pathway (Megalin/Cubilin)

An important task of the proximal tubule is to reabsorb filtered proteins, including peptide hormones, as well as small carrier proteins binding fat-soluble vitamins and trace elements. Therefore, by reabsorbing filtered proteins the proximal tubule actively participates in the homeostasis of hormones, trace elements and vitamins. In addition, some lipoproteins, such as apolipoprotein A-I and A-IV are also reabsorbed in the proximal tubule [89]. Reabsorption of the vast majority of filtered proteins is mediated by two endocytic receptors: megalin and cubilin (reviewed in [90, 91]). These receptors contain several protein-binding domains and protrude from the microvilli, which make up the brush border of the proximal tubule, into the tubular lumen. Once a protein is attached, the receptor-ligand complex moves towards the base of the microvilli into clathrin-coated pits, which then bud off into the cytoplasm to form endosomes (see Fig. 35.1). Subsequently, the receptors are recycled back to the membrane to mediate further uptake. The fate of the protein ligands is different: most are degraded by acid hydrolysis after fusion of the endosome to a lysosome, while others, such as vitamins, are released back into the blood circulation across the basolateral membrane. In this fashion, the megalin/cubilin complex assumes a role in the regulation of several hormonal pathways, the importance of which becomes apparent, when considering, for

instance, calcium-regulation: Megalin competes with the PTH receptor for the binding of filtered PTH and renders it non-functional by endocytosis and subsequent delivery to a lysosome for degradation [93]. In contrast, megalin/cubilin facilitates activation of Vitamin D by binding of filtered 25-OH vitamin D-Vitamin D binding protein and thus allowing uptake into the proximal tubule cell and activation by 1α-hydroxylase [43, 94].

Megalin is a large transmembrane protein belonging to the family of low-density lipoprotein receptors and was originally identified as the target of antibodies causing Heymann nephritis in rats [95]. It is expressed in epithelial cells of a variety of other tissues active in endocytosis [92]. Megalin-deficient mice mostly die in utero, but those that survive indeed show Fanconi-type low-molecular weight proteinuria, confirming the central role of megalin in endocytosis in the proximal tubule [96]. Interestingly, mutations in *LRP2*, the gene encoding megalin, were identified as the cause of Donnai-Barrow syndrome [97]. Donnai-Barrow syndrome is characterized by facial and ocular anomalies, sensorineural hearing loss and proteinuria. However, whilst these patients have, as expected, low-molecular weight proteinuria, there is no generalized proximal tubular dysfunction [98].

Cubilin is a peripheral membrane protein and is dependent on megalin to initiate endocytosis after ligand binding. These two proteins are co-expressed in proximal tubule and along the endocytic pathway and work in tandem to mediate protein uptake [90, 91]. Cubilin is otherwise known as the intrinsic factor-vitamin B12 receptor [99]. Loss-of-function mutations are associated with juvenile megaloblastic anemia or Imerslund-Graesbeck disease [100, 101]. The anemia is caused by deficient intestinal endocytosis of intrinsic factor-vitamin B12. In addition, some of these patients also have a selective low-molecular weight proteinuria that identifies those proteins requiring cubilin for endocytosis, such as albumin, transferrin, immunoglobulin light chains and α1- and β2-microglobulin [102]. Yet, as with Megalin, mutations in Cubilin are not associated with complete RFS.

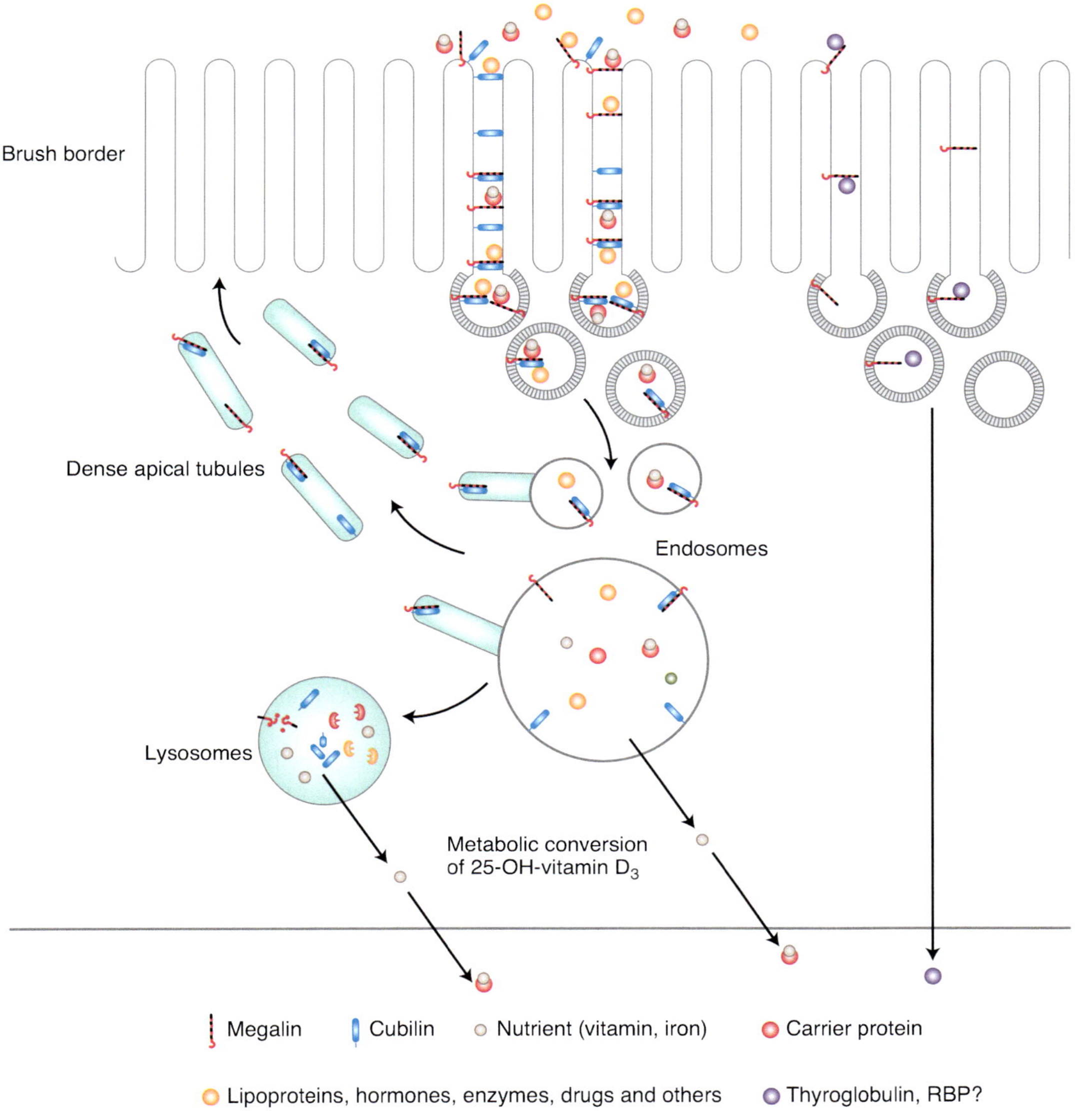

Brush border

Dense apical tubules

Endosomes

Lysosomes

Metabolic conversion
of 25-OH-vitamin D$_3$

| Megalin | Cubilin | ○ Nutrient (vitamin, iron) | ● Carrier protein |

○ Lipoproteins, hormones, enzymes, drugs and others   ● Thyroglobulin, RBP?

Fig. 35.1 Role of Megalin and Cubilin in proximal tubular transport. The receptors Megalin and Cubilin stick out from the brush border into the lumen of the proximal tubule. Once bound to a ligand (such as LMWP, nutrients etc.), the complex is endocytosed and ligand and receptor are separated by the low pH in the endosomes. The receptors are subsequently recycled to the membrane. (From [92])

Decreased expression of both megalin and cubilin at the brush border has been described in a mouse model of Dent disease [103]. Decreased levels of megalin have also been found in the urine of patients with Dent disease and Lowe syndrome, suggesting defective trafficking of the receptors as a mechanism of the low-molecular weight proteinuria seen in affected patients [104, 105]. The loss of vitamins, hormones and trace elements associated with endocytic dysfunction may explain some of the clinical heterogeneity seen in RFS.

Primary Renal Fanconi Syndromes

Sometimes, RFS appears in patients without an identified cause. The majority of these primary or idiopathic cases occur in adulthood, but some have also been reported in children [106]. A small number of cases occur in families and different modes of inheritance have been reported [47, 107–111]. Amongst the families with autosomal-dominant inheritance two distinct forms are recognized: (1) RFS with progressive chronic kidney disease (OMIM 134600), which is related to mutations in *GATM* [75] and (2) RFS with preserved GFR into advanced age (OMIM 615605) [88]. *GATM* encodes arginine-glycine amidinotransferase, an enzyme involved in creatine synthesis and recessive mutations are associated with a neurological disorder, cerebral creatine deficiency (OMIM 612718). However, the dominant mutations associated with RFS do not cause creatine deficiency and affected patients have no associated neurological manifestations. Instead, these dominant mutations cause linear aggregates of GATM in mitochondria, which are visible on electron microscopy in biopsy specimen. These aggregates appear to affect mitochondrial fission with consequent elongation of mitochondria, enhanced reactive oxygen species production and activation of the inflammasome, which in turn, is thought to contribute to tubulointerstitial fibrosis and progressive chronic kidney disease [75].

In RFS with preserved GFR so far only one specific dominant mutation in *EHHADH* has been identified (c.7G>A). *EHHADH* encodes a peroxisomal enzyme involved in fatty acid oxidation and, similar to *GATM*, this mutation does not lead to enzyme deficiency. Instead, the variant creates a novel mitochondrial targeting motif, leading to misrouting of the enzyme from the peroxisome to the mitochondria, where it interferes with fatty acid oxidation [74, 112]. While EHHADH is expressed in all organ systems, clinical manifestations appear restricted to the proximal tubule only, highlighting the dependence of the proximal tubule on mitochondrial fatty acid

oxidation, rather than glucose metabolism [74, 112–114].

Another dominantly inherited form of RFS is associated with impaired insulin secretion (initially hyperinsulinism, later maturity onset diabetes in the young, OMIM 616026) and due to a specific missense mutation in *HNF4A* (p.Arg85Trp, also annotated as p.Arg63Trp or p.Arg76Trp, depending on reference sequence), encoding a transcription factor expressed in liver, pancreas and kidney [115, 116]. Interestingly, other dominant mutations in *HNF4A* are only associated with impaired insulin secretion, but not RFS. The exact mechanisms of how this particular mutations causes RFS are unclear, but impaired phosphorylation with subsequent changes in localization of HNF4A has been reported [76].

An autosomal recessive form of an incomplete RFS in two siblings has been attributed to a specific mutation in the phosphate transporter NaPi2a (*SLC34A1*), an in-frame 21bp duplication g.2061_2081dup; p.I154_V160dup [88]. It is yet to be clarified, how exactly this specific defect in proximal tubular phosphate transport causes a more generalized proximal tubular dysfunction, especially when considering that recessive mutations in *SLC34A1* have since been identified as the cause of a different disorder, infantile hypercalcaemia [117]. Interestingly, the specific mutation initially linked to proximal tubular dysfunction was subsequently linked also to infantile hypercalcaemia [118].

Treatment of these primary forms is symptomatic and in those with kidney failure, transplantation is an option.

Secondary Forms of Inherited Renal Fanconi Syndromes

Cystinosis

Nephropathic cystinosis, the most common cause of RFS in children, is covered in Chap. 30.

Tyrosinemia

The tyrosinemias are a group of disorders affecting the metabolism of tyrosine. The most severe one is tyrosinemia type 1, due to a defect in the enzyme fumarylacetoacetate hydrolase. Severity of clinical symptoms is variable but typically includes hepatic dysfunction with progression to cirrhosis and risk of hepatic cancer, as well as a porphyria-like neuropathy. In addition, patients can develop a severe RFS and chronic renal impairment may eventually ensue. The enzymatic defect in tyrosinemia leads to an accumulation of succinylacetone, which is thought to cause the symptoms. In experimental models succinylacetone inhibits transport in the proximal tubule, potentially by inhibition of mitochondrial function [77–79]. In addition, it inhibits porphobilinogen synthetase, which may explain the porphyria-like neuropathy [119]. Further evidence for the pathogenic role of succinylacetone comes from the discovery that blockade of tyrosine metabolism further upstream effectively remedies the symptoms of tyrosinemia: mice deleted for the gene encoding fumarylacetoacetate hydrolase die in the neonatal period, but are rescued by the additional deletion of the 4-OH-phenylpyruvate dioxygenase (HPD) gene (the basis for tyrosinemia type 3) which prevents the accumulation of succinylacetone [120]. Similarly, administration of nitisinone, a blocker of HPD effectively prevents and even reverses the symptoms of tyrosinemia in the vast majority of patients [121]. Consequently, nitisinone is now the first line therapy for tyrosinemia together with a tyrosine- and phenylalanine-restricted diet [122]. In the roughly 10% of patients where this fails, liver transplantation is an option. However, even though transplantation corrects the enzymatic defect in the liver, elevated levels of succinylacetone are still found in the urine of these patients and some of them have persisting tubular defects [123, 124].

Mitochondrial Cytopathies

The proximal tubule has a high energy requirement in order to reabsorb the bulk of filtered solutes. Cellular energy is provided in the form of ATP, produced by the respiratory chain in mitochondria. Therefore, proximal tubular cells are rich in mitochondria and it is not surprising that the proximal tubule is particularly susceptible to mitochondrial dysfunction. Indeed, RFS is the most common renal manifestation of mitochondrial cytopathies [60]. The clinical manifestations of mitochondrial disorders are highly variable, but those with RFS typically have severe multi-organ involvement and present during infancy [60]. Neuromuscular manifestations usually predominate and the prognosis is often poor. Mitochondrial DNA mutations are inherited through the maternal line, as mitochondria derive from the maternal egg. An egg contains several mitochondria, each carrying their own DNA. Mutations in mitochondrial DNA can therefore be present in some mitochondria, but not in others within the same cell, a state termed heteroplasmy. Depending on the number of mitochondria with mutations passed on during cell division the ratio of mutated to healthy mitochondria can be highly variable within different tissues and cells, which may explain some of the clinical variability [125]. However, the majority of genes encoding the respiratory chain enzymes are encoded in the nuclear genome and mutations in these genes are typically inherited in autosomal-recessive fashion and affect all mitochondria uniformly.

An initial investigation in suspected mitochondrial cytopathies is typically to determine the ratio of lactate to pyruvate in the serum. However, in patients with RFS, this ratio is often normal, due to the grossly increased loss of organic acids in the urine [60]. Therefore, measurement of activity of respiratory chain enzymes should be performed in those patients with high suspicion of a mitochondrial cytopathy. Renal histology is typically non-specific, showing tubular damage, but may show giant mitochondria [126, 127]. Some forms of mitochondrial cytopathies can be improved by supplementation with certain vitamins, especially those with a deficiency in the coenzyme Q10 [128]. Otherwise, no definitive treatment exists and management is only supportive for the renal manifestations.

Fanconi-Bickel-Syndrome

Fanconi-Bickel-syndrome is a rare autosomal-recessive glycogen-storage disease, caused by mutations in the gene *SLC2A2* encoding the glucose transporter GLUT2 [62, 129]. Patients typically present in infancy with hepatomegaly, failure-to-thrive and renal Fanconi-syndrome with excessive glucosuria [130]. GLUT2 is expressed in liver, intestine, pancreatic β-cells and proximal tubule cells. In hepatocytes, the transporter facilitates glucose uptake, as well as release. The impaired release leads to hepatomegaly and hypoglycemia during fasting, while the defective uptake causes post-prandial hyperglycemia. In the pancreas, it leads to impaired glucose sensing and insulin release [130, 131]. In the kidney, GLUT2 localizes to the basolateral membrane of the proximal tubule, easily explaining the excessive glucosuria, which has been reported to exceed 300 g per day [132] The RFS is less well understood, but may be due to impaired mitochondrial function [133]. Interestingly, *GLUT2*-deleted mice reproduce the hepatic and pancreatic phenotype and also have glucosuria, but RFS has not been reported [131]. The mouse model is therefore not helpful in understanding the mechanisms responsible for the RFS.

Mutations in *SLC2A2* associated with Fanconi-Bickel are typically severe, expected to completely abrogate GLUT2 function, although mutations with a milder phenotype with only mild glycosuria and LMWP have recently been described [134]. Interestingly, some heterozygous carriers of *SLC2A2* mutations can have isolated renal glucosuria and some milder recessive mutations, associated only with glucosuria and LMWP have also been described [134, 135].

Treatment consists of frequent feedings of slowly absorbed carbohydrates, as well as replacement of renal losses of water and solutes [136].

Fructose Intolerance

Fructose intolerance is due to a deficiency in the enzyme fructose-1-phosphate aldolase B, also simply called aldolase. Affected infants typically become symptomatic at weaning, with the introduction of fructose-containing food, such as fruits and vegetables. Patients develop nausea, vomiting and diarrhea and can progress to hypoglycemia, convulsions and shock. Proximal tubule dysfunction develops and is most obvious in the form of a renal tubular acidosis, which is compounded by accumulation of lactic acid in the blood. The mechanism of cellular dysfunction is thought to be intracellular phosphate depletion due to phosphorylation of accumulating fructose. Phosphate is required for the generation of the cellular fuel ATP [137]. Moreover, a direct association between aldolase and the vacuolar proton pump V-H$^+$-ATPase has been shown [138]. This pump is involved in bicarbonate reabsorption in the proximal tubule, as well as acid secretion in the distal tubule and an inhibition by defective aldolase may explain the pronounced acidosis seen in patients. Treatment consists of a fructose-free diet, which completely reverses the renal symptoms.

Galactosemia

A reversible and incomplete form of proximal tubular dysfunction can be seen in infants with classical galactosemia, an autosomal-recessive disorder due to loss-of-function of the enzyme galactose-1-phosphate uridyl transferase [139]. This is a key enzyme for the conversion of galactose to glucose. Affected infants typically present with failure-to-thrive and develop vomiting, diarrhea and jaundice after ingestion of galactose-containing feeds. Untreated, hepatomegaly with progression to cirrhosis, cataracts and mental retardation develop. Renal manifestation are aminoaciduria, albuminuria, acidosis and galactosuria, the latter due to the elevated blood galactose levels [140]. The mechanism of tubular dysfunction is unclear, but may be related to intracellular depletion of free phosphate, due to phosphorylation of the accumulating galactose.

The diagnosis is made by increased blood galactose levels and confirmed by demonstration of enzyme deficiency. Importantly, the RFS is completely reversible with treatment, which is the elimination of galactose from the diet.

ARC-Syndrome

The combination of arthrogryposis, renal dysfunction and cholestasis constitutes a rare autosomal recessive disorder, due to mutations in genes encoding vacuolar sorting protein involved in intracellular transport, including *VPS33B and VIPAR* [141, 142]. Affected neonates are identified by their contractures, conjugated hyperbilirubinemia and severe failure to thrive. In addition, giant platelets with a bleeding diathesis are observed. Renal manifestations include severe proximal tubular dysfunction, but nephrocalcinosis, nephrogenic diabetes insipidus and dysplasia have also been described [143]. No specific treatment exists and the prognosis is poor with patients typically dying in their first year of life [141, 143–146]. However, milder forms have been described [147].

Membranous Nephropathy with Anti-proximal Tubule Basement Membrane Antibodies

Several reports exist about an association between membranous nephropathy and RFS [30–38, 148]. In most cases, antibodies have been found directed against the basement membrane of the proximal tubule. In some cases, pulmonary symptoms associated with anti-alveolar basement membrane antibodies are also present [34]. Most likely the antibodies are directed against an antigen expressed in the glomerulus, as well, explaining the combination of glomerular and proximal tubular dysfunction. In two families the syndrome has been linked to a region on the X-chromosome, but no gene has yet been identified [36].

Dent Disease

Clinical Features

Dent disease is an X-linked recessive proximal tubulopathy, characterized by low-molecular weight proteinuria (LMWP) and hypercalciuria with nephrocalcinosis and nephrolithiasis, as well as progressive renal failure [149]. Patients may also have aminoaciduria, glucosuria and phosphaturia, consistent with generalized proximal tubular dysfunction. It was first described as hypercalciuric rickets by Dent and Friedman [150]. Clinical manifestations can vary enormously and once an underlying gene, *CLCN5*, was identified in 1996, it was realized that mutations in the same gene also caused related tubulopathies, previously thought to be distinct, namely X-linked recessive nephrolithiasis and Japanese idiopathic low-molecular-weight proteinuria [151–157]. Patients typically manifest with complications of hypercalciuria, such as hematuria, nephrocalcinosis or stones. Progression to ESKD is rare in childhood. Women very rarely can be affected, probably due to skewed X-chromosome inactivation [158]. The diagnosis is made by the presence of hypercalciuria and low-molecular weight proteinuria (see above: proteinuria) and typically a family history on the maternal side. Renal histology is non-specific, showing features of interstitial nephritis and calcium deposits and is thus not useful in establishing the diagnosis.

Genetics

The first gene identified to underlie Dent disease was *CLCN5*, encoding a proton-chloride antiporter expressed in the proximal tubule and especially on late endosomes and lysosomes [151]. Mutations in this gene are identified in approximately 60% of patients with a clinical diagnosis of Dent disease. A second gene, *OCRL*, encoding a phosphatidylinositol 4,5-bisphosphate 5-phosphatase (PIP_2-5-phosphatase), was identified later and mutations in this gene are found in approximately 15% of patients [159]. These patients are often referred to as having Dent2 disease, to distinguish them from CLCN5-based Dent disease. In the remaining approximately 25% of patients, no mutation in either gene is found, indicating that other genes may be responsible.

The identification of *OCRL* underlying Dent disease was surprising, as this gene also underlies Lowe syndrome, which besides renal proximal tubular dysfunction includes cataracts and developmental delay (see below). A genotype-phenotype effect has been hypothesized, as frameshift, splice site and nonsense mutations in *OCRL* causing Dent disease all cluster in exons 1–7, whereas those associated with Lowe syndrome mostly localize to the exons further downstream [160]. Use of potential alternate start codons in exons 7 and 8, which maintain the *OCRL* frame and, presumably, some functionality, could explain the milder phenotype in Dent disease. However, this hypothesis cannot explain, why some missense mutations in OCRL are associated with multiorgan disease (the Lowe phenotype) in some patients and predominant kidney involvement (the Dent phenotype) in others [160].

Pathophysiology

Whilst the identification of underlying genes has provided great insights, the pathogenesis of Dent disease is still incompletely understood. *CLCN5* clearly plays an important part in endocytosis in the proximal tubule. It is highly expressed in endosomes and lysosomes, where it co-localizes with endocytosed proteins [103]. *CLCN5* is likely to provide an electric shunt in the lysosome that neutralizes the electrical gradient otherwise created by the H^+-ATPase, to allow its efficient operation. However, *CLCN5* is not a voltage-gated chloride channel, as initially described, but in fact a Cl^-/H^+ antiporter, which thus would remove protons from the lysosomal lumen [161, 162]. However, the net effect of CLCN5 function still appears to favor lysosomal acidification, as loss of function of *CLCN5* has been shown to impair this process in mice and also in cultured human proximal tubular cells *in vitro* [103, 163]. Initially, the LMWP was thought to be a consequence of the impaired lysosomal function, but there is evidence for a role of CLCN5 beyond the lysosome. CLCN5 is also expressed at the apical surface of proximal tubule cells, where it is important in the assembly of the endocytic complex containing megalin and cubilin (see above) [104, 164–166]. Indeed, megalin and cubilin expression at the brush border is dramatically reduced in *CLCN5*-deleted mice, as is the excretion of megalin in the urine in Dent patients and the mouse model [104, 105]. Therefore, the proteinuria seen in this disease likely reflects impaired receptor-mediated endocytosis [163]. This is consistent also with the involvement of OCRL in endocytosis (see Lowe syndrome, below). Indeed, the renal phenotype of Lowe syndrome strongly resembles that of Dent disease [39] and proteomic analysis of the urine of patients with Dent disease shows a similar pattern as in Lowe syndrome, suggesting that *CLCN5* and *OCRL* may participate in similar endocytic pathways [167]. Potentially, in patients with Dent2 disease, other PIP_2-5-phosphatases can compensate for the loss of *OCRL* except with respect to endocytosis and hypercalciuria. Redundancy in PIP_2-5-phosphatases is suggested by the fact that *OCRL*-deleted mice do not show any clinical phenotype [168]. Interestingly, children with Dent2 disease frequently have some extra-renal manifestations in the form of elevated plasma levels of LDH and CK and poorer growth [169]. In addition, mild developmental delay is noted in some patients and it has been suggested that Dent2 disease is just a milder form of Lowe syndrome [170].

The hypercalciuria of Dent disease is poorly understood. One hypothesis is based on altered endocytosis of PTH and vitamin D-binding protein and a subsequently altered balance of calciotropic hormones [171]. Others propose a more direct role of CLCN5 in calcium handling by the kidney and bone [172, 173]. This discrepancy may in part be due to the fact that there are two different mouse strains with deleted *CLCN5* function, one of which has LMWP but no hypercalciuria [103].

Treatment

Treatment is mainly symptomatic and includes a large fluid intake to dilute urinary calcium and 1-α-OH vitamin D supplementation, to normalize PTH levels, so as to treat or prevent rickets. This needs to be monitored carefully, as excessive supplementation would worsen the hypercalciuria. Citrate supplementation has been helpful in a mouse model of the disease [174]. Thiazide diuretics have been shown to reduce calcium excretion at least in the short term and thus reduce the stone-forming risk in Dent disease [175] but are sometimes poorly tolerated. The reduction in urinary calcium excretion by thiazides in this disorder is surprising, as thiazides are thought to enhance calcium reabsorption in the proximal tubule, the segment affected in these patients [176].

Lowe Syndrome

Clinical Features

Lowe syndrome (oculo-cerebro-renal syndrome) was first described in 1952 as a clinical entity comprising "organic aciduria, decreased renal ammonia production, hydrophthalmus and mental retardation" [177]. Severity of symptoms varies, but in its complete form, patients are profoundly hypotonic with absent reflexes, have

severe mental impairment, congenital cataracts, glaucoma and RFS [178, 179]. There is often a delay in establishing the diagnosis and the renal manifestations can be minimal in early years but gross LMWP is characteristic [44]. Most patients first present to the ophthalmologist due to congenital cataracts [180–182]. Interestingly, individual patients with pathogenic variants in *OCRL* and brain and kidney involvement, but without cataracts, have been described recently, further blurring the distinction between Dent2 disease and Lowe syndrome [160, 183, 184].

Motor development is typically delayed and most patients do not achieve independent walking before 3 years of age. Mental impairment can be very variable, but in one study most patients had IQ measured around 50, yet with 25% in the normal range (>70). Seizures have been reported in about a third of patients [185]. Brain imaging, if performed, may show white matter changes, cerebral atrophy or periventricular cysts [186–188]. Behavioral abnormalities in the form of temper tantrums, negativism and obsessive behavior are another typical feature that can be extremely difficult for the families [189, 190].

The renal phenotype, as discussed above, is predominated by LMWP and hypercalciuria, but can involve more generalized proximal dysfunction, such as a metabolic acidosis and phosphate wasting [39]. Hypercalciuria is presumably due to impaired proximal reabsorption, but may be compounded by increased intestinal absorption, which OCRL may be involved in regulating [191]. Associated with the hypercalciuria is nephrocalcinosis/lithiasis with is seen in about two thirds of Lowe patients.

Renal histology is non-specific, showing some distortion of proximal tubular architecture and later also glomerular changes [192]. Most patients exhibit a slow progression of renal insufficiency with ESKD typically reported during the fourth and fifth decade of life [193, 194]. Using the Schwartz-Haycock formula with usual k-values substantially overestimates the GFR in children with Lowe syndrome from serum creatinine when compared to formal GFR measurements, probably due to the low muscle mass of these patients [39].

In addition to the manifestations in eyes, brain and kidneys, other clinical symptoms can occur. These include:

- platelet dysfunction with increased bleeding risk [195]
- a debilitating arthropathy [196]
- growth failure [178], which is independent of GFR [170]
- skeletal abnormalities, such as kyphosis, scoliosis, joint hypermobility and hip dislocation [197]. Some of these features may be secondary to the neurological features, such as the muscular hypotonia
- dental abnormalities, such as eruption and dental cysts [198]
- dermal cysts [199]

Genetics

The gene underlying Lowe syndrome was cloned in 1992 and named OCRL [200].

Mutations are identified in approximately 80–90% of cases suspected of Lowe syndrome and in one study roughly one third of these occurred de novo [160]. About two thirds of mutations in patients diagnosed with Lowe syndrome are nonsense, frameshift and splice site changes, the remainder missense plus a few gross deletions. The presence of lens opacities has been suggested to identify female mutation carriers, although the reported sensitivity is variable [44, 181, 201–204].

Pathophysiology

Since identification of the underlying gene, much progress has been made towards understanding the pathophysiology. The OCRL protein contains several functional domains, including PIP_2-5-phosphatase located in the Golgi apparatus. Impairment of this phosphatase function results in elevated cellular levels of PIP_2. PIP_2 levels affect vesicle trafficking at the Golgi [205] and may also account for alterations in the actin cytoskeleton seen in fibroblasts from patients with Lowe's syndrome [206], resulting in altered endosomal membrane trafficking [207] (Fig. 35.2). Besides, the phosphatase domain, the

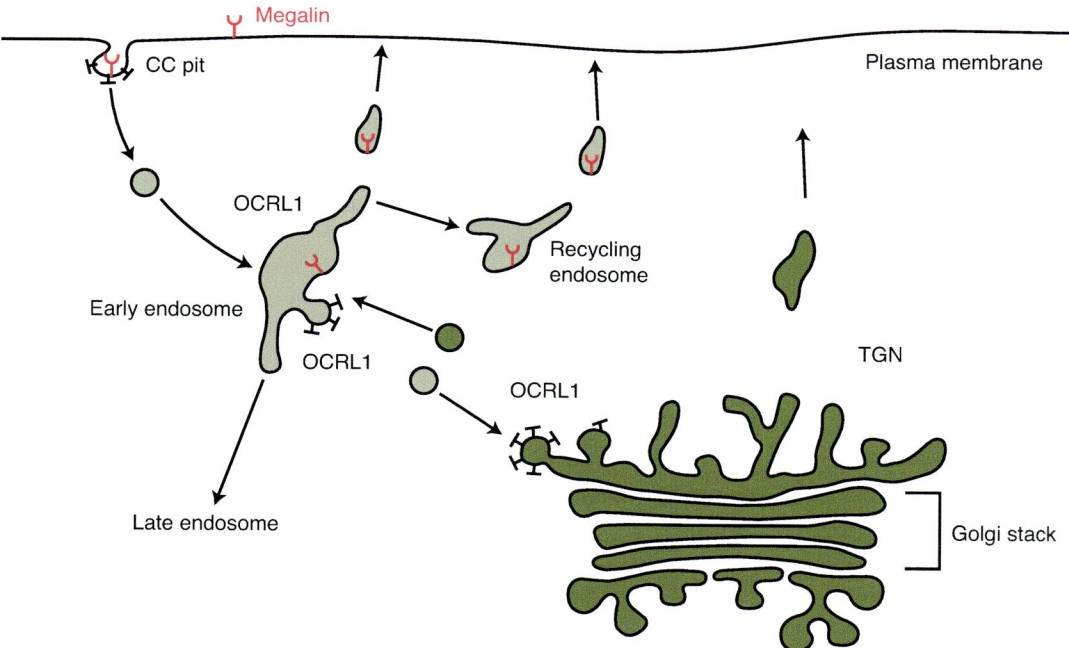

Fig. 35.2 Role of OCRL in regulation of traffic between apical membrane, endosomes and the trans-Golgi network. OCRL is present in clathrin-coated pits (CC) on the apical membrane of proximal tubular epithelial cells, early endosomes and the trans-Golgi network (TGN). (Adapted from [208])

OCRL protein also contains several other domains that are important for endosomal trafficking via protein-protein interactions, including an N-terminal PH (pleckstrin homology) domain, an ASH (ASPM-SPD2-Hydin) domain, and a C-terminal RhoGAP (Rho GTPase activating) domain [209]. Missense mutations within the RhoGAP domain were identified in some patients with Lowe syndrome, highlighting its importance for OCRL function [210].

Beyond the role in endocytosis, intracellular trafficking and regulation of the actin skeleton, OCRL has also been implicated in a wide range of cellular processes, including cell migration, cell polarity, cell-cell interaction, cytokinesis, mitochondrial function and cilia formation. Indeed, it has been suggested that Lowe syndrome could be considered a mitochondrial cytopathy [211] or, more recently, a ciliopathy [212]. It remains to be determined, to what degree these multiple mechanisms are clinically relevant and contribute to the variable phenotype associated with OCRL mutations.

Treatment

There is no specific treatment of Lowe syndrome and thus, management is symptomatic. Supplementation of electrolytes, alkali and vitamin D is based on biochemistries, and vitamin D is usually needed in 1-α- hydroxylated forms. Oversupplementation could worsen the hypercalciuria, so monitoring parathyroid hormone (PTH) and calcium levels is advised. Nutritional support with tube feeding may be helpful in the more severely affected patients.

The bleeding diathesis from the platelet dysfunction may be ameliorated with tranexamic acid and this should be considered prior to elective surgeries.

Cataract surgery is usually performed in the first year of life, but vision is nevertheless typically impaired and rarely better than 20/70 [213]. Anti-epileptic drugs can help in those patients suffering from recurrent seizures [187].

Acquired RFS

Many exogenous causes of RFS have been reported and are listed in Table 35.2. The mechanism of tubular damage is often unclear, although mitochondrial dysfunction has been implicated in some forms (see below).

Treatment, aside from supportive measures, is always the removal of the offending agent, which typically reverses the symptoms. Except for those compounds, where blood levels can be measured (such as lead or aminoglycosides), no specific diagnostic tests exist. Thus, the diagnosis is typically made through suspicion of an exogenous cause and its subsequent removal.

Chemotherapeutic Agents

Ifosfamide is the chemotherapeutic agent most commonly associated with RFS, which is seen in up to 10% of patients. Risk factors include total dose, reduced renal mass, young age or the combination with other nephrotoxic agents, such as cisplatin [214–218]. Symptoms typically reverse within weeks after cessation of the drug, but in some cases persist for several years and chronic impaired kidney function is possible [219, 220]. A mechanism has been proposed implicating specific ifosfamide uptake and metabolization in the proximal tubular cells [84].

Antibiotics and Antiretrovirals

Aminoglycosides are well known for their nephrotoxic side effects. In a small percentage of patients, they can also induce RFS. In fact, aminoaciduria has been proposed as a highly sensitive marker for aminoglycoside-induced renal injury, at least in the rat model [221]. The mechanism of damage is thought to be mitochondrial dysfunction: aminoglycosides target bacterial ribosomes where they induce faulty protein synthesis and since mitochondrial ribosomes bear structural resemblances to those of bacteria, they are vulnerable to the toxicity [222]. The risk appears to be related to the dosage and length of treatment and symptoms typically reverse after cessation of the drug (reviewed in [223]).

With the advent of retroviral treatment, tenofovir has become an increasingly common cause of RFS, although rarely seen in children as risk factors for tenofovir toxicity include older age, pre-existing kidney disease and low body mass [11, 224]. The exact mechanism is unclear, but histology, if obtained, typically shows dysmorphic mitochondria [224].

Treatment

Specific therapy of RFSs depends on the underlying cause. The renal features of galactosemia and hereditary fructose intolerance are reversed by appropriate dietary therapy. Removal of the causative toxin or drug usually ameliorates the tubulopathy although some drugs (e.g. ifosfamide) can cause long-term dysfunction. Nitisinone (NTBC (2-(2-nitro-4-trifluoromethylbenzoyl)-1,3-cyclohexanedione)), reverses the RFS in tyrosinemia (see above). Otherwise, treatment of RFS is mainly supportive. In severe cases, rehydration initially with 0.9% saline and careful electrolyte correction is necessary and can be hazardous if not monitored and managed by experts. Historically, fatalities occurred during rehydration with glucose-containing solutions, which exacerbated the profound hypokalemia. Rapid correction of acidosis can precipitate hypocalcemic seizures, exacerbated by the "hungry bone" phenomenon [225]. Once stabilized, large amounts of alkali (3–20 mmol/kg/day) are often needed to maintain acid-base homeostasis. As so often in tubular disorders, the more supplementation is given, the higher the filtered load and consequently, the more is lost in the urine. Smaller, but frequent dosing can help to maintain more consistent plasma levels and to reduce urinary losses from brief spikes in filtered load, associated with intermittent large doses, as well as side effects, such as diarrhoea. Alkali supplementation is typically prescribed in the form of

sodium or potassium bicarbonate or citrate, or as a compound preparation. Supplements of sodium chloride may also be needed. For some children, provision of all the above supplements fails to correct the biochemical disturbances and growth failure persists. Indomethacin or an alternative non-steroidal anti-inflammatory agent may be helpful in such cases [226]. Carnitine supplements have been used to correct the plasma and muscle carnitine deficiencies that can occur due to renal losses. Hypophosphataemic rickets is treated with phosphate supplementation and 1-α-calcidol or calcitriol.

References

1. Fanconi G. Die nicht diabetischen Glykosurien und Hyperglykaemien des aelteren Kindes. Jahrbuch fuer Kinderheilkunde. 1931;133:257–300.
2. Lucas RC. On a form of late rickets associated with albuminuria, rickets of adolescence. Lancet. 1883;121(3119):993–4.
3. de Toni G. Remarks on the relationship between renal rickets (renal Dwarfism) and renal diabetes. Acta Paediatr. 1933;16:479–84.
4. Debre R, Marie J, Cleret F, Messimy R. Rachitisme tardif coexistant avec une Nephrite chronique et une Glycosurie. Archive de Medicine des Enfants. 1934;37:597–606.
5. G F. Der nephrotisch-glykosurische Zwergwuchs mit hypophosphataemischer Rachitis. Deutsche medizinische Wochenschrift. 1936;62:1169–71.
6. van't Hoff W. Renal tubular disorders. In: Postlethwaite RJ, editor. Clinical paediatric nephrology. 3rd ed. p. 103–12.
7. Kintzel PE. Anticancer drug-induced kidney disorders. Drug Saf. 2001;24(1):19–38.
8. Sadoff L. Nephrotoxicity of streptozotocin (NSC-85998). Cancer Chemother Rep. 1970;54(6):457–9.
9. Montoliu J, Carrera M, Darnell A, Revert L. Lactic acidosis and Fanconi's syndrome due to degraded tetracycline. Br Med J (Clin Res Ed). 1981;283(6306):1576–7.
10. Cleveland WW, Adams WC, Mann JB, Nyhan WL. Acquired fanconi syndrome following degraded tetracycline. J Pediatrics. 1965;66:333–42.
11. Hall AM. Update on tenofovir toxicity in the kidney. Pediatr Nephrol. 2013;28(7):1011–23.
12. Izzedine H, Hulot JS, Villard E, Goyenvalle C, Dominguez S, Ghosn J, et al. Association between ABCC2 gene haplotypes and tenofovir-induced proximal tubulopathy. J Infect Dis. 2006;194(11):1481–91.

13. Earle KE, Seneviratne T, Shaker J, Shoback D. Fanconi's syndrome in HIV+ adults: report of three cases and literature review. J Bone Miner Res. 2004;19(5):714–21.

14. Verhelst D, Monge M, Meynard JL, Fouqueray B, Mougenot B, Girard PM, et al. Fanconi syndrome and renal failure induced by tenofovir: a first case report. Am J Kidney Dis. 2002;40(6):1331–3.

15. Vittecoq D, Dumitrescu L, Beaufils H, Deray G. Fanconi syndrome associated with cidofovir therapy. Antimicrob Agents Chemother. 1997;41(8):1846.

16. Izzedine H, Launay-Vacher V, Deray G. Fanconi syndrome associated with didanosine therapy. AIDS. 2005;19(8):844–5.

17. Crowther MA, Callaghan W, Hodsman AB, Mackie ID. Dideoxyinosine-associated nephrotoxicity. AIDS. 1993;7(1):131–2.

18. Chisolm JJ Jr, Harrison HC, Eberlein WR, Harrison HE. Amino-aciduria, hypophosphatemia, and rickets in lead poisoning; study of a case. AMA Am J Dis Child. 1955;89(2):159–68.

19. Kazantzis G, Flynn FV, Spowage JS, Trott DG. Renal tubular malfunction and pulmonary emphysema in cadmium pigment workers. Q J Med. 1963;32:165–92.

20. Lande MB, Kim MS, Bartlett C, Guay-Woodford LM. Reversible Fanconi syndrome associated with valproate therapy. J Pediatrics. 1993;123(2):320–2.

21. Hong YT, Fu LS, Chung LH, Hung SC, Huang YT, Chi CS. Fanconi's syndrome, interstitial fibrosis and renal failure by aristolochic acid in Chinese herbs. Pediatr Nephrol. 2006;21(4):577–9.

22. Lee S, Lee T, Lee B, Choi H, Yang M, Ihm CG, et al. Fanconi's syndrome and subsequent progressive renal failure caused by a Chinese herb containing aristolochic acid. Nephrology. 2004;9(3):126–9.

23. Yang SS, Chu P, Lin YF, Chen A, Lin SH. Aristolochic acid-induced Fanconi's syndrome and nephropathy presenting as hypokalemic paralysis. Am J Kidney Dis. 2002;39(3):E14.

24. Moss AH, Gabow PA, Kaehny WD, Goodman SI, Haut LL. Fanconi's syndrome and distal renal tubular acidosis after glue sniffing. Ann Intern Med. 1980;92(1):69–70.

25. Raschka C, Koch HJ. Longterm treatment of psoriasis using fumaric acid preparations can be associated with severe proximal tubular damage. Hum Exp Toxicol. 1999;18(12):738–9.

26. Rago RP, Miles JM, Sufit RL, Spriggs DR, Wilding G. Suramin-induced weakness from hypophosphatemia and mitochondrial myopathy. Association of suramin with mitochondrial toxicity in humans. Cancer. 1994;73(7):1954–9.

27. Gil HW, Yang JO, Lee EY, Hong SY. Paraquat-induced Fanconi syndrome. Nephrology (Carlton). 2005;10(5):430–2.

28. Lo JC, Chertow GM, Rennke H, Seifter JL. Fanconi's syndrome and tubulointerstitial nephritis in association with L-lysine ingestion. Am J Kidney Dis. 1996;28(4):614–7.

29. Igarashi T, Kawato H, Kamoshita S, Nosaka K, Seiya K, Hayakawa H. Acute tubulointerstitial nephritis with uveitis syndrome presenting as multiple tubular dysfunction including Fanconi's syndrome. Pediatr Nephrol. 1992;6(6):547–9.

30. Shenoy M, Krishnan R, Moghal N. Childhood membranous nephropathy in association with interstitial nephritis and Fanconi syndrome. Pediatr Nephrol. 2006;21(3):441.

31. Dumas R, Dumas ML, Baldet P, Bascoul S. [Membranous glomerulonephritis in two brothers associated in one with tubulo-interstitial disease, Fanconi syndrome and anti-TBM antibodies (author's transl)]. Arch Fr Pediatr. 1982;39(2):75–78.

32. Griswold WR, Krous HF, Reznik V, Lemire J, Wilson NW, Bastian J, et al. The syndrome of autoimmune interstitial nephritis and membranous nephropathy. Pediatr Nephrol. 1997;11(6):699–702.

33. Katz A, Fish AJ, Santamaria P, Nevins TE, Kim Y, Butkowski RJ. Role of antibodies to tubulointerstitial nephritis antigen in human anti-tubular basement membrane nephritis associated with membranous nephropathy. Am J Med. 1992;93(6):691–8.

34. Levy M, Gagnadoux MF, Beziau A, Habib R. Membranous glomerulonephritis associated with anti-tubular and anti-alveolar basement membrane antibodies. Clin Nephrol. 1978;10(4):158–65.

35. Makker SP, Widstrom R, Huang J. Membranous nephropathy, interstitial nephritis, and Fanconi syndrome—glomerular antigen. Pediatr Nephrol. 1996;10(1):7–13.

36. Tay AH, Ren EC, Murugasu B, Sim SK, Tan PH, Cohen AH, et al. Membranous nephropathy with anti-tubular basement membrane antibody may be X-linked. Pediatr Nephrol. 2000;14(8–9):747–53.

37. Wood EG, Brouhard BH, Travis LB, Cavallo T, Lynch RE. Membranous glomerulonephropathy with tubular dysfunction and linear tubular basement membrane IgG deposition. J Pediatr. 1982;101(3):414–7.

38. Yagame M, Tomino Y, Miura M, Suga T, Nomoto Y, Sakai H. An adult case of Fanconi's syndrome associated with membranous nephropathy. Tokai J Exp Clin Med. 1986;11(2):101–6.

39. Bockenhauer D, Bokenkamp A, van't Hoff W, Levtchenko E, Kist-van Holthe JE, Tasic V, et al. Renal phenotype in Lowe syndrome: a selective proximal tubular dysfunction. Clin J Am Soc Nephrol. 2008;3(5):1430–6.

40. Kleta R. Fanconi or not Fanconi? Lowe syndrome revisited. Clin J Am Soc Nephrol. 2008;3(5):1244–5.

41. Bockenhauer D, van't Hoff W, Dattani M, Lehnhardt A, Subtirelu M, Hildebrandt F, et al. Secondary nephrogenic diabetes insipidus as a complica-

tion of inherited renal diseases. Nephron Physiol. 2010;116(4):23–9.

42. Bockenhauer D, Bichet DG. Inherited secondary nephrogenic diabetes insipidus: concentrating on humans. Am J Physiol Renal Physiol. 2013;304(8):F1037–42.

43. Nykjaer A, Dragun D, Walther D, Vorum H, Jacobsen C, Herz J, et al. An endocytic pathway essential for renal uptake and activation of the steroid 25-(OH) vitamin D3. Cell. 1999;96(4):507–15.

44. Laube GF, Russell-Eggitt IM, van't Hoff WG. Early proximal tubular dysfunction in Lowe's syndrome. Arch Dis Child. 2004;89(5):479–80.

45. Norden AG, Scheinman SJ, Deschodt-Lanckman MM, Lapsley M, Nortier JL, Thakker RV, et al. Tubular proteinuria defined by a study of Dent's (CLCN5 mutation) and other tubular diseases. Kidney Int. 2000;57(1):240–9.

46. Norden AG, Lapsley M, Lee PJ, Pusey CD, Scheinman SJ, Tam FW, et al. Glomerular protein sieving and implications for renal failure in Fanconi syndrome. Kidney Int. 2001;60(5):1885–92.

47. Tolaymat A, Sakarcan A, Neiberger R. Idiopathic Fanconi syndrome in a family. Part I. Clinical aspects. J Am Soc Nephrol. 1992;2(8):1310–7.

48. Birn H, Christensen EI. Renal albumin absorption in physiology and pathology. Kidney Int. 2006;69(3):440–9.

49. Mogensen CE, Solling. Studies on renal tubular protein reabsorption: partial and near complete inhibition by certain amino acids. Scand J Clin Lab Invest. 1977;37(6):477–86.

50. Dickson LE, Wagner MC, Sandoval RM, Molitoris BA. The proximal tubule and albuminuria: really! J Am Soc Nephrol. 2014;25(3):443–53.

51. Ovunc B, Otto EA, Vega-Warner V, Saisawat P, Ashraf S, Ramaswami G, et al. Exome sequencing reveals cubilin mutation as a single-gene cause of proteinuria. J Am Soc Nephrol. 2011;22(10):1815–20.

52. Cramer MT, Charlton JR, Fogo AB, Fathallah-Shaykh SA, Askenazi DJ, Guay-Woodford LM. Expanding the phenotype of proteinuria in Dent disease. A case series. Pediatr Nephrol. 2014;29(10):2051–4.

53. van Berkel Y, Ludwig M, van Wijk JA, Bokenkamp A. Proteinuria in Dent disease: a review of the literature. Pediatr Nephrol. 2017;32(10):1851–9.

54. Preston R, Naylor RW, Stewart G, Bierzynska A, Saleem MA, Lowe M, et al. A role for OCRL in glomerular function and disease. Pediatr Nephrol. 2020;35(4):641–8.

55. Bazzi C, Petrini C, Rizza V, Arrigo G, D'Amico G. A modern approach to selectivity of proteinuria and tubulointerstitial damage in nephrotic syndrome. Kidney Int. 2000;58(4):1732–41.

56. Valles P, Peralta M, Carrizo L, Martin L, Principi I, Gonzalez A, et al. Follow-up of steroid-resistant nephrotic syndrome: tubular proteinuria and enzymuria. Pediatr Nephrol. 2000;15(3-4):252–8.

57. Cogan MG. Disorders of proximal nephron function. Am J Med. 1982;72(2):275–88.

58. Unwin RJ, Capasso G, Shirley DG. An overview of divalent cation and citrate handling by the kidney. Nephron Physiol. 2004;98(2):15–20.

59. Roch-Ramel F. Renal transport of organic anions. Curr Opin Nephrol Hypertens. 1998;7(5):517–24.

60. Niaudet P, Rotig A. Renal involvement in mitochondrial cytopathies. Pediatr Nephrol. 1996;10(3):368–73.

61. Elsas LJ, Rosenberg LE. Familial renal glycosuria: a genetic reappraisal of hexose transport by kidney and intestine. J Clin Invest. 1969;48(10):1845–54.

62. Santer R, Calado J. Familial renal glucosuria and SGLT2: from a mendelian trait to a therapeutic target. Clin J Am Soc Nephrol. 2010;5(1):133–41.

63. Walton RJ, Bijvoet OL. Nomogram for derivation of renal threshold phosphate concentration. Lancet. 1975;2(7929):309–10.

64. Kruse K, Kracht U, Gopfert G. Renal threshold phosphate concentration (TmPO4/GFR). Arch Dis Child. 1982;57(3):217–23.

65. Bistarakis L, Voskaki I, Lambadaridis J, Sereti H, Sbyrakis S. Renal handling of phosphate in the first six months of life. Arch Dis Child. 1986;61(7):677–81.

66. Shaw NJ, Wheeldon J, Brocklebank JT. Indices of intact serum parathyroid hormone and renal excretion of calcium, phosphate, and magnesium. Arch Dis Child. 1990;65(11):1208–11.

67. Pajor AM. Citrate transport by the kidney and intestine. Semin Nephrol. 1999;19(2):195–200.

68. Houston IB, Boichis H, Edelmann CM Jr. Fanconi syndrome with renal sodium wasting and metabolic alkalosis. Am J Med. 1968;44(4):638–46.

69. Lemire J, Kaplan BS. The various renal manifestations of the nephropathic form of cystinosis. Am J Nephrol. 1984;4(2):81–5.

70. Yildiz B, Durmus-Aydogdu S, Kural N, Bildirici K, Basmak H, Yarar C. A patient with cystinosis presenting transient features of Bartter syndrome. Turk J Pediatr. 2006;48(3):260–2.

71. Gahl WA, Bernardini IM, Dalakas MC, Markello TC, Krasnewich DM, Charnas LR. Muscle carnitine repletion by long-term carnitine supplementation in nephropathic cystinosis. Pediatr Res. 1993;34(2):115–9.

72. Nissenkorn A, Korman SH, Vardi O, Levine A, Katzir Z, Ballin A, et al. Carnitine-deficient myopathy as a presentation of tyrosinemia type I. J Child Neurol. 2001;16(9):642–4.

73. Moestrup SK, Verroust PJ. Megalin- and cubilin-mediated endocytosis of protein-bound vitamins, lipids, and hormones in polarized epithelia. Annu Rev Nutr. 2001;21:407–28.

74. Klootwijk ED, Reichold M, Helip-Wooley A, Tolaymat A, Broeker C, Robinette SL, et al. Mistargeting of peroxisomal EHHADH and inherited renal Fanconi's syndrome. N Engl J Med. 2014;370(2):129–38.

75. Reichold M, Klootwijk ED, Reinders J, Otto EA, Milani M, Broeker C, et al. Glycine amidinotrans-

ferase (GATM), renal Fanconi syndrome, and kidney failure. J Am Soc Nephrol. 2018;29(7): 1849–58.

76. Marchesin V, Perez-Marti A, Le Meur G, Pichler R, Grand K, Klootwijk ED, et al. Molecular basis for autosomal-dominant renal Fanconi syndrome caused by HNF4A. Cell Rep. 2019;29(13):4407–21.e5.

77. Spencer PD, Medow MS, Moses LC, Roth KS. Effects of succinylacetone on the uptake of sugars and amino acids by brush border vesicles. Kidney Int. 1988;34(5):671–7.

78. Wyss PA, Boynton SB, Chu J, Spencer RF, Roth KS. Physiological basis for an animal model of the renal Fanconi syndrome: use of succinylacetone in the rat. Clin Sci. 1992;83(1):81–7.

79. Roth KS, Carter BE, Higgins ES. Succinylacetone effects on renal tubular phosphate metabolism: a model for experimental renal Fanconi syndrome. Proc Soc Exp Biol Med. 1991;196(4):428–31.

80. Eiam-ong S, Spohn M, Kurtzman NA, Sabatini S. Insights into the biochemical mechanism of maleic acid-induced Fanconi syndrome. Kidney Int. 1995;48(5):1542–8.

81. Rossi R, Kleta R, Ehrich JH. Renal involvement in children with malignancies. Pediatr Nephrol. 1999;13(2):153–62.

82. Sener G, Sehirli O, Yegen BC, Cetinel S, Gedik N, Sakarcan A. Melatonin attenuates ifosfamide-induced Fanconi syndrome in rats. J Pineal Res. 2004;37(1):17–25.

83. Schwerdt G, Freudinger R, Mildenberger S, Silbernagl S, Gekle M. The nephrotoxin ochratoxin A induces apoptosis in cultured human proximal tubule cells. Cell Biol Toxicol. 1999;15(6):405–15.

84. Ciarimboli G, Holle SK, Vollenbrocker B, Hagos Y, Reuter S, Burckhardt G, et al. New clues for nephrotoxicity induced by ifosfamide: preferential renal uptake via the human organic cation transporter 2. Mol Pharm. 2011;8(1):270–9.

85. Haviv YS, Wald H, Levi M, Dranitzki-Elhalel M, Popovtzer MM. Late-onset downregulation of NaPi-2 in experimental Fanconi syndrome. Pediatr Nephrol. 2001;16(5):412–6.

86. Pontoglio M, Barra J, Hadchouel M, Doyen A, Kress C, Bach JP, et al. Hepatocyte nuclear factor 1 inactivation results in hepatic dysfunction, phenylketonuria, and renal Fanconi syndrome. Cell. 1996;84(4):575–85.

87. Cheret C, Doyen A, Yaniv M, Pontoglio M. Hepatocyte nuclear factor 1 alpha controls renal expression of the Npt1-Npt4 anionic transporter locus. J Mol Biol. 2002;322(5):929–41.

88. Magen D, Berger L, Coady MJ, Ilivitzki A, Militianu D, Tieder M, et al. A loss-of-function mutation in NaPi-IIa and renal Fanconi's syndrome. N Engl J Med. 2010;362(12):1102–9.

89. Graversen JH, Castro G, Kandoussi A, Nielsen H, Christensen EI, Norden A, et al. A pivotal role of the human kidney in catabolism of HDL protein components apolipoprotein A-I and A-IV but not of A-II. Lipids. 2008;43(5):467–70.

90. Verroust PJ, Birn H, Nielsen R, Kozyraki R, Christensen EI. The tandem endocytic receptors megalin and cubilin are important proteins in renal pathology. Kidney Int. 2002;62(3):745–56.

91. Christensen EI, Gburek J. Protein reabsorption in renal proximal tubule-function and dysfunction in kidney pathophysiology. Pediatr Nephrol. 2004;19(7):714–21.

92. Christensen EI, Birn H. Megalin and cubilin: multifunctional endocytic receptors. Nat Rev Mol Cell Biol. 2002;3(4):256–66.

93. Hilpert J, Nykjaer A, Jacobsen C, Wallukat G, Nielsen R, Moestrup SK, et al. Megalin antagonizes activation of the parathyroid hormone receptor. J Biol Chem. 1999;274(9):5620–5.

94. Nykjaer A, Fyfe JC, Kozyraki R, Leheste JR, Jacobsen C, Nielsen MS, et al. Cubilin dysfunction causes abnormal metabolism of the steroid hormone 25(OH) vitamin D(3). Proc Natl Acad Sci U S A. 2001;98(24):13895–900.

95. Raychowdhury R, Niles JL, McCluskey RT, Smith JA. Autoimmune target in Heymann nephritis is a glycoprotein with homology to the LDL receptor. Science. 1989;244(4909):1163–5.

96. Leheste JR, Rolinski B, Vorum H, Hilpert J, Nykjaer A, Jacobsen C, et al. Megalin knockout mice as an animal model of low molecular weight proteinuria. Am J Pathol. 1999;155(4):1361–70.

97. Kantarci S, Al-Gazali L, Hill RS, Donnai D, Black GC, Bieth E, et al. Mutations in LRP2, which encodes the multiligand receptor megalin, cause Donnai-Barrow and facio-oculo-acoustico-renal syndromes. Nat Genet. 2007;39(8):957–9.

98. Storm T, Tranebjaerg L, Frykholm C, Birn H, Verroust PJ, Neveus T, et al. Renal phenotypic investigations of megalin-deficient patients: novel insights into tubular proteinuria and albumin filtration. Nephrol Dial Transplant. 2013;28(3): 585–91.

99. Moestrup SK, Kozyraki R, Kristiansen M, Kaysen JH, Rasmussen HH, Brault D, et al. The intrinsic factor-vitamin B12 receptor and target of teratogenic antibodies is a megalin-binding peripheral membrane protein with homology to developmental proteins. J Biol Chem. 1998;273(9):5235–42.

100. Imerslund O. Idiopathic chronic megaloblastic anemia in children. Acta Paediatr Suppl. 1960;49(Suppl 119):1–115.

101. Grasbeck R, Gordin R, Kantero I, Kuhlback B. Selective vitamin B12 malabsorption and proteinuria in young people. A syndrome. Acta Med Scand. 1960;167:289–96.

102. Wahlstedt-Froberg V, Pettersson T, Aminoff M, Dugue B, Grasbeck R. Proteinuria in cubilin-deficient patients with selective vitamin B12 malabsorption. Pediatr Nephrol. 2003;18(5):417–21.

103. Piwon N, Gunther W, Schwake M, Bosl MR, Jentsch TJ. ClC-5 Cl− -channel disruption impairs endocy-

tosis in a mouse model for Dent's disease. Nature. 2000;408(6810):369–73.

104. Christensen EI, Devuyst O, Dom G, Nielsen R, Van der Smissen P, Verroust P, et al. Loss of chloride channel ClC-5 impairs endocytosis by defective trafficking of megalin and cubilin in kidney proximal tubules. Proc Natl Acad Sci U S A. 2003;100(14):8472–7.

105. Norden AG, Lapsley M, Igarashi T, Kelleher CL, Lee PJ, Matsuyama T, et al. Urinary megalin deficiency implicates abnormal tubular endocytic function in Fanconi syndrome. J Am Soc Nephrol. 2002;13(1):125–33.

106. Haffner D, Weinfurth A, Seidel C, Manz F, Schmidt H, Waldherr R, et al. Body growth in primary de Toni-Debre-Fanconi syndrome. Pediatr Nephrol. 1997;11(1):40–5.

107. Friedman AL, Trygstad CW, Chesney RW. Autosomal dominant Fanconi syndrome with early renal failure. Am J Med Genet. 1978;2(3):225–32.

108. Neimann N, Pierson M, Marchal C, Rauber G, Grignon G. [Familial glomerulo-tubular nephropathy with the de Toni-Debre-Fanconi syndrome]. Archives francaises de pediatrie. 1968;25(1):43–69.

109. Tieder M, Arie R, Modai D, Samuel R, Weissgarten J, Liberman UA. Elevated serum 1,25-dihydroxyvitamin D concentrations in siblings with primary Fanconi's syndrome. N Engl J Med. 1988;319(13):845–9.

110. Patrick A, Cameron JS, Ogg CS. A family with a dominant form of idiopathic Fanconi syndrome leading to renal failure in adult life. Clin Nephrol. 1981;16(6):289–92.

111. Wen SF, Friedman AL, Oberley TD. Two case studies from a family with primary Fanconi syndrome. Am J Kidney Dis. 1989;13(3):240–6.

112. Assmann N, Dettmer K, Simbuerger JM, Broeker C, Nuernberger N, Renner K, et al. Renal Fanconi syndrome is caused by a mistargeting-based mitochondriopathy. Cell Rep. 2016;15(7):1423–9.

113. Schmidt U, Dubach UC, Guder WG, Funk B, Paris K. Metabolic patterns in various structures of the rat nephron. The distribution of enzymes of carbohydrate metabolism. Curr Prob Clin Biochem. 1975;4:22–32.

114. Balaban RS, Mandel LJ. Metabolic substrate utilization by rabbit proximal tubule. An NADH fluorescence study. Am J Physiol. 1988;254(3 Pt 2):F407–16.

115. Hamilton AJ, Bingham C, McDonald TJ, Cook PR, Caswell RC, Weedon MN, et al. The HNF4A R76W mutation causes atypical dominant Fanconi syndrome in addition to a beta cell phenotype. J Med Genet. 2014;51(3):165–9.

116. Improda N, Shah P, Guemes M, Gilbert C, Morgan K, Sebire N, et al. Hepatocyte nuclear factor-4 alfa mutation associated with hyperinsulinaemic hypoglycaemia and atypical renal fanconi syndrome: expanding the clinical phenotype. Horm Res Paediatr. 2016;86(5):337–41.

117. Schlingmann KP, Ruminska J, Kaufmann M, Dursun I, Patti M, Kranz B, et al. Autosomal-recessive mutations in SLC34A1 encoding sodium-phosphate cotransporter 2A cause idiopathic infantile hypercalcemia. J Am Soc Nephrol. 2016;27(2):604–14.

118. Demir K, Yildiz M, Bahat H, Goldman M, Hassan N, Tzur S, et al. Clinical heterogeneity and phenotypic expansion of NaPi-IIa-associated disease. J Clin Endocrinol Metab. 2017;102(12):4604–14.

119. Sassa S, Kappas A. Hereditary tyrosinemia and the heme biosynthetic pathway. Profound inhibition of delta-aminolevulinic acid dehydratase activity by succinylacetone. J Clin Invest. 1983;71(3):625–34.

120. Endo F, Sun MS. Tyrosinaemia type I and apoptosis of hepatocytes and renal tubular cells. J Inherit Metab Dis. 2002;25(3):227–34.

121. Holme E, Lindstedt S. Tyrosinaemia type I and NTBC (2-(2-nitro-4-trifluoromethylbenzoyl)-1,3-cyclohexanedione). J Inherit Metab Dis. 1998;21(5):507–17.

122. McKiernan PJ. Nitisinone in the treatment of hereditary tyrosinaemia type 1. Drugs. 2006;66(6):743–50.

123. Tuchman M, Freese DK, Sharp HL, Ramnaraine ML, Ascher N, Bloomer JR. Contribution of extrahepatic tissues to biochemical abnormalities in hereditary tyrosinemia type I: study of three patients after liver transplantation. J Pediatr. 1987;110(3):399–403.

124. Pierik LJ, van Spronsen FJ, Bijleveld CM, van Dael CM. Renal function in tyrosinaemia type I after liver transplantation: a long-term follow-up. J Inherit Metab Dis. 2005;28(6):871–6.

125. Govers LP, Toka HR, Hariri A, Walsh SB, Bockenhauer D. Mitochondrial DNA mutations in renal disease: an overview. Pediatr Nephrol. 2021;36(1):9–17.

126. Thorner PS, Balfe JW, Becker LE, Baumal R. Abnormal mitochondria on a renal biopsy from a case of mitochondrial myopathy. Pediatr Pathol. 1985;4(1–2):25–35.

127. Hall AM, Unwin RJ. The not so 'mighty chondrion': emergence of renal diseases due to mitochondrial dysfunction. Nephron Physiol. 2007;105(1):1–10.

128. Montini G, Malaventura C, Salviati L. Early coenzyme Q10 supplementation in primary coenzyme Q10 deficiency. N Engl J Med. 2008;358(26):2849–50.

129. Peduto A, Spada M, Alluto A, La Dolcetta M, Ponzone A, Santer R. A novel mutation in the GLUT2 gene in a patient with Fanconi-Bickel syndrome detected by neonatal screening for galactosaemia. J Inherit Metab Dis. 2004;27(2):279–80.

130. Santer R, Schneppenheim R, Suter D, Schaub J, Steinmann B. Fanconi-Bickel syndrome—the original patient and his natural history, historical steps leading to the primary defect, and a review of the literature. Eur J Pediatr. 1998;157(10):783–97.

131. Guillam MT, Hummler E, Schaerer E, Yeh JI, Birnbaum MJ, Beermann F, et al. Early diabetes and abnormal postnatal pancreatic islet development in mice lacking Glut-2. Nat Genet. 1997;17(3):327–30.

132. Brivet M, Moatti N, Corriat A, Lemonnier A, Odievre M. Defective galactose oxidation in a patient with glycogen storage disease and Fanconi syndrome. Pediatr Res. 1983;17(2):157–61.

133. Odievre MH, Lombes A, Dessemme P, Santer R, Brivet M, Chevallier B, et al. A secondary respiratory chain defect in a patient with Fanconi-Bickel syndrome. J Inherit Metab Dis. 2002;25(5):379–84.

134. Grunert SC, Schwab KO, Pohl M, Sass JO, Santer R. Fanconi-Bickel syndrome: GLUT2 mutations associated with a mild phenotype. Mol Genet Metab. 2012;105(3):433–7.

135. Sakamoto O, Ogawa E, Ohura T, Igarashi Y, Matsubara Y, Narisawa K, et al. Mutation analysis of the GLUT2 gene in patients with Fanconi-Bickel syndrome. Pediatr Res. 2000;48(5):586–9.

136. Lee PJ, Van't Hoff WG, Leonard JV. Catch-up growth in Fanconi-Bickel syndrome with uncooked cornstarch. J Inherit Metab Dis. 1995;18(2):153–6.

137. Morris RC Jr, Nigon K, Reed EB. Evidence that the severity of depletion of inorganic phosphate determines the severity of the disturbance of adenine nucleotide metabolism in the liver and renal cortex of the fructose-loaded rat. J Clin Invest. 1978;61(1):209–20.

138. Lu M, Holliday LS, Zhang L, Dunn WA Jr, Gluck SL. Interaction between aldolase and vacuolar H+-ATPase: evidence for direct coupling of glycolysis to the ATP-hydrolyzing proton pump. J Biol Chem. 2001;276(32):30407–13.

139. Reichardt JK, Woo SL. Molecular basis of galactosemia: mutations and polymorphisms in the gene encoding human galactose-1-phosphate uridylyltransferase. Proc Natl Acad Sci U S A. 1991;88(7):2633–7.

140. Golberg L, Holzel A, Komrower GM, Schwarz V. A clinical and biochemical study of galactosaemia; a possible explanation of the nature of the biochemical lesion. Arch Dis Child. 1956;31(158):254–64.

141. Gissen P, Johnson CA, Morgan NV, Stapelbroek JM, Forshew T, Cooper WN, et al. Mutations in VPS33B, encoding a regulator of SNARE-dependent membrane fusion, cause arthrogryposis-renal dysfunction-cholestasis (ARC) syndrome. Nat Genet. 2004;36(4):400–4.

142. Cullinane AR, Straatman-Iwanowska A, Zaucker A, Wakabayashi Y, Bruce CK, Luo G, et al. Mutations in VIPAR cause an arthrogryposis, renal dysfunction and cholestasis syndrome phenotype with defects in epithelial polarization. Nat Genet. 2010;42(4):303–12.

143. Eastham KM, McKiernan PJ, Milford DV, Ramani P, Wyllie J, van't Hoff W, et al. ARC syndrome: an expanding range of phenotypes. Arch Dis Child. 2001;85(5):415–20.

144. Horslen SP, Quarrell OW, Tanner MS. Liver histology in the arthrogryposis multiplex congenita, renal dysfunction, and cholestasis (ARC) syndrome: report of three new cases and review. J Med Genet. 1994;31(1):62–4.

145. Di Rocco M, Callea F, Pollice B, Faraci M, Campiani F, Borrone C. Arthrogryposis, renal dysfunction and cholestasis syndrome: report of five patients from three Italian families. Eur J Pediatr. 1995;154(10):835–9.

146. Gissen P, Tee L, Johnson CA, Genin E, Caliebe A, Chitayat D, et al. Clinical and molecular genetic features of ARC syndrome. Hum Genet. 2006;120(3):396–409.

147. Smith H, Galmes R, Gogolina E, Straatman-Iwanowska A, Reay K, Banushi B, et al. Associations among genotype, clinical phenotype, and intracellular localization of trafficking proteins in ARC syndrome. Hum Mutat. 2012;33(12):1656–64.

148. Kazama I, Matsubara M, Michimata M, Suzuki M, Hatano R, Sato H, et al. Adult onset Fanconi syndrome: extensive tubulo-interstitial lesions and glomerulopathy in the early stage of Chinese herbs nephropathy. Clin Exp Nephrol. 2004;8(3):283–7.

149. Wrong OM, Norden AG, Feest TG. Dent's disease; a familial proximal renal tubular syndrome with low-molecular-weight proteinuria, hypercalciuria, nephrocalcinosis, metabolic bone disease, progressive renal failure and a marked male predominance. QJM. 1994;87(8):473–93.

150. Dent CE, Friedman M. Hypercalcuric rickets associated with renal tubular damage. Arch Dis Child. 1964;39:240–9.

151. Lloyd SE, Pearce SH, Fisher SE, Steinmeyer K, Schwappach B, Scheinman SJ, et al. A common molecular basis for three inherited kidney stone diseases. Nature. 1996;379(6564):445–9.

152. Igarashi T, Inatomi J, Ohara T, Kuwahara T, Shimadzu M, Thakker RV. Clinical and genetic studies of CLCN5 mutations in Japanese families with Dent's disease. Kidney Int. 2000;58(2):520–7.

153. Thakker RV. Pathogenesis of Dent's disease and related syndromes of X-linked nephrolithiasis. Kidney Int. 2000;57(3):787–93.

154. Scheinman SJ, Cox JP, Lloyd SE, Pearce SH, Salenger PV, Hoopes RR, et al. Isolated hypercalciuria with mutation in CLCN5: relevance to idiopathic hypercalciuria. Kidney Int. 2000;57(1):232–9.

155. Langlois V, Bernard C, Scheinman SJ, Thakker RV, Cox JP, Goodyer PR. Clinical features of X-linked nephrolithiasis in childhood. Pediatr Nephrol. 1998;12(8):625–9.

156. Akuta N, Lloyd SE, Igarashi T, Shiraga H, Matsuyama T, Yokoro S, et al. Mutations of CLCN5 in Japanese children with idiopathic low molecular weight proteinuria, hypercalciuria and nephrocalcinosis. Kidney Int. 1997;52(4):911–6.

157. Lloyd SE, Pearce SH, Gunther W, Kawaguchi H, Igarashi T, Jentsch TJ, et al. Idiopathic low molecular weight proteinuria associated with hypercalciuric nephrocalcinosis in Japanese children is due to mutations of the renal chloride channel (CLCN5). J Clin Invest. 1997;99(5):967–74.

158. Hoopes RR Jr, Hueber PA, Reid RJ Jr, Braden GL, Goodyer PR, Melnyk AR, et al. CLCN5 chloride-

channel mutations in six new North American families with X-linked nephrolithiasis. Kidney Int. 1998;54(3):698–705.

159. Hoopes RR Jr, Shrimpton AE, Knohl SJ, Hueber P, Hoppe B, Matyus J, et al. Dent disease with mutations in OCRL1. Am J Hum Genet. 2005;76(2):260–7.

160. Hichri H, Rendu J, Monnier N, Coutton C, Dorseuil O, Poussou RV, et al. From Lowe syndrome to Dent disease: correlations between mutations of the OCRL1 gene and clinical and biochemical phenotypes. Hum Mutat. 2011;32(4):379–88.

161. Scheel O, Zdebik AA, Lourdel S, Jentsch TJ. Voltage-dependent electrogenic chloride/proton exchange by endosomal CLC proteins. Nature. 2005;436(7049):424–7.

162. Accardi A, Miller C. Secondary active transport mediated by a prokaryotic homologue of ClC Cl− channels. Nature. 2004;427(6977):803–7.

163. Gorvin CM, Wilmer MJ, Piret SE, Harding B, van den Heuvel LP, Wrong O, et al. Receptor-mediated endocytosis and endosomal acidification is impaired in proximal tubule epithelial cells of Dent disease patients. Proc Natl Acad Sci U S A. 2013;110(17):7014–9.

164. Wang Y, Cai H, Cebotaru L, Hryciw DH, Weinman EJ, Donowitz M, et al. ClC-5: role in endocytosis in the proximal tubule. Am J Physiol Renal Physiol. 2005;289(4):F850–62.

165. Hryciw DH, Ekberg J, Ferguson C, Lee A, Wang D, Parton RG, et al. Regulation of albumin endocytosis by PSD95/Dlg/ZO-1 (PDZ) scaffolds. Interaction of Na+-H+ exchange regulatory factor-2 with ClC-5. J Biol Chem. 2006;281(23):16068–77.

166. Hryciw DH, Ekberg J, Pollock CA, Poronnik P. ClC-5: a chloride channel with multiple roles in renal tubular albumin uptake. Int J Biochem cell Biol. 2006;38(7):1036–42.

167. Norden AG, Sharratt P, Cutillas PR, Cramer R, Gardner SC, Unwin RJ. Quantitative amino acid and proteomic analysis: very low excretion of polypeptides >750 Da in normal urine. Kidney Int. 2004;66(5):1994–2003.

168. Janne PA, Suchy SF, Bernard D, MacDonald M, Crawley J, Grinberg A, et al. Functional overlap between murine Inpp5b and Ocrl1 may explain why deficiency of the murine ortholog for OCRL1 does not cause Lowe syndrome in mice. J Clin Invest. 1998;101(10):2042–53.

169. Utsch B, Bökenkamp A, Benz MR, Besbas N, Dotsch J, Franke I, Frund S, Gok F, Hoppe B, Karle S, Kuwertz-Broking E, Laube G, Neb M, Nuutinen M, Ozaltin F, Rascher W, Ring T, Tasic V, van Wijk JA, Ludwig M. Novel OCRL1 mutations in patients with the phenotype of Dent disease. Am J Kidney Dis. 2006;48(6):942–56.

170. Bokenkamp A, Bockenhauer D, Cheong HI, Hoppe B, Tasic V, Unwin R, et al. Dent-2 disease: a mild variant of Lowe syndrome. J Pediatrics. 2009;155(1):94–9.

171. Gunther W, Piwon N, Jentsch TJ. The ClC-5 chloride channel knock-out mouse—an animal model for Dent's disease. Pflugers Archiv. 2003;445(4):456–62.

172. Silva IV, Cebotaru V, Wang H, Wang XT, Wang SS, Guo G, et al. The ClC-5 knockout mouse model of Dent's disease has renal hypercalciuria and increased bone turnover. J Bone Miner Res. 2003;18(4):615–23.

173. Devuyst O, Jouret F, Auzanneau C, Courtoy PJ. Chloride channels and endocytosis: new insights from Dent's disease and ClC-5 knockout mice. Nephron Physiol. 2005;99(3):p69–73.

174. Cebotaru V, Kaul S, Devuyst O, Cai H, Racusen L, Guggino WB, et al. High citrate diet delays progression of renal insufficiency in the ClC-5 knockout mouse model of Dent's disease. Kidney Int. 2005;68(2):642–52.

175. Raja KA, Schurman S, D'Mello RG, Blowey D, Goodyer P, Van Why S, et al. Responsiveness of hypercalciuria to thiazide in Dent's disease. J Am Soc Nephrol. 2002;13(12):2938–44.

176. Nijenhuis T, Vallon V, van der Kemp AW, Loffing J, Hoenderop JG, Bindels RJ. Enhanced passive Ca2+ reabsorption and reduced Mg2+ channel abundance explains thiazide-induced hypocalciuria and hypomagnesemia. J Clin Invest. 2005;115(6):1651–8.

177. Lowe CU, Terrey M, Mac LE. Organic-aciduria, decreased renal ammonia production, hydrophthalmos, and mental retardation; a clinical entity. AMA Am J Dis Child. 1952;83(2):164–84.

178. Charnas LR, Bernardini I, Rader D, Hoeg JM, Gahl WA. Clinical and laboratory findings in the oculocerebrorenal syndrome of Lowe, with special reference to growth and renal function. N Engl J Med. 1991;324(19):1318–25.

179. Abbassi V, Lowe CU, Calcagno PL. Oculocerebro-renal syndrome. A review. Am J Dis Child. 1968;115(2):145–68.

180. Loi M. Lowe syndrome. Orphanet J Rare Dis. 2006;1:16.

181. Roschinger W, Muntau AC, Rudolph G, Roscher AA, Kammerer S. Carrier assessment in families with lowe oculocerebrorenal syndrome: novel mutations in the OCRL1 gene and correlation of direct DNA diagnosis with ocular examination. Mol Genet Metab. 2000;69(3):213–22.

182. Walton DS, Katsavounidou G, Lowe CU. Glaucoma with the oculocerebrorenal syndrome of Lowe. J Glaucoma. 2005;14(3):181–5.

183. Keilhauer CN, Gal A, Sold JE, Zimmermann J, Netzer KO, Schramm L. [Clinical findings in a patient with Lowe syndrome and a splice site mutation in the OCRL1 gene]. Klin Monbl Augenheilkd. 2007;224(3):207–209.

184. Pasternack SM, Bockenhauer D, Refke M, Tasic V, Draaken M, Conrad C, et al. A premature termination mutation in a patient with Lowe syndrome without congenital cataracts: dropping the "O" in OCRL. Klinische Padiatrie. 2013;225(1):29–33.

185. Recker F, Reutter H, Ludwig M. Lowe syndrome/Dent-2 disease: a comprehensive review of known and novel aspects. J Pediatr Genet. 2013;2(2):53–68.

186. Charnas L, Bernar J, Pezeshkpour GH, Dalakas M, Harper GS, Gahl WA. MRI findings and peripheral neuropathy in Lowe's syndrome. Neuropediatrics. 1988;19(1):7–9.

187. Ono J, Harada K, Mano T, Yamamoto T, Okada S. MR findings and neurologic manifestations in Lowe oculocerebrorenal syndrome. Pediatr Neurol. 1996;14(2):162–4.

188. Schneider JF, Boltshauser E, Neuhaus TJ, Rauscher C, Martin E. MRI and proton spectroscopy in Lowe syndrome. Neuropediatrics. 2001;32(1):45–8.

189. Kenworthy L, Charnas L. Evidence for a discrete behavioral phenotype in the oculocerebrorenal syndrome of Lowe. Am J Med Genet. 1995;59(3):283–90.

190. Kenworthy L, Park T, Charnas LR. Cognitive and behavioral profile of the oculocerebrorenal syndrome of Lowe. Am J Med Genet. 1993;46(3):297–303.

191. Wu G, Zhang W, Na T, Jing H, Wu H, Peng JB. Suppression of intestinal calcium entry channel TRPV6 by OCRL, a lipid phosphatase associated with Lowe syndrome and Dent disease. Am J Physiol Cell Physiol. 2012;302(10):C1479–91.

192. Witzleben CL, Schoen EJ, Tu WH, McDonald LW. Progressive morphologic renal changes in the oculo-cerebro-renal syndrome of Lowe. Am J Med. 1968;44(2):319–24.

193. Tricot L, Yahiaoui Y, Teixeira L, Benabdallah L, Rothschild E, Juquel JP, et al. End-stage renal failure in Lowe syndrome. Nephrol Dialysis Transplant. 2003;18(9):1923–5.

194. Schramm L, Gal A, Zimmermann J, Netzer KO, Heidbreder E, Lopau K, et al. Advanced renal insufficiency in a 34-year-old man with Lowe syndrome. Am J Kidney Dis. 2004;43(3):538–43.

195. Lasne D, Baujat G, Mirault T, Lunardi J, Grelac F, Egot M, et al. Bleeding disorders in Lowe syndrome patients: evidence for a link between OCRL mutations and primary haemostasis disorders. Br J Haematol. 2010;150(6):685–8.

196. Athreya BH, Schumacher HR, Getz HD, Norman ME, Borden ST, Witzleben CL. Arthropathy of Lowe's (oculocerebrorenal) syndrome. Arthritis Rheum. 1983;26(6):728–35.

197. Holtgrewe JL, Kalen V. Orthopedic manifestations of the Lowe (oculocerebrorenal) syndrome. J Pediatr Orthop. 1986;6(2):165–71.

198. Rodrigues Santos MT, Watanabe MM, Manzano FS, Lopes CH, Masiero D. Oculocerebrorenal Lowe syndrome: a literature review and two case reports. Spec Care Dentist. 2007;27(3):108–11.

199. Won JH, Lee MJ, Park JS, Chung H, Kim JK, Shim JS. Multiple epidermal cysts in lowe syndrome. Ann Dermatol. 2010;22(4):444–6.

200. Attree O, Olivos IM, Okabe I, Bailey LC, Nelson DL, Lewis RA, et al. The Lowe's oculocerebrorenal syndrome gene encodes a protein highly homologous to inositol polyphosphate-5-phosphatase. Nature. 1992;358(6383):239–42.

201. Lin T, Lewis RA, Nussbaum RL. Molecular confirmation of carriers for Lowe syndrome. Ophthalmology. 1999;106(1):119–22.

202. Brown N, Gardner RJ. Lowe syndrome: identification of the carrier state. Birth Defects Orig Artic Ser. 1976;12(3):579–95.

203. Delleman JW, Bleeker-Wagemakers EM, van Veelen AW. Opacities of the lens indicating carrier status in the oculo-cerebro-renal (Lowe) syndrome. J Pediatr Ophthalmol. 1977;14(4):205–12.

204. Cibis GW, Waeltermann JM, Whitcraft CT, Tripathi RC, Harris DJ. Lenticular opacities in carriers of Lowe's syndrome. Ophthalmology. 1986;93(8):1041–5.

205. Dressman MA, Olivos-Glander IM, Nussbaum RL, Suchy SF. Ocrl1, a PtdIns(4,5)P(2) 5-phosphatase, is localized to the trans-Golgi network of fibroblasts and epithelial cells. J Histochem Cytochem. 2000;48(2):179–90.

206. Suchy SF, Nussbaum RL. The deficiency of PIP2 5-phosphatase in Lowe syndrome affects actin polymerization. Am J Hum Genet. 2002;71(6):1420–7.

207. Apodaca G. Endocytic traffic in polarized epithelial cells: role of the actin and microtubule cytoskeleton. Traffic. 2001;2(3):149–59.

208. Lowe M. Structure and function of the Lowe syndrome protein OCRL1. Traffic. 2005;6(9):711–9.

209. Pirruccello M, De Camilli P. Inositol 5-phosphatases: insights from the Lowe syndrome protein OCRL. Trends Biochem Sci. 2012;37(4):134–43.

210. McCrea HJ, Paradise S, Tomasini L, Addis M, Melis MA, De Matteis MA, et al. All known patient mutations in the ASH-RhoGAP domains of OCRL affect targeting and APPL1 binding. Biochem Biophys Res Commun. 2008;369(2):493–9.

211. Gobernado JM, Lousa M, Gimeno A, Gonsalvez M. Mitochondrial defects in Lowe's oculocerebrorenal syndrome. Arch Neurol. 1984;41(2):208–9.

212. Madhivanan K, Mukherjee D, Aguilar RC. Lowe syndrome: between primary cilia assembly and Rac1-mediated membrane remodeling. Commun Integr Biol. 2012;5(6):641–4.

213. Kruger SJ, Wilson ME Jr, Hutchinson AK, Peterseim MM, Bartholomew LR, Saunders RA. Cataracts and glaucoma in patients with oculocerebrorenal syndrome. Arch Ophthalmol. 2003;121(9):1234–7.

214. Rossi R, Pleyer J, Schafers P, Kuhn N, Kleta R, Deufel T, et al. Development of ifosfamide-induced nephrotoxicity: prospective follow-up in 75 patients. Med Pediatr Oncol. 1999;32(3):177–82.

215. Rossi R, Ehrich JH. Partial and complete de Toni-Debre-Fanconi syndrome after ifosfamide chemotherapy of childhood malignancy. Eur J Clin Pharmacol. 1993;44(Suppl 1):S43–5.

216. Loebstein R, Koren G. Ifosfamide-induced nephrotoxicity in children: critical review of predictive risk factors. Pediatrics. 1998;101(6):E8.

217. Skinner R, Pearson AD, English MW, Price L, Wyllie RA, Coulthard MG, et al. Cisplatin dose rate as a risk factor for nephrotoxicity in children. Br J Cancer. 1998;77(10):1677–82.

218. Skinner R, Pearson AD, English MW, Price L, Wyllie RA, Coulthard MG, et al. Risk factors for ifosfamide nephrotoxicity in children. Lancet. 1996;348(9027):578–80.

219. Loebstein R, Atanackovic G, Bishai R, Wolpin J, Khattak S, Hashemi G, et al. Risk factors for long-term outcome of ifosfamide-induced nephrotoxicity in children. J Clin Pharmacol. 1999;39(5):454–61.

220. Skinner R, Cotterill SJ, Stevens MC. Risk factors for nephrotoxicity after ifosfamide treatment in children: a UKCCSG Late Effects Group study. United Kingdom Children's Cancer Study Group. Br J Cancer. 2000;82(10):1636–45.

221. Macpherson NA, Moscarello MA, Goldberg DM. Aminoaciduria is an earlier index of renal tubular damage than conventional renal disease markers in the gentamicin-rat model of acute renal failure. Clin Invest Med. 1991;14(2):101–10.

222. Spahn CM, Prescott CD. Throwing a spanner in the works: antibiotics and the translation apparatus. J Mol Med. 1996;74(8):423–39.

223. Izzedine H, Launay-Vacher V, Isnard-Bagnis C, Deray G. Drug-induced Fanconi's syndrome. Am J Kidney Dis. 2003;41(2):292–309.

224. Hall AM, Hendry BM, Nitsch D, Connolly JO. Tenofovir-associated kidney toxicity in HIV-infected patients: a review of the evidence. Am J Kidney Dis. 2011;57(5):773–80.

225. Frisch LS, Mimouni F. Hypomagnesemia following correction of metabolic acidosis: a case of hungry bones. J Am Coll Nutr. 1993;12(6):710–3.

226. Haycock GB, Al-Dahhan J, Mak RH, Chantler C. Effect of indomethacin on clinical progress and renal function in cystinosis. Arch Dis Child. 1982;57(12):934–9.

Bartter-, Gitelman-, and Related Syndromes

36

Siegfried Waldegger, Karl Peter Schlingmann, and Martin Konrad

Basic Principles of Ion Transport in the TAL and the Early DCT

With respect to their role in sodium reabsorption, the TAL and early DCT form a functional unit that separates tubular sodium chloride from water. Compared to sodium reabsorption in the other nephron segments, which occurs via sodium hydrogen exchange or by sodium channels in the proximal nephron and in the ASDN, respectively, TAL and early DCT sodium transport is accomplished primarily by the active reabsorption of sodium together with chloride from the tubular fluid. These nephron segments are relatively water-tight and thus prevent osmotically driven absorptive flow of water. About 30% of the total sodium load provided by glomerular filtration is absorbed along the TAL and—via counter current multiplication—contribute to medullary interstitial hypertonicity. TAL sodium reabsorption thus not only accounts for the—in quantitative terms—most important mechanism of sodium retention (apart from the proximal neph-

S. Waldegger
Department of Pediatrics I, Innsbruck Medical University, Innsbruck, Austria
e-mail: siegfried.waldegger@tirol-kliniken.at

K. P. Schlingmann · M. Konrad (✉)
Department of General Pediatrics, University Hospital Münster, Münster, Germany
e-mail: karlpeter.schlingmann@ukmuenster.de; konradma@uni-muenster.de

ron, which reabsorbs about 60% of the filtered sodium load), but also generates the osmotic driving force for water reabsorption along the CD. For this reason, disturbances in TAL salt reabsorption result in both salt-wasting and severely reduced urinary concentrating capacity (i.e. water loss). In contrast, DCT mediated salt reabsorption accounts for only about 5% of the filtered sodium load and does not contribute to the urinary concentrating mechanisms. Impaired DCT salt reabsorption therefore does not interfere with urinary concentrating capability, although the accompanying saluresis indirectly increases renal water excretion even with normal urine osmolalities.

Transepithelial sodium chloride reabsorption in the TAL and DCT is driven by secondary active transport processes that depend on a low intracellular sodium concentration maintained by active extrusion of sodium by the basolateral sodium-potassium-ATPase (sodium pump). By far the majority of TAL sodium reabsorption depends upon the operation of the furosemide-sensitive sodium-potassium-chloride cotransporter (NKCC2) with about half of the sodium taking the transcellular route and half taking a paracellular route by cation-selective intercellular pathways (Fig. 36.1a). Potassium that enters the TAL cell by sodium-potassium-chloride cotransport (1 potassium ion being transported with 1 sodium and 2 chloride ions) recycles back to the tubular urine through KCNJ1 (ROMK).

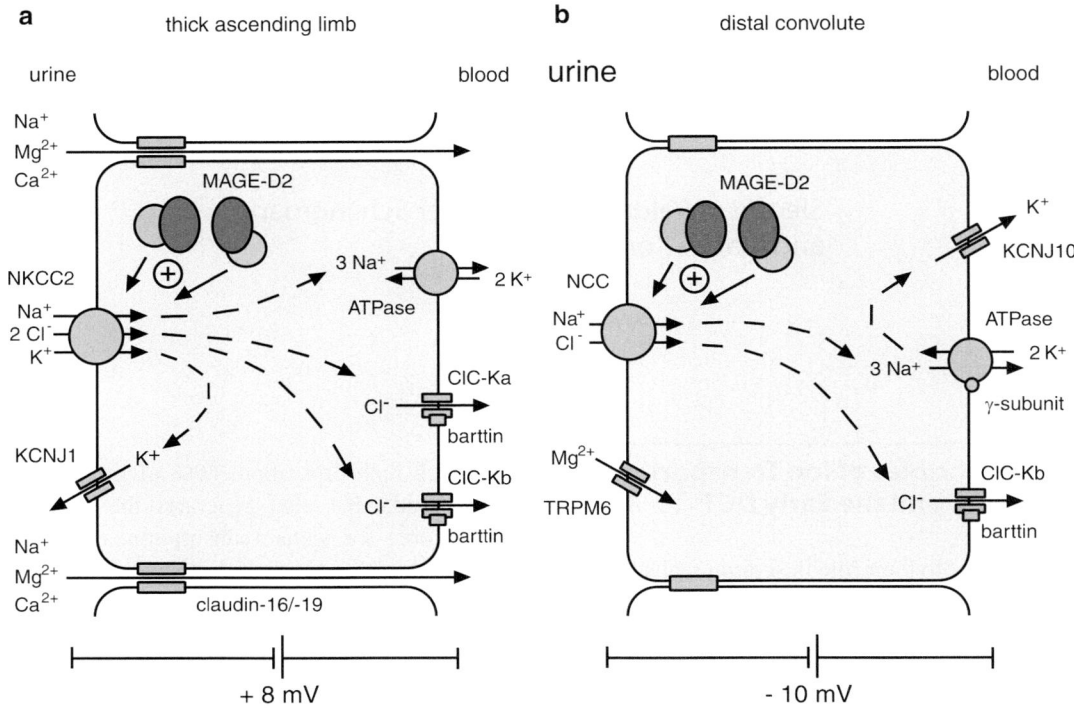

Fig. 36.1 Mechanisms of sodium reabsorption along the distal nephron. The key transport proteins and ion channels are shown for the thick ascending limb (**a**) and the distal convolute (**b**), for details please see text

This not only guarantees proper activity of NKCC2-mediated transport along the entire length of the TAL by replenishment of urinary potassium that otherwise would rapidly decrease along the TAL through reabsorption by NKCC2. Even more important, luminal potassium secretion in addition establishes a lumen-positive transepithelial voltage gradient that provides—in terms of energy recovery—a low-priced driving force for paracellular transport of cations like sodium, calcium, and magnesium. The essential functions of the TAL thus not only include the reabsorption of sodium chloride but also that of magnesium and calcium. Noteworthy, all of the TAL chloride reabsorption occurs by the transcellular route. Overall parity of sodium (with ~50% transcellular and ~50% paracellular) and chloride (100% transcellular) reabsorption is due to the stoichiometry of the apical NKCC2 cotransporter that transports two chloride ions for each sodium ion (Fig. 36.1a).

Taken together, the initial step of transcellular sodium chloride and paracellular sodium transport across the TAL epithelium critically depends on the proper activity of NKCC2 and KCNJ1.

In contrast to the TAL, sodium chloride reabsorption in the DCT occurs almost exclusively by the transcellular route (Fig. 36.1b). Luminal sodium chloride uptake is mediated by the electroneutral thiazide-sensitive sodium chloride cotransporter NCC that is structurally related to the NKCC2 protein, but transports 1 sodium ion together with 1 chloride ion without potassium. A relevant apical potassium conductance seems not to exist in early DCT cells, that instead express TRPM6 cation channels that permit apical magnesium entry. Inhibition of NCC transport by long term administration of thiazides or by genetic ablation in animal models has been shown to reduce the number of DCT cells, which might explain impaired renal magnesium reabsorption with consequent hypomagnesemia observed in human diseases caused by impaired NCC mediated transport.

DCT and TAL cells differ with respect to the apical entry step for sodium chloride, however, as mentioned above, basolateral sodium release in both cell types is accounted for by the sodium pump. Moreover, epithelial cells in TAL and early DCT share similar pathways for basolateral chloride exit. In both cell types two highly homologous ClC-K type chloride channel proteins (ClC-Ka and ClC-Kb) associate with their beta subunit barttin to form a basolateral chloride conductance, which accounts for the release of the majority of reabsorbed chloride ions (Fig. 36.1a, b).

Taken together, NCC mediates early DCT cell sodium chloride uptake and ClC-K channels in association with barttin account for basolateral chloride release.

In the transition zone between the TAL and DCT a plaque of closely packed epithelial cells morphologically different from TAL- and DCT-cells forms the *macula densa*. Together with closely adjacent extraglomerular mesangial cells and granular cells of the afferent arterioles appendant to the same nephron, these specialized tubular cells assemble the juxtaglomerular apparatus. *Macula densa* cells serve an important function in coupling renal hemodynamics with tubular reabsorption in that they monitor the sodium chloride concentration of the tubular fluid. Via paracrine signalling molecules like prostaglandin E_2 (PGE_2), ATP, adenosin, and NO, the *macula densa* provides a feed-back mechanism, which adapts glomerular filtration to tubular reabsorption (tubuloglomerular feedback, TGF). In case of an increased sodium chloride concentration at the *macula densa* the TGF induces afferent arteriole vasoconstriction and decreases renin release, whereas a decreased *macula densa* sodium chloride concentration dilates the afferent arteriole and increases renin release. To sense the tubular sodium chloride concentration the *macula densa* takes advantage of essentially the same repertoire of transport proteins as found in salt-reabsorbing TAL cells. Via apical sodium chloride uptake (NKCC2 and KCNJ1) and baso-

lateral chloride release (ClC-K and barttin) changes in luminal sodium chloride concentration are translated in alterations of basolateral transmembrane voltage. This again results from recycling of potassium into the tubular lumen, which guarantees an asymmetric - hence electrogenic - transcellular transport of sodium chloride, which results in basolateral membrane depolarization. This in turn regulates among other processes voltage-sensitive calcium entry, which triggers a series of intracellular signalling events eventually resulting in the release of the above mentioned paracrine signals. Owing to these combined functions in transepithelial transport and sensing of tubular sodium chloride, impaired activity of one of the participating proteins not only results in salt-wasting due to reduced TAL salt-reabsorbing capacity, but also abrogates the TGF as an important safety valve, which otherwise would reduce the filtered sodium chloride load by decreasing glomerular filtration. In fact, blinding of the *macula densa* for the tubular sodium chloride concentration with resultant disinhibition of glomerular filtration might constitute the single most important mechanism underlying the severe salt-wasting observed in impaired TAL salt transport.

Taken together, NKCC2, KCNJ1, ClC-K chloride channels, and barttin participate in the salt sensing-mechanism of the *macula densa*. Impaired function of one of these proteins affects the TGF and prevents adjustment of glomerular filtration with tubular salt-reabsorbing capacity, which further aggravates renal salt wasting [1].

Hypokalemic Salt-Wasting Tubular Disorders

With the exception of the medullary collecting duct that is primarily responsible for the reabsorption of water, reabsorption of sodium chloride from the glomerular filtrate at least in quantitative terms constitutes the key function of all nephron segments. Given the normal daily amount of 170 liters of glomerular filtrate produced by adult kidneys, at a normal plasma sodium concentration of 140 mmol/L and plasma chloride concentration of 105 mmol/L the filtered load of sodium and chloride per 24 h amounts to 23.8 mols (about 550 g) and 17.9 mols (about 630 g), respectively. Healthy kidneys manage the reabsorption of more than 99% of the filtered load, with about 60% by the proximal tubule, 30% by the TAL, 5% by the early DCT, and the remainder by the aldosterone-sensitive distal nephron (ASDN). Impairment of sodium transport in any of these nephron segments causes a permanent reduction in extracellular fluid volume, which in turn causes compensatory activation of sodium conserving mechanisms, i.e. stimulation of renin secretion and aldosterone synthesis. Accordingly, with intact ASDN function, the primary symptoms of renal salt-wasting like hypovolemia with tendency for reduced arterial blood pressure mix with those of secondary hyperaldosteronism, which increases ASDN sodium retention at the expense of an increased potassium excretion eventually resulting in hypokalemia. In case of renal salt-wasting, hypokalemia thus indicates proper function of the ASDN and points to the involvement of nephron segments upstream to the ASDN.

As mentioned above, sodium reabsorption along the TAL and early DCT is coupled to the reabsorption of chloride. Sodium-wasting caused by defects in these nephron segments hence is accompanied by decreased reabsorption of chloride. Unlike sodium, which at least partially may be recovered by increased reabsorption along the ASDN, chloride irretrievably gets lost with the urine. Accordingly, the urinary chloride-loss exceeds that of sodium and for the sake of electroneutrality has to be balanced by other cations like ammonium or potassium. Loss of ammonium, the main carrier of protons in the urine, results in metabolic alkalosis, potassium loss in addition aggravates hypokalemia caused by secondary hyperaldosteronism. For this reason, hypochloremia with metabolic alkalosis, in addition to severe hypokalemia characterizes salt-wasting due to defects along the TAL and early DCT.

Finally, sodium reabsorption along the proximal tubule via the sodium proton exchanger and

the carboanhydrase is indirectly coupled to the reabsorption of bicarbonate. Proximal tubular salt-wasting thus—in addition to hypokalemia—is accompanied by urinary loss of bicarbonate resulting in hyperchloremic metabolic acidosis.

Taken together, in the state of renal salt-wasting the determination of plasma potassium, chloride, and bicarbonate concentrations allows for the rapid assessment of the affected nephron segment. Of note, in this context the determination of the plasma sodium concentration is not very helpful, since changes in plasma sodium—the more or less exclusive extracellular cation accounting for plasma osmolality—reflects disturbances in the osmoregulation (i.e. water balance) rather than in the regulation of sodium balance.

Apart from more general disturbances of proximal tubular function which among other transport processes affect proximal tubular sodium reabsorption (as seen in Fanconi syndrome), no hereditary defects specifically affecting the proximal tubular sodium proton exchanger have been described in humans. By contrast, several genetic defects affect sodium chloride transport along the TAL and DCT and will be the focus of the following section.

Renal Salt-Wasting with Hypokalemia and Hypochloremic Metabolic Alkalosis

Historical Overview and Nomenclature

In 1957, two pediatricians described an infant with congenital hypokalemic alkalosis, failure to thrive, dehydration, and hyposthenuria, who finally died at the age of 7.5 months [2]. Some years later, two patients with normotensive hyperaldosteronism, hyperplasia of the juxtaglomerular apparatus, metabolic alkalosis and severe renal potassium wasting were characterized by the endocrinologist Frederic Bartter [3]. Other features of this syndrome were increased activity of the renin-angiotensin system and a relative vascular resistance to the pressor effect of exogenously applied angiotensin II. Following these original reports, hundreds of such Bartter syndrome (BS) cases have been described. While all shared the findings of hypokalemia and hypochloremic alkalosis, patients differed with respect to age of onset, severity of symptoms, degree of growth retardation, urinary concentration capacity, magnitude of urinary excretion of potassium and prostaglandins, presence of hypomagnesemia, and extents of urinary calcium excretion.

Gitelman and colleagues pointed to the susceptibility to carpopedal spasms and tetany in three BS cases [4]. Tetany was attributed to low plasma magnesium levels secondary to impaired renal conservation of magnesium. Further examination of these patients in addition revealed low urinary calcium excretion [5]. Consequently, the association of hypocalciuria with renal magnesium-wasting was regarded as a hallmark to separate the then defined Gitelman syndrome (GS) from other forms of BS [6]. Interestingly, both patients in Bartter's original report displayed positive Chvostek's sign and carpopedal spasms. Indeed, in a review of the original observations described by Bartter et al., one of the coauthors conceded that the majority of patients seen by both endocrinologists perfectly matched the later description of Gitelman [7].

Phenotypic homogeneity of BS was challenged even more seriously when the pediatricians Fanconi and McCredie described high urinary calcium excretion and medullary nephrocalcinosis in preterm infants initially suspected of having BS [8, 9]. Descriptions of this variant in the literature became more frequent in the 1980s, most likely because advances in neonatal medicine resulted in higher survival rates of extremely preterm born babies. The neonatologist Ohlsson finally described the antenatal history with maternal polyhydramnios, which likely predisposed to premature birth [10]. Immediately after birth, profound polyuria puts such patients at great risk for life-threatening dehydration. Contraction of the extracellular fluid (ECF) volume is accompanied by markedly elevated renal and extrarenal prostaglandin E_2 (PGE_2) production. Treatment with prostaglandin synthesis inhibitors effectively reduced polyuria, ameliorated hypokalemia, and improved growth [11, 12]. Another variant of this severe, prenatal-onset salt-wasting disorder was first described in a Bedouin family. It differs from the above mentioned antenatal variant of BS by the presence of sensorineural deafness, absence of medullary nephrocalcinosis, and slowly deteriorating renal function [13]. The last variant that has been described is X-linked transient antenatal BS. This disorder is of peculiar interest because at onset the clinical course is very severe and still many patients die from complications. Interestingly, the disease phenotype is self-limited and clinical symptoms disappear within a few weeks to months of life [14].

Taken together, renal salt-wasting syndromes associated with hypokalemia and hypochloremic metabolic alkalosis (frequently subsumed as "Bartter syndrome" in a broader sense) present with marked clinical variability. Severe, early onset forms (**antenatal Bartter syndrome, aBS**) with symptoms directly arising from profound salt-wasting with extracellular volume depletion contrast with milder late onset forms primarily characterized by the features of secondary hyperaldosteronism (**Gitelman syndrome, GS**). In between these two extremes, the Bartter syndrome *sensu stricto* (**classic Bartter syndrome, cBS**) presents as a disorder of intermediate severity. Variable extents of extracellular volume depletion and secondary electrolyte disturbances contribute to a rather variable disease phenotype, which in its extremes may mimic aBS or GS.

This classification based on clinical criteria was enriched by clarification of the underlying *genetic* defects, of which all but one follow an autosomal recessive mode of inheritance. As disclosed by molecular genetic analyses, aBS results from disturbed salt reabsorption along the TAL due to defects either in NKCC2 [15], KCNJ1 (ROMK) [16], Barttin [17], or both ClC-Ka and ClC-Kb [18]. X-linked transient aBS is caused by mutations in MAGE-D2, a chaperone-like molecule affecting the expression of NKCC2 and NCC during fetal life [14]. The cBS is caused by dysfunction of ClC-Kb [19], which impairs salt transport to some extent along the TAL and in

Table 36.1 Molecular genetics of renal salt wasting disorders

	BS1	BS2	BS3	BS4a	BS4b	BS5	GS	EAST/SeSAME
OMIM	601678	241200	607364	602522	613090	300971	263800	612780
Gene	*SLC12A1*	*KCNJ1*	*CLCNKB*	*BSND*	*CLCNKA + CLCNKB*	*MAGED2*	*SLC12A3*	*KCNJ10*
Protein	NKCC2	KCNJ1 (ROMK)	ClC-Kb	Barttin	ClC-Ka + ClC-Kb	MAGE-D2	NCC	KCNJ10
Inheritance	AR	AR	AR	AR	AR	XLR	AR	AR

OMIM Online Mendelian Inheritance in Man, *AR* autosomal recessive, *XLR* X-linked recessive

particular along the DCT. A pure defect of salt reabsorption in the DCT due to dysfunction of NCC finally results in GS [20].

Given the significant clinical overlap within the different subtypes of BS and also with GS, it is more and more accepted to describe the subtypes by the underlying genetic abnormality (Table 36.1). According to this molecular genetic classification, Bartter syndrome type 1 (**BS1**) refers to a defect in NKCC2 (gene name *SLC12A1*), **BS2** in KCNJ1 (*KCNJ1*), **BS3** in ClC-Kb (*CLCNKB*), **BS4a** in Barttin (*BSND*), **BS4b** to a digenic defect in ClC-Ka and ClC-Kb, and **BS5** in MAGE-D2. Previously patients with a Bartter-like phenotype with gain of function mutations in the calcium sensing receptor (CaSR) have been described [21, 22] and sometimes referred to as BS5, but this designation has been abandoned in accordance with the current OMIM nomenclature. **GS**, owing to disturbed NCC (*SLC12A3*) function, was not included in this classification despite its apparent relatedness to this group of disorders.

Another facet of the clinical and genetic heterogeneity of inherited renal salt wasting disorders unsurfaced in 2009, when a new autosomal recessive clinical syndrome characterized by epilepsy, ataxia, sensorineural deafness and renal salt wasting with or without mental retardation was described under the acronyms EAST or SeSAME syndrome [23, 24]. **EAST/SeSAME** syndrome is caused by loss-of-function mutations in the *KCNJ10* gene encoding the inwardly-rectifying potassium channel KCNJ10 (Kir4.1). The renal tubular defect disturbs the reabsorption of sodium chloride in the DCT and thus symptoms closely resemble GS with hypokalemic alkalosis, hypomagnesemia and hypocalciuria.

Taken together, renal salt-wasting with hypokalemia and hypochloremic metabolic alkalosis becomes manifest in three clinically defined syndromes: BS, GS, and EAST syndrome.

Genetic Disorders with Hypokalemic Salt-Wasting

Bartter Syndrome Type 1 (BS1)

Disruption of sodium chloride reabsorption in the TAL due to inactivating mutations of the *SLC12A1* gene which encodes NKCC2 causes BS1, a severe disorder with onset *in utero*. Within the second trimester, fetal polyuria leads to progressive maternal polyhydramnios. Untreated, premature delivery occurs around 32 weeks of gestation. The most striking abnormality of the newborns is profound polyuria. With adequate fluid replacement, daily urinary outputs can easily exceed half of the body weight of the newborn (>20 mL/kg/h). Despite ECF volume contraction and presence of high AVP levels, urine osmolality hardly approaches that of plasma, indicating a severe renal concentrating defect. Salt reabsorption along the TAL segment is also critical for urine dilution, which explains that urine osmolality on the other hand typically does not decrease below 160 mosmol/kg. Some preserved ability to dilute urine might be explained by an adaptive increase of salt reabsorption in the DCT which functions as the most distal portion of the diluting segment. This moderate hyposthenuria clearly separates NKCC2-deficient patients from polyuric patients with nephrogenic diabetes insipidus, who typically display urine osmolalities below 100 mosmol/kg.

Within the first months of life, nearly all patients develop medullary nephrocalcinosis in parallel with persistently high urinary calcium excretion. Remarkably, conservation of magnesium is not affected to a similar extent and

NKCC2-deficient patients usually do not develop hypomagnesemia. This is even more surprising given that mutations in either *CLDN16* or *CLDN19* which both encode tight junction proteins that mediate paracellular transport of divalent cations along the TAL, invariably cause both hypercalciuria and hypermagnesiuria with subsequent hypomagnesemia [25, 26]. With respect to magnesium transport, the difference between both disorders might be explained by an upregulation of magnesium reabsorption parallel to a compensatory increase of sodium chloride reabsorption in DCT cells in case of a NKCC2 defect [27].

Bartter Syndrome Type 2 (BS2)

Patients with mutations in the *KCNJ1* gene encoding the ATP-sensitive inwardly rectifying potassium channel KCNJ1 (ROMK) similarly show a history of maternal polyhydramnios, prematurity with a median age of gestation of 33 weeks, vasopressin-insensitive polyuria, isosthenuria, and hypercalciuria with secondary nephrocalcinosis. As in the case of NKCC2 dysfunction, the severity of the symptoms argues for a complete defect of sodium chloride reabsorption along the TAL. The mechanism of RAAS activation is virtually identical to that proposed for NKCC2-deficient patients. However, despite the presence of high plasma aldosterone levels, KCNJ1-deficient patients exhibit transient hyperkalemia in the first days of life [28]. The simultaneous appearance of hyperkalemia and hyponatremia resembles the clinical picture of mineralocorticoid-deficiency (which however shows low aldosterone levels) or that of pseudohypoaldosteronism type I (PHA-I; high aldosterone levels). Indeed, several published cases of PHA-I turned out to be misdiagnosed and subsequent genetic analysis revealed KCNJ1 mutations as the underlying defect [29]. The severity of initial hyperkalemia decreases with gestational age [30]. Hyperkalemia may be attributed to the additional role of KCNJ1 in the cortical collecting duct (CCD) where it participates in the process of potassium secretion. Although less pronounced as compared to NKCC2-deficiency, the majority of KCNJ1-deficient patients develop hypokalemia in the later course of the disease. The transient nature of hyperkalemia may be explained by the upregulation of alternative pathways for potassium secretion in the CCD.

Bartter Syndrome Type 3 (BS3)

BS3, previously often designated as "classic Bartter syndrome", is caused by mutations in *CLCNKB* (encoding the basolateral chloride channel ClC-Kb). This subtype of BS is characterized by a very high clinical variability which might be partly explained by an alternative chloride extrusion pathway in the basolateral membrane of TAL cells, namely ClC-Ka. Several studies have indicated that the clinical variability is not related to a certain type of mutation [31, 32]. Even the most deleterious mutation, which implies the absence of the complete *CLCNKB* gene and which affects nearly 50% of patients, can cause varying degrees of disease severity. Features of tubular dysfunction distal from the TAL predominate, suggesting a major role of ClC-Kb along the DCT. Although TAL salt transport can be impaired to a variable extent, its function is never completely perturbed.

With respect to renal function, the neonatal period in ClC-Kb-deficient patients usually passes without major problems. Maternal polyhydramnios is observed in only one fourth of the patients and usually is mild. Accordingly, duration of pregnancy is not substantially shortened. More than half of the patients are diagnosed within the first year of life. Symptoms at initial presentation include failure to thrive, dehydration, muscular hypotonia, and lethargy. Laboratory examination typically reveals low plasma chloride concentrations (down to 60 mmol/L), decreased plasma sodium concentration, and severe hypokalemic alkalosis. At first presentation, electrolyte derangement is usually more pronounced as compared to the other variants of BS. However, because renal salt wasting progresses slowly and polyuria may be absent, medical consultation may be delayed. Plasma renin activity is greatly increased, whereas plasma aldosterone concentration is only slightly elevated. This discrepancy might be attributed to negative feed-back regulation of aldosterone incretion by hypokalemia and alkalosis. Therefore, normal or slightly elevated aldosterone levels under conditions of profound hypokalemic alkalosis are in fact inappropriately low.

Urinary concentrating ability is preserved at least to a certain extent and a number of patients with BS3 achieve urinary osmolalities above 700 mosmol/kg in morning urine samples. Because renal medullary interstitial hypertonicity is critically dependent on sodium chloride reabsorption in the TAL, the ability to concentrate urine above 700 mosmol/kg indicates nearly intact TAL function despite of ClC-Kb deficiency. Moreover, the integrity of TAL function is also reflected by the finding that hypercalciuria is not a typical feature of ClC-Kb dysfunction and—if present—occurs only temporarily. The majority of patients exhibit normal or even low urinary calcium excretion. Accordingly, medullary nephrocalcinosis—a hallmark of pure TAL dysfunction—is rare. The plasma magnesium concentration gradually decreases over time owing to impaired renal magnesium conservation, as is observed in other forms of abnormal DCT function. Accordingly, several ClC-Kb deficient patients exhibit both hypomagnesemia and hypocalciuria, a constellation which usually is thought to be highly indicative for an NCC-defect. ClC-Kb deficiency thus may mimic GS.

Bartter Syndrome Type 4a (BS4a)

In 2001, a new player in the process of salt reabsorption along the TAL and DCT was identified—the ClC-K channel beta-subunit barttin—following the discovery of molecular defects in *BSND* in patients with a very rare variant of BS with sensorineural deafness [17]. Because Barttin had no homology to any known protein, its physiologic function remained unclear until its role as an essential beta-subunit of the ClC-K channels was demonstrated [33, 34].

Two ClC-K isoforms of the ClC family of chloride channels are highly expressed along the distal nephron, with ClC-Ka being primarily expressed in the thin ascending limb and decreasing expression levels along the adjacent distal nephron. Its close homologue, ClC-Kb, is predominantly expressed in the DCT. Along the TAL, both channel isoforms are equally expressed. Barttin, which is found in all ClC-K expressing nephron segments, is essential for proper ClC-K channel function in that it facilitates the transport of ClC-K channels to the cell surface and modulates biophysical properties of the assembled channel complex.

In affected individuals, the Barttin defect seems to completely disrupt chloride exit across the basolateral membrane in TAL as well as DCT cells. Accordingly, patients display the severest salt-wasting kidney disorder described so far. As with defects of NKCC2 and KCNJ1, the first symptom of a Barttin defect is maternal polyhydramnios due to fetal polyuria beginning at approximately 22 weeks of gestation. Again, polyhydramnios accounts for preterm labor and extreme prematurity. Postnatally, patients are at high risk of volume depletion. Plasma chloride levels fall to approximately 80 mmol/l, a further decrease usually can be avoided by close laboratory monitoring and rapid intervention. Polyuria again is resistant to vasopressin and urine osmolalities range between 200 and 400 mOsmol/kg.

Unlike patients with loss-of-function mutations in KCNJ1 and NKCC2, Barttin-deficient patients exhibit only transitory hypercalciuria [35]. Medullary nephrocalcinosis is absent, yet progressive renal failure is common with histologic signs of pronounced tissue damage like glomerular sclerosis, tubular atrophy, and mononuclear infiltration. The mechanisms underlying the deterioration of renal function are not yet understood. The lack of hypercalciuria, however, may be explained by disturbed sodium chloride reabsorption along the DCT. Isolated DCT dysfunction as seen in GS (see below) or after long-term inhibition of NCC-mediated transport by thiazides is known to induce hypocalciuria. This effect might counter-balance the hypercalciuric effect of TAL-dysfunction in case of a combined impairment of salt reabsorption along the TAL and DCT. In contrast to calcium, the renal conservation of magnesium is impaired, leading to hypomagnesemia. This might be explained by the disruption of both magnesium reabsorption pathways, the paracellular one in the TAL and the transcellular one in the DCT, respectively.

Barttin defects are invariably associated with sensorineurinal deafness. Elucidation of the pathogenesis of this rare disorder has provided a deeper insight into the mechanisms of potassium rich endolymph secretion in the inner ear: Marginal cells of the *stria vascularis* contribute to the endolymph formation by apical potassium secretion. Transcellular potassium transport is mediated by the furosemide-sensitive Na-K-2Cl-cotransporter type 1 (NKCC1) ensuring basolateral potassium entry into the marginal cells. Voltage-dependent potassium channels mediate apical potassium secretion into the endolymph. Proper function of NKCC1 requires basolateral recycling of chloride. Deafness associated with Barttin defects suggests that this recycling is enabled by the ClC-K/barttin channel complex.

A Digenic Disorder: Bartter Syndrome Type 4b (BS4b)

The concept of the physiologic role of Barttin as a common beta-subunit of ClC-K channels was substantiated by the description of patients harbouring inactivating mutations in both the ClC-Ka and ClC-Kb chloride channels, respectively [18]. The clinical symptoms resulting from this digenic disease are indistinguishable from those of Barttin-deficient patients. This observation not only proves the concept of the functional interaction of Barttin with both ClC-K isoforms but also excludes important other functions of Barttin not related to ClC-K channel interaction.

X-Linked Transient Bartter Syndrome (BS5)

Transient forms of antenatal BS have been first described in the 1990s [36, 37]. The clinical course is characterized by early development of severe polyhydramnios, high prenatal mortality and excessive neonatal salt wasting in the surviving infants. This disease condition is mainly observed in male infants and surprisingly the disease manifestations spontaneously resolve within a few weeks to several months of life. Mutations in *MAGED2* encoding the melanoma-associated antigen-D2 have been identified to underlie the disorder [14]. As expected for an X-linked disease, transient BS (BS5) is almost exclusively observed in boys. Only two female infants have been described to date [38]. Functional data indicate that MAGED2 regulates the expression of NKCC2 and NCC, especially during fetal life. Because of the transient character of the disease, it is of crucial importance to establish the exact diagnosis in order to avoid therapies such as NSAIDs which are no longer necessary by nature of the disease.

Gitelman Syndrome (GS)

DCT epithelia contain two cell types: early DCT cells (DCT1) which express the thiazide-sensitive sodium chloride cotransporter (NCC) as its predominant apical sodium entry pathway, and further distal residing late DCT cells (DCT2), which express the epithelial sodium channel (ENaC) as the main pathway for apical sodium reabsorption. Both sodium entry pathways are inducible by aldosterone. Early DCT and late DCT cells probably also differ with respect to their function in divalent cation transport.

Genetic defects in *SLC12A3* encoding NCC result in only mild renal salt wasting. Initial presentation frequently occurs at school age or later with the characteristic symptoms being muscular weakness, cramps, and fatigue. Whereas a history of salt craving is common, urinary concentrating ability typically is preserved. Laboratory examination shows a typical constellation of metabolic alkalosis, low normal chloride levels, hypokalemia, and hypomagnesemia, urine analysis shows hypocalciuria. Family studies revealed that electrolyte imbalances are present from infancy, although most of the affected infants displayed no obvious clinical signs. Of note, the combination of hypokalemia and hypomagnesemia exerts an exceptionally unfavorable effect on cardiac excitability, which puts these patients at high risk for cardiac arrhythmia.

The pathognomonic feature of GS is the dissociation of renal calcium and magnesium handling, with low urinary calcium and high urinary magnesium levels. Subsequent hypomagnesemia causes neuromuscular irritability and tetany. Decreased renal calcium elimination together with magnesium deficiency favors deposition of mineral calcium as demonstrated by increased bone density as well as chondrocalcinosis. Although the combination of hypomagnesemia and hypocalciuria is typical for GS, it is neither a specific nor universal finding. Clinical observations in GS patients disclosed intra- and inter-individual variations in urinary calcium concentrations which can be attributed to gender, age-related conditions of bone metabolism, intake of magnesium supplements, changes in diuresis and urinary osmolality, respectively. Likewise, hypomagnesemia might not be present from the beginning. Because less than one percent of total body magnesium is circulating in the blood, renal magnesium loss can be balanced temporarily by magnesium release from bone and muscle stores as well as by an increase of intestinal magnesium reabsorption. Accordingly, the strict definition of hypomagnesemia with coincident hypocalciuria in order to separate GS from BS3 appears arbitrary.

The mechanisms compromising distal magnesium reabsorption and favoring reabsorption of calcium are not yet completely understood. The occasional co-existence of hypomagnesemia and hypocalciuria in ClC-Kb deficient patients indicates that this phenomenon is not restricted to NCC defects but is rather a consequence of impaired transcellular sodium chloride reabsorption along the early DCT. It is tempting to speculate, that with a functional defect of early DCT cells, which in addition to sodium chloride normally reabsorb magnesium by apical TRPM6 magnesium channels, these cells are replaced by late DCT cells, which reabsorb sodium via ENaC channels and calcium via epithelial calcium channels (TRPV5). Accordingly, reabsorption of magnesium would decrease and that of calcium increase. Moreover, other phenomena like for example the redistribution of renal tubular sodium chloride reabsorption to more proximal nephron segments (proximal tubule and TAL) might contribute to alterations in renal calcium and magnesium handling.

EAST/SeSAME Syndrome

In 2009, a newly described autosomal recessive clinical syndrome characterized by epilepsy, ataxia, sensorineural deafness and renal salt wasting with/without mental retardation was described under the acronyms EAST or SeSAME syndrome

[23, 24]. EAST/SeSAME syndrome is caused by loss of function mutations in the *KCNJ10* gene encoding the inwardly-rectifying potassium channel KCNJ10 (Kir4.1). The expression pattern of KCNJ10 fits the disease phenotype with high expression levels in brain, the stria vascularis of the inner ear, and in the distal nephron, especially in the DCT. Here, KCNJ10 is localized at the basolateral membrane of DCT cells where it is thought to function in collaboration with the Na^+K^+-ATPase as it might allow for a recycling of potassium ions entering the tubular cells in countermove for the extruded sodium [24]. Loss of KCNJ10 function most likely leads to a depolarization of the basolateral membrane and thereby to a reduction of the driving force for basolateral anion channels as well as sodium-coupled exchangers. By this mechanism, KCNJ10 defects could also affect the putative Na^+/Mg^{2+} exchanger and possibly explain the magnesium wasting observed in EAST/SeSAME syndrome. Moreover, it could be demonstrated that lack of KCNJ10 decreases basolateral chloride conductance and results in a diminished expression of NCC in the apical membrane [39]. These results could explain the salt loss observed in EAST/SeSAME patients. Interestingly, the renal phenotype of KCNJ10 knockout mice had not been thoroughly studied until the description of the human disease [40]. However, the reevaluation of KCNJ10 knockout mice clearly demonstrated renal salt wasting leading to significant growth retardation [23].

Patients usually present early in infancy with generalized tonic-clonic seizures, speech and motor delay, as well as severe ataxia leading to an inability to walk, intention tremor, and dysdiadochokinesis. In addition they exhibit a severe hearing impairment. Renal salt wasting may develop or be recognized only later during the course of the disease [41]. Closely resembling GS, the renal phenotype includes the combination of hypokalemic alkalosis, hypomagnesemia and hypocalciuria.

A summary of the most important clinical features and the ordinary age of disease manifestation is given in Table 36.2.

Table 36.2 Main clinical and biochemical characteristics of different renal salt wasting disorders

	BS1	BS2	BS3	BS4a	BS4b	BS5	GS	EAST/SeSAME
Age at onset	Prenatally	Prenatally	0–5 years	Prenatally		Prenatally	>5 years	Infancy
Polyhydramnios	Severe	Severe	Absent-mild	Severe		Very severe	Absent	Absent
Leading symptoms	Polyuria Hypochloremia Alkalosis Hypokalemia	Polyuria Hypochloremia Alkalosis Transient neonatal hyperkalemia	Hypokalemia Hypochloremia Alkalosis Failure to thrive	Polyuria Hypochloremia Alkalosis Hypokalemia		Polyuria Hypochloremia Alkalosis Hypokalemia	Hypokalemia Alkalosis Hypomagnesemia	Hypokalemia Alkalosis Hypomagnesemia
Calcium excretion	High	High	Variable	Variable		High	Low	Low
Nephrocalcinosis	Very frequent	Very frequent	Rare, mild	Rare, mild		Rare, mild	Rare, mild	Rare, mild
Other findings			Mild Hypomagnesemia	Deafness Risk for CKD Risk of ESKD		Large for gestational age Transient disease	Growth retardation Chondrocalcinosis	Ataxia Deafness Seizures Mental retardation

CKD chronic kidney disease, *ESKD* end stage kidney disease

Treatment

As with other hereditary diseases the desirable correction of the primary genetic defects is not yet feasible. In the case of salt-wasting kidney disorders, however, the correction of secondary phenomena like increased renal prostaglandin synthesis or disturbed electrolyte homeostasis have been part of treatment virtually from the first description of the diseases. To the present, the cornerstones in the treatment of renal salt-wasting are non-steroidal anti-inflammatory drugs (NSAID) and long-term salt and electrolyte substitution [1].

In all subtypes of BS inhibition of renal and systemic prostaglandin synthesis leads to reduced urinary prostaglandin E_2 (PGE_2) excretion, dramatically decreases polyuria, converts hyposthenuria to isosthenuria, reduces hypercalciuria, and stimulates catch up growth [11, 12, 30]. Maintenance of euvolemia in the immediate postnatal period by meticulous replacement of renal fluid and salt loss is of central importance before starting NSAID therapy, which might precipitate acute renal failure if extracellular volume is depleted. There is long standing experience with the unselective cyclooxygenase (COX) inhibitor indomethacin which is started at 0.05 mg/kg per day and may be gradually increased to 1.5 mg/kg per day according to its effects on urinary output, renal PGE_2-synthesis and blood aldosterone levels. However, the potential benefit of indomethacin in preterm infants and neonates should be weighed against potential risks of severe gastrointestinal complications, i.e. ulcers, perforation and necrotizing enterocolitis [42, 43]. In particular, indomethacin therapy of newborns with KCNJ1 defects (BS2) may be complicated by oliguric renal failure and severe hyperkalemia. At any age, KCNJ1-deficient patients are particularly sensitive to indomethacin, with doses well below 1mg/kg/day being sufficient to maintain normal plasma potassium levels.

Gastrointestinal side effects (gastritis and peptic ulcers) are also the main drawbacks of longterm indomethacin therapy. These might be reduced by the use of COX-2 specific inhibitors (e.g. celecoxib), which show a comparable effect on renal salt wasting but adversely affect blood pressure [44]. A convincing explanation for these unsurpassed effects of NSAIDs is still missing although a reduction of glomerular filtration and blockage of an aberrant tubulo-glomerular feedback certainly are important contributors. Despite these beneficial effects of NSAIDs, lifelong substitution of potassium chloride usually is required to prevent life-threatening episodes of hypokalemia. Additional potassium supplementation is more often required for NKCC2-deficient (BS1) than KCNJ1-deficient (BS2) patients [1, 30]. In single patients, treatment with a potassium-sparing diuretic (i.e. spironolactone) has been shown to effectively increase serum potassium levels. Also ACE inhibitors have been used in a few patients with success but should be used with caution because ACE inhibitors could impair the compensatory mechanisms for sodium reabsorption in the more distal nephron. Thiazides should not be used to reduce hypercalciuria, since they interfere with compensatory mechanisms in the DCT and further aggravate salt and fluid losses.

Patients with BSND (BS4) are managed primarily with intravenous fluids in neonatal intensive care units. In contrast to other forms of BS, and despite high levels of urinary PGE_2, the effect of indomethacin on growth and correction of electrolyte disorders is rather poor [35, 45]. Hypokalemic metabolic alkalosis persists despite high doses of sodium chloride and potassium chloride supplementation [35]. In a single patient, combined therapy with indomethacin and captopril was needed to discontinue intravenous fluids and improve weight gain [46]. A pre-emptive nephrectomy for refractory electrolyte and fluid losses and persistent failure to thrive, followed by peritoneal dialysis and successful renal transplantation has been reported in a 1-year-old child with BS4 [47].

Patients with cBS (BS3) are typically treated with NSAIDs. Indomethacin is the most frequently used drug, usually started within the first years of life at doses ranging from 1 to 2.5 mg/kg/day. Potassium supplementation (usually KCl, 1–3 mmol/kg/day) is mandatory in BS3, as hypokalemia is often severe at presentation and is not fully corrected by indomethacin. If potassium chloride alone fails to correct hypokalemia, then addition of spironolactone (1–1.5 mg/kg/day) may be considered. ACE-inhibitors should be given with caution because of the risk of hypotension. Magnesium supplementation should be added when hypomagnesemia is present, but the correction is typically difficult [30].

In patients with GS, unrestricted salt intake as well as magnesium and potassium supplementations are the main therapeutic measures. Magnesium supplementation should be considered first, since magnesium repletion will facilitate potassium repletion and reduce the risk of tetany and other complications related to hypomagnesemia [48, 49]. All types of magnesium salts are effective, but their bioavailability is variable. Magnesium chloride, magnesium lactate and magnesium aspartate show higher bioavailability [48]. Magnesium chloride is recommended since it will also correct the urinary loss of chloride. The dose of magnesium must be adjusted individually in 3–4 daily administrations, with diarrhea being the limiting factor. In addition to magnesium, high doses of oral potassium chloride supplements are necessary in the majority of patients with GS [50]. Importantly, magnesium and potassium supplementation results in catchup growth [51, 52]. Spironolactone or amiloride can be useful, both to increase serum potassium levels in patients resistant to potassium chloride supplements and to treat magnesium depletion that is worsened by elevated aldosterone levels [53]. Both drugs should be started cautiously to avoid hypotension. Patients should be encouraged not to deny their usual salt craving, particularly if they practice regular physical activity. Following the pathophysiology with salt loss distal to the *macula densa* and thus not involving disturbances of the tubuloglomerular feeback, prostaglandin inhibitors are less frequently used in GS, since urinary PGE_2 levels are usually normal. However, in a recent controlled, randomized crossover study, Blanchard et al. demonstrated that indomethacin in GS effectively increases potassium levels. In this study, it was even more effective than amiloride or eplere-

none [54]. Considering the occurrence of prolonged QT interval in up to 50% GS patients [55, 56], QT-prolonging medications should be used with caution.

Although GS adversely affects the quality of life [57], information about the long-term outcome of these patients are lacking. Renal function and growth appear to be normal, provided lifelong supplementation. Progression to renal failure is extremely rare in GS: only 2 patients with GS who developed end-stage renal disease have been reported [58, 59].

For further details, please see two recent expert consensus statements summarizing the current knowledge on diagnosis and management of BS and GS [60, 61].

References

1. Jeck N, Schlingmann KP, Reinalter SC, et al. Salt handling in the distal nephron: lessons learned from inherited human disorders. Am J Physiol Regul Integr Comp Physiol. 2005;288(4):R782–95.
2. Rosenbaum P, Hughes M. Persistent, probably congenital, hypokalemic metabolic alkalosis with hyaline degeneration of renal tubules and normal urinary aldosterone. Am J Dis Child. 1957;94:560.
3. Bartter FC, Pronove P, Gill JR, MacCardle RC. Hyperplasia of the juxtaglomerular complex with hyperaldosteronism and hypokalemic alkalosis. A new syndrome. Am J Med. 1962;33:811–28.
4. Gitelman HJ, Graham JB, Welt LG. A new familial disorder characterized by hypokalemia and hypomagnesemia. Trans Assoc Am Physicians. 1966;79:221–35.
5. Rodriguez-Soriano J, Vallo A, Garcia-Fuentes M. Hypomagnesaemia of hereditary renal origin. Pediatr Nephrol. 1987;1(3):465–72.
6. Bettinelli A, Bianchetti MG, Girardin E, et al. Use of calcium excretion values to distinguish two forms of primary renal tubular hypokalemic alkalosis: Bartter and Gitelman syndromes. J Pediatr. 1992;120(1):38–43.
7. Bartter FC, Pronove P, Gill JR Jr, MacCardle RC. Hyperplasia of the juxtaglomerular complex with hyperaldosteronism and hypokalemic alkalosis. A new syndrome. 1962. J Am Soc Nephrol. 1998;9(3):516–28.
8. Fanconi A, Schachenmann G, Nüssli R, Prader A. Chronic hypokalaemia with growth retardation, normotensive hyperrenin-hyperaldosteronism ("Bartter's syndrome"), and hypercalciuria. Report of two cases with emphasis on natural history and on catch-up growth during treatment. Helv Paediatr Acta. 1971;26(2):144–63.

9. McCredie DA, Blair-West JR, Scoggins BA, Shipman R. Potassium-losing nephropathy of childhood. Med J Aust. 1971;1(3):129–35.

10. Ohlsson A, Sieck U, Cumming W, Akhtar M, Serenius F. A variant of Bartter's syndrome. Bartter's syndrome associated with hydramnios, prematurity, hypercalciuria and nephrocalcinosis. Acta Paediatr Scand. 1984;73(6):868–74.

11. Seyberth HW, Rascher W, Schweer H, Kühl PG, Mehls O, Schärer K. Congenital hypokalemia with hypercalciuria in preterm infants: a hyperprostaglandinuric tubular syndrome different from Bartter syndrome. J Pediatr. 1985;107(5):694–701.

12. Seyberth HW, Königer SJ, Rascher W, Kühl PG, Schweer H. Role of prostaglandins in hyperprostaglandin E syndrome and in selected renal tubular disorders. Pediatr Nephrol. 1987;1(3):491–7.

13. Landau D, Shalev H, Ohaly M, Carmi R. Infantile variant of Bartter syndrome and sensorineural deafness: a new autosomal recessive disorder. Am J Med Genet. 1995;59(4):454–9.

14. Laghmani K, Beck BB, Yang SS, et al. Polyhydramnios, transient antenatal Bartter's syndrome, and MAGED2 mutations. N Engl J Med. 2016;374(19):1853–63.

15. Simon DB, Karet FE, Hamdan JM, DiPietro A, Sanjad SA, Lifton RP. Bartter's syndrome, hypokalaemic alkalosis with hypercalciuria, is caused by mutations in the Na-K-2Cl cotransporter NKCC2. Nat Genet. 1996;13(2):183–8.

16. Simon DB, Karet FE, Rodriguez-Soriano J, et al. Genetic heterogeneity of Bartter's syndrome revealed by mutations in the K+ channel, ROMK. Nat Genet. 1996;14(2):152–6.

17. Birkenhäger R, Otto E, Schürmann MJ, et al. Mutation of BSND causes Bartter syndrome with sensorineural deafness and kidney failure. Nat Genet. 2001;29(3):310–4.

18. Schlingmann KP, Konrad M, Jeck N, et al. Salt wasting and deafness resulting from mutations in two chloride channels. N Engl J Med. 2004;350(13):1314–9.

19. Simon DB, Bindra RS, Mansfield TA, et al. Mutations in the chloride channel gene, CLCNKB, cause Bartter's syndrome type III. Nat Genet. 1997;17(2):171–8.

20. Simon DB, Nelson-Williams C, Bia MJ, et al. Gitelman's variant of Bartter's syndrome, inherited hypokalaemic alkalosis, is caused by mutations in the thiazide-sensitive Na-Cl cotransporter. Nat Genet. 1996;12(1):24–30.

21. Watanabe S, Fukumoto S, Chang H, et al. Association between activating mutations of calcium-sensing receptor and Bartter's syndrome. Lancet. 2002;360(9334):692–4.

22. Hebert SC. Bartter syndrome. Curr Opin Nephrol Hypertens. 2003;12(5):527–32.

23. Bockenhauer D, Feather S, Stanescu HC, et al. Epilepsy, ataxia, sensorineural deafness, tubulopathy, and KCNJ10 mutations. N Engl J Med. 2009;360(19):1960–70.

24. Scholl UI, Choi M, Liu T, et al. Seizures, sensorineural deafness, ataxia, mental retardation, and electrolyte imbalance (SeSAME syndrome) caused by mutations in KCNJ10. Proc Natl Acad Sci U S A. 2009;106(14):5842–7.

25. Simon DB, Lu Y, Choate KA, et al. Paracellin-1, a renal tight junction protein required for paracellular Mg2+ resorption. Science. 1999;285(5424):103–6.

26. Konrad M, Schaller A, Seelow D, et al. Mutations in the tight-junction gene claudin 19 (CLDN19) are associated with renal magnesium wasting, renal failure, and severe ocular involvement. Am J Hum Genet. 2006;79(5):949–57.

27. Kamel KS, Oh MS, Halperin ML. Bartter's, Gitelman's, and Gordon's syndromes. From physiology to molecular biology and back, yet still some unanswered questions. Nephron. 2002;92(Suppl 1):18–27.

28. Jeck N, Derst C, Wischmeyer E, et al. Functional heterogeneity of ROMK mutations linked to hyperprostaglandin E syndrome. Kidney Int. 2001;59(5):1803–11.

29. Finer G, Shalev H, Birk OS, et al. Transient neonatal hyperkalemia in the antenatal (ROMK defective) Bartter syndrome. J Pediatr. 2003;142(3):318–23.

30. Peters M, Jeck N, Reinalter S, et al. Clinical presentation of genetically defined patients with hypokalemic salt-losing tubulopathies. Am J Med. 2002;112(3):183–90.

31. Konrad M, Vollmer M, Lemmink HH, et al. Mutations in the chloride channel gene CLCNKB as a cause of classic Bartter syndrome. J Am Soc Nephrol. 2000;11(8):1449–59.

32. Zelikovic I, Szargel R, Hawash A, et al. A novel mutation in the chloride channel gene, CLCNKB, as a cause of Gitelman and Bartter syndromes. Kidney Int. 2003;63(1):24–32.

33. Estévez R, Boettger T, Stein V, et al. Barttin is a Cl− channel beta-subunit crucial for renal Cl− reabsorption and inner ear K+ secretion. Nature. 2001;414(6863):558–61.

34. Waldegger S, Jeck N, Barth P, et al. Barttin increases surface expression and changes current properties of ClC-K channels. Pflugers Arch. 2002;444(3):411–8.

35. Jeck N, Reinalter SC, Henne T, et al. Hypokalemic salt-losing tubulopathy with chronic renal failure and sensorineural deafness. Pediatrics. 2001;108(1):E5.

36. Engels A, Gordjani N, Nolte S, Seyberth HW. Angeborene passagere hyperprostaglandinurische Tubulopathie bei zwei frühgeborenen Geschwistern. Mschr Kinderheilk. 1991;139:185.

37. Reinalter S, Devlieger H, Proesmans W. Neonatal Bartter syndrome: spontaneous resolution of all signs and symptoms. Pediatr Nephrol. 1998;12(3):186–8.

38. Legrand A, Treard C, Roncelin I, et al. Prevalence of novel. Clin J Am Soc Nephrol. 2018;13(2):242–50.

39. Zhang C, Wang L, Zhang J, et al. KCNJ10 determines the expression of the apical Na-Cl cotransporter (NCC) in the early distal convoluted tubule (DCT1). Proc Natl Acad Sci U S A. 2014;111(32):11864–9.

40. Neusch C, Rozengurt N, Jacobs RE, Lester HA, Kofuji P. Kir4.1 potassium channel subunit is crucial

for oligodendrocyte development and in vivo myelination. J Neurosci. 2001;21(15):5429–38.

41. Scholl UI, Dave HB, Lu M, et al. SeSAME/EAST syndrome—phenotypic variability and delayed activity of the distal convoluted tubule. Pediatr Nephrol. 2012;27(11):2081–90.

42. Rodriguez-Soriano J. Bartter's syndrome comes of age. Pediatrics. 1999;103(3):663–4.

43. Vaisbich MH, Fujimura MD, Koch VH. Bartter syndrome: benefits and side effects of long-term treatment. Pediatr Nephrol. 2004;19(8):858–63.

44. Reinalter SC, Jeck N, Brochhausen C, et al. Role of cyclooxygenase-2 in hyperprostaglandin E syndrome/antenatal Bartter syndrome. Kidney Int. 2002;62(1):253–60.

45. Shalev H, Ohali M, Kachko L, Landau D. The neonatal variant of Bartter syndrome and deafness: preservation of renal function. Pediatrics. 2003;112(3 Pt 1):628–33.

46. Zaffanello M, Taranta A, Palma A, Bettinelli A, Marseglia GL, Emma F. Type IV Bartter syndrome: report of two new cases. Pediatr Nephrol. 2006;21(6):766–70.

47. Chaudhuri A, Salvatierra O, Alexander SR, Sarwal MM. Option of pre-emptive nephrectomy and renal transplantation for Bartter's syndrome. Pediatr Transplant. 2006;10(2):266–70.

48. Knoers NV. Gitelman syndrome. Adv Chronic Kidney Dis. 2006;13(2):148–54.

49. Rodríguez-Soriano J. Bartter and related syndromes: the puzzle is almost solved. Pediatr Nephrol. 1998;12(4):315–27.

50. Shaer AJ. Inherited primary renal tubular hypokalemic alkalosis: a review of Gitelman and Bartter syndromes. Am J Med Sci. 2001;322(6):316–32.

51. Riveira-Munoz E, Chang Q, Godefroid N, et al. Transcriptional and functional analyses of SLC12A3 mutations: new clues for the pathogenesis of Gitelman syndrome. J Am Soc Nephrol. 2007;18(4):1271–83.

52. Godefroid N, Riveira-Munoz E, Saint-Martin C, Nassogne MC, Dahan K, Devuyst O. A novel splicing mutation in SLC12A3 associated with Gitelman syndrome and idiopathic intracranial hypertension. Am J Kidney Dis. 2006;48(5):e73–9.

53. Colussi G, Rombola G, De Ferrari ME, Macaluso M, Minetti L. Correction of hypokalemia with anti-aldosterone therapy in Gitelman's syndrome. Am J Nephrol. 1994;14(2):127–35.

54. Blanchard A, Vargas-Poussou R, Vallet M, et al. Indomethacin, amiloride, or eplerenone for treating hypokalemia in Gitelman syndrome. J Am Soc Nephrol. 2015;26(2):468–75.

55. Bettinelli A, Tosetto C, Colussi G, Tommasini G, Edefonti A, Bianchetti MG. Electrocardiogram with prolonged QT interval in Gitelman disease. Kidney Int. 2002;62(2):580–4.

56. Foglia PE, Bettinelli A, Tosetto C, et al. Cardiac work up in primary renal hypokalaemia-hypomagnesaemia (Gitelman syndrome). Nephrol Dial Transplant. 2004;19(6):1398–402.

57. Cruz DN, Shaer AJ, Bia MJ, Lifton RP, Simon DB, Yale Gitelman's and Bartter's Syndrome Collaborative Study Group. Gitelman's syndrome revisited: an evaluation of symptoms and health-related quality of life. Kidney Int. 2001;59(2):710–7.

58. Bonfante L, Davis PA, Spinello M, et al. Chronic renal failure, end-stage renal disease, and peritoneal dialysis in Gitelman's syndrome. Am J Kidney Dis. 2001;38(1):165–8.

59. Calò LA, Marchini F, Davis PA, Rigotti P, Pagnin E, Semplicini A. Kidney transplant in Gitelman's syndrome. Report of the first case. J Nephrol. 2003;16(1):144–7.

60. Konrad M, Nijenhuis T, Ariceta G, et al. Diagnosis and management of Bartter syndrome: executive summary of the consensus and recommendations from the European Rare Kidney Disease Reference Network Working Group for Tubular Disorders. Kidney Int. 2021;99(2):324–35.

61. Blanchard A, Bockenhauer D, Bolignano D, et al. Gitelman syndrome: consensus and guidance from a Kidney Disease: Improving Global Outcomes (KDIGO) controversies conference. Kidney Int. 2017;91(1):24–33.

Disorders of Calcium and Magnesium Metabolism

37

Karl Peter Schlingmann and Martin Konrad

Calcium Physiology

Approximately one kilogram of the adult human body consists of elemental Ca^{2+}, of which 99% are bound in bone. The extracellular fluid contains only ~1000 mg of Ca^{2+}. Following national boards of nutrition, a daily uptake of 1000–1200 mg of elemental Ca^{2+} with a normal diet is recommended [1]. The intestine reabsorbs approximately 25–33% of the nutritional Ca^{2+} content [2]. In the kidney, ~800 mg of Ca^{2+} are filtered per day in the glomeruli of which 99% are reabsorbed along the renal tubule. Only ~10 mg (~0.1 mg/kg/day) are excreted with the urine. In plasma, ~50% of Ca^{2+} is present in the free ionized form, ~35% is protein-bound, and ~15% is complexed to bicarbonate, citrate or phosphate. The physiological range for blood Ca^{2+} equals 1.1–1.35 mmol/L for free, ionized Ca^{2+} and 2.2–2.6 mmol/L for total Ca^{2+} (in the presence of physiological whole protein levels) [3]. Only the free, ionized fraction is responsible for the biological Ca^{2+} effects.

The blood Ca^{2+} level is kept within a narrow physiological range by the concerted action of endocrine systems controlling intestinal Ca^{2+} uptake, renal Ca^{2+} excretion, and Ca^{2+} transport in bone and soft tissues. These comprise the parathyroid gland, active 1,25-$(OH)_2$-vitamin D_3, and the bone-derived phosphaturic hormone FGF-23 [4]. All three systems are tightly linked and influence each other's activity. Parathyroid hormone (PTH) increases intestinal Ca^{2+} absorption and Ca^{2+} release from bone, it promotes renal Ca^{2+} reabsorption while stimulating renal phosphate excretion. In contrast, active 1,25-$(OH)_2$-vitamin D_3 promotes intestinal Ca^{2+} and phosphate absorption as well as renal Ca^{2+} and phosphate conservation thereby ensuring sufficient Ca^{2+} and phosphate supply for bone mineralization. Finally, FGF-23 together with its co-factor klotho increases renal phosphate excretion by inhibiting proximal tubular phosphate reabsorption, but also negatively regulates active 1,25-$(OH)_2$-vitamin D_3 by inhibiting its activation and promoting its degradation [5]. The common aim of this endocrine interplay is to keep extracellular Ca^{2+} levels constant while supplying sufficient amounts of Ca^{2+} for soft tissues and bone mineralization.

At the glomerulus, the ionized fraction of serum Ca^{2+} is freely filtered. The majority of filtered Ca^{2+} (60–70%) is reabsorbed in the proximal tubule (Fig. 37.1) [6]. Classically, Ca^{2+} transport in the proximal tubule is considered to occur via the paracellular pathway driven by active transcellular Na^+ reabsorption and paracellular water flow [7]. Apical uptake of Na^+ into the

K. P. Schlingmann · M. Konrad (✉)
Department of General Pediatrics, Pediatric Nephrology, University Hospital Münster, Münster, Germany
e-mail: karlpeter.schlingmann@ukmuenster.de; konradma@uni-muenster.de

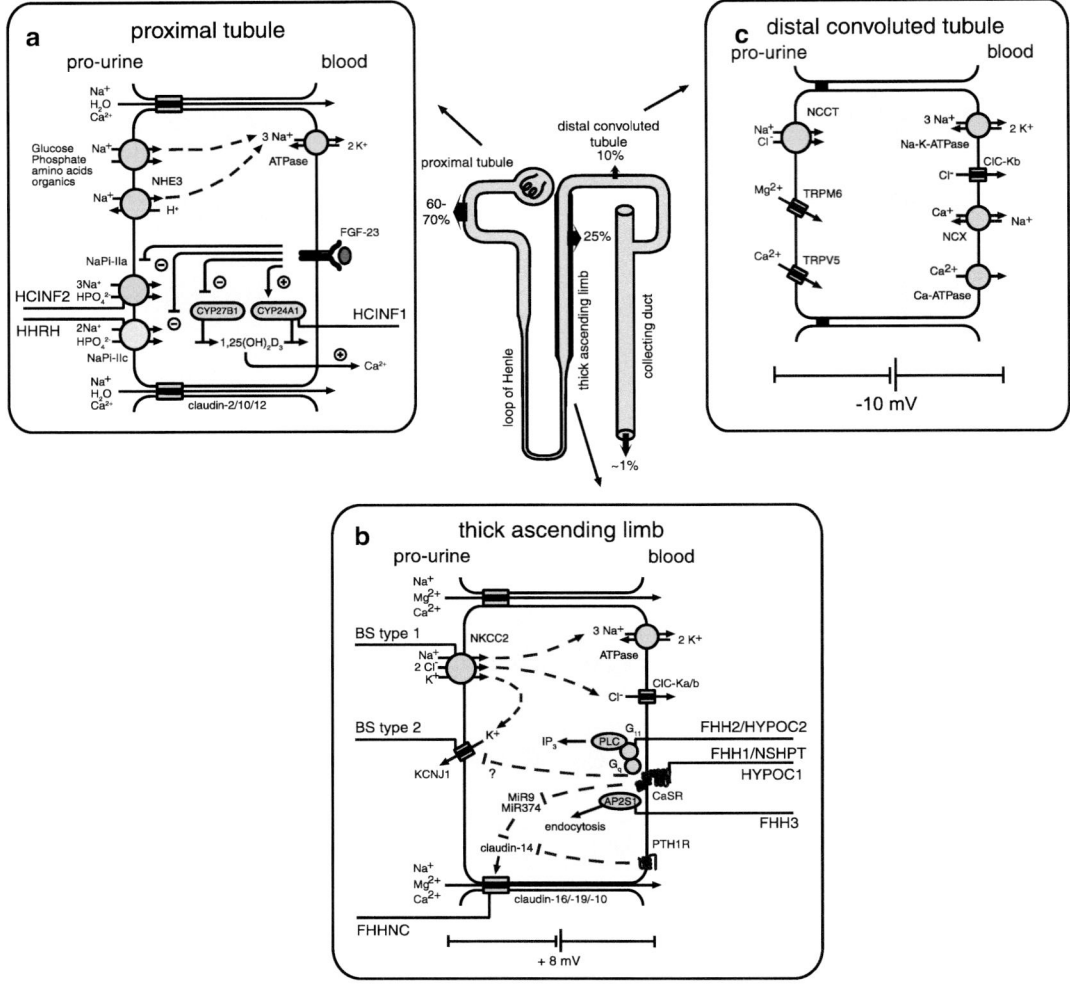

Fig. 37.1 Ca^{2+} reabsorption along the kidney tubule. (**a**) In the proximal tubule (PT), Ca^{2+} is reabsorbed via a paracellular pathway through tight junctions containing claudin-2. Also, the enzymes responsible for vitamin D activation, 1a-hydroxylase (CYP27B1), and vitamin D inactivation, 24-hydroxylase (*CYP24A1*), are expressed in PT cells and functionally linked to PO$_4^{3-}$ reabsorption via NaPi-IIa (*SLC34A1*) and NaPi-IIc (*SLC34A3*). (**b**) In the thick ascending limb (TAL), Ca^{2+} is reabsorbed together with Mg^{2+} through paracellular tight junctions composed by claudin-16 and -19. This process is negatively regulated by basolateral Ca^{2+}-sensing receptor (CaSR) and PTH. Mutations in the CaSR and its associated proteins lead to mirror-like changes in calcium metabolism. (**c**) In the distal convoluted tubule (DCT), Ca^{2+} is actively reabsorbed via the transcellular pathway involving an apical entry through TRPV5 and a basolateral exit via Ca^{2+}-ATPase and Na^{+}/Ca^{2+}-exchanger (NCX). Hereditary defects affecting tubular Ca^{2+} reabsorption are indicated

proximal tubular cell is achieved via the Na^{+}/H^{+}-exchanger NHE3 (*SLC9A3*) followed by basolateral extrusion via Na^{+}/K^{+}-ATPase [8]. The paracellular space in the proximal tubule has a high permeability for ions and water that is conferred by tight junctions composed of claudin-2, claudin-10, and claudin-12 [9, 10]. Interestingly,

recent data also indicate transcellular Ca^{2+} transport in the proximal tubule involving apically expressed Ca^{2+}-sensing receptor (CaSR) and the Ca^{2+}-permeable ion channel TRPC3 (transient receptor potential family C member 3) [11].

Around 25% of filtered Ca^{2+} is reabsorbed in the thick ascending limb (TAL) of the loop of

Henle. Here, Ca^{2+} transport is passive and paracellular in nature and occurs together with magnesium (Fig. 37.1). It is driven by a lumen-positive transepithelial voltage generated by active transcellular salt reabsorption. Next to changes in transcellular NaCl reabsorption, the permeability and cation selectivity of the paracellular pathway play a critical role in determining Ca^{2+} and Mg^{2+} reabsorption. Paracellular tight junctions in the TAL are composed of a complex set of claudin proteins conferring different properties: Claudin-16 and claudin-19 facilitate paracellular Ca^{2+} and Mg^{2+} transport, but also influence Na^+ permeability while sealing the paracellular space for Cl^- [12]. Furthermore, paracellular movement of Ca^{2+} and Mg^{2+} is modified by claudin-10 which is thought to form a paracellular Na^+ pore [13]. Paracellular Ca^{2+} and Mg^{2+} transport in the TAL is regulated by a complex network involving claudin-14 as well as the CaSR and PTH receptor, both expressed at the basolateral membrane [14–16]. Claudin-14 interacts with claudin-16 and diminishes paracellular cation permeability in vitro. Under physiologic conditions, the expression of claudin-14 is suppressed via a microRNA pathway [17]. By activation of the CaSR, extracellular Ca^{2+} is able to relieve this suppression and to induce claudin-14 expression, thus inhibiting paracellular divalent cation reabsorption [15]. The CaSR is a G-protein-coupled receptor that stimulates phospholipase C through G-proteins G_q and G_{11} resulting in the production of inositol 1,4,5-trisphosphate. This in turn leads to a reduction in PTH secretion from the parathyroid gland as well as increased urinary Ca^{2+} and Mg^{2+} excretion rates [18]. Finally, claudin-14 expression and therefore paracellular cation transport are also directly regulated by PTH via basolaterally expressed PTH-receptor PTH1R [16].

The distal convoluted tubule (DCT) only reabsorbs a small proportion of filtered Ca^{2+} (10–15%), however, as for Mg^{2+}, the DCT determines the final urinary excretion as there is no Ca^{2+} reabsorption beyond this segment. Transcellular Ca^{2+} reabsorption in the DCT is a sequential process of three steps: apical entry into the epithelial cell through Ca^{2+}-permeable ion channels (TRPV5), binding to calbindin-D_{28k} for diffusion through the cytoplasm, and basolateral exit through either a Ca^{2+}-ATPase (PMCA1b, ATP2B1), or a Na^+/Ca^{2+}-exchanger (NCX1, SLC8A1) [19]. Transcellular Ca^{2+} reabsorption in the DCT is critically influenced by PTH and active 1,25-OH_2-vit D_3 that regulate the expression levels of all the mentioned transport proteins [20]. In addition, Ca^{2+} (as well as Mg^{2+}) handling in the DCT appears to depend on dietary K^+ and the rate of active transcellular salt reabsorption [21, 22].

Disturbances of Calcium Homeostasis

Disturbances in Ca^{2+} metabolism comprise states of Ca^{2+} deficiency as well as Ca^{2+} excess usually detected in the form of hypo- or hypercalcemia. Whereas hypocalcemia represents a more common finding and is usually apparent by typical clinical signs and symptoms, hypercalcemia in infancy and childhood is a rare event and may remain unrecognized as clinical symptoms are rather unspecific. An overview on symptoms, causes, and the diagnostic work-up of pediatric hypocalcemia and hypercalcemia is provided in Chap. 31. Here, we focus on hereditary disorders of Ca^{2+} metabolism. These typically manifest with characteristic changes in serum and urine Ca^{2+} levels. As for acquired disorders of Ca^{2+} homeostasis, the diagnostic work-up, next to the parallel measurement of serum and urine electrolytes and creatinine, comprises the determination of parathyroid hormone (PTH) and vitamin D metabolites.

Hypercalciuria

The assessment of urinary Ca^{2+} excretion rates provides important information on alterations of renal Ca^{2+} conservation. Reference values for urinary Ca^{2+} excretion rates in infants and children are provided in Table 37.1 [23]. An increased urinary Ca^{2+} excretion may either reflect a primary disturbance in renal calcium handling or may reflect changes in renal Ca^{2+} handling in order to

Table 37.1 Reference ranges for urinary calcium excretion in children

Age (years)	Urinary Ca/Crea mg/mg (mol/mol)	
	5th percentile	95th percentile
0–1	0.03 (0.09)	0.81 (2.2)
1–2	0.03 (0.07)	0.56 (1.5)
2–3	0.02 (0.06)	0.50 (1.4)
3–5	0.02 (0.05)	0.41 (1.1)
5–7	0.01 (0.04)	0.30 (0.8)
7–10	0.01 (0.04)	0.25 (0.7)
10–14	0.01 (0.04)	0.24 (0.7)
14–17	0.01 (0.04)	0.24 (0.7)

Used with permission of Nature Publishing Group from Matos et al. [23]

compensate for disturbances in body Ca^{2+} homeostasis or its hormonal regulation.

Hypercalciuria is the most common risk factor for nephrocalcinosis and stone formation in children [24]. The etiology is assumed to be multifactorial with a complex interaction of environmental and genetic factors. Still, despite an increased knowledge in the underlying genetic causes, the majority of patients are classified as having idiopathic hypercalciuria. A detailed overview on hypercalciuria and its role in the etiology of nephrocalcinosis and kidney stone disease is also provided in Chap. 44 "Renal Calculi".

In the past two decades, genetic studies have identified variants in an increasing number of genes involved in tubular Ca^{2+} reabsorption in patients with hypercalciuria, nephrocalcinosis and kidney stone disease. Classic examples of disturbed renal tubular calcium (and magnesium) reabsorption are hereditary defects in the tight junction proteins claudin-16 and -19 in patients with FHHNC (HOMG3, HOMG5), as well as activating and inactivating mutations in the CaSR producing mirror images of disturbed calcium homeostasis (ADH1, FHH1, NSHPT) (see below).

Disorders affecting proximal tubular Ca^{2+} reabsorption comprise Dent's disease (DENT1, DENT2) and Lowe syndrome (see Chaps. 32 and 44). Both disorders affect endosomal function in proximal tubular epithelial cells resulting in a complex dysfunction characterized by tubular proteinuria, hypercalciuria, renal Fanconi syndrome, and progressive renal failure [25, 26].

Next to different metabolic disorders affecting proximal tubular function leading to renal Fanconi syndrome (see Table 37.2), Fanconi-Bickel syndrome due to mutations in *SLC2A2* [27] is another generalized defect of proximal tubular function with hypercalciuria. Moreover, an isolated renal phenotype without hepatic symptoms and disturbance in glucose metabolism has been described in families with bi-allelic *SLC2A2* mutations [28].

Detailed descriptions of differential diagnoses for hereditary renal Fanconi syndrome and proximal tubulopathies are also provided in Chap. 32.

Hereditary defects of proximal tubular phosphate reabsorption and vitamin D degradation are discussed below (section "Hypercalcemia").

A recent study directly implicated defective paracellular Ca^{2+} reabsorption in the proximal tubule in the pathogenesis of hypercalciuria and renal calcifications since deletion of claudin-2 in mice resulted in hypercalciuria and renal calcifications [29]. The same study also identified a potentially pathogenic heterozygous variant in *CLDN2* in a family with multiple members affected by kidney stones and associated common genetic variants near the *CLDN2* locus with kidney stone risk [29]. No primary defects in transcellular Ca^{2+} reabsorption in the DCT have been linked to monogenic human disease to date. Deletion of the epithelial Ca^{2+} channel TRPV5 in mice resulted in severe hypercalciuria, compensatory intestinal hyperabsorption of Ca^{2+}, and reduced bone thickness [30]. A TRPV5 missense mutation was identified in a mouse model with dominant hypercalciuria [31]. In contrast, homozygous knock-out of basolateral NCX1 (SLC8A1) and PMCA1b (ATP2B1) in mice is embryonically lethal [32, 33].

Finally, hypercalciuria is observed in other renal tubular disorders including Bartter syndrome (see Chap. 33) and renal tubular acidosis (see Chap. 36).

Table 37.2 Monogenic disorders associated with hypercalciuria

Proximal tubule	OMIM #	Inheritance	Gene	Protein
Dent's disease type 1	300009	XLR	*CLCN5*	ClC-5 chloride channel
Dent disease type 2/Lowe syndrome	309000	XLR	*OCRL*	Inositol-polyphosphate-5-phosphatase
Nephropathic cystinosis	219800	AR	*CTNS*	Cystinosin cystine transporter
Tyrosinemia 1	276700	AR	*FAH*	Fumarylacetoacetate hydrolase
Fanconi renotubular syndrome 3	615605	AD	*EHHADH*	Enoyl-CoA-hydratase
Fanconi renotubular syndrome with MODY	600281	AD	*HNF4A*	Hepatocyte nuclear factor 4α
Fanconi-Bickel syndrome	227810	AR	*SLC2A2*	GLUT2 glucose transporter
Infantile hypercalcemia 1 (HCINF1), nephrocalcinosis, calcium nephrolithiasis	143880	AR, AD	*CYP24A1*	25-OH-vitamin D_3-24-hydroxylase
Infantile hypercalcemia 2 (HCINF2), nephrocalcinosis, calcium nephrolithiasis	616963	AR, AD	*SLC34A1*	Na-Po$_4$ co-transporter NaPi-IIa
Hypophosphatemic rickets with hypercalciuria (HHRH), nephrocalcinosis, calcium nephrolithiasis	241530	AR, AD	*SLC34A3*	Na-Po$_4$ co-transporter NaPi-IIc
Thick ascending limb	**OMIM #**	**Inheritance**	**Gene**	**Protein**
Bartter syndrome type 1	601678	AR	*SLC12A1*	NKCC2 co-transporter
Bartter syndrome type 2	241200	AR	*KCNJ1*	ROMK potassium channel
Bartter syndrome type 3	607364	AR	*CLCNKB*	ClC-Kb chloride channel
Bartter syndrome type 4a	602522	AR	*BSND*	Barttin subunit
Bartter syndrome type 4b	613090	DR	*CLCNKA/B*	ClC-Ka/ClC-Kb chloride channels
Bartter syndrome type 5	300971	XLR	*MAGED2*	MAGE-D2
Familial hypomagnesemia with hypercalciuria/nephrocalcinosis (FHHNC)(HOMG3)	248250	AR	*CLDN16*	Claudin-16 (paracellin-1), tight junction protein
Familial hypomagnesemia with hypercalciuria/nephrocalcinosis (FHHNC) and severe ocular involvement (HOMG5)	248190	AR	*CLDN19*	Claudin-19, tight junction protein
Autosomal dominant hypoparathyroidism 1 (ADH1)	601198	AD	*CASR*	CaSR, Ca^{2+}/Mg^{2+} sensing receptor
Autosomal dominant hypoparathyroidism 2 (ADH2)	615361	AD	*GNA11*	G-protein α-11
Collecting duct (CD)	**OMIM #**	**Inheritance**	**Gene**	**Protein**
dRTA 1	179800	AD	*SLC4A1*	AE1 anion echanger
dRTA 4	611590	AR		
dRTA 2 with progressive sensorineural deafness	267300	AR	*ATP6V1B1*	H⁺-ATPase subunit B1
dRTA with/without sensorineural deafness	602722	AR	*ATP6V0A4*	H⁺-ATPase subunit A4
dRTA with early onset sensorineural deafness	600791	AR	*FOXI1*	Forkhead box I1 transcription factor

Hypocalcemia

A detailed description of clinical symptoms and signs of hypocalcemia is provided in Chap. 31 (see Table 30.18). Following the approach outlined there (Table 30.19), the etiology of Ca^{2+} deficiency and hypocalcemia can be categorized according to the serum level of PTH [34]. Low levels of PTH indicate primary dysfunction of the parathyroid gland with impaired or absent PTH production or release. Hereditary disorders involving abnormal parathyroid gland function include **primary hypoparathyroidism** due to mutations in the *PTH* gene (**isolated familial hypoparathyroidism 1**, OMIM #146200), due to **Di George syndrome** caused by microdeletions on chromosome 22q11 (OMIM #188400), or due to **HDR syndrome** (hypoparathyroidism, sensorineural deafness, renal dysplasia, OMIM #146255) caused by mutations in the transcription factor GATA3.

However, inappropriately low or normal levels of PTH may also point to an activating mutation in the *CASR* gene encoding the Ca^{2+} sensing receptor (CaSR) or in the *GNA11* gene encoding the accessory G-protein G-alpha-11 causing **autosomal-dominant hypocalcemia type 1 and 2**, respectively (ADH1, ADH2). These entities will be discussed in more detail below. ADH1 might be differentiated from the above mentioned disorders by determination of urinary Ca^{2+} excretion: In contrast to low urinary Ca^{2+} excretion found in primary forms of parathyroid dysfunction, urinary Ca^{2+} excretion is inappropriately high in face of hypocalcemia in patients with ADH1.

Elevated levels of PTH in the presence of normal renal function are also found in **acquired Ca^{2+}- and vitamin D-deficient rickets**. Whereas hypocalcemia might also be an associated finding in **renal Fanconi syndrome**, it is rather uncommon in other disorders of the proximal tubule such as hypophosphatemic rickets, Dent's disease or Lowe syndrome. These disorders are discussed in detail in Chaps. 32 and 44.

Pseudohypoparathyroidism represents a heterogeneous group of rare hereditary disorders with the common feature of PTH end-organ resistance and hypocalcemia despite elevated serum PTH levels (PHP1A OMIM #103580; PHP1B, OMIM #612462; PHP1C, OMIM #203330). Different (epi)genetic defects have been discovered as underlying causes, including loss of function mutations in the *GNAS* gene encoding the Gs-alpha isoform or methylation defects of the *GNAS* gene locus [35].

Autosomal Dominant Hypocalcemia

The extracellular **Ca^{2+}-sensing receptor (CaSR)** plays an essential role in Ca^{2+} and Mg^{2+} homeostasis by modulating PTH secretion and by directly regulating the rate of Ca^{2+} and Mg^{2+} reabsorption in the kidney [36]. The CaSR, a dimeric cell-surface protein of the G-protein receptor family, has a large extracellular domain that can bind extracellular Ca^{2+} at multiple sites [37]. Activation of the CaSR induces G_q and $G_{alpha-11}$ dependent phospholipase C signaling [18, 38], resulting in an inhibition of PTH release from the parathyroid gland and of renal tubular Ca^{2+} absorption. The function of the CaSR is inhibited by non-competitive binding of PO_4^{3-} to anion binding sites at the extracellular domain, leading to increased PTH secretion from the parathyroid gland [39]. Ca^{2+} sensing is also influenced by the level of CaSR surface expression. The CaSR is internalized from the plasma membrane by clathrin-mediated endocytosis. A central component of these clathrin-coated vesicles (CCVs) is the adaptor protein 2 (AP2) that forms a heterotetrameric complexes of α, β, μ, and σ (*AP2S1*) subunits [40]. Several diseases associated with both activating and inactivating mutations in the *CASR* gene, *GNA11*, and *AP2S1* have been described.

In the kidney, the CaSR is expression and basolateral localized in TAL, DCT, and intercalated cells of the cortical collecting duct (CCD) [41]. In addition, the CaSR is expressed in the apical membrane of the collecting duct as a putative sensor of urine Ca^{2+} levels [42]. Here, by adjusting aquaporin-2 expression, the CaSR is thought to adjust water diuresis to Ca^{2+} load, minimizing the risk of stone formation in the face of an increased urine Ca^{2+} excretion [43].

Autosomal dominant hypocalcemia 1 (ADH1) is caused by activating mutations in the *CASR* gene. Affected individuals typically manifest during childhood with seizures or carpopedal spasms. Laboratory evaluation reveals the typical combination of hypocalcemia and low PTH levels. Serum Ca^{2+} levels are usually in a range of 6–7 mg/

dL. In addition, many patients also exhibit moderate hypomagnesemia [44, 45]. Patients are often given the incorrect diagnosis of primary hypoparathyroidism on the basis of inappropriately low PTH levels. As indicated above, the differential diagnosis can be established by determination of urinary Ca^{2+} excretion which is low in primary hypoparathyroidism but usually increased in ADH1 patients. The differentiation of ADH from primary hypoparathyroidism is of particular importance because treatment with active vitamin D in ADH may result in a dramatic increase in hypercalciuria with subsequent nephrocalcinosis and impairment of renal function. Therefore, therapy with active vitamin D or Ca^{2+} supplementation should be reserved for symptomatic patients with the aim to maintain serum Ca^{2+} levels just sufficient for the relief of symptoms [45].

Activating *CASR* mutations lead to a lower setpoint of the receptor or an increased affinity for extracellular Ca^{2+} and Mg^{2+}. This inadequate activation by physiological extracellular Ca^{2+} and Mg^{2+} levels results in a diminished PTH secretion in the parathyroid gland as well as a decreased reabsorption of both divalent cations in the TAL. A severe degree of hypocalcemia and hypomagnesemia is observed in patients with complete activation of the CaSR at physiologic serum Ca^{2+} and Mg^{2+} concentrations who may also exhibit a Bartter-like phenotype [46]. In these patients, CaSR activation inhibits TAL-mediated salt and divalent cation reabsorption to an extent that cannot be compensated in more distal nephron segments [46].

Genetic heterogeneity in autosomal-dominant hypocalcemia (**ADH2**) was demonstrated by the discovery of heterozygous missense mutations in *GNA11* encoding the accessory G-protein $G_{alpha\text{-}11}$ of the CaSR [47, 48].

Hypercalcemia

Clinical Findings

In contrast to hypocalcemia, hypercalcemia represents a rather uncommon finding in infancy and childhood but requires prompt diagnostic work-up and targeted therapy [49, 50]. Hypercalcemia is defined as ionized Ca^{2+} above 1.35 mmol/L, usually with concomitant elevation of total serum Ca^{2+} levels above 2.7 mmol/L. While most children with a mild degree of hypercalcemia remain asymptomatic, more severe hypercalcemia can lead to a serious clinical disease pattern that may even be life-threatening, especially in infants. Symptoms of hypercalcemia include failure to thrive, weight loss, dehydration, fever, muscular hypotonia, constipation, irritability, lethargy, and disturbed consciousness. Cardiovascular findings may comprise bradycardia, shortened QT interval, and arterial hypertension (Table 37.3).

An impairment of renal function by volume contraction can further limit renal Ca^{2+} elimination and therefore aggravate hypercalcemia. On the other hand, the increase of renal Ca^{2+} excretion in hypercalcemic conditions is a risk factor for the development of nephrocalcinosis and kidney stone formation.

Table 37.3 Symptoms of acute hypercalcemia

Neurology
  Muscle weakness
  Irritability/confusion
  Somnolence, stupor, coma
  Abnormal behaviour
  Headache
Gastrointestinal tract
  Loss of appetite
  Nausea/vomiting
  Constipation
  Abdominal cramping
  Pancreatitis
Kidneys and urinary tract
  Polyuria/polydipsia
  Dehydratation
  Nephrocalcinosis
  Nephro-/urolithiasis
Musculoskeletal system
  Bone pain
  Ectopic calcifications
Heart/cardiovascular system
  Shortened QT interval
  Cardiac arrhythmia
  Arterial hypertension

Diagnostic Workup

The assessment of past medical history should comprise medications including over-the-counter vitamin preparations and family history with a focus on disturbances in Ca^{2+} metabolism, renal disease and urolithiasis.

The etiology of hypercalcemia in children and especially infants significantly differs from that in adulthood where primary hyperparathyroidism and malignancy represent the most common underlying causes [51]. Especially in infants, rare hereditary disorders should be considered in the differential diagnosis [49].

The diagnostic work-up requires comprehensive laboratory testing including molecular genetics. Next to the parallel measurement of serum and urine electrolytes, the determination of PTH and vitamin D metabolites represents the most important element. Potential diagnostic parameters are summarized in Table 37.4.

Inappropriately normal or elevated levels of PTH point to a primary defect in the parathyroid

Table 37.4 Evaluation of hypercalcemia in children

Laboratory tests

Blood Ionized and total calcium
        Sodium, potassium, chloride, magnesium, phosphate
        Renal function tests
        Alkaline phosphatase
        Blood gases
        Intact parathyroid hormone (iPTH)
        Vitamin D metabolites (25-OH-D_3, 1,25-$(OH)_2$-D_3)
        Optional: PTH-related peptide (PTHrP)
        Vitamin A
        Angiotensin converting enzyme (ACE)
        FISH (Williams-Beuren-Syndrom)

Urine Calcium
        Sodium, potassium, chloride, magnesium, phosphate
        Creatinine
        ->Ca^{2+}/Crea ratio and tubular phosphate reabsorption (TRP)

Imaging studies

        Ultrasound examination of kidneys and urinary tract
        Optional:
        X-ray studies (long bones, thorax)
        Ultrasound of parathyroid glands

gland (Fig. 37.2). Next to primary hyperparathyroidism, which is extremely rare in infancy and childhood, hypercalcemia with elevated PTH might be caused by a hereditary disorder of the CaSR or associated proteins. In contrast to dominant activating CaSR mutations as present in ADH1 (see above), inactivating CaSR mutations may be present in either heterozygous or homozygous/compound-heterozygous state leading to Familial Hypocalciuric Hypercalcemia 1 (FHH1) and Neonatal Severe Hyperparathyroidism (NSHPT), respectively (see below). Genetic heterogeneity in FHH was demonstrated in 2013 by discovery of heterozygous mutations in *GNA11* (FHH2) and *AP2S1* (FHH3) [40, 47].

In face of an appropriate suppression of PTH, vitamin D metabolites should be evaluated. The determination of 25-OH-vitamin D_3 primarily helps to exclude overt vitamin D intoxication. While cut-off values vary in the literature, levels above 200 ng/mL are usually considered toxic [52]. Next, serum levels of active 1,25-$(OH)_2$-vitamin D_3 are of critical importance for further diagnostic considerations (Fig. 37.2). Elevated levels are not only observed in vitamin D poisoning, but also in disorders with extra-renal expression of 1α-hydroxylase including granulomatous disease or subcutaneous fat necrosis. In these disorders, 1α-hydroxylase (CYP27B1) is expressed by monocytes and, in contrast to renal tissue, not regulated by serum Ca^{2+}, PO_4^{3-}, PTH, and 1,25-$(OH)_2$-vitamin D_3. Finally, in hypercalcemic individuals with high levels of active 1,25-$(OH)_2$-vitamin D_3, hereditary disorders of vitamin D metabolism or renal phosphate handling should be considered (see below).

Treatment

Acute therapeutic measures in hypercalcemic patients primarily aim at the lowering of serum Ca^{2+} levels into the reference range resulting in a rapid relief of clinical symptoms. For this purpose, different pharmacologic approaches have been considered (Table 37.5).

Even before clarification of the underlying etiology, vitamin D supplements need to be

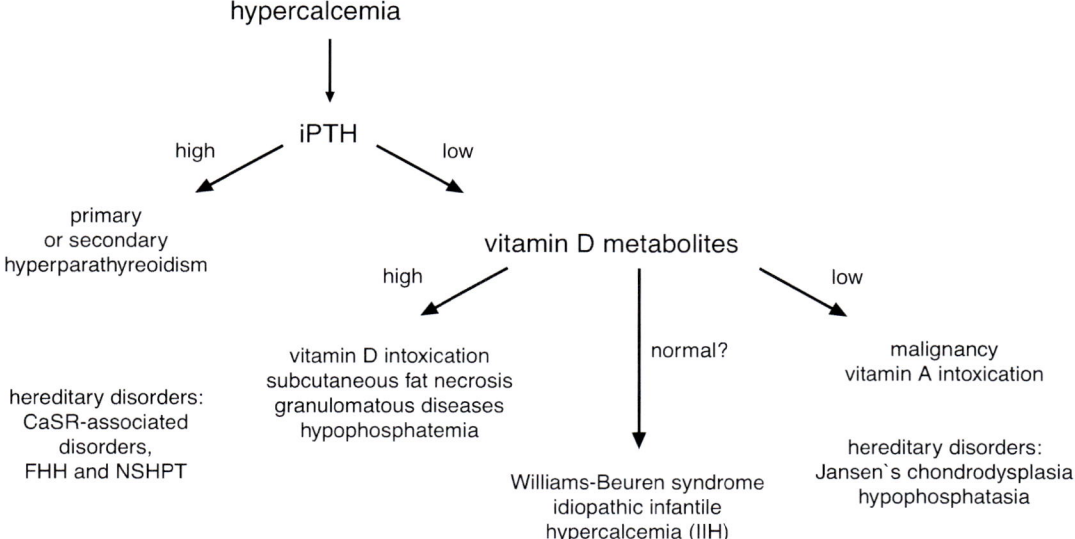

hypercalcemia

iPTH

high   low

primary
or secondary
hyperparathyreoidism

vitamin D metabolites

high   low

vitamin D intoxication   normal?   malignancy
subcutaneous fat necrosis   vitamin A intoxication
granulomatous diseases
hereditary disorders: hypophosphatemia
CaSR-associated
disorders,   hereditary disorders:
FHH and NSHPT   Jansen`s chondrodysplasia
                                                                        hypophosphatasia

Williams-Beuren syndrome
idiopathic infantile
hypercalcemia (IIH)

Fig. 37.2 Diagnostic approach in hypercalcemia in childhood. Central diagnostic steps are the determination of parathyroid hormone (PTH) and vitamin D-metabolites. Following this diagnostic approach, three major entities can be discerned: PTH-dependent hypercalcemia as pres-ent in primary hyperparathyroidism and in disorders due to inactivating mutation of the CaSR, vitamin D-induced hypercalcemia including idiopathic infantile hypercalcemia, and hypercalcemia due to third causes including also hypophosphatasia

Table 37.5 Therapy of hypercalcemia in children

General measures
  Stop of vitamin D supplementation
  Ca^{2+} restriction in enteral and parenteral nutrition
Specific measures
  Promotion of renal Ca^{2+} excretion
  – Furosemide 0.5–1 mg per kg body weight q6h
  Inhibition of enteral Ca^{2+} absorption/inhibition of vitamin D-conversion
  – Glucocorticoids, i.e. methylprednisolone ~1 mg/kg q.6h
  – Na$^+$-cellulose phosphate
  Inhibition of Ca^{2+} release from bone
  – Bisphosphonates, i.e. pamidronate 0.5–1 mg/kg over 4–6 h
  – Calcitonin 4–8 IU/kg body weight
  Inhibition of vitamin D-activation by 1α-hydroxylase
  – Imidazole derivates, i.e. ketoconazole 3–9 mg per kg body weight per day
  Hemodialysis/hemofiltration

stopped and, if appropriate, a low-Ca^{2+} diet should be implemented. Vigorous rehydration, usually performed via the intravenous route, is a key therapeutic strategy in hypercalcemia independent of etiology. Quantities up to twice the daily fluid requirements have been described.

Pharmacological treatment includes measures to decrease Ca^{2+} absorption from the intestine, to promote renal Ca^{2+} excretion, and to inhibit Ca^{2+} release from bone. To increase renal Ca^{2+} elimination loop diuretics that inhibit paracellular Ca^{2+} reabsorption in the TAL (such as furosemide) are widely used. A fast and effective approach to inhibit enteral Ca^{2+} absorption is the administration of glucocorticoids, i.e. prednisolone. Next to this intestinal effect, glucocorticoids also inhibit the conversion of 25-OH-vitamin D$_3$ into active 1,25-(OH)$_2$-vitamin D$_3$, an effect that is of special importance in vitamin D-mediated hypercalcemia. Sodium cellulose phosphate (SCP) is a non-absorbable cation exchange resin used for the removal of excess Ca^{2+} from the body [53]. It was initially used in patients with so-called absorptive hypercalciuria in order to decrease renal Ca^{2+} excretion and prevent stone formation [54]. In the acute phase of hypercalcemia calcitonin may be used because of its prompt and pronounced effect on serum Ca^{2+} levels, however, its therapeutic usefulness is limited by its short duration of action due to the development of end organ resistance. In the presence of intermediate to severe symptomatic hypercalcemia, bisphosphonates such as pamidronate may be used [55]. If bisphosphonate therapy is considered, it is important to have the diagnostic work-up completed in advance to avoid misinterpretation of diagnostic tests for PTH and vitamin D metabolites. A class of drugs that are specifically used in vitamin D-mediated hypercalcemia are imidazole derivates, such as ketoconazole [56]. Next to their antifungal effect these compounds also inhibit mammalian cytochrome P450 enzymes. Via inhibition of 1α-hydroxylase (CYP27B1) they are able to effectively lower serum levels of active $1,25\text{-}(OH)_2\text{-vitamin } D_3$ and consecutively normalize serum Ca^{2+} levels. In individual patients with extremely high serum Ca^{2+} levels hemofiltration and hemodialysis have been applied sucessfully [57].

Hypercalcemia with Inappropriately High PTH

Familial Hypocalciuric Hypercalcemia/ Neonatal Severe Hyperparathyroidism

Familial hypocalciuric hypercalcemia 1 (FHH1) and **neonatal severe hyperparathyroidism** (NSHPT) result from inactivating mutations of the CaSR present in either mono-allelic or bi-allelic state, respectively [58]. Genetic heterogeneity has been described in FHH with heterozygous variants in *GNA11* (**FHH2**) encoding accessory G-protein $G_{\alpha 11}$ of the CaSR and in *AP2S1* (**FHH3**) encoding adaptor protein σ1 involved in CaSR recycling from the plasma membrane [40, 47]. Therefore, all three subtypes of FHH share the pathophysiology of a decreased CaSR-mediated Ca^{2+} sensing. FHH patients typically present with mild to moderate hypercalcemia, accompanied by few if any symptoms, and often do not require treatment. However, the occurrence of pancreatitis and chondrocalcinosis has been described [59]. Urinary Ca^{2+} and Mg^{2+} excretion rates are markedly reduced and serum PTH levels are inappropriately high. In addition, affected individuals also show mild hypermagnesemia [60].

In contrast to FHH, patients with **NSHPT** with two mutant CaSR alleles usually present in early infancy with polyuria and dehydration due to severe symptomatic hypercalcemia (Table 37.9). Unrecognized and untreated, hyperparathyroidism and hypercalcemia result in skeletal deformities, extraosseous calcifications, and also severe neurodevelopmental deficit. Early treatment with partial to total parathyroidectomy therefore seems to be essential for outcome [61]. Serum PO_4^{3-} levels are typically low due to increased iPTH levels. Data on serum Mg^{2+} in NSHPT is sparse and contradictory [62]. However, elevations to levels around 50% above the reference range have been reported.

Hypercalcemia with Suppressed PTH and Inappropriately High $1,25\text{-}(OH)_2$- Vitamin D_3

Idiopathic Infantile Hypercalcemia

Idiopathic Infantile Hypercalcemia (IIH) was first decribed in the 1950s after an endemic occurrence in the United Kingdom (UK) [63, 64]. Affected infants present with typical symptoms of severe hypercalcemia. Concomitant hypercalciuria typically leads to the development of early nephrocalcinosis (Table 37.9). The laboratory analysis reveals serum Ca^{2+} levels up to 5 mmol/L. Intact PTH is suppressed while levels of active $1,25\text{-}(OH)_2\text{-vitamin } D_3$ are usually elevated or in the upper normal range. A role of exogenously administered vitamin D was suspected early on [65–67]. Some children exhibited a complex phenotype that became later known as the Williams Beuren syndrome [68, 69]. However, most hypercalcemic infants did not have syndromic features and were considered to be affected by a milder variant of the syndrome that was termed idiopathic infantile hypercalcemia (IIH) [63, 64].

The pathophysiology of IIH remained elusive until the discovery of loss-of-function mutations in the vitamin D catabolizing enzyme

25-OH-vitamin D_3-24-hydroxylase (CYP24A1) [70]. CYP24A1 is responsible for several sequential degradation steps that convert active 1,25-$(OH)_2$-vitamin D_3 into water soluble calcitroic acid [71, 72]. Loss-of-function mutations of *CYP24A1* lead to an accumulation and increased action of active 1,25-$(OH)_2$-vitamin D_3. Functional studies in vitro demonstrated a complete loss of enzyme function for most of the identified *CYP24A1* mutations [70]. In addition to the genetic analysis of the *CYP24A1* gene, the determination of 24-hydroxylated vitamin D metabolites by liquid chromatography/mass spectrometry (LC/MS) represents a quick and reliable test in the diagnosis of the disease [73].

The critical role of the cumulative dose of exogenous vitamin D is underscored by the following observations: Under the most commonly used dose of 500 IU vitamin D_3 per day, symptoms usually develop after several months. Higher doses of supplemental vitamin D most likely lead to an increased incidence of the disease in infancy and an earlier manifestation. Regimens using oral bolus doses of up to 600.000 IU provoke symptoms of acute vitamin D toxicity in infants with CYP24A1 deficiency while being tolerated well by healthy individuals [74]. Finally, omitting vitamin D supplementation in a genetically affected infant due to symptomatic disease in the older sibling prevented hypercalcemic episodes and the development of nephrocalcinosis [70].

After diagnosis of symptomatic hypercalcemia with inappropriately high levels of 1,25-$(OH)_2$-vitamin D_3, vitamin D prophylaxis is usually stopped and a low-Ca^{2+} diet might be instituted. The restriction of dietary Ca^{2+} has to be carefully monitored as it might lead to a defective mineralization of bone as well as an increased intestinal absorption of oxalate with subsequent risk of stone formation. Next to these immediate therapeutic measures, vigorous intravenous rehydration and a repertoire of strategies to reduce serum Ca^{2+} levels as described above are used (Table 37.5).

Currently, it remains an unanswered question, why many of the affected individuals after acute treatment in infancy do not show recurrence of symptomatic hypercalcemia during later life. Potentially, compensatory mechanisms, i.e. a down-regulation of 1α-hydroxylase (CYP27B1) are able to prevent an excessive activation of vitamin D. Laboratory parameters, i.e. suppressed PTH and inappropriately high values of 1,25-$(OH)_2$-vitamin D_3, are detectable for a long time during follow-up. However, nephrocalcinosis persists and together with recurrent nephrolithiasis might result in an impairment of renal function. Interestingly, since the initial description of *CYP24A1* mutations, several groups identified *CYP24A1* mutations also in adult patients with mild hypercalcemia, nephrocalcinosis, and recurrent kidney stone disease [75–77].

Genetic heterogeneity in IH was demonstrated by discovery of recessive mutations in *SLC34A1* encoding proximal-tubular sodium-phosphate co-transporter NaPi-IIa [78]. Patients with NaPi-IIa defects share phenotypic and biochemical features of patients with *CYP24A1* mutations but hypercalcemia is usually milder. In addition, they exhibit phosphate depletion and hypophosphatemia. The pathophysiology involves primary renal phosphate wasting, phosphate depletion, and suppression of the phosphaturic hormone FGF-23. FGF-23, next to its role in proximal-tubular phosphate reabsorption, negatively regulates vitamin D metabolism by inhibiting 1α-hydroxylase (*CYP27B1*) and promoting the degradation of active 1,25-$(OH)_2$-vitamin D_3 by 24-hydroxylase (*CYP24A1*) [78].

In addition to acute therapeutic measures also applied in patients with *CYP24A1* defects, hypercalcemic patients potentially benefit from PO_4^{3-} supplementation in order to control Ca^{2+} metabolism.

A significant subset of patients with NaPi-IIa defects may also be diagnosed with isolated early nephrocalcinosis or present later in childhood or adolescence with nephrolithiasis [79]. Of note, prenatally diagnosed renal calcifications due to *SLC34A1* mutations have even been described as a differential diagnosis for fetal hyperechogenic kidneys [80].

Very similar biochemical changes as in NaPi-IIa deficiency have also been reported in patients with *SLC34A3* defects encoding the closely related proximal-tubular sodium-phosphate co-transporter NaPi-IIc [81]. Mutations in *SLC34A3* have initially been described in patients with **hypophosphatemic rickets with hypercalciuria** (HHRH) [82, 83]. Whereas a clinical manifestation with hypercalcemia in infancy has not been reported yet in a patient with *SLC34A3* defect, patients with bi-allelicas well as mono-allelic *SLC34A3* mutations appear to commonly present with nephrocalcinosis and/or kidney stones [81]. As individuals with CYP24A1 defects, patients with NaPi-IIa and NaPI-IIc defects are at risk to develop chronic renal failure [84].

Magnesium Physiology

Mg^{2+} is the second most abundant intracellular cation in the body. As a cofactor for many enzymes, it is involved in energy metabolism and protein and nucleic acid synthesis. It also plays a critical role in the modulation of membrane transporters and in signal transduction. Under physiologic conditions, serum Mg^{2+} levels are maintained at almost constant values. Homeostasis depends on the balance between intestinal absorption and renal excretion. Mg^{2+} deficiency can result from reduced dietary intake, intestinal malabsorption or renal loss. The control of body Mg^{2+} homeostasis is primarily accomplished in the kidney tubules.

The daily dietary intake of Mg^{2+} varies substantially. Within physiologic ranges, diminished Mg^{2+} intake is balanced by enhanced Mg^{2+} absorption in the intestine and reduced renal excretion. These transport processes are regulated by metabolic and hormonal influences [85, 86]. The principal site of Mg^{2+} absorption is the small intestine, with smaller amounts being absorbed in the colon. Intestinal Mg^{2+} absorption occurs via two different pathways: a saturable active transcellular transport and a nonsaturable paracellular passive transport (Fig. 37.3a) [86, 87]. Saturation kinetics of the transcellular transport system are explained by the limited transport capacity of active transport. At low intraluminal concentrations Mg^{2+} is absorbed primarily via the active transcellular route and with rising concentrations via the paracellular pathway, yielding a curvilinear function for total absorption (Fig. 37.3b).

In the kidney, approximately 80% of total serum Mg^{2+} is filtered in the glomeruli, of which more than 95% is reabsorbed along the nephron. Mg^{2+} reabsorption differs in quantity and kinetics depending on the different nephron segments. 15–20% are reabsorbed in the proximal tubule of the adult kidney. Interestingly, the premature kidney of the newborn is able to reabsorb up to 70% of the filtered Mg^{2+} in this nephron segment [88].

From early childhood onward, the majority of Mg^{2+} (around 70%) is reabsorbed in the loop of Henle, especially in the cortical TAL. Transport in this segment is passive and paracellular, driven by the lumen-positive transepithelial voltage (Fig. 37.4a). Although only 5–10% of the filtered Mg^{2+} is reabsorbed in the distal convoluted tubule (DCT), this is the part of the nephron where the fine adjustment of renal excretion is accomplished. The reabsorption rate in the DCT defines the final urinary Mg^{2+} excretion as there is no significant uptake of Mg^{2+} in the collecting duct. Mg^{2+} transport in this part of the nephron is an active transcellular process (Fig. 37.4b). The apical entry into DCT cells is mediated by a specific and regulated Mg^{2+} channel driven by a favorable transmembrane voltage [89]. The mechanism of basolateral transport into the interstitium is unknown. Here, Mg^{2+} has to be extruded against an unfavourable electrochemical gradient. Most physiologic studies favor a Na^+-dependent exchange mechanism [90]. Mg^{2+} entry into DCT cells appears to be the rate-limiting step and the site of regulation. Finally, 3–5% of the filtered Mg^{2+} is excreted in the urine.

Fig. 37.3 Intestinal Mg²⁺ reabsorption. (**a**) Model of intestinal Mg²⁺ absorption via two independent pathways: passive absorption via the paracellular pathway and active, transcellular transport consisting of an apical entry through a putative Mg²⁺ channel and a basolateral exit mediated by a putative Na⁺–coupled exchange. (**b**) Kinetics of intestinal Mg²⁺ absorption in humans. Paracellular transport linearly rising with intraluminal concentrations (dotted line) and saturable active transcellular transport (dashed line) together yield a curvilinear function for net Mg²⁺ absorption (solid line)

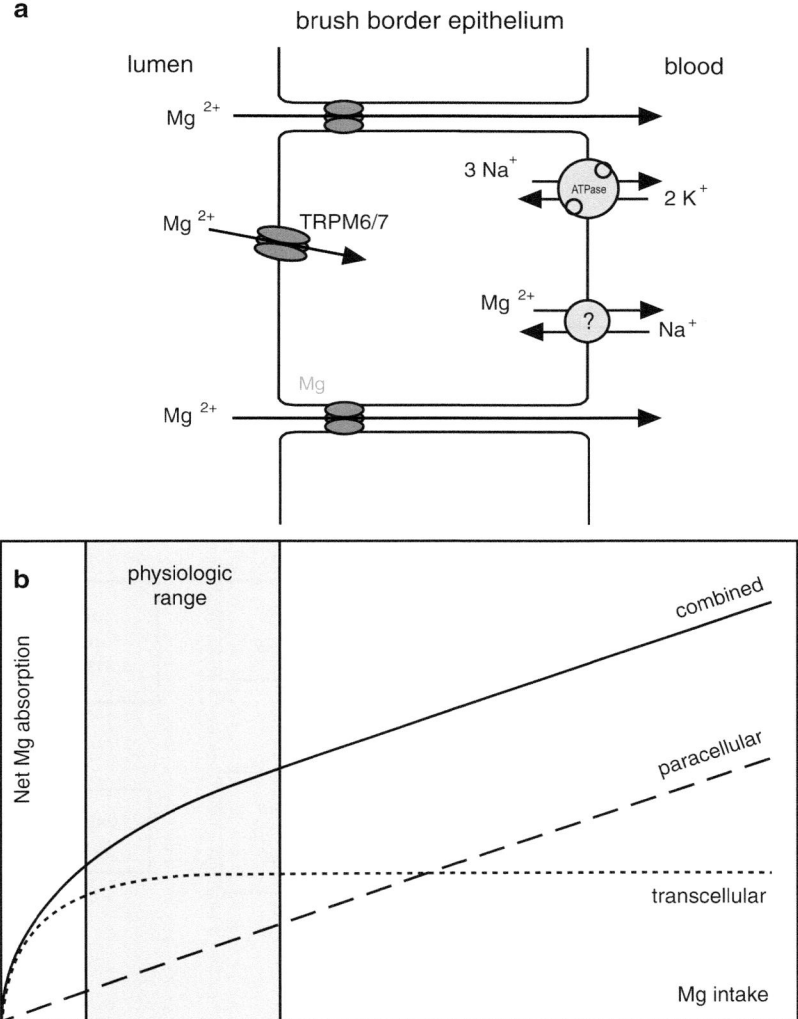

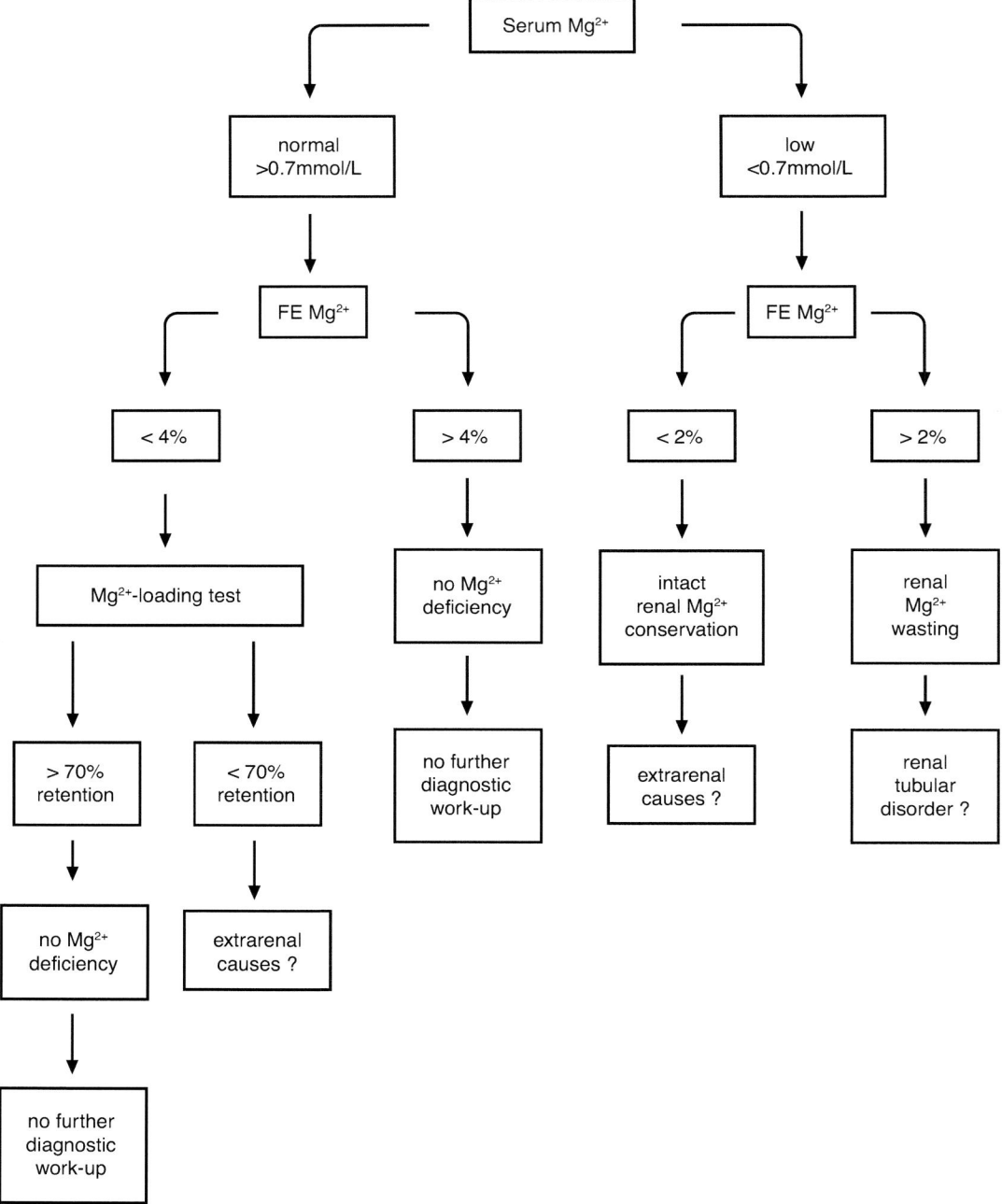

Fig. 37.4 Diagnostic workup in patients with suspected magnesium deficiency. In face of hypomagnesemia, the determination of urinary Mg^{2+} excretion allows for a distinction between renal Mg^{2+} wasting and extrarenal losses. In normomagnesemic individuals with low urinary magne-sium excretions, an increased retention of Mg^{2+} in the Mg^{2+}-loading test might indicate Mg^{2+} deficiency. This test, however, requires an intact renal Mg^{2+} conservation process

Magnesium Depletion

Mg^{2+} depletion usually occurs secondarily to another disease process or to a therapeutic agent. Some disorders that can be associated with Mg^{2+} depletion are summarized in Table 37.6 [91]. Mg^{2+} may be lost via the gastrointestinal tract, either by excessive loss of secreted fluids or impaired absorption of both dietary and endogenous Mg^{2+}. Mg^{2+} depletion is common in patients with acute or chronic diarrhea. Malabsorption syndromes such as celiac disease may also result in Mg^{2+} deficiency. Also, acute severe pancreatitis may be associated with hypomagnesemia.

Excessive excretion of Mg^{2+} into the urine is another cause of Mg^{2+} depletion. Renal Mg^{2+} excretion is proportional to tubular fluid flow as well as to Na^+ and Ca^{2+} excretion. Therefore, both chronic intravenous fluid therapy with Na^+-

Table 37.6 Main causes of magnesium deficiency

Gastrointestinal loss
    Prolonged nasogastric suction/vomiting
    Acute and chronic diarrhea
    Malabsorption syndromes (e.g., celiac disease)
    Extensive bowel resection
    Intestinal and biliary fistulas
    Acute hemorrhagic pancreatitis
Renal loss
    Chronic parenteral fluid therapy
    Osmotic diuresis (e.g. due to presence of glucose in diabetes mellitus)
    Hypercalcemia
    Drugs (e.g. diuretics, aminoglycosides, calcineurin inhibitors)
    Alcohol
    Metabolic acidosis
    Renal diseases
    – Chronic pyelonephritis, interstitial nephritis, and glomerulonephritis
    – Polyuria after acute renal failure
    – Post-obstructive nephropathy
    – Renal tubular acidosis
    – After kidney transplantation
    Inherited tubular diseases
    Endocrine disorders
    – Hyperparathyroidism
    – Hyperthyroidism
    – Hyperaldosteronism
    Syndrome of inappropriate secretion of antidiuretic hormone (SIADH)

containing fluids and disorders in which there is extracellular volume expansion may result in Mg^{2+} depletion. Hypercalcemia and hypercalciuria have been shown to decrease renal Mg^{2+} reabsorption and are probably the cause of excessive renal Mg^{2+} excretion and hypomagnesemia observed in many hypercalcemic states. A large variety of pharmacological agents also cause renal Mg^{2+} wasting and Mg^{2+} depletion (see below). Various renal diseases, e.g. chronic pyelonephritis or post-obstructive nephropathy may also be accompanied by Mg^{2+} losses.

During infancy and childhood, a substantial proportion of patients receiving medical attention for signs of hypomagnesemia are affected by inherited renal disorders associated with Mg^{2+} wasting. In these disorders, hypomagnesemia may either be the leading symptom or may be part of a complex phenotype resulting from tubular dysfunction. Finally, Mg^{2+} wasting may be caused by endocrine disorders, e.g. by hyperparathyroidism because of the hypercalcemia or within the context of a SIADH state. In SIADH, Mg^{2+} losses are explained by the volume expansion.

Manifestations of Hypomagnesemia

Mg^{2+} deficiency and hypomagnesemia often remain asymptomatic. Clinical symptoms are mostly not very specific and Mg^{2+} deficiency is frequently associated with other electrolyte abnormalities. The biochemical and physiologic manifestations of severe Mg^{2+} depletion are summarized in Table 37.7.

Hypokalemia

A common accompanying feature of Mg^{2+} depletion is hypokalemia [91]. During Mg^{2+} depletion, there is loss of K^+ from the cell with intracellular K^+ depletion, which is enhanced due to the inability of the kidney to conserve K^+. Attempts to replete the K^+ deficit with K^+ therapy alone may not be successful without simultaneous Mg^{2+}

Table 37.7 Major manifestations of magnesium depletion

Biochemical
   Hypokalemia
   Excessive renal potassium excretion
   Decreased intracellular potassium
   Hypocalcemia
   Impaired parathyroid hormone (PTH) secretion
   Renal and skeletal resistance to PTH
   Resistance to vitamin D
Neuromuscular
   Positive Chvostek's and Trousseau's sign
   Spontaneous carpal-pedal spasm
   Seizures
   Vertigo, ataxia, nystagmus, athetoid and chorioform movements
   Muscular weakness, tremor, fasciculation and wasting
   Psychiatric: depression, psychosis
Cardiovascular
   Electrocardiographic abnormalities
      Prolonged PR- and QT-intervals
      U-waves
Cardiac arrhythmia
   Atrial tachycardia, fibrillations
   "Torsades de pointes"
Gastrointestinal
   Nausea, vomiting
   Anorexia

supplementation. K^+ depletion may contribute to the electrocardiographic findings and cardiac arrhythmias observed in Mg^{2+} deficiency. Secondary K^+ depletion in the presence of Mg^{2+} deficiency must be differentiated from renal tubular disorders mainly affecting the distal convoluted tubule (DCT) that lead to combined losses of both cations, such as Gitelman syndrome (see below).

Hypocalcemia

Hypocalcemia is a common finding in moderate to severe Mg^{2+} depletion and may be a major contributing factor to the increased neuromuscular excitability often present in Mg^{2+}-depleted patients. The pathogenesis of hypocalcemia is multifactorial. Impaired parathyroid hormone (PTH) secretion appears to be a major factor in hypomagnesemia-induced hypocalcemia. Serum

PTH concentrations are usually low in these patients, and Mg^{2+} administration will immediately stimulate PTH secretion. Patients with hypocalcemia due to Mg^{2+} depletion also exhibit both renal and skeletal resistance to exogenously administered PTH, as manifested by subnormal urinary cyclic AMP (cAMP) and phosphate excretion and a diminished calcemic response. All these effects are reversed following several days of Mg^{2+} therapy. The paradoxical inhibition of PTH secretion in patients with severe hypomagnesemia was already described in the 1970s [92]. Later, the failure of the parathyroid gland to synthesize and secrete PTH was attributed to a defect in G-protein signaling within parathyroid cells [93]. As a functional consequence, the intracellular signaling pathways responsible for Ca^{2+}-sensing Receptor (CaSR)-mediated inhibition of PTH secretion are enhanced including the generation of inositol phosphates and the inhibition of cAMP. Because cAMP is also an important second messenger mediating PTH effects in kidney and bone, it was also postulated that there may be a defect in adenylate cyclase function as Mg^{2+} is both an essential part of the substrate (Mg-ATP) as well as an important co-factor for catalytic activity [94].

Vitamin D metabolism and action may also be abnormal in hypocalcemic Mg^{2+}-deficient patients. Resistance to vitamin D therapy has been reported in such cases. This resistance may be due to impaired metabolism of vitamin D because plasma concentrations of 1,25-dihydroxyvitamin D_3 are low. Because PTH is a major stimulator of 1,25-dihydroxyvitamin D_3 synthesis, the decrease in PTH secretion observed in hypomagnesemia and hypocalcemia may also be a cause of the impaired metabolism of vitamin D.

Neuromuscular Manifestations

Neuromuscular hyperexcitability may be the prominent complaint of patients with Mg^{2+} deficiency. Tetany and muscle cramps may be present. Generalized seizures may also occur. Other neuromuscular signs may include dizziness, disequilibrium, muscular tremor, wasting, and weakness [91]. Although hypocalcemia often contributes to the neurologic signs, hypomagnesemia without hypocalcemia has also been reported to result in neuromuscular hyperexcitability.

Cardiovascular Manifestations

Mg^{2+} depletion may also result in electrocardiographic abnormalities as well as in cardiac arrhythmias [95], which may be manifested by tachycardia, premature beats, or a totally irregular cardiac rhythm (fibrillation). Cardiac arrhythmia is also known to occur during K^+ depletion; therefore, the effect of Mg^{2+} deficiency on K^+ loss may be a contributing factor (see section on Gitelman syndrome below) [91].

Clinical Assessment of Magnesium Deficiency

Although Mg^{2+} is an abundant cation in the body, more than 99% of it are located either intracellularly or in bone. The less than 1% of total Mg^{2+} present in the body fluids is the most easily accessible compartment for clinical testing, and the total serum Mg^{2+} concentration is the most widely used measure of Mg^{2+} status, although its limitations in reflecting Mg^{2+} deficiency are well recognized [96]. The reference range for normal total serum Mg^{2+} concentration is a subject of ongoing debate, but concentrations of 0.7–1.1 mmol/L are widely accepted. Because the measurement of serum Mg^{2+} concentration does not necessarily reflect the true total body Mg^{2+} content, it has been suggested that measurement of ionized serum Mg^{2+} or intracellular Mg^{2+} concentrations might provide more precise information on Mg^{2+} status. However, the relevance of such measurements to body Mg^{2+} stores has been questioned because the ionized serum Mg^{2+} and intracellular Mg^{2+} did not correlate with tissue Mg^{2+} and the correlation with the results of Mg^{2+} retention tests was contradictory [97–99].

Hypomagnesemia develops late in the course of Mg^{2+} deficiency and intracellular Mg^{2+} depletion may be present despite normal serum Mg^{2+} levels. Due to the kidney's ability to sensitively adapt its Mg^{2+} transport rate to imminent deficiency, the urinary Mg^{2+} excretion rate is important in the assessment of the Mg^{2+} status. In hypomagnesemic patients, urinary Mg^{2+} excretion rates help to discern renal Mg^{2+} wasting from extrarenal losses. In the presence of hypomagnesemia, the 24-h Mg^{2+} excretion is expected to decrease below 1 mmol [100]. Mg^{2+}/creatinine ratios and fractional Mg^{2+} excretions have also been advocated as indicators of evolving Mg^{2+} deficiency [101, 102]. However, the interpretation of these results seems to be limited due to intra- and inter-individual variability [103, 104].

In patients at risk for Mg^{2+} deficiency but with normal serum Mg^{2+} levels, the Mg^{2+} status can be further evaluated by determining the amount of Mg^{2+} excreted in the urine following an intravenous infusion of Mg^{2+}. This procedure has been described as "parenteral Mg^{2+} loading test" and is still the gold standard for the evaluation of the body Mg^{2+} status [96, 98]. Normal subjects excrete at least 80% of an intravenous Mg^{2+} load within 24 h, whereas patients with Mg^{2+} deficiency excrete much less. The Mg^{2+} loading test, however, requires normal renal handling of Mg^{2+}.

Hereditary Disorders of Mg^{2+} Handling

Recent advances in molecular genetics of hereditary hypomagnesemia substantiated the role of a variety of genes and their encoded proteins in human epithelial Mg^{2+} transport (Table 37.8). The knowledge of underlying genetic defects helps to distinguish different clinical subtypes of hereditary disorders of Mg^{2+} homeostasis.

By careful clinical observation and additional biochemical parameters, the different disease entities can already be distinguished clinically and biochemically in many cases, even if there might be a considerable overlap in phenotypic characteristics (Table 37.9).

Table 37.8 Inherited disorders of renal Ca^{2+} and Mg^{2+} handling

Thick ascending limb (TAL)	OMIM #	Inheritance	Gene	Protein
Autosomal dominant hypoparathyroidism 1 (ADH1)	601198	AD	CASR	CaSR, Ca^{2+}/Mg^{2+} sensing receptor
Autosomal dominant hypoparathyroidism 2 (ADH2)	615361	AD	GNA11	G-protein α-11
Familial hypocalciuric hypercalcemia 1 (FHH1)	145980	AD	CASR	CaSR, Ca^{2+}/Mg^{2+} sensing receptor
Familial hypocalciuric hypercalcemia 2 (FHH2)	145981	AD	GNA11	G-protein α-11
Familial hypocalciuric hypercalcemia 3 (FHH3)	600740	AD	AP2S1	Adaptor protein 2 σ-subunit
Neonatal severe hyperparathyroidism (NSHPT)	239200	AR	CASR	CaSR, Ca^{2+}/Mg^{2+} sensing receptor
Familial hypomagnesemia with hypercalciuria/ nephrocalcinosis (FHHNC) (HOMG3)	248250	AR	CLDN16	Claudin-16, tight junction protein
Familial hypomagnesemia with hypercalciuria/ nephrocalcinosis (FHHNC) and severe ocular involvement (HOMG5)	248190	AR	CLDN19	Claudin-19, tight junction protein
Hypohidrosis, electrolyte imbalance, lacrimal gland dysfunction, ichthyosis, and xerodermia (HELIX)	617671	AR	CLDN10	Claudin-10, tight junction protein
Distal convoluted tubule (DCT)	**OMIM #**	**Inheritance**	**Gene**	**Protein**
Gitelman syndrome (GS)	263800	AR	SLC12A3	NCC, NaCl cotransporter
EAST/SeSAME syndrome	612780	AR	KCNJ10	KCNJ10, basolateral potassium channel
Hypomagnesemia with secondary hypocalcemia (HSH) (HOMG1)	602014	AR	TRPM6	TRPM6, ion channel subunit
Hypomagnesemia, seizures, and mental retardation 2 (HOMGSMR2)	618314	AD	ATP1A1	α1-subunit of the Na^+-K^+-ATPase
Isolated dominant hypomagnesemia (IDH) (HOMG2)	154020	AD	FXYD2	γ-subunit of the Na^+-K^+-ATPase
Hypomagnesemia, episodic ataxia/myokymia syndrome	160120	AD	KCNA1	Kv1.1, apical potassium channel
Isolated recessive hypomagnesemia (IRH)(HOMG4)	611718	AR	EGF	Pro-EGF (epidermal growth factor)
Hypomagnesemia, seizures, and mental retardation 1 (HOMGSMR1)	616418	AR, AD	CNNM2	CNNM2, Cyclin M2
HNF1α nephropathy	137920	AD	HNF1B	HNF1beta, transcription factor
Transient neonatal hyperphenylalaninemia	264070	AR	PCBD1	PCBD1, tetrahydrobioterin metabolism
Hypomagnesemia/metabolic syndrome	500005	mito	MTTI	Mitochondrial tRNA (Isoleucin)

Table 37.9 Clinical and biochemical characteristics of inherited Ca^{2+} and Mg^{2+} disorders

Disorder	Age at onset	Serum Mg^{2+}	Serum Ca^{2+}	Serum K^+	Blood pH	Urine Mg^{2+}	Urine Ca^{2+}	Nephro-calcinosis	Renal stones
Autosomal dominant hypoparathyroidism (ADH)	Infancy	↓	↓	N	N or ↑	↑	↑–↑↑	Yes[a]	Yes[a]
Familial hypocalciuric hypercalcemia (FHH)	Often asymptomatic	N to ↑	↑	N	N	↓	↓	No	?
Neonatal severe hyperparathyroidism (NSHPT)	Infancy	N to ↑	↑↑↑	N	N	↓	↓	No	?
Infantile hypercalcemia	Infancy	N	↑↑↑	N	N	?	↑↑	Yes	Yes
Familial hypomagnesemia with hypercalciuria/ nephrocalcinosis (FHHNC)	Childhood	↓	N	N	N or ↓	↑↑	↑↑	Yes	Yes
HELIX syndrome, CLDN10 tubulopathy	Childhood to adulthood	↓	N or ↑	↓	↑	↓	↓	No	No
Gitelman syndrome (GS)	Adolescence	↓	N	↓	↑	↑	↓	No	No
EAST/SeSAME syndrome	Infancy	↓	N	↓	↑	↑	↓	No	No
Hypomagnesemia with secondary hypocalcemia (HSH)	Infancy	↓↓↓	↓	N	N	↑	N	No	No
Hypomagnesemia, seizures, and mental retardation 2	Infancy	↓↓↓	N	N or ↓	N	↑↑	N	No	No
Isolated dominant hypomagnesemia (IDH)	Childhood	↓	N	N	N	↑	↓	No	No
Isolated recessive hypomagnesemia (IRH)	Childhood	↓	N	N	N	↑	N	No	No
Hypomagnesemia, seizures, and mental retardation 1	Infancy to adolescence	↓↓	N	N	N	↑	N	No	No
HNF1B nephropathy	Childhood	↓	N	N	N	↑	↓	No	No
Transient neonatal hyperphenylalaninemia	Adulthood	↓	N	N	N	↑	↓	No	No
Hypomagnesemia/metabolic syndrome	Adulthood	↓	N	↓	N	↑	↓	No	No

[a] Frequent complication under therapy with Ca^{2+} and vitamin D

Familial Hypomagnesemia with Hypercalciuria and Nephrocalcinosis

Familial hypomagnesemia with hypercalciuria and nephrocalcinosis (**FHHNC**) is an autosomal recessive disorder caused by mutations in two members of the claudin gene family which encode the tight junction proteins claudin-16 and claudin-19 [105, 106]. More than 150 patients have been reported to date, allowing a comprehensive characterization of the clinical spectrum [107–111]. Due to excessive renal Mg^{2+} and Ca^{2+} wasting, affected individuals almost uniformly develop the characteristic triad of hypomagnesemia, hypercalciuria, and nephrocalcinosis that gave the disease its name. Additional biochemical abnormalities include elevated PTH levels before the onset of chronic renal failure, hypocitraturia, and hyperuricemia. The majority of patients clinically present during early childhood with recurrent urinary tract infections, polyuria/polydipsia, nephrolithiasis, and/or failure to thrive. Clinical symptoms of severe hypomagnesemia such as seizures and muscular tetany are less common. The clinical course of FHHNC patients is complicated by the development of chronic renal failure (CRF) early in life. A considerable number of patients exhibit a marked decline in GFR (<60 mL/min per 1.73 m^2) already at the time of diagnosis and about one third of patients develops ESRD during adolescence. Hypomagnesemia may completely disappear with the decline of GFR due to a reduction in filtered Mg^{2+} that limits urinary Mg^{2+} losses. Whereas the renal phenotype is almost identical in carriers of *CLDN16* and *CLDN19* mutations, ocular involvement including severe myopia, nystagmus, or macular coloboma are observed only in patients with *CLDN19* mutations [106, 107, 109, 110].

Claudins are crucial components of tight junctions and the individual composition of tight junctions strands with different claudin members confers the characteristic properties of different epithelia regarding paracellular permeability and/or transepithelial resistance. Within the tight junction barrier, claudins positioned on neigbouring cells are thought to form charge-selective pores.

Claudin-16 and claudin-19 colocalize at tight junctions of the TAL [106]. Tight-junction strands in this part of the renal tubule also express other members of the claudin family including claudin-3, claudin-10 and claudin-18. These other claudins maintain the barrier function of the tight junction complex also in the absence of claudin-16 and -19, however, claudin-16 and -19 depleted tight junctions display a loss in cation permselectivity [112]. Mice deficient in Claudin-16 or claudin-19 also exhibit increased renal Na^+ and K^+ losses in addition to impaired renal Mg^{2+} and Ca^{2+} handling [113].

The majority of *CLDN16* and *CLDN19* mutations reported in FHHNC are missense mutations affecting the transmembrane domains and the extracellular loops with a particular clustering in the first extracellular loop. Within this domain, patients originating from Germany or Eastern European countries exhibit a common mutation (p.L151F) due to a founder effect [108].

Progressive renal failure in FHHNC is thought to be a consequence of massive urinary Ca^{2+} wasting and nephrocalcinosis. Individuals with bi-allelic loss-of-function mutations in *CLDN16* exhibit a younger age at manifestation and a more rapid renal function loss compared to patients with at least one allele with residual claudin-16 function [114]. Of note, first degree relatives of FHHNC patients appear to have a high incidence of hypercalciuria, nephrolithiasis and/or nephrocalcinosis [107, 108]. Moreover, a tendency towards mild hypomagnesemia has been observed in these heterozygous family members [115]. Thus, one might speculate that *CLDN16* mutations could be involved in idiopathic hypercalciuric stone formation. Finally, a homozygous *CLDN16* mutation (p.T303R) affecting the C-terminal PDZ domain has been identified in two families with isolated hypercalciuria and nephrocalcinosis without abnormalities in renal Mg^{2+} handling [116]. Notably, hypercalciuria disappeared during follow-up and urinary Ca^{2+} levels reached normal values beyond puberty.

In addition to oral Mg^{2+} supplementation, **therapy** aims at a reduction of Ca^{2+} excretion in order to prevent the progression of nephrocalcinosis and stone formation because the degree of renal calcifications has been correlated with progression of chronic renal failure [107]. In a short term study, thiazides effectively reduced urinary Ca^{2+} excretion in FHHNC patients [117]. However, these therapeutic strategies have not been shown yet to significantly influence the progression of renal failure. Supportive therapy is important for the protection of kidney function and should include provision of sufficient fluids and effective treatment of stone formation and bacterial colonization. As expected, renal transplantation is performed without evidence of recurrence of the disease because the primary defect resides in the kidney.

Gitelman Syndrome

Gitelman syndrome (GS) is the most frequent inherited salt wasting disorder with an estimated prevalence of approximately 1:40.000 [118]. It is caused by mutations in the *SLC12A3* gene coding for the thiazide-sensitive NaCl- cotransporter, NCC [119]. The NCC is exclusively expressed at the apical membrane of the DCT where it reabsorbs approximately 5–10% of the filtered NaCl (Fig. 37.5). The cardinal biochemical features of GS are persistent hypokalemia and metabolic alkalosis together with hypomagnesemia and hypocalciuria [120, 121]. Hundreds of GS patients have been reported to date, allowing for a thorough clinical description of the phenotype as well as for an extensive analysis of the mutational spectrum in the *SLC12A3* gene [122–126].

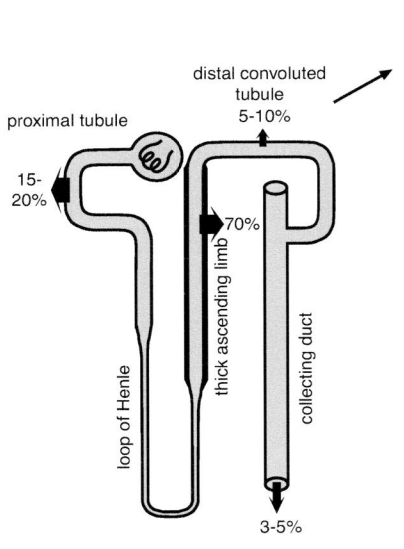

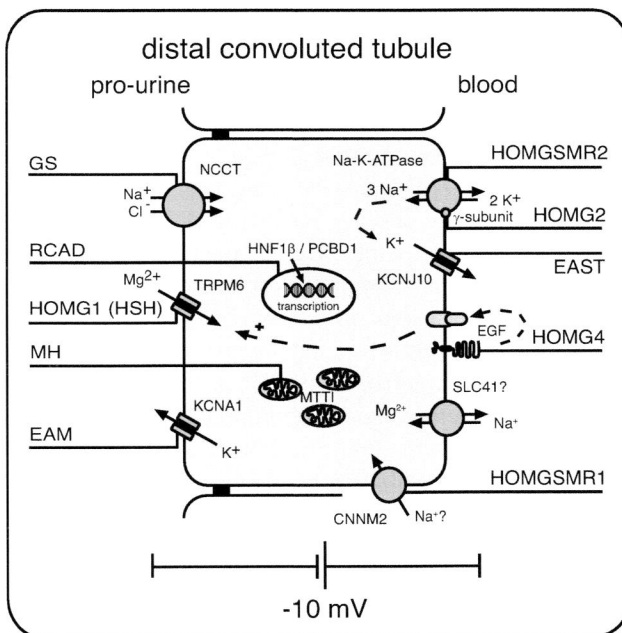

Fig. 37.5 Mg^{2+} reabsorption in the distal convoluted tubule. Mg^{2+} is actively reabsorbed via the transcellular pathway involving an apical entry step through a Mg^{2+}-permeable ion channel (TRPM6) and a basolateral exit, presumably mediated by a Na^+-coupled exchange mechanism. Mg^{2+} reabsorption in the DCT is dependent on transcellular salt reabsorption via NCC, basolateral Na^+/ K^+-ATPase activity, and K^+ recycling. It is regulated by basolateral EGF and the putative Mg^{2+} sensor CNNM2. Furthermore, Mg^{2+} transport rates are influenced by cellular energy metabolism (mitochondrial function) and expression levels of transport proteins (regulated by HNF1B). The respective hereditary defects are indicated

A consensus and guidance document concerning the diagnostic criteria, clinical workup, genetic testing, treatment, and long-term follow-up of patients with GS was recently published to which the reader should refer if diagnosing or treating a GS patient [127].

The initial presentation of GS most frequently occurs at school age or later with the characteristic symptoms being muscular weakness, cramps, and fatigue [128]. However, severe manifestations with early onset of disease, growth retardation, chondrocalcinosis, tetany, rhabdomyolysis, seizures, or ventricular arrhythmia have been reported [122, 129]. On the other hand, patients are frequently diagnosed accidentally while searching medical consultation for unrelated reasons, because of growth retardation, constipation or enuresis. A thorough past medical history of such patients commonly reveals long-standing salt craving [122]. Typically, urinary concentrating ability is not affected. Laboratory examination shows the characteristic constellation of metabolic alkalosis, low-normal Cl^- levels, hypokalemia, and hypomagnesemia; urine analysis reveals hypocalciuria [130]. Family studies demonstrated electrolyte imbalances present since infancy despite the absence of obvious clinical signs and symptoms in the affected infant [131].

Of note, the combination of hypokalemia and hypomagnesemia exerts an exceptionally unfavorable effect on cardiac excitability, which puts these patients at high risk for cardiac arrhythmia [132, 133]. Therefore, next to appropriate potassium and magnesium supplementation, the recognition of other possible triggering mechanisms as well as the avoidance of drugs that aggravate K^+ and Mg^{2+} depletion or prolong the QT-interval appears to be critical. Respective tables of drugs that should be avoided are available online (www.crediblemeds.org).

The pathognomonic feature of Gitelman syndrome is the dissociation of renal Ca^{2+} and Mg^{2+} handling, with low urinary Ca^{2+} and high urinary Mg^{2+} levels. Subsequent hypomagnesemia causes neuromuscular irritability and tetany. Decreased renal Ca^{2+} elimination together with Mg^{2+} deficiency favors deposition of mineral Ca^{2+} as demonstrated by increased bone density as well as chondrocalcinosis [134].

Although the combination of hypomagnesemia and hypocalciuria is typical for NCC deficiency, this finding is neither specific nor universal. Clinical observations in NCC deficient patients disclosed intra- and inter-individual variations in urinary Ca^{2+} concentrations which can be attributed to gender, age-related conditions of bone metabolism, intake of Mg^{2+} supplements, changes in diuresis and urinary osmolality, respectively. Likewise, hypomagnesemia might not be present from the beginning. Renal Mg^{2+} loss can be balanced temporarily by Mg^{2+} release from bone and muscle stores as well as by an increase of intestinal Mg^{2+} reabsorption. The mechanisms compromising distal Mg^{2+} reabsorption and favoring reabsorption of Ca^{2+} are not yet completely understood.

In contrast to TAL defects, disturbed salt reabsorption along the DCT does not affect the tubulo-glomerular feedback and thus is not associated with increased renal prostaglandin synthesis [135]. Accordingly, NSAIDs are of little benefit in Gitelman syndrome. Substitution of KCl and Mg^{2+} is therefore of prime importance in the treatment of this disorder. As pointed out above, avoidance of factors which in addition to hypokalemia and hypomagnesemia might affect cardiac excitability (in particular QT-time prolonging drugs) is mandatory to prevent life-threatening cardiac arrhythmia.

EAST/SeSAME Syndrome

A clinical syndrome with autosomal recessive inheritance combining epilepsy, ataxia, sensorineural deafness and renal salt wasting with/without mental retardation was first described in 2009 under the acronyms EAST or SeSAME syndrome [136, 137]. Patients usually present early in infancy with generalized tonic–clonic seizures, speech and motor delay, as well as ataxia leading to an inability to walk, intention tremor, and dysdiadochokinesis. In addition, they exhibit a variable degree of hearing impairment [138]. The neurological features and hearing impairment are usually non-progressive [139]. Renal salt wasting is often recognized later during the course of the disease. Closely resembling GS, the renal phenotype includes the combination of hypokalemic alkalosis, hypomagnesemia and hypocalciuria.

EAST/SeSAME syndrome is caused by loss-of-function mutations in the *KCNJ10* gene encoding the inwardly-rectifying K⁺-channel KCNJ10 (Kir4.1) [136, 137]. The expression pattern of KCNJ10 fits to the disease phenotype with highest expression in brain, the stria vascularis of the inner ear, and in the distal nephron, especially in the DCT (Fig. 37.5). Here, KCNJ10 is localized at the basolateral membrane of DCT cells and supposed to function in collaboration with Na⁺-K⁺-ATPase as it might allow for a recycling of K⁺ ions entering the tubular cells in countermove for the extruded Na⁺ [137]. Loss of KCNJ10 function most likely leads to a depolarization of the basolateral membrane and thereby to a reduction of the driving force for basolateral anion channels as well as sodium-coupled exchangers. By this mechanism, KCNJ10 defects might also affect the putative Na⁺/Mg²⁺ exchanger and possibly explain the Mg²⁺ wasting observed in EAST/SeSAME syndrome.

As in patients with Gitelman syndrome, medical treatment of EAST/SeSAME patients regarding the renal phenotype mainly comprises potassium and magnesium supplementation. In individual adult patients, persistent hypokalemia despite supplementation has been treated with spironolactone in order to prevent frequent hospitalisations [140]. Seizures typically respond well to initial anti-epileptic treatment but may recur at later age. Finally, ataxia remains a major debilitating disease feature.

Hypomagnesemia with Secondary Hypocalcemia

Hypomagnesemia with secondary hypocalcemia (HSH) is a rare recessive disorder that manifests in early infancy with generalized seizures or other symptoms of increased neuromuscular excitability [141]. Biochemical abnormalities include extremely low serum Mg²⁺ (about 0.2 mmol/L) and low serum Ca²⁺ levels. Hypocalcemia is thought to result from an impaired synthesis and/or release of PTH in the presence of severe hypomagnesemia [92]. The failure of the parathyroid gland to synthesize and secrete parathyroid hormone has been attributed to a defect in g-protein signalling within parathyroid cells required for CaSR-mediated stimulation of PTH release [93].

Transport studies in HSH patients pointed to a primary defect in intestinal Mg²⁺ absorption [142, 143]. However, in some patients an additional renal leak for Mg²⁺ was suspected [144]. In 2002, recessive loss of function mutations in TRPM6 encoding a member of the transient receptor potential (TRP) family of ion channels were discovered as the underlying genetic defect [145, 146]. To date, mutations in *TRPM6* have been identified in more than 50 families affected by HSH [145–149]. The mutational spectrum mainly comprises truncating mutations. In addition, a number of missense mutations have been described for which functional analyses also indicated a complete loss-of-function [145, 147, 149, 150].

TRPM6 is expressed along the intestine (duodenum, jejunum, ileum, colon) as well as in the DCT of the kidney (Fig. 37.5) [145].

In the intestine, intraluminal Mg²⁺ concentrations and rates of Mg²⁺ absorption show a curvilinear relationship presumably reflecting two transport processes working in-parallel: an active and saturable transcellular transport essential at low intraluminal Mg²⁺ concentrations and a passive paracellular Mg²⁺ absorption gaining importance at higher intraluminal Mg²⁺ concentrations [87]. The observation that in HSH patients the substitution of high oral doses of Mg²⁺ achieves at least subnormal serum Mg²⁺ levels supports the hypothesis of two independent intestinal transport systems for Mg²⁺. By participating in the formation of apical magnesium-permeable ion channels, TRPM6 probably represents a molecular component of active transcellular Mg²⁺ transport. An increased intraluminal Mg²⁺ concentration (by increased oral intake) enables to compensate for the defect in active transcellular transport by increasing absorption via the passive paracellular pathway (Fig. 37.1).

In the kidney, TRPM6 is expressed predominantly in the DCT arguing for an important role of renal Mg^{2+} wasting for the pathogenesis of HSH [151]. This is also supported by intravenous Mg^{2+} loading tests in HSH patients, which disclosed a considerable renal Mg^{2+} leak albeit still being hypomagnesemic [146].

Hypocalcemia in patients with HSH is resistant to treatment with Ca^{2+} or vitamin D. Relief of clinical symptoms, normocalcemia, and normalization of PTH levels are only achieved by administration of high doses of Mg^{2+} [152]. Oral magnesium supplementation is preferentially performed with organic magnesium compounds (i.e. Mg-citrate, -aspartate, or -gluconate), doses vary between 0.5 and 4 mmol/kg/day. Serum magnesium levels usually remain in the subnormal range despite adequate treatment, but usually enable an undisturbed physical and mental development. However, delayed diagnosis or noncompliance with treatment can be fatal or result in permanent neurological damage.

Hypomagnesemia, Refractory Seizures and Mental Retardation Type 2

Heterozygous de-novo mutations in the *ATP1A1* gene encoding the α1-subunit of Na^+K^+-ATPase have recently been described in three children with severe hypomagnesemia due to renal magnesium wasting [153]. The affected children presented in infancy with cerebral seizures that were refractory to antiepileptic medication and also did not respond to high dose magnesium supplementation. All three children developed a significant degree of mental retardation and global developmental delay. Serum magnesium concentrations remained low despite adequate oral supplementation.

The α1-subunit (ATP1A1) is one of four different α-subunits of Na^+K^+-ATPase in human, but it represents the exclusive α-subunit in kidney. Along the kidney tubule, the DCT represents the segment with the highest energy consumption and density of Na^+K^+-ATPase expression [154]. Here, basolaterally expressed Na^+K^+-ATPase generates favorable electrochemical gradients for transcellular salt and magnesium reabsorption (Fig. 37.5). The critical role of Na^+K^+-ATPase for magnesium reabsorption had previously been demonstrated by discovery of mutations in its γ-subunit (*FXYD2*) in patients with isolated dominant hypomagnesemia (see below). In the central nervous system, the α1-subunit is ubiquitously expressed and thought to maintain neuronal housekeeping functions by generating the resting membrane potential and clearing extracellular K^+ during neuronal activity [155].

The ATP1A1 mutations discovered in hypomagnesemic children were shown to not only lead to a loss of ATPase function, but also to result in abnormal ion permeabilities and leak currents [153]. Therefore, the severe hypomagnesemia phenotype might not be the result of a simple ATP1A1 haploinsufficiency. Whereas a homozygous loss of ATP1A1 function is not compatible with life, heterozygous germline ATP1A1 mutations have also been described in patients with Charcot-Marie-Tooth disease type 2 and hereditary spastic paraplegia [156, 157]. Originally, somatic ATP1A1 mutations had been identified in patients with primary hyperaldosteronism due to aldosterone producing adenomas [158].

Isolated Dominant Hypomagnesemia

A first variant of isolated dominant hypomagnesemia (**IDH**) was described in 1999 in two related families by Meij et al. who discovered a mutation in the *FXYD2* gene encoding the γ-subunit of renal Na^+K^+-ATPase [159]. The γ-subunit of Na^+K^+-ATPase is a member of the FXYD family of small single transmembrane proteins that constitute regulatory, tissue-specific subunits of the Na^+K^+-ATPase. Along the kidney tubule, *FXYD2* is preferentially expressed in the DCT, where it is thought to increase the affinity of Na^+K^+-ATPase for ATP while decreasing its Na^+ affinity thereby providing a mechanism for balancing energy utilization and maintaining appropriate salt gradients [160, 161] The reported G41R mutation in the γ-subunit leads to retention of the γ-subunit within the cell.

Urinary Mg^{2+} wasting together with the expression pattern of the *FXYD2* gene point to a defect in transcellular Mg^{2+} reabsorption in the DCT in IDH patients. Affected children present with cerebral seizures and hypomagnesemia around 0.5 mmol/L. [162] Hypomagnesemia is due to renal losses while intestinal Mg^{2+} absorption is preserved or even stimulated [162]. Low Ca^{2+} excretion, hypokalemia and metabolic alkalosis reminiscent of Gitelman syndrome have also been reported in some families [163]. Selective magnesium supplementation partially corrects hypomagnesemia and normalizes serum potassium levels [163].

Hypomagnesemia, Episodic Ataxia/ Myokymia Syndrome

Another form of dominant hypomagnesemia was established by the identification of a heterozygous missense mutation in *KCNA1,* which encodes the voltage-gated potassium channel KCNA1 (Kv1.1) [164]. The clinical phenotype associated with the reported p.N255D mutation in Kv1.1 includes muscle cramps, tetany, tremor, and muscle weakness starting during infancy.

Originally, dominant *KCNA1* mutations had been identified in patients with episodic ataxia with myokymia (OMIM #160120), a neurologic disorder characterized by an intermittent appearance of incoordination and imbalance as well as myokymia, an involuntary, spontaneous, and localized trembling of muscles [165]. In addition to muscle cramps and tetany attributed to Mg^{2+} deficiency, these symptoms were also present in hypomagnesemic patients with the p.N255D mutant. Urine analyses in these patients revealed a renal Mg^{2+} leak without alterations in renal Ca^{2+} handling.

Co-expression studies of the mutant and wild-type Kv1.1 channel subunits indicate a dominant-negative effect of the mutant [166]. Kv1.1 is expressed at the apical membrane of the DCT. As

Kit is co-localized there with TRPM6, Kv1.1 may allow for hyperpolarization of the apical membrane of DCT cells as a prerequisite for TRPM6-mediated Mg^{2+} entry (Fig. 37.4b), thereby linking Mg^{2+} reabsorption to K+ secretion in the DCT [164].

Isolated Recessive Hypomagnesemia

In the 1980s Geven et al. first reported a form of isolated hypomagnesemia in a consanguineous family indicating autosomal recessive inheritance [167]. Two affected sisters presented in infancy with generalized seizures. Unfortunately, a late diagnosis resulted in neurodevelopmental deficits in both girls. A thorough clinical and laboratory workup at 4 and 8 years of age, respectively, revealed serum Mg^{2+} levels around 0.5–0.6 mmol/L with no other associated serum electrolyte abnormality. Of note, renal Ca^{2+} excretion rates were in the normal range. A ^{28}Mg-retention test in one patient indicated a primary defect in renal Mg^{2+} conservation [167].

Groenestege et al. identified a homozygous missense mutation in the *EGF* gene leading to a nonconservative amino acid exchange in the encoded pro-EGF protein (pro-epidermal growth factor) in the two sisters [168]. In the kidney, co-expression with key proteins of transcellular Mg^{2+} reabsorption including TRPM6 in the DCT was demonstrated. Pro-EGF is a transmembrane protein that is inserted in both the luminal and basolateral membrane of polarized epithelia. After the soluble EGF peptide is cleaved, it binds to and activates specialized EGF receptors (EGFRs). In case of the DCT, these EGFRs are exclusively expressed at the basolateral membrane (Fig. 37.5). Their activation leads to increased trafficking of TRPM6 to the luminal membrane and increased Mg^{2+} reabsorption [169]. The mutation described in IRH (p.P1070L) disrupts the basolateral sorting motif in pro-EGF leading to a mistargeting of pro-EGF [168]. Therefore, the activation of basolateral EGFRs is compromised which ultimately causes impaired active transcellular Mg^{2+} reabsorption. Despite acting in a paracrine fashion in the DCT, the authors speculate on a role of EGF as a first selectively acting magnesiotropic hormone [168].

Hypomagnesemia, Refractory Seizures, and Mental Retardation 1

Another form of hereditary Mg^{2+} wasting has been linked to mutations in *CNNM2* encoding the transmembrane protein CNNM2 or Cyclin M2 [170]. CNNM2 was identified by differential expression in murine DCT cells exposed to varying Mg^{2+} concentrations and by transcriptome studies in mice lacking claudin-16 [170, 171]. In addition, common variants in CNNM2 were found to be associated with serum Mg^{2+} levels in a genome-wide association study [172]. The precise physiological function of CNNM2 is still elusive. CNNM2 is ubiquitously expressed in mammalian tissues, most prominently in kidney, brain and lung [173, 174]. In the kidney, CNNM2 is expressed at the basolateral membrane of TAL and DCT. Whereas CNNM2 had initially been proposed as a Mg^{2+} transporter, more recent data point to a role in Mg^{2+}-sensing [171, 174].

CNNM2-associated disease shows a wide phenotypic as well as genetic spectrum. Most patients identified thus far carry heterozygous de novo mutations in *CNNM2*. These patients mainly present in infancy with generalized convulsions and display a mild to moderate degree of neurodevelopmental delay with a disturbed speech development and dysarthria as prominent features [175]. Cerebral seizures tend to subside during follow-up in the majority of patients. A considerable number of patients of both genders develops severe obesity as the most prominent extraneurological symptom [175]. Serum magnesium levels are typically in the range of 0.5–0.6 mmol/L and remain in the subnormal range upon oral magnesium supplementation.

A milder clinical phenotype without significant intellectual disability was originally described in members of two families with dominant inheritance [170]. By contrast, patients with bi-allelic *CNNM2* mutations exhibit profound hypomagnesemia and a severe neurological phenotype with refractory epilepsy, microcephaly, global developmental delay, and severe intellectual disability [176, 177]. Brain MR imaging in these patients demonstrate widened outer cerebrospinal liquor spaces indicative of cerebral atrophy as well as myelinization defects.

HNF1B Nephropathy

Hepatocyte nuclear factor 1β (HNF1B) is a transcription factor critical for the development of the kidney and the pancreas. *HNF1B* mutations are present in heterozygous state, either inherited or de novo, and comprise point mutations as well as whole-gene deletions [178]. *HNF1B* mutations were first implicated in a subtype of maturity-onset diabetes of the young (MODY5) [179]. Later, an association with anomalous kidney development was reported. The renal phenotype is highly variable comprising enlarged hyperechogenic kidneys, multicystic kidney disease, renal agenesis, renal hypoplasia, cystic dysplasia, as well as hyperuricemic nephropathy (see Chap. 8). Since neither a renal cystic phenotype nor diabetes are constant clinical findings, the neutral term HNF1B nephropathy has been introduced [180]. Interestingly, 25–50% of patients present with hypomagnesemia due to impaired renal Mg^{2+} conservation [181, 182]. As *HNF1B* regulates the expression of *FXYD2* (see above), defective basolateral Na^+K^+-ATPase function potentially explains renal Mg^{2+} wasting in patients with HNF1B mutations [182]. In agreement with this assumption, renal Mg^{2+} wasting in HNF1B nephropathy can be part of a Gitelman syndrome-like picture with hypokalemia, metabolic alkalosis and hypocalciuria, compatible with dysfunction of the DCT [182, 183].

The observed variable prevalence of hypomagnesemia in children with HNF1B nephropathy suggests that this phenotypic feature of HNF1B nephropathy may represent an age-dependent phenomenon and develop over time [184]. Indeed, a study from Poland reports an increasing fraction of hypomagnesemic HNF1B patients during follow-up [185].

Transient Neonatal Hyperphenylalaninemia

Renal Mg^{2+} wasting has been demonstrated in transient neonatal hyperphenylalaninemia due to recessive mutations in the *PCBD1* gene [186]. Affected patients developed hypomagnesemia and a MODY type diabetes in adulthood. Functional studies revealed that PCBD1 is an essential dimerization cofactor of HNF1B. Defective dimerization of PCBD1 with HNF1B abrogates the HNF1B-mediated stimulation of *FXYD2* promoter activity in the DCT [186].

Mitochondrial Hypomagnesemia

A mutation in the mitochondrial tRNA gene for Isoleucine, tRNA[Ile] or MTTI, has been discovered in a single large Caucasian kindred [187]. An extensive clinical evaluation of this family was prompted after the discovery of hypomagnesemia in the index patient. Pedigree analysis was compatible with mitochondrial inheritance as the phenotype was exclusively transmitted by affected females. The phenotype included hypomagnesemia, hypercholesterolemia, and hypertension. Of the adults on the maternal lineage, the majority of offspring exhibited at least one of the mentioned symptoms, approximately half of the individuals showed a combination of two or more symptoms, and around 1/6 had all three features [187]. Serum Mg^{2+} levels of family members on the maternal lineage greatly varied ranging from 0.3 to 1.0 mmol/L with approximately 50% of individuals being hypomagnesemic. Hypomagnesemic individuals showed higher fractional excretions (median around 7.5%) than their normomagnesemic relatives on the maternal lineage (median around 3%) clearly pointing to renal Mg^{2+} wasting as causative for hypomagnesemia. Interestingly, hypomagnesemia was accompanied by decreased urinary Ca^{2+} levels, a finding pointing to the DCT as the affected tubular segment. As ATP consumption along the tubule is highest in the DCT, energy metabolism of DCT cells may be impaired as a consequence of the mitochondrial defect which in turn could lead to disturbed transcellular Mg^{2+} reabsorption [187].

Acquired Hypomagnesemia

Cisplatin and Carboplatin

The cytostatic agent cisplatin and the newer antineoplastic drug, carboplatin, are widely used in various protocols for the therapy of solid tumors. Among different side effects, nephrotoxicity receives most attention as the major dose-limiting factor. Carboplatin has been reported to have less severe side effects than cisplatin [188–190].

Hypomagnesemia due to renal Mg^{2+} wasting is regularly observed in patients treated with cisplatin [189, 191]. The incidence of Mg^{2+} deficiency is greater than 30% and even increases to over 70% with extended cisplatin usage and greater cumulative doses. Notably, cisplatin-induced Mg^{2+} wasting is relatively selective [189]. Hypocalcemia and hypokalemia may be observed but only with prolonged and severe Mg^{2+} deficiency [192]. The influence of Mg^{2+} deficiency on PTH secretion and end-organ resistance is a possible explanation for enhanced urinary Ca^{2+} excretion and diminished mobilization resulting in low serum Ca^{2+} concentrations [193]. The effects on K^+ balance are more difficult to explain. The hypokalemia observed with Mg^{2+} deficiency is refractory to K^+ supplementation. The effects of cisplatin may persist for months or years, long after the inorganic platinum has disappeared from the renal tissue [194, 195].

In the rat model cisplatin treatment resulted in EGF and TRPM6 downregulation in the DCT [196]. Nephrotoxicity was effectively prevented by Mg^{2+} supplementation either during or even before cisplatin administration, demonstrating the close relationship between cisplatin-induced Mg^{2+} deficiency and nephrotoxicity [197].

Aminoglycosides

Aminoglycosides, such as gentamicin, induce renal impairment in up to 35% patients dependent on the dose and duration of administration. In addition, aminoglycosides cause hypermagnesiuria and hypomagnesemia [198]. As many as 25% of patients receiving gentamicin develop hypomagnesemia [198]. The hypermagnesiuric response occurs soon after the onset of therapy; it is dose-dependent and readily reversible upon withdrawal. As with adults, neonates also display an immediate increase of Ca^{2+} and Mg^{2+} excretion after gentamicin infusion [199, 200]. Mg^{2+} wasting is associated with hypercalciuria that may lead to diminished plasma Ca^{2+} concentrations. This would suggest that aminoglycosides affect renal Mg^{2+} and Ca^{2+} transport in the distal tubule where both are reabsorbed. The cellular mechanisms are not completely understood but hypermagnesiuria and hypercalciuria are observed in the absence of histopathological changes. Because gentamicin is a polyvalent cation it has been postulated that it may interfere with the function of the Ca^{2+}-sensing receptor (CaSR) [89, 201]. CaSR activation by polyvalent cations would inhibit passive absorption of Mg^{2+} and Ca^{2+} in the loop of Henle and active hormone-mediated transport in the DCT, leading to renal Mg^{2+} and Ca^{2+} wasting. The observation that gentamicin treatment results in an up-regulation of Ca^{2+} and Mg^{2+} transport proteins in the DCT, namely TRPV5, TRPM6 and calbindin-D28k, suggests that this adaptation represents an attempt to counter upstream losses, i.e. in the TAL [202]. This would be in accordance with the hypothesis that gentamicin affects Na^+ reabsorption in TAL leading to a reduced lumen-positive voltage and a subsequent reduction in Ca^{2+} and Mg^{2+} reabsorption.

Calcineurin Inhibitors

The calcineurin inhibitors cyclosporine and tacrolimus are widely prescribed as immunosuppressants to organ transplant recipients and in numerous immunologic disorders. Under this therapy, patients are at high risk of developing renal injury and hypertension. Tubular dysfunction with subsequent disturbance of mineral metabolism is another common side effect. Both drugs commonly lead to renal Mg^{2+} wasting and hypomagnesemia [203]. Unlike the other agents mentioned above, these drugs also cause modest hypercalcemia with hypercalciuria and hypokalemia [203]. The hypomagnesemic effect is probably attenuated by the fall in GFR and reduction in filtered Mg^{2+} but this defect appears to be specific for Mg^{2+}. Calcineurin inhibitor therapy is associated with an inappropriately high fractional excretion rate of Mg^{2+}, suggesting impaired passive reabsorption in the TAL or active Mg^{2+} transport in the DCT [204]. Cyclosporine reduces claudin-16 expression in the TAL [205]. Moreover, tacrolimus downregulates specific Ca^{2+} and Mg^{2+} transport proteins in the DCT. In an animal study, tacrolimus suppressed the expression of TRPV5, calbindin-D28k and TRPM6 [206]. In accordance with these observations, urinary EGF levels were found decreased in adult and pediatric hypomagnesemic renal allograft recipients treated with cyclosporin pointing to a defect of transcellular magnesium reabsorption in the DCT [207, 208].

EGF Receptor Antibodies

The EGF hormone axis has been implicated in renal Mg^{2+} handling by the identification of a homozygous mutation in the *EGF* gene in a family with isolated recessive hypomagnesemia (see below) [168]. The way for this discovery was paved by the observation that anticancer treatments with monoclonal antibodies against the EGF receptor (EGFR) resulted in renal Mg^{2+} wasting and hypomagnesemia [209]. Of note, patients treated with EGFR targeting antibodies (cetuximab, panitumumab) for colorectal cancer usually receive a combination therapy with platinum compounds potentially aggravating the effects on serum Mg^{2+} levels. A significant number of patients receiving such a chemotherapeutic regimen shows decreasing serum Mg^{2+} concentrations over time [209–211]. 24-h urine collections as well as Mg^{2+} loading tests in single patients demonstrated defective renal Mg^{2+} conservation [209]. Together with the genetic findings in patients with isolated recessive hypomagnesemia due to a pro-EGF mutation, these observations imply a selective effect of EGF-receptor targeting on transcellular Mg^{2+} transport in the DCT. There, TRPM6 mediated Mg^{2+} uptake into DCT cells is stimulated by basolaterally secreted EGF via its receptor (EGFR) [168]. It is still controversial If the development of hypomagnesemia correlates with the efficacy of anti-EGF receptor treatment [212, 213].

Proton-Pump Inhibitors (PPIs)

Over the past two decades, PPIs for the reduction of gastric acidity have emerged to one of the most widely prescribed classes of drugs worldwide [214]. Symptomatic hypomagnesemia has been observed in a small but significant number of patients receiving PPIs [215]. A systematic review of the published cases showed severe hypomagnesemia (below 0.4 mmol/L) with concomitant hypocalcemia, a laboratory constellation reminiscent of Hypomagnesemia with Secondary Hypocalcemia (HSH) due to TRPM6 defects (see below) [214]. The initial report on hypomagnesemia following PPI treatment had already described suppressed PTH levels during episodes of severe hypomagnesemia as a probable cause of hypocalcemia [215]. Although a number of patients additionally receive diuretics, this finding does not explain the profound degree of Mg^{2+} deficiency observed in patients receiving PPIs.

Unfortunately, the molecular link between proton-pump inhibition and hypomagnesemia still remains unclear. Data regarding renal Mg^{2+} losses in hypomagnesemic patients receiving PPIs are inconclusive. Fractional Mg^{2+} excretion was reported to be low in face of profound hypomagnesemia, possibly pointing to an intact tubular Mg^{2+} reabsorption [215, 216]. However, as observed in HSH patients, a renal Mg^{2+} leak might only become apparent if serum Mg^{2+} levels reach a certain threshold. An alternative explanation could involve disturbed intestinal reabsorption of Mg^{2+}. Possible molecular mechanisms include an inhibition of TRPM6 leading to a combined intestinal and renal defect, but also a disturbance of ATPases or ATPase-subunits other than gastric H^+-K^+-ATPase involved in epithelial Mg^{2+} transport.

It is recommended to monitor serum Mg^{2+} levels patients receiving PPIs, particularly on those with concomitant cardiac disease at risk for arrhythmia.

Miscellaneous Agents

A number of antibiotics, tuberculostatics, and antiviral drugs may result in renal Mg^{2+} wasting [198]. The cellular basis and molecular mechanisms by which these agents lead to abnormal Mg^{2+} reabsorption are largely unknown. Many are associated with general cytotoxicity. Amphotericin B may lead to an acquired distal tubular acidosis which in turn reduces renal Mg^{2+} reabsorption. Pamidronate used in the treatment of acute symptomatic hypercalcemia of various origin has also been reported to cause transient hypomagnesemia. Again, the cellular mechanisms are difficult to predict since this drug is used in patients with hypercalcemia that may aggravate renal Mg^{2+} wasting [217].

Particular attention should be given to these medications in patients with pre-existing hypomagnesemia and especially hereditary disorders of magnesium metabolism.

Therapy of Hypomagnesemia

The substitution of Mg^{2+} in patients with hypomagnesemia is primarily aimed at the relief of clinical symptoms. Unfortunately, in patients with renal Mg^{2+} wasting, normal values for total serum Mg^{2+} are hardly achieved by oral substitution without considerable side effects, mainly resulting from the cathartic effects of Mg^{2+} salts.

The primary route of administration depends on the severity of the clinical findings. Acute intravenous infusion is usually reserved for patients with symptomatic hypomagnesemia, i.e. with cerebral convulsions or tetany [218]. Intravenous administration should be preferred to painful intramuscular injections, especially in children.

In neonates and children, the initial treatment usually consists of 25–50 mg Mg^{2+} sulphate (0.1–0.2 mmol Mg^{2+}) per kilogram body weight slowly given intravenously (over 20 min) (up to a maximum of 2 g Mg^{2+} sulphate, which is the adult dosage). This dose can be repeated every 6–8 h or can be followed by a continuous infusion of 100–200 mg Mg^{2+} sulphate (0.4–0.8 mmol Mg^{2+}) per kilogram body weight given over 24 h [178, 219].

In the presence of hypocalcemia, this regimen can be continued for 3–5 days. When Mg^{2+} is administered intravenously, Ca^{2+} gluconate (i.v.) should be available as an antidote. Control of blood pressure, heart rate, and respiration is important as well as a close monitoring of serum Mg^{2+} levels. Before administration, normal renal function has to be ascertained.

In asymptomatic hypomagnesemic or Mg^{2+}-deficient patients, oral replacement represents the preferred route of administration. Exact dosages required to correct Mg^{2+} deficiency are largely unknown. For the pediatric population, 10–20 mg Mg^{2+} (0.4–0.8 mmol) per kg body weight given three to four times a day have been recommended to correct hypomagnesemia [220]. Dosages for maintenance therapy (i.e. in hereditary disorders (see below)) vary between 10 and 100 mg Mg^{2+} (0.4–4 mmol) per kg per day.

Due to the laxative effect of oral magnesium and due to rapid renal excretion especially in case of high peak serum levels, the required daily amount should be given in two to four divided doses preferentially with meals. Solubility, intestinal absorption, and side effects greatly differ depending on the Mg^{2+} salt used for oral treatment. The bioavailability and pharmacokinetics of diverse Mg^{2+} salts have been reviewed [221]. Considering solubility, intestinal absorption and bioavailability, organic Mg^{2+} salts such as Mg^{2+} citrate or aspartate appear most suitable for oral replacement therapy. In addition, the laxative effect of these preparations seems to be less pronounced compared with inorganic Mg^{2+} salts. Moreover, slow-release formulations might be used if available. In our personal experience continuous administration of Mg^{2+}, for example dissolved in mineral water, has proven useful, as peak Mg^{2+} blood levels are avoided. When initiating therapy, dosages should be titrated based on blood levels and intestinal tolerance.

In addition to replacement therapy, the use of certain diuretics has been proposed for the reduction of renal Mg^{2+} excretion. The aldosterone antagonist spironolactone, as well as K^+-sparing diuretics such as amiloride, exert Mg^{2+}-sparing effects [222, 223]. Studies in patients with hereditary Mg^{2+} wasting disorders showed beneficial effects of these diuretics on renal Mg^{2+} excretions, serum Mg^{2+} levels, and clinical manifestations [224, 225].

References

1. Institute of Medicine (US) Committee to Review Dietary Reference Intakes for Vitamin D and Calcium. Dietary reference intakes for calcium and vitamin D, vol. 1. The National Academies; 2011.
2. Gueguen L, Pointillart A. The bioavailability of dietary calcium. J Am Coll Nutr. 2000;19(2 Suppl):119s–36s.
3. Moe SM. Confusion on the complexity of calcium balance. Semin Dial. 2010;23(5):492–7.
4. Martin A, David V, Quarles LD. Regulation and function of the FGF23/klotho endocrine pathways. Physiol Rev. 2012;92(1):131–55. https://doi.org/10.1152/physrev.00002.2011.
5. Kumar R, Tebben PJ, Thompson JR. Vitamin D and the kidney. Arch Biochem Biophys. 2012;523(1):77–86. https://doi.org/10.1016/j.abb.2012.03.003.
6. Suki WN. Calcium transport in the nephron. Am J Physiol. 1979;237(1):F1–6. https://doi.org/10.1152/ajprenal.1979.237.1.F1.
7. Wright FS, Bomsztyk K. Calcium transport by the proximal tubule. Adv Exp Med Biol. 1986;208:165–70. https://doi.org/10.1007/978-1-4684-5206-8_18.
8. Alexander RT, Dimke H, Cordat E. Proximal tubular NHEs: sodium, protons and calcium? Am J Physiol Renal Physiol. 2013;305(3):F229–36. https://doi.org/10.1152/ajprenal.00065.2013.
9. Kiuchi-Saishin Y, Gotoh S, Furuse M, Takasuga A, Tano Y, Tsukita S. Differential expression patterns of claudins, tight junction membrane proteins, in mouse nephron segments. J Am Soc Nephrol. 2002;13(4):875–86.

10. Lee JW, Chou CL, Knepper MA. Deep sequencing in microdissected renal tubules identifies nephron segment-specific transcriptomes. J Am Soc Nephrol. 2015;26(11):2669–77. https://doi.org/10.1681/ASN.2014111067.

11. Ibeh CL, Yiu AJ, Kanaras YL, et al. Evidence for a regulated Ca2+ entry in proximal tubular cells and its implication in calcium stone formation. J Cell Sci. 2019;132(9):jcs225268. https://doi.org/10.1242/jcs.225268.

12. Hou J, Renigunta A, Konrad M, et al. Claudin-16 and claudin-19 interact and form a cation-selective tight junction complex. J Clin Invest. 2008;118(2):619–28. https://doi.org/10.1172/jci33970.

13. Breiderhoff T, Himmerkus N, Stuiver M, et al. Deletion of claudin-10 (Cldn10) in the thick ascending limb impairs paracellular sodium permeability and leads to hypermagnesemia and nephrocalcinosis. Proc Natl Acad Sci U S A. 2012;109(35):14241–6. https://doi.org/10.1073/pnas.1203834109.

14. Gong Y, Renigunta V, Himmerkus N, et al. Claudin-14 regulates renal Ca(+)(+) transport in response to CaSR signalling via a novel microRNA pathway. EMBO J. 2012;31(8):1999–2012. https://doi.org/10.1038/emboj.2012.49.

15. Dimke H, Desai P, Borovac J, Lau A, Pan W, Alexander RT. Activation of the Ca(2+)-sensing receptor increases renal claudin-14 expression and urinary Ca(2+) excretion. Am J Physiol Renal Physiol. 2013;304(6):F761–9. https://doi.org/10.1152/ajprenal.00263.2012.

16. Sato T, Courbebaisse M, Ide N, et al. Parathyroid hormone controls paracellular Ca(2+) transport in the thick ascending limb by regulating the tight-junction protein Claudin14. Proc Natl Acad Sci U S A. 2017;114(16):E3344–53. https://doi.org/10.1073/pnas.1616733114.

17. Gong Y, Himmerkus N, Plain A, Bleich M, Hou J. Epigenetic regulation of microRNAs controlling CLDN14 expression as a mechanism for renal calcium handling. J Am Soc Nephrol. 2015;26(3):663–76. https://doi.org/10.1681/asn.2014020129.

18. Hofer AM, Brown EM. Extracellular calcium sensing and signalling. Nat Rev Mol Cell Biol. 2003;4(7):530–8. https://doi.org/10.1038/nrm1154.

19. Lambers TT, Bindels RJ, Hoenderop JG. Coordinated control of renal Ca2+ handling. Kidney Int. 2006;69(4):650–4. https://doi.org/10.1038/sj.ki.5000169.

20. Hoenderop JG, Nilius B, Bindels RJ. Calcium absorption across epithelia. Physiol Rev. 2005;85(1):373–422. https://doi.org/10.1152/physrev.00003.2004.

21. Terker AS, Zhang C, McCormick JA, et al. Potassium modulates electrolyte balance and blood pressure through effects on distal cell voltage and chloride. Cell Metab. 2015;21(1):39–50. https://doi.org/10.1016/j.cmet.2014.12.006.

22. van der Wijst J, Tutakhel OAZ, Bos C, et al. Effects of a high-sodium/low-potassium diet on renal calcium, magnesium, and phosphate handling. Am J Physiol Renal Physiol. 2018;315(1):F110–22. https://doi.org/10.1152/ajprenal.00379.2017.

23. Matos V, van Melle G, Boulat O, Markert M, Bachmann C, Guignard JP. Urinary phosphate/creatinine, calcium/creatinine, and magnesium/creatinine ratios in a healthy pediatric population. J Pediatr. 1997;131(2):252–7.

24. Bergsland KJ, Coe FL, White MD, et al. Urine risk factors in children with calcium kidney stones and their siblings. Kidney Int. 2012;81(11):1140–8. https://doi.org/10.1038/ki.2012.7.

25. Blanchard A, Curis E, Guyon-Roger T, et al. Observations of a large Dent disease cohort. Kidney Int. 2016;90(2):430–9. https://doi.org/10.1016/j.kint.2016.04.022.

26. Zaniew M, Bökenkamp A, Kolbuc M, et al. Long-term renal outcome in children with OCRL mutations: retrospective analysis of a large international cohort. Nephrol Dial Transplant. 2018;33(1):85–94. https://doi.org/10.1093/ndt/gfw350.

27. Santer R, Schneppenheim R, Dombrowski A, Götze H, Steinmann B, Schaub J. Mutations in GLUT2, the gene for the liver-type glucose transporter, in patients with Fanconi-Bickel syndrome. Nat Genet. 1997;17(3):324–6. https://doi.org/10.1038/ng1197-324.

28. Mannstadt M, Magen D, Segawa H, et al. Fanconi-Bickel syndrome and autosomal recessive proximal tubulopathy with hypercalciuria (ARPTH) are allelic variants caused by GLUT2 mutations. J Clin Endocrinol Metab. 2012;97(10):E1978–86. https://doi.org/10.1210/jc.2012-1279.

29. Curry JN, Saurette M, Askari M, et al. Claudin-2 deficiency associates with hypercalciuria in mice and human kidney stone disease. J Clin Invest. 2020;130(4):1948–60. https://doi.org/10.1172/JCI127750.

30. Hoenderop JG, van Leeuwen JP, van der Eerden BC, et al. Renal Ca2+ wasting, hyperabsorption, and reduced bone thickness in mice lacking TRPV5. J Clin Invest. 2003;112(12):1906–14. https://doi.org/10.1172/jci19826.

31. Loh NY, Bentley L, Dimke H, et al. Autosomal dominant hypercalciuria in a mouse model due to a mutation of the epithelial calcium channel, TRPV5. PLoS One. 2013;8(1):e55412. https://doi.org/10.1371/journal.pone.0055412.

32. Wakimoto K, Kobayashi K, Kuro-O M, et al. Targeted disruption of Na+/Ca2+ exchanger gene leads to cardiomyocyte apoptosis and defects in heartbeat. J Biol Chem. 2000;275(47):36991–8. https://doi.org/10.1074/jbc.M004035200.

33. Okunade GW, Miller ML, Pyne GJ, et al. Targeted ablation of plasma membrane Ca2+-ATPase

(PMCA) 1 and 4 indicates a major housekeeping function for PMCA1 and a critical role in hyperactivated sperm motility and male fertility for PMCA4. J Biol Chem. 2004;279(32):33742–50. https://doi.org/10.1074/jbc.M404628200.

34. Singh J, Moghal N, Pearce SH, Cheetham T. The investigation of hypocalcaemia and rickets. Arch Dis Child. 2003;88(5):403–7.

35. Bastepe M. Genetics and epigenetics of parathyroid hormone resistance. Endocr Dev. 2013;24:11–24. https://doi.org/10.1159/000342494.

36. Brown EM, Pollak M, Chou YH, Seidman CE, Seidman JG, Hebert SC. Cloning and functional characterization of extracellular Ca(2+)-sensing receptors from parathyroid and kidney. Bone. 1995;17(2 Suppl):7S–11S.

37. Zhang C, Zhang T, Zou J, et al. Structural basis for regulation of human calcium-sensing receptor by magnesium ions and an unexpected tryptophan derivative co-agonist. Sci Adv. 2016;2(5):e1600241. https://doi.org/10.1126/sciadv.1600241.

38. Wettschureck N, Lee E, Libutti SK, Offermanns S, Robey PG, Spiegel AM. Parathyroid-specific double knockout of Gq and G11 alpha-subunits leads to a phenotype resembling germline knockout of the extracellular Ca2+ -sensing receptor. Mol Endocrinol. 2007;21(1):274–80. https://doi.org/10.1210/me.2006-0110.

39. Centeno PP, Herberger A, Mun HC, et al. Phosphate acts directly on the calcium-sensing receptor to stimulate parathyroid hormone secretion. Nat Commun. 2019;10(1):4693. https://doi.org/10.1038/s41467-019-12399-9.

40. Nesbit MA, Hannan FM, Howles SA, et al. Mutations in AP2S1 cause familial hypocalciuric hypercalcemia type 3. Nat Genet. 2013;45(1):93–7. https://doi.org/10.1038/ng.2492.

41. Yasuoka Y, Sato Y, Healy JM, Nonoguchi H, Kawahara K. pH-sensitive expression of calcium-sensing receptor (CaSR) in type-B intercalated cells of the cortical collecting ducts (CCD) in mouse kidney. Clin Exp Nephrol. 2015;19(5):771–82. https://doi.org/10.1007/s10157-014-1063-1.

42. Sands JM, Naruse M, Baum M, et al. Apical extracellular calcium/polyvalent cation-sensing receptor regulates vasopressin-elicited water permeability in rat kidney inner medullary collecting duct. J Clin Invest. 1997;99(6):1399–405. https://doi.org/10.1172/JCI119299.

43. Ranieri M, Di Mise A, Tamma G, Valenti G. Calcium sensing receptor exerts a negative regulatory action toward vasopressin-induced aquaporin-2 expression and trafficking in renal collecting duct. Vitam Horm. 2020;112:289–310. https://doi.org/10.1016/bs.vh.2019.08.008.

44. Pollak MR, Brown EM, Estep HL, et al. Autosomal dominant hypocalcaemia caused by a Ca(2+)-sensing receptor gene mutation. Nat Genet. 1994;8(3):303–7. https://doi.org/10.1038/ng1194-303.

45. Pearce SH, Williamson C, Kifor O, et al. A familial syndrome of hypocalcemia with hypercalciuria due to mutations in the calcium-sensing receptor. N Engl J Med. 1996;335(15):1115–22. https://doi.org/10.1056/NEJM199610103351505.

46. Watanabe S, Fukumoto S, Chang H, et al. Association between activating mutations of calcium-sensing receptor and Bartter's syndrome. Lancet. 2002;360(9334):692–4. https://doi.org/10.1016/S0140-6736(02)09842-2. S0140-6736(02)09842-2 [pii]

47. Nesbit MA, Hannan FM, Howles SA, et al. Mutations affecting G-protein subunit α11 in hypercalcemia and hypocalcemia. N Engl J Med. 2013;368(26):2476–86. https://doi.org/10.1056/NEJMoa1300253.

48. Mannstadt M, Harris M, Bravenboer B, et al. Germline mutations affecting Gα11 in hypoparathyroidism. N Engl J Med. 2013;368(26):2532–4. https://doi.org/10.1056/NEJMc1300278.

49. Rodd C, Goodyer P. Hypercalcemia of the newborn: etiology, evaluation, and management. Pediatr Nephrol. 1999;13(6):542–7.

50. Davies JH. A practical approach to problems of hypercalcaemia. Endocr Dev. 2009;16:93–114. https://doi.org/10.1159/000223691. 000223691 [pii]

51. Davies JH, Shaw NJ. Investigation and management of hypercalcaemia in children. Arch Dis Child. 2012;97(6):533–8. https://doi.org/10.1136/archdischild-2011-301284.

52. Vieth R. The mechanisms of vitamin D toxicity. Bone Miner. 1990;11(3):267–72.

53. Mizusawa Y, Burke JR. Prednisolone and cellulose phosphate treatment in idiopathic infantile hypercalcaemia with nephrocalcinosis. J Paediatr Child Health. 1996;32(4):350–2.

54. Pak CY. Clinical pharmacology of sodium cellulose phosphate. J Clin Pharmacol. 1979;19(8–9 Pt 1):451–7.

55. Skalova S, Cerna L, Bayer M, Kutilek S, Konrad M, Schlingmann KP. Intravenous pamidronate in the treatment of severe idiopathic infantile hypercalcemia. Iran J Kidney Dis. 2013;7(2):160–4.

56. Nguyen M, Boutignon H, Mallet E, et al. Infantile hypercalcemia and hypercalciuria: new insights into a vitamin D-dependent mechanism and response to ketoconazole treatment. J Pediatr. 2010;157(2):296–302. https://doi.org/10.1016/j.jpeds.2010.02.025. S0022-3476(10)00149-6 [pii]

57. Fencl F, Blahova K, Schlingmann KP, Konrad M, Seeman T. Severe hypercalcemic crisis in an infant with idiopathic infantile hypercalcemia caused by mutation in CYP24A1 gene. Eur J Pediatr. 2013;172(1):45–9. https://doi.org/10.1007/s00431-012-1818-1.

58. Pollak MR, Brown EM, Chou YH, et al. Mutations in the human Ca(2+)-sensing receptor gene cause familial hypocalciuric hypercalcemia and neonatal severe hyperparathyroidism. Cell. 1993;75(7):1297–303. 0092-8674(93)90617-Y [pii].

59. Thakker RV. Diseases associated with the extracellular calcium-sensing receptor. Cell Calcium. 2004;35(3):275–82. https://doi.org/10.1016/j.ceca.2003.10.010.

60. Marx SJ, Attie MF, Levine MA, Spiegel AM, Downs RW, Lasker RD. The hypocalciuric or benign variant of familial hypercalcemia: clinical and biochemical features in fifteen kindreds. Medicine (Baltimore). 1981;60(6):397–412.

61. Cole DE, Janicic N, Salisbury SR, Hendy GN. Neonatal severe hyperparathyroidism, secondary hyperparathyroidism, and familial hypocalciuric hypercalcemia: multiple different phenotypes associated with an inactivating Alu insertion mutation of the calcium-sensing receptor gene. Am J Med Genet. 1997;71(2):202–10.

62. Gunn IR, Gaffney D. Clinical and laboratory features of calcium-sensing receptor disorders: a systematic review. Ann Clin Biochem. 2004;41(Pt 6):441–58. https://doi.org/10.1258/0004563042466802.

63. Lightwood R, Stapleton T. Idiopathic hypercalcaemia in infants. Lancet. 1953;265(6779):255–6.

64. Fanconi G. [Chronic disorders of calcium and phosphate metabolism in children]. Schweiz Med Wochenschr. 1951;81(38):908–913.

65. Morgan HG, Mitchell RG, Stowers JM, Thomson J. Metabolic studies on two infants with idiopathic hypercalcaemia. Lancet. 1956;270(6929):925–31.

66. Fraser D. The relation between infantile hypercalcemia and vitamin D—public health implications in North America. Pediatrics. 1967;40(6):1050–61.

67. Pronicka E, Rowińska E, Kulczycka H, Lukaszkiewicz J, Lorenc R, Janas R. Persistent hypercalciuria and elevated 25-hydroxyvitamin D3 in children with infantile hypercalcaemia. Pediatr Nephrol. 1997;11(1):2–6.

68. Williams JC, Barratt-Boyes BG, Lowe JB. Supravalvular aortic stenosis. Circulation. 1961;24:1311–8.

69. Beuren AJ, Apitz J, Harmjanz D. Supravalvular aortic stenosis in association with mental retardation and a certain facial appearance. Circulation. 1962;26:1235–40.

70. Schlingmann KP, Kaufmann M, Weber S, et al. Mutations in CYP24A1 and idiopathic infantile hypercalcemia. N Engl J Med. 2011;365(5):410–21. https://doi.org/10.1056/NEJMoa1103864.

71. Makin G, Lohnes D, Byford V, Ray R, Jones G. Target cell metabolism of 1,25-dihydroxyvitamin D3 to calcitroic acid. Evidence for a pathway in kidney and bone involving 24-oxidation. Biochem J. 1989, 262;(1):173–80.

72. Reddy GS, Tserng KY. Calcitroic acid, end product of renal metabolism of 1,25-dihydroxyvitamin D3 through C-24 oxidation pathway. Biochemistry. 1989;28(4):1763–9.

73. Kaufmann M, Gallagher JC, Peacock M, et al. Clinical utility of simultaneous quantitation of 25-Hydroxyvitamin D and 24,25-Dihydroxyvitamin D by LC-MS/MS involving derivatization with DMEQ-TAD. J Clin Endocrinol Metab. 2014;99(7):2567–74. https://doi.org/10.1210/jc.2013-4388.

74. Misselwitz J, Hesse V. [Hypercalcemia following prophylactic vitamin D administration]. Kinderarztl Prax. 1986;54(8):431–438.

75. Streeten EA, Zarbalian K, Damcott CM. CYP24A1 mutations in idiopathic infantile hypercalcemia. N Engl J Med. 2011;365(18):1741–2; author reply 1742–3. https://doi.org/10.1056/NEJMc1110226#SA2.

76. Tebben PJ, Milliner DS, Horst RL, et al. Hypercalcemia, hypercalciuria, and elevated calcitriol concentrations with autosomal dominant transmission due to CYP24A1 mutations: effects of ketoconazole therapy. J Clin Endocrinol Metab. 2012;97(3):E423–7. https://doi.org/10.1210/jc.2011-1935. jc.2011-1935 [pii]

77. Nesterova G, Malicdan MC, Yasuda K, et al. 1,25-(OH)2D-24 hydroxylase (CYP24A1) deficiency as a cause of nephrolithiasis. Clin J Am Soc Nephrol. 2013;8(4):649–57. https://doi.org/10.2215/cjn.05360512.

78. Schlingmann KP, Ruminska J, Kaufmann M, et al. Autosomal-recessive mutations in SLC34A1 encoding sodium-phosphate cotransporter 2A cause idiopathic infantile hypercalcemia. J Am Soc Nephrol. 2016;27(2):604–14. https://doi.org/10.1681/asn.2014101025.

79. Daga A, Majmundar AJ, Braun DA, et al. Whole exome sequencing frequently detects a monogenic cause in early onset nephrolithiasis and nephrocalcinosis. Kidney Int. 2018;93(1):204–13. https://doi.org/10.1016/j.kint.2017.06.025.

80. Hureaux M, Molin A, Jay N, et al. Prenatal hyperechogenic kidneys in three cases of infantile hypercalcemia associated with SLC34A1 mutations. Pediatr Nephrol. 2018;33(10):1723–9. https://doi.org/10.1007/s00467-018-3998-z.

81. Dasgupta D, Wee MJ, Reyes M, et al. Mutations in SLC34A3/NPT2c are associated with kidney stones and nephrocalcinosis. J Am Soc Nephrol. 2014;25(10):2366–75. https://doi.org/10.1681/asn.2013101085.

82. Lorenz-Depiereux B, Benet-Pages A, Eckstein G, et al. Hereditary hypophosphatemic rickets with hypercalciuria is caused by mutations in the sodium-phosphate cotransporter gene SLC34A3. Am J Hum Genet. 2006;78(2):193–201. https://doi.org/10.1086/499410.

83. Bergwitz C, Roslin NM, Tieder M, et al. SLC34A3 mutations in patients with hereditary hypophosphatemic rickets with hypercalciuria predict a key role for the sodium-phosphate cotransporter NaPi-IIc in maintaining phosphate homeostasis. Am J Hum Genet. 2006;78(2):179–92. https://doi.org/10.1086/499409.

84. Janiec A, Halat-Wolska P, Obrycki Ł, et al. Long-term outcome of the survivors of infantile hypercalcaemia with CYP24A1 and SLC34A1 mutations. Nephrol Dial Transplant. 2021;36(8):1484–92. https://doi.org/10.1093/ndt/gfaa178.

85. Quamme GA, de Rouffignac C. Epithelial magnesium transport and regulation by the kidney. Front Biosci. 2000;5:D694–711.

86. Kerstan D, Quamme GA. Physiology and pathophysiology of intestinal absorption of magnesium. In: Massry SGMH, Nishizawa Y, editors. Calcium in internal medicine. Springer; 2002. p. 171–83.

87. Fine KD, Santa Ana CA, Porter JL, Fordtran JS. Intestinal absorption of magnesium from food and supplements. J Clin Invest. 1991;88(2):396–402. https://doi.org/10.1172/jci115317.

88. de Rouffignac C, Quamme G. Renal magnesium handling and its hormonal control. Physiol Rev. 1994;74(2):305–22.

89. Dai LJ, Ritchie G, Kerstan D, Kang HS, Cole DE, Quamme GA. Magnesium transport in the renal distal convoluted tubule. Physiol Rev. 2001;81(1):51–84.

90. Quamme GA. Renal magnesium handling: new insights in understanding old problems. Kidney Int. 1997;52(5):1180–95.

91. Whang R, Hampton EM, Whang DD. Magnesium homeostasis and clinical disorders of magnesium deficiency. Ann Pharmacother. 1994;28(2):220–6.

92. Anast CS, Mohs JM, Kaplan SL, Burns TW. Evidence for parathyroid failure in magnesium deficiency. Science. 1972;177(4049):606–8.

93. Quitterer U, Hoffmann M, Freichel M, Lohse MJ. Paradoxical block of parathormone secretion is mediated by increased activity of G alpha subunits. J Biol Chem. 2001;276(9):6763–9. https://doi.org/10.1074/jbc.M007727200.

94. Zimmermann G, Zhou D, Taussig R. Mutations uncover a role for two magnesium ions in the catalytic mechanism of adenylyl cyclase. J Biol Chem. 1998;273(31):19650–5.

95. Hollifield JW. Magnesium depletion, diuretics, and arrhythmias. Am J Med. 1987;82(3a):30–7.

96. Elin RJ. Magnesium: the fifth but forgotten electrolyte. Am J Clin Pathol. 1994;102(5):616–22.

97. Arnold A, Tovey J, Mangat P, Penny W, Jacobs S. Magnesium deficiency in critically ill patients. Anaesthesia. 1995;50(3):203–5.

98. Hébert P, Mehta N, Wang J, Hindmarsh T, Jones G, Cardinal P. Functional magnesium deficiency in critically ill patients identified using a magnesium-loading test. Crit Care Med. 1997;25(5):749–55.

99. Hashimoto Y, Nishimura Y, Maeda H, Yokoyama M. Assessment of magnesium status in patients with bronchial asthma. J Asthma. 2000;37(6):489–96.

100. Sutton RA, Domrongkitchaiporn S. Abnormal renal magnesium handling. Miner Electrolyte Metab. 1993;19(4–5):232–40.

101. Elisaf M, Panteli K, Theodorou J, Siamopoulos KC. Fractional excretion of magnesium in normal subjects and in patients with hypomagnesemia. Magnes Res. 1997;10(4):315–20.

102. Tang NL, Cran YK, Hui E, Woo J. Application of urine magnesium/creatinine ratio as an indicator for insufficient magnesium intake. Clin Biochem. 2000;33(8):675–8. S0009912000001739 [pii].

103. Nicoll GW, Struthers AD, Fraser CG. Biological variation of urinary magnesium. Clin Chem. 1991;37(10 Pt 1):1794–5.

104. Djurhuus MS, Gram J, Petersen PH, Klitgaard NA, Bollerslev J, Beck-Nielsen H. Biological variation of serum and urinary magnesium in apparently healthy males. Scand J Clin Lab Invest. 1995;55(6):549–58.

105. Simon DB, Lu Y, Choate KA, et al. Paracellin-1, a renal tight junction protein required for paracellular Mg2+ resorption. Science. 1999;285(5424):103–6. 7616 [pii].

106. Konrad M, Schaller A, Seelow D, et al. Mutations in the tight-junction gene claudin 19 (CLDN19) are associated with renal magnesium wasting, renal failure, and severe ocular involvement. Am J Hum Genet. 2006;79(5):949–57. S0002-9297(07)60838-6 [pii]. https://doi.org/10.1086/508617.

107. Praga M, Vara J, González-Parra E, et al. Familial hypomagnesemia with hypercalciuria and nephrocalcinosis. Kidney Int. 1995;47(5):1419–25.

108. Weber S, Schneider L, Peters M, et al. Novel paracellin-1 mutations in 25 families with familial hypomagnesemia with hypercalciuria and nephrocalcinosis. J Am Soc Nephrol. 2001;12(9):1872–81.

109. Godron A, Harambat J, Boccio V, et al. Familial hypomagnesemia with hypercalciuria and nephrocalcinosis: phenotype-genotype correlation and outcome in 32 patients with CLDN16 or CLDN19 mutations. Clin J Am Soc Nephrol. 2012;7(5):801–9. CJN.12841211 [pii]. https://doi.org/10.2215/CJN.12841211.

110. Claverie-Martin F, Garcia-Nieto V, Loris C, et al. Claudin-19 mutations and clinical phenotype in Spanish patients with familial hypomagnesemia with hypercalciuria and nephrocalcinosis. PLoS One. 2013;8(1):e53151. https://doi.org/10.1371/journal.pone.0053151.

111. Sikora P, Zaniew M, Haisch L, et al. Retrospective cohort study of familial hypomagnesaemia with hypercalciuria and nephrocalcinosis due to CLDN16 mutations. Nephrol Dial Transplant. 2015;30(4):636–44. https://doi.org/10.1093/ndt/gfu374.

112. Hou J, Goodenough DA. Claudin-16 and claudin-19 function in the thick ascending limb. Curr Opin

Nephrol Hypertens. 2010;19(5):483–8. https://doi.org/10.1097/MNH.0b013e32833b7125.

113. Hou J, Renigunta A, Gomes AS, et al. Claudin-16 and claudin-19 interaction is required for their assembly into tight junctions and for renal reabsorption of magnesium. Proc Natl Acad Sci U S A. 2009;106(36):15350–5. https://doi.org/10.1073/pnas.0907724106. 0907724106 [pii].

114. Konrad M, Hou J, Weber S, et al. CLDN16 genotype predicts renal decline in familial hypomagnesemia with hypercalciuria and nephrocalcinosis. J Am Soc Nephrol. 2008;19(1):171–81. ASN.2007060709 [pii]. https://doi.org/10.1681/ASN.2007060709.

115. Blanchard A, Jeunemaitre X, Coudol P, et al. Paracellin-1 is critical for magnesium and calcium reabsorption in the human thick ascending limb of Henle. Kidney Int. 2001;59(6):2206–15. kid736 [pii]. https://doi.org/10.1046/j.1523-1755.2001.00736.x.

116. Müller D, Kausalya PJ, Claverie-Martin F, et al. A novel claudin 16 mutation associated with childhood hypercalciuria abolishes binding to ZO-1 and results in lysosomal mistargeting. Am J Hum Genet. 2003;73(6):1293–301. S0002-9297(07)63982-2 [pii]. https://doi.org/10.1086/380418.

117. Zimmermann B, Plank C, Konrad M, et al. Hydrochlorothiazide in CLDN16 mutation. Nephrol Dial Transplant. 2006;21(8):2127–32. https://doi.org/10.1093/ndt/gfl144.

118. Knoers NV, Levtchenko EN. Gitelman syndrome. Orphanet J Rare Dis. 2008;3:22. https://doi.org/10.1186/1750-1172-3-22.

119. Simon DB, Nelson-Williams C, Bia MJ, et al. Gitelman's variant of Bartter's syndrome, inherited hypokalaemic alkalosis, is caused by mutations in the thiazide-sensitive Na-Cl cotransporter. Nat Genet. 1996;12(1):24–30. https://doi.org/10.1038/ng0196-24.

120. Gitelman HJ, Graham JB, Welt LG. A new familial disorder characterized by hypokalemia and hypomagnesemia. Trans Assoc Am Phys. 1966;79:221–35.

121. Peters N, Bettinelli A, Spicher I, Basilico E, Metta MG, Bianchetti MG. Renal tubular function in children and adolescents with Gitelman's syndrome, the hypocalciuric variant of Bartter's syndrome. Nephrol Dial Transplant. 1995;10(8):1313–9.

122 Cruz DN, Shaer AJ, Bia MJ, Lifton RP, Simon DB, Yale Gitelman's and Bartter's Syndrome Collaborative Study Group. Gitelman's syndrome revisited: an evaluation of symptoms and health-related quality of life. Kidney Int. 2001;59(2):710–7. kid540 [pii]. https://doi.org/10.1046/j.1523-1755.2001.059002710.x.

123. Vargas-Poussou R, Dahan K, Kahila D, et al. Spectrum of mutations in Gitelman syndrome. J Am Soc Nephrol. 2011;22(4):693–703. https://doi.org/10.1681/ASN.2010090907.

124. Glaudemans B, Yntema HG, San-Cristobal P, et al. Novel NCC mutants and functional analysis in a new cohort of patients with Gitelman syndrome. Eur J Hum Genet. 2012;20(3):263–70. https://doi.org/10.1038/ejhg.2011.189.

125. Lee JW, Lee J, Heo NJ, Cheong HI, Han JS. Mutations in SLC12A3 and CLCNKB and their correlation with clinical phenotype in patients with Gitelman and Gitelman-like syndrome. J Korean Med Sci. 2016;31(1):47–54. https://doi.org/10.3346/jkms.2016.31.1.47.

126. Fujimura J, Nozu K, Yamamura T, et al. Clinical and genetic characteristics in patients with Gitelman syndrome. Kidney Int Rep. 2019;4(1):119–25. https://doi.org/10.1016/j.ekir.2018.09.015.

127. Blanchard A, Bockenhauer D, Bolignano D, et al. Gitelman syndrome: consensus and guidance from a Kidney Disease: Improving Global Outcomes (KDIGO) Controversies Conference. Kidney Int. 2017;91(1):24–33. https://doi.org/10.1016/j.kint.2016.09.046.

128. Peters M, Jeck N, Reinalter S, et al. Clinical presentation of genetically defined patients with hypokalemic salt-losing tubulopathies. Am J Med. 2002;112(3):183–90. S0002934301010865 [pii].

129. Pachulski RT, Lopez F, Sharaf R. Gitelman's not-so-benign syndrome. N Engl J Med. 2005;353(8):850–1. https://doi.org/10.1056/NEJMc051040.

130. Bianchetti MG, Edefonti A, Bettinelli A. The biochemical diagnosis of Gitelman disease and the definition of "hypocalciuria". Pediatr Nephrol. 2003;18(5):409–11.

131. Tammaro F, Bettinelli A, Cattarelli D, et al. Early appearance of hypokalemia in Gitelman syndrome. Pediatr Nephrol. 2010;25(10):2179–82. https://doi.org/10.1007/s00467-010-1575-1.

132. Bettinelli A, Tosetto C, Colussi G, Tommasini G, Edefonti A, Bianchetti MG. Electrocardiogram with prolonged QT interval in Gitelman disease. Kidney Int. 2002;62(2):580–4. https://doi.org/10.1046/j.1523-1755.2002.00467.x.

133. Scognamiglio R, Negut C, Calò LA. Aborted sudden cardiac death in two patients with Bartter's/Gitelman's syndromes. Clin Nephrol. 2007;67(3):193–7. https://doi.org/10.5414/cnp67193.

134. Calo L, Punzi L, Semplicini A. Hypomagnesemia and chondrocalcinosis in Bartter's and Gitelman's syndrome: review of the pathogenetic mechanisms. Am J Nephrol. 2000;5:347–50.

135. Luthy C, Bettinelli A, Iselin S, et al. Normal prostaglandinuria E2 in Gitelman's syndrome, the hypocalciuric variant of Bartter's syndrome. Am J Kidney Dis. 1995;25(6):824–8.

136. Bockenhauer D, Feather S, Stanescu HC, et al. Epilepsy, ataxia, sensorineural deafness, tubulopathy, and KCNJ10 mutations. N Engl J Med. 2009;360(19):1960–70. 360/19/1960 [pii]. https://doi.org/10.1056/NEJMoa0810276.

137. Scholl UI, Choi M, Liu T, et al. Seizures, sensorineural deafness, ataxia, mental retardation, and electrolyte imbalance (SeSAME syndrome) caused by

mutations in KCNJ10. Proc Natl Acad Sci U S A. 2009;106(14):5842–7. 0901749106 [pii]. https://doi.org/10.1073/pnas.0901749106.

138. Celmina M, Micule I, Inashkina I, et al. EAST/SeSAME syndrome: review of the literature and introduction of four new Latvian patients. Clin Genet. 2019;95(1):63–78. https://doi.org/10.1111/cge.13374.

139. Cross JH, Arora R, Heckemann RA, et al. Neurological features of epilepsy, ataxia, sensorineural deafness, tubulopathy syndrome. Dev Med Child Neurol. 2013;55(9):846–56. https://doi.org/10.1111/dmcn.12171.

140. Suzumoto Y, Columbano V, Gervasi L, et al. A case series of adult patients affected by EAST/SeSAME syndrome suggests more severe disease in subjects bearing. Intract Rare Dis Res. 2021;10(2):95–101. https://doi.org/10.5582/irdr.2020.03158.

141. Paunier L, Radde IC, Kooh SW, Conen PE, Fraser D. Primary hypomagnesemia with secondary hypocalcemia in an infant. Pediatrics. 1968;41(2):385–402.

142. Lombeck I, Ritzl F, Schnippering HG, et al. Primary hypomagnesemia. I. Absorption studies. Z Kinderheilkd. 1975;118(4):249–58.

143. Milla PJ, Aggett PJ, Wolff OH, Harries JT. Studies in primary hypomagnesaemia: evidence for defective carrier-mediated small intestinal transport of magnesium. Gut. 1979;20(11):1028–33.

144. Matzkin H, Lotan D, Boichis H. Primary hypomagnesemia with a probable double magnesium transport defect. Nephron. 1989;52(1):83–6.

145. Schlingmann KP, Weber S, Peters M, et al. Hypomagnesemia with secondary hypocalcemia is caused by mutations in TRPM6, a new member of the TRPM gene family. Nat Genet. 2002;31(2):166–70. ng889 [pii]. https://doi.org/10.1038/ng889.

146. Walder RY, Landau D, Meyer P, et al. Mutation of TRPM6 causes familial hypomagnesemia with secondary hypocalcemia. Nat Genet. 2002;31(2):171–4. ng901 [pii]. https://doi.org/10.1038/ng901.

147. Jalkanen R, Pronicka E, Tyynismaa H, Hanauer A, Walder R, Alitalo T. Genetic background of HSH in three Polish families and a patient with an X;9 translocation. Eur J Hum Genet. 2006;14(1):55–62. 5201515 [pii]. https://doi.org/10.1038/sj.ejhg.5201515.

148. Guran T, Akcay T, Bereket A, et al. Clinical and molecular characterization of Turkish patients with familial hypomagnesaemia: novel mutations in TRPM6 and CLDN16 genes. Nephrol Dial Transplant. 2012;27(2):667–73. gfr300 [pii]. https://doi.org/10.1093/ndt/gfr300.

149. Lainez S, Schlingmann KP, van der Wijst J, et al. New TRPM6 missense mutations linked to hypomagnesemia with secondary hypocalcemia. Eur J Hum Genet. 2014;22(4):497–504. https://doi.org/10.1038/ejhg.2013.178.

150. Chubanov V, Schlingmann KP, Wäring J, et al. Hypomagnesemia with secondary hypocalcemia due to a missense mutation in the putative pore-forming region of TRPM6. J Biol Chem. 2007;282(10):7656–67. M611117200 [pii]. https://doi.org/10.1074/jbc.M611117200.

151. Cole DE, Kooh SW, Vieth R. Primary infantile hypomagnesaemia: outcome after 21 years and treatment with continuous nocturnal nasogastric magnesium infusion. Eur J Pediatr. 2000;159(1–2):38–43.

152. Shalev H, Phillip M, Galil A, Carmi R, Landau D. Clinical presentation and outcome in primary familial hypomagnesaemia. Arch Dis Child. 1998;78(2):127–30.

153. Schlingmann KP, Bandulik S, Mammen C, et al. Germline de novo mutations in ATP1A1 cause renal hypomagnesemia, refractory seizures, and intellectual disability. Am J Hum Genet. 2018;103(5):808–16. https://doi.org/10.1016/j.ajhg.2018.10.004.

154. Lucking K, Nielsen JM, Pedersen PA, Jorgensen PL. Na-K-ATPase isoform (alpha 3, alpha 2, alpha 1) abundance in rat kidney estimated by competitive RT-PCR and ouabain binding. Am J Phys. 1996;271(2 Pt 2):F253–60.

155. Munzer JS, Daly SE, Jewell-Motz EA, Lingrel JB, Blostein R. Tissue- and isoform-specific kinetic behavior of the Na,K-ATPase. J Biol Chem. 1994;269(24):16668–76.

156. Lassuthova P, Rebelo AP, Ravenscroft G, et al. Mutations in ATP1A1 cause dominant Charcot-Marie-tooth type 2. Am J Hum Genet. 2018;102(3):505–14. https://doi.org/10.1016/j.ajhg.2018.01.023.

157. Stregapede F, Travaglini L, Rebelo AP, et al. Hereditary spastic paraplegia is a novel phenotype for germline de novo ATP1A1 mutation. Clin Genet. 2020;97(3):521–6. https://doi.org/10.1111/cge.13668.

158. Beuschlein F, Boulkroun S, Osswald A, et al. Somatic mutations in ATP1A1 and ATP2B3 lead to aldosterone-producing adenomas and secondary hypertension. Nat Genet. 2013;45(4):440–4., , 444. e1–2. https://doi.org/10.1038/ng.2550.

159. Meij IC, Koenderink JB, van Bokhoven H, et al. Dominant isolated renal magnesium loss is caused by misrouting of the Na(+),K(+)-ATPase gamma-subunit. Nat Genet. 2000;26(3):265–6. https://doi.org/10.1038/81543.

160. Arystarkhova E, Wetzel RK, Sweadner KJ. Distribution and oligomeric association of splice forms of Na(+)-K(+)-ATPase regulatory gamma-subunit in rat kidney. Am J Physiol Renal Physiol. 2002;282(3):F393–407. https://doi.org/10.1152/ajprenal.00146.2001.

161. Arystarkhova E, Donnet C, Asinovski NK, Sweadner KJ. Differential regulation of renal Na,K-ATPase by splice variants of the gamma subunit. J Biol Chem.

2002;277(12):10162–72. M111552200 [pii]. https://doi.org/10.1074/jbc.M111552200.

162. Geven WB, Monnens LA, Willems HL, Buijs WC, ter Haar BG. Renal magnesium wasting in two families with autosomal dominant inheritance. Kidney Int. 1987;31(5):1140–4.

163. de Baaij JH, Dorresteijn EM, Hennekam EA, et al. Recurrent FXYD2 p.Gly41Arg mutation in patients with isolated dominant hypomagnesaemia. Nephrol Dial Transplant. 2015;30(6):952–7. https://doi.org/10.1093/ndt/gfv014.

164. Glaudemans B, van der Wijst J, Scola RH, et al. A missense mutation in the Kv1.1 voltage-gated potassium channel-encoding gene KCNA1 is linked to human autosomal dominant hypomagnesemia. J Clin Invest. 2009;119(4):936–42. 36948 [pii]. https://doi.org/10.1172/JCI36948.

165. Browne DL, Gancher ST, Nutt JG, et al. Episodic ataxia/myokymia syndrome is associated with point mutations in the human potassium channel gene, KCNA1. Nat Genet. 1994;8(2):136–40. https://doi.org/10.1038/ng1094-136.

166. van der Wijst J, Glaudemans B, Venselaar H, et al. Functional analysis of the Kv1.1 N255D mutation associated with autosomal dominant hypomagnesemia. J Biol Chem. 2010;285(1):171–8. M109.041517 [pii]. https://doi.org/10.1074/jbc.M109.041517.

167. Geven WB, Monnens LA, Willems JL, Buijs W, Hamel CJ. Isolated autosomal recessive renal magnesium loss in two sisters. Clin Genet. 1987;32(6):398–402.

168. Groenestege WM, Thébault S, van der Wijst J, et al. Impaired basolateral sorting of pro-EGF causes isolated recessive renal hypomagnesemia. J Clin Invest. 2007;117(8):2260–7. https://doi.org/10.1172/JCI31680.

169. Thebault S, Alexander RT, Tiel Groenestege WM, Hoenderop JG, Bindels RJ. EGF increases TRPM6 activity and surface expression. J Am Soc Nephrol. 2009;20(1):78–85. ASN.2008030327 [pii]. https://doi.org/10.1681/ASN.2008030327.

170. Stuiver M, Lainez S, Will C, et al. CNNM2, encoding a basolateral protein required for renal Mg2+ handling, is mutated in dominant hypomagnesemia. Am J Hum Genet. 2011;88(3):333–43. S0002-9297(11)00053-X [pii]. https://doi.org/10.1016/j.ajhg.2011.02.005.

171. Goytain A, Quamme GA. Functional characterization of ACDP2 (ancient conserved domain protein), a divalent metal transporter. Physiol Genomics. 2005;22(3):382–9. 00058.2005 [pii]. https://doi.org/10.1152/physiolgenomics.00058.2005.

172. Meyer TE, Verwoert GC, Hwang SJ, et al. Genome-wide association studies of serum magnesium, potassium, and sodium concentrations identify six Loci influencing serum magnesium levels. PLoS Genet. 2010;6(8):e1001045. https://doi.org/10.1371/journal.pgen.1001045.

173. Wang CY, Shi JD, Yang P, et al. Molecular cloning and characterization of a novel gene family of four ancient conserved domain proteins (ACDP). Gene. 2003;(306):37–44.

174. de Baaij JH, Stuiver M, Meij IC, et al. Membrane topology and intracellular processing of cyclin M2 (CNNM2). J Biol Chem. 2012;287(17):13644–55. https://doi.org/10.1074/jbc.M112.342204.

175. Franken GAC, Müller D, Mignot C, et al. Phenotypic and genetic spectrum of patients with heterozygous mutations in cyclin M2 (CNNM2). Hum Mutat. 2021;42(4):473–86. https://doi.org/10.1002/humu.24182.

176. Arjona FJ, de Baaij JH, Schlingmann KP, et al. CNNM2 mutations cause impaired brain development and seizures in patients with hypomagnesemia. PLoS Genet. 2014;10(4):e1004267. https://doi.org/10.1371/journal.pgen.1004267.

177. Accogli A, Scala M, Calcagno A, et al. CNNM2 homozygous mutations cause severe refractory hypomagnesemia, epileptic encephalopathy and brain malformations. Eur J Med Genet. 2019;62(3):198–203. https://doi.org/10.1016/j.ejmg.2018.07.014.

178. Cronan K, ME N. Renal and electrolyte emergencies. In: Fleisher G, S L, eds. Pediatric emergency medicine. 4th ed. Lippincott, Williams & Wilkins; 2000.

179. Horikawa Y, Iwasaki N, Hara M, et al. Mutation in hepatocyte nuclear factor-1 beta gene (TCF2) associated with MODY. Nat Genet. 1997;17(4):384–5. https://doi.org/10.1038/ng1297-384.

180. Faguer S, Decramer S, Chassaing N, et al. Diagnosis, management, and prognosis of HNF1B nephropathy in adulthood. Kidney Int. 2011;80(7):768–76. https://doi.org/10.1038/ki.2011.225.

181. Heidet L, Decramer S, Pawtowski A, et al. Spectrum of HNF1B mutations in a large cohort of patients who harbor renal diseases. Clin J Am Soc Nephrol. 2010;5(6):1079–90. CJN.06810909 [pii]. https://doi.org/10.2215/CJN.06810909.

182. Adalat S, Woolf AS, Johnstone KA, et al. HNF1B mutations associate with hypomagnesemia and renal magnesium wasting. J Am Soc Nephrol. 2009;20(5):1123–31. ASN.2008060633 [pii]. https://doi.org/10.1681/ASN.2008060633.

183. Adalat S, Hayes WN, Bryant WA, et al. HNF1B mutations are associated with a Gitelman-like Tubulopathy that develops during childhood. Kidney Int Rep. 2019;4(9):1304–11. https://doi.org/10.1016/j.ekir.2019.05.019.

184. Raaijmakers A, Corveleyn A, Devriendt K, et al. Criteria for HNF1B analysis in patients with congenital abnormalities of kidney and urinary tract. Nephrol Dial Transplant. 2015;30(5):835–42. https://doi.org/10.1093/ndt/gfu370.

185. Kołbuc M, Leßmeier L, Salamon-Słowińska D, et al. Hypomagnesemia is underestimated in children with HNF1B mutations. Pediatr Nephrol. 2020;35(10):1877–86. https://doi.org/10.1007/s00467-020-04576-6.

186. Ferre S, de Baaij JH, Ferreira P, et al. Mutations in PCBD1 cause hypomagnesemia and renal magnesium

wasting. J Am Soc Nephrol. 2014;25(3):574–86. https://doi.org/10.1681/asn.2013040337.

187. Wilson FH, Hariri A, Farhi A, et al. A cluster of metabolic defects caused by mutation in a mitochondrial tRNA. Science. 2004;306(5699):1190–4. 1102521 [pii]. https://doi.org/10.1126/science.1102521.

188. English MW, Skinner R, Pearson AD, Price L, Wyllie R, Craft AW. Dose-related nephrotoxicity of carboplatin in children. Br J Cancer. 1999;81(2):336–41. https://doi.org/10.1038/sj.bjc.6690697.

189. Goren MP. Cisplatin nephrotoxicity affects magnesium and calcium metabolism. Med Pediatr Oncol. 2003;41(3):186–9. https://doi.org/10.1002/mpo.10335.

190. Boulikas T, Vougiouka M. Recent clinical trials using cisplatin, carboplatin and their combination chemotherapy drugs (review). Oncol Rep. 2004;11(3):559–95.

191. Lajer H, Daugaard G. Cisplatin and hypomagnesemia. Cancer Treat Rev. 1999;25(1):47–58. S0305-7372(99)90097-X [pii]. https://doi.org/10.1053/ctrv.1999.0097.

192. Mavichak V, Coppin CM, Wong NL, Dirks JH, Walker V, Sutton RA. Renal magnesium wasting and hypocalciuria in chronic cis-platinum nephropathy in man. Clin Sci (Lond). 1988;75(2):203–7.

193. Puchalski AR, Hodge MB. Parathyroid hormone resistance from severe hypomagnesaemia caused by cisplatin. Endokrynol Pol. 2020;71(6):577–8. https://doi.org/10.5603/EP.a2020.0061.

194. Bianchetti MG, Kanaka C, Ridolfi-Lüthy A, Hirt A, Wagner HP, Oetliker OH. Persisting renotubular sequelae after cisplatin in children and adolescents. Am J Nephrol. 1991;11(2):127–30.

195. Markmann M, Rothman R, Reichman B, et al. Persistent hypomagnesemia following cisplatin chemotherapy in patients with ovarian cancer. J Cancer Res Clin Oncol. 1991;117(2):89–90.

196. Ledeganck KJ, Boulet GA, Bogers JJ, Verpooten GA, De Winter BY. The TRPM6/EGF pathway is downregulated in a rat model of cisplatin nephrotoxicity. PLoS One. 2013;8(2):e57016. https://doi.org/10.1371/journal.pone.0057016.

197. Yoshida T, Niho S, Toda M, et al. Protective effect of magnesium preloading on cisplatin-induced nephrotoxicity: a retrospective study. Jpn J Clin Oncol. 2014;44(4):346–54. https://doi.org/10.1093/jjco/hyu004.

198. Shah GM, Kirschenbaum MA. Renal magnesium wasting associated with therapeutic agents. Miner Electrolyte Metab. 1991;17(1):58–64.

199. Elliott C, Newman N, Madan A. Gentamicin effects on urinary electrolyte excretion in healthy subjects. Clin Pharmacol Ther. 2000;67(1):16–21. S0009-9236(00)47829-X [pii]. https://doi.org/10.1067/mcp.2000.103864.

200. Giapros VI, Cholevas VI, Andronikou SK. Acute effects of gentamicin on urinary electrolyte excretion in neonates. Pediatr Nephrol. 2004;19(3):322–5. https://doi.org/10.1007/s00467-003-1381-0.

201. Ward DT, McLarnon SJ, Riccardi D. Aminoglycosides increase intracellular calcium levels and ERK activity in proximal tubular OK cells expressing the extracellular calcium-sensing receptor. J Am Soc Nephrol. 2002;13(6):1481–9.

202. Lee CT, Chen HC, Ng HY, Lai LW, Lien YH. Renal adaptation to gentamicin-induced mineral loss. Am J Nephrol. 2012;35(3):279–86. https://doi.org/10.1159/000336518.

203. Rob PM, Lebeau A, Nobiling R, et al. Magnesium metabolism: basic aspects and implications of ciclosporine toxicity in rats. Nephron. 1996;72(1):59–66.

204. Lote CJ, Thewles A, Wood JA, Zafar T. The hypomagnesaemic action of FK506: urinary excretion of magnesium and calcium and the role of parathyroid hormone. Clin Sci (Lond). 2000;99(4):285–92.

205. Chang CT, Hung CC, Tian YC, Yang CW, Wu MS. Ciclosporin reduces paracellin-1 expression and magnesium transport in thick ascending limb cells. Nephrol Dial Transplant. 2007;22(4):1033–40. https://doi.org/10.1093/ndt/gfl817.

206. Nijenhuis T, Hoenderop JG, Bindels RJ. Downregulation of Ca(2+) and Mg(2+) transport proteins in the kidney explains tacrolimus (FK506)-induced hypercalciuria and hypomagnesemia. J Am Soc Nephrol. 2004;15(3):549–57.

207. Ledeganck KJ, De Winter BY, Van den Driessche A, et al. Magnesium loss in cyclosporine-treated patients is related to renal epidermal growth factor downregulation. Nephrol Dial Transplant. 2014;29(5):1097–102. https://doi.org/10.1093/ndt/gft498.

208. Ledeganck KJ, Anné C, De Monie A, et al. Longitudinal study of the role of epidermal growth factor on the fractional excretion of magnesium in children: effect of calcineurin inhibitors. Nutrients. 2018;10(6):677. https://doi.org/10.3390/nu10060677.

209. Tejpar S, Piessevaux H, Claes K, et al. Magnesium wasting associated with epidermal-growth-factor receptor-targeting antibodies in colorectal cancer: a prospective study. Lancet Oncol. 2007;8(5):387–94. S1470-2045(07)70108-0 [pii]. https://doi.org/10.1016/S1470-2045(07)70108-0.

210. Cao Y, Liao C, Tan A, Liu L, Gao F. Meta-analysis of incidence and risk of hypomagnesemia with cetuximab for advanced cancer. Chemotherapy. 2010;56(6):459–65. 000321011 [pii]. https://doi.org/10.1159/000321011.

211. Kimura M, Usami E, Teramachi H, Yoshimura T. Identifying optimal magnesium replenishment points based on risk of severe hypomagnesemia in colorectal cancer patients treated with cetuximab or panitumumab. Cancer Chemother Pharmacol. 2020;86(3):383–91. https://doi.org/10.1007/s00280-020-04126-9.

212. Fujii H, Iihara H, Suzuki A, et al. Hypomagnesemia is a reliable predictor for efficacy of anti-EGFR monoclonal antibody used in combination with first-line chemotherapy for metastatic colorectal cancer.

Cancer Chemother Pharmacol. 2016;77(6):1209–15. https://doi.org/10.1007/s00280-016-3039-1.

213. Vickers MM, Karapetis CS, Tu D, et al. Association of hypomagnesemia with inferior survival in a phase III, randomized study of cetuximab plus best supportive care versus best supportive care alone: NCIC CTG/AGITG CO.17. Ann Oncol. 2013;24(4):953–60. https://doi.org/10.1093/annonc/mds577.

214. Cundy T, Mackay J. Proton pump inhibitors and severe hypomagnesaemia. Curr Opin Gastroenterol. 2011;27(2):180–5. https://doi.org/10.1097/MOG.0b013e32833ff5d6.

215. Epstein M, McGrath S, Law F. Proton-pump inhibitors and hypomagnesemic hypoparathyroidism. N Engl J Med. 2006;355(17):1834–6. 355/17/1834 [pii]. https://doi.org/10.1056/NEJMc066308.

216. Shabajee N, Lamb EJ, Sturgess I, Sumathipala RW. Omeprazole and refractory hypomagnesaemia. BMJ. 2008;337:a425. https://doi.org/10.1136/bmj.39505.738981.BE.

217. Ahmad ASR. Disorders of magnesium metabolism. The kidney: physiology and pathophysiology. New York: Raven Press; 2000. p. 1732–48.

218. Agus ZS. Hypomagnesemia. J Am Soc Nephrol. 1999;10(7):1616–22.

219. Koo W, RC T. Calcium and magnesium homeostasis. In: Avery G, Fletcher M, MacDonald M, eds. Neonatology—pathophysiology and management of the newborn. 5th ed. Lippincott Williams & Wilkins; 1999. p. 730.

220. P G, Reed M. Medications. In: Behrman R, Kliegman R, Jenson H, eds. Textbook of pediatrics. 16th ed. WB Saunders; 2000.

221. Ranade VV, Somberg JC. Bioavailability and pharmacokinetics of magnesium after administration of magnesium salts to humans. Am J Ther. 2001;8(5):345–57.

222. Ryan MP. Magnesium and potassium-sparing diuretics. Magnesium. 1986;5(5–6):282–92.

223. Netzer T, Knauf H, Mutschler E. Modulation of electrolyte excretion by potassium retaining diuretics. Eur Heart J. 1992;13 Suppl G:22–7.

224. Colussi G, Rombola G, De Ferrari ME, Macaluso M, Minetti L. Correction of hypokalemia with anti-aldosterone therapy in Gitelman's syndrome. Am J Nephrol. 1994;14(2):127–35.

225. Bundy JT, Connito D, Mahoney MD, Pontier PJ. Treatment of idiopathic renal magnesium wasting with amiloride. Am J Nephrol. 1995;15(1):75–7.

Disorders of Phosphorus Metabolism

38

Dieter Haffner and Siegfried Waldegger

Introduction

The underlying pathophysiological mechanisms of hypophosphatemic disorders have been unraveled during the last decade, although some puzzles remain to be solved. In 1937, Albright first reported on a patient with rickets and severe hypophosphatemia not responding to high doses of vitamin D. The term vitamin D resistant rickets was coined, and later the disease was named X-linked hypophosphatemic rickets respective X-linked hypophosphatemia (XLH) [1].

In recent years several underlying genes have been identified in distinct forms of hypophosphatemic rickets [2, 3]. Rickets is a disease of the growth plate and therefore only growing children are affected [4]. Whereas in the past rickets was thought to be a disease of calcium and vitamin D metabolism, there is growing evidence that rickets is due to insufficient availability of phosphate which is required for normal bone metabolism [5].

In principle, phosphate deficiency may result from inappropriate absorption in the gut or reabsorption in the kidney. The latter situation can be further divided between defects in the tubular reabsorption apparatus and abnormalities of circulating factors which regulate phosphate reabsorption [6]. The major breakthrough in our understanding of hypophosphatemic disorders was the discovery of fibroblast growth factor 23 (FGF23), a member of the FGF family, which mediates the combined renal tubular defects in phosphate reabsorption and altered vitamin D metabolism observed in patients with hypophosphatemic rickets [7].

Currently, specific disease-causing mutations in genes involved in the regulation of phosphate homeostasis can be identified in approx. 85% of familial or sporadic cases of hypophosphatemic rickets [8–11]. This chapter focuses on the etiology, pathogenesis, clinical presentation, differential diagnosis and treatment of hypophosphatemic disorders due to a reduction of renal tubular reabsorption.

D. Haffner (✉)
Department of Pediatric Kidney, Liver and Metabolic Diseases, Hannover Medical School, Hannover, Germany
e-mail: haffner.dieter@mh-hannover.de

S. Waldegger
Department of Pediatric Nephrology, Medical University of Innsbruck, Innsbruck, Austria
e-mail: siegfried.waldegger@uki.at

Phosphate Homeostasis

Inorganic phosphate (Pi) is a key player in cellular metabolism and skeletal mineralization. It accounts for about 0.6 and 1% of body weight of a neonate and an adult, respectively. Approximately 85% of total body Pi content is deposited as hydroxyl-apatite [Ca$_5$(PO$_4$)$_3$OH] in the skeleton and the teeth. About 14% distributes within the intracellular compartment. There, Pi participates in as diverse cellular processes as cell membrane function (phospholipids), energy metabolism (ATP), cell signaling (phosphorylation by kinases), and DNA- or RNA-biosynthesis (phosphorylated nucleotides). Only 1% of the total body Pi content is found as a soluble fraction in the extracellular compartment. There, Pi contributes to the acid-base buffering capacity of the plasma and even more important of the urine. Solely this tip of the iceberg is amenable to conventional laboratory investigations from blood and urine samples. Moreover, circulatory Pi is the central mediator between bone, the parathyroid glands, the gut and the kidneys, which are fine-tuned by numerous hormonal signals to keep the serum phosphate concentration within close limits.

In a steady state condition, as it is the case after completion of skeletal growth, the serum Pi concentration is determined by the balance between intestinal absorption of phosphate from the diet (16 mg/kg per day), bone-turnover of phosphate in the skeleton (3 mg/kg per day), and excretion of phosphate through the urine (16 mg/kg per day), (Fig. 38.1). In growing individuals, the balance of Pi must be positive to meet the needs of skeletal growth and consolidation. A typical Western diet commonly provides plenty of alimentary Pi, most of which provided by protein-rich foods like meat, milk and eggs. In contrast to plant-derived phosphate in the form of phytate (hexa-phospho-inosite), the animal derived phosphate is easily absorbed by the intestine, where roughly two thirds of the ingested phosphate are absorbed. Intestinal Pi absorption in growing infants is higher than in adults and can exceed 90% of dietary intake. Absorbed Pi first distributes in the extracellular compartment and then equilibrates with the bone and intracellular compartment. Within the kidney, Pi is freely filtered at the glomerular capillaries and is reabsorbed mainly along the proximal nephrons according to the actual requirements of the organism. The majority of the transepithelial Pi transport in the intestine

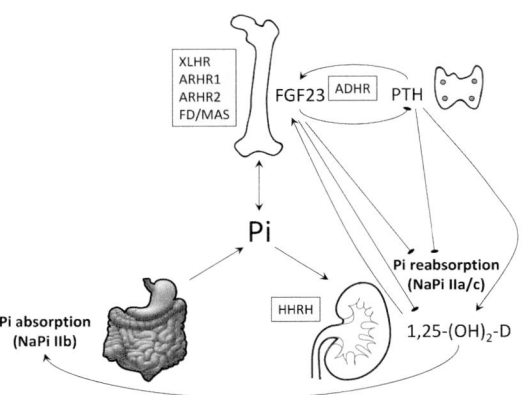

Fig. 38.1 Regulation of phosphate (P$_i$) homeostasis. FGF23 and PTH reduce renal tubular phosphate reabsorption via a decrease in apical expression of the sodium-phosphate cotransporters NaPi IIa and NaPi IIc. In contrast to FGF23, which inhibits 1,25-(OH)$_2$D synthesis, PTH stimulates 1,25-(OH)$_2$D production. 1,25-(OH)$_2$D increases intestinal absorption of dietary P$_i$ via increased expression of NaPi IIb and activates FGF23 production. PTH and FGF23 affect each other's production through a negative feedback loop that is not yet fully elucidated. The mode of action of the therapeutic antibody burosumab is indicated. Note, burosumab is currently licensed for treatment of XLH and tumor induced osteomalacia (TIO), only. The sites of defect of the different genetic forms of hypophosphatemic disorders are given. *XLH* X-linked hypophosphatemia, *ARHR1/2* autosomal recessive hypophosphatemic rickets 1/2, *Raine S.* Raine syndrome, *FD/MAS* Fibrous dysplasia/McCune-Albright syndrome, *HHRH* hereditary hypophosphatemic rickets with hypercalciuria, *ADHR* X-linked dominant hypophosphatemic rickets. *FGF23 protein resistant to degradation

and the kidney is mediated by the type II family of sodium-coupled phosphate transporters, i.e. NaPi-IIa (NPT2a; *SLC34A1*), NaPi-IIb (NPT2b; *SLC34A2*), and NaPi-IIc (NPT2c; *SLC34A3*) [12]. NaPi-IIa is primarily localized at the brush border of proximal tubular epithelial cells and accounts for roughly 90% of renal phosphate reabsorption. Reabsorption of the remaining 10% is accomplished by NaPi-IIc exclusively expressed along proximal tubules of deep nephrons. Its critical contribution to Pi homeostasis is demonstrated by loss-of-function mutations, which leads to renal phosphate wasting resulting in the rare syndrome of hypophosphatemic rickets with hypercalcemia (HHRH) [13].

In contrast to NaPi-IIa and NaPi-IIc, NaPi-IIb shows a broader expression pattern including pulmonary alveolar type II cells, where it participates in Pi uptake from the alveolar fluid for surfactant production. *SLC34A2* mutations cause pulmonary alveolar microlithiasis, a disease characterized by the deposition of calcium-phosphate crystals throughout the lungs [14]. In the intestine, NaPi-IIb is expressed in the brush border membrane of enterocytes and mediates absorption of ingested phosphate.

Regulators of Phosphate Homeostasis

The amount of intestinal phosphate absorption directly correlates with dietary supply. Only 30% of intestinal Pi absorption occurs in a regulated, 1,25-dihydroxyvitamin D [1,25-(OH)$_2$D] dependent manner. This poor regulation at the uptake level contrasts with the meticulous regulation of phosphate excretion within the kidney. Proximal tubular reabsorption of phosphate, mainly via regulation of expression of NaPi-IIa and NaPi-IIc within proximal tubular brush border membranes, thus plays a key role in maintaining serum phosphate homeostasis. The amount of renal phosphate reabsorption is tightly regulated primarily by dietary Pi intake, parathyroid hormone (PTH) and fibroblast growth factor 23 (FGF23). Other factors like insulin, human growth hormone, and possibly FGF7 also affect renal phosphate handling, but their actions are less well understood [15].

Dietary Pi intake directly affects the amount of renal phosphate reabsorption. An increase or decrease in dietary Pi induces an increase or decrease, respectively, in renal Pi excretion independent of vitamin D, PTH or FGF23. Part of this effect might be explained by a phosphate-responsive element in the promoter of the *SLC34A1* gene [16].

Parathyroid hormone is a major hormonal regulator of proximal tubular Pi reabsorption. PTH synthesis and secretion are up-regulated by low serum calcium and increased serum phosphate levels, and down-regulated by increased serum calcium and 1,25(OH)$_2$D levels. Its binding to proximal tubular PTH receptors results in an inhibition of NaPi-cotransport through mechanisms that involve rapid clearance of NaPi-IIa from the tubular epithelial brush border membrane [17]. On the other hand, PTH stimulates the synthesis of 1,25-(OH)$_2$D. The net effect of these actions is an increase of serum calcium levels and a decrease in serum phosphate levels.

Fibroblast Growth Factor 23 is a glycoprotein primarily synthesized in osteocytes and osteoblasts. FGF23 expression is induced by increased serum phosphate and 1,25(OH)$_2$D levels. In the presence of Klotho, a membrane bound protein with ß-glucuronidase activity, FGF23 binds with high affinity to the FGF receptor FGFR1 [15]. Klotho/FGFR1 mediated renal effects of FGF23 result in inhibition of proximal tubular Pi reabsorption and 1,25(OH)$_2$D synthesis. Its net effect thus is a reduction in serum phosphate and 1,25-(OH)$_2$D levels, which may result in hypocalcemia (Fig. 38.1).

Hypophosphatemic Disorders

Clinical, Biochemical, and Radiological Manifestations

Clinical Findings

The clinical and radiological features of the various types of hypophosphatemic rickets are similar, although not identical. In children, the primary clinical symptoms are rickets, skeletal pain and deformity, disproportionate short stature, and dental abscesses' (Figs. 38.2 and 38.3) [19]. In adults, osteomalacia, bone pain and stiffness, pseudofractures, enthesopathy and poor dental condition including periodontitis are typical findings. With medical therapy these abnormalities can be improved, but usually do not entirely resolve [18, 20]. Most children with hypophosphatemic rickets are identified in the first year of life if there is a known family history of the disorder. By 6 months of age, classic skeletal deformities may already appear including frontal bossing with flattening at the back of the head. In the absence of a family history, children often present at 2–3 years of age with delayed walking, muscle weakness, a waddling gait and

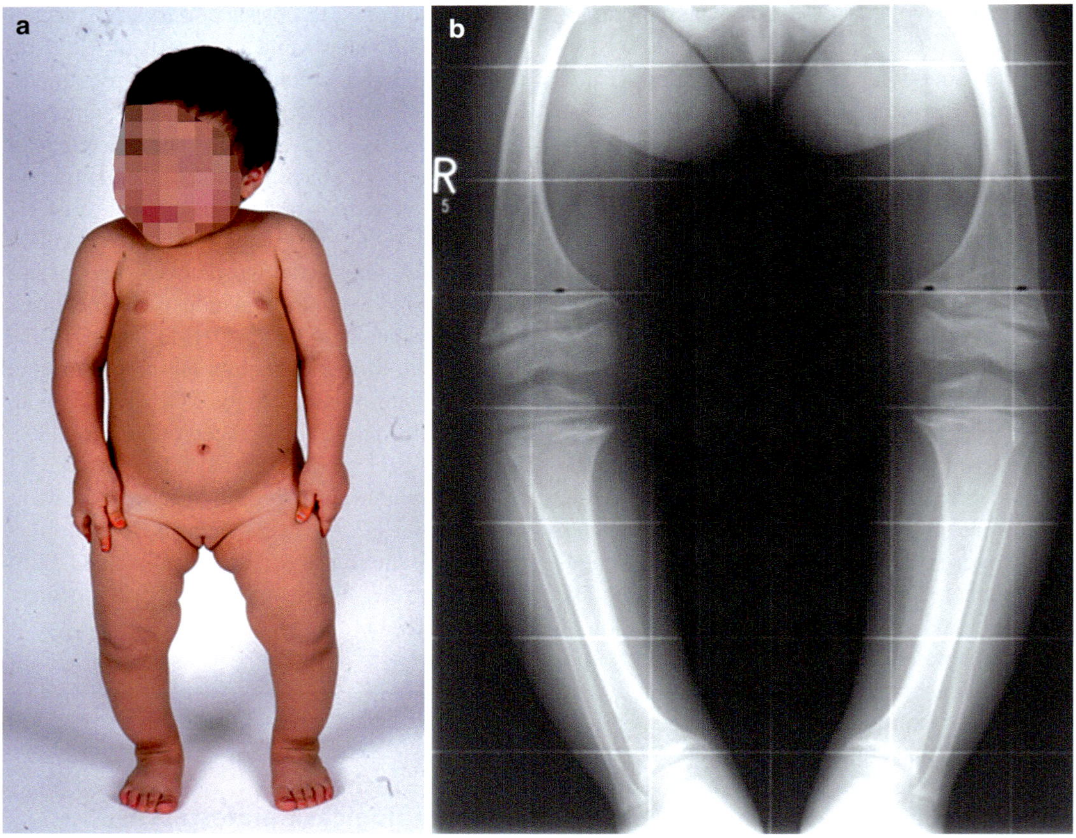

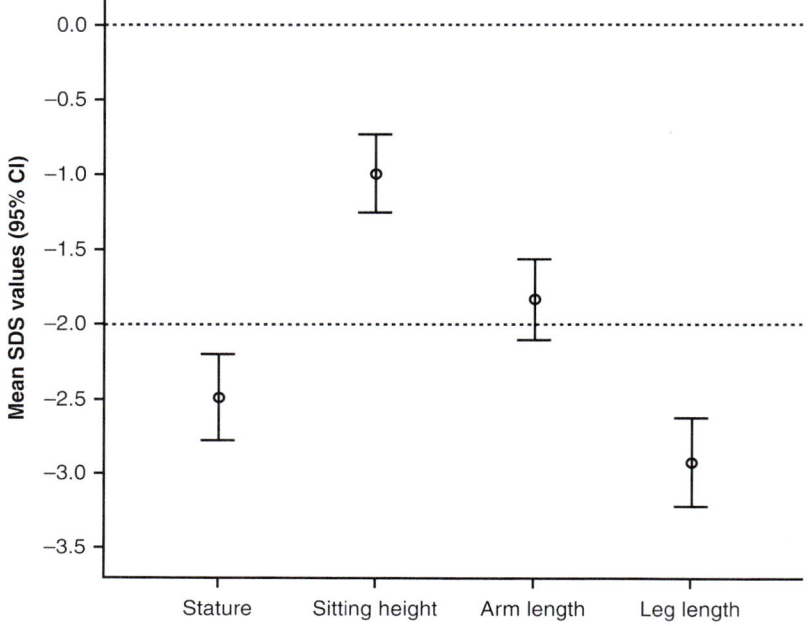

Fig. 38.2 Photograph (**a**) and radiograph of the lower extremities (**b**) of a 3-year-old girl with X-linked hypophosphatemia. The patient shows disproportionate stunting with bowed legs. The radiograph reveals severe leg bowing, partial fraying and irregularity of the distal femoral and proximal tibial growth plates

Fig. 38.3 Mean standard deviation scores (SDS) and 95% confidence intervals (CI) of stature, sitting height, and arm and leg length in 76 children with X-linked hypophosphatemia. Patients showed disproportionate stunting. Leg length was the most impaired and trunk length the most preserved linear body dimension (Used with permission of Nature/ Springer from Zivicnjak et al. [18])

progressive lower extremity deformities (bow-legged). Leg growth is often more impaired than trunk growth resulting in disproportionate short stature [18]. Patients may present with abnormal skull shape, i.e. dolichocephaly, characterized by frontal bossing, parietal flattening and widened sutures due to premature cranial synostosis [21]. Common misdiagnoses are metaphyseal dysplasia and nutritional rickets. Long-term outcomes are substantially better when treatment is applied at an early age, i.e. in the first year of life [22–24]. In adults, the occurrence of pseudofractures of the long bones and enthesopathies may result in additional pain and substantially compromised quality of life [25].

Bone histology is influenced by the pathophysiology of the disease. In general, pure hypophosphatemia results in accumulation of unmineralized osteoid (Fig. 38.4), while the concomitant presence of hyperparathyroidism adds the component of enhanced bone resorption by osteoclasts [27]. However, establishing a diagnosis of phosphopenic osteomalacia requires histopathological proof that the abundant osteoid results from abnormal mineralization and not increased osteoid production. Thus, histopathological detection of an increase in the bone-forming cell surface by incompletely covered mineralized osteoid, an increase in osteoid volume and thickness and a decrease in the mineralization front (the percentage of osteoid-covered bone-forming surface

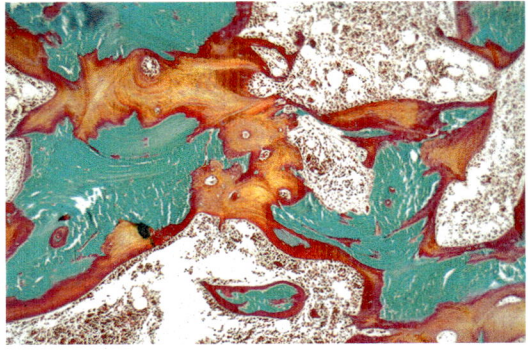

Fig. 38.4 Bone biopsy in a patient with X-linked hypophosphatemia showing abundance of unmineralized osteoid (orange), and decreased mineralization of trabecular and cortical bone (Used with permission of Nature/Springer from Schnabel and Haffner [26])

undergoing calcification) or the mineral apposition rate is a prerequisite [27].

In addition to these skeletal defects, dental abnormalities contribute to considerable clinical morbidity. Tooth eruption may be delayed and teeth may exhibit inadequate dentine calcification [28–32]. As a result, the pulp chambers expand, and the overall barrier to external pathogens is compromised, thereby predisposing to dental abscesses. The prevalence of dental abscesses is about 25% in children and more than 85% in adults [33]. Individuals who present with one abscess usually develop multiple abscesses during follow-up, indicating that the development of one abscess predicts future abscesses. It is important to note that dental abscesses usually occur in the absence of caries. Finally, hypertension, left ventricular hypertrophy, nephrocalcinosis, and hearing loss have been identified in patients suffering from hypophosphatemic rickets, although it is not clear if these abnormalities are due to the disease itself or to the treatment [34–36].

Radiological Findings

The rachitic abnormalities in children with phosphopenic disease result in a variety of characteristic radiological findings in the skeleton. The growth plates of the long bones are cupped and show increased thickness and irregular, hazy appearance at the diaphyseal line (Fig. 38.2). The latter is due to an irregular invasion of recently calcified cartilage in bone tissue. These abnormalities preferentially occur at sites of rapid growth. Therefore, widening of the forearm at the wrist and thickening of the costochondral junctions frequently occur. For clinical confirmation, an x-ray of the knees and/or the wrist is usually sufficient to diagnose rickets [19]. In addition, other typical signs of rickets such as rachitic rosary and Harrison's groove may also develop.

Biochemical Findings

In general, the primary diagnosis of rickets is based on typical clinical and radiological findings (see above) in combination with an elevated serum alkaline phosphatase activity. Physicians often overlook the latter abnormality in children, since normal levels in young children are high. On the other hand, in some affected patients, normal alkaline phosphatase activity might be observed. Moreover, in adults, the alkaline phosphatase levels are often inexplicably normal. For differential diagnosis of the various forms of rickets, additional biochemical parameters are needed. Phosphorus is the common denominator of all types of rickets [5, 6]. Therefore, the diagnostic approach focuses on the mechanisms leading to hypophosphatemia, i.e. (1) high PTH activity, (2) inadequate phosphate absorption from the gut, or (3) renal phosphate wasting. The latter may be due to either intrinsic tubular defects or high circulating FGF23 levels (Fig. 38.5) [5, 6, 19].

Renal phosphate loss can be evaluated through the tubular reabsorption of phosphate per glomerular filtration rate (TmP/GFR) as: $TmP/GFR = P_p - (U_p \times P_{cr}/U_{cr})$, where P_p, U_p, P_{cr} and U_{cr} refer to plasma and urine concentration of phosphate and creatinine, respectively. All values must be expressed in the same units, e.g. in milligrams per deciliter [37]. The normal range of TmP/GFR in infants and children (6 months – 6 years)

ranges from 1.2 to 2.6 mmol/L and in adults from 0.6 to 1.7 mmol/L. An important pitfall to recognize is that in patients with insufficient intake or absorption of phosphate from the gut TmP/GFR might be falsely low when serum phosphate levels have not been restored to normal. This can usually be assumed in the presence of low urinary phosphate levels. In such cases, TmP/GFR should only be calculated after phosphate supplementation when serum and urine phosphate concentrations are raised.

Typically, in cases of hypophosphatemic rickets due to renal tubular abnormalities or elevated serum levels of FGF23, serum concentrations of calcium and PTH are normal before initiation of treatment. Circulating $1,25(OH)_2D$ levels are low or inappropriately normal in the setting of hypophosphatemia. Plasma FGF23 levels are usually elevated with the exception of HHRH patients. Measurement of serum $1,25(OH)_2D$ levels may be a useful tool for diagnosis in HHRH patients. In Table 38.1, the main biochemical features of the various forms of hypophosphatemic rickets due to perturbations in proximal tubule phosphate reabsorption compared to vitamin D defi-

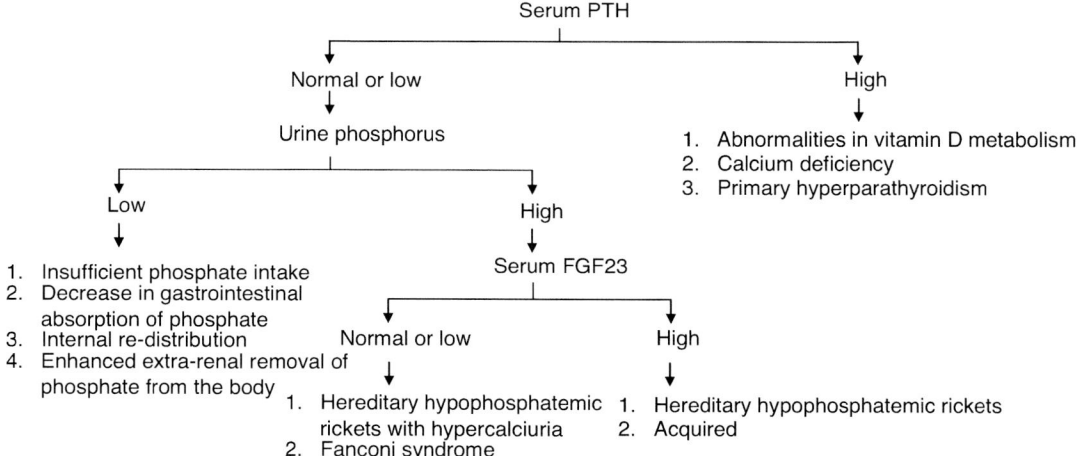

Fig. 38.5 Algorithm for the evaluation of the child with rickets presenting with hypophosphatemia. The differential diagnoses are based on the mechanisms leading to hypophosphatemia, namely high parathyroid hormone (PTH) activity, inadequate phosphate absorption from the gut, or renal phosphate wasting. The latter may be due to

either primary tubular defects or high levels of circulating FGF23. Further details of individual entities can be found in Table 38.1; *FGF-23* fibroblast growth factor 23 (Used with permission of Nature/Springer from Haffner et al. [19])

Table 38.1 Molecular genetic and biochemical characteristics of inherited or acquired causes of phosphopenic rickets in comparison to calcipenic rickets. (Adapted from [19])

Disorder (abbreviation; OMIM#)	Gene (location)	Ca	P	ALP	U_{Ca}	U_P	TmP/GFR	FGF23	PTH	25(OH)D[a]	1,25(OH)$_2$D	Pathogenesis
Rickets and/or osteomalacia with high PTH levels (calcipenic rickets)												
Nutritional rickets (vitamin D and/or calcium deficiency)	NA	N, ↓	N, ↓	↑↑↑	↓	Varies	↓	N	↑↑↑	↓↓, N	varies	Vitamin D deficiency
Vitamin D dependent rickets type 1A (VDDR1A; OMIM#264700)	CYP27B1 (12q14.1)	↓	N, ↓	↑↑↑	↓	Varies	↓	N, ↓	↑↑↑	N	↓	Impaired synthesis of 1,25 (OH)$_2$D
Vitamin D dependent rickets type 1B (VDDR1B; OMIM#600081)	CYP2R1 (11p15.2)	↓	N, ↓	↑↑↑	↓	Varies	↓	N	↑↑↑	↓↓	varies	Impaired synthesis of 25 (OH)D
Vitamin D dependent rickets type 2A (VDDR2A; OMIM#277440)	VDR (12q13.11)	↓	N, ↓	↑↑↑	↓	Varies	↓	N, ↓	↑↑↑	N	↑↑	Impaired signaling of the VDR
Vitamin D dependent rickets type 2B (VDDR2B; OMIM#264700)	HNRNPC	↓	N, ↓	↑↑↑	↓	Varies	↓	N	↑↑↑	N	↑↑	Impaired signaling of the VDR
Vitamin D dependent rickets type 3 (VDDR3; OMIM# pending)	CYP3A4	↓	N, ↓	↑↑↑	↓	Varies	↓	?	↑↑↑	↓	↓	↑ inactivation of 1,25 (OH)$_2$D
Phosphopenic rickets												
Rickets and/or osteomalacia due to dietary phosphate deficiency or impaired bioavailability												
Breastfed very low birthweight infants	NA	N, ↑	↓	↑, ↑↑	?	↓	N[b]	N, ↓	N	N	N, ↑	Phosphate deficiency
Use of elemental or hypoallergenic formula diet or parental nutrition												
Excessive use of phosphate binders												
Gastrointestinal surgery or disorders												
Rickets and/or osteomalacia with renal tubular phosphate wasting due to elevated FGF23 levels and/or signaling												
X-linked hypophosphatemia (XLH; OMIM#307800)	PHEX (Xp22.1)	N	↓	↑, ↑↑	↓	↑	↓	↑, N	N, ↑[c]	N	N[d]	↑FGF23 expression in bone and impaired FGF23 cleavage
Autosomal dominant hypophosphatemic rickets (ADHR; OMIM#193100)	FGF23 (12p13.3)	N	↓	↑, ↑↑	↓	↑	↓	↑, N	N, ↑[c]	N	N[d]	FGF23 protein resistant to degradation
Autosomal recessive hypophosphatemic rickets 1 (ARHR1; OMIM#241520)	DMP1 (4q22.1)	N	↓	↑, ↑↑	↓	↑	↓	↑, N	N, ↑[c]	N	N[d]	↑FGF23 expression in bone
Autosomal recessive hypophosphatemic rickets 2 (ARHR2; OMIM#613312)	ENPP1 (6q23.2)	N	↓	↑, ↑↑	↓	↑	↓	↑, N	N, ↑[c]	N	N[d]	↑FGF23 expression in bone
Raine syndrome associated (ARHR3; OMIM#259775)	FAM20C (7q22.3)	N	↓	↑, ↑↑	?	↑	↓	↑, N	N, ↑[c]	N	N[d]	↑FGF23 expression in bone

(continued)

Table 38.1 (continued)

Disorder (abbreviation; OMIM#)	Gene (location)	Ca	P	ALP	U_{Ca}	U_P	TmP/GFR	FGF23	PTH	25(OH)D[a]	1,25(OH)$_2$D	Pathogenesis
Fibrous dysplasia (FD: OMIM#174800)	GNAS (20q13.3)	N, ↓	↓	↑, ↑↑	↓	↑	↓	N, ↑	N, ↑[c]	N	N[d]	↑ FGF23 expression in bone
Tumor induced osteomalacia (TIO)	NA	N, ↓	↓	↑, ↑↑	↓	↑	↓	N, ↑	N, ↑[c]	N	N[d]	↑ FGF23 express-ion in tumoral cells
Cutaneous skeletal Hypophosphatemia syndrome (SFM; OMIM#163200)	RAS (1p13.2)	N, ↓	↓	↑, ↑↑	↓	↑	↓	N, ↑	N, ↑[c]	N	N[d]	?
Osteoglophonic dysplasia (OGD) (OMIM#166250)	FGFR1 (8p11.23)	N	↓	↑, N	N	↑	↓	N	N, ↑[c]	N	N[d]	↑ FGF23 expression in bone
Hypophosphatemic rickets and hyperparathyroidism (OMIM#612089)	KLOTHO (13q13.1)	N	↓	↑, ↑↑	↓	↑	↓	↑	↑↑	N	N[d]	Unknown; translocation of the KLOTHO promoter
Rickets and/or osteomalacia due to primary renal tubular phosphate wasting												
Hereditary hypophosphatemic rickets with hypercalciuria (HHRH; OMIM#241530)	SLC34A3 (9q34.3)	N	↓	↑ (↑↑)	N, ↑	↑	↓	↓	Low N, ↓	N	↑↑	Loss of function of NaPi2c in the proximal tubule
X-linked recessive hypophosphatemic rickets (OMIM#300554)	CLCN5 (Xp11.23)	N	↓	↑ (↑↑)	N, ↑	↑	↓	varies	varies	N	↑	Loss of function of CLCN5 in the proximal tubule
Hypophosphatemia and nephrocalcinosis (NPHLOP1; OMIM#612286) Fanconi reno-tubular syndrome 2 (FRTS2; OMIM#613388)	SLC34A1 (5q35.3)	N	↓	↑ (↑↑)	↑	↑	↓	↓	varies	N	↑	Loss of function of NaPi2a in the proximal tubule
Cystinosis (OMIM#219800) and other hereditary forms of Fanconi syndrome)	CTNS (17p13.2)	N, ↓	↓	↑ (↑↑)	N, ↑	↑	N, ↓	N, ↑[e]	N, ↑[e]	N	N[d]	Cysteine accumulation in the proximal tubule
Iatrogenic proximal tubulopathy	NA	N	↓	↑ (↑↑)	varies	↑	↓	↓	N	↑	varies	Drug toxicity

N normal, ↑ elevated, ↑↑ or ↑↑↑ very elevated, ↑ (↑↑) may range widely: Ca, serum levels of calcium, *P* serum levels of phosphate, *ALP* alkaline phosphatase, U_{Ca} urinary calcium excretion, *TmP/GFR* maximum rate of renal tubular reabsorption of phosphate normalized to the glomerular filtration rate, *FGF23* fibroblast growth factor 23, *PTH* parathyroid hormone, *1,25(OH)$_2$D* 1,25-dihydroxyvitamin, *25(OH)D* cholecalciferol, *NA* not applicable

[a] Cave: prevalence of vitamin D deficiency was reported to be up-to 50% in healthy children

[b] Normal after restoration of P, but falsely reduced before restoration

[c] PTH may be moderately elevated

[d] Decreased relative to the serum phosphate concentration

[e] Depending on the stage of chronic kidney disease

ciency rickets are summarized. Extended molecular genetic analysis may be required to establish diagnosis in unclear cases [38].

Hypophosphatemic Disorders with Increased FGF23 Activity

X-Linked Hypophosphatemia (*PHEX* Mutation)

X-linked hypophosphatemia (XLH) is the most frequent inherited phosphate wasting disorder, accounting for about 80% of familial cases with an incidence of 1:20,000 individuals. It typically presents within the first 2 years of life. Males usually show the full manifestation of the disease and females show a wide spectrum ranging from one identical to males to one with no clinical symptoms but only isolated hypophosphatemia. The characteristic laboratory results are hypophosphatemia, hyperphosphaturia, hyperphosphatasia and normocalcemia. Serum 25(OH)D and 1,25(OH)$_2$D levels are in the normal range [19]. However, the level of the latter appears to be decreased relative to the diminished serum phosphate concentrations. Elevated serum levels of FGF23 and mutations in the *PHEX* gene (phosphate regulating gene with homologies to endopeptidases on the X-chromosome) are found in most patients [11, 19, 39]. Of note, serum levels of phosphate, TmP/GFR and alkaline phosphatase activity might be in the normal range within the first 3 months of life in XLH patients. Therefore, in the case of a positive family history, affected patients should undergo mutation analysis of the *PHEX* gene in order to establish the diagnosis and treatment of XLH as early as possible [19]. More than 350 different PHEX mutations have been reported so far including nonsense, missense, frame shift, splice site, deletion and duplication mutations. Mutations were reported in all 22 *PHEX* exons without a hot spot and no genotype-phenotype correlations were found in children with XLH [8].

Although the genetic cause of XLH is well established, the exact pathogenic mechanisms of how mutations in the *PHEX* gene result in elevated plasma FGF23 levels remains to be elucidated. *PHEX* encodes for a membrane-bound endopeptidase and is primarily expressed in osteoblasts, osteocytes, odontoblasts, muscle, lung and ovary [40]. The finding that hypophosphatemia recurs in XLH patients undergoing kidney transplantation with prior parathyreoidectomy strongly suggested a circulating factor causing phosphate wasting in the kidney transplant [41]. Likewise, studies in *Hyp* mice, an orthologic animal model of XLH employing parabiosis and cross-transplantation of the kidneys between *Hyp* and normal mice, also showed recurrence of hypophosphatemia [42]. After it became clear that FGF23 is the cause of ADHR, FGF23 levels were measured in patients with XLH and *Hyp* mice. The majority of XLH patients as well as *Hyp* mice show elevated FGF23 levels [43, 44]. The normal FGF23 serum levels found in some XLH patients might still be viewed as inappropriately high in relation to the degree of hypophosphatemia. Administration of neutralizing antibodies to FGF23 corrects hypophosphatemia and decreases 1,25(OH)$_2$D levels in *Hyp* mice and patients with XLH and thus confirms the pathogenic role of FGF23 in XLH [45, 46]. Although PHEX is an enzyme, it is thought that *PHEX* affects the expression of FGF23 rather than its degradation [7, 47]. PHEX may regulate serum FGF23 indirectly via cleavage by proprotein convertases such as subtilisin/kexin-type 2 (PC2). In addition, *PHEX* malfunction results in increased skeletal synthesis of osteopontin and acid serine aspartate-rich-MEPE-associated protein (ASARM) peptide, both of which also contribute to impaired bone mineralization in XLH [7, 48]. Thus, XLH results from a complex osteoblast/odontoblast defect. Therefore, it remains to be seen whether therapeutic FGF23 blockade in patients with XLH (*vide infra*) will result in complete healing of bone and teeth abnormalities as well as prevention of rare complications like sensorineural hearing loss.

ADHR (*FGF23* Mutation)

Autosomal-dominant hypophosphatemic rickets (ADHR) is a rare disorder that was first described by Bianchine et al. in 1971 [49]. ADHR and XLH have marked clinical similarities but differ in their modes of inheritance. ADHR is due to activating mutations of the *FGF23* gene. The mutated protein is resistant to cleavage by proteolytic activity, which in turn leads to elevated, circulating FGF23 level [50]. Elevated FGF23 levels result in phosphaturia, hypophosphatemia, and inappropriately low levels of $1,25(OH)_2D$. The penetrance of ADHR is incomplete, with a highly variable phenotype and, thus, variable symptomatology and biological findings. In contrast to XLH, patients suffering from ADHR may become symptomatic in adolescence or even during adulthood. During childhood, the clinical symptoms are similar to that observed in XLH, i.e. rickets with bone deformities, disproportionately short stature, and dental abnormalities (abscesses) [51]. If patients become symptomatic after puberty, complications due to osteomalacia, e.g. weakness, fatigue, bone pain and pseudofractures are the major symptoms. Adults present with symptoms similar to those with tumor induced osteomalacia (TIO), as discussed below. Interestingly, some children show improvement of phosphate wasting during puberty [52]. Studies in ADHR mice and humans suggest that iron status is an important regulator of FGF23 metabolic pathways [52–54]. Therefore, the onset of ADHR is the product of gene-environment interactions. Serum iron levels are negatively associated with FGF23 plasma level both in ADHR patients and in healthy subjects, indicating increased expression of FGF23 in the setting of a low iron status. A recent study in iron deficient adult ADHR patients demonstrated normalization of both serum FGF23 and phosphate levels by oral iron repletion [55]. Therefore, the standard approach to ADHR patients should also include the recognition and correction of iron deficiency.

ARHR (1, *DMP1* Mutation; 2, *ENPP1* Mutation)

The finding of hypophosphatemic rickets in consanguineous kindreds suggested an autosomal recessive form of hypophosphatemia (ARHR) [56]. Clinical symptoms are similar to those observed in XLH patients and affected individuals present with elevated FGF23 serum levels, renal phosphate wasting and inappropriately normal levels of $1,25(OH)_2D$. One characteristic radiological feature of this disorder is the relatively high bone density of the vertebral bodies.

ARHR is either due to mutations in the *DMP1* gene encoding for dentin matrix acidic phosphoprotein 1 (ARHR1) or to mutations in the *ENPP1* gene encoding for ectonucleotide pyrophosphatase/phosphodiesterase 1 (ARHR2) [57–60].

DMP1 is a member of the short integrin-binding ligand interacting N-linked glycoprotein (SIBLING) family of skeletal matrix proteins and is highly expressed in mineralized tissues, e.g. in osteoblasts and osteocytes. It is an important regulator of the development of bone, cartilage, and teeth. How mutations in *DMP1* result in elevated FGF23 serum levels in ADHR1 patients is unclear.

Levi-Litan et al. identified an inactivating mutation in the *ENPP1* gene (later named ARHR2) that caused ARHR in a Bedouin family [60]. ENPP1 is a cell surface protein that catalyzes phosphoester cleavage of adenosine triphosphate, generating the mineralization inhibitor pyrophosphate. Mutations in *ENPP1* were initially reported in patients with infantile arterial calcifications [61] but clinical and biochemical manifestations can markedly differ even in patients presenting with the same biallelic *ENPP1* pathogenic variants and include enthesopathy and primary hyperparathyroidism [62]. It remains to be elucidated how inactivating *ENPP1* gene mutations result in increased FGF23 synthesis from bone.

Raine Syndrome Associated (*FAM20C* Mutation)

Raine syndrome is a rare skeletal disorder with highly variable clinical phenotype ranging from lethal to isolated teeth and/or bone phenotypes [63]. It is caused by biallelic mutations in the *FAM20C* gene coding for a protein kinase which phosphorylates FGF23 and thereby promotes FGF23 cleavage. Therefore, *FAM20C* mutations result in high serum FGF23 concentrations causing renal phosphate wasting with consecutive hypophosphatemic rickets [64, 65]. The majority of patients die in early life from respiratory failure [63].

Tumor-Induced Osteomalacia and Tumor-Induced Rickets (TIO)

Tumor-induced osteomalacia (TIO), also called tumor-induced rickets, is a rare disorder characterized by hypophosphatemia, hyperphosphaturia, low 1,25(OH)$_2$D serum levels, and osteomalacia which develops in previously healthy individuals [66–68]. Therefore, in any patients presenting with hypophosphatemic rickets beyond the second year of life TIO should be excluded. Clinical symptoms are similar to that in XLHR or ADHR patients. TIO is caused by usually small, often difficult to locate, tumors. Most histologic diagnoses have been classified as phosphaturic mesenchymal tumors of the mixed connective tissue type. A characteristic histologic feature of these tumors is a background of spindle cells that tend to have low mitotic activity [66, 68]. Once the tumor is removed, the clinical symptoms quickly resolve, which has led to the notion that circulating factors produced by the tumor (phosphatonins) are causing renal phosphate loss in these patients. Later, TIO tumors were shown to contain high levels of FGF23 mRNA and protein, and TIO patients revealed elevated circulating FGF23 levels, which rapidly declined after removal of the tumor in parallel with resolution of clinical symptoms. The tumors are benign, but may recur. The paranasal sinuses, neck and mandible are common sites of these tumors. Newer imaging techniques such as nuclear magnetic resonance and positron emission tomography are helpful in establishing diagnosis of TIO. If tumor resection is not possible, treatment with the anti-FGF23 antibody Burosumab results in improvement of bone lesions [68].

Hypophosphatemic Rickets and Hyperparathyroidism

This is an extremely rare disorder caused by increased synthesis of α-Klotho. Patients reveal both hypophosphatemic rickets and hyperparathyroidism due to parathyroid hyperplasia. It is caused by *de novo* translocation resulting in elevated plasma α-Klotho levels [69]. Recently it was demonstrated that α-Klotho enhances FGF23-stimulated FGF receptor activation, and consequently inhibition of sodium phosphate transporter and hyperphosphaturia [70]. It is thought that the concomitant suppression of calcitriol production by α-Klotho/FGF23 action may cause increased production of FGF23 and PTH in these patients.

Fibrous Dysplasia (FD) and McCune-Albright Syndrome (MAS)

Fibrous dysplasia (FD) is characterized by fibrous skeletal lesions and localized mineralization defects. Patients may present with solitary or multiple bone lesions. When the skeletal findings occur in combination with abnormal skin pigmentation (e.g. café-au-lait spots), premature sexual development and/or thyrotoxicosis, the disease is called McCune-Albright syndrome (MAS) [71]. FD/MAS is a rare disorder due to post-zygotic gain-of-function mutations in the *GNAS1* gene, encoding for the α subunit of a stimulatory G protein [72]. G proteins function to couple specific receptors to intracellular signaling molecules. Phosphate wasting is due to increased secretion of FGF23 from bone lesions and the severity of hypophosphatemia correlates with the number of fibrous dysplasia lesions. However, how *GNAS1* mutations result in elevated FGF23 secretion is currently unknown.

Hypophosphatemic Disorders with Normal or Suppressed FGF23 Activity

HHRH (*SLC34A3* Mutation)

In 1985 Tieder et al. described an unusual case of hypophosphatemic rickets in a consanguineous Bedouin tribe [73]. In contrast to XLH, hypophosphatemia and phosphate wasting was associated with elevated 1,25(OH)$_2$D serum levels resulting in hypercalciuria and suppressed PTH plasma concentrations. The disorder was later shown to be caused by mutations in the *SLC34A3* gene encoding for the NaPi-IIc renal phosphate cotransporter in the proximal tubule, and many more patients were identified [74]. The reported mutations were all loss-of-function mutations and, most likely, reduced renal phosphate absorption through decreasing the apical membrane expression of NaPi-IIc or the uncoupling of sodium-phosphate co-transport in the proximal tubule [75]. Thus, in contrast to XLH and ADHR hypophosphatemia is not due to enhanced FGF23 serum levels in HHRH. The normal physiological reaction to hypophosphatemia resulting in increased serum elevated 1,25(OH)$_2$D levels results in increased intestinal calcium absorption, hypercalciuria and suppression of PTH. Consequent to hypercalciuria, patients developed nephrocalcinosis and nephrolithiasis. Milder forms may be under-diagnosed and therefore careful evaluation of urinary calcium excretion before and during medical treatment is strongly recommended in all patients with hypophosphatemic rickets, especially in those without a proven underlying genetic cause [76].

Hypophosphatemia and Nephrocalcinosis (*SLC34A1* Mutation)

The *SLC34A1* gene is located on chromosome 5q34 and encodes for the NaPi-IIa renal phosphate cotransporter in the proximal tubule. *SLC34A1* mutations can lead to a wide range of clinical phenotypes including infantile hypercalcemia, kidney stones and rickets, all of which are accompanied by reduced serum phosphate levels [77, 78].

Nephrolithiasis and Osteoporosis Associated with Hypophosphatemia

Two different heterozygous mutations (A48P and V147M) in *NPT2a*, a gene encoding a sodium dependent phosphate transporter, have been reported in patients suffering from urolithiasis or osteoporosis and persistent hypophosphatemia due to decreased tubular phosphate reabsorption [79].

Fanconi Syndrome

Fanconi syndrome is characterized by generalized proximal tubular dysfunction with impaired ability to absorb water, phosphate, glucose, urate, amino acids and low molecular weight proteins. Other common features include increased excretion of sodium, potassium, calcium and bicarbonate. Clinical consequences result mainly from hypophosphatemia and metabolic acidosis, i.e. rickets and osteomalacia. The syndrome may be due to both genetic defects and acquired disorders (see Chap. 31).

Treatment of XLH

For more than four decades treatment of XLH patients was based on oral supplementation of inorganic phosphate salts and treatment with active vitamin D metabolites (calcitriol or alfacalcidol) [80]. Recently, a fully humanized anti-FGF23 antibody (burosumab) has become available for the treatment for XLH, which represents a major breakthrough and paradigm shift in the treatment of this disorder (Fig. 38.1). The advantages of burosumab over conventional treatment are (1) the removal of the burden to take medications several times a day as required with conventional treatment, which frequently leads to non-adherence particularly in adolescents and adults, (2) its greater efficacy in ameliorating rickets compared to conventional treatment, and (3) its excellent safety profile and removal of the typical side effects of conventional therapy such as diarrhea and nephrocalcinosis.

However, one has to keep in mind that the disease spectrum, and thus the medication requirement, is heterogeneous—some individuals are only minimally affected even without treatment [81]. Adults need less treatment than children or even no treatment depending on the clinical symptoms. Other forms of FGF23-dependent hypophosphatemic rickets like ADHR are usually treated with phosphate salts and active vitamin D, whereas FGF23-independent forms require disease specific therapeutic approaches (*vide infra*).

The European Medicines Agency (EMA) and the U.S. Food and Drug Administration (FDA) approved burosumab to treat children ≥1 year and adults with XLH and TIO showing radiographic evidence of bone disease. If available, burosumab treatment should be considered in children with XLH ≥ 1 year and in adolescents with growing skeletons in the following situations: radiographic evidence of overt bone disease; disease that is refractory to conventional therapy; complications related to conventional therapy; or patient's inability to adhere to conventional therapy, presumed that adequate monitoring is feasible [19]. Evidence-based recommendations for the treatment of XLH were recently published and will be outlined below [19].

Phosphate Supplementation and Active Vitamin D Metabolites

Children in affected families should be screened for abnormal serum and urine phosphorus levels and serum alkaline phosphatase activity within the first month of life and at 3 and 6 months, and if available should undergo *PHEX* gene mutation analysis [19]. In case of confirmed diagnosis, therapy with active vitamin D metabolites and phosphate should be started immediately. The required dosages differ largely depending on the severity of rickets (*vide infra*). In patients with negative family history for XLH, hypercalciuria should be excluded before initiation of calcitriol treatment. The latter would suggest the diagnosis of HHRH where calcitriol treatment is contraindicated.

Administration of phosphate increases the plasma phosphate concentration, which lowers the plasma ionized calcium concentration, and further reduces the plasma calcitriol concentration (by removing the hypophosphatemic stimulus of its synthesis). This causes secondary hyperparathyroidism [19, 82]. The latter can aggravate the bone disease and increase urinary phosphate excretion, thereby defeating the aim of phosphate therapy. Secondary hyperparathyroidism can be prevented by additional treatment with calcitriol. Calcitriol increases intestinal calcium absorption, and to a lesser degree phosphate, and consequently suppresses secondary hyperparathyroidism. In addition, it also directly suppresses PTH release.

The recommended starting dose of phosphate based on elemental phosphorus is 20–60 mg/kg/day (0.7–2.0 mmol/kg per day) in infants and preschool children, which should be adjusted according to the improvements of rickets, growth, alkaline phosphatase and parathyroid hormone levels [19]. Doses above 80 mg/kg per day should be avoided to prevent gastrointestinal discomfort and hyperparathyroidism. In infants diagnosed before they develop bone changes, the goal of the treatment is to prevent rickets. Important to note, serum phosphate levels increase rapidly after oral intake but return to baseline levels within 1.5 h. Therefore, phosphorus should be administered at least four times a day. Especially in infants and young children, a nighttime dose may be required to achieve satisfactory results. Liquid formulations may improve adherence and allow for more precise dosing in young children. Powders and crushed tablets may also be employed. Powders/tablets can be dissolved in water and the child may drink the solution at intervals during the day. It is important not to administer the phosphate preparation with dairy products, since their calcium content interferes with intestinal phosphate absorption. In general, phosphorus absorption is slower in capsule or tablet formulations than in liquid ones. Therefore, when possible, it is better to use the former. The recommended starting dose of calcitriol and alfacalcidiol is 20–30 ng/kg body weight and 30–50 ng/kg body weight daily respectively. Alternatively, treatment may be started empirically at 0.5 µg daily of calcitriol or 1 µg daily of alfacalcidiol in patients aged above 12 months and adjusted on the basis of clinical and biochemical response. In addition, supplementation with native vitamin D is recommended in case of vitamin D deficiency [19].

Monitoring and Dose Adjustments During Conventional Treatment

The primary goals of treatment are to correct or minimize rickets/osteomalacia, as assessed by clinical, biochemical and radiological findings. Serum alkaline phosphatase activity is a useful surrogate marker for bone healing. With adequate treatment, serum levels of alkaline phosphatase decrease, reaching normal or slightly elevated levels. A common misconception is that successful conventional treatment requires normalization of serum phosphate concentration, which is not a practical goal in these patients, since this could only be reached by excessive phosphate doses and paying the price of severe side effects like nephrocalcinosis and secondary hyperparathyroidism. Therefore, important measures of therapeutic efficacy include enhanced growth velocity, improvement in lower extremity bowing and associated abnormalities, and radiological evidence of epiphyseal healing.

Children should be seen every 2–4 months to monitor growth, serum concentrations of calcium, phosphate, alkaline phosphatase activity, creatinine, PTH and urinary calcium excretion. A random "spot" urine collection can be used to monitor urinary calcium excretion. The goal is to maintain a spot calcium/creatinine ratio < 0.3 mg/mg. Renal ultrasound should be performed at yearly intervals to detect nephrocalcinosis. The etiology of nephrocalcinosis, shown by kidney biopsies to be composed of calcium phosphate precipitates, was thought to be due either to hypercalciuria, hyperphosphaturia, hyperoxaluria, hyperparathyroidism or any combination of these [19, 83–85]. However, the reported prevalence of nephrocalcinosis in XLH patients ranges between 17 and 80% and is clearly related to the dose of phosphate medication [18, 86, 87]. In addition, other soft-tissue calcifications, e.g. ocular, myocardial, and aortic valve calcifications, have been reported in XLH patients with persistent hyperparathyroidism and/or high dose treatment [34, 88]. Therefore, the calcitriol doses should be adjusted according to the serum levels of PTH and urinary calcium excretion. A high PTH level requires an increase in the calcitriol dose and/or a decrease of the phosphate dose.

The main side effect of an excessive dose of calcitriol is the development of hypercalciuria. In the presence of hypercalciuria the calcitriol dose should be reduced or thiazide diuretics added. The latter not only reduces urinary calcium excretion but also raises the TmP/GFR, most likely secondary to some degree of volume contraction.

Calcitriol and phosphate treatment increases FGF23 levels, thereby further stimulating urinary phosphate excretion [34]. Therefore, high dose treatment should not only be avoided to prevent hypercalciuria and nephrocalcinosis but also to prevent a vicious circle of therapy driven phosphate wasting. When secondary hyperparathyroidism cannot be adequately controlled by calcitriol treatment, i.e. persistent hypercalcemia and/or hypercalciuria, autonomous (tertiary) hyperparathyroidism can occur, necessitating surgical intervention.

It is often necessary to increase dosages of phosphate and calcitriol during the pubertal growth spurt as this may result in greater mineral demands and worsening of bowing defects so that a transient increase in dosage can be advantageous. Therapy with phosphate and calcitriol is maintained as long as the growth plates are open.

Burosumab

Efficacy and Safety

The efficacy and safety of burosumab has been investigated in three clinical trials in children with XLH [46, 89, 90]. In two open-label uncon-

trolled trials in a total of 65 children aged 1–12 years with severe XLH treated for 12–16 months, burosumab resulted in normalized TmP/GFR, near normal serum phosphate levels, increased $1,25(OH)_2$ vitamin D levels and significantly improved radiological rickets, bone pain and functional abilities [46, 91]. A head-on comparison between burosumab and conventional treatment was performed in an open-label phase 3 trial including 61 children aged 1–12 over 64 weeks [90]. After 40 weeks children treated with burosumab had significantly greater improvement in rickets severity scores than patients on conventional therapy (Fig. 38.6). Biochemical parameters such as serum alkaline phosphatase and serum phosphate levels were also rapidly normalized during burosumab treatment. Two-weekly dosing was superior to four-weekly dosing with respect to normalization of serum levels of phosphate and radiological improvement of rickets. The most common adverse reactions observed with burosumab were injection site reactions, headache and pain in the extremities.

Two open-label, uncontrolled trials and one randomized, double blind, placebo-controlled studies (including a total of 176 patients) have investigated burosumab in adult XLH patients, the majority of whom presented with skeletal pain associated with XLH and/or osteomalacia [91–95]. Four-weekly doses of burosumab given for 4–12 months yielded the following outcomes: significantly increased TmP/GFR and consequently raised serum levels of phosphate into the lower normal range and increased $1,25(OH)_2$ vitamin D levels; healed osteomalacia, and accelerated healing of active fractures and pseudofractures; and significantly reduced stiffness. It is important to note that conventional treatment with oral phosphate and active vitamin D metabolites should be stopped at least one week before the start of burosumab therapy for wash-out and to prove that fasting serum phosphate levels are below the normal reference for age.

Monitoring and Dose Adjustments During Burosumab Treatment

Burosumab should be started at a dose of 0.8 mg/kg body weight, given every 2 weeks subcutane-

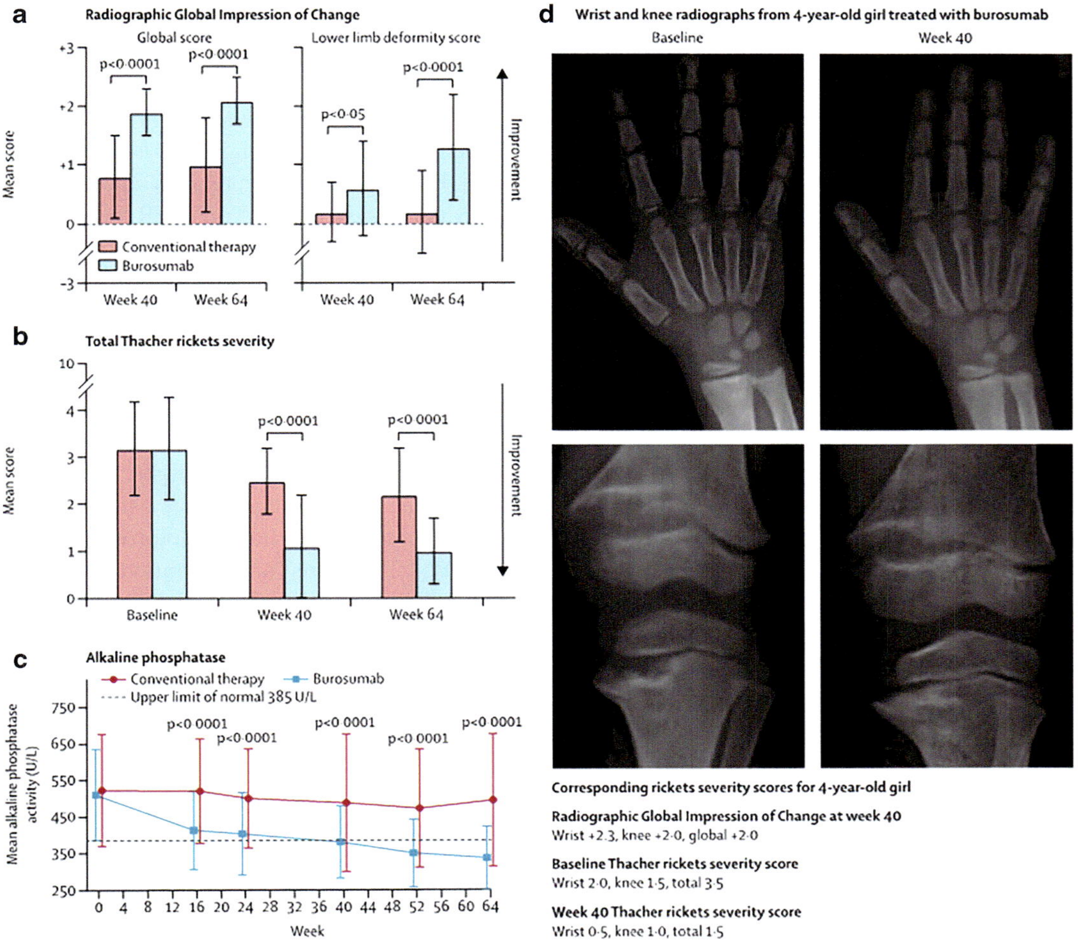

a

Radiographic Global Impression of Change

b

Total Thacher rickets severity

c

Alkaline phosphatase

d Wrist and knee radiographs from 4-year-old girl treated with burosumab

Corresponding rickets severity scores for 4-year-old girl

Radiographic Global Impression of Change at week 40
Wrist +2.3, knee +2.0, global +2.0

Baseline Thacher rickets severity score
Wrist 2.0, knee 1.5, total 3.5

Week 40 Thacher rickets severity score
Wrist 0.5, knee 1.0, total 1.5

Fig. 38.6 Improvements in rickets severity in children on burosumab versus conventional therapy with phosphate and active vitamin D metabolites. Data in panels **a**, **b**, and **c** are reported as mean (SD). p values are based on the comparison between treatment groups in the least squares mean change from baseline, using the ANCOVA model for the week 40 Radiographic Global Impression of Change global score and week 40 Thacher rickets severity score assessments, and the generalized estimating equation model for alkaline phosphatase assessments, lower limb deformity assessments, and week 64 rickets assessments. The upper limit of normal for alkaline phosphatase varies by age and sex: girls aged 1–4 years 317 U/L, 4–7 years 297 U/L, 7–10 years 325 U/L, and 10–15 years 300 U/L; boys aged 1–4 years 383 U/L, 4–7 years 345 U/L, 7–10 years 309 U/L, and 10–15 years 385 U/L. These ranges were provided by Covance laboratories. Radiographs in panel **d** show improvement in rickets with burosumab in a 4-year-old girl who previously received conventional therapy for approximately 26 months (Used with permission of Elsevier from Imel et al. [90])

ously. Burosumab should be titrated in 0.4 mg/kg increments to raise fasting serum phosphate levels to the lower end of the normal reference range for age, to a maximum dosage of 2 mg/kg body weight (maximum dose 90 mg).

The half-life of burosumab is approximately 19 days and the peak serum concentration of burosumab occurs at 7–11 days after injection. Therefore, it is recommended to monitor fasting serum phosphate levels during the titration period between injections, ideally 7–11 days after last injection in order to detect hyperphosphatemia. After achievement of a steady-state, which can be assumed after 3 months of a stable dosage, fasting serum phosphate levels should be assessed directly before injections in order to detect hypophosphatemia. In some patients burosumab might initially improve TmP/GFR while serum level of phosphate is still below the normal range owing to the high demand for phosphate of the bone. Therefore, TmP/GFR should be monitored together with fasting serum phosphate levels as a measure of drug efficacy. Serum levels of $1,25(OH)_2$ vitamin D might increase under burosumab therapy and should be monitored together with urinary calcium excretion.

Burosumab should be withdrawn if fasting serum phosphate level is above the upper range of normal. Burosumab can be restarted at approximately half of the previous dose when serum phosphate concentration is back within the normal range. Important to note, burosumab must not be given in conjunction with conventional treatment, when fasting phosphate levels are within the age-related normal range before initiation of treatment, or in the presence of severe renal impairment.

Adjunctive Therapies

Growth Hormone

Adult height is reduced in up to 60% of XLH patients and burosumab did not substantially improve longitudinal growth in pediatric XLH patients in clinical trials [19]. Although an impairment of the somatotropic hormone axis is not the primary cause of short stature in XLH patients, the physiological antiphosphaturic effect of growth hormone (GH) by stimulation of phosphate retention may be a useful adjunct to conventional treatment in improving growth in poorly growing XLH patients. Several mostly uncontrolled studies and a placebo-controlled randomized trial have documented sustained increases in age-standardized height during treatment periods of up to 3 years, and prepubertal patients responded better to GH than pubertal patients [96–102]. In a randomized trial on 3-year

rhGH treatment in severely short prepubertal XLH patients, standardized height increased in the rhGH group by 1.1 SD scores with no change in body disproportion, whereas no significant change in standardized height was noted in controls [102]. In line with previous uncontrolled studies, a transient rise in TmP/GFR, and consequently of serum phosphate concentrations, was noted during the first 6 months of GH treatment but not in controls. Importantly, the degree of leg bowing tended to be higher in GH treated patients. Long-term follow-up of the same study failed to show significant benefits on the adult height, most likely due to the low number of patients followed up to adult height. In another study mean final height was significantly increased compared to non-randomized controls [97, 103]. Therefore, administration of rhGH should be considered in XLH patients with persistent short stature despite adequate metabolic control [19].

Calcimimetics

The calcimimetic compound cinacalcet reduces PTH levels in XLH patients, leading to increases in TmP/GFR and serum phosphate [104, 105]. The cinacalcet-induced decrease in serum PTH was accompanied by a slight decrease in serum-ionized calcium concentrations and was not associated with clinical symptoms. Similarly, Geller et al. proved the efficacy of cinacalcet in increasing serum phosphate levels in patients with TIO [106]. It has been suggested that long-term adjunctive treatment of XLH patients with cinacalcet may allow for lower doses of phosphate and calcitriol and thus may minimize the risk of secondary hyperparathyroidism, hypercalcemia, hypercalciuria and nephrocalcinosis caused by high-dose phosphate and calcitriol treatment [19]. However, randomized controlled trials on the long-term efficacy and safety of this drug in XLH patients are lacking.

Surgical Management

Many patients require surgical corrections of severe bowing, regardless of adequate medical treatment [19, 107]. In general, it is recommended that patients presenting with persisting deformity despite optimized medical treatment and/or the presence of symptoms interfering with function should be considered for surgical treatment [19, 107–109]. The age of the child should be considered as an important factor in the decision-making process. Corrective osteotomies are not usually performed in children aged less than 6 years, as medical therapy often improves bone deformities in this age group. Newer, less-invasive approaches include epiphysiodesis, which induces differential corrective growth of the growth plate. Guided growth techniques depend on the remaining growth potential of the child and must therefore be carried out at least 2–3 years before skeletal maturity (age 14 in girls and age 16 in boys). By contrast, the complications associated with osteotomy reduce when the surgery is performed later in childhood or after skeletal maturity. Calcitriol medication should be adjusted during times of immobilization to avoid hypercalcemic episodes [19].

Dental Care

Children and adult patients with XLH might present with spontaneous endodontic infections on apparently intact teeth [19, 30]. Dental abscesses can develop on deciduous as well as on permanent teeth. The endodontic infection might be asymptomatic for months or years or it might evolve into dental abscesses, causing pain and swelling. Dental complications in patients with XLH are secondary to poorly mineralized dentin. On dental radiographs, the pulp chambers of deciduous or permanent teeth are larger than usual with long pulp horns extending to the dentino-enamel junction. In addition, the frequency and severity of periodontitis is increased in adult patients with XLH and can lead to tooth loss.

Conventional treatment improves dentin mineralization, reduces the number of dental abscesses, and decreases the frequency and severity of periodontitis [110, 111]. The effect of burosumab on dental health in XLH patients is currently unknown.

In children, in addition to standard preventative care, dental visits every 6 months are recommended and sealing of pits and fissures with flowable resin composite on both temporary and permanent teeth should be considered, as soon and as frequently as required. In adults, twice-yearly visits are recommended to perform conventional supportive periodontal therapy. Visits should include a thorough clinical investigation searching for pulp necrosis (color changes, fistula, swelling, abscess, cellulitis or pain), and performance of retrocoronal and/or periapical radiographs or orthopantomogram to search for enlarged pulp chambers and periapical bone loss depending on findings from a clinical examination. Finally, optimized conventional medical treatment of XLH is recommended before initiation of orthodontic treatment [19].

Expected Outcomes

Children with XLH have normal length at birth and show growth retardation, hypophosphatemia and rickets during the first year of life [112, 113]. With conventional treatment, growth and skeletal deformities generally improve. Height velocity commonly increases during the first year of treatment. Leg deformities may correct spontaneously obviating the need for surgery, although this is not always the case. Despite general growth improvement during treatment, correction is limited and adult height is often compromised. Median adult height in XLH patients on calcitriol and phosphate supplements (median age at start 2.3 years) published during the last two decades amounted to −2.3 SDS (range −2.7 to −1.2 SDS) [20, 22, 24, 103, 112–115]. However, growth outcome is significantly better if treatment is initiated early (<1 year). In three studies the mean standardized height after average treatment periods of 10 years was substantially higher in XLH patients with early compared to late treatment (−0.7 SDS versus −2.0 SDS, p < 0.01; −1.3 SDS versus −2.0 SDS, p = 0.06; Fig. 38.7; −0.7 SDS versus −2.0 SDS, p < 0.01) [22–24]. However, even early treatment does not completely normalize skeletal development, and the main effect of early treatment was the prevention of a severe height deficit during early childhood.

A recent North American cross-sectional study in 232 adult XLH patients treated with conventional therapy during childhood and adoles-

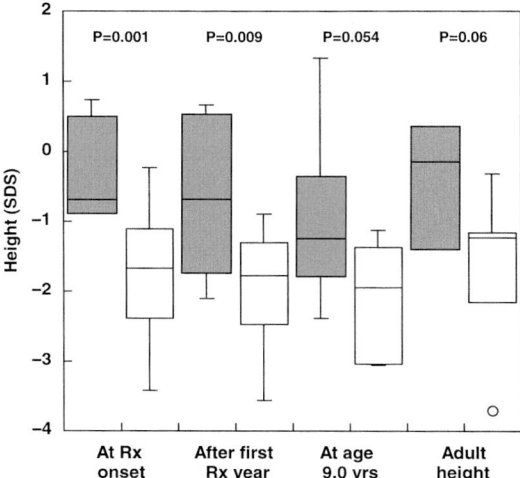

Fig. 38.7 Height z-scores in XLH patients started on calcitriol and phosphate treatment within the first 12 months of life 1 (■) and after the age of 12 months (□) at treatment onset, at the end of first treatment year, at age 9 years, and at final height (adult height or predicted adult height). The bottom of each box indicates the 25th, the cross line the 50th, and the top the 75th percentile; the bottom and top lines indicate the minimum and maximum values. P values refer to the difference between groups. *Rx* Treatment (Used with permission of Makitie et al. [23])

cence revealed a high prevalence of short stature (80%), bone or joint pain/stiffness (97%), and history of pseudofractures (44%) [116]. In addition, osteophytes, enthesopathy and spinal stenosis were reported in 46%, 27%, and 19% of patients, respectively. Similar results were reported in several European studies [25, 117, 118]. Reduced quality of life was shown in 84% of adult patients and associated with age and presence of structural lesions such as enthesopathy [25].

Zivicnjak et al reported on age-related stature and linear body dimensions in 76 children with XLH [18]. Despite calcitriol and phosphate treatment XLH patients showed progressive stunting and body disproportion during childhood, which was mainly due to diminished growth in the legs; growth of the trunk was less affected (Fig. 38.8). This resulted in an ever-increasing sitting height index (i.e. ratio between sitting height to stature).

Treatment with burosumab results in substantial improvement of ricketic bone lesions and degree of leg deformities but only minor changes in standardized height in children aged 1–12 years treated for up to 16 months. The observed limited growth improvement may be due to rather short observation periods and/or the primary osteoblast defect in XLH. Long-term outcome data on the impact of burosumab on linear growth and final height, dental health and rare complications such as hearing loss are urgently required, and multinational patient registries have been initiated to address this issue.

Treatment of Other Forms of Hypophosphatemic Rickets

Limited experience is available regarding the treatment of other forms of hypophosphatemic rickets. In general, hypophosphatemic conditions associated with elevated FGF23 and low/inappropriately low $1,25(OH)_2D$ levels, i.e. **ADHR and ARHR** are treated similarly as XLH. However, burosumab is currently not licensed for treatment of these FGF23 driven diseases.

In patients with **FD/MAS**, treatment with bisphosphonates results in decreased serum FGF23 levels and improves TmP/GFR [18, 119]. Treatment with bisphosphonates in combination with cabergoline, a synthetic ergot alkaloid which acts as a long-acting D2-selective dopamine agonist, successfully arrested both dysplastic bone growth and endocrine malfunction in a female patient with FD/MAS and severe facial involvement [119, 120]. This approach might be a suitable option in order to circumvent surgical interventions that might be of particular risk in patients suffering from polyostotic FD involving the skull base.

In patients with **TIO**, tumor removal usually results in a rapid clinical improvement but tumors might recur. Before surgery, patients are treated similarly to XLH patients. Cinacalcet was successfully used in TIO patients resulting in increased TmP/GFR and serum phosphate concentrations, thereby allowing the use of significantly lower doses of phosphate and calcitriol before surgery [106]. If available, patients may

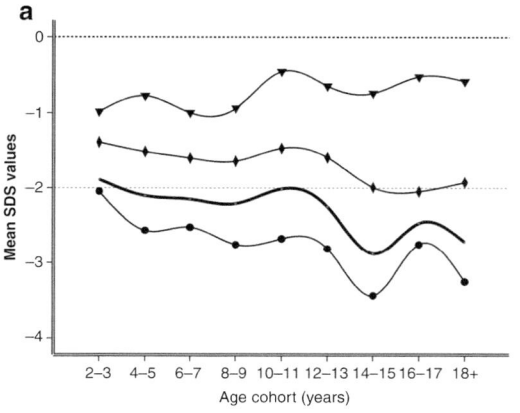
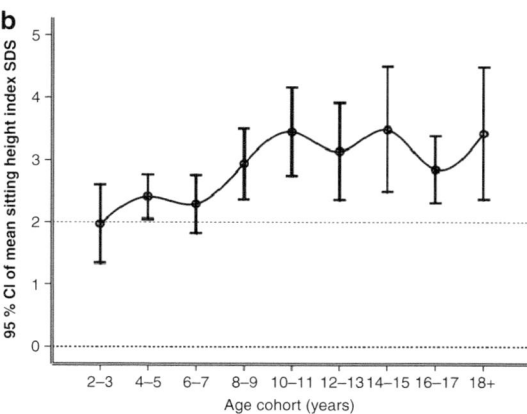

Fig. 38.8 Stature, sitting height, and arm and leg length (**a**) as well as the sitting height index (**b**) as a function of age in 76 children with XLH on conventional treatment. To assess age-related changes in body dimensions, all measurements were grouped according to age at the time of examination. Each age cohort comprised eight up to 26 children with 16 up to 38 measurements. A spline function was used to fit age-related changes. Unmarked solid line Stature, solid line with filled circles leg length, solid line with filled rhombuses arm length, solid line with filled inverted triangles sitting height. The 95% CI is indicated for sitting height index [18]

also be effectively treated by burosumab, which should be the preferred treatment option if tumor resection is not possible [68].

Treatment of **HHRH** usually requires the administration of phosphate salts alone. In fact, treatment with calcitriol may lead to nephrocalcinosis and chronic renal failure. The treatment goal is to provide sufficient phosphorus to improve mineralization of osteoid. In addition, oral phosphate supplementation is supposed to normalize decreased FGF23 levels and thereby suppress elevated circulating $1,25(OH)_2D$ level and consequently reduce intestinal calcium resorption and hypercalciuria [19, 121].

References

1. Winters RW, Graham JB, Williams TF, McFalls VW, Burnett CH. A genetic study of familial hypophosphatemia and vitamin D resistant rickets with a review of the literature. Medicine (Baltimore). 1958;37:97–142.
2. Imel EA, Carpenter TO. A practical clinical approach to paediatric phosphate disorders. Endocr Dev. 2015;28:134–61.
3. Marcucci G, Masi L, Ferrari S, Haffner D, Javaid MK, Kamenický P, Reginster JY, Rizzoli R, Brandi ML. Phosphate wasting disorders in adults. Osteoporos Int. 2018;29:2369–87.
4. Carpenter TO, Shaw NJ, Portale AA, Ward LM, Abrams SA, Pettifor JM. Rickets. Nat Rev Dis Primers. 2017;3:17101.
5. Tiosano D, Hochberg Z. Hypophosphatemia: the common denominator of all rickets. J Bone Miner Metab. 2009;27:392–401.
6. Penido MG, Alon US. Phosphate homeostasis and its role in bone health. Pediatr Nephrol. 2012;27:2039–48.
7. Beck-Nielsen SS, Mughal Z, Haffner D, Nilsson O, Levtchenko E, Ariceta G, de Lucas Collantes C, Schnabel D, Jandhyala R, Mäkitie O. FGF23 and its role in X-linked hypophosphatemia-related morbidity. Orphanet J Rare Dis. 2019;14:58.
8. Zheng B, Wang C, Chen Q, Che R, Sha Y, Zhao F, Ding G, Zhou W, Jia Z, Huang S, Chen Y, Zhang A. Functional characterization of PHEX gene variants in children with X-linked hypophosphatemic rickets shows no evidence of genotype-phenotype correlation. J Bone Miner Res. 2020;35(9):1718–25.
9. Gaucher C, Walrant-Debray O, Nguyen TM, Esterle L, Garabedian M, Jehan F. PHEX analysis in 118 pedigrees reveals new genetic clues in hypophosphatemic rickets. Hum Genet. 2009;125:401–11.
10. A gene (PEX) with homologies to endopeptidases is mutated in patients with X-linked hypophosphatemic rickets. the HYP consortium. Nat Genet. 1995;11:130–136.
11. Beck-Nielsen SS, Brixen K, Gram J, Brusgaard K. Mutational analysis of PHEX, FGF23, DMP1, SLC34A3 and CLCN5 in patients with hypophosphatemic rickets. J Hum Genet. 2012;57:453–8.
12. Biber J, Hernando N, Forster I. Phosphate transporters and their function. Annu Rev Physiol. 2013;75:535–50.

13. Bergwitz C, Roslin NM, Tieder M, Loredo-Osti JC, Bastepe M, Abu-Zahra H, Frappier D, Burkett K, Carpenter TO, Anderson D, Garabedian M, Sermet I, Fujiwara TM, Morgan K, Tenenhouse HS, Juppner H. SLC34A3 mutations in patients with hereditary hypophosphatemic rickets with hypercalciuria predict a key role for the sodium-phosphate cotransporter NaPi-IIc in maintaining phosphate homeostasis. Am J Hum Genet. 2006;78:179–92.

14. Huqun IS, Miyazawa H, Ishii K, Uchiyama B, Ishida T, Tanaka S, Tazawa R, Fukuyama S, Tanaka T, Nagai Y, Yokote A, Takahashi H, Fukushima T, Kobayashi K, Chiba H, Nagata M, Sakamoto S, Nakata K, Takebayashi Y, Shimizu Y, Kaneko K, Shimizu M, Kanazawa M, Abe S, Inoue Y, Takenoshita S, Yoshimura K, Kudo K, Tachibana T, Nukiwa T, Hagiwara K. Mutations in the SLC34A2 gene are associated with pulmonary alveolar microlithiasis. Am J Respir Crit Care Med. 2007;175:263–8.

15. Bergwitz C, Juppner H. Regulation of phosphate homeostasis by PTH, vitamin D, and FGF23. Annu Rev Med. 2010;61:91–104.

16. Kido S, Miyamoto K, Mizobuchi H, Taketani Y, Ohkido I, Ogawa N, Kaneko Y, Harashima S, Takeda E. Identification of regulatory sequences and binding proteins in the type II sodium/phosphate cotransporter NPT2 gene responsive to dietary phosphate. J Biol Chem. 1999;274:28256–63.

17. Murer H, Biber J. Molecular mechanisms of renal apical na/phosphate cotransport. Annu Rev Physiol. 1996;58:607–18.

18. Zivicnjak M, Schnabel D, Billing H, Staude H, Filler G, Querfeld U, Schumacher M, Pyper A, Schroder C, Bramswig J, Haffner D, Hypophosphatemic Rickets Study Group of Arbeitsgemeinschaft fur Padiatrische Endokrinologie and Gesellschaft fur Padiatrische Nephrologie. Age-related stature and linear body segments in children with X-linked hypophosphatemic rickets. Pediatr Nephrol. 2011;26:223–31.

19. Haffner D, Emma F, Eastwood DM, Duplan MB, Bacchetta J, Schnabel D, Wicart P, Bockenhauer D, Santos F, Levtchenko E, Harvengt P, Kirchhoff M, Di Rocco F, Chaussain C, Brandi ML, Savendahl L, Briot K, Kamenicky P, Rejnmark L, Linglart A. Clinical practice recommendations for the diagnosis and management of X-linked hypophosphataemia. Nat Rev Nephrol. 2019;15:435–55.

20. Beck-Nielsen SS, Brusgaard K, Rasmussen LM, Brixen K, Brock-Jacobsen B, Poulsen MR, Vestergaard P, Ralston SH, Albagha OM, Poulsen S, Haubek D, Gjorup H, Hintze H, Andersen MG, Heickendorff L, Hjelmborg J, Gram J. Phenotype presentation of hypophosphatemic rickets in adults. Calcif Tissue Int. 2010;87:108–19.

21. Vega RA, Opalak C, Harshbarger RJ, Fearon JA, Ritter AM, Collins JJ, Rhodes JL. Hypophosphatemic rickets and craniosynostosis: a multicenter case series. J Neurosurg Pediatr. 2016;17:694–700.

22. Kruse K, Hinkel GK, Griefahn B. Calcium metabolism and growth during early treatment of children with X-linked hypophosphataemic rickets. Eur J Pediatr. 1998;157:894–900.

23. Makitie O, Doria A, Kooh SW, Cole WG, Daneman A, Sochett E. Early treatment improves growth and biochemical and radiographic outcome in X-linked hypophosphatemic rickets. J Clin Endocrinol Metab. 2003;88:3591–7.

24. Quinlan C, Guegan K, Offiah A, Neill RO, Hiorns MP, Ellard S, Bockenhauer D, Hoff WV, Waters AM. Growth in PHEX-associated X-linked hypophosphatemic rickets: the importance of early treatment. Pediatr Nephrol. 2012;27:581–8.

25. Che H, Roux C, Etcheto A, Rothenbuhler A, Kamenicky P, Linglart A, Briot K. Impaired quality of life in adults with X-linked hypophosphatemia and skeletal symptoms. Eur J Endocrinol. 2016;174:325–33.

26. Schnabel D, Haffner D. Rickets. diagnosis and therapy. Orthopade. 2005;34:703–6.

27. Robinson ME, AlQuorain H, Murshed M, Rauch F. Mineralized tissues in hypophosphatemic rickets. Pediatr Nephrol. 2020;35(10):1843–54.

28. Lee BN, Jung HY, Chang HS, Hwang YC, Oh WM. Dental management of patients with X-linked hypophosphatemia. Restor Dent Endod. 2017;42:146–51.

29. Gjørup H, Beck-Nielsen SS, Haubek D. Craniofacial and dental characteristics of patients with vitamin-D-dependent rickets type 1A compared to controls and patients with X-linked hypophosphatemia. Clin Oral Investig. 2018;22:745–55.

30. Coyac BR, Falgayrac G, Baroukh B, Slimani L, Sadoine J, Penel G, Biosse-Duplan M, Schinke T, Linglart A, McKee MD, Chaussain C, Bardet C. Tissue-specific mineralization defects in the periodontium of the hyp mouse model of X-linked hypophosphatemia. Bone. 2017;103:334–46.

31. Coyac BR, Falgayrac G, Penel G, Schmitt A, Schinke T, Linglart A, McKee MD, Chaussain C, Bardet C. Impaired mineral quality in dentin in X-linked hypophosphatemia. Connect Tissue Res. 2018;59:91–6.

32. Hanisch M, Bohner L, Sabandal MMI, Kleinheinz J, Jung S. Oral symptoms and oral health-related quality of life of individuals with x-linked hypophosphatemia. Head Face Med. 2019;15:8.

33. Andersen MG, Beck-Nielsen SS, Haubek D, Hintze H, Gjorup H, Poulsen S. Periapical and endodontic status of permanent teeth in patients with hypophosphatemic rickets. J Oral Rehabil. 2012;39:144–50.

34. Sun GE, Suer O, Carpenter TO, Tan CD, Li-Ng M. Heart failure in hypophosphatemic rickets: complications from high-dose phosphate therapy. Endocr Pract. 2013;19:e8–e11.

35. Fishman G, Miller-Hansen D, Jacobsen C, Singhal VK, Alon US. Hearing impairment in familial X-linked hypophosphatemic rickets. Eur J Pediatr. 2004;163:622–3.

36. Alon US, Monzavi R, Lilien M, Rasoulpour M, Geffner ME, Yadin O. Hypertension in

hypophosphatemic rickets—role of secondary hyperparathyroidism. Pediatr Nephrol. 2003;18:155–8.

37. Brodehl J, Krause A, Hoyer PF. Assessment of maximal tubular phosphate reabsorption: comparison of direct measurement with the nomogram of Bijvoet. Pediatr Nephrol. 1988;2:183–9.

38. Ma SL, Vega-Warner V, Gillies C, Sampson MG, Kher V, Sethi SK, Otto EA. Whole exome sequencing reveals novel PHEX splice site mutations in patients with hypophosphatemic rickets. PLoS One. 2015;10:e0130729.

39. Carpenter TO, Insogna KL, Zhang JH, Ellis B, Nieman S, Simpson C, Olear E, Gundberg CM. Circulating levels of soluble klotho and FGF23 in X-linked hypophosphatemia: Circadian variance, effects of treatment, and relationship to parathyroid status. J Clin Endocrinol Metab. 2010;95:352.

40. Du L, Desbarats M, Viel J, Glorieux FH, Cawthorn C, Ecarot B. cDNA cloning of the murine pex gene implicated in X-linked hypophosphatemia and evidence for expression in bone. Genomics. 1996;36:22–8.

41. Morgan JM, Hawley WL, Chenoweth AI, Retan WJ, Diethelm AG. Renal transplantation in hypophosphatemia with vitamin D-resistant rickets. Arch Intern Med. 1974;134:549–52.

42. Meyer RA Jr, Tenenhouse HS, Meyer MH, Klugerman AH. The renal phosphate transport defect in normal mice parabiosed to X-linked hypophosphatemic mice persists after parathyroidectomy. J Bone Miner Res. 1989;4:523–32.

43. Liu S, Zhou J, Tang W, Jiang X, Rowe DW, Quarles LD. Pathogenic role of Fgf23 in hyp mice. Am J Physiol Endocrinol Metab. 2006;291:38.

44. Yamazaki Y, Okazaki R, Shibata M, Hasegawa Y, Satoh K, Tajima T, Takeuchi Y, Fujita T, Nakahara K, Yamashita T, Fukumoto S. Increased circulatory level of biologically active full-length FGF-23 in patients with hypophosphatemic rickets/osteomalacia. J Clin Endocrinol Metab. 2002;87:4957–60.

45. Aono Y, Yamazaki Y, Yasutake J, Kawata T, Hasegawa H, Urakawa I, Fujita T, Wada M, Yamashita T, Fukumoto S, Shimada T. Therapeutic effects of anti-FGF23 antibodies in hypophosphatemic rickets/osteomalacia. J Bone Miner Res. 2009;24:1879–88.

46. Carpenter TO, Whyte MP, Imel EA, Boot AM, Högler W, Linglart A, Padidela R, Van't Hoff W, Mao M, Chen CY, Skrinar A, Kakkis E, San Martin J, Portale AA. Burosumab therapy in children with X-linked hypophosphatemia. N Engl J Med. 2018;378:1987–98.

47. Gattineni J, Baum M. Regulation of phosphate transport by fibroblast growth factor 23 (FGF23): implications for disorders of phosphate metabolism. Pediatr Nephrol. 2010;25:591–601.

48. Barros NM, Hoac B, Neves RL, Addison WN, Assis DM, Murshed M, Carmona AK, McKee MD. Proteolytic processing of osteopontin by PHEX and accumulation of osteopontin fragments in hyp mouse bone, the murine model of X-linked hypophosphatemia. J Bone Miner Res. 2013;28:688–99.

49. Bianchine JW, Stambler AA, Harrison HE. Familial hypophosphatemic rickets showing autosomal dominant inheritance. Birth Defects Orig Artic Ser. 1971;7:287–95.

50. Gribaa M, Younes M, Bouyacoub Y, Korbaa W, Ben Charfeddine I, Touzi M, Adala L, Mamay O, Bergaoui N, Saad A. An autosomal dominant hypophosphatemic rickets phenotype in a tunisian family caused by a new FGF23 missense mutation. J Bone Miner Metab. 2010;28:111–5.

51. Econs MJ, McEnery PT. Autosomal dominant hypophosphatemic rickets/osteomalacia: clinical characterization of a novel renal phosphate-wasting disorder. J Clin Endocrinol Metab. 1997;82: 674–81.

52. Kruse K, Woelfel D, Strom TM. Loss of renal phosphate wasting in a child with autosomal dominant hypophosphatemic rickets caused by a FGF23 mutation. Horm Res. 2001;55:305–8.

53. Farrow EG, Yu X, Summers LJ, Davis SI, Fleet JC, Allen MR, Robling AG, Stayrook KR, Jideonwo V, Magers MJ, Garringer HJ, Vidal R, Chan RJ, Goodwin CB, Hui SL, Peacock M, White KE. Iron deficiency drives an autosomal dominant hypophosphatemic rickets (ADHR) phenotype in fibroblast growth factor-23 (Fgf23) knock-in mice. Proc Natl Acad Sci U S A. 2011;108:1146.

54. Imel EA, Peacock M, Gray AK, Padgett LR, Hui SL, Econs MJ. Iron modifies plasma FGF23 differently in autosomal dominant hypophosphatemic rickets and healthy humans. J Clin Endocrinol Metab. 2011;96:3541–9.

55. Imel EA, Biggin A, Schindeler A, Munns CF. FGF23, hypophosphatemia, and emerging treatments. JBMR Plus. 2019;3:e10190.

56. Perry W, Stamp TC. Hereditary hypophosphataemic rickets with autosomal recessive inheritance and severe osteosclerosis. A report of two cases. J Bone Joint Surg Br. 1978;60-B:430–4.

57. Feng JQ, Ward LM, Liu S, Lu Y, Xie Y, Yuan B, Yu X, Rauch F, Davis SI, Zhang S, Rios H, Drezner MK, Quarles LD, Bonewald LF, White KE. Loss of DMP1 causes rickets and osteomalacia and identifies a role for osteocytes in mineral metabolism. Nat Genet. 2006;38:1310–5.

58. Lorenz-Depiereux B, Bastepe M, Benet-Pages A, Amyere M, Wagenstaller J, Muller-Barth U, Badenhoop K, Kaiser SM, Rittmaster RS, Shlossberg AH, Olivares JL, Loris C, Ramos FJ, Glorieux F, Vikkula M, Juppner H, Strom TM. DMP1 mutations in autosomal recessive hypophosphatemia implicate a bone matrix protein in the regulation of phosphate homeostasis. Nat Genet. 2006;38:1248–50.

59. Lorenz-Depiereux B, Schnabel D, Tiosano D, Hausler G, Strom TM. Loss-of-function ENPP1 mutations cause both generalized arterial calcification of infancy and autosomal-recessive hypophosphatemic rickets. Am J Hum Genet. 2010;86:267–72.

60. Levy-Litan V, Hershkovitz E, Avizov L, Leventhal N, Bercovich D, Chalifa-Caspi V, Manor E, Buriakovsky S, Hadad Y, Goding J, Parvari R. Autosomal-recessive hypophosphatemic rickets is associated with an inactivation mutation in the ENPP1 gene. Am J Hum Genet. 2010;86:273–8.

61. Rutsch F, Ruf N, Vaingankar S, Toliat MR, Suk A, Hohne W, Schauer G, Lehmann M, Roscioli T, Schnabel D, Epplen JT, Knisely A, Superti-Furga A, McGill J, Filippone M, Sinaiko AR, Vallance H, Hinrichs B, Smith W, Ferre M, Terkeltaub R, Nurnberg P. Mutations in ENPP1 are associated with 'idiopathic' infantile arterial calcification. Nat Genet. 2003;34:379–81.

62. Kotwal A, Ferrer A, Kumar R, Singh RJ, Murthy V, Schultz-Rogers L, Zimmermann M, Lanpher B, Zimmerman K, Stabach PR, Klee E, Braddock DT, Wermers RA. Clinical and biochemical phenotypes in a family with ENPP1 mutations. J Bone Miner Res. 2020;35:662–70.

63. Faundes V, Castillo-Taucher S, Gonzalez-Hormazabal P, Chandler K, Crosby A, Chioza B. Raine syndrome: an overview. Eur J Med Genet. 2014;57:536–42.

64. Eltan M, Alavanda C, Yavas Abali Z, Ergenekon P, Yalındag Ozturk N, Sakar M, Dagcinar A, Kirkgoz T, Kaygusuz SB, Gokdemir Y, Elcioglu HN, Guran T, Bereket A, Ata P, Turan S. A rare cause of hypophosphatemia: Raine syndrome changing clinical features with age. Calcif Tissue Int. 2020;107:96–103.

65. Tagliabracci VS, Engel JL, Wiley SE, Xiao J, Gonzalez DJ, Nidumanda Appaiah H, Koller A, Nizet V, White KE, Dixon JE. Dynamic regulation of FGF23 by Fam20C phosphorylation, GalNAc-T3 glycosylation, and furin proteolysis. Proc Natl Acad Sci U S A. 2014;111:5520–5.

66. Chong WH, Andreopoulou P, Chen CC, Reynolds J, Guthrie L, Kelly M, Gafni RI, Bhattacharyya N, Boyce AM, El-Maouche D, Crespo DO, Sherry R, Chang R, Wodajo FM, Kletter GB, Dwyer A, Collins MT. Tumor localization and biochemical response to cure in tumor-induced osteomalacia. J Bone Miner Res. 2013;28:1386–98.

67. Weidner N, Santa Cruz D. Phosphaturic mesenchymal tumors. A polymorphous group causing osteomalacia or rickets. Cancer. 1987;59:1442–54.

68. Florenzano P, Hartley IR, Jimenez M, Roszko K, Gafni RI, Collins MT. Tumor-induced osteomalacia. Calcif Tissue Int. 2021;108(1):128–42.

69. Brownstein CA, Adler F, Nelson-Williams C, Iijima J, Li P, Imura A, Nabeshima Y, Reyes-Mugica M, Carpenter TO, Lifton RP. A translocation causing increased alpha-klotho level results in hypophosphatemic rickets and hyperparathyroidism. Proc Natl Acad Sci U S A. 2008;105:3455–60.

70. Kovesdy CP, Quarles LD. Fibroblast growth factor-23: what we know, what we don't know, and what we need to know. Nephrol Dial Transplant. 2013;28:2228–36.

71. Boyce AM, Glover M, Kelly MH, Brillante BA, Butman JA, Fitzgibbon EJ, Brewer CC, Zalewski CK, Cutler Peck CM, Kim HJ, Collins MT. Optic neuropathy in McCune-albright syndrome: effects of early diagnosis and treatment of growth hormone excess. J Clin Endocrinol Metab. 2013;98:126.

72. Narumi S, Matsuo K, Ishii T, Tanahashi Y, Hasegawa T. Quantitative and sensitive detection of GNAS mutations causing mccune-albright syndrome with next generation sequencing. PLoS One. 2013;8:e60525.

73. Tieder M, Modai D, Samuel R, Arie R, Halabe A, Bab I, Gabizon D, Liberman UA. Hereditary hypophosphatemic rickets with hypercalciuria. N Engl J Med. 1985;312:611–7.

74. Lorenz-Depiereux B, Benet-Pages A, Eckstein G, Tenenbaum-Rakover Y, Wagenstaller J, Tiosano D, Gershoni-Baruch R, Albers N, Lichtner P, Schnabel D, Hochberg Z, Strom TM. Hereditary hypophosphatemic rickets with hypercalciuria is caused by mutations in the sodium-phosphate cotransporter gene SLC34A3. Am J Hum Genet. 2006;78:193–201.

75. Jaureguiberry G, Carpenter TO, Forman S, Juppner H, Bergwitz C. A novel missense mutation in SLC34A3 that causes hereditary hypophosphatemic rickets with hypercalciuria in humans identifies threonine 137 as an important determinant of sodium-phosphate cotransport in NaPi-IIc. Am J Physiol Renal Physiol. 2008;295:371.

76. Dasgupta D, Wee MJ, Reyes M, Li Y, Simm PJ, Sharma A, Schlingmann KP, Janner M, Biggin A, Lazier J, Gessner M, Chrysis D, Tuchman S, Baluarte HJ, Levine MA, Tiosano D, Insogna K, Hanley DA, Carpenter TO, Ichikawa S, Hoppe B, Konrad M, Sävendahl L, Munns CF, Lee H, Jüppner H, Bergwitz C. Mutations in SLC34A3/NPT2c are associated with kidney stones and nephrocalcinosis. J Am Soc Nephrol. 2014;25:2366–75.

77. Segawa H, Kaneko I, Takahashi A, Kuwahata M, Ito M, Ohkido I, Tatsumi S, Miyamoto K. Growth-related renal type II na/pi cotransporter. J Biol Chem. 2002;277:19665–72.

78. Ma Y, Lv H, Wang J, Tan J. Heterozygous mutation of SLC34A1 in patients with hypophosphatemic kidney stones and osteoporosis: a case report. J Int Med Res. 2020;48:300060519896146.

79. Prie D, Huart V, Bakouh N, Planelles G, Dellis O, Gerard B, Hulin P, Benque-Blanchet F, Silve C, Grandchamp B, Friedlander G. Nephrolithiasis and osteoporosis associated with hypophosphatemia caused by mutations in the type 2a sodium-phosphate cotransporter. N Engl J Med. 2002;347:983–91.

80. Carpenter TO, Imel EA, Holm IA, Jan de Beur SM, Insogna KL. A clinician's guide to X-linked hypophosphatemia. J Bone Miner Res. 2011;26:1381–8.

81. Emma F, Haffner D. FGF23 blockade coming to clinical practice. Kidney Int. 2018;94:846–8.

82. Schmitt CP, Mehls O. The enigma of hyperparathyroidism in hypophosphatemic rickets. Pediatr Nephrol. 2004;19:473–7.

83. Reusz GS, Latta K, Hoyer PF, Byrd DJ, Ehrich JH, Brodehl J. Evidence suggesting hyperoxaluria as a cause of nephrocalcinosis in phosphate-treated hypophosphataemic rickets. Lancet. 1990;335:1240–3.

84. Patzer L, van't Hoff W, Shah V, Hallson P, Kasidas GP, Samuell C, de Bruyn R, Barratt TM, Dillon MJ. Urinary supersaturation of calcium oxalate and phosphate in patients with X-linked hypophosphatemic rickets and in healthy schoolchildren. J Pediatr. 1999;135:611–7.

85. Alon U, Donaldson DL, Hellerstein S, Warady BA, Harris DJ. Metabolic and histologic investigation of the nature of nephrocalcinosis in children with hypophosphatemic rickets and in the hyp mouse. J Pediatr. 1992;120:899–905.

86. Friedman NE, Lobaugh B, Drezner MK. Effects of calcitriol and phosphorus therapy on the growth of patients with X-linked hypophosphatemia. J Clin Endocrinol Metab. 1993;76:839–44.

87. Verge CF, Lam A, Simpson JM, Cowell CT, Howard NJ, Silink M. Effects of therapy in X-linked hypophosphatemic rickets. N Engl J Med. 1991;325:1843–8.

88. Lecoq AL, Chaumet-Riffaud P, Blanchard A, Dupeux M, Rothenbuhler A, Lambert B, Durand E, Boros E, Briot K, Silve C, Francou B, Piketty M, Chanson P, Brailly-Tabard S, Linglart A, Kamenický P. Hyperparathyroidism in patients with X-linked hypophosphatemia. J Bone Miner Res. 2020;35:1263–73.

89. Whyte MP, Carpenter TO, Gottesman GS, Mao M, Skrinar A, San Martin J, Imel EA. Efficacy and safety of burosumab in children aged 1-4 years with X-linked hypophosphataemia: a multicentre, open-label, phase 2 trial. Lancet Diabetes Endocrinol. 2019;7:189–99.

90. Imel EA, Glorieux FH, Whyte MP, Munns CF, Ward LM, Nilsson O, Simmons JH, Padidela R, Namba N, Cheong HI, Pitukcheewanont P, Sochett E, Högler W, Muroya K, Tanaka H, Gottesman GS, Biggin A, Perwad F, Mao M, Chen CY, Skrinar A, San Martin J, Portale AA. Burosumab versus conventional therapy in children with X-linked hypophosphataemia: a randomised, active-controlled, open-label, phase 3 trial. Lancet. 2019;393:2416–27.

91. Imel EA, Zhang X, Ruppe MD, Weber TJ, Klausner MA, Ito T, Vergeire M, Humphrey JS, Glorieux FH, Portale AA, Insogna K, Peacock M, Carpenter TO. Prolonged correction of serum phosphorus in adults with X-linked hypophosphatemia using monthly doses of KRN23. J Clin Endocrinol Metab. 2015;100:2565–73.

92. Ruppe MD, Zhang X, Imel EA, Weber TJ, Klausner MA, Ito T, Vergeire M, Humphrey JS, Glorieux FH, Portale AA, Insogna K, Peacock M, Carpenter TO. Effect of four monthly doses of a human monoclonal anti-FGF23 antibody (KRN23) on quality of life in X-linked hypophosphatemia. Bone Rep. 2016;5:158–62.

93. Insogna KL, Briot K, Imel EA, Kamenický P, Ruppe MD, Portale AA, Weber T, Pitukcheewanont P, Cheong HI, Jan de Beur S, Imanishi Y, Ito N, Lachmann RH, Tanaka H, Perwad F, Zhang L, Chen CY, Theodore-Oklota C, Mealiffe M, San Martin J, Carpenter TO, AXLES 1 Investigators. A randomized, double-blind, placebo-controlled, phase 3 trial evaluating the efficacy of burosumab, an anti-FGF23 antibody, in adults with X-linked hypophosphatemia: week 24 primary analysis. J Bone Miner Res. 2018;33:1383–93.

94. Portale AA, Carpenter TO, Brandi ML, Briot K, Cheong HI, Cohen-Solal M, Crowley R, Jan De Beur S, Eastell R, Imanishi Y, Imel EA, Ing S, Ito N, Javaid M, Kamenicky P, Keen R, Kubota T, Lachmann R, Perwad F, Pitukcheewanont P, Ralston SH, Takeuchi Y, Tanaka H, Weber TJ, Yoo HW, Zhang L, Theodore-Oklota C, Mealiffe M, San Martin J, Insogna K. Continued beneficial effects of burosumab in adults with X-linked hypophosphatemia: results from a 24-week treatment continuation period after a 24-week double-blind placebo-controlled period. Calcif Tissue Int. 2019;105:271–84.

95. Insogna KL, Rauch F, Kamenický P, Ito N, Kubota T, Nakamura A, Zhang L, Mealiffe M, San Martin J, Portale AA. Burosumab improved histomorphometric measures of osteomalacia in adults with X-linked hypophosphatemia: a phase 3, single-arm, international trial. J Bone Miner Res. 2019;34:2183–91.

96. Wilson DM. Growth hormone and hypophosphatemic rickets. J Pediatr Endocrinol Metab. 2000;13(Suppl 2):993–8.

97. Baroncelli GI, Bertelloni S, Ceccarelli C, Saggese G. Effect of growth hormone treatment on final height, phosphate metabolism, and bone mineral density in children with X-linked hypophosphatemic rickets. J Pediatr. 2001;138:236–43.

98. Haffner D, Nissel R, Wuhl E, Mehls O. Effects of growth hormone treatment on body proportions and final height among small children with X-linked hypophosphatemic rickets. Pediatrics. 2004;113:593.

99. Reusz GS, Miltenyi G, Stubnya G, Szabo A, Horvath C, Byrd DJ, Peter F, Tulassay T. X-linked hypophosphatemia: effects of treatment with recombinant human growth hormone. Pediatr Nephrol. 1997;11:573–7.

100. Seikaly MG, Brown R, Baum M. The effect of recombinant human growth hormone in children with X-linked hypophosphatemia. Pediatrics. 1997;100:879–84.

101. Rothenbuhler A, Esterle L, Gueorguieva I, Salles JP, Mignot B, Colle M, Linglart A. Two-year recombinant human growth hormone (rhGH) treatment is more effective in pre-pubertal compared to pubertal short children with X-linked hypophosphatemic rickets (XLHR). Growth Horm IGF Res. 2017;36:11–5.

102. Zivicnjak M, Schnabel D, Staude H, Even G, Marx M, Beetz R, Holder M, Billing H, Fischer DC, Rabl W, Schumacher M, Hiort O, Haffner D, Hypophosphatemic Rickets Study Group of the Arbeitsgemeinschaft fur Padiatrische Endokrinologie and Gesellschaft fur Padiatrische Nephrologie. Three-year growth hormone treatment in short children with X-linked hypophosphatemic rickets: effects on linear growth and body disproportion. J Clin Endocrinol Metab. 2011;96:2097.

103. Meyerhoff N, Haffner D, Staude H, Wühl E, Marx M, Beetz R, Querfeld U, Holder M, Billing H, Rabl W, Schröder C, Hiort O, Brämswig JH, Richter-Unruh A, Schnabel D, Živičnjak M, Hypophosphatemic Rickets Study Group of the "Deutsche Gesellschaft für Kinderendokrinologie und -diabetologie" and "Gesellschaft für Pädiatrische Nephrologie". Effects of growth hormone treatment on adult height in severely short children with X-linked hypophosphatemic rickets. Pediatr Nephrol. 2018;33:447–56.

104. Yavropoulou MP, Kotsa K, Gotzamani Psarrakou A, Papazisi A, Tranga T, Ventis S, Yovos JG. Cinacalcet in hyperparathyroidism secondary to X-linked hypophosphatemic rickets: case report and brief literature review. Hormones (Athens). 2010;9:274–8.

105. Alon US, Levy-Olomucki R, Moore WV, Stubbs J, Liu S, Quarles LD. Calcimimetics as an adjuvant treatment for familial hypophosphatemic rickets. Clin J Am Soc Nephrol. 2008;3:658–64.

106. Geller JL, Khosravi A, Kelly MH, Riminucci M, Adams JS, Collins MT. Cinacalcet in the management of tumor-induced osteomalacia. J Bone Miner Res. 2007;22:931–7.

107. Gizard A, Rothenbuhler A, Pejin Z, Finidori G, Glorion C, de Billy B, Linglart A, Wicart P. Outcomes of orthopedic surgery in a cohort of 49 patients with X-linked hypophosphatemic rickets (XLHR). Endocr Connect. 2017;6:566–73.

108. Horn A, Wright J, Bockenhauer D, Van't Hoff W, Eastwood DM. The orthopaedic management of lower limb deformity in hypophosphataemic rickets. J Child Orthop. 2017;11:298–305.

109. Petje G, Meizer R, Radler C, Aigner N, Grill F. Deformity correction in children with hereditary hypophosphatemic rickets. Clin Orthop Relat Res. 2008;466:3078–85.

110. Chaussain-Miller C, Sinding C, Wolikow M, Lasfargues JJ, Godeau G, Garabedian M. Dental abnormalities in patients with familial hypophosphatemic vitamin D-resistant rickets: prevention by early treatment with 1-hydroxyvitamin D. J Pediatr. 2003;142:324–31.

111. Biosse Duplan M, Coyac BR, Bardet C, Zadikian C, Rothenbuhler A, Kamenicky P, Briot K, Linglart A, Chaussain C. Phosphate and vitamin D prevent periodontitis in X-linked hypophosphatemia. J Dent Res. 2017;96:388–95.

112. Mao M, Carpenter TO, Whyte MP, Skrinar A, Chen CY, San Martin J, Rogol AD. Growth curves for children with X-linked hypophosphatemia. J Clin Endocrinol Metab. 2020;105(10):3243–9.

113. Cagnoli M, Richter R, Böhm P, Knye K, Empting S, Mohnike K. Spontaneous growth and effect of early therapy with calcitriol and phosphate in X-linked hypophosphatemic rickets. Pediatr Endocrinol Rev. 2017;15:119–22.

114. Berndt M, Ehrich JH, Lazovic D, Zimmermann J, Hillmann G, Kayser C, Prokop M, Schirg E, Siegert B, Wolff G, Brodehl J. Clinical course of hypophosphatemic rickets in 23 adults. Clin Nephrol. 1996;45:33–41.

115. Haffner D, Weinfurth A, Manz F, Schmidt H, Bremer HJ, Mehls O, Scharer K. Long-term outcome of paediatric patients with hereditary tubular disorders. Nephron. 1999;83:250–60.

116. Skrinar A, Dvorak-Ewell M, Evins A, Macica C, Linglart A, Imel EA, Theodore-Oklota C, San Martin J. The lifelong impact of X-linked hypophosphatemia: results from a burden of disease survey. J Endocr Soc. 2019;3:1321–34.

117. Chesher D, Oddy M, Darbar U, Sayal P, Casey A, Ryan A, Sechi A, Simister C, Waters A, Wedatilake Y, Lachmann RH, Murphy E. Outcome of adult patients with X-linked hypophosphatemia caused by PHEX gene mutations. J Inherit Metab Dis. 2018;41:865–76.

118. Lo SH, Lachmann R, Williams A, Piglowska N, Lloyd AJ. Exploring the burden of X-linked hypophosphatemia: a European multi-country qualitative study. Qual Life Res. 2020;29:1883–93.

119. Silverman SL. Bisphosphonate use in conditions other than osteoporosis. Ann N Y Acad Sci. 2011;1218:33–7.

120. Classen CF, Mix M, Kyank U, Hauenstein C, Haffner D. Pamidronic acid and cabergoline as effective long-term therapy in a 12-year-old girl with extended facial polyostotic fibrous dysplasia, prolactinoma and acromegaly in McCune-Albright syndrome: a case report. J Med Case Rep. 2012;6:32.

121. Bergwitz C, Miyamoto KI. Hereditary hypophosphatemic rickets with hypercalciuria: pathophysiology, clinical presentation, diagnosis and therapy. Pflugers Arch. 2019;471:149–63.

Renal Tubular Acidosis

39

R. Todd Alexander and Detlef Bockenhauer

Introduction

Plasma pH is maintained in a very tight range, from 7.35 to 7.45, via multiple regulatory mechanisms including buffering, altered respiration and ultimately fine regulation by the kidney. This tight control of plasma pH is essential for many physiological functions including but not limited to: proper folding and functioning of proteins, neural transmission and cardiac contractility. Typically, perturbations in plasma pH are caused by alterations in respiration or the presence of exogenous acids, which overwhelm the remarkable underlying capacity of the body to regulate plasma pH. However, less commonly, excess loss of bicarbonate from the gut or kidney, or the failure of the renal tubule to excrete acid is at fault. It is these less common causes of metabolic acidosis that are the subject of this chapter.

In order to understand the molecular pathogenesis of renal tubular acidosis, it is a prerequisite to know both the role of the kidney in the maintenance and regulation of plasma pH and its interrelation to other processes that participate in acid-base homeostasis. Proteins and phosphate mediate buffering in the cell. In the extracellular compartment bicarbonate is the predominant buffer preventing decreases in pH in response to an acid load. This is followed by an increase in respiratory rate and depth (respiratory compensation). Finally, the kidneys respond by increasing bicarbonate reabsorption, a process that leads to increased ammoniagenesis and ultimately facilitates increased acid secretion from the distal nephron. A detailed discussion of buffering and respiratory control of acid-base status is beyond the scope of this chapter. However, in order to inform the discussion of the pathophysiology of altered tubular handling of acid, we will begin by detailing the current understanding of how the kidney participates in acid-base homeostasis.

Physiology of Renal Acid-Base Handling

Bicarbonate Reabsorption

A significant amount of bicarbonate is filtered and consequently reabsorbed daily in order to preserve extracellular buffering capacity [1, 2]. Assuming a GFR of 120 mL/min in the average adult male and a plasma bicarbonate concentration of 24 mM, this amounts to approximately

R. T. Alexander (✉)
Department of Pediatrics, Edmonton Clinic Health Academy, University of Alberta, Edmonton, AB, Canada
e-mail: todd2@ualberta.ca

D. Bockenhauer
UCL Department of Renal Medicine and Great Ormond Street Hospital for Children NHS Foundation Trust, London, UK
e-mail: d.bockenhauer@ucl.ac.uk

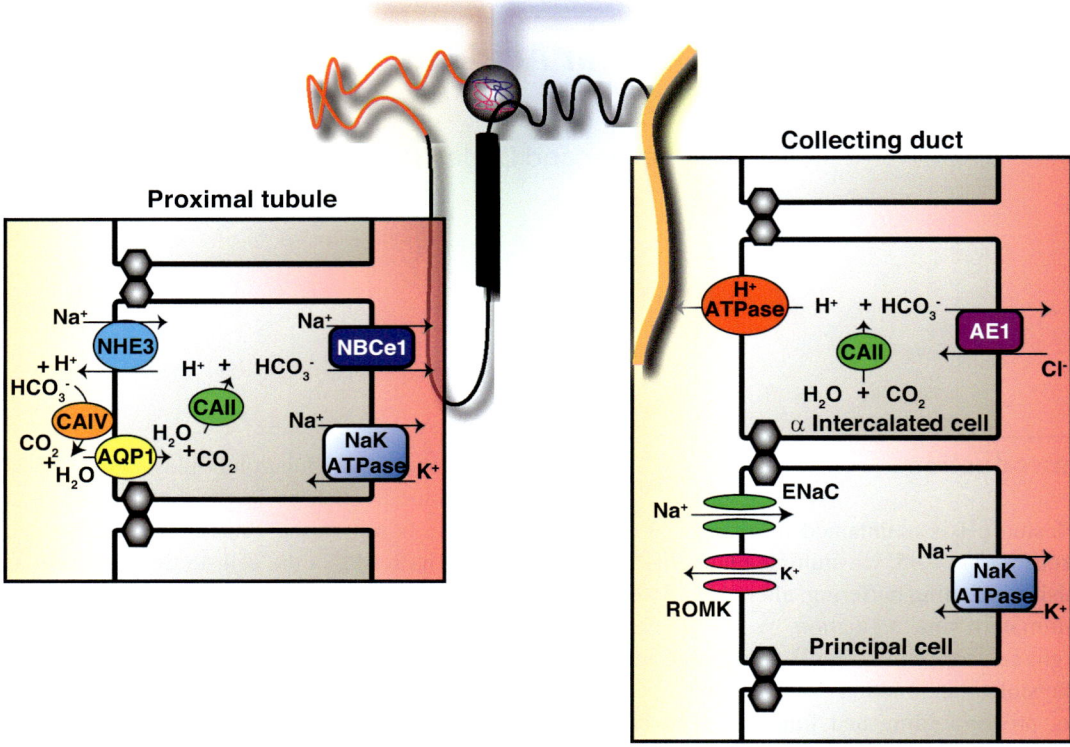

Fig. 39.1 Renal handling of bicarbonate and acid. The majority of filtered bicarbonate (HCO_3^-) is reabsorbed from the proximal tubule, after enzymatic (carbonic anhydrase IV, CAIV) conversion to water and carbon dioxide (CO_2). This is facilitated by proton excretion through the sodium proton exchanger isoform 3 (NHE3). In the cytosol carbonic anhydrase II (CAII), converts the water and CO_2 back into a proton, which is recycled through NHE3, and HCO_3^-, which is effluxed back into the blood through the sodium bicarbonate cotransporter NBCe1. In the col-

lecting duct, H^+ is secreted from the α-intercalated cell via the apically expressed H^+ATPase. The proton is generated via the catalysis, by CAII, of water and CO_2. This also generates HCO_3^-, which is exchanged for Cl⁻ by the basolateral anion exchanger (AE1). In principle, cell sodium is reabsorbed through the epithelial sodium channel (ENaC). As this is an electrogenic process, either potassium (K^+) excretion trough ROMK or proton secretion via the H^+ATPase is required to maintain a permissive potential difference across the luminal membrane

4150 mmoles of bicarbonate that is filtered daily. Under normal circumstances the urine is free of bicarbonate, which means that all filtered bicarbonate is reabsorbed by the nephron [3] (Fig. 39.1). The vast majority is reabsorbed from the proximal tubule [4, 5]. Animal experiments provide evidence for bicarbonate reabsorption also in the thick ascending limb and the collecting duct, albeit to a much lesser degree [6–11]. The relative amount of bicarbonate absorbed from these sites varies depending on physiological status but in normal physiologic conditions is never more than a fraction of the proximal tubule's contribution to this process [3].

Proximal Tubule

There is no known bicarbonate transporter in the apical membrane of the proximal tubule. Consequently filtered bicarbonate is converted to water and carbon dioxide by a brush border membrane carbonic anhydrase [12]. Carbonic anhydrase IV and likely also the transmembrane isoform carbonic anhydrase XIV mediate this function [13–15]. The water channel, aquaporin-1, permits the rapid influx of water into the proximal tubular epithelial cell [16–19] and may also facilitate the permeation of carbon dioxide [20–22], in addition to diffusion across the membrane down its concentration gradient [23]. Cytoplasmic carbonic anhydrase II, which interacts directly with aquaporin-1 enhancing water flux, then converts intracellular water and carbon dioxide back into bicarbonate and a proton (through the intermediate carbonic acid) [24–29]. The proton is exchanged for a sodium ion, predominantly by the apical sodium proton exchanger isoform 3 (NHE3) [30–33], while the bicarbonate is extruded back into the circulation across the basolateral membrane via the electrogenic sodium dependent bicarbonate transporter (NBCe1) [34, 35]. Yet, while mutations in *SLC4A4* (encoding NBCe1) are associated with a severe form of inherited pRTA, mutations in *SLC9A3* (encoding NHE3) cause congenital sodium diarrhea with only mild renal bicarbonate wasting [36–39]. This likely reflects redundancy provided by other NHE isoforms, such as NHE8 [40].

There is also a proton pump, H^+ ATPase which effluxes protons into the lumen of the proximal tubule [41, 42], although its contribution to proximal tubular bicarbonate reabsorption is minimal relative to that of NHE3 [32]. The majority of bicarbonate transport occurs in the first part of the proximal tubule [43]. This results in a slightly lumen negative transepithelial potential difference which is believed to be responsible for driving paracellular chloride reabsorption from the latter part of the proximal tubule [44, 45].

Thick Ascending Limb of Henle's Loop

NHE3, the epithelial sodium proton exchanger, is also expressed in the apical membrane of the thick ascending limb of Henle's loop (TAL) [46]. Consequently, bicarbonate reabsorption from this segment is felt to occur via a similar process as in the proximal tubule [47, 48]. The absence of aquaporin-1 from this segment may explain the decreased efficiency of bicarbonate reabsorption from the thick ascending limb relative to the proximal tubule [16]. Efflux across the basolateral membrane is mediated by the anion exchanger isoform 2 [49–51].

Collecting Duct

Any remaining bicarbonate reaching the collecting duct is reabsorbed by an analogous process [7, 8]. Efflux of a proton into the lumen permits the titration of bicarbonate back into carbonic acid and then carbon dioxide and water. Proton efflux is achieved via a luminally situated V-type H^+ ATPase, also called a proton pump [52]. Apically expressed proton pumps are only found in α-intercalated cells [41, 53, 54], whose apical membranes are largely impermeable to water, although carbon dioxide could diffuse into the epithelial cells of the collecting duct including α-intercalated cells. Intracellular carbon dioxide is hydrated, generating a proton and bicarbonate. This is achieved by cytosolic carbonic anhydrase II [54, 55]. The *de novo* generated bicarbonate is then extruded into the circulation via the basolateral anion-exchanger (AE1) [56]. This is the same mechanism permitting the trapping of ammonium in the distal nephron described below.

Acid Secretion

Acid secretion is achieved in the collecting duct via the mechanism described above for the titration of bicarbonate. The luminal H^+ ATPase in α-intercalated cells secretes a proton that is trapped by converting ammonia into ammonium, or by titrating another acid [57, 58]. These so-called titratable acids include: bicarbonate, phosphate and sulphate. The proton is generated from cytosolic carbon dioxide and water via the action of carbonic anhydrase II [24, 55]. The bicarbonate generated by this process is extruded back into the circulation in exchange for a chloride via AE1 [59, 60]. Moreover, there is a potassium-proton pump in the apical membrane of collecting duct α-intercalated cells, which also participates in acid secretion, although to a lesser extent [61–63].

Beta-intercalated cells exhibit essentially reverse polarity to α-intercalated cells and thus have an opposite function, as they can generate and secrete bicarbonate into the urine and a proton back into the circulation [8, 41, 53]. They contain a chloride bicarbonate exchanger in their apical membrane, Pendrin, and a proton pump in the basolateral membrane [54, 64–66]. They also contain a cytosolic carbonic anhydrase, CAII [60, 64]. Importantly, recent evidence has implicated this cell type in sodium and chloride reabsorption [67, 68]. ß-intercalated cells nearly completely lack the expression of the Na⁺/K⁺ ATPase, instead the basolateral H⁺ ATPase appears to drive transport across this cell type [69]. This facilitative role of the H⁺ ATPase may contribute to the polyuria and volume contraction often observed in patients with distal renal tubular acidosis due to mutations in this pump [70, 71].

Ammonia Genesis and Recycling

Ammonia (NH_3) is the major urinary buffer and consequently its protonation to ammonium (NH_4^+) is essential for the efficient urinary excretion of acid [57, 72].

Ammonia Genesis

Ammonium is produced in the proximal tubule from glutamine and then secreted into the lumen [73]. Free circulating glutamine in the plasma enters the proximal tubular epithelial cell across the basolateral membrane via the LAT2 amino acid transporter [74]. Glutamine in the cytosol then enters the mitochondria via an electroneutral uniporter [75] where it is first converted to glutamate by glutaminase, then to ammonium by a glutamate dehydrogenase [76]. These enzyme-catalyzed reactions produce bicarbonate, which is returned to the circulation via the sodium-dependent bicarbonate transporter NBCe1. Of note, hyperkalemia inhibits the generation of ammonia [77].

Ammonia Recycling

Ammonium has been thought to be secreted into the proximal tubule by substituting for sodium on the apical sodium proton exchanger NHE3 [78–81]. However, a study employing a proximal tubular *Nhe3* knockout mouse argues against this role for the exchanger [39]. Alternatively, another EIPA (Ethylisopropyl-amiloride) sensitive sodium proton exchanger that is expressed in the apical membrane of the proximal tubule such as NHE8 may play this role [32, 82, 83], or free

ammonia may diffuse into the lumen where proton excretion may trap it by conversion to ammonium.

Luminal ammonium then travels down the thin descending limb. In TAL, a nephron segment largely impermeant to ammonia, luminal ammonium is absorbed into the tubular epithelial cell across the apical membrane via the sodium potassium chloride co-transporter NKCC2 [84]. Ammonium is approximately the size of potassium and consequently can substitute for it. Thus hyperkalemia can inhibit ammonium excretion, as increased luminal concentrations of potassium will compete with ammonium for the transport site on NKCC2, preventing its influx into the tubular epithelial cell [85, 86]. Once transported across the luminal membrane of TAL cells, it diffuses across the basolateral membrane into the interstitium in the form of ammonia. Accumulation in the interstitium occurs as the apical membrane is impermeable to ammonia, preventing a back leak of ammonia into the tubular lumen [87].

This medullary interstitial accumulation of ammonia is essential to the efficient excretion of acid as it provides a concentration difference, from interstitium to lumen of the collecting duct for ammonia diffusion into the lumen. Consequently, ammonia diffuses into the lumen of the collecting duct where it is trapped via the excretion of protons as ammonium [88, 89]. The collecting duct is relatively impermeable to ammonium [90]. There is evidence implicating RhCG, a rhesus glycoprotein homologue, in this process as it forms a pore in the apical and basolateral membranes of the collecting duct epithelial cells permitting the passage of ammonia, but not ammonium [91–94]. Proton excretion is achieved as described above via apically expressed ATPases, predominantly the V-type H⁺ ATPase and to a lesser extent the H⁺K⁺-ATPase. Ultimately, ammonium generation in the proximal tubule, recycling in the loop of Henle and finally trapping in the collecting duct permit significant and efficient proton excretion in the urine (Fig. 39.2).

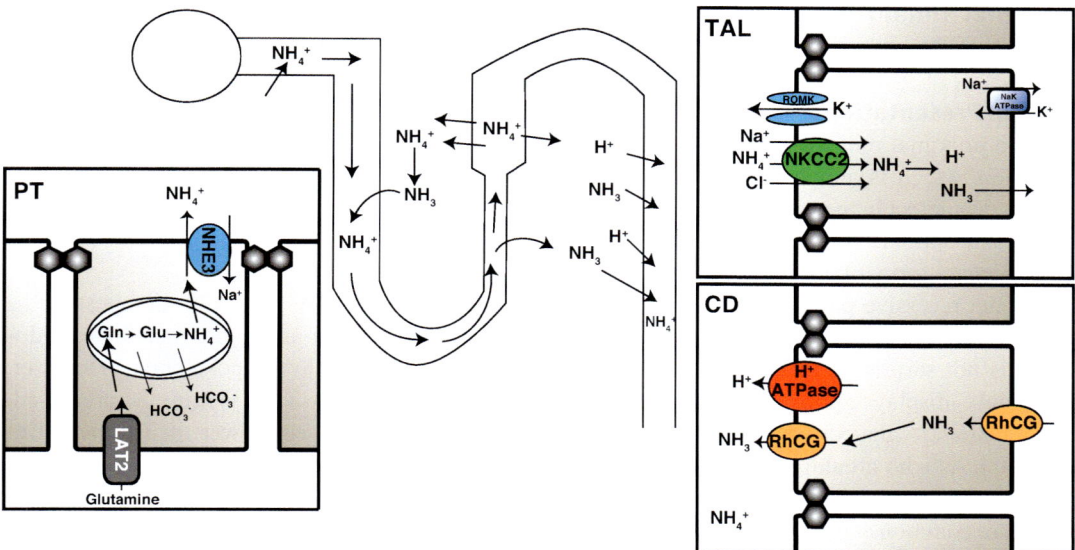

Fig. 39.2 Ammonia generation and recycling. Ammonium is generated in the proximal tubule (PT) and secreted into the lumen in exchange for sodium (Na^+) by the sodium proton exchanger isoform 3 (NHE3). It then travels down the nephron to the thick ascending limb (TAL) where it is reab-sorbed by the sodium potassium chloride cotransporter, (NKCC2). Ammonia then diffuses into the interstitium where it either undergoes recycling in the loop or permeates the collecting duct through RhCG and is trapped by a proton secreted through the H^+-ATPase

Pathophysiology of Renal-Acid Base Handling

Definitions

The principles of renal tubular acid-base handling discussed above provide the foundation of the classification of renal tubular acidosis. Defects in bicarbonate reabsorption, which occurs predominantly in the proximal nephron, are referred to as proximal renal tubular acidosis, or pRTA [95]. Historically, pRTA has also been classified as type II RTA. Defects in distal tubular proton secretion are referred to as distal renal tubular acidosis, dRTA [95]. This type of RTA has also been referred to as Type I. Clinical syndromes with features of both proximal and distal renal tubular acidosis, *i.e.* a failure to reclaim both filtered bicarbonate and excrete acid in the urine, are known as mixed renal tubular acidosis or type III RTA. All these types of RTA are typi-cally accompanied by normal or low plasma potassium levels, and are distinguished by the presence of bicarbonaturia and/or the failure to acidify the urine in the presence of an acid load. Due to the molecular link between sodium and acid-base homeostasis, RTA can also occur as a secondary consequence of impaired sodium reab-sorption in the collecting duct, as sodium uptake by ENaC provides a favorable electrical gradient for proton secretion. The salt-wasting tubulopa-thy related to impaired ENaC activity is also referred to as aldosterone insufficient or resistant RTA, or type IV RTA. Since ENaC activity also facilitates potassium secretion, this type of RTA is distinguished from the other types by being associated with hyperkalemia. All forms of RTA are associated with a non-anion gap acidosis, consistent with loss of bicarbonate. For pRTA, this is obvious, as bicarbonate reabsorption is impaired. In dRTA the mechanism is indirect: bicarbonate is consumed for buffering the protons the distal tubule fails to excrete.

Proximal Renal Tubular Acidosis (Type II RTA)

Clinical Presentations

Isolated proximal renal tubular acidosis is a rare condition, which is almost exclusively due to a single gene defect in the sodium dependent bicarbonate transporter, NBCe1 (*SLC4A4*) [96–98]. This genetic form of pRTA is inherited in an autosomal recessive pattern [99]. Given that the renal isoform of NBCe1 is also expressed in the eye it is not surprising that affected individuals commonly display eye abnormalities, such as band cataracts, glaucoma or band keratopathy [99–101]. As with all untreated renal tubular acidosis, failure to thrive and hypomineralized bones are common at presentation [99]. There are also pancreatic and brain isoforms of NBCe1 and consequently, some patients with mutations affecting these isoforms also have increased circulating amylase levels (without evidence of pancreatitis) and there are reports of associated intellectual impairment [99].

Autosomal dominant pRTA has been described in two separate families. The responsible gene accounting for this syndrome has yet to be determined. The first family identified is Costa Rican. One affected brother presented with short stature, bilateral coloboma and subaortic stenosis, while another brother showed limited clinical symptoms, except metabolic acidosis with a urinary pH < 5.0 as did the affected sibling [102]. They both had evidence of hypomineralized bones. The other family described includes a father and all 4 of his children who have metabolic acidosis with increased bicarbonate excretion following bicarbonate loading. Despite sequencing a number of candidate genes the cause of their disease is yet to be defined [97]. As detailed above, mutations in NHE3 have not been reported to cause pRTA, but instead congenital sodium diarrhea [38]. Interestingly, affected patients have either absent or only mild acidosis. Similarly, mice with proximal tubule-specific knock out of Nhe3, also only have marginally lower serum bicarbonate levels compared to wild type [39]. There are some data suggesting compensatory upregulation of Nhe8 [103].

Other genetic and acquired forms of pRTA usually occur as part of the renal Fanconi syndrome [104], which is characterized by complex proximal tubular dysfunction due to genetic defects or proximal tubular toxicity from a drug, toxin or metabolite. Renal Fanconi syndrome causes are listed and described in Chap. 31.

Diagnosis

Patients with pRTA typically demonstrate a hyperchloremic non-anion gap metabolic acidosis, accompanied by hypokalemia. However, since the ability to acidify urine is preserved, patients with pRTA can lower their urine pH to less than 5.5 when plasma bicarbonate levels are lower than their renal threshold for tubular bicarbonate absorption. This distinguishes pRTA from dRTA. A definitive means of diagnosing pRTA is by assessing renal tubular bicarbonate absorption (or the fractional excretion of bicarbonate) across a range of plasma bicarbonate levels. A fractional excretion of bicarbonate greater than 15% in the context of a metabolic acidosis definitively diagnoses pRTA [104, 105]. Some authors have suggested an even lower cut off level, i.e. 5% [41]. In case of doubt, the diagnosis can be ascertained by assessing tubular bicarbonate handling as an alkali is given to the patient, resulting in a gradual increase in plasma pH [106]. Practically this can be done by measuring the fractional excretion of bicarbonate repeatedly while normalizing plasma bicarbonate levels with increasing doses of alkali (e.g., administration of intravenous bicarbonate at a rate predicted to increase blood bicarbonate by 2 mmol/L/h, until urine pH is >6.8 [103]). A marked increase in urinary bicarbonate excretion normally occurs at a specific serum bicarbonate level. This is called the bicarbonate threshold. A normal bicarbonate threshold is around 22 mmol/L in infants and 25 mmol/L in older children/adults [107]. A bicarbonate threshold less than 20 indicates pRTA. In practical terms, a pRTA patient with a bicarbonate threshold of 16 will stop wasting bicarbonate and be able to acidify the urine to <5.5 at a plasma bicarbonate at or below 16 [108].

In clinical practice, the fractional excretion of bicarbonate is rarely performed, due to technical considerations especially relevant in children: when urine is exposed to air, CO_2 diffuses out, lowering urinary bicarbonate concentration, while at the same time increasing the pH (CO_2 + H_2O <<<=> H^+ + HCO_3^-). Thus, fresh urine should be obtained and ideally under oil to minimize CO_2 loss. This is obviously challenging in non-toilet trained children, unless a catheter is inserted. Similarly, the lab should be alerted to handle these samples urgently and not every biochemical lab will measure urinary bicarbonate. From a practical point of view: isolated pRTA is exceedingly rare and virtually always associated with eye abnormalities. Otherwise, pRTA occurs in the context of a more generalized proximal tubulopathy. Thus, if pRTA is suspected, an eye examination and a screen for renal Fanconi syndrome (glycosuria, phosphaturia, low molecular weight proteinuria, amino- and organic aciduria, see Chap. 31) should be performed and is usually sufficient to establish a diagnosis. If typical abnormalities are present, a genetic diagnosis can be established by sequencing *SLC4A4* [96]. An algorithm for the diagnosis of RTA is presented in Fig. 39.3.

Treatment

For treatment of renal Fanconi syndrome, please see Chap. 31. For isolated pRTA, alkali replacement is the main line of therapy [109, 110]. This is especially important in prepubertal children as persistent metabolic acidosis will impair growth [109]. Given the pathophysiology, with bicarbonate wasting when plasma bicarbonate levels are above the threshold, it is not surprising that even with prodigious quantities (5–15 mEq/kg/day) of bicarbonate supplementation, plasma levels may remain low [104]. This is another distinguishing factor from dRTA, where normal plasma bicarbonate levels can be achieved with doses of usually 2–5 mEq/kg/day [111]. It is recommended to administer smaller doses of alkali replacement frequently, as the larger the dose, the higher the peak in subsequent plasma bicarbonate concentration which, in turn, will increase urinary bicarbonate losses [112]. The use of long-acting alkali replacement formulations has not been reported in pRTA, but should help to maintain more consistent plasma bicarbonate levels, while minimizing the frequency of daily doses.

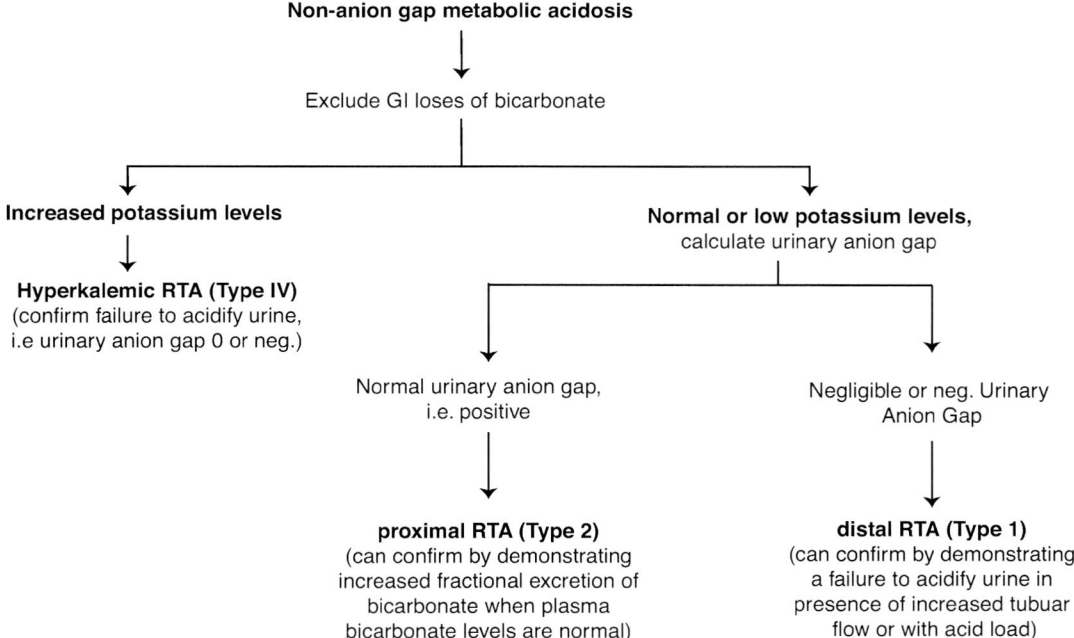

Fig. 39.3 Algorithm for diagnosis of RTA

Prognosis

Due to the extreme rarity of the disease, little information on the long-term outcomes of children with isolated pRTA is available. So far, renal failure has not been reported in contrast to dRTA, and growth can be improved with alkali supplementation [109, 113].

Distal Renal Tubular Acidosis (Type I RTA)

Clinical Presentation

Distal renal tubular acidosis is more common than the proximal form. Biochemically, it also presents as a hyperchloremic non-anion-gap metabolic acidosis, typically in association with hypokalemia, hypercalciuria and nephrocalcinois, although these features are not always present [114]. Some patients will also display renal cysts, although these typically develop later [115].

Mutations in at least 5 different genes have been identified and found to cause dRTA [116]. Moreover, a number of conditions, drugs and toxins can cause dRTA (see Table 39.1), yet this is more commonly seen in adults. In particular drugs targeting the distal nephron, autoimmune diseases and conditions characterized by hypercalciuria can be associated with dRTA [117].

Distal RTA with Mutations in AE1 (SLC4A1)

Mutations in the anion exchanger isoform 1, AE1, have been found to cause dRTA [118–120]. The encoding gene, *SLC4A1*, is expressed in both red blood cells as well as in α-intercalated cells of the collecting duct [121]. Some mutations in AE1 cause congenital forms of anemia including hereditary spherocytosis and ovalocytosis [122–126]. These mutations are predominantly found in regions of Southeast Asia with a historically high incidence of *plasmodium falciparum* infections, against which ovalocytosis provides protection [127]. Interestingly, mutations in AE1 that cause blood dyscrasias generally do not result in dRTA and conversely, mutations causing

Table 39.1 Causes of distal renal tubular acidosis

Genetic
  H+ATPase, α4 (*ATPV0A4*)
  H+ATPase, ß1 (*ATPV1B1*)
  AE1 (*SLC4A1*)
  FOXI1 (*FOXI1*)
  WDR72 (*WDR72*, tryptophan-aspartate repeat domain 72)
  CAII (*CA2*)[a]
Autoimmune
  Cryoglobulinemia
  Sjorgren syndrome
  Thyroiditis
  HIV-nephropathy
  Chronic active hepatitis
  Primary bilary cirrhosis
  Polyarthritis nodosa
Hypercalciuria/nephrocalcinosis
  Primary hyperparathyroidism
  Hyperthyroidism
  Medullary sponge kidney
Drug induced
  Amphotericin B
  Cyclamate
  Vanadate
  Ifosfamide
  Toluene
  Mercury
  Lithium
  Foscarnet
  Analgesic nephropathy
Miscellaneous causes
  Sickle cell disease
  Marfan syndrome
  Ehlers-Danlos syndrome
  Carnitine palmitoyltransferase deficiency

[a]CAII deficiency causes a combined pRTA and dRTA i.e. type III RTA

dRTA often do not cause anemia. Most mutations associated with dRTA are missense variants leading to aberrant trafficking (e.g. to the apical membrane) or ER retention. AE1 functions as a dimer, so that these mutations can have a dominant negative effect [127–129]. Since red cells are not polarized, aberrant trafficking is less of a problem. Moreover, red cells express glycophorin and other chaperones responsible for trafficking AE1 to the plasma membrane that are absent in renal epithelial cells. This explains how some mutations cause dRTA and not anemia [130]. In contrast, mutations causing isolated red cell disorders typically affect transport function, suggesting a susceptibility of red cells to AE1 haploinsufficiency [128]. In addition, the isoforms of AE1 expressed in red cells and kidney are different; the latter lacks the first 65 amino acids, so that mutations in this region are not expected to cause kidney disease [131]. In a minority of patients both dRTA and anemia are present [132–136].

Mutations in AE1 were originally reported to only be transmitted in an autosomal dominant fashion [118]. Such families have been reported globally [118–120, 133, 137, 138]. Autosomal dominant mutations can cause complete or incomplete dRTA (note incomplete dRTA is evidence of a failure to acidify urine when challenged with an acid load in an individual *without* metabolic acidosis at baseline) [139]. Typically, patients with autosomal dominant dRTA present in adolescence or even at adult age. In general, biochemical abnormalities are less severe than in patients with recessive disease due to mutations in subunits of the H^+-ATPase, potentially explaining the later presentation [115]. Hypercalciuria, nephrocalcinosis and nephrolithiasis have been associated with this disease [120, 130, 138]. The frequency of these associations appears to increase with patient age.

Later, patients with mutations in AE1 inherited in an autosomal recessive fashion were reported [125, 130, 140–144]. Such recessive mutations typically cause a milder trafficking defect, so that both alleles need to be mutated to cause a clinically relevant problem. Patients who are compound heterozygous for one mutation causing ovalocytosis and one causing dRTA can have both disorders [128].

Distal RTA with Mutations in Proton Pump Subunits a4 (ATP6V0A4) and B1 (ATP6V1B1)

Mutations in at least two of the subunits of the vacuolar H^+-ATPase also cause dRTA [70, 145–149]. This 14-subunit proton pump is expressed in the luminal membrane of the α-intercalated cell and is responsible for the secretion of protons

into the collecting duct. Mutations in the a4 (*ATP6V0A4*) and B1 (*ATP6V1B1*) subunit have been reported to cause complete dRTA [149]. These mutations are inherited in an autosomal recessive pattern, although a specific mutation in the B1 subunit (p. Arg394Gln) has been reported recurrently in heterozygous form without an identified mutation on the other allele [111, 150]. Both the a4 and B1 subunits are also expressed in the inner ear, so it is not surprising that they are also associated with sensorineural hearing loss [149]. Nevertheless, some genotype-phenotype correlations exist: mutations in *ATP6V0A4* are associated with more severe dRTA, as assessed by a trend to earlier presentation, increased frequency of nephrocalcinosis and higher prescribed daily alkali dose [111, 115]. Yet, only about a third of patients with mutations in the a4 subunit have documented sensorineural hearing loss, compared to almost 90% in patients with B1 mutations [111]. Moreover, age at diagnosis of hearing loss and prescription of hearing aids or cochlear implants is significantly younger in patients with *ATP6V1B1* mutations compared to *ATP6V0A4*. [146, 149, 151]. The vast majority of patients with mutations in the a4 and B1 subunits have nephrocalcinosis (98% with *ATP6V1B1* and 90% with *ATP6V0A4*), which is typically present already at diagnosis [116].

Distal RTA with Mutations in FOXI1

FOXI1 is a transcription factor expressed in acid secreting epithelia important for the regulation of several genes involved in acid secretion, including *SLC4A1*, *ATP6V1B1* and *ATP6V0A4* [152]. Foxi1 knock out mice had already been reported in 2004 to have dRTA with sensorineural deafness [153]. It took another 14 years until two families with recessive mutations in FOXI1 were identified, suggesting that this is a very rare cause of dRTA [154]. Reported patients also have sensorineural deafness with massive enlargement of the endolymphatic sac [154]. Of note, male Foxi1 knock out mice are infertile, due to insufficient acidification of the luminal fluid in the epididymis with consequent pathologic post-testicular sperm maturation [153]. Whether male infertility is also a clinical problem in human FOXI1-related dRTA remains to be seen.

Distal RTA with Mutations in WDR72

WDR72 (tryptophan-aspartate repeat domain 72) is a protein presumed to be involved in intracellular vesicle transport that was initially identified as a cause of autosomal recessive amelogenesis imperfecta [155]. In 2018, two families with dRTA were reported with recessive mutations in WDR72 [156]. Subsequently, more families have been reported [157, 158]. Whether some families only exhibit dRTA, others only amelogenesis imperfecta and others both features is not clear. Potentially, the report of only one manifestation may betray the focus of the reporting specialist (dentist versus nephrologist). Interestingly, in one report, reverse phenotyping of patients with WDR72 mutations and a clinical diagnosis of dRTA revealed that all patients also had findings of amelogenesis imperfecta [158]. Interestingly, not all family members with WDR72-associated amelogenesis imperfecta have clear evidence of dRTA [157]. This suggests that WDR72-associated dRTA is typically milder than the forms associated with the other recessive disease genes.

Candidate Genes

Currently, about 60–80% of families with a clinical diagnosis of inherited dRTA have identifiable pathogenic variants in the known disease-causing genes described above, suggesting that there are more yet unidentified dRTA disease genes [115, 150, 158]. Further, subunits of the vacuolar H+-ATPase expressed in the kidney, such as C2, G3 and d3 have been suggested as candidates, but thus far, evidence definitively linking them to dRTA is limited [158–160].

Diagnosis

The presence of a hypokalemic, hyperchloremic, non-anion gap metabolic acidosis in the absence of intestinal losses and in the presence of a normal GFR should make one suspect RTA [161, 162]. Notably, substantially reduced GFR (CKD stage >3) can cause a normal anion gap metabolic acidosis due to insufficient nephron mass to excrete sufficient protons to maintain normal plasma pH. This cause of metabolic acidosis due to renal insufficiency is not traditionally labeled as dRTA, and can be easily distinguished by assessment of global renal function and the presence of the other clinical consequences of kidney disease.

Urinary pH will be inappropriately elevated with dRTA. Unfortunately, this finding can also be observed with pRTA when plasma pH is above the bicarbonate threshold. Definitive diagnosis of dRTA is made by demonstrating an inability to acidify the urine. Since ammonium is the major component of acid secretion it should be measured, ideally directly. However, most clinical laboratories do not offer urinary ammonium determination, but excretion can be estimated indirectly, using the **urine anion gap** [163]. This is in analogy to the plasma anion gap, although it would better be termed "cation gap", as it serves to estimate the unmeasured cation ammonium [164]. It is calculated using the formula: $U_{AG} = [Na^+]_U + [K^+]_U - [Cl^-]_U$.

The unmeasured urinary anions sulphate and phosphate are generally constant and at low levels. Moreover bicarbonate is not typically present in urine. Similarly, the urinary excretion of calcium and magnesium is relatively low and constant relative to sodium and potassium. Consequently, the urinary excretion of ammonium (NH_4^+) represents the greatest unmeasured urinary cation, making this equation a useful estimate of ammonium excretion. In the presence of metabolic acidosis there should be significant urinary ammonium excretion and consequently a negative anion gap. An alkaline urine pH in the presence of a negative urinary anion gap is consistent with the diagnosis of pRTA. An anion gap >10 mmol/L reflects the inappropriate absence of ammonium excretion and supports a diagnosis of dRTA [165]. Alternatively (or additionally), the urinary osmolality gap can be used [166].

In clinical practice, in the absence of intestinal losses of bicarbonate, hypokalaemic hyperchloremic metabolic acidosis with elevated urine pH is most likely caused by dRTA. In contrast, generalized proximal tubular dysfunction is consistent with pRTA. It is important to remember though, that approximately a third of patients with dRTA have evidence of proximal tubular dysfunction at presentation, confounding an accurate diagnosis [115]. This is likely related to the acidosis, as proximal dysfunction resolves with resolution of the acidosis. The complete **normalization of plasma bicarbonate levels with alkali supplementation** suggests a diagnosis of dRTA. In contrast, the ongoing bicarbonate wasting present in pRTA usually **precludes complete normalization of plasma bicarbonate levels. Further, a diagnosis of dRTA is confirmed by the later resolution of proximal dysfunction with adequate alkali treatment. The diagnosis can be secured by genetic testing in the vast majority of cases.**

The diagnosis can be challenging in milder (incomplete) forms, as these patients typically have normal plasma biochemistries at baseline.

Further **diagnostic procedures to assess distal acidification** can help. Two such procedures are commonly employed to this end. The first is the administration of an acid load typically as ammonium [167]. This is to induce an actual metabolic acidosis, so that appropriate urinary acidification can be assessed. Unfortunately, ammonium has a foul taste and may not be tolerated by patients. Alternatively, distal acidification can be stimulated by co-administration of a loop diuretic and mineralocorticoid, such as furosemide and fludrocortisone [168, 169]. Sodium reabsorption via the epithelial sodium channel ENaC (see Fig. 39.1) provides a favorable electrical gradient for acid secretion in the collecting duct. In patients with normal distal tubular function this results in an acidification of the urine (as sodium absorption stimulates the secretion of a counter ion, *i.e.* H^+ and K^+). Patients with dRTA will not acidify their urine under these conditions either. The tests are described in Fig. 39.4.

Once a diagnosis of dRTA has been made, identification of clinical conditions and/or toxins causing dRTA is important and their treatment or removal often effective therapy. In pediatric prac-

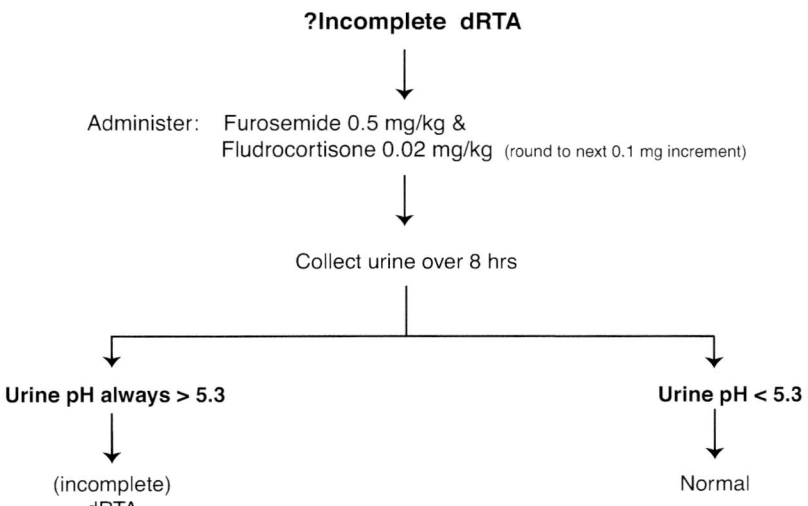

Fig. 39.4 Approach to diagnosis of incomplete dRTA. Note that one can substitute 100 mg/kg NH_4Cl for furosemide and fludrocortisone, however the described test is better tolerated and consequently preferable. Urine pH will be increased by sample exposure to air, due to diffusion of CO_2 and NH_3 from the sample. Thus, the test is difficult to do in non-toilet trained children, unless catheterised. Samples are ideally collected under oil and need to be analyzed straight away

tice, the etiology is almost always primary dRTA. A formal **hearing examination** is recommended. Patients with mutations in AE1 typically have normal hearing, patients with mutations in carbonic anhydrase II may have conductive hearing loss while patients with mutations in the H$^+$ ATPase often have sensorineural hearing loss, especially those with mutations in the B1 subunit [70, 111, 170].

Treatment

The goal of therapy is to ensure adequate growth, heal or prevent bony abnormalities and normalization of urinary calcium excretion to prevent worsening of nephrocalcinosis and the (re) occurrence of nephrolithiasis [161]. Treatment is simple in principle: provision of sufficient doses of alkali supplementation. Yet, in a large international study of 340 patients with primary dRTA, more than half had inadequate metabolic control, as judged by plasma bicarbonate and urinary calcium at last follow-up [111]. Importantly, inadequate metabolic control was associated with lower final height and lower eGFR at last follow-up, highlighting the importance of good treatment. Impediments to proper treatment likely include the need for frequent dosing, lack of approved alkali supplementation and poor taste of available preparations. Of note, more than 30 different preparations were prescribed and there was no apparent difference in outcome whether bicarbonate or citrate preparations were employed [165].

The key to optimal therapy is to provide a sufficient quantity of alkali frequently enough to maintain sustained control of the acidosis. The dose of alkali equivalents to compensate alkalosis decreases with age and is typically 3–6 mEq/kg/day below the age of 6 years (but up to 10 mEq/kg/day in infancy) and declines to 1–2 mEq/kg/day in adulthood [103, 115, 161]. Alkali supplementation reflects the renal acid load, which is derived primarily from dietary protein, specifically from sulfur-containing amino-acids which are metabolized to sulfuric acid [171]. Animal proteins have a higher content of sulfuric amino acids than plant proteins and consequently, a reduction in animal protein intake reduces the dose of alkali supplementation required for buffering. Nevertheless, sufficient protein intake (the recommended daily intake) is needed for normal growth and development in children.

In pRTA, because of the ongoing bicarbonate wasting, sustained normal plasma bicarbonate levels may not be achievable, despite often enormous prescribed doses. As detailed above, more frequent provision of smaller doses will provide more stable plasma levels and less wastage. However, this may be difficult for some patients and there families. Finally, the management of kidney stones, coexisting hearing loss or anemia may require other subspecialty support.

Prognosis

In dRTA, if the diagnosis is made early and alkali therapy provided consistently the prognosis is good, with final height in the normal range, albeit slightly below average [111]. While mild CKD is common, ESKD is exceedingly rare and was not observed in the cohort of 340 dRTA patients, which included 83 adults up to the age of 70 years [163]. Unfortunately, due to the non-specific nature of presenting symptoms, diagnosis is often delayed [151] and in these or non-compliant patients progression to renal failure and or significant growth impairment can occur [172, 173]. Importantly, alkali therapy does not prevent hearing loss [174].

When pRTA occurs in association with renal Fanconi syndrome, the prognosis depends primarily on the underlying condition. For isolated pRTA with eye findings, not enough patients have been reported to make meaningful statements on prognosis.

Mixed Proximal and Distal Renal Tubular Acidosis (Type III RTA)

Carbonic anhydrase II (CAII) is a metalloenzyme that catalyzes the reversible hydration of carbon dioxide into a proton and bicarbonate. This cytosolic enzyme is expressed in renal tubular epithelial cells along the nephron. The highest level of expression is in the intercalated cells with reduced levels of expression in the proximal tubule and thick ascending limb. In both the proximal tubule and the α-intercalated cells it provides protons for secretion into the lumen (via NHE3 and the H$^+$-ATPase respectively). Its other product bicarbonate is effluxed into the peritubular interstitium via NBCe1 and AE1 respectively. Mutations in CAII lead to mixed proximal and distal RTA, or Type III RTA, which can be variable in severity and is often associated with nephrocalcinosis and nephrolithiasis [37, 175]. Carbonic anhydrase II is also essential for osteoclast function, and loss-of-function is therefore associated with excessive mineralization (osteopetrosis) accompanied by cerebral calcification, developmental delay, facial dysmorphism (low set ears, hypertelorism and a depressed nasal bridge), conductive hearing loss and cognitive impairment [145, 176–178]. This rare condition is inherited in an autosomal recessive fashion [179]. Bone marrow or stem cell transplantation has been used to prevent the progression of osteopetrosis although it may not be completely curative [180]. Alkali supplementation remains the mainstay of treatment for metabolic acidosis.

Hyperkalemic Renal Tubular Acidosis (Type IV RTA)

Clinical Presentation

Hyperkalemic renal tubular acidosis is typically the result of actual or functional (pseudo-)hypoaldosteronism [181]. This condition is primarily a salt-wasting tubulopathy of the collecting duct. Since sodium reabsorption and potassium and proton secretion are coupled in this nephron segment, hyperkalemic acidosis occurs as a secondary consequence. Aldosterone is required for sodium reabsorption through the epithelial sodium channel, ENaC, which generates the negative transmembrane potential required to drive both potassium and proton secretion across this nephron segment. While several rare genetic disorders are associated with hyperkalemic RTA, this type of RTA more commonly results from acquired causes such as renal damage from obstructive uropathy, due to an autoimmune dis-

order, drug therapy or interstitial renal disease (Table 39.2). Drugs such as amiloride, triamterene and spironolactone either directly or indirectly inhibit sodium absorption from the collecting duct through ENaC. Due to the coupling of sodium absorption to either potassium or proton excretion in this segment, these drugs also cause hyperkalemic metabolic acidosis. Ascending infections and urinary obstruction disproportionately affect collecting duct function resulting in Type 4 RTA, while autoimmune diseases can produce autoantibodies targeting col-

Table 39.2 Causes of hyperkalemic renal tubular acidosis

Genetic	
Pseudohypoaldosteronism type 1	MR
	ENaC, α, ß and γ subunits
Pseudohypoaldosteronism type 2	WNK1 (PHA2)
	WNK4 (PHA2)
Bartter syndrome type 2[a]	KCNJ1/ROMK (Bartter Type 2)
Congenital adrenal insufficiency	21 hydroxylase deficiency
Drug induced	
Spironolactone	
Heparin	
Amiloride	
Prostaglandin inhibitors	
Triamterene	
ACE inhibitors and ARBs	
Calcineurin inhibitors	
Methicillin	
Intrinsic renal disease	
Obstructive uropathy	
Pylonephritis	
Interstitial nephritis	
Nephrosclerosis	
Post renal transplant	
Lupus nephritis	
Renal amyloidosis	
Miscellaneous causes	
Addison's disease	
Diabetes	
Gout	
Renal venous thrombosis	

[a] Note KCNJ1/ROMK mutations can cause type IV RTA in infancy that evolves into a hypokalemic metabolic alkalosis as a young child

lecting duct epithelial cells thereby causing the disease.

Notably, hyperkalemia in type IV RTA is not only a consequence of impaired distal sodium reabsorption, due to aldosterone insufficiency or resistance. Hyperkalemia also appears to inhibit ammonia production in the proximal tubule, thereby reducing ammonium excretion and exacerbating the renal tubular acidosis [182, 183].

An important cause of hyperkalemic RTA is **pseudohypoaldosteronism (PHA)**, both type 1 and type 2 [184]. **Type 1** is associated with lower blood pressure, hyponatremia and renal salt wasting, despite elevated circulating levels of aldosterone and renin. The condition results from mineralocorticoid resistance. Patients typically present as infants with dehydration, hypotension, weight loss and vomiting. There are two clinically and genetically distinct subtypes of this disorder. A milder renal-limited form, which is inherited in an autosomal dominant fashion, is due to loss-of-function mutations in the mineralocorticoid receptor [185, 186]. These patients typically present in the first few months of life with growth failure and subsequent work-up reveals the hyperkalaemic acidosis. Interestingly, plasma electrolytes spontaneously normalize with age, although renin and aldosterone levels usually remain elevated life-long [184, 187]. Genetic analysis of parents in the absence of a family history suggests that some cases may go undetected [150].

The more severe form of PHA type 1 is inherited in an autosomal recessive fashion and often displays evidence of multiple organ dysfunction, including increased sodium concentration in sweat, saliva and airway liquid with consequent pulmonary manifestations that can mimic cystic fibrosis [188]. This form of pseudohypoaldosteronism type 1 is caused by mutations in one of the three epithelial sodium channel subunits, α, ß or γ [189–192]. Affected patients typically present in the first days of life with failure to gain weight. Electrolyte abnormalities can be severe, with plasma potassium levels around 10 mmol/L or higher at presentation [193].

Pseudohypoaldosteronism type II, also known as hyperkalemic hypertension or Gordon's syndrome, describes a disorder characterized by hyperkalemic renal tubular acidosis and hypertension with variable aldosterone and low renin levels. In contrast to the salt-wasting hypovolemic disorder PHA type 1, type 2 is characterized by hypervolemia due to salt-retention in the distal convoluted tubule [194]. The consequent lack of delivery of sodium to the collecting duct causes the hyperkalemic acidosis. Consequently, PHA type 2 is highly sensitive to therapy with thiazide diuretics, whose target is the apically expressed sodium chloride co-transporter, NCC, which is expressed in the apical membrane of the distal convoluted tubule. Mutations in several genes have been identified to cause this disorder, including *WNK1*, *WNK4*, *CUL3* and *KLHL3* [195–197], (Table 39.3). Most patients with inherited PHA type 2 present during adolescence or even adulthood and especially hypertension may not be present until adulthood [194]. However, mutations in KLHL3 can be dominantly or recessively inherited and the latter ones can present already in infancy. Moreover, mutations in CUL3 appear to be associated with a more severe course with earlier presentation, early hypertension and failure-to-thrive [196].

Investigations into PHA have provided fascinating insights into the so-called "aldosterone paradox", i.e. the fact that the two key functions of aldosterone, regulation of volume and of potassium, can sometimes be competing. For instance, in a fasting state, the body may need to conserve volume (sodium) without sacrificing potassium. Conversely, in the presence of a high serum potassium, aldosterone is released to enhance potassium excretion, but without necessarily changing salt reabsorption [198]. The answer to this conundrum was provided by the identification of the WNK kinases and their associated regulatory proteins. If volume needs to be preserved without affecting potassium secretion, salt reabsorption is shifted to the distal convoluted tubule, so less sodium is delivered to the collecting duct where it could be exchanged for potassium. If potassium needs to be excreted without affecting sodium reabsorption, the process is shifted to the collecting duct, such that less sodium is reabsorbed in the distal convoluted

Table 39.3 Genetic causes of RTA

Gene name	Protein name	MIM #	Inheritance	Typical clinical features	Type of RTA
SLC4A4	NBCe1	603345, 604278	AR	Glaucoma, cataracts, band keratopathy	pRTA, Type II
?	?	?179830	AD	Short stature?	pRTA, Type II
ATP6V1B1	B1 subunit of the H⁺ATPase	267300	AR	Sensorineural hearing loss, nephrocalcinosis or nephrolithiasis	dRTA, Type I
ATP6V0A4	A4 subunit of H⁺ATPase	602722, 605239	AR	Late onset sensorineural hearing loss, nephrocalcinosis or nephrolithiasis	dRTA, Type I
SLC4A1	AE1	109270, 179800, 611590	AD (less commonly AR)	Nephrocalcinosis, osteomalacia, hemolytic anemia with AR Inheritence	dRTA, Type I
FOXI1	FOXI1	601093	AR	Deafness with enlarged vestibular aquaduct	dRTA, Type I
WDR72	WDR72	613214	AR	Amelogenesis imperfecta	dRTA, Type I
CA2	CAII	611492, 259730	AR	Osteopetrosis	Mixed or Type III
NR3C2	Mineralo-corticoid receptor	600983, 177735	AD	Pseudo-hypoaldosteronism Type 1	Hyperkalemic RTA, Type IV
SCNN1A, SCNN1B, SCNN1G	α, ß or γ subunit of ENaC	264350, 600228, 600761, 600760	AR	Pseuodo-hypoaldosterism Type 1	Hyperkalemic RTA, Type IV
WNK1	WNK1	6052323, 614492	AD	Pseudo-hypoaldosterism Type 2, Hypertension	Hyperkalemic RTA, Type IV
WNK4	WNK4	145260	AD	Pseudo-hypoaldosterism Type 2, Hypertension	Hyperkalemic RTA, Type IV
CUL3	Cullin 3	603136, 614496	AD	Pseudo-hypoaldosterism Type 2, Hypertension	Hyperkalemic RTA, Type IV
KLHL3	Kelch-Like 3	614495	AD or AR	Pseudo-hypoaldosterism Type 2, Hypertension	Hyperkalemic RTA, Type IV

[a] Mutations of the genes in grey are primarily disorders of renal sodium handling and may not always cause RTA

tubule and therefore available for exchange with potassium. Mutations causing PHA type 2 shift this regulatory response towards salt reabsorption in the distal convoluted tubule, leading to hypervolameia and hyperkalaemic acidosis. The actual regulation is quite complicated, involving further kinases, such as SPAK and OSR1 [199, 200]. The final consequence of the mutations identified in affected individuals is increased phosphorylation and cell surface expression of NCC with increased sodium reabsorption. The volume expansion caused by increased NCC activity suppresses renin and the reduced delivery of sodium to the collecting duct impairs the distal secretion of potassium and protons leading to a hyperkalemic metabolic acidosis. Aldosterone levels can be variable, as aldosterone is also stimulated by hyperkalaemia. While inherited PHA type 2 is rare, a much more common acquired form, associated with calcineurin inhibitor treatment, has been described [201]. Typically, this complication occurs with large doses of tacrolimus, as commonly prescribed for instance in heart transplants. The exact mechanism is unclear, but in the mouse model, tacrolimus exposure leads to increased abundance of SPAK and WNK4 kinases and consequent increased phosphorylation and surface expression of NCC, analogous to inherited PHA type 2 [201]. Most imnportantly, this acquired form of PHA type 2 responds just as well to thiazides as the inherited form (see "treatment" below), providing an elegant and simple treatment, if reduction of tacrolimus is deemed clinically unacceptable.

Diagnosis

The initial diagnosis of type IV RTA is rather straightforward. The combination of hyperchloremic normal anion gap metabolic acidosis with hyperkalemia is pathognomonic for the diagnosis. In the context of clinical hypovolemia and elevated aldosterone levels, this is PHA type 1, whereas normal or elevated blood pressure is consistent with type 2. The diagnosis of type 2 PHA can be further confirmed by the excellent response to thiazide diuretics.

Investigations to determine the underlying cause are guided by patient history and physical examination and may include serum and urinary biochemistry to screen for nephritis, as well as renal ultrasound to assess urinary tract obstruction. Potential inciting drugs should be identified. Ambiguous genitalia point to congenital adrenal hyperplasia. Genetic testing should be sought whenever available to confirm hereditary disorders. As most mutations causing PHA are inherited in a dominant fashion, a careful family history should be obtained and frequently, further family members are identified, who have often been given a diagnosis of treatment-resistant hypertension or may even have suffered complications, such as stroke or myocardial infarction.

Treatment

The treatment of type IV RTA is largely etiology dependent. Offending drugs should be discontinued and any underlying renal disease treated. This often leads to complete resolution of the hyperkalemic metabolic acidosis. In the case of obstructive uropathy adequate urinary flow should be achieved by catheterization or an appropriate urologic procedure. Unfortunately, the metabolic acidosis associated with some cases of congenital obstruction may be irreversible, especially if associated with marked GFR impairment, and continued alkali supplementation is required.

In PHA type 1, especially the recessive form, immediate supplementation with sodium chloride, such as infusion of 0.9% saline will help stabilize intravascular volume. Correction of the acidosis with sodium bicarbonate will also lower plasma potassium levels. For longer term control, oral supplementation with sodium chloride and bicarbonate is often needed in doses >10 mmol/kg/day. Sodium resonium is helpful to eliminate potassium and provide sodium supplementation [193]. In the dominant form, oral supplementation with sodium chloride and/or bicarbonate is typically needed only in the first year of life or so.

In the case of pseudohyperaldosteronism type 2, thiazide diuretics are very effective and resolve the biochemical abnormalities, as well as the hypertension [202–204].

References

1. Maren TH. Chemistry of the renal reabsorption of bicarbonate. Can J Physiol Pharmacol. 1974;52(6):1041–50.
2. Rector FC Jr. Renal regulation of acid-base balance. Aust NZ J Med. 1981;11(Suppl 1):1–5.
3. DuBose TD Jr. Reclamation of filtered bicarbonate. Kidney Int. 1990;38(4):584–9.
4. Cogan MG, Maddox DA, Lucci MS, Rector FC Jr. Control of proximal bicarbonate reabsorption in normal and acidotic rats. J Clin Invest. 1979;64(5):1168–80.
5. Cogan MG. Disorders of proximal nephron function. Am J Med. 1982;72(2):275–88.
6. Lombard WE, Kokko JP, Jacobson HR. Bicarbonate transport in cortical and outer medullary collecting tubules. Am J Physiol. 1983;244(3):F289–96.
7. McKinney TD, Burg MB. Bicarbonate transport by rabbit cortical collecting tubules. Effect of acid and alkali loads in vivo on transport in vitro. J Clin Invest. 1977;60(3):766–8.
8. Atkins JL, Burg MB. Bicarbonate transport by isolated perfused rat collecting ducts. Am J Physiol. 1985;249(4 Pt 2):F485–9.
9. Capasso G, Unwin R, Agulian S, Giebisch G. Bicarbonate transport along the loop of Henle. I. Microperfusion studies of load and inhibitor sensitivity. J Clin Invest. 1991;88(2):430–7.
10. Good DW. Sodium-dependent bicarbonate absorption by cortical thick ascending limb of rat kidney. Am J Physiol. 1985;248(6 Pt 2):F821–9.
11. Good DW, Knepper MA, Burg MB. Ammonia and bicarbonate transport by thick ascending limb of rat kidney. Am J Physiol. 1984;247(1 Pt 2):F35–44.
12. Rector FC Jr, Carter NW, Seldin DW. The mechanism of bicarbonate reabsorption in the proximal and distal tubules of the kidney. J Clin Invest. 1965;44:278–90.
13. Brown D, Zhu XL, Sly WS. Localization of membrane-associated carbonic anhydrase type IV in kidney epithelial cells. Proc Natl Acad Sci U S A. 1990;87(19):7457–61.

14. Zhu XL, Sly WS. Carbonic anhydrase IV from human lung. Purification, characterization, and comparison with membrane carbonic anhydrase from human kidney. J Biol Chem. 1990;265(15):8795–801.

15. Kaunisto K, Parkkila S, Rajaniemi H, Waheed A, Grubb J, Sly WS. Carbonic anhydrase XIV: luminal expression suggests key role in renal acidification. Kidney Int. 2002;61(6):2111–8.

16. Nielsen S, Smith BL, Christensen EI, Agre P. Distribution of the aquaporin CHIP in secretory and resorptive epithelia and capillary endothelia. Proc Natl Acad Sci U S A. 1993;90(15):7275–9.

17. Preston GM, Carroll TP, Guggino WB, Agre P. Appearance of water channels in Xenopus oocytes expressing red cell CHIP28 protein. Science. 1992;256(5055):385–7.

18. Schnermann J, Chou CL, Ma T, Traynor T, Knepper MA, Verkman AS. Defective proximal tubular fluid reabsorption in transgenic aquaporin-1 null mice. Proc Natl Acad Sci U S A. 1998;95(16):9660–4.

19. Vallon V, Verkman AS, Schnermann J. Luminal hypotonicity in proximal tubules of aquaporin-1-knockout mice. Am J Physiol Renal Physiol. 2000;278(6):F1030–3.

20. Cooper GJ, Boron WF. Effect of PCMBS on CO2 permeability of Xenopus oocytes expressing aquaporin 1 or its C189S mutant. Am J Physiol. 1998;275(6 Pt 1):C1481–6.

21. Endeward V, Musa-Aziz R, Cooper GJ, Chen LM, Pelletier MF, Virkki LV, et al. Evidence that aquaporin 1 is a major pathway for CO2 transport across the human erythrocyte membrane. FASEB J. 2006;20(12):1974–81.

22. Nakhoul NL, Davis BA, Romero MF, Boron WF. Effect of expressing the water channel aquaporin-1 on the CO2 permeability of Xenopus oocytes. Am J Physiol. 1998;274(2 Pt 1):C543–8.

23. de Groot BL, Hub JS. A decade of debate: significance of CO2 permeation through membrane channels still controversial. Chemphyschem. 2011;12(5):1021–2.

24. Spicer SS, Sens MA, Tashian RE. Immunocytochemical demonstration of carbonic anhydrase in human epithelial cells. J Histochem Cytochem. 1982;30(9):864–73.

25. Sly WS, Hewett-Emmett D, Whyte MP, Yu YS, Tashian RE. Carbonic anhydrase II deficiency identified as the primary defect in the autosomal recessive syndrome of osteopetrosis with renal tubular acidosis and cerebral calcification. Proc Natl Acad Sci U S A. 1983;80(9):2752–6.

26. Sly WS, Whyte MP, Sundaram V, Tashian RE, Hewett-Emmett D, Guibaud P, et al. Carbonic anhydrase II deficiency in 12 families with the autosomal recessive syndrome of osteopetrosis with renal tubular acidosis and cerebral calcification. N Engl J Med. 1985;313(3):139–45.

27. Pitts RF, Lotspeich WD. Bicarbonate and the renal regulation of acid base balance. Am J Physiol. 1946;147:138–54.

28. Pitts RF, Lotspeich WD. The renal excretion and reabsorption of bicarbonate. Federation Proceedings. 1946;5(1 Pt 2):82.

29. Vilas G, Krishnan D, Loganathan SK, Malhotra D, Liu L, Beggs MR, et al. Increased water flux induced by an aquaporin-1/carbonic anhydrase II interaction. Mol Biol Cell. 2015;26(6):1106–18.

30. Lorenz JN, Schultheis PJ, Traynor T, Shull GE, Schnermann J. Micropuncture analysis of single-nephron function in NHE3-deficient mice. Am J Physiol. 1999;277(3 Pt 2):F447–53.

31. Schultheis PJ, Clarke LL, Meneton P, Miller ML, Soleimani M, Gawenis LR, et al. Renal and intestinal absorptive defects in mice lacking the NHE3 Na+/H+ exchanger. Nat Genet. 1998;19(3):282–5.

32. Wang T, Yang CL, Abbiati T, Schultheis PJ, Shull GE, Giebisch G, et al. Mechanism of proximal tubule bicarbonate absorption in NHE3 null mice. Am J Physiol. 1999;277(2 Pt 2):F298–302.

33. Berry CA, Warnock DG, Rector FC Jr. Ion selectivity and proximal salt reabsorption. Am J Physiol. 1978;235(3):F234–45.

34. Krapf R, Alpern RJ, Rector FC Jr, Berry CA. Basolateral membrane Na/base cotransport is dependent on CO2/HCO3 in the proximal convoluted tubule. J Gen Physiol. 1987;90(6):833–53.

35. Damkier HH, Nielsen S, Praetorius J. Molecular expression of SLC4-derived Na+-dependent anion transporters in selected human tissues. Am J Physiol Regul Integr Comp Physiol. 2007;293(5):R2136–46.

36. Igarashi T, Sekine T, Inatomi J, Seki G. Unraveling the molecular pathogenesis of isolated proximal renal tubular acidosis. J Am Soc Nephrol. 2002;13(8):2171–7.

37. Alper SL. Familial renal tubular acidosis. J Nephrol. 2010;23(Suppl 16):S57–76.

38. Janecke AR, Heinz-Erian P, Yin J, Petersen BS, Franke A, Lechner S, et al. Reduced sodium/proton exchanger NHE3 activity causes congenital sodium diarrhea. Hum Mol Genet. 2015;24(23):6614–23.

39. Li HC, Du Z, Barone S, Rubera I, McDonough AA, Tauc M, et al. Proximal tubule specific knockout of the Na(+)/H(+) exchanger NHE3: effects on bicarbonate absorption and ammonium excretion. J Mol Med. 2013;91(8):951–63.

40. Goyal S, Mentone S, Aronson PS. Immunolocalization of NHE8 in rat kidney. Am J Physiol Renal Physiol. 2005;288(3):F530–8.

41. Brown D, Hirsch S, Gluck S. Localization of a proton-pumping ATPase in rat kidney. J Clin Invest. 1988;82(6):2114–26.

42. Zimolo Z, Montrose MH, Murer H. H+ extrusion by an apical vacuolar-type H(+)-ATPase in rat renal proximal tubules. J Membr Biol. 1992;126(1):19–26.

43. Liu FY, Cogan MG. Axial heterogeneity of bicarbonate, chloride, and water transport in the rat proximal convoluted tubule. Effects of change in luminal flow rate and of alkalemia. J Clin Invest. 1986;78(6):1547–57.

44. Fromter E, Rumrich G, Ullrich KJ. Phenomenologic description of Na+, Cl− and HCO-3 absorption from proximal tubules of rat kidney. Pflugers Arch. 1973;343(3):189–220.

45. Rector FC Jr. Sodium, bicarbonate, and chloride absorption by the proximal tubule. Am J Physiol. 1983;244(5):F461–71.

46. Biemesderfer D, Rutherford PA, Nagy T, Pizzonia JH, Abu-Alfa AK, Aronson PS. Monoclonal antibodies for high-resolution localization of NHE3 in adult and neonatal rat kidney. Am J Physiol. 1997;273(2 Pt 2):F289–99.

47. Capasso G, Rizzo M, Pica A, Ferrara D, Di Maio FS, Morelli F, et al. Physiology and molecular biology of tubular bicarbonate transport. Nephrol Dial Transplant. 2000;15(Suppl 6):36–8.

48. Capasso G, Unwin R, Rizzo M, Pica A, Giebisch G. Bicarbonate transport along the loop of Henle: molecular mechanisms and regulation. J Nephrol. 2002;15(Suppl 5):S88–96.

49. Quentin F, Eladari D, Frische S, Cambillau M, Nielsen S, Alper SL, et al. Regulation of the Cl−/HCO3− exchanger AE2 in rat thick ascending limb of Henle's loop in response to changes in acid-base and sodium balance. J Am Soc Nephrol. 2004;15(12):2988–97.

50. Alper SL, Stuart-Tilley AK, Biemesderfer D, Shmukler BE, Brown D. Immunolocalization of AE2 anion exchanger in rat kidney. Am J Physiol. 1997;273(4 Pt 2):F601–14.

51. Leviel F, Eladari D, Blanchard A, Poumarat JS, Paillard M, Podevin RA. Pathways for HCO-3 exit across the basolateral membrane in rat thick limbs. Am J Physiol. 1999;276(6 Pt 2):F847–56.

52. Bastani B, Haragsim L. Immunocytochemistry of renal H-ATPase. Miner Electrolyte Metab. 1996;22(5–6):382–95.

53. Brown D, Hirsch S, Gluck S. An H+-ATPase in opposite plasma membrane domains in kidney epithelial cell subpopulations. Nature. 1988;331(6157):622–4.

54. Teng-umnuay P, Verlander JW, Yuan W, Tisher CC, Madsen KM. Identification of distinct subpopulations of intercalated cells in the mouse collecting duct. J Am Soc Nephrol. 1996;7(2):260–74.

55. Brown D, Roth J, Kumpulainen T, Orci L. Ultrastructural immunocytochemical localization of carbonic anhydrase. Presence in intercalated cells of the rat collecting tubule. Histochemistry. 1982;75(2):209–13.

56. Stehberger PA, Shmukler BE, Stuart-Tilley AK, Peters LL, Alper SL, Wagner CA. Distal renal tubular acidosis in mice lacking the AE1 (band3) Cl−/HCO3− exchanger (slc4a1). J Am Soc Nephrol. 2007;18(5):1408–18.

57. Hamm LL, Simon EE. Roles and mechanisms of urinary buffer excretion. Am J Physiol. 1987;253(4 Pt 2):F595–605.

58. Wagner CA, Devuyst O, Bourgeois S, Mohebbi N. Regulated acid-base transport in the collecting duct. Pflugers Arch. 2009;458(1):137–56.

59. Han JS, Kim GH, Kim J, Jeon US, Joo KW, Na KY, et al. Secretory-defect distal renal tubular acidosis is associated with transporter defect in H(+)-ATPase and anion exchanger-1. J Am Soc Nephrol. 2002;13(6):1425–32.

60. Kim J, Kim YH, Cha JH, Tisher CC, Madsen KM. Intercalated cell subtypes in connecting tubule and cortical collecting duct of rat and mouse. J Am Soc Nephrol. 1999;10(1):1–12.

61. Campbell-Thompson ML, Verlander JW, Curran KA, Campbell WG, Cain BD, Wingo CS, et al. In situ hybridization of H-K-ATPase beta-subunit mRNA in rat and rabbit kidney. Am J Physiol. 1995;269(3 Pt 2):F345–54.

62. Nakamura S. H+-ATPase activity in selective disruption of H+-K+-ATPase alpha 1 gene of mice under normal and K-depleted conditions. J Lab Clin Med. 2006;147(1):45–51.

63. Lynch IJ, Rudin A, Xia SL, Stow LR, Shull GE, Weiner ID, et al. Impaired acid secretion in cortical collecting duct intercalated cells from H-K-ATPase-deficient mice: role of HKalpha isoforms. Am J Physiol Renal Physiol. 2008;294(3):F621–7.

64. Kim YH, Kwon TH, Frische S, Kim J, Tisher CC, Madsen KM, et al. Immunocytochemical localization of pendrin in intercalated cell subtypes in rat and mouse kidney. Am J Physiol Renal Physiol. 2002;283(4):F744–54.

65. Wall SM, Hassell KA, Royaux IE, Green ED, Chang JY, Shipley GL, et al. Localization of pendrin in mouse kidney. Am J Physiol Renal Physiol. 2003;284(1):F229–41.

66. Wagner CA, Mohebbi N, Capasso G, Geibel JP. The anion exchanger pendrin (SLC26A4) and renal acid-base homeostasis. Cell Physiol Biochem. 2011;28(3):497–504.

67. Leviel F, Hubner CA, Houillier P, Morla L, El Moghrabi S, Brideau G, et al. The Na+-dependent chloride-bicarbonate exchanger SLC4A8 mediates an electroneutral Na+ reabsorption process in the renal cortical collecting ducts of mice. J Clin Invest. 2010;120(5):1627–35.

68. Gueutin V, Vallet M, Jayat M, Peti-Peterdi J, Corniere N, Leviel F, et al. Renal beta-intercalated cells maintain body fluid and electrolyte balance. J Clin Invest. 2013;123(10):4219–31.

69. Chambrey R, Kurth I, Peti-Peterdi J, Houillier P, Purkerson JM, Leviel F, et al. Renal intercalated cells are rather energized by a proton than a sodium pump. Proc Natl Acad Sci U S A. 2013;110(19):7928–33.

70. Karet FE, Finberg KE, Nelson RD, Nayir A, Mocan H, Sanjad SA, et al. Mutations in the gene encoding B1 subunit of H+-ATPase cause renal tubular acidosis with sensorineural deafness. Nat Genet. 1999;21(1):84–90.

71. Smith AN, Skaug J, Choate KA, Nayir A, Bakkaloglu A, Ozen S, et al. Mutations in ATP6N1B, encoding a new kidney vacuolar proton pump 116-kD subunit, cause recessive distal renal tubular acidosis with preserved hearing. Nat Genet. 2000;26(1):71–5.

72. Eladari D, Chambrey R. Ammonium transport in the kidney. J Nephrol. 2010;23(Suppl 16):S28–34.

73. Good DW, Burg MB. Ammonia production by individual segments of the rat nephron. J Clin Invest. 1984;73(3):602–10.

74. Rossier G, Meier C, Bauch C, Summa V, Sordat B, Verrey F, et al. LAT2, a new basolateral 4F2hc/CD98-associated amino acid transporter of kidney and intestine. J Biol Chem. 1999;274(49):34948–54.

75. Sastrasinh S, Sastrasinh M. Glutamine transport in submitochondrial particles. Am J Physiol. 1989;257(6 Pt 2):F1050–8.

76. Taylor L, Curthoys NP. Glutamine metabolism: role in acid-base balance*. Biochem Mol Biol. 2004;32(5):291–304.

77. Harris AN, Grimm PR, Lee HW, Delpire E, Fang L, Verlander JW, et al. Mechanism of hyperkalemia-induced metabolic acidosis. J Am Soc Nephrol. 2018;29(5):1411–25.

78. Aronson PS, Suhm MA, Nee J. Interaction of external H+ with the Na+-H+ exchanger in renal microvillus membrane vesicles. J Biol Chem. 1983;258(11):6767–71.

79. Kinsella JL, Aronson PS. Interaction of NH4+ and Li+ with the renal microvillus membrane Na+-H+ exchanger. Am J Physiol. 1981;241(5):C220–6.

80. Nagami GT. Luminal secretion of ammonia in the mouse proximal tubule perfused in vitro. J Clin Invest. 1988;81(1):159–64.

81. Nagami GT. Net luminal secretion of ammonia by the proximal tubule. Contrib Nephrol. 1988;63:1–5.

82. Choi JY, Shah M, Lee MG, Schultheis PJ, Shull GE, Muallem S, et al. Novel amiloride-sensitive sodium-dependent proton secretion in the mouse proximal convoluted tubule. J Clin Invest. 2000;105(8):1141–6.

83. Baum M, Twombley K, Gattineni J, Joseph C, Wang L, Zhang Q, et al. Proximal tubule Na+/H+ exchanger activity in adult NHE8−/−, NHE3−/−, and NHE3−/−/NHE8−/− mice. Am J Physiol Renal Physiol. 2012;303(11):F1495–502.

84. Good DW. Ammonium transport by the thick ascending limb of Henle's loop. Annu Rev Physiol. 1994;56:623–47.

85. Good DW. Effects of potassium on ammonia transport by medullary thick ascending limb of the rat. J Clin Invest. 1987;80(5):1358–65.

86. Good DW. Active absorption of NH4+ by rat medullary thick ascending limb: inhibition by potassium. Am J Physiol. 1988;255(1 Pt 2):F78–87.

87. Kikeri D, Sun A, Zeidel ML, Hebert SC. Cell membranes impermeable to NH3. Nature. 1989;339(6224):478–80.

88. Flessner MF, Wall SM, Knepper MA. Permeabilities of rat collecting duct segments to NH3 and NH4+. Am J Physiol. 1991;260(2 Pt 2):F264–72.

89. Flessner MF, Wall SM, Knepper MA. Ammonium and bicarbonate transport in rat outer medullary collecting ducts. Am J Physiol. 1992;262(1 Pt 2):F1–7.

90. Flessner MF, Knepper MA. Ammonium transport in collecting ducts. Miner Electrolyte Metab. 1990;16(5):299–307.

91. Liu Z, Chen Y, Mo R, Hui C, Cheng JF, Mohandas N, et al. Characterization of human RhCG and mouse Rhcg as novel nonerythroid Rh glycoprotein homologues predominantly expressed in kidney and testis. J Biol Chem. 2000;275(33):25641–51.

92. Yip KP, Kurtz I. NH3 permeability of principal cells and intercalated cells measured by confocal fluorescence imaging. Am J Physiol. 1995;269(4 Pt 2):F545–50.

93. Biver S, Belge H, Bourgeois S, Van Vooren P, Nowik M, Scohy S, et al. A role for Rhesus factor Rhcg in renal ammonium excretion and male fertility. Nature. 2008;456(7220):339–43.

94. Bourgeois S, Bounoure L, Christensen EI, Ramakrishnan SK, Houillier P, Devuyst O, et al. Haploinsufficiency of the ammonia transporter Rhcg predisposes to chronic acidosis: Rhcg is critical for apical and basolateral ammonia transport in the mouse collecting duct. J Biol Chem. 2013;288(8):5518–29.

95. Rodriguez-Soriano J, Edelmann CM Jr. Renal tubular acidosis. Annu Rev Med. 1969;20:363–82.

96. Seki G, Horita S, Suzuki M, Yamazaki O, Usui T, Nakamura M, et al. Molecular mechanisms of renal and extrarenal manifestations caused by inactivation of the electrogenic Na-HCO cotransporter NBCe1. Front Physiol. 2013;4:270.

97. Katzir Z, Dinour D, Reznik-Wolf H, Nissenkorn A, Holtzman E. Familial pure proximal renal tubular acidosis—a clinical and genetic study. Nephrol Dial Transplant. 2008;23(4):1211–5.

98. Inatomi J, Horita S, Braverman N, Sekine T, Yamada H, Suzuki Y, et al. Mutational and functional analysis of SLC4A4 in a patient with proximal renal tubular acidosis. Pflugers Arch. 2004;448(4):438–44.

99. Igarashi T, Inatomi J, Sekine T, Cha SH, Kanai Y, Kunimi M, et al. Mutations in SLC4A4 cause permanent isolated proximal renal tubular acidosis with ocular abnormalities. Nat Genet. 1999;23(3):264–6.

100. Demirci FY, Chang MH, Mah TS, Romero MF, Gorin MB. Proximal renal tubular acidosis and ocular pathology: a novel missense mutation in the gene (SLC4A4) for sodium bicarbonate cotransporter protein (NBCe1). Mol Vis. 2006;12:324–30.

101. Dinour D, Chang MH, Satoh J, Smith BL, Angle N, Knecht A, et al. A novel missense mutation in the sodium bicarbonate cotransporter (NBCe1/SLC4A4) causes proximal tubular acidosis and glaucoma through ion transport defects. J Biol Chem. 2004;279(50):52238–46.

102. Lemann J Jr, Adams ND, Wilz DR, Brenes LG. Acid and mineral balances and bone in familial proximal renal tubular acidosis. Kidney Int. 2000;58(3):1267–77.

103. Xu H, Li J, Chen R, Zhang B, Wang C, King N, et al. NHE2X3 DKO mice exhibit gender-specific NHE8

compensation. Am J Physiol Gastrointest Liver Physiol. 2011;300(4):G647–53.

104. Haque SK, Ariceta G, Batlle D. Proximal renal tubular acidosis: a not so rare disorder of multiple etiologies. Nephrol Dial Transplant. 2012;27(12):4273–87.

105. McSherry E, Sebastian A, Morris RC Jr. Renal tubular acidosis in infants: the several kinds, including bicarbonate-wasting, classic renal tubular acidosis. J Clin Invest. 1972;51(3):499–514.

106. Soriano JR, Boichis H, Edelmann CM Jr. Bicarbonate reabsorption and hydrogen ion excretion in children with renal tubular acidosis. J Pediatr. 1967;71(6):802–13.

107. Edelmann CM, Soriano JR, Boichis H, Gruskin AB, Acosta MI. Renal bicarbonate reabsorption and hydrogen ion excretion in normal infants. J Clin Invest. 1967;46(8):1309–17.

108. Soriano JR. Renal tubular acidosis: the clinical entity. J Am Soc Nephrol. 2002;13(8):2160–70.

109. McSherry E, Morris RC Jr. Attainment and maintenance of normal stature with alkali therapy in infants and children with classic renal tubular acidosis. J Clin Invest. 1978;61(2):509–27.

110. Nash MA, Torrado AD, Greifer I, Spitzer A, Edelmann CM Jr. Renal tubular acidosis in infants and children. Clinical course, response to treatment, and prognosis. J Pediatr. 1972;80(5):738–48.

111. Lopez-Garcia SC, Emma F, Walsh SB, Fila M, Hooman N, Zaniew M, et al. Treatment and long-term outcome in primary distal renal tubular acidosis. Nephrol Dial Transplant. 2019;34(6):981–91.

112. Kari J, El Desoky S, Singh AK, Gari M, Kleta R, Bockenhauer D. Renal tubular acidosis and eye findings. Kidney Int. 2014;86:217–8.

113. Shiohara M, Igarashi T, Mori T, Komiyama A. Genetic and long-term data on a patient with permanent isolated proximal renal tubular acidosis. Eur J Pediatr. 2000;159(12):892–4.

114. Rodriguez-Soriano J, Vallo A. Renal tubular acidosis. Pediatr Nephrol. 1990;4(3):268–75.

115. Besouw MT, Bienias M, Walsh P, Kleta R, Van't Hoff WG, Ashton E, et al. Clinical and molecular aspects of distal renal tubular acidosis in children. Pediatr Nephrol. 2017;32(6):987–96.

116. Downie ML, Lopez Garcia SC, Kleta R, Bockenhauer D. Inherited tubulopathies of the kidney: insights from genetics. Clin J Am Soc Nephrol. 2020;16:620–30.

117. Reddy P. Clinical approach to renal tubular acidosis in adult patients. Int J Clin Pract. 2011;65(3):350–60.

118. Karet FE, Gainza FJ, Gyory AZ, Unwin RJ, Wrong O, Tanner MJ, et al. Mutations in the chloride-bicarbonate exchanger gene AE1 cause autosomal dominant but not autosomal recessive distal renal tubular acidosis. Proc Natl Acad Sci U S A. 1998;95(11):6337–42.

119. Bruce LJ, Cope DL, Jones GK, Schofield AE, Burley M, Povey S, et al. Familial distal renal tubular acidosis is associated with mutations in the red cell anion exchanger (Band 3, AE1) gene. J Clin Invest. 1997;100(7):1693–707.

120. Jarolim P, Shayakul C, Prabakaran D, Jiang L, Stuart-Tilley A, Rubin HL, et al. Autosomal dominant distal renal tubular acidosis is associated in three families with heterozygosity for the R589H mutation in the AE1 (band 3) Cl–/HCO3– exchanger. J Biol Chem. 1998;273(11):6380–8.

121. Fejes-Toth G, Chen WR, Rusvai E, Moser T, Naray-Fejes-Toth A. Differential expression of AE1 in renal HCO3-secreting and -reabsorbing intercalated cells. J Biol Chem. 1994;269(43):26717–21.

122. Jarolim P, Rubin HL, Liu SC, Cho MR, Brabec V, Derick LH, et al. Duplication of 10 nucleotides in the erythroid band 3 (AE1) gene in a kindred with hereditary spherocytosis and band 3 protein deficiency (band 3PRAGUE). J Clin Invest. 1994;93(1):121–30.

123. Maillet P, Vallier A, Reinhart WH, Wyss EJ, Ott P, Texier P, et al. Band 3 Chur: a variant associated with band 3-deficient hereditary spherocytosis and substitution in a highly conserved position of transmembrane segment 11. Br J Haematol. 1995;91(4):804–10.

124. Mohandas N, Winardi R, Knowles D, Leung A, Parra M, George E, et al. Molecular basis for membrane rigidity of hereditary ovalocytosis. A novel mechanism involving the cytoplasmic domain of band 3. J Clin Invest. 1992;89(2):686–92.

125. Jarolim P, Palek J, Amato D, Hassan K, Sapak P, Nurse GT, et al. Deletion in erythrocyte band 3 gene in malaria-resistant southeast Asian ovalocytosis. Proc Natl Acad Sci U S A. 1991;88(24):11022–6.

126. Tanner MJ, Bruce L, Martin PG, Rearden DM, Jones GL. Melanesian hereditary ovalocytes have a deletion in red cell band 3. Blood. 1991;78(10):2785–6.

127. Wrong O, Bruce LJ, Unwin RJ, Toye AM, Tanner MJ. Band 3 mutations, distal renal tubular acidosis, and southeast Asian ovalocytosis. Kidney Int. 2002;62(1):10–9.

128. Reithmeier RA, Casey JR, Kalli AC, Sansom MS, Alguel Y, Iwata S. Band 3, the human red cell chloride/bicarbonate anion exchanger (AE1, SLC4A1), in a structural context. Biochim Biophys Acta. 2016;1858(7 Pt A):1507–32.

129. Devonald MA, Smith AN, Poon JP, Ihrke G, Karet FE. Non-polarized targeting of AE1 causes autosomal dominant distal renal tubular acidosis. Nat Genet. 2003;33(2):125–7.

130. Tanphaichitr VS, Sumboonnanonda A, Ideguchi H, Shayakul C, Brugnara C, Takao M, et al. Novel AE1 mutations in recessive distal renal tubular acidosis. Loss-of-function is rescued by glycophorin A. J Clin Invest. 1998;102(12):2173–9.

131. Parker MD, Boron WF. The divergence, actions, roles, and relatives of sodium-coupled bicarbonate transporters. Physiol Rev. 2013;93(2):803–959.

132. Vasuvattakul S, Yenchitsomanus PT, Vachuanichsanong P, Thuwajit P, Kaitwatcharachai

C, Laosombat V, et al. Autosomal recessive distal renal tubular acidosis associated with southeast Asian ovalocytosis. Kidney Int. 1999;56(5):1674–82.

133. Bruce LJ, Wrong O, Toye AM, Young MT, Ogle G, Ismail Z, et al. Band 3 mutations, renal tubular acidosis and South-East Asian ovalocytosis in Malaysia and Papua New Guinea: loss of up to 95% band 3 transport in red cells. Biochem J. 2000;350(Pt 1):41–51.

134. Chu C, Woods N, Sawasdee N, Guizouarn H, Pellissier B, Borgese F, et al. Band 3 Edmonton I, a novel mutant of the anion exchanger 1 causing spherocytosis and distal renal tubular acidosis. Biochem J. 2010;426(3):379–88.

135. Shmukler BE, Kedar PS, Warang P, Desai M, Madkaikar M, Ghosh K, et al. Hemolytic anemia and distal renal tubular acidosis in two Indian patients homozygous for SLC4A1/AE1 mutation A858D. Am J Hematol. 2010;85(10):824–8.

136. Fawaz NA, Beshlawi IO, Al Zadjali S, Al Ghaithi HK, Elnaggari MA, Elnour I, et al. dRTA and hemolytic anemia: first detailed description of SLC4A1 A858D mutation in homozygous state. Eur J Haematol. 2012;88(4):350–5.

137. Rungroj N, Devonald MA, Cuthbert AW, Reimann F, Akkarapatumwong V, Yenchitsomanus PT, et al. A novel missense mutation in AE1 causing autosomal dominant distal renal tubular acidosis retains normal transport function but is mistargeted in polarized epithelial cells. J Biol Chem. 2004;279(14):13833–8.

138. Cheidde L, Vieira TC, Lima PR, Saad ST, Heilberg IP. A novel mutation in the anion exchanger 1 gene is associated with familial distal renal tubular acidosis and nephrocalcinosis. Pediatrics. 2003;112(6 Pt 1):1361–7.

139. Rysava R, Tesar V, Jirsa M Jr, Brabec V, Jarolim P. Incomplete distal renal tubular acidosis coinherited with a mutation in the band 3 (AE1) gene. Nephrol Dial Transplant. 1997;12(9):1869–73.

140. Ribeiro ML, Alloisio N, Almeida H, Gomes C, Texier P, Lemos C, et al. Severe hereditary spherocytosis and distal renal tubular acidosis associated with the total absence of band 3. Blood. 2000;96(4):1602–4.

141. Sritippayawan S, Sumboonnanonda A, Vasuvattakul S, Keskanokwong T, Sawasdee N, Paemanee A, et al. Novel compound heterozygous SLC4A1 mutations in Thai patients with autosomal recessive distal renal tubular acidosis. Am J Kidney Dis. 2004;44(1):64–70.

142. Yenchitsomanus PT, Sawasdee N, Paemanee A, Keskanokwong T, Vasuvattakul S, Bejrachandra S, et al. Anion exchanger 1 mutations associated with distal renal tubular acidosis in the Thai population. J Hum Genet. 2003;48(9):451–6.

143. Choo KE, Nicoli TK, Bruce LJ, Tanner MJ, Ruiz-Linares A, Wrong OM. Recessive distal renal tubular acidosis in Sarawak caused by AE1 mutations. Pediatr Nephrol. 2006;21(2):212–7.

144. Kittanakom S, Cordat E, Akkarapatumwong V, Yenchitsomanus PT, Reithmeier RA. Trafficking defects of a novel autosomal recessive distal renal tubular acidosis mutant (S773P) of the human kidney anion exchanger (kAE1). J Biol Chem. 2004;279(39):40960–71.

145. Borthwick KJ, Kandemir N, Topaloglu R, Kornak U, Bakkaloglu A, Yordam N, et al. A phenocopy of CAII deficiency: a novel genetic explanation for inherited infantile osteopetrosis with distal renal tubular acidosis. J Med Genet. 2003;40(2):115–21.

146. Feldman M, Prikis M, Athanasiou Y, Elia A, Pierides A, Deltas CC. Molecular investigation and long-term clinical progress in Greek Cypriot families with recessive distal renal tubular acidosis and sensorineural deafness due to mutations in the ATP6V1B1 gene. Clin Genet. 2006;69(2):135–44.

147. Hahn H, Kang HG, Ha IS, Cheong HI, Choi Y. ATP6B1 gene mutations associated with distal renal tubular acidosis and deafness in a child. Am J Kidney Dis. 2003;41(1):238–43.

148. Ruf R, Rensing C, Topaloglu R, Guay-Woodford L, Klein C, Vollmer M, et al. Confirmation of the ATP6B1 gene as responsible for distal renal tubular acidosis. Pediatr Nephrol. 2003;18(2):105–9.

149. Stover EH, Borthwick KJ, Bavalia C, Eady N, Fritz DM, Rungroj N, et al. Novel ATP6V1B1 and ATP6V0A4 mutations in autosomal recessive distal renal tubular acidosis with new evidence for hearing loss. J Med Genet. 2002;39(11):796–803.

150. Ashton EJ, Legrand A, Benoit V, Roncelin I, Venisse A, Zennaro MC, et al. Simultaneous sequencing of 37 genes identified causative mutations in the majority of children with renal tubulopathies. Kidney Int. 2018;93(4):961–7.

151. Vivante A, Lotan D, Pode-Shakked N, Landau D, Svec P, Nampoothiri S, et al. Familial autosomal recessive renal tubular acidosis: importance of early diagnosis. Nephron Physiol. 2011;119(3):31–9.

152. Vidarsson H, Westergren R, Heglind M, Blomqvist SR, Breton S, Enerback S. The forkhead transcription factor Foxi1 is a master regulator of vacuolar H-ATPase proton pump subunits in the inner ear, kidney and epididymis. PLoS One. 2009;4(2):e4471.

153. Blomqvist SR, Vidarsson H, Fitzgerald S, Johansson BR, Ollerstam A, Brown R, et al. Distal renal tubular acidosis in mice that lack the forkhead transcription factor Foxi1. J Clin Invest. 2004;113(11):1560–70.

154. Enerback S, Nilsson D, Edwards N, Heglind M, Alkanderi S, Ashton E, et al. Acidosis and deafness in patients with recessive mutations in FOXI1. J Am Soc Nephrol. 2018;29(3):1041–8.

155. El-Sayed W, Parry DA, Shore RC, Ahmed M, Jafri H, Rashid Y, et al. Mutations in the beta propeller WDR72 cause autosomal-recessive hypomaturation amelogenesis imperfecta. Am J Hum Genet. 2009;85(5):699–705.

156. Rungroj N, Nettuwakul C, Sawasdee N, Sangnual S, Deejai N, Misgar RA, et al. Distal renal tubular acidosis caused by tryptophan-aspartate repeat domain 72 (WDR72) mutations. Clin Genet. 2018;94(5):409–18.

157. Zhang H, Koruyucu M, Seymen F, Kasimoglu Y, Kim JW, Tinawi S, et al. WDR72 mutations associated with Amelogenesis imperfecta and acidosis. J Dent Res. 2019;98(5):541–8.

158. Jobst-Schwan T, Klambt V, Tarsio M, Heneghan JF, Majmundar AJ, Shril S, et al. Whole exome sequencing identified ATP6V1C2 as a novel candidate gene for recessive distal renal tubular acidosis. Kidney Int. 2020;97(3):567–79.

159. Smith AN, Borthwick KJ, Karet FE. Molecular cloning and characterization of novel tissue-specific isoforms of the human vacuolar H(+)-ATPase C, G and d subunits, and their evaluation in autosomal recessive distal renal tubular acidosis. Gene. 2002;297(1–2):169–77.

160. Ashton E, Bockenhauer D. Diagnosis of uncertain significance: can next-generation sequencing replace the clinician? Kidney Int. 2020;97(3):455–7.

161. Batlle D, Haque SK. Genetic causes and mechanisms of distal renal tubular acidosis. Nephrol Dial Transplant. 2012;27(10):3691–704.

162. Unwin RJ, Capasso G. The renal tubular acidoses. J R Soc Med. 2001;94(5):221–5.

163. Rodriguez-Soriano J, Vallo A. Pathophysiology of the renal acidification defect present in the syndrome of familial hypomagnesaemia-hypercalciuria. Pediatr Nephrol. 1994;8(4):431–5.

164. Batlle DC, Hizon M, Cohen E, Gutterman C, Gupta R. The use of the urinary anion gap in the diagnosis of hyperchloremic metabolic acidosis. N Engl J Med. 1988;318(10):594–9.

165. Sisson D, Batlle D. Aquaporin-2 as a biomarker of distal renal tubular function using lithium as an experimental model. Ren Fail. 1999;21(3–4):331–6.

166. Kim GH, Han JS, Kim YS, Joo KW, Kim S, Lee JS. Evaluation of urine acidification by urine anion gap and urine osmolal gap in chronic metabolic acidosis. Am J Kidney Dis. 1996;27(1):42–7.

167. Wrong O, Davies HE. The excretion of acid in renal disease. Q J Med. 1959;28(110):259–313.

168. Walsh SB, Shirley DG, Wrong OM, Unwin RJ. Urinary acidification assessed by simultaneous furosemide and fludrocortisone treatment: an alternative to ammonium chloride. Kidney Int. 2007;71(12):1310–6.

169. Smulders YM, Frissen PH, Slaats EH, Silberbusch J. Renal tubular acidosis. Pathophysiology and diagnosis. Arch Intern Med. 1996;156(15):1629–36.

170. Batlle D, Ghanekar H, Jain S, Mitra A. Hereditary distal renal tubular acidosis: new understandings. Annu Rev Med. 2001;52:471–84.

171. Passey C. Reducing the dietary acid load: how a more alkaline diet benefits patients with chronic kidney disease. J Renal Nutr. 2017;27(3):151–60.

172. Santos F, Chan JC. Renal tubular acidosis in children. Diagnosis, treatment and prognosis. Am J Nephrol. 1986;6(4):289–95.

173. Bajpai A, Bagga A, Hari P, Bardia A, Mantan M. Long-term outcome in children with primary distal renal tubular acidosis. Indian Pediatr. 2005;42(4):321–8.

174. Bajaj G, Quan A. Renal tubular acidosis and deafness: report of a large family. Am J Kidney Dis. 1996;27(6):880–2.

175. Bolt RJ, Wennink JM, Verbeke JI, Shah GN, Sly WS, Bokenkamp A. Carbonic anhydrase type II deficiency. Am J Kidney Dis. 2005;46(5):A50, e71–3, Quiz Page November 2005.

176. Shah GN, Bonapace G, Hu PY, Strisciuglio P, Sly WS. Carbonic anhydrase II deficiency syndrome (osteopetrosis with renal tubular acidosis and brain calcification): novel mutations in CA2 identified by direct sequencing expand the opportunity for genotype-phenotype correlation. Hum Mutat. 2004;24(3):272.

177. Ismail EA, Abul Saad S, Sabry MA. Nephrocalcinosis and urolithiasis in carbonic anhydrase II deficiency syndrome. Eur J Pediatr. 1997;156(12):957–62.

178. Muzalef A, Alshehri M, Al-Abidi A, Al-Trabolsi HA. Marble brain disease in two Saudi Arabian siblings. Ann Trop Paediatr. 2005;25(3):213–8.

179. Fathallah DM, Bejaoui M, Lepaslier D, Chater K, Sly WS, Dellagi K. Carbonic anhydrase II (CA II) deficiency in Maghrebian patients: evidence for founder effect and genomic recombination at the CA II locus. Hum Genet. 1997;99(5):634–7.

180. McMahon C, Will A, Hu P, Shah GN, Sly WS, Smith OP. Bone marrow transplantation corrects osteopetrosis in the carbonic anhydrase II deficiency syndrome. Blood. 2001;97(7):1947–50.

181. Karet FE. Mechanisms in hyperkalemic renal tubular acidosis. J Am Soc Nephrol. 2009;20(2):251–4.

182. DuBose TD Jr, Good DW. Effects of chronic hyperkalemia on renal production and proximal tubule transport of ammonium in rats. Am J Physiol. 1991;260(5 Pt 2):F680–7.

183. Jaeger P, Bonjour JP, Karlmark B, Stanton B, Kirk RG, Duplinsky T, et al. Influence of acute potassium loading on renal phosphate transport in the rat kidney. Am J Physiol. 1983;245(5 Pt 1):F601–5.

184. Riepe FG. Pseudohypoaldosteronism. Endocr Dev. 2013;24:86–95.

185. Geller DS, Rodriguez-Soriano J, Vallo Boado A, Schifter S, Bayer M, Chang SS, et al. Mutations in the mineralocorticoid receptor gene cause autosomal dominant pseudohypoaldosteronism type I. Nat Genet. 1998;19(3):279–81.

186. Sartorato P, Lapeyraque AL, Armanini D, Kuhnle U, Khaldi Y, Salomon R, et al. Different inactivating mutations of the mineralocorticoid receptor in fourteen families affected by type I pseudohypoaldosteronism. J Clin Endocrinol Metab. 2003;88(6):2508–17.

187. Dillon MJ, Leonard JV, Buckler JM, Ogilvie D, Lillystone D, Honour JW, et al. Pseudohypoaldosteronism. Arch Dis Child. 1980;55(6):427–34.

188. Hanukoglu A, Bistritzer T, Rakover Y, Mandelberg A. Pseudohypoaldosteronism with increased sweat

and saliva electrolyte values and frequent lower respiratory tract infections mimicking cystic fibrosis. J Pediatr. 1994;125(5 Pt 1):752–5.

189. Chang SS, Grunder S, Hanukoglu A, Rosler A, Mathew PM, Hanukoglu I, et al. Mutations in subunits of the epithelial sodium channel cause salt wasting with hyperkalaemic acidosis, pseudohypoaldosteronism type 1. Nat Genet. 1996;12(3):248–53.

190. Kerem E, Bistritzer T, Hanukoglu A, Hofmann T, Zhou Z, Bennett W, et al. Pulmonary epithelial sodium-channel dysfunction and excess airway liquid in pseudohypoaldosteronism. N Engl J Med. 1999;341(3):156–62.

191. Saxena A, Hanukoglu I, Saxena D, Thompson RJ, Gardiner RM, Hanukoglu A. Novel mutations responsible for autosomal recessive multisystem pseudohypoaldosteronism and sequence variants in epithelial sodium channel alpha-, beta-, and gamma-subunit genes. J Clin Endocrinol Metab. 2002;87(7):3344–50.

192. Strautnieks SS, Thompson RJ, Gardiner RM, Chung E. A novel splice-site mutation in the gamma subunit of the epithelial sodium channel gene in three pseudohypoaldosteronism type 1 families. Nat Genet. 1996;13(2):248–50.

193. Savage MO, Jefferson IG, Dillon MJ, Milla PJ, Honour JW, Grant DB. Pseudohypoaldosteronism: severe salt wasting in infancy caused by generalized mineralocorticoid unresponsiveness. J Pediatr. 1982;101(2):239–42.

194. O'Shaughnessy KM. Gordon syndrome: a continuing story. Pediatr Nephrol. 2015;30(11):1903–8.

195. Wilson FH, Disse-Nicodeme S, Choate KA, Ishikawa K, Nelson-Williams C, Desitter I, et al. Human hypertension caused by mutations in WNK kinases. Science. 2001;293(5532):1107–12.

196. Boyden LM, Choi M, Choate KA, Nelson-Williams CJ, Farhi A, Toka HR, et al. Mutations in kelch-like 3 and cullin 3 cause hypertension and electrolyte abnormalities. Nature. 2012;482(7383):98–102.

197. Louis-Dit-Picard H, Barc J, Trujillano D, Miserey-Lenkei S, Bouatia-Naji N, Pylypenko O, et al. KLHL3 mutations cause familial hyperkalemic hypertension by impairing ion transport in the distal nephron. Nat Genet. 2012;44(4):456–60, S1–3

198. Arroyo JP, Ronzaud C, Lagnaz D, Staub O, Gamba G. Aldosterone paradox: differential regulation of ion transport in distal nephron. Physiology (Bethesda). 2011;26(2):115–23.

199. Shibata S, Zhang J, Puthumana J, Stone KL, Lifton RP. Kelch-like 3 and Cullin 3 regulate electrolyte homeostasis via ubiquitination and degradation of WNK4. Proc Natl Acad Sci U S A. 2013;110(19):7838–43.

200. Hadchouel J, Ellison DH, Gamba G. Regulation of renal electrolyte transport by WNK and SPAK-OSR1 kinases. Annu Rev Physiol. 2016;78:367–89.

201. Hoorn EJ, Walsh SB, McCormick JA, Furstenberg A, Yang CL, Roeschel T, et al. The calcineurin inhibitor tacrolimus activates the renal sodium chloride cotransporter to cause hypertension. Nat Med. 2011;17(10):1304–9.

202. Achard JM, Disse-Nicodeme S, Fiquet-Kempf B, Jeunemaitre X. Phenotypic and genetic heterogeneity of familial hyperkalaemic hypertension (Gordon syndrome). Clin Exp Pharmacol Physiol. 2001;28(12):1048–52.

203. Gordon RD, Geddes RA, Pawsey CG, O'Halloran MW. Hypertension and severe hyperkalaemia associated with suppression of renin and aldosterone and completely reversed by dietary sodium restriction. Australas Ann Med. 1970;19(4):287–94.

204. Schambelan M, Sebastian A, Rector FC Jr. Mineralocorticoid-resistant renal hyperkalemia without salt wasting (type II pseudohypoaldosteronism): role of increased renal chloride reabsorption. Kidney Int. 1981;19(5):716–27.

Diabetes Insipidus

40

Detlef Bockenhauer and Daniel G. Bichet

History

Diabetes insipidus derives from the Greek word *diabinein* for "flow-through" and the Latin word *insapere* for "non-sweet tasting", separating it from another polyuric disorder, diabetes mellitus ("like honey"). A familial form affecting "chiefly males on the female side of the house" was first described by McIlraith in 1892 [1]. De Lange in 1935 reported a family with diabetes insipidus and no male-to-male transmission unresponsive to injections of posterior lobe extracts [2]. Forssman [3] and Waring [4] in 1945 recognized the disorder in these families as a renal problem. In 1947 Williams and Henry established the unresponsiveness to arginine-vasopressin (AVP) in these patients and coined the term nephrogenic diabetes insipidus (NDI) [5]. In 1969 the "Hopewell Hypothesis" was proposed by Bode and Crawford, proposing that most cases of NDI in the USA and Canada could be traced to descendants of Ulster Scots, who arrived on the ship Hopewell in Novia Scotia in 1761 [6]. Bichet later refuted this by molecular analysis [7]. In 1992 the *AVPR2* gene encoding the AVP2 receptor was cloned and mutations identified in patients with X-linked NDI [8–11]. Shortly after, the *AQP2* gene encoding the vasopressin-regulated water channel aquaporin-2 (*AQP2*) was cloned [12, 13] and in 1994 mutations in *AQP2* were found to underlie autosomal recessive DI [14].

Clinic

Presentation in Infancy

Patients with congenital NDI typically present in the first weeks to months of life with dehydration [15]. Sometimes, patients receive repeated investigations for sepsis, as the dehydration can be associated with low-grade temperatures, until a set of serum electrolytes is obtained, revealing hypernatraemia. Failure-to-thrive with irritability are further symptoms. Often, patients suck vigorously, but develop vomiting shortly after starting to feed. Vomiting may be due to reflux exacerbated by the large volumes of fluid necessary to compensate for the renal losses. Interestingly, breast-fed infants with NDI typically thrive better

D. Bockenhauer (✉)
Great Ormond Street Hospital, London, UK

Department of Renal Medicine, University College London, London, UK
e-mail: d.bockenhauer@ucl.ac.uk

D. G. Bichet
Department of Medicine and Pharmacology, Université de Montréal, Montréal, QC, Canada

Department of Physiology, Université de Montréal, Montréal, QC, Canada

Unité de Recherche Clinique, Centre de Recherche et Service de Néphrologie, Hôpital du Sacré-Coeur de Montréal, Montréal, QC, Canada
e-mail: daniel.bichet@umontreal.ca

© The Author(s), under exclusive license to Springer Nature Switzerland AG 2023
F. Schaefer, L. A. Greenbaum (eds.), *Pediatric Kidney Disease*,
https://doi.org/10.1007/978-3-031-11665-0_40

than formula-fed ones, as breast milk presents a lower osmolar load than most standard formulas (see below). Of note, pregnancies with babies afflicted with NDI are not complicated by poly-hydramnios, since the AVP-dependent mechanisms for urinary concentration are not fully developed until after birth and the osmolar load is cleared by the placenta [16].

Clinical Features and Long-Term Prognosis

Symptoms typically improve with advancing age, especially once food intake has changed to mainly solids, so that caloric and fluid intake are separated. Free access to water allows for self-regulation of serum osmolality. Patients remain polyuric, however and the frequency of voiding and drinking, especially during the night is useful information to assess the severity of the problem. Constipation is a common complication, presumably due to maximal extraction of water from the gut and should be discussed with the families and treated appropriately. Nocturnal enuresis is a frequent concern in childhood, obviously aggravated by the large urine volumes (parents often refer to it as "bed flooding" rather than bed wetting) and the average age at which patients achieve nocturnal continence is between 10 and 12 years [17, 18]. Parents also often report problems with concentration and attention span in their children and in one study almost half the patients were diagnosed with attention deficit hyperactivity disorder [19]. The reason for this is unclear, but maybe partly due to the constant need to drink and void. In an international multi-centre study of 315 patients with primary NDI, 16% were reported to have ADHD and an additional 20% to have other mental health problems [17]. Nevertheless, with treatment, patients with NDI can function well and while the proportion of adults with a university degree (27%) was lower than in the overall population, the rate of full-time employment and independent living in adulthood was similar [17, 19]. Impaired mental development with intracranial calcifications used to be a common feature in NDI [20–22]. This likely reflected

repeated episodes of severe hypernatraemic dehydration and with appropriate treatment of NDI this devastating complication is essentially no longer seen. And while failure to thrive is a common problem in infancy, final height is typically in the normal range [17]. Indeed, a surprising finding from the international cohort study was the increased incidence of obesity in adult NDI patients (41%), which may be an unintended consequence of the intense efforts in childhood to maximise caloric intake [17].

Some patients develop dilatation of the urinary tract from the high urinary flow, especially if they have poor voiding habits [20, 23, 24]. However, in those with hydronephrosis, anatomic causes of obstruction need also be considered, as these are potentially remediable and even minor impediments to flow can cause severe dilatation in this polyuric disorder [25]. In the international cohort study, 38% of patients had evidence of flow uropathy which may contribute to the increased prevalence of CKD Stage ≥ 2 in children (32%) and adults (48%) [17].

Physiologic Principles

Tubular Concentration/Dilution Mechanism (Countercurrent Mechanism with Figure)

The kidney creates a concentration gradient via a so-called countercurrent multiplication system [26, 27]. The tonicity (osmolality) of urine as it proceeds along the nephron is depicted in Fig. 40.1. In the proximal tubule the urine remains isotonic to plasma because of the high water permeability of this segment, mediated by aquaporin 1 (AQP1) [28–30]. Urine then enters the tubular segment most important for countercurrent multiplication: the loop of Henle. First, urine is concentrated as it descends the thin descending limb (TDL). The precise mechanism of concentration are still debated: initially, it was thought that the TDL also expresses AQP1, allowing water exit into the medullary interstitium [31]. More recent data, however, show that only about 10–15% of TDL (the "long-looped" nephrons) express AQP1, whereas the other ones do not [32].

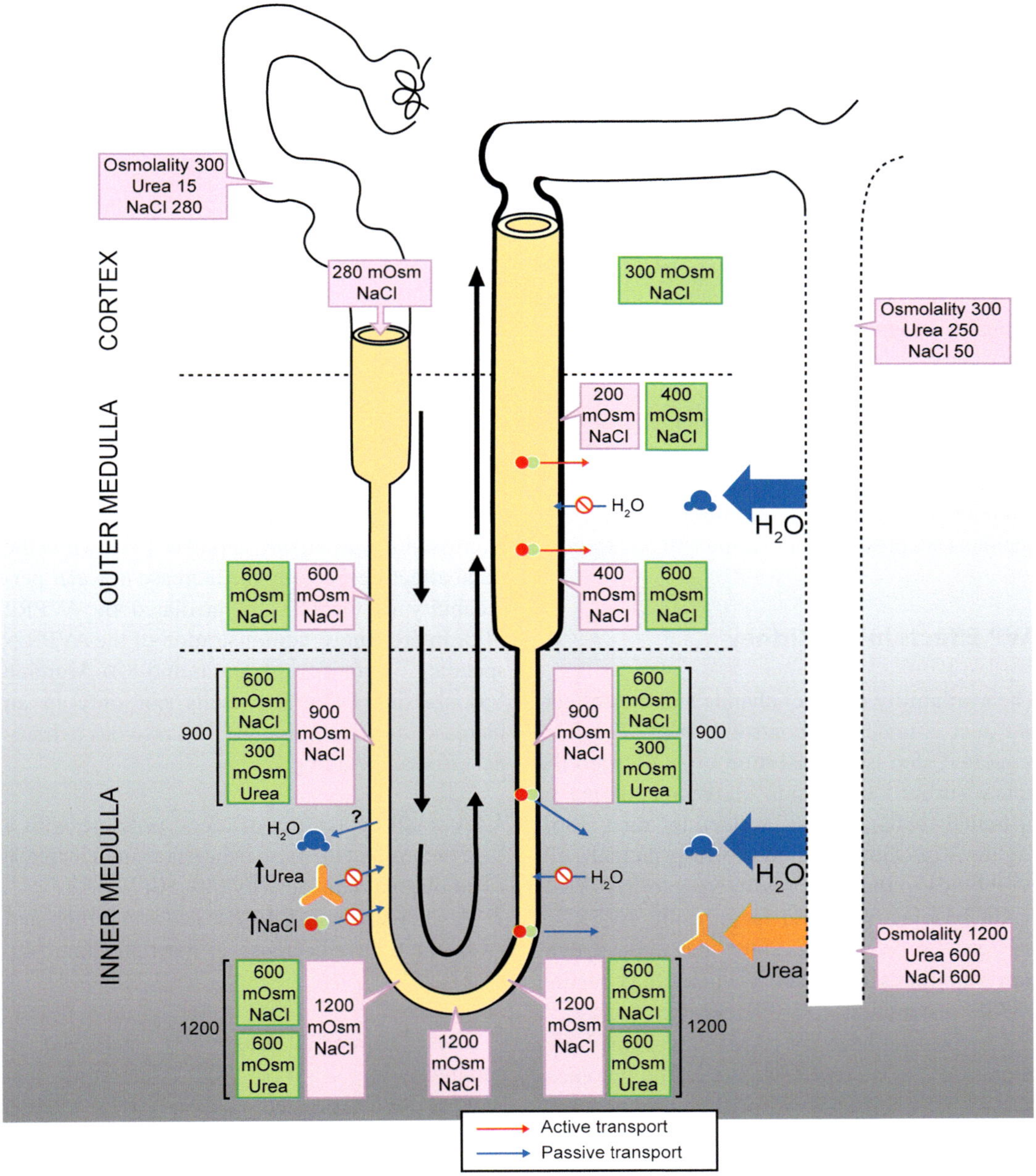

Fig. 40.1 Diagram of the renal concentration and dilution mechanism. The numbers indicate approximate osmolalities of the tubular and interstitial fluids. The names of the relevant transport proteins are indicated. The concentration gradient is mainly generated by the active reabsorption of solutes in the thick ascending limb by the transporter NKCC2. Note that urine exiting the loop of Henle is hypotonic. Final urine concentration is then dependent on the availability of AQP2 water channels in the collecting duct. For further details, see text

Consequently, concentration of the tubular fluid in TDL of these nephrons is assumed to occur via passive sodium influx [33]. Urine subsequently enters the thick ascending limb (TAL), which is impermeable for water, but actively removes sodium chloride, via the co-transporter NKCC2 [34]. Therefore, urine is diluted on its way up the TAL by active removal of solutes. The accumulation of solutes in the interstitium in turn generates the driving force for the removal of water from the thin descending limb (in the long-looped nephrons) and the entry of sodium chloride (into the short-looped majority of nephrons), completing the countercurrent multiplier.

There is further removal of sodium chloride in the distal convoluted tubule via the thiazide-sensitive co-transporter NCC and at entry in the collecting duct, urinary osmolality is typically around 50–100 mOsm/kg. The final osmolality of the urine is now solely dependent on the water permeability of the collecting duct and thus the availability of water channels. If water channels are present, water will exit the tubule following the interstitial concentration gradient and the urine is concentrated. If no water channels are present, dilute urine will be excreted.

AVP Effects in the Kidney

The availability of water channels in the collecting duct is under the control of AVP. The final regulated step is the insertion of AQP2 into the apical (urine-facing) side of the membrane of principal cells in the collecting duct [35]. Figure 40.2 shows a model of a principal cell. AVP binds to the vasopressin receptor (AVPR2) on the basolateral (blood-facing) side. AVPR2 is a G-protein coupled receptor that upon activation stimulates adenylate cyclase, thus raising cAMP production [36–39]. Protein kinase A (PKA) is stimulated by cAMP and phosphorylates AQP2 at a consensus site in the cytoplasmic carboxy-terminal tail of the protein, serine 256 (S256) [12, 40, 41]. Unphosphorylated AQP2 is present in intracellular vesicles, which upon phosphorylation at S256 are fused in the apical membrane [42]. Of note, AQP2 water channels are homotetramers, i.e. consisting of four subunits. In vitro evidence suggests that minimally three subunits need to be phosphorylated for the channel to be fused in the plasma membrane [43].

After insertion of AQP2 in the apical membrane water can enter from the tubular lumen into the cell and exit via the basolateral water channels AQP3 and AQP4. While AQP4 appears to be constitutively expressed in collecting duct, there is some evidence that AVP may also regulate the expression of AQP3 [44–46].

Extrarenal Effects of AVP

The vasopressive and glycogenolytic effects of AVP are mediated through AVP1 receptors expressed in vasculature and liver [47], while the renal effects, especially the increase in water permeability of the CD are mediated by AVPR2 [48]. Interestingly, administration of the AVPR2-specific agonist 1-Desamino-8-D-Arginine Vasopressin (DDAVP) results not only in an increase in urine osmolality, but also has extrarenal effects, including:

1. A small depression of blood pressure with a concomitant increase in heart rate and increase in plasma renin activity [49, 50].
2. An increase in factor VIIIc and von Willebrand factor with a decrease in bleeding time [49, 51, 52].

These extrarenal effects are abolished in patients with X-linked NDI, suggesting that AVPR2 is expressed beyond the kidney. Clinically, this can be used to differentiate between X-linked and autosomal recessive NDI (see below).

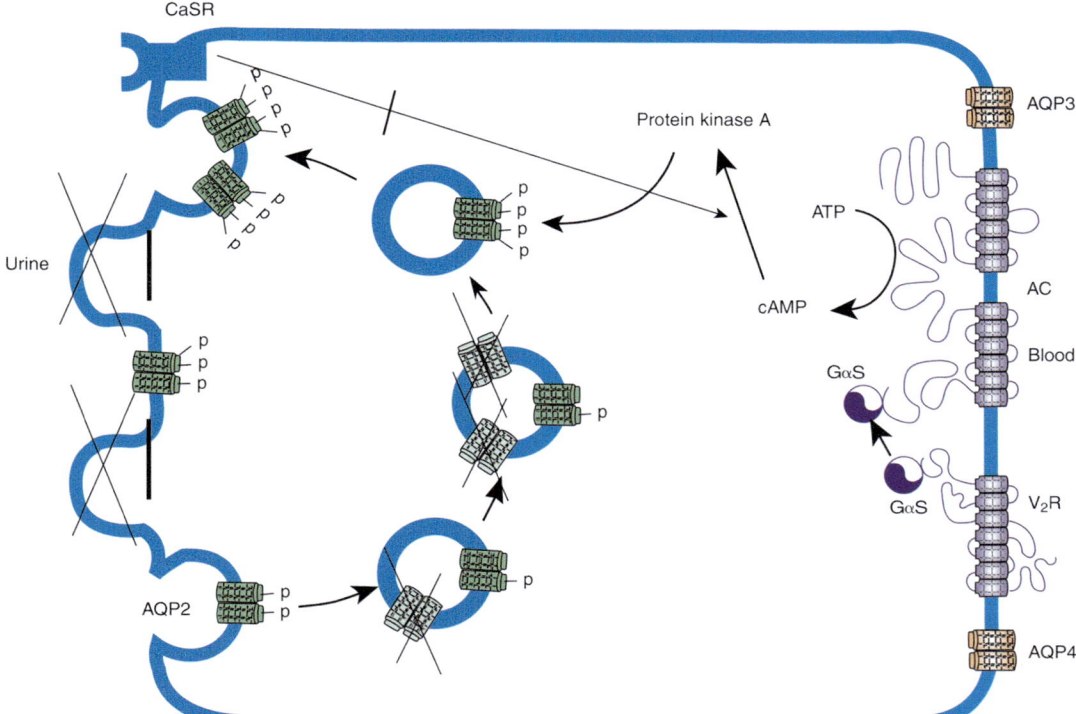

Fig. 40.2 Diagram of a principal cell. Depicted is a schematic of a principal cell with relevant proteins for water transport. AVP binds to the AVR2 receptor (depicted in green), expressed on the basolateral side of the cell. AVPR2 is a G-protein-coupled receptor and AVP binding releases the stimulatory G-protein GαS, which, in turn, stimulates adenylcylase. The increased production of cycline adenosine monophosphate (cAMP) stimulates protein kinase A (PKA), which phosphorylates the water channel AQP2, leading to insertion of these channels into the apical membrane. Water can then enter the cell from the tubular lumen and exit into the interstitium via the constitutively expressed water channels AQP3 and AQP4

Diagnosis

The presence of inappropriately dilute urine in the face of an elevated serum osmolality defines DI. Dehydration in a child with good urine output should always prompt consideration of a urinary concentrating defect. The diagnosis is easily made by obtaining serum and urine biochemistries. Maximal urinary concentrating ability increases with age, but a urine osmolality below plasma osmolality in a dehydrated child establishes a diagnosis of DI [53]. In classic NDI the urine osmolality is always below 200 mOsm/kg.

Diagnostic Procedures

Water Deprivation Test

The aim of the water-deprivation test is to induce mild dehydration and thus challenge the kidney to preserve water. Water is withheld until serum osmolality is just above the upper limit of normal (>295 mOsm/kg). Obviously, no child presenting with hypernatraemia and inappropriately dilute urine needs to undergo this test, as the challenge had already presented naturally. A water deprivation test carries the risk of severe hypernatraemic dehydration, especially in infants, as there may be delays in obtaining and reacting to laboratory results. It is useful to distinguish habitual polydipsia from central DI in patients with a good response to DDAVP, and is usually reserved for those particular patients: those with habitual polydipsia will be able to increase urine osmolality with water deprivation, whilst those with central DI will not. For a first assessment, a simple and informal water deprivation test is to ask the parents to obtain the first morning urine on their child and note the last time the child has drunk (water should not be withheld from the child). This can be used as an initial screening test in polyuric patients, as a concentrated urine excludes a diagnosis of DI.

DDAVP Test

The kidney concentrates the urine in response to the pituitary hormone AVP. Failure to concentrate can therefore be due to a deficiency in AVP (central DI or CDI) or an inability of the kidney to respond to it (NDI). AVP effects are mediated via two different receptors: the vasoconstriction ("vasopressin") is mediated by AVP receptor 1 (AVPR1), while the antidiuretic response is mediated by receptor type 2 (AVPR2). DDAVP has a high specificity for AVPR2 and can there-fore be used to assess the renal response while avoiding the systemic effects mediated by AVPR1. Different protocols exist in the literature with respect to dosage and route of administration of DDAVP. Some authors use intranasal DDAVP, others oral, subcutaneous (sc), intramuscular (im) or intravenous (iv) administration [49, 54, 55]. While oral or intranasal DDAVP is less invasive, absorption is less reliable. Thus, if the result of the test is inconclusive, it may need to be repeated using injected DDAVP. DDAVP given iv requires a shorter observation period (2 h) than other modes of administration (4–6 h), where absorption is more protracted. Moreover, DDAVP at the dose commonly used in von Willebrand disease (0.3 µg/kg iv) induces some systemic side effects in the form of a mild decrease in blood pressure and concomitant increase in heart rate via AVPR2 (see above). Consequently, patients with mutated AVPR2 (X-linked NDI) do not experience these haemodynamic changes, while patients with intact AVPR2, but mutated AQP2 (autosomal DI) do. The DDAVP test can therefore help differentiate between these two forms. A typical protocol, modified from [49] is given in Table 40.1. A commonly feared, but actually rare complication of

Table 40.1 Protocol of a DDAVP test

Time	-30	-15	0	10	15	20	30	40	50	60	75	90	110	130	150
Actual time (example: 09:00)	_:_	_:_	_:_	_:_	_:_	_:_	_:_	_:_	_:_	_:_	_:_	_:_	_:_	_:_	_:_
dDAVP infusion															
Blood pressure (mmHg)															
Pulse (b/min)															
Fluid intake (ml)															
Urine: volume (ml)															
Osmolality															
Na															
Plasma: U&E															
Osmolality															

Patients should be observed for a minimum of 2 h (iv) to 6 h (oral and nasal) after DDAVP administration. Volume of fluid intake during the test must be limited to the volume of urine produced in order to avoid hyponatremia
See text for more information and interpretation of results

the DDAVP test is hyponatraemia. Patients with intact thirst mechanism who respond to DDAVP will stop drinking water, due to their stable serum osmolality. Yet patients with habitual polydipsia, who will keep on drinking despite lowered serum osmolality, and infants, who continue to be fed by their caregivers throughout the test are at risk for hyponatraemia. Thus, close observation and strict limitation of fluid intake to a volume equal to urine output during the test period is critical to prevent this complication.

A urine osmolality after DDAVP below 200 mOsm/kg is consistent with a diagnosis of NDI, while patients with intact urinary concentrating ability typically achieve urine osmolalities greater than 800 mOsm/kg (>300 in infants) [53]. Patients with intermediate values should be assessed for inaccurate test results (especially when DDAVP was administered intranasally) or intrinsic renal disease limiting the urinary concentrating capacity (including chronic renal failure and obstructive uropathy, see below).

Differential Diagnosis

Central DI

A urinary concentrating defect can be due to a lack of AVP (central DI) or the inability of the kidney to respond to it (NDI). A DDAVP test helps to differentiate between the two (see above). Central DI is most commonly the consequence of head trauma, or other diseases affecting the hypothalamus or pituitary, but there are some rare cases of hereditary DI due to mutations in the gene encoding *AVP* [56–58]. In addition, loss-of-function variants in the *PCSK1* gene, encoding Proprotein Convertase 1, an endopeptidase involved in cleaving of precursor proteins into active peptide hormones have a complex endocrine phenotype that can include polyuria-polydipsia [59].

X-Linked and Autosomal NDI

A careful family history and assessment of systemic effects in the DDAVP test can discriminate the more common X-linked (90% of patients with identified mutations) from the rare autosomal NDI (10%). In approximately 10% of patients with presumed primary NDI, no mutation in either AVPR2 or AQP2 is identified [60]. Thus, these patients either have mutations in genes not yet identified to cause primary NDI, or in regions of the two known genes not assayed (e.g. introns or promoter), or have been misdiagnosed and actually have a secondary form of NDI (see below).

Partial NDI

An intermediate urine osmolality, that is between 200 and 800 mOsm/kg after administration of DDAVP is referred to as partial NDI. As discussed above, children less than 3 years of age, and especially in the first months of life, may not be able to maximally concentrate their urine yet and a value below 800 can be physiologic [53]. Further, technical problems with the DDAVP test should be excluded, especially if administration was intranasally, before a diagnosis of partial NDI is considered.

Inherited forms of partial DI are typically due to mutations in the *AVPR2* gene, that allow proper expression of the receptor at the cell membrane, but decrease the affinity to AVP, thus shifting the dose-response curve and requiring higher amounts of AVP to increase urinary concentration [61, 62]. However, mutations in *AQP2* with some retained urinary concentrating ability have also been identified [63]. Obviously, since these patients have a partially retained ability to concentrate their urine, their clinical symptoms are milder.

Secondary NDI

The defining feature of NDI is a pathologic deficiency of AQP2 in the apical membrane of the collecting duct. This can be primary inherited, i.e. due to mutations in either *AQP2* itself or in *AVPR2*, or occur as a secondary phenomenon: as a side effect of medications, anatomical problems or in the context of other tubulopathies [64]. The distinction is important, as misclassification as primary NDI may miss the opportunity to identify a remediable cause, such as urinary obstruction, or to make the correct diagnosis, which may result in potentially harmful treatment. Thus, in any patient with clinical NDI who displays unusual features, such as a history of polyhydramnios or hypercalciuria/nephrocalcinosis or hypokalaemia (before thiazide treatment), a secondary form of NDI should be considered and consequently a primary diagnosis sought.

Secondary Inherited NDI

A secondary form of NDI has been observed in other inherited tubulopathies, which can lead to misdiagnosis [65]. This seems to occur most commonly in Bartter syndrome types 1 and 2 [66–68]. Whilst isosthenuria (i.e. an impaired ability to either concentrate or dilute the urine with a urine osmolality similar to that of plasma) is an expected feature of Bartter syndrome (see section "Disorders Impairing the Generation of a Medullary Concentration Gradient" below), some of the affected patients clearly have hyposthenuria (i.e. a urine osmolality persistently below that of plasma). Indeed, in the laboratory in Montreal, the genes underlying type 1 and type 2 Bartter syndrome, *NKCC2* and *KCNJ1*, are tested next if no mutations were identified in *AVPR2* or *AQP2* in the DNA of patients referred with a clinical diagnosis of NDI [64].

Secondary NDI has also been described in many other inherited diseases affecting the kidney, including renal Fanconi syndromes, especially cystinosis, distal renal tubular acidosis (dRTA), apparent mineralocorticoid excess (AME) and ciliopathies [64, 65].

The precise etiology of this secondary NDI is unclear, but may be related to the electrolyte abnormalities inherent in these disorders, especially hypercalciuria and hypokalaemia (see below). Regardless of the etiology, establishing the correct diagnosis is obviously important: some of the primary disorders can be treated specifically (e.g. cystinosis, dRTA or AME). Moreover, the thiazide treatment commonly used in NDI could compound the defect in tubular salt reabsorption inherent to some of these disorders (e.g. renal Fanconi syndromes, Bartter syndrome) resulting potentially in serious hypovolaemia.

Obstructive Uropathy

Polyuria after release of urinary tract obstruction is a well-recognized phenomenon (post-obstructive diuresis). However, if obstruction is incomplete, it is often associated with polyuria, as well. Animal studies show a decreased level of AQP2 expression with bilateral ureteric obstruction [69]. Experiments with unilateral obstruction show a marked decrease in AQP2 in the obstructed kidney, consistent with the view that local factors, such as increased pressure, affect AQP2 expression [70]. Supporting this view is also the fact that other signs of distal tubular dysfunction are usually present in obstructive uropathies, like hyperkalaemia and acidosis. The downregulation of AQP2 persists up to 30 days after release of obstruction, explaining the post-obstructive diuresis [35].

Interstitial Renal Disease

Polyuria is frequently seen in renal failure, especially if the underlying aetiology primarily affects the interstitium, such as in renal dysplasia (see Chap. 9), nephronophthisis (see Chap. 12) or tubulointerstitial nephritis (see Chap. 37). It is also commonly seen after ischemic renal failure [71, 72]. However, these patients will typically have isosthenuria. This is in contrast to the hyposthenuria, i.e. a urine osmolality persistently below that of plasma that characterizes NDI.

Lithium

While rarely used in children, lithium therapy is a common treatment for manic-depressive disease in adults and roughly a fifth of patients develop polyuria [73]. Animal studies have shown decreased expression of AQP2 in principal cells, probably due to inhibition of cAMP formation in the collecting duct [38, 74–76].

Hypercalcaemia and Hypercalciuria

Hypercalcaemia can be associated with polyuria and two mechanisms have been proposed to explain the AVP-resistant concentrating defect; both likely involving the calcium-sensing receptor (CaSR). This receptor is expressed on the basolateral (blood) side of thick ascending limb cells and indirectly inhibits the NKCC2 co-transporter, thus impairing the generation of a medullary concentration gradient [77–79]. Second, this receptor is also expressed on the luminal (urine) side of collecting duct cells and thought to affect AQP2 trafficking [80, 81]. The latter mechanism would thus be mediated by hypercalciuria and has been proposed to constitute a protective measure against the formation of calcium-containing stones [82]. It would also provide an explanation for the hypercalciuric forms of secondary NDI, such as in Bartter syndrome (see above). However, doubts have been raised about the clinical relevance of this mechanism, as the protection against stones would come at the risk of dehydration. Indeed, in healthy control subjects the highest urine calcium concentrations were found in the most concentrated urine samples, arguing against a clinically relevant effect of urine calcium on urine concentration [83].

Hypokalaemia

Hypokalaemia causes an AVP-resistant concentration defect. As in the other forms of acquired NDI, reduced expression of AQP2 has been demonstrated [84]. Thus, downregulation of AQP2 seems to be a common feature in acquired NDI [35]. However, the mechanism by which hypokalaemia affects this remains to be elucidated.

Disorders Impairing the Generation of a Medullary Concentration Gradient

Bartter Syndrome

As discussed above, the loop of Henle and active salt reabsorption in thick ascending limb are necessary for the generation of a medullary concentration gradient. Therefore, factors impairing salt reabsorption in the thick ascending limb will lead to a urinary concentration defect (hypo- or isosthenuria). Patients with Bartter syndrome have inherited defects in thick ascending limb salt transport and symptoms include polyuria and episodes of hypernatraemic dehydration (see Chap. 29), similar to patients with NDI. However, the presence of a hypokalaemic alkalosis and elevated urinary electrolytes, particularly chloride, help differentiate it from NDI, although the former may be absent in young infants [67]. A history of polyhydramnios further helps to exclude a diagnosis of NDI.

Urea Transporter

Urea is an important constituent of the medullary interstitial concentration gradient. Urea is a bipolar molecule and thus can only diffuse slowly through membranes [85]. Diffusion is facilitated by urea transporters and two genes encoding these transporters have been identified in humans [86]. A mild urinary concentrating defect has been described in patients not expressing the minor blood group antigen Kidd (Jk) [87]. Later, this antigen was identified to be identical with the urea transporter UT-1, encoded by *SLC14A1* and several mutations in this gene have been identified in Kidd-negative individuals [88–90]. Recent evidence suggests that UT-1 is also expressed in the endothelium of the vasa recta and that the combined defect in red cell and vascular urea diffusion impairs countercurrent concentration [91, 92]. Interestingly, no mutations have been found so far in the gene encoding the urea transporter expressed in renal tubule UT-2 (*SLC14A2*).

Genetics

AVPR2

The majority of cases of NDI (90%) are due to mutations in the *AVPR2* gene [93, 94]. The gene is located on chromosome region Xq28 and the mode of inheritance is X-linked recessive. Therefore, the majority of patients with NDI are male, but due to skewed X-inactivation (lionization), females can be affected with variable degrees of polyuria and polydipsia [20, 95–97]. Indeed, in some families, X-inactivation is strongly biased leading to a pseudo-dominant inheritance pattern [98]. X-inactivation may be strongly biased because of (a) chance, (b) a co-existent mutation on the affected X-chromosome affecting cell survival or (c) a co-existing mutation in a gene regulating X-inactivation [99].

So far, more than 211 distinct putative disease-causing mutations have been described in more than 326 families [93, 100]. When investigated in vitro, these mutations can be classified according to their effect [101–118]:

Class 1 mutations result in frame-shifts, premature stop-codons and aberrant splicing and prevent translation of the receptor protein.

Class 2 mutations are missense mutations that allow for translation of the protein, but lead to aberrant trafficking. Typically, these mutations induce improper folding with subsequent trapping in the endoplasmic reticulum (ER).

Class 3 mutations allow the mutated protein to reach the cell-surface, but impair the receptor's signaling, typically by affecting binding of AVP.

The majority of mutations identified in X-linked NDI belong to class 2 [119]. Conversely, mutations identified in inherited partial NDI fall into class 3: these mutated receptors reach the cell membrane, but have a decreased affinity for AVP [54, 61].

Interestingly, three distinct class 3 mutation have been identified in the *AVPR2* gene, leading to gain-of-function with constitutive activation of the receptor and thus to a "nephrogenic syndrome of inappropriate antidiuresis" [120, 121].

AQP2

The analysis of a pedigree with affected females and the presence of intact extrarenal responses to DDAVP in some patients with NDI lead to the postulation of an autosomal inherited "post-receptor" defect in these individuals [122–124]. The molecular basis for this distinct form of NDI was identified in 1994 to be the water channel aquaporin-2, which is expressed in collecting duct [14]. Approximately 10% of all patients with NDI carry mutations in the *AQP2*. As expected for a loss-of-function defect, inheritance is usually recessive and—similar to AVPR2—the majority of mutations fall into class 2 with retention in the endoplasmic reticulum

[119, 125]. Interestingly, there are some families with autosomal dominant inheritance of NDI. Molecular analysis has shown that affected members carry mutations in the c-terminus of AQP2 [43, 126–128]. So why does this lead to a dominant inheritance? The final waterchannel is a homotetramer, meaning it consists of four AQP2 subunits (see Fig. 40.2). Dominant mutations in the C-terminus lead to aberrant trafficking (class 2), but are able to oligomerize with wild-type protein to form the tetramer. As tetramerization takes place before export to the plasma membrane, these mutations exert a dominant-negative effect on AQP2 function, by misguiding trafficking of the assembled tetramer. Interestingly, specific mutations direct AQP2 trafficking to distinct cellular compartments, such as the Golgi complex [43], late endosomes/lysosomes [126] or the basolateral membrane [128, 129].

Treatment

General Aspects of Treatment

The importance of prompt treatment of NDI is highlighted by the fact that mental retardation used to be an invariable feature, but can be completely prevented by proper treatment. Caring for a patient with NDI is most difficult during infancy, when the babies are dependent on their caregivers for access to fluids. Therefore fluids should be offered in 2-h intervals, placing a considerable burden on the caregivers, particularly at night. Feeding per nasogastric tube is often helpful in this period. A continuous overnight feed delivered by a pump will provide fluid and calories to the baby and much needed rest to the parents. Families also need to be instructed to bring the child to immediate medical attention, when there are increased extra-renal fluid losses, such as when diarrhoea, vomiting or fever are present. It is often helpful for the parents to have a letter detailing the condition of their child and the need for prompt physical and biochemical assessment, that they can present in these instances in order to avoid being sent home by medical personnel with no experience in this condition. There should be a low threshold for admission and intravenous hydration in these instances to prevent dehydration. When in hospital, hypotonic fluids, such as 5% Dextrose or 0.22% saline are usually appropriate for intravenous hydration, because of the obligate water losses in the urine. Replacement fluids with a higher osmolality than urine osmolality will exacerbate hypernatraemia. For instance, 0.45% saline results in an osmotic load of 154 mOsm/L (77 mOsm Na and 77 mOsm Cl). A patient with a maximal urine osmolality of 100 mOsm/kg will need to excrete 1.54 L of urine for each litre of 0.45% saline received in order to excrete the osmotic load presented by the replacement fluid (see below). Thus, in patients with NDI, the administration of fluids that are hypertonic compared to urine can lead to hypernatraemic dehydration, even though the fluid may be hypotonic to plasma. However, if there are increased salt losses, as can occur with diarrhea, or if hypotonic fluids are administered at a rate higher than the urine losses, hyponatraemia could ensue. Close monitoring of the patient with respect to weight, fluid balance, clinical symptoms and biochemistries is therefore imperative to prevent complications.

Osmotic Load Reduction

The most important part in the treatment of patients with NDI is a reduction in their osmotic load, also called renal solute load, which determines urine volume. Therefore close involvement of a dietician with experience in the management of children with kidney problems is necessary. The osmotic load consists of osmotically active substances that need to be excreted in the urine, i.e. proteins, as they are metabolized to urea, and salts. A typical western diet contains about 800 mOsm per day. Thus, an individual with a urine osmolality of 800 mOsm/kg only needs 1 L of water to excrete that load. Yet a patient with NDI and a maximal urine osmolality of 100 mOsm/kg needs at least 8 L of water for excretion and if the urine osmolality is 50 mOsm/kg then 16 L of water are required. One gram of table salt is equivalent to about 18 mmol NaCl,

providing an osmolar load of 36 mOsm (18 mOsm Na and 18 mOsm Cl). Consequently, for a patient with a urine osmolality of 100 mOsm/kg, each gram of salt ingested increases obligatory urine output by 360 mL. The osmolar load of a diet can be roughly estimated by the following formula: twice the millimolar amount of sodium and potassium (to account for the accompanying anions) plus protein [g] times 4 (as metabolisation of each g of protein yields approximately 4 mmol of urea) [130]. Since lipids and sugars are metabolized without byproducts requiring renal excretion, only protein intake needs to be limited, but should still meet the recommended daily allowance to enable normal growth and development. A reasonable goal is a diet containing about 15 mOsm/kg/day. A child with a urine osmolality of 100 mOsm will need a fluid intake of 150 mL/kg/day to be able to excrete that load, which is achievable. Enriching the fluid intake with carbohydrates will provide additional calories without increasing the osmolar load.

Diuretics

The use of a diuretic in a polyuric disorder appears at first glance counterintuitive, but does make physiologic sense. The successful use of thiazides in NDI with a subsequent increase in urine osmolality and concomitant decrease in urine output was first reported in 1959 [131, 132]. Thiazides inhibit reabsorption of sodium and chloride in the distal convoluted tubule (part of the section "Tubular Concentration/Dilution Mechanism (Countercurrent Mechanism with Figure)"—see above) and thus increase the salt concentration and osmolality of the urine. The increased salt losses decrease intravascular volume with a subsequent up-regulation of proximal tubular reabsorption of salt and water. Consequently, less volume is delivered to the collecting duct and lost in the urine. Typically used is hydrochlorothiazide at 2 mg/kg/day in two divided doses. The more long-acting Bendroflumethiazide (50–100 μg/kg/day) can be given as a single daily dose. Hypokalaemia is a common complication of thiazide administration, but supplementation with potassium salts increases the osmolar load. Therefore, combination of the thiazide with a potassium-sparing diuretic, such as amiloride (0.1–0.3 mg/kg/day) is advantageous, but the latter can cause gastrointestinal side effects, especially nausea.

Non-steroidal Anti-inflammatory Drugs (NSAID)

Like in many other tubular disorders NSAID (prostaglandin synthesis inhibitors) are used in NDI. Initially, it was thought that these worked by reducing GFR and thus a "partial chemical nephrectomy" to minimize losses. However, observations in animals and humans suggest that NSAID can increase urine osmolality without decreasing GFR. In fact, an improvement in GFR can be observed, presumably reflecting improved volume status [66]. The exact mechanism remains to be elucidated, but appears to be ADH-independent [133–135]. Some evidence suggests that activation of basolateral prostaglandin receptors by prostaglandin E2 inhibits Adenylcyclase and/or the shuttling of AQP2 to the apical membrane [136–138].

Typically used is Indomethacin (1–3 mg/kg/day in three to four divided doses). The long-term use of this drug is associated with deterioration of renal function and haematological, as well as gastro-intestinal side effects including life-threatening haemorrhage [139, 140]. The latter may be avoided by using a selective COX-2 inhibitor and the successful use of these in NDI has been reported [141, 142]. However, there are concerns about cardiotoxic side effects of these drugs, as evident by the removal of Rofecoxib from the marketplace [143]. In our experience, the combination of Hydrochlorothiazide with an NSAID is useful during the first years of life, with a subsequent switch to Bendroflumethiazide with or without Amiloride. Key is the close observation of the individual patient for side effects and for changes in urine output or growth percentiles.

The concurrent use of antacids can help with the vomiting often seen in infants with NDI and help prevent gastro-intestinal side effects of NSAID.

Future Perspectives

An increasing understanding of the molecular mechanisms of the (patho)physiology of urinary concentration opens up perspectives for novel treatments [144].

Molecular Chaperones

The vast majority of mutations identified in the *AVPR2* gene lead to improper folding of the resultant protein with entrapment in the endoplasmic reticulum (see section "AVPR2"). Retention is dependent on specialized endoplasmic reticulum proteins, many of which require calcium for optimal function. Therefore, depletion of endoplasmic reticulum calcium stores by inhibiting the sarcoplasmatic calcium pump may be useful to overcome entrapment [145]. Indeed, this approach has been successfully used in vitro to induce surface expression of an AVPR2 mutant [146]. More specific, is the idea to use small pharmacological chaperones that can enter the cell, bind to the mutant receptor and thus induce proper folding with subsequent release from the endoplasmic reticulum [147, 148]. With the development of small membrane-permeable AVPR2-receptor antagonists, designed to fit neatly into the binding fold of the receptor, this approach has become feasible and indeed successful in vitro [149–151]. More importantly, a recent trial of a AVP antagonist in five patients with NDI, bearing either the mutation del62-64, R137H or W164S (all of which lead to ER retention), has shown a significant decrease in urine output with a concomitant increase in urine osmolality [152]. Total 24-h urine volume decreased from a mean of 11.9–8.2 L and mean urine osmolality rose from 98 to 170 mOsm/kg and thus the observed effect was modest. Nevertheless, these results hold the promise of a targeted, mutation-specific therapy in patients with NDI. Increasingly, gene therapy is becoming a reality, either by provision of the wild-type gene or by correcting the specific genetic mutation through gene editing [153]. Once safe and efficacious methods to deliver such treatments to the kidney have been developed, these obviously would provide specific treatments for inherited NDI.

Prostaglandin Receptor Agonists

The identification of cAMP as a key messenger in urinary concentration has led to the search for compounds that could increase cAMP in the principal cell independent of AVPR2. Recently, it was shown that agonists for the prostaglandin receptor EP2 and EP4, such as prostaglandin E2 could provide such an alternative pathway [154]. Indeed, in a rat model of NDI these compounds were able to reduce urine output significantly. Yet, giving prostaglandins to treat NDI is in apparent contradiction to the clinically proven efficacy of prostaglandin synthesis inhibition (see above) and more data are needed to resolve this conundrum.

References

1. McIlraith CH. Notes on some cases of diabetes insipidus with marked family and hereditary tendencies. Lancet. 1892;2:767.
2. de Lange C. Ueber erblichen Diabetes Insipidus. Jahrbuch fuer Kinderheilkunde. 1935;145(1):135.
3. Forssman HH. On hereditary diabetes insipidus. Acta Med Scand. 1945;121(Suppl 159):9.
4. Waring AJK, Tappan LV. A congenital defect of water metabolism. Am J Dis Childhood. 1945;69:323–4.
5. Williams RH, Henry C. Nephrogenic diabetes insipidus: transmitted by females and appearing during infancy in males. Ann Intern Med. 1947;27:84–95.
6. Bode HH, Crawford JD. Nephrogenic diabetes insipidus in North America—the Hopewell hypothesis. N Engl J Med. 1967;280:750–4.
7. Seibold A, Rosenthal W, Bichet DG, Birnbaumer M. The vasopressin type 2 receptor gene. Chromosomal localization and its role in nephrogenic diabetes insipidus. Regul Pept. 1993;45(1–2):67–71.
8. Lolait SJ, O'Carroll AM, McBride OW, Konig M, Morel A, Brownstein MJ. Cloning and characterization of a vasopressin V2 receptor and possible link to nephrogenic diabetes insipidus. Nature. 1992;357(6376):336–9.
9. Rosenthal W, Seibold A, Antaramian A, Lonergan M, Arthus MF, Hendy GN, et al. Molecular identification of the gene responsible for congenital nephrogenic diabetes insipidus. Nature. 1992;359(6392):233–5.
10. van den Ouweland AM, Dreesen JC, Verdijk M, Knoers NV, Monnens LA, Rocchi M, et al. Mutations in the vasopressin type 2 receptor gene (AVPR2) associated with nephrogenic diabetes insipidus. Nat Genet. 1992;2(2):99–102.
11. Pan Y, Metzenberg A, Das S, Jing B, Gitschier J. Mutations in the V2 vasopressin receptor gene are associated with X-linked nephrogenic diabetes insipidus. Nat Genet. 1992;2(2):103–6.
12. Fushimi K, Uchida S, Hara Y, Hirata Y, Marumo F, Sasaki S. Cloning and expression of apical membrane water channel of rat kidney collecting tubule. Nature. 1993;361(6412):549–52.
13. Sasaki S, Fushimi K, Saito H, Saito F, Uchida S, Ishibashi K, et al. Cloning, characterization, and chromosomal mapping of human aquaporin of collecting duct. J Clin Invest. 1994;93(3):1250–6.
14. Deen PM, Verdijk MA, Knoers NV, Wieringa B, Monnens LA, van Os CH, et al. Requirement of human renal water channel aquaporin-2 for vasopressin-dependent concentration of urine. Science. 1994;264(5155):92–5.
15. Bockenhauer D, Bichet DG. Pathophysiology, diagnosis and management of nephrogenic diabetes insipidus. Nat Rev Nephrol. 2015;11(10):576–88.
16. Bonilla-Felix M. Development of water transport in the collecting duct. Am J Physiol Renal Physiol. 2004;287(6):F1093–101.
17. Lopez-Garcia SC, Downie ML, Kim JS, Boyer O, Walsh SB, Nijenhuis T, et al. Treatment and long-term outcome in primary nephrogenic diabetes insipidus. Nephrol Dial Transplant. 2020;2020:gfaa243.
18. Sharma S, Ashton E, Iancu D, Arthus MF, Hayes W, Van't Hoff W, et al. Long-term outcome in inherited nephrogenic diabetes insipidus. Clin Kidney J. 2019;12(2):180–7.
19. Hoekstra JA, van Lieburg AF, Monnens LA, Hulstijn-Dirkmaat GM, Knoers VV. Cognitive and psychosocial functioning of patients with congenital nephrogenic diabetes insipidus. Am J Med Genet. 1996;61(1):81–8.
20. van Lieburg AF, Knoers NV, Monnens LA. Clinical presentation and follow-up of 30 patients with congenital nephrogenic diabetes insipidus. J Am Soc Nephrol. 1999;10(9):1958–64.
21. Hillman DA, Neyzi O, Porter P, Cushman A, Talbot NB. Renal (vasopressin-resistant) diabetes insipidus; definition of the effects of a homeostatic limitation in capacity to conserve water on the physical, intellectual and emotional development of a child. Pediatrics. 1958;21(3):430–5.
22. Vest M, Talbotnb, Crawford JD. Hypocaloric dwarfism and hydronephrosis in diabetes insipidus. Am J Dis Child. 1963;105:175–81.
23. Yoo TH, Ryu DR, Song YS, Lee SC, Kim HJ, Kim JS, et al. Congenital nephrogenic diabetes insipidus presented with bilateral hydronephrosis: genetic analysis of V2R gene mutations. Yonsei Med J. 2006;47(1):126–30.
24. Stevens S, Brown BD, McGahan JP. Nephrogenic diabetes insipidus: a cause of severe nonobstructive urinary tract dilatation. J Ultrasound Med. 1995;14(7):543–5.
25. Jaureguiberry G, Van't Hoff W, Mushtaq I, Desai D, Mann NP, Kleta R, et al. A patient with polyuria and hydronephrosis: question. Pediatr Nephrol. 2011;26(11):1977–8, 9–80.

26. Stephenson JL. Concentration of urine in a central core model of the renal counterflow system. Kidney Int. 1972;2(2):85–94.

27. Kokko JP, Rector FC Jr. Countercurrent multiplication system without active transport in inner medulla. Kidney Int. 1972;2(4):214–23.

28. Zhang R, Skach W, Hasegawa H, van Hoek AN, Verkman AS. Cloning, functional analysis and cell localization of a kidney proximal tubule water transporter homologous to CHIP28. J Cell Biol. 1993;120(2):359–69.

29. Sabolic I, Valenti G, Verbavatz JM, Van Hoek AN, Verkman AS, Ausiello DA, et al. Localization of the CHIP28 water channel in rat kidney. Am J Phys. 1992;263(6 Pt 1):C1225–33.

30. Nielsen S, Smith BL, Christensen EI, Knepper MA, Agre P. CHIP28 water channels are localized in constitutively water-permeable segments of the nephron. J Cell Biol. 1993;120(2):371–83.

31. Nielsen S, Pallone T, Smith BL, Christensen EI, Agre P, Maunsbach AB. Aquaporin-1 water channels in short and long loop descending thin limbs and in descending vasa recta in rat kidney. Am J Phys. 1995;268(6 Pt 2):F1023–37.

32. Zhai XY, Fenton RA, Andreasen A, Thomsen JS, Christensen EI. Aquaporin-1 is not expressed in descending thin limbs of short-loop nephrons. J Am Soc Nephrol. 2007;18(11):2937–44.

33. Halperin ML, Kamel KS, Oh MS. Mechanisms to concentrate the urine: an opinion. Curr Opin Nephrol Hypertens. 2008;17(4):416–22.

34. Obermuller N, Kunchaparty S, Ellison DH, Bachmann S. Expression of the Na-K-2Cl cotransporter by macula densa and thick ascending limb cells of rat and rabbit nephron. J Clin Invest. 1996;98(3):635–40.

35. Nielsen S, Frokiaer J, Marples D, Kwon TH, Agre P, Knepper MA. Aquaporins in the kidney: from molecules to medicine. Physiol Rev. 2002;82(1):205–44.

36. Eggena P, Christakis J, Deppisch L. Effect of hypotonicity on cyclic adenosine monophosphate formation and action in vasopressin target cells. Kidney Int. 1975;7(3):161–9.

37. Edwards RM, Jackson BA, Dousa TP. ADH-sensitive cAMP system in papillary collecting duct: effect of osmolality and PGE2. Am J Phys. 1981;240(4):F311–8.

38. Nielsen S, Chou CL, Marples D, Christensen EI, Kishore BK, Knepper MA. Vasopressin increases water permeability of kidney collecting duct by inducing translocation of aquaporin-CD water channels to plasma membrane. Proc Natl Acad Sci U S A. 1995;92(4):1013–7.

39. Knepper MA, Nielsen S, Chou CL, DiGiovanni SR. Mechanism of vasopressin action in the renal collecting duct. Semin Nephrol. 1994;14(4):302–21.

40. Katsura T, Gustafson CE, Ausiello DA, Brown D. Protein kinase A phosphorylation is involved in regulated exocytosis of aquaporin-2 in trans-fected LLC-PK1 cells. Am J Phys. 1997;272(6 Pt 2):F817–22.

41. Fushimi K, Sasaki S, Marumo F. Phosphorylation of serine 256 is required for cAMP-dependent regulatory exocytosis of the aquaporin-2 water channel. J Biol Chem. 1997;272(23):14800–4.

42. Christensen BM, Zelenina M, Aperia A, Nielsen S. Localization and regulation of PKA-phosphorylated AQP2 in response to V(2)-receptor agonist/antagonist treatment. Am J Physiol Renal Physiol. 2000;278(1):F29–42.

43. Mulders SM, Bichet DG, Rijss JP, Kamsteeg EJ, Arthus MF, Lonergan M, et al. An aquaporin-2 water channel mutant which causes autosomal dominant nephrogenic diabetes insipidus is retained in the Golgi complex. J Clin Invest. 1998;102(1):57–66.

44. Ecelbarger CA, Terris J, Frindt G, Echevarria M, Marples D, Nielsen S, et al. Aquaporin-3 water channel localization and regulation in rat kidney. Am J Phys. 1995;269(5 Pt 2):F663–72.

45. Terris J, Ecelbarger CA, Nielsen S, Knepper MA. Long-term regulation of four renal aquaporins in rats. Am J Phys. 1996;271(2 Pt 2):F414–22.

46. Terris J, Ecelbarger CA, Marples D, Knepper MA, Nielsen S. Distribution of aquaporin-4 water channel expression within rat kidney. Am J Phys. 1995;269(6 Pt 2):F775–85.

47. Hua Li J, Jain S, McMillin SM, Cui Y, Gautam D, Sakamoto W, et al. A novel experimental strategy to assess the metabolic effects of selective activation of a Gq-coupled receptor in hepatocytes in vivo. Endocrinology. 2013;154(10):3539–51.

48. Holmes CL, Landry DW, Granton JT. Science review: Vasopressin and the cardiovascular system Part 1—Receptor physiology. Crit Care. 2003;7(6):427–34.

49. Bichet DG, Razi M, Lonergan M, Arthus MF, Papukna V, Kortas C, et al. Hemodynamic and coagulation responses to 1-desamino[8-D-arginine] vasopressin in patients with congenital nephrogenic diabetes insipidus. N Engl J Med. 1988;318(14):881–7.

50. Williams TD, Lightman SL, Leadbeater MJ. Hormonal and cardiovascular responses to DDAVP in man. Clin Endocrinol. 1986;24(1):89–96.

51. Mannucci PM, Canciani MT, Rota L, Donovan BS. Response of factor VIII/von Willebrand factor to DDAVP in healthy subjects and patients with haemophilia A and von Willebrand's disease. Br J Haematol. 1981;47(2):283–93.

52. Mannucci PM, Aberg M, Nilsson IM, Robertson B. Mechanism of plasminogen activator and factor VIII increase after vasoactive drugs. Br J Haematol. 1975;30(1):81–93.

53. Winberg J. Determination of renal concentration capacity in infants and children without renal disease. Acta Paediatr. 1958;48:318–28.

54. Vargas-Poussou R, Forestier L, Dautzenberg MD, Niaudet P, Dechaux M, Antignac C. Mutations in the vasopressin V2 receptor and aquaporin-2 genes

in 12 families with congenital nephrogenic diabetes insipidus. J Am Soc Nephrol. 1997;8(12):1855–62.

55. Monnens L, Smulders Y, van Lier H, de Boo T. DDAVP test for assessment of renal concentrating capacity in infants and children. Nephron. 1981;29(3–4):151–4.

56. Ito M, Mori Y, Oiso Y, Saito H. A single base substitution in the coding region for neurophysin II associated with familial central diabetes insipidus. J Clin Invest. 1991;87(2):725–8.

57. Ghirardello S, Malattia C, Scagnelli P, Maghnie M. Current perspective on the pathogenesis of central diabetes insipidus. J Pediatr Endocrinol Metab. 2005;18(7):631–45.

58. Christensen JH, Rittig S. Familial neurohypophyseal diabetes insipidus—an update. Semin Nephrol. 2006;26(3):209–23.

59. Pepin L, Colin E, Tessarech M, Rouleau S, Bouhours-Nouet N, Bonneau D, et al. A new case of PCSK1 pathogenic variant with congenital proprotein convertase 1/3 deficiency and literature review. J Clin Endocrinol Metab. 2019;104(4):985–93.

60. Sasaki S, Chiga M, Kikuchi E, Rai T, Uchida S. Hereditary nephrogenic diabetes insipidus in Japanese patients: analysis of 78 families and report of 22 new mutations in AVPR2 and AQP2. Clin Exp Nephrol. 2013;17(3):338–44.

61. Sadeghi H, Robertson GL, Bichet DG, Innamorati G, Birnbaumer M. Biochemical basis of partial nephrogenic diabetes insipidus phenotypes. Mol Endocrinol. 1997;11(12):1806–13.

62. Bockenhauer D, Carpentier E, Rochdi D, Van't Hoff W, Breton B, Bernier V, et al. Vasopressin type 2 receptor V88M mutation: molecular basis of partial and complete nephrogenic diabetes insipidus. Nephron Physiol. 2009;114(1):p1–p10.

63. Canfield MC, Tamarappoo BK, Moses AM, Verkman AS, Holtzman EJ. Identification and characterization of aquaporin-2 water channel mutations causing nephrogenic diabetes insipidus with partial vasopressin response. Hum Mol Genet. 1997;6(11):1865–71.

64. Bockenhauer D, Bichet DG. Inherited secondary nephrogenic diabetes insipidus: concentrating on humans. Am J Physiol Renal Physiol. 2013;304(8):F1037–42.

65. Bockenhauer D, Van't Hoff W, Dattani M, Lehnhardt A, Subtirelu M, Hildebrandt F, et al. Secondary nephrogenic diabetes insipidus as a complication of inherited renal diseases. Nephron Physiol. 2010;116(4):23–9.

66. Bockenhauer D, Cruwys M, Kleta R, Halperin LF, Wildgoose P, Souma T, et al. Antenatal Bartter's syndrome: why is this not a lethal condition? QJM. 2008;101(12):927–42.

67. Bettinelli A, Ciarmatori S, Cesareo L, Tedeschi S, Ruffa G, Appiani AC, et al. Phenotypic variability in Bartter syndrome type I. Pediatr Nephrol. 2000;14(10–11):940–5.

68. Lee EH, Heo JS, Lee HK, Han KH, Kang HG, Ha IS, et al. A case of Bartter syndrome type I with atypical presentations. Korean J Pediatr. 2010;53(8):809–13.

69. Frokiaer J, Marples D, Knepper MA, Nielsen S. Bilateral ureteral obstruction downregulates expression of vasopressin-sensitive AQP-2 water channel in rat kidney. Am J Phys. 1996;270(4 Pt 2):F657–68.

70. Frokiaer J, Christensen BM, Marples D, Djurhuus JC, Jensen UB, Knepper MA, et al. Downregulation of aquaporin-2 parallels changes in renal water excretion in unilateral ureteral obstruction. Am J Phys. 1997;273(2 Pt 2):F213–23.

71. Kwon TH, Frokiaer J, Fernandez-Llama P, Knepper MA, Nielsen S. Reduced abundance of aquaporins in rats with bilateral ischemia-induced acute renal failure: prevention by alpha-MSH. Am J Phys. 1999;277(3 Pt 2):F413–27.

72. Johnston PA, Rennke H, Levinsky NG. Recovery of proximal tubular function from ischemic injury. Am J Phys. 1984;246(2 Pt 2):F159–66.

73. Boton R, Gaviria M, Batlle DC. Prevalence, pathogenesis, and treatment of renal dysfunction associated with chronic lithium therapy. Am J Kidney Dis. 1987;10(5):329–45.

74. Carney SL, Ray C, Gillies AH. Mechanism of lithium-induced polyuria in the rat. Kidney Int. 1996;50(2):377–83.

75. Christensen S, Kusano E, Yusufi AN, Murayama N, Dousa TP. Pathogenesis of nephrogenic diabetes insipidus due to chronic administration of lithium in rats. J Clin Invest. 1985;75(6):1869–79.

76. Trepiccione F, Christensen BM. Lithium-induced nephrogenic diabetes insipidus: new clinical and experimental findings. J Nephrol. 2010;23(Suppl 16):S43–8.

77. Watanabe S, Fukumoto S, Chang H, Takeuchi Y, Hasegawa Y, Okazaki R, et al. Association between activating mutations of calcium-sensing receptor and Bartter's syndrome. Lancet. 2002;360(9334):692–4.

78. Hebert SC. Bartter syndrome. Curr Opin Nephrol Hypertens. 2003;12(5):527–32.

79. Wang W, Kwon TH, Li C, Frokiaer J, Knepper MA, Nielsen S. Reduced expression of Na-K-2Cl cotransporter in medullary TAL in vitamin D-induced hypercalcemia in rats. Am J Physiol Renal Physiol. 2002;282(1):F34–44.

80. Sands JM, Naruse M, Baum M, Jo I, Hebert SC, Brown EM, et al. Apical extracellular calcium/polyvalent cation-sensing receptor regulates vasopressin-elicited water permeability in rat kidney inner medullary collecting duct. J Clin Invest. 1997;99(6):1399–405.

81. Earm JH, Christensen BM, Frokiaer J, Marples D, Han JS, Knepper MA, et al. Decreased aquaporin-2 expression and apical plasma membrane delivery in kidney collecting ducts of polyuric hypercalcemic rats. J Am Soc Nephrol. 1998;9(12):2181–93.

82. Hebert SC, Brown EM, Harris HW. Role of the Ca(2+)-sensing receptor in divalent mineral ion homeostasis. J Exp Biol. 1997;200(Pt 2):295–302.

83. Lam GS, Asplin JR, Halperin ML. Does a high concentration of calcium in the urine cause an important renal concentrating defect in human subjects? Clin Sci. 2000;98(3):313–9.

84. Marples D, Frokiaer J, Dorup J, Knepper MA, Nielsen S. Hypokalemia-induced downregulation of aquaporin-2 water channel expression in rat kidney medulla and cortex. J Clin Invest. 1996;97(8):1960–8.

85. Gallucci E, Micelli S, Lippe C. Non-electrolyte permeability across thin lipid membranes. Arch Int Physiol Biochim. 1971;79(5):881–7.

86. Sands JM. Renal urea transporters. Curr Opin Nephrol Hypertens. 2004;13(5):525–32.

87. Gillin AG, Sands JM. Urea transport in the kidney. Semin Nephrol. 1993;13(2):146–54.

88. Sidoux-Walter F, Lucien N, Nissinen R, Sistonen P, Henry S, Moulds J, et al. Molecular heterogeneity of the Jk(null) phenotype: expression analysis of the Jk(S291P) mutation found in Finns. Blood. 2000;96(4):1566–73.

89. Lucien N, Sidoux-Walter F, Olives B, Moulds J, Le Pennec PY, Cartron JP, et al. Characterization of the gene encoding the human Kidd blood group/urea transporter protein. Evidence for splice site mutations in Jknull individuals. J Biol Chem. 1998;273(21):12973–80.

90. Olives B, Mattei MG, Huet M, Neau P, Martial S, Cartron JP, et al. Kidd blood group and urea transport function of human erythrocytes are carried by the same protein. J Biol Chem. 1995;270(26):15607–10.

91. Pallone TL, Turner MR, Edwards A, Jamison RL. Countercurrent exchange in the renal medulla. Am J Physiol Regul Integr Comp Physiol. 2003;284(5):R1153–75.

92. Promeneur D, Rousselet G, Bankir L, Bailly P, Cartron JP, Ripoche P, et al. Evidence for distinct vascular and tubular urea transporters in the rat kidney. J Am Soc Nephrol. 1996;7(6):852–60.

93. Sands JM, Bichet DG. Nephrogenic diabetes insipidus. Ann Intern Med. 2006;144(3):186–94.

94. Bichet DG, Oksche A, Rosenthal W. Congenital nephrogenic diabetes insipidus. J Am Soc Nephrol. 1997;8(12):1951–8.

95. Sato K, Fukuno H, Taniguchi T, Sawada S, Fukui T, Kinoshita M. A novel mutation in the vasopressin V2 receptor gene in a woman with congenital nephrogenic diabetes insipidus. Intern Med. 1999;38(10):808–12.

96. Arthus MF, Lonergan M, Crumley MJ, Naumova AK, Morin D, De Marco LA, et al. Report of 33 novel AVPR2 mutations and analysis of 117 families with X-linked nephrogenic diabetes insipidus. J Am Soc Nephrol. 2000;11(6):1044–54.

97. Kinoshita K, Miura Y, Nagasaki H, Murase T, Bando Y, Oiso Y. A novel deletion mutation in the arginine vasopressin receptor 2 gene and skewed X chromosome inactivation in a female patient with congenital nephrogenic diabetes insipidus. J Endocrinol Investig. 2004;27(2):167–70.

98. Friedman E, Bale AE, Carson E, Boson WL, Nordenskjold M, Ritzen M, et al. Nephrogenic diabetes insipidus: an X chromosome-linked dominant inheritance pattern with a vasopressin type 2 receptor gene that is structurally normal. Proc Natl Acad Sci U S A. 1994;91(18):8457–61.

99. Puck JM, Willard HF. X inactivation in females with X-linked disease. N Engl J Med. 1998;338(5):325–8.

100. Spanakis E, Milord E, Gragnoli C. AVPR2 variants and mutations in nephrogenic diabetes insipidus: review and missense mutation significance. J Cell Physiol. 2008;217(3):605–17.

101. Holtzman EJ, Kolakowski LF Jr, Geifman-Holtzman O, O'Brien DG, Rasoulpour M, Guillot AP, et al. Mutations in the vasopressin V2 receptor gene in two families with nephrogenic diabetes insipidus. J Am Soc Nephrol. 1994;5(2):169–76.

102. Pan Y, Wilson P, Gitschier J. The effect of eight V2 vasopressin receptor mutations on stimulation of adenylyl cyclase and binding to vasopressin. J Biol Chem. 1994;269(50):31933–7.

103. Tsukaguchi H, Matsubara H, Mori Y, Yoshimasa Y, Yoshimasa T, Nakao K, et al. Two vasopressin type 2 receptor gene mutations R143P and delta V278 in patients with nephrogenic diabetes insipidus impair ligand binding of the receptor. Biochem Biophys Res Commun. 1995;211(3):967–77.

104. Tsukaguchi H, Matsubara H, Inada M. Expression studies of two vasopressin V2 receptor gene mutations, R202C and 804insG, in nephrogenic diabetes insipidus. Kidney Int. 1995;48(2):554–62.

105. Tsukaguchi H, Matsubara H, Taketani S, Mori Y, Seido T, Inada M. Binding-, intracellular transport-, and biosynthesis-defective mutants of vasopressin type 2 receptor in patients with X-linked nephrogenic diabetes insipidus. J Clin Invest. 1995;96(4):2043–50.

106. Yokoyama K, Yamauchi A, Izumi M, Itoh T, Ando A, Imai E, et al. A low-affinity vasopressin V2-receptor gene in a kindred with X-linked nephrogenic diabetes insipidus. J Am Soc Nephrol. 1996;7(3):410–4.

107. Oksche A, Schulein R, Rutz C, Liebenhoff U, Dickson J, Muller H, et al. Vasopressin V2 receptor mutants that cause X-linked nephrogenic diabetes insipidus: analysis of expression, processing, and function. Mol Pharmacol. 1996;50(4):820–8.

108. Wenkert D, Schoneberg T, Merendino JJ Jr, Rodriguez Pena MS, Vinitsky R, Goldsmith PK, et al. Functional characterization of five V2 vasopressin receptor gene mutations. Mol Cell Endocrinol. 1996;124(1–2):43–50.

109. Sadeghi HM, Innamorati G, Birnbaumer M. An X-linked NDI mutation reveals a requirement for cell surface V2R expression. Mol Endocrinol. 1997;11(6):706–13.

110. Schoneberg T, Schulz A, Biebermann H, Gruters A, Grimm T, Hubschmann K, et al. V2 vasopressin

receptor dysfunction in nephrogenic diabetes insipidus caused by different molecular mechanisms. Hum Mutat. 1998;12(3):196–205.

111. Ala Y, Morin D, Mouillac B, Sabatier N, Vargas R, Cotte N, et al. Functional studies of twelve mutant V2 vasopressin receptors related to nephrogenic diabetes insipidus: molecular basis of a mild clinical phenotype. J Am Soc Nephrol. 1998;9(10):1861–72.

112. Wildin RS, Cogdell DE, Valadez V. AVPR2 variants and V2 vasopressin receptor function in nephrogenic diabetes insipidus. Kidney Int. 1998;54(6):1909–22.

113. Pasel K, Schulz A, Timmermann K, Linnemann K, Hoeltzenbein M, Jaaskelainen J, et al. Functional characterization of the molecular defects causing nephrogenic diabetes insipidus in eight families. J Clin Endocrinol Metab. 2000;85(4):1703–10.

114. Albertazzi E, Zanchetta D, Barbier P, Faranda S, Frattini A, Vezzoni P, et al. Nephrogenic diabetes insipidus: functional analysis of new AVPR2 mutations identified in Italian families. J Am Soc Nephrol. 2000;11(6):1033–43.

115. Postina R, Ufer E, Pfeiffer R, Knoers NV, Fahrenholz F. Misfolded vasopressin V2 receptors caused by extracellular point mutations entail congenital nephrogenic diabetes insipidus. Mol Cell Endocrinol. 2000;164(1–2):31–9.

116. Knoers NV, Deen PM. Molecular and cellular defects in nephrogenic diabetes insipidus. Pediatr Nephrol. 2001;16(12):1146–52.

117. Hermosilla R, Oueslati M, Donalies U, Schonenberger E, Krause E, Oksche A, et al. Disease-causing V(2) vasopressin receptors are retained in different compartments of the early secretory pathway. Traffic. 2004;5(12):993–1005.

118. Robben JH, Knoers NV, Deen PM. Characterization of vasopressin V2 receptor mutants in nephrogenic diabetes insipidus in a polarized cell model. Am J Physiol Renal Physiol. 2005;289(2):F265–72.

119. Fujiwara TM, Bichet DG. Molecular biology of hereditary diabetes insipidus. J Am Soc Nephrol. 2005;16(10):2836–46.

120. Feldman BJ, Rosenthal SM, Vargas GA, Fenwick RG, Huang EA, Matsuda-Abedini M, et al. Nephrogenic syndrome of inappropriate antidiuresis. N Engl J Med. 2005;352(18):1884–90.

121. Carpentier E, Greenbaum LA, Rochdi D, Abrol R, Goddard WA III, Bichet DG, et al. Identification and characterization of an activating F229V substitution in the V2 vasopressin receptor in an infant with NSIAD. J Am Soc Nephrol. 2012;23(10):1635–40.

122. Brenner B, Seligsohn U, Hochberg Z. Normal response of factor VIII and von Willebrand factor to 1-deamino-8D-arginine vasopressin in nephrogenic diabetes insipidus. J Clin Endocrinol Metab. 1988;67(1):191–3.

123. Knoers N, Monnens LA. A variant of nephrogenic diabetes insipidus: V2 receptor abnormality restricted to the kidney. Eur J Pediatr. 1991;150(5):370–3.

124. Langley JM, Balfe JW, Selander T, Ray PN, Clarke JT. Autosomal recessive inheritance of vasopressin-

125. Marr N, Bichet DG, Hoefs S, Savelkoul PJ, Konings IB, De Mattia F, et al. Cell-biologic and functional analyses of five new Aquaporin-2 missense mutations that cause recessive nephrogenic diabetes insipidus. J Am Soc Nephrol. 2002;13(9):2267–77.

126. Marr N, Bichet DG, Lonergan M, Arthus MF, Jeck N, Seyberth HW, et al. Heteroligomerization of an Aquaporin-2 mutant with wild-type Aquaporin-2 and their misrouting to late endosomes/lysosomes explains dominant nephrogenic diabetes insipidus. Hum Mol Genet. 2002;11(7):779–89.

127. Kuwahara M, Iwai K, Ooeda T, Igarashi T, Ogawa E, Katsushima Y, et al. Three families with autosomal dominant nephrogenic diabetes insipidus caused by aquaporin-2 mutations in the C-terminus. Am J Hum Genet. 2001;69(4):738–48.

128. Kamsteeg EJ, Bichet DG, Konings IB, Nivet H, Lonergan M, Arthus MF, et al. Reversed polarized delivery of an aquaporin-2 mutant causes dominant nephrogenic diabetes insipidus. J Cell Biol. 2003;163(5):1099–109.

129. Bichet DG, el Tarazi A, Matar J, Lussier Y, Arthus MF, Lonergan M, et al. Aquaporin-2: new mutations responsible for autosomal-recessive nephrogenic diabetes insipidus—update and epidemiology. Clin Kidney J. 2012;5:195–202.

130. Coleman J. Diseases of organ system: the kidney. In: Shaw V, Lawson M, editors. Clinical paediatric dietetics. 2nd ed. Oxford: Blackwell Science Ltd; 2001.

131. Kennedy GC, Crawford JD. Treatment of diabetes insipidus with hydrochlorothiazide. Lancet. 1959;1(7078):866–7.

132. Crawford JD, Kennedy GC. Chlorothiazid in diabetes insipidus. Nature. 1959;183(4665):891–2.

133. Stoff JS, Rosa RM, Silva P, Epstein FH. Indomethacin impairs water diuresis in the DI rat: role of prostaglandins independent of ADH. Am J Phys. 1981;241(3):F231–7.

134. Walker RM, Brown RS, Stoff JS. Role of renal prostaglandins during antidiuresis and water diuresis in man. Kidney Int. 1982;21(2):365–70.

135. Usberti M, Pecoraro C, Federico S, Cianciaruso B, Guida B, Romano A, et al. Mechanism of action of indomethacin in tubular defects. Pediatrics. 1985;75(3):501–7.

136. Tamma G, Wiesner B, Furkert J, Hahm D, Oksche A, Schaefer M, et al. The prostaglandin E2 analogue sulprostone antagonizes vasopressin-induced antidiuresis through activation of Rho. J Cell Sci. 2003;116(Pt 16):3285–94.

137. Huber TB, Simons M, Hartleben B, Sernetz L, Schmidts M, Gundlach E, et al. Molecular basis of the functional podocin-nephrin complex: mutations in the NPHS2 gene disrupt nephrin targeting to lipid raft microdomains. Hum Mol Genet. 2003;12(24):3397–405.

138. Hebert RL, Breyer RM, Jacobson HR, Breyer MD. Functional and molecular aspects of prostaglandin E receptors in the cortical collecting duct. Can J Physiol Pharmacol. 1995;73(2):172–9.

139. Langman MJ, Weil J, Wainwright P, Lawson DH, Rawlins MD, Logan RF, et al. Risks of bleeding peptic ulcer associated with individual non-steroidal anti-inflammatory drugs. Lancet. 1994;343(8905):1075–8.

140. Garcia Rodriguez LA, Jick H. Risk of upper gastrointestinal bleeding and perforation associated with individual non-steroidal anti-inflammatory drugs. Lancet. 1994;343(8900):769–72.

141. Soylu A, Kasap B, Ogun N, Ozturk Y, Turkmen M, Hoefsloot L, et al. Efficacy of COX-2 inhibitors in a case of congenital nephrogenic diabetes insipidus. Pediatr Nephrol. 2005;20(12):1814–7.

142. Pattaragarn A, Alon US. Treatment of congenital nephrogenic diabetes insipidus by hydrochlorothiazide and cyclooxygenase-2 inhibitor. Pediatr Nephrol. 2003;18(10):1073–6.

143. Dogne JM, Hanson J, Supuran C, Pratico D. Coxibs and cardiovascular side-effects: from light to shadow. Curr Pharm Des. 2006;12(8):971–5.

144. Bockenhauer D, Bichet DG. Urinary concentration: different ways to open and close the tap. Pediatr Nephrol. 2014;29(8):1297–303.

145. Egan ME, Glockner-Pagel J, Ambrose C, Cahill PA, Pappoe L, Balamuth N, et al. Calcium-pump inhibitors induce functional surface expression of Delta F508-CFTR protein in cystic fibrosis epithelial cells. Nat Med. 2002;8(5):485–92.

146. Robben JH, Sze M, Knoers NV, Deen PM. Rescue of vasopressin V2 receptor mutants by chemical chaperones: specificity and mechanism. Mol Biol Cell. 2006;17(1):379–86.

147. Romisch K. A cure for traffic jams: small molecule chaperones in the endoplasmic reticulum. Traffic. 2004;5(11):815–20.

148. Ulloa-Aguirre A, Janovick JA, Brothers SP, Conn PM. Pharmacologic rescue of conformationally-defective proteins: implications for the treatment of human disease. Traffic. 2004;5(11):821–37.

149. Morello JP, Salahpour A, Laperriere A, Bernier V, Arthus MF, Lonergan M, et al. Pharmacological chaperones rescue cell-surface expression and function of misfolded V2 vasopressin receptor mutants. J Clin Invest. 2000;105(7):887–95.

150. Tan CM, Nickols HH, Limbird LE. Appropriate polarization following pharmacological rescue of V2 vasopressin receptors encoded by X-linked nephrogenic diabetes insipidus alleles involves a conformation of the receptor that also attains mature glycosylation. J Biol Chem. 2003;278(37):35678–86.

151. Wuller S, Wiesner B, Loffler A, Furkert J, Krause G, Hermosilla R, et al. Pharmacochaperones post-translationally enhance cell surface expression by increasing conformational stability of wild-type and mutant vasopressin V2 receptors. J Biol Chem. 2004;279(45):47254–63.

152. Bernier V, Morello JP, Zarruk A, Debrand N, Salahpour A, Lonergan M, et al. Pharmacologic chaperones as a potential treatment for X-linked nephrogenic diabetes insipidus. J Am Soc Nephrol. 2006;17(1):232–43.

153. WareJoncas Z, Campbell JM, Martinez-Galvez G, Gendron WAC, Barry MA, Harris PC, et al. Precision gene editing technology and applications in nephrology. Nat Rev Nephrol. 2018;14(11):663–77.

154. Olesen ET, Rutzler MR, Moeller HB, Praetorius HA, Fenton RA. Vasopressin-independent targeting of aquaporin-2 by selective E-prostanoid receptor agonists alleviates nephrogenic diabetes insipidus. Proc Natl Acad Sci U S A. 2011;108(31):12949–54.

Part VIII

Renal Neoplasia and Tubulointerstitial Disease

Pediatric Renal Tumors

41

Kathryn S. Sutton and Andrew L. Hong

Introduction

Pediatric renal tumors include a heterogeneous group of diagnoses that vary greatly in both required treatment and long-term outcome. This chapter will review both benign and malignant renal masses, with a particular emphasis on pediatric kidney cancers given their impact on morbidity and mortality. Approximately 600 children are diagnosed with renal cancer each year in the United States, accounting for 7% of all pediatric malignancies. The predominant renal tumor pathology in young children is Wilms tumor, although renal cell carcinoma overtakes Wilms tumor in older adolescents [1, 2]. Additional tumor types of varying malignant potential arising in the kidney include renal medullary carcinoma, malignant rhabdoid tumor, clear cell sarcoma of the kidney, and congenital mesoblastic nephroma (Table 41.1) [3]. Pediatric leukemia and lymphoma can also present as a renal mass, although often there are additional sites of disease [4–6]. Benign kidney masses include metanephric neoplasms and cystic nephroma [3]. Rounding out the differential diagnosis of a pediatric renal mass are tumors that are adjacent to, but not arising from the kidney, most commonly adrenal tumors such as neuroblastoma and adrenal cortical carcinoma, or kidney malformations such as multicystic dysplastic kidneys.

Typical presentations of each diagnosis will be discussed in detail below; however, in general presenting symptoms of pediatric renal tumors may include painless abdominal masses or swelling, abdominal pain, hypertension, and hematuria. The initial workup for pediatric abdominal masses includes ultrasonography and laboratory evaluation, with further imaging recommended based on preliminary findings. Laboratory testing can both help to rule in and classify a renal tumor and to rule out other common pediatric abdominal cancers (Table 41.2).

K. S. Sutton (✉)
Aflac Cancer and Blood Disorders Center, Children's Healthcare of Atlanta, Atlanta, GA, USA

Department of Pediatrics, Emory University School of Medicine, Atlanta, GA, USA
e-mail: Kathryn.sutton@choa.org

A. L. Hong
Aflac Cancer and Blood Disorders Center, Children's Healthcare of Atlanta, Atlanta, GA, USA

Department of Pediatrics, Emory University School of Medicine, Atlanta, GA, USA

Winship Cancer Institute, Atlanta, GA, USA
e-mail: andrew.hong2@emory.edu

Table 41.1 Pediatric renal tumors

Malignant	Wilms tumor (nephroblastoma)
	Nephroblastomatosis (pre-malignant)
	Clear cell sarcoma of the kidney
	Renal cell carcinoma
	Renal medullary carcinoma
	Malignant rhabdoid tumor
	Ewing sarcoma of the kidney
Low malignant potential	Angiomyolipoma/malignant epithelial angiomyolipoma
	Congenital mesoblastic nephroma
Benign	Cystic nephroma
	Ossifying renal tumor of infancy
	Metanephric adenoma/metanephric stromal tumor/metanephric adenofibroma
Secondary tumors	Leukemia/Lymphoma
	Neuroblastoma (suprarenal)

Table 41.2 Initial laboratory evaluation for pediatric renal masses

Lab	Possible findings/interpretation
Complete Blood Count with differential	Anemia due subcapsular hemorrhage
	Pancytopenia or blast cells due to leukemia/lymphoma
	Polycythemia in metanephric adenoma/adenofibroma or renal cell carcinoma
Complete Metabolic Panel	Renal dysfunction
	Hypercalcemia in congenital mesoblastic nephroma
	Liver dysfunction in the setting of metastatic disease
Urinalysis	Hematuria
Coagulation studies (PT/PTT)	Acquired Von Willebrand's Disease in Wilms tumor
Urine catecholamines	Elevated in neuroblastoma (arises in suprarenal region)
LDH/Uric acid	Elevated in tumor lysis syndrome, especially in leukemia/lymphoma

Wilms Tumor

Epidemiology

Wilms tumor (WT), also known as nephroblastoma, is named for Max Wilms, a German pathologist and surgeon, who described the tumor in 1899 [7]. Wilms tumor represents the vast majority of pediatric renal tumors, accounting for 85–90% of kidney tumors diagnosed in children younger than age 14 [1]. There are approximately 600 new cases of WT in the United States annually, and worldwide the incidence approaches 1:10,000 children. There is a very slight female predominance, and WT is more common in Blacks and Whites than Asians [8].

Wilms tumor presents most commonly in preschool aged children, with the majority of cases diagnosed before the age of 5 years and nearly all before 10 years. Boys tend to present at a younger age than girls. Approximately 5–10% of WTs are bilateral at diagnosis, and these patients present earlier, with a median age at diagnosis of 31 months as compared to 44 months for patients with unilateral tumors [8]. Ten to 15% of WT are associated with an underlying predisposition syndrome (Table 41.3) [9, 10].

Predisposition Syndromes

The majority of Wilms tumor predisposition syndromes are associated with two genes, *WT1* and *WT2*, both located on chromosome 11 [9]. Patients with predisposition syndromes are more likely to present at a younger age and with bilateral disease [8]. The treatment approach to WT arising in patients with underlying predisposition syndromes requires modification to preserve

Table 41.3 Wilms tumor predisposition syndromes [9–11, 20, 22, 23]

Syndrome	Gene (locus)	Wilms tumor risk
WAGR	*WT1* (11p13)	50%
Denys-Drash	*WT1* (11p13)	>90%
Frasier	*WT1* (11p13)	8%
Beckwith-Weidemann	WT2 locus: *CDKN1C, H19, LIT1, IGF2* (11p15.5)	5% (Can be higher depending on specific genetic finding)
Simpson-Golabi-Behmel	*GPC3* (Xq26), *GPC4* (Xq26), *OFD1* (Xp22)	8%
Sotos	*NSD1* (5q35.3)	<5%
Perlman	*DIS3L2* (2q37.1)	50–75%
Trisomy 13	Chromosome 13	Rare
Trisomy 18	Chromosome 18	>1%
Mulibrey nanism	*TRIM37* (17q22)	7%
Bohring-Optiz	*ASXL1* (20q11.21)	7%
Isolated hemihypertrophy	WT2 locus (11p15.5), among others	5%
Familial Wilms	*FWT1* (17q12-21), *FWT2* (19q13)	Variable, approximately 15–30%
Gorlin (9q22.3 Microdeletion)	*PTCH1* (9q22.3)	<5%
Mosaic Variegated Aneuploidy/Premature Chromatid Separation	*BUB1* (2q13), *TRIP13* (5p15.33)	>20%
Bloom	*RECQL3* (15q26.1)	<5%
Fanconi Anemia with Bialleic BRCA2/PALB2 mutations	*BRCA2* (13q13.1), *PALB2* (16p12.2)	>20%
DICER1	*DICER1* (14q32.13)	<5%
Li Fraumeni	*TP53* (17p13.1)	<5%
Hyperparathyroidism-Jaw Tumor	*HPRT2* (1q31.2)	<5%
PIK3CA-related Segmental Overgrowth (CLOVE)	*PI3KCA* (3q26.32)	<5%
2q37 microdeletion	2q37.1	3%

normal kidney tissue and function and will be discussed later.

WT1, found at chromosome 11p13, encodes for a transcription factor associated with kidney and gonadal development [9]. Mutations of *WT1* are typically autosomal dominant and the majority arise *de novo* [11]. Deletion of *WT1* results in Wilms tumor-Aniridia-Genitourinary anomalies- Intellectual disability (formerly mental Retardation) (WAGR) Syndrome first described in 1964 [12]. Patients with WAGR Syndrome have an approximately 50% lifetime incidence of Wilms tumor [13]. Aniridia is nearly universal and is due to deletion of the neighboring *PAX6* gene, and developmental delay is present in the majority of patients. Renal failure can occur secondary to nephropathy and glomerulonephritis and occurs in 20–40% of patients [14, 15]. Variable screening recommendations for WT in patients with WAGR Syndrome have been proposed. All groups recommend renal ultrasounds every 3–4 months beginning at the time of diagnosis of the underlying syndrome; however, recommended duration varies from through age 5 to through age 8 years [11, 14, 16, 17]. Point mutations of *WT1* result in multiple syndromes, including Denys-Drash and Frasier Syndromes [10, 18, 19]. Denys-Drash Syndrome portends a greater than 90% incidence of WT [10]. On the contrary, patients with Frasier Syndrome have only an 8% likelihood of developing WT [20]. Both may present with nephropathy and genitourinary abnormalities. Males with Denys-Drash Syndrome may present with hypospadias, ambiguous genitalia, or streak gonads. The associated nephropathy (mesangial sclerosis) commonly progresses to end stage kidney disease (ESKD) by the second decade of life. Frasier Syndrome is associated with focal segmental glomerulosclerosis with later onset of renal failure. Patients with Frasier Syndrome have gonadal dysgenesis and a propensity for development of gonadoblastoma in addition to WT [20].

Syndromes associated with the *WT2* gene found at chromosome 11p15 are associated with imprinting or hypermethylation of *WT2* as well as neighboring genes, including *IGF2* and *CDKN1C*. Due to effects on *IGF2*, these syndromes are frequently associated with body and visceral overgrowth [11, 21]. Beckwith-Weidemann Syndrome (BWS) may present with hemihypertrophy, omphalocele or abdominal hernia, macroglossia, ear creases or pits, and neonatal hypoglycemia [20]. Patients with BWS are at increased risk of multiple embryonal tumors, including Wilms tumor, neuroblastoma, hepatoblastoma, and embryonal rhabdomyosarcoma, as well as adrenal cortical carcinoma. The overall malignancy rate approaches 10%, with WT making up approximately 50% of those cancers. Cancer screening recommendations in BWS may be further tailored depending on the specific genes affected; however, general recommendations include ultrasound every 3 months through age 7: abdominal ultrasound until the fourth birthday to also screen for hepatoblastoma followed by renal ultrasounds until the seventh birthday. In addition, alpha fetoprotein (AFP) and urine catecholamines are employed to screen for hepatoblastoma and neuroblastoma, respectively [11, 21]. Table 41.3 provides a complete list of syndromes predisposing to WT.

Pathology

Wilms tumor is an embryonal tumor, arising from pluripotent fetal metanephric tissue. WTs display triphasic histology, including epithelial, stromal, and blastemal components, though monophasic and biphasic tumors can occur (Fig. 41.1). The epithelial component often resembles rudimentary renal tubules; whereas, the blastemal component consists of undifferentiated small blue cells favoring embryonic renal mesenchyme [24]. The compilation of histologic subtypes is a key feature in defining prognosis and occurs along a continuum with epithelial-predominant tumors behaving less aggressively and blastemal-predominant portending increased risk [25–28].

Wilms tumor histology is further classified as favorable histology Wilms tumor (FHWT) versus anaplastic Wilms tumor (AWT) by the presence or absence of anaplasia, described as large, pleomorphic, hyperchromatic tumor cell nuclei with abnormal multipolar mitotic figures (Fig. 41.1) [25]. Anaplasia may be focal or diffuse, and is present in the tumors of 6–8% of patients. Anaplastic Wilms tumor is more common in older patients and in patients of African descent. Anaplasia, especially when diffuse, is associated with chemotherapy resistance and overall poor prognosis [25, 28–30]. Anaplastic Wilms tumors frequently express aberrant *TP53*, a prominent

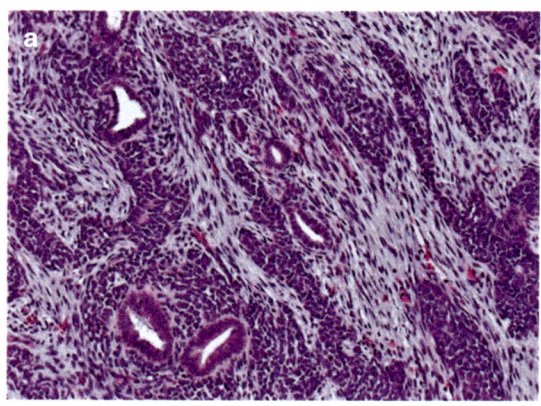
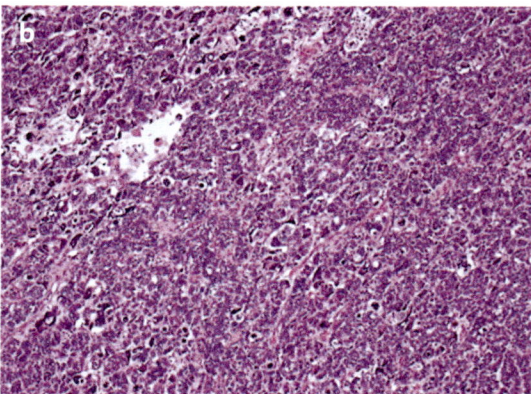

Fig. 41.1 Histology of Wilms tumor—(**a**) Triphasic histology of favorable histology Wilms tumor showing tubule formation by the epithelial component surrounded by blastemal cells separated by pale-colored stroma (200×), (**b**) diffuse anaplastic histology (100×). (Courtesy of Hong Yin, MD; Children's Healthcare of Atlanta)

tumor suppressor gene known to be somatically mutated in many aggressive cancers and associated with the cancer predisposition syndrome, Li Fraumeni Syndrome, when mutated in the germline [31].

Further pathologic characteristics critical for appropriate staging and, therefore, treatment of WT include tumor size and weight; the extent of tumor including involvement of the renal sinus, renal vein, or extension through the renal capsule; margin status following resection; pathologic status of resected peri-renal lymph nodes; and evaluation of additional somatic mutations.

In addition to germline syndromes, somatic mutations commonly found in WTs have both prognostic and therapeutic implications. The most commonly mutated genes in WT include *WT1*, Wnt-signaling pathway genes such as *CTNNB1*, and the oncogene *MYCN*. Therapies targeting several of these frequent mutations are in development [9]. In addition, specific genomic findings, including copy number variations and loss of heterozygosity (LOH), are prognostic in WT, allowing for therapeutic risk-stratification in clinical trials. Adverse biologic markers include LOH of chromosome 1p and 16q, LOH or loss of imprinting at 11p15, gain of 1q, and loss of 17p [9, 31–42].

Nephrogenic Rests and Nephroblastomatosis

Nephrogenic rests and nephroblastomatosis are pre-malignant lesions associated with Wilms tumor. Fetal metanephric cells typically disappear by 36 weeks gestation. Nephrogenic rests are clusters of pluripotent embryonal cells persisting past that developmental time point and into post-natal life [43]. They are common, being incidentally found in 1% of unselected pediatric kidneys at autopsy, 35–40% of kidneys with unilateral WT, and nearly 100% of kidneys with bilateral WTs. Nephroblastomatosis is the presence of multiple or diffuse nephrogenic rests and can be perilobar or intralobar. Nephrogenic rests and nephroblastomatosis may self-resolve, persist, or undergo malignant transformation into

WT [44]. Diffuse hyperplastic perilobar nephroblastomatosis (DHPLN) is a specific form of nephroblastomatosis, strictly defined as "massive enlargement of the kidney with a rind-like expansion of the renal cortex of homogeneous signal intensity, and preservation of the renal shape." DHPLN carries an incredibly high likelihood of malignant transformation and treatment with chemotherapy should be strongly considered even before the development of frank WT [43].

Presentation

Wilms tumor most commonly presents as a painless abdominal mass in a young child, although a minority of patients may present with abdominal pain, gross hematuria, fever, or constipation. Rarely, patients will report anorexia or weight loss. Approximately 25–67% of patients are hypertensive at presentation, predominantly secondary to renin-angiotensin system activation in the setting of renal ischemia. These patients frequently require anti-hypertensive medications prior to nephrectomy which can often be weaned in the weeks following tumor removal [45–48]. Quite rarely, male patients with left-sided renal tumors can present with a left-sided varicocele secondary to compression of the left renal and testicular veins. (The right testicular vein does not arise from the right renal vein, so right-sided varicoceles do not occur) [49]. Although not common, patients can present acutely following subcapsular hemorrhage of their tumor. This can lead to rapid abdominal enlargement, acute anemia, blood pressure abnormalities (hyper- or hypotension), and fever and often requires urgent surgical intervention [50–52]. Patients with WT should be assessed for findings of an associated predisposition syndrome as described previously, including hemihypertrophy, macroglossia, aniridia, genitourinary anomalies, and developmental delay.

Metastatic disease is present in approximately 12% of patients at the time of diagnosis. The lungs are by far the most common site of spread (80%), followed by lymph nodes (15–20%) and the liver (15%), with other sites being extremely rare at the time of presentation. The likelihood of metastatic disease increases with increasing age at diagnosis and with signs of aggressiveness at the primary tumor site [53]. It is rare for a child to present with symptoms related to metastases, which are often only discovered during a thorough staging evaluation.

Evaluation and Staging

Following initial history and physical, pediatric abdominal masses are typically evaluated via ultrasonography. On ultrasound, Wilms tumor can frequently be identified as a well-circumscribed mass of varying echogenicity arising from the kidney. The classic finding is a "claw sign" where the renal parenchyma is seen wrapping around the mass like an open hand or claw [54]. Recommended initial laboratory evaluation includes a complete blood count with differential, complete metabolic panel, urinalysis, coagulation studies, and tumor markers to rule out other common pediatric abdominal tumors (Table 41.2). The complete blood count is important for the evaluation of intra-tumoral hemorrhage, the urinalysis for the evaluation of hematuria, and coagulation studies to evaluate for paraneoplastic acquired Von Willebrand Disease which can accompany WT [55].

Once a renal tumor is suspected on ultrasound, further anatomic imaging of the chest, abdomen, and pelvis should be completed along with consultation of a pediatric oncologist. Abdominopelvic computed tomography (CT) and magnetic resonance imaging (MRI) are both appropriate for further evaluation of renal tumors, although CT is often more facile to obtain at the time of diagnosis (Fig. 41.2). MRI is preferred in cases of suspected bilateral Wilms tumor and in patients with known predisposition syndromes due to improved ability to detect small tumors and nephrogenic rests [54]. In comparison to neuroblastoma, the other most common pediatric abdominal tumor, WTs lack calcifications and push away rather than encase surrounding structures [56]. In addition to further description of the renal mass, including measurement of vol-

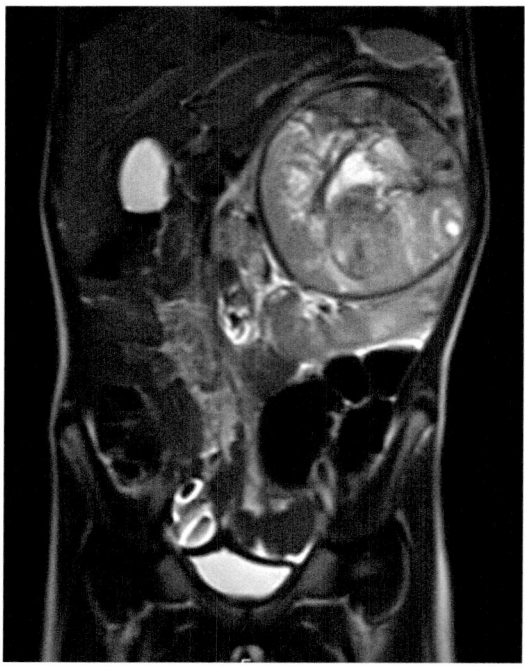

Fig. 41.2 Abdominopelvic T2 sequence magnetic resonance image displaying a left-sided Wilms tumor with left kidney displaced inferiorly and displaying a characteristic "claw sign"

ume and extent of disease, CT/MRI serve to evaluate for tumor thrombus in the renal vein and inferior vena cava (IVC), assess for pathologic adenopathy, and screen the contralateral kidney and liver for additional sites of disease. Finally, a CT of the chest should be obtained to assess for pulmonary metastases [54].

Two different staging systems are employed for Wilms tumor. The varied approaches correspond with the opposing schools of thought regarding treatment approach between the North American and European pediatric oncology cooperative groups. While these differences will be discussed in more detail in the subsequent section "Treatment", it is imperative to understand that the North American (Children's Oncology Group [COG], formerly National Wilms Tumor Study Group [NWTS]) approach to WT includes up front nephrectomy when feasible. This lends itself to a pre-chemotherapy staging system based on extent of local and distant disease, as well as operative findings, including margin

Table 41.4 Renal tumors staging (Children's Oncology Group), applicable to Wilms tumor, clear cell sarcoma of the kidney, malignant rhabdoid tumor, and congenital mesoblastic nephroma; renal cell carcinoma staging discussed separately

Stage	Description
I	Completely resected primary tumor with negative margins
	Tumor limited to the kidney with renal capsule intact
II	Completely resected primary tumor with negative margins, but with extension outside of the kidney via penetration of the capsule, invasion of soft tissue or renal sinus, involvement of extra-renal blood vessels
III	Residual tumor confined to the abdomen
	• Incomplete resection/positive margins
	• Penetration through the peritoneal surface or peritoneal implants
	• Tumor rupture/spillage
	• Pre-operative chemotherapy
	• Pre-operative biopsy
	• Tumor removed in multiple pieces
	• Positive lymph nodes in the abdomen/pelvis
	Tumor excised from the thoracic vena cava or heart
IV	Distant metastases (lung, liver, bone, brain, other)
	Positive lymph nodes beyond the abdomen/pelvis
V	Bilateral renal tumors

status after nephrectomy and the presence of tumor spill into the peritoneal cavity. In addition, patients are up-staged in this system if pre-nephrectomy biopsy or neoadjuvant chemotherapy are undertaken (Table 41.4). On the contrary, the European equivalent to COG, the International Society for Pediatric Oncology (SIOP), uniformly recommends neoadjuvant chemotherapy and utilizes a staging system incorporating post-chemotherapy response. Additionally, pre-operative biopsy does not necessarily require up-staging of the patient in the SIOP system [57].

Treatment

The treatment of Wilms tumor has evolved over the past half century through the efforts of large collaborative groups. In North America this effort was undertaken initially by the NWTS, which has now become COG, while the European approach was developed by SIOP. The treatment paradigms now practiced by both groups espouse multimodal therapy (surgery, chemotherapy, and radiation) tailored by tumor risk classification. SIOP risk assignment is based upon stage, patient age, and post-chemotherapy histology, including extent of tumor necrosis, degree of blastemal tissue, and the presence of focal or diffuse anaplasia. In comparison, COG risk definitions include

additional prognostic factors such as tumor weight and adverse biomarkers such as LOH of 1p and 16q, in addition to stage and histology (favorable vs. anaplastic) [57–59].

In general, the surgical approach for Wilms tumor is radical nephrectomy with sampling of the most proximal draining retroperitoneal lymph nodes. Ideally, the tumor is removed via a trans-abdominal incision with the capsule intact and tumor thrombus removed *en bloc* [58]. COG advocates for nephrectomy at the time of diagnosis whenever feasible. Reasons to delay nephrectomy in the setting of unilateral disease may include tumor thrombus extending above the hepatic veins, tumor invading contiguous organs, high risk of tumor spill or gross residual disease, or pulmonary compromise at the time of diagnosis. In such cases, biopsy is acceptable, although this does up-stage the patient. Nephrectomy should then be performed by weeks 6–12 of therapy. As discussed previously, the European standard is delayed nephrectomy regardless of initial tumor characteristics. This method allows for the incorporation of histologic chemotherapy response into further treatment decisions [57]. Despite their differences, both groups have achieved overall excellent response rates (see section "Prognosis and Outcomes" below).

In the setting of bilateral disease or a known Wilms tumor predisposition syndrome, focus changes to preservation of normal renal parenchyma. This nephron-sparing approach includes neoadjuvant chemotherapy, which may proceed with or without upfront biopsy, followed by partial nephrectomy(ies) with a surgeon with such expertise depending upon tumor response [58, 60, 61].

A small subset of very low-risk patients may be cured by surgery alone, including patients younger than 2 years of age with small stage I tumors. This approach was initially established in the early NWTS trials and confirmed through a later COG trial for low-risk FHWT [40].

The vast majority of patients require chemotherapy in addition to surgery for cure of Wilms tumor. The goal of chemotherapy is to shrink known tumors and prevent the development of distant metastatic disease. Chemotherapy for FHWT builds upon a backbone of two drugs, vincristine and dactinomycin initially established in the first NWTS trial completed in 1975 [62]. Patients with low-stage disease have excellent cure rates with these two drugs alone [42]. Treatment for stage III–IV tumors or tumors with adverse prognostics markers such as combined LOH at 1p and 16q, includes at minimum the addition of the anthracycline doxorubicin and treatment for longer duration [39]. Additional agents such as cyclophosphamide and etoposide may be required for stage IV patients based on response of pulmonary metastatic disease and the presence of extra-pulmonary metastases [63]. Anaplastic Wilms tumor routinely requires aggressive chemotherapy, especially in the setting of diffuse anaplasia [30].

In patients with FHWT, radiation is reserved for patients with stage III–IV disease. Radiation to the primary renal tumor site is confined to the flank unless there is concern for gross tumor spill or peritoneal spread and is given at modest doses of 10.5–10.8 Gy. Radiation is also indicated for local control of extra-abdominal sites of metastatic disease, except that pulmonary radiation may be avoided in patients with a complete response of pulmonary disease to chemotherapy by week 6 [63]. Patients with stage II–IV AWT also require radiotherapy, while results from both COG and SIOP suggest omission of radiation for patients with stage I disease is possible in the setting of three-drug chemotherapy including doxorubicin [64, 65].

Prognosis and Outcomes

The overall prognosis for Wilms tumor has improved significantly since the adoption of multimodal therapy from 0% overall survival in the early twentieth century to 90% today; however, there remain a significant number of patients with more guarded outcomes [2, 58, 62, 66, 67]. In addition, the excellent outcomes for patients with low-risk disease require evaluation of when and where therapy can be further de-escalated.

Prognosis depends mostly upon stage and histology. Patients with low stage and favorable histology with epithelial predominance fare best even with limited therapy, while patients with higher stage and blastemal predominance or anaplasia fare the worst [26, 27, 30, 40, 63, 68]. Additional indicators of poor prognosis include older age at diagnosis, larger tumor size, and adverse chromosomal abnormalities including LOH at 1p and 16q, gain of 1q, loss of 11p15 (specific to very low-risk WT), and loss of 17p [9, 31–41, 57, 69–73]. Outcomes based on the most recently completed series of COG clinical trials are reviewed in Table 41.5. SIOP results have been similar. Salvage after relapse is possible, with a 5-year overall survival of 50%. Outcomes following relapse depend upon initial stage and treatment with patients initially receiving fewer chemotherapy agents faring better than those who required more aggressive treatment up front [74–76].

Late Effects

The multimodal therapy required to produce such excellent cure rates for Wilms tumor leads to significant late effects, with approximately 20% of long-term survivors reporting severe (grade 3–5) late effects at 20 years after diagnosis [78, 79]. In general, the adverse effects expected vary significantly based upon the presence of bilateral renal

Table 41.5 Results of COG renal tumors studies

Study	Stage/histology	Subgroup	Chemotherapy	Outcomes	Reference
AREN0532	Stage I FHWT	Very low-risk (age < 2 years, tumor < 550 g)	None	4-year EFS: 89.7% 4-year OS: 100%	[40]
	Stage I/II FHWT	LOH 1p + 16q	EE4A → DD4A	4-year EFS: 87.3% 4-year OS: 100%	[39]
	Stage III FHWT	No LOH 1p + 16q	DD4A	4-year EFS: 88% 4-year OS: 97%	[41]
		Negative LN and no LOH 1p or 16q	DD4A	4-year EFS: 96.7% 4-year OS: 99.4%	[41]
		Positive LN and either LOH 1p or 16q	DD4A	4-year EFS: 74% 4-year OS 92.4%	[41]
AREN0533	Stage III/IV FHWT	LOH 1p + 16q	DD4A → Regimen M	4-year EFS: 90.2% 4-year OS: 96.1%	[39]
	Stage IV FHWT	All	DD4A or DD4A→ Regimen M	4-year EFS: 85.4% 4-year OS: 95.6%	[63]
		LOH 1p + 16q	DD4A → Regimen M	4-year EFS: 100% 4-year OS: 100%	[63]
		No LOH, isolated lung mets, RCR	DD4A	4-year EFS: 79.5% 4-year OS: 96.1%	[63]
		No LOH, isolated lung mets, SIR	DD4A→ Regimen M	4-year EFS: 88.5% 4-year OS: 95.4%	[63]
		Isolated lung mets, RCR, gain of 1q	DD4A	4-year EFS: 57% 4-year OS: 89%	[63]
		Isolated lung mets, RCR, no gain of 1q	DD4A	4-year EFS: 86% 4-year OS: 97%	[63]
		Isolated lung mets, SIR, gain of 1q	DD4A → Regimen M	4-years EFS: 86% 4-years OS: 93%	[63]
		Isolated lung mets, SIR, no gain of 1q	DD4A → Regimen M	4-year EFS: 92% 4-year OS: 96%	[63]
AREN0534	Stage V (bilateral) FHWT	All	Most VAD → then per histology	4-year EFS: 82.1% 4-year OS: 94.9% 39% retained parts of both kidneys	[61]
	Variable	Unilateral tumors, multicentric or in predisposed patients	Variable	4-year EFS: 94% 4-year OS: 100%	[77]

(continued)

Table 41.5 (continued)

Study	Stage/histology	Subgroup	Chemotherapy	Outcomes	Reference
AREN0321	Stage I FAWT or DAWT	All	DD-4A	4-year EFS: 100% 4-year OS: 100%	[65]
	Stage II DAWT	All	Regimen UH-1	4-year EFS: 86.7% 4-year OS: 86.2%	[30]
	Stage III DAWT	All	Regimen UH-1	4-year EFS: 80.9% 4-year OS: 88.6%	[30]
	Stage IV DAWT	All	Regimen UH-1 or VI + Regimen UH-2	4-year EFS: 41.7% 4-year OS: 49.2%	[30]

FHWT favorable histology Wilms tumor, *DAWT* diffuse anaplastic Wilms tumor, *EFS* event free survival, *OS* overall survival, *Mets* metastases, *RCR* rapid complete response, *SIR* slow incomplete response, *EE4A* vincristine/actinomycin, *DD4A* vincristine/actinomycin/doxorubicin, *Regimen M* vincristine/actinomycin/doxorubicin/etoposide/cyclophosphamide, *VAD* vincristine/actinomycin/doxorubicin, *Regimen UH-1* vincristine/actinomycin/doxorubicin/carboplatin/etoposide/cyclophosphamide, *VI* vincristine/irinotecan, *Regimen UH-2* vincristine/actinomycin/doxorubicin/carboplatin/etoposide/cyclophosphamide/irinotecan

tumors, chemotherapy regimen, and use of radiation.

The cumulative incidence of ESKD in patients with unilateral WT at 20 years after diagnosis is less than 1%; whereas, the incidence increases to 12% in patients with bilateral WT [80]. The rate is increased in patients with metachronous presentation of bilateral disease and is as high as 19.3% [81]. The risk of renal disease is also impacted by underlying predisposition syndromes associated with nephropathy such as WAGR, Denys-Drash, and Frasier Syndromes, as well as the presence of intralobar nephrogenic rests [13, 80, 81]. Lower-stage chronic kidney disease occurs, however, in 23–55% of patients, and a significant proportion of patients have chronic hypertension by their mid-20s [82–84]. Patients requiring only unilateral nephrectomy without nephrotoxic chemotherapy or radiation have a much lower risk of chronic kidney disease and hypertension [85].

Renal toxicity can occur due to nephron loss during surgical resection and secondary to chemotherapy and ionizing radiation. The etiology of renal failure is more commonly surgical for patients with bilateral disease who require either bilateral nephrectomies or partial nephrectomies resulting in less than 25% residual renal parenchyma [80]. Patients requiring only unilateral nephrectomy are typically able to maintain renal function through compensatory hypertrophy of the remaining kidney [86]. The frequency of nephron-sparing surgery in patients with bilateral disease and those with WT arising in a solitary kidney is an on-going focus of research. On the COG study AREN0534, 39% of patients with bilateral WT retained parts of both kidneys and only 2.5% required bilateral nephrectomies following neoadjuvant chemotherapy [61].

The chemotherapy agents required for the majority of Wilms tumor patients (vincristine, dactinomycin, and doxorubicin) are rarely implicated in long-term renal toxicity; however, the alkylating agent ifosfamide and platinum agent carboplatin utilized for augmentation of therapy in more aggressive disease or in the setting of relapse may adversely affect renal function [87]. This risk is higher in younger patients and when combined with other nephrotoxic exposures, including additional nephrotoxic medications, renal radiation, and nephrectomy [88]. Radiation nephritis is the cause of renal failure in a minority of patients and is rare at the typical radiation doses used in the treatment of WT [88, 89]. Recommendations for screening for renal late effects is variable based on treatment received. Most patients treated for WT will require annual blood pressure monitoring, creatinine assessment, and urinalysis, with electrolyte monitoring recommended at the time of entry into long-term follow-up and then as needed. Counseling is required regarding risk of renal injury in the setting of a single kidney and use of nephrotoxic medication should be limited [90].

The most notable non-renal late effects for these patients include cardiac toxicity in the setting of doxorubicin exposure, secondary malignancies and poor growth due to both chemotherapy and radiation exposure, and infertility for patients requiring alkylating agents or carboplatin [91].

Clear Cell Sarcoma of the Kidney

Epidemiology

Clear cell sarcoma of the kidney (CCSK) is the second most common renal neoplasm in young children, accounting for 2–5% of primary kidney cancers in this demographic [92, 93]. It was first described by Kidd in 1970 and subsequently noted to be distinct from Wilms tumor due to its propensity to metastasize to bone [25, 92–95]. It presents more commonly in males than females at a 2:1 ratio. Clear cell sarcoma of the kidney is seen most commonly in toddlers with a median age at diagnosis of 36 months, and 50% arising in 2–3 year olds in the NTWS trials. It is incredibly rare in infants less than 6 months [92, 93, 96]. There are no known predisposition syndromes, although there is at least one case reported in a patient with Fanconi anemia [97].

Pathology

Clear cell sarcoma of the kidney typically presents as a large, unilateral, well-circumscribed mass. CCSK displays heterogeneous histology, with upwards of nine different histologic types described. Most tumors include the classic variant described as nests and cords of round or oval cells separated by fibrovascular septae. The clear cell appearance arises from extracellular mucopolysaccharide matrix located between the cord cells. Additional variants include: myxoid, sclerosing, cellular, epithelioid, palisading, spindle cell, storiform, and anaplastic patterns [92, 93, 98]. Most tumors contain a mixture of subtypes and, unlike WT, histologic subtypes are not used for risk stratification. There are two predominant known somatic genetic findings in CCSK which are mutually exclusive: a translocation involving *YWHAE* and *NUTM2B/E* (previously *FAM22*), t(10;17)(q22;p13), and internal tandem duplications of the BCL-6 co-receptor, *BCOR*. A third subset of patients displays neither event [92, 99, 100]. *TP53* is located at 17p13 and is overexpressed in the small subset of anaplastic CCSK, but does not seem to be a predominant driver in CCSK. A BCOR fusion has also been identified in a small case series of CCSK [99, 101]. Like histology, to date specific genetic findings have not been utilized for risk classification.

Presentation and Evaluation

Similar to WT, CCSK presents in young children as a painless abdominal mass or distension, although abdominal pain, hematuria, vomiting, anorexia, fever, constipation, and hypertension have all been reported. In addition, patients with metastatic disease may present with symptoms of bone pain or mass [92, 100, 102]. The initial workup mimics that of WT, including ultrasound followed by cross sectional imaging with CT or MRI. There are no defining imaging characteristics to differentiate CCSK from the much more common WT, and the diagnosis is often not made until postoperative pathologic review of the nephrectomy specimen.

The staging of CCSK is similar to that for WT. A minority (4–7%) of cases of CCSK are metastatic at diagnosis. The pattern of metastatic spread differs from WT, with CCSK having a strong propensity for bone and brain, although like WT can also affect regional lymph nodes and liver. Bilateral tumors are exceedingly rare [92, 93, 96]. As a result, in addition to a chest CT, the metastatic workup includes a brain MRI and systemic imaging for bony disease such as nuclear medicine bone scan or positron emission tomography scan.

Treatment

The treatment of CCSK is multimodal and includes surgery, chemotherapy, and radiation. The chemotherapy and radiation is more aggressive than that required for many patients with WT.

The surgical approach mimics that for WT, with COG advocating for upfront nephrectomy when feasible while SIOP recommends delayed nephrectomy following neoadjuvant chemotherapy [100, 103]. As in WT, sampling of lymph nodes is important for accurate staging [96, 104]. Given the rarity of bilateral disease, the focus on nephron-sparing surgery is less consequential in CCSK. Surgical metastasectomy is considered for feasible sites and level of disease burden.

Chemotherapy recommendations for CCSK are similar to those for high-risk WT. In the SIOP approach, patients with localized disease are treated initially with vincristine and dactinomycin, with doxorubicin added for patients with distant metastatic disease at diagnosis [103]. Both SIOP and NWTS/COG have demonstrated improved survival when doxorubicin is included in the treatment of CCSK, so the anthracycline is started or continued after nephrectomy once the diagnosis of CCSK is confirmed [93, 103]. In addition, the alkylating agents ifosfamide and cyclophosphamide along with etoposide are added for all stages [103]. In North America, patients with CCSK have been treated with a regimen of cyclophosphamide and etoposide alternating with vincristine, doxorubicin, and cyclophosphamide since the study NWTS-5 in the mid-1990s [92, 104].

Most patients with CCSK require additional local control with radiation. In Europe, stage I CCSK patients have been spared radiation. A study in the United Kingdom omitted radiation for stage II patients, but revealed a high rate of local treatment failures, emphasizing the importance of radiotherapy in this group [92, 96]. Both collaborative groups recommend radiation for local control of metastatic disease [103, 104].

Prognosis and Outcomes

Outcomes for patients with CCSK are more guarded, leading to its label as a high-risk renal tumor. Prognosis depends most notably upon stage, with 5-year event-free survival (EFS) of 91% and overall survival (OS) of 98% for patients with stage I/II disease on the COG trial NWTS-5, compared with 79% and 90% for stage III/IV patients. The relatively poor prognosis is most pronounced in the metastatic patients, who when evaluated individually had a 5-year EFS of only 29% and OS of 36% [104]. Results by stage follow a similar trend in SIOP trials, with the 5-year EFS and OS for stage I patients reported as 79% and 87%, respectively, and that for stage IV being 59% and 73%, respectively [96]. Patients who fall outside of the typical age-range of 2–3 years at diagnosis also seem to fare more poorly [93, 96]. Clear cell sarcoma of the kidney differs from other pediatric renal tumors concerning the timing of relapse. Although most relapses occur by 3 years, a small subset of patients present with recurrent tumor 5–10 years after initial presentation, necessitating prolonged surveillance. The frequency of late relapses does, however, appear to be decreasing in the era of modern chemotherapy regimens [92, 100, 103, 104]. Most relapses are to metastatic sites, including brain, lung, and bone. Patients with relapsed disease are potentially salvageable with aggressive multimodal therapy; therefore, long-term follow-up to detect potentially treatable relapses is critical [105].

Late Effects

The late effects following treatment for CCSK are less well studied than that of WT due to the significantly smaller patient population. In general, the renal long-term complications of unilateral nephrectomy are the same as for WT, and the need for bilateral renal surgeries is essentially non-existent. However, the chemotherapy used up front, most notably ifosfamide and carboplatin, is more nephrotoxic than the therapy required for the majority of WT patients, and most patients require radiation. Nearly all patients will require routine monitoring of renal function and blood pressure. The risk for non-renal late effects is higher secondary to the augmented therapy required for all patients with CCSK and includes cardiac toxicity, secondary malignancies, poor growth, and fertility concerns.

Malignant Rhabdoid Tumor

Malignant rhabdoid tumor (MRT) of the kidney was identified in the late 1970s and early 1980s as part of the NWTS [106]. This tumor is an aggressive cancer with poor prognosis despite intensive chemotherapy, radiation therapy, and surgical management. These cancers share biology with renal medullary carcinomas (below), atypical teratoid rhabdoid tumors, and epithelioid sarcomas through the loss of *SMARCB1* and less commonly *SMARCA4*, both members of the SWI/SNF chromatin-remodeling complex. Rhabdoid tumor only causes 3% of pediatric renal tumors [107]. Studies have shown that children with rhabdoid tumors were demographically similar to case controls [108] and usually presented in the first year of life [109–111].

There are two known predisposition syndromes associated with MRT: rhabdoid tumor predisposition syndromes 1 and 2 (RTPS1/2). Patients have germline pathogenic variants in *SMARCB1* and *SMARCA4* [112]. These patients usually develop cancer at a median age of 4–7 months; whereas, those with sporadic MRT have a median age of presentation of 18 months. There are other germline variants of *SMARCB1* and *SMARCA4* that lead to Coffin-Siris Syndrome, but these mutations are not known to lead to cancer. Recently, SIOP has put forth a set of recommendations for patients/probands with RTPS [112].

SMARCB1 is part of the SWI/SNF complex and serves as a tumor suppressor. This complex is preserved across species and affects many cancer related pathways such as the Hedgehog-Gli, Wnt/b-catenin, and retinoblastoma pathways along with pathways involving cell motility and differentiation [113–115].

Patients present similarly to others with abdominal masses, but in some cases disease progression is swift, prompting emergent chemotherapy. Staging of MRT is the same as for WT and CCSK. Currently, therapy is a combination of chemotherapy, surgery, and radiation therapy (depending on the age of the patient). There is suggestion that lower-stage MRTs are able to achieve cure with a 4-year overall survival in the 40% range. Yet, many patients have higher-stage disease, with 4-year overall survival <20% [109–111, 116, 117].

Pediatric Renal Cell Carcinoma

Renal cell carcinomas (RCC) are a group of heterogenous kidney tumors predominantly seen in adults. However, RCCs occur in children and young adults as well [118].

Pediatric and adolescent/young adult (AYA) renal cell carcinomas (pRCCs) account for 2–4% of childhood kidney cancers [119]. When further subtyped, MiT-RCC (or translocation RCC) are the most common RCC in childhood, causing 42% of RCCs. Other RCCs include papillary, chromophobe, clear-cell (the most common kidney cancer in adults), renal medullary carcinomas (RMC; further discussed below), fumarate hydratase-deficient, succinate dehydrogenase-deficient, TSC-associated (further discussed below), ALK-rearranged, thyroid-like, and myoepithelial carcinomas (see Fig. 41.3) [118]. Another 7–8% of RCCs are unclassified.

A number of predisposition genes have been implicated in this group of heterogenous cancers [120]. These include *VHL* (Von Hippel-Lindau disease and clear cell RCCs), *MET* (hereditary

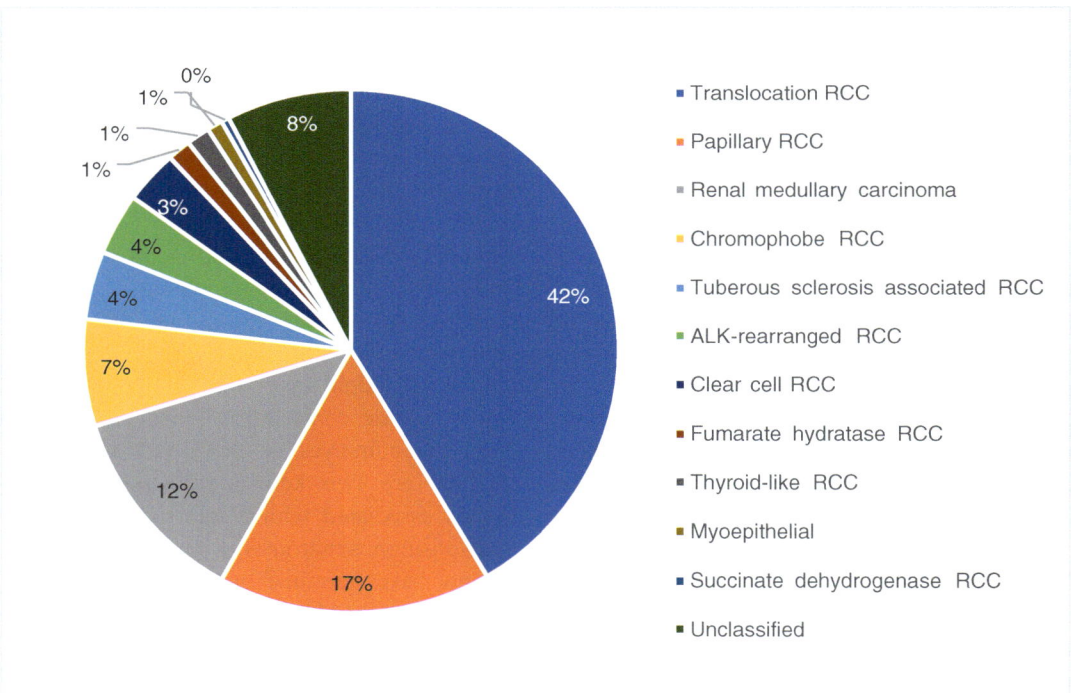

Fig. 41.3 Distribution of 212 pediatric and young adult RCCs from Cajaiba et al. [118]

papillary renal carcinoma; HPRC), *FLCN* (Birt-Hogg-Dube syndrome and various RCCs), *FH* (hereditary leiomyomatosis and renal cell carcinoma; HLRCC), *SDHB/C/D* (Succinate dehydrogenase-deficient renal cell carcinoma), *TSC1/2* (tuberous sclerosis complex; TSC), and mutations in *BAP1* and *MiTF*. Presentations of such tumors can occur in the second decade, but some are not seen until the sixth or seventh decade (e.g., HPRC). While the pathogenesis of cancer predisposition syndromes such as VHL have been well characterized [121], other genes of importance remain an area of study.

The clinical presentation of most pRCCs is similar to that of a child or young adult with any new renal tumor. Usually, the patient will have a painless but enlarging abdominal mass. Occasionally, there will be microscopic or gross hematuria depending on the location of the tumor, unexplained hypertension, or polycythemia. As described for WT, workup usually proceeds with imaging of the abdomen via ultrasound followed by a CT of the chest and CT or MRI of the abdomen and pelvis. Outside of a classical "claw sign," which usually is suggestive of a WT, the COG approach is to either request a pediatric surgical consultation to determine the feasibility of a nephrectomy or biopsy. In cases with bilateral tumors and depending on the patient's age, further discussions are needed to determine if upfront chemotherapy is preferred over biopsy.

Staging of pRCCs is based on the adult RCC staging system, the American Joint Committee on Cancer (AJCC)—TNM Staging System for Kidney Cancer [122]. The primary tumor is assessed by size in greatest dimension (T1 is 7.0 cm or less while T2 is greater than 7.0 cm) and whether the tumor has invaded or extended into the renal veins or above the diaphragm (T3a–c) or beyond Gerota's fascia (T4). Regional lymph nodes are then assessed as the lack of lymph node involvement (N0); involvement of a single lymph node (N1); or of more than one (N2). Metastasis is a binary categorization (M0 for no distant metastasis and M1 for distant metastasis). Based on the TNM status, stage grouping is assigned. Primary tumors at or less than 7.0 cm in dimension are classified as stage I,

while stage II is larger than 7.0 cm in dimension. Single regional lymph node involvement (N1) or invasion of the renal veins (T3a–c) is considered stage III. Stage IV disease includes any T1–3 which has multiple regional lymph node involvement (N2) or distant metastasis (M1) and includes tumors that invade Gerota's fascia (T4).

While it is unclear whether the biology of pRCCs is similar to adult RCCs, there is evidence that outcomes are different. COG AREN0321, a phase II study, prospectively assessed outcomes in children and young adults with pRCCs. If complete resection was done, there was no further therapy. For those who had incomplete resections, given the generally poor outcomes and lack of definitive therapies, institutional preference dictated treatment options (e.g. immunotherapy or tyrosine kinase inhibitors). Those with stage I, II, and III disease had 96%, 100% and 88% 4-year overall survival, respectively [123]. However, those with stage IV disease had poor outcomes, with a 29% 4-year overall survival. Primary deaths occurred in patients with either translocation RCC or renal medullary carcinoma.

In summary, pRCCs are a heterogeneous group of kidney cancers for which some have an underlying cancer predisposition syndrome. This group of cancers make up the second most common kidney cancers in children, with the majority occurring in adolescent patients. Short-term outcomes for stage I–III pRCCs remain good with a 4-year overall survival in the 88–100% range. However, stage IV pRCCs (primarily translocation RCCs and renal medullary carcinomas) have poor outcomes.

Renal Medullary Carcinoma

Renal medullary carcinoma (RMC) is a subtype of renal cell carcinoma driven by loss of *SMARCB1*. Unlike malignant rhabdoid tumor, RMC occurs primarily in adolescents and young adults of African descent with sickle cell trait [124–128]. Estimated prevalence based on United States data is 5 in 100,000 patients with sickle cell trait [126, 129]. Although sickle cell trait is the primary hemoglobinopathy associated with this cancer, there are case reports of other hemoglobinopathies such as sickle cell disease (HbSC and HbSS). There is no known predisposition syndrome other than the association with sickle cell trait. The gene implicated in RMC is *SMARCB1*, which has been discussed in reference to MRT above. Here, the primary mode of disruption is through a translocation event.

Currently, there is no standard of care treatment for RMC given the rarity of this disease and age of presentation (around 10–40 years). However, general consensus among physicians involved in the care of patients with RMC has been to treat with a platinum agent along with other chemotherapy, nephrectomy, and radiation therapy [130, 131]. Despite this aggressive approach, outcomes for RMC remain very poor as overall survival ranges from 4–5 months to 17–18 months for those with or without metastatic disease, respectively [129, 132].

Renal Angiomyolipoma and Epithelioid Angiomyolipoma

Renal angiomyolipomas (AML) are another rare kidney tumor which are considered benign tumors, but may lead to complications given the location [133]. First identified in 1900, AML describes the histopathological features of abnormal blood vessels with components of smooth muscle and adipose tissue [134]. Even more rare is epithelioid angiomyolipoma (EAML), a subtype of angiomyolipoma which is defined by having >10% epithelioid cells by histopathology. Renal AML, depending on the populations studied, affects women more than men [134, 135]. There is a bimodal distribution for the time of presentation. For those with an underlying genetic predisposition, they usually present during the first several decades, while sporadic renal AMLs tend to occur in the fourth or fifth decade [134–136].

Predisposition for renal AML has been associated with tuberous sclerosis complex (TSC) or lymphangioleiomyomatosis (LAM). Genes involved in TSC or LAM include *TSC1* and *TSC2*. TSC1 and TSC2 form a complex which inhibits downstream targets of mechanistic target of rapamycin (mTOR) [137]. For patients with TSC diagnosed in childhood, renal AML occur in over 50% of patients, typically arising in adolescents/young adults [138].

The clinical presentation for renal AMLs differs slightly from other renal tumors as hemorrhage is more commonly seen as compared to microscopic or gross hematuria [134]. Patients also present with abdominal pain or flank pain. AML is likely in a child with TSC presenting with a new renal mass.

Prior management was a complete or partial nephrectomy, but as the natural history of this tumor has been studied for the past century, more conservative approaches are being taken [139]. These lesions grow slowly so surveillance may be used as an initial approach in many patients. Medical therapy with an mTOR inhibitor, everolimus, is an option in select patients (sirolimus is also effective). Outstanding questions remain regarding the duration of therapy as lesions may regrow after a year of treatment. Recent studies have looked at extending therapy to 2 years with minimal regrowth during the second year of therapy. Overall response rate was 44% in patients with TSC or LAM [140]. These findings were further validated in the phase III EXIST-2 trial and the follow-up extension phase where patients received treatment for up to 4 years [141, 142]. Currently, surgery is not recommended, particularly for those with TSC given the potential growth of new renal AMLs in the remaining tissue, thereby compromising renal function further. Another approach is embolization of the vascular supply for the renal AMLs, but this is considered second-line therapy. For EAMLs, little is available to suggest a standard of care. Furthermore, for patients with a known history of TSC, abdominal imaging (ideally MRI) is recommended every 1–3 years throughout the patient's lifetime.

Ewing Sarcoma of the kidney

Ewing sarcoma of the kidney is a rare renal tumor with few cases in the literature. As the name implies, this renal tumor has a fusion oncoprotein between *EWS* and members of the

ETS family such as *FLI1* or *ERG*. Furthermore, these tumors express CD99, which can be detected by immunohistochemistry. The epidemiology of this cancer is not well described given the rarity and is limited to single institution experiences. Furthermore, there is no known predisposition syndrome related to this particular renal tumor.

Here, we will describe the M.D. Anderson experience as it is the most comprehensive institutional review to date of patients presenting with this renal tumor over 23 years [143]. Patients with Ewing sarcoma of the kidney presented with new flank or abdominal pain and/or hematuria. Age of presentation ranged from 8 to 69 years, with a median age at diagnosis of 30.5 years.

Staging was as follows: Group I had tumor confined to the kidney, Group II had local extension, and Group III had metastatic disease. Therapy included nephrectomy (Groups I and II primarily had upfront surgery, whereas Group III patients had biopsy initially and then subsequent nephrectomy with or without neoadjuvant chemotherapy), chemotherapy, and in some cases radiation therapy. Chemotherapy regimens included those utilized to treat extra-renal Ewing sarcomas, but a limitation noted by the authors was that this was inconsistent over the 23-year experience.

Overall, outcomes were poor. Four-year event free survival was 43% and overall survival was 63%. Those with metastatic disease had poorer outcomes. For those with Group I disease, nephrectomy followed by chemotherapy had a more favorable outcome, suggestive of potential for cure.

Congenital Mesoblastic Nephroma

Congenital mesoblastic nephroma (CMN) is a renal tumor that occurs in infancy. It has a low malignant potential and accounts for 2–3% of all pediatric renal tumors [144–146]. With respect to predisposition syndromes, there has been a rare association of Beckwith-Wiedemann syndrome in several case reports. Otherwise, congenital anomalies have been identified in several patients,

but there have been no other constitutional syndromes identified. There are three subtypes of CMNs: classic, cellular and mixed (both classic and cellular) type. The genomics of the classic and mixed type of CMNs have not been well characterized. However in cellular, the most common genetic aberration is a translocation of t(12;15)(p13;q25) leading to a fusion of *ETV6* and *NTRK3* [147, 148]. Furthermore, trisomy 11 has been identified in this group.

CMN may present as either a mass detected during a prenatal ultrasound or in an infant found to have a new abdominal mass, hypertension, or hematuria. There may also be polyhydramnios, hypercalcemia, and hyperreninemia, with the latter two resolving following resection of the tumor [146]. Staging for CMNs follows that of WT, MRT, and CCSK. Please refer to staging in those sections. Treatment for these patients has primarily been surgical, with less consensus on postoperative therapies such as chemotherapy and radiation therapy.

The SIOP/German Society of Oncology and Hematology (GPOH) experience with CMNs showed that 5-year relapse free survival and overall survival were 93.8% and 96.1%, respectively [144]. Those with cellular or mixed MN had inferior relapse free survival as compared to classic MN, but overall survival was similar across these subtypes. This experience was similar to that of the United Kingdom Children's Cancer and Leukaemia Group [149]. Similar to that of other renal tumors, long-term issues relate to caring for a patient with a solitary kidney.

Cystic Tumors

Cystic tumors are rare and usually benign renal tumors which account for <1% of pediatric renal tumors [150]. These are further sub-categorized into cystic nephromas (CN) or cystic partially differentiated nephroblastoma (CPDN). In the case of CNs, there is an association with *DICER1* [151] and *DICER1* syndromes which may lead to tumors in the lungs, ovaries, thyroid and kidneys. Patients usually present with CNs in the first few years of life or during the AYA period. There is a skew toward females being affected. For CPDN, there is no known genetic predisposition.

Children present with a new abdominal mass (may be an incidental finding unless there is a known personal or family history for *DICER1*). Bosniak imaging scores (based on classifying adult renal cysts from a benign simple cyst to a malignant cystic mass) allows one to assess concerns for malignancy based on imaging [152]. Staging in CNs or CPDNs requires chest to pelvis imaging given risks of identifying an underlying *DICER1* syndrome. Pathology and treatment is primarily surgical in nature and, given the rarity, it is unclear if chemotherapy plays a role in these relatively benign tumors [150]. However, there is an association with *DICER1*-renal sarcomas in CNs suggestive that similar to pleuropulmonary blastoma in the lungs, there is a range of potential tumors that can develop in the kidney for those with *DICER1* syndrome [153].

Overall outcomes from small patient cohorts in national or international trials suggests that CNs or CPDNs are benign in nature. Given the potential risk of additional malignancies in patients with CNs in particular, referral to a cancer predisposition clinic is warranted.

Ossifying Renal Tumor of Infancy

Ossifying renal tumor of infancy (ORTI) was first described in 1980 [154]. It is extremely rare, with well under 50 cases reported in the literature [155]. Approximately 90% present in the first year of life and the oldest reported patient presented at 30 months. There is a strong male predominance [156, 157]. It most commonly presents with gross hematuria, although rarely a palpable abdominal mass is appreciated [156, 158]. Reported cases have been exclusively unilateral, and ORTI carries no known risk of metastasis [155, 156]. Imaging reveals an intact renal outline with a calcified intrapelvic mass which is hypointense on T2-weighted MRI [159]. Upon resection, ORTI is typically attached to a papilla within the calyceal lumen. On histopathologic examination, ORTI are composed of osteoid, osteoblastic cells, and spindle cells. The degree

of ossification increases with older age at presentation. Interestingly, the spindle cell component may represent hyperplastic intralobar nephrogenic rests (see section "Nephrogenic Rests and Nephroblastomatosis" under Wilms Tumor) while the osseous component may be urothelial in origin [157]. No predisposition syndromes are known to be associated with ORTI. Clonal trisomy 4 has been detected in multiple tumor specimens [156, 160].

Although quite rare, knowledge of ORTI, including the typical presentation and imaging appearance, is important. Treatment for ORTI is surgical and may be via complete or partial nephrectomy as dictated by size and location within the kidney. There is no requirement for systemic therapy and to date no recurrences have been reported [155, 156]. The late effects of treatment are limited to the risk of nephron loss due to nephrectomy.

Metanephric Tumors

Metanephric adenoma (MA), metanephric adenofibroma (MAF), and metanephric stromal tumor (MST) are described together as metanephric tumors in the 2016 World Health Organization Classification of tumors of the kidney [161]. These three neoplasms share morphologic features with WT and are considered by some authors to represent differentiated tumors along the same spectrum [162]. Metanephric adenoma is purely epithelial and can closely resemble epithelial-predominant WT, MST is purely stromal, and MAF is biphasic, containing both epithelial and stromal elements. There are no reliable distinguishing imaging features allowing separation of these mostly benign tumors from WT, and as such, they may inadvertently be treated with neoadjuvant chemotherapy.

Metanephric adenoma was first described in detail in 1995. It can occur across the age spectrum, and when compared with MST and MAF, is the most common of the three in adult patients. There is a female predominance. In nearly 50% of cases, it is identified incidentally; however, it can present with polycythemia, hypertension, hematuria, abdominal pain, or a palpable abdominal mass. It is routinely unilateral. Histologically, MA is described as small acinar cells within an acellular stroma, and the majority of cases express BRAF V600E mutations [163–165]. It is considered a benign lesion, although several reports of metastatic disease do exist [166]. In addition, there are overlap lesions between MA and epithelial WT [167]. Treatment is nephrectomy or partial nephrectomy followed by observation excepting in cases overlapping with WT or with metastases, and outcomes are typically excellent.

A purely stromal metanephric neoplasm coined metanephric stromal tumor was first noted by Beckwith in 1998 and further described in a review of 31 cases by Argani and Beckwith in 2000. In this initial review, the median age at diagnosis was 13 months, ranging from newborns to 11 years [168]. A more recent review reported a median age of 2 years and included three adult patients. There does not appear to be a strong gender predilection. Most patients present with an asymptomatic abdominal mass, although hematuria, hypertension, and abdominal pain have been reported. All cases are unilateral, although multifocal disease does occur [169]. Under the microscope these tumors develop a characteristic "onion skin" pattern of rings of cells surrounding renal tubules or blood vessels [168, 169]. A majority of MST have BRAF V600E mutations which can serve to differentiate them from other renal stromal tumors and provides further link to MA [170]. Despite one report of metastatic disease, most MST are cured with nephrectomy alone. As such, care must be taken to distinguish these tumors from more aggressive stromal renal tumors such as CCSK, which require much more aggressive intervention [168, 169].

The mixed lesion, metanephric adenofibroma, was originally reported in 1992 [171]. The stromal component of these tumors resembles, although is distinct from, mesoblastic nephroma, and is identical to MST, while the epithelial component favors nephroblastomatosis and epithelial WT and is identical to MA. Additionally, some tumors are described as MAF transitioning to epithelial-predominant WT. Finally, there may also be a component of low-grade papillary carcinoma or adenosarcoma present. Similar to MA and MST, patients presented with polycythemia, hypertension, or hematuria which resolved following nephrectomy [171, 172]. The median age at diagnosis in a series of 25 patients from the NWTS studies was 30 months, although MAF can present in adolescents and young adults [173]. This tumor is more common in males at a ratio of 2:1 [172]. Historically, all patients were treated similar to WT, with nephrectomy and adjuvant chemotherapy. More recently, patients with MAF without evidence of a malignant component are typically observed after nephrectomy with good outcomes [172].

Summary

Although overall uncommon, within the context of pediatric extra-cranial solid tumors pediatric renal tumors make up a large proportion of diagnoses. Accurate diagnosis is critical as the necessary treatment and prognosis varies greatly. Pediatric nephrologists may be involved at many points during the care of these patients, including initial diagnosis in a patient who presents with hematuria, early management in a patient with hypertension, and long-term in patients with significant nephron-loss or treatment-induced nephropathy.

References

1. SEER Cancer Statistics Review, 1975–2017 [Internet]. SEER. [cited 2021 Jan 21]. Available from: https://seer.cancer.gov/csr/1975_2017/index.html.
2. Dome JS, Fernandez CV, Mullen EA, Kalapurakal JA, Geller JI, Huff V, et al. Children's Oncology Group's 2013 blueprint for research: renal tumors. Pediatr Blood Cancer. 2013;60(6):994–1000.
3. Lowe LH, Isuani BH, Heller RM, Stein SM, Johnson JE, Navarro OM, et al. Pediatric renal masses: Wilms tumor and beyond. Radiographics. 2000;20(6):1585–603.
4. Arranz Arija JA, Carrion JR, Garcia FR, Tejedor A, Pérez-Manga G, Tardio J, et al. Primary renal lymphoma: report of 3 cases and review of the literature. Am J Nephrol. 1994;14(2):148–53.

5. Dhull VS, Mukherjee A, Karunanithi S, Durgapal P, Bal C, Kumar R. Bilateral primary renal lymphoma in a pediatric patient: staging and response evaluation with ^{18}F-FDG PET/CT. Rev Esp Med Nucl Imagen Mol. 2015;34(1):49–52.

6. Fujiki T, Nishimura R, Mase S, Kuroda R, Ikawa Y, Araki R, et al. Accurate detection of renal leukemic involvement in children using 3-D computed tomography modeling. Pediatr Int. 2019;61(7):679–87.

7. Raffensperger J. Max Wilms and his tumor. J Pediatr Surg. 2015;50(2):356–9.

8. Breslow N, Olshan A, Beckwith JB, Green DM. Epidemiology of Wilms tumor. Med Pediatr Oncol. 1993;21(3):172–81.

9. Treger TD, Chowdhury T, Pritchard-Jones K, Behjati S. The genetic changes of Wilms tumour. Nat Rev Nephrol. 2019;15(4):240–51.

10. Capasso M, Montella A, Tirelli M, Maiorino T, Cantalupo S, Iolascon A. Genetic predisposition to solid pediatric cancers. Front Oncol. 2020;10:590033.

11. Kalish JM, Doros L, Helman LJ, Hennekam RC, Kuiper RP, Maas SM, et al. Surveillance recommendations for children with overgrowth syndromes and predisposition to Wilms tumors and hepatoblastoma. Clin Cancer Res. 2017;23(13):e115–22.

12. Miller RW, Fraumeni JF, Manning MD. Association of Wilms's tumor with aniridia, Hemihypertrophy and other congenital malformations. N Engl J Med. 1964;270(18):922–7.

13. Hol JA, Jongmans MCJ, Sudour-Bonnange H, Ramírez-Villar GL, Chowdhury T, Rechnitzer C, et al. Clinical characteristics and outcomes of children with WAGR syndrome and Wilms tumor and/or nephroblastomatosis: the 30-year SIOP-RTSG experience. Cancer. 2020;2020:cncr.33304.

14. Fischbach BV. WAGR syndrome: a clinical review of 54 cases. Pediatrics. 2005;116(4):984–8.

15. Breslow NE, Takashima JR, Ritchey ML, Strong LC, Green DM. Renal failure in the Denys-Drash and Wilms' tumor-aniridia syndromes. Cancer Res. 2000;60(15):4030–2.

16. Scott RH, Walker L, Olsen ØE, Levitt G, Kenney I, Maher E, et al. Surveillance for Wilms tumour in at-risk children: pragmatic recommendations for best practice. Arch Dis Child. 2006;91(12):995–9.

17. About WAGR - W is for Wilms Tumor [Internet]. [cited 2021 Jan 25]. Available from: https://wagr.org/wilms-tumor.

18. Pelletier J, Bruening W, Kashtan CE, Mauer SM, Manivel JC, Striegel JE, et al. Germline mutations in the Wilms' tumor suppressor gene are associated with abnormal urogenital development in Denys-Drash syndrome. Cell. 1991;67(2):437–47.

19. Barbaux S, Niaudet P, Gubler M-C, Grünfeld J-P, Jaubert F, Kuttenn F, et al. Donor splice-site mutations in WT1 are responsible for Frasier syndrome. Nat Genet. 1997;17(4):467–70.

20. Scott RH, Stiller CA, Walker L, Rahman N. Syndromes and constitutional chromosomal abnormalities associated with Wilms tumour. J Med Genet. 2006;43(9):705–15.

21. Mussa A, Molinatto C, Baldassarre G, Riberi E, Russo S, Larizza L, et al. Cancer risk in Beckwith-Wiedemann syndrome: a systematic review and meta-analysis outlining a novel (epi)genotype specific histotype targeted screening protocol. J Pediatr. 2016;176:142–149.e1.

22. OMIM - Online Mendelian Inheritance in Man [Internet]. [cited 2021 Feb 1]. Available from: https://www.omim.org/.

23. Rahman N, Arbour L, Houlston R, Bonaïti-Pellié C, Abidi F, Tranchemontagne J, et al. Penetrance of mutations in the familial Wilms tumor gene FWT1. J Natl Cancer Inst. 2000;92(8):650–2.

24. Rivera MN, Haber DA. Wilms' tumour: connecting tumorigenesis and organ development in the kidney. Nat Rev Cancer. 2005;5(9):699–712.

25. Beckwith JB, Palmer NF. Histopathology and prognosis of Wilms tumors: results from the First National Wilms' Tumor Study. Cancer. 1978;41(5):1937–48.

26. Parsons LN, Mullen EA, Geller JI, Chi Y-Y, Khanna G, Glick RD, et al. Outcome analysis of stage I epithelial-predominant favorable-histology Wilms tumors: a report from Children's Oncology Group study AREN03B2. Cancer. 2020;126(12):2866–71.

27. Verschuur AC, Vujanic GM, Van Tinteren H, Jones KP, de Kraker J, Sandstedt B. Stromal and epithelial predominant Wilms tumours have an excellent outcome: the SIOP 93 01 experience. Pediatr Blood Cancer. 2010;55(2):233–8.

28. Reinhard H, Semler O, Bürger D, Bode U, Flentje M, Göbel U, et al. Results of the SIOP 93-01/GPOH trial and study for the treatment of patients with unilateral nonmetastatic Wilms Tumor. Klin Padiatr. 2004;216(3):132–40.

29. Dome JS, Cotton CA, Perlman EJ, Breslow NE, Kalapurakal JA, Ritchey ML, et al. Treatment of anaplastic histology Wilms' tumor: results from the fifth National Wilms' Tumor Study. J Clin Oncol. 2006;24(15):2352–8.

30. Daw NC, Chi Y-Y, Kalapurakal JA, Kim Y, Hoffer FA, Geller JI, et al. Activity of vincristine and irinotecan in diffuse anaplastic Wilms tumor and therapy outcomes of stage II to IV disease: results of the Children's Oncology Group AREN0321 Study. J Clin Oncol. 2020;38(14):1558–68.

31. Ooms AHAG, Gadd S, Gerhard DS, Smith MA, Guidry Auvil JM, Meerzaman D, et al. Significance of TP53 mutation in Wilms tumors with diffuse anaplasia: a report from the Children's Oncology Group. Clin Cancer Res. 2016;22(22):5582–91.

32. Lu Y-J, Hing S, Williams R, Pinkerton R, Shipley J, Pritchard-Jones K, et al. Chromosome 1q expression profiling and relapse in Wilms' tumour. Lancet. 2002;360(9330):385–6.

33. Bown N, Cotterill SJ, Roberts P, Griffiths M, Larkins S, Hibbert S, et al. Cytogenetic abnormalities and clinical outcome in Wilms tumor: a study by the U.K. cancer cytogenetics group and the

U.K. Children's Cancer Study Group. Med Pediatr Oncol. 2002;38(1):11–21.

34. Hing S, Lu YJ, Summersgill B, King-Underwood L, Nicholson J, Grundy P, et al. Gain of 1q is associated with adverse outcome in favorable histology Wilms' tumors. Am J Pathol. 2001;158(2):393–8.

35. Natrajan R, Little SE, Sodha N, Reis-Filho JS, Mackay A, Fenwick K, et al. Analysis by array CGH of genomic changes associated with the progression or relapse of Wilms' tumour. J Pathol. 2007;211(1):52–9.

36. Segers H, van den Heuvel-Eibrink MM, Williams RD, van Tinteren H, Vujanic G, Pieters R, et al. Gain of 1q is a marker of poor prognosis in Wilms' tumors. Genes Chromosomes Cancer. 2013;52(11): 1065–74.

37. Gratias EJ, Jennings LJ, Anderson JR, Dome JS, Grundy P, Perlman EJ. Gain of 1q is associated with inferior event-free and overall survival in patients with favorable histology Wilms tumor: a report from the Children's Oncology Group. Cancer. 2013;119(21):3887–94.

38. Gratias EJ, Dome JS, Jennings LJ, Chi Y-Y, Tian J, Anderson J, et al. Association of chromosome 1q gain with inferior survival in favorable-histology Wilms tumor: a report from the Children's Oncology Group. J Clin Oncol. 2016;34(26):3189–94.

39. Dix DB, Fernandez CV, Chi Y-Y, Mullen EA, Geller JI, Gratias EJ, et al. Augmentation of therapy for combined loss of heterozygosity 1p and 16q in favorable histology Wilms tumor: a Children's Oncology Group AREN0532 and AREN0533 Study Report. J Clin Oncol. 2019;37(30):2769–77.

40. Fernandez CV, Perlman EJ, Mullen EA, Chi Y-Y, Hamilton TE, Gow KW, et al. Clinical outcome and biological predictors of relapse after nephrectomy only for very low-risk Wilms tumor. Ann Surg. 2017;265(4):835–40.

41. Fernandez CV, Mullen EA, Chi Y-Y, Ehrlich PF, Perlman EJ, Kalapurakal JA, et al. Outcome and prognostic factors in stage III favorable-histology Wilms tumor: a report from the Children's Oncology Group Study AREN0532. J Clin Oncol. 2018;36(3):254–61.

42. Grundy PE, Breslow NE, Li S, Perlman E, Beckwith JB, Ritchey ML, et al. Loss of heterozygosity for chromosomes 1p and 16q is an adverse prognostic factor in favorable-histology Wilms tumor: a report from the National Wilms Tumor Study Group. J Clin Oncol. 2005;23(29):7312–21.

43. Perlman EJ, Faria P, Soares A, Hoffer F, Sredni S, Ritchey M, et al. Hyperplastic perilobar nephroblastomatosis: long-term survival of 52 patients. Pediatr Blood Cancer. 2006;46(2):203–21.

44. Beckwith JB. Nephrogenic rests and the pathogenesis of Wilms tumor: developmental and clinical considerations. Am J Med Genet. 1998;79(4):268–73.

45. Sukarochana K, Tolentino W, Klesewetter WB. Wilms' tumor and hypertension. J Pediatr Surg. 1972;7(5):573–8.

46. Steinbrecher HA, Malone PS. Wilms' tumour and hypertension: incidence and outcome. Br J Urol. 1995;76(2):241–3.

47. Maas MH, Cransberg K, van Grotel M, Pieters R, van den Heuvel-Eibrink MM. Renin-induced hypertension in Wilms tumor patients. Pediatr Blood Cancer. 2007;48(5):500–3.

48. Jastaniah W, Elimam N, Alluhaibi RS, Alharbi AT, Abbas AA, Abrar MB. The prognostic significance of hypertension at diagnosis in children with Wilms tumor. Saudi Med J. 2017;38(3):262–7.

49. Idowu BM, Tanimola AG. Wilm's tumor presenting with scrotal varicocele in an 11-month-old boy. Indian J Radiol Imaging. 2018;28(2):247–9.

50. Ramsay NK, Dehner LP, Coccia PF, D'Angio GJ, Nesbit ME. Acute hemorrhage into Wilms tumor: a cause of rapidly developing abdominal mass with hypertension, anemia, and fever. J Pediatr. 1977;91(5):763–5.

51. Baig MR. Radiological case of the month. Arch Pediatr Adolesc Med. 1981;135(3):267.

52. Byerly D, Coley B, Ruymann F. Perirenal hemorrhage as first presentation of Wilms tumor. Pediatr Radiol. 2006;36(7):714–7.

53. Breslow NE, Churchill G, Nesmith B, Thomas PR, Beckwith JB, Othersen HB, et al. Clinicopathologic features and prognosis for Wilms' tumor patients with metastases at diagnosis. Cancer. 1986;58(11):2501–11.

54. Servaes SE, Hoffer FA, Smith EA, Khanna G. Imaging of Wilms tumor: an update. Pediatr Radiol. 2019;49(11):1441–52.

55. Jonge Poerink-Stockschlader AB, Dekker I, Risseeuw-Appel IM, Hählen K. Acquired Von Willebrand disease in children with a Wilms' tumor. Med Pediatr Oncol. 1996;26(4):238–43.

56. Dickson PV, Sims TL, Streck CJ, McCarville MB, Santana VM, McGregor LM, et al. Avoiding misdiagnosing neuroblastoma as Wilms tumor. J Pediatr Surg. 2008;43(6):1159–63.

57. Dome JS, Perlman EJ, Graf N. Risk stratification for Wilms tumor: current approach and future directions. Am Soc Clin Oncol Educ Book. 2014;2014: 215–23.

58. Irtan S, Ehrlich PF, Pritchard-Jones K. Wilms tumor: "State-of-the-art" update, 2016. Semin Pediatr Surg. 2016;25(5):250–6.

59. Nelson MV, van den Heuvel-Eibrink MM, Graf N, Dome JS. New approaches to risk stratification for Wilms tumor. Curr Opin Pediatr [Internet]. 2020 Dec 29 [cited 2021 Feb 6]; Publish Ahead of Print. Available from: https://journals.lww.com/10.1097/MOP.0000000000000988.

60. Murphy AJ, Davidoff AM. Bilateral Wilms tumor: a surgical perspective. Children (Basel). 2018;5(10):134.

61. Ehrlich PF, Chi Y-Y, Chintagumpala MM, Hoffer FA, Perlman EJ, Kalapurakal JA, et al. Results of the first prospective multi-institutional treatment study in children with bilateral Wilms tumor (AREN0534):

a report from the Children's Oncology Group. Ann Surg. 2017;266(3):470–8.

62. D'Angio GJ, Evans AE, Breslow N, Beckwith B, Bishop H, Feigl P, et al. The treatment of Wilms' tumor: results of the national Wilms' tumor study. Cancer. 1976;38(2):633–46.

63. Dix DB, Seibel NL, Chi Y-Y, Khanna G, Gratias E, Anderson JR, et al. Treatment of stage IV favorable histology Wilms tumor with lung metastases: a report from the Children's Oncology Group AREN0533 Study. J Clin Oncol. 2018;36(16):1564–70.

64. Fajardo RD, van den Heuvel-Eibrink MM, van Tinteren H, Spreafico F, Acha T, Bergeron C, et al. Is radiotherapy required in first-line treatment of stage I diffuse anaplastic Wilms tumor? A report of SIOP-RTSG, AIEOP, JWiTS, and UKCCSG. Pediatr Blood Cancer. 2020;67(2):e28039.

65. Daw NC, Chi Y-Y, Kim Y, Mullen EA, Kalapurakal JA, Tian J, et al. Treatment of stage I anaplastic Wilms' tumour: a report from the Children's Oncology Group AREN0321 study. Eur J Cancer. 1990;2019(118):58–66.

66. Smith MA, Altekruse SF, Adamson PC, Reaman GH, Seibel NL. Declining childhood and adolescent cancer mortality. Cancer. 2014;120(16):2497–506.

67. D'Angio GJ. The National Wilms Tumor Study: a 40 year perspective. Lifetime Data Anal. 2007;13(4):463–70.

68. Vujanić GM, Gessler M, Ooms AHAG, Collini P, Coulomb-l'Hermine A, D'Hooghe E, et al. The UMBRELLA SIOP-RTSG 2016 Wilms tumour pathology and molecular biology protocol. Nat Rev Urol. 2018;15(11):693–701.

69. Hol JA, Lopez-Yurda MI, Van Tinteren H, Van Grotel M, Godzinski J, Vujanic G, et al. Prognostic significance of age in 5631 patients with Wilms tumour prospectively registered in International Society of Paediatric Oncology (SIOP) 93-01 and 2001. PLoS One. 2019;14(8):e0221373.

70. Pritchard-Jones K, Kelsey A, Vujanic G, Imeson J, Hutton C, Mitchell C, et al. Older age is an adverse prognostic factor in stage I, favorable histology Wilms' tumor treated with vincristine monochemotherapy: a study by the United Kingdom Children's Cancer Study Group, Wilm's Tumor Working Group. J Clin Oncol. 2003;21(17):3269–75.

71. Green DM, Beckwith JB, Weeks DA, Moksness J, Breslow NE, D'Angio GJ. The relationship between microsubstaging variables, age at diagnosis, and tumor weight of children with stage I/favorable histology Wilms' tumor. A report from the National Wilms' Tumor study. Cancer. 1994;74(6):1817–20.

72. Breslow N, Sharples K, Beckwith JB, Takashima J, Kelalis PP, Green DM, et al. Prognostic factors in nonmetastatic, favorable histology Wilms' tumor. Results of the Third National Wilms' Tumor Study. Cancer. 1991;68(11):2345–53.

73. Tang F, Zhang H, Lu Z, Wang J, He C, He Z. Prognostic factors and nomograms to predict overall and cancer-specific survival for children with Wilms' tumor. Dis Markers. 2019;2019:1092769.

74. Green DM, Cotton CA, Malogolowkin M, Breslow NE, Perlman E, Miser J, et al. Treatment of Wilms tumor relapsing after initial treatment with vincristine and actinomycin D: a report from the National Wilms Tumor Study Group. Pediatr Blood Cancer. 2007;48(5):493–9.

75. Malogolowkin M, Cotton CA, Green DM, Breslow NE, Perlman E, Miser J, et al. Treatment of Wilms tumor relapsing after initial treatment with vincristine, actinomycin D, and doxorubicin. A report from the National Wilms Tumor Study Group. Pediatr Blood Cancer. 2008;50(2):236–41.

76. Reinhard H, Schmidt A, Furtwängler R, Leuschner I, Rübe C, Von Schweinitz D, et al. Outcome of relapses of nephroblastoma in patients registered in the SIOP/GPOH trials and studies. Oncol Rep. 2008;20(2):463–7.

77. Ehrlich PF, Chi Y-Y, Chintagumpala MM, Hoffer FA, Perlman EJ, Kalapurakal JA, et al. Results of treatment for patients with multicentric or bilaterally predisposed unilateral Wilms Tumor (AREN0534): a report from the Children's Oncology Group. Cancer. 2020;126(15):3516–25.

78. Oeffinger KC, Mertens AC, Sklar CA, Kawashima T, Hudson MM, Meadows AT, et al. Chronic health conditions in adult survivors of childhood cancer. N Engl J Med. 2006;355(15):1572–82.

79. Termuhlen AM, Tersak JM, Liu Q, Yasui Y, Stovall M, Weathers R, et al. Twenty-five year follow-up of childhood Wilms tumor: a report from the Childhood Cancer Survivor study: twenty-five year follow-up of Wilms tumor. Pediatr Blood Cancer. 2011;57(7):1210–6.

80. Breslow NE, Collins AJ, Ritchey ML, Grigoriev YA, Peterson SM, Green DM. End stage renal disease in patients with Wilms tumor: results from the National Wilms Tumor Study Group and the United States Renal Data System. J Urol. 2005;174(5):1972–5.

81. Lange J, Peterson SM, Takashima JR, Grigoriev Y, Ritchey ML, Shamberger RC, et al. Risk factors for end stage renal disease in non-WT1-syndromic Wilms tumor. J Urol. 2011;186(2):378–86.

82. Bárdi E, Oláh AV, Bartyik K, Endreffy E, Jenei C, Kappelmayer J, et al. Late effects on renal glomerular and tubular function in childhood cancer survivors. Pediatr Blood Cancer. 2004;43(6):668–73.

83. Neu MA, Russo A, Wingerter A, Alt F, Theruvath J, El Malki K, et al. Prospective analysis of long-term renal function in survivors of childhood Wilms tumor. Pediatr Nephrol. 2017;32(10):1915–25.

84. Mavinkurve-Groothuis AMC, van de Kracht F, Westland R, van Wijk JAE, Loonen JJ, Schreuder MF. Long-term follow-up of blood pressure and glomerular filtration rate in patients with a solitary functioning kidney: a comparison between Wilms tumor survivors and nephrectomy for other reasons. Pediatr Nephrol. 2016;31(3):435–41.

85. Interiano RB, Delos Santos N, Huang S, Srivastava DK, Robison LL, Hudson MM, et al. Renal function in survivors of nonsyndromic Wilms tumor treated with unilateral radical nephrectomy. Cancer. 2015;121(14):2449–56.

86. Wikstad I, Pettersson BA, Elinder G, Sökücü S, Aperia A. A comparative study of size and function of the remnant kidney in patients nephrectomized in childhood for Wilms' tumor and hydronephrosis. Acta Paediatr Scand. 1986;75(3):408–14.

87. Daw NC, Gregornik D, Rodman J, Marina N, Wu J, Kun LE, et al. Renal function after ifosfamide, carboplatin and etoposide (ICE) chemotherapy, nephrectomy and radiotherapy in children with Wilms tumour. Eur J Cancer. 2009;45(1):99–106.

88. Jones DP, Spunt SL, Green D, Springate JE. Renal late effects in patients treated for cancer in childhood: a report from the Children's Oncology Group. Pediatr Blood Cancer. 2008;51(6):724–31.

89. Ritchey ML, Green DM, Thomas PR, Smith GR, Haase G, Shochat S, et al. Renal failure in Wilms' tumor patients: a report from the National Wilms' Tumor Study Group. Med Pediatr Oncol. 1996;26(2):75–80.

90. Children's Oncology Group (COG). Long-term follow-up guidelines for survivors of childhood, adolescent, and young adult cancers. [Internet]. Monravia, CA: Children's Oncology Group Data Center; 2018 [cited 2021 Feb 19]. Available from: http://www.survivorshipguidelines.org/pdf/2018/COGLTFUGuidelinesv5.pdf.

91. Wright KD, Green DM, Daw NC. Late effects of treatment for Wilms tumor. Pediatr Hematol Oncol. 2009;26(6):407–13.

92. Gooskens SLM, Furtwängler R, Vujanic GM, Dome JS, Graf N, van den Heuvel-Eibrink MM. Clear cell sarcoma of the kidney: a review. Eur J Cancer. 2012;48(14):2219–26.

93. Argani P, Perlman EJ, Breslow NE, Browning NG, Green DM, D'Angio GJ, et al. Clear cell sarcoma of the kidney: a review of 351 cases from the National Wilms Tumor Study Group Pathology Center. Am J Surg Pathol. 2000;24(1):4–18.

94. Marsden HB, Lawler W, Kumar PM. Bone metastasizing renal tumor of childhood: morphological and clinical features, and differences from Wilms' tumor. Cancer. 1978;42(4):1922–8.

95. Marsden HB, Lennox EL, Lawler W, Kinnier-Wilson LM. Bone metastases in childhood renal tumours. Br J Cancer. 1980;41(6):875–9.

96. Furtwängler R, Gooskens SL, van Tinteren H, de Kraker J, Schleiermacher G, Bergeron C, et al. Clear cell sarcomas of the kidney registered on International Society of Pediatric Oncology (SIOP) 93-01 and SIOP 2001 protocols: a report of the SIOP Renal Tumour Study Group. Eur J Cancer. 2013;49(16):3497–506.

97. Trejo Bittar HE, Radder JE, Ranganathan S, Srinivasan A, Madan-Khetarpal S, Reyes-Múgica M. Clear cell sarcoma of the kidney in a child with Fanconi anemia. Pediatr Dev Pathol. 2014;17(4):297–301.

98. Balarezo FS, Joshi VV. Clear cell sarcoma of the pediatric kidney: detailed description and analysis of variant histologic patterns of a tumor with many faces. Adv Anat Pathol. 2001;8(2):98–108.

99. Wong MK, Ng CCY, Kuick CH, Aw SJ, Rajasegaran V, Lim JQ, et al. Clear cell sarcomas of the kidney are characterised by BCOR gene abnormalities, including exon 15 internal tandem duplications and BCOR–CCNB3 gene fusion. Histopathology. 2018;72(2):320–9.

100. Aldera AP, Pillay K. Clear cell sarcoma of the kidney. Arch Pathol Lab Med. 2020;144(1):119–23.

101. Han H, Bertrand KC, Patel KR, Fisher KE, Roy A, Muscal JA, et al. BCOR-CCNB3 fusion-positive clear cell sarcoma of the kidney. Pediatr Blood Cancer. 2020;67(4):e28151.

102. Wood DP, Kay R, Norris D. Renal sarcomas of childhood. Urology. 1990;36(1):73–8.

103. Gooskens SL, Graf N, Furtwängler R, Spreafico F, Bergeron C, Ramírez-Villar GL, et al. Rationale for the treatment of children with CCSK in the UMBRELLA SIOP–RTSG 2016 protocol. Nat Rev Urol. 2018;15(5):309–19.

104. Seibel NL, Chi Y-Y, Perlman EJ, Tian J, Sun J, Anderson JR, et al. Impact of cyclophosphamide and etoposide on outcome of clear cell sarcoma of the kidney treated on the National Wilms Tumor Study-5 (NWTS-5). Pediatr Blood Cancer. 2019;66(1):e27450.

105. Gooskens SL, Furtwängler R, Spreafico F, van Tinteren H, de Kraker J, Vujanic GM, et al. Treatment and outcome of patients with relapsed clear cell sarcoma of the kidney: a combined SIOP and AIEOP study. Br J Cancer. 2014;111(2):227–33.

106. Haas JE, Palmer NF, Weinberg AG, Beckwith JB. Ultrastructure of malignant rhabdoid tumor of the kidney: a distinctive renal tumor of children. Hum Pathol. 1981;12(7):646–57.

107. Mullen EA, Geller JI, Gratias EJ, Perlman EJ, Ehrlich PF, Khanna G, et al. Real-time central review: a report of the first 3,000 patients enrolled on the Children's Oncology Group Renal Tumor Biology and Risk Stratification protocol AREN03B2. J Clin Oncol. 2014;32(15_Suppl):10000.

108. Heck JE, Lombardi CA, Cockburn M, Meyers TJ, Wilhelm M, Ritz B. Epidemiology of rhabdoid tumors of early childhood. Pediatr Blood Cancer. 2013;60(1):77–81.

109. van den Heuvel-Eibrink MM, van Tinteren H, Rehorst H, Coulombe A, Patte C, de Camargo B, et al. Malignant rhabdoid tumours of the kidney (MRTKs), registered on recent SIOP protocols from 1993 to 2005: a report of the SIOP renal tumour study group. Pediatr Blood Cancer. 2011;56(5):733–7.

110. Tomlinson GE, Breslow NE, Dome J, Guthrie KA, Norkool P, Li S, et al. Rhabdoid tumor of the kidney in the National Wilms' Tumor Study: age

at diagnosis as a prognostic factor. J Clin Oncol. 2005;23(30):7641–5.

111. Oue T, Fukuzawa M, Okita H, Mugishima H, Horie H, Hata J, et al. Outcome of pediatric renal tumor treated using the Japan Wilms Tumor Study-1 (JWiTS-1) protocol: a report from the JWiTS Group. Pediatr Surg Int. 2009;25(11):923–9.

112. Frühwald MC, Nemes K, Boztug H, Cornips MCA, Evans DG, Farah R, et al. Current recommendations for clinical surveillance and genetic testing in rhabdoid tumor predisposition: a report from the SIOPE Host Genome Working Group. Fam Cancer [Internet]. 2021 Feb 3 [cited 2021 Feb 15]; Available from: https://doi.org/10.1007/s10689-021-00229-1.

113. Hodges C, Kirkland JG, Crabtree GR. The many roles of BAF (mSWI/SNF) and PBAF complexes in cancer. Cold Spring Harb Perspect Med. 2016;6(8):a026930.

114. Wang X, Haswell JR, Roberts CWM. Molecular pathways: SWI/SNF (BAF) complexes are frequently mutated in cancer—mechanisms and potential therapeutic insights. Clin Cancer Res. 2014;20(1):21.

115. Biegel JA, Busse TM, Weissman BE. SWI/SNF chromatin remodeling complexes and cancer. Am J Med Genet C Semin Med Genet. 2014;166(3):350–66.

116. Pastore G, Znaor A, Spreafico F, Graf N, Pritchard-Jones K, Steliarova-Foucher E. Malignant renal tumours incidence and survival in European children (1978–1997): report from the Automated Childhood Cancer Information System project. Eur J Cancer. 2006;42(13):2103–14.

117. Brennan B, Salvo GLD, Orbach D, Paoli AD, Kelsey A, Mudry P, et al. Outcome of extracranial malignant rhabdoid tumours in children registered in the European Paediatric Soft Tissue Sarcoma Study Group Non-Rhabdomyosarcoma Soft Tissue Sarcoma 2005 Study-EpSSG NRSTS 2005. Eur J Cancer. 2016;60:69–82.

118. Cajaiba MM, Dyer LM, Geller JI, Jennings LJ, George D, Kirschmann D, et al. The classification of pediatric and young adult renal cell carcinomas registered on the children's oncology group (COG) protocol AREN03B2 after focused genetic testing. Cancer. 2018;124(16):3381–9.

119. Geller JI, Ehrlich PF, Cost NG, Khanna G, Mullen EA, Gratias EJ, et al. Characterization of adolescent and pediatric renal cell carcinoma: a report from the Children's Oncology Group study AREN03B2. Cancer. 2015;121(14):2457–64.

120. Schmidt LS, Linehan WM. Genetic predisposition to kidney cancer. Semin Oncol. 2016;43(5):566–74.

121. Gnarra JR, Tory K, Weng Y, Schmidt L, Wei MH, Li H, et al. Mutations of the VHL tumour suppressor gene in renal carcinoma. Nat Genet. 1994;7(1):85–90.

122. Paner GP, Stadler WM, Hansel DE, Montironi R, Lin DW, Amin MB. Updates in the eighth edition of the tumor-node-metastasis staging classification for urologic cancers. Eur Urol. 2018;73(4):560–9.

123. Geller JI, Cost NG, Chi Y-Y, Tornwall B, Cajaiba M, Perlman EJ, et al. A prospective study of pediatric and adolescent renal cell carcinoma: a report from the Children's Oncology Group AREN0321 study [Internet]. Cancer. John Wiley & Sons, Ltd; 2020 [cited 2020 Nov 2]. Available from: https://acsjournals-onlinelibrary-wiley-com.proxy.library.emory.edu/doi/abs/10.1002/cncr.33173.

124. Davis CJ Jr, Mostofi FK, Sesterhenn IA. Renal medullary carcinoma. The seventh sickle cell nephropathy. Am J Surg Pathol. 1995;19(1):1–11.

125. Cheng JX, Tretiakova M, Gong C, Mandal S, Krausz T, Taxy JB. Renal medullary carcinoma: rhabdoid features and the absence of INI1 expression as markers of aggressive behavior. Mod Pathol. 2008;21(6):647–52.

126. Alvarez O, Rodriguez MM, Jordan L, Sarnaik S. Renal medullary carcinoma and sickle cell trait: a systematic review. Pediatr Blood Cancer. 2015;62(10):1694–9.

127. Calderaro J, Masliah-Planchon J, Richer W, Maillot L, Maille P, Mansuy L, et al. Balanced translocations disrupting SMARCB1 are hallmark recurrent genetic alterations in renal medullary carcinomas. Eur Urol. 2016;69(6):1055–61.

128. Msaouel P, Malouf GG, Su X, Yao H, Tripathi DN, Soeung M, et al. Comprehensive molecular characterization identifies distinct genomic and immune hallmarks of renal medullary carcinoma. Cancer Cell. 2020;37(5):720–734.e13.

129. Ezekian B, Englum B, Gilmore BF, Nag UP, Kim J, Leraas HJ, et al. Renal medullary carcinoma: a national analysis of 159 patients. Pediatr Blood Cancer. 2017; https://doi.org/10.1002/pbc.26609.

130. Beckermann KE, Sharma D, Chaturvedi S, Msaouel P, Abboud MR, Allory Y, et al. Renal medullary carcinoma: establishing standards in practice. J Oncol Pract. 2017;13(7):414–21.

131. Msaouel P, Hong AL, Mullen EA, Atkins MB, Walker CL, Lee C-H, et al. Updated recommendations on the diagnosis, management, and clinical trial eligibility criteria for patients with renal medullary carcinoma. Clin Genitourin Cancer. 2019; 17(1):1–6.

132. Iacovelli R, Modica D, Palazzo A, Trenta P, Piesco G, Cortesi E. Clinical outcome and prognostic factors in renal medullary carcinoma: a pooled analysis from 18 years of medical literature. Can Urol Assoc J. 2015;9(3–4):172.

133. Flum AS, Nabeel H, Said MA, Yang XJ, Casalino DD, McGuire BB, et al. Update on the diagnosis and management of renal angiomyolipoma. J Urol. 2016;195(4 Part 1):834–46.

134. Oesterling JE, Fishman EK, Goldman SM, Marshall FF. The management of renal angiomyolipoma. J Urol. 1986;135(6):1121–4.

135. Fujii Y, Ajima J-I, Oka K, Tosaka A, Takehara Y. Benign renal tumors detected among healthy adults by abdominal ultrasonography. Eur Urol. 1995;27:124–7.

136. Seyam RM, Bissada NK, Kattan SA, Mokhtar AA, Aslam M, Fahmy WE, et al. Changing trends in presentation, diagnosis and management of renal angiomyolipoma: comparison of sporadic and tuberous sclerosis complex-associated forms. Urology. 2008;72(5):1077–82.

137. Inoki K, Li Y, Zhu T, Wu J, Guan K-L. TSC2 is phosphorylated and inhibited by Akt and suppresses mTOR signalling. Nat Cell Biol. 2002;4(9):648–57.

138. Curatolo P, Bombardieri R, Jozwiak S. Tuberous sclerosis. Lancet. 2008;372(9639):657–68.

139. Samuels JA. Treatment of renal angiomyolipoma and other hamartomas in patients with tuberous sclerosis complex. Clin J Am Soc Nephrol. 2017;12(7):1196–202.

140. Dabora SL, Franz DN, Ashwal S, Sagalowsky A, DiMario FJ, Miles D, et al. Multicenter phase 2 trial of sirolimus for tuberous sclerosis: kidney angiomyolipomas and other tumors regress and VEGF-D levels decrease. PLoS One. 2011;6(9):e23379.

141. Bissler JJ, Kingswood JC, Radzikowska E, Zonnenberg BA, Frost M, Belousova E, et al. Everolimus for angiomyolipoma associated with tuberous sclerosis complex or sporadic lymphangioleiomyomatosis (EXIST-2): a multicentre, randomised, double-blind, placebo-controlled trial. Lancet. 2013;381(9869):817–24.

142. Bissler JJ, Kingswood JC, Radzikowska E, Zonnenberg BA, Belousova E, Frost MD, et al. Everolimus long-term use in patients with tuberous sclerosis complex: four-year update of the EXIST-2 study. PLoS One. 2017;12(8):e0180939.

143. Tarek N, Said R, Andersen CR, Suki TS, Foglesong J, Herzog CE, et al. Primary Ewing sarcoma/primitive neuroectodermal tumor of the kidney: the MD Anderson Cancer Center Experience. Cancers. 2020;12(10):2927.

144. van den Heuvel-Eibrink MM, Grundy P, Graf N, Pritchard-Jones K, Bergeron C, Patte C, et al. Characteristics and survival of 750 children diagnosed with a renal tumor in the first seven months of life: a collaborative study by the SIOP/GPOH/SFOP, NWTSG, and UKCCSG Wilms tumor study groups. Pediatr Blood Cancer. 2008;50(6):1130–4.

145. Bolande RP, Brough AJ, Izant RJ. Congenital mesoblastic nephroma of infancy: a report of eight cases and the relationship to Wilms' tumor. Pediatrics. 1967;40(2):272–8.

146. Gooskens SL, Houwing ME, Vujanic GM, Dome JS, Diertens T, Coulomb-l'Herminé A, et al. Congenital mesoblastic nephroma 50 years after its recognition: a narrative review. Pediatr Blood Cancer. 2017;64(7).

147. Knezevich SR, Garnett MJ, Pysher TJ, Beckwith JB, Grundy PE, Sorensen PHB. ETV6-NTRK3 gene fusions and trisomy 11 establish a histogenetic link between mesoblastic nephroma and congenital fibrosarcoma. Cancer Res. 1998;58(22):5046–8.

148. Vokuhl C, Nourkami-Tutdibi N, Furtwängler R, Gessler M, Graf N, Leuschner I. ETV6–NTRK3 in congenital mesoblastic nephroma: a report of the SIOP/GPOH nephroblastoma study. Pediatr Blood Cancer. 2018;65(4):e26925.

149. England RJ, Haider N, Vujanic GM, Kelsey A, Stiller CA, Pritchard-Jones K, et al. Mesoblastic nephroma: a report of the United Kingdom children's cancer and leukaemia group (CCLG). Pediatr Blood Cancer. 2011;56(5):744–8.

150. Tobias L, Philipp S, Rhoikos F, Norbert G, Jörg F. Treatment of cystic nephroma and cystic partially differentiated nephroblastoma—a report from the SIOP/GPOH Study Group. J Urol. 2007;177(1):294–6.

151. Cajaiba MM, Khanna G, Smith EA, Gellert L, Chi Y-Y, Mullen EA, et al. Pediatric cystic nephromas: distinctive features and frequent DICER1 mutations. Hum Pathol. 2016;48:81–7.

152. Silverman SG, Pedrosa I, Ellis JH, Hindman NM, Schieda N, Smith AD, et al. Bosniak classification of cystic renal masses, Version 2019: an update proposal and needs assessment. Radiology. 2019;292(2):475–88.

153. Doros LA, Rossi CT, Yang J, Field A, Williams GM, Messinger Y, et al. DICER1 mutations in childhood cystic nephroma and its relationship to DICER1-renal sarcoma. Mod Pathol. 2014;27(9):1267–80.

154. Chatten J, Cromie WJ, Duckett JW. Ossifying tumor of infantile kidney: report of two cases. Cancer. 1980;45(3):609–12.

155. Hajiran A, Jessop M, Werner Z, Crigger C, Barnard J, Vos J, et al. Ossifying renal tumor of infancy: laparoscopic treatment and literature review. Case Rep Urol. 2018;2018:1935657.

156. Guan W, Yan Y, He W, Qiao M, Liu Y, Wang Y, et al. Ossifying renal tumor of infancy (ORIT): the clinicopathological and cytogenetic feature of two cases and literature review. Pathol Res Pract. 2016;212(11):1004–9.

157. Sotelo-Avila C, Beckwith JB, Johnson JE. Ossifying renal tumor of infancy: a clinicopathologic study of nine cases. Pediatr Pathol Lab Med. 1995;15(5):745–62.

158. Vazquez JL, Barnewolt CE, Shamberger RC, Chung T, Perez-Atayde AR. Ossifying renal tumor of infancy presenting as a palpable abdominal mass. Pediatr Radiol. 1998;28(6):454–7.

159. Lee SH, Choi YH, Kim WS, Cheon J-E, Moon KC. Ossifying renal tumor of infancy: findings at ultrasound, CT and MRI. Pediatr Radiol. 2014;44(5):625–8.

160. Liu J, Guzman MA, Pawel BR, Pezanowski DM, Patel DM, Roth JA, et al. Clonal trisomy 4 cells detected in the ossifying renal tumor of infancy: study of 3 cases. Mod Pathol. 2013;26(2):275–81.

161. Moch H, Cubilla AL, Humphrey PA, Reuter VE, Ulbright TM. The 2016 WHO classification of tumours of the urinary system and male genital organs—Part A: Renal, penile, and testicular tumours. Eur Urol. 2016;70(1):93–105.

162. Argani P. Metanephric neoplasms: the hyper-differentiated, benign end of the Wilms tumor spectrum? Clin Lab Med. 2005;25(2): 379–92.

163. Davis CJ, Barton JH, Sesterhenn IA, Mostofi FK. Metanephric adenoma. Clinicopathological study of fifty patients. Am J Surg Pathol. 1995;19(10):1101–14.

164. Jones EC, Pins M, Dickersin GR, Young RH. Metanephric adenoma of the kidney. A clinicopathological, immunohistochemical, flow cytometric, cytogenetic, and electron microscopic study of seven cases. Am J Surg Pathol. 1995;19(6):615–26.

165. Choueiri TK, Cheville J, Palescandolo E, Fay AP, Kantoff PW, Atkins MB, et al. BRAF mutations in metanephric adenoma of the kidney. Eur Urol. 2012;62(5):917–22.

166. Renshaw AA, Freyer DR, Hammers YA. Metastatic metanephric adenoma in a child. Am J Surg Pathol. 2000;24(4):570–4.

167. Wobker SE, Matoso A, Pratilas CA, Mangray S, Zheng G, Lin M-T, et al. Metanephric adenoma-epithelial Wilms tumor overlap lesions: an analysis of BRAF status. Am J Surg Pathol. 2019;43(9):1157–69.

168. Argani P, Beckwith JB. Metanephric stromal tumor: report of 31 cases of a distinctive pediatric renal neoplasm. Am J Surg Pathol. 2000;24(7):917–26.

169. Zhang X, Yadav PK, Niu Q, Cheng H, Xiao Y, Wang Y, et al. Reevaluation of metanephric stromal tumor two decades after it was named: a narrative review. J Pediatr Urol. 2020;16(6):822–9.

170. Marsden L, Jennings LJ, Gadd S, Yu M, Perlman EJ, Cajaiba MM. BRAF exon 15 mutations in pediatric renal stromal tumors: prevalence in metanephric stromal tumors. Hum Pathol. 2017;60:32–6.

171. Hennigar RA, Beckwith JB. Nephrogenic adenofibroma. A novel kidney tumor of young people. Am J Surg Pathol. 1992;16(4):325–34.

172. Arroyo MR, Green DM, Perlman EJ, Beckwith JB, Argani P. The spectrum of metanephric adenofibroma and related lesions: clinicopathologic study of 25 cases from the National Wilms Tumor Study Group Pathology Center. Am J Surg Pathol. 2001;25(4):433–44.

173. Yao D-W, Qu F, Hu S-W, Zheng J-Y, Wang J-M, Zhu X-Y, et al. Metanephric adenofibroma in a 10-year-old boy: report of a case and review of the literature. Int J Clin Exp Pathol. 2015;8(3):3250–6.

Tubulointerstitial Nephritis in Children

42

Priya S. Verghese, Kera E. Luckritz, and Allison A. Eddy

Introduction and Historical Perspective

An estimated 85% of the kidney consists of tubules and their surrounding interstitial space. Given their preeminence, it is crucial to understand the contribution of the tubulointerstitium in all renal disease processes. Despite its anatomical dominance, current understanding of the role of the interstitium in both primary and secondary disease processes remains incomplete.

The term acute interstitial nephritis (AIN) was coined by Councilman in 1898 when he provided the first and now classic description of

Priya S. Verghese, Kera E. Luckritz and Allison A. Eddy contributed equally with all other contributors.

P. S. Verghese
Ann & Robert H. Lurie Children's Hospital, Northwestern University Feinberg School of Medicine, Chicago, IL, USA
e-mail: pverghese@luriechildrens.org

K. E. Luckritz
C.S. Mott Children's Hospital, University of Michigan Health System, Ann Arbor, MI, USA
e-mail: keral@med.umich.edu

A. A. Eddy (✉)
Department of Pediatrics, University of British Columbia, Vancouver, BC, Canada

BC Children's Hospital, Vancouver, BC, Canada
e-mail: allison.eddy@cw.bc.ca; allison.eddy@ubc.ca

the histopathologic changes following an investigation of autopsy specimens from patients with diphtheria, scarlet fever and other infectious diseases [1, 2]. Primary AIN is typically an immunologically-mediated disease characterized by tubular injury and interstitial inflammation, with relative sparing of the glomeruli and vessels, initiated by drugs, infections or other causes mentioned in detail in section "Etiology" [3]. Councilman's early description still has merit, though it may be more accurate to categorize the disease process as acute tubulointerstitial nephritis (TIN) since the renal tubules are also involved in all cases, both clinically and histopathologically.

In the pre-antibiotic era, systemic infections were the most common cause of tubulointerstitial disease. Today, a drug hypersensitivity reaction is a more common inciting event. Ironically many of these drugs were developed to treat the infectious disorders that had often been implicated as causes of AIN. In kidney transplant allografts, TIN can occur due to drugs, but also due to infections such as BK polyomavirus and adenovirus [4, 5] that often necessitate drastic reduction in immunosuppression to enable viral clearance.

Progressive chronic kidney disease (CKD), irrespective of the primary disease process, is characterized by significant chronic TIN indicating that TIN is a spectrum of pathologies, ranging from acute and reversible nephritis to chronic and

© The Author(s), under exclusive license to Springer Nature Switzerland AG 2023
F. Schaefer, L. A. Greenbaum (eds.), *Pediatric Kidney Disease*,
https://doi.org/10.1007/978-3-031-11665-0_42

irreversible disease with fibrosis. For each individual patient, it is critical to try to identify and discontinue the offending toxin or agent before acute injury progresses to the chronic stage.

Epidemiology

Acute injury to the interstitium and the surrounding tubules is an important cause of renal dysfunction, currently accounting for 5–27% of kidney biopsies performed for acute kidney injury [6–9]. Reliable data on the incidence and prevalence of TIN are lacking, especially in the pediatric population. Within available biopsy registries, TIN represents approximately 1–3% of all biopsy diagnoses [7, 10]. Often the diagnosis is made clinically without performing a renal biopsy to confirm the diagnosis. Furthermore, it is likely that many cases are self-limited and remain clinically silent. Thus, the estimated numbers are likely conservative and lower than the true incidence. The incidence of TIN in kidney transplant allografts is also unknown [4, 5].

Histology and Pathogenesis

By definition, TIN is characterized by interstitial cellular infiltrates, usually sparing the vessels and glomeruli (Fig. 42.1a), although it is noted that severe primary glomerular injury rarely occurs without concurrent tubulointerstitial injury. Tubular cell damage may be manifest as epithelial proliferation and/or tubular dilatation. Intratubular cast deposition is often present as well [11]. Interstitial fibrosis and tubular atrophy, often accompanied by the persistent mononuclear cell infiltrate [11], can be representative of chronic TIN. The infiltrate is composed predominantly of T cells with some macrophages and plasma cells [6, 11, 12]. An impressive number of eosinophils may be present and suggests a drug-induced etiology (Fig. 42.1d). These lymphohematopoietic cells are a rich source of cytokines that contribute to kidney injury. Granuloma formation is a feature of biopsies in 6% of the patients and can occur in any form of AIN; granulomas are considered common in drug-induced TIN, infection-associated TIN and renal vasculitis

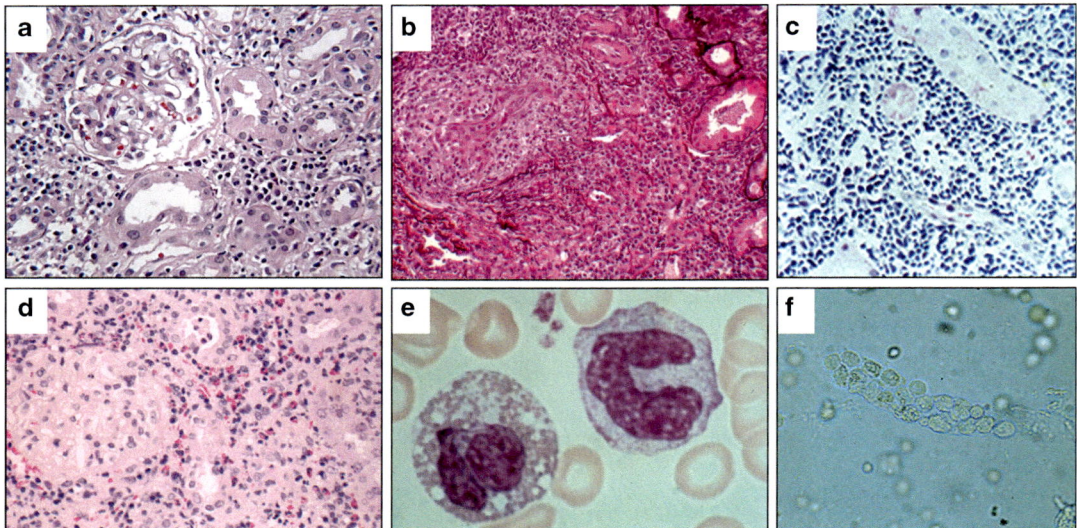

Fig. 42.1 Histological and urinary sediment features of acute tubulointerstitial nephritis (TIN). Histological photomicrographs illustrate an interstitial infiltrate of mononuclear cells, interstitial edema and tubular dilatation in acute TIN (**a**); acute TIN with granuloma formation (**b**); TIN characterized by an infiltrate of monomorphic interstitial mononuclear cell due to lymphoma (**c**); acute drug-induced TIN with numerous polymorphonuclear eosinophils (**d**). Examination of the urinary sediment may show eosinophils in drug-induced TIN (**e**), white blood cells and while blood cell casts (**f**)

[13] (Fig. 42.1b). Some studies have suggested that the degree of tubulointerstitial inflammation may be predictive of renal functional outcome, even in primary glomerular diseases [3, 8, 14, 15]. However, other studies have suggested the extent of chronic changes such as tubular atrophy on the initial biopsy are more predictive of long-term outcomes [8, 16]. Interestingly, in kidney transplant allografts, inflammation in areas of interstitial fibrosis is associated with decreased graft survival with or without concurrent evidence of rejection [17], once again supporting the prior theory that the degree of inflammation is more predictive of long-term outcomes.

In primary TIN, immunofluorescence staining for antibodies and complement proteins are typically negative. Occasionally, linear or granular deposits of IgG or IgM may be present along the tubular basement membranes [3]. Electron microscopy may reveal loss of continuity of basement membranes as well as thickened and multilaminated areas indicative of chronic damage [3].

These histopathologic findings, together with the apparent clinical response to corticosteroid therapy, supports a role for immune-mediated pathogenic mechanisms. Though the specific mechanisms remain unclear, an important role of chemokines and other inflammatory mediators is presumed [18]. A reliable animal model that faithfully mimics human acute drug or infection associated TIN is not available to elucidate specific pathways. Animal studies have shown that three endogenous kidney antigens (uromodulin, megalin, and a tubular basement membrane glycoprotein named TIN antigen) can elicit TIN, but the relevance of these findings to human acute TIN is unknown [9]. Isolated case reports describe autoantibodies to aquaporin 2 and HOXB7 [19], mitochondrial M2 protein [20] and two unidentified brush border antigens [21]. Current concepts suggest that an antigen, be it a hapten derived from a drug or microbe, can mimic a yet-to-be identified antigen normally present in renal tubules. When this antigen is presented to T-helper cells, an immune response is triggered. Macrophage and natural killer cell recruitment and activation follows. Evidence of a primary pathogenic role of T cells is supported by a study that demonstrated the presence of drug-specific sensitized T cells in the peripheral blood of patients with acute drug-induced TIN [22]. Four non-mutually exclusive theories of immune pathogenesis have been proposed [23]. (1) A component of the drug may be trapped along the tubular basement membrane (TBM) where it acts as a hapten, becoming the target of immune attack by sensitized T-cells, or less commonly, antibody producing B-cells. (2) A component of the circulating drug may be recognized as a foreign antigen that triggers an immune response. The antigen may be structurally similar (molecular "mimic") to a normal component of the tubulointerstitium (endogenous antigen) that becomes a target of the immune attack. (3) A drug-derived antigen may first be trapped "in situ" in the tubulointerstitium where immunologically reactive cells and/or antibodies are recruited. (4) Circulating antibodies generated against a drug-derived antigen may form immune complexes within the circulation that are subsequently trapped within the tubulointerstitium and initiate inflammation. Similar theories of pathogenesis have been proposed for "reactive" acute TIN triggered by an infectious agent.

A related drug-induced hypersensitivity syndrome is DRESS (drug reaction with eosinophilia and systemic symptoms), which is more common in adults than children. DRESS is characterized by a severe rash and visceral involvement that includes TIN in 10–30% of cases [24].

There is an animal model of anti-tubular basement membrane disease that has been well-characterized and thought to be mediated by an immune response to an endogenous TBM antigen [25]. However, human anti-TBM nephritis is distinctly rare; it is most commonly encountered in association with anti-GBM disease. Of interest, a patient harboring a deletion in the gene that encodes the human TIN antigen has been reported with CKD [26]. Three patients with autoimmune polyendocrine syndrome type 1 developed end-stage kidney disease (ESKD) due to TIN associated with autoantibodies to aquaporin 2 and HOXB7 [19]. Despite several studies, it is not clear that specific phenotyping studies of the infiltrating interstitial cells can differentiate the antigenic trigger. The one exception is TIN due to lymphoma/lymphoproliferative disease where a single monomorphic cellular population invades the interstitium (Fig. 42.1c). The kidney is the most common solid organ to be infiltrated (60–90%) in patients with hematological malignancies [27].

Overlooked for many years, it is increasingly appreciated that many drug-induced nephrotoxic reactions triggered by tubular epithelial cell damage are associated with significant interstitial inflammation that also contributes to renal functional impairment. Recent studies have elucidated mechanisms that define "necroinflammation", which is distinct from the hypersensitivity-type responses that cause acute TIN

(Fig. 42.2). Necroinflammation is defined pathologically as a pattern of injury associated with an auto-amplification loop that is triggered by a specific form of cell death called necroptosis—characterized by the release of intracellular debris into the interstitial space. This "debris" includes "danger-associated molecular patterns" or DAMPS that bind to unique pattern recognition receptors; an interstitial inflammatory response ensues. It is curious that a few drugs such as vancomycin [29], ciprofloxacin [30] and non-steroidal anti-inflammatory drugs are able to initiate either response. The nephrotoxic effects of some drugs are linked with intratubular crystal or cast formation that trigger necroinflammation (Fig. 42.2).

Spectrum of Drug-Induced Tubulointerstitial Injury

Primary tubular damage → inflammation

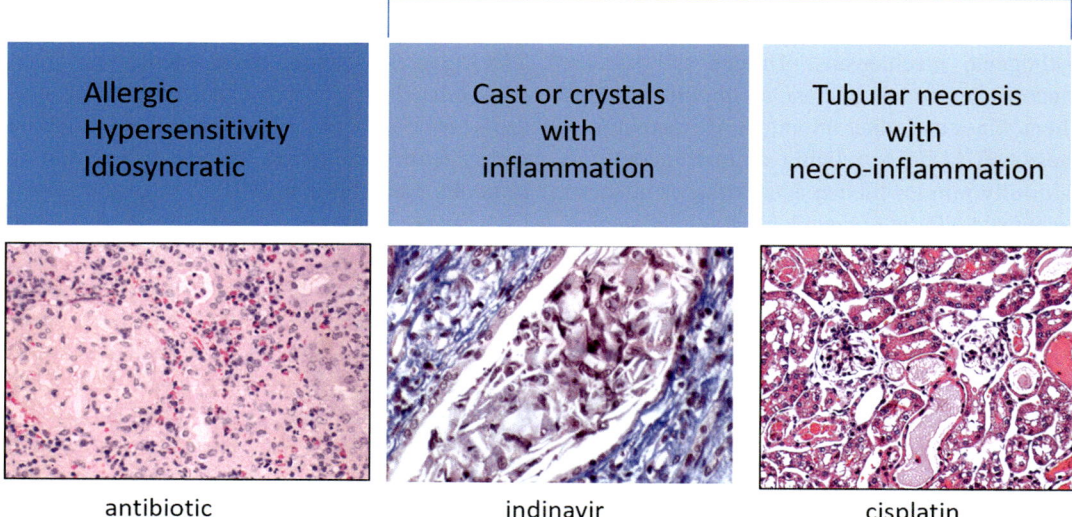

| Allergic Hypersensitivity Idiosyncratic | Cast or crystals with inflammation | Tubular necrosis with necro-inflammation |

antibiotic   indinavir   cisplatin

Fig. 42.2 Mechanisms of drug-induced TIN. Classical acute TIN results from an idiosyncratic allergic reaction with a primary interstitial inflammatory response (left). The nephrotoxic effects of some drugs such as indinavir are linked with intratubular crystal or cast formation, which causes tubular injury followed by interstitial inflammation (middle). Necroinflammation is a more recently recognized mechanism of tubular injury that can be initiated by drugs and is characterized by an auto-amplification loop of interstitial inflammation (right). Tubular death is caused by a specific mechanism called necroptosis, characterized by the release of intracellular debris into the interstitial space that activates unique pro-inflammatory signaling pathways. (The indinavir photomicrograph was reproduced from Fogo et al. [28] with copyright permission. The cisplatin photomicrograph was provided by Dr. Prasad Devarajan, University of Cincinnati College of Medicine)

In kidney transplant allografts, viral TIN secondary to BK polyomavirus or adenovirus is likely secondary to viral transmission via the donor organ [31].

Clinical Findings

When TIN was originally described, it was typically associated with systemic signs of inflammation. A "classic" triad of fever, eosinophilia and rash was observed in a third of the patients with methicillin-induced TIN. Recently, based on European studies of children with severe biopsy-confirmed TIN, clinical manifestations are frequently encountered but heterogenous and often non-specific [6, 8, 32–34]. When TIN occurs as a manifestation of a multi-system disease process, associated systemic symptoms may be present.

The classical clinical presentation of drug-induced TIN is acute kidney injury that begins after exposure to the offending drug. The kinetics of the onset of TIN varies depending upon the exposure history. Symptoms typically begin 3–5 days after re-exposure to the inciting drug, with a mean of 10 days until diagnosis, while it may take several weeks for the symptoms to develop with first-time drug exposure. The TIN risk is not dose-dependent, an observation that supports the theory that the pathogenesis of this disease is a 'hypersensitivity-type' immunological reaction. TIN recurrence following drug re-challenge also supports this hypothesis. Extra-renal symptoms and signs of hypersensitivity, including low-grade fever, a maculopapular rash and mild arthralgias, are more common in TIN associated with infectious and autoimmune diseases. Today, hypersensitivity symptoms are rare in drug-induced TIN and their presence does not exclude the possibility of drug-induced nephrotoxicity and/or acute tubular necrosis (ATN) rather than TIN as the primary kidney lesion. Nonspecific symptoms due to acute kidney injury including anorexia, nausea, vomiting and malaise were frequently reported in a significant number of the 106 children with a biopsy confirmed diagnoses of TIN [mean/median age ranged from 11.6–14 years; 22%

males] published in five separate European studies (Table 42.1) [6, 8, 32–34]. Unlike limited studies in North America, however, a significant number of these children had tubulointerstitial nephritis and uveitis (TINU) syndrome. Kidney interstitial edema may cause renal enlargement and capsular swelling, thought to be the cause of flank pain that is present in some patients with AIN (33–79% of children as reported in the European studies) [6, 8, 32–34]. Adults (121 cases with 91% drug-induced TIN) [9, 35, 36] had similar clinical features as pediatric TIN patients, but with an increased reporting of skin rash and arthralgia.

Antimicrobials and non-steroidal anti-inflammatory drugs (NSAIDS) are most frequently suspected as the cause of drug-induced TIN, but the list of potential offending pharmacological agents is endless (Table 42.2). The risk of acute TIN is very low for an individual drug, despite a long list of single published case reports. The hallmark of TIN is an acute decline in renal function as evidenced by the rise in serum creatinine. This may be the only laboratory abnormality [3]. Acute TIN may also present as one of several more complex clinical scenarios:

1. Acute kidney injury. The absence of hypertension, significant albuminuria and red blood cell casts are clues to a diagnosis of TIN rather than glomerular or vascular disease, though in a given patient clinical manifestations may overlap considerably. Recent exposure to a potentially offending agent, significant pyuria in the absence of bacteriuria, a good urine output and evidence of tubular dysfunction suggest a diagnosis of TIN. Distinguishing between acute TIN and ATN may be challenging, although the presence of many renal tubular cells and muddy brown casts in the urine sediment is more suggestive of a diagnosis of ATN.

2. Chronic renal failure. When evaluating a new patient, the diagnostic challenge may be differentiating acute from chronic TIN. Small kidneys with increased echogenicity and anemia suggest a long-standing process. Many of the causes of chronic TIN in the pediatric population are associated with extra-renal

Table 42.1 Clinical features of TIN in pediatric patients

First author	Howell [32]	Jahnukainen [8]	Taktak [34]	Clavé [6]	Roy [33]	Extrapolated total
Year	2016	2011	2015	2017	2020	
Country	England (GOSH)	Finland	Turkey	France	England (Liverpool)	
N	27	26	19	25	10	
Years	1990–2012	1995–2007	1999–2014	2006–2016	2007–2014	
Anorexia	81%	54%		28%	Yes	43/78 = 55%
Vomiting	59%	35%	27%		70%	37/82 = 9%
Nausea	48%		21%			4/46 = 9%
Fever	41%	92%		28%	30%	45/88 = 51%
Loin/abdominal pain	33%	46%	79%	44%	Yes	47/97 = 48%
Uveitis	65%	46%	5%	28%	60%	43/107 = 41%
Initial creatinine[a] (μmol/L)	263	253	188	183	303	–
Follow up duration (months)	21	35	6	12	18.5	–
Abnormal renal function at last follow up (μmol/L)	56% have eGFR <80 mL/min/1.73 m²	15% have eGFR <80 mL/min/1.73 m²	Mean creatinine 49 μmol/L (35–73)	40% have eGFR <80 mL/min/1.73 m²	50% have eGFR <80 mL/min/1.73 m²	34/88 = 39%[b]
Proportion treated with steroids	96%	88%	32%	72%	80%	82/107 = 77%

[a] Median values reported (except for Taktak study in which mean value is reported)

[b] Taktak study excluded (follow-up renal functional data not provided)

Table 42.2 Drugs most commonly reported to cause acute TIN

Antimicrobials	Analgesics and narcotics	Diuretics	Others
Beta-lactams	NSAIDs	Furosemide	Allopurinol
Methicillin	5-Amino-salicylic acid [41]	Thiazides	Azathioprine [40]
Ampicillin	Mesalazine [42, 43]	Triamterene	Ifosfamide
Penicillin	COX-2 inhibitors		H2 blocker
Oxacillin	Acetaminophen		Ranitidine
Nafcillin	*Drugs of Abuse*	*Biologics*	PPIs
Amoxicillin	Cocaine [54–57]	Nivolumab (anti-PD1)	Omeprazole
Cephalosporins	Synthetic cannabinoids [58]	Vedolizumab [64]	Lansoprazole
Sulfonamides	Anabolic steroids [59]	Pembrolixumab (anti-PD1)	Pantoprazole [44]
Macrolides	Inhaled solvents/toluene	[65]	Antihypertensives
Erythromycin	[60–63]	Infliximab	Amlodipine
Clarithromycin		Adalimumab (anti-TNF)	Diltiazem
Other antibiotics		Atezolizumab (anti-PD-L1)	Captopril
Colistin		Bortezomib [66]	Valsartan [45]
Rifampin			Nifedipine [46]
Polymyxin			Anti-epileptics
Ethambutol			Carbamazepine
Tetracycline			Phenytoin
Vancomycin [37]			Levetiracetam
Linezolid [38]			Clozapine [47]
Ciprofloxacin			Miscellaneous
Isoniazid			Apixaban [48]
Piperacillin-Tazobactam			Cetirizine
Clindamycin [39]			Clozapine
Fluoroquinolone			Ergotamine
Anti-virals			Etanercept
Acyclovir			Glucosamine [49]
Indinavir			Immune checkpoint
Tenofovir			inhibitors [50, 51]
Alpha-interferon			Isotretinoin [52]
Direct-acting antiviral			IVIG [53]
agents for hepatitis C [40]			Lenalidomide
			Exenatide
			Mercury
			Rosuvastatin
			Warfarin
			Zoledronate

Citations are selected from recent publications. Unreferenced medications were cited in prior editions of this chapter
Abbreviations: *NSAID* non-steroidal anti-inflammatory drug, *COX-2* cyclo-oxygenase-2, *PPI* proton pump inhibitor

manifestations such as cystinosis, certain inborn errors of metabolism, and inflammatory bowel disease (IBD). More recently, chronic TIN has become a major cause of CKD in agricultural communities and is thought to be associated with heavy metal and/or pesticide exposure.

3. Tubulopathy. Patients may come to medical attention due to signs and symptoms of tubular dysfunction. The specific manifestations of tubular cell injury/dysfunction vary depending on the primary site of injury. Proximal tubular injury may cause Fanconi's syndrome with glucosuria, proteinuria, and phosphaturia, or it may present as a proximal renal tubular acidosis (RTA). Distal tubular cell injury may manifest as acidosis and hyperkalemia (type 4 RTA) while collecting duct damage typically results in a urinary concentrating defect (nephrogenic diabetes insipidus) (Fig. 42.3). Tubular cell injury may also manifest as potassium wasting. The pediatric case series by Howell et al. reported 7/10 with potassium wasting, 8/13 with reduced phosphate reabsorption and 7/16 with metabolic acidosis [32].

Tubular Cell Injury and Dysfunction Patterns

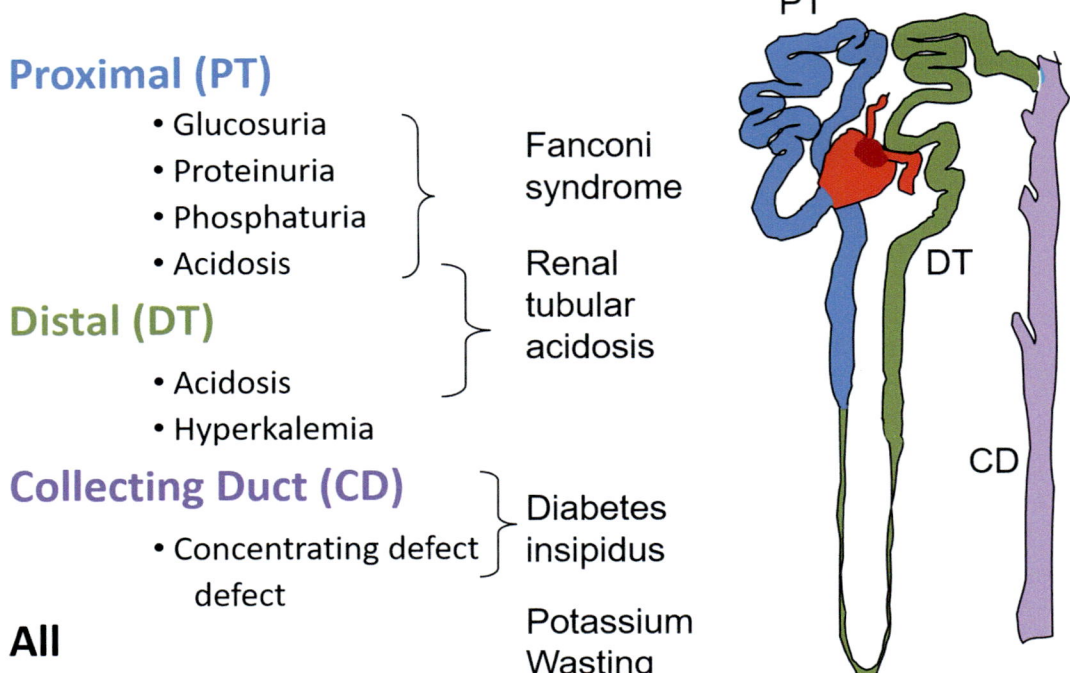

Fig. 42.3 Variable patterns of renal tubular functional defects present in patients with TIN, depending on which nephron segments (proximal, distal or collecting ducts) are injured because of the primary disease process and/or the associated interstitial inflammation

Diagnosis

Often diagnosed clinically, the sensitivity and specificity of the non-invasive diagnostic studies that are performed to diagnose TIN are poor.

Urinary Sediment

The urinary sediment often shows red cells, white cells and white cell casts (Fig. 42.1f) [3]. Sterile pyuria may or may not be associated with eosinophiluria. Urinary eosinophils (Fig. 42.1e) were once considered helpful, but more recent studies and a review of published data by Lusica et al. [67] conclude that urinary eosinophil counts lack adequate sensitivity or specificity. It is also important to remember that a bland urinary sediment does not exclude the diagnosis of acute TIN [15]. Proteinuria may be present, but is typically less than 1 g/24 h. Nephrotic range proteinuria is rare except in NSAID-induced TIN, where it is thought to be mediated by cytokine-induced glomerular injury.

Low Molecular Weight Proteinuria

Beta 2-microglobulin is a low molecular weight (~12 kDa) protein used in the evaluation of the re-absorptive capacity of the proximal kidney tubule. Its daily production is constant and its clearance is almost exclusively by glomerular filtration followed by 99.9% reabsorption by the proximal tubule. Therefore, urinary beta 2-microglobulin levels are often elevated in patients with proximal tubular dysfunction, as frequently observed in TIN; an elevated urinary beta 2-microglobulin/creatinine ratio can help support a diagnosis of TIN [8]. Recent studies suggest that quantitative assessment of other low molecular weight urinary proteins such as α1 microglobulin, retinol binding globulin and vitamin D binding protein may also be informative [68, 69].

Blood Work

In the five most recent pediatric retrospective case series of biopsy-confirmed acute kidney injury due to TIN, the initial serum creatine (median in 4 series, mean in 1 series) ranged from 183 to 303 μmol/L (2.1–3.4 mg/dL). Anemia and elevated serum inflammatory markers (C-reactive protein and erythrocyte sedimentation rate) are common in patients with severe disease [6, 8, 32–34] (Table 42.1). Peripheral eosinophilia may be present in patients with TIN; and was described frequently in the era of methicillin-induced TIN.

Urinary TIN Biomarkers

There is considerable interest in the use of biomarkers to both differentiate causes of kidney disease non-invasively and to follow the disease course. A recent study of adult patients undergoing a kidney biopsy reported that patients with AIN have significantly higher urinary TNF-alpha and IL-9 levels than those with other causes of acute kidney injury [70]. Other promising urinary biomarkers include kidney injury molecule-1 (KIM-1) [71], N-acetyl-beta-D-glucosaminidase (NAG), complement C5b-9 [72] and increased urinary magnesium excretion [73].

Radiology

The renal ultrasound usually demonstrates increased echogenicity, often associated with an increased renal bipolar length, but these findings are non-specific [2, 3]. Gallium scanning has been proposed to differentiate between acute TIN and ATN, but the findings are often non-conclusive and the study is rarely performed now [2].

Biopsy

Since none of the non-invasive studies are both specific and sensitive for TIN, kidney biopsy remains the only definitive diagnostic study. For details on biopsy findings, see the section "Histology".

Causes, Treatment and Outcomes

The causes of TIN are numerous, but can be broadly divided into acute and chronic disorders, though there may be considerable overlap for any single etiology. Most of the larger case series have been conducted in adults and conclude that the majority (approximately 70%) are drug-related, followed by infections (16%) [12, 74]. In the five pediatric case series published since 2010 (*n* = 106 cases), 39% were due to drugs, followed by 36% due to TINU (5% in the adult series) and 17% associated with infections [6, 8, 32–34]. In a systematic review of 592 published TINU cases, it was reported that the median age was 17 years (interquartile range 13–46); 51% were under the age of 18 years [75]. The most common causes of acute TIN in pediatric patients are summarized in Fig. 42.4 and discussed in more detail in the following sections and Tables 42.2, 42.3 and 42.4.

Drugs

In the current era, drugs clearly surpass infections as the most commonly implicated cause of

Fig. 42.4 Causes of pediatric acute TIN. Data are based on five European pediatric case series published since 2010, that also from the basis for Table 42.1. (n = 106 individual patients; etiology counted twice for 8 patients in the series by Howell et al. who had TINU plus a secondary etiology identified) [6, 8, 32–34]

Etiology of Pediatric Acute Tubulointerstitial Nephritis

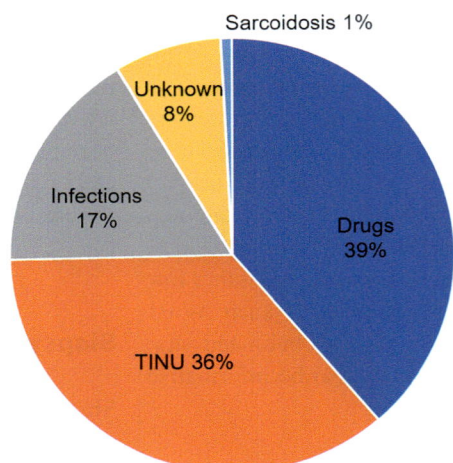

acute TIN. In the adult literature, where there are more data, 35% are caused by PPIs, 35% by antibiotics and 20% by NSAIDS [78]. However, the list of potentially causative agents is extensive, expanding, and variable over time as drug prescribing practices change (Table 42.2).

Methicillin was long considered the prototypical cause of drug-induced TIN, as first reported in 1968 [79]. In fact, due to its infamy, its use has declined worldwide and it is no longer available in most countries. Methicillin and other beta-lactam antibiotics (penicillins and cephalosporins) are still more commonly associated with systemic signs of hypersensitivity, including the classic triad of rash, fever, and eosinophilia than any other group of drugs.

Rifampin has frequently been implicated as a cause of acute TIN. Affected patients fall into two groups: (1) Patients who receive short duration therapy with rifampin and (2) patients who have had prior or intermittent exposure to the drug. The first group typically lacks anti-rifampin antibodies and the onset of clinical symptoms is insidious. The second group may develop antibodies and clinical symptoms often begin abruptly [23]. Associated with certain agents such as rifampin and allopurinol, hemolysis or hepatitis may also be present [23].

NSAID-induced TIN may be associated with nephrotic syndrome in as many as 70% of the

cases [23]. It is reported to occur more frequently in older patients, but it is unclear whether this is due to under-reporting in pediatrics, lower exposure rates or other factors. In NSAID-induced TIN, hematuria is almost always microscopic and extra-renal symptoms such as fever and rash occur in less than 10% of the patients [23]. The degree of interstitial inflammation is often less with NSAID-induced TIN. In addition to the classic TIN accompanied by "minimal change" glomerular disease, NSAIDs can also cause membranous nephropathy. Therefore, all patients with nephrotic syndrome associated with NSAID use should undergo a diagnostic renal biopsy [80].

The epidemiology of drug-induced TIN has changed significantly in the past two decades, especially following the first published report of PPI-induced TIN in 1992 [81]. In adults taking PPIs, a three times increased risk of developing TIN [82], a four times increased risk of acute kidney injury and a 20% increased risk for CKD [83] were reported. A meta-analysis also identified a 1.2 increased risk of CKD among PPI users, but no increased risk among H2 receptor antagonists [84]. Additionally, there is evidence that the duration of exposure to PPI is associated with increased risk and progression of CKD [85]. As newer therapies and drugs are introduced, one must maintain a high index of suspicion for drugs

Table 42.3 Infectious causes of acute TIN

Bacteria
Brucella
Campylobacter
Corynebacterium diphtheria
E. coli
Enterococcus
Legionella
Leptospira
Mycobacteria
Mycoplasma
Salmonella
Staphylococci
Streptococci
Syphilis
Yersinia
Viruses
Adenovirus [76]
BK polyoma
Cytomegalovirus
Epstein Barr virus
Hantavirus
Hepatitis A
Herpes simplex
Human immunodeficiency virus [77]
Influenza H1N1
Mumps
Rubeola
SARS-COV-2
Fungi
Cryptococcus
Histoplasmosis
Parasites
Babesiosis
Encephalitozoon cuniculi
Hydatid Disease
Leishmaniasis
Toxoplasmosis
Rickettsia
R. diaporica
R. rickettsii

Table 42.4 Causes of acute tubulointerstitial nephritis in the pediatric age-group (drugs and infections excluded)

Autoimmune disorders with TIN as typical renal manifestation
Tubulointerstitial nephritis and uveitis syndrome (TINU)
Sjögren's syndrome
Sarcoidosis
Anti-TBM nephritis (rare)
Autoimmune disorders with TIN usually associated with glomerular disease
Systemic lupus erythematosus
ANCA+ vasculitis
Many types of primary glomerulonephritis
Autoimmune disorders with TIN as rare manifestation
Inflammatory bowel disease
Ankylosing spondylitis
Malignant infiltration
Lymphoma
Leukemia
Other
Amanita mushrooms
Sickle cell nephropathy
Snake bites
Wasp and hornet stings (usually multiple)
Radiation nephritis
Renal allograft rejection
Xanthogranulomatous pyelonephritis
Idiopathic

as a cause of acute renal dysfunction without relying on the presence of the historically "classical" clinical features [86]. Future pharmacogenomic studies may identify patients at higher risk of TIN in association with the use of specific medications. One study failed to show that individuals with the CYP2C19 slower metabolizer genotype were at increased risk of omeprazole-induced AIN [87].

The primary treatment of drug-induced TIN is to identify and stop the offending agent. The immunologic trigger must be removed, particularly since persistent tubulointerstitial injury can progress to chronic irreversible damage. Early removal of the offending agent alone frequently leads to complete reversal of renal injury. Kidney biopsies are not performed and additional therapy is not required, if the drug exposure time was short and renal function improves quickly. After drug-induced acute TIN, the mean recovery time to the nadir creatinine is 1.5 months [23]. There are an increasing number of long-term follow-up studies in adults reporting an increased risk of CKD after PPI-induced TIN [85, 88].

Therapy with corticosteroids has been used for several decades to treat severe acute drug-induced TIN, but indications for treatment and evidence of efficacy are problematic due to the lack of prospective randomized controlled clinical trials. Earlier case series have suggested faster rates of renal recovery with steroids, but their benefit to long-term kidney function is still debated. A systematic review of all studies published between 1975 and 2016 concluded: (1) Findings suggest that the evidence for the use of corticosteroids in the treatment of drug-induced AIN remains uncertain, (2) Given the shortage of proven treatments for drug-induced AIN to ameliorate the burden and consequences of acute kidney injury, suitably designed studies should be prioritized [89]. In the interim, there is a growing consensus of expert opinions that a course of corticosteroids is reasonable to treat acute kidney

injury secondary to biopsy-proven acute TIN (in the absence of significant tubular atrophy and interstitial fibrosis) when kidney function does not improve within 3–6 days after the offending drug is withdrawn [90]. Studies by Gonzales et al. [36] and Fernandez-Juarez et al. [91] report worse renal functional outcome if treatment is delayed for more than a few weeks after the diagnosis is made (Fig. 42.5).

While older studies may have argued against the use of routine corticosteroids for severe drug-induced TIN, there are several possible explanations for a lack of glucocorticoid efficacy in

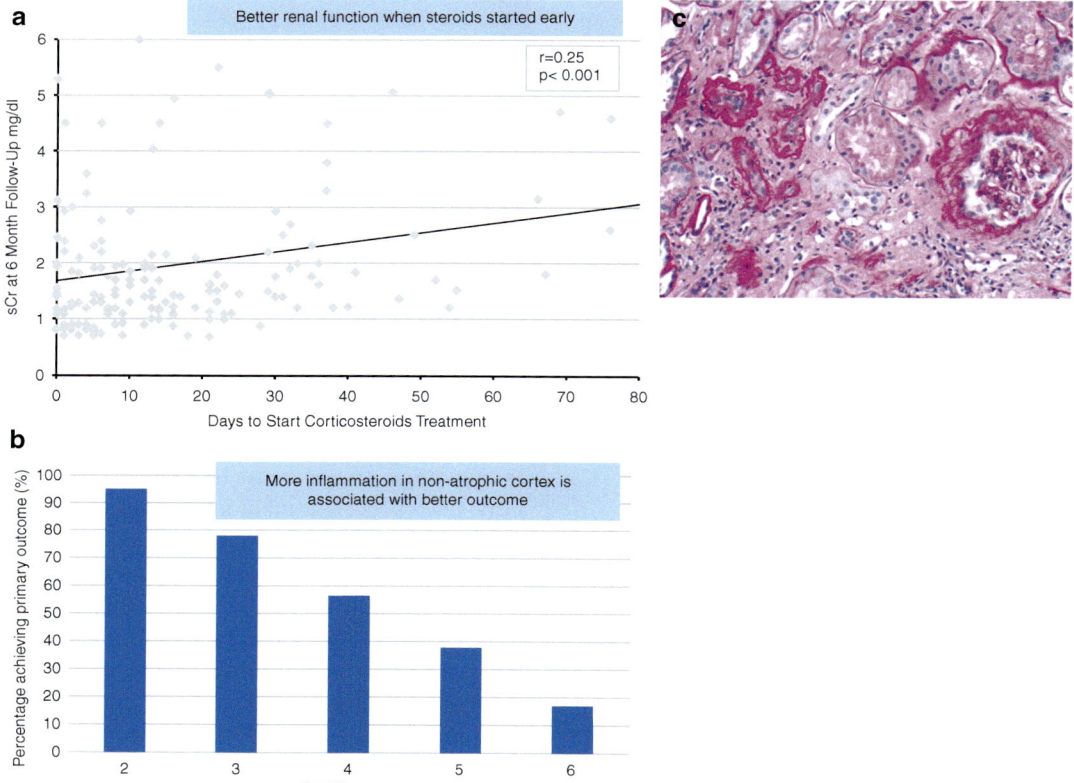

Fig. 42.5 Prognostic impact of early steroid initiation, and degree of tubulointerstitial inflammation and fibrosis/tubular atrophy on TIN outcomes. In a study of 182 adults with severe drug-induced TIN treated in Spain (mean peak creatinine 504 ± 309 μmol/L), the serum creatinine level 6 months after diagnosis was better when corticosteroid treatment was started early [91] (**a**). A kidney injury chronicity score applied to 120 adult kidney biopsies with primary acute TIN reported better clinical outcomes (50% reduction in serum creatinine or eGFR greater than 60 mL/min/1.73 m^2 at 1 year) in patients with low cortical tubular atrophy and with higher interstitial inflammation in non-fibrotic cortex scores. These data were combined into a single score called TANFI, calculated as the tubular atrophy score pulse the inverse of the non-fibrotic cortex with inflammation [92] (**b**). Representative photomicrograph of renal biopsy illustrating the features of chronic TIN—tubular atrophy, thickened tubular basement membranes and an expanded interstitial space occupied by scar tissue (**c**). (**a**, **b** were originally published in *Histopathology* and *CJASN*, respectively, and are reproduced with copyright permission)

earlier studies, including a bias towards treating the patients with worse disease, the possibility that a significant proportion of the patients had NSAID-associated TIN, which appears to be less likely to respond to glucocorticoid therapy, and the negative impact of delayed therapy onset [9, 23, 35]. Future studies will also need to control for the degree of chronic damage as quantified on the kidney biopsy (tubular atrophy and interstitial fibrosis), which negatively impacts reversibility and long-term prognosis [92]. When indicated, the leading experts recommend treating acute drug-induced TIN with prednisone 1 mg/kg/day for 2–4 weeks, followed by tapering to discontinuation over 3–4 weeks. The retrospective study by Fernandez-Juraz et al. with 182 adults from 13 centers in Spain reported that using high dose corticosteroids for longer than 3 weeks and total therapy duration longer than 8 weeks has a non-significant effect on renal recovery and may increase the risk for adverse steroid therapy effects [91]. Data on the use of immunosuppressive agents such as mycophenolate mofetil are too sparse to draw any conclusions.

While the serum creatinine at the time of biopsy is a poor prognostic indicator [36], evidence is emerging to suggest that patients with acute systemic inflammation (elevated ESR and CRP) [93] and low chronicity scores on biopsy [92] have better renal function outcome (Fig. 42.5).

Drugs have also been implicated in unusual cases of TIN. For example, anti-carbonic anhydrase II antibodies were detected in a patient with TIN associated with the use of famotidine [94].

Tubulointerstitial Nephritis with Uveitis

An association between TIN and anterior uveitis, occasionally associated with bone marrow granulomas, was first reported in 1975 and called TINU [95]. While anterior uveitis is more common, posterior uveitis can also occur. When first described, there was a female predominance; recent studies also indicate that 65% are female. The median age of onset is 17 years (55% are under 18 years of age) [75]. TINU is a syndrome of multiple etiologies. Though often idiopathic and presumed to be autoimmune in pathogenesis, it is important to search for evidence of the known causes of TIN with uveitis that are summarized in Fig. 42.6. It is speculated that disease pathogenesis involves an immunological response triggered by a recent drug exposure (often an

TINU Syndrome

Differential Diagnosis
- Sarcoidosis
- Sjögren's syndrome
- SLE
- ANCA-associated vasculits
- Behcet's disease
- Infections
  (TB, brucellosis, toxoplasmosis, histoplasmosis, EBV, HIV, chlamydia, mycoplasma)

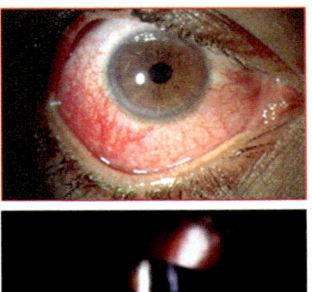
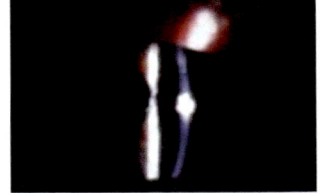

Slit lamp exam for uveitis

Fig. 42.6 Tubulointerstitial nephritis with uveitis syndrome (TINU). While often idiopathic, the known secondary causes of TINU listed in this figure should be considered in the differential diagnosis as specific therapy is available for many of them. The ocular photomicrographs, taken from patients with acute uveitis, serve as a reminder of the importance of performing a slit lamp examination as part of the evaluation of a patient with suspected acute TIN of unknown etiology

antimicrobial agent), an infection or an unknown agent. The systematic review of 592 cases, reported an association with drugs in 21%, infections in 6% and no identified trigger in 63% [75]. Some patients have serum auto-antibodies such as antinuclear antibodies, rheumatoid factor, antineutrophil cytoplasmic antibodies and/or anticardiolipin antibodies. One study posits that modified C-reactive protein might be a target antigen [96]. Some patients have associated autoimmune diseases such as hyperthyroidism [97], hyperparathyroidism, or rheumatoid arthritis. Patients may also have a history of recent insect bites [98].

The report of TINU in monozygotic male twins separated in onset by 2 years suggests the possibility of a genetic predisposition to the syndrome [99], as does a report in 1994 of identical female twins with the onset of TINU syndrome 1 year apart [100]. However, the lack of reports of multiple affected family members and the lack of geographic clustering questions the influence of environment and genetic factors. Reviewed by Cline and Vanguri [101], several small studies (2–20 patients from several countries), have suggested different HLA associations (especially some DRB1* alleles), but ethnic diversity among the cohorts prevents broader extrapolation of the findings.

Several of the non-specific symptoms associated with TIN may be present in patients with TINU syndrome. These include fever, weight loss, fatigue, malaise, loss of appetite, weakness, asthenia, abdominal or flank pain, arthralgias and myalgias. Less commonly, headache, polyuria, lymphadenopathy, edema, pharyngitis or rash may occur. The ocular manifestations commonly include eye pain and redness (77%), decreased visual acuity (20%) and photophobia (14%) [98], but recent studies have suggested that up to 58% of patients with TINU have reported no ocular symptoms despite slit-lamp confirmation of uveitis, making it critical that patients with acute TIN undergo regular eye examinations [8]. Onset of uveitis varies from several weeks before the onset of renal involvement, concurrent with the TIN, or up to 15 months after the onset of TIN. The systematic review by Regusci et al.

reported the onset of uveitis after renal involvement in 52% of the patients [75]. Both recurrent acute and chronic uveitis are commonly described. The timing of uveitis recurrence has varied from 3 months after steroid tapering to 2 years after the first episode. The renal and ocular manifestations of TINU have also been reported to recur years after initial presentation, even after transplantation, further supporting a role for systemic immunological factors in the disease pathogenesis [102].

Laboratory findings may include elevated serum creatinine, evidence of tubular dysfunction, anemia, slightly abnormal liver function tests, eosinophilia, hypergammaglobulinemia and elevated erythrocyte sedimentation rate. A variety of serological markers have been reported without evidence of the associated diseases in 15% of patients (such as SLE, ANCA-associated vasculitis, anti-phospholipid syndrome, rheumatoid arthritis). However, definitive diagnosis requires a renal biopsy and a formal ophthalmologic slit-lamp examination to diagnose uveitis. Bone marrow and lymph node granulomas have been reported, but these studies are rarely performed now that TINU syndrome has become recognized as a distinct clinical entity.

The tubulointerstitial disease is self-limited in most patients, but there are reports of individuals progressing to ESKD [8, 102]. In the 2021 systematic review, 11% of the patients under 18 years had CKD at a median follow-up of 18 months [75]. The ocular disease usually requires treatment, with both topical and systemic steroids. There are anecdotal reports of utilizing other immunomodulatory therapies in the treatment of recalcitrant eye disease. While the acute eye disease usually improves, recurrences, complications, and chronic ocular disease are not uncommon. Most of the long-term complications of TINU have been ocular, estimated to occur in 20% of patients. These include posterior synechiae, optic disc swelling, cystoid macular edema, chorio-retinal scar formation, cataracts and glaucoma [95, 98]. Fortunately, the risk of visual loss appears low. Due to the morbidity associated with the ocular manifestations, early detection by slit lamp examination is essential.

Infections

Numerous infectious agents have been implicated in the pathogenesis of TIN, both acute and chronic. TIN was first recognized as a unique clinical entity in 1860 in a patient with scarlet fever. However, it was several decades later before Councilman introduced the term "interstitial nephritis" and described the histologic lesions. To quote his landmark paper "Acute interstitial lesions of the kidneys have been considered as common in scarlet fever, and are regarded by some authors as constituting the most frequent pathological alteration of the kidney in this disease. This has also been described in diphtheria and in other infectious diseases" [1]. The 1939–1945 era saw the eradication of serious and fatal streptococcal infections due to the introduction of antibiotics. In the current era, the infections implicated as causes of TIN vary from Councilman's time due to childhood immunizations and the use of effective antibiotics. In fact, since 1960 antibiotics rather than infections are a more common cause of acute TIN (Table 42.3, Fig. 42.4).

The infectious microorganisms may directly invade the renal parenchyma to cause a specific form of TIN (pyelonephritis). TIN is the most frequent renal biopsy finding in patients with renal tuberculosis [103]. Rare infectious processes may induce emphysematous or necrotizing interstitial parenchymal lesions [104, 105]. However, the traditional form of acute TIN is associated with infection at an extrarenal site and the tubulointerstitial inflammation is thought to represent a secondary or "reactive" immunological response to the infection. In the latter, the infectious agent is not cultured from the kidney or urine and cytokines derived from inflammatory cells are key kidney disease mediators.

When a renal biopsy is performed in a patient with pyelonephritis (not typically required or recommended), the interstitial lesion is often localized to a single pyramid and characterized by neutrophil predominance. In contrast, "reactive" TIN associated with a systemic infection is characterized histologically as either patchy or diffuse lesions that are associated with interstitial edema and a predominance of mononuclear cells. The pathogenic microbial antigens that initiate the immune response to cause TIN are largely unknown. One exception is leptospirosis, where an isolated outer membrane protein has been shown to interact in vitro with Toll-like receptor 2 to stimulate synthesis of inflammatory cytokines, chemokines and collagen by renal tubules [106]. The primary therapeutic measure is to treat the infection, preferably with non-nephrotoxic antimicrobials.

Viral infections are an important cause of TIN. Epstein-Barr virus (EBV) may have a pathogenetic role in certain forms of "idiopathic" TIN based on the detection of EBV genome in the proximal tubules in one case series [107]. HIV-1-associated nephropathy is typically characterized by significant glomerular pathology, but co-existent TIN is common and more severe than observed in other primary glomerular disorders. This is likely related to the ability of HIV-1 to infect and damage tubular cells [108]. In a kidney biopsy series of 222 HIV-infected patients, 27% had TIN as the predominant lesion [77]. However, in at least half of the latter patient group, the concurrent use of nephrotoxic agents such as antiretroviral drugs may have contributed to the TIN. TIN has also been reported as a feature of the immune reconstitution syndrome in the HIV-infected population [109].

BK polyomavirus is an important cause of TIN in immunocompromised patients, especially following kidney transplantation, though it has been reported in other transplants recipients as well and rarely in children with a lymphoid malignancy [4, 110–112]. Adenovirus DNA has also been identified in a few kidney allografts with granulomatous TIN [5, 76]. Many other viruses listed in Table 42.3 have been associated with reported cases of TIN.

Granulomatous Interstitial Nephritis

TIN may be associated with the presence of granulomas on renal biopsy (Fig. 42.1b). Granulomatous TIN is found in approximately 6% of renal biopsies with TIN [13]. The differential diagnosis of this histologically distinct variant includes drug-induced TIN (~25% of cases), infectious causes (tuberculosis, brucellosis, histoplasmosis, adenovirus, fungal), ANCA-associated vasculitis, sarcoidosis, TINU syndrome, multiple myeloma, IBD [113] and other dyspro-teinemias; it may be idiopathic in as many as 50% of the patients [114]. While TIN has been reported in up to 20% of renal biopsies performed in patients with IBD [41], granulomatous TIN is exceptionally rare and limited to a few IBD case reports [115].

Additionally, there is the frequent challenge of distinguishing between drug-induced AIN associ-ated with IBD treatment and extra-intestinal mani-festations of IBD primary disease. There are reports of biopsy proven AIN in IBD patients before they have started IBD treatment, suggesting a pathogen-esis distinct from drug-induced AIN [116].

There are several systemic diseases that may cause acute TIN even in the pediatric age group (Table 42.4). A few of the more common exam-ples are discussed briefly in the next sections.

Sarcoidosis

Sarcoidosis is a multisystem disease character-ized by non-caseating granuloma formation in various organs, including the kidney. While the exact incidence of granulomatous TIN among patients with sarcoidosis is unknown, studies have cited an incidence up to 30% [114]. Although histologic evidence of renal involve-ment is said to be common in sarcoidosis, iso-lated renal sarcoidosis is rare [117, 118].

Patients with sarcoidosis tend to avidly absorb dietary calcium, leading to hypercalciuria and, less commonly, hypercalcemia. The clinical manifestations of calcium hyperabsorption may be silent or may cause nephrolithiasis, nephrocal-cinosis, renal insufficiency or polyuria. Nephrocalcinosis is the most common cause of chronic renal failure in sarcoidosis [119]. Polyuria may be the result of hypercalcemia and hypercalciuria that decreases tubular responsive-ness to antidiuretic hormone, or it may be a mani-festation of diabetes insipidus or primary polydipsia as a consequence of granulomatous

infiltration of the hypothalamus. It is important to recognize that the abnormalities in calcium metabolism can occur in other chronic granulo-matous diseases due to increased calcitriol pro-duced by activated mononuclear cells [120].

The urinary manifestations of sarcoid granu-lomatous TIN are similar to other forms of chronic TIN, often associated with a bland urine sediment, sterile pyuria and/or mild proteinuria. The serum creatinine is usually normal and CKD is rare. The renal biopsy findings may include TIN with mononuclear cell infiltration and non-caseating granulomas in the interstitium [121]. When glomerular disease is present, it is most frequently membranous nephropathy; however, granulomatous TIN is present in 2/3 of the cases with glomerular disease [122]. Chronic injury, manifest as interstitial fibrosis and tubular dam-age, is common in the primary sarcoidosis-associated glomerulopathies.

Corticosteroids remain the treatment of choice, with slowly tapered protocols to prevent disease recurrence [122–125]. While there are currently no large trials of therapeutic protocols for renal sarcoidosis, there are reports of tumor necrosis factor-α blocking agents improving renal function, supporting the theory that TNF-α may play a pathogenetic role [119, 126]. In the rare patient who develops ESKD, it is usually due to hypercal-cemia and hypercalciuria rather than TIN [119]. Renal sarcoidosis has been reported to recur in approximately 15% of renal allografts [127, 128].

Sjögren's Syndrome

Sjögren's syndrome is classically described as a sicca syndrome that occurs as a consequence of lymphocytic (mainly activated CD4+ cells and B cells) and plasmacytic infiltrates in the exocrine glands, especially the salivary, parotid and lacri-mal glands. This causes dry mouth and dry eyes. These sicca symptoms are less common in chil-dren; recurrent parotitis is a common presenting symptom [129]. The pathogenic immune process may also affect non-exocrine organs, including the skin, lung, gastrointestinal tract, central and peripheral nervous systems, musculoskeletal system and the kidney. The most common renal manifestation is TIN with associated tubular dysfunction (Fanconi syndrome); glomerular disease has also been reported [130–132]. Though the presence of renal disease in patients with Sjögren's syndrome was first reported in the 1960s, its prevalence and primary pathogenesis remain ill-defined. In the literature, the frequency of renal abnormalities varies widely from 16% to 67% [130, 133]. The diagnosis of idiopathic Sjögren's syndrome is based on clinical and/or histopathological evidence of ocular, oral or salivary involvement and the presence of anti-Ro/SSA and/or anti-La/SSB auto-antibodies. Symptoms due to renal disease, such as polyuria and renal tubular acidosis, may precede sicca syndrome-related symptoms [133]. TIN is the most common renal finding in Sjögren's syndrome and carries the best prognosis [134], although one case series reported four patients with isolated TIN and primary Sjogren's disease that progressed to ESKD [131]. While steroids remain the mainstay of therapy for the renal manifestations, other medications such as rituximab have shown improvement in the extrarenal manifestations [131, 132, 135, 136].

Other Systemic Autoimmune Diseases

Renal involvement is common when systemic lupus erythematosus begins in the pediatric age group: 20–80% within a year of diagnosis and 48–100% at some point during the course of the disease [137]. Isolated TIN associated with tubular basement membrane (TBM) immune deposits can occur, but is extremely rare. Conversely, focal or diffuse interstitial inflammation in association with glomerular disease is relatively common and does not typically show a clear association with TBM immune deposits and the presence of TIN is not considered in the primary classification of lupus nephritis (Classes 1–VI) [138]. The severity of interstitial inflammation and, in particular, its association with tubular atrophy and interstitial fibrosis, are strong predictors of renal outcome [139].

The majority of pediatric patients with ANCA-associated systemic vasculitis have renal involvement (75–88%) [140]. TIN is typically present in association with focal necrotizing glomerulonephritis, though isolated cases of TIN have been reported [141]. The "signature" interstitial granuloma is only present in 6–12% of renal biopsies performed in patients with granulomatosis with polyangiitis [142].

Over the past decade, an increasing number of adults have been diagnosed with TIN due to an autoimmune multisystem disease referred to as IgG4-related disease [143], but there are very few published pediatric cases [144]. It is noted that IgG4+ cells can be detected in other forms of TIN [145]. Other causes of primary TIN include IBD [115, 116] and ankylosing spondylitis [113, 146]. In a study of native kidney biopsies performed in Finland, 13.3% of the patients with TIN had IBD [147]. Both IBD and some of the drug treatments (5-aminosalicylic acid, infliximab, vedolizumab) have been implicated as TIN triggers. Since many patients with systemic autoimmune disorders have complicated medical courses, it is always important to consider alternative causes for their TIN such as drugs and infection.

TIN has been reported in young boys with immunodysregulation, polyendocrinopathy. Enteropathy X-linked (IPEX), a rare genetic disease caused by an inherited mutation in the gene encoding forkhead box P3 (FOXP3) [148].

Xanthogranulomatous TIN

Xanthogranulomatous pyelonephritis (XGP) is a rare entity usually occurring in the fifth or sixth decade of life, though neonatal and childhood cases have been reported [149–151]. In a review of 66 children who underwent nephrectomy in Ireland between 1963 and 2016 for XPN, the median age was 4.84 years (range 1.1–14.8 years) [151]. It is a chronic destructive granulomatous inflammation of the renal parenchyma first described in 1916 by Schlagenhaufer in association with *Escherichia coli* and *Proteus mirabilis* urinary tract infections [152]. The exact etiology remains unknown, but it is thought to be a result of chronic obstruction with persistent urinary infection [150, 153]. The disease may be mistaken for malignancy, with the consequence that diagnosis is often made on histology after nephrectomy. Medical management of the suppurative infection is possible when an early diagnosis is made, but this is unusual. Nephrectomy is not uncommon due to irreversible parenchymal destruction [154, 155].

Idiopathic TIN

Approximately 8–10% of cases of acute TIN remain idiopathic [6–8, 12, 32–34]. This diagnosis can only be made after all other possible causes have been eliminated by a thorough history, clinical examination, and relevant laboratory investigations.

Chronic Interstitial Nephritis

Epidemiology

The exact incidence and prevalence of primary chronic TIN is poorly documented. This topic is complicated by the fact that chronic interstitial changes typify virtually all chronic renal disorders that eventually progress to CKD stage 5.

Pathology

The early phase of chronic TIN shares histopathologic features with acute TIN, including interstitial inflammation and tubular cell activation. However, as the disease progresses, interstitial fibrosis and chronic tubular injury (dilated tubules with/without cast formation, atrophied tubules and thickened tubular basement membrane) appear (Fig. 42.5) [156, 157]. In the advanced stages, glomerulosclerosis may occur as a secondary consequence of the tubular damage or periglomerular interstitial fibrosis. For all chronic kidneys diseases, whether initially a glomerular or tubulointerstitial disorder, interstitial

fibrosis severity is a strong predictor of renal functional loss and risk of progressive renal disease, as illustrated by a recent study of 1022 patients with IgA nephropathy [158].

Clinical Findings

The clinical findings in chronic TIN are similar to those in acute TIN, but tend to be more subtle and often go undetected until the patient develops signs and symptoms due to chronic renal insufficiency. Compared to chronic glomerular disease, in patients with chronic TIN hypertension is less common, daily protein excretion rates rarely exceeds 1.5 g/day and anemia may be disproportionately worse than the degree of renal functional impairment due to the loss of erythropoietin-producing cells in the peritubular interstitium. Bone disease may also be more prominent as a result of chronic phosphate wasting due to proximal tubular dysfunction.

Etiology

As in acute TIN, there are numerous causes of chronic TIN. In addition to diseases that may progress from acute TIN to chronic TIN, several diseases more typically present as chronic TIN. In the pediatric population, the causes of chronic TIN that are not sequelae of acute TIN can be broadly grouped into the following categories that are also summarized in Table 42.5; many are reviewed in greater detail in other chapters.

Genetic Kidney Diseases, especially the ciliopathies (nephronophthisis) and polycystic kidney disease, are associated with significant tubular damage and interstitial inflammation and fibrosis. Another group of inherited diseases that are increasingly recognized since first reported in 2002 are now classified as autosomal dominant tubulointerstitial kidney disease (ADTKD) [159]. They are rare diseases that are largely undetected in childhood, as the kidney disease is typically silent until clinical manifestations of chronic renal failure develop. Some patients provide a history of polyuria and/or enuresis due to a uri-

Table 42.5 Common causes of chronic TIN in childhood and adolescence

Category	Specific entity
Persistent TIN	All categories (late diagnosis)
Inherited kidney disease	Autosomal Dominant Tubulointerstitial Kidney Diseases (ADTKD) (*UMOD, MUC1, REN* and other less common gene mutations)
	Karyomegalic TIN (*FAN1* mutation)
	Nephronophthisis (ciliopathies)
	Polycystic kidney diseases
Inherited metabolic disease	Cystinosis
	Oxalosis
	Methylmalonic acidemia
	Mitochondrial cytopathies
	Adenine phosphoribosyltransferase (APRT) deficiency
Acquired metabolic disease	Nephrocalcinosis
	Uric acid-induced injury
	Potassium deficiency (anorexia nervosa)
Chronic nephrotoxicity	Chronic interstitial nephritis in agricultural communities (CINAC)
	Heavy metals (lead, cadmium)
	Calcineurin inhibitors
	Analgesic nephropathy
	Chinese herbs (Aristolochia fangchi)
	Chemotherapy (cisplatinum, isophosphamide)
Structural renal disease	Dysplasia
	Obstruction
	Reflux

nary concentrating defect. The first cases reported were caused by autosomal dominant mutations in *UMOD*, the gene that encodes the kidney-specific protein uromodulin (also known as Tamm-Horsfall protein). Patients often present with symptoms of gout between 15 and 40 years of age due to hyperuricemia (present in ~70% of affected patients) [160]. Stage 5 CKD due to chronic TIN develops between ages 30–60 years; the rate of progression may be decreased in the hyperuricemic patients with the use of allopurinol. Mutations in the *MUC1* gene, which encodes the glycoprotein mucin-1, were first reported in 2013. Mutations in *UMOD* and *MUC1* are the most prevalent etiologies of ADTKD [161]. It is estimated that ~50% of the ADTKD patients currently lack a genetic diagnosis [160]. Eight mutations have been reported in the *REN* gene that encodes prorenin [162, 163]. These patients may develop transient childhood anemia, have a tendency for hyperkalemia, defective urinary concentration and gout. Additional diseases have been classified as ADTKD, although the kidney phenotype may include features in addition to

chronic TIN. These include patients with mutations in the genes *HNF1B* encoding hepatocyte nuclear factor 1 beta, and *SEC61A1* that encodes the alpha 1 subunit of SEC61 [161].

There is another rare genetic disease that resembles nephronophthisis histologically except for the presence of hyperchromatic and abnormally enlarged tubular epithelial cell nuclei that causes ESKD in the third or fourth decade of life. It was first recognized as a distinct entity and named karyomegalic interstitial nephritis (KIN) in 1979 [164]. In 2012 Zhou et al. [165] identified an autosomal recessive mutation in *FAN1* as a cause of TIN.

Other causes of chronic TIN include:

1. ***Congenital anomalies of the kidney and urinary tract.***
2. ***Inborn error of metabolism***, including cystinosis, oxalosis, methylmalonic acidemia, the mitochondrial cytopathies, adenine phosphoribosyltransferase (APRT) deficiency.
3. ***Chronic nephrotoxin exposure***, especially the calcineurin inhibitors, lithium, heavy met-

als (cadmium, mercury, and lead), chemotherapeutic agents (cisplatinum, ifosfamide), antimicrobials (amphotericin B, antiretroviral drugs), NSAIDs and certain Chinese herbs.

4. **Chronic interstitial nephritis in agricultural communities (CINAC)**. This disease entity is increasing in endemic areas of the world, characterized as agricultural communities in hot tropical communities (patients in Sri Lanka and Central America are best studied) [166]. While male agricultural workers in the 20s to 40s age group are most frequently reported, it has also been reported in women, and markers of kidney damage can be found in children [167]. Histopathologically CINAC is a chronic TIN. The etiology is unclear and likely multifactorial. A recent kidney biopsy study by Vervaet et al. [168] reported abnormal proximal tubular lysosomes; by electron microscopy they contained electron-dense aggregates suggestive of a toxin-associate proximal tubulopathy. Several toxic agrochemicals and pesticides have been identified as candidates, but definitive proof of their role is still lacking. Exposure might be direct or may occur from contaminated water consumption or by inhalation. Heat stress and recurrent dehydration may be a contributing factor.

5. *Chronic allograft nephropathy.*

Treatment and Prognosis

Treatment of chronic TIN is based on the treatment of the primary disease process. In addition, there is increasing evidence that correction of anemia, reduction of proteinuria and suppression of inflammation may also slow the rate of the kidney disease progression [156]. Angiotensin converting-enzyme inhibitors and angiotensin receptor type 1 blockers are being used with increasing frequency for a variety of chronic renal diseases, especially when associated with hypertension and/or proteinuria. It is believed that in addition to decreasing intraglomerular pressure, these drugs reduce proteinuria and may also have an anti-fibrotic role related to angiotensin II blockade [169].

Outcomes

Patients with chronic TIN and CKD stage III (GFR 30–59 mL/min/1.73 m^2) or stage IV (GFR between 15 and 29 mL/min/1.73 m^2) are destined to progress to ESKD (GFR < 15 mL/min/1.73 m^2). Numerous comorbid factors correlate with a faster rate of renal functional decline, including hypertension, high-grade proteinuria, diabetes, smoking, obesity, dyslipidemia and anemia [12, 96].

While definitive therapy may not be available for the primary disease process that is responsible for chronic TIN, many of these comorbidities can be addressed therapeutically to preserve residual nephrons and slow the rate of CKD progression. Landmark studies by Risdon and Shainuck, more than half a century ago, highlighted the central importance of chronic TIN, assessed as the degree of tubular atrophy and interstitial fibrosis, to renal functional outcomes irrespective of the primary etiology of the CKD. Since then, advances in the field of cellular and molecular biology and genome sciences have utilized animal models and human kidney tissue biorepositories to decipher fundamental mechanisms that cause the chronic TIN component in human CKD. A major priority for ongoing and future studies is the identification of new therapeutic targets, development of safe therapeutic agents based on these "candidate" targets and subsequent randomized prospective clinical trials to establish their efficacy in patients with CKD. Analogous to current cancer treatment protocols, a multi-agent approach will almost certainly be necessary, taking into consideration specific genetic and molecular disease markers that get us closer to personalized medicine. Based on the current state of knowledge, several interrelated pathogenic pathways are potentially amenable to drug therapies [157]:

1. Preserving tubular epithelial cell integrity (and thus intact nephrons) by minimizing tubular injury/death/senescence and enhancing the repair of damaged tubules. Reactivating key kidney developmental pathways has been promising in experimental models. Permanent

tubular loss is a key predictor of irreversible CKD.

2. Blocking the numbers and/or function of a unique population of interstitial myofibroblasts that are the primary source of the scar-forming extracellular matrix proteins.

3. Regulating the interstitial cell inflammatory response that has multiple consequences—some harmful and others healing. The role of macrophages appears to be particularly important.

4. Disrupting the vicious circle of hypoxia and oxidant stress that develops at least in part because of the lack of preservation of a healthy interstitial capillary network vital for adequate kidney oxygenation.

5. Reducing the progressive accumulation of extracellular matrix proteins in the interstitium. Despite the identification of several matrix-degrading proteases in kidneys, there is still no convincing evidence that renal fibrosis can be reversed in humans. Effective therapies will need to target the extracellular matrix production pathways.

Further laboratory and clinical studies are needed to identify new evidence-based therapeutic options to improve long-term outcomes for patients with chronic TIN.

References

1. Councilman WT. Acute interstitial nephritis. J Exp Med. 1898; https://doi.org/10.1084/jem.3.4-5.393.
2. Kodner CM, Kudrimoti A. Diagnosis and management of acute interstitial nephritis. Am Fam Physician. 2003;67(12):2527–34.
3. Michel DM, Kelly CJ. Acute interstitial nephritis. J Am Soc Nephrol. 1998; https://doi.org/10.5005/jp/books/12074_52.
4. Hirsch HH, Vincenti F, Friman S, Tuncer M, Citterio F, Wiecek A, Scheuermann EH, Klinger M, Russ G, Pescovitz MD, Prestele H. Polyomavirus BK replication in de novo kidney transplant patients receiving tacrolimus or cyclosporine: a prospective, randomized, multicenter study. Am J Transplant. 2013;13(1):136–45. https://doi.org/10.1111/j.1600-6143.2012.04320.x.
5. Moreira LC, Rocha J, Silva M, Silva J, Almeida M, Pedroso S, Vizcaíno R, Martins LS, Dias L,

Henriques AC, Cabrita A. Adenovirus infection-a rare cause of interstitial nephritis in kidney transplant. Nefrologia. 2019;39(1):106–7. https://doi.org/10.1016/j.nefro.2018.06.001.
6. Clavé S, Rousset-Rouvière C, Daniel L, Tsimaratos M. Acute tubulointerstitial nephritis in children and chronic kidney disease. Arch Pediatr. 2019;26(5):290–4. https://doi.org/10.1016/j.arcped.2019.05.002.
7. Goicoechea M, Rivera F, López-Gómez JM. Increased prevalence of acute tubulointerstitial nephritis. Nephrol Dial Transplant. 2013; https://doi.org/10.1093/ndt/gfs143.
8. Jahnukainen T, Ala-Houhala M, Karikoski R, Kataja J, Saarela V, Nuutinen M. Clinical outcome and occurrence of uveitis in children with idiopathic tubulointerstitial nephritis. Pediatr Nephrol. 2011; https://doi.org/10.1007/s00467-010-1698-4.
9. Praga M, González E. Acute interstitial nephritis. Kidney Int. 2012; https://doi.org/10.1038/ki.2010.89.
10. Lanewala A, Mubarak M, Akhter F, Aziz S, Bhatti S, Kazi JI. Pattern of pediatric renal disease observed in native renal biopsies in Pakistan. J Nephrol. 2009;22(6):739–46.
11. Braden GL, O'Shea MH, Mulhern JG. Tubulointerstitial diseases. Am J Kidney Dis. 2005; https://doi.org/10.1053/j.ajkd.2005.03.024.
12. Baker RJ, Pusey CD. The changing profile of acute tubulointerstitial nephritis. Nephrol Dial Transplant. 2004; https://doi.org/10.1093/ndt/gfg464.
13. Viero RM, Cavallo T. Granulomatous interstitial nephritis. Hum Pathol. 1995; https://doi.org/10.1016/0046-8177(95)90300-3.
14. Cameron JS. Tubular and interstitial factors in the progression of glomerulonephritis. Pediatr Nephrol. 1992; https://doi.org/10.1007/BF00878382.
15. Ulinski T, Sellier-Leclerc AL, Tudorache E, Bensman A, Aoun B. Acute tubulointerstitial nephritis. Pediatr Nephrol. 2012; https://doi.org/10.1007/s00467-011-1915-9.
16. Buysen JGM, Houthoff HJ, Krediet RT, Arisz L. Acute interstitial nephritis: a clinical and morphological study in 27 patients. Nephrol Dial Transplant. 1990; https://doi.org/10.1093/ndt/5.2.94.
17. Halloran PF, Matas A, Kasiske BL, Madill-Thomsen KS, Mackova M, Famulski KS. Molecular phenotype of kidney transplant indication biopsies with inflammation in scarred areas. Am J Transplant. 2019;19(5):1356–70. https://doi.org/10.1111/ajt.15178.
18. Harris DCH. Tubulointerstitial renal disease. Curr Opin Nephrol Hypertension. 2001; https://doi.org/10.1097/00041552-200105000-00003.
19. Landegren N, Pourmousa Lindberg M, Skov J, Hallgren Å, Eriksson D, Lisberg Toft-Bertelsen T, MacAulay N, Hagforsen E, Räisänen-Sokolowski A, Saha H, Nilsson T, Nordmark G, Ohlsson S, Gustafsson J, Husebye ES, Larsson E, Anderson MS, Perheentupa J, Rorsman F, et al. Autoantibodies

targeting a collecting duct-specific water channel in tubulointerstitial nephritis. J Am Soc Nephrol. 2016;27(10):3220–8. https://doi.org/10.1681/ASN.2015101126.

20. Nakamori A, Akagaki F, Yamaguchi Y, Sugiura T. Relapsing tubulointerstitial nephritis with anti-mitochondrial M2 antibody accompanied by pulmonary involvement. Intern Med (Tokyo, Japan). 2020;59(9):1179–87. https://doi.org/10.2169/internalmedicine.4048-19.

21. Rosales IA, Collins AB, do Carmo PAS, Tolkoff-Rubin N, Smith RN, Colvin RB. Immune complex tubulointerstitial nephritis due to autoantibodies to the proximal tubule brush border. J Am Soc Nephrol. 2016;27(2):380–4. https://doi.org/10.1681/ASN.2015030334.

22. Spanou Z, Keller M, Britschgi M, Yawalkar N, Fehr T, Neuweiler J, Gugger M, Mohaupt M, Pichler WJ. Involvement of drug-specific t cells in acute drug-induced interstitial nephritis. J Am Soc Nephrol. 2006; https://doi.org/10.1681/ASN.2006050418.

23. Rossert J. Drug-induced acute interstitial nephritis. Kidney Int. 2001; https://doi.org/10.1046/j.1523-1755.2001.060002804.x.

24. Metterle L, Hatch L, Seminario-Vidal L. Pediatric drug reaction with eosinophilia and systemic symptoms: a systematic review of the literature. Pediatr Dermatol. 2020;37(1):124–9. https://doi.org/10.1111/pde.14044.

25. Heeger PS, Smoyer WE, Saad T, Albert S, Kelly CJ, Neilson EG. Molecular analysis of the helper T cell response in murine interstitial nephritis. T cells recognizing an immunodominant epitope use multiple T cell receptor Vβ genes with similarities across CDR3. J Clin Investig. 1994; https://doi.org/10.1172/jci117563.

26. Takemura Y, Koshimichi M, Sugimoto K, Yanagida H, Fujita S, Miyazawa T, Miyazaki K, Okada M, Takemura T. A tubulointerstitial nephritis antigen gene defect causes childhood-onset chronic renal failure. Pediatr Nephrol. 2010; https://doi.org/10.1007/s00467-010-1463-8.

27. Luciano RL, Brewster UC. Kidney involvement in leukemia and lymphoma. Adv Chronic Kidney Dis. 2014; https://doi.org/10.1053/j.ackd.2013.07.004.

28. Fogo AB, Lusco MA, Najafian B, Alpers CE. AJKD atlas of renal pathology: indinavir nephrotoxicity. Am J Kidney Dis. 2017;69(1):e3.

29. Madigan LM, Fox LP. Vancomycin-associated drug-induced hypersensitivity syndrome. J Am Acad Dermatol. 2019;81(1):123–8. https://doi.org/10.1016/j.jaad.2019.02.002.

30. Goli R, Mukku KK, Raju SB, Uppin MS. Acute ciprofloxacin-induced crystal nephropathy with granulomatous interstitial nephritis. Indian J Nephrol. 2017;27(3):231–3. https://doi.org/10.4103/0971-4065.200522.

31. Verghese PS, Schmeling DO, Filtz EA, Matas AJ, Balfour HH. The impact of recipient BKV shedding before transplant on BKV viruria, DNAemia,

and nephropathy post-transplant: a prospective study. Pediatr Transplant. 2017;21(5) https://doi.org/10.1111/petr.12942.

32. Howell M, Sebire NJ, Marks SD, Tullus K. Biopsy-proven paediatric tubulointerstitial nephritis. Pediatr Nephrol. 2016;31(10):1625–30. https://doi.org/10.1007/s00467-016-3374-9.

33. Roy S, Awogbemi T, Holt RCL. Acute tubulointerstitial nephritis in children—a retrospective case series in a UK tertiary paediatric centre. BMC Nephrol. 2020;21(1):17. https://doi.org/10.1186/s12882-020-1681-7.

34. Taktak A, Uncu N, Acar B, Çaycı Ş, Ensari A, Gür G, Köksoy A, Çakar N. Acute tubulointerstitial nephritis: a case series and long-term renal outcomes. Turk J Pediatr. 2015;57(6):566–71.

35. Clarkson MR, Giblin L, O'Connell FP, O'Kelly P, Walshe JJ, Conlon P, O'Meara Y, Dormon A, Campbell E, Donohoe J. Acute interstitial nephritis: clinical features and response to corticosteroid therapy. Nephrol Dial Transplant. 2004; https://doi.org/10.1093/ndt/gfh485.

36. González E, Gutiérrez E, Galeano C, Chevia C, De Sequera P, Bernis C, Parra EG, Delgado R, Sanz M, Ortiz M, Goicoechea M, Quereda C, Olea T, Bouarich H, Hernández Y, Segovia B, Praga M. Early steroid treatment improves the recovery of renal function in patients with drug-induced acute interstitial nephritis. Kidney Int. 2008; https://doi.org/10.1038/sj.ki.5002776.

37. Minhas JS, Wickner PG, Long AA, Banerji A, Blumenthal KG. Immune-mediated reactions to vancomycin: a systematic case review and analysis. Ann Allergy Asthma Immunol. 2016;116(6):544–53. https://doi.org/10.1016/j.anai.2016.03.030.

38. Nayak S, Nandwani A, Rastogi A, Gupta V. Acute interstitial nephritis and drug rash with secondary to Linezolid. Indian J Nephrol. 2012; https://doi.org/10.4103/0971-4065.103918.

39. Xie H, Chen H, Hu Y, Xu S, He Q, Liu J, Hu W, Liu Z. Clindamycin-induced acute kidney injury: large biopsy case series. Am J Nephrol. 2013; https://doi.org/10.1159/000354088.

40. Duque JC, Dejman A, Venkat V, Hernandez M, Roth D, Ladino MA. Acute interstitial nephritis following treatment with direct-acting antiviral agents in hepatitis C virus-infected patients: a case series. Clin Nephrol. 2021;95(1):22–7. https://doi.org/10.5414/CN110276.

41. Ambruzs JM, Walker PD, Larsen CP. The histopathologic spectrum of kidney biopsies in patients with inflammatory bowel disease. Clin J Am Soc Nephrol. 2014;9(2):265–70. https://doi.org/10.2215/CJN.04660513.

42. Skalova S, Dedek P, Pozler O, Podhola M. Mesalazine-induced interstitial nephritis. Ren Fail. 2009; https://doi.org/10.1080/08860220802595922.

43. Vasanth P, Parmley M, Torrealba J, Hamdi T. Interstitial nephritis in a patient with inflamma-

tory bowel disease. Case Rep Nephrol. 2016;2016:4260365. https://doi.org/10.1155/2016/4260365.

44. Al-Aly Z, Maddukuri G, Xie Y. Proton pump inhibitors and the kidney: implications of current evidence for clinical practice and when and how to deprescribe. Am J Kidney Dis. 2020;75(4):497–507. https://doi.org/10.1053/j.ajkd.2019.07.012.

45. Chen T, Xu P-C, Hu S-Y, Yan T-K, Jiang J-Q, Jia J-Y, Wei L, Shang W-Y. Severe acute interstitial nephritis induced by valsartan: a case report. Medicine. 2019b;98(6):e14428. https://doi.org/10.1097/MD.0000000000014428.

46. Golbin L, Dolley-Hitze T, Lorcy N, Rioux-Leclercq N, Vigneau C. Drug-induced acute interstitial nephritis with nifedipine. Case Rep Nephrol. 2016;2016:1971465. https://doi.org/10.1155/2016/1971465.

47. Lally J, Al Kalbani H, Krivoy A, Murphy KC, Gaughran F, MacCabe JH. Hepatitis, interstitial nephritis, and pancreatitis in association with clozapine treatment: a systematic review of case series and reports. J Clin Psychopharmacol. 2018;38(5):520–7. https://doi.org/10.1097/JCP.0000000000000922.

48. Abdulhadi B, Mulki R, Goyal A, Rangaswami J. Novel oral anticoagulant and kidney injury: apixaban-related acute interstitial nephritis. BMJ Case Rep. 2017; https://doi.org/10.1136/bcr-2017-221641.

49. Gueye S, Saint-Cricq M, Coulibaly M, Goumri N, Guilbeau-Frugier C, Quentin H, Ged E, Sidi Aly A, Rostaing L. Chronic tubulointerstitial nephropathy induced by glucosamine: a case report and literature review. Clin Nephrol. 2016;86(2):106–10. https://doi.org/10.5414/cn108781.

50. Manohar S, Albright RC. Interstitial nephritis in immune checkpoint inhibitor therapy. Kidney Int. 2019;96(1):252. https://doi.org/10.1016/j.kint.2018.11.009.

51. Shingarev R, Glezerman IG. Kidney complications of immune checkpoint inhibitors: a review. Am J Kidney Dis. 2019;74(4):529–37. https://doi.org/10.1053/j.ajkd.2019.03.433.

52. Kaya Aksoy G, Koyun M, Akkaya B, Comak E, Gemici A, Akman S. Eosinophilic tubulointerstitial nephritis on treatment with isotretinoin. Eur J Pediatr. 2016;175(12):2005–6. https://doi.org/10.1007/s00431-016-2778-7.

53. Sugimoto K, Nishi H, Miyazawa T, Wada N, Izu A, Enya T, Okada M. Takemura T. Tubulointerstitial nephritis complicating IVIG therapy for X-linked agammaglobulinemia. BMC Nephrol. 2014;15:109. https://doi.org/10.1186/1471-2369-15-109.

54. Bahaa Aldeen M, Talibmamury N, Alalusi S, Nadham O, Omer AR, Smalligan RD. When coke is not hydrating: cocaine-induced acute interstitial nephritis. J Investig Med High Impact Case Rep. 2014;2(3):2324709614551557. https://doi.org/10.1177/2324709614551557.

55. Decelle L, Cosyns JP, Georges B, Jadoul M, Lefebvre C. Acute interstitial nephritis after cocaine sniffing. Clin Nephrol. 2007;67(2):105–8. https://doi.org/10.5414/cnp67105.

56. Inayat F, Bokhari SRA, Roberts L, Rosen RM. Cocaine-induced acute interstitial nephritis: a comparative review of 7 cases. J Investig Med High Impact Case Rep. 2020;8:2324709620932450. https://doi.org/10.1177/2324709620932450.

57. Wojciechowski D, Kallakury B, Nouri P. A case of cocaine-induced acute interstitial nephritis. Am J Kidney Dis. 2008; https://doi.org/10.1053/j.ajkd.2008.03.018.

58. Riederer AM, Campleman SL, Carlson RG, Boyer EW, Manini AF, Wax PM, Brent JA, Toxicology Investigators Consortium (ToxIC). Acute poisonings from synthetic cannabinoids—50 U.S. Toxicology Investigators Consortium Registry sites, 2010–2015. MMWR Morb Mortal Wkly Rep. 2016;65(27):692–5. https://doi.org/10.15585/mmwr.mm6527a2.

59. Daher EF, Silva Júnior GB, Queiroz AL, Ramos LMA, Santos SQ, Barreto DMS, Guimarães AAC, Barbosa CA, Franco LM, Patrocínio RMSV. Acute kidney injury due to anabolic steroid and vitamin supplement abuse: report of two cases and a literature review. Int Urol Nephrol. 2009;41(3):717–23. https://doi.org/10.1007/s11255-009-9571-8.

60. Gupta RK, van der Meulen J, Johny KV. Oliguric acute renal failure due to glue-sniffing. Case report. Scand J Urol Nephrol. 1991;25(3):247–50. https://doi.org/10.3109/00365599109107958.

61. Nanavati A, Herlitz LC. Tubulointerstitial injury and drugs of abuse. Adv Chronic Kidney Dis. 2017;24(2):80–5. https://doi.org/10.1053/j.ackd.2016.09.008.

62. Patel R, Benjamin J. Renal disease associated with toluene inhalation. J Toxicol Clin Toxicol. 1986;24(3):213–23. https://doi.org/10.3109/15563658608990459.

63. Taverner D, Harrison DJ, Bell GM. Acute renal failure due to interstitial nephritis induced by "glue-sniffing" with subsequent recovery. Scott Med J. 1988;33(2):246–7. https://doi.org/10.1177/003693308803300208.

64. Bailly E, Von Tokarski F, Beau-Salinas F, Picon L, Miquelestorena-Standley E, Rousseau G, Jonville-Bera A-P, Halimi J-M. Interstitial nephritis secondary to vedolizumab treatment in Crohn disease and safe rechallenge using steroids: a case report. Am J Kidney Dis. 2018;71(1):142–5. https://doi.org/10.1053/j.ajkd.2017.08.008.

65. Escandon J, Peacock S, Trabolsi A, Thomas DB, Layka A, Lutzky J. Interstitial nephritis in melanoma patients secondary to PD-1 checkpoint inhibitor. J Immunother Cancer. 2017;5:3. https://doi.org/10.1186/s40425-016-0205-2.

66. Cheungpasitporn W, Leung N, Rajkumar SV, Cornell LD, Sethi S, Angioi A, Fervenza FC. Bortezomib-induced acute interstitial nephritis. Nephrol Dial Transplant. 2015;30(7):1225–9. https://doi.org/10.1093/ndt/gfv222.

67. Lusica M, Rondon-Berrios H, Feldman L. Urine eosinophils for acute interstitial nephritis. J Hosp Med. 2017;12(5):343–5. https://doi.org/10.12788/jhm.2737.

68. Mirković K, Doorenbos CRC, Dam WA, Lambers Heerspink HJ, Slagman MCJ, Nauta FL, Kramer AB, Gansevoort RT, van den Born J, Navis G, de Borst MH. Urinary vitamin D binding protein: a potential novel marker of renal interstitial inflammation and fibrosis. PLoS One. 2013; https://doi.org/10.1371/journal.pone.0055887.

69. Robles NR, Lopez-Gomez J, Garcia-Pino G, Ferreira F, Alvarado R, Sanchez-Casado E, Cubero JJ. Use of α1-microglobulin for diagnosing chronic interstitial nephropathy. Clin Exp Med. 2014; https://doi.org/10.1007/s10238-013-0242-9.

70. Moledina DG, Wilson FP, Pober JS, Perazella MA, Singh N, Luciano RL, Obeid W, Lin H, Kuperman M, Moeckel GW, Kashgarian M, Cantley LG, Parikh CR. Urine TNF-α and IL-9 for clinical diagnosis of acute interstitial nephritis. JCI Insight. 2019;4(10):e127456. https://doi.org/10.1172/jci.insight.127456.

71. Zhang Y, Li A, Wen J, Zhen J, Hao Q, Zhang Y, Hu Z, Xiao X. Kidney injury molecule-1 level is associated with the severity of renal interstitial injury and prognosis in adult Henoch-Schönlein purpura nephritis. Arch Med Res. 2017;48(5):449–58. https://doi.org/10.1016/j.arcmed.2017.10.005.

72. Zhao W-T, Huang J-W, Sun P-P, Su T, Tang J-W, Wang S-X, Liu G, Yang L. Diagnostic roles of urinary kidney injury molecule 1 and soluble C5b-9 in acute tubulointerstitial nephritis. Am J Physiol Renal Physiol. 2019;317(3):F584–92. https://doi.org/10.1152/ajprenal.00176.2019.

73. Noiri C, Shimizu T, Takayanagi K, Tayama Y, Iwashita T, Okazaki S, Hatano M, Matsumura O, Kato H, Matsuda A, Mitarai T, Hasegawa H. Clinical significance of fractional magnesium excretion (FEMg) as a predictor of interstitial nephropathy and its correlation with conventional parameters. Clin Exp Nephrol. 2015;19(6):1071–8. https://doi.org/10.1007/s10157-015-1099-x.

74. Perazella MA, Markowitz GS. Drug-induced acute interstitial nephritis. Nat Rev Nephrol. 2010; https://doi.org/10.1038/nrneph.2010.71.

75. Regusci A, Lava SAG, Milani GP, Bianchetti MG, Simonetti GD, Vanoni F. Tubulointerstitial nephritis and uveitis syndrome: a systematic review. Nephrol Dial Transplant. 2021; https://doi.org/10.1093/ndt/gfab030.

76. Storsley L, Gibson IW. Adenovirus interstitial nephritis and rejection in an allograft. J Am Soc Nephrol. 2011; https://doi.org/10.1681/ASN.2010090941.

77. Zaidan M, Lescure FX, Brochériou I, Dettwiler S, Guiard-Schmid JB, Pacanowski J, Rondeau E, Pialoux G, Girard PM, Ronco P, Plaisie E. Tubulointerstitial nephropathies in HIV-infected patients over the past 15 years: a clinico-pathological study. Clin J Am Soc Nephrol. 2013; https://doi.org/10.2215/CJN.10051012.

78. Valluri A, Hetherington L, Mcquarrie E, Fleming S, Kipgen D, Geddes CC, Mackinnon B, Bell S. Acute tubulointerstitial nephritis in Scotland. QJM. 2015;108(7):527–32. https://doi.org/10.1093/qjmed/hcu236.

79. Baldwin DS, Levine BB, McCluskey RT, Gallo GR. Renal failure and interstitial nephritis due to penicillin and methicillin. N Engl J Med. 1968; https://doi.org/10.1056/nejm196812052792302.

80. Nawaz FA, Larsen CP, Troxell ML. Membranous nephropathy and nonsteroidal anti-inflammatory agents. Am J Kidney Dis. 2013; https://doi.org/10.1053/j.ajkd.2013.03.045.

81. Ruffenach SJ, Siskind MS, Lien YHH. Acute interstitial nephritis due to omeprazole. Am J Med. 1992; https://doi.org/10.1016/0002-9343(92)90181-A.

82. Antoniou T, Macdonald EM, Hollands S, Gomes T, Mamdani MM, Garg AX, Paterson JM, Juurlink DN. Proton pump inhibitors and the risk of acute kidney injury in older patients: a population-based cohort study. CMAJ Open. 2015;3(2):E166–71. https://doi.org/10.9778/cmajo.20140074.

83. Hart E, Dunn TE, Feuerstein S, Jacobs DM. Proton pump inhibitors and risk of acute and chronic kidney disease: a retrospective cohort study. Pharmacotherapy. 2019;39(4):443–53. https://doi.org/10.1002/phar.2235.

84. Wijarnpreecha K, Thongprayoon C, Chesdachai S, Panjawatanana P, Ungprasert P, Cheungpasitporn W. Associations of proton-pump inhibitors and H2 receptor antagonists with chronic kidney disease: a meta-analysis. Dig Dis Sci. 2017;62(10):2821–7. https://doi.org/10.1007/s10620-017-4725-5.

85. Xie Y, Bowe B, Li T, Xian H, Balasubramanian S, Al-Aly Z. Proton pump inhibitors and risk of incident CKD and progression to ESRD. J Am Soc Nephrol. 2016;27(10):3153–63. https://doi.org/10.1681/ASN.2015121377.

86. Klassen S, Krepinsky JC, Prebtani APH. Pantoprazole-induced acute interstitial nephritis. CMAJ. 2013; https://doi.org/10.1503/cmaj.120954.

87. Helsby NA, Lo WY, Simpson IJ, Voss DM, Logan KE, Searle M, Schollum JBW, De Zoysa JR. Omeprazole-induced acute interstitial nephritis is not related to CYP2C19 genotype or CYP2C19 phenotype. Br J Clin Pharmacol. 2010; https://doi.org/10.1111/j.1365-2125.2010.03623.x.

88. Rodríguez-Poncelas A, Barceló MA, Saez M, Coll-de-Tuero G. Duration and dosing of Proton Pump Inhibitors associated with high incidence of chronic kidney disease in population-based cohort. PLoS One. 2018;13(10):e0204231. https://doi.org/10.1371/journal.pone.0204231.

89. Quinto LR, Sukkar L, Gallagher M. Effectiveness of corticosteroid compared with non-corticosteroid therapy for the treatment of drug-induced acute interstitial nephritis: a systematic review. Intern

Med J. 2019;49(5):562–9. https://doi.org/10.1111/imj.14081.

90. Moledina DG, Perazella MA. Drug-induced acute interstitial nephritis. Clin J Am Soc Nephrol. 2017; https://doi.org/10.2215/CJN.07630717.

91. Fernandez-Juarez G, Perez JV, Caravaca-Fontán F, Quintana L, Shabaka A, Rodriguez E, Gadola L, de Lorenzo A, Cobo MA, Oliet A, Sierra M, Cobelo C, Iglesias E, Blasco M, Galeano C, Cordon A, Oliva J, Praga M, Spanish Group for the Study of Glomerular Diseases (GLOSEN). Duration of treatment with corticosteroids and recovery of kidney function in acute interstitial nephritis. Clin J Am Soc Nephrol. 2018;13(12):1851–8. https://doi.org/10.2215/CJN.01390118.

92. Rankin AJ, Cannon E, Gillis K, Crosby J, Mark PB, Geddes CC, Fox JG, Mackinnon B, McQuarrie EP, Kipgen D. Predicting outcome in acute interstitial nephritis: a case-series examining the importance of histological parameters. Histopathology. 2020;76(5):698–706. https://doi.org/10.1111/his.14031.

93. Zheng X-Z, Gu Y-H, Su T, Zhou X-J, Huang J-W, Sun P-P, Jia Y, Xu D-M, Wang S-X, Liu G, Yang L. Elevation of erythrocyte sedimentation rate and C-reactive protein levels reflects renal interstitial inflammation in drug-induced acute tubulointerstitial nephritis. BMC Nephrol. 2020;21(1):514. https://doi.org/10.1186/s12882-020-02175-z.

94. Tojo A, Miyashita K, Kinugasa S, Takemura T, Goto A. Acute tubulointerstitial nephritis with an autoantibody response against carbonic anhydrase II. Am J Med Sci. 2013; https://doi.org/10.1097/MAJ.0b013e318272f1a6.

95. Dobrin RS, Vernier RL, Fish AJ. Acute eosinophilic interstitial nephritis and renal failure with bone marrow-lymph node granulomas and anterior uveitis. A new syndrome. Am J Med. 1975; https://doi.org/10.1016/0002-9343(75)90390-3.

96. Tan Y, Yu F, Qu Z, Su T, Xing GQ, Wu LH, Wang FM, Liu G, Yang L, Zhao MH. Modified C-reactive protein might be a target autoantigen of TINU syndrome. Clin J Am Soc Nephrol. 2011; https://doi.org/10.2215/CJN.09051209.

97. Yasuda K, Sasaki K, Yamato M, Rakugi H, Isaka Y, Hayashi T. Tubulointerstitial nephritis and uveitis syndrome with transient hyperthyroidism in an elderly patient. Clin Exp Nephrol. 2011; https://doi.org/10.1007/s10157-011-0505-2.

98. Mandeville JTH, Levinson RD, Holland GN. The tubulointerstitial nephritis and uveitis syndrome. Surv Ophthalmol. 2001; https://doi.org/10.1016/S0039-6257(01)00261-2.

99. Howarth L, Gilbert RD, Bass P, Deshpande PV. Tubulointerstitial nephritis and uveitis in monozygotic twin boys. Pediatr Nephrol. 2004; https://doi.org/10.1007/s00467-004-1518-9.

100. Gianviti A, Greco M, Barsotti P, Rizzoni G. Acute tubulointerstitial nephritis occurring with 1-year lapse in identical twins. Pediatr Nephrol. 1994; https://doi.org/10.1007/BF00856521.

101. Clive DM, Vanguri VK. The syndrome of tubulointerstitial nephritis with uveitis (TINU). Am J Kidney Dis. 2018;72(1):118–28. https://doi.org/10.1053/j.ajkd.2017.11.013.

102. Onyekpe I, Shenoy M, Denley H, Riad H, Webb NJA. Recurrent tubulointerstitial nephritis and uveitis syndrome in a renal transplant recipient. Nephrol Dial Transplant. 2011; https://doi.org/10.1093/ndt/gfr352.

103. Chapagain A, Dobbie H, Sheaff M, Yaqoob MM. Presentation, diagnosis, and treatment outcome of tuberculous-mediated tubulointerstitial nephritis. Kidney Int. 2011; https://doi.org/10.1038/ki.2010.482.

104. Alsaad KO, Tobar A, Belanger E, Ahmad M, Cattran DC, Herzenberg AM. Late-onset acute haemorrhagic necrotizing granulomatous adenovirus tubulointerstitial nephritis in a renal allograft. Nephrol Dial Transplant. 2007; https://doi.org/10.1093/ndt/gfl843.

105. Ubee SS, McGlynn L, Fordham M. Emphysematous pyelonephritis. BJU Int. 2011; https://doi.org/10.1111/j.1464-410X.2010.09660.x.

106. Tian YC, Chen YC, Hung CC, Chang CT, Wu MS, Phillips AO, Yang CW. Leptospiral outer membrane protein induces extracellular matrix accumulation through a TGF-β1/Smad-dependent pathway. J Am Soc Nephrol. 2006; https://doi.org/10.1681/ASN.2006020159.

107. Becker JL, Miller F, Nuovo GJ, Josepovitz C, Schubach WH, Nord EP. Epstein-Barr virus infection of renal proximal tubule cells: possible role in chronic interstitial nephritis. J Clin Investig. 1999; https://doi.org/10.1172/JCI7286.

108. Medapalli RK, He JC, Klotman PE. HIV-associated nephropathy: pathogenesis. Curr Opin Nephrol Hypertension. 2011; https://doi.org/10.1097/MNH.0b013e328345359a.

109. Martin-Blondel G, Debard A, Laurent C, Pugnet G, Modesto A, Massip P, Chauveau D, Marchou B. Mycobacterial-immune reconstitution inflammatory syndrome: a cause of acute interstitial nephritis during HIV infection. Nephrol Dial Transplant. 2011; https://doi.org/10.1093/ndt/gfr197.

110. Balba GP, Javaid B, Timpone JG. BK polyomavirus infection in the renal transplant recipient. Infect Dis Clin North Am. 2013; https://doi.org/10.1016/j.idc.2013.02.002.

111. Filler G, Licht C, Haig A. Native kidney BK virus nephropathy associated with acute lymphocytic leukemia. Pediatr Nephrol. 2013; https://doi.org/10.1007/s00467-013-2438-3.

112. Verghese PS, Finn LS, Englund JA, Sanders JE, Hingorani SR. BK nephropathy in pediatric hematopoietic stem cell transplant recipients. Pediatr Transplant. 2009;13(7):913–8. https://doi.org/10.1111/j.1399-3046.2008.01069.x.

113. Colvin RB, Traum AZ, Taheri D, Jafari M, Dolatkhah S. Granulomatous interstitial nephritis as a manifestation of Crohn disease. Arch Pathol Lab Med. 2014; https://doi.org/10.5858/arpa.2012-0224-CR.

114. Joss N, Morris S, Young B, Geddes C. Granulomatous interstitial nephritis. Clin J Am Soc Nephrol. 2007; https://doi.org/10.2215/CJN.01790506.

115. Timmermans SAMEG, Christiaans MHL, Abdul-Hamid MA, Stifft F, Damoiseaux JGMC, van Paassen P. Granulomatous interstitial nephritis and Crohn's disease. Clin Kidney J. 2016;9(4):556–9. https://doi.org/10.1093/ckj/sfw041.

116. Izzedine H, Simon J, Piette A-M, Lucsko M, Baumelou A, Charitanski D, Kernaonet E, Baglin A-C, Deray G, Beaufils H. Primary chronic interstitial nephritis in Crohn's disease. Gastroenterology. 2002;123(5):1436–40. https://doi.org/10.1053/gast.2002.36613.

117. Ghani AA, Al Waheeb S, Al Homoud E. Isolated sarcoid renal granulomatous tubulointerstitial disease. Saudi J Kidney Dis Transplant. 2011;22(6):1208–10.

118. Nagaraja P, Davies MR. Granulomatous interstitial nephritis causing acute renal failure: a rare presenting feature of sarcoidosis. QJM. 2014; https://doi.org/10.1093/qjmed/hcr263.

119. Thumfart J, Müller D, Rudolph B, Zimmering M, Querfeld U, Haffner D. Isolated sarcoid granulomatous interstitial nephritis responding to infliximab therapy. Am J Kidney Dis. 2005;45(2):411–4. https://doi.org/10.1053/j.ajkd.2004.10.011.

120. Inui N, Murayama A, Sasaki S, Suda T, Chida K, Kato S, Nakamura H. Correlation between 25-hydroxyvitamin D3 1α-hydroxylase gene expression in alveolar macrophages and the activity of sarcoidosis. Am J Med. 2001; https://doi.org/10.1016/S0002-9343(01)00724-0.

121. Nasr SH, Koscica J, Markowitz GS, D'Agati VD. Granulomatous interstitial nephritis. Am J Kidney Dis. 2003; https://doi.org/10.1053/ajkd.2003.50143.

122. Stehlé T, Joly D, Vanhille P, Boffa JJ, Rémy P, Mesnard L, Hoffmann M, Grimbert P, Choukroun G, Vrtovsnik F, Verine J, Desvaux D, Walker F, Lang P, Mahevas M, Sahali D, Audard V. Clinicopathological study of glomerular diseases associated with sarcoidosis: a multicenter study. Orphanet J Rare Dis. 2013; https://doi.org/10.1186/1750-1172-8-65.

123. Vorselaars AD, van Moorsel CH, Deneer VH, Grutters JC. Current therapy in sarcoidosis, the role of existing drugs and future medicine. Inflamm Allergy Drug Targets. 2013;12(6):369–77.

124. Correia FASC, Marchini GS, Torricelli FC, Danilovic A, Vicentini FC, Srougi M, Nahas WC, Mazzucchi E. Renal manifestations of sarcoidosis: from accurate diagnosis to specific treatment. Int Braz J Urol. 2020;46(1):15–25. https://doi.org/10.1590/S1677-5538.IBJU.2019.0042.

125. Zammouri A, Barbouch S, Najjar M, Aoudia R, Jaziri F, Kaaroud H, Hedri H, Abderrahim E, Goucha R, Hamida FB, Harzallah A, Abdallah TB. Tubulointerstitial nephritis due to sarcoidosis: clinical, laboratory, and histological features and outcome in a cohort of 24 patients. Saudi J Kidney Dis Transplant. 2019; https://doi.org/10.4103/1319-2442.275471.

126. Saha MK, Tarek H, Sagar V, Abraham P. Role of tumor necrosis factor inhibitor in granulomatous interstitial nephritis secondary to Crohn's disease. Int Urol Nephrol. 2014; https://doi.org/10.1007/s11255-012-0362-2.

127. Aouizerate J, Matignon M, Kamar N, Thervet E, Randoux C, Moulin B, Raffray L, Buchler M, Villar E, Mahevas M, Desvaux D, Dahan K, Diet C, Audard V, Lang P, Grimbert P. Renal transplantation in patients with sarcoidosis: a French multicenter study. Clin J Am Soc Nephrol. 2010; https://doi.org/10.2215/CJN.03970510.

128. Mann DM, Fyfe B, Osband AJ, Lebowitz J, Laskow DA, Jones J, Mann RA. Sarcoidosis within a renal allograft: a case report and review of the literature. Transplant Proc. 2013; https://doi.org/10.1016/j.transproceed.2012.11.008.

129. Igarashi T, Itoh Y, Shimizu A, Igarashi T, Yoshizaki K, Fukunaga Y. A case of juvenile Sjögren's syndrome with interstitial nephritis. J Nippon Med Sch. 2012; https://doi.org/10.1272/jnms.79.286.

130. Bossini N, Savoldi S, Franceschini F, Mombelloni S, Baronio M, Cavazzana I, Viola BF, Valzorio B, Mazzucchelli C, Cattaneo R, Scolari F, Maiorca R. Clinical and morphological features of kidney involvement in primary Sjögren's syndrome. Nephrol Dial Transplant. 2001; https://doi.org/10.1093/ndt/16.12.2328.

131. Jasiek M, Karras A, Le Guern V, Krastinova E, Mesbah R, Faguer S, Jourde-Chiche N, Fauchais A-L, Chiche L, Dernis E, Moulis G, Fraison J-B, Lazaro E, Jullien P, Hachulla E, Le Quellec A, Rémy P, Hummel A, Costedoat-Chalumeau N, Terrier B. A multicentre study of 95 biopsy-proven cases of renal disease in primary Sjögren's syndrome. Rheumatology (Oxford). 2017;56(3):362–70. https://doi.org/10.1093/rheumatology/kew376.

132. Maripuri S, Grande JP, Osborn TG, Fervenza FC, Matteson EL, Donadio JV, Hogan MC. Renal involvement in primary Sjögren's syndrome: a clinicopathologic study. Clin J Am Soc Nephrol. 2009; https://doi.org/10.2215/CJN.00980209.

133. Jain A, Srinivas BH, Emmanuel D, Jain VK, Parameshwaran S, Negi VS. Renal involvement in primary Sjogren's syndrome: a prospective cohort study. Rheumatol Int. 2018;38(12):2251–62. https://doi.org/10.1007/s00296-018-4118-x.

134. Goules AV, Tatouli IP, Moutsopoulos HM, Tzioufas AG. Clinically significant renal involvement in primary Sjögren's syndrome: clinical presentation and outcome. Arthritis Rheum. 2013; https://doi.org/10.1002/art.38100.

135. Kassan SS, Moutsopoulos HM. Clinical manifestations and early diagnosis of Sjögren syndrome.

Arch Intern Med. 2004; https://doi.org/10.1001/archinte.164.12.1275.

136. Pijpe J, Van Imhoff GW, Spijkervet FKL, Roodenburg JLN, Wolbink GJ, Mansour K, Vissink A, Kallenberg CGM, Bootsma H. Rituximab treatment in patients with primary Sjögren's syndrome: an open-label phase II study. Arthritis Rheum. 2005; https://doi.org/10.1002/art.21260.

137. Silverman E, Eddy A. Systemic erythematosus. In: Textbook of pediatric rheumatology. 6th ed. Amsterdam: Elsevier; 2011. p. 315–43.

138. Lan-Ting H, You-Ming C, Li-Xin W, Chen W, Xiao-Yan Z, Hong-Yan H. Clinicopathological factors for tubulointerstitial injury in lupus nephritis. Clin Rheumatol. 2020;39(5):1617–26. https://doi.org/10.1007/s10067-019-04909-3.

139. Yu F, Wu LH, Tan Y, Li LH, Wang CL, Wang WK, Qu Z, Chen MH, Gao JJ, Li ZY, Zheng X, Ao J, Zhu SN, Wang SX, Zhao MH, Zou WZ, Liu G. Tubulointerstitial lesions of patients with lupus nephritis classified by the 2003 International Society of Nephrology and Renal Pathology Society system. Kidney Int. 2010; https://doi.org/10.1038/ki.2010.13.

140. Cabral D, Benseler S. Granulomatous vasculitis, microscopic polyangiitis and primary angiitis of the central nervous system. In: Textbook of pediatric rheumatology. Amsterdam: Elsevier; 2011. https://doi.org/10.1016/B978-1-4160-6581-4.10034-2.

141. Plafkin C, Zhong W, Singh T. ANCA vasculitis presenting with acute interstitial nephritis without glomerular involvement. Clin Nephrol Case Stud. 2019;7:46–50. https://doi.org/10.5414/CNCS109805.

142. Javaud N, Belenfant X, Stirnemann J, Laederich J, Ziol M, Callard P, Ronco P, Rondeau E, Fain O. Renal granulomatoses: a retrospective study of 40 cases and review of the literature. Medicine. 2007;86(3):170–80. https://doi.org/10.1097/MD.0b013e3180699f55.

143. Mann S, Seidman MA, Barbour SJ, Levin A, Carruthers M, Chen LYC. Recognizing IgG4-related tubulointerstitial nephritis. Can J Kidney Health Dis. 2016;3:34. https://doi.org/10.1186/s40697-016-0126-5.

144. Şahin Akkelle B. IgG4 related disease in a 7 year old girl with multiple organ involvement: a rare presentation. Türk Pediatri Arşivi. 2019; https://doi.org/10.14744/TurkPediatriArs.2019.83435.

145. Houghton DC, Troxell ML. An abundance of IgG4 plasma cells is not specific for IgG4-related tubulointerstitial nephritis. Mod Pathol. 2011; https://doi.org/10.1038/modpathol.2011.101.

146. Wen YK. Tubulointerstitial nephritis and uveitis with Fanconi syndrome in a patient with ankylosing spondylitis. Clin Nephrol. 2009; https://doi.org/10.5414/cnp72315.

147. Pohjonen J, Nurmi R, Metso M, Oksanen P, Huhtala H, Pörsti I, Mustonen J, Kaukinen K, Mäkelä S. Inflammatory bowel disease in patients undergoing renal biopsies. Clin Kidney J. 2019;12(5):645–51. https://doi.org/10.1093/ckj/sfz004.

148. Sheikine Y, Woda CB, Lee PY, Chatila TA, Keles S, Charbonnier L-M, Schmidt B, Rosen S, Rodig NM. Renal involvement in the immunodysregulation, polyendocrinopathy, enteropathy, X-linked (IPEX) disorder. Pediatr Nephrol (Berlin, Germany). 2015;30(7):1197–202. https://doi.org/10.1007/s00467-015-3102-x.

149. Busto Castanon L, Gomez Castro A, Candal Alonso J, Gonzalez Martin M. Pielonefritis xantogranolomatosa (Y displasia quistica) en un recien nacido. Arch Esp Urol. 1980;(3):33, 303–314.

150. Li L, Parwani AV. Xanthogranulomatous pyelonephritis. Arch Pathol Lab Med. 2011; https://doi.org/10.2223/jped.692.

151. Stoica I, O'Kelly F, McDermott MB, Quinn FMJ. Xanthogranulomatous pyelonephritis in a paediatric cohort (1963–2016): outcomes from a large single-center series. J Pediatr Urol. 2018;14(2):169.e1–7. https://doi.org/10.1016/j.jpurol.2017.10.017.

152. Schlagenhaufer F. Uber eigentumliche staphylomykosen der Nieren und des pararenalen Bindegewebes. Frankf Zt Pathol. 1916;19:139–48.

153. Kim SW, Yoon BI, Ha US, Sohn DW, Cho YH. Xanthogranulomatous pyelonephritis: clinical experience with 21 cases. J Infect Chemother. 2013; https://doi.org/10.1007/s10156-013-0611-z.

154. Brown PS, Dodson M, Weintrub PS. Xanthogranulomatous pyelonephritis: report of nonsurgical management of a case and review of the literature. Clin Infect Dis. 1996; https://doi.org/10.1093/clinids/22.2.308.

155. Hughes PM, Gupta SC, Thomas NB. Xanthogranulomatous pyelonephritis in childhood. Clin Radiol. 1990;41(5):360–2. https://doi.org/10.1016/s0009-9260(05)81705-2.

156. Eddy A, Yamaguchi I. Chronic tubulointerstitial nephritis. In: Schrier's diseases of the kidney, vol. 2. 9th ed. Philadelphia, PA: Wolters Kluwer/Lippincott Williams & Wilkins; 2013. p. 1626–58.

157. Ruiz-Ortega M, Rayego-Mateos S, Lamas S, Ortiz A, Rodrigues-Diez RR. Targeting the progression of chronic kidney disease. Nat Rev Nephrol. 2020;16(5):269–88. https://doi.org/10.1038/s41581-019-0248-y.

158. Chen T, Li X, Li Y, Xia E, Qin Y, Liang S, Xu F, Liang D, Zeng C, Liu Z. Prediction and risk stratification of kidney outcomes in IgA nephropathy. Am J Kidney Dis. 2019a;74(3):300–9. https://doi.org/10.1053/j.ajkd.2019.02.016.

159. Eckardt K-U, Alper SL, Antignac C, Bleyer AJ, Chauveau D, Dahan K, Deltas C, Hosking A, Kmoch S, Rampoldi L, Wiesener M, Wolf MT, Devuyst O, Kidney Disease: Improving Global Outcomes. Autosomal dominant tubulointerstitial kidney disease: diagnosis, classification, and management—a KDIGO consensus report. Kidney

Int. 2015;88(4):676–83. https://doi.org/10.1038/ki.2015.28.

160. Olinger E, Hofmann P, Kidd K, Dufour I, Belge H, Schaeffer C, Kipp A, Bonny O, Deltas C, Demoulin N, Fehr T, Fuster DG, Gale DP, Goffin E, Hodaňová K, Huynh-Do U, Kistler A, Morelle J, Papagregoriou G, et al. Clinical and genetic spectra of autosomal dominant tubulointerstitial kidney disease due to mutations in UMOD and MUC1. Kidney Int. 2020;98(3):717–31. https://doi.org/10.1016/j.kint.2020.04.038.

161. Devuyst O, Olinger E, Weber S, Eckardt KU, Kmoch S, Rampoldi L, Bleyer AJ. Autosomal dominant tubulointerstitial kidney disease. Nat Rev Dis Primers. 2019; https://doi.org/10.1038/s41572-019-0109-9.

162. Schaeffer C, Olinger E. Clinical and genetic spectra of kidney disease caused by REN mutations. Kidney Int. 2020;98(6):1397–400. https://doi.org/10.1016/j.kint.2020.08.013.

163. Živná M, Kidd K, Zaidan M, Vyleťal P, Barešová V, Hodaňová K, Sovová J, Hartmannová H, Votruba M, Trešlová H, Jedličková I, Sikora J, Hůlková H, Robins V, Hnízda A, Živný J, Papagregoriou G, Mesnard L, Beck BB, et al. An international cohort study of autosomal dominant tubulointerstitial kidney disease due to REN mutations identifies distinct clinical subtypes. Kidney Int. 2020;98(6):1589–604. https://doi.org/10.1016/j.kint.2020.06.041.

164. Mihatsch MJ, Gudat F, Zollinger HU, Heierli C, Thölen H, Reutter FW. Systemic karyomegaly associated with chronic interstitial nephritis. A new disease entity? Clin Nephrol. 1979;12(2):54–62.

165. Zhou W, Otto EA, Cluckey A, Airik R, Hurd TW, Chaki M, Diaz K, Lach FP, Bennett GR, Gee HY, Ghosh AK, Natarajan S, Thongthip S, Veturi U, Allen SJ, Janssen S, Ramaswami G, Dixon J, Burkhalter F, et al. FAN1 mutations cause karyomegalic interstitial nephritis, linking chronic kidney failure to defective DNA damage repair. Nat Genet. 2012; https://doi.org/10.1038/ng.2347.

166. Jayasumana C, Orantes C, Herrera R, Almaguer M, Lopez L, Silva LC, Ordunez P, Siribaddana S, Gunatilake S, De Broe ME. Chronic interstitial nephritis in agricultural communities: a worldwide epidemic with social, occupational and environmental determinants. Nephrol Dial Transplant. 2017;32(2):234–41. https://doi.org/10.1093/ndt/gfw346.

167. Ramírez-Rubio O, Amador JJ, Kaufman JS, Weiner DE, Parikh CR, Khan U, McClean MD, Laws RL, López-Pilarte D, Friedman DJ, Kupferman J, Brooks DR. Urine biomarkers of kidney injury among adolescents in Nicaragua, a region affected by an epidemic of chronic kidney disease of unknown aetiology. Nephrol Dial Transplant. 2016;31(3):424–32. https://doi.org/10.1093/ndt/gfv292.

168. Vervaet BA, Nast CC, Jayasumana C, Schreurs G, Roels F, Herath C, Kojc N, Samaee V, Rodrigo S, Gowrishankar S, Mousson C, Dassanayake R, Orantes CM, Vuiblet V, Rigothier C, D'Haese PC, De Broe ME. Chronic interstitial nephritis in agricultural communities is a toxin-induced proximal tubular nephropathy. Kidney Int. 2020;97(2):350–69. https://doi.org/10.1016/j.kint.2019.11.009.

169. Rodríguez-Iturbe B, Johnson RJ, Herrera-Acosta J. Tubulointerstitial damage and progression of renal failure. Kidney Int. 2005; https://doi.org/10.1111/j.1523-1755.2005.09915.x.

Part IX

Urinary Tract Disorders

Diagnosis and Management of Urinary Tract Infections

43

Ian K. Hewitt and Giovanni Montini

Introduction

Urinary tract infection (UTI) represents colonisation and invasion of the urinary tract by bacteria. The term cystitis is used when the organisms are confined to the bladder and urethra, and usually accompanied by localized symptoms such as dysuria, frequency, malodorous urine, day time and night time urinary incontinence. They occur most predominantly in girls older than 3 years of age and are easily treated. Acute pyelonephritis, considered by many to be the most common serious bacterial illness in childhood, is an infection that involves the renal parenchyma. Most affected children, particularly infants, present systemically unwell with symptoms including high fever, which may be the only indicative feature, lethargy, abdominal pain, nausea, vomiting and irritability. These infections have been considered of most concern for their potential to result in renal scarring, with the potential for long-term morbidity. Asymptomatic bacteriuria is a further type of urinary tract infection whereby a significant growth of organisms from the urine occurs in the absence of any illness or symptoms. It has been found in approximately 1% of school-aged girls on screening, and does not warrant treatment or investigation, as trials have demonstrated a good outcome, uninfluenced by any intervention.

Approximately 2% of boys and 7–8% of girls will experience a urinary tract infection in the first 8 years of life [1]. Febrile urinary tract infections suggestive of acute pyelonephritis are most common in the first year of life with a male predominance in the first 6 months, after which they are more often seen in girls (Fig. 43.1). Non-febrile UTI, typically cystitis, is seen more commonly in girls as they get older.

I. K. Hewitt
Department of Nephrology, Perth Children's
Hospital, Perth, WA, Australia
e-mail: ian.hewitt@health.wa.gov.au

G. Montini (✉)
Pediatric Nephrology, Dialysis and Transplant Unit,
Fondazione IRCCS Ca' Granda, University of Milan,
Milan, Italy
e-mail: giovanni.montini@unimi.it

© The Author(s), under exclusive license to Springer Nature Switzerland AG 2023
F. Schaefer, L. A. Greenbaum (eds.), *Pediatric Kidney Disease*,
https://doi.org/10.1007/978-3-031-11665-0_43

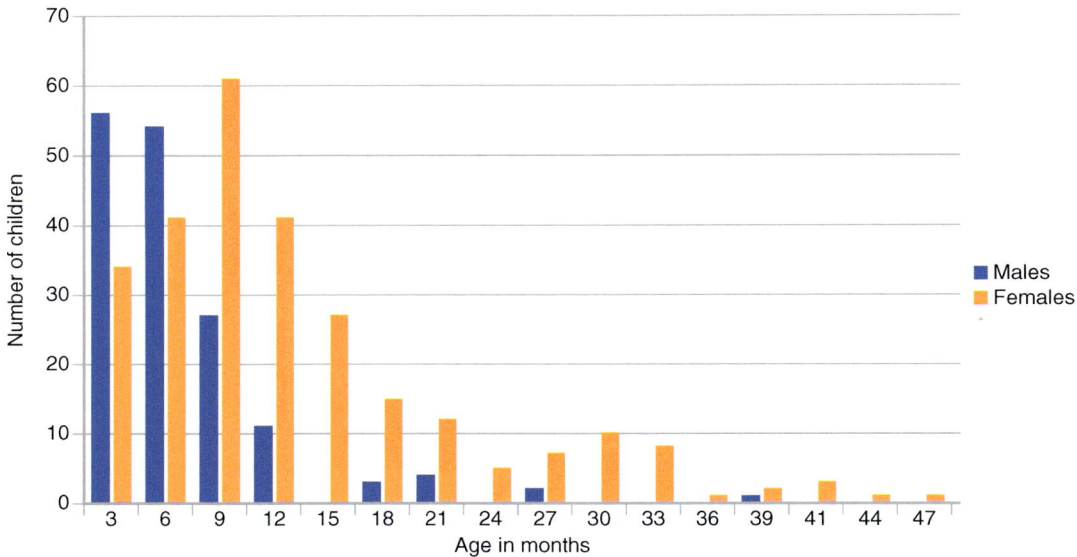

Fig. 43.1 Distribution by age (months) and sex of a cohort of 427 children (269 F, 158 M), aged 1 month to 4 years, at the first febrile urinary tract infection

Background

In recent years there has been a re-evaluation of the potential for UTI to culminate in severe long term renal parenchymal damage. In the past children usually came to attention only after experiencing UTIs, and were investigated with invasive imaging modalities, such as intravenous pyelography and voiding cystourethrograms. Small hypodysplastic and scarred kidneys, often in association with vesicoureteral reflux (VUR), were occasionally found, and were thought to be the consequence of previous episodes of unrecognized pyelonephritis. This led to the concept of reflux nephropathy, linking VUR to ascending infection and pyelonephritis, with subsequent renal scarring [2]. Consequent upon this, children with reflux were often placed on long term antibiotic prophylaxis or underwent surgical correction (Fig. 43.2a). Already at this time, not all agreed with this view. A French paper demonstrated that 11 of 12 nephrectomies performed because of severe reflux nephropathy were congenital small kidneys, with the remaining kidney showing isolated and specific histologic signs of chronic pyelonephritis [3]. Two early studies randomized children with VUR detected following a UTI to either antibiotic prophylaxis with surgical correction alone or combined with adjuvant prophylaxis [4, 5]. In one study the rate of scarring was 38% at presentation, while subsequent rates of scarring were low (2% and 9%) and unrelated to the presence or absence of VUR or breakthrough infection [4]. These two studies already demonstrated the difference between congenital renal mal-development and acquired scarring as a consequence of pyelonephritis. The introduction of routine antenatal ultrasound from the mid1980s onward, led to the recognition that much of the significant renal damage, often familial and seen in association with high grade VUR was the consequence of congenital abnormalities of the kidney and urinary tract (CAKUT) (Fig. 43.2b) [6]. This has led to questioning the role of acquired renal damage as a consequence of pyelonephritis as the major contributor to chronic kidney damage.

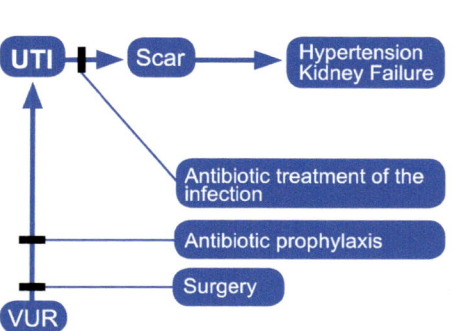

The old concept   **The new concept**

Fig. 43.2 The old concept (**a**). A casual relationship between febrile urinary tract infections and chronic renal failure was believed in the past to be the cause of major scarring. Vesicoureteric reflux was thought to be a major predisposing factor. Prompt antibiotic treatment of the acute infection was suggested to prevent renal scarring. Long term antibiotic prophylaxis and surgical correction of vesicoureteric reflux were employed to prevent recurrent urinary infections. The new concept (**b**). An enhanced understanding of genetic and immunologic mechanisms and prenatal ultrasound have revealed that major kidney damage appears to be congenital in origin. Trials have demonstrated surgery and antibiotic prophylaxis to be of limited if any benefit in preventing kidney damage. New treatments, such as the use of steroids and vitamin A, show promise in reducing the burden of post-infectious scarring

Clinical Presentation

Symptomatology of urinary tract infection varies considerably and is influenced by the child's age, level of infection, virulence of the organism and the inflammatory immune response. In newborns and infants, nonspecific symptoms such as prolonged neonatal jaundice, labile temperature, slow feeding and poor weight gain, irritability or listlessness with the infant unusually floppy are all hallmarks of infection. There is a propensity for infection in the very young to result in septicemia and sepsis, with possible adverse consequences such as seeding of infection at other sites, including meningitis.

Symptoms directly referable to the urinary tract such as frequency and pain on micturition are not usually recognised until around 2 years of age and beyond. Loin pain as a consequence of pyelonephritis, even if present, is not generally commented on by the child until 4–5 years of age. Cystitis can be associated with fever, how-

ever when this is 38.5 °C and above the likelihood of renal parenchymal infection is increased.

In older children, recurrent cystitis and, less frequently recurrent febrile UTIs, may be a feature of voiding disturbances, including hyperactivity and dysfunctional bladder emptying. Therefore, in these children, it is important to obtain a precise history of voiding patterns including incontinence, enuresis, frequency of micturition, urgency and bowel habits (see Chap. 47 for further discussion).

Diagnosis of Urinary Tract Infection

The diagnosis of urinary tract infection is contingent upon the culture of a single organism in significant numbers from an appropriately collected urine specimen. Laboratories use a standardized technique taking 0.001–0.002 mL (1–2 μL) of urine in a sterile loop, plating it out and on a culture medium and incubating in air at 35 °C with the plates checked for the nature and number of colonies (Fig. 43.3). Dipslide cultures (Fig. 43.4) are an alternative to the loop technique, particularly when specimens are collected after hours, thus allowing earlier reporting of culture results. While urinalysis is a useful adjunct in the diagnosis, particularly as culture results may take 24–48 h, it can never be a substitute for urine culture. The cut-off level for significant growth of organisms was first set by Kass 60 years ago at $\geq 10^5$ organisms/mL studying pyelonephritis in pregnant women [7]. It was apparent to Kass at the time that such a cut-off would by necessity miss UTIs. This is no less so in the childhood population. A recent study of infants <1 year with a

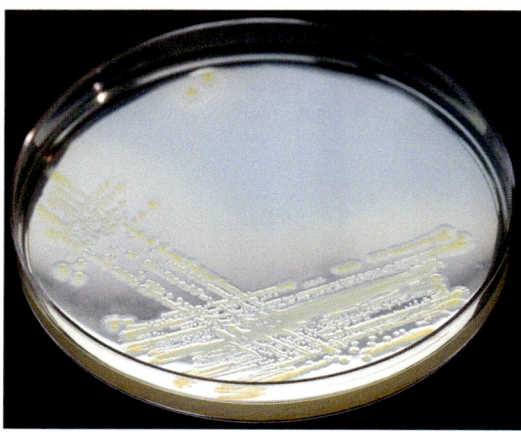

Fig. 43.3 This image shows bacterial colonies growing on an agar plate incubated at 35°C

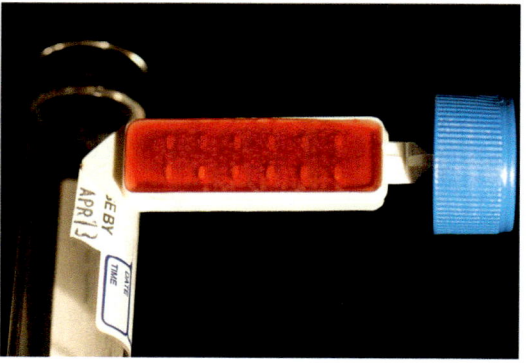

Fig. 43.4 Dipslide culture, which consists of a sterile culture medium on a plastic carrier that is dipped into the urine to be sampled and then incubated at 30°C for 48 h

symptomatic UTI diagnosed by supra-pubic aspirate demonstrated 19% to have colony counts <10⁵ of whom 87% had counts $<5 \times 10^4$ [8]. In an editorial comment on the paper it was noted that diagnosing a UTI on a strict cut-off level was inappropriate [9]. Most guidelines on investigation and management of UTI in children have avoided a detailed discussion of what constitutes an infection. Recently the Diagnosis of Urinary Tract infection in Young children (DUTY) study aimed at validating a clinical algorithm for the diagnosis of a UTI in children presenting with an acute illness to primary care. Collection was by pads in infants and clean-catch in older children. Agreement on UTI diagnosis was lower than expected between government and research laboratories and clean-catch encouraged as the preferred collection method [10]. A particular problem that creates difficulty with interpretation of urine cultures, resulting in false positive tests, is contamination during collection, which can be influenced by a number of factors. Contamination occurs when organisms from the genitalia, surrounding skin, urethra or periurethral area infect the specimen during collection. *Suprapubic aspiration* of urine and samples obtained by percutaneous nephrostomy are considered to be the "gold" standard for diagnosis of UTI, as they are the least likely to be contaminated, with the culture of any organism generally considered to be significant. Ideally suprapubic aspiration should be performed under ultrasound guidance, even then the invasive nature and lack of skill in the procedure often preclude its use. *Urethral catheterization* is the next most effective method of obtaining a reliable specimen for culture with a growth of 10^3–10^4 colonies per mL considered significant. Once again parents may consider this invasive and distressing for the child, with concerns that infection may be introduced by the procedure. A *voided clean catch midstream urine collection* has been long been considered the most practical method, particularly when children are toilet trained and can void on request. Colony counts of a single organism $\geq 50,000$ colonies per mL accompanied by pyuria are considered diagnostically significant [11]. In our experience, mainly using midstream samples, we believe that both urinary leucocytes and a significant colony count are needed for the diagnosis of UTI [12]. The presence of pyuria is a useful means to assist in the differentiation between contamination, colonization and clinically significant infection. When sterile pyuria is detected with leukocyte counts $>100 \times 10^6$/L, the urine should be tested for antibacterial activity, if negative, consideration should be given to the culture of fastidious organisms such as *Ureaplasma* and *Gardnerella* species that require specific growth media. When multiple organisms are cultured, there is an increased likelihood of contamination and the culture should be repeated.

Clean catch urine specimens can be obtained on occasion in infants and the very young, with the diaper removed and the parent waiting patiently for voiding to occur, however this is not always successful. One study described a success rate of 86.3% for obtaining a midstream urine specimen within 5 min in infants up to 30 days of age, using a bladder and lumbar stimulation technique [13]. *Bag collections* are practiced in a variety of settings and are of use as a screening procedure when the risk of infection is considered low or the child is afebrile. Controversy exists when bags are employed as the sole method of collection, with many claiming contamination rates are too high [14], such that a single positive specimen should be repeated, preferably with a catheter collection or supra-pubic aspirate. From a practical viewpoint, the use of bag collections is widespread, particularly in the primary care setting, where practitioners often do not have formal training in how to perform a suprapubic or catheter collection [15]. A bag specimen is particularly useful if negative for leukocytes on dipstick, in which case culture is unnecessary. If positive for leukocytes then a clean catch or catheter specimen for culture is appropriate. It has to be empha-

sized that if bag collection is the only method employed, strict protocols for the procedure are mandatory to reduce the contamination risk (how to wash the genitalia, how to apply the bag, the need to change the bag every 20–30 min). In our experience, when a count $>10^5$ of the same single organism in two consecutive carefully collected bag specimens is obtained, the likelihood of a genuine infection is extremely high.

Because of the delay in obtaining a urine culture result, the initial diagnosis and treatment is often guided by results of preliminary urinalysis and clinical symptoms. If a UTI is strongly suspected, particularly when accompanied by fever, antibiotic treatment should be initiated, based on the knowledge of local drug sensitivities, prior to availability of culture results. When urine microscopy is available this can be used to determine the number of white cells per mL in an un-spun urine specimen as well as document the presence of bacteria and non-glomerular hematuria that may occur with cystitis. Urine dipsticks provide a rapid, easy and cost-effective way of guiding initial management and treatment (Table 43.1). Leukocyte esterase activity in the urine is a sensitive indicator of pyuria while the nitrite test is based on the ability of most uropathogens to convert nitrite to nitrate. While a positive nitrite test is a good indicator of infection, it can be positive with asymptomatic bacteriuria and thus requires significant pyuria for confirmation [12], in addition, up to 4 h is required for the organisms to generate sufficient nitrite such that infants and those with urine frequency often have a false negative test. When more than one abnormality is found on urinalysis the likelihood of UTI is increased. Difficulties can arise with a single abnormality and subsequent borderline culture result, particularly when antibiotics have already been commenced.

Table 43.1 Interpretation and suggested practical approach following the result of nitrite and leukocyte esterase urine dipstick testing, performed immediately following collection (Adapted from Ammenti et al. [12] with permission)

Nitrite positive Leucocyte esterase positive	UTI very likely	Perform urine culture and start antibiotics empirically
Nitrite negative Leucocyte esterase positive	UTI likely	Perform urine culture and start antibiotics empirically
Nitrite negative Leucocyte esterase negative	UTI quite unlikely	Search for alternative diagnosis

Abbreviation: *UTI* urinary tract infection

There is a need for studies on appropriate urine sampling, interpretation of urine culture results (in particular the appropriate cut-offs for various methods of urine collection in children) and to determine if a negative urine leucocyte test can safely rule out a UTI or whether a culture is required.

Differentiating Upper from Lower Urinary Tract Infections

Differentiating between lower tract cystitis and upper tract pyelonephritis can be difficult in the acute setting. While fever and loin pain can result in a presumptive diagnosis of renal parenchymal infection it is not always the case. Currently there is no marker that can reliably predict the presence of acute pyelonephritis. While C-reactive protein and white cell count are often elevated they are insufficiently sensitive and specific for the diagnosis of renal parenchymal infection. Procalcitonin, a precursor of calcitonin, produced by the thyroid gland, and released in response to bacterial infections, appears to be the most robust blood test, but not a perfect predictor, of pyelonephritis and propensity for subsequent renal scarring [16]. Urinary markers that differ in pyelonephritis compared with cystitis include chemokine ligand CXCL1, CXCL9, CXCL12, INF gamma and IL15, however none has proved better than Procalcitonin [17]. Technetium-99m-labelled DimercaptoSuccinic Acid (DMSA) scans are considered the "gold standard" for confirmation of acute pyelonephritis (Fig. 43.5). DMSA scanning had been recommended as an initial investigation in the past, but did not receive wide uptake as it causes a significant radiation dose, needs to be performed within a week of the infection and is not available in many non-tertiary centers. Fever associated with the UTI has become indicative of likely pyelonephritis for clinical purposes [18, 19].

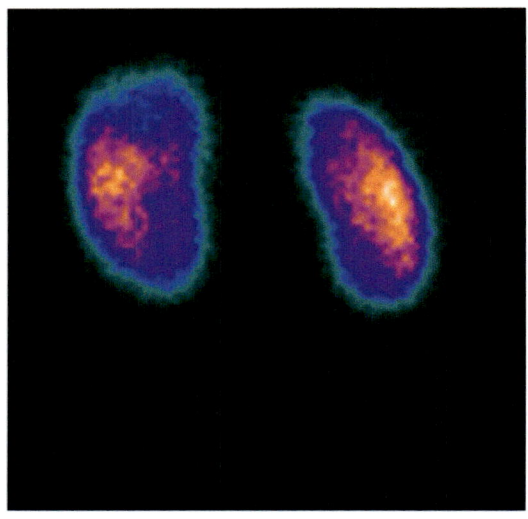

Fig. 43.5 Renal DMSA scintigraphy during the acute phase of a febrile urinary tract infection, showing acute pyelonephritis involving the left kidney

Pathogenesis

The kidneys and urinary tract are germ free environments under normal circumstances, while some infections may be blood born in origin, the majority are considered to be ascending in nature. When bacteria enter the bladder they are frequently washed out without causing infection [20]. Some develop asymptomatic bacteriuria while others develop cystitis with inflammation of the bladder mucosa. A few children will experience febrile UTIs with systemic activation of the immune inflammatory process.

A variety of host factors are thought to contribute to UTI in early childhood in the absence of significant renal tract anatomical abnormalities, these include dysfunctional bladder emptying prior to and after the development of urinary continence [21, 22], detrusor instability [23], constipation and fecal soiling prior to establishing bowel continence. Children with primary immunodeficiency do not appear particularly prone to

UTI, even those with frequent bacterial infections elsewhere, secondary to primary antibody deficiency states [24–26]. Information on UTIs in this group is scarce as the majority of infections are respiratory, gastrointestinal and skin. In the few instances where mention is made of UTIs in primary immunodeficiency diseases, associated renal tract abnormalities appear a feature. Similarly, with acquired immunodeficiency, such as organ transplantation, immunosuppression with steroids and chemotherapy, the issue of UTIs arises only in the context of catheterisation, instrumentation, stents involving the renal tract and not isolated immunosuppression per se. These observations support the contention that urine flow and integrity of the uroepithelium are the important factors in preventing infection. In addition, the intact uroepithelium appears to have an innate immune system with the intercalated cells secreting antimicrobial peptides that demonstrate potent bactericidal activity toward uropathogens [27]. Recent interest has focussed on uromodulin (UMOD), a glycoprotein secreted by the kidney into the urine. Eighty percent of humans have a UMOD promoter variant that results in a doubling of the urinary UMOD concentration, resulting in a reduced predisposition to UTIs [28, 29]. UMOD protein filaments aggregate around uropathogens causing bacterial clumping; it is likely that this inhibits adhesion, allowing clearance of the organisms by micturition [30].

Certain bacterial characteristics predispose to infection. In excess of 80% of infections are caused by *Escherichia coli*. These are the predominant bowel organisms found in close proximity to the urethral orifice. In addition, they have P fimbriae that enable uroepithelial adherence even in the presence of adequate urine flow. When children have neurogenic bladders or renal tract malformations that lead to urine stasis or residual urine after voiding, non-attaching bacteria may cause infection.

When uropathogens infect kidney parenchyma localized inflammation occurs, triggering the innate immune system through a variety of pathways. Recognition of bacteria initiates toll like receptor signalling that in turn causes an immune response involving nuclear factor κβ, cytokines and chemokines. Interleukin 8 (IL-8) is an important chemokine that activates neutrophils via receptors CXCR1 and CXCR2. Children with polymorphisms of IL-8, CXCR1 and CXCR2 have reduced trans-epithelial migration of neutrophils, defective clearance of bacteria and demonstrate a predisposition to recurrent pyelonephritis [31–33].

Full recovery can occur, however if the inflammation is prolonged, scarring can result, though the exact predisposing factors and mechanisms remain ill understood, a number of possible genetic determinants have been identified [34]. Interleukin 6 is one factor that plays a role in the immune response and has been shown to be a marker of children who develop later scarring [35]. Functional variants in genes that encode for vascular endothelial growth factor and transforming growth factor β1 and factors that regulate fibrosis in response to tissue inflammation have also been implicated in renal parenchymal scarring following pyelonephritis in children [36]. Ethnicity has been proposed as an additional risk factor: a meta-analysis demonstrated that post pyelonephritic scarring in children varied by region from 27% in Australia to 49% in Asia [37].

Several pharmacological approaches to limit renal scarring have been explored. Three randomized controlled trials (RCTs) on the use of **steroids** yielded conflicting results. One study of oral methylprednisolone compared with placebo in 84 children with a first episode of pyelonephritis on DMSA scan demonstrated a significant reduction in scarring at 6 months (33% vs. 60% $p < 0.05$) in those given steroid [38]. The second study comparing dexamethasone with placebo in 52 children with pyelonephritis showed no benefit in scarring [39]. The most recent double blind RCT evaluated the efficacy of an oral 3-day course of dexamethasone in reducing kidney scarring in children 2 months to 6 years of age [40]. Unfortunately, only 254 of the 546 children randomized had the primary outcome evaluated with a late DMSA scan. The absolute risk reduction was 5.9% (95% confidence interval: −2.2; 14.1), which did not reach statistical significance.

Vitamin A has been promoted as an agent that might alleviate scarring following acute pyelonephritis. It has also been demonstrated to impact urinary tract morphogenesis, with a deficiency or excess resulting in CAKUT [41]. A meta-analysis including 4 RCTs of 248 children concluded that Vitamin A may be of benefit, however the studies were of low methodologic quality [42]. A recent high-quality double-blind placebo RCT assigned 90 girls (mean age 5, range 2–12 years) with DMSA scan-confirmed acute PN to a 10-day course of oral vitamin A (1500 U/kg/day) or placebo. Symptoms were briefer in the treatment group. A late DMSA scan demonstrated worsening in 8 (21%) on vitamin A vs. 17 (48%) on placebo (P = 0.003), while 23 (64%) on vitamin A and 8 (21%) on placebo demonstrated improvement in photopenia (P < 0.0001) [43].

In experimental models a variety of agents including montelukast, a leukotriene CysLT1 receptor antagonist that reverses oxidative effects [44], COX-2 inhibitors [45], melatonin [46], an inhibitor of neutrophil infiltration, and losartan, that down regulates TGFβ production [47], have all shown potential as therapeutic agents, though all lack clinical corroboration. More needs to be understood regarding the renal parenchymal inflammatory response and mechanisms of scar formation if effective strategies are to be developed to prevent or reduce scarring.

Bacterial Virulence

Uropathogenic *Escherichia coli* (UPEC) are a subgroup of the *Escherichia coli* that form the normal bowel flora. They express a range of virulence mechanisms that make them well suited to invade the renal tract and kidneys, resist the innate immune responses and initiate a damaging inflammatory cascade. Specific adhesins that form part of fimbriae or pili on the external surface of the organism facilitate attachment to uroepithelial cells [48]. Type 1 pili found on virtually all UPEC predispose to bladder infection, while P pili are associated with acute pyelonephritis [49]. Once they invade the uroepithelial cells, additional virulence factors, termed autoinducers,

can coordinate the formation of an intracellular biofilm like cluster of rapidly multiplying organisms, that are protected from the host immune system. The bacteria can go on to infect other cells or remain dormant for a period with the ability to cause recurrent infections [50]. Additional virulence factors transmitted by plasmids promote tolerance to antibiotics [51]. Understanding these host pathogen interactions is of increasing importance at a time where drug resistance is a serious issue. Strategies specifically targeting virulence factors are being investigated as an alternative to antibiotics [52–54] as is the colonization of at-risk patients with non-pathogenic *Escherichia coli* in the hope that they might keep uropathogenic organisms at bay [55].

Organisms Causing Infection

Escherichia coli is the causative organism in 80–90% of UTIs that occur in the outpatient setting [56, 57]. The remaining 10–20% of infections are caused by a variety of organisms including *Klebsiella, Enterococcus, Enterobacter, Proteus* and *Pseudomonas species*. Infection with atypical organisms such as *Pseudomonas* increase the risk that underlying renal pathology exists, such as a neurogenic bladder or significant anatomic abnormalities [58]. In the inpatient setting *E. coli* account for approximately 60% of infections with the higher incidence of atypical organisms a reflection of underlying pathology as well as urinary tract procedures undertaken in this context [59].

Candida UTIs are predominantly a concern for neonatal intensive care units. The infections are associated with prematurity, respiratory distress, congenital heart disease, major renal tract abnormalities and sepsis, while systemic corticosteroids use is a probable additional risk factor. Mortality has been reported as high as 30% and is more likely when systemic spread has occurred, with the co-morbid conditions also playing a role [60].

Granulomatous interstitial tuberculous nephritis is a recognised entity that can occur on rare occasions in children, almost always in developing countries, and often associated with co-morbid conditions such as human immunodeficiency virus (HIV) [61] or underlying renal disease that predisposes to the infection [62]. It should be considered when sterile pyuria occurs in association with tuberculosis elsewhere in the body [63]. *Schistosomiasis* is a common tropical blood fluke infection, particularly in sub-Saharan Africa. A fresh water snail is the intermediate host, with infection following exposure to the infected water; children have the highest burden of disease [64]. The organism enters through the skin and can infect the ureters and bladder causing hematuria. It is being seen with increasing frequency in high income countries with the arrival of travellers and refugees from endemic areas [65].

Treatment of the Acute Episode

With their advent, antibiotics have become the cornerstone of treatment for UTIs resulting in dramatically improved outcomes. In the early twentieth century infants and young children hospitalized with acute pyelonephritis frequently died as a consequence [66]. Despite the recognized effectiveness of antibiotics in treating UTIs and impeding their parenchymal localization, until the mid-1990s there was a lack of research regarding the appropriate agent, manner of administration and duration of treatment required. Uncomplicated afebrile UTIs were and remain for the most part treated with oral antibiotics that have a high renal excretion and a restricted spectrum of activity. A recent systematic review of antibiotic treatment for uncomplicated lower UTI in children concluded that short course oral therapy (3–7 days) was as effective as long course (7–10 days) treatment with single dose therapy not recommended until further studies are undertaken to determine its effectiveness [67]. In contrast, for febrile UTIs, particularly when occurring in infants and younger children, hospital admission and broad-spectrum intravenous antibiotics became the norm. Between 1995 and 2004 five trials demonstrated that short courses of intravenous antibiotics (up to 4 days) followed by oral therapy, were as

Table 43.2 Treatment of complicated and uncomplicated febrile urinary tract infections

Uncomplicated febrile UTI ↓	Complicated febrile UTI ↓
Oral antibiotic on an outpatient basis	Parenteral antibiotic—hospital admission
Good general condition	Septic child
Able to drink	Vomiting
Absent to mild dehydration	Moderate to severe dehydration
Good compliance	Possible poor compliance

effective as longer courses of intravenous treatment (7–14 days) [68–72]. Four studies involving a total of 1344 infants and children as young as 1 month of age with a first febrile UTI went further, demonstrating that oral antibiotics alone were as effective as intravenous antibiotics followed by oral antibiotics, the studies showed no difference in time to resolution of fever or subsequent renal damage [56, 57, 73, 74]. Current guidelines for treatment of a febrile UTI recommend oral antibiotic administration on an outpatient basis, with hospital admission and parenteral administration restricted to those children who appear to be severely ill, vomiting or where poor compliance is a risk (Table 43.2) [75, 76]. The choice of antibiotic should be guided by local resistance patterns and the lead organism, *E. coli*. Where good β lactam and cephalosporin sensitivity has been demonstrated, these are the preferred antibiotics. Of concern, there is an increased prevalence of *E. coli* producing extended spectrum beta-lactamase (ESBL) [77]. Commonly used antibiotics are listed in Table 43.3. Provided an organism is sensitive to the drug chosen, no antibiotic has been shown as superior to another. Hence, we encourage cephalosporins (cefixime or ceftibuten for the oral route and cefotaxime or ceftriaxone for iv administration) in children with severe infections. Cephalosporins are recognized to have a more rapid onset of action, making the possibility of resistance a less important issue. When a febrile infection occurs in children receiving antibiotic prophylaxis, a different antibiotic is required, because of an almost certain resistance to the prophylactic agent.

Table 43.3 Antibiotics commonly used for the treatment of febrile urinary tract infections in children. (Adapted from Montini et al. [6] and Ammenti et al. [12]). Antibiotic choice should be based on local antimicrobial sensitivity patterns

Intravenous treatment	Dose	Comments
Penicillins		
Ampicillin-Sulbactam	100 mg/kg/day of ampicillin in 3–4 doses	
Amoxicillin-clavulanic acid	100 mg/kg/day of amoxicillin in 3–4 doses	
Cephalosporin		
Cefotaxime	20–40 mg/kg four times per day	Increasing resistance
Ceftazidime	30–50 mg/kg three times per day	Good coverage for Pseudomonas
Ceftriaxone	50 mg/kg once per day	Advantage of once daily dosing Contraindicated in neonates, especially prematures
Aminoglycoside		Useful if beta-lactam allergy.
Gentamycin	6–7.5 mg/kg once per day or 2–2.5 mg/kg three times per day	Nephrotoxic. Must monitor with serum levels and adjust dosage
Amikacin	15 mg/kg once per day or 7.5 mg/kg twice per day	accordingly. A recent meta-analysis supports single daily dosage[a]
Oral treatment	Dose	Comments
Trimethoprim-sulfamethoxazole	4 mg/kg twice per day (dose expressed as trimethoprim)	High resistance rates Risk of allergic reaction
Amoxicillin-clavulanic acid	25–50 mg/kg twice per day (dose expressed as amoxicillin)	Increasing resistance
Cephalosporin		Increasing resistance
Ceftibuten	9 mg/kg twice per day the first day, once daily thereafter	
Cefixime	8 mg/kg twice per day the first day, once daily thereafter	
Quinolone		Treatment of complicated UTIs as a
Ciprofloxacin	10–20 mg/kg twice per day (maximum 750 mg per dose)	second choice. Increasing resistance Increased risk of musculoskeletal adverse events

[a]Contopoulos-Ioannidis DG, Giotis ND, Baliatsa DV, Ioannidis JP. Extended interval aminoglycoside administration for children: a meta-analysis. Pediatrics 2004;114(1):e111–e118

Infants in the first month of life who present unwell with unstable temperature, lethargy, poor feeding or prolonged jaundice, and are thought to be septic, are a particular group that warrants intravenous antibiotics after appropriate cultures, including blood and urine, are taken. Sepsis in the first 72 h is most commonly group B streptococcus, although *E. coli* infections can occur in this period and become more common thereafter. There is a lack of controlled trials in this age group, as neonatal sepsis is recognized as a serious illness, particularly when it occurs in low birth weight preterm infants. Contributing factors to the potential severity of bacterial infection in infants include an immature immune system, and in the case of preterm infants, reduced placental transfer of protective maternal antibodies. Thus,

intravenous penicillins combined with aminoglycosides are commonly used on an empiric basis. Care should be taken to monitor aminoglycoside levels because of their potential nephrotoxicity, particularly in infants with impaired renal function secondary to renal dysplasia.

Imaging After a Febrile Urinary Tract Infection

There is a lack of consensus as to the recommendations for imaging after a fUTI, although recent improved understanding of UTIs and their sequelae has resulted in a lessening of the nature and number of procedures indicated (Table 43.4). Published protocols give guidance on the investi-

Table 43.4 Imaging tests routinely recommended by the most recent published guidelines in children following a first febrile urinary tract infection

Guideline	Ultrasound	VCUG	DMSA	Prophylaxis
NICE (2007, updated 2017)	Atypical, <6/12 age	No unless <6 months of age with positive US or atypical UTI	Yes >6/12 post UTI	No
AAP (2011)	Yes	No unless abnormal US	No	No
ISPN (2020)	Yes	No unless abnormal US or bacteria other than UPEC	Consider if major abnormalities at US	Considered for VUR IV–V
CARI (2014)	Yes, if: no second or third trimester US, <3/12 age or atypical UTI	No unless abnormal US	No	No
Canadian (2014)	Yes	No unless abnormal US	No	No

gation of febrile UTIs in infants and younger children; however, there is little advice regarding afebrile UTIs or infections occurring in older children.

Ultrasonography

Ultrasonography is a non-invasive procedure that can detect a variety of anatomical abnormalities, but is dependent on the expertise of the radiologist. In recent years antenatal ultrasound has proved of value in detecting most of the significant CAKUT prior to birth, including renal hypodysplasia, pelviureteric junction obstruction, vesicoureteric obstruction often as a result of ureteroceles and posterior urethral valves [78]. In three prospective trials involving 864 children investigated after a first febrile UTI, ultrasonography did not reliably detect changes associated with reflux or predict subsequent scarring. Minor abnormalities were found in 12–14% of cases that had little influence on subsequent outcomes [79–81].

The American Academy of Pediatrics (AAP) recommends ultrasonography in all children under 2 years of age after an initial febrile UTI [11], as does the Italian Society of Pediatric Nephrology (ISPN) [75]. The recently published Italian guideline identifies specific ultrasound abnormalities which represent an indication to perform VCUG: mono- or bilateral renal hypoplasia, abnormal parenchymal echogenicity, ureteral dilatation, kidney pelvis epithelial thickening, pelvi-calyceal dilatation, and bladder abnormalities [12].

The National Institute for Health and Care Excellence (NICE) guidelines restrict ultrasonography further to those <6 months of age, unless the infection is atypical or additional risk factors are present [76]. The Australian guidelines even restrict ultrasound to <3 months of life or to children with an atypical UTI or absent antenatal ultrasound [82]. Given the low detection rate of clinically significant findings following an uncomplicated UTI in childhood, we enquire as to whether a reliable second or third trimester antenatal ultrasound is available to be reviewed and limit ultrasound to those where this is not the case (Fig. 43.6). If the infection appears atypical, there is evidence of renal function impairment, inadequate urine stream or repeated infection, we believe ultrasonography to be indicated [83, 84]. For older children ultrasonography is indicated for repeated febrile and nonfebrile UTIs after a precise history of voiding patterns has been taken, particularly in girls.

The ultrasound examination should assess bladder filling and emptying, post-micturition residual urine and bladder wall thickness when full and empty. Normal values are usually less than 3 mm when the bladder is full and less than 5 mm when empty. In case of significant abnormal findings on bladder ultrasound, urodynamic studies should be considered.

Voiding Cystourethrography

Voiding cystourethrography generally requires the bladder instillation of a radiopaque, radioactive or echogenic contrast medium via urethral

Fig. 43.6 Treatment of complicated and uncomplicated febrile urinary tract infections

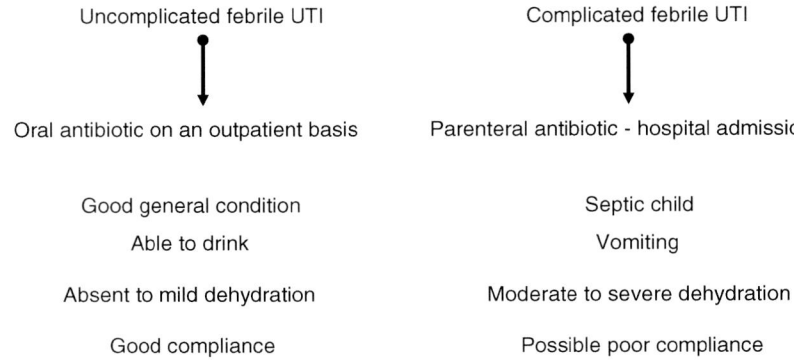

catheterization, followed by serial imaging. It can demonstrate VUR during the filling and voiding phases, as well as demonstrate urethral obstruction due to posterior urethral valves in boys. Much controversy has centred on the need or otherwise for this study, given the distress this invasive procedure can cause children. Those advocating cystourethrography cite a strong association between the severity of reflux and presence of renal damage [83], which is being increasingly recognized as congenital rather than acquired in origin [85, 86]. As there is a lack of evidence that intervention is beneficial for all but those few children with high grade dilating reflux, in terms of medical or surgical procedures [87], published protocols support a selective approach to this investigation. In children following a febrile UTI in the first 2–3 years of life, they recommend this study if the ultrasound is positive or the UTI atypical (Table 43.4). We believe that this investigation is rarely indicated following a first febrile UTI and should be restricted to those few children with significant bladder abnormalities, ureteric dilatation on ultrasound or inadequate urine stream (Fig. 43.6). For older children with febrile UTIs and those with recurrent cystitis, we believe voiding cystourethrography is rarely indicated, as a precise history of voiding patterns and an ultrasound are usually sufficient to establish the diagnosis and treatment (see Chap. … for further discussion).

Renal Scintigraphy

Renal imaging with DMSA requires the intravenous administration of a radio-active isotope which localizes to the renal parenchyma, the procedure is highly sensitive, with decreased uptake that may represent inflammation as seen in acute pyelonephritis (Fig. 43.5) or may represent scarring (Fig. 43.8a). The main concern is the radiation dose of approximately 1 mSv. The procedure has been used to confirm pyelonephritis when performed in close proximity to a febrile UTI, or from 6 to 12 months after to determine if scarring has resulted. The delay is important for the determination of scarring, as uptake defects can persist for some months following the acute infection, without necessarily indicating scarring. The technique may also detect congenital renal hypodysplasia (Fig. 43.8b), which can sometimes be difficult to differentiate from acquired scarring, however the former usually appears as a small kidney with uniform uptake of isotope while the latter is more likely to present as a loss of smooth contour with a focal uptake defect (Fig. 43.8a, b).

The AAP guidelines do not recommend an acute or late DMSA scan following a febrile UTI [11], while a late DMSA scan is recommended by NICE when the infection is atypical [76] and by the ISPN where ultrasound shows abnormalities or there is evidence of VUR [75]. In both cases the purpose is to detect any scarring. An

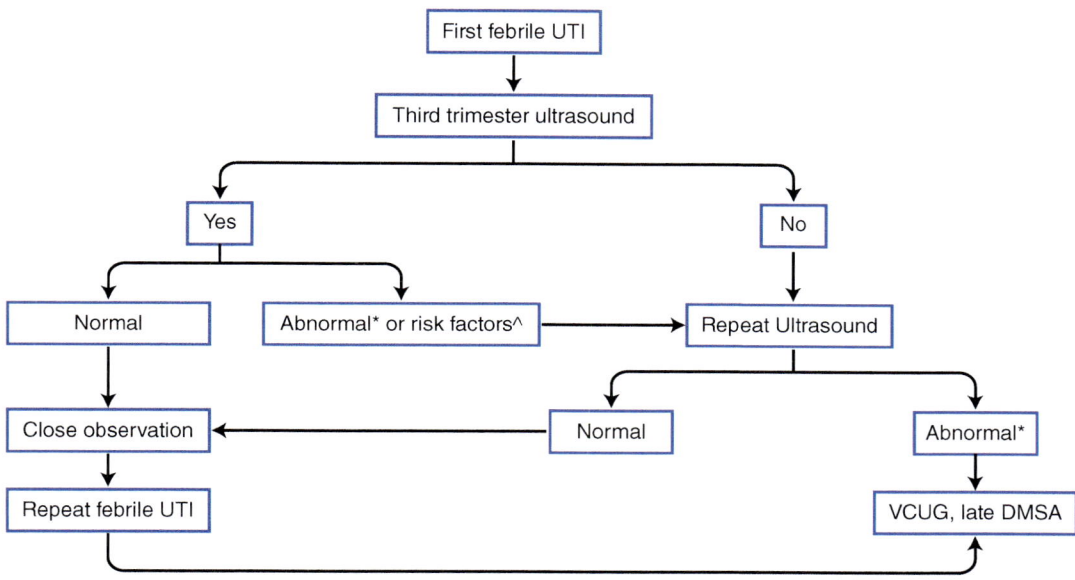

Fig. 43.7 Diagnostic flow chart of the suggested diagnostic protocol in a child 2 months to 3 years of age, following a first febrile urinary tract infection

alternative that was never widely accepted was the "top down" approach whereby a DMSA scan is performed in the acute phase of the illness, followed by cystourethrography if the scan is positive. Two studies claimed a strong correlation between high grade dilating VUR and abnormal scans. In contrast, a later study demonstrated 14/46 children with grade III–IV reflux to have a normal DMSA scan during the acute infection [88]. Some investigators have recommended a DMSA scan 6–12 months following an infection as the most appropriate investigation, as this would detect those children with permanent renal scarring that requires follow-up [81, 89]. When UTIs are afebrile, DMSA scans are not indicated.

Technetium-99m-labelled diethylenetriamine-pentaacetic acid (DTPA) and technetium-99m-mercaptoacetyltriglycine (MAG 3) are radionuclides that as well as being taken up by the kidney have an early excretory phase. As such that they are useful for assessing the presence and severity of any obstruction, and are indicated when other imaging raises this possibility. They are not used primarily for the detection of pyelonephritis or scarring.

Other Imaging Modalities

Plain abdominal X-ray may detect radio-opaque renal calculi, however most calculi can now be detected on ultrasound. **Intravenous pyelography** has for the most part been superseded by ultrasound and radionuclide scintigraphy. **Magnetic resonance urography** is a newer modality that gives excellent anatomical detail as well functional imaging without an attendant radiation dose. It appears to have some ability to indirectly assess obstruction, by measuring cortical transit times, when used in conjunction with contrast material. While at the present time it cannot be recommended as a first line procedure, in future as the technology becomes more available and cost effective, it may supplant a range of current imaging procedures (Fig. 43.8) [90]. A major limitation in younger children is the need for sedation or general anesthesia.

Impact of Reduced Imaging

Some concern has been expressed that the trend toward reduced imaging may be accompanied by adverse risks, with voiding cystourethrography being the most contentious procedure. Several studies have addressed this issue.

a

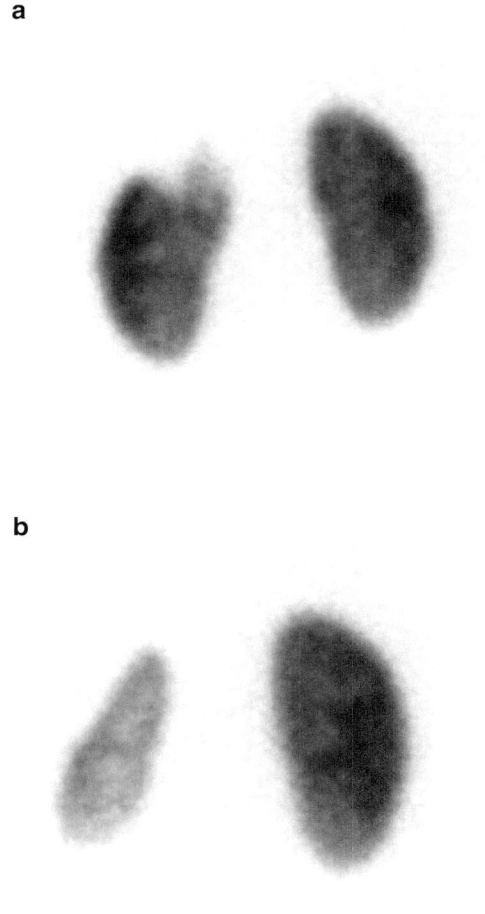

b

Fig. 43.8 Renal DMSA scintigraphy demonstrating a left upper pole scar (panel a) and a left hypodysplastic kidney (panel b)

Following publication of the NICE guidelines, two studies assessed their impact [91, 92]. Schroeder et al. compared the more selective imaging algorithm (NICE) with the formerly employed comprehensive algorithm (AAP 1999) [76, 91, 93]. The change led to a reduction in cystourethrograms performed following a febrile UTI from 99% to 13% and ultrasounds from 99% to 67%. The recurrence rate of UTI and detection rate of grade 4 and 5 VUR did not change, and the use of prophylactic antibiotics diminished. Deader et al. performed a retrospective analysis of 346 children who had an ultrasound performed at their institution fol-

lowing a UTI, to determine if significant renal pathology would have been overlooked had the procedure been restricted to those <6 months of age in accordance with NICE. Three scars confirmed on DMSA and one ureterocele would have been missed, such that the more restrictive guidelines regarding ultrasound appeared safe and provided significant cost savings [92]. Similarly, Jerardi et al. instituted a rapid uptake of the revised AAP guidelines [11] that significantly reduced the number of investigations performed, without any significant difference in the rate of abnormalities detected pre and post-intervention [94]. La Scola et al. evaluated the yield, cost and radiation dose of five different investigative guidelines if they had been applied to 304 children 2–36 months of age with a first febrile UTI that had been comprehensively evaluated in a RCT [95]. Scarring would have been detected by those that recommend a late DMSA scan in all cases [18], while guidelines that recommend a late DMSA in selected circumstances missed approximately half of the scars [75, 76] and all scars were missed in those guidelines that do not recommend a DMSA scan [11, 96]. Four of the five protocols failed to reliably detect high grade VUR, and proved even less effective when all grades of reflux were considered [11, 75, 76, 96]. Conversely the protocol that would detect all scarring had the highest cost and radiation burden [18], while the more selective protocols including the AAP guidelines, are the least costly with the lowest radiation dose.

Antibiotic Prophylaxis

Recent prospective studies have demonstrated antibiotic prophylaxis to be of little or no benefit in preventing recurrent infections, or reducing the risk of scarring in the majority of children following an uncomplicated first febrile UTI. Antibiotic prophylaxis has been widely recommended in the past following pyelonephritis, particularly where VUR was present, on the assumption that it would reduce the recurrence rate of infections and prevent renal scarring [93]. Eight randomised prospective studies involving 2390 children and adolescents evaluating the effectiveness of prophylaxis have been published between 2006 and 2015 [97–104]. While a direct comparison between the studies is not possible, due to their disparate populations, duration of follow-up and investigations undertaken, it is reasonable to draw a number of conclusions. All studies had recurrent UTI as a primary end-point. Four studies in patients with absent or predominantly low grade reflux showed rates of recurrence to be similar in the prophylactic compared with no treatment groups [97–100], two of these studies demonstrating a trend toward increased infections in the children with grade III reflux who were not on prophylaxis [99, 100]. One smaller study demonstrated an increase in UTIs on prophylaxis compared with controls [104]. A further study, the Swedish Reflux Trial, restricted to 203 infants with higher grade (III–IV) dilating reflux, demonstrated a clinically significant reduction in febrile UTIs on prophylaxis compared with controls (19% vs. 57%, p < 0.001) over a 2 year period in girls, but not boys [102]. The two largest and only studies to be placebo controlled, the PRIVENT and RIVUR trials involving 1183 children showed prophylaxis to result in a statistically significant though clinically insignificant reduction in UTIs, with 14–16 patient years of prophylaxis needed to prevent one symptomatic infection and 22 patient years of treatment to prevent one febrile infection [101, 103]. In both studies the maximum benefit of prophylaxis occurred in the initial 6 months. A systematic review of antibiotic prophylaxis for prevention of recurrent UTI in children demonstrated a small benefit of low dose antibiotic prophylaxis in preventing recurrent UTI, at the expense of increasing bacterial resistance to the treatment drug with subsequent infections. The analysis did not address the severity of VUR as a risk factor neither did it evaluate scarring as an adverse outcome [105].

Seven studies looked at late renal scarring on DMSA scan as a secondary endpoint. Only one paper, restricted to infants with high grade reflux, demonstrated a benefit of prophylaxis in preventing scarring, once again only in girls [87]. This benefit was not confirmed in the larger RIVUR trial, comparing antibiotic prophylaxis to placebo, which recruited 607 children (92% female) following a UTI, 46% of whom had grade III–IV dilating reflux [103]. No study was sufficiently powered to detect a possible benefit of prophylaxis in prevention of renal scarring. To address this, a systematic review and meta-analysis of 1427 subjects from 7 RCTs was undertaken and demonstrated no prevention of renal scarring by antibiotic prophylaxis, as did a sub-analysis restricted to the 1004 subjects with VUR [106].

These findings suggest that antibiotic prophylaxis is of minimal if any benefit in infants and children with absent or grades I–III reflux with a low recurrence rate for infection [101]. In a single study prophylaxis appeared to be of benefit in reducing recurrent pyelonephritis and scarring in the female infants and young children with high grade (III–IV) dilating reflux [102], although the finding in relation to scarring was not confirmed in the RIVUR trial with larger numbers of randomised girls who had the same degree of reflux [103]. In the few children with recurrent febrile UTIs who might benefit from prophylaxis, there is no consensus at what age or for what duration it should be prescribed.

Based on current evidence, we believe that antibiotic prophylaxis should be prescribed for 2 years in young girls and for 1 year in young boys with high grade reflux. Nitrofurantoin appears the most effective agent; however, the side effect profile and risk of poor compliance appear to outweigh any benefit of the medication, such that cotrimoxazole, amoxiclavulanate and the cephalosporins are generally preferred.

Antibiotic Prophylaxis in Children with Major Urologic Malformation, Spina Bifida, Neurogenic Bladder and Intermittent Catheterisation

Urinary tract infections are common in children with major urologic malformations that pertain particularly to the bladder. Children with ongoing bladder dysfunction for a variety of reasons including surgical resolution of posterior urethral valves, those with neurogenic bladders as a consequence of spina bifida or spinal cord injury, and children with bladder exstrophy, many of whom have undergone multiple surgical procedures and are on clean intermittent catheterisation, are at risk of long-term bladder colonisation and recurrent UTIs. The role of antibiotics and prophylaxis remains unclear in these patients. In the only RCT of antibiotic prophylaxis in children on clean intermittent catheterization, those that continued prophylaxis had a significantly higher incidence of UTIs when compared with those that ceased treatment [107]. Furthermore, a meta-analysis of adolescents and adults with spinal cord dysfunction did not support the use of prophylactic antibiotics [108]. Despite these findings, there is a lack of uniformity in management of children with neurogenic bladder dysfunction, with a remarkable variation in the prescription of prophylactic and therapeutic antibiotics in this population.

Given the difficulty of eradicating organisms from the bladder of patients on long-term intermittent catheterization, an alternative approach with some promise is to colonize the bladder with an avirulent strain of *E. coli* using infected catheters [55]. A further study of children with neurogenic bladder showed they most commonly carried avirulent commensal clones [109]. Uropathogenic clones, when present, were associated with prolonged carriage, however this was not associated with symptomatic disease or deterioration of the upper urinary tract. Thus, urine culture and antibiotic treatment of any infection detected in these children should on current evidence be restricted to those with definite symptoms.

Infants and young children with chronic kidney disease due to dysplasia are at particular risk of early deterioration to the point of requiring kidney replacement therapy, with some evidence that the rate of deterioration is accelerated in those with recurrent febrile UTIs [110]. A large multicentre RCT, the PREDICT trial, is currently underway evaluating the usefulness of antibiotic prophylaxis in this at risk population.

Surgical Correction of VUR

Surgical correction of VUR can be achieved by either re-implanting a tunnelled ureter through the bladder wall or endoscopic injection of a bulking agent adjacent to the vesicoureteral ori-

fice. The reported success rate for re-implantation is 98% (95% CI 95–99) and 83% for a single attempt at endoscopic treatment, with uncertainty regarding the permanency of the endoscopic approach [111]. Surgical correction is no longer routinely recommended, but may be considered when breakthrough febrile UTIs occur on prophylaxis, particularly in association with high grade dilating reflux in females.

A recent study, the Swedish infant high-grade reflux trial, randomized 77 infants <8 months of age with VUR grade IV–V to antibiotic prophylaxis or endoscopic correction of VUR with prophylaxis until VUR resolution was confirmed. The study showed no benefit of surgical intervention over prophylaxis in the risk of UTI recurrence or renal function deterioration. The study did not include a no-treatment control group to assess whether the interventions were of benefit. Of interest, over the 1-year follow-up 21% of the infants on antibiotic prophylaxis had a reduction in VUR severity to grades 0–II [112].

Additional Therapies

Circumcision

There are no RCTs on routine neonatal circumcision for the prevention of UTIs in males [113]. Two systematic reviews including predominantly cohort studies, reached opposite conclusions. One review concluded that routine circumcision to prevent UTI was not indicated in normal boys with the number needed to treat to prevent one UTI calculated at 111, however it could be considered in those with recurrent UTIs or high grade reflux, where the benefits appear to outweigh risks of the procedure [114]. A second review concluded that circumcision was indicated in all boys, as it reduced the lifetime risk of UTI, with a little over four low risk operative procedures to prevent one infection [115].

Cranberry Juice

Some studies suggest that cranberry juice may be of benefit in reducing recurrent UTIs, presumably by inhibiting bacterial adhesion to uroepithelial cells. A Cochrane review of 24 randomized controlled or quasi randomized controlled trials failed to demonstrate any significant benefit of cranberry juice, concentrate or capsules/tablets in the management of recurrent UTI in a variety of circumstances, including children and those with neuropathic bladder or spinal injury [116].

Probiotics

Studies have been undertaken to assess the possible benefit of probiotics in reducing or preventing recurrent UTIs. Most studies have been undertaken in women with variable results [117]. The studies are difficult to assess, as they use different strains of organisms, predominantly lactobacilli that have a variable effect on intestinal flora. One retrospective study demonstrated a possible benefit of probiotic prophylaxis similar to antibiotic prophylaxis in prevention of UTIs over a 6 month period, however the paper had significant methodologic shortcomings such that further studies are needed before any recommendations can be made on probiotic use [118]. Given the low quality of studies, a systematic review failed to show a role of probiotics in reducing recurrent UTIs, however a benefit cannot be ruled out prior to larger scale prospective RCTs [119].

The treatment of **constipation** and soiling in at risk children, as well as strategies to manage **dysfunctional voiding**, are considered by many to be worthwhile in the prevention of recurrent UTI. Unfortunately, there are no RCTs that assess the efficacy of any particular intervention.

Long-Term Clinical Consequences

Uncomplicated UTIs are common in children. When associated with fever there is an increased probability of renal parenchymal involvement, which can result in permanent renal scarring. In the absence of scarring there is no documentation of any adverse long-term outcomes. The frequency and severity of scarring as a consequence of acute pyelonephritis, the age at which it occurs and the long-term sequelae have been points of conjecture, as has the risk of consequent chronic kidney disease (CKD), hypertension and preeclampsia. The introduction of routine antenatal

ultrasound over the past 20–30 years, has demonstrated that much of the renal parenchymal damage previously attributed to pyelonephritis, is the result of congenital mal-development of the kidneys, often associated with significant urinary tract abnormalities such as high grade VUR or obstruction (Fig. 43.2b).

This recognition has led to a critical re-evaluation of the potential for pyelonephritis to cause scarring and result in adverse outcomes. A systematic review of renal scarring reported a prevalence of 15% following a UTI [120]. The risk and severity of scarring as a consequence of a single episode of pyelonephritis appears unrelated to age, when infants and young children are compared with older children [121]. In a meta-analysis involving 1280 children and adolescents following a UTI from 9 studies, a scar developed in 191, those with an abnormal ultrasound, fever >39 °C or an organism other than *E. coli* were at higher risk of kidney damage [122]. A review looking at long term consequences of UTI in children noted that despite numerous publications there are no clear data as to the outcomes [123]. They noted that earlier publications, often retrospective and from selected populations, had a tendency to record frequent adverse outcomes. More recent studies, particularly those that are population based, and with the benefit of prenatal ultrasound to exclude congenital kidney disease, reported a much lower incidence of harmful sequelae. In regard to kidney function they reported that only 0.4% of the 1029 children in prospective studies with normal function at the outset reported a decrease on follow-up. Conversely, virtually all the children with decreased kidney function at the conclusion of studies had scarring or kidney dysplasia at the beginning. There was a low risk of hypertension. In five studies involving 713 children where blood pressure was measured at the beginning and completion of follow-up (which ranged from 5 to 20 years), the incidence of hypertension increased from 2.4% to 4.6% [124–128]. In the studies reporting a high incidence of hypertension, up to 35%, scarring and kidney damage was almost always present on enrolment. In contrast, one study that followed two groups of children after a first UTI for 16–26 years found no significant differences in ambulatory blood pressure monitoring between the 53 individuals with scars when compared with 51 controls without scars [129]. A further paper addressing the obstetric outcome of 72 parous women followed from their first UTI in childhood to a median age of 41 years noted that pregnancy complications were few. Irrespective of the presence or absence of kidney damage, none were diagnosed with hypertension prior to their first pregnancy. Hypertension was diagnosed in 10 of 151 pregnancies, all in women with renal damage of whom 4 experienced preeclampsia [130]. A well conducted population based controlled study evaluated pregnancy-related complications in 260 women who experienced childhood UTIs compared to a control group of 500 mothers without a childhood UTI [131]. There was no difference in essential or gestational hypertension, pre-eclampsia or pyelonephritis during their first pregnancy between the UTI group (40%) and the controls (41%). Thus, the data appears to exclude a major influence of childhood UTIs on subsequent growth and pregnancy related complications.

Summary

Children with normal kidneys at birth and no obstruction to drainage would appear to be the ones at minimal risk of developing chronic kidney insufficiency or other adverse outcomes following an uncomplicated febrile UTI. The infection can be treated with oral antibiotics and the child monitored to ensure recurrent episodes do not occur. Children with significant congenital abnormalities of the kidneys and urinary tract, appear at risk of progressive kidney impairment. Whether dysplastic kidneys are more prone to severe damage as a consequence of pyelonephritis remains to be determined. Further research is underway that will clarify a number of unresolved issues: the need for antibiotic prophylaxis in children with high grade reflux with and without kidney hypodysplasia, the use of new biomarkers to diagnose UTI and to differentiate upper from lower tract infections, the optimal duration of antibiotic treatment during the acute phase, and the appropriate cut-offs for culture results in children. Long term follow-up of children who have been prospectively studied following a first febrile UTI with normal kidneys, as well as those with prenatally diagnosed hypodysplasia, will be important to determine the late risks such as hypertension, pre-eclampsia, and chronic kidney insufficiency.

References

1. Hellstrom A, et al. Association between urinary symptoms at 7 years old and previous urinary tract infection. Arch Dis Child. 1991;66(2):232–4.
2. Bailey RR. The relationship of vesico-ureteric reflux to urinary tract infection and chronic pyelonephritis-reflux nephropathy. Clin Nephrol. 1973;1(3):132–41.
3. Boccon-Gibod L, Galian P, Boccon-Gibod L. [Renal atrophy due to reflux. Myth or realities. 12 cases]. Nouv Press Med. 1972;1(8):507–10.
4. Prospective trial of operative versus non-operative treatment of severe vesicoureteric reflux: two years' observation in 96 children. Br Med J (Clin Res Ed). 1983;287(6386):171–4.
5. Medical versus surgical treatment of primary vesicoureteral reflux: report of the International Reflux Study Committee. Pediatrics. 1981;67(3):392–400.
6. Montini G, Tullus K, Hewitt I. Febrile urinary tract infections in children. N Engl J Med. 2011;365(3):239–50.
7. Kass EH. Bacteriuria and pyelonephritis of pregnancy. Arch Intern Med. 1960;105:194–8.
8. Swerkersson S, et al. Urinary tract infection in infants: the significance of low bacterial count. Pediatr Nephrol. 2016;31(2):239–45.
9. Tullus K. Low urinary bacterial counts: do they count? Pediatr Nephrol. 2016;31(2):171–4.
10. Hay AD, et al. The Diagnosis of Urinary Tract infection in Young children (DUTY): a diagnostic prospective observational study to derive and validate a clinical algorithm for the diagnosis of urinary tract infection in children presenting to primary care with an acute illness. Health Technol Assess. 2016;20(51):1–294.
11. Subcommittee on Urinary Tract Infection, S.C.o.Q.I., Management, Roberts KB. Urinary tract infection: clinical practice guideline for the diagnosis and management of the initial UTI in febrile infants and children 2 to 24 months. Pediatrics. 2011;128(3):595–610.
12. Ammenti A, et al. Updated Italian recommendations for the diagnosis, treatment and follow-up of the first febrile urinary tract infection in young children. Acta Paediatr. 2020;109(2):236–47.
13. Herreros Fernandez ML, et al. A new technique for fast and safe collection of urine in newborns. Arch Dis Child. 2013;98(1):27–9.

14. Al-Orifi F, et al. Urine culture from bag specimens in young children: are the risks too high? J Pediatr. 2000;137(2):221–6.

15. Kennedy KM, Glynn LG, Dineen B. A survey of the management of urinary tract infection in children in primary care and comparison with the NICE guidelines. BMC Fam Pract. 2010;11:6.

16. Leroy S, et al. Association of procalcitonin with acute pyelonephritis and renal scars in pediatric UTI. Pediatrics. 2013;131(5):870–9.

17. Shaikh N, et al. Host and bacterial markers that differ in children with cystitis and pyelonephritis. J Pediatr. 2019;209:146–153.e1.

18. Preda I, et al. Normal dimercaptosuccinic acid scintigraphy makes voiding cystourethrography unnecessary after urinary tract infection. J Pediatr. 2007;151(6):581–4, 584.e1.

19. Hansson S, et al. Dimercapto-succinic acid scintigraphy instead of voiding cystourethrography for infants with urinary tract infection. J Urol. 2004;172(3):1071–3; discussion 1073–4.

20. Cox CE, Hinman F Jr. Experiments with induced bacteriuria, vesical emptying and bacterial growth on the mechanism of bladder defense to infection. J Urol. 1961;86:739–48.

21. van Gool JD, et al. Historical clues to the complex of dysfunctional voiding, urinary tract infection and vesicoureteral reflux. The International Reflux Study in Children. J Urol. 1992;148(5 Pt 2): 1699–702.

22. Sillen U, et al. The Swedish reflux trial in children: V. Bladder dysfunction. J Urol. 2010;184(1):298–304.

23. Ramamurthy HR, Kanitkar M. Recurrent urinary tract infection and functional voiding disorders. Indian Pediatr. 2008;45(8):689–91.

24. Sideras P, Smith CI. Molecular and cellular aspects of X-linked agammaglobulinemia. Adv Immunol. 1995;59:135–223.

25. Forbes GS, et al. Genitourinary involvement in chronic granulomatous disease of childhood. AJR Am J Roentgenol. 1976;127(4):683–6.

26. The International Nijmegen Breakage Syndrome Study Group. Nijmegen breakage syndrome. Arch Dis Child. 2000;82(5):400–6.

27. Becknell B, et al. Amplifying renal immunity: the role of antimicrobial peptides in pyelonephritis. Nat Rev Nephrol. 2015;11(11):642–55.

28. Trudu M, et al. Common noncoding UMOD gene variants induce salt-sensitive hypertension and kidney damage by increasing uromodulin expression. Nat Med. 2013;19(12):1655–60.

29. Ghirotto S, et al. The uromodulin gene locus shows evidence of pathogen adaptation through human evolution. J Am Soc Nephrol. 2016;27(10): 2983–96.

30. Weiss GL, et al. Architecture and function of human uromodulin filaments in urinary tract infections. Science. 2020;369(6506):1005–10.

31. Javor J, et al. Genetic variations of interleukin-8, CXCR1 and CXCR2 genes and risk of acute pyelonephritis in children. Int J Immunogenet. 2012;39(4):338–45.

32. Sheu JN, et al. The role of serum and urine interleukin-8 on acute pyelonephritis and subsequent renal scarring in children. Pediatr Infect Dis J. 2009;28(10):885–90.

33. Hussein A, et al. Impact of cytokine genetic polymorphisms on the risk of renal parenchymal infection in children. J Pediatr Urol. 2017;13(6):593. e1–593.e10.

34. Zaffanello M, et al. Genetic susceptibility to renal scar formation after urinary tract infection: a systematic review and meta-analysis of candidate gene polymorphisms. Pediatr Nephrol. 2011;26(7): 1017–29.

35. Tramma D, et al. Interleukin-6 and interleukin-8 levels in the urine of children with renal scarring. Pediatr Nephrol. 2012;27(9):1525–30.

36. Hussein A, et al. Functional polymorphisms in transforming growth factor-beta-1 (TGFbeta-1) and vascular endothelial growth factor (VEGF) genes modify risk of renal parenchymal scarring following childhood urinary tract infection. Nephrol Dial Transplant. 2010;25(3):779–85.

37. Faust WC, Diaz M, Pohl HG. Incidence of post-pyelonephritic renal scarring: a meta-analysis of the dimercapto-succinic acid literature. J Urol. 2009;181(1):290–7; discussion 297–8.

38. Huang YY, et al. Adjunctive oral methylprednisolone in pediatric acute pyelonephritis alleviates renal scarring. Pediatrics. 2011;128(3):e496–504.

39. Ghaffari J, et al. Assessment the effect of dexamethasone on urinary cytokines and renal scar in children with acute pyelonephritis. Iran J Kidney Dis. 2019;13(4):244–50.

40. Shaikh N, et al. Corticosteroids to prevent kidney scarring in children with a febrile urinary tract infection: a randomized trial. Pediatr Nephrol. 2020;35(11):2113–20.

41. Jackson AR, et al. Roles for urothelium in normal and aberrant urinary tract development. Nat Rev Urol. 2020;17(8):459–68.

42. Zhang GQ, Chen JL, Zhao Y. The effect of vitamin A on renal damage following acute pyelonephritis in children: a meta-analysis of randomized controlled trials. Pediatr Nephrol. 2016;31(3):373–9.

43. Kahbazi M, et al. Vitamin A supplementation is effective for improving the clinical symptoms of urinary tract infections and reducing renal scarring in girls with acute pyelonephritis: a randomized, double-blind placebo-controlled, clinical trial study. Complement Ther Med. 2019;42:429–37.

44. Tugtepe H, et al. Oxidative renal damage in pyelonephritic rats is ameliorated by montelukast, a selective leukotriene CysLT1 receptor antagonist. Eur J Pharmacol. 2007;557(1):69–75.

45. Gurocak S, et al. Renal tissue damage after experimental pyelonephritis: role of antioxidants and selective cyclooxygenase-2 inhibitors. Urology. 2010;76(2):508.e1–5.

46. Imamoglu M, et al. Effects of melatonin on suppression of renal scarring in experimental model of pyelonephritis. Urology. 2006;67(6):1315–9.

47. Khalil A, et al. Angiotensin II type 1 receptor antagonist (losartan) down-regulates transforming growth factor-beta in experimental acute pyelonephritis. J Urol. 2000;164(1):186–91.

48. Tullus K, et al. Relative importance of eight virulence characteristics of pyelonephritogenic Escherichia coli strains assessed by multivariate statistical analysis. J Urol. 1991;146(4):1153–5.

49. Mulvey MA. Adhesion and entry of uropathogenic Escherichia coli. Cell Microbiol. 2002;4(5):257–71.

50. Mysorekar IU, Hultgren SJ. Mechanisms of uropathogenic Escherichia coli persistence and eradication from the urinary tract. Proc Natl Acad Sci U S A. 2006;103(38):14170–5.

51. Hussain A, et al. Multiresistant uropathogenic Escherichia coli from a region in India where urinary tract infections are endemic: genotypic and phenotypic characteristics of sequence type 131 isolates of the CTX-M-15 extended-spectrum-beta-lactamase-producing lineage. Antimicrob Agents Chemother. 2012;56(12):6358–65.

52. Cegelski L, et al. The biology and future prospects of antivirulence therapies. Nat Rev Microbiol. 2008;6(1):17–27.

53. Ribic R, et al. Proposed dual antagonist approach for the prevention and treatment of urinary tract infections caused by uropathogenic Escherichia coli. Med Hypotheses. 2019;124:17–20.

54. Dadi BR, et al. Distribution of virulence genes and phylogenetics of uropathogenic Escherichia coli among urinary tract infection patients in Addis Ababa, Ethiopia. BMC Infect Dis. 2020;20(1):108.

55. Darouiche RO, Hull RA. Bacterial interference for prevention of urinary tract infection. Clin Infect Dis. 2012;55(10):1400–7.

56. Montini G, et al. Antibiotic treatment for pyelonephritis in children: multicentre randomised controlled non-inferiority trial. BMJ. 2007;335(7616):386.

57. Neuhaus TJ, et al. Randomised trial of oral versus sequential intravenous/oral cephalosporins in children with pyelonephritis. Eur J Pediatr. 2008;167(9):1037–47.

58. Prelog M, et al. Febrile urinary tract infection in children: ampicillin and trimethoprim insufficient as empirical mono-therapy. Pediatr Nephrol. 2008;23(4):597–602.

59. Alberici I, et al. First urinary tract infections in children: the role of the risk factors proposed by the Italian recommendations. Acta Paediatr. 2019;108(3):544–50.

60. Robinson JL, et al. Characteristics and outcome of infants with candiduria in neonatal intensive care - a Paediatric Investigators Collaborative Network on Infections in Canada (PICNIC) study. BMC Infect Dis. 2009;9:183.

61. Nourse PJ, Cotton MF, Bates WD. Renal manifestations in children co-infected with HIV and disseminated tuberculosis. Pediatr Nephrol. 2010;25(9):1759–63.

62. Chebotareva AA, et al. [Extrapulmonary tuberculosis in risk-group children: detection methods and clinical characteristics]. Probl Tuberk Bolezn Legk. 2008;(4):11–7.

63. Arora N, Saha A, Kaur M. Tuberculous pyelonephritis in children: three case reports. Paediatr Int Child Health. 2017;37(4):292–7.

64. MacConnachie A. Schistosomiasis. J R Coll Physicians Edinb. 2012;42(1):47–9; quiz 50.

65. Morgan OW, et al. Schistosomiasis among recreational users of Upper Nile River, Uganda, 2007. Emerg Infect Dis. 2010;16(5):866–8.

66. Thomson J, McDonald S. On acute pyelitis due to bacillus coli as it occurs in infancy. QJM. 2010;3:251–68.

67. Fitzgerald A, et al. Antibiotics for treating lower urinary tract infection in children. Cochrane Database Syst Rev. 2012;8:CD006857.

68. Francois P, et al. [Comparative study of cefixime versus amoxicillin-clavulanic acid combination in the oral treatment of urinary tract infections in children]. Arch Pediatr. 1995;2(2):136–42.

69. Benador D, et al. Randomised controlled trial of three day versus 10 day intravenous antibiotics in acute pyelonephritis: effect on renal scarring. Arch Dis Child. 2001;84(3):241–6.

70. Levtchenko E, et al. Treatment of children with acute pyelonephritis: a prospective randomized study. Pediatr Nephrol. 2001;16(11):878–84.

71. Vilaichone A, Watana D, Chaiwatanarat T. Oral ceftibuten switch therapy for acute pyelonephritis in children. J Med Assoc Thail. 2001;84(Suppl 1):S61–7.

72. Noorbakhsh S, et al. Comparison of intravenous aminoglycoside therapy with switch therapy to cefixime in urinary tract infections. Saudi Med J. 2004;25(10):1513–5.

73. Hoberman A, et al. Oral versus initial intravenous therapy for urinary tract infections in young febrile children. Pediatrics. 1999;104(1 Pt 1):79–86.

74. Bocquet N, et al. Randomized trial of oral versus sequential IV/oral antibiotic for acute pyelonephritis in children. Pediatrics. 2012;129(2):e269–75.

75. Ammenti A, et al. Febrile urinary tract infections in young children: recommendations for the diagnosis, treatment and follow-up. Acta Paediatr. 2012;101(5):451–7.

76. Urinary tract infection in children: diagnosis, treatment and long-term management. National Institute for Health and Clinical Excellence: Guidance. London. 2007. Available from: http://www.nice.org.uk/cg54.

77. Delbet JD, Lorrot M, Ulinski T. An update on new antibiotic prophylaxis and treatment for urinary tract infections in children. Expert Opin Pharmacother. 2017;18(15):1619–25.

78. Hogan J, et al. Renal outcome in children with antenatal diagnosis of severe CAKUT. Pediatr Nephrol. 2012;27(3):497–502.

79. Hoberman A, et al. Imaging studies after a first febrile urinary tract infection in young children. N Engl J Med. 2003;348(3):195–202.

80. Zamir G, et al. Urinary tract infection: is there a need for routine renal ultrasonography? Arch Dis Child. 2004;89(5):466–8.

81. Montini G, et al. Value of imaging studies after a first febrile urinary tract infection in young children: data from Italian renal infection study 1. Pediatrics. 2009;123(2):e239–46.

82. McTaggart S, et al. KHA-CARI guideline: diagnosis and treatment of urinary tract infection in children. Nephrology (Carlton). 2015;20(2):55–60.

83. Wan J, et al. Section on Urology response to new guidelines for the diagnosis and management of UTI. Pediatrics. 2012;129(4):e1051–3.

84. Rensing A, Austin P. The diagnosis and treatment of vesicoureteral reflux: an update. Open J Urol Nephrol. 2015;8(suppl 3:M3):96–103.

85. Wennerstrom M, et al. Primary and acquired renal scarring in boys and girls with urinary tract infection. J Pediatr. 2000;136(1):30–4.

86. Broyer M, et al. The paediatric registry of the European Dialysis and Transplant Association: 20 years' experience. Pediatr Nephrol. 1993;7(6):758–68.

87. Brandstrom P, et al. The Swedish reflux trial in children: IV. Renal damage. J Urol. 2010;184(1):292–7.

88. Fouzas S, et al. DMSA scan for revealing vesicoureteral reflux in young children with urinary tract infection. Pediatrics. 2010;126(3):e513–9.

89. Marks SD, Gordon I, Tullus K. Imaging in childhood urinary tract infections: time to reduce investigations. Pediatr Nephrol. 2008;23(1):9–17.

90. Jones RA, Grattan-Smith JD, Little S. Pediatric magnetic resonance urography. J Magn Reson Imaging. 2011;33(3):510–26.

91. Schroeder AR, et al. Impact of a more restrictive approach to urinary tract imaging after febrile urinary tract infection. Arch Pediatr Adolesc Med. 2011;165(11):1027–32.

92. Deader R, et al. Will the implementation of the 2007 National Institute for Health and Clinical Excellence (NICE) guidelines on childhood urinary tract infection (UTI) in the UK miss significant urinary tract pathology? BJU Int. 2012;110(3):454–8.

93. Practice parameter: the diagnosis, treatment, and evaluation of the initial urinary tract infection in febrile infants and young children. American Academy of Pediatrics. Committee on Quality Improvement. Subcommittee on Urinary Tract Infection. Pediatrics. 1999;103(4 Pt 1):843–52.

94. Jerardi KE, et al. Rapid implementation of evidence-based guidelines for imaging after first urinary tract infection. Pediatrics. 2013;132(3):e749–55.

95. La Scola C, et al. Different guidelines for imaging after first UTI in febrile infants: yield, cost, and radiation. Pediatrics. 2013;131(3):e665–71.

96. Royal Children's Hospital. Clinical practice guidelines. Urinary tract infection. Available from: http://www.rch.org.au/clinicalguide/guideline_index/Urinary_Tract_Infection_Guideline/.

97. Garin EH, et al. Clinical significance of primary vesicoureteral reflux and urinary antibiotic prophylaxis after acute pyelonephritis: a multicenter, randomized, controlled study. Pediatrics. 2006;117(3):626–32.

98. Pennesi M, et al. Is antibiotic prophylaxis in children with vesicoureteral reflux effective in preventing pyelonephritis and renal scars? A randomized, controlled trial. Pediatrics. 2008;121(6):e1489–94.

99. Roussey-Kesler G, et al. Antibiotic prophylaxis for the prevention of recurrent urinary tract infection in children with low grade vesicoureteral reflux: results from a prospective randomized study. J Urol. 2008;179(2):674–9; discussion 679.

100. Montini G, et al. Prophylaxis after first febrile urinary tract infection in children? A multicenter, randomized, controlled, noninferiority trial. Pediatrics. 2008;122(5):1064–71.

101. Craig JC, et al. Antibiotic prophylaxis and recurrent urinary tract infection in children. N Engl J Med. 2009;361(18):1748–59.

102. Brandstrom P, et al. The Swedish reflux trial in children: III. Urinary tract infection pattern. J Urol. 2010;184(1):286–91.

103. RIVUR Trial Investigators, et al. Antimicrobial prophylaxis for children with vesicoureteral reflux. N Engl J Med. 2014;370(25):2367–76.

104. Hari P, et al. Antibiotic prophylaxis in the management of vesicoureteric reflux: a randomized double-blind placebo-controlled trial. Pediatr Nephrol. 2015;30(3):479–86.

105. Williams G, Craig JC. Long-term antibiotics for preventing recurrent urinary tract infection in children. Cochrane Database Syst Rev. 2019;4:CD001534.

106. Hewitt IK, et al. Antibiotic prophylaxis for urinary tract infection-related renal scarring: a systematic review. Pediatrics. 2017;139(5):e20163145.

107. Clarke SA, Samuel M, Boddy SA. Are prophylactic antibiotics necessary with clean intermittent catheterization? A randomized controlled trial. J Pediatr Surg. 2005;40(3):568–71.

108. Morton SC, et al. Antimicrobial prophylaxis for urinary tract infection in persons with spinal cord dysfunction. Arch Phys Med Rehabil. 2002;83(1):129–38.

109. Schlager TA, et al. Escherichia coli colonizing the neurogenic bladder are similar to widespread clones causing disease in patients with normal bladder function. Spinal Cord. 2008;46(9):633–8.

110. Gonzalez Celedon C, Bitsori M, Tullus K. Progression of chronic renal failure in children with dysplastic kidneys. Pediatr Nephrol. 2007;22(7):1014–20.

111. American Urological Association. Clinical guidelines. Vesicoureteral reflux. Available from: http://www.auanet.org/education/guidelines/vesicoureteral-reflux-a.cfm.

112. Nordenstrom J, et al. The Swedish infant high-grade reflux trial: UTI and renal damage. J Pediatr Urol. 2017;13(2):146–54.

113. Jagannath VA, et al. Routine neonatal circumcision for the prevention of urinary tract infections in infancy. Cochrane Database Syst Rev. 2012;11:CD009129.

114. Singh-Grewal D, Macdessi J, Craig J. Circumcision for the prevention of urinary tract infection in boys: a systematic review of randomised trials and observational studies. Arch Dis Child. 2005;90(8):853–8.

115. Morris BJ, Wiswell TE. Circumcision and lifetime risk of urinary tract infection: a systematic review and meta-analysis. J Urol. 2013;189(6):2118–24.

116. Jepson RG, Williams G, Craig JC. Cranberries for preventing urinary tract infections. Cochrane Database Syst Rev. 2012;10:CD001321.

117. Stapleton AE, et al. Randomized, placebo-controlled phase 2 trial of a Lactobacillus crispatus probiotic given intravaginally for prevention of recurrent urinary tract infection. Clin Infect Dis. 2011;52(10):1212–7.

118. Lee SJ, Cha J, Lee JW. Probiotics prophylaxis in pyelonephritis infants with normal urinary tracts. World J Pediatr. 2016;12(4):425–9.

119. Schwenger EM, Tejani AM, Loewen PS. Probiotics for preventing urinary tract infections in adults and children. Cochrane Database Syst Rev. 2015;12:CD008772.

120. Shaikh N, et al. Risk of renal scarring in children with a first urinary tract infection: a systematic review. Pediatrics. 2010;126(6):1084–91.

121. Hewitt IK, et al. Early treatment of acute pyelonephritis in children fails to reduce renal scarring: data from the Italian Renal Infection Study Trials. Pediatrics. 2008;122(3):486–90.

122. Shaikh N, et al. Identification of children and adolescents at risk for renal scarring after a first urinary tract infection: a meta-analysis with individual patient data. JAMA Pediatr. 2014;168(10):893–900.

123. Toffolo A, Ammenti A, Montini G. Long-term clinical consequences of urinary tract infections during childhood: a review. Acta Paediatr. 2012;101(10):1018–31.

124. Jansen H, Scholtmeijer RJ. Results of surgical treatment of severe vesicoureteric reflux. Retrospective study of reflux grades 4 and 5. Br J Urol. 1990;65(4):413–7.

125. Weiss R, Duckett J, Spitzer A. Results of a randomized clinical trial of medical versus surgical management of infants and children with grades III and IV primary vesicoureteral reflux (United States). The International Reflux Study in Children. J Urol. 1992;148(5 Pt 2):1667–73.

126. Smellie JM, et al. Childhood reflux and urinary infection: a follow-up of 10–41 years in 226 adults. Pediatr Nephrol. 1998;12(9):727–36.

127. Smellie JM, et al. Medical versus surgical treatment in children with severe bilateral vesicoureteric reflux and bilateral nephropathy: a randomised trial. Lancet. 2001;357(9265):1329–33.

128. Jodal U, et al. Ten-year results of randomized treatment of children with severe vesicoureteral reflux. Final report of the International Reflux Study in Children. Pediatr Nephrol. 2006;21(6):785–92.

129. Wennerstrom M, et al. Renal function 16 to 26 years after the first urinary tract infection in childhood. Arch Pediatr Adolesc Med. 2000;154(4):339–45.

130. Geback C, et al. Obstetrical outcome in women with urinary tract infections in childhood. Acta Obstet Gynecol Scand. 2016;95(4):452–7.

131. Honkila M, et al., Childhood urinary tract infections and pregnancy-related complications in adult women. Pediatrics, 2020. 146(2):e20200610.

Vesicoureteral Reflux

44

Ranjiv Mathews, Tiffany L. Damm,
and Sverker Hansson

Introduction

Vesicoureteral reflux (VUR) is the retrograde flow of urine from the bladder to the kidneys. VUR may be classified as primary, which is a congenital defect in the vesicoureteral junction anatomy, or secondary, which is the result of persistent high intravesical pressures that overwhelm the vesicoureteral junction. VUR has been implicated in renal injury prior to birth as well as postnatal development of urinary tract infections (UTIs) and further renal damage. Primary VUR is most commonly identified in infants and children, and historically has been most prevalent in infants 0–24 months of age. Although much is known about the diagnosis, medical, and surgical management of VUR, many questions remain regarding the potential of VUR to cause infections and renal injury.

R. Mathews (✉) · T. L. Damm
Division of Urology, Department of Surgery,
Southern Illinois University School of Medicine,
Springfield, IL, USA
e-mail: rmathews94@siumed.edu;
tdamm84@siumed.edu

S. Hansson
Pediatric Uronephrologic Center, The Queen Silvia
Children's Hospital, Sahlgrenska Academy,
Gothenburg University, Gothenburg, Sweden
e-mail: sverker.hansson@gu.se

Embryology

Anatomic Factors

Ureteral development has been studied to understand the anatomic factors that may lead to primary VUR. The development of periureteral sheaths, intravesical ureteral muscles and trigonal muscles have been studied for potential contribution in VUR [1]. Based on observations in 11–27 week fetuses, it has been determined that the superficial trigone is derived from the intravesical ureteral muscles and the deep trigone is derived from the deep periureteral sheath of the ureter. Fixation of the ureters in the appropriate location is important for the development of a normal trigone and non-refluxing ureters. The intravesical submucosal length of the ureter and the oblique path of entry of the ureter into the bladder have been identified as critical factors in the prevention of VUR (Fig. 44.1).

Development of renal scarring in children appears to be independent of the presence or absence of VUR. Anatomic factors in the ureterovesical junction, however, may play a role in the degree of renal injury produced by VUR in that higher grade VUR that occurs with lower bladder pressure is associated with increased risk of nephropathy [2].

Other anatomic anomalies outside the ureterovesical junction anti-reflux mechanism, such as periureteral diverticula or duplications of the

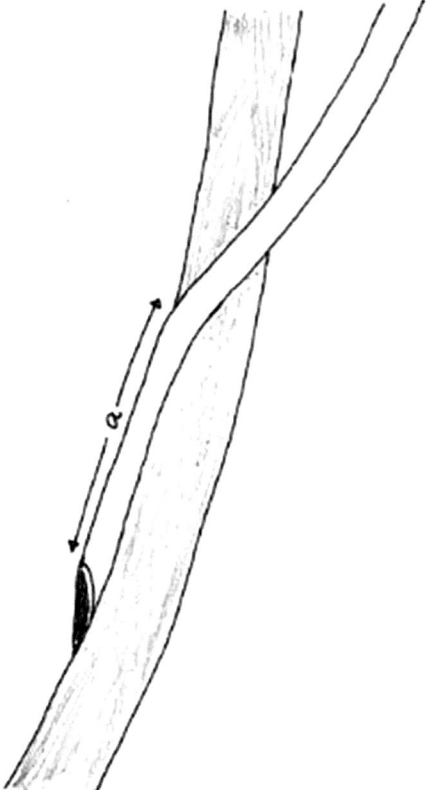

Fig. 44.1 Ureterovesical junction anatomy contributes to the anti-reflux mechanism of the compression valve, which includes the length of the tunneled ureter, angle of the ureteral insertion, and fixation of inlet and outlet points

collecting system, can contribute to persistence of VUR, increasing the risk of renal damage and the requirement for surgical correction.

Extra-anatomic Factors

Embryological development of the ureteral bud from the mesonephric duct is dependent on multiple factors. Signaling by glial cell line derived neurotrophic factor (GDNF)has been shown in the mouse model to induce the formation of ureteral buds [3]. Misexpression of GDNF has been shown to be associated with the development of multiple ureteral buds. Additionally, GDNF is focally expressed in the appropriate location of ureteral bud development. If GDNF is expressed

in an ectopic location, the ureteral bud will develop in this ectopic location, leading to lateral or medial localization of the ureter in the bladder predisposing to VUR or obstruction. Additionally, trigonal development is dependent on apoptosis induced by a vitamin A signaling pathway [4]. Normal development of the trigone is also necessary to provide appropriate support to the distal ureter. Studies have shown that symmetric muscle contractions and unidirectional peristalsis also play a significant role in the competence of the ureterovesical junction [5].

Associated Conditions

Many anatomic and genetic conditions are associated with the presence of VUR in children. The most commonly noted anatomic conditions are multicystic dysplastic kidney (MCDK), renal agenesis and renal or ureteral ectopia and duplication. VUR is also a common occurrence with many syndromic conditions.

Multicystic Dysplastic Kidney (MCDK)

Contralateral VUR is the most common abnormality present in children with MCDK [6]. VUR has been noted in 12–28% of contralateral kidneys in children with MCDK [7]. The impact of this contralateral VUR continues to be debated. One study has indicated that contralateral renal growth is compromised in the presence of VUR [8]; however, other studies have revealed that VUR into the contralateral renal unit is usually low grade and does not lead to renal compromise [9]. Study of the natural history of VUR in the presence of MCDK indicates that in most boys and 40% of girls there will be eventual spontaneous resolution.

Renal Agenesis

As with MCDK, VUR is the most common abnormality noted in the contralateral kidney in children with unilateral renal agenesis.

Management of VUR in the context of a solitary kidney is not different from that in patients with two kidneys [10].

Ectopia and Duplication

Dilating VUR occurs in up to 26% of children with renal ectopia and hydronephrosis [11]. VUR is the most commonly associated anomaly noted in children with renal ectopia. The presence of renal ectopia does not seem to reduce the potential for VUR to resolve spontaneously [12].

Ureteral duplication is also associated with the presence of VUR, typically into the lower pole of the duplex system. The ureteral orifice is displaced proximally and laterally in children with duplex systems and plays a role in the development of VUR into the lower pole moiety. Following endoscopic management of ureteroceles associated with duplex systems, VUR into the lower poles unilaterally or bilaterally may be unmasked, and may even occur into the upper pole as an iatrogenic entity. Many patients with duplex systems will eventually require surgical management for their VUR [13]. Typically, surgery in these patients is indicated for the associated conditions that are present (i.e. ureteroceles, ectopic ureters, etc.).

Ureteral ectopia may also be noted into the bladder neck and urethra, leading to VUR during voiding. Bilateral or single system ureteral ectopia is associated with reduction in bladder growth and capacity and requires surgical management with ureteral reimplantation and possible later bladder neck reconstruction to provide continence [14]. Prognosis in this condition is based on development of adequate bladder capacity.

Syndromes

Syndromes that have been associated with the presence of VUR include the VATER-VACTERL syndrome, Townes-Brock syndrome (*SALL1* mutation), cat-eye Syndrome (tetrasomy, chromosome 22), Casamassima-Morton-Nance syndrome, renal coloboma syndrome (*PAX2*

mutation), branchio-oto-renal syndrome (*EYE1* mutation) and Frasier syndrome (*WT1* mutation).

Incidence

Although it is difficult to quantify a disease process that has the ability to be transient, several studies have sought to estimate the prevalence of VUR among children. In a meta-analysis, the incidence of VUR was classified based on initial presentation. The prevalence of VUR in children undergoing cystography for UTI was 30%, as compared to 17% in children who underwent radiographic imaging for other reasons such as hydronephrosis [15].

Guidelines from the American Academy of Pediatrics (AAP) and the National Institute for Health and Care Excellence (NICE) appear to have had an impact on the evaluation of children with UTI. A reduction in the utilization of voiding cystourethrogram (VCU) has led to decreases in the rates of VUR identified. This was reflected in a study that demonstrated a decline in the incidence of VUR in children 0–2 years of age from 38/100,000, to 25/100,000, following publication of the 2011 AAP guidelines. Additionally, reduction in the performance of VCUs was also noted in children 3–10 years of age [16], suggesting a reluctance to screen older children as well.

Age

VUR is more commonly identified in younger children. In a retrospective review of 15,504 children, the incidence of VUR was 35.3% in children less than 2 years of age, 22.7% in those 2–6 years of age, 15.3% in those 7–11 years of age, and 7.9% in those 12–21 years of age [17].

Gender and Race

There is a gender disparity between the patients diagnosed following identification of hydronephrosis on antenatal ultrasonography and those diagnosed following initial UTI. The majority of infants with VUR following identification of antenatal hydronephrosis are male [18]. It has also been noted that the incidence of dysplasia is greater in male infants with VUR. Girls form a majority of patients presenting with VUR identified following UTIs, except for the first 6 months of life, when UTI is more common in boys [19].

African-American girls have a lower potential for development of VUR as compared to Caucasian girls. This difference in incidence was also noted in infants diagnosed with VUR following identification of antenatal hydronephrosis [20]. Additionally, few African American girls presenting with VUR following a UTI have high grade VUR [17]. The incidence of scarring, however, is higher in African-American girls than Caucasian girls, although progression of scarring is less in African American girls. Additionally, time to spontaneous resolution of VUR is shorter in African American girls [21]. The incidence of VUR in Hispanic girls is comparable to Caucasian girls [22].

Presentation

VUR is identified in four groups of children—those identified during evaluation of antenatally identified hydronephrosis, those with other congenital anomalies, those following a febrile or symptomatic UTI and those evaluated due to VUR in a child or parent.

Antenatal Diagnosis

The widespread utilization of antenatal ultrasonography has made early detection of hydronephrosis and subsequent diagnosis of VUR possible prior to the occurrence of UTIs. Fetal pelvic diameter of 7 mm during the third trimester or 10 mm at postnatal examination is considered an indication for further investigation, including possible evaluation for VUR. About 10% of such patients evaluated for hydronephrosis on antenatal ultrasonography are diagnosed with VUR [23]. Cohorts of infants with VUR

diagnosed following antenatal identification of hydronephrosis have greater numbers of boys [24]. Additionally, compared to children with VUR following a UTI, there are more patients that have low grade VUR, with greater propensity for spontaneous resolution. Boys with even high grades of VUR (IV–V) have a 29–37% rate of spontaneous resolution in the first year of life [25]. This potential for VUR resolution is attributed to the resolution of a mixed pattern of voiding, with coordinated voiding interspersed with high pressure voiding due to increased sphincteric activity.

Urinary Tract Infections

Most children are diagnosed with VUR following an initial febrile UTI. Since UTIs are most prevalent during the first 2 years of life, the majority of VUR diagnosis is made in infants and young children. In a cohort of 1953 patients with UTI <2 years of age undergoing VCU, VUR was noted in 30% [26]. This incidence was similar to that noted by Hoberman et al. [27]. In more recent studies, the overall incidence of VUR has been 15–20% [28].

Siblings with VUR

There remains debate on the benefit of routine screening of siblings of index patients with VUR. In one study, 88% of siblings had VUR. However, index patients had high grade VUR, and siblings screened were less than 3 years old, and were generally symptomatic with UTI [29]. Therefore, restricting evaluation for VUR to siblings that present with an infection may have a better yield in identifying children with VUR that may benefit from intervention.

Genetics of Reflux

There is increasing evidence for a genetic basis for primary VUR. The reported incidence of VUR in siblings of an affected patient varies from 27% to 45% [30]. A higher incidence of VUR has also been reported in children of parents with a history of VUR [31]. VUR is most certainly genetically heterogenous. Autosomal dominant inheritance with variable expression or multifactorial inheritance has been implicated for VUR and reflux nephropathy (RN). In a study of 88 families with at least one individual with primary VUR, the authors concluded that a single major locus was the most important causal factor [32]. Kaefer and colleagues found 100% concordance in monozygotic twins and 50% concordance among dizygotic twins [33]. One gene associated with apparent autosomal dominant VUR has been mapped to chromosome 1 [34], though two of the families studied showed negative linkage to this locus, further confirming the genetic heterogeneity of VUR.

Association of Urinary Tract Infections

VUR is believed to be the primary risk factor for pyelonephritis, although some studies dispute this association [35]. The International Reflux Study in Children (IRSC) reported recurrent UTI in 28% of children with medically managed severe VUR [36]. The risk of UTI recurrence is related to the degree of VUR: 6–8% for VUR grade I and II; 27% for grade III; and 43% for grade IV [37]. The usual organisms that cause UTI originate from fecal flora that colonize the perineum, and the organisms that cause recurrent UTI can be found on perineal cultures prior to the onset of UTI [38]. Escherichia coli (E. coli) is the most frequent organism, being responsible for approximately 80% of UTIs, the rest being due to Klebsiella, Enterobacter, Citrobacter, Proteus, Providencia, Morganella, Serratia and Salmonella species [39]. In prospective study of infants with a first UTI, the incidence of non-E. coli bacteria were associated with an increased VUR severity (12% with VUR I–II, 30% with VUR III–V) [28]. A variety of bacterial virulence factors increase the ability of E. coli to cause a UTI. The presence of P fimbriae allows E. coli to adhere to the epithelial cells of the urinary tract, while other virulence factors increase tissue damage and protect E. coli from serum bactericidal activity [35].

Diagnosis

There remains significant debate regarding which children should be evaluated for VUR, both those identified following antenatally identified hydronephrosis, and those that had a UTI. This is partially due to concerns about the efficacy of antibiotics in the prevention of UTI. Multiple radiographic modalities have been successfully utilized for the diagnosis of VUR.

Renal Bladder Ultrasound

The AAP guidelines recommend ultrasonography as the first imaging modality for evaluation of children ages 2–24 months presenting with UTI. Ultrasound is the initial modality for evaluation of *any* child that is being evaluated for possible VUR. This permits evaluation of the upper tracts to determine the presence of anomalies (e.g., duplication, hydronephrosis, MCDK, agenesis). Ultrasound should always include evaluation of the ureters and bladder before and after voiding to determine if there are lower tract changes that might suggest the possibility of VUR (i.e. diverticula, ureteral dilation) or other lower tract anomalies (ureteroceles, megaureter) that may predispose to UTI. Although the presence of abnormalities on ultrasound may increase the likelihood of VUR, there are no specific findings that have a definite correlation [40].

Voiding Cystourethrogram

The gold standard for the diagnosis of VUR is the radiographic voiding cystourethrogram (VCU). VCU requires urethral catheterization and fluoroscopy. This modality allows grading of VUR as standardized by the IRSC. The AAP and NICE UTI Guidelines have suggested limiting further evaluation of children presenting with a first UTI. This has led to a significant decrease in the utilization of VCU since the publication of the guidelines. Although VCU is the best procedure for the identification of VUR, discrepancy can be noted in the grading of VUR even among experienced readers and when multiple filling cycles are utilized [41]. The timing for the performance of VCU has been debated. It was felt that early VCU may lead to increase in the diagnosis of VUR due to the "instability" of the VUR in the child with a recent UTI. Recent studies have demonstrated that performing the VCU within a week of presenting with a UTI leads to improved compliance with performing the study and does not change the potential for the identification of VUR [42].

The discomfort of catheterization is a contributor to the reluctance to perform VCUs. The use of sedation improves the tolerance for the procedure without changing the potential for the diagnosis of VUR [43]. Intermittent fluoroscopic evaluation reduces the exposure of radiation during the procedure, further improving the safety of the study [44]. The use of one or a few doses of antibiotics may help to prevent UTI due to catheterisation.

VCU is also used for the follow-up of VUR to determine its persistence or improvement. There is a trend to reduce the frequency of performance of VCU during follow-up of children with VUR. Additionally, VCU has been typically omitted following surgical correction of VUR, due to the high success rates achieved with most techniques.

In an effort to reduce the radiation associated with the use of standard (conventional) VCU, radionuclide cystogram (RNC) has been performed. This study uses technetium-99m (Tc-99m) sodium pertechnetate. It requires catheterization, but utilizes less radiation than a standard VCU. RNC has excellent correlation to conventional VCU [45]. The major limitation of this procedure is the inability to grade VUR as recommended by the IRSC. Using RNC, grading is limited to mild, moderate and severe. It is an excellent modality for the follow-up of VUR and for the determination of resolution of VUR. It is also used as the modality of choice for the identification of surgical success in the correction of VUR.

Dimercaptosuccinic Acid Scan

The major concern with the presence of VUR is the development of infections and subsequent renal scarring [46]. A nuclear scan with Tc-99m dimercaptosuccinic acid (DMSA) is the best modality for identifying renal scarring in the kidneys [47]. The difficulty is to determine if the scars that are identified are the result of prenatal hypodysplasia or secondary to recurrent UTI [48]. Some have suggested using a DMSA scan as the primary test for the evaluation of children presenting with UTI. The absence of renal involvement on DMSA scan performed during the acute phase of a febrile UTI makes higher grades of VUR unlikely [28].

Experimental Diagnosis Modalities

Voiding Ultrasonography

Another alternative to VCU is contrast-enhanced voiding urosonography with intravesical contrast, a method increasingly used in Europe. This method has the advantages of not using ionizing radiation and obtaining simultaneous images of the renal parenchyma. However, the use of this method for the evaluation of the male urethra is controversial [49, 50]. Urosonography has been recommended as a primary diagnostic modality for the diagnosis of VUR to reduce radiation exposure [51]. This modality is not widely available; the reduction in radiation exposure with current fluoroscopic techniques and the requirement for catheterization have limited its utilization.

Magnetic Resonance Imaging

Magnetic resonance imaging (MRI) may be used in the diagnosis of renal scarring, and less frequently is used in the setting of voiding imaging. MR voiding cystography (MR VCU) has the benefits of not requiring catheterization, simultaneously imaging the upper tract, and no radiation exposure. However, in younger children sedation may be required. In a small study, MR VCU was found to be 90% sensitive and 96% specific for detecting VUR [52]. When compared to the gold standard DMSA scan for detecting renal scars, magnetic resonance urography has a much higher interobserver agreement and may provide superior detection of renal scars due to its ability to differentiate swelling from renal scarring [53].

Grading of VUR

Grading of VUR was standardized in 1982 [54] using the radiographic VCU, by the International Reflux Study Committee (IRSC). This system of grading divides VUR into five grades (Fig. 44.2). Grading of VUR correlates with the degree of renal scarring as well as the potential for spontaneous resolution. Lower grades of VUR have greater potential for spontaneous resolution independent of the age at diagnosis [55]. In addition, the grade of VUR is a consideration in the appro-

priate choice of management (endoscopic vs. open surgical reconstruction) [56]. Unfortunately, there is significant interobserver variability when grading VUR by VCU. In an analysis comparing a local radiologist with the interpretations of two blinded reference radiologists, VUR grade was agreed upon unanimously in only 59% of ureters [57]. The ureter may also be dilated without renal calyx dilation, which could lead to inconsistent grading.

Bladder and Bowel Dysfunction

Bladder and bowel dysfunction (BBD) is the combination of lower urinary tract symptoms (urgency, frequency, hesitation, straining, and withholding maneuvers) with bowel symptoms such as painful defecation, encopresis and constipation [58]. At baseline this is a common disorder. In a prospective study of children diagnosed

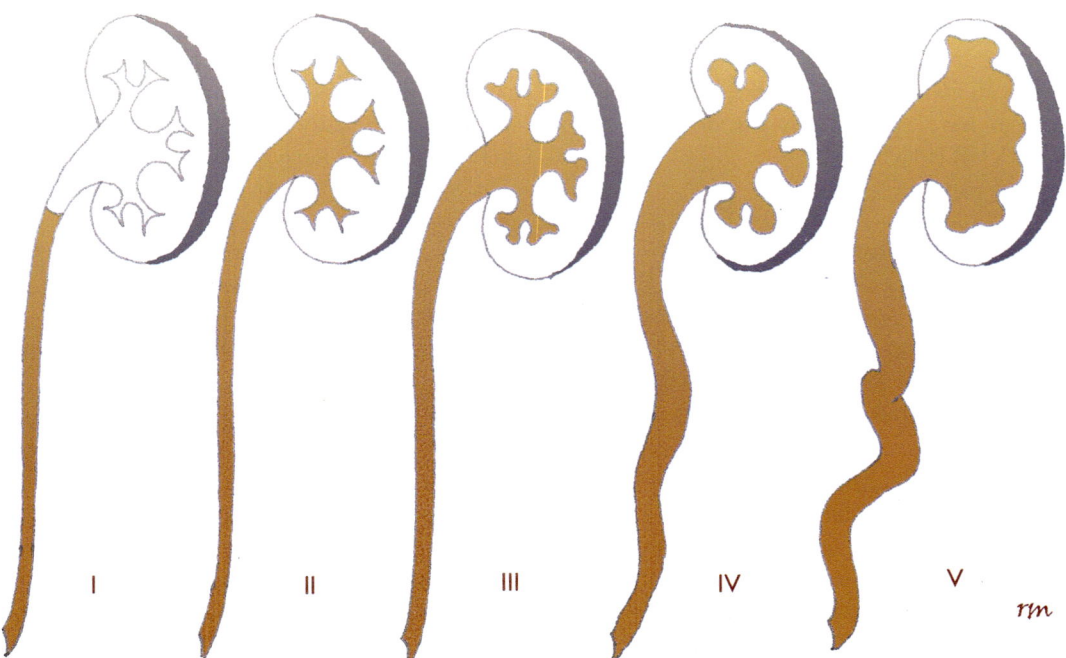

Fig. 44.2 International grading system for vesicoureteral reflux. Grade *I*—contrast in the non-dilated ureter; Grade *II*—contrast in the non-dilated ureter and renal pelvis; Grade *III*—mild dilation of the ureter and renal pelvis with minimal blunting; Grade *IV*—moderate tortuosity of the ureter and dilation of the renal pelvis and calyces; Grade *V*—gross dilation of the renal pelvis and calyces with significant ureteral tortuosity. (Grading based on International Reflux Study. *Pediatrics* 1981; 67:392–400; Figure copyrighted by Dr. Ranjiv Mathews)

with VUR, the presence of BBD significantly increased the rate of recurrent UTIs from 20% to 51% [59].

Potential for Reflux Resolution

The potential for spontaneous resolution of VUR is the basis for its conservative non-operative management. All grades of VUR have the potential for resolution, although the likelihood of resolution is based on the grade and presentation of VUR [60]. Overall 39% of refluxing ureters will have spontaneous resolution [61].

Multiple studies have evaluated the rate of resolution of the various grades of VUR. In one study, resolution of Grade I VUR was 82%, Grade II VUR was 80% and Grade III was 46% [62]. Similar rates of resolution have been noted in other studies evaluating the medical management of VUR [63]. Resolution rates over 5 years of Grade IV and V VUR were 30% and 11%, respectively [60]. In a study from Sweden, a negative correlation was found between bladder dysfunction and spontaneous improvement of VUR grades III and IV [64]. Boys are more likely than girls to have spontaneous resolution of high-grade VUR [61].

Potential for Renal Injury

A variety of factors influence the probability of scarring in children with VUR and UTI. The role of VUR, initially proven in piglets [65], has been shown in multiple clinical studies [66, 67]. Moreover, children with higher grades of VUR have an increased likelihood of developing renal scarring [68, 69]. Renal damage is more common in infants with UTI and VUR because of their unique kidney papillary morphology [70].

Factors affecting the probability of renal scarring in children with VUR and UTI include delay in the treatment of UTI, recurrent UTI and bacterial virulence [71]. Finally, there is evidence that genetic factors predispose patients with VUR to scarring as demonstrated by studies of angiotensin converting enzyme gene polymorphisms [72],

and by studies of the IL-8 receptor CXCR1, which have identified a genetic innate immune deficiency with a strong link to acute pyelonephritis and renal scarring [73, 74].

Reflux Nephropathy

Several studies have shown that scarring develops at the same site as previous infection [75]. The pathogenesis of renal scarring following acute pyelonephritis is not well understood. The process is an inflammatory response, with chemotaxis and phagocytosis, release of lysosomal enzymes and superoxides, production of peroxide and hydroxyl radicals, tubular ischemia and reperfusion injury [76, 77].

Reflux nephropathy (RN) is the primary diagnosis in 5.2% of children undergoing renal transplantation according to a North American registry [78]. High grade VUR confers the greatest risk for kidney damage [79], and males with RN appear to have a poorer outcome than females [79, 80]. It is likely that the most severe renal damage associated with VUR is congenital hypoplasia/dysplasia and not postinfectious scarring. In a study from Sweden, boys were more inclined to have congenital lesions while girls were more likley to have acquired RN associated with prior infections [80]. While previous literature reported that younger children had the highest risk for new kidney scacrring, the Randomized Intervention for Vesicoureteral Reflux (RIVUR) trial and other studies reported that the risk for aquired scarring is higher in older children [79, 81, 82]. A lower threshold for identification of VUR in younger children may potentially have a protective role in preventing renal scarring. Despite succesful surgical management, patients with higher grades of VUR at diagnosis are more likely to progress to chronic kidney disease as compared to those with mild or moderate VUR, reflecting the possible role of prenatal dysplasia [83]. Long-term consequences from acquired renal damage, such as renal insufficency, hypertension and pregnancy complications, are considerably less than previously thought [84–86].

Management of VUR

A close relationship between pyelonephritis and VUR was demonstrated by Hodson and Edwards in 1960 [87]. VUR was believed to be detrimental to the kidneys and surgical procedures to correct VUR were developed during the 1960s [88]. However, the high rate of spontaneous resolution of VUR led to more limited surgical intervention [89]. Long-term antibiotic prophylaxis was implemented to protect children with VUR from renal damage induced by infection [90].

The potential for VUR to resolve spontaneously in many patients has changed the paradigm of management from one of immediate surgical correction to initial medical management with antibiotic prophylaxis [91]. Another alternative is watchful waiting. In current clinical practice, treatment decisions are made individually based on VUR grade, previous febrile UTIs, renal damage, bladder and bowel function, adherence to prophylaxis if given, and the parents' preferences. Surgical treatment is typically reserved for patients without spontaneous resolution and with recurrent infections.

Antibiotic Prophylaxis

The main objective of treatment in children with VUR is the prevention of recurrent UTI and renal parenchymal damage. Antibiotic prophylaxis was introduced in 1975 [91]. Controlled trials demonstrated the effectiveness of daily, low dose trimethoprim-sulfamethoxazole (TMP-SMZ) or nitrofurantoin in preventing UTIs [92]. Breakthrough infections are common in children with VUR, with rates ranging from 25% to 38% [93]. Side effects are not uncommon; these include gastrointestinal disturbances, skin rashes, hepatotoxicity and hematological complications [94].

There is no significant outcome difference between medical and surgical management in the incidence of renal scarring. The IRSC European cohort included 300 children with VUR randomly allocated to medical or surgical management. Follow-up with intravenous urography and DMSA scintigraphy over 5 years revealed no difference in the development of new renal scars or the progression of existing scars [95]. Similar results were reported by the Birmingham Study [96].

Recently, several randomized, controlled studies comparing antibiotic prophylaxis and no treatment were performed [97–101]. The results of these studies were summarized in a meta-analysis published in the latest AAP clinical practice guidelines [102]. These studies were unable to show a beneficial effect of antibiotic prophylaxis. However, most children in these studies had no VUR or low grades of VUR, underlining the fact that for most patients, prophylaxis is unnecessary. For children with higher grades of VUR, especially grades IV–V, there may be a benefit. The RIVUR trial, which randomized children with VUR to placebo or prophylaxis, demonstrated a 50% reduction in the risk of recurrent infections with the use of prophylaxis (TMP-SMZ). Additionally, the RIVUR trial showed that in children presenting with a second UTI, older children and those with grade IV VUR, there was greater potential for development of new renal scarring. Given these risk factors, it would suggest that there is a role for prevention of UTIs as a means to prevent new renal scarring [79]. A reanalysis of the RIVUR study divided patients into low risk and high-risk categories (high risk defined as grade IV VUR, female grade I–III, and uncircumcised males with grade I–III, with concurrent BBD) and showed that antibiotic prophylaxis significantly decreased UTI recurrence in the high risk patients. Thus, the treatment of high-risk patients confers greater benefit [103]. The necessity to analyze boys and girls separately was illustrated in the Swedish Reflux Trial, where a beneficial effect of prophylaxis was seen in girls with grades III–IV VUR, but not in boys [101].

Treatment of Bladder and Bowel Dysfunction

Since children with BBD have a higher risk of recurrent UTIs, it is imperative to treat BBD. Adequate hydration, timed voiding, pelvic floor muscle awareness and a bowel regimen alleviate the urinary and bowel symptoms associated with BBD [58]. BBD increases the risk of UTI in VUR patients regardless of antimicrobial prophylaxis, decreases the likelihood of spontaneous VUR resolution, and may decrease the efficacy of surgical treatment of VUR [59, 64].

Surgical Management

The major indications for surgical intervention in children with VUR include recurrent UTI despite appropriate antibiotic prophylaxis, worsening of renal scarring during follow-up, and grade V VUR, which is unlikely to resolve spontaneously. Surgical correction of VUR may be more important in patients with a single renal system. Surgical management decisions, however, should be individualized based on potential risk to the renal units.

Minimally Invasive Treatment Options

Minimally invasive options for the treatment of VUR are endoscopic and laparoscopic techniques, with robotic techniques applied to improve the results with laparoscopy.

Endoscopic Treatment

Endoscopic techniques use bulking agents to increase resistance at the ureteral orifice to prevent VUR. Polytetrafluoroethylene (Polytef) has been used successfully for correction of VUR since the early 1980s [104]. Polytef had excellent surgical success that was maintained over time; however, the concern of particle migration prevented approval in the United States (US) and led to the gradual decline in use worldwide. Polydimethylsiloxane has been utilized in Canada and has been associated with no migration and high success rates [105], but this agent has also not been approved for use in the US. Bovine cross-linked collagen has been used in the US and, although initial results were acceptable, long-term recurrence of VUR was frequent due to absorption of collagen over time [106, 107]. Other agents that have been tried include expanded chondrocytes and placement of balloons; however, these techniques require multiple procedures [108, 109].

Dextranomer hyaluronidase (Dx/HA, Deflux™) has been utilized for bulking of the ureters for treatment of VUR (Fig. 44.3a, b). Initially reported by Stenberg and Lackgren in 1995 [110], worldwide experience has grown rapidly. The overall cure rates with Dx/HA are 94% for grade 1, 85% for grade II, 78% for grade

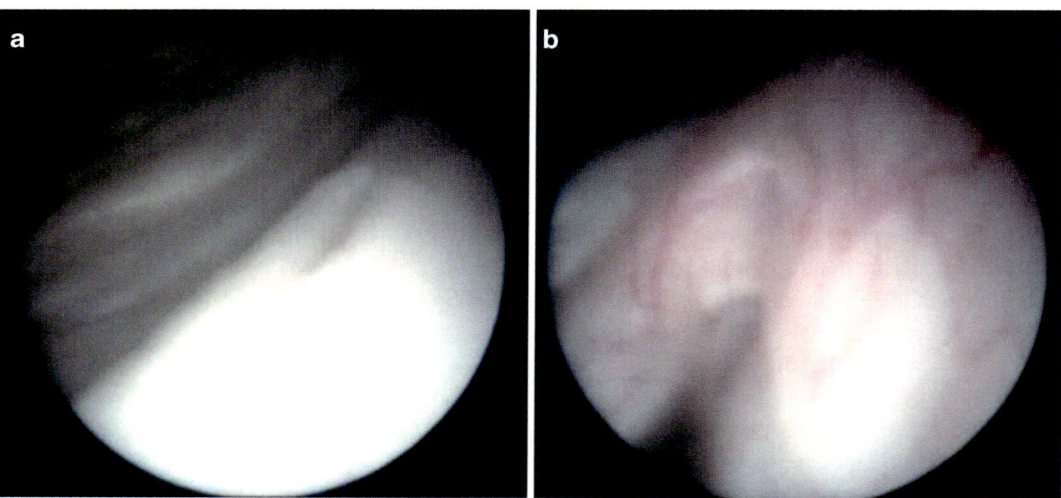

Fig. 44.3 (a, b) Injections are placed in one of several locations either within or near the ureter to increase coaptation of the ureterovesical junction. a depicts a ureteral orifice before injection, and b depicts after injection

III and 71% for grade IV VUR [111]. Dx/HA is effective in patients that fail prior treatment and in those that have associated urologic anomalies like ureteroceles and duplex systems. Patients that fail endoscopic management are still candidates for open surgical reconstruction. Late recurrence of VUR was noted in 20% of patients that had follow-up [112].

The efficacy and relative simplicity of the use of Dx/HA for the correction of VUR has led some to question the current paradigm of VUR management [113]. It has been suggested that Dx/HA should be used as a first line treatment for VUR. This procedure requires the use of general anesthesia, which is a significant consideration in infants.

Laparoscopic and Robotic Treatment

Laparoscopy has been successfully utilized for the surgical correction of VUR [114]. Laparoscopic techniques allow small incisions to be used and have the potential to reduce discomfort and length of hospital stays. The technique initially involved an extravesical approach for the correction of VUR [115]. Intravesical and transvesical techniques have since been reported [116]. The presumed benefit of reduction in hospital stay and smaller incisions have been eclipsed by the advent of improved endoscopic management with Dx/HA. The recent advent of the use of robotic techniques has shortened the length of the procedure and has made laparoscopic surgery for VUR more universally accepted. In a single surgeon direct comparison of open versus robotic approach to ureteral reimplant, surgical complications did not differ between the groups. There was a decrease in pain medication usage in the robotic group, albeit a 12% longer operative time in the robotic group [117]. However, in larger comparisons, there is more variation in reports of surgical complications in the robotic approach [118]. Wide variation in usage, success and complication rates of robotic surgery can be attributed to a learning curve and reported outcomes [119].

Open Surgical Techniques

Open surgery remains the gold standard for the surgical correction of VUR. The technique devised by Politano-Leadbetter combined an intra and extravesical technique and has been used widely with great success [87]. This technique, however, has been supplanted by the two techniques described below. In general, open surgical techniques are associated with 90–95% success rates and most can now be performed with a 1–3 day hospital stay. The success rates are so consistent across multiple studies that the use of routine post-procedure VCU has been abandoned. Despite high success rates for the correction of VUR, along with a decrease in the incidence of pyelonephritis [120], there has been no reduction in the incidence of renal scarring during follow-up.

Intravesical (Cohen) Cross-trigonal Reimplantation

Since the initial description of this technique, it has been rapidly adopted by most pediatric urologists due to the consistency of surgical outcomes and low rates of complications [121]. This technique involves the dissection of the ureters within the bladder and then the ureters are placed in submucosal tunnels created across the trigone of the bladder. Over time, significant improvement in pain management has permitted reduction in hospital stays, reduction in the need for stenting and suprapubic tube placement, and high patient satisfaction rates [121]. Because of the high rate of success, this technique is the most frequently performed and taught procedure for the correction of VUR. It is routinely used for the correction of bilateral VUR. It also allows for other bladder anomalies (e.g., ureteroceles, bladder diverticula) to be corrected concurrently. Potential complications associated with this technique are the development of contralateral VUR following correction of unilateral VUR, ureteral obstruction and residual VUR [122].

Extravesical (Lich-Gregoir) Reimplantation

This technique allows reimplantation without entry into the bladder. The ureters are dissected prior to the entry into the bladder and reimplantation is performed by placing the ureters into troughs created in the bladder wall [123]. It has been utilized most frequently for the management of unilateral VUR as there is a concern that some patients that have had bilateral reimplantation using this technique have had secondary transient neuropathic bladder dysfunction requiring temporary intermittent catheterization [124]. This technique also has a high success rate for the correction of VUR. Many patients can be managed with a 24 h hospitalization as bladder spasms are less frequently noted.

Controversies and Conclusions

The routine use of antenatal ultrasound has increased identification of hydronephrosis. This has permitted early identification of high grade VUR, potentially permitting reduction in renal injury from postnatal infection. In children with VUR identified during the evaluation of antenatal hydronephrosis, there is a pattern of boys with dilating VUR and renal dysplasia and girls with mild VUR and normal renal units [125]. A similar pattern of renal injury has also been noted in a population-based cohort of children followed after a first episode of UTI [80]. However, it remains unclear if the renal damage identified is congenital or acquired. The ability to distinguish renal scarring from dysplasia on DMSA renal scan is at the center of this debate. Newer imaging modalities will potentially help to differentiate these two entities.

The AAP and NICE guidelines have recommended limiting evaluation for diagnosis of VUR to those children presenting with recurrent infections, or those with abnormalities identified on ultrasound. These recommendations have led to a significant reduction in the numbers of children being identified with VUR. Additionally, studies have demonstrated that these recommendations have led to some children with high grade VUR being missed [126]. The long-term impact of this remains a concern.

The role of antibiotic prophylaxis in the prevention of recurrent infections also remains debated. We would certainly recommend prophylactic regimens for those children in higher risk groups as identified by the RIVUR study and other studies.

Surgical management of VUR has been shown to have high success rates for the resolution of VUR, but patients with BBD may continue to develop lower tract infections despite abatement of VUR.

References

1. Itatani H, Koide T, Okuyama A, Sonoda T. Development of the ureterovesical junction in human fetus: in consideration of the vesicoureteral reflux. Investig Urol. 1977;15(3):232–8.
2. Nielsen JB. The clinical significance of the reflux producing intrinsic bladder pressure and bladder volume in reflux and reflux nephropathy. Scand J Urol Nephrol Suppl. 1989;125:9–13.
3. Shakya R, Watanabe T, Costantini F. The role of GDNF/Ret signaling in ureteric bud cell fate and branching morphogenesis. Dev Cell. 2005;8(1): 65–74. https://doi.org/10.1016/j.devcel.2004. 11.008.
4. Batourina E, Tsai S, Lambert S, Sprenkle P, Viana R, Dutta S, et al. Apoptosis induced by vitamin A signaling is crucial for connecting the ureters to the bladder. Nat Genet. 2005;37(10):1082–9. https://doi. org/10.1038/ng1645.
5. Schwentner C, Oswald J, Lunacek A, Fritsch H, Deibl M, Bartsch G, et al. Loss of interstitial cells of Cajal and gap junction protein connexin 43 at the vesicoureteral junction in children with vesicoureteral reflux. J Urol. 2005;174(5):1981–6. https://doi. org/10.1097/01.ju.0000176818.71501.93.
6. Atiyeh B, Husmann D, Baum M. Contralateral renal abnormalities in multicystic-dysplastic kidney disease. J Pediatr. 1992;121(1):65–7. https://doi. org/10.1016/s0022-3476(05)82543-0.
7. Flack CE, Bellinger MF. The multicystic dysplastic kidney and contralateral vesicoureteral reflux: protection of the solitary kidney. J Urol. 1993;150(6):1873–4. https://doi.org/10.1016/ s0022-5347(17)35919-0.
8. Zerin JM, Leiser J. The impact of vesicoureteral reflux on contralateral renal length in infants with multicystic dysplastic kidney. Pediatr Radiol. 1998;28(9):683–6. https://doi.org/10.1007/ s002470050439.
9. Miller DC, Rumohr JA, Dunn RL, Bloom DA, Park JM. What is the fate of the refluxing contralateral kidney in children with multicystic dysplastic kidney? J Urol. 2004;172(4 Pt 2):1630–4. https://doi. org/10.1097/01.ju.0000138818.10910.1f.
10. Palmer LS, Andros GJ, Maizels M, Kaplan WE, Firlit CF. Management considerations for treating vesicoureteral reflux in children with solitary kidneys. Urology. 1997;49(4):604–8. https://doi. org/10.1016/s0090-4295(97)00007-1.

11. Gleason PE, Kelalis PP, Husmann DA, Kramer SA. Hydronephrosis in renal ectopia: incidence, etiology and significance. J Urol. 1994;151(6):1660–1. https://doi.org/10.1016/s0022-5347(17)35338-7.

12. Guarino N, Casamassima MG, Tadini B, Marras E, Lace R, Bianchi M. Natural history of vesicoureteral reflux associated with kidney anomalies. Urology. 2005;65(6):1208–11. https://doi.org/10.1016/j.urology.2005.01.044.

13. Jee LD, Rickwood AM, Williams MP, Anderson PA. Experience with duplex system anomalies detected by prenatal ultrasonography. J Urol. 1993;149(4):808–10. https://doi.org/10.1016/s0022-5347(17)36213-4.

14. Noseworthy J, Persky L. Spectrum of bilateral ureteral ectopia. Urology. 1982;19(5):489–94. https://doi.org/10.1016/0090-4295(82)90605-7.

15. Sargent MA. What is the normal prevalence of vesicoureteral reflux? Pediatr Radiol. 2000;30(9):587–93. https://doi.org/10.1007/s002470000263.

16. Lee T, Ellimoottil C, Marchetti KA, Banerjee T, Ivančić V, Kraft KH, et al. Impact of clinical guidelines on voiding cystourethrogram use and vesicoureteral reflux incidence. J Urol. 2018;199(3):831–6. https://doi.org/10.1016/j.juro.2017.08.099.

17. Chand DH, Rhoades T, Poe SA, Kraus S, Strife CF. Incidence and severity of vesicoureteral reflux in children related to age, gender, race and diagnosis. J Urol. 2003;170(4 Pt 2):1548–50. https://doi.org/10.1097/01.ju.0000084299.55552.6c.

18. Visuri S, Kivisaari R, Jahnukainen T, Taskinen S. Postnatal imaging of prenatally detected hydronephrosis-when is voiding cystourethrogram necessary? Pediatr Nephrol. 2018;33(10):1751–7. https://doi.org/10.1007/s00467-018-3938-y.

19. Arena F, Romeo C, Cruccetti A, Centonze A, Basile M, Arena S, et al. Fetal vesicoureteral reflux: neonatal findings and follow-up study. Pediatr Med Chir. 2001;23(1):31–4.

20. Horowitz M, Gershbein AB, Glassberg KI. Vesicoureteral reflux in infants with prenatal hydronephrosis confirmed at birth: racial differences. J Urol. 1999;161(1):248–50.

21. Skoog SJ, Belman AB. Primary vesicoureteral reflux in the black child. Pediatrics. 1991;87(4):538–43.

22. Pinto KJ. Vesicoureteral reflux in the Hispanic child with urinary tract infection. J Urol. 2004;171(3):1266–7. https://doi.org/10.1097/01.ju.0000113002.57543.34.

23. Chiodini B, Ghassemi M, Khelif K, Ismaili K. Clinical outcome of children with antenatally diagnosed hydronephrosis. Front Pediatr. 2019;7:103. https://doi.org/10.3389/fped.2019.00103.

24. Penido Silva JM, Oliveira EA, Diniz JS, Bouzada MC, Vergara RM, Souza BC. Clinical course of prenatally detected primary vesicoureteral reflux. Pediatr Nephrol. 2006;21(1):86–91. https://doi.org/10.1007/s00467-005-2058-7.

25. Sjöström S, Sillén U, Bachelard M, Hansson S, Stokland E. Spontaneous resolution of high grade infantile vesicoureteral reflux. J Urol. 2004;172(2):694–8; discussion 9. https://doi.org/10.1097/01.ju.0000130747.89561.cf.

26. Hansson S, Bollgren I, Esbjörner E, Jakobsson B, Mårild S. Urinary tract infections in children below two years of age: a quality assurance project in Sweden. The Swedish Pediatric Nephrology Association. Acta Paediatr. 1999;88(3):270–4. https://doi.org/10.1080/08035259950170015.

27. Hoberman A, Charron M, Hickey RW, Baskin M, Kearney DH, Wald ER. Imaging studies after a first febrile urinary tract infection in young children. N Engl J Med. 2003;348(3):195–202. https://doi.org/10.1056/NEJMoa021698.

28. Preda I, Jodal U, Sixt R, Stokland E, Hansson S. Normal dimercaptosuccinic acid scintigraphy makes voiding cystourethrography unnecessary after urinary tract infection. J Pediatr. 2007;151(6):581–4, 4.e1. https://doi.org/10.1016/j.jpeds.2007.05.008.

29. Menezes M, Puri P. Familial vesicoureteral reflux—is screening beneficial? J Urol. 2009;182(4 Suppl):1673–7. https://doi.org/10.1016/j.juro.2009.02.087.

30. Wan J, Greenfield SP, Ng M, Zerin M, Ritchey ML, Bloom D. Sibling reflux: a dual center retrospective study. J Urol. 1996;156(2 Pt 2):677–9.

31. Noe HN, Wyatt RJ, Peeden JN Jr, Rivas ML. The transmission of vesicoureteral reflux from parent to child. J Urol. 1992;148(6):1869–71. https://doi.org/10.1016/s0022-5347(17)37053-2.

32. Chapman CJ, Bailey RR, Janus ED, Abbott GD, Lynn KL. Vesicoureteric reflux: segregation analysis. Am J Med Genet. 1985;20(4):577–84. https://doi.org/10.1002/ajmg.1320200403.

33. Kaefer M, Curran M, Treves ST, Bauer S, Hendren WH, Peters CA, et al. Sibling vesicoureteral reflux in multiple gestation births. Pediatrics. 2000;105(4 Pt 1):800–4. https://doi.org/10.1542/peds.105.4.800.

34. Feather SA, Malcolm S, Woolf AS, Wright V, Blaydon D, Reid CJ, et al. Primary, nonsyndromic vesicoureteric reflux and its nephropathy is genetically heterogeneous, with a locus on chromosome 1. Am J Hum Genet. 2000;66(4):1420–5. https://doi.org/10.1086/302864.

35. Majd M, Rushton HG, Jantausch B, Wiedermann BL. Relationship among vesicoureteral reflux, P-fimbriated Escherichia coli, and acute pyelonephritis in children with febrile urinary tract infection. J Pediatr. 1991;119(4):578–85. https://doi.org/10.1016/s0022-3476(05)82407-2.

36. Piepsz A, Tamminen-Möbius T, Reiners C, Heikkilä J, Kivisaari A, Nilsson NJ, et al. Five-year study of medical or surgical treatment in children with severe vesico-ureteral reflux dimercaptosuccinic acid findings. International Reflux Study Group in Europe. Eur J Pediatr. 1998;157(9):753–8. https://doi.org/10.1007/s004310050929.

37. Roberts KB. Urinary tract infection: clinical practice guideline for the diagnosis and management of the initial UTI in febrile infants and children 2 to 24

months. Pediatrics. 2011;128(3):595–610. https://doi.org/10.1542/peds.2011-1330.

38. Bollgren I, Winberg J. The periurethral aerobic bacterial flora in healthy boys and girls. Acta Paediatr Scand. 1976;65(1):74–80. https://doi.org/10.1111/j.1651-2227.1976.tb04410.x.

39. Rushton HG Jr. Vesicoureteral reflux—new concepts and techniques. J Urol. 1997;157(4):1414–5. https://doi.org/10.1016/s0022-5347(01)65005-5.

40. Logvinenko T, Chow JS, Nelson CP. Predictive value of specific ultrasound findings when used as a screening test for abnormalities on VCUG. J Pediatr Urol. 2015;11(4):176.e1–7. https://doi.org/10.1016/j.jpurol.2015.03.006.

41. Jequier S, Jequier JC. Reliability of voiding cystourethrography to detect reflux. AJR Am J Roentgenol. 1989;153(4):807–10. https://doi.org/10.2214/ajr.153.4.807.

42. Mahant S, To T, Friedman J. Timing of voiding cystourethrogram in the investigation of urinary tract infections in children. J Pediatr. 2001;139(4):568–71. https://doi.org/10.1067/mpd.2001.118188.

43. Stokland E, Andréasson S, Jacobsson B, Jodal U, Ljung B. Sedation with midazolam for voiding cystourethrography in children: a randomised double-blind study. Pediatr Radiol. 2003;33(4):247–9. https://doi.org/10.1007/s00247-003-0874-0.

44. Ward VL, Strauss KJ, Barnewolt CE, Zurakowski D, Venkatakrishnan V, Fahey FH, et al. Pediatric radiation exposure and effective dose reduction during voiding cystourethrography. Radiology. 2008;249(3):1002–9. https://doi.org/10.1148/radiol.2492062066.

45. Unver T, Alpay H, Biyikli NK, Ones T. Comparison of direct radionuclide cystography and voiding cystourethrography in detecting vesicoureteral reflux. Pediatr Int. 2006;48(3):287–91. https://doi.org/10.1111/j.1442-200X.2006.02206.x.

46. Caione P, Ciofetta G, Collura G, Morano S, Capozza N. Renal damage in vesico-ureteric reflux. BJU Int. 2004;93(4):591–5. https://doi.org/10.1111/j.1464-410x.2003.04673.x.

47. Merguerian PA, Jamal MA, Agarwal SK, McLorie GA, Bägli DJ, Shuckett B, et al. Utility of SPECT DMSA renal scanning in the evaluation of children with primary vesicoureteral reflux. Urology. 1999;53(5):1024–8. https://doi.org/10.1016/s0090-4295(99)00049-7.

48. Stock JA, Wilson D, Hanna MK. Congenital reflux nephropathy and severe unilateral fetal reflux. J Urol. 1998;160(3 Pt 2):1017–8. https://doi.org/10.1097/00005392-199809020-00013.

49. Darge K. Voiding urosonography with US contrast agent for the diagnosis of vesicoureteric reflux in children: an update. Pediatr Radiol. 2010;40(6):956–62. https://doi.org/10.1007/s00247-010-1623-9.

50. Duran C, del Riego J, Riera L, Martin C, Serrano C, Palaña P. Voiding urosonography including urethrosonography: high-quality examinations with an optimised procedure using a second-generation US contrast agent. Pediatr Radiol. 2012;42(6):660–7. https://doi.org/10.1007/s00247-012-2360-z.

51. Piaggio G, Degl' Innocenti ML, Tomà P, Calevo MG, Perfumo F. Cystosonography and voiding cystourethrography in the diagnosis of vesicoureteral reflux. Pediatr Nephrol. 2003;18(1):18–22. https://doi.org/10.1007/s00467-002-0974-3.

52. Takazakura R, Johnin K, Furukawa A, Nitta N, Takahashi M, Okada Y, et al. Magnetic resonance voiding cystourethrography for vesicoureteral reflux. J Magn Reson Imaging. 2007;25(1):170–4. https://doi.org/10.1002/jmri.20822.

53. Cerwinka WH, Grattan-Smith JD, Jones RA, Haber M, Little SB, Blews DE, et al. Comparison of magnetic resonance urography to dimercaptosuccinic acid scan for the identification of renal parenchyma defects in children with vesicoureteral reflux. J Pediatr Urol. 2014;10(2):344–51. https://doi.org/10.1016/j.jpurol.2013.09.016.

54. Duckett JW, Bellinger MF. A plea for standardized grading of vesicoureteral reflux. Eur Urol. 1982;8(2):74–7. https://doi.org/10.1159/000473484.

55. Papachristou F, Printza N, Kavaki D, Koliakos G. The characteristics and outcome of primary vesicoureteric reflux diagnosed in the first year of life. Int J Clin Pract. 2006;60(7):829–34. https://doi.org/10.1111/j.1742-1241.2006.00859.x.

56. Routh JC, Vandersteen DR, Pfefferle H, Wolpert JJ, Reinberg Y. Single center experience with endoscopic management of vesicoureteral reflux in children. J Urol. 2006;175(5):1889–92; discussion 92–3. https://doi.org/10.1016/s0022-5347(05)00926-2.

57. Schaeffer AJ, Greenfield SP, Ivanova A, Cui G, Zerin JM, Chow JS, et al. Reliability of grading of vesicoureteral reflux and other findings on voiding cystourethrography. J Pediatr Urol. 2017;13(2):192–8. https://doi.org/10.1016/j.jpurol.2016.06.020.

58. Santos JD, Lopes RI, Koyle MA. Bladder and bowel dysfunction in children: an update on the diagnosis and treatment of a common, but underdiagnosed pediatric problem. Can Urol Assoc J. 2017;11(1–2Suppl 1):S64–s72. https://doi.org/10.5489/cuaj.4411.

59. Shaikh N, Hoberman A, Keren R, Gotman N, Docimo SG, Mathews R, et al. Recurrent urinary tract infections in children with bladder and bowel dysfunction. Pediatrics. 2016;137(1):e20152982. https://doi.org/10.1542/peds.2015-2982.

60. McLorie GA, McKenna PH, Jumper BM, Churchill BM, Gilmour RF, Khoury AE. High grade vesicoureteral reflux: analysis of observational therapy. J Urol. 1990;144(2 Pt 2):537–40; discussion 45. https://doi.org/10.1016/s0022-5347(17)39516-2.

61. Skoog SJ, Belman AB, Majd M. A nonsurgical approach to the management of primary vesicoureteral reflux. J Urol. 1987;138(4 Pt 2):941–6. https://doi.org/10.1016/s0022-5347(17)43465-3.

62. Arant BS Jr. Medical management of mild and moderate vesicoureteral reflux: followup studies of infants and young children. A preliminary

report of the Southwest Pediatric Nephrology Study Group. J Urol. 1992;148(5 Pt 2):1683–7. https://doi.org/10.1016/s0022-5347(17)37002-7.

63. Huang FY, Tsai TC. Resolution of vesicoureteral reflux during medical management in children. Pediatr Nephrol. 1995;9(6):715–7. https://doi.org/10.1007/bf00868720.

64. Sillén U, Brandström P, Jodal U, Holmdahl G, Sandin A, Sjöberg I, et al. The Swedish reflux trial in children: v. Bladder dysfunction. J Urol. 2010;184(1):298–304. https://doi.org/10.1016/j.juro.2010.03.063.

65. Ransley PG, Risdon RA, Godley ML. High pressure sterile vesicoureteral reflux and renal scarring: an experimental study in the pig and minipig. Contrib Nephrol. 1984;39:320–43. https://doi.org/10.1159/000409261.

66. Smellie JM, Normand IC. Bacteriuria, reflux, and renal scarring. Arch Dis Child. 1975;50(8):581–5. https://doi.org/10.1136/adc.50.8.581.

67. Rolleston GL, Shannon FT, Utley WL. Relationship of infantile vesicoureteric reflux to renal damage. Br Med J. 1970;1(5694):460–3. https://doi.org/10.1136/bmj.1.5694.460.

68. Ozen HA, Whitaker RH. Does the severity of presentation in children with vesicoureteric reflux relate to the severity of the disease or the need for operation? Br J Urol. 1987;60(2):110–2. https://doi.org/10.1111/j.1464-410x.1987.tb04943.x.

69. Verber IG, Meller ST. Serial 99mTc dimercaptosuccinic acid (DMSA) scans after urinary infections presenting before the age of 5 years. Arch Dis Child. 1989;64(11):1533–7. https://doi.org/10.1136/adc.64.11.1533.

70. Ransley PG, Risdon RA. Renal papillary morphology and intrarenal reflux in the young pig. Urol Res. 1975;3(3):105–9. https://doi.org/10.1007/bf00256030.

71. Lomberg H, Hellström M, Jodal U, Leffler H, Lincoln K, Svanborg Edén C. Virulence-associated traits in Escherichia coli causing first and recurrent episodes of urinary tract infection in children with or without vesicoureteral reflux. J Infect Dis. 1984;150(4):561–9. https://doi.org/10.1093/infdis/150.4.561.

72. Hohenfellner K, Hunley TE, Brezinska R, Brodhag P, Shyr Y, Brenner W, et al. ACE I/D gene polymorphism predicts renal damage in congenital uropathies. Pediatr Nephrol. 1999;13(6):514–8. https://doi.org/10.1007/s004670050649.

73. Lundstedt AC, McCarthy S, Gustafsson MC, Godaly G, Jodal U, Karpman D, et al. A genetic basis of susceptibility to acute pyelonephritis. PLoS One. 2007;2(9):e825. https://doi.org/10.1371/journal.pone.0000825.

74. Ragnarsdóttir B, Fischer H, Godaly G, Grönberg-Hernandez J, Gustafsson M, Karpman D, et al. TLR- and CXCR1-dependent innate immunity: insights into the genetics of urinary tract infections. Eur J Clin Investig. 2008;38(Suppl 2):12–20. https://doi.org/10.1111/j.1365-2362.2008.02004.x.

75. Rushton HG, Majd M, Jantausch B, Wiedermann BL, Belman AB. Renal scarring following reflux and nonreflux pyelonephritis in children: evaluation with 99mtechnetium-dimercaptosuccinic acid scintigraphy. J Urol. 1992;147(5):1327–32. https://doi.org/10.1016/s0022-5347(17)37555-9.

76. Kaack MB, Dowling KJ, Patterson GM, Roberts JA. Immunology of pyelonephritis. VIII. E. coli causes granulocytic aggregation and renal ischemia. J Urol. 1986;136(5):1117–22. https://doi.org/10.1016/s0022-5347(17)45235-9.

77. Roberts JA. Mechanisms of renal damage in chronic pyelonephritis (reflux nephropathy). Curr Top Pathol. 1995;88:265–87. https://doi.org/10.1007/978-3-642-79517-6_9.

78. Feld LG, Stablein D, Fivush B, Harmon W, Tejani A. Renal transplantation in children from 1987–1996: the 1996 Annual Report of the North American Pediatric Renal Transplant Cooperative Study. Pediatr Transplant. 1997;1(2):146–62.

79. Mattoo TK, Chesney RW, Greenfield SP, Hoberman A, Keren R, Mathews R, et al. Renal scarring in the Randomized Intervention for Children with Vesicoureteral Reflux (RIVUR) trial. Clin J Am Soc Nephrol. 2016;11(1):54–61. https://doi.org/10.2215/cjn.05210515.

80. Wennerström M, Hansson S, Jodal U, Stokland E. Primary and acquired renal scarring in boys and girls with urinary tract infection. J Pediatr. 2000;136(1):30–4. https://doi.org/10.1016/s0022-3476(00)90045-3.

81. Shaikh N, Craig JC, Rovers MM, Da Dalt L, Gardikis S, Hoberman A, et al. Identification of children and adolescents at risk for renal scarring after a first urinary tract infection: a meta-analysis with individual patient data. JAMA Pediatr. 2014;168(10):893–900. https://doi.org/10.1001/jamapediatrics.2014.637.

82. Snodgrass WT, Shah A, Yang M, Kwon J, Villanueva C, Traylor J, et al. Prevalence and risk factors for renal scars in children with febrile UTI and/or VUR: a cross-sectional observational study of 565 consecutive patients. J Pediatr Urol. 2013;9(6 Pt A):856–63. https://doi.org/10.1016/j.jpurol.2012.11.019.

83. Matsuoka H, Tanaka M, Yamaguchi T, Miyazato M, Kihara T, Nakagawa M, et al. The long-term prognosis of nephropathy in operated reflux. J Pediatr Urol. 2019;15(6):605.e1–8. https://doi.org/10.1016/j.jpurol.2019.08.015.

84. Wennerström M, Hansson S, Hedner T, Himmelmann A, Jodal U. Ambulatory blood pressure 16–26 years after the first urinary tract infection in childhood. J Hypertens. 2000;18(4):485–91. https://doi.org/10.1097/00004872-200018040-00019.

85. Gebäck C, Hansson S, Martinell J, Milsom I, Sandberg T, Jodal U. Obstetrical outcome in women with urinary tract infections in childhood. Acta Obstet Gynecol Scand. 2016;95(4):452–7. https://doi.org/10.1111/aogs.12853.

86. Gebäck C, Hansson S, Martinell J, Sandberg T, Sixt R, Jodal U. Renal function in adult women with uri-

nary tract infection in childhood. Pediatr Nephrol. 2015;30(9):1493–9. https://doi.org/10.1007/s00467-015-3084-8.

87. Politano VA, Leadbetter WF. An operative technique for the correction of vesicoureteral reflux. J Urol. 1958;79(6):932–41. https://doi.org/10.1016/s0022-5347(17)66369-9.

88. Baker R, Maxted W, Maylath J, Shuman I. Relation of age, sex, and infection to reflux: data indicating high spontaneous cure rate in pediatric patients. J Urol. 1966;95(1):27–32. https://doi.org/10.1016/s0022-5347(17)63403-7.

89. Edwards D, Normand IC, Prescod N, Smellie JM. Disappearance of vesicoureteric reflux during long-term prophylaxis of urinary tract infection in children. Br Med J. 1977;2(6082):285–8. https://doi.org/10.1136/bmj.2.6082.285.

90. Senekjian HO, Suki WN. Vesicoureteral reflux and reflux nephropathy. Am J Nephrol. 1982;2(5):245–50. https://doi.org/10.1159/000166654.

91. Grüneberg RN, Leakey A, Bendall MJ, Smellie JM. Bowel flora in urinary tract infection: effect of chemotherapy with special reference to cotrimoxazole. Kidney Int Suppl. 1975;4:S122–9.

92. Smellie JM, Katz G, Grüneberg RN. Controlled trial of prophylactic treatment in childhood urinary-tract infection. Lancet. 1978;2(8082):175–8. https://doi.org/10.1016/s0140-6736(78)91919-0.

93. Tamminen-Möbius T, Brunier E, Ebel KD, Lebowitz R, Olbing H, Seppänen U, et al. Cessation of vesicoureteral reflux for 5 years in infants and children allocated to medical treatment. The International Reflux Study in Children. J Urol. 1992;148(5 Pt 2):1662–6. https://doi.org/10.1016/s0022-5347(17)36997-5.

94. Karpman E, Kurzrock EA. Adverse reactions of nitrofurantoin, trimethoprim and sulfamethoxazole in children. J Urol. 2004;172(2):448–53. https://doi.org/10.1097/01.ju.0000130653.74548.d6.

95. Smellie JM, Tamminen-Möbius T, Olbing H, Claesson I, Wikstad I, Jodal U, et al. Five-year study of medical or surgical treatment in children with severe reflux: radiological renal findings. The International Reflux Study in Children. Pediatr Nephrol. 1992;6(3):223–30. https://doi.org/10.1007/bf00878353.

96. Prospective trial of operative versus non-operative treatment of severe vesicoureteric reflux in children: five years' observation. Birmingham Reflux Study Group. Br Med J (Clin Res Ed). 1987;295(6592):237–41. https://doi.org/10.1136/bmj.295.6592.237.

97. Garin EH, Olavarria F, Garcia Nieto V, Valenciano B, Campos A, Young L. Clinical significance of primary vesicoureteral reflux and urinary antibiotic prophylaxis after acute pyelonephritis: a multicenter, randomized, controlled study. Pediatrics. 2006;117(3):626–32. https://doi.org/10.1542/peds.2005-1362.

98. Roussey-Kesler G, Gadjos V, Idres N, Horen B, Ichay L, Leclair MD, et al. Antibiotic prophylaxis for the prevention of recurrent urinary tract infection in children with low grade vesicoureteral reflux: results from a prospective randomized study. J Urol. 2008;179(2):674–9; discussion 9. https://doi.org/10.1016/j.juro.2007.09.090.

99. Pennesi M, Travan L, Peratoner L, Bordugo A, Cattaneo A, Ronfani L, et al. Is antibiotic prophylaxis in children with vesicoureteral reflux effective in preventing pyelonephritis and renal scars? A randomized, controlled trial. Pediatrics. 2008;121(6):e1489–94. https://doi.org/10.1542/peds.2007-2652.

100. Craig JC, Simpson JM, Williams GJ, Lowe A, Reynolds GJ, McTaggart SJ, et al. Antibiotic prophylaxis and recurrent urinary tract infection in children. N Engl J Med. 2009;361(18):1748–59. https://doi.org/10.1056/NEJMoa0902295.

101. Brandström P, Esbjörner E, Herthelius M, Swerkersson S, Jodal U, Hansson S. The Swedish reflux trial in children: III. Urinary tract infection pattern. J Urol. 2010;184(1):286–91. https://doi.org/10.1016/j.juro.2010.01.061.

102. Roberts KB. Revised AAP guideline on UTI in febrile infants and young children. Am Fam Physician. 2012;86(10):940–6.

103. Wang ZT, Wehbi E, Alam Y, Khoury A. A reanalysis of the RIVUR trial using a risk classification system. J Urol. 2018;199(6):1608–14. https://doi.org/10.1016/j.juro.2017.11.080.

104. O'Donnell B, Puri P. Technical refinements in endoscopic correction of vesicoureteral reflux. J Urol. 1988;140(5 Pt 2):1101–2. https://doi.org/10.1016/s0022-5347(17)41971-9.

105. Smith DP, Kaplan WE, Oyasu R. Evaluation of polydimethylsiloxane as an alternative in the endoscopic treatment of vesicoureteral reflux. J Urol. 1994;152(4):1221–4. https://doi.org/10.1016/s0022-5347(17)32552-1.

106. Leonard MP, Canning DA, Peters CA, Gearhart JP, Jeffs RD. Endoscopic injection of glutaraldehyde cross-linked bovine dermal collagen for correction of vesicoureteral reflux. J Urol. 1991;145(1):115–9. https://doi.org/10.1016/s0022-5347(17)38264-2.

107. Frankenschmidt A, Katzenwadel A, Zimmerhackl LB, Sommerkamp H. Endoscopic treatment of reflux by subureteric collagen injection: critical review of 5 years' experience. J Endourol. 1997;11(5):343–8. https://doi.org/10.1089/end.1997.11.343.

108. Atala A, Peters CA, Retik AB, Mandell J. Endoscopic treatment of vesicoureteral reflux with a self-detachable balloon system. J Urol. 1992;148(2 Pt 2):724–7. https://doi.org/10.1016/s0022-5347(17)36704-6.

109. Atala A, Cima LG, Kim W, Paige KT, Vacanti JP, Retik AB, et al. Injectable alginate seeded with chondrocytes as a poten-

tial treatment for vesicoureteral reflux. J Urol. 1993;150(2 Pt 2):745–7. https://doi.org/10.1016/s0022-5347(17)35603-3.

110. Stenberg A, Läckgren G. A new bioimplant for the endoscopic treatment of vesicoureteral reflux: experimental and short-term clinical results. J Urol. 1995;154(2 Pt 2):800–3. https://doi.org/10.1097/00005392-199508000-00127.

111. Kirsch AJ, Perez-Brayfield M, Smith EA, Scherz HC. The modified sting procedure to correct vesicoureteral reflux: improved results with submucosal implantation within the intramural ureter. J Urol. 2004;171(6 Pt 1):2413–6. https://doi.org/10.1097/01.ju.0000127754.79866.7f.

112. Holmdahl G, Brandström P, Läckgren G, Sillén U, Stokland E, Jodal U, et al. The Swedish reflux trial in children: II. Vesicoureteral reflux outcome. J Urol. 2010;184(1):280–5. https://doi.org/10.1016/j.juro.2010.01.059.

113. Aaronson IA. Does deflux alter the paradigm for the management of children with vesicoureteral reflux? Curr Urol Rep. 2005;6(2):152–6. https://doi.org/10.1007/s11934-005-0085-3.

114. Atala A, Kavoussi LR, Goldstein DS, Retik AB, Peters CA. Laparoscopic correction of vesicoureteral reflux. J Urol. 1993;150(2 Pt 2):748–51. https://doi.org/10.1016/s0022-5347(17)35604-5.

115. Kawauchi A, Fujito A, Soh J, Ukimura O, Mizutani Y, Miki T. Laparoscopic correction of vesicoureteral reflux using the Lich-Gregoir technique: initial experience and technical aspects. Int J Urol. 2003;10(2):90–3. https://doi.org/10.1046/j.1442-2042.2003.00570.x.

116. Yeung CK, Sihoe JD, Borzi PA. Endoscopic cross-trigonal ureteral reimplantation under carbon dioxide bladder insufflation: a novel technique. J Endourol. 2005;19(3):295–9. https://doi.org/10.1089/end.2005.19.295.

117. Smith RP, Oliver JL, Peters CA. Pediatric robotic extravesical ureteral reimplantation: comparison with open surgery. J Urol. 2011;185(5):1876–81. https://doi.org/10.1016/j.juro.2010.12.072.

118. Kurtz MP, Leow JJ, Varda BK, Logvinenko T, Yu RN, Nelson CP, et al. Robotic versus open pediatric ureteral reimplantation: costs and complications from a nationwide sample. J Pediatr Urol. 2016;12(6):408.e1–6. https://doi.org/10.1016/j.jpurol.2016.06.016.

119. Satyanarayan A, Peters CA. Advances in robotic surgery for pediatric ureteropelvic junction obstruction and vesicoureteral reflux: history, present, and future. World J Urol. 2020;38(8):1821–6. https://doi.org/10.1007/s00345-019-02753-3.

120. Duckett JW, Walker RD, Weiss R. Surgical results: International Reflux Study in Children—United States branch. J Urol. 1992;148(5 Pt 2):1674–5. https://doi.org/10.1016/s0022-5347(17)36999-9.

121. Kennelly MJ, Bloom DA, Ritchey ML, Panzl AC. Outcome analysis of bilateral Cohen cross-trigonal ureteroneocystostomy. Urology. 1995;46(3):393–5. https://doi.org/10.1016/s0090-4295(99)80226-x.

122. Diamond DA, Rabinowitz R, Hoenig D, Caldamone AA. The mechanism of new onset contralateral reflux following unilateral ureteroneocystostomy. J Urol. 1996;156(2 Pt 2):665–7. https://doi.org/10.1097/00005392-199608001-00026.

123. Linn R, Ginesin Y, Bolkier M, Levin DR. Lich-Gregoir anti-reflux operation: a surgical experience and 5–20 years of follow-up in 149 ureters. Eur Urol. 1989;16(3):200–3. https://doi.org/10.1159/000471569.

124. Barrieras D, Lapointe S, Reddy PP, Williot P, McLorie GA, Bägli D, et al. Urinary retention after bilateral extravesical ureteral reimplantation: does dissection distal to the ureteral orifice have a role? J Urol. 1999;162(3 Pt 2):1197–200.

125. Yeung CK, Godley ML, Dhillon HK, Gordon I, Duffy PG, Ransley PG. The characteristics of primary vesico-ureteric reflux in male and female infants with pre-natal hydronephrosis. Br J Urol. 1997;80(2):319–27. https://doi.org/10.1046/j.1464-410x.1997.00309.x.

126. Suson KD, Mathews R. Evaluation of children with urinary tract infection—impact of the 2011 AAP guidelines on the diagnosis of vesicoureteral reflux using a historical series. J Pediatr Urol. 2014;10(1):182–5. https://doi.org/10.1016/j.jpurol.2013.07.025.

Obstructive Uropathies

45

Benedetta D. Chiodini, Khalid Ismaili,
David A. Diamond, and Michael P. Kurtz

Introduction

Obstructive uropathy is the partial or complete blockage to the flow of urine, which can occur as the consequence of an anomaly at any level of the urinary system: the ureteropelvic junction, distal ureter, ureterocele, urethra, or extrinsic compression by other structures (e.g., blood vessels, tumors).

As most of these conditions are congenital, they are currently routinely diagnosed on prenatal ultrasound (US) in developed countries. Early in fetal development, urinary tract obstruction starts a complex sequence of events affecting renal growth and development, and eventually leading to renal impairment. Congenital urinary tract obstruction is associated with a significant reduction in the number of nephrons and is the primary cause of end-stage renal disease (ESRD) in children [1, 2].

Detection of these conditions during pregnancy varies according to gestational timing at which screening is performed. Thanks to its safety, excellent anatomical resolution, wide accessibility and low-cost, US is the first examination to perform before and after birth [3].

From the beginning of the second trimester of gestation, the renal pelvis becomes detectable and appears as a sonolucent area in the middle of the kidney. Pyelectasis and hydronephrosis are the most common signs of obstruction detected on US. Other signs of obstructive uropathies are cysts, abnormal corticomedullary differentiation, increased echogenicity of the renal parenchyma, ureteral dilatation, pelvic or ureteral wall thickening, increased bladder size or wall thickness or presence of ureterocele [4–6].

Pyelectasis, defined as the dilation of the renal pelvis, and hydronephrosis, defined as the dilation of both the pelvis and calices, are evaluated in the sections of fetal abdominal transverse planes by measuring the anteroposterior diameter (APD) of the renal pelvis. APD may vary depending on the gestational week.

A third-trimester renal pelvis APD diameter of 7 mm is the most widely used criterion to select patients requiring postnatal investigation [4, 7]. Fetal distension of the urinary collecting system is often a dynamic and physiologic process which resolves spontaneously after birth [3, 8–10]. Among the prenatal mild pyelectasis cases, only a small proportion are associated with a serious problem in the postnatal period. However, in some cases pyelectasis can signal

B. D. Chiodini (✉) · K. Ismaili
Department of Pediatric Nephrology, Hôpital des Enfants Reine-Fabiola, Université Libre de Bruxelles, Brussels, Belgium
e-mail: benedetta.chiodini@huderf.be; khalid.ismaili@huderf.be

D. A. Diamond · M. P. Kurtz
Department of Urology, Boston Children's Hospital, Harvard Medical School, Boston, MA, USA
e-mail: david.diamond@children.harvard.edu; michael.kurtz@childrens.harvard.edu

Fig. 45.1 Algorithm for antenatally detected urinary tract dilation and postnatal imaging strategy

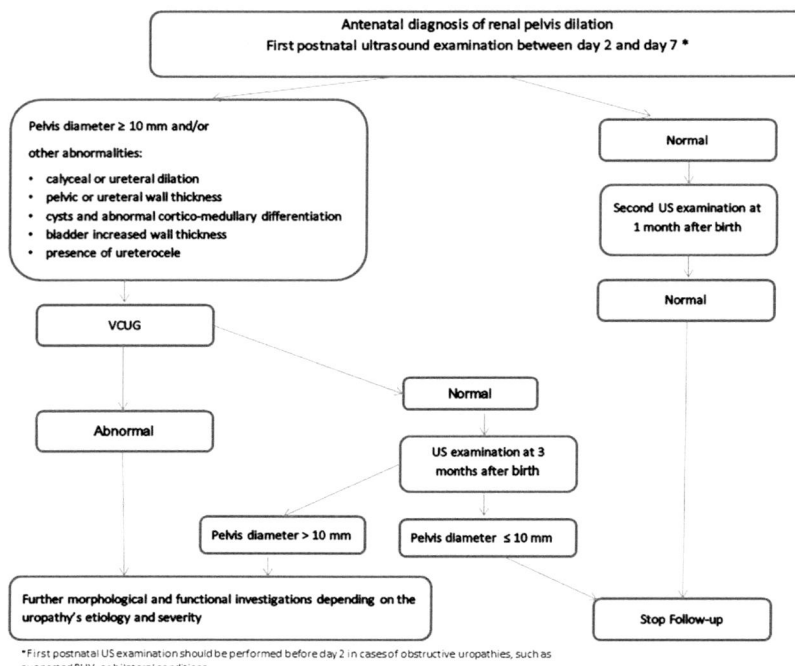

*First postnatal US examination should be performed before day 2 in cases of obstructive uropathies, such as suspected PUV, or bilateral conditions.

the presence of severe urinary tract pathology [11], especially in patients with significant hydronephrosis [7]. Renal pathology is confirmed postnatally in 12–14% of mild, 45% of moderate and 90% of severe pyelectasis cases detected in the second and third trimesters of pregnancy [12].

After birth, a renal pelvis APD of 10 mm is the most commonly accepted upper limit threshold value of normal [5] while a renal pelvis APD >15 mm is often associated with significant uronephropathies [4, 6, 13]. Based on the American [4] and European recommendations [14] and on our experience [3, 6, 7], we have suggested an algorithm for a pragmatic postnatal imaging strategy [15] (Fig. 45.1).

Common Obstructive Uropathies

The presentation and management may be divided into upper and lower urinary tract obstruction. Upper urinary tract obstruction is often unilateral and therefore less critical for overall renal function. Lower urinary tract obstruction, especially of the bladder outlet, is

usually associated with a more serious prognosis.

The most frequent congenital upper urinary tract conditions are ureteropelvic junction obstruction (UPJO), ureterovesical junction obstruction (also referred to as primary megaureter) and renal duplication anomalies. Posterior urethral valves (PUV) in boys are the most common cause of lower urinary tract obstruction.

The clinical management of these pathologies remains a challenge for nephrologists and urologists, due to the wide spectrum of severity and clinical progression and the difficulty in predicting long-term prognosis [1].

The different imaging and clinical features as well as current treatment options of the most common obstructive uropathies are reported below.

Ureteropelvic Junction Obstruction

UPJO is the most common cause of persistent prenatal hydronephrosis, occurring in 5–20% of children with antenatally diagnosed renal pelvis dilation [3]. It is usually unilateral, more common on the left side and more often observed in males [16]. Bilateral UPJO has a higher risk of additional kidney anomalies and potential renal function impairment, and often has a poor prognosis when associated with oligohydramnios and hyperechoic renal parenchyma in utero. UPJO is primarily caused by an aperistaltic segment, or crossing vessels at the level of junction between the pelvis and the ureter [17]. Rarely, obstruction is caused by an epithelial polyp, a benign growth of urothelium blocking the lumen at, or distal to, the UPJ. UPJO is highly suspected when there is significant pyelectasis, often >15 mm, in the absence of any dilation of the ureter (Fig. 45.2), and once vesicoureteral reflux (VUR) has been excluded by voiding cystourethrography (VCUG). In severe obstruction, caliceal dilation, hyperechoic parenchyma and sometimes a perirenal urinoma may be seen. On US, perirenal urinoma appears as a perinephric pseudocyst confined to the Gerota's fascia [12, 18]. Although the development of a urinoma is rare, it is most common when there is an ipsilateral dysplastic kidney [12].

The postnatal management of children with antenatally detected UPJO remains controversial [19, 20]. The primary question is how to identify asymptomatic children with hydronephrosis at risk for loss of renal function if managed by observation alone. To date, there is no consensus about the criteria for surgery, even within the same center [21, 22].

In 2016, the Cochrane review by Weitz et al. [23] focusing on unilateral UPJO evaluated the effects of surgical versus conservative management in newborns and children under 2 years of age. Unfortunately, the study was limited by the small sample size and short follow-up time and therefore was unable to clarify the optimal therapy for young children with unilateral UPJO. One year later, Weitz published a systematic review [21] on more than 1083 patients from 20 studies, with the aim of determining the effect of non-surgical management of unilateral UPJO. Although this review was also biased by the great heterogeneity of the included studies, it showed that more than 80% of the cases had improved drainage pattern over time, that about 20% of the patients were at risk for split renal function deterioration, and that nearly 30% underwent surgical intervention [21]. In order to definitively resolve the ongoing controversy and define the optimal management of unilateral UPJO, a randomized controlled trial with sufficient statistical power and adequate follow-up would be required.

A major challenge is that children with UPJO are often clinically asymptomatic and the criteria for surgery are primarily related to sonographic and isotopic parameters. In addition to the severity of the hydronephrosis on US, important predictors of the need for intervention are impaired differential renal function (DRF) and renal drainage on renogram [19, 21, 24]. MAG3 renogram is the gold standard for the evaluation of differential renal function and severity of obstruction. The Society of Fetal Urology and the Pediatric Nuclear Medicine Council of the Society of Nuclear Medicine have provided a consistent methodology for renography [25]. The Paediatric Committee of the European Association of Nuclear Medicine guidelines [26] has underlined the potential pitfalls in the acquisition, processing and interpretation of isotopic examinations.

Pediatric urologists decide on the need for pyeloplasty primarily based on poor drainage [25, 27–29] as indicated by delayed cortical transit time, which is the passage of the tracer from

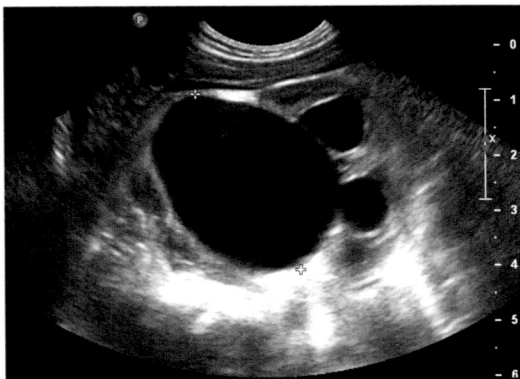

Fig. 45.2 Ultrasound of severe dilatation in a ureteropelvic junction obstruction

the outer cortex to the collecting system [30]. The cortical transit is generally fast, and fairly homogeneous kidney filling can be observed in approximately 2 min. In cases of delayed cortical transit, the tracer is retained in the outer cortical rim and the remaining kidney remains hypoactive for several minutes. Severely delayed cortical transit is an important indication for surgery to avoid renal function deterioration [24, 31].

A sensible clinical approach can be summarized as follows:

- Absolute indications for surgical treatment include symptoms such as febrile urinary tract infections (UTIs), hematuria, and kidney stones. Surgery is also indicated in a solitary kidney with evidence of reduced overall renal function.
- For unilateral UPJO, observation with close monitoring is the prudent approach for the large majority of cases, even in those with severe hydronephrosis initially on US.
- A MAG3 renogram should be performed to exclude worsening drainage in the event of a significant increase of the pelvic diameter on US.
- Early surgical intervention is recommended in cases of severe hydronephrosis with impaired split renal function and/or delayed cortical transit.

Megaureter

Megaureter is a ureteral diameter greater than 8 mm [32] and represents nearly one fourth of all causes of urinary tract obstruction in children [32], with cases presenting initially on prenatal US. In utero, megaureter appears as a serpentine fluid-filled structure with or without dilatation of the renal pelvis and calices [6]. Primary megaureter (pMU) is a ureteral dilation caused by an obstruction at the junction between ureter and bladder. pMU can be caused by both an aperistaltic (adynamic) segment in the terminal ureter causing a functional obstruction or, less commonly, by anatomic causes such as congenital distal ureteral strictures or valves [32]. Secondary

megaureter represents an obstructive process due to elevated intravesical pressure associated with an underlying bladder or bladder outlet condition. Common causes include high-grade VUR, neurogenic bladder and PUV. It is important to distinguish between primary and secondary megaureter, as in the latter treatment is directed at the underlying pathology and not at the ureter itself [32]. Differentiating primary and secondary megaureter relies on a VCUG.

With the exception of cases associated with the highest grades of hydroureteronephrosis, the prognosis of pMU is generally good and spontaneous resolution usually occurs within the first 3 years of life. The likelihood of requiring surgical correction increases with ureteral diameter exceeding 10 mm [33]. Regarding the management of pMU, two controversies remain. The first relates to the need for continuous antibacterial prophylaxis (CAP) to prevent UTIs while awaiting resolution. The second relates to indications for surgery.

Some authors recommend CAP in the first 6 months of life [34], although for others CAP is not considered mandatory, in the absence of recurrent UTIs and/or VUR [7]. Unfortunately, the risk of pyelonephritis in newborns with pMU is not clear [35]. A systematic review [36], including 16 studies and 749 patients, found a prevalence of UTIs in patients with pMU greater than 14% and a calculated number needed to treat for patients on CAP to prevent one UTI over the course of 1–2 years of 4.3. The authors recommended CAP in children with pMU selected for non-surgical management, at least in patients with poor emptying or greater ureteral dilatation, and for children in the first months of life [36].

When considering indications for surgery, Rubenwolf et al. reviewed a two-decade experience of pMU, and showed a constant decline of surgical interventions due to the favorable outcomes of conservative management in the majority of children [34]. However, in cases of severe hydronephrosis or a retrovesical ureteral diameter greater than 10 mm, resolution may take longer, and more commonly requires surgery [6]. The British Association of Pediatric Urologists (BAPU) recommends surgical intervention only in case of recurrent febrile UTIs, impaired renal function associated with severe or progressive hydronephrosis, or a drop in differential function on serial renograms [37]. In these cases, the BAPU recommends megaureter repair in patients over 1 year of age even though the procedure may be challenging in small children [37].

A sensible clinical approach can be summarized as follow:

- For a patient with a megaureter, VCUG should be performed in order to differentiate between primary and secondary megaureter.
- In children with asymptomatic pMU, close surveillance is recommended.
- Continuous antibiotic prophylaxis can be recommended in newborns with the highest grades of hydronephrosis and children with a history of a febrile UTI.
- Surgical intervention is mainly required in case of recurrent febrile UTIs, impaired renal function associated with progressive hydronephrosis and/or deteriorating split renal function on serial renograms.

Duplex Kidney

Duplication of the renal collecting system is a congenital defect that involves a kidney drained by two ureters that may be completely or partially separated [38]. Most patients with duplex kidneys have no significant clinical symptoms. When there is no hydronephrosis or renal impairment, a duplex kidney should be considered a normal variant [39]. However, it can also be pathological, associated with the presence of VUR and/or obstruction. Fetal urinary tract dilatation is associated with renal duplication anomalies in under 5% of cases [39]. In those, VUR classically involves the lower pole ureter and tends to be of higher grade as compared to single system reflux [38, 40]. Obstruction of the upper pole may also present secondary to an ectopic insertion, or more often due to a ureterocele, which on US appears as a thin-walled anechoic cystic dilation of the intravesical submucosal ureter (Fig. 45.3). However, ureteroceles can sometimes escape

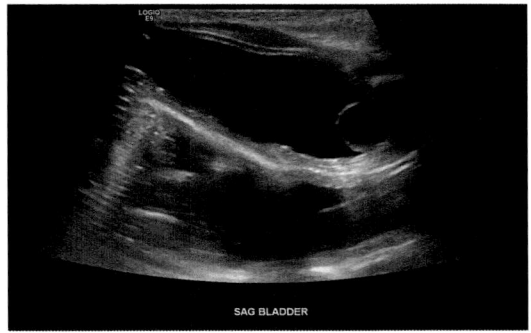

Fig. 45.3 Ultrasound of a ureterocele appearing as a thin-walled anechoic cystic dilation of the intravesical submucosal ureter

sonographic detection, as an overdistended bladder can compress the ureterocele or occasionally the ureterocele itself may be mistaken for the bladder.

In utero, duplex kidneys may be seen as two noncommunicating renal pelves, dilated structures within one pole, and a cystic dilation in the bladder, representing a ureterocele [41].

Postnatal investigations are US and VCUG [42]. Most authors agree that the surgical approach to pathological duplex systems is largely dictated by the anatomic etiology, clinical evolution, and the degree of function in the affected renal moiety [39, 42]. Children with a pathological duplex collecting system and/or ureterocele are also at higher risk of UTIs despite the use of prophylactic antibiotics [43].

A practical clinical approach can be summarized as follows:

- In children with dilated duplex system, US and VCUG are recommended after birth in order to diagnose VUR, assess renal parenchymal anatomy, and detect the presence of a ureterocele.
- In complex cases, prophylactic antibiotics should be started. Isotopic studies are recommended in order to evaluate renal function in the affected renal moiety.
- Decompressive surgery should be planned in cases of an obstructive ureterocele associated with good function, albeit depending on the clinical circumstance. Surgical options include

ureterocele puncture, ureteral reimplantation, and connecting an obstructed ureter to a non-obstructed, non-refluxing ureter. Poor renal function associated with a ureterocele may be an indication for removal of the affected moiety in cases with recurrent UTIs or lower urinary tract obstruction.

Posterior Urethral Valves

PUV are membranous folds fanning distally from the prostatic urethra to the external urinary sphincter and represent the most common cause of lower urinary tract obstruction in boys, affecting 1 in 4000–8000 infants [44]. This congenital malformation, depending on the severity of obstruction and the time of diagnosis, causes a wide spectrum of clinical manifestations. When suspected very early in pregnancy, as in the first or early second trimester, PUV carry a very poor prognosis [45] and are associated with high fetal and neonatal mortality. Impaired urine output leads to oligohydramnios and, ultimately, pulmonary hypoplasia and renal failure [46, 47]. With milder obstruction, the outcome is less predictable. In general, the obstruction leads to hypertrophy of the detrusor muscle, which often affects compliance and raises intravesical pressure. This elevated bladder pressure may be transmitted to the ureters, with or without VUR. This predisposes patients to an increased risk of UTIs, incontinence, and progressive renal impairment [44].

In utero, PUV should be suspected with the following findings: bilateral hydroureteronephrosis, abnormal renal cortex, failure of the bladder to empty, oligohydramnios, and an enlarged, thick-walled bladder with a dilated posterior urethra producing a keyhole configuration (Fig. 45.4). In rare cases, extravasation of urine can be recognized as a urinoma or urinary ascites due to bladder rupture [48] (Fig. 45.5).

Fetal urinary electrolytes and β-2 microglobulin are the most used biological markers to predict postnatal renal function. Fetal urine should be hypotonic, with osmolality less than 210 mEq/L. The combination of raised osmolality and a β-2 microglobulin greater than 4 mg/L

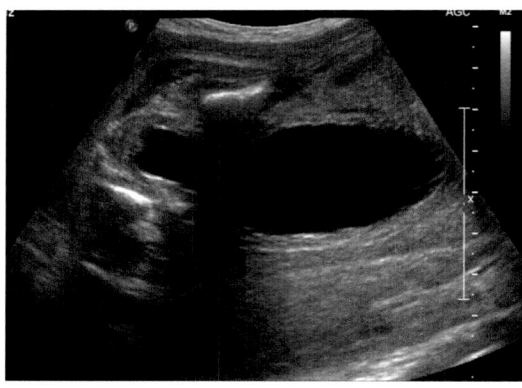

Fig. 45.4 Ultrasound of posterior urethral valves in a 32 weeks gestation fetus. It shows an enlarged thick-walled bladder with a dilated posterior urethra producing a keyhole configuration

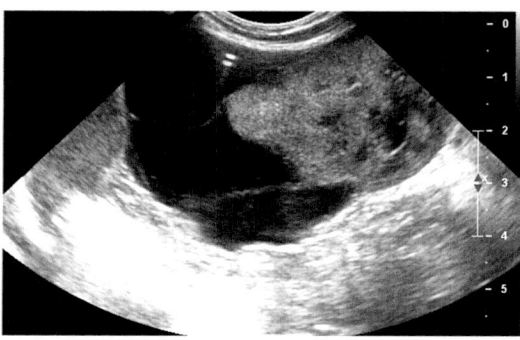

Fig. 45.5 Ultrasound of a perinephric urinoma in the context of severe posterior urethral valves

suggests irreversible renal dysfunction, and is a contraindication of shunt placement to restore amniotic volume [49].

Once PUV are suspected prenatally, management warrants the prompt involvement of a multidisciplinary team in a fetal and pediatric urology referral center. Various options can be discussed according to the severity of presentation, including termination of pregnancy, in utero therapy or follow-up with planned (active or palliative) postnatal management.

For decades, a variety of in utero approaches to therapeutically relieve obstructing posterior urethral valves have been utilized: open surgical technique of fetal vesicostomy [50], direct fetoscopic valve resection [51, 52], and vesicoamniotic shunting [53].

Vesicoamniotic shunting is the method most commonly used for bladder drainage. It involves the placement of a double pig-tailed catheter under US guidance with the distal end in the fetal bladder and the proximal end in the amniotic cavity to allow drainage of fetal urine [54, 55]. Its principal benefit is prevention of early neonatal pulmonary insufficiency and death. However, the risks of premature labor, perforation of fetal bowel or bladder, and fetal or maternal hemorrhage or infection are significant [56]. In 2013, the PLUTO (Percutaneous vesicoamniotic shunting in Lower Urinary Tract Obstruction) study was completed [57]. In this trial, fetuses diagnosed with lower urinary tract obstruction were randomly assigned to either vesicoamniotic shunting or conservative management. Despite its small sample size, PLUTO's results suggest that survival in the neonatal period was higher with vesicoamniotic shunting than with conservative management. However, there was substantial morbidity in both groups, with only two out of seven shunted survivors having normal renal function at 1 year of age. These results indicate a low likelihood of patients with severe PUV surviving with normal renal function, irrespective of management [58].

In summary, the experience with the intrauterine shunting technique as currently practiced suggests that postnatal survival may be increased, but that a significant improvement of postnatal renal function cannot be expected. Hence, the goals of care in patients with PUV are prompt urological care following a full gestation delivery with the aim of maximizing bladder and renal function.

The long-term outcome of PUV is far from satisfactory, with 15–30% of patients reaching ESRD during childhood [59, 60]. Indeed, PUV are the most frequent cause of chronic renal disease in boys and account for about 17% of children with ESRD [61]. In a retrospective study of more than 100 patients with PUV, the factors associated with a higher risk of CKD and ESRD were antenatal diagnosis, prematurity, abnormal renal cortex with loss of corticomedullary differentiation on initial US and elevated plasma creatinine at 1 year of age [62]. The decreased number of total nephrons present at birth leads to hyperfiltration injury, exacerbation of the underlying inflammatory process, renal fibrosis and, ultimately, renal failure.

In addition to renal impairment, the severity of bladder dysfunction in PUV patients varies widely, as the clinical spectrum ranges from severely pathological, high pressure bladders to late presentation with mild lower urinary tract symptoms, incontinence and recurrent UTIs. Indeed, children not diagnosed prenatally may present in infancy with urosepsis, poor urinary stream and/or failure to thrive. Older children may also present with urinary symptoms of incontinence, poor flow or retention. In a systematic review [63] of the outcomes of PUV in nearly 1500 patients, urodynamic bladder dysfunction was seen in more than half of the patients after endoscopic treatment of PUV, and nearly one in five cases had urinary incontinence.

A reasonable clinical approach can be summarized as follows:

- All cases antenatally suspected with PUV should be discussed by a multidisciplinary team, including obstetrician or maternal fetal medicine specialist, radiologist, pediatric nephrologist and urologist. All cases should then be referred to a pediatric center with a neonatal intensive care unit with nephro-urological expertise.
- Once the risks and benefits have been assessed, if an antenatal therapeutic intervention is proposed, the procedure should be performed selectively in qualified centers.
- In all children suspected of PUV, catheter drainage of the bladder should be performed at birth. Fluid status, serum electrolytes, and renal function should be monitored closely. Prophylactic antibiotics should be started.
- VCUG should be performed as soon as possible after birth. A voiding view of the urethra with the catheter removed is crucial for definitive evaluation of the urethra. Antibiotics should be administered 1 day prior and 1 day after the VCUG to prevent UTIs.
- The standard of care for PUV is endoscopic valve ablation when the child is medically

stable. Circumcision is also recommended to reduce the risk of infection.

- If catheter drainage improves hydronephrosis and plasma creatinine, then valve ablation is all that is necessary.
- If catheter drainage improves hydronephrosis, but renal function does not improve, this suggests renal dysplasia.
- If with catheter drainage the hydronephrosis and renal function do not improve, an upper tract diversion should be considered.
- If the newborn is too small (under 2 kg), the urethra might not safely allow standard resectoscope introduction. In these cases, alternative techniques such as vesicostomy, Fogarty balloon-based intervention, or laser ablation can be performed in order to alleviate or bypass the obstruction until the child is large enough for definitive treatment.
- Due to the high risk of chronic kidney disease in this patient population, patients should have close, long-term follow-up of renal function.
- Urodynamic studies are particularly valuable in order to evaluate bladder storage, pressure, compliance, emptying, and post-void residual volume, and help guide medical and surgical management.
- In children with ESRD, full assessment of the bladder is crucial before transplantation in order to prevent a hostile bladder from damaging the renal allograft. Moreover, with immunosuppression, the risks of transplant pyelonephritis and subsequent renal allograft damage need to be considered. If urological intervention is required, then reconstruction, such as bladder augmentation, should be performed pretransplant.

References

1. Chevalier RL. Congenital urinary tract obstruction: the long view. Adv Chronic Kidney Dis. 2015;22:312–9.
2. Mong Hiep TT, Ismaili K, Collart F, Van Damme-Lombaerts R, Godefroid N, Ghuysen MS, Van Hoeck K, Raes A, Janssen F, Robert A. Clinical characteristics and outcomes of children with stage 3–5 chronic kidney disease. Pediatr Nephrol. 2010;25:935–40.
3. Ismaili K, Avni FE, Wissing KM, Hall M. Long-term clinical outcome of infants with mild and moderate fetal pyelectasis: validation of neonatal ultrasound as a screening tool to detect significant nephrouropathies. J Pediatr. 2004;144:759–65.
4. Nguyen HT, Benson CB, Bromley B, Campbell JB, Chow J, Coleman B, Cooper C, Crino J, Darge K, Herndon CD, Odibo AO, Somers MJ, Stein DR. Multidisciplinary consensus on the classification of prenatal and postnatal urinary tract dilation (UTD classification system). J Pediatr Urol. 2014;10:982–99.
5. Avni EF, Ayadi K, Rypens F, Hall M, Schulman CC. Can careful ultrasound examination of the urinary tract exclude vesicoureteric reflux in the neonate? Br J Radiol. 1997;70:977–82.
6. Ismaili K, Cassart M, Avni FE, Hall M. Antenatal assessment of kidney morphology and function. In: Geary D, Schaefer F, editors. Pediatric kidney disease. 2nd ed. Berlin: Springer; 2016. p. 49–76.
7. Ismaili K, Hall M, Piepsz A, Alexander M, Schulman C, Avni FE. Insights into the pathogenesis and natural history of fetuses with renal pelvis dilatation. Eur Urol. 2005;48:207–14.
8. Sherer DM. Is fetal hydronephrosis overdiagnosed? Ultrasound Obstet Gynecol. 2000;16:601–6.
9. Persutte WH, Hussey M, Chyu J, Hobbins JC. Striking findings concerning the variability in the measurement of the fetal renal collecting system. Ultrasound Obstet Gynecol. 2000;15:186–90.
10. Sairam S, Al-Habib A, Sasson S, Thilaganathan B. Natural history of fetal hydronephrosis diagnosed on mid-trimester ultrasound. Ultrasound Obstet Gynecol. 2001;17:191–6.
11. Chudleigh T. Mild pyelectasis. Prenat Diagn. 2001;21:936–41.
12. Has R, Sarac Sivrkoz T. Prenatal diagnosis and findings in ureteropelvic junction type hydronephrosis. Front Pediatr. 2020;8:492.
13. Zhang L, Li Y, Liu C, Li X, Sun H. Diagnostic value of anteroposterior diameter of renal pelvis for predicting postnatal surgery: a systematic review and meta-analysis. J Urol. 2018;200:1346–53.
14. Riccabona M, Avni FE, Blickmann JG, Dacher JN, Darge K, Lobo ML, Willi U. Imaging recommendations in pediatric uroradiology: minutes of the ESPR work group session on urinary tract infection, fetal hydronephrosis, urinary tract ultrasonography and voiding cystourethrograhy, Barcelona, Spain, June 2007. Pediatr Radiol. 2008;38:138–45.
15. Chiodini B, Ghassemi M, Khelif K, Ismaili K. Clinical outcome of children with antenatally diagnosed hydronephrosis. Front Pediatr. 2019;7:103.
16. Johnston JH, Evans JP, Glassberg KI, Shapiro SR. Pelvic hydronephrosis in children: a review of 219 personal cases. J Urol. 1977;117:97–101.
17. Koff SA. Requirements for accurately diagnosing chronic partial upper urinary tract obstruction in children with hydronephrosis. Pediatr Radiol. 2008;38(Suppl 1):S41–8.

18. Piepsz A, Gordon I, Brock J III, Koff S. Round table on the management of renal pelvic dilatation in children. J Pediatr Urol. 2009;5:437–44.

19. Caldamone AA, Palmer JS, Mouriquand P, Koyle M, Jorgensen TM. Ureteropelvic junction obstruction: contemporary approaches to several case scenarios. Dialog Pediatr Urol. 2010;31:1–7.

20. Ismaili K, Avni FE, Piepsz A, Wissing KM, Cochat P, Aubert D, Hall M. Current management of infants with fetal renal pelvis dilation: a survey by French-speaking pediatric nephrologists and urologists. Pediatr Nephrol. 2004;19:966–71.

21. Weitz M, Schmidt M, Laube G. Primary non-surgical management of unilateral ureteropelvic junction obstruction in children: a systematic review. Pediatr Nephrol. 2017;32:2203–13.

22. Passoni NM, Peters CA. Managing ureteropelvic junction obstruction in the young infant. Front Pediatr. 2020;8:242.

23. Weitz M, Portz S, Laube GF, Meerpohl JJ, Bassler D. Surgery versus non-surgical management for unilateral ureteric-pelvic junction obstruction in newborns and infants less than two years of age. Cochrane Database Syst Rev. 2016;7:CD010716.

24. Ismaili K, Piepsz A. The antenatally detected pelvi-ureteric stenosis: advances in renography and strategy of management. Pediatr Radiol. 2013;43: 428–35.

25. Gordon I, Piepsz A, Sixt R. Guidelines for standard and diuretic renogram in children. Eur J Nucl Med Mol Imaging. 2011;38:1175–88.

26. Tondeur M, Nogarede C, Donoso G, Piepsz A. Inter- and intra-observer reproducibility of quantitative renographic parameters of differential function and renal drainage in children. Scand J Clin Lab Invest. 2013;73:414–21.

27. Conway JJ, Maizels M. The "well-tempered" diuretic renogram: a standard method to examine the asymptomatic neonate with hydronephrosis or hydroureteronephrosis. A report from combined meetings of The Society for Fetal Urology and members of The Pediatric Nuclear Medicine Council-The Society of Nuclear Medicine. J Nucl Med. 1992;33: 2047–51.

28. Ulman I, Jayanthi VR, Koff SA. The long-term follow-up of newborns with severe unilateral hydronephrosis initially treated nonoperatively. J Urol. 2000;164:1101–5.

29. Nogarède C, Tondeur M, Piepsz A. Normalized residual activity and output efficiency in case of early furosemide injection in children. Nucl Med Commun. 2010;31:355–8.

30. Piepsz A, Tondeur M, Nogarède C, Collier F, Ismaili K, Hall M, Dobbeleir A, Ham H. Can severely impaired cortical transit predict which children with pelvi-ureteric junction stenosis detected antenatally might benefit from pyeloplasty? Nucl Med Commun. 2011;32:199–205.

31. Duong HP, Piepsz A, Collier F, Khelif K, Christophe C, Cassart M, Janssen F, Hall M, Ismaili K. Predicting the clinical outcome of antenatally detected unilateral pelviureteric junction stenosis. Urology. 2013;82:691–6.

32. Hodges SJ, Werle D, McLorie G, Atala A. Megaureter. ScientificWorldJournal. 2010;10:603–12.

33. McLellan DL, Retik AB, Bauer SB, Diamond DA, Atala A, Mandell J, Lebowitz RL, Borer JG, Peters CA. Rate and predictors of spontaneous resolution of prenatally diagnosed primary nonrefluxing megaureter. J Urol. 2002;168:2177–80.

34. Rubenwolf J, Herrmann, Nuber M, Schreckenberger R, Stein R, Beetz R. Primary non-refluxive megaureter in children: single center experience and follow-up of 212 patients. Int Urol Nephrol. 2016;48: 1743–9.

35. Gimpel C, Masioniene L, Djakovic N, Schenk JP, Haberkorn U, Tönshoff B. Complications and long-term outcome of primary obstructive megaureter in childhood. Pediatr Nephrol. 2010;25:1679–86.

36. Rohner K, Mazzi S, Buder K, Weitz M. Febrile urinary tract infections in children with primary non-refluxing megaureter: a systematic review and meta-analysis. Klin Padiatr. 2022;234(1):5–13.

37. Farrugia MK, Hitchcock R, Radford A, Burki T, Robb A, Murphy F. British Association of Paediatric Urologists consensus statement on the management of the primary obstructive megaureter. J Pediatr Urol. 2014;10:26–33.

38. Whitten SM, Wilcox DT. Duplex systems. Prenat Diagn. 2001;21:952–7.

39. Ismaili K, Hall M, Ham H, Piepsz A. Evolution of individual renal function in children with unilateral complex renal duplication. J Pediatr. 2005;147: 208–12.

40. Peppas DS, Skoog SJ, Canning DA, Belman AB. Nonsurgical management of primary vesicoureteric reflux in complete ureteral duplication. Is it justified? J Urol. 1991;146:1594–5.

41. Avni FE, Dacher JN, Stallenberg B, Collier F, Hall M, Schulman CC. Renal duplications: the impact of perinatal US on diagnosis and management. Eur Urol. 1991;20:43–8.

42. Decter RM. Renal duplication and fusion anomalies. Pediatr Clin N Am. 1997;44:1323–41.

43. Visuri S, Jahnukainen T, Taskinen S. Prenatal complicated duplex collecting system and ureterocele-important risk factors for urinary tract infection. J Pediatr Surg. 2018;53:813–7.

44. Krishnan A, De Souza A, Konijeti R, Baskin LS. The anatomy and embryology of posterior urethral valves. J Urol. 2006;175:1214–20.

45. Jouannic JM, Hyett JA, Pandya PP, Gulbis B, Rodeck CH, Jauniaux E. Perinatal outcome in foetuses with megacystis in the first half of pregnancy. Prenat Diagn. 2003;23:340–4.

46. Morris RK, Malin GL, Khan KS, Kilby MD. Antenatal ultrasound to predict postnatal renal function in congenital lower urinary tract obstruction: systematic review of test accuracy. BJOG. 2009;116: 1290–9.

47. Housley HT, Harrisson MR. Fetal urinary tract abnormalities. Natural history, pathophysiology, and treatment. Urol Clin North Am. 1998;25: 63–73.

48. Spaggiari E, Dreux S, Czerkiewicz I, Favre R, Schmitz T, Guimiot F, Laurichesse Delmas H, Verspyck E, Oury JF, Ville Y, Muller F. Fetal obstructive uropathy complicated by urinary ascites: outcome and prognostic value of fetal serum β-2-microglobulin. Ultrasound Obstet Gynecol. 2013;41:185–9.

49. Sharma S, Joshi M, Gupta DK, Abraham M, Mathur P, Mahajan JK, Gangopadhyay AN, Rattan SK, Vora R, Prasad GR, Bhattacharya NC, Samuj R, Rao KLN, Basu AK. Consensus on the management of posterior urethral valves from antenatal period to puberty. J Indian Assoc Pediatr Surg. 2019;24:4–14.

50. Holmes N, Harrison MR, Baskin LS. Fetal surgery for posterior urethral valves: long term postnatal outcomes. Pediatrics. 2001;108:36–42.

51. Quintero RA, Hume R, Smith C, Johnson MP, Cotton DB, Romero R, Evans MI. Percutaneous fetal cystoscopy and endoscopic fulguration of posterior urethral valves. Am J Obstet Gynecol. 1995;172:206–9.

52. Agarwal SK, Fisk NM. In utero therapy for lower urinary tract obstruction. Prenat Diagn. 2001;21: 970–6.

53. Golbus MS, Harrison MR, Filly RA. In utero treatment of urinary tract obstruction. Am J Obstet Gynecol. 1982;142:383–8.

54. Clark TJ, Martin WL, Divakaran TG, Whittle MJ, Kilby MD, Khan KS. Prenatal bladder drainage in the management of fetal lower urinary tract obstruction: a systematic review and metaanalysis. Obstet Gynecol. 2003;102:367–82.

55. Coplen DE. Prenatal intervention for hydronephrosis. J Urol. 1997;157:2270–7.

56. Lee RS, Diamond DA. Perinatal urology. In: Avner E, Harmon W, Niaudet P, Yoshikawa N, editors. Pediatric nephrology. Berlin: Springer; 2009.

57. Morris RK, Malin GL, Quinlan-Jones E, Middleton LJ, Diwakar L, Hemming K, for the Percutaneous vesicoamniotic shunting in Lower Urinary Tract Obstruction (PLUTO) Collaborative Group. Percutaneous vesicoamniotic shunting versus conservative management for fetal lower urinary tract obstruction (PLUTO): a randomised trial. Lancet. 2013;382:1496–506.

58. Van Mieghem T, Ryan G. The PLUTO trial: a missed opportunity (comment). Lancet. 2013;382:1471–3.

59. Dinneen MD, Duffy PG. Posterior urethral valves. Br J Urol. 1996;78:275–81.

60. Caione P, Nappo SG. Posterior urethral valves: long-term outcome. Pediatr Surg Int. 2011;27:1027–35.

61. Hodges SJ, Patel B, McLorie G, Atala A. Posterior urethral valves. ScientificWorldJournal. 2009;9:1119–26.

62. Bilgutay A, Roth D, Gonzales E, Janzen N, Zhang W, Koh C, et al. Posterior urethral valves: risk factors for progression to renal failure. J Pediatr Urol. 2016;12:179.

63. Hennus PM, van der Heijden GJ, Bosch JL, de Jong TP, de Kort LM. A systematic review on renal and bladder dysfunction after endoscopic treatment of infravesical obstruction in boys. PLoS One. 2012;7:e44663.

Renal Calculi

46

Larisa Kovacevic and Paul Goodyer

Introduction

Pediatric nephrolithiasis has shown a dramatic increase in incidence [1], hospitalization and complication rates over the past two decades [2], and is no longer considered a rare or benign disease. Shifts in epidemiology, etiology, and stone composition have been noted and are related, at least in part, to the modern life-style [3, 4]. New trends include: an increasing annual incidence among two specific age groups (young and adolescent children), and among girls and African-Americans [5]; a change in the etiology from infectious to metabolic [6], and in the main metabolic focus from hypercalciuria to hypocitraturia [7], along with alterations in stone composition (ammonium and urate to calcium) [8]. Additionally, there is an increasing body of evidence supporting the association of nephrolithiasis with other conditions such as hypertension, coronary heart disease, atherosclerosis, diabetes and low bone mineral density, supporting the hypothesis that nephrolithiasis has a multisystemic involvement rather than being a single disease [9–11]. Moreover, the serious consequences of kidney stones are increasingly recognized based on new data on its association with chronic kidney disease (CKD) [12, 13]. Altogether, this emphasizes the need for comprehensive re-evaluation of pediatric stone management, which will help identify the modifiable risk factors at an early stage, guide treatment, and allow better prevention strategy.

There are several unique characteristic features of pediatric stone disease compared to adult stone formers: heterogeneous clinical presentation, high frequency of an underlying etiology (anatomic and genetic in infants and younger children, metabolic in older children), great variability of risk factors in relation to age, gender and race, and high rate of recurrence.

In this chapter, we will address the differences between children and adults and recently observed trends in pediatric nephrolithiasis, as well as advances in pathophysiology and treatment strategies, and future directions.

L. Kovacevic (✉)
Pediatric Urology, Children's Hospital of Michigan, Detroit, MI, USA
e-mail: lkovacev@dmc.org

P. Goodyer
Division of Pediatric Nephrology, McGill University Health Centre, Montreal, QC, Canada
e-mail: paul.goodyer@mcgill.ca

Epidemiology

The true incidence of pediatric nephrolithiasis is not known because many cases are either misinterpreted or undiagnosed due to the lack of symptoms. The estimates obtained from population-based observational studies indicate a range from 36 to 57 stone cases per 100,000 children

[14, 15]. Overall, the incidence of pediatric neph-rolithiasis is lower than in adults, and this may be due to higher concentration of urinary inhibitors of stone formation such as citrate and magnesium [16]. The presence of certain urinary macromol-ecules (UMM) in children, containing higher proportions of fibronectin and glycosaminogly-cans, also exhibit crystal-cell adhesion inhibitory activity compared with adult UMMs [17].

A change in epidemiology and a 4–16% annual increase in incidence of pediatric nephrolithiasis were noted over the past two decades, with the greatest increased rates among children between 12 and 17 years old, females, and African-Americans. Although the cause of the increasing incidence of pediatric nephrolithi-asis is not entirely clear, potential explanations focus on changes in dietary habits (increased intake of sodium and decreased water intake), an increase in antibiotic usage and other lithogenic drugs, and the increased use and sensitivity of imaging.

The prevalence, incidence and risk of nephrolithiasis varies with gender, race, climate/geographic location, dietary habits and socioeco-nomic factors.

Gender

The strong male gender predominance found in adults with nephrolithiasis is not seen in children [18]. An age-dependent gender distribution was reported in the United States, with boys being more affected in the first decade of life and girls in the second decade [19]. This could be due to the main risk factor of stones identified in these groups, namely obstructive urinary malforma-tions in boys and urinary tract infections in post-pubertal, sexually active girls. Recent data show a higher prevalence in girls compared with boys (52% versus 48%) [20], and a male-to-female ratio of 1:1.4, a difference that becomes more pronounced in adolescence [2, 20]. Additionally, female gender imposes a relative risk (RR) of 1.5 for hospitalization for nephrolithiasis [21, 22]. This marked increase seen in females has special significance due to the association of nephroli-thiasis with cardiovascular disease and fractures. The incidence of stone disease shifts towards a male predominance around 26 years of age, which continues throughout adulthood.

Age

During a 12-year period, one study reported the lowest incidence in children aged 0–3 years (0.6 per 100,000) and the highest in children aged 14–18 years (34.9 per 100,000) [6]. The same study showed that children aged 14–18 years had a 10.2-fold greater risk for nephrolithiasis and hospitalization compared to children 0–13 years of age [7]. Ureteral stones are more common in older children, whereas younger children are more likely to develop renal stones [19, 20]. Moreover, it seems that age is not predictive of spontaneous passage of stones, but stones less than 5 mm in size are more likely to pass com-pared to stones more than 5 mm [23, 24].

Race/Ethnicity

Nephrolithiasis is more common in non-Hispanic white children [5, 15, 17], followed by Hispanic and African American children [5, 7, 8, 14, 15]. However, it is unclear whether these differences are due to genetic differences or dietary habits.

Regional Differences

The incidence of pediatric nephrolithiasis varies by geographic area (rural vs. urban), and among countries, and is due to differences in climate, diet, socio-economic factors, and genetics. A higher incidence of kidney stones was found in children living in western countries (5–10% of that in adults) and in rural communities. In devel-oped countries, stones are found mainly in the kidney and ureter, and are predominantly calcium-oxalate or calcium phosphate. In under-developed and developing countries, bladder stones are commonly seen, and usually consist of uric acid or ammonium [25].

Turkey and Thailand are endemic areas with the highest incidence of renal stones. "Stone belts" have been described in different parts of the world, and include Southeast US (Virginia, North Carolina, Georgia, Tennessee, and Kentucky), Sudan, Egypt, Saudi Arabia, the United Arab Emirates, Iran, Pakistan, India, Turkey, Myanmar, Thailand, Indonesia and Philippines. This is probably due to the hot, dry climate causing dehydration, and high rates of consanguinity.

Pathogenesis

The initiation and growth of calculi requires high urinary solute concentration (supersaturation) and low urinary volume. Supersaturation represents the ratio of a salt's concentration in urine to its solubility; a ratio of more than 1 favors crystal formation, while a ratio less than 1 allows the crystals to dissolve. Further growth and aggregation is favored by ionic strength, urinary pH, and the concentration of promoters and inhibitors of crystallization (Table 46.1). These aggregates may occlude the tubular lumen and serve as an initial nidus (the free particle theory) [26]. This mechanism is particularly important for stone formation in cystinuria, where high urinary levels of cystine initiate intratubular nucleation. Adherence to the epithelial renal tubule cells of the urinary tract is required to allow for crystal growth (the fixed particle theory) [27], a process especially important in patients with brushite and apatite stones. Injured renal tubular cells by either toxins, infection or medication (e.g., calcineurin inhibitors and gentamycin) favor crystal attachment. The expected urine washout of crystal aggregates is impaired by stasis caused by congenital anomalies of the urinary tract.

In the Randall's hypothesis, apatite plaques or other sources of uroepithelial damage (infection, foreign body) represent the nidus for calcium oxalate stone formation [28]. Randall's plaque originates from the basal membrane of the thin loops of Henle, expands through the interstitium and protrudes into the papillary vasculature causing injury and repair in an atherosclerotic like fashion (vascular theory of Randall's plaque formation) [29]. This theory accounts for stones which appear to be embedded in the papillary wall and is supported by the physiology of renal papilla: turbulent flow, high osmolality and hypoxia [30, 31]. The reported association between vascular disease (hypertension, atherosclerosis, myocardial infarction) and nephrolithiasis [32] and the tendency of unilateral stones to develop on the sleeping side due to increased renal flow [33] are additional evidence supportive of the vascular theory.

Initial Presentation, Evaluation and Management

The presenting symptoms of nephrolithiasis in children differs from that in adults and depends on the child's age. Typical renal colic and gross hematuria are more often seen in older children and adolescents, who have higher rates of ureteral stones and spontaneous passage [6]. Flank pain may identify the position of stones: trapped at ureteropelvic junction (costovertebral angle tenderness), passing down the ureter (lateral flank tenderness) or trapped at the ureterovesical junction (lower abdomen or groin pain). In contrast, younger children may present with irritability, vomiting, failure to thrive, nonspecific

Table 46.1 Promoters and inhibitors of stone formation

Promoting factors	Inhibiting factors
Calcium	Citrate
Oxalate	Magnesium
Sodium	Pyrophosphate
Urate	Tamm-Horsfall protein
Cystine	Osteopontin
	Prothrombin fragment-1
	Bikunin
	Inter-alpha-inhibitor
	Alpha-1-microglobulin
	Calgranulin
	Fibronectin
	Matrix Gla protein
	Renal lithostathine
	Glycosaminoglycans (i.e. heparan sulfate)

Table 46.2 Initial evaluation of a child with nephrolithiasis

Medical history

Diuretic use in premature newborns, urinary tract abnormalities, urinary tract infections, intestinal malabsorption (Crohn's disease, bowel resection, cystic fibrosis), immobilization, diabetes mellitus, hypertension

Medications (antibiotics, anticonvulsants, diuretics, corticosteroids, chemotherapy, antacids, protease inhibitors)

Dietary history

Daily intake of fluid, sodium, potassium, calcium, oxalate and protein; special diets (vegetarian, meat). Use of vitamins C or D, herbal products, special therapeutic diets (e.g. ketogenic diet)

Family history of stone, hematuria, or renal failure (pedigree to establish mode of genetic transmission)

Physical examination: obesity, growth failure (distal renal tubular acidosis), dysmorphic features (William's syndrome), rickets (Dent disease), lower urinary tract stasis (spina bifida)

Urine

Urinalysis (pH[a], specific gravity or osmolality, glucose[b], protein[c]) and culture

Urine solute to creatinine ratios in random urine: spot urine

Qualitative cystine screening

Urine solute concentrations and excretion rates in timed 24-h urine collection (volume, calcium, phosphorus, oxalate, citrate, uric acid, sodium, potassium)

Serum chemistry: calcium, phosphorus, magnesium, alkaline phosphatase, sodium, potassium, chloride, bicarbonate, uric acid, creatinine, urea nitrogen

[a] Urine pH higher than 6 favors calcium phosphate precipitation; higher than 7 suggests urease producing organisms and struvite stones; lower than 6 favors cystine or uric acid stones
[b] Glycosuria and proteinuria indicates tubular dysfunction
[c] Low-molecular weight proteinuria is consistent with Dent disease

abdominal pain, microscopic hematuria and urinary tract infection [34].

Some form of hematuria is present in about half of children with stones [35]. Dysuria or frequency is seen in about 10%, while urinary retention/bladder pain may be seen in others. Other features include failure to thrive, hypertension and kidney failure; stones are occasionally reported in association with enuresis, penile edema, and anorexia. Rarely, children present with acute anuria caused by bilateral obstructive stones.

The initial assessment of children with nephrolithiasis is presented in Table 46.2; a proposed algorithm for the initial management of suspected nephrolithiasis is shown in Fig. 46.1. At presentation in the emergency room or during primary outpatient consultation, patients should have a careful medical history, family history and physical examination as outlined in Table 46.2. Blood should be drawn for measurement of serum creatinine, urea nitrogen, electrolytes, uric acid, calcium, alkaline phosphatase, parathyroid hormone and 1,25-dihydroxy vitamin D. Urine should be obtained for standard urinalysis and microscopy to screen for specific crystals in the urinary sediment (Table 46.3). Urine should also be screened for the ratio of calcium, oxalate, uric acid and cystine to creatinine (measures of excess excretion of these solutes) and for the ratio of citrate and magnesium to creatinine (measures of suboptimal levels of these stone inhibitors) (Table 46.4). Fractional excretion of sodium can be calculated to identify renal salt-losing states.

Diagnostic Imaging

The goals of initial imaging are to confirm the presence of a stone, detect whether it is obstructing urinary flow, estimate stone size (and likelihood of passing), ascertain whether the stone contains calcium and identify any anatomic abnormality (congenital or acquired) which might cause local urinary stasis. Ultrasonography and a plain abdominal radiograph showing kidney/ureter/bladder (KUB) are the mainstay of radiological imaging in children (Table 46.5) [36, 37]. Color Doppler ultrasonography provides information about the "twinkling effect" that is characteristic of small stones and should be used in patients who show no stones by B mode ultrasonography. A simultaneous KUB should be performed to identify ureteral stones and assess the calcium content of the stone.

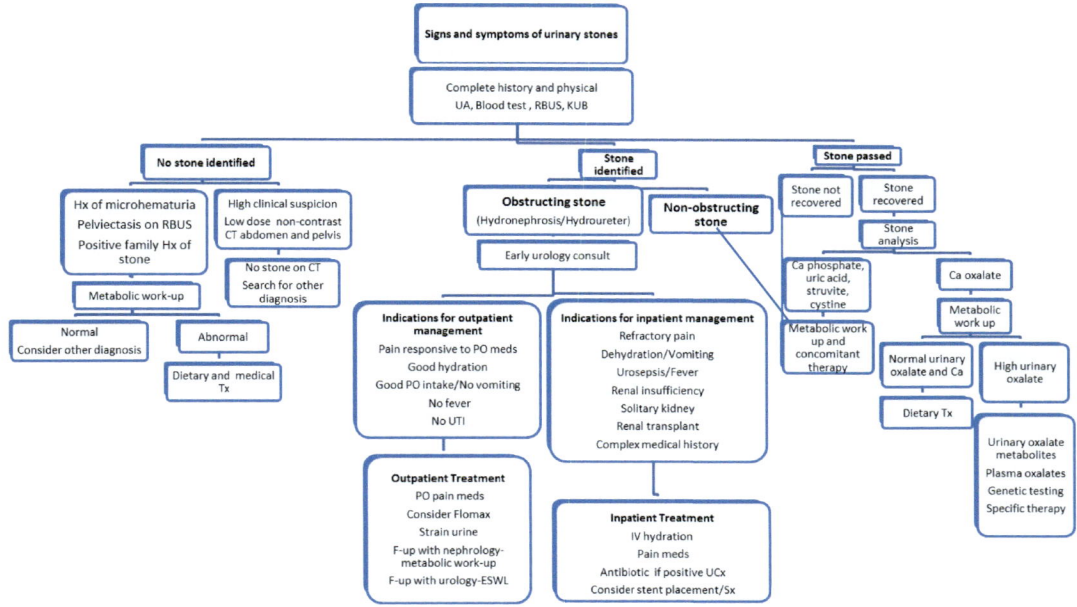

Fig. 46.1 Algorithm for the initial management of suspected nephrolithiasis

Table 46.3 Stone composition in children

Crystal type (stone incidence)	Possible causes	Appearance	Urine pH	Appearance
Calcium oxalate Monohydrate (Whewellite-80%)	Primary hyperoxaluria	Dumbbell or oval	Acidic	
Calcium oxalate dehydrate (Whedellite-20%)	Hypercalciuria Hyperoxaluria Hypocitraturia	Envelope	Acidic	
Uric acid (0.5–1%)	Hyperuricosuria (primary or secondary)	Varying sizes and shapes—rhomboids, parallelograms and rosettes	Acidic	
Struvite (triple phosphate) (Struvite 5–7%, Calcium phosphate 0.5–6%)	Infection	"Coffin lid"	Alkaline	
Cystine (1–5%)	Cystinuria	Hexagonal	Acidic	
2,8 dihydroxyadenine	Adenine phosphoribosyltransferase deficiency	Round, reddish brown with dark outlines and central spicules	Acidic	
Drug related -sulfa -acyclovir		Needle like crystals		

Table 46.4 Normal value for urinary excretion of metabolites

	Age	Random (mg/mg)	Random (mmol/mmol)	Timed (all ages)
Calcium	0–6 months	<0.8	<0.8	<4 mg/kg per 24 h (<0.1 mmol/kg per 24 h)
	7–12 months	<0.6	<0.6	
	>2 years	<0.2	<0.2	
Oxalate	0–6 months	<0.26	<0.26	<40 mg/1.73 m^2 per 24 h (<0.5 mmol/1.73 m^2 per 24 h)
	7–24 months	<0.11	<0.11	
	2–5 years	<0.08	<0.08	
	5–14 years	<0.06	<0.06	
	>16 years	<0.32	<0.32	
Cystine	>6 months	<0.075	<0.075	<60 mg/1.73 m^2 per 24 h (<250 μmol/1.73 m^2 per 24 h)
Uric acid	<1 year	<2.2	<1.5	<815 mg/1.73 m^2 per 24 h (<486 mmol/1.73 m^2 per 24 h)
	1–3 years	<1.9	<1.3	
	3–5 years	<1.5	<1.0	
	5–10 years	<0.9	<0.6	
	>10 years	<0.6	<0.4	
Citrate[a]	0–5 years	>0.2–0.42	>0.12–0.25	>310 mg/1.73 m^2 per 24 h (>1.6 mmol/1.73 m^2 per 24 h) in girls and
	>5 years	>0.14–0.25	>0.08–0.15	>365 mg/1.73 m^2 per 24 h (>1.9 mmol/1.73 m^2 per 24 h) in boys
Magnesium	>2 years	>0.13	>0.13	>0.8 mg/kg (>0.04 mmol/kg)

[a] A range for normal random citrate values is presented in the table to account for regional variations

Table 46.5 Radiologic imaging of the urinary tract

Radiologic imaging	Advantages	Disadvantages
Ultrasonography[a] (Sensitivity 77–90% Specificity 88–94%)	Wide availability, easy to perform, no pain, no radiation, no anesthesia, can be repeated, low cost. Shows stones of all compositions. Shows the anatomy of the kidney and bladder. Identifies associated hydronephrosis	Operator dependent. Body habitus and bowel gas may affect stone visualization. Can miss ureteral calculi. Can miss papillary or calyceal stones, and small calculi (<5 mm). Overestimates stone size
Plain abdominal radiography (Sensitivity 45–58%)	Detects large ureteral stones not seen on ultrasonography: Detects calcium (radiodense), struvite and cystine stones (intermediate radiodensity)	Misses radiolucent stones: uric acid, xanthine and indinavir. Risk of malignancy with radiation
Noncontrast computed tomography[b,c] (Sensitivity and specificity 90–100%)	Detects radiolucent and small stones. Provides anatomic details	Can miss indinavir and small distal stones. Risk of malignancy with radiation. Potential need for sedation
Intravenous pyelogram	Indicated in medullary sponge kidney	

[a] First choice in the initial assessment
[b] Gold standard
[c] New pediatric protocols have decreased the radiation exposure by 60–90%

Although computed tomography (CT) scan without contrast is the gold standard for assessing nephrolithiasis in adults, it is used sparingly during the initial evaluation in children to minimize radiation and to avoid the need for sedation. However, low radiation dose, non-contrast CT scan protocols have been developed for pediatrics and are mainly indicated when the patient is symptomatic and stones are suspected but not seen by ultrasound. A single center study found that a history of previous stones, vomiting, and the presence of blood on urinalysis were the strongest predictors for finding kidney stones on unenhanced CT scans [38]. Contrast agents can mask the presence of a stone and should be avoided on the initial CT scan; however, contrast may be useful in defining additional anatomical abnormalities.

Stone Analysis

If acute nephrolithiasis is suspected, patients should be asked to pass urine through a sieve to capture stones for analysis. This should continue until acute symptoms have resolved and/or passage of the stones are confirmed by repeat imaging. The composition of all recovered stone fragments should be analyzed by either infrared spectroscopy or X-ray diffraction, and components exceeding 5% should be reported. This should be done with each passage of stone since the composition may differ from the initial presentation. About two thirds of stones are composed of more than one substance. The composition of stones varies in children, although calcium oxalate is the most common [39, 40] (Table 46.3).

Differential Diagnosis

Abdominal or flank pain may be found in children with infections, such as gastroenteritis, urinary tract infections (UTI), appendicitis, ovarian torsion, intussusception, constipation, and pneumonia. UTI can concomitantly exist with nephrolithiasis. Worsening UTI or failure to improve within 24–48 h following antibiotic therapy may indicate the presence of renal stone, renal abscess, or underlying anatomic abnormalities/obstruction, and requires imaging of the urinary tract.

Gross hematuria may be caused by UTI, irritation of the meatus or perineum, trauma, and glomerular disease. Cola-colored urine, urinary sediment, and the possible presence of hypertension and/or edema indicate glomerulonephritis.

Acute Management

When a child presents with an acute stone episode, the immediate treatment goals are pain relief, nausea/vomiting control, rehydration, and treatment of associated infection if present. Nonsteroidal anti-inflammatory medications may be used with caution, provided renal function and hydration are adequate. If this is insufficient, oral or intravenous narcotics (e.g. morphine 0.3 mg/kg oral q3–4 h or 0.05 mg/kg intravenous q2–4 h) can be used for pain control, depending on oral tolerance. The preferred antiemetic agent is ondansetron due to its minimal side effects; metoclopramide hydrochloride or prochlorperazine are acceptable alternatives.

Once the diagnosis of nephrolithiasis is established, it must be determined if the patient can pass the stone spontaneously or whether surgical intervention is required. The size of the stone and its orientation are the critical determinants, with stones up to 5 mm having a high likelihood of spontaneous passage in children of all ages. With adequate pain control, uncomplicated unilateral stones causing only minimal or partial obstruction can be managed conservatively for several weeks before surgical intervention is considered. During this period, medical expulsive therapy (MET) for smaller ureteral stones has been used, especially in older children, with some success. However, the evidence to support this form of therapy in children is conflicting. There are a few randomized trials showing no efficacy in children [41] or adults [42]. In contrast, others concluded that MET is effective in pediatric patients [8, 43]. The most commonly used agent is tamsulosin, which causes relaxation of ureteral smooth muscle with inhibition of ureteral spasm and dilatation of the ureter. A prospective cohort study by Mokhless et al. demonstrated that ibuprofen and tamsulosin administered at bedtime (0.2 mg for children <4 years of age, and 0.4 mg for children >4 years of age) to children with distal ureteral stones led to significantly increased percentage of stone passage (88% vs. 64%), shorter passage time (8 vs. 14 days), and less need for analgesia (0.7 vs. 1.4 days) [44]. Tamsulosin is safe and has been approved by the US Food and Drug

Administration in pediatric patients. Alternatively, alpha blockers or calcium channel blockers can be used to facilitate the passage of ureteral stones under 10 mm in size [45]. Calcium channel blockers act by decreasing the intracellular calcium concentration, which induces relaxation of the ureteral smooth muscle. Alpha adrenergic receptors are abundant in the smooth muscle of the distal third of the ureter and ureterovesical junction and their blockage promotes relaxation of the ureteral wall.

In most cases, passage of the stone takes days or weeks and is usually managed as an outpatient, with careful medical oversight of pain control, expulsive therapy when stones are in the ureter and treatment of UTI if indicated. However, some children may need hospitalization. In general, this is restricted to those with an urgent need for upper tract decompression (nephrostomy tube or a lower tract stent), severe pain requiring intravenous analgesia, or need for intravenous antibiotic therapy for a UTI, as in urosepsis.

Evaluation for Risk of Recurrent Nephrolithiasis

Following the initial presentation and management, children with suspected or proven stones should be referred for evaluation of primary factors that might predispose to recurrence of nephrolithiasis, and provided with appropriate preventative measures. Ideally, this involves a clinic setting that can provide access to urologic expertise, genetic testing, nutritionist support and appropriate metabolic laboratory investigation. The risk of recurrent renal stones in children is high, with approximately 50% presenting with recurrent symptomatic stone within 3 years from the first episode of nephrolithiasis [46]. Those who have an identifiable metabolic abnormality are at fivefold higher risk compared to those without [23]. The rate of recurrence is also higher in those with a positive family history of stones in first-degree relatives.

Compared to adults, a predisposing cause for stone formation is found in about 2/3 of children and includes metabolic (33–95%), anatomic

(8–32%) and infectious factors (2–24%), alone or in combination [47–49]. About 50% of children under 10 years of age with stone disease have an underlying metabolic condition [23] caused by a renal, enteric or endocrinologic abnormality. The chance of finding a metabolic risk factor is higher in infants, patients with a positive family history or consanguinity, and those with recurrent kidney stones [25]. The risk of CKD and end-stage kidney disease (ESKD) is doubled in recurrent stone-formers compared to non-stone formers [8].

Thus, the primary goal of the "stone work-up" in children is to identify hyperexcretion of specific solutes that are likely to drive stone formation and to characterize the urinary content of inhibitors that normally protect against precipitation of lithogenic salts. When possible, a timed 24-h urine collection should be obtained to confirm the results of initial screening with spot urine samples.

Due to day-to-day variation in diet and fluid intake, at least two initial 24-h urine collections should be done. Urine creatinine should be checked for the completeness of urine collection (>15 mg/kg/day). The timed collection should be performed without altering the child's usual fluid intake, diet or activity, in the absence of a urinary tract infection, and at least a month after the spontaneous passage of stone or surgical intervention. Results can be interpreted with respect to weight, body surface area and urine creatinine (Table 46.4). When 24-h timed urine collections are not possible, shorter collection periods or repeat spot urine specimens measuring solute to creatinine ratios are acceptable. Normal values vary by age and prandial state (Table 46.4).

Blood analyses for calcium, uric acid, parathyroid hormone (PTH) and for assessment of renal tubular function (Table 46.2) should be performed at the time of the urine evaluation. Calcium homeostasis should be assessed in detail among children with hypercalcemia or hypercalciuria. Primary hyperparathyroidism is rare in children, but suppression of PTH offers a clue to states of vitamin D excess.

A fundamental assumption underlying the management of recurrent nephrolithiasis is that stones form when the urine is supersaturated with certain lithogenic salts (e.g. calcium oxalate, calcium phosphate). A 24-h urine identifies conditions that cause the urine to be supersaturated: (a) excessive excretion of calcium, oxalate, uric acid and cystine; (b) suboptimal excretion of citrate and magnesium; (c) unfavorable urinary factors such as pH, electrolyte concentrations. Supersaturation for calcium oxalate, calcium phosphate and uric acid are predicted by the well-established Equil2 program. Cystine saturation of the urine is established empirically by measuring the capacity of the urine to dissolve cystine crystals after 48 h. Serial determinations of supersaturation might be predictive of recurrence risk and, therefore, useful in monitoring successful interventions. Reduction of initial calcium oxalate supersaturation by 50% in stone-formers is a reasonable target. There are several publications supporting the utility of this approach in adults [50], but clinical trials in children are lacking, with the exception of cystinuria [51].

Other programs for calculating supersaturation of urine have been developed and adapted for use on personal computer platforms and smartphones [52]. A new web-based platform offers (for a fee) individual access to software that estimates supersaturation for calcium oxalate, struvite (NH_4MgPO_4-$6H_2O$), brushite ($CaHPO_4$-$2H_2O$), uric acid and cystine, using urinary parameters widely available in clinical labs.

Surveillance

Repeat renal ultrasound is needed to diagnose stone recurrence or increasing size of previous stones. The frequency of these tests depends on the presence and severity of the metabolic abnormality, the number of stones and recurrence rate. A child with a single stone and no evidence of an underlying metabolic abnormality will require less frequent monitoring than a child with multiple stones and a significant metabolic problem known to be at greater risk for recurrent nephrolithiasis (primary hyperoxaluria or cystinuria). Compliance with high fluid intake should be monitored by measuring the urine specific gravity.

In an asymptomatic child, a repeat kidney ultrasound is usually done 6 months after the initial episode. If the ultrasound shows no stone recurrence or change in residual stone size, the study can be performed yearly. Metabolic workup is repeated 4–6 weeks after therapy has been initiated. If the metabolic abnormality was corrected, repeat studies should be done at 6 months, and then yearly. Re-evaluation is needed if metabolic abnormalities persist. A multidisciplinary approach through a combined "Stone Clinic" including nephrology, urology, and dietary services serves these children well for long-term management.

Types of Kidney Stones

Calcium-Based Stones

Isolated hypercalciuria (excretion of >4 mg calcium/kg/day) is the most common cause of stones in children (Table 46.4). Early work in adults by Coe and Pak led to the suggestion that patients with calcium nephrolithiasis could be subdivided into those with "renal hypercalciuria" (decreased calcium reabsorption in the renal tubules), those with "absorptive hypercalciuria" (excessive vitamin D-dependent hyperabsorption), and those with "resorptive hypercalciuria" (parathyroid hormone-driven resorption of calcium from bone). While these classifications refer to important mechanisms in calcium homeostasis, it has become increasingly clear that the majority of patients don't fit easily into one category, and the stone work-up has shifted to other approaches.

Urinary stones develop about three times more often in adults with a family history of nephrolithiasis [53]. Twin studies indicate that the heritability of stone disease ranges from 46% to 63% [53, 54]. In a family study of children with hypercalciuria, Goldfarb et al. noted evidence of heritability in more than 50% [13]. However, it has been difficult to identify a primary genetic cause in most patients with calcium stones. Large genome-wide association studies in adults suggest that the heritable calcium stone trait is complex, influenced by multiple common variants of genes implicated in rare monogenic forms of nephrolithiasis. Among 3773 adult calcium stone-formers from Denmark and Iceland, homozygosity for a single nucleotide polymorphism (SNP) close to the claudin-14 gene conferred a 1.64 RR of developing stones among Icelanders [55], but could not be confirmed in the Danish group [56]. In large Japanese [57], Chinese [58] and British/Japanese cohorts, multiple SNPs were identified that conferred modest increased risk of nephrolithiasis (RR usually about 1.2), but there was little overlap between studies. Thus, the genetic factors predisposing to calcium nephrolithiasis in humans appear to be complex and remain elusive.

Increasingly, there is a focus on urinary factors that influence the saturation of lithogenic calcium salts. One major risk factor is urinary citrate excretion [7]. Hypocitraturia is defined in children as a urinary citrate excretion rate <310 mg/1.73 m^2/day in girls and 365 mg/1.73 m^2/day in boys, or less than 400 mg/g of creatinine in a 24-h urine collection (Table 46.4). Others have suggested even lower limit values (250 mg/1.73 m^2/day in girls and 180 mg/1.73 m^2/day in boys) due to decreased urinary citrate excretion per kg body weight with increasing age. Citrate is best interpreted in a 24-h urine collection because urinary citrate excretion appears to be influenced by diet and prandial state. It should not be measured during an active UTI because it may be artifactually low. Children have more citrate excretion than adults. Citrate combines with calcium in the tubular lumen to form a soluble complex resulting in less free calcium available to combine with oxalate. Moreover, citrate exerts a direct or indirect inhibitory effect on crystal aggregation, growth, and adherence to renal tubular cells. The indirect effect is due to enhancement of the inhibitory effect of Tamm-Horsfall protein on stone formation. Hypocitraturia is seen in patients with metabolic acidosis and hypokalemia, as well as in those with complete form of distal renal tubular acidosis (RTA).

Oral citrate supplementation is an effective strategy for treating adults with calcium-based kidney stones [59]. Two prospective studies in children showed that oral potassium citrate reduces the risk of stone recurrence by about 50% [60, 61]. Doses typically range from 0.5 to 1.0 mEq/kg/day in hypercalciuric patients; doses up to 2–3 mEq/kg/day may be required in children with dRTA. It is available in tablet and oral solution; a palatable, flavored form is commercially available.

The rationale for this approach is based on the well-established affinity of calcium for citrate (vs. oxalate or phosphate) and the relative solubility of calcium citrate. Individuals excreting suboptimal urinary citrate have increased risk of nephrolithiasis [62]. Srivastava et al. showed that hypercalciuric children with stones have higher calcium/citrate ratios (0.65 mg/mg) in urine than hypercalciuric non-stone formers (0.23 mg/mg) or controls (0.17 mg/mg) [63]. The authors suggested that calcium/citrate ratios of <0.33 mg/mg might decrease stone risk.

However, the decision to introduce citrate therapy for hypercalciuric children is sometimes complicated. There is theoretic concern about the potentially deleterious effect of citrate in raising urinary pH. Shen et al. found that oral supplements with potassium citrate (2 mEq/kg/day) for 5 days had marginal effect on urinary citrate levels, but did increase urinary pH [64]. An interesting resolution to this conundrum was proposed by Rodgers et al. who reported that the therapeutic effect of oral citrate may be due to formation of a pH-dependent soluble calcium/citrate/phosphate complex, and that clinical benefit is derived from the increase in urine pH, rather than from a change in citrate concentration [65].

Another well-established treatment for calcium stones is the use of a thiazide diuretic, sometimes with a potassium-sparing diuretic. The rationale for this therapy is to generate a mild volume deficit, which stimulates paracellular calcium reabsorption in the thick ascending limb of the loop of Henle. A thiazide diuretic consistently reduces urine calcium level in children [61, 66–68]. The RR of recurrent stones (3.3), episodes of hematuria (2.5) and osteopenia (3.0) are increased in those with hypercalciuria [68]. Interestingly, thiazide diuretics reduce stone recurrence even when the pre-treatment urinary calcium is within the normal range [67, 69]. However, while hydrochlorothiazide (0.5 mg/kg bid) reliably decreases urinary calcium, long-term adherence is reported in only one third of patients and hypercalciuria recurs in 44% [68]. Furthermore, a thiazide diuretic may induce hypokalemia, requiring oral potassium supplements or the addition of a potassium-sparing diuretic.

Uric Acid Stones

The oldest known urinary tract stone was a bladder stone found in a 7000 year-old mummy in upper Egypt; the stone had a mixed composition, including uric acid [70]. About 11.7% and 7% of stones in adult males and females, respectively contain uric acid and it may be the dominant component, but it is often mixed with calcium salts [71]. In middle eastern regions, uric acid accounts for up to one third of stones [72], but only 1% in India [73].

On a typical Western diet, humans excrete about 10 mg/kg/day of uric acid, 50% derived from turnover of nucleic acids and 50% from the diet [70]. However, the dietary component can be doubled on diets containing high amounts of meat, fish and certain vegetables (e.g. asparagus, mushrooms) [70]. Since the pKa of uric acid is about 5.3, it tends to precipitate in acidic urine to form identifiable geometric crystals (Table 46.3). However, uric acid crystals easily dissolve at the higher urine pHs during the normal "alkaline tide" each day. Thus, it has been proposed that uric stones may form in those with sustained acidic urine, perhaps among individuals with blunted renal ammoniagenesis.

In children, pure uric acid stones are rare, and are seen mostly in settings where there is over-production of uric acid such as tumor lysis syndrome, lymphoproliferative and myeloproliferative disorders, and genetic disorders (Lesch-Nyhan syndrome and glycogen storage disorders). However, mixed composition stones containing some uric acid are seen in 2–8% of children with nephrolithiasis and hyper-

uricosuria (>815 mg/1.73 m^2/day) (Table 46.4). Uric acid excretion is highest in infancy; pinkish-brown uric acid crystals may precipitate in the diaper and are often mistaken for blood, but are not associated with stone formation.

Children with uric acid-containing stones can be managed with oral citrate (0.5–1.0 mEq/day in divided doses) to maintain urine pH above 6.5, while also offsetting lithogenic calcium salt supersaturation. Sometimes an extra evening dose is required to manage overnight aciduria. In children with malignancy, use of a xanthine oxidase inhibitor (e.g. allopurinol or febuxostat) and recombinant rasburicase are remarkably effective, and have largely eliminated elevated uric acid as a cause of complications in tumour lysis syndrome.

Monogenic Forms of Nephrolithiasis

In a study of children (age at first stone <18 years) consecutively referred to a kidney stone clinic, patients were screened for 30 genetic disorders predisposing to kidney stones. In 20.8% of these cases, a causative mutant gene was identified. Thus, the work-up of pediatric patients presenting with urinary tract stones should include a focused effort to diagnose monogenic forms of nephrolithiasis.

Primary hyperoxalurias (incidence 1:120,000) are recessive, hereditary errors of glyoxylate metabolism, leading to overproduction and excessive urinary excretion of oxalate [74]. Hyperoxaluria is defined as a urinary oxalate excretion rate that is greater than 40 mg/1.73 m^2 per 24 h (Table 46.4), and is found in about 10–20% of children. The oxalate to creatinine ratio on a spot urine sample can also be used, but the normal values are age- and assay-dependent. Primary hyperoxaluria, type 1 (PH1), caused by biallelic mutations of *AGXT*, is the most common (80%), and about one third of these are responsive to oral pyridoxine (5–10 mg/kg/day). Excess oxalate in urine drives calcium oxylate crystallization within tubules, while elevated plasma oxalate causes tissue deposition in many tissues, including the renal parenchyma (nephrocalcinosis), leading to progressive renal insufficiency [75]. About one quarter of PH1 patients develop ESKD by 20 years of age. Most develop kidney stones in early childhood, and sometimes present with failure to thrive and stones in the first year of life. Those with milder mutations may be relatively asymptomatic until middle age. PH1 stones have a pale, yellowish surface, unlike the darker surface of those with idiopathic calcium oxalate stones.

PH2 (biallelic mutations of *GHPRH*) constitutes about 10% of the primary hyperoxalurias and is milder than PH1. PH2 patients usually excrete excess oxalate and glycerate in the urine [76]. PH3 (about 12% of hyperoxalurias), due to biallelic mutations of *HOGA1*, results from mutations of a mitochondrial enzyme that normally generates glyoxylate from 4-hydroxy-2-oxoglutarate (HOG). Although the pathomechanism is not entirely understood, PH3 urine has excessive oxalate and HOG [77].

Screening for the hyperoxalurias should be performed in all children with early onset nephrolithiasis. Normal urine oxalate/creatinine ratio ranges are age dependent (Table 46.4). Genetic diagnosis of primary hyperoxalurias involves mutation screening for the panel of *AGXT*, *GRHPR* and *HOAG1*.

Cystinuria is caused by mutations of the recessively inherited *SLC3A1* or the incompletely dominant *SLC7A9*, found in about 5% of children with renal calculi. These genes encode the two protein partners of the luminal reabsorptive transport mechanism for cystine and the dibasic amino acids in the renal proximal convoluted tubule. Cystinuria genotype can often be inferred from the level of urinary cystine in parents of affected children, since *SLC3A1* is recessive (urine cystine is normal in the heterozygote), whereas loss of one *SLC7A9* allele partially compromises cystine reabsorption (heterozygotes have moderate cystinuria).

Children with biallelic mutations of *SLC3A1* or *SLC7A9* excrete cystine in the range of 3000–5000 μmol half-cystine/g creatinine vs. normal levels of <150 μmol/g creatinine. Over 24 h, normal cystine excretion is <60 mg half-cystine/1.73 m^2/day. Microscopic hexagonal

cystine crystals are pathognomonic. Crystal volume is thought to correlate with stone risk and commonly give rise to asymptomatic bladder debris visible on ultrasound. In one cohort, 1.1% required dialysis at a mean age of 35 years and 15.6% had an estimated glomerular filtration rate (eGFR) <60 mL/min/1.73 m^2 [78].

During the first 1–2 years, children who have heterozygous mutations in *SLC7A9* excrete cystine in the homozygous range, but with tubular maturation and elongation over the first 2 years, it decreases to an intermediate level, varying between 300 and 1500 μmol half-cystine/g creatinine. Although their urine cystine levels are usually below the threshold of solubility, *SLC7A9* heterozygotes may occasionally form stones in childhood during periods of dehydration. Halbritter et al. found that *SLC7A9* heterozygotes were the most common cause of nephrolithiasis among 101 pediatric stone-formers recruited from a stone clinic [79]; adult heterozygotes may comprise nearly half of the cystinuria patients in a stone clinic.

Pre-symptomatic children who excrete cystine in the stone-forming range (>1200 μmol/L) should be monitored carefully by annual ultrasonography and serial urine cystine/L measurements [80], but interventions are usually restricted to increased fluid intake (2–2.5 L/m^2/day) and avoidance of excessive salt intake. Among stone formers, alkalinization of the urine is usually initiated (particularly overnight), and some clinicians recommend low salt intake and limited animal protein diet. With frequent or obstructive stones, tiopronin (10–15 mg/kg/day in divided doses), which reduces free cystine, should be introduced. Malieckal et al. have shown in adults that a dose of 1 g/day reduces excretion of free cystine and increases cystine capacity of urine from −39 to +130 mg cystine/L [81].

Distal RTA is caused by dysfunction of the transport mechanism in alpha-intercalated cells of the cortical collecting tubule that pumps hydrogen ions (H$^+$) into the lumen and normally allows excretion of the daily metabolic acid load (about 2 mEq/kg/day). In adults, dRTA is seen with various autoimmune diseases (e.g. Sjögren syndrome and systemic lupus erythematosus) and acquired tubular injury from drugs (e.g. lithium). In children, however, dRTA is usually the result of mutations in genes encoding subunits of the "vacuolar type" ATPase (*ATP6V1B1, ATP6V0A4, ATP6V1C2*) that secretes H⁺ out of the cell across the apical membrane, the basolateral anion exchanger (*SLC4A1*) that pumps bicarbonate across the basolateral cell surface or the transcription factors that regulate the process (*FOX1, WDR72*) [31]. Mutations of *ATP6V1B1* and *FOX1* are associated with early deafness, while *ATP6V0A4* mutations cause later onset deafness. Heterozygous mutations of the *ATP6V1B1* [82] and *ATP6V0A4* have been linked to "incomplete" (mild) dRTA and kidney stones in adults, but this has not been described in children with nephrolithiasis.

dRTA presents in infancy, with normal anion gap, hyperchloremic metabolic acidosis and failure to thrive. Urine pH is inappropriately high (6–8) and urinary anion gap is inappropriately positive in the setting of a metabolic acidosis (reflecting absence of urinary NH4⁺). Sustained acidosis causes dissolution of bone mineral and hypercalciuria. The acidosis also causes consumption of citrate by the mitochondrial citric acid cycle, so that urinary citrate levels are low. Thus, as the tubular fluid is progressively concentrated in the collecting ducts, when pH is high and citrate levels are low, urine becomes supersaturated with lithogenic calcium salts, particularly calcium phosphate (brushite). Brushite crystals are unusually large and may completely obstruct individual renal papillae, accounting for the characteristic medullary nephrocalcinosis on ultrasound. Crystals arriving in the renal calyces may coalesce to produce stones.

Given the pathogenesis of calcium phosphate stones in dRTA, management involves correction of acidosis, hypokalemia and hypocitraturia with potassium citrate 1–2 mEq/kg/day in 3–4 divided doses. In early infancy, slightly higher doses (2–3 mEq/kg/day) may be needed. In children with mild dRTA and erythrocyte abnormalities caused by heterozygous mutations of *SLC4A1*, lower doses of potassium citrate (0.5–1.5 mEq/kg/day) are needed.

Dent Disease is an X-linked recessive form of nephrocalcinosis and nephrolithiasis caused by mutations of *CLCN5* (Dent1, about 60% of cases) or *OCRL* (Dent2, about 15–20% of cases), causing endolysosome dysfunction in the kidney [83, 84]. Progressive proximal tubule damage leads to a partial Fanconi syndrome, with low molecular weight proteinuria in affected males, with some developing rickets. Hypercalciuria and nephrocalcinosis are common (99%) in young males, but only about 25% develop stones (calcium oxalate and calcium phosphate) in childhood [85]. Urinary oxalate and citrate are usually within the normal range [85]. About half develop ESKD between the third and fifth decades of life. Females may be mildly affected, but kidney stone and progressive renal insufficiency are uncommon.

The optimal treatment of Dent disease is unclear but, since hypercalciuria, nephrocalcinosis and nephrolithiasis are prominent early features, Raja et al. tested a combination of chlorthalidone and amiloride to treat a cohort of Dent disease patients. They found that the diuretics reduced hypercalciuria and decreased calcium phosphate and calcium oxalate supersaturation by 35% and 25%, respectively [86]. However, it is unclear whether this strategy can slow the progressive loss of GFR [86].

Bartter Syndrome, a recessively inherited disorder, is caused by mutations in genes (*SLC12A1, KCNJ1, ROMK, CLCNKB, BSND*) that cause dysfunction of the apical transport mechanism for sodium, potassium and chloride in the thick ascending limb of the loop of Henle (TALH). Massive salt and water loss may cause polyhydramnios, hyponatremia and failure to thrive in infancy and hyperreninemic hypokalemic alkalosis due to compensatory mechanisms in the distal nephron. Since TALH dysfunction causes hypercalciuria by blocking paracellular reabsorption of calcium, Bartter syndrome patients may develop stones in childhood, but this is rare. Halbritter found no mutant Bartter genes in their screen of 106 serial children with nephrolithiasis recruited from specialized stone clinics [79]. However, nephrocalcinosis is common.

Adenine Phosphoribosyl Transferase Deficiency is due to biallelic mutations of *APRT*, which causes recurrent stones from high urinary levels of 2,8 dihydroxy adenine (DHA) and progressive renal insufficiency [87]. The stones are radiolucent and urinary crystals have a Maltese cross pattern [88]. Excessive DHA production is treated with xanthine oxidase inhibitors (allopurinol and febuxostat) and these therapies can reduce new stone formation [89]. Patients with mistargeting mutations are often responsive to pyridoxal phosphate (10 mg/kg/day).

Idiopathic Infantile Hypercalcemia is a syndrome of 1,25-dihydroxy vitamin D excess caused by biallelic mutations of *CYP24A1* (encoding a key enzyme of the renal vitamin D degradative pathway) or *SLC34A1* (encoding the sodium-phosphate co-transporter, NaPi2). Infants with *CYP24A1 mutations* present with hypercalcemia due to 1,25-dihydroxy vitamin D excess, failure to thrive, episodes of vomiting and dehydration and sterile pyuria. Initial treatment usually involves strategies to limit intestinal calcium absorption such as prednisone (0.5–2.0 mg/kg/day) to suppress vitamin D receptor expression in the small intestine, oral phosphate supplements (25–50 mg phosphate/kg/day) to bind dietary calcium. Oral supplements of vitamin D should be discontinued. As a longer-term strategy, bisphosphonates can be used to limit the flux of calcium from bone. Infants usually show marked clinical improvement and normal weight gain once serum calcium is normalized. Calcium stone formation presumably correlates with normalization of urinary calcium excretion, but this has not been formally studied. Interestingly, the need for medical therapy tends to diminish in the first years of life, although the mechanism is unknown.

Hereditary hypophosphatemic rickets with hypercalciuria (HHRH) is caused by biallelic mutations of *SLC34A3*, which encodes the sodium-phosphate co-transporter NPT2c in the renal proximal tubule. Infants present with metabolic bone disease resembling X-linked hypophosphatemic rickets (hypophosphatemia, bowing of legs) but with higher levels of 1,25-dihydroxy vitamin D. The latter drives hyperabsorption of dietary calcium, suppression of PTH and hypercalciuria. About one third of these patients develop calcium phosphate (brushite) stones [90]. Treatment usually consists of oral phosphate supplements to repair bone (without oral vitamin D as would be given in X-linked hypophosphatemic rickets) but the long-term effect on nephrolithiasis has not been studied.

Stones and Structural Abnormalities of the Urinary Tract

Conditions associated with urinary stasis cause crystal and stone formation, and include primary megaureter, polymegacalicosis, medullary sponge disease, autosomal dominant polycystic kidney disease, ureteropelvic junction obstruction, ureterocele, horseshoe kidney, bladder exstrophy, neuropathic bladder and surgically reconstructed or augmented bladders. Polymegacalicosis is a congenital abnormality with a higher number (more than 12) and larger in size calyces, and can be isolated or part of a syndrome.

Stones and Urinary Tract Infection

UTIs occur in about 1/4 of children with nephrolithiasis and may be either the cause or the effect of a kidney stone. The distinction between the two is important for further management, but can be difficult to distinguish, but the stone analysis may provide helpful clues. Usually, the stone associated with infection has a mixed composition, with the surface made of struvite and the core containing calcium-oxalate. In contrast, the stone induced by infection (so-called infectious or triple-phosphate stone) is entirely made of struvite (magnesium ammonium phosphate). The infectious stone is commonly seen in boys younger than 5 years of age with obstructive uropathy (e.g. ureteropelvic junction obstruction, urethral valves, primary megaureter). Urease produced by bacteria such as Proteus, Klebsiella, Pseudomonas, and enterococci metabolizes urea into ammonium and bicarbonate. This creates a favorable milieu for struvite stones, which can further grow into the renal calyces, and produce "staghorn" calculi with high morbidity. It is important to note that patients with struvite stones and negative urine culture should be evaluated for Ureaplasma urealyticum infection. Other patients prone to struvite stones are those with a neurogenic bladder.

An important consideration in children with urinary tract stones and urinary tract infections is that organisms within the stone may produce a biofilm that excludes certain antibiotics. Therapeutic options include a protracted course of an antibiotic, an antibiotic with good biofilm penetration and aggressive efforts to remove the stone.

Drug-Induced Nephrolithiasis

Drug-induced nephrolithiasis is uncommon in children, and causes 1–2% of stones, but its recognition is important for optimal management. Besides the specific drug, other contributory risk factors include higher drug dose, prolonged duration of treatment, poor hydration, the urine pH (which will affect the drug solubility), and the age of the patient (younger patients are at higher risk).

The responsible drugs are classified based on the mechanism involved in stone formation. The first category involves poorly soluble drugs that directly or through their metabolites induce urine supersaturation and increase the risk of crystallization. More common examples are triamterene (used in the treatment of Liddle syndrome), indinavir (used in HIV treatment) and antibacterial drugs, including third-generation cephalosporins (such as ceftriaxone and cefotaxime), sulfa drugs, nitrofurantoin, broad-spectrum penicillins, and fluoroquinolones. Usually these stones are radiolucent and therefore cannot be seen on plain X-rays unless they also contain calcium. The sec-

ond category are drugs that cause metabolic changes in the urine, such as furosemide, acetazolamide, topiramate, zonisamide and allopurinol. Furosemide causes inhibition of calcium reabsorption and hence hypercalciuria, while acetazolamide inhibits the proximal tubular reabsorption of bicarbonate leading to metabolic acidosis, alkaline urine and hypocitraturia. Anticonvulsants such as topiramate and zonisamide have carbonic anhydrase inhibitory activity causing acidosis that leads to bone resorption and hypercalciuria, as well as hypocitraturia. Allopurinol increases urinary excretion of xanthine, which has low urinary solubility (Fig. 46.2).

Intoxication with ethylene glycol following accidental or intentional ingestion of antifreeze leads to excessive production of oxalic acid causing calcium oxalate deposition in the kidneys and resulting in acute renal failure. Other substances reported to cause similar problems include xylitol (a constituent of parenteral nutrition), methoxyflurane (anesthetic agent), ascorbic acid, piridoxilate, and food high in oxalate (carambola or start fruit, sorrel and rhubarb).

Specific Pediatric Populations at Risk for Nephrolithiasis

Premature and low birth weight infants have an increased risk for nephrolithiasis and nephrocalcinosis for several reasons: metabolic disturbances related to parenteral nutrition (hypercalciuria and hyperoxaluria), use of loop diuretic (e.g. furosemide) and nephrotoxic drugs [25], and renal tubular immaturity causing changes in urine composition. About half of these patients show spontaneous resolution of nephrocalcinosis within several years, although a few patients may have persistent hypercalciuria.

Inflammatory bowel disease and other diseases of the gastrointestinal tract associated with malabsorption can cause metabolic disturbances leading to stone formation. These patients can develop hyperoxaluria (due to increased enteric

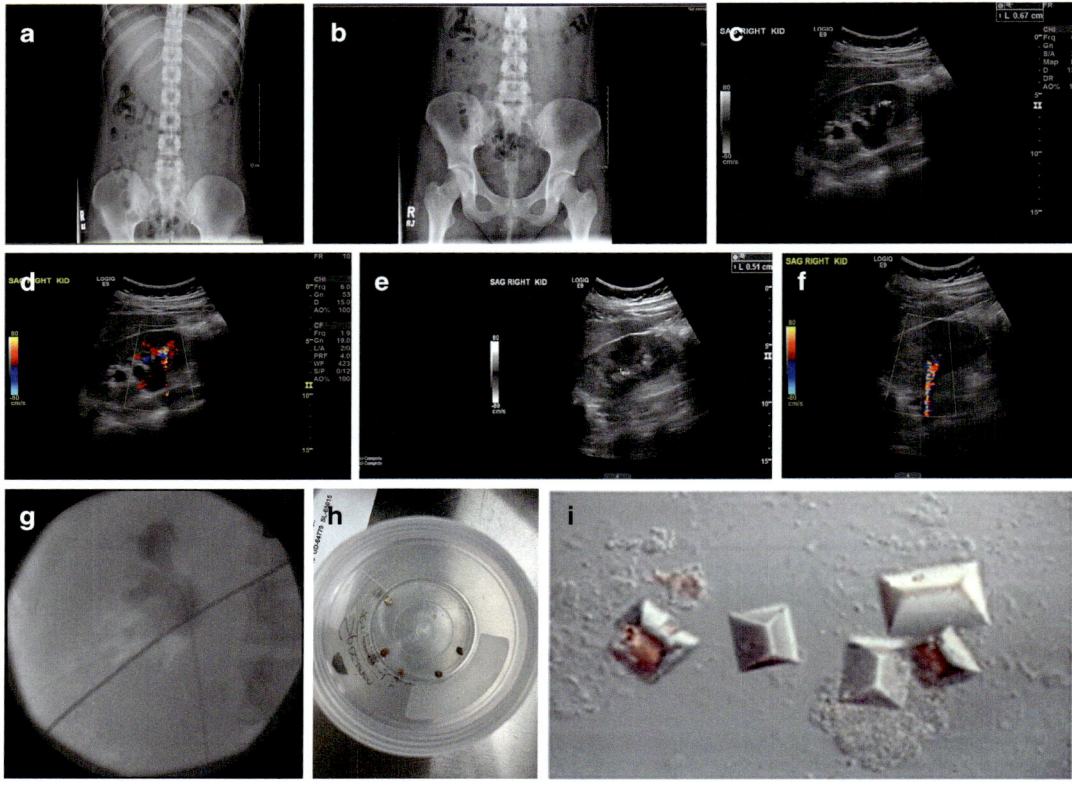

Fig. 46.2 Plain X-ray in an 18-year-old girl showing a 5 mm calcific density overlying the mid to lower pole of the right kidney consistent with calculus (**a**), and a 4 mm calcific density in the pelvis on the right side presumably in the distal ureter or bladder (**b**). Renal ultrasound showed moderate hydronephrosis of the right collecting system (**c**) and a 0.67 cm in the lower pole (**c**). Color ultrasound demonstrated acoustic shadowing behind the stone, creating the "twinkle artifact" (**d**). An additional stone was noted in the mid-polar region of the right kidney (**e**, **f**). Despite right hydronephrosis, no ureteral stones were detected by ultrasound. However, cystoscopy confirmed that there was a right obstructing ureterovesical junction stone and this required ureteral stent placement (**g**). Retrieved stones were composed of 80% calcium phosphate and 20% calcium oxalate (**h**). Urinalysis showed triple phosphate crystals (**i**). (**a**) A 5 mm calcific density overlying the mid to lower pole of the right kidney consistent with calculus (arrow). (**b**) A 4 mm calcific density in the pelvis on the right side presumably in the distal ureter or bladder (arrow). (**c**) Stone measuring 0.67 cm in the lower pole of the right kidney and right hydronephrosis. (**d**) Acoustic shadowing behind the stone creating the "twinkle artifact". (**e**) Stone measuring 0.51 cm in the midpole of the right kidney. (**f**) Acoustic shadowing behind the stone creating the "twinkle artifact." (**g**) Cystoscopy demonstrating placement of a right ureteral stent with its proximal pigtail in the region of the right renal pelvis, and the injection of contrast into a dilated right renal collecting system. (**h**) Macroscopic appearance of the surgically removed stones that showed mixed calcium phosphate and calcium oxalate composition. (**i**) Triple phosphate crystals on contrast microscopy (160× magnification)

absorption of oxalate), decreased urine citrate and hypomagnesuria (due to stool loses of bicarbonate and magnesium), hyperuricosuria (due to increased cell turnover), and low urinary volume induced by diarrhea. Patients with cystic fibrosis can develop calcium oxalate nephrolithiasis and nephrocalcinosis. Uric acid stones may also form due to acidic urine.

Patients with neurological disease represent another category at risk for renal stones. Risk factors in this population include reduced fluid intake, medications that predispose to stones (anticonvulsants), ketogenic diet used for the treatment of seizures, and decreased or absent ambulation.

Obesity has been associated with lower urine pH and volume, and increased urinary excretion of uric acid, oxalate, sodium and phosphate, indicating that these children may be at higher risk for renal stones in general and uric acid stones in particular. Additionally, insulin resistance causes impaired renal ammonia production. While some studies found an association between body mass index and pediatric nephrolithiasis, others believe that additional lithogenic risk factors are necessary in order to develop a stone [5, 11, 91].

Management

Dietary Considerations

High intake of fluid, vegetables and fruit, and salt restriction should be recommended in all patients with nephrolithiasis regardless of cause [92]. Aggressive fluid intake at 1.5 times "maintenance" is aimed to prevent tubular precipitation of renal stone promoters. Targeted fluid goal can be calculated using either body surface area (minimum 2 L/m^2) or desired age-related daily urinary volume: infants ≥750 mL; children below 5 years of age ≥1000 mL; children 5–10 years of age ≥1500 mL; children >10 years of age ≥2000 mL. Water should be encouraged because other beverages may contribute to increased calorie intake, an undesired effect in overweight children. Additionally, the fructose found in sugary drinks could further enhance the stone risk by increasing urinary excretion of calcium and oxalate.

High intake of fruit and vegetables is desirable in all patients because they represent a good source of potassium (which facilitates urinary citrate excretion) and phytates (which increase calcium salt solubility). Sodium should be restricted to <3 mEq/kg/day. Patients should be advised to avoid adding salt or sodium-rich seasoning to food during preparation or consumption. Families should be educated to read food labels, and to choose food with low sodium High-salt foods such as processed and canned food, fast food, pickles and olives, salt crackers and pizza should be avoided.

Restriction of calcium and protein intake is not recommended in children because they are both needed for growth and bone health, and should be consumed at 100% of the daily allowance. Moreover, calcium binds to free oxalate in the digestive tract and prevents hyperoxaluria. If not consumed with meals, calcium supplements may increase the risk of calcium oxalate stones. Vitamin D should be monitored and supplemented if low.

Urinary alkalinization to achieve a pH >7.0 can be achieved with oral potassium citrate or high lemon extract intake ("Lemon Protocol") and is useful in patients with dRTA, hypercalciuria, hyperoxaluria, hyperuricosuria, hypocitraturia and cystinuria. This can be achieved with a diet rich in whole grains and with cranberry extract. However, high intake of lemon or cranberry may not be well tolerated by children leading to non-compliance.

The renal dietitian has a key role in identifying the nutritive risk factors for nephrolithiasis, which is important for both treatment and prevention of stone recurrence. Patients should be asked to complete a dietary diary at the same time as the 24-h urine collection. The diary should include the type and amount of each consumed food and drink. Disease-specific dietary considerations are addressed in Table 46.6.

Surgical Treatment

Surgical management is indicated for larger, obstructing and infected stones, and in those who develop sepsis, acute kidney injury and have pain refractory to analgesics. A retrospective pediatric study of 129 patients found it to be extremely rare for stones >5 mm to pass spontaneously [23]. Despite revolutionary advances in pediatric endourological techniques and the development of small endoscopic instruments such as Miniperc and Microperc, surgical management of stones continues to pose technical challenges and requires a skilled pediatric urologist. A shift in the surgical approach has been noted in recent years. While the majority of stones were treated by open surgery in the past, now this is mainly reserved for patients with

Table 46.6 Dietary and pharmacologic intervention in pediatric nephrolithiasis

Condition	Dietary	Pharmacologic
Hypercalciuria	• High fluid intake • Restricted sodium • High potassium diet • RDA for calcium intake • Moderate animal protein • High fiber and low in oxalate	• Hydrochlorothiazide (1–2 mg/kg per day, older children 25–100 mg/day)-may need potassium supplementation if hypokalemia occurs • Potassium citrate in dRTA (2–4 mEq/kg/day, older children 30–90 mEq/day)
Hypocitraturia	• High fluid intake • RDA for animal protein intake • High lemon intake • High in fruit and vegetables	• Potassium citrate (2–4 mEq/kg/day, older children 30–90 mEq/day)
Hyperoxaluria	• Very high fluid intake (>3 L/1.73/m^2/day) • Moderate oxalate restriction (avoid spinach, nuts) • High magnesium and potassium • Low-fat diet • Avoid excessive vitamin C • RDA for calcium intake	• Potassium citrate (2–4 mEq/kg/day, older children 30–90 mEq/day) • Pyridoxine (8–10 mg/kg per day) for primary hyperoxaluria • Neutral phosphate (25–30 mg/kg/day of elemental phosphate divided into 3–4 doses) • Magnesium
Hyperuricosuria	• High fluid intake • RDA for animal protein intake • Restricted sodium • Avoid red meats	• Potassium citrate (2–4 mEq/kg/day, older children 30–90 mEq/day) • Allopurinol (4–10 mg/kg/day, older children 300 mg per day)[a]
Cystinuria	• Very high fluid intake (day and night) • Low protein diet (avoid excessive consumption of eggs, fish, meat, cheese)	• Potassium citrate (2–4 mEq/kg/day, older children 30–90 mEq/day)[b] • Alpha-mercapto-propionyl-glycine (Thiola) (10–15 mg/kg/day) • D-Penicillamine (30 mg/kg/day divided in 4 doses) • Captopril (0.5–1.5 mg/kg/day divided in 4 doses)

Abbreviations: *RDA* recommended daily allowance, *dRTA* distal renal tubular acidosis
[a] Reserved for children with a known disorder of uric acid metabolism
[b] Dose targeted to achieve a urine pH equal to or above 7.0

associated congenital renal anomalies requiring anatomical repair combined with stone removal (such as ureteropelvic or ureterovesical junction obstruction), for infected and staghorn stones, and for patients with previous multiple abdominal surgeries (augmented bladder with large bladder calculus).

Various minimally invasive surgery (MIS) techniques have been developed and are increasingly being used. These include extracorporeal shock wave lithotripsy (ESWL), ureteroscopy (URS), percutaneous nephrolithotomy (PCNL), and laparoscopic and robotic surgery (pyelolithotomy and nephrolithotomy). Their specific indications, advantages and complications are presented in Table 46.7.

MIS allows faster recovery and less pain than open surgery, but has an increased risk for the need for repeated procedures.

The choice of surgical intervention depends on the child's age and body habitus, stone characteristics (composition, size, and location), number of calculi (single vs. multiple), presence of obstruction or infection, the anatomy of the urinary tract, associated conditions (bladder dysfunction), patient or family preference, and the surgeon's experience and skills. Careful patient selection for the best choice of MIS ensures a better outcome for stone treatment and renal preservation as well as increased safety. Complete stone clearance is crucial for the prevention of stone recurrence, known to be high in children [8, 93, 94]. The remaining stone fragments can facilitate bacteria growth and become a nidus for a new struvite stone. Each MIS technique can cause gross hematuria, UTI or urosepsis, renal subcapsular hematoma, renal parenchymal injuries and injury to surrounding structures.

Table 46.7 Surgical management of pediatric nephrolithiasis

Indications and advantages	Specific complications
Extracorporeal shock wave lithotripsy	Ureteric obstruction with stone fragments causing pain
First line treatment of small renal and proximal ureteral stones<1.5 cm	Debate on the long-term effect on the kidney development
Non-invasive outpatient approach	
High safety, minimal morbidity	
Overall success range 81–96%	
Ureteroscopy/retrograde intrarenal surgery	Shorter operative time and in-hospital stay due to less invasive approach
Best choice for stones located in the lower pole calices (<1.5–2 cm) and for mid- or distal ureteral stones (<1 cm)	Ureteral injury, which may be prevented by a double stent placement for
Overall success rate 47–100%	2–3 weeks before the treatment to induce passive ureteral dilatation
Good visualization due to their fiber optic and video systems	
Wide range in size scopes 4.5–12 Fr, allowing use in children of all ages and sizes	
The stone can be directly extracted (using basket or grasping forceps), or can be fragmented (by laser or electrohydraulic or ultrasonic probes)	
Percutaneous nephrolithotomy	Longer operative time and in-hospital stay due to more invasive approach
Kidney stones >1.5 cm	Hemorrhage (0.4–23.9% cases) (can be severe requiring blood transfusion)
Staghorn stones	Can be difficult in patients with obesity, hemorrhagic diathesis and renal tumors
Overall success range 67–100%	Renal pelvis perforation
Laparoscopic and robotic surgery (pyelolithotomy and nephrolithotomy)	Shorter operative time and in-hospital stay due to less invasive approach
Hard stones difficult to fragment (staghorn calculi, stone in calyceal diverticulum)	Lower rate of bleeding and sepsis
When simultaneous reconstruction and repair is needed (concurrent ureteropelvic junction obstruction)	
Stones in ectopic kidney	
Failed previous endourological procedures; stones containing gas	
Excellent clearance rate up to 96% due to complete stone removal without fragmentation	
Reduced need for repeat procedures	
It can be done retroperitoneally	
Improving suturing and reconstruction	

Extracorporeal Shock Wave Lithotripsy

ESWL is usually successful in children and is becoming the first-line intervention in many centers. The likelihood of success depends on stone size (lower with larger stones), stone location (poorer with calyceal stones located in the lower pole compared to those located in the upper and mid-pole), stone composition (lower with struvite, cystine and calcium oxalate monohydrate), and the number of previous ESWL sessions. Struvite fragments in particular are friable facilitating stone fragment retention. Decreased urine output in CKD may also compromise the stone clearance. Success rates are lower in children with abnormal anatomy of the urinary tract or obesity.

During the procedure, it is important that the shock waves pass into the body and hit the stone with minimal loss of energy. New generation instruments that use a smaller focal area and provide less energy have been developed. The shock waves fragment the stones and the patient passes fragments spontaneously, although some need a stent placed at the time of ESWL. An ESWL method called ramping decreases the risk of complications. It starts with low energy shockwaves, followed by a stepwise increase in the power. This allows the surgeon to find the lowest energy level at which a stone starts to disintegrate, therefore avoiding overtreatment and decreasing the risk of tissue injury and bleeding. Repeated ESWL may be needed for stones >1.5 cm, and nomograms and scoring systems for prediction of outcomes after ESWL have been developed [93, 95, 96]. Younger children require the insertion of a ureteral stent. One major concern with ESWL use is the potential for damaging the developing kidney. In a small study of 16 children, no significant changes in serum creatinine and kidney morphology were found on ultrasound imaging post ESWL. Subsequent studies showed no significant impairment in kidney growth, loss of kidney function or the development of parenchymal scarring or hypertension after ESWL/PCNL. However, transient enzymuria and elevated urinary β2-microglobulin indicating proximal renal tubular dysfunction can be found post ESWL, but resolves 14 days following the procedure [46] (Fig. 46.3).

Stones >1.5–2 cm are not usually amenable to ESWL, and will require other surgical techniques including PCNL, URS/retrograde intrarenal surgery (RIS) and robotic-assisted pyelolithotomy (RPL) [97]. Nephrectomy may be a consideration if renal function is markedly decreased, in association with a large stone burden and recurrent UTIs. Infected stones require careful antibiotic treatment because bacteria may be released during stone fragmentation following any surgical procedure. Bladder stones are managed endoscopically via the urethra (per-urethral cystolith-

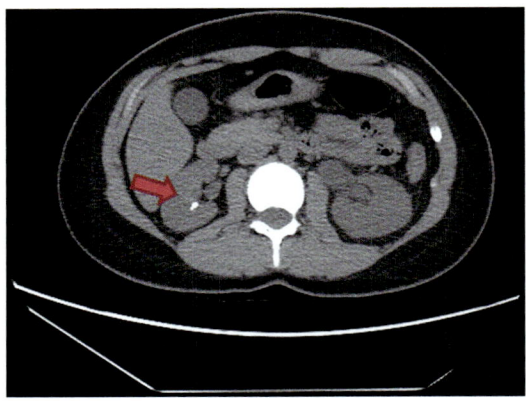

Fig. 46.4 CT imaging of stone: Non-obstructive 5 mm radiopaque calculus is demonstrated at the inferior polar region of the right kidney

otripsy), or via percutaneous cystolithotripsy. Open surgery may be needed in patients with reconstructed urinary bladders (Fig. 46.4).

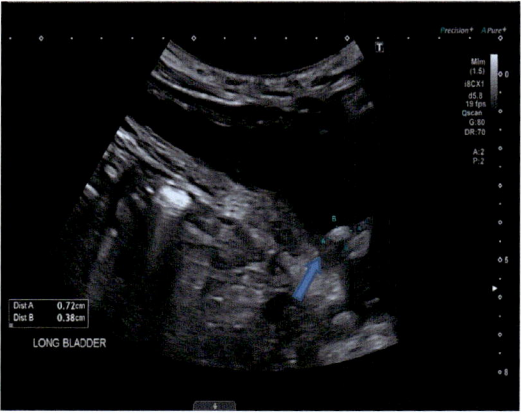

Fig. 46.3 Real time gray scale ultrasound of the urinary bladder in a 20-year-old male with history of neurogenic bladder. Echogenic debris is noted within the bladder. A shadowing calculus that measures approximately 0.7 cm is noted within the dependent portion of the urinary bladder (arrow)

References

1. Dwyer ME, et al. Temporal trends in incidence of kidney stones among children: a 25-year population based study. J Urol. 2012;188(1):247–52.
2. Sas DJ, et al. Increasing incidence of kidney stones in children evaluated in the emergency department. J Pediatr. 2010;157(1):132–7.
3. Bush NC, et al. Hospitalizations for pediatric stone disease in United States, 2002–2007. J Urol. 2010;183(3):1151–6.
4. Bowen DK, Tasian GE. Pediatric stone disease. Urol Clin North Am. 2018;45(4):539–50.
5. Sas DJ. An update on the changing epidemiology and metabolic risk factors in pediatric kidney stone disease. Clin J Am Soc Nephrol. 2011;6(8):2062–8.
6. Schissel BL, Johnson BK. Renal stones: evolving epidemiology and management. Pediatr Emerg Care. 2011;27(7):676–81.
7. Kovacevic L, et al. From hypercalciuria to hypocitraturia—a shifting trend in pediatric urolithiasis? J Urol. 2012;188(4 Suppl):1623–7.
8. Tasian GE, et al. Annual incidence of nephrolithiasis among children and adults in South Carolina from 1997 to 2012. Clin J Am Soc Nephrol. 2016;11(3):488–96.
9. Grases F, Sohnel O, Costa-Bauza A. Renal stone formation and development. Int Urol Nephrol. 1999;31(5):591–600.
10. Ferraro PM, et al. Soda and other beverages and the risk of kidney stones. Clin J Am Soc Nephrol. 2013;8(8):1389–95.

11. Gambaro G, et al. Crystals, Randall's plaques and renal stones: do bone and atherosclerosis teach us something? J Nephrol. 2004;17(6):774–7.

12. Gambaro G, Ferraro PM, Capasso G. Calcium nephrolithiasis, metabolic syndrome and the cardiovascular risk. Nephrol Dial Transplant. 2012;27(8):3008–10.

13. Goldfarb DS. Kidney stones and the risk of coronary heart disease. Am J Kidney Dis. 2013;62(6):1039–41.

14. Reiner AP, et al. Kidney stones and subclinical atherosclerosis in young adults: the CARDIA study. J Urol. 2011;185(3):920–5.

15. Sakhaee K. Nephrolithiasis as a systemic disorder. Curr Opin Nephrol Hypertens. 2008;17(3):304–9.

16. Taylor EN, Stampfer MJ, Curhan GC. Diabetes mellitus and the risk of nephrolithiasis. Kidney Int. 2005;68(3):1230–5.

17. Jungers P, et al. ESRD caused by nephrolithiasis: prevalence, mechanisms, and prevention. Am J Kidney Dis. 2004;44(5):799–805.

18. Valentini RP, Lakshmanan Y. Nephrolithiasis in children. Adv Chronic Kidney Dis. 2011;18(5):370–5.

19. Li Y, et al. Stone formation in patients less than 20 years of age is associated with higher rates of stone recurrence: results from the Registry for Stones of the Kidney and Ureter (ReSKU). J Pediatr Urol. 2020;16(3):373.e1–6.

20. Routh JC, Graham DA, Nelson CP. Epidemiological trends in pediatric urolithiasis at United States freestanding pediatric hospitals. J Urol. 2010;184(3):1100–4.

21. Novak TE, et al. Sex prevalence of pediatric kidney stone disease in the United States: an epidemiologic investigation. Urology. 2009;74(1):104–7.

22. Edvardsson V, et al. High incidence of kidney stones in Icelandic children. Pediatr Nephrol. 2005;20(7):940–4.

23. Pietrow PK, et al. Clinical outcome of pediatric stone disease. J Urol. 2002;167(2 Pt 1):670–3.

24. Kalorin CM, et al. Pediatric urinary stone disease—does age matter? J Urol. 2009;181(5):2267–71; discussion 2271.

25. Marra G, et al. Pediatric nephrolithiasis: a systematic approach from diagnosis to treatment. J Nephrol. 2019;32(2):199–210.

26. Finlayson B, Reid F. The expectation of free and fixed particles in urinary stone disease. Invest Urol. 1978;15(6):442–8.

27. Kok DJ, Khan SR. Calcium oxalate nephrolithiasis, a free or fixed particle disease. Kidney Int. 1994;46(3):847–54.

28. Randall A. The origin and growth of renal calculi. Ann Surg. 1937;105(6):1009–27.

29. Evan AP, et al. Randall's plaque of patients with nephrolithiasis begins in basement membranes of thin loops of Henle. J Clin Invest. 2003;111(5):607–16.

30. Kwon MS, Lim SW, Kwon HM. Hypertonic stress in the kidney: a necessary evil. Physiology (Bethesda). 2009;24:186–91.

31. Alexander RT, et al. Hereditary distal renal tubular acidosis. In: Adam MP, et al., editors. GeneReviews((R)). Seattle, WA: University of Washington; 1993.

32. Bagga HS, et al. New insights into the pathogenesis of renal calculi. Urol Clin North Am. 2013;40(1):1–12.

33. Shekarriz B, Lu HF, Stoller ML. Correlation of unilateral urolithiasis with sleep posture. J Urol. 2001;165(4):1085–7.

34. Dogan HS, Tekgul S. Management of pediatric stone disease. Curr Urol Rep. 2007;8(2):163–73.

35. Dursun I, et al. Pediatric urolithiasis: an 8-year experience of single centre. Int Urol Nephrol. 2008;40(1):3–9.

36. Smith SL, et al. The role of the plain radiograph and renal tract ultrasound in the management of children with renal tract calculi. Clin Radiol. 2000;55(9):708–10.

37. Vrtiska TJ, et al. Role of ultrasound in medical management of patients with renal stone disease. Urol Radiol. 1992;14(3):131–8.

38. Persaud AC, et al. Pediatric urolithiasis: clinical predictors in the emergency department. Pediatrics. 2009;124(3):888–94.

39. McKay CP. Renal stone disease. Pediatr Rev. 2010;31(5):179–88.

40. Stapleton FB. Clinical approach to children with urolithiasis. Semin Nephrol. 1996;16(5):389–97.

41. Aydogdu O, et al. Effectiveness of doxazosin in treatment of distal ureteral stones in children. J Urol. 2009;182(6):2880–4.

42. Pickard R, et al. Medical expulsive therapy in adults with ureteric colic: a multicentre, randomised, placebo-controlled trial. Lancet. 2015;386(9991):341–9.

43. Velazquez N, et al. Medical expulsive therapy for pediatric urolithiasis: systematic review and meta-analysis. J Pediatr Urol. 2015;11(6):321–7.

44. Mokhless I, et al. Tamsulosin for the management of distal ureteral stones in children: a prospective randomized study. J Pediatr Urol. 2012;8(5):544–8.

45. Seitz C, et al. Medical therapy to facilitate the passage of stones: what is the evidence? Eur Urol. 2009;56(3):455–71.

46. Ranabothu S, Bernstein AP, Drzewiecki BA. Diagnosis and management of non-calcium-containing stones in the pediatric population. Int Urol Nephrol. 2018;50(7):1191–8.

47. Bergsland KJ, et al. Urine risk factors in children with calcium kidney stones and their siblings. Kidney Int. 2012;81(11):1140–8.

48. Cameron MA, Sakhaee K, Moe OW. Nephrolithiasis in children. Pediatr Nephrol. 2005;20(11):1587–92.

49. Gurgoze MK, Sari MY. Results of medical treatment and metabolic risk factors in children with urolithiasis. Pediatr Nephrol. 2011;26(6):933–7.

50. Prochaska M, et al. Relative supersaturation of 24-hour urine and likelihood of kidney stones. J Urol. 2018;199(5):1262–6.

51. Friedlander JI, et al. Do urinary cystine parameters predict clinical stone activity? J Urol. 2018;199(2):495–9.

52. Marangella M, et al. LITHORISK.COM: the novel version of a software for calculating and visualizing the risk of renal stone. Urolithiasis. 2021;49(3):211–7.

53. Resnick M, Pridgen DB, Goodman HO. Genetic predisposition to formation of calcium oxalate renal calculi. N Engl J Med. 1968;278(24):1313–8.

54. McGeown MG. Heredity in renal stone disease. Clin Sci. 1960;19:465–71.

55. Howles SA, et al. Genetic variants of calcium and vitamin D metabolism in kidney stone disease. Nat Commun. 2019;10(1):5175.

56. Palsson R, et al. Genetics of common complex kidney stone disease: insights from genome-wide association studies. Urolithiasis. 2019;47(1):11–21.

57. Urabe Y, et al. A genome-wide association study of nephrolithiasis in the Japanese population identifies novel susceptible Loci at 5q35.3, 7p14.3, and 13q14.1. PLoS Genet. 2012;8(3):e1002541.

58. Renkema KY, et al. TRPV5 gene polymorphisms in renal hypercalciuria. Nephrol Dial Transplant. 2009;24(6):1919–24.

59. Phillips R, et al. Citrate salts for preventing and treating calcium containing kidney stones in adults. Cochrane Database Syst Rev. 2015;10:CD010057.

60. Tekin A, et al. Oral potassium citrate treatment for idiopathic hypocitruria in children with calcium urolithiasis. J Urol. 2002;168(6):2572–4.

61. Sarica K. Pediatric urolithiasis: etiology, specific pathogenesis and medical treatment. Urol Res. 2006;34(2):96–101.

62. van der Voort PH, et al. Furosemide does not improve renal recovery after hemofiltration for acute renal failure in critically ill patients: a double blind randomized controlled trial. Crit Care Med. 2009;37(2):533–8.

63. Srivastava T, et al. Urine calcium/citrate ratio in children with hypercalciuric stones. Pediatr Res. 2009;66(1):85–90.

64. Shen J, Zhang X. Potassium citrate is better in reducing salt and increasing urine pH than oral intake of lemonade: a cross-over study. Med Sci Monit. 2018;24:1924–9.

65. Rodgers A, Allie-Hamdulay S, Jackson G. Therapeutic action of citrate in urolithiasis explained by chemical speciation: increase in pH is the determinant factor. Nephrol Dial Transplant. 2006;21(2):361–9.

66. Voskaki I, et al. Effect of hydrochlorothiazide on renal hypercalciuria. Child Nephrol Urol. 1992;12(1):6–9.

67. Parvin M, et al. The most important metabolic risk factors in recurrent urinary stone formers. Urol J. 2011;8(2):99–106.

68. Liern M, Bohorquez M, Vallejo G. Treatment of idiopathic hypercalciuria and its impact on associated diseases. Arch Argent Pediatr. 2013;111(2):110–4.

69. Reilly RF, Peixoto AJ, Desir GV. The evidence-based use of thiazide diuretics in hypertension and nephrolithiasis. Clin J Am Soc Nephrol. 2010;5(10):1893–903.

70. Wiederkehr MR, Moe OW. Uric acid nephrolithiasis: a systemic metabolic disorder. Clin Rev Bone Miner Metab. 2011;9(3–4):207–17.

71. Knoll T, et al. Urolithiasis through the ages: data on more than 200,000 urinary stone analyses. J Urol. 2011;185(4):1304–11.

72. Zaidman JL, Pinto N. Studies on urolithiasis in Israel. J Urol. 1976;115(6):626–7.

73. Ansari MS, et al. Spectrum of stone composition: structural analysis of 1050 upper urinary tract calculi from northern India. Int J Urol. 2005;12(1):12–6.

74. Cochat P, Groothoff J. Primary hyperoxaluria type 1: practical and ethical issues. Pediatr Nephrol. 2013;28(12):2273–81.

75. Hopp K, et al. Phenotype-genotype correlations and estimated carrier frequencies of primary hyperoxaluria. J Am Soc Nephrol. 2015;26(10):2559–70.

76. Cramer SD, et al. The gene encoding hydroxypyruvate reductase (GRHPR) is mutated in patients with primary hyperoxaluria type II. Hum Mol Genet. 1999;8(11):2063–9.

77. Greed L, et al. Metabolite diagnosis of primary hyperoxaluria type 3. Pediatr Nephrol. 2018;33(8):1443–6.

78. Prot-Bertoye C, et al. CKD and its risk factors among patients with cystinuria. Clin J Am Soc Nephrol. 2015;10(5):842–51.

79. Halbritter J, et al. Fourteen monogenic genes account for 15% of nephrolithiasis/nephrocalcinosis. J Am Soc Nephrol. 2015;26(3):543–51.

80. Parvex P, Pippi-Salle JL, Goodyer PR. Rapid loss of renal parenchyma after acute obstruction. Pediatr Nephrol. 2001;16(12):1076–9.

81. Malieckal DA, et al. Effect of increasing doses of cystine-binding thiol drugs on cystine capacity in patients with cystinuria. Urolithiasis. 2019;47(6):549–55.

82. Zhang J, et al. Incomplete distal renal tubular acidosis from a heterozygous mutation of the V-ATPase B1 subunit. Am J Physiol Renal Physiol. 2014;307(9):F1063–71.

83. Ehlayel AM, Copelovitch L. Update on dent disease. Pediatr Clin North Am. 2019;66(1):169–78.

84. Devuyst O, Thakker RV. Dent's disease. Orphanet J Rare Dis. 2010;5:28.

85. Anglani F, et al. Dent disease: a window into calcium and phosphate transport. J Cell Mol Med. 2019;23(11):7132–42.

86. Raja KA, et al. Responsiveness of hypercalciuria to thiazide in Dent's disease. J Am Soc Nephrol. 2002;13(12):2938–44.

87. Bollee G, et al. Phenotype and genotype characterization of adenine phosphoribosyltransferase deficiency. J Am Soc Nephrol. 2010;21(4):679–88.

88. Harambat J, et al. Adenine phosphoribosyltransferase deficiency in children. Pediatr Nephrol. 2012;27(4):571–9.

89. Runolfsdottir HL, et al. Long-term renal outcomes of APRT deficiency presenting in childhood. Pediatr Nephrol. 2019;34(3):435–42.

90. Dasgupta D, et al. Mutations in SLC34A3/NPT2c are associated with kidney stones and nephrocalcinosis. J Am Soc Nephrol. 2014;25(10):2366–75.

91. Van Batavia JP, Tasian GE. Clinical effectiveness in the diagnosis and acute management of pediatric nephrolithiasis. Int J Surg. 2016;36(Pt D):698–704.

92. Copelovitch L. Urolithiasis in children: medical approach. Pediatr Clin North Am. 2012;59(4): 881–96.

93. Sultan S, et al. Update on surgical management of pediatric urolithiasis. Front Pediatr. 2019;7:252.

94. Tasker RC, Acerini CL. Cerebral edema in children with diabetic ketoacidosis: vasogenic rather than cellular? Pediatr Diabetes. 2014;15(4):261–70.

95. Colleran GC, et al. Imaging in the diagnosis of pediatric urolithiasis. Pediatr Radiol. 2017;47(1):5–16.

96. Young BJ, et al. Is the economic impact and utilization of imaging studies for pediatric urolithiasis across the United States increasing? Urology. 2016;94:208–13.

97. Ghani KR, et al. Robotic nephrolithotomy and pyelolithotomy with utilization of the robotic ultrasound probe. Int Braz J Urol. 2014;40(1):125–6; discussion 126.

Voiding Disorders in Children

47

Johan Vande Walle and Søren Rittig

Abbreviations

AVP	Arginine vasopressin
CAKU	Congenital abnormalities of kidney and urinary tract
CKD	Chronic kidney disease
FBC	Functional bladder capacity
LUTS	Lower urinary tract symptoms
MNE	Monosymptomatic nocturnal enuresis
MVV	Maximal voided volume
NE	Nocturnal enuresis
OAB	Overactive bladder
PD	Pharmacodynamic
PK	Pharmacokinetic
PLMS	Periodic limb movements during sleep
UTI	Urinary tract infection
VCUG	Voiding cystourethrography
VUR	Vesicoureteral reflux

J. V. Walle (✉)
Department of Pediatrics, Section of Pediatric
Nephrology, Ghent University Hospital, Ghent
University, Ghent, Belgium
e-mail: Johan.Vandewalle@uzgent.be

S. Rittig
Department of Pediatrics and Adolescence Medicine,
Nephrology Section, Aarhus University Hospital,
Aarhus, DENMARK
e-mail: Rittig@clin.au.dk

Introduction

Wetting either the bed or pants is still one of the most feared events among children, especially when school age is reached, resulting in poor self-esteem and burden for child and parents [1–4]. It is one of the most common chronic disorders of childhood [5, 6]. Despite the high prevalence and negative psychological consequences, enuresis as a disease has not been of much interest to medical doctors, and there is little good clinical research, leading to a deficiency in medical training and absence of the subject in pediatric nephrology courses and handbooks [7–9]. Consequently, in most areas of the world the perception of pathophysiology and treatment are too simplified and guidelines insufficient, all resulting in a variety of non-evidence based approaches [10–16].

Voiding problems are often not benign, self-limiting conditions restricted to delayed acquirement of continence (daytime incontinence) and enuresis (bedwetting), but play a major role in many conditions in the interface between paediatric nephrology and urology. Voiding disorders include a complexity of conditions in children, caused by abnormalities in bladder function and diuresis. Bladder dysfunction is a well-known pathogenic or comorbid factor in urinary tract infections (UTIs) [17–19], in many congenital anomalies of the kidney and urinary tract (CAKUT) (uropathies) [20], constipation [21,

22] and neurogenic bladder [22–25]. The prevalence and importance of bladder dysfunction in children with chronic kidney disease (CKD) prior to and after transplantation is underestimated [26–28]. It is associated with hypertension, sleep disturbances, and cognitive dysfunction. Deficient concentrating capacity as well as circadian rhythm abnormalities of renal function, have been documented in patients with enuresis, but are also an essential characteristic of glomerular as well as tubular renal pathophysiology.

The International Children's Continence Society (ICCS) has standardized both the terminology and management of various aspects of incontinence in children, including enuresis, bladder overactivity, dysfunctional voiding, and psychological comorbidities. A number of guidelines have been published to aid those involved in the care of children with lower urinary tract (LUT) symptoms [8, 23, 29–35].

Nocturnal Enuresis

Definition and Epidemiology

Nocturnal enuresis (NE) is defined as intermittent incontinence that occurs exclusively during periods of sleep. Enuresis can be qualified as frequent (≥4 per week) or infrequent (<4 per week) [32, 36]. There is ample evidence that children with NE and concomitant symptoms of LUT dysfunction differ clinically and therapeutically from children without daytime symptoms [32, 34, 36, 37]. There is less evidence that the pathogenesis and genetic predisposition are different [38].

However, since enuresis is a common disorder and many patients can benefit from simple therapies (desmopressin, alarm and urotherapy), a strategy has been developed to identify patients who can be treated with a high success rate in primary care, thereby avoiding unnecessary exposure to secondary and tertiary care [2, 32, 36].

Enuresis without other LUT symptoms (nocturia excluded), and without bladder dysfunction, is defined as *monosymptomatic enuresis*. Children with enuresis and any LUT symptom have *non-monosymptomatic enuresis* (Fig. 47.1). Subtyping of NE in this manner is promoted in all guidelines, and helps direct the patient to the right therapy [33]. The rationale for this approach is the observation that non-monosymptomatic enuresis has a lower response rate to first line treatment with desmopressin, although the evidence is weak. Once daytime LUT symptoms have abated, the enuresis can be reclassified from the non-monosymptomatic to the monosymptomatic subgroup [33, 34] (Fig. 47.1). It is unclear if other LUTS symptoms beyond daytime incontinence have the same negative predictive value for therapy response.

In *primary* NE, the child has never been dry for a period longer than 6 months, whereas in *secondary* NE there has been such a period. Most

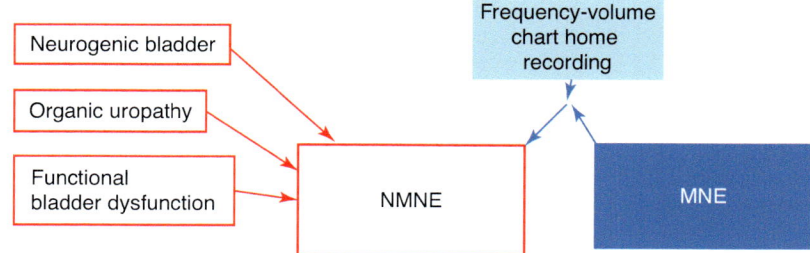

Fig. 47.1 Nocturnal enuresis can be subdivided into monosymptomatic enuresis (in absence of daytime symptoms) and non-monosymptomatic enuresis, when daytime symptoms (LUTS) are present. Children with daytime symptoms likely have underlying bladder dysfunction, and in the differential diagnosis, we should always exclude congenital uropathies and neurogenic bladder dysfunction, before considering it as functional bladder dysfunction

countries regard NE as pathological when it is present after the age of 5 years, but in practice it may be appropriate to delay treatment to 6–7 years of age. Although major importance was previously given to differences between primary and secondary enuresis, where secondary was more related to psychological problems [39, 40], there is an increase in the view that the diagnostic and treatment algorithm do not differ between the two subtypes.

NE is the most frequent disease in children after asthma, with a prevalence of 5–10% at the age of 7 years and of 0.5–1% during adulthood [5, 6, 9, 41–49]. More boys than girls have NE, although this difference tends to diminish after the age of 10 years. The spontaneous cure rate has been estimated to be approximately 15% annually between the age of 5 and 19 years, but is much lower in children with frequent bedwetting, making a 'wait and see' attitude unacceptable [5, 6].

Although only 15–30% of enuretic children were reported to experience daytime incontinence [8, 49] and were labelled non-monosymptomatic according to the old ICCS definition [50], a recent epidemiological, population-based study analyzed children aged 7.5 years and found that 15.5% wet the bed and 2.6% had a frequency of 2 or more wet episodes per week [51]. Of those children with 2 or more wet nights per week, 68.5% were classified as monosymptomatic and 31.5% as non-monosymptomatic. Other studies have estimated that more patients have subtle daytime symptoms of bladder dysfunction such as urgency or decreased or increased voiding frequency and thus qualify for the label non-monosymptomatic NE (NMNE) [34], leaving the subgroup of enuretic children who are truly monosymptomatic to less half of all bedwetting children [52–54]. The majority of guidelines and standardisation papers recommend to differentiate between MNE and NMNE, with the major aim to treat concurrent LUT symptoms before the enuresis. Thus, it has been documented that NMNE patients who have been resistant to desmopressin treatment become desmopressin responders after successful treatment of daytime LUT symptoms [52]. The prevalence of specific subtypes of NE is still unclear, since most of the available epidemiological studies either did not differentiate between MNE and NMNE, or used the previous pre-2006 ICCS definitions. After inclusion of all daytime LUT symptoms as qualifiers for NMNE, 30–50% of previously labeled MNE patients would be classified as NMNE [32, 55].

Pathophysiology

The pathophysiology of enuresis is complex, involving the central nervous system, circadian rhythm regulation (sleep, arousal, hormones), the kidney (diuresis, renal function), and bladder function disorders. It is widely accepted that the central nervous system, and especially dysregulation in control of biorhythms and bladder capacity, plays a major role. Several neurotransmitters and receptors may be involved. There is also a strong correlation with a variety of comorbidities, where it remains to be elucidated if there might be common pathways in pathogenesis and reciprocal effects (constipation, sleep, psychology, neurocognitive functions) [33].

NE in the majority of patients is caused by a mismatch between nocturnal diuresis and functional bladder capacity overnight in the presence of a deficient arousal mechanism [8, 56, 57]. Although some authors have proposed decreased arousability to be a primary mechanism in enuresis, direct evidence for this is rather week since only a minority of children (4.1%) acquire continence by waking them during the night [49]. Multiple mechanisms, discussed below, are involved in the pathogenesis.

Nocturnal Urine Production

In humans, a marked circadian rhythm of urine production is present from early childhood, with a pronounced nocturnal reduction in diuresis to approximately 50% of daytime levels [58–65]. This nyctohemeral rhythm of diuresis in children is controlled by increased nocturnal release of hormones that regulate free water excretion (arginine vasopressin, AVP) [58] as well as solute excretion (renin, angiotensin II, aldosterone, and atrial natriuretic peptide). These mechanisms are associated with multiple other circadian rhythms: sleep, melatonin, and blood pressure. Circumstances such as light/dark, sleep/awake, activity/rest, body posture, fluid and food intake, and temperature as well as several drugs may interfere with the circadian rhythm of diuresis [66–70]. Interestingly, acute sleep deprivation results in elevated blood pressures and increased solute and water excretion overnight [71].

The initial description by Poulton in the 1950s that children with NE have significantly larger nocturnal urine productions than non-enuretic children [64] has been confirmed by multiple authors [58, 59, 65, 72–74]. Consensus has been obtained that the optimal method of measuring this variable is diaper weighing and measurement of morning voided volume [33]. Nocturnal diuresis has significant night-to-night variation, making nocturnal polyuria only present intermittently [75]. The demonstration that nocturnal urine volume is significantly larger on wet nights compared with dry nights has emphasized that nocturnal polyuria should only be evaluated during nights where enuresis is experienced [76]. Patients with nocturnal polyuria are likely to be desmopressin responders, in absence of associated bladder dysfunction [59, 77–79]. Nocturnal polyuria is defined as nocturnal diuresis >130% of expected bladder capacity for age ((expected bladder capacity = age + 1)*30 mL)

One NE archetype is the patient without an increase in plasma arginine vasopressin (AVP) level during the early night, correlating with the occurrence of increased nocturnal diuresis (nocturnal polyuria) with low urinary osmolality as well as a good response to the AVP analogue desmopressin. Whether this deficit in AVP is always the primary cause or if it is in some cases secondary remains to be elucidated.

There is, however, growing evidence from studies in children who are refractory to desmopressin that the pathogenesis of nocturnal polyuria might be much more complex. Increased solute and sodium excretion overnight has been documented, both in absolute values, as a loss of circadian rhythm in a subpopulation of children with nocturnal polyuria and is probably multifactorial [80–83]. High osmotic load, especially in the evening, is associated with high diuresis rate overnight, but whether dietary intervention would be beneficial in such patients remains to be elucidated [82, 83]. Indirect evidence may have been provided by reports of an association between enuresis and metabolic syndrome and obesity. The increased sodium and osmotic excretion overnight may be caused by increased osmotic load (due to increased caloric intake) as well as abnormal circadian rhythm of osmole excretion [84–86].

Vasoactive hormones also play a potential role in NE pathogenesis, but results have so far not been convincing except for prostaglandins (PGs). Kamperis et al. found an abnormal circadian rhythm of urine PGs. Intervention with a PG inhibitor was, however, not superior to placebo [65, 80, 87]. Increased sodium excretion overnight may be secondary to increased sodium retention during daytime [81], a mechanism described in adults with nocturia. There is certainly a continuum between the pathogenesis of enuresis in adolescence and nocturia in adulthood [88–90]. The role of hypercalciuria has been overestimated, and is secondary to nutritional intake and renal sodium handling [81, 91–93].

Many pharmacokinetic (PK) and pharmacodynamic (PD) studies with desmopressin demonstrate that only 75% of enuresis patients reach >850 mosmol/L on therapeutic desmopressin doses, which is clearly a lower percentage than in control studies. This does not indicate a renal diabetes insipidus diagnosis, but might reflect the lower end of the normal spectrum, where a 20% loss of maximal concentrating capacity results in a 20% higher diuresis rate (the difference between 300 and 360 mL, or possibly between a dry and wet night) [94–96]. Since none of the studied PK/PD enuresis populations received intravenous vasopressin to study their maximal concentrating capacity, the question remains open if a subpopulation of enuresis patients have suboptimal ability to maximally concentrate the urine.

Glomerular dysfunction and specifically an abnormal circadian rhythm of glomerular filtration rate (GFR) might also play a pathogenic role. In healthy children and young adolescents, GFR decreases overnight by approximately 25%, a phenomenon that is absent in a subgroup of refractory enuresis patients [97]. This observation is in line with the decreased nocturnal dipping of blood pressure in children with nocturnal polyuria. The relationship between hypertension and absent circadian rhythm of blood pressure and nocturnal polyuria is well-known in adults and renal transplant patients [28, 70].

Bladder Function

Bladder function comprises a storage phase and a micturition phase. Micturition in infants and young children, until the age of 2–4 years, is involuntary. The functional bladder volume increases with age, and reaches a maximum at teenage. This maturation requires intact pathways in the central, pontine, spinal, and peripheral nervous systems. The innervation of the bladder is complex, with an interplay between the voluntary motor system and the ortho- and parasympathetic nervous systems.

The pathogenic role of functional abnormalities of the bladder in the pathogenesis of daytime LUTS and NMNE is accepted, but remains unclear in children with MNE. Organic abnormalities and neurogenic bladder are rare in children presenting with MNE, but should always be considered in the presence of daytime symptoms, history of UTI or enuresis refractory to conventional therapy.

In MNE, most evidence points towards a deficient development of nocturnal bladder reservoir function, at least in a subgroup of patients. Nocturnal bladder capacity in normal children is significantly larger than daytime capacity, probably due to inhibitory effects of sleep on the micturition centers. Nocturnal bladder capacity is not easy to measure in enuretic patients, even with diaper weighing, as many enuresis episodes are incomplete voids associated with significant residual urine [98]. However, when estimated as maximal voided volume (MVV) during daytime and excluding the first morning void, daytime bladder capacity is also reduced in many enuretics, even in MNE patients. Clinically, an esti-

mate of daytime bladder capacity is relatively easy to obtain and it has been shown to be of value when selecting a treatment modality in the individual patient. Thus, a MVV that is below 70% of the predicted MVV for age (age × 30 + 30 mL) has been shown to predict a poor response to desmopressin treatment [99–101]. This corroborates very closely the fact that alarm treatment, which that is highly effective in this patient subgroup, increases nocturnal bladder capacity, whereas nocturnal urine production does not change [101, 102].

Comorbidities

Voiding abnormalities are strongly associated with various comorbidities.

Constipation

The coexistence of LUT symptoms and functional constipation and/or faecal incontinence in children is not uncommon, and was previously identified as dysfunctional elimination syndrome (DES) [103–106] and more recently as 'bladder and bowel dysfunction' (BBD) [22]. Although the association with dysfunctional voiding, decreased voiding frequency and underactivity is obvious, there is also a clear comorbidity between bladder overactivity (urge), increased voiding frequency, bladder underactivity and constipation [21]. It is a well-established that treatment of defecation problems in children with BBD enhances successful management of LUT disturbances such as daytime urinary incontinence (DUI), enuresis, and UTIs [21, 22, 103]. Treatment of the bowel dysfunction ameliorates the voiding disorder and should be first-line treatment [21].

Psychological/Behavioural Problems: Attention Deficit, Neurocognitive Dysfunction

Psychological comorbidity among children with functional urinary incontinence is high: 20–30% of children with NE, 20–40% of children with DUI, and 30–50% of children with fecal incontinence (FI) [107–110]. Both internalizing and externalizing characteristics are represented [109, 111]. The best documented comorbidity conditions are attention deficit-hyperactivity disorder

(ADHD) and oppositional defiant disorder (ODD). Children with attention deficit disorders have a higher prevalence of enuresis (both MNE and NMNE), whereas the prevalence of ADHD in the enuresis population is up to four times higher than the background population. The association of abnormal prepulse inhibition (Startle reflex) in both ADHD and enuresis patients might suggest a common central nervous pathogenic pathway, but it is far from fully understood [109, 112–114].

Sleep
Regardless of the cause of the mismatch between nocturnal bladder capacity and nocturnal diuresis, enuresis only occurs when the child is unable to wake up; hence, lack of arousal is a prerequisite for NE. This has caused many to conclude that sleep disturbance *per se* is the major pathophysiological factor in enuresis and it is still a general belief in the general population that enuretic children are deep sleepers. However, this hypothesis has been questioned due to the inability to convincingly show abnormalities in sleep EEG patterns together with the observation that a considerable proportion of non-enuretic children also are unable to wake up when polyuria is induced overnight [11, 115–120].

It was documented that enuretic children did not exhibit deep sleep, but rather a disturbed sleep with increased periodic limb movements during sleep (PLMS), cortical arousals, and awakenings [66, 67, 121]. Polysomnography studies documented a significant difference in PLMS index, arousal index, and awakening index compared with healthy control subjects. The presence of sleep fragmentation does not exclude a high sleep pressure or high arousal threshold. The role of sleep fragmentation in children with NE was earlier emphasised using sleep actigraphy [122]. Obstructive sleep airway syndrome causes nocturnal polyuria in both children and adults, eventually resulting in enuresis [123–125]. The prevalence of this NE subtype in patients primarily consulting for NE is not known, but the anti-enuretic response to therapy to address obstructive sleep airway syndrome suggests that in refractory cases this might be considered [126–129].

In conclusion, albeit there is little doubt that sleep and/or arousal plays a role in the pathophysiology of NE, the clinical relevance and possible implications are still unclear and so far sleep investigation is not part of routine evaluation of enuretic children.

Hypertension
One of the first characteristics of arterial hypertension is the loss of nocturnal dipping and patients without nocturnal dipping have a poor cardiovascular prognosis. The association between hypertension and increased nocturnal diuresis is well-documented [28, 70].

Renal Diseases
Many renal diseases are associated with disrupted circadian rhythms of renal water and solute handling [60, 81, 83, 87, 97]. Thus, the kidney disease may have a role in causing the NE. However, such patients may have the same predisposition to NE as other children. Hence, they should have the same workup as any child with NE.

Drug Induced Changes in Circadian Rhythm
Many drugs result in disrupted circadian rhythms. The best known are the steroids, certainly when given twice a day or in high doses. Even a low dose at 08.00 h induces a shift in circadian rhythm, since the normal physiologic cortisol peak is 4 h earlier. Diuretics have of course a major effect on water and sodium excretion, especially long-acting thiazides, or loop-diuretics when they are given twice a day.

Genetics
NE has a strong hereditary component given that approximately 70% of NE patients have a positive family history and that monozygotic twin studies find concordance rates of 80%. Positive linkage was established between enuresis and several gene loci on different chromosomes (4p, 12q, 8q, 13q, and 22q). However, although several candidate genes have been proposed, no specific pathogenic variant has been identified. Moreover, it is unknown whether there is a

genotype-phenotype correlation to specific NE subtypes [38]. Interestingly, a recent genome wide association study in a large Danish population identified common genetic variants associated with NE. The study pinpointed potential NE risk genes, among which *PRDM13*, *SIM1*, and *EDNRB* might affect sleep, urine production, and bladder function, respectively. It also identified for the first time a significant genetic overlap between NE and ADHD [130].

Evaluation

In the child with *primary* NE, evaluation should not be initiated before 5 years of age. In contrast, children with *secondary* NE should be evaluated for an underlying etiology (e.g. diabetes mellitus, constipation, and UTI) when the wetting reappears. The initial approach to primary NE should avoid unnecessary investigations if there are no concerning symptoms (Fig. 47.1).

Evaluation should comprise a detailed history, with a focus on the duration and severity of the night wetting, but also inquire about LUT symptom such as daytime incontinence, increased or decreased daytime voiding frequency, urgency, voiding postponement, holding maneuvers, constant dribbling, and intermittent urinary stream. It is important to ask specific questions regarding LUT and bowel symptoms. A history of uropathy, UTI, and constipation suggests possible bladder dysfunction.

The physical examination should comprise the external genitalia (e.g. congenital anomalies, phimosis), the lumbar region (e.g. deformations, pigmentations, and hair growth), and neurological examination (e.g. ano-cutaneous and cremaster reflexes, lower extremity reflexes, muscle tone, and gait). Laboratory evaluation should include a urinalysis of a morning or spot urine sample, with examination for glucose, leukocytes, nitrite, and albumin. In the majority of children with NE, these investigations will be normal.

A cornerstone in the further evaluation of a child or adolescent with NE is an estimation of their bladder capacity and nocturnal urine pro-

duction. For this purpose, a frequency-volume chart (registration of the time and volume of all micturitions and fluid intakes during daytime) during two weekends and a recording of nighttime urine production (weight of diaper in the morning (g) − weight of diaper before bedtime (g) = volume of morning micturition (mL)) during 1 week are very useful approaches for obtaining this information. Compliance is usually good when the purpose is explained to the parents. Measurement of MVV (excluding the first morning void) needs to be made over a minimum of 3–4 days for accuracy: weekends or school holidays are ideal, but have the disadvantage that lifestyle is significantly different and often less structured than on schooldays [33, 76].

Treatment

The simplified evaluation process enables the identification of two archetypes of NE that correlate with their pathophysiologic characteristics (Fig. 47.2). The first archetype is children with MNE and no apparent LUTS; the mismatch between nocturnal diuresis and functional bladder capacity is caused by nocturnal polyuria. The majority of these patients will have low urinary osmolality overnight due to low vasopressin levels [18, 19], and will be desmopressin responsive. The second archetype is the "small for age" bladder capacity. These patients will likely be desmopressin resistant, and are expected to have a good response to the enuresis alarm [33]. A combination of both types is not uncommon and such patients generally respond well to combined therapy with desmopressin and an alarm [33]. If patients do not respond to one of these treatments, a more complicated underlying mechanism might be present and referral to a tertiary multidisciplinary centre should be considered.

Thus, a simple "trial and error" treatment strategy for enuresis is no longer recommended as it may even have an adverse psychological effect on the child [2]. A rational therapeutic approach as outlined in the ICCS standardization document [31, 33] leads to higher success rates.

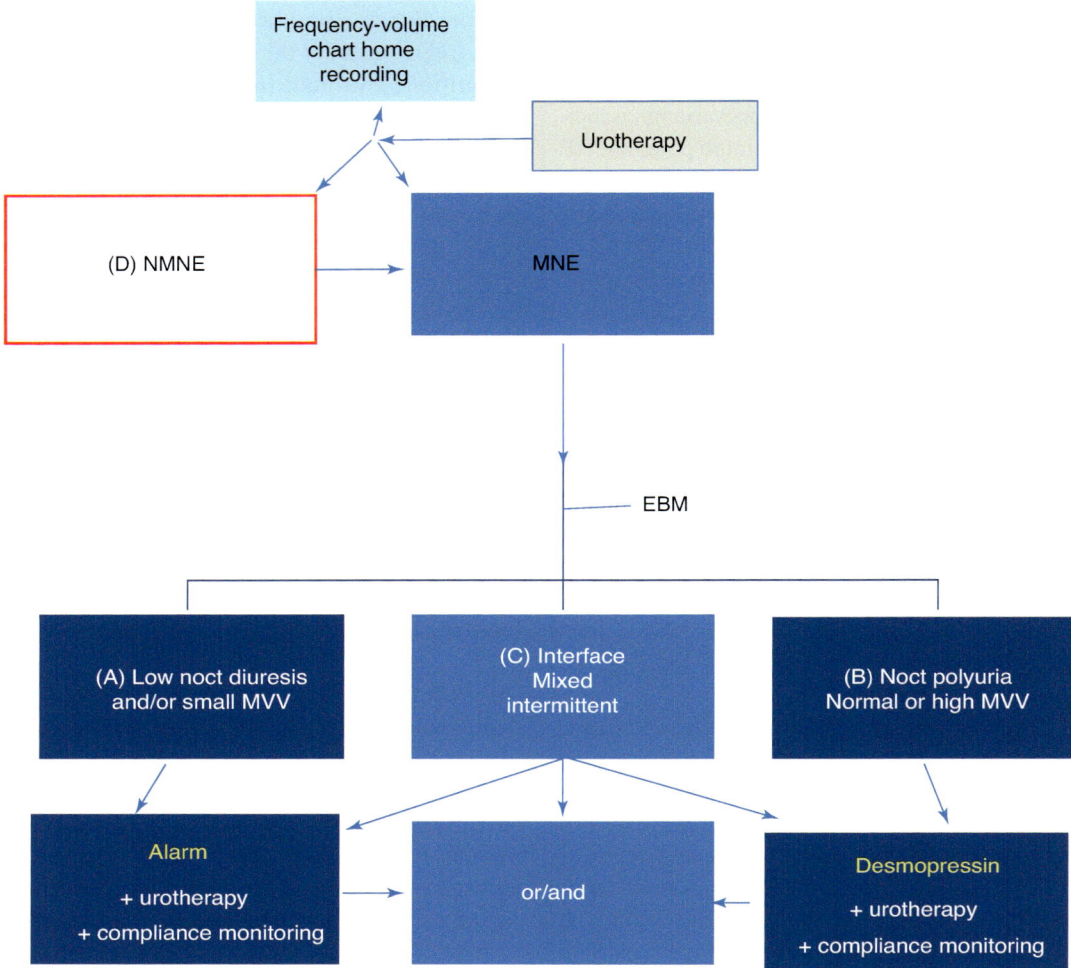

Fig. 47.2 A simple flow chart illustrating that noninvasive screening, identifying the subgroup of patients with monosymptomatic enuresis, may lead to a rationalized therapeutic approach in primary and secondary care avoiding unnecessary invasive investigations. All children should receive urotherapy according to the ICCS guidelines, including normalization of fluid- and nutritional intake, voiding pattern and sleep hygiene. If despite this urotherapy, enuresis persists, according to the ICCS standardization papers, children should only receive EBM therapies: the alarm and desmopressin. Although both therapies reach EBM IA levels, success rates vary between 30% and 60%, with high relapse rates. Targeting the underlying pathophysiological characteristics of the enuresis, and especially the mismatch between nocturnal diuresis volume and functional bladder capacity (MVV) overnight might lead to increased success rates. Patients can be subdivided into two archetypes, children with nocturnal polyuria (B) and children with overactive bladder (A). Children with low diuresis-rate overnight (and high osmolality) and/or small bladder capacity (MVV), are likely desmopressin resistant, and should receive the alarm as primary therapy. Children with nocturnal polyuria (+low osmolality) and normal bladder capacity (MVV) for age will likely benefit from antidiuretic therapy rather than from the alarm. Desmopressin should be first line therapy. For some there is a continuum between the two archetypes (C), where some children have only a mild, often intermittent mismatch, between diuresis and bladder, where each characteristic does not reach the level of abnormality as defined by the ICCS. In these children both therapy options are defendable. In cases, refractory to therapy or in the subgroup where we identify a combination of nocturnal polyuria and overactive bladder, combination therapy should be advocated. (D) NMNE-children with successful therapy of the LUTS symptoms can subsequently be treated as MNE patients

Therapy is often initiated at the age of 6–7 years, although enuresis is considered abnormal in children ≥5 years of age. Reasons for a proactive attitude towards treatment include the distress caused to child and family, difficulty with "sleeping over" on holiday or at friends' houses, social withdrawal, reduced self-esteem [2], disrupted sleep with possible secondary effects on cognitive function and health [119, 131–134], and the burden [3] and costs associated with frequent laundering of bedsheets and clothing [135, 136]. In addition, spontaneous resolution is low in children >5 years with frequent bedwetting; the negative impact on the child and family induces a risk for intolerance of some parents [137]. Whether early treatment reduces the prevalence in adulthood is unclear [5, 6, 88, 138–141].

Treatment [8–11]

Step 1: Demystification

Explanation of the pathophysiological mechanisms that are involved in enuresis is essential. Children and families should be convinced that bedwetting is a common problem, that they should not be embarrassed or feel guilt, and that it is definitely not a primary psychological problem. Patients should understand that the primary cause is a mismatch between nocturnal diuresis volume and the bladder capacity overnight.

Parents and children should be warned that success rates of monotherapy vary from 30% to 60%, leaving up to 1/3 with persistent symptoms after 1 year. This message is obligatory to prevent early frustration during therapy [8, 31, 33].

Step 2: Urotherapy [35, 142, 143] includes all nonspecific advice, including toilet habits, frequency, fluid intake, and nutrition advice. This is a well-accepted first line therapy in children with enuresis, especially in children with associated bladder dysfunction. Recently there is increasing evidence that urotherapy might not be effective at all in treatment of the enuresis component. Increased fluid intake might be beneficial in some patients, but might worsen enuresis in other patients. This data does not support starting with full spectrum urotherapy in all enuresis patients, but rather as an individualized modality in therapy refractory patients [144].

Advice on fluid and nutritional intake:

Many children have both their maximum fluid intake and main meal in the evening, and the high sodium and protein load may result in high osmotic excretion and polyuria overnight, as has been demonstrated in children with desmopressin refractory polyuria. Opinion leaders empirically advise that fluid and nutritional intake should be normalised, with fluid intake spread during the whole day, and avoiding caffeinated beverages and high fluid intake in the evening [8, 31, 33, 145]. This should be accompanied with healthy food intake in the evening, avoiding high protein and sodium load, to reduce osmotic diuresis [82, 83]. However, the evidence level for this strategy is weak.

Sleep advice is suggested due to the close interaction between sleep and several renal, hemodynamic, and endocrine circadian rhythms. Children should be encouraged to develop good sleep habits, including sufficient time for sleeping. Hyperstimulation of the brain (e.g. bright light exposure, computer games, television, music) should be avoided before sleeping, since it might have profound effects on the regulation of circadian rhythms, potentially affecting melatonin secretion and sleep patterns. Children should void immediately before going to bed, and lights should be turned off, once children are in bed. There is ample evidence that the overall sleep quality of children and teenagers is decreasing. There are also issues with timing and duration. The use of mobile devices once in bed is a big challenge, and should be discouraged. Children should not drink during the night [96, 146], and definitely not during therapy. However, the evidence supporting these interventions is weak.

Step 3: Non-medical behavioural management:

If urotherapy and lifestyle interventions are unsuccessful, more intensive treatment modalities are recommended. The alarm and desmopressin are the only two evidence-based management level I, grade A recommended treatments. The choice between the two options should ideally be individualised based upon patient characteristics identified during the evaluation [33]. There is evidence that the response to these treatments is highly dependent on the underlying pathogenic mechanism: The alarm is the treatment of choice in the archetype patient with *small* bladder capacity (i.e. MVV) and *normal* nocturnal urine production on wet nights. Such patients are usually desmopressin resistance. In contrast, desmopressin is the treatment of choice in the patient with *large* nocturnal urine production on wet nights and *normal* bladder capacity. Such patients will likely not respond to the alarm, unless they are developing nocturia. In general, desmopressin and the alarm should not be regarded as competing modalities, but as complementary or even supplementary to each other and targeting different patient subtypes. If, however, initial evaluation of the underlying enuresis mechanism is not possible, or the clinical pattern is unclear, other factors such as family motivation and preferences, availability of close follow-up, cost, and frequency of enuretic episodes, should all be included in the decision process.

Enuresis alarms have a level 1, grade A International Consultation on Incontinence (ICI) recommendation [8, 31, 33, 147–149]. Different types of alarms exist, but the common feature is a sensor placed in the sheets or nightclothes that is triggered when it becomes wet, setting off an auditory or vibration signal and causing the child to awaken, cease voiding, and arise to finish the void at the toilet. Parents are advised to wake their child when the alarm is activated; otherwise, children are prone to ignore it or turn it off and go back to sleep. The first weeks are a burden for the child and parents, and thus appropriate education prior to initiation and close follow-up are essential. The alarm should be worn every night. Response is usually not immediate and treatment should be continued for 2–3 months or until the child is dry for 14 consecutive nights (whichever comes first). Often compared to Pavlov training mechanisms, the true mechanism remains poorly understood. However, successful alarm treatment has been associated with a significant increase in bladder capacity [101, 150], whereas nocturnal urine production and sleep is unchanged. There may be cultural differences in its acceptability, as it may be highly disruptive for the household. The family must be motivated and adhere to the regimen to be successful. Doctors should monitor the child's progress early to address any problems and facilitate adherence. The response rate is high in families who continue treatment for a sufficient period, with relatively low relapse rates, though the lasting cure rate is still <50% [147]. Poor compliance and early withdrawal from treatment are common [14, 151, 152], which may exacerbate parental intolerance. Identifying the motivated patient in the right family is essential, and in cases where the child or the family is reluctant to accept the alarm, desmopressin is the alternative [149]. Alarm therapy has high failure rates when the buzzer is activated more than once a night. The goal is to obtain continence without waking up, although up to 25% develop nocturia. Relapse rates vary from 30% to 60% [147].

Desmopressin (DDAVP) [78, 153–156]

Desmopressin also received a level 1, grade A recommendation from the ICI in 2009 [49]. Desmopressin is a synthetic analogue of arginine vasopressin, the naturally occurring antidiuretic hormone. One of its major actions via the renal V2 receptor is to reduce the volume of urine produced overnight to a normal amount. Since the demonstration of nocturnal polyuria in patients with MNE, and the lack of the normal rise in plasma AVP levels during night, the use of DDAVP became a logical choice [58, 59]. Beyond the major effect on free water reabsorption, DDAVP has been claimed to have additional effects in enuresis, including detrusor muscle activity, central control of micturition, tubular sodium handling [157], and sleep, or arousal function, but the evidence in unselected enuretic populations is very low. The direct effect on sleep and arousal is controversial since it is unclear if DDAVP crosses the blood-brain barrier. Several formulations are available: rhinal nasal solution, nasal spray, oral tablet and oral lyophilisate (sublingual MELT formulation), all characterized by low bioavailability with large intra-individual variability (0.08–0.16% in adults), but only the oral tablet and lyophilisate formulations are labelled for treatment of NE in children. The low bioavailability is related to the peptide structure compromising oral and intestinal reabsorption. It is available for the treatment of enuresis as a tablet (dosage, 0.2–0.6 mg) or a fast-melting oral lyophilisate (MELT formulation, dosage, 120–360 µg). The latter is a recommended formulation for all children and is preferred for children under 12 years [94, 95, 158, 159]. Unlike other preparations, the MELT formulation is not affected by nasal congestion or gastrointestinal transit and does not require fluid intake. Since tablets usually require 1–200 mL of fluid intake, which is a significant percentage of a 7-year-old's bladder capacity and nocturnal diuresis, the MELT formulation seems more suited to the antidiuretic indication of desmopressin. Good pharmacodynamic data are available for the MELT formulation and its dosing in children with enuresis [94].

The efficacy of desmopressin in the treatment of NE is well documented. In a Cochrane analysis, 17 controlled trials all showed superiority of desmopressin compared to placebo regardless of the route of administration [153]. An estimated 70% of the NE population has full or partial response [95]; the response to desmopressin is highly dependent on factors such as nocturnal urine production and bladder capacity. The few studies that have tried to compare different doses of the drug reveal comparable efficacies [160–162]. Several key issues should be taken in consideration. First, 200–400 µg tablets are considered to be bioequivalent to 120–240 µg of the MELT formulation and represents the therapeutic range for children between 7 and 18 years with MNE. However, higher doses might be needed in larger children [159].

Desmopressin should be taken 1 h before the last void at bedtime to allow timely enhanced concentration of urine to occur. Fluid intake should be reduced from 1 h before desmopressin administration and for 8 subsequent hours to optimize concentrating capacity and treatment response, as well as to reduce the risk of hyponatremia due to water intoxication [94, 95]. Desmopressin is only effective on the day it is taken; full adherence is required to avoid wet nights [151, 152].There are different initial dosing regimens with comparable efficacy such as gradual dose escalation over a few weeks or starting with a high dose followed by gradual tapering to the lowest effective dose. If desmopressin is effective, then treatment can be continued for an additional 3 months; country-specific regulations regarding treatment breaks should be followed. If patients are dry on desmopressin treatment, breaks are recommended to ascertain whether the problem has resolved and therapy is no longer needed. If the child does not achieve complete dryness, or if wetting resumes once treatment is withdrawn, it should be continued or resumed, respectively. There is some evidence that structured withdrawal of medication may reduce relapse rates following its discontinuation [163, 164]. Desmopressin is well-tolerated, but clinicians should be aware that it is a potent antidiuretic and families must be educated regarding the rare possibility of developing hyponatremia due to water intoxication with symptoms including headache, nausea, and vomiting [155]. Self-titration of medication should be avoided.

Adherence to the management plan is crucial, especially for a drug whose action covers only the first night after intake. It is estimated that approximately 30% of non-responders are not taking medication correctly [151, 152]. Non-adherence to recommendations regarding timing of medication, voiding before bedtime, and limiting evening fluids can decrease treatment success [100]. Moreover, compliance is often overestimated by patients and caregivers; therefore, it should be documented in a diary. Regular contacts between caregiver and patient are necessary to maintain compliance. Patients who appear treatment-resistant should be advised of the importance of full adherence and asked if they have had any difficulty complying with recommendations.

Desmopressin has higher success rates in children with large bladder capacity and nocturnal polyuria [100]. The response rates in the initial studies of >70% decreased to 20–30% in subsequent studies. This lower response rate is likely due to local referral patterns and the use of desmopressin among general practitioners and consequent selection of more challenging patients at tertiary referral centers, and higher incidence of patients with overactive bladder (OAB) since the prevalence of occult OAB patients with small bladder volume and low nocturnal diuresis volume was high in these populations [54].

There are several unanswered questions regarding desmopressin therapy. It is still unclear whether desmopressin treatment leads to better long-term outcome than the spontaneous cure rate. The long-term cure rate of 15–30% annually with desmopressin in unselected populations is higher than the spontaneous cure rate [79, 154, 165], but depends on the severity of the study population. Long-term follow-up showed persistent LUT symptoms in the patients with NMNE and not in the MNE patients [88]. The suggestion that tapering of the dose and the structured withdrawal program should be beneficial is still unproven [163, 164].

It is obvious that many renal patients (CKD, and tubulopathies) with NE have impaired response to desmopressin, and do not reach maximal concentrating capacity, but this does not exclude at least some antidiuretic effect overnight, not normalizing but at least optimizing antidiuresis [166].

Tricyclic antidepressants were among the first drugs widely used in NE [167–172]. They act on adrenergic and serotonergic receptors in the central nervous system. Although the exact mechanism of action remains unclear, imipramine reduces both urinary sodium and the overall urinary osmolar excretion, decreasing the nocturnal urine output in children with nocturnal polyuria. Imipramine has potential to modulate sleep and increase arousability and it has a parasympatholytic effect on the detrusor and an alpha-mimetic activity on the sphincter. Side effects are the major drawback, ranging from postural hypotension, mouth dryness, and constipation to hepatotoxicity and cardiotoxicity in large doses [173]. Hence, imipramine is currently not recommended as a first line enuresis treatment but, has been suggested in treatment of refractory patients. Some recommend a pre-treatment ECG to exclude long QT-syndrome, but there is no evidence of benefit in children, and few MD's follow this strategy,

Anti-muscarinic Therapy

Anti-muscarinic therapy (e.g. oxybutynin, tolterodine, propiverine, solifenacin) has not been proven effective mono-therapy for patients with MNE, but may have a role in combination with first line modalities [174, 175]. These drugs are widely prescribed in children with NMNE for the daytime symptoms and are suggested to have beneficial effect on NE [175], but prospective there is no supportive evidence from randomized clinical trials. They might be indicated as add-on therapy in the subgroup of patients with MNE and small for age bladder capacity.

Cognitive Training and Psychotherapy

Cognitive training and psychotherapy was more widely used before desmopressin was available, and when physicians were less involved in treatment. Cognitive training and psychotherapy may still have value as an adjuvant to conventional therapy, although the evidence is weak. Most of studies were performed in patient groups defined by criteria from the Diagnostic and Statistical Manual of Mental Disorders, fourth edition, which does not differentiate between MNE and NMNE, and with a higher incidence of psychopathology [33].

Alternative Treatments

There are multiple alternative treatments for NE, but little or no evidence. There is no evidence supporting the efficacy of hypnosis [13, 176, 177], chiropractic [178–180], and reflexology. There is weak evidence demonstrating benefit from traditional acupuncture [181, 182]. There is insufficient evidence supporting acupuncture variations such as manual acupuncture, acupressure, and electro- and laser-acupuncture [183]. Transcutaneous electrical nerve stimulation (TENS) may have benefit, but mainly in a NMNE population [184, 185].

Treatment Refractory MNE (Fig. 47.3)

The major reasons that patients with MNE are non or partial responders to first line treatment modalities are that (1) the initial evaluation was not sufficient and the patient was a NMNE patient, (2) non-adherence to the treatment prescribed (3) a complex phenotype with more

than one underlying mechanism (e.g. both nocturnal polyuria and low bladder capacity) and (4) rare types of enuresis with underlying mechanisms not influenced by treatment (e.g. polyuria caused by large osmotic excretion) (Fig. 47.2).

In such patients, a repeat, extended evaluation should be performed, including detailed history of LUTS with particular emphasis on daytime OAB symptoms and constipation (classification of constipation according to the Rome IV criteria) [269]. The patient should keep a bladder diary with recordings of daytime intake and output and nighttime urine volume (diaper

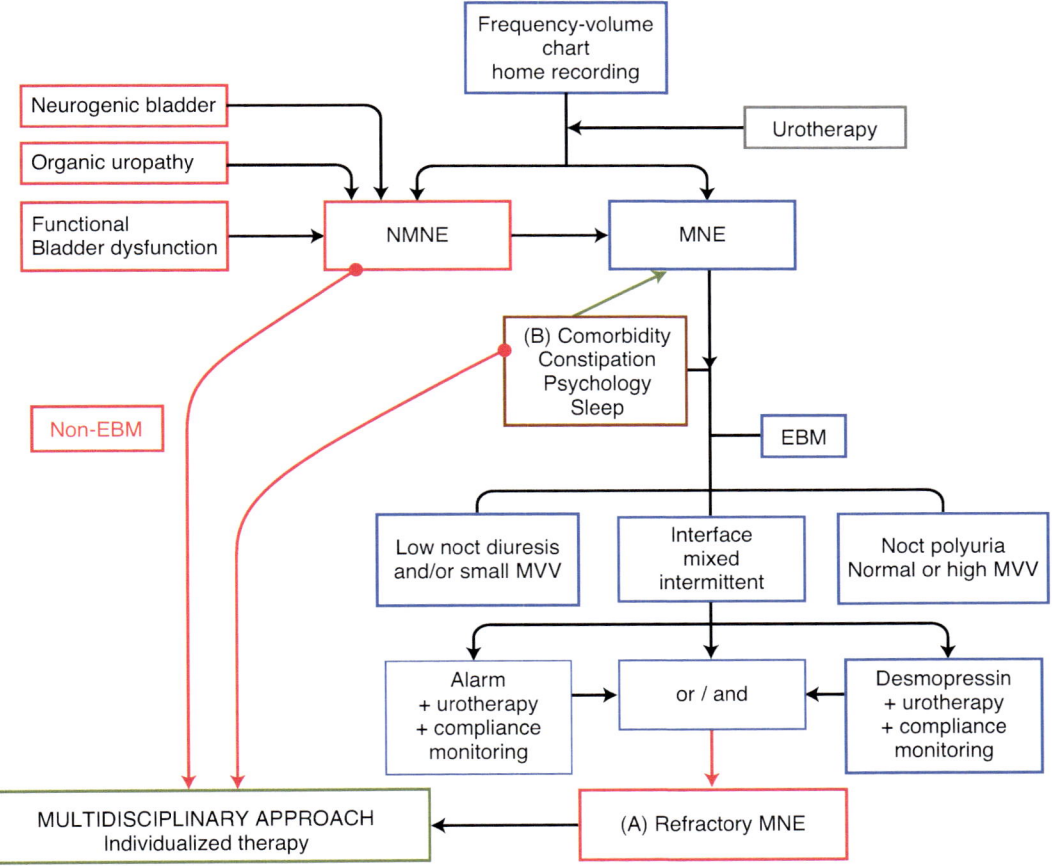

Fig. 47.3 Illustrates further the flow chart when children are refractory to initial therapy. (A) In these patients EBM therapy is insufficient and a multidisciplinary diagnostic and therapeutic approach should be offered, resulting in individualized therapy regimens. This multidisciplinary therapeutic approach should involve experts in pediatric nephrology and urology, as well as targeting psychological characteristics, compliance issues and comorbidities. Since the majority of comorbidities associated with therapy-resistance are easy to identify by simple questionnaires, we advocate not only to search for them in refractory cases, but also in the early stages of evaluation (B)

weighing). Advice the patient to keep the diary during a day with standardized fluid intake (1.5 L/1.73 m²/day), since low fluid intake might mask frequency and daytime incontinence. The night-time recording can be repeated during 1 week of desmopressin treatment in order to verify whether the patient has the intended reduction in urine production. Spontaneous low fluid intake suggests a defence mechanism, and may mask OAB symptoms. These symptoms are often not mentioned by parents, and thus deserve repeated questioning or documentation in a bladder diary. Uroflowmetry, bladder ultrasonography and rectal diameter measurement can give additional information on the voiding pattern, bladder emptying, bladder wall thickness (OAB), and constipation.

In desmopressin refractory patients without bladder dysfunction, alternative explanations for the lack of efficacy may include (1) anti-enuretic effect = number of wet nights, (2) anti-diuretic effect (= nocturnal diuresis rate), and (3) concentrating capacity (= urinary osmolality). Partial response to desmopressin in MNE (anti-enuretic effect) is related to persistent nocturnal polyuria on wet nights [75] (Fig. 47.4).

Poor compliance should be excluded [152], including not taking the drug (record in drug-diary). Determine the number of filled prescriptions to monitor compliance. Other causes for suboptimal effect of desmopressin are:

1. The child forgets to void and empty the bladder before sleeping thereby increasing the risk of exceeding maximal bladder capacity during the night.
2. Fluid intake overnight or even the hour before desmopressin administration reduces both the maximum and duration of the anti-diuretic effect.
3. Intermittent polyuria might also be related to the PK/PD characteristics of desmopressin [94, 95, 159], but the phenomenon might be intermittent, varying from night to night. Factors which influence PK/PD include;
   (a) The recommended formulations (tablet, MELT formulation), but also the nasal spray, have poor bioavailability, ranging 0.2–2%, but with a large intra-individual variability. Only for the MELT formulation are dose-response and PK/PD data available in children. The MELT

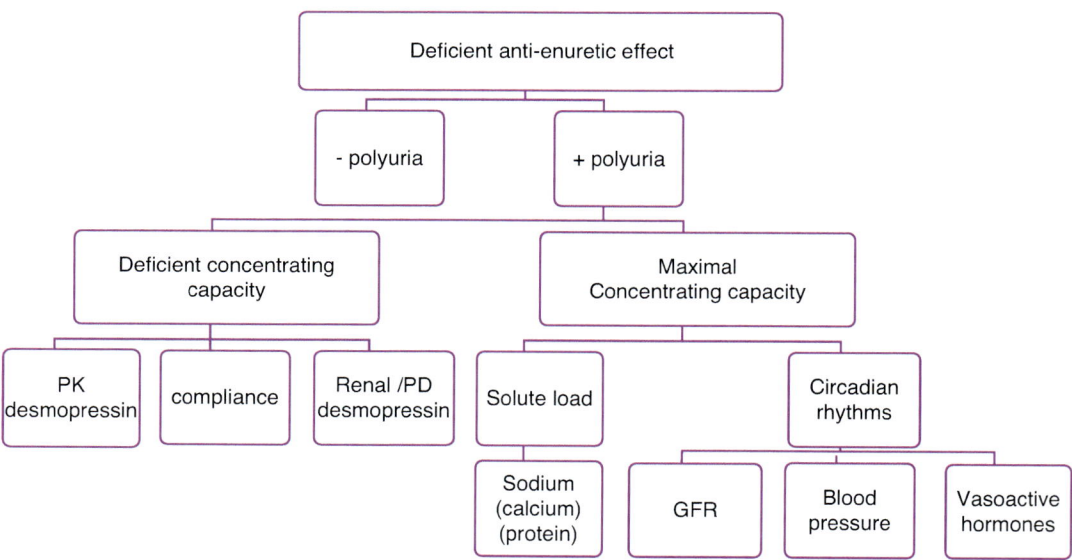

Fig. 47.4 Patients with desmopressin resistant monosymptomatic enuresis can be subtyped according to persistence or not of nocturnal polyuria and ability to reach maximal concentrating capacity. An individualized treatment choice is possible when by considering the different pathophysiologic mechanisms involved

formulation had superior PK and PD profile, better compliance, and some indices of higher response rates than the tablet, although there have been no randomized trials comparing the anti-enuretic effect of the two preparations. In treatment resistant patients on tablets, a switch to the MELT formulation should be considered.

(b) The child takes desmopressin just before sleeping time. Since the time to reach maximum concentrating capacity and anti-diuretic effect is 1–3 h, the drug should be taken at least 1 h before the last void at bedtime [94].

(c) Even in the therapeutic range of 120–240 μg, there are large standard deviations in maximal concentrating capacity and antidiuresis, as well as duration of action. Better understanding of this PK/PD, can lead to more personalized medicine, with individualized dose schemes. The PK/PD data demonstrate that at least 25% of patients might benefit from higher doses; these patients can be identified by a PD test in an ambulatory setting, especially the older patient (24 h concentration-profile). Increasing the dose should only be done following this test, typically done in expert centers, due to the risk of toxicity.

In desmopressin refractory nocturnal polyuria with low urinary osmolality, nephrogenic diabetes insipidus (NDI) should be excluded. The X-linked NDI in boys does not usually present as enuresis, but female carriers might have a more subtle phenotype with enuresis as the major symptom. Many renal diseases (CKD, tubulopathies, renal dysplasia, uropathy) may present with enuresis. Hypertension, especially nighttime hypertension, coincides with nocturnal polyuria, and should be considered in refractory patients.

Desmopressin resistant nocturnal polyuria might be associated with high urinary osmolality overnight. This can be caused by an increased solute load only in the evening or during all 24 h [82, 83]. Sodium is the major osmotic agent [80, 81, 83, 87, 186]. Although nutritional intake plays a major role, abnormalities of several circadian rhythms like prostaglandins [65, 80, 87], GFR [187], blood pressure [70] and sleep pattern [66, 67] may also have a significant impact. Extrapolation to primary care enuresis patients remains premature, but these findings suggest future treatment options. Some pilot studies had promising results such as sodium restricted diet, diuretics (furosemide [186]), nonsteroidal antiinflammatory drugs (NSAIDs), and melatonin [127, 188–190]. There was a focus on the role of calcium [91], and the efficacy of a calcium restricted diet [92]. However, hypercalciuria might be a secondary phenomenon, unrelated to diet.

Therapy resistance may be related to the *presence of comorbidities* [33], and addressing them, when possible, might increase the response rate. Constipation and FI should be treated before treating MNE, but are often underestimated and underreported. Psychological comorbidities, both internalizing as well as externalizing, are more frequent in NE patients. Attention deficit disorder and autism seem to have common central nervous pathways with enuresis. Renal dysfunction, hypertension, diabetes mellitus and sleep disturbances may worsen NE, and should be treated. NE may also be exacerbated by drug interfering with circadian rhythms, including diuretics, steroids, cyclosporine A, and neurotropic drugs.

In conclusion, children with MNE the two first-line treatment options are desmopressin and the enuresis alarm, as monotherapy or in combination. Outcomes are less favorable if therapy is not guided by patient characteristics, with initial success rates of monotherapy potentially below 30% and a relapse rate of up to 50%.

In summary, the optimal strategy is as follows:

1. The initial treatment choice should be guided by the family's level of motivation and their preference.
2. Based on the information from diaries, one can identify subtypes of MNE that should

allow further fine-tuning of treatment according to the child's characteristics and family motivation.

1. Children with a normal urine output during the night and normal bladder capacity can be given either the alarm or desmopressin.
2. Children with smaller than expected bladder capacity for age will likely be desmopressin-resistant and more responsive to the alarm.
3. Children with nocturnal polyuria and normal bladder capacity will be more sensitive to desmopressin.
4. Children with both nocturnal polyuria and reduced bladder capacity may have a successful outcome with the combination of alarm and desmopressin.

Other Forms of Urinary Incontinence (Fig. 47.5)

The classification of daytime LUT conditions is more complex than enuresis because of the heterogeneity of symptoms of LUT dysfunction and the considerable overlap between the conditions. Although there is a significant overlap with enuresis, not all LUT patients have enuresis, and not all enuresis patients have apparent LUT symptoms. Additionally, borderline cases are common and the rationale for grouping of symptom complexes into specific LUT dysfunction conditions is often not fully evidence-based. The ICCS has standardized the terminology and approach [31].

Epidemiology

Most children are toilet trained by 2 years of age, although there are important country and cultural differences. Early interventions might speed up toilet training, but have not been shown to decrease the prevalence of any LUTS at 5–7 years [191, 192]. Daytime symptoms from the LUT are very common in childhood, especially urgency and frequency (approximately 5–20% of 7-year olds), rapidly decreasing during the following years. As outlined above, the majority of these children have non monosymptomatic enuresis. Urinary incontinence is also relatively common, with a prevalence of approximately 3% of 7-year olds [49]. Voiding complaints, such as dysuria and interrupted stream, are far less frequent. Five years of age is the usual cutoff for reporting symptoms and LUT conditions. The prevalence of the various subtypes of LUTs, especially OAB, versus dysfunctional voiding is not known.

Definitions and Characteristics

Assessment

To classify daytime LUT dysfunction conditions, we recommend assessment and documentation be based on the following parameters:

1. Incontinence (presence or absence, and symptom frequency)
2. Voiding frequency
3. Urgency (presence or absence)
4. Voided volumes
5. Fluid intake

This is more important than subgrouping the children into the various recognized conditions listed below.

There are several archetypes, but with large overlap. Rather than forcing children into an archetype as was done historically (*non-neuropathic* bladder-sphincter dysfunction, *urge incontinence, dysfunctional voiding, lazy bladder syndrome, Hinman bladder*) *it is advised to start with a detailed clinical history and using a diary and uroflowmetry to describe the characteristics of the bladder during the filling phase (storage) and the emptying phase.* Urgency, holding manoeuvres and daytime incontinence are frequent with an overactive bladder, but infrequent in an underactive bladder.

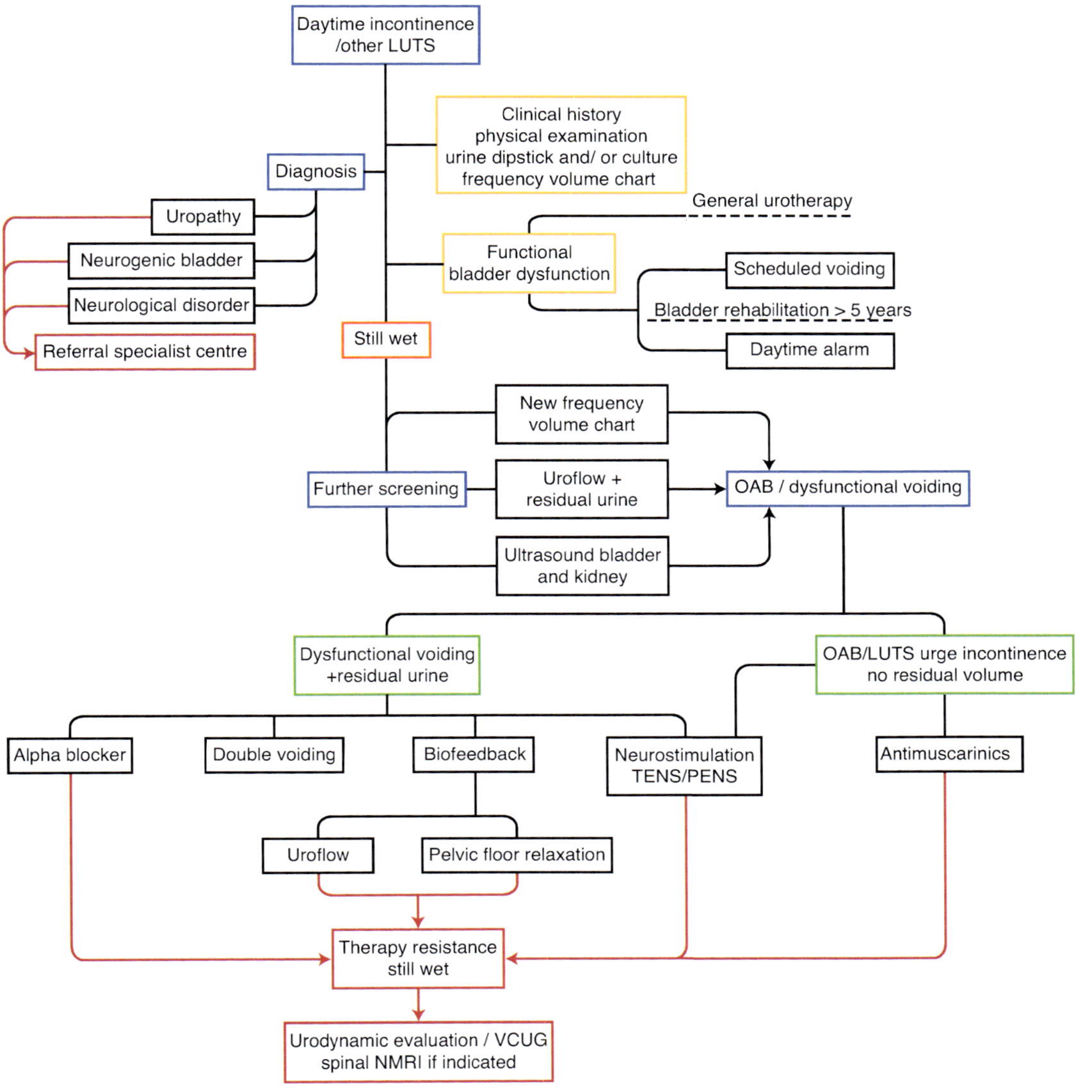

Fig. 47.5 Flow chart illustrating the evaluation and treatment of daytime incontinence/LUTS in children. The initial evaluation in children with LUTS starts at the age of 4–5 years. Clinical evaluation should focus not only on the bladder symptoms, but also on comorbidities such as constipation, neurologic disorders, neurologic bladder, and anatomical abnormalities uropathies. If these are excluded, we can conclude to a functional bladder dysfunction. Initial therapeutic approach, consists of treatment of constipation, and subsequent urotherapy. Bladder rehabilitation regimens and daytime alarm might be add on therapies. If this therapy fails, additional screening should be performed, including frequency-voiding chart during normalized fluid intake, uroflowmetry with US evaluation of residual volume, and ultrasound of kidney and the bladder. This non-invasive approach may lead to identification of the two archetypes, OAB and dysfunctional voiding, although there is a certain overlap between the two. In children with OAB, antimuscarinics are the treatment of choice, although neurostimulation offers an alternative treatment option. Patients with dysfunctional voiding benefit from a variety of urotherapy regimens, including pelvic floor relaxation- and uroflow biofeedback. In refractory cases, video-urodynamic investigation is mandatory. In cases where the videourodynamics give further indication for a neurologic disorder, spinal NMRI should be performed

Comorbidities: Dysfunctional voiding (previously called bladder-sphincter dysfunction), such as OAB with defence mechanisms, is associated with recurrent UTI, asymptomatic bacteriuria, vesicoureteral reflux and constipation and/or faecal incontinence (30–50% of children with urge incontinence). Furthermore, urinary incontinence is highly associated with increase in body mass index, constipation and/or faecal incontinence (10–15% of children with urge incontinence), neuropsychiatric conditions (e.g. ADHD, oppositional defiant disorder) and intellectual disabilities.

Urinary Incontinence Classification

Several structural congenital abnormalities (e.g. ectopic ureter, congenital urethral valve), and neurogenic bladder (e.g. spina bifida, sacral agenesis) often present with therapy refractory LUTS. Urinary incontinence can be divided into separate subtypes based upon the underlying mechanism [193]. The two subtypes that pose the greatest threat to the upper urinary tract and therefore should be identified and treated as early as possible are *neuropathic* bladder sphincter dysfunction and *structural* incontinence (organic). These two groups comprise only a few percent of incontinent children as most have no underlying neurological or anatomic cause. In *non-neuropathic* bladder-sphincter dysfunction, it is possible to further subtype the type of bladder dysfunction based upon clinical history, voiding pattern, uroflowmetry and residual urine. Continuous incontinence is often due to an organic disorder.

Bladder and bowel dysfunction (BBD): BBD is a condition of combined bladder and bowel disturbances that encompasses LUT and bowel function. *Severe BBD* is LUT and bowel dysfunction that is characteristic of the dysfunction seen in children with neurologic conditions, yet have no identifiable neurologic abnormality. This is almost synonymous with the historical term Hinman syndrome.

Overactive Bladder

OAB manifests as urinary urgency, usually accompanied by frequency and nocturia, with or without daytime incontinence, in the absence of UTI or other alternative etiology. Some patients may have minimal symptoms because they limit fluid intake during the day in an effort to decrease symptoms.

OAB is the most frequent cause of LUTS, with daytime incontinence, urgency, frequency, and small voided volumes as symptoms. Parents often notice efforts to prevent daytime enuresis, which they interpret as delaying micturition ("postponement"), but these children have high micturition frequency, in contrast with the typical postponers, who have low frequency of large voided volumes. Children with OAB usually have *detrusor overactivity*, but this should not be assumed without cystometric evaluation (see above). *Urgency incontinence* is involuntary loss of urine associated with urgency and is applicable to many children with OAB.

Voiding Postponement

Children who habitually postpone micturition using holding maneuvers have *voiding postponement*, which is diagnosed by clinical history. It is often associated with a low micturition frequency, and a feeling of urgency and possibly incontinence, due to a full bladder. Some children restrict fluid intake to reduce incontinence. The rationale for delineating this entity lies in the observation that these children often suffer from psychological comorbidity or behavioral disturbances such as oppositional defiant disorder (ODD).

Underactive Bladder

Children with underactive bladder need to strain with increased intra-abdominal pressure to void. The children may have low voiding frequency despite adequate hydration, but may also have frequency due to incomplete emptying with prompt refilling of the bladder. These children often produce an interrupted uroflow pattern, and have *detrusor underactivity* during invasive urodynamics. Flow patterns may also be plateau-shaped; pressure–flow studies will distinguish it from bladder outlet obstruction. The prevalence is higher in females and increases with age.

Dysfunctional Voiding

The child with *dysfunctional voiding* habitually contracts the urethral sphincter or pelvic floor during voiding and demonstrates a staccato pattern with or without an interrupted flow on repeated uroflowmetry when concomitantly recording electromyography (EMG) activity. There is a clear correlation with UTI and constipation, and in rare cases high intravesical pressure during voiding might lead to VUR and renal damage with or without UTI.

Bladder Outlet Obstruction

Bladder outlet obstruction has to some extent comparable symptoms as dysfunctional voiding, but it can only be diagnosed during urodynamic investigation.

Stress Incontinence

Stress incontinence is the involuntary leakage of small amounts of urine when intraabdominal pressure is increased. It is rare in children, in contrast to adult females, and can only be diagnosed during urodynamic investigation. This rare type of incontinence is occasionally seen in female elite athletes [194]. The underlying mechanisms are not fully understood, but may involve a hypermobile pelvic floor.

Vaginal Reflux

Vaginal reflux is frequent in young girls after they complete toilet training. They experience daytime incontinence in moderate amounts shortly after normal voiding and have no underlying mechanism other than obvious vaginal entrapment of urine. This is not associated with other LUT symptoms or enuresis. It is worsened by voiding with the legs closed, leading to urine entrapment inside the introitus. It may be seen in girls with labial adhesions and chronic, recurrent vaginitis.

Giggle Incontinence

Giggle incontinence is a rare condition in which complete voiding occurs specifically during or immediately after laughing in girls. Bladder function is normal when the child is not laughing. Giggle incontinence is not linked to any other disturbance of LUT function. It is often familial, and has a proven hereditary predisposition. It should be differentiated from giggling incontinence as a symptom, where the leakage is secondary to contraction of an overactive bladder, induced not exclusively by laughing but also by physical activity and coughing.

Extraordinary Daytime Urinary Frequency

Extraordinary daytime urinary frequency is seen in toilet-trained children who void very often and with very small volumes during the daytime only. The daytime voiding frequency is at least once per hour and average voided volumes are less than 50% of expected bladder capacity age for age (usually much smaller). Nocturia is absent, and it is not usually associated with incontinence.

Bladder Neck Dysfunction

Bladder neck dysfunction is impaired or delayed opening of the bladder neck, resulting in impaired flow despite an adequate or elevated detrusor contraction [195]. The prolonged opening time, which is the time between the start of a voiding detrusor contraction and the start of urine flow, can be seen on videourodynamics. Alternatively, bladder neck dysfunction can be diagnosed noninvasively with a uroflow/EMG when there is a prolonged EMG lag time, which is the time interval between the start of pelvic floor relaxation and the actual start of flow.

Evaluation

If a wetting child has daytime symptoms, initial evaluation should be started from the age of 4 to 5 years due to the importance of excluding neurological and structural causes. The history is very important, including the psychomotor development, the type of incontinence (e.g. constant dribbling indicating a structural cause), recurrent UTI, constipation, and FI. Information about the family situation, motivation and behavioral problems should be included in a structured history. The physical examination should focus on the same areas as in a child with NE (above); urinalysis is also indicated. If the initial evaluation raises suspicion of an underlying disease, e.g. a neurological disorder or anatomical anomaly, the child should be referred to a secondary or tertiary referral center. The cornerstone in the initial evaluation of an incontinent child is a frequency-volume chart, as described for enuresis, with documentation of all incontinence episodes as well as the time and volume of all intake and voids during 2 days, typically during a weekend. This gives very valuable information about the severity of symptoms, drinking habits, voiding pattern and bladder capacity. Occasionally, just filling out a frequency-volume chart enables the parents to adjust an inappropriate voiding or drinking pattern, resulting in a continent child before the next clinic visit.

In a child with recurrent UTI, prophylactic antibiotics should be instituted and an ultrasound of the urinary tract obtained. If there is suspicion of constipation, and in all children with soiling or FI, this should be treated aggressively. If, however, no underlying disease is suspected, further evaluation is not necessary at this stage and treatment can be reduced to general advice about good voiding habits and awareness about signs of constipation and UTI. In the motivated child, bladder rehabilitation with scheduled voids can be commenced. If the incontinence symptoms persist after 5–6 years of age, the initial evaluation should be supplemented with an ultrasound examination of the urinary tract, uroflowmetry and measurement of postvoid residual urine by ultrasound. These investigations usually require referral to a specialist. These simple urodynamic evaluations characterize the voiding and bladder emptying and will enable differentiate between types of incontinence, e.g. urge syndrome and dysfunctional voiding, and may raise suspicion of a urinary tract obstruction. More invasive evaluations such as conventional transurethral cystometry, natural fill ambulatory continuous bladder pressure monitoring, and voiding cystourethrography are only indicated if there is suspicion of neuropathic or structural incontinence (abnormal uroflow, residual urine) or if the patient does not respond to the initial therapy.

Treatment

Overactive Bladder (Formerly Urge Incontinence)

1. Two to three percent of 7-year-olds have incontinence with concomitant signs of an overactive bladder, and up to one third of 7-year-olds have urgency with increased voiding frequency. This syndrome has undergone a conceptual change over the last decade. Previously, there was a clear-cut urodynamic definition of the "unstable" bladder, with bladder contractions during the filling phase of a cystometry; it has expanded to a diagnosis based on clinical history and diary.

   There is evidence that cystometry at screening adds no value to the initial therapeutic approach. Moreover, the majority of patients with OAB on cystometry had the typical clinical pattern of OAB (urgency, frequency, small voided volume). Hence, a clinical diagnosis and a cystometry diagnosis of OAB are viewed as equivalent on initial evaluation. OAB probably does not have a single pathogenic explanation. Rather, mechanisms include hypersensitivity of the bladder wall (efferent), low compliance of the bladder wall, and an imbalance between ortho and parasympathetic tone (documented in refractory patients by the therapeutic action of anticholinergics and beta-3-adrenoceptor mimetics).

   Because the clinical picture of this incontinence is so typical, the diagnosis can be made with confidence by a structured approach as described above and no further urodynamic testing is necessary unless the child fails to respond to initial therapy. The urodynamic definition, however, has been widened to include bladder and urethral dysfunction. Clinically, urge syndrome is characterized by frequent attacks of a need to void, countered by holding manoeuvres such as squatting, eventually resulting in usually small leaks of urine.

2. Treatment:
   (a) Urotherapy [143, 196]:
       Treatment of urge incontinence begins with elimination of concomitant

constipation and UTI followed by behavioural treatment (bladder rehabilitation).

- Standard urotherapy [143]
- Standard urotherapy (ICCS, ICI level 3C) will cure at least 50% of children and can be started by primary care physicians. The cornerstone of urotherapy is to establish the child's awareness about his/her particular voiding habits. Different specific strategies are utilized, but most include a normalisation of fluid intake and elimination of caffeine intake. The evidence is weak [145, 197]. Standard urotherapy also includes an initial increase in the number of voids, followed by a gradual decrease to normal frequency [35]. Based on a randomized study, it is helpful to use a programmable watch that gives a signal to the child when it is time to void. Inappropriate posture during voiding, if present, should be corrected. At referral centres, the clinical team should include a specialized team of doctors, specialist nurses (urotherapists), psychologists and eventually physiotherapists [198].
- Although the majority of urotherapy regimens concentrate mainly on the quality and quantity of fluid intake, elevated nutritional intake of sodium and protein will result in higher sodium and acid load in the urine [82, 83]. High urinary acidity and osmolality might trigger bladder overactivity [199, 200]. Furthermore, in patients with CKD, (who may have a deficit in concentrating capacity, a high osmotic load) will result in higher diuresis rate and therefore more OAB symptoms [201, 202].

(b) Anticholinergics/antimuscarinics
   If urotherapy for a couple of months does not eliminate the symptoms, antimuscarinics should be initiated [203, 204].
   There are only a few medications with substantiated effect in children, and some have significant side effects, especially in children with ADHD. More recently developed antimuscarinics seem to have less influence on cognitive function and are therefore better tolerated [205, 206]. Antimuscarinic therapy should not be instituted in a child with significant post-void residual urine and many centres monitor bladder emptying 4–5 weeks after initiation of treatment.

- Oxybutynin hydrochloride
  - Oxybutynin hydrochloride, a tertiary amine, is a moderately potent anticholinergic agent with strong musculotropic relaxant and local anaesthetic activity. In animal studies, it has weak anticholinergic activities, but strong spasmolytic effects [13, 207, 208]. It is worldwide the most prescribed drug for OAB.
  - The side effects are those of all antimuscarinic agents and include inhibition of salivary secretion (dry mouth), blockade of the ciliary muscle of the lens (disturbed accommodation, blurred vision), facial flushing during exercise, tachycardia, drowsiness and inhibition of gut motility, leading to constipation. Central nervous system side-effects, especially in children with ADHD, are quite important, including pronounced attention deficit and behavioural problems, and are related to ability of oxybutynin and its metabolites to pass the central blood barrier.
  - The half-life of the drug is low, necessitating at least three doses a day. One dose in the morning for daytime symptoms or one dose in the evening for OAB, is ineffective, based on this PK characteristics. Oxybutynin XL is absorbed in the large intestine, thereby bypassing the first pass liver metabolism

[209]. However, the tablets must be swallowed intact, and thus cannot be used in many young children. Transdermal administration has been proposed as an alternative, but data in children are absent [210]. Intravesical administration has been promoted, but is only feasible in neurogenic bladders with intermittent catheterisation [211–213].

- Although widely prescribed, the therapeutic evidence in children as monotherapy is rather weak (Evidence 3C), certainly for the enuresis symptom, though it is mentioned in all guidelines [196, 214]. Many studies report the use of combination therapy (desmopressin, imipramine, urotherapy, neurostimulation) [175, 215–218].

- Tolterodine
  - Tolterodine is a selective antimuscarinic drug, which has a more pronounced antimuscarinic effect on the urinary bladder than on salivary gland, and there is less penetration through the blood-brain barrier, potentially decreasing side-effect [219]. This was supported by EEG measurements [203].
  - In adults, tolterodine effectively decreased the symptoms of detrusor overactivity and caused fewer side-effects than oxybutynin. Studies in neurogenic bladder were promising, but this was not confirmed in pediatric OAB studies. There were three explanations given for this failure: (a) the chosen primary endpoints in the study design, (b) pediatric OAB has never been proven to have the same pathophysiology as in adults, and (c) the large difference in metabolism of the drug, dependent of genetic differences in cytochrome P450 (CYP)-metabolism, resulting in underdosing in 1/3 of children.

Therefore, the drug was never approved in children [220–222].
  - The extended-release form was developed for the adult indication, evaluated in two pediatric studies, but without clinically significant benefit [223, 224].
  - Although the evidence level 3C is in line with other available drugs, the large intra-individual PK variation related to the CYP-polymorphisms for metabolism of the drug suggests that it should not be first line therapy [220, 225, 226].

- Propiverine hydrochloride is an antimuscarinic drug with proven efficacy and better tolerability than oxybutynin in children with OAB. This was documented in a phase 3 trial. Both ICI and ICCS classifies this drug as evidence level 1 B/C, but there were never confirmatory data with propiverine as monotherapy [227–229].

- Solifenacin is a recently developed antimuscarinic with some interesting characteristics [206, 230–233]. Given once daily, it significantly decreased urgency episodes in a pooled analysis of four pivotal trials including more than 2800 adults. PK/PD data in adults demonstrated a long half-life, enabling once daily administration with a potential of increasing therapy compliance [234]. Additional studies showed promising results [205, 232]. The side effect profile, with a high affinity for the M3 muscarinic receptor, is more favourable than that of some nonspecific antimuscarinics. In children with neurogenic bladder and OAB, studies documented a good safety profile and a half-life almost comparable to adults [205, 235, 236].

- Preliminary PK data show that metabolism of the drug is even higher than expected from adult data. Recent PK/PD data in children with neurogenic bladder and OAB are in line with the

PK predicted data based on adult studies. The clinical effect seems to be better in neurogenic bladder than in OAB in the paediatric population, although the evidence is limited. The drug has a very acid taste, which makes crushing the pills to individualize the dose to the size of the child challenging. Moreover, the drug powder is very irritative, especially to the eye, if the pills are cut or crushed.

- Several drugs have been proposed off-label as alternatives to anticholinergics such as calcium channel blockers, NSAIDs, alpha-adrenergic blockers, and beta-3-adrenoceptor mimetics. However, none have enough evidence to recommend as first line OAB therapy in children.
- Calcium channel blockers and alpha-adrenergic blockers have common side effects, including hypotension, facial flushing, headache, dizziness, constipation, and nausea.
- Fesoterodine [237] has documented antimuscarinic PD-effect on OAB in adults, and comparable PK characteristics in children [238], but more side-effects than solifenacin, without improved efficacy [203, 225, 239–241]. Darifenacin is approved for adults, but without convincing data in children [203, 242].
- If one anticholinergic is not effective or has intolerable side effects, it is reasonable to switch to another given different PK and side effect profiles. However, combination therapy of two anti-muscarinics is not recommended since there are no clinical data regarding efficacy or side effects.

(c) Tricyclic antidepressants are useful agents for facilitating urine storage, by both decreasing detrusor contractility and increasing outlet resistance. They are no longer recommended as first line treatment for MNE. The mechanism of action

NE remains unclear, but might involve anticholinergic effects on the bladder, effects on sleep patterns and reduced nocturnal polyuria (through reduced natriuresis) [169]. Many expert consensus papers consider imipramine as a third-line therapy for OAB after urotherapy and anticholinergics for LUTS. Imipramine has weak anticholinergic effects as well as adrenergic effects on bladder muscle. It may exert a local anaesthetic-like action on the bladder. Clinically, imipramine is effective by decreasing bladder contractility and increasing outlet resistance. Stimulation of the beta-receptor by peripheral blockade of noradrenaline reuptake could account for the decrease in bladder contractility, and stimulation of the alpha-receptors in the smooth muscle of the bladder base and proximal urethra increases bladder outlet resistance [203, 215, 243]. Some favour reboxetine because of efficacy and safety reasons, although convincing data are lacking [244, 245].

(d) The beta3-adrenoreceptor agonist mirabegron is the first of a new type of drugs targeting the orthosympathetic pathway [145, 246, 247]. In controlled randomised trials in adults mirabegron had a positive effect on OAB symptoms [145, 234]. A few limited studies have supported this effect in children [234, 248–251]. The tablets cannot be crushed or chewed because of major changes in bioavailability, and this limits their use in smaller children [231].

(e) Electro neuromodulation

Electro neuromodulation using cutaneous stimulation of either the sacral or peripheral nerves is a treatment modality in children, gaining interest over the last decade despite some controversy regarding efficacy. The devices and techniques are very heterogeneous, using skin surface or percutaneous electrodes (TENS or percutaneous electrical nerve stimulation), but also anal or intravesical electrodes. The devices have varying frequencies, waveforms and intensities, but there is no evidence regarding the optimal choice for each subtype of patients. The major proposed indication is in OAB patients refractory to antimuscarinic drug therapy, either alone or in combination with the drug. If percutaneous needle sacral stimulation is beneficial, an implantable pacemaker is a possible option in very treatment-resistant patients.

(f) Botulinum toxin

There is increasing evidence to support the use of botulinum A-toxin in the detrusor for treatment-refractory OAB (EB 3C). It was approved by the Food and Drug Administration in 2021 for neurogenic bladder detrusor overactivity. The safety and efficacy is well-documented. Small, single center studies show promising results in children with OAB, but prospective controlled studies are ongoing.

Dysfunctional Voiding (Staccato Voiding)

Voiding dysfunction in children is rare. Approximately 1% of 7-year-olds will have a uroflowmetry clearly deviating from normal [55, 252]. The predominant pattern is that of staccato voiding, which consists of frequent interruptions of detrusor initiated voiding. Dysfunctional voiding has many names, including non-neuropathic bladder-sphincter dyscoordination and overactive urethra another, but ICCS recommends the term 'dysfunctional voiding' [36]. The symptoms are to some extent similar to those of the urge syndrome, although recurrent UTI, constipation and soiling are more prevalent in this patient group. It is generally agreed that diagnosis requires a consistent pattern of three consecutive characteristic uroflowmetry results. The aetiology of dysfunctional voiding is not fully elucidated. The simplest theory is that it can be a long-term effect caused by voiding pains following a UTI, where the child learns to protect the urethra from the full urine stream by contracting the sphincter and continues to do so after the urethral pain has disappeared. This may lead to overtraining of the pelvic floor and the urethral sphincter during holding. It is also hypothesized that it is a sign of a delayed maturation of the interaction between the detrusor and the pelvic floor or an increased nociceptive receptor response in the proximal part of urethra.

Besides elimination of UTI and constipation, initial treatment consists of bladder rehabilitation with timed voids and double voiding twice a day. If insufficient, uroflow-biofeedback training may provide additional pelvic floor relaxation [143]. A treatment trial with an alpha-adrenergic blocker can be considered in refractory cases, although the evidence is weak [252, 253]. This approach is based on the fact that the physiological internal sphincter is controlled by alpha-adrenergic receptors in the smooth musculature of the bladder neck and proximal urethra. Although the theoretical expected effect would be best in those patients with bladder neck obstruction, good results are described in patients with detrusor sphincter dyssynergia, suggesting that there may also be an effect on striated sphincter tone [254–257]. To date, alpha-adrenergic blockers have no approved indication in children. Terazosin, alfuzosin and other similar new alpha-adrenergic blockers are more selective for the urinary tract. The side effects are orthostatic hypotension, tachycardia and a possible first-dose phenomenon with faintness, dizziness, palpitations and syncope. Effectiveness can be monitored with a combination uroflowmetry and residual urine measurement. Special techniques have been used in therapy-resistant cases, like training in voiding schools, as well as intermittent catheterisation.

Underactive Bladder

This entity is characterized by few (≤3) daily voids with unusually large volumes, poor bladder emptying, and a very high prevalence of UTI, constipation, and vesicoureteral reflux; it is more frequent in girls [258, 259]. The child typically strains during micturition and leakage occurs secondary to overflow incontinence. The aetiology is multifactorial but one hypothesis suggests that it is the result of sustained bladder-sphincter dyscoordination. In some children, the syndrome is associated with a prior history of previous infravesical obstruction. In order to establish the correct diagnosis, it is often necessary to perform a urodynamic examination to exclude an associated underlying neuropathy. The cystometry shows large bladder capacity, most often a weak detrusor, a negative bethanechol test and no signs of obstruction on the pressure-flow examination. The treatment is similar to that described for dysfunctional voiding except that a larger proportion of patients require a period of clean intermittent catheterisation [270]. Structured training programs offer a non-invasive alternative.

Neuropathic Incontinence

Although incontinence secondary to neuropathy is rare, it is associated with significant risks of serious long-term injury to the urinary tract as well as decreased renal function [260, 261]. This chapter will not provide details of the different types of incontinence due to neuropathic causes, but emphasize the importance of close and thorough long-term monitoring of bladder and renal function in such patients. The variability of urodynamic abnormalities and their ability to change over time in children with congenital neurological defects such as myelomeningocele illustrates the need for life-long specialist follow-up [9, 29]. Treatment of severe neuropathic incontinence usually requires a large interdisciplinary team, including pediatric nephrology, urology, neurology, neurosurgery, orthopedics, psychology, and physiotherapy. Furthermore, all incontinent children should be screened for neurological defects as outlined above. If a suspicion of neuropathy is raised, an MRI of the spinal canal should be performed together with urodynamic evaluation, cystourethrogram, and ultrasound of the urinary tract. Conservative treatment includes antimuscarinics, either peroral or intravesical, clean intermittent catheterization, laxatives, and prophylactic antibiotics. Surgical treatments include bladder augmentation, cutaneous vesicostomy, anti-reflux surgery, and continence preserving surgery. Intravesical injection of botulinum toxin represents a newer method of detrusor relaxant therapy.

Structural Incontinence

Anatomical abnormalities can also be associated with significant voiding symptoms and are potentially damaging forms of incontinence [262]. Although not all are visible by physical examination, it is mandatory to inspect the genital region of the incontinent child for a possible cause of the incontinence.

Sphincter by-pass: Dribbling incontinence should always raise suspicion of a structural defect in the urinary tract, such as an ectopic ureter, often arising from the upper segment of a duplex kidney. Other forms of structural incontinence with sphincter by-pass are the exstrophy complex and epispadia, where diagnosis is much less complicated than the subsequent complex treatment.

Urinary tract obstruction: Voiding dysfunction and incontinence resulting from congenital malformations that cause LUT obstruction is much more common in boys than girls. The classical example is a posterior urethral valve, which most often arises from the colliculus and forms a membrane that obstructs urinary flow. In the severe forms, the diagnosis may be detected by prenatal ultrasound showing a distended bladder, bilateral hydronephrosis, and hydroureter. In milder cases, the diagnosis is often obtained by urodynamic evaluation, either by reduced flow rate on a uroflowmetry or by detrusor hyperactivity during filling and high pressures during voiding on invasive urodynamic investigation in a boy with treatment resistant day-time incontinence. Valve patients have long-lasting bladder dysfunction that often requires treatment and should be followed to adulthood [7]. Another problem in these patients is polyuria caused by post-obstructive renal tubular damage. Especially at night, this can result in bladder retention and a nocturnal catheter may be necessary. Other forms of LUT obstructions exist ranging from bladder neck obstruction, syringocele, meatal stenosis, and in rare cases a stenosis caused by phimosis.

Other Types of Incontinence

Giggle Incontinence

Giggle incontinence typically occurs during pre-puberty and more commonly in girls [259, 263]. The aetiology is unknown [264]. Physical and urodynamic examination are most often normal. It has been postulated that the giggling, via central nervous system centres, triggers a reflex relaxation of the urethral sphincter, which starts a bladder contraction and micturition. The syndrome is often very disturbing for the affected child, and it is of little comfort to the child that the condition generally improves over time. Many different treatment modalities have been tried, but no controlled trials exist. No treatment is documented as effective, and most are ineffective. Sympathicomimetic agents, such as methylphenidate, and imipramine, together with biofeedback training for better pelvic floor control and for control of the sphincter are some of the treatment options. Others have tried anticholinergics. Only 50% of patients benefit from medication [263, 265–268].

Vaginal Voiding

In a substantial number of girls, the hymen is funnel-shaped or the labia are partly fused, and during voiding part of the stream will enter the vagina so that the urine will dribble after the patient has left the toilet. In addition, some girls, especially obese ones, tend to sit on the toilet with the thighs close together, which will obstruct normal urine flow and direct some urine into the vagina during micturition. Symptoms are diagnostic, with dribbling just after leaving the toilet and the treatment is simple in most cases: the child changes to a backward position on the toilet, with one leg on each side of the toilet so that she will be forced to spread her legs widely.

Summary

NE and voiding dysfunction are very common disorders of childhood and adolescence that despite their benign nature are often chronic and cause significant negative effects on the child's well-being. Furthermore, although the large majority of patients have a non-organic etiology, some have an underlying structural or neurogenic anomaly that causes not only resistance to standard therapy but also poses a threat to renal function. With a structured approach based mainly on a thorough history and physical examination and a frequency-volume chart, it is possible to identify subjects at risk for having underlying pathology and to obtain the correct diagnosis in the majority of cases. Only a minority of patients need invasive urodynamic investigation and imaging. In patients with NE, knowledge about functional bladder capacity and nocturnal urine volume facilitate the choice of treatment modality. The initial conservative treatment of daytime incontinence is based primarily upon bladder rehabilitation and only some patients need pharmacological treatment, biofeedback, or more aggressive treatment. Although there have been advances in our understanding of the mechanisms behind non-neuropathic bladder-sphincter dysfunction, there are still many unanswered questions and good evidence-based treatment modalities are still needed.

References

1. Hagglof B, et al. Self-esteem in children with nocturnal enuresis and urinary incontinence: improvement of self-esteem after treatment. Eur Urol. 1998;33(Suppl 3):16–9.
2. Theunis M, et al. Self-image and performance in children with nocturnal enuresis. Eur Urol. 2002;41(6):660–7; discussion 667.
3. De Bruyne E, et al. Problem behavior, parental stress and enuresis. J Urol. 2009;182(4 Suppl):2015–20.
4. Warzak WJ. Psychosocial implications of nocturnal enuresis. Clin Pediatr (Phila). 1993;Spec No:38–40.
5. Yeung CK, et al. Characteristics of primary nocturnal enuresis in adults: an epidemiological study. BJU Int. 2004;93(3):341–5.
6. Yeung CK, et al. Differences in characteristics of nocturnal enuresis between children and adoles-

cents: a critical appraisal from a large epidemiological study. BJU Int. 2006;97(5):1069–73.

7. Djurhuus JC, Rittig S. Nocturnal enuresis. Curr Opin Urol. 2002;12(4):317–20.

8. Hjalmas K, et al. Nocturnal enuresis: an international evidence based management strategy. J Urol. 2004;171(6 Pt 2):2545–61.

9. Forsythe WI, Redmond A. Enuresis and spontaneous cure rate. Study of 1129 enuretis. Arch Dis Child. 1974;49(4):259–63.

10. Evans PR. The treatment of enuresis in childhood. Nurs Mirror Midwives J. 1976;142(13):62–3.

11. Evans JI. Sleep of enuretics. Br Med J. 1971;3(5766):110.

12. Alexander L. Tackling the problem of enuresis. RN. 1966;29(6):46–50.

13. Edwards SD, van der Spuy HI. Hypnotherapy as a treatment for enuresis. J Child Psychol Psychiatry. 1985;26(1):161–70.

14. Wagner WG, Johnson JT. Childhood nocturnal enuresis - the prediction of premature withdrawal from behavioral conditioning. J Abnorm Child Psychol. 1988;16(6):687–92.

15. Stark M. Assessment and management of the care of children with nocturnal enuresis: guidelines for primary care. Nurse Pract Forum. 1994;5(3):170–6.

16. Poulton EM, Hinden E. The classification of enuresis. Arch Dis Child. 1953;28(141):392–7.

17. van Gool JD, et al. Multi-center randomized controlled trial of cognitive treatment, placebo, oxybutynin, bladder training, and pelvic floor training in children with functional urinary incontinence. Neurourol Urodyn. 2014;33(5):482–7.

18. De Paepe H, et al. Pelvic-floor therapy in girls with recurrent urinary tract infections and dysfunctional voiding. Br J Urol. 1998;81(Suppl 3):109–13.

19. Hellstrom A, et al. Association between urinary symptoms at 7 years old and previous urinary tract infection. Arch Dis Child. 1991;66(2):232–4.

20. Capitanucci ML, et al. Long-term bladder function followup in boys with posterior urethral valves: comparison of noninvasive vs invasive urodynamic studies. J Urol. 2012;188(3):953–7.

21. Borch L, et al. Bladder and bowel dysfunction and the resolution of urinary incontinence with successful management of bowel symptoms in children. Acta Paediatr. 2013;102(5):e215–20.

22. Burgers RE, et al. Management of functional constipation in children with lower urinary tract symptoms: report from the Standardization Committee of the International Children's Continence Society. J Urol. 2013;190(1):29–36.

23. Bauer SB, et al. Standardizing terminology in pediatric urology. J Pediatr Urol. 2007;3(2):163.

24. Bauer SB. Neurogenic bladder dysfunction. Pediatr Clin N Am. 1987;34(5):1121–32.

25. Bauer SB. Special considerations of the overactive bladder in children. Urology. 2002;60(5 Suppl 1):43–8; discussion 49.

26. Song M, et al. Bladder capacity in kidney transplant patients with end-stage renal disease. Int Urol Nephrol. 2015;47(1):101–6.

27. Dion M, et al. Debilitating lower urinary tract symptoms in the post-renal transplant population can be predicted pretransplantation. Transplantation. 2013;95(4):589–94.

28. Alstrup K, et al. Abnormal diurnal rhythm of urine output following renal transplantation: the impact of blood pressure and diuretics. Transplant Proc. 2010;42(9):3529–36.

29. Norgaard JP, et al. Standardization and definitions in lower urinary tract dysfunction in children. International Children's Continence Society. Br J Urol. 1998;81(Suppl 3):1–16.

30. Neveus T. The new International Children's Continence Society's terminology for the paediatric lower urinary tract—why it has been set up and why we should use it. Pediatr Nephrol. 2008;23(11):1931–2.

31. Neveus T, et al. Evaluation of and treatment for monosymptomatic enuresis: a standardization document from the International Children's Continence Society. J Urol. 2010;183(2):441–7.

32. Austin PF, et al. The standardization of terminology of lower urinary tract function in children and adolescents: update report from the Standardization Committee of the International Children's Continence Society. J Urol. 2014;191(6): 1863–1865.e13.

33. Vande Walle J, et al. Practical consensus guidelines for the management of enuresis. Eur J Pediatr. 2012;171(6):971–83.

34. Franco I, et al. Evaluation and treatment of non-monosymptomatic nocturnal enuresis: a standardization document from the International Children's Continence Society. J Pediatr Urol. 2013;9(2):234–43.

35. Neveus T, et al. Management and treatment of nocturnal enuresis-an updated standardization document from the International Children's Continence Society. J Pediatr Urol. 2020;16(1):10–9.

36. Neveus T, et al. The standardization of terminology of lower urinary tract function in children and adolescents: report from the Standardisation Committee of the International Children's Continence Society. J Urol. 2006;176(1):314–24.

37. Neveus T. The evaluation and treatment of therapy-resistant enuresis: a review. Ups J Med Sci. 2006;111(1):61–71.

38. Loeys B, et al. Does monosymptomatic enuresis exist? A molecular genetic exploration of 32 families with enuresis/incontinence. BJU Int. 2002;90(1):76–83.

39. Collier J, et al. An investigation of the impact of nocturnal enuresis on children's self-concept. Scand J Urol Nephrol. 2002;36(3):204–8.

40. Robson WL, Leung AK. Secondary nocturnal enuresis. Clin Pediatr (Phila). 2000;39(7):379–85.

41. Feehan M, et al. A 6 year follow-up of childhood enuresis: prevalence in adolescence and consequences for mental health. J Paediatr Child Health. 1990;26(2):75–9.
42. Sakamoto K, Blaivas JG. Adult onset nocturnal enuresis. J Urol. 2001;165(6 Pt 1):1914–7.
43. Rawashdeh YF, et al. Demographics of enuresis patients attending a referral centre. Scand J Urol Nephrol. 2002;36(5):348–53.
44. Jarvelin MR, et al. Enuresis in seven-year-old children. Acta Paediatr Scand. 1988;77(1):148–53.
45. Hirasing RA, et al. Enuresis nocturna in adults. Scand J Urol Nephrol. 1997;31(6):533–6.
46. Hsu CC, Chiu Y. An epidemiological study on enuresis among school age children: 2nd report. A study on the reliability of information obtained through questionnaires regarding the presence and absence of enuresis. Taiwan Yi Xue Hui Za Zhi. 1969;68(1):35–9.
47. Serel TA, et al. Epidemiology of enuresis in Turkish children. Scand J Urol Nephrol. 1997;31(6):537–9.
48. Moilanen I, et al. A follow-up of enuresis from childhood to adolescence. Br J Urol. 1998;81(Suppl 3):94–7.
49. Hellstrom AL, et al. Micturition habits and incontinence in 7-year-old Swedish school entrants. Eur J Pediatr. 1990;149(6):434–7.
50. Norgaard JP, Rittig S, Djurhuus JC. Nocturnal enuresis: an approach to treatment based on pathogenesis. J Pediatr. 1989;114(4 Pt 2):705–10.
51. Butler RJ, et al. Nocturnal enuresis at 7.5 years old: prevalence and analysis of clinical signs. BJU Int. 2005;96(3):404–10.
52. Rittig N, et al. Outcome of a standardized approach to childhood urinary symptoms-long-term follow-up of 720 patients. Neurourol Urodyn. 2014;33(5):475–81.
53. Van Herzeele C, et al. Predictive parameters of response to desmopressin in primary nocturnal enuresis. J Pediatr Urol. 2015;11(4):200.e1–8.
54. Lottmann H, et al. Long-term desmopressin response in primary nocturnal enuresis: open-label, multinational study. Int J Clin Pract. 2009;63(1):35–45.
55. Franco I. New ideas in the cause of bladder dysfunction in children. Curr Opin Urol. 2011;21(4):334–8.
56. Neveus T. The role of sleep and arousal in nocturnal enuresis. Acta Paediatr. 2003;92(10):1118–23.
57. Neveus T, et al. Enuresis—background and treatment. Scand J Urol Nephrol Suppl. 2000;206:1–44.
58. Rittig S, et al. Abnormal diurnal rhythm of plasma vasopressin and urinary output in patients with enuresis. Am J Phys. 1989;256(4 Pt 2):F664–71.
59. Rittig S, et al. The circadian defect in plasma vasopressin and urine output is related to desmopressin response and enuresis status in children with nocturnal enuresis. J Urol. 2008;179(6):2389–95.
60. Kamperis K, et al. Excess diuresis and natriuresis during acute sleep deprivation in healthy adults. Am J Physiol Renal Physiol. 2010;299(2):F404–11.
61. Rittig S, et al. Age related nocturnal urine volume and maximum voided volume in healthy children: reappraisal of International Children's Continence Society definitions. J Urol. 2010;183(4):1561–7.
62. Rittig S, et al. Age-related changes in the circadian control of urine output. Scand J Urol Nephrol Suppl. 1995;173:71–4; discussion 74–5.
63. Rittig S, et al. Adult enuresis. The role of vasopressin and atrial natriuretic peptide. Scand J Urol Nephrol Suppl. 1989;125:79–86.
64. Poulton EM. Relative nocturnal polyuria as a factor in enuresis. Lancet. 1952;2(6741):906–7.
65. Kamperis K, et al. The circadian rhythm of urine production, and urinary vasopressin and prostaglandin E2 excretion in healthy children. J Urol. 2004;171(6 Pt 2):2571–5.
66. Dhondt K, et al. Sleep fragmentation and increased periodic limb movements are more common in children with nocturnal enuresis. Acta Paediatr. 2014;103(6):e268–72.
67. Dhondt K, et al. Abnormal sleep architecture and refractory nocturnal enuresis. J Urol. 2009;182(4 Suppl):1961–5.
68. Mahler B, et al. Puberty alters renal water handling. Am J Physiol Renal Physiol. 2013;305(12):F1728–35.
69. Rittig S. Neuroendocrine response to supine posture in healthy children and patients with nocturnal enuresis. Clin Endocrinol. 2010;72(6):781–6.
70. Kruse A, et al. Increased nocturnal blood pressure in enuretic children with polyuria. J Urol. 2009;182(4 Suppl):1954–60.
71. Mahler B, et al. Sleep deprivation induces excess diuresis and natriuresis in healthy children. Am J Physiol Renal Physiol. 2012;302(2):F236–43.
72. Hunsballe JM, et al. Polyuric and non-polyuric bedwetting—pathogenic differences in nocturnal enuresis. Scand J Urol Nephrol Suppl. 1995;173:77–8; discussion 79.
73. Rittig S, et al. Long-term home studies of water balance in patients with nocturnal enuresis. Scand J Urol Nephrol Suppl. 1997;183:25–6; discussion 26–7.
74. Norgaard JP, et al. Nocturnal studies in enuretics. A polygraphic study of sleep-EEG and bladder activity. Scand J Urol Nephrol Suppl. 1989;125:73–8.
75. Raes A, et al. Partial response to intranasal desmopressin in children with monosymptomatic nocturnal enuresis is related to persistent nocturnal polyuria on wet nights. J Urol. 2007;178(3 Pt 1):1048–51; discussion 1051–2.
76. Hansen MN, et al. Intra-individual variability in nighttime urine production and functional bladder capacity estimated by home recordings in patients with nocturnal enuresis. J Urol. 2001;166(6):2452–5.
77. Tauris LH, et al. Reduced anti-diuretic response to desmopressin during wet nights in patients with monosymptomatic nocturnal enuresis. J Pediatr Urol. 2012;8(3):285–90.

78. Knudsen UB, et al. Long-term treatment of nocturnal enuresis with desmopressin. A follow-up study. Urol Res. 1991;19(4):237–40.

79. Rittig S, Knudsen UB, Sorensen S. Longterm doubleblind crossover study of DDAVP intranasal spray in the management of nocturnal enuresis. In: Desmopresin in nocturnal enuresis. Sutton Coldfield, England: Horus Medical Publications; 1989.

80. Kamperis K, et al. Nocturnal polyuria in monosymptomatic nocturnal enuresis refractory to desmopressin treatment. Am J Physiol Renal Physiol. 2006;291(6):F1232–40.

81. Raes A, et al. Abnormal circadian rhythm of diuresis or nocturnal polyuria in a subgroup of children with enuresis and hypercalciuria is related to increased sodium retention during daytime. J Urol. 2006;176(3):1147–51.

82. Vande Walle J, et al. Nocturnal polyuria is related to 24-hour diuresis and osmotic excretion in an enuresis population referred to a tertiary center. J Urol. 2007;178(6):2630–4.

83. Dehoorne JL, et al. Desmopressin resistant nocturnal polyuria secondary to increased nocturnal osmotic excretion. J Urol. 2006;176(2):749–53.

84. Guven A, Giramonti K, Kogan BA. The effect of obesity on treatment efficacy in children with nocturnal enuresis and voiding dysfunction. J Urol. 2007;178(4 Pt 1):1458–62.

85. Merhi BA, et al. Mono-symptomatic nocturnal enuresis in lebanese children: prevalence, relation with obesity, and psychological effect. Clin Med Insights Pediatr. 2014;8:5–9.

86. Weintraub Y, et al. Enuresis—an unattended comorbidity of childhood obesity. Int J Obes. 2013;37(1):75–8.

87. Kamperis K, et al. Effect of indomethacin on desmopressin resistant nocturnal polyuria and nocturnal enuresis. J Urol. 2012;188(5):1915–22.

88. Goessaert AS, et al. Long-term followup of children with nocturnal enuresis: increased frequency of nocturia in adulthood. J Urol. 2014;191(6):1866–70.

89. Goessaert AS, et al. Nocturnal enuresis and nocturia, differences and similarities - lessons to learn? Acta Clin Belg. 2014;2014:2295333714Y0000000055.

90. Goessaert AS, et al. Diagnosing the pathophysiologic mechanisms of nocturnal polyuria. Eur Urol. 2015;67(2):283–8.

91. Aceto G, et al. Enuresis subtypes based on nocturnal hypercalciuria: a multicenter study. J Urol. 2003;170(4 Pt 2):1670–3.

92. Valenti G, et al. Low-calcium diet in hypercalciuric enuretic children restores AQP2 excretion and improves clinical symptoms. Am J Physiol Renal Physiol. 2002;283(5):F895–903.

93. Valenti G, et al. Urinary aquaporin 2 and calciuria correlate with the severity of enuresis in children. J Am Soc Nephrol. 2000;11(10):1873–81.

94. Vande Walle JG, et al. A new fast-melting oral formulation of desmopressin: a pharmacodynamic study in children with primary nocturnal enuresis. BJU Int. 2006;97(3):603–9.

95. De Guchtenaere A, et al. Oral lyophylizate formulation of desmopressin: superior pharmacodynamics compared to tablet due to low food interaction. J Urol. 2011;185(6):2308–13.

96. De Guchtenaere A, et al. Evidence of partial antienuretic response related to poor pharmacodynamic effects of desmopressin nasal spray. J Urol. 2009;181(1):302–9; discussion 309.

97. De Guchtenaere A, et al. Nocturnal polyuria is related to absent circadian rhythm of glomerular filtration rate. J Urol. 2007;178(6):2626–9.

98. Hagstroem S, et al. Monosymptomatic nocturnal enuresis is associated with abnormal nocturnal bladder emptying. J Urol. 2004;171(6 Pt 2):2562–6; discussion 2566.

99. Rushton HG, et al. The influence of small functional bladder capacity and other predictors on the response to desmopressin in the management of monosymptomatic nocturnal enuresis. J Urol. 1996;156(2 Pt 2):651–5.

100. Rushton HG, et al. Predictors of response to desmopressin in children and adolescents with monosymptomatic nocturnal enuresis. Scand J Urol Nephrol Suppl. 1995;173:109–10; discussion 110–1.

101. Oredsson AF, Jorgensen TM. Changes in nocturnal bladder capacity during treatment with the bell and pad for monosymptomatic nocturnal enuresis. J Urol. 1998;160(1):166–9.

102. Hvistendahl GM, et al. The relationship between desmopressin treatment and voiding pattern in children. BJU Int. 2002;89(9):917–22.

103. Koff SA, Wagner TT, Jayanthi VR. The relationship among dysfunctional elimination syndromes, primary vesicoureteral reflux and urinary tract infections in children. J Urol. 1998;160(3 Pt 2): 1019–22.

104. Joensson IM, et al. 24-hour rectal manometry for overactive bladder. J Urol. 2009;182(4 Suppl):1927–32.

105. Joensson IM, et al. Transabdominal ultrasound of rectum as a diagnostic tool in childhood constipation. J Urol. 2008;179(5):1997–2002.

106. Chase JW, et al. Functional constipation in children. J Urol. 2004;171(6 Pt 2):2641–3.

107. Niemczyk J, et al. Prevalence of incontinence, attention deficit/hyperactivity disorder and oppositional defiant disorder in preschool children. Eur Child Adolesc Psychiatry. 2015;24(7):837–43.

108. von Gontard A, et al. Association of attention deficit and elimination disorders at school entry: a population based study. J Urol. 2011;186(5): 2027–32.

109. Von Gontard A, et al. Central nervous system involvement in nocturnal enuresis: evidence of general neuromotor delay and specific brainstem dysfunction. J Urol. 2001;166(6):2448–51.

110. Baeyens D, et al. The prevalence of ADHD in children with enuresis: comparison between a

tertiary and non-tertiary care sample. Acta Paediatr. 2006;95(3):347–52.

111. Van Hoecke E, et al. Internalizing and externalizing problem behavior in children with nocturnal and diurnal enuresis: a five-factor model perspective. J Pediatr Psychol. 2006;31(5):460–8.

112. Ornitz EM, et al. Prepulse inhibition of startle, intelligence and familial primary nocturnal enuresis. Acta Paediatr. 2000;89(4):475–81.

113. Ornitz EM, et al. Prepulse inhibition of startle and the neurobiology of primary nocturnal enuresis. Biol Psychiatry. 1999;45(11):1455–66.

114. Baeyens D, et al. The impact of attention deficit hyperactivity disorders on brainstem dysfunction in nocturnal enuresis. J Urol. 2006;176(2):744–8.

115. Norgaard JP, et al. Simultaneous registration of sleep-stages and bladder activity in enuresis. Urology. 1985;26(3):316–9.

116. Hunsballe JM, Rittig S, Djurhuus JC. Sleep and arousal in adolescents and adults with nocturnal enuresis. Scand J Urol Nephrol Suppl. 1995;173: 59–60; discussion 60–1.

117. Watanabe H. Sleep patterns in children with nocturnal enuresis. Scand J Urol Nephrol Suppl. 1995;173:55–6; discussion 56–7.

118. Pedersen MJ, et al. The role of sleep in the pathophysiology of nocturnal enuresis. Sleep Med Rev. 2020;49:101228.

119. Ertan P, et al. Relationship of sleep quality and quality of life in children with monosymptomatic enuresis. Child Care Health Dev. 2009;35(4):469–74.

120. Wolfish NM. Sleep/arousal and enuresis subtypes. J Urol. 2001;166(6):2444–7.

121. Van Herzeele C, et al. Periodic limb movements during sleep are associated with a lower quality of life in children with monosymptomatic nocturnal enuresis. Eur J Pediatr. 2015;174(7):897–902.

122. Cohen-Zrubavel V, et al. Sleep and sleepiness in children with nocturnal enuresis. Sleep. 2011;34(2):191–4.

123. Ferrara P, et al. Association among nocturnal enuresis, body weight and obstructive sleep apnea in children of south Italy: an observational study. Minerva Pediatr. 2019;71(6):511–4.

124. Weissbach A, et al. Adenotonsilectomy improves enuresis in children with obstructive sleep apnea syndrome. Int J Pediatr Otorhinolaryngol. 2006;70(8):1351–6.

125. Kaditis AG, et al. Obstructive sleep disordered breathing in 2- to 18-year-old children: diagnosis and management. Eur Respir J. 2016;47(1):69–94.

126. Kovacevic L, et al. Why does adenotonsillectomy not correct enuresis in all children with sleep disordered breathing? J Urol. 2014;191(5 Suppl):1592–6.

127. Neveus T, et al. Respiration during sleep in children with therapy-resistant enuresis. Acta Paediatr. 2014;103(3):300–4.

128. Kovacevic L, et al. Adenotonsillectomy improves quality of life in children with sleep-disordered breathing regardless of nocturnal enuresis outcome. J Pediatr Urol. 2015;11(5):269.e1–5.

129. Kovacevic L, et al. Adenotonsillectomy normalizes hormones and urinary electrolytes in children with nocturnal enuresis and sleep-disordered breathing. Urology. 2015;86(1):158–61.

130. Jorgensen CS, et al. Identification of genetic loci associated with nocturnal enuresis: a genome-wide association study. Lancet Child Adolesc Health. 2021;5(3):201–9.

131. Carskadon MA. Sleep deprivation: health consequences and societal impact. Med Clin North Am. 2004;88(3):767–76.

132. Culpepper L. Secondary insomnia in the primary care setting: review of diagnosis, treatment, and management. Curr Med Res Opin. 2006;22(7): 1257–68.

133. Hislop J, Arber S. Sleepers wake! The gendered nature of sleep disruption among mid-life women. Sociology. 2003;37(4):695–711.

134. Yeung CK, Diao M, Sreedhar B. Cortical arousal in children with severe enuresis. N Engl J Med. 2008;358(22):2414–5.

135. Kanaheswari Y, Poulsaeman V, Chandran V. Self-esteem in 6- to 16-year-olds with monosymptomatic nocturnal enuresis. J Paediatr Child Health. 2012;48(10):E178–82.

136. Natale N, et al. Quality of life and self-esteem for children with urinary urge incontinence and voiding postponement. J Urol. 2009;182(2):692–8.

137. Butler R, McKenna S. Overcoming parental intolerance in childhood nocturnal enuresis: a survey of professional opinion. BJU Int. 2002;89(3): 295–7.

138. Pugner K, Holmes J. Nocturnal enuresis: economic impacts and self-esteem preliminary research results. Scand J Urol Nephrol Suppl. 1997;183:65–9.

139. Schulpen TW. The burden of nocturnal enuresis. Acta Paediatr. 1997;86(9):981–4.

140. Hagglof B, et al. Self-esteem before and after treatment in children with nocturnal enuresis and urinary incontinence. Scand J Urol Nephrol Suppl. 1997;183:79–82.

141. Longstaffe S, Moffatt ME, Whalen JC. Behavioral and self-concept changes after six months of enuresis treatment: a randomized, controlled trial. Pediatrics. 2000;105(4 Pt 2):935–40.

142. Maternik M, Krzeminska K, Zurowska A. The management of childhood urinary incontinence. Pediatr Nephrol. 2015;30(1):41–50.

143. Nieuwhof-Leppink AJ, et al. Definitions, indications and practice of urotherapy in children and adolescents: a standardization document of the International Children's Continence Society (ICCS). J Pediatr Urol. 2021;17(2):172–81.

144. Cederblad M, et al. No effect of basic bladder advice in enuresis: a randomized controlled trial. J Pediatr Urol. 2015;11(3):153.e1–5.

145. Olivera CK, et al. Nonantimuscarinic treatment for overactive bladder: a systematic review. Am J Obstet Gynecol. 2016;215(1):34–57.

146. Riley KE. Evaluation and management of primary nocturnal enuresis. J Am Acad Nurse Pract. 1997;9(1):33–9; quiz 40–1.

147. Glazener CM, Evans JH, Peto RE. Alarm interventions for nocturnal enuresis in children. Cochrane Database Syst Rev. 2005;(2):CD002911.

148. Glazener CM, Evans JH, Cheuk DK. Complementary and miscellaneous interventions for nocturnal enuresis in children. Cochrane Database Syst Rev. 2005;(2):CD005230.

149. Woo SH, Park KH. Enuresis alarm treatment as a second line to pharmacotherapy in children with monosymptomatic nocturnal enuresis. J Urol. 2004;171(6 Pt 2):2615–7.

150. Hvistendahl GM, et al. The effect of alarm treatment on the functional bladder capacity in children with monosymptomatic nocturnal enuresis. J Urol. 2004;171(6 Pt 2):2611–4.

151. Baeyens D, et al. Adherence in children with nocturnal enuresis. J Pediatr Urol. 2009;5(2):105–9.

152. Van Herzeele C, et al. Poor compliance with primary nocturnal enuresis therapy may contribute to insufficient desmopressin response. J Urol. 2009;182(4 Suppl):2045–9.

153. Glazener CM, Evans JH. Desmopressin for nocturnal enuresis in children. Cochrane Database Syst Rev. 2002;(3):CD002112.

154. Lackgren G, et al. Desmopressin in the treatment of severe nocturnal enuresis in adolescents—a 7-year follow-up study. Br J Urol. 1998;81(Suppl 3):17–23.

155. Vande Walle J, et al. Desmopressin 30 years in clinical use: a safety review. Curr Drug Saf. 2007;2(3):232–8.

156. Robson WL. Clinical practice. Evaluation and management of enuresis. N Engl J Med. 2009;360(14):1429–36.

157. Kamperis K, et al. The effect of desmopressin on renal water and solute handling in desmopressin resistant monosymptomatic nocturnal enuresis. J Urol. 2008;180(2):707–13; discussion 713–4.

158. Lottmann H, et al. A randomised comparison of oral desmopressin lyophilisate (MELT) and tablet formulations in children and adolescents with primary nocturnal enuresis. Int J Clin Pract. 2007;61(9):1454–60.

159. De Bruyne P, et al. Pharmacokinetics of desmopressin administered as tablet and oral lyophilisate formulation in children with monosymptomatic nocturnal enuresis. Eur J Pediatr. 2014;173(2):223–8.

160. Hjalmas K, Bengtsson B. Efficacy, safety, and dosing of desmopressin for nocturnal enuresis in Europe. Clin Pediatr (Phila). 1993;Spec No:19–24.

161. Kjoller SS, Hejl M, Pedersen PS. Enuresis treated with minurin (DDAVP). A controlled clinical study. Ugeskr Laeger. 1984;146(43):3281–2.

162. Janknegt RA, Smans AJ. Treatment with desmopressin in severe nocturnal enuresis in childhood. Br J Urol. 1990;66(5):535–7.

163. Butler RJ, Holland P, Robinson J. Examination of the structured withdrawal program to prevent relapse of nocturnal enuresis. J Urol. 2001;166(6):2463–6.

164. Marschall-Kehrel D, Harms TW, Surve EAM. Structured desmopressin withdrawal improves response and treatment outcome for monosymptomatic enuretic children. J Urol. 2009;182(4):2022–6.

165. Hjalmas K, et al. Long-term treatment with desmopressin in children with primary monosymptomatic nocturnal enuresis: an open multicentre study. Swedish Enuresis Trial (SWEET) Group. Br J Urol. 1998;82(5):704–9.

166. Keenswijk W, Walle JV. A 4-year-old boy presenting with persistent urinary incontinence: Questions. Pediatr Nephrol (Berlin, Germany). 2017;32(5):767–8.

167. Hall H, Sallemark M, Wedel I. Acute effects of atypical antidepressants on various receptors in the rat brain. Acta Pharmacol Toxicol (Copenh). 1984;54(5):379–84.

168. Labay P, Boyarsky S. The action of imipramine on the bladder musculature. J Urol. 1973;109(3):385–7.

169. Hunsballe JM, et al. Single dose imipramine reduces nocturnal urine output in patients with nocturnal enuresis and nocturnal polyuria. J Urol. 1997;158(3 Pt 1):830–6.

170. Kales A, et al. Effects of imipramine on enuretic frequency and sleep stages. Pediatrics. 1977;60(4):431–6.

171. Esperanca M, Gerrard JW. Nocturnal enuresis: comparison of the effect of imipramine and dietary restriction on bladder capacity. Can Med Assoc J. 1969;101(12):65–8.

172. Puri VN. Increased urinary antidiuretic hormone excretion by imipramine. Exp Clin Endocrinol. 1986;88(1):112–4.

173. Rohner TJ Jr, Sanford EJ. Imipramine toxicity. J Urol. 1975;114(3):402–3.

174. Montaldo P, et al. Desmopressin and oxybutynin in monosymptomatic nocturnal enuresis: a randomized, double-blind, placebo-controlled trial and an assessment of predictive factors. BJU Int. 2012;110(8 Pt B):E381–6.

175. Austin PF, et al. Combination therapy with desmopressin and an anticholinergic medication

for nonresponders to desmopressin for monosymptomatic nocturnal enuresis: a randomized, double-blind, placebo-controlled trial. Pediatrics. 2008;122(5):1027–32.

176. Iglesias A, Iglesias A. Secondary diurnal enuresis treated with hypnosis: a time-series design. Int J Clin Exp Hypn. 2008;56(2):229–40.

177. Seabrook JA, Gorodzinsky F, Freedman S. Treatment of primary nocturnal enuresis: a randomized clinical trial comparing hypnotherapy and alarm therapy. Paediatr Child Health. 2005;10(10):609–10.

178. Leboeuf C, et al. Chiropractic care of children with nocturnal enuresis: a prospective outcome study. J Manip Physiol Ther. 1991;14(2):110–5.

179. Reed WR, et al. Chiropractic management of primary nocturnal enuresis. J Manip Physiol Ther. 1994;17(9):596–600.

180. van Poecke AJ, Cunliffe C. Chiropractic treatment for primary nocturnal enuresis: a case series of 33 consecutive patients. J Manip Physiol Ther. 2009;32(8):675–81.

181. Huang T, et al. Complementary and miscellaneous interventions for nocturnal enuresis in children. Cochrane Database Syst Rev. 2011;(12):CD005230.

182. Bower WF, Diao M. Acupuncture as a treatment for nocturnal enuresis. Auton Neurosci. 2010;157(1–2):63–7.

183. Radvanska E, et al. Effect of laser acupuncture for monosymptomatic nocturnal enuresis on bladder reservoir function and nocturnal urine output. J Urol. 2011;185(5):1857–61.

184. Lordelo P, et al. Treatment of non-monosymptomatic nocturnal enuresis by transcutaneous parasacral electrical nerve stimulation. J Pediatr Urol. 2010;6(5):486–9.

185. Barroso U Jr, et al. Nonpharmacological treatment of lower urinary tract dysfunction using biofeedback and transcutaneous electrical stimulation: a pilot study. BJU Int. 2006;98(1):166–71.

186. De Guchtenaere A, et al. Desmopressin resistant nocturnal polyuria may benefit from furosemide therapy administered in the morning. J Urol. 2007;178(6):2635–9; discussion 2639.

187. De Guchtenaere A, et al. Abnormal circadian rhythm of diuresis is related to absence of circadian variation in GFR. Pediatr Nephrol. 2007;22:1639.

188. Merks BT, et al. Melatonin treatment in children with therapy-resistant monosymptomatic nocturnal enuresis. J Pediatr Urol. 2012;8(4):416–20.

189. Kovacevic L, et al. Enuretic children with obstructive sleep apnea syndrome: should they see otolaryngology first? J Pediatr Urol. 2013;9(2):145–50.

190. Neveus T, et al. Orthodontic widening of the palate may provide a cure for selected children with therapy-resistant enuresis. Acta Paediatr. 2014;103(11):1187–91.

191. Kaerts N, et al. Toilet training in daycare centers in Flanders, Belgium. Eur J Pediatr. 2012;171(6):955–61.

192. van Nunen K, et al. Parents' views on toilet training (TT): a quantitative study to identify the beliefs and attitudes of parents concerning TT. J Child Health Care. 2015;19(2):265–74.

193. van Gool JD, et al. Subtypes in monosymptomatic nocturnal enuresis. II. Scand J Urol Nephrol Suppl. 1999;202:8–11.

194. Whitney KE, et al. Low energy availability and impact sport participation as risk factors for urinary incontinence in female athletes. J Pediatr Urol. 2021;17(3):290.e1–7.

195. Combs AJ, et al. Primary bladder neck dysfunction in children and adolescents I: Pelvic floor electromyography lag time—a new noninvasive method to screen for and monitor therapeutic response. J Urol. 2005;173(1):207–10; discussion 210–1.

196. Chase J, et al. The management of dysfunctional voiding in children: a report from the Standardisation Committee of the International Children's Continence Society. J Urol. 2010;183(4):1296–302.

197. Wells MJ, et al. The effect of caffeinated versus decaffeinated drinks on overactive bladder: a double-blind, randomized, crossover study. J Wound Ostomy Continence Nurs. 2014;41(4):371–8.

198. Dossche L, et al. The long-term added value of voiding school for children with refractory non-neurogenic overactive bladder: an inpatient bladder rehabilitation program. J Pediatr Urol. 2020;16(3):350 e1–8.

199. Everaerts W, De Ridder D. Unravelling the underactive bladder: a role for TRPV4? BJU Int. 2013;111(2):353–4.

200. Everaerts W, et al. On the origin of bladder sensing: Tr(i)ps in urology. Neurourol Urodyn. 2008;27(4):264–73.

201. Mawla I, et al. Natural bladder filling alters resting brain function at multiple spatial scales: a proof-of-concept MAPP Network Neuroimaging Study. Sci Rep. 2020;10(1):19901.

202. Yeung CK, et al. Natural filling cystometry in infants and children. Br J Urol. 1995;75(4):531–7.

203. Nijman RJ. Role of antimuscarinics in the treatment of nonneurogenic daytime urinary incontinence in children. Urology. 2004;63(3 Suppl 1):45–50.

204. Bogaert G, et al. Practical recommendations of the EAU-ESPU guidelines committee for monosymptomatic enuresis-Bedwetting. Neurourol Urodyn. 2020;39(2):489–97.

205. Hoebeke P, et al. Solifenacin for therapy resistant overactive bladder. J Urol. 2009;182(4 Suppl):2040–4.

206. Newgreen D, et al. Solifenacin in children and adolescents with overactive bladder: results of a phase 3 randomised clinical trial. Eur Urol. 2017;71(3):483–90.

207. Diokno AC, Lapides J. Oxybutynin: a new drug with analgesic and anticholinergic properties. J Urol. 1972;108(2):307–9.

208. Glazener CM, Evans JH, Peto RE. Tricyclic and related drugs for nocturnal enuresis in children. Cochrane Database Syst Rev. 2003;(3): CD002117.

209. Youdim K, Kogan BA. Preliminary study of the safety and efficacy of extended-release oxybutynin in children. Urology. 2002;59(3):428–32.

210. Gleason JM, et al. Single center experience with oxybutynin transdermal system (patch) for management of symptoms related to non-neuropathic overactive bladder in children: an attractive, well tolerated alternative form of administration. J Pediatr Urol. 2014;10(4):753–7.

211. Kretschmar M, et al. A population pharmacokinetic model of (R)- and (S-) oxybutynin and its active metabolites after oral and intravesical administration to healthy volunteers. J Clin Pharmacol. 2021;61(7):961–71.

212. Schroder A, et al. Efficacy, safety, and tolerability of intravesically administered 0.1% oxybutynin hydrochloride solution in adult patients with neurogenic bladder: a randomized, prospective, controlled multi-center trial. Neurourol Urodyn. 2016;35(5): 582–8.

213. Molina Caballero A, et al. Intravesical oxybutynin for urgent bladder rescue in a newborn with posterior urethral valves. Eur J Pediatr Surg Rep. 2019;7(1):e90–2.

214. Van Kampen M, et al. High initial efficacy of full-spectrum therapy for nocturnal enuresis in children and adolescents. BJU Int. 2002;90(1):84–7.

215. Sureshkumar P, et al. Treatment of daytime urinary incontinence in children: a systematic review of randomized controlled trials. J Urol. 2003;170(1):196–200; discussion 200.

216. De Grazia E, Cimador M. Oxybutinin-desmopressin association in the treatment of primary nocturnal enuresis with diurnal urination disorders. Minerva Pediatr. 1999;51(5):149–52.

217. Azarfar A, et al. Comparison of combined treatment with desmopressin plus oxybutynin and desmopressin plus tolterodine in treatment of children with primary nocturnal enuresis. J Renal Inj Prev. 2015;4(3):80–6.

218. Tahmaz L, et al. Combination therapy of imipramine with oxybutynin in children with enuresis nocturna. Urol Int. 2000;65(3):135–9.

219. Hjalmas K, et al. The overactive bladder in children: a potential future indication for tolterodine. BJU Int. 2001;87(6):569–74.

220. Ellsworth PI, et al. Use of tolterodine in children with neurogenic detrusor overactivity: relationship between dose and urodynamic response. J Urol. 2005;174(4 Pt 2):1647–51; discussion 1651.

221. Nijman RJ, et al. Tolterodine treatment for children with symptoms of urinary urge incontinence suggestive of detrusor overactivity: results from 2 randomized, placebo controlled trials. J Urol. 2005;173(4):1334–9.

222. Reddy PP, et al. Long-term efficacy and safety of tolterodine in children with neurogenic detrusor overactivity. J Pediatr Urol. 2008;4(6):428–33.

223. Nijman RJ, et al. Long-term tolerability of tolterodine extended release in children 5-11 years of age: results from a 12-month, open-label study. Eur Urol. 2007;52(5):1511–6.

224. Reinberg Y, et al. Therapeutic efficacy of extended release oxybutynin chloride, and immediate release and long acting tolterodine tartrate in children with diurnal urinary incontinence. J Urol. 2003;169(1):317–9.

225. Malhotra B, et al. The design and development of fesoterodine as a prodrug of 5-hydroxymethyl tolterodine (5-HMT), the active metabolite of tolterodine. Curr Med Chem. 2009;16(33):4481–9.

226. Oh M, et al. Genotype-based enrichment study design for minimizing the sample size in bioequivalence studies using tolterodine and CYP2D6 genotype. Int J Clin Pharmacol Ther. 2019;57(2): 110–6.

227. Marschall-Kehrel D, et al. Treatment with propiverine in children suffering from nonneurogenic overactive bladder and urinary incontinence: results of a randomized placebo-controlled phase 3 clinical trial. Eur Urol. 2009;55(3):729–36.

228. Alloussi S, et al. Efficacy, tolerability and safety of propiverine hydrochloride in comparison to oxybutynin in children with urge incontinence due to overactive bladder: results of a multicentre observational cohort study. BJU Int. 2010;106(4):550–6.

229. Kim WJ, et al. Efficacy and safety of propiverine in children with overactive bladder. Korean J Urol. 2012;53(4):275–9.

230. Fujinaga S, Nishizaki N, Ohtomo Y. Initial combination therapy with desmopressin, solifenacin, and alarm for monosymptomatic nocturnal enuresis. Pediatr Int. 2017;59(3):383–4.

231. Abrams P, et al. Combination treatment with mirabegron and solifenacin in patients with overactive bladder: exploratory responder analyses of efficacy and evaluation of patient-reported outcomes from a randomized, double-blind, factorial, dose-ranging, Phase II study (SYMPHONY). World J Urol. 2017;35(5):827–38.

232. Bolduc S, et al. Prospective open label study of solifenacin for overactive bladder in children. J Urol. 2010;184(4 Suppl):1668–73.

233. Nadeau G, et al. Long-term use of solifenacin in pediatric patients with overactive bladder: extension of a prospective open-label study. Can Urol Assoc J. 2014;8(3–4):118–23.

234. Krauwinkel WJ, et al. Evaluation of the pharmacokinetic interaction between the beta3-adrenoceptor agonist mirabegron and the muscarinic receptor antagonist solifenacin in healthy subjects. Clin Pharmacol Drug Dev. 2013;2(3):255–63.

235. Tannenbaum S, et al. Pharmacokinetics of solifenacin in pediatric populations with overactive bladder

or neurogenic detrusor overactivity. Pharmacol Res Perspect. 2020;8(6):e00684.

236. Franco I, et al. Long-term efficacy and safety of solifenacin in pediatric patients aged 6 months to 18 years with neurogenic detrusor overactivity: results from two phase 3 prospective open-label studies. J Pediatr Urol. 2020;16(2):180.e1–8.

237. van den Heijkant M, et al. Can oral fesoterodine be an alternative for intravesical oxybutynin instillations in children with neuropathic bladder dysfunction? Urol Int. 2019;103(2):202–10.

238. Kim TH, et al. Safety and efficacy of fesoterodine fumarate in patients with overactive bladder: results of a post-marketing surveillance study in Korea. Curr Med Res Opin. 2016;32(8):1361–6.

239. Ramsay S, et al. A randomized, crossover trial comparing the efficacy and safety of fesoterodine and extended-release oxybutynin in children with overactive bladder with 12-month extension on fesoterodine: the FOXY study. Can Urol Assoc J. 2020;14(6):192–8.

240. Vella M, Cardozo L. Review of fesoterodine. Expert Opin Drug Saf. 2011;10(5):805–8.

241. Malhotra B, et al. Dose-escalating study of the pharmacokinetics and tolerability of fesoterodine in children with overactive bladder. J Pediatr Urol. 2012;8(4):336–42.

242. Humphreys MR, Reinberg YE. Contemporary and emerging drug treatments for urinary incontinence in children. Paediatr Drugs. 2005;7(3):151–62.

243. Meadow R, Berg I. Controlled trial of imipramine in diurnal enuresis. Arch Dis Child. 1982;57(9):714–6.

244. Neveus T. Reboxetine in therapy-resistant enuresis: results and pathogenetic implications. Scand J Urol Nephrol. 2006;40(1):31–4.

245. Lundmark E, Neveus T. Reboxetine in therapy-resistant enuresis: a retrospective evaluation. Scand J Urol Nephrol. 2009;43(5):365–8.

246. Andersson KE, Martin N, Nitti V. Selective beta(3)-adrenoceptor agonists for the treatment of overactive bladder. J Urol. 2013;190(4):1173–80.

247. Rossanese M, et al. Critical analysis of phase II and III randomised control trials (RCTs) evaluating efficacy and tolerability of a beta(3)-adrenoceptor agonist (Mirabegron) for overactive bladder (OAB). BJU Int. 2015;115(1):32–40.

248. Park JS, et al. Efficacy and safety of mirabegron, a beta3-adrenoceptor agonist, for treating neurogenic bladder in pediatric patients with spina bifida: a retrospective pilot study. World J Urol. 2019;37(8):1665–70.

249. Fryer S, et al. Effectiveness and tolerability of mirabegron in children with overactive bladder: a retrospective pilot study. J Pediatr Surg. 2020;55(2):316–8.

250. Blais AS, et al. Prospective pilot study of mirabegron in pediatric patients with overactive bladder. Eur Urol. 2016;70(1):9–13.

251. Rittig S, et al. The pharmacokinetics, safety, and tolerability of mirabegron in children and adolescents with neurogenic detrusor overactivity or idiopathic overactive bladder and development of a population pharmacokinetic model-based pediatric dose estimation. J Pediatr Urol. 2020;16(1):31 e1–31 e10.

252. Homsy YL. Dysfunctional voiding syndromes and vesicoureteral reflux. Pediatr Nephrol. 1994;8(1):116–21.

253. Cain MP, et al. Alpha blocker therapy for children with dysfunctional voiding and urinary retention. J Urol. 2003;170(4 Pt 2):1514–5; discussion 1516–7.

254. Donohoe JM, Combs AJ, Glassberg KI. Primary bladder neck dysfunction in children and adolescents II: results of treatment with alpha-adrenergic antagonists. J Urol. 2005;173(1):212–6.

255. Van Batavia JP, et al. Primary bladder neck dysfunction in children and adolescents III: results of long-term alpha-blocker therapy. J Urol. 2010;183(2):724–30.

256. Austin P. The role of alpha blockers in children with dysfunctional voiding. TheScientificWorldJournal. 2009;9:880–3.

257. Austin PF, et al. alpha-Adrenergic blockade in children with neuropathic and nonneuropathic voiding dysfunction. J Urol. 1999;162(3 Pt 2):1064–7.

258. Tarcan T, et al. Do the definitions of the underactive bladder and detrusor underactivity help in managing patients: International Consultation on Incontinence Research Society (ICI-RS) Think Tank 2017? Neurourol Urodyn. 2018;37(S4):S60–8.

259. Austin PF, et al. The standardization of terminology of lower urinary tract function in children and adolescents: update report from the standardization committee of the International Children's Continence Society. Neurourol Urodyn. 2016;35(4):471–81.

260. Bauer SB, et al. International Children's Continence Society standardization report on urodynamic studies of the lower urinary tract in children. Neurourol Urodyn. 2015;34(7):640–7.

261. Bauer SB. Neurogenic bladder: etiology and assessment. Pediatr Nephrol. 2008;23(4):541–51.

262. Gumus B, et al. Prevalence of nocturnal enuresis and accompanying factors in children aged 7–11 years in Turkey. Acta Paediatr. 1999;88(12):1369–72.

263. Richardson I, Palmer LS. Successful treatment for giggle incontinence with biofeedback. J Urol. 2009;182(4 Suppl):2062–6.

264. Logan BL, Blais S. Giggle incontinence: evolution of concept and treatment. J Pediatr Urol. 2017;13(5):430–5.

265. Berry AK, Zderic S, Carr M. Methylphenidate for giggle incontinence. J Urol. 2009;182(4 Suppl):2028–32.

266. Chang JH, et al. Clinical and urodynamic effect of methylphenidate for the treatment of giggle incontinence (enuresis risoria). Neurourol Urodyn. 2011;30(7):1338–42.

267. Sher PK, Reinberg Y. Successful treatment of giggle incontinence with methylphenidate. J Urol. 1996;156(2 Pt 2):656–8.

268. Haciislamoglu A, et al. Evaluation of the efficacies of methylphenidate and biofeedback treatments in giggle incontinence: one-year follow-up study. J Pediatr Urol. 2021;17(5):646.e1–5.

269. Benninga MA, Faure C, Hyman PE, St James Roberts I, Schechter NL, Nurko S. Childhood functional gastrointestinal disorders: neonate/toddler. Gastroenterology. 2016;150:1443–1455.e2.

270. Tekgul S, Stein R, Bogaert G, Undre S, Nijman RJM, Quaedackers J, 't Hoen L, Kocvara R, Silay MS, Radmayr C, Dogan HS. EAU-ESPU guidelines recommendations for daytime lower urinary tract conditions in children. Eur J Pediatr. 2020;179(7):1069–77. https://doi.org/10.1007/s00431-020-03681-w.

Part X

Hypertension

Hypertension: Epidemiology, Evaluation, and Blood Pressure Monitoring

48

Ian Macumber and Andrew M. South

Abbreviations

2016 ESH guidelines	2016 European Society of Hypertension guidelines for the management of high blood pressure in children and adults
2017 CPG	2017 American Academy of Pediatrics Clinical Practice Guideline for Screening and Management of High Blood Pressure in Children and Adolescents

ABPM	Ambulatory blood pressure monitoring
BSA	Body surface area
CKD	Chronic kidney disease
CTA	Computed tomographic angiography
Fourth Report	2004 Fourth Report on the Diagnosis, Evaluation, and Treatment of High Blood Pressure in Children and Adolescents
HTN	Hypertension
LVH	Left ventricular hypertrophy
LVMI	Left ventricular mass index
MRA	Magnetic resonance angiography

I. Macumber (✉)
Section of Nephrology, Department of Pediatrics, Children's Hospital Los Angeles, Keck School of Medicine of the University of Southern California, Los Angeles, CA, USA
e-mail: imacumber@chla.usc.edu

A. M. South
Section of Nephrology, Department of Pediatrics, Brenner Children's, Wake Forest University School of Medicine, Winston-Salem, NC, USA

Department of Epidemiology and Prevention, Division of Public Health Services, Wake Forest University School of Medicine, Winston-Salem, NC, USA

Department of Surgery – Hypertension and Vascular Research, Wake Forest University School of Medicine, Winston-Salem, NC, USA
e-mail: asouth@wakehealth.edu

Introduction and Importance

Hypertension (HTN) remains an important but underappreciated medical condition in youth. In the short term, acute and chronic HTN rarely are associated with increased morbidity and mortality during childhood, though specific sub-populations of youth with secondary HTN (e.g., patients with kidney failure on dialysis) have an increased incidence of morbidity and mortality during childhood. Youth-onset HTN predicts persistent adult HTN and cardiovascular disease [1] and is associated with target organ damage both in childhood and adulthood [2]. While long-term outcome data remain limited [3], it is paramount that children and adolescents continue to be appropriately screened for HTN and that patients with HTN are accurately diagnosed, evaluated, and treated by health care providers with sufficient expertise in pediatric HTN [4]. In this chapter, we will discuss blood pressure screening recommendations and high-risk populations, compare the different methods of blood pressure assessment, and review diagnosis and evaluation recommendations for children and adolescents with HTN.

Morbidity and Mortality During Childhood

Cardiac Complications

Subclinical cardiovascular disease is detectable in children and young adults with HTN. Left ventricular hypertrophy (LVH), defined by an elevated left ventricular mass index (LVMI) relative to body size, is detectable in approximately 40% of children and young adults with HTN [5–7]. Children with HTN had impaired ventricular relaxation and diastolic dysfunction compared to healthy peers with normal blood pressure [8]. Higher blood pressure was associated with fatty streaks and fibrous plaques in the coronary arteries and aorta of deceased children and young adults in the Bogalusa Heart Study [9]. Congestive heart failure may develop, presenting with peripheral or pulmonary edema, dyspnea, chest pain, or a gallop rhythm. Some or all of these symptoms can occur in up to 29% of patients with acute severe HTN [10]. Cardiomegaly may be detected on imaging, though chest radiographs have poor sensitivity and specificity and should not be used to screen for cardiomegaly in this setting [11]. LVH was found in 43% of pediatrics patients presenting with hypertensive emergency [12], suggesting a high prevalence of chronic HTN.

Neuropathy/Retinopathy

Neurologic manifestations are the most common symptoms and include headache and dizziness, with seizures occurring in up to 20% of patients [13]. Facial nerve palsy secondary to acute severe HTN is most commonly seen in children and can occur in 5% of cases [14]. Additional neurologic signs include vomiting, mental status changes and lethargy (i.e., encephalopathy), and visual disturbances including cortical blindness. The constellation of mental status changes, headache, visual disturbances, and seizures, coupled with radiographic findings, constitutes reversible posterior leukoencephalopathy syndrome. Increased blood pressure over time was strongly associated with development of reversible posterior leukoencephalopathy syndrome in children and adolescents at high risk [15]. Visual changes may be a sign of hypertensive retinopathy and can be due to ischemic neuropathy, retinal infarcts, optic disk edema, cortical blindness, or increased intracranial pressure. A careful physical exam can reveal papilledema or retinal hemorrhages, which indicate target organ damage in the eyes, and it is important to note that lack of visual changes does not exclude hypertensive retinopathy [16].

Cognitive Dysfunction

Increasing evidence suggests that HTN affects neurocognition during childhood and into adulthood. Multiple studies have shown that children with HTN perform worse in tests of neurocognitive function compared to normotensive controls, though of note these individuals still test in the normal range [17–19]. Recent evidence suggests that uric acid may play a role in HTN-associated neurocognitive changes [20]. Neurocognitive test results improve with successful HTN treatment [21, 22].

Kidney Disease

Kidney disease—both acute and chronic—remains one of the most common etiologies of acute severe HTN in children and adolescents [13]. Less robust evidence suggests that acute severe HTN may contribute to kidney dysfunction as well. In adults, hypertensive crisis has been associated with elevated levels of urine neutrophil gelatinase-associated lipocalin [23], an early urinary marker of acute kidney injury. The data in children are less clear, though hyponatremic hypertensive syndrome—severe HTN and natriuresis thought to be due to increased renin-angiotensin-aldosterone system activity—has been described in children with acute severe HTN [24, 25], particularly those with unilateral renal artery stenosis.

Risk Across Life Course

Numerous clinical and epidemiological studies with long-term follow up have consistently demonstrated that, across diverse populations, childhood blood pressure tracks with blood pressure throughout adulthood and that youth-onset HTN increases the risk of HTN, cardiovascular disease, and kidney disease, including associated mortality, in later adulthood [1, 26, 27]. Data from the Fels Longitudinal Study demonstrated that even a single childhood systolic blood pressure measurement that exceeded age- and sex-specific criteria (at approximately the 50th percentile) increased the odds of HTN and metabolic syndrome at ≥30 years of age [28]. This association increased exponentially with increasing numbers of blood pressure measurements [28, 29]. Individuals with higher blood pressure trajectories during childhood were more likely to have HTN as adults, a relationship that was more pronounced during adolescence in individuals who were Black and in females [30–32]. In the Childhood Determinants of Adult Health Study, children with high blood pressure had a 35% increased risk of having high blood pressure as adults compared to those with normal childhood blood pressure [27]. Higher blood pressure trajectories were also associated with the presence of more cardiovascular disease risk factors at age 38 years [32].

Pediatric blood pressure consistently has been shown to be associated with several intermediate markers of cardiovascular disease risk. Individuals with higher blood pressure during both childhood and adulthood had an increased risk of higher pulse wave velocity and higher carotid intima-media thickness (a marker of subclinical arteriosclerosis) as older adults [33–39]. Further, individuals who decreased their number of cardiovascular disease risk factors from childhood into adulthood, including resolution of prior pediatric high blood pressure, had a decreased risk of higher pulse wave velocity and higher carotid intima-media thickness compared to individuals whose risk factors did not improve into adulthood [40, 41]. Moreover, higher childhood blood pressure (12–18 years) and greater blood pressure trajectories in young adulthood (18–

30 years) were associated with higher coronary artery calcification scores 25 years later [42, 43].

Higher blood pressure trajectories during childhood and adolescence were associated with greater left ventricular mass index and LVH in later adulthood [36, 44]. Cumulative exposure to higher blood pressure in childhood and young adulthood—defined by the total and incremental areas under the curve—were significantly associated with concentric LVH, eccentric LVH, and left ventricular systolic and diastolic dysfunction in later adulthood [45–47]. In the Bogalusa Heart Study, higher blood pressure beginning in childhood was associated with greater premature mortality due to coronary artery disease (mean age 45 years) [48]. In large population-based studies from Sweden, higher blood pressure in adolescents and young adults was associated with an increased risk of coronary heart disease, myocardial infarction, stroke, and death from cardiovascular causes [49, 50]. In the Harvard Alumni Health Study, high blood pressure at young adult age was associated with increased risk of death from coronary heart disease and cardiovascular disease in later adulthood (mean age 46 years) [51]. Compared to normal or elevated blood pressure, HTN in young adults was associated with shortened life expectancy of at least 2.2 years and accounted for 58.5% excess deaths from cardiovascular disease [52].

Blood pressure during childhood is also associated with the development of kidney disease later in life. In the Hanzhong Adolescent Hypertension Cohort, worse blood pressure trajectory starting in childhood (mean age 12 years) was associated with chronic kidney disease (CKD) in adults 30 years later, defined as either an estimated glomerular filtration rate 30–60 mL/min/1.73 m^2 or albuminuria [53]. In a study of over 2.6 million healthy adolescents in Israel (mean age 17 years), adolescents with HTN had double the risk of kidney failure and triple the risk of stroke mortality after a median of 20 years of follow up [54, 55].

As summarized by the 2020 U.S. Preventive Services Task Force, "there is adequate evidence about the longitudinal association between high blood pressure in children and adolescents and high blood pressure and other intermediate outcomes in adults" [3]. Despite this wealth of evidence, long-term interventional trials are lacking due in large part to the difficulty to perform such studies. Hence, it remains unknown whether identifying or treating youth-onset HTN improves long-term outcomes.

Definition and Epidemiology

In adults, normative blood pressure thresholds and definitions for hypertensive disorders are based on robust outcomes data, including cardiovascular and all-cause mortality and morbidity [56]. However in children there is a lack of clinical outcome data, and pediatric blood pressure thresholds and definitions are instead based on epidemiological data from normative blood pressure distributions obtained from approximately 50,000 healthy children [57]. Normative distributions are based upon age, sex, and height, as these factors strongly influence blood pressure values.

In 2017, the American Academy of Pediatrics released a clinical practice guideline (CPG) for the diagnosis, evaluation, and treatment of high blood pressure in children and adolescents [4]. According to this guideline, normative blood pressure values should be based on age, sex, and height-based percentile distributions for children aged 1–13 years (tables can be found in [4]). These normative values are based on reference populations from which children with overweight or obesity were excluded since these individuals have higher blood pressure than their normal-weight peers [58–61]. Thresholds based on absolute blood pressure values were instituted for adolescents 13 years and older to integrate with the 2017 American College of Cardiology/American Heart Association (AHA) Guideline for the Prevention, Detection, Evaluation, and Management of High Blood Pressure in Adults [56].

Definition and Classification

Children and Adolescents Aged 1–17 Years of Age

The 2017 CPG instituted several changes in how it defined hypertensive disorders (Table 48.1).

Table 48.1 Blood pressure classification by casual (office) measurement. Adapted from [4]

Classification	Age <13 Years[a]	Age ≥13 Years (mmHg)
Normal BP	<90th %ile or <120/80 mmHg	<120/80
High BP	≥90th %ile or ≥120/80 mmHg	≥120/80
Elevated BP	≥90th to <95th %ile or 120–129/<80 mmHg	120–129/<80
HTN	≥95th %ile or ≥130/80 mmHg	≥130/80
Stage 1 HTN	≥95th to <95th %ile + 12 mmHg or 130–139/80–89 mmHg	130–139/80–89
Stage 2 HTN	≥95th %ile + 12 mmHg or ≥140/90 mmHg	≥140/90

BP blood pressure
[a] Whichever is lower between the percentile-based or absolute blood pressure

"Prehypertension" was replaced with "elevated blood pressure" to be consistent with adult guidelines and to emphasize the importance of lifestyle measures in preventing HTN development. Stage 2 HTN in children <13 years of age is defined as "≥95th percentile plus 12 mmHg". In adolescents 13 years of age and older, the definitions are now based only on absolute blood pressure values to be harmonious with the 2017 adult guidelines.

Infants Under a Year of Age

The normative blood pressure tables in the 2017 CPG start at age 1 year [4]. For infants under a year of age, the definition of HTN is less clear due to a paucity of normative data and increased difficulty in obtaining accurate and consistent blood pressure measurements. The 2017 CPG recommended using data compiled in Dionne et al. 2012 to define high blood pressure values in neonates up to 44 weeks postmenstrual age [62] and the published blood pressure curves provided in the 1987 Second Task Force for infants aged 1–12 months of age [63]. However, important caveats remain and warrant further study, including validation in larger and more diverse populations and normative values for infants born preterm, small for gestational age, or who have additional early-life risk factors.

Hypertensive Emergency

Acute severe HTN—also termed hypertensive emergency, a type of hypertensive crisis—describes any episode of acute, symptomatic HTN with severely high blood pressure and is associated with acute target organ damage, including acute neurologic injury, acute kidney injury, and hypertensive cardiomyopathy/congestive heart failure [4]. There exist a wide variety of symptoms—and symptom severity—that may occur with acute severe HTN. There is no established, evidenced-based definition for what constitutes severely high blood pressure. According to the 2017 CPG, clinicians should be concerned when blood pressure is 30 mmHg or more above the 95th percentile for age, sex, and height [4]. Among pediatric patients presenting to the emergency department with hypertensive crisis, 98–100% had blood pressure at or above the stage 2 HTN threshold, and patients with hypertensive emergency had higher systolic and diastolic blood pressure ratios (blood pressure indexed to the stage 2 HTN threshold) compared to those with hypertensive urgency (i.e., severely high blood pressure without symptoms or evidence of target organ damage) [10, 64, 65]. Blood pressure equal to the stage 2 HTN threshold strongly predicted development of reversible posterior leukoencephalopathy syndrome in children and adolescents at high risk [15]. Future studies are warranted to better define acute severe HTN in children, including at which blood pressure thresholds predict organ or life-threatening injury, and to develop more specific criteria to define "symptomatic" HTN with adequate predictive capabilities.

Incidence and Prevalence

True HTN incidence in the general pediatric population has not been well described historically or after publication of the 2017 CPG. In the United States, a Houston, Texas school-based screening study estimated the yearly incidence of HTN in adolescents to be approximately 0.5% [66]. In that study, HTN incidence was significantly higher in at-risk groups, including 1.4%

per year in adolescents who had a prior elevated blood pressure reading that normalized at follow up and 6.6% per year in adolescents with persistent elevated blood pressure [66]. Future investigation is needed to better define the true HTN incidence in the general pediatric population and select high-risk groups.

Prior to the 2017 CPG, multiple studies estimated youth-onset HTN prevalence to be 2–5% [67–69], while a recent meta-analysis reported the global prevalence to be 4% [70]. HTN is more common in certain pediatric populations: up to 50% of youth with CKD [71] and 24% of youth with obesity [72]. Several studies have assessed the change in prevalence of pediatric hypertensive disorders due to the 2017 CPG compared to the Fourth Report [59, 61, 73–76]. Due in part to the slightly lower threshold to define HTN in the 2017 CPG, high blood pressure prevalence increased in 6–17-year-olds in a large study in China compared to the Fourth Report [74]. A large, retrospective cohort study found prevalence of HTN to be 4.9% and of elevated blood pressure to be 4.3% [77]. Bell et al. found that high blood pressure prevalence (defined as elevated blood pressure plus HTN [78]) increased using the 2017 CPG criteria, while HTN prevalence decreased [59]. This was due, in part, to a large proportion of adolescent participants aged 13–14 years who were categorized using absolute thresholds rather than percentiles.

Screening Recommendations

There is a plethora of data demonstrating that youth-onset HTN increases the risk of morbidity and mortality in childhood (see section "Morbidity and Mortality During Childhood") and persists into adulthood and increases the future risk of cardiovascular disease, kidney disease, and related mortality across the life course (see section "Risk Across Life Course"). However, there remains insufficient evidence regarding which blood pressure thresholds predict future risk, the appropriate age to start blood pressure screening, or if screening is even efficacious [3]. Despite this, numerous organizations

and Drug Administration device approval only indicates that the device is as good as previous devices already on the market, and less than 20% of all devices have undergone validation testing for accuracy.

For these reasons, oscillometric blood pressure readings obtained with devices—validated in children—are acceptable to use as a screening method but should not be used alone to diagnose hypertensive disorders in children [4]. High blood pressures obtained via the oscillometric method should be confirmed by auscultation [4, 124].

Technical Considerations

Appropriate measurement technique is critical for accurate blood pressure assessment and HTN diagnosis. Errors in technique are especially common in children and include incorrect positioning, improper cuff bladder size, inadequate equipment, or poor provider technique.

Best practice mandates that the patient should sit calmly in a quiet room for a minimum of 5 min prior to blood pressure measurement [4, 85]. The patient's back should be supported and their feet flat on the floor and uncrossed. Unless there is a contraindication, blood pressure should be measured in the upper portion of the right upper extremity. In addition to normative blood pressures being defined in the right upper extremity, this approach also avoids falsely normal blood pressures in the setting of coarctation of the aorta. Repeated blood pressure measurements should be taken in the same extremity at each visit.

Incorrect cuff size is a common source of error, especially in children; cuffs that are too small can provide a falsely high reading, while cuffs that are too large can provide a falsely low reading [125]. Health care providers must ensure that they have the full range of cuff sizes, including thigh cuffs. The provider should measure the mid-arm circumference, located at the midpoint between the acromion and the olecranon. The cuff's bladder length should cover 75–100% of the arm circumference, without overlapping itself, and the width should be 37–50% of the arm circumference. The cuff should be placed on bare skin—avoiding tightly rolled clothing proximally—and should fit snuggly but not too tightly approximately 2 cm above the antecubital fossa. The middle of the bladder cuff should be placed over the brachial artery proximal to the antecubital fossa; most cuffs have a line or marker to assist with lining the cuff up with the artery. The extremity should be supported at heart level (i.e., the midpoint of the sternum) by the provider or a table. The patient should remain calm and still during measurement, and both the provider and the patient should avoid talking.

For manual measurements, the provider should first palpate and locate the brachial artery, which is often just proximal and medial to the antecubital fossa. They should palpate the radial artery pulse as they inflate the cuff, up to 20–30 mmHg above the point at which the pulse is no longer palpable and avoiding over-inflation. Either the diaphragm or bell of the stethoscope should be placed over the brachial artery below the lower edge of the cuff, ensuring that the diaphragm or bell is not under the cuff itself. The provider should ensure a steady and appropriate rate of cuff deflation, typically 2–3 mmHg per second. The first audible sound (phase I Korotkoff) and last audible sound (phase V Korotkoff) should be noted as the systolic and diastolic blood pressures to the nearest even number (i.e., by 2 mmHg). If the Korotkoff sounds are heard at 0 mmHg, the point at which the sound is muffled (phase IV Korotkoff) should be taken as the diastolic blood pressure.

If the patient's initial blood pressure is high, it should be repeated at least two additional times separated by 1–2 min and the subsequent readings should be averaged. If the initial blood pressures were taken manually, this averaged value is used to classify the patient's blood pressure category. If measured via an oscillometric device, then two manual blood pressure measurements should be taken and averaged [4].

Lower Extremity Measurement

For blood pressure screening and HTN diagnosis, blood pressure measurement in the lower extremities should generally be avoided as blood pressures measured in the lower extremities have been shown to correlate poorly and unreliably with blood pressures measured in the upper extremities and centrally [126–129]. However, there may be times that upper extremity blood pressures are medically contraindicated or four-extremity blood pressures are indicated (e.g., screening for coarctation of the aorta). For lower extremity measurements, the patient should be in the prone position and the appropriately sized cuff should be placed on the middle of the upper portion of the lower extremity. Cuff size recommendations are the same as for the upper extremity, and the stethoscope's diaphragm or bell is placed over the popliteal artery in the popliteal fossa [4].

Measurement in Infants

Infants provide a challenge to accurate and reliable blood pressures measurement [62]. Oscillometric readings are recommended, at least until the child's upper extremity is large enough to appropriately fit the smallest auscultatory cuff [4]. Ideally, the cuff should be left undisturbed for 15 min after placement and the measurement should not be taken within 90 min of a feed or medical intervention. Once the patient is in a relatively calm state, the blood pressure should be taken three times at 2-min intervals with the patient in the prone or supine position [62]. While these guidelines provide a standardized approach to measurement of infantile blood pressures, they are cumbersome and may be difficult to follow in practice, especially in an outpatient setting.

Importance of Repeated Measurements

As stated previously, high initial blood pressures need to be repeated at least two times at the same visit and the values averaged. Ample evidence has shown that misclassification of high blood pressure status occurs when based on only a single blood pressure reading [130, 131]. Studies in adult patients have consistently found a mean decrease in systolic blood pressure on repeat blood pressure measurements that can reclassify

many patients to a lower blood pressure category [132–134]. In a cohort study of over 800,000 children in the United States, among children with an initially high blood pressure value 71% had normal blood pressure value when rechecked at the same visit; 51% had a mean blood pressure below the 95th percentile when the two blood pressure values were averaged [130].

Repeating blood pressure measurements at subsequent visits is also critical in order to appropriately classify children. Large, population-based studies have found that 63–66% of children with initial blood pressure measurements meeting criteria for HTN will have normal blood pressures when rechecked at subsequent visits [135, 136]. Unfortunately, many children do not have appropriate follow-up visits for repeat blood pressure checks within the recommended time period. A large, retrospective study found that among 6108 individuals that had initial blood pressure values at the HTN threshold by office measurement, only 45% had a repeat measurement obtained within 6 months of the original blood pressure measurement [135].

Blood Pressure Follow-Up and Diagnosis Protocol

No additional action needs to be taken if a patient's averaged manual blood pressure is normal (Fig. 48.1). The patient should continue to have their blood pressure measured at least yearly, depending on their specific factors. However, if a screening blood pressure value is high, specific follow-up recommendations to repeat and monitor blood pressure should be followed [4]. All patients with a confirmed high blood pressure measurement should undergo lifestyle counseling (see Chap. XX).

Elevated Blood Pressure

For patients whose initial blood pressure is in the 'elevated' category, blood pressure should be checked again in 6 months. If the blood pressure remains in the elevated category at the 6-month follow-up visit, a more thorough examination should be conducted, including blood pressure

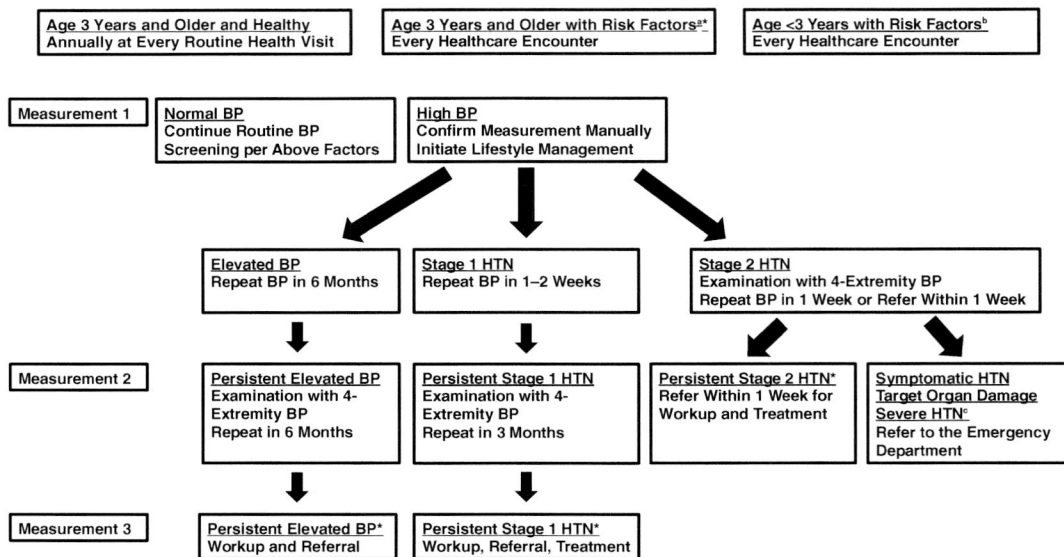

Fig. 48.1 Blood pressure screening and follow-up protocol. Recommendations based on the 2017 CPG [4]. Flow diagram based on classification of each BP measurement; a hypertension disorder diagnosis requires at least three BP measurements—obtained with appropriate methods—from different days. If BP changes classification on repeated measurement, follow flow diagram for most recent values. ABPM can be used to more accurately assess follow-up BP. [a]Obesity, chronic kidney disease, history of aortic arch obstruction or coarctation (regardless of repair status), diabetes mellitus, or taking medication known to increase BP; [b]see Table 48.2; [c]systolic or diastolic BP >30 mmHg above the 95th percentile for age, sex, and height if age <13 years or >180/120 mmHg if age ≥13 years; *indicates consideration for obtaining ABPM. ABPM, ambulatory blood pressure monitoring; *BP* blood pressure; *HTN* hypertension

measurements in both upper extremities and at least one lower extremity. The patient should be evaluated again in 6 months for another blood pressure assessment [4]. If at that point the blood pressure remains in the elevated blood pressure category—now persistent for at least 1 year—the patient should undergo ambulatory blood pressure monitoring (ABPM) under the direction of a qualified provider if available (see section "Ambulatory Blood Pressure Monitoring"), an initial workup (see section "Evaluation"), and/or referral to a HTN specialist. If at any point during this time the blood pressure normalizes, the patient can resume the standard screening regimen based on their individual risk. However, if their blood pressure worsens to the HTN category, follow-up measurements should occur more frequently as discussed below.

Stage 1 Hypertension

Patients with an initial blood pressure in the stage 1 HTN category should have their blood pressure

rechecked in 1–2 weeks and, if still high, should include both upper extremities and at least one lower extremity. If stage 1 HTN persists, blood pressure should be rechecked in 3 months. If at the third blood pressure check, the patient has persistent stage 1 HTN, they should be referred to a HTN specialist for ABPM, further evaluation, and treatment. As before, if the blood pressure improves or worsens, the provider should follow the appropriate follow-up protocol.

Stage 2 Hypertension

Patients with an initial blood pressure value in the stage 2 HTN category require more urgent follow up and evaluation. The blood pressure should be measured in the bilateral upper extremities and at least one lower extremity at the first visit. A repeat blood pressure should be obtained within 1 week, or the patient should be referred to a HTN specialist to be seen within 1 week. If the second measurement remains in the stage 2 HTN category, the patient should be referred to and seen by a HTN specialist within 1 week, in order to initiate a thorough evaluation, ABPM, and to determine if the patient warrants treatment.

Importantly, patients whose blood pressure at any point is at the stage 2 HTN category and who are symptomatic, have signs of target organ damage, or whose blood pressure is >30 mmHg above the 95th percentile for age, sex, and height (or >180/120 mmHg for adolescents), should be sent right away to the emergency department.

Ambulatory Blood Pressure Monitoring

ABPM has become a critical tool in the diagnosis and management of HTN. It more accurately predicts intermediate cardiovascular outcome measures [137] and development of future HTN [138] compared to other blood pressure measurement methods, may better distinguish primary from secondary causes of HTN [139], and is the only modality to formally evaluate for white coat HTN or masked HTN. It also has greater intra-individual reproducibility compared to in-office or out-of-office blood pressure measurement [140, 141]. The 2016 European Society of Hypertension (2016 ESH) guidelines and the 2017 CPG recognize the increasing importance of ABPM and provide specific recommendations for its use in children and adolescents at risk of HTN and as a screening tool in specific patient populations [4, 86].

Technical Considerations

The AHA has published detailed guidelines for ABPM in children and adolescents [2, 142]. The following is a brief summary, and the latest version of the AHA guidelines should be referred to for more detail.

To ensure that the data are properly collected and analyzed, ABPM should be administered by clinical staff who have sufficient training and expertise. Use of ABPM devices validated in children is essential [117, 123]. The cuff should be placed on the upper portion of the non-dominant upper extremity to minimize disruption of daily activities, unless medically contraindi-

cated. However, if there is a significant discrepancy in office blood pressure measurement (e.g., approximately >10 mmHg) between the two upper extremities, the cuff should be placed on the upper extremity with the higher blood pressure. Proper cuff size is determined using the same guidelines that are used for office blood pressure measurement [4].

Prior to having the ABPM placed, the patient and family should receive education about the study. Patients should be instructed to keep their arm still during blood pressure measurements whenever possible [2]. Patients should record major activities in a provided diary, including the patient's sleep and awake times, episodes of physical activity, stress, or pain, and medication doses. The device should only be taken off during bathing or swimming. The monitor should be programmed to record blood pressures every 15–20 min while awake and every 20–30 min while asleep.

An ABPM study is considered adequate for interpretation if there is at least one valid reading every hour and at least 40–50 valid readings in the 24-h period [2]. Interpretation should be based on the recorded sleep and awake times as opposed to the preset times to decrease the risk of misclassification [143]. When interpreting the results, it is important to determine how well the patient tolerated wearing the cuff. Reported intolerance during both awake and sleep are common [144, 145], and may influence the results of the study [146]. Some monitors use actigraphy to measure patient activity at night, and this may be a more accurate method to determine the patient's sleep time and quality [147]. The provider should screen all recorded blood pressures to identify and exclude outlier values that are above the preset parameters for values that are likely out of the normal physiologic range; most software packages do this automatically.

Classifications Incorporating Ambulatory Blood Pressure Monitoring

ABPM classifications recommended by the AHA and the 2017 CPG are primarily based on blood pressure percentiles for age, sex, and height that are distinct from those based on manual blood pressure measurement. However, important caveats remain regarding the available normative ABPM data in children. The generally accepted normative ABPM data in use are from a study of the German Working Group in 949 healthy individuals aged 5–20 years [148]. While this is widely used for ABPM interpretation, there are legitimate concerns regarding the data. The study was comprised of Caucasian children from Mid-Europe, and it is not clear how generalizable the data are to other populations. There have been few robust attempts thus far to address this issue [149], and it remains one of the most pressing issues for pediatric ABPM. There is also surprisingly little variability in the mean diastolic blood pressures among children of different heights, unlike that seen with casual blood pressures. The data also do not account for children under 120 cm in height, which may be problematic in young children with chronic conditions such as CKD in whom short stature is common.

As opposed to adult ABPM, which classifies blood pressure according to mean ambulatory blood pressure values, pediatric ABPM classification is based upon ambulatory blood pressure mean values (Table 48.3). The device software calculates and reports mean ambulatory blood pressure values for the 24-h period and for the awake and asleep periods. Mean values at or above the 95th percentile for sex and either age or height confirm a diagnosis of ambulatory HTN (Table 48.4). Adolescent patients who are tall—whose 95th percentile ambulatory blood pressure values are higher than the absolute values used in adults—are often categorized according to the adult criteria. Prior recommendations included the blood pressure load (the proportion of ABPM readings that are at or above the 95th percentile) in the diagnostic classification [2].

Table 48.3 Ambulatory blood pressure parameters

Variable	Definition	Abnormal threshold
Mean BP	Mean BP over each time period	≥95th %ile
% dipping	[Mean awake − mean sleep BP]/[mean awake BP] × 100	<10%
BP index	Mean BP/95th %ile per time period	≥1

BP blood pressure

Table 48.4 Ambulatory blood pressure classification. Adapted from [261]

Category	Casual (office) BP Age <13 years[a] Age ≥13 years	Mean ambulatory BP Age <13 years[a] Age ≥13 years
Normal BP	<95th %ile or <130/80 mmHg <130/80 mmHg	<95th %ile <130/80 wake, <110/65 sleep, <125/75 24 h
White coat hypertension	≥95th %ile or ≥130/80 mmHg ≥130/80 mmHg	<95th %ile <130/80 wake, <110/65 sleep, <125/75 24 h
Masked hypertension	<95th %ile or <130/80 mmHg <130/80 mmHg	≥95th %ile ≥130/80 wake, ≥110/65 sleep, ≥125/75 24 h
Ambulatory hypertension	≥95th or ≥130/80 mmHg ≥130/80 mmHg	≥95th %ile ≥130/80 wake, ≥110/65 sleep, ≥125/75 24 h

BP blood pressures
[a] Whichever is lower between the percentile of absolute blood pressure

However, more recent data suggest that blood pressure load does not provide prognostic value in children [150, 151], and it is no longer recommended to be included in the classification.

White Coat Hypertension

White coat HTN is a condition in which the patient's office blood pressure is in the HTN category but ambulatory blood pressure is normal (Table 48.4). White coat HTN is common in children, occurring in up to 30–50% of patients who are referred for HTN evaluation [152, 153].

Traditionally thought to be a benign condition, increasing evidence supports that white coat HTN may be associated with progression to sustained HTN [152, 154]. Although the prevalence of LVH between children who are normotensive and children with white coat HTN is not significantly different, there is evidence that patients with white coat HTN have higher LVMI [153]. The presence of obesity complicates the interpretation of these and similar data, as children with white coat HTN are more likely to have obesity, and obesity is associated with higher LVMI [155]. Studies of associations with other intermediate outcomes, such as increased carotid intima-media thickness, have provided mixed results [152, 156]. In adults, white coat HTN is associated with increased risks of cardiovascular and all-cause mortality compared to patients with normal blood pressure [157, 158], although controversy exists as to whether this increased mortality is due to white coat HTN or is due to confounding bias from common comorbidities [159].

Given the uncertainty regarding the clinical implications of white coat HTN, the optimal approach to management of these patients remains undefined. The 2017 CPG recommend that children with white coat HTN have repeat ABPM in 1–2 years to assess for improvement or progression to ambulatory HTN [4]. Further investigation is warranted to better delineate these relationships and the risk white coat HTN confers and to develop evidence-based management strategies.

Masked Hypertension

Patients whose office blood pressure is normal but who have ambulatory HTN on ABPM are classified as having masked HTN (Table 48.4). Due to the fact that patients with normal blood pressures in the office, masked HTN is generally only diagnosed in high-risk patients that undergo ABPM screening. This ascertainment bias makes it difficult to accurately estimate masked HTN prevalence in children and adolescents; several studies have estimated an 8–10% prevalence [160–162]. Masked HTN is more strongly associated with target organ damage than white coat HTN [156]. It is more common in children with secondary HTN and may help in determining HTN etiology.

Isolated nocturnal HTN, a specific form of masked HTN in which ambulatory blood pressure is only in the HTN range during sleep and office blood pressure is normal, has been strongly associated with cardiovascular outcomes in adults [163, 164]. The few studies in children have shown associations with obesity, CKD, insulin resistance, and proteinuria [165–168].

Indications for Ambulatory Blood Pressure Monitoring

While ABPM is recommended for all children and adolescents who are being evaluated for

Table 48.5 Indications for ambulatory blood pressure monitoring and associated hypertensive disorders

Clinical condition	Hypertensive disorder
Chronic kidney disease	Nocturnal HTN, masked HTN [71]
Kidney failure on dialysis	Masked HTN, worse HTN on non-dialysis days [262]
Solid-organ transplant recipient	Nocturnal HTN, masked HTN [263, 264]
Solitary kidney	Ambulatory HTN, non-dipping [265]
Type 1 or type 2 diabetes mellitus	Nocturnal HTN, masked HTN [266, 267]
Coarctation of the aorta	Masked HTN, post-repair HTN [268]
Sickle cell disease	Non-dipping [269]
History of prematurity	Ambulatory HTN, non-dipping [102, 270]

HTN, certain patient populations who are at high-risk for HTN (including those with masked HTN) may benefit from more frequent ABPM screening (Table 48.5) [4]. In particular, the 2017 CPG recommends annual ABPM screening in patients with CKD and patients with coarctation of the aorta starting no later than 12 years post-repair.

Evaluation

Once a diagnosis of HTN is established, careful and thorough evaluation, including a complete history and physical exam, is necessary to determine the etiology, detect target organ damage, and identify co-morbid conditions that may increase the risk of cardiovascular disease. In addition, emerging evidence suggests that children and adolescents with HTN may have specific cardiovascular phenotypes that stratify their risk of future cardiovascular disease. The history and physical exam in particular can detect causes of secondary HTN and can help avoid expensive and unnecessary testing.

History

With the widespread use of electronic health records, it is important to verify a patient's history recorded in their chart with what they and their caregiver report. This includes reconciling records from other practices and hospital systems. The history should evaluate for risk factors for systemic disease that may cause secondary HTN as well as risk factors for primary HTN (see Table 48.6 and Chap. XX). These include, but are not limited to, acute kidney injury or CKD (gross hematuria, edema, poor growth), rheumatologic diseases (fever, weight loss, rashes, arthritis), hyper- or hypothyroidism/endocrine disease, including pheochromocytomas/paragangliomas, (weight changes, sweating, flushing, hair changes, palpitations, tachycardia, anxiety), and sleep-disordered breathing (snoring, daytime somnolence). A careful review of medications, supplements, and recreational substance use is important. Most patients with HTN are asymptomatic, but some patients describe nonspecific symptoms such as fatigue and sleep disturbances [169]. It is vitally important to detect symptoms associated with severe HTN, including headaches, visual changes, mental status changes, seizures, chest pain, shortness of breath, and edema (Table 48.7). In infants, severe, symptomatic HTN may present as irritability, poor feeding, or poor weight gain.

Table 48.6 Key components of a history relevant to pediatric hypertension. Adapted from [271]

History	Risk factor

Birth history	Gestational age and birth weight
	    Preterm birth (<37 weeks' completed gestational age)
	    Small for gestational age

	Fetal risk factors
	    Intrauterine growth restriction
	    Abnormal fetal ultrasound including oligohydramnios

	Maternal risk factors Chronic hypertension/gestational hypertension, preeclampsia, maternal diabetes/gestational diabetes, maternal medications (including antenatal corticosteroids), maternal recreational drugs, maternal tobacco or alcohol

	Birth risk factors:
	    Cesarean section
	    Asphyxia
	    Resuscitation

	Postnatal risk factors:
	    Neonatal Intensive Care Unit admission
	    Umbilical catheters
	    Intubation with mechanical ventilation

Medical history	Kidney disease
	    Congenital anomalies of the kidney and urinary tract (including hydronephrosis and vesicoureteral reflux), solitary kidney
	    Urinary tract infection, including pyelonephritis
	    Acute kidney injury (including in neonatal period)
	    Chronic kidney disease, kidney failure on dialysis

	Prior hypertension (including in neonatal period)

	Congenital and inherited conditions
	    Congenital heart disease, including coarctation of the aorta
	    Genetic variants and syndromes

	Bronchopulmonary dysplasia, chronic lung disease, asthma
	Growth history and trajectories, overweight or obesity

	Systemic disease
	    Rheumatologic (systemic lupus erythematosus)
	    Endocrinologic (diabetes mellitus of any type, hyperthyroidism, hypothyroidism)
	    Hematologic (sickle cell disease)

	Malignancy (remission or active)
	    Chemotherapy and which regimen
	    Complications

Table 48.6   (continued)

History	Risk factor
	Transplantation: Solid organ, stem cell
	Medication regimen including immunosuppression
	Complications
	Mental/behavioral health
	Attention deficit hyperactivity disorder
	Anxiety
	Depression
	Post-traumatic stress disorder
	Sleep-disordered breathing
	Dyslipidemia, insulin resistance, hyperglycemia
Surgical history	Repaired congenital heart disease or coarctation of the aorta or vascular malformations
	Gender identity surgery
Medications/drugs	Decongestants (pseudoephedrine, phenylpropanolamine)
	Corticosteroids (short-term or chronic)
	Non-steroidal anti-inflammatory drugs
	Stimulants
	Methylphenidate
	Methylxanthines (caffeine, theophylline, aminophylline)
	Recreational drugs (marijuana, amphetamines, cocaine)
	Immunosuppressants (tacrolimus, cyclosporine)
	Tricyclic antidepressants
	Oral contraceptives
	Nicotine
Family history[a]	Hypertension (and cause)
	Overweight or obesity, dyslipidemia, diabetes mellitus of any type
	Cardiovascular disease[b]
	Coronary heart disease (myocardial infarction, angina pectoris, heart failure, and coronary death)
	Heart surgery
	Sudden cardiac death
	Cerebrovascular disease (stroke, transient ischemic attack)
	Peripheral artery disease
	Aortic atherosclerosis
	Thoracic or abdominal aortic aneurysm
	Chronic kidney disease, kidney failure on dialysis
	Congenital or inherited disease, including genetic variants and syndromes
	Systemic disease: rheumatologic, endocrinologic, hematologic, etc.
Nutritional history	Sodium intake
	Fruit and vegetable intake
	Fruit juice and sugar-sweetened beverages
	Caffeine, black licorice
Physical activity history	Organized sports or activities
	Access to physical activity resources (playground, gym, physical education in school)
Social history	More than one home and whose homes
	Who lives at home
	Who is (are) the primary caregiver(s)
	School environment (nurse available to check blood pressure)
	Unmet social needs
	Food insecurity
	Transportation insecurity
	Financial insecurity

[a] Immediate biological family members, including parents, siblings, grandparents, aunts, and uncles
[b] Especially in men before 55 years and women before 65 years

Table 48.7 Key signs and symptoms associated with hypertensive crisis

Symptoms	Physical exam findings
Visual changes	Papilledema
Headaches	Retinal hemorrhages or exudates
Mental status changes	Facial palsy
Shortness of breath	Tachypnea, crackles
Chest pains	Cardiac findings: gallop, new murmur
Gross hematuria	Peripheral edema
Seizures	Abdominal mass

Increasing and substantial evidence has demonstrated that a thorough antenatal and neonatal history should be obtained (see section "Screening Recommendations"), including maternal and fetal conditions, abnormal fetal ultrasounds (including cystic kidneys, hydronephrosis, oligohydramnios), gestational age and birth weight (including intrauterine/fetal growth restriction, small for gestational age), delivery mode and indication, and maternal medication exposure. A detailed review of any hospitalizations and medical conditions in the neonatal period is important, including admission to the Neonatal Intensive Care Unit, umbilical artery/vein catheter placement, intubation and mechanical ventilation, bronchopulmonary dysplasia, asphyxia, head or body cooling, antimicrobial exposure, nonsteroidal anti-inflammatory drug exposure, urinary tract infections, acute kidney injury, and HTN in the neonatal period.

Family history may give clues to the risk of primary HTN or select heritable forms of secondary HTN or CKD. Questions should center around family members who have HTN and at what age they were diagnosed, as well as for other conditions that are associated with HTN, such as CKD, diabetes, obesity, and sleep-disordered breathing. A specific surgical history should be obtained, with emphasis on surgeries involving the heart, intra-abdominal and retroperitoneal organs, or vasculature.

A general nutrition history should be obtained, focusing on aspects of the diet known to be associated with HTN. There is strong evidence in adults linking high dietary sodium intake with increased risk of HTN, and while the evidence in children is not as robust, numerous associations have been described, particularly in children with overweight and obesity [170]. Potassium intake is an important nutritional component, as higher potassium intake has been associated with lower blood pressures in adults [171]. This is thought to be related to the interplay between sodium and potassium, with potassium depletion increasing blood pressure sensitivity to sodium intake [172]. In children and adolescents, the relationship between potassium and blood pressure is less clear. Some studies have found an association between higher long-term potassium intake and lower risk of HTN, particularly in adolescent females [173, 174].

A comprehensive social history should be carefully obtained, as one can acquire important information about risk factors for HTN as well as barriers that may hinder the patient's ability to access and adhere to lifestyle counseling and medication. Providers should understand the patient's home and school environment, including who are the primary caregivers and if a school nurse is available to check blood pressure. Providers should assess a patient's current physical activity status, including organized sports and activities, physical education in school, and access to parks, playgrounds, and gyms. Increasing evidence in children and adults demonstrates that health disparities and unmet social needs—including limited access to health care, food, and transportation as well as financial insecurity—contribute to poor health outcomes in the short and long term [78, 175–182]. Importantly, these risk factors and barriers preferentially affect under-represented populations [183]. Providers should be cognizant of how systemic and implicit bias can affect patients' health, including HTN [184]. Further investigation into these important relationships is strongly needed, including mitigating barriers to equitable health care and social needs.

Physical Exam

The physical exam will be normal in the majority of children and adolescents with HTN. Blood pressures should be measured at all four extremi-

Table 48.8 Physical exam findings associated with secondary hypertension. Adapted from [4]

System	Exam finding	Associated condition
Growth	Overweight, obesity, central adiposity	Cushing syndrome, hypothyroidism
	Low body mass index for age and sex	Hyperthyroidism, neuroblastoma, pheochromocytoma, paraganglioma
	Short stature and poor growth velocity	Systemic disease, including chronic kidney disease, kidney failure on dialysis, inherited condition/syndrome
Dermatologic	Café-au-lait spots	Neurofibromatosis
	Neurofibromas	Neurofibromatosis
	Ash-leaf spots	Tuberous sclerosis complex
	Malar rash	Systemic lupus erythematosus
	Striae, acne	Cushing syndrome
	Flushing, diaphoresis	Pheochromocytoma, paraganglioma, neuroblastoma
	Acanthosis nigricans	Insulin resistance, type 2 diabetes mellitus, Cushing syndrome
	Spaced nipples	Turner syndrome
HEENT	Round/moon facies	Cushing syndrome
	Proptosis	Hyperthyroidism
	Adenotonsillar hypertrophy	Sleep-disordered breathing
	Elfin facies	William syndrome
	Thyromegaly	Hyperthyroidism
	Webbed neck	Turner syndrome
Cardiovascular	Tachycardia	Hyperthyroidism, neuroblastoma, pheochromocytoma/paraganglioma
	Decreased femoral pulses	Coarctation of the aorta
	Friction rub	Pericarditis (systemic lupus erythematosus, kidney failure)
	Murmur	Coarctation of the aorta
Abdomen	Mass	Wilm's tumor, pheochromocytoma/paraganglioma, neuroblastoma
	Palpable kidney	Polycystic kidney disease, hydronephrosis
	Hepatosplenomegaly	Infantile polycystic disease
	Bruit	Renovascular disease
	Edema	Kidney/renovascular disease, liver disease, heart disease, protein-losing enteropathy
Back/Flank	Flank tenderness	Pyelonephritis, obstruction, acute nephritis
Genitourinary	Ambiguous genitalia	Congenital adrenal hyperplasia
Extremities	Disparity in BPs	Aortic coarctation
	Edema	Kidney disease
	Joint swelling/stiffness	Systemic lupus erythematosus, collagen vascular disease
	Muscle weakness	Hyperaldosteronism, monogenenic hypertension
	Rickets	Chronic kidney disease, X-linked hypophosphatemia

ties to assess for coarctation of the aorta and mid-aortic syndrome. Classically, coarctation is associated with systolic HTN in the upper extremities, low blood pressure in the lower extremities, and delayed or diminished femoral pulses (also called the brachial-femoral delay) [185]. Certain physical exam findings are associated with various causes of secondary HTN and may help with diagnosis (Table 48.8). In addition, the patient should be evaluated for potential signs of HTN-induced target organ damage (Table 48.7).

Secondary Causes and Target Organ Damage

Laboratory Workup

Laboratory evaluation is performed to investigate for secondary causes of HTN and to assess for HTN-induced target organ damage, most commonly in the heart and kidneys (Table 48.9). Up to 20% of all children with HTN have CKD [4] so generally all pediatric patients with HTN should have a chemistry panel to evaluate kidney function and electrolytes. Further laboratory

Table 48.9 Recommended laboratory evaluation in patients with hypertension. Adapted from [4]

Standard assessment	Secondary assessment
Blood	*Blood*
Metabolic panel, including phosphorus, AST, ALT	Uric acid
Complete blood count with differential	Vitamin D 25-hydroxy and vitamin D-1,25-dihydroxy
Lipid profile	Complements 3 and 4
Hemoglobin A1c	Antistreptolysin O antibody
Plasma renin activity and serum aldosterone	Anti-DNase B antibody
Thyroid stimulating hormone and free thyroxine	Antinuclear antibody
	Antineutrophil cytoplasmic antibodies with proteinase 3 and myeloperoxidase antibodies
	Serum cortisol and precursors
	Plasma fractionated metanephrine
Urine	*Urine*
Urinalysis	Drug screen
Albumin, protein, and creatinine	24-h stone profile
Sodium and potassium	24-h fractionated metanephrines and catecholamines
Calcium	Vanillylmandelic acid and homovanillic acid

ALT alanine aminotransferase, *AST* aspartate aminotransferase

Table 48.10 Laboratory abnormalities in monogenic forms of hypertension. Adapted from [271]

Condition	Pota	PRA	Aldosterone	ARR
Glucocorticoid remediable aldosteronism/Familial hyperaldosteronism type I	N or ↓	↓	N or ↑	↑
Familial hyperaldosteronism type II–IV	N or ↓	↑	↑	↑
Liddle syndrome	N or ↓	↓	↓	–
Gordon syndrome	N or ↑	↓	N or ↑	↑
Apparent mineralocorticoid excess	N or ↓	↓	↓	–
Congenital adrenal hyperplasia	N or ↓	↓	↓	–
Familial glucocorticoid resistance	N or ↓	↓	↓	–

ARR aldosterone-to-renin ratio, *PRA* plasma renin activity

evaluation will depend on the specific history, physical exam, and screening study results, but may include thyroid studies, plasma renin activity, serum aldosterone levels, neurohormones, and genetic testing.

Serum electrolytes are commonly normal in children with HTN, but abnormal results may assist in identifying secondary causes of HTN including primary or secondary hyperaldosteronism or monogenic HTN [186]. These can often be distinguished from each other via serum potassium levels, plasma renin activity, and serum aldosterone levels; genetic testing is usually necessary to confirm the diagnosis (Table 48.10, Chap. XX). It is important to note that serum potassium can be normal in aldosterone-mediated HTN and that these diagnoses should be considered if an adherent patient's blood pressure is poorly controlled on multiple anti-hypertensive medications that are optimally dosed [187].

A urinalysis with urine microscopy should be performed on all children and adolescents who have HTN to investigate for secondary causes, and it may play a role in identifying target organ damage. Microscopic hematuria, defined as at least six red blood cells per high-powered field, may indicate glomerular disease—including acute glomerulonephritis of various etiologies—particularly if it confirms dysmorphic red blood cells or red blood cell casts. Proteinuria is concerning for acute kidney injury or CKD and can be a sign of target organ damage to the kidneys. A spot urine sample to quantify urine protein is highly predictive of 24-h concentrations [188] and, if positive (>0.2 mg protein/mg creatinine), should be repeated on a first-morning urine sample to differentiate orthostatic proteinuria—a common and benign condition wherein the first-morning sample is normal [189]—from pathologic proteinuria that is persistently positive.

Albuminuria

Albuminuria is defined as >30 mg albumin/g creatinine in a spot urine sample. In adults it is considered a marker of HTN-induced target organ damage to the kidneys and predicts cardiovascular disease [190]. However, there is inadequate data in children to confirm a causal relationship between albuminuria and HTN [191], and the 2017 CPG does not recommended screening for albuminuria in youth with primary HTN. Thus, the role of urine albumin testing as a marker of HTN-induced kidney-specific target organ damage warrants further study.

Renin-Angiotensin-Aldosterone System

Of note, there may be increasing utility in measuring components of the renin-angiotensin-aldosterone system in circulation and in the urine in patients with HTN. Classically, plasma renin activity and serum aldosterone have been measured to assist in screening for renal artery stenosis and secondary and primary aldosteronism (which can occur in up to 15% of adults with HTN). In adults, a suppressed plasma renin activity, elevated serum aldosterone concentration, and aldosterone-to-renin ratio >20–30 (in [ng/dL]/[ng angiotensin I/mL/h])—even in the absence of hypokalemia—increase the likelihood of an aldosterone-mediated form of HTN [192–197]. Specific diagnostic criteria to screen for and diagnose primary aldosteronism in children do not exist, though some studies suggest an ARR >10 may have utility [198].

Baseline plasma renin activity and serum aldosterone are correlated with HTN severity, and higher values predict greater improvements in blood pressure and LVMI in response to treatment in youth with primary HTN [199]. Among 47 pediatric patients with HTN, higher values of baseline urine sodium-to-potassium ratio (a proxy measure of increased dietary sodium intake relative to potassium) were associated with lower plasma renin activity and higher aldosterone-to-renin ratio values [200]. These findings suggest that these measures of the renin-angiotensin-aldosterone system may distinguish emerging HTN phenotypes such as salt-sensitive blood pressure and renin-angiotensin-aldosterone system activation vs. suppression-mediated HTN.

However, renin and aldosterone measurements have limited clinical value in part because they only represent proximal and distal aspects of the renin-angiotensin-aldosterone system. It is crucially important to consider both pathways of the renin-angiotensin-aldosterone system: angiotensin-converting enzyme/angiotensin II and angiotensin-converting enzyme 2/angiotensin-(1–7) [201]. Emerging evidence supports the value of fully assessing both pathways of the renin-angiotensin-aldosterone system in individuals with HTN. Adults with untreated primary HTN had lower urinary angiotensin-(1–7) concentrations and 24-h excretion rates compared to control participants with normal blood pressure [202]. Children with primary HTN had higher plasma angiotensin-(1–7) levels compared to peers with normal blood pressure [203]. Adolescents born preterm with very low birth weight, who are at increased risk for HTN, had a higher ratio of angiotensin II to angiotensin-(1–7) in plasma compared to term-born peers, an association that was greater in individuals with obesity and in females [105, 204]. In addition, lower urinary angiotensin-(1–7) concentrations corrected for urine creatinine were associated with higher blood pressure in adolescents and adults and predicted higher blood pressure approximately 5 years later [106, 202]. However, accurate and reproducible measurement of the renin-angiotensin-aldosterone system depends upon adhering to rigorous methods [205, 206], and reliable normative data have not been fully defined for children or adults. Further research into the role of the renin-angiotensin-aldosterone system in pediatric HTN is ongoing.

Uric Acid

The utility of obtaining serum uric acid concentrations remains controversial. Observational studies consistently demonstrate that uric acid levels are associated with HTN in cross-section and predict development of HTN, CKD, and cardiovascular mortality over time, and that lowering uric acid (e.g., with allopurinol) reduces the risk of these outcomes [109, 207–216]. However, data from clinical trials to lower uric acid levels remain conflicting [217, 218]. Evidence suggests that younger patients with shorter duration of HTN and better cardiovascular health may benefit from pharmacologic uric acid reduction [219, 220]. The reasons for these conflicting data are complex and include inadequate study design and variable patient populations/experimental disease models. Further, uric acid pathophysiology remains poorly described. The renin-angiotensin-aldosterone system likely mediates, in part, uric acid's deleterious effects, and uric acid can have anti-oxidant as well as pro-oxidant properties depending upon which tissue one investigates [109, 221–223]. The 2017 CPG concluded that there remains insufficient evidence to support or refute routine uric acid measurement when evaluating and managing youth with high blood pressure. This area remains an important area of further investigation, including the role of pharmacologic uric acid lowering.

Kidney Imaging

A **kidney ultrasound** should be considered when evaluating a patient for HTN, especially in those under 6 years of age or those who have an abnormal urinalysis or chemistry panel, have proteinuria, or who have a history of kidney abnormalities, acute kidney injury, urinary tract infections, or a family history of congenital anomalies of the kidney and urinary tract [4]. Ultrasonography can detect secondary HTN associated with CKD and aid in the diagnosis of renal artery stenosis; findings of note can include hypodysplasia, size discrepancy between both kidneys, solitary kidney or horseshoe kidney, cystic kidney disease, hydronephrosis, masses, increased echogenicity relative to the liver, and decreased corticomedullary differentiation.

For patients with a history of recurrent urinary tract infections (especially pyelonephritis), dimercaptosuccinic acid scintigraphy has historically been deemed helpful to identify scarring of the affected kidney, though it has well documented limitations [224]. To evaluate for scarring, it is recommended to wait at least 6 months after the most recent infection to allow for resolution of acute inflammation to avoid false-positive results [225]. HTN development may be delayed for years in patients who develop kidney scarring from urinary tract infections and vesicoureteral reflux [226].

Renovascular Imaging

Doppler ultrasonography can be used to screen for possible renal artery stenosis in normal-weight youth at least 8 years of age who are suspected of having renovascular HTN and can cooperate with the procedure [4]. Doppler studies are often the first-line imaging modality of choice to evaluate for renovascular HTN. However, sensitivity (64–90%) and specificity (68–70%) are low to detect or rule out renal artery stenosis and can be highly variable between sonographers and across institutions, particularly in patients with obesity and in younger children less than 8 years of age, and require extensive observer experience [227–229].

Further investigation is required when the Doppler study is normal but suspicion for renovascular disease remains high. **Computed tomographic angiography** (CTA) and **magnetic resonance angiography** (MRA) are commonly used non-invasive imaging modalities that have significantly higher sensitivity and specificity to detect renal artery stenosis compared to Doppler ultrasonography. Data in children are limited, but recent studies have estimated 88–100% sensitivity and 81–100% specificity for CTA [229–231]. For MRA, data are even more scarce, but one study estimated 81% sensitivity and 63% specificity [231]. Both CTA and MRA have additional advantages and limitations. CTA is less expensive and quicker to perform but involves significant radiation and contrast exposure, an important consideration in young patients. MRA is a longer, more expensive test that often requires sedation or general anesthesia in young children or patients with behavioral or developmental conditions that limit their ability to remain still during the test and involves exposure to contrast such as gadolinium.

The gold standard for diagnosis of renovascular HTN remains angiography [231]. Angiography may be therapeutic as well as diagnostic, but requires anesthesia, involves exposure to contrast and radiation, and is an invasive, higher risk procedure compared to CTA and MRA. A detailed description of the recommended diagnostic workflow for suspected renovascular hypertension is provided in Chap. XX.

Cardiac Imaging

Echocardiography is a useful and recommended test to diagnose cardiac causes of HTN—such as coarctation of the aorta—and HTN-induced target organ damage in the heart. The 2017 CPG recommends that echocardiography be performed when considering pharmacologic treatment of HTN [4], but many programs obtain echocardiograms for the majority of patients referred for HTN due to the fact that it is difficult to predict which patients have target organ damage. Recent evidence suggests that echocardiographic changes including LVH occur in youth with elevated blood pressure.

HTN can induce several deleterious changes to heart mass, structure, and function, including LVH, left ventricular remodeling, left atrial dilation, and, rarely, left ventricular systolic or diastolic dysfunction. Target organ damage in the heart occurs in approximately 40% of youth with HTN [5–7]. LVH is the most prominent evidence of target organ damage in children with HTN, and LVH should be defined by standardized left ventricular mass due to its correlation with body size [232]. Methods by which to calculate left ventricular mass are discussed in detail in Chap. 61.

Echocardiography should be repeated every 6–12 months to monitor for interval changes, including in patients with difficult-to-control HTN, concentric LVH, or reduced left ventricular ejection fraction. In patients with an initially normal echocardiogram, yearly repeated echocardiograms can be considered, especially for patients with stage 2 HTN, secondary HTN, or stable stage 1 HTN that is not well controlled.

While **electrocardiography** is low-cost and easy to perform, it has poor sensitivity and specificity for identifying LVH in children with HTN [233] and is therefore not recommended for use in the evaluation of pediatric HTN [4, 86].

Additional Considerations
Patients with a concern for HTN-related retinal findings should be referred to a pediatric ophthal-

mologist. The role of routine screening ophthalmologic exams by pediatric ophthalmologists in all patients with HTN remains unknown and warrants further study; however, availability of a pediatric ophthalmologist is a concern. Patients with HTN who have additional indications should undergo evaluation by a pediatric nephrologist for kidney biopsy; indications include presence of persistent proteinuria, hematuria, and acute kidney injury in addition to HTN. Patients with concern for or confirmed secondary causes of HTN should be referred to the relevant specialists for co-management with the HTN specialist (e.g., endocrinologist, cardiologist).

Co-morbidities

Patients with obesity or other risk factors for insulin resistance and diabetes mellitus should have a hemoglobin A1c assessed to screen for diabetes and liver enzymes (aspartate aminotransferase, alanine aminotransferase) to screen for non-alcoholic fatty liver disease, which is associated with HTN in children [4, 166, 234, 235]. A lipid profile should be obtained in all patients to evaluate for dyslipidemia; initial testing may be fasting or non-fasting [4]. Patients with obesity who are at higher risk should have a fasting lipid profile obtained.

Patients who have signs or symptoms of sleep-disordered breathing should be referred for polysomnography [4]. Potential symptoms include snoring, daytime somnolence, or reports of poor sleep quality. Adenotonsillar hypertrophy is a common cause of obstructive sleep apnea in children, and affected patients should be referred even in the absence of obvious symptoms. Unfortunately, access to centers with sufficient expertise in pediatric polysomnography and sleep medicine specialists is commonly limited and an area of pressing need in pediatrics.

Cardiovascular Phenotyping

There is increasing evidence that youth with HTN likely have a spectrum of cardiovascular abnormalities that may affect their HTN trajectory in the short term as well as their long-term risk of cardiovascular disease across the life course [236, 237]. Newer, non-invasive imaging modalities are under investigation to assess cardiovascular target organ damage, including arterial structure and function, and to provide valuable normative data in children [238]. Measures of central arterial stiffness include pulse wave velocity and augmentation index. Pulse wave velocity estimates the speed at which the wave produced by ventricular systole propagates through the arterial circulation, while augmentation index is an indirect measure of central aortic pressure augmentation [239, 240]. Higher pulse wave velocity and augmentation index can indicate greater arterial stiffness associated with HTN; device-specific normative data exist for youth with and without HTN [241–244]. Carotid intima-media thickness—measured by high-spacial ultrasonography—quantifies the combined thickness of the intimal and medial layer of the carotid artery and is an established marker of subclinical arteriosclerosis [245]. Pediatric normative data are available [246]. Several pediatric studies have shown an association between HTN and higher carotid intima-media thickness [247], including in children with CKD [248, 249] (see Chap. 61 for a detailed review). Additional though less utilized studies include arterial flow-mediated dilation and distensibility [237].

Finally, abnormal autonomic function—characterized by abnormal heart rate or blood pressure variability and baroreflex sensitivity—associates with HTN in children and adults and predicts cardiovascular disease [108, 250–256]. At this time, however, these modalities are not yet recommended for routine use in the diagnosis or management of pediatric HTN [4, 86] and are not widely available in clinical practice, even to HTN specialists. More research is needed, including establishment of normative data and evidence-based cut-offs for abnormal values in diverse patient and healthy control populations.

Follow Up for Patients with Hypertension

All patients with HTN require close follow up with their HTN specialist and primary care pro-

vider to monitor their blood pressure and target organ damage response to lifestyle counseling and pharmacologic treatment. Youth treated with an anti-hypertensive medication should be followed up every 4–6 weeks until blood pressure is controlled and then every 2–6 months thereafter, while patients treated only with lifestyle counseling should be followed every 3–6 months. Follow-up periods and modality (HTN specialist clinic, primary care provider clinic, home, school) should be tailored to each individual patient and the resources available to them. ABPM has increasing importance in monitoring patients' response to treatment, especially in patients with CKD or kidney transplant recipients (see section "Ambulatory Blood Pressure Monitoring"). Specific recommendations for long-term follow up and transition of care when patients become adults remain undefined and are a major topic for further research.

Out-of-Office Measurement

Home

Home blood pressure monitoring with an oscillometric device or via manual measurement is not recommended to diagnose HTN in children, due in part to lack of normative data and heterogeneous technique [140], but may be a useful approach to blood pressure follow up to complement office and ABPM measurement [4]. Much like ABPM, home blood pressure measurement has the advantage of occurring in a familiar, calm environment that partially mitigates falsely high blood pressure readings and white coat HTN. Home blood pressure measurement often demonstrates better reproducibility compared to office-based blood pressure measurement [141].

School

Blood pressure measurements taken at school can be useful to monitor children with HTN. However, data on the accuracy of these measurements is limited, and universal protocols have yet to be developed. In addition, it is difficult to evaluate the skill and technique of the person taking the blood pressure. For these reasons, school blood pressure measurements are not recommended for use in the diagnosis of HTN [4].

As with office-based blood pressure measurement using oscillometric devices, it is crucial to use only those devices that are validated in children. Additional considerations include inter-device variation and difficulty in obtaining the correct cuff size [257].

Transition of Care

Health care transition from adolescence into adulthood is an underappreciated but crucially important aspect of care [258]. Exact transition recommendations and risk profiles for long-term outcomes for children with HTN remain undefined. Adolescents with HTN—and arguably those with other hypertension disorders such as elevated blood pressure and white coat HTN—regardless of whether they are receiving pharmacologic treatment should transition their care from a pediatric to an adult health care provider as they enter adulthood [4]. The specific age for transition can vary widely across centers and should be tailored to each individual patient based on their circumstances. The pediatric specialist managing their HTN should transfer all relevant information regarding etiology, target organ damage, co-morbidity evaluation and management history. Generally, adult primary care providers have sufficient experience to manage the majority of young adults with HTN, though certain populations may require adult specialist care, including patients with CKD or secondary HTN. It is extremely important, however, that the patients themselves and all adult providers caring for these transitioned patients be educated about the importance of pediatric HTN, especially the long-term cardiovascular risk conferred.

Conclusions and Future Directions

Pediatric HTN remains an important but under-appreciated medical condition that has short and long-term implications for health during childhood and across the life course. Much progress has been made in recent years to better understand pediatric HTN risk factors, pathophysiology, detection, diagnosis, and related target organ damage. It remains critically important that primary care providers and HTN specialists—pediatric and adult providers alike—remain up-to-date on clinical care of youth with HTN and recognize its importance to long-term cardiovascular health. However, there are many areas that warrant further investigation to improve patients' cardiovascular health.

There is a pressing need for updated normative blood pressure data in youth of all ages and from diverse, international populations that can demonstrate intra-individual change over time as those individuals age and enter adulthood. This will allow for the transition of HTN definitions from more traditional, statistical/epidemiological-based normative blood pressure values to cardiovascular outcome-based approaches. Similarly, there is a need for robustly validated normative ABPM data from diverse populations that, ideally, will include cardiovascular outcome measures across the life course. This is especially true for populations with short stature or chronic medical conditions such as CKD. It remains unknown if ABPM data obtained during childhood is associated with increased risk of morbidity or mortality in later adulthood. There is no consensus regarding the appropriate blood pressure cutoffs for ABPM to confirm HTN, particularly in adolescents who are tall. The 2016 ESH guidelines recommend using adult ABPM values in cases in which pediatric thresholds exceed adult thresholds [86]. However, even the adult thresholds are not consistent, as different adult guidelines utilize different values to diagnose HTN [56, 259]. Clarification regarding the optimal thresholds is necessary for children and adolescents, as these competing guidelines can result in significantly different blood pressure classifications in pediatric patients [260]. Finally, rigorous validation and comparison of oscillometric and ABPM devices is a pressing need.

It is critically important to better understand how established and emerging early-life risk factors contribute to pediatric HTN and its short and long-term complications, including antenatal and neonatal exposures as well as social and health disparities. The long-term effects of the COVID-19 pandemic should be considered, including indirect effects from social/structural changes and direct effects via severe infection and multisystem inflammatory syndrome in children. This new knowledge will allow for more targeted and appropriate blood pressure screening guidelines.

High-quality studies are required to determine if routine blood pressure screening practices can improve short and long-term outcomes. Further investigation is required to determine the optimal approach to defining cardiovascular phenotypes (e.g., pulse wave velocity, carotid intima-media thickness), the utility of biomarkers such as angiotensin-(1–7) and other components of the renin-angiotensin-aldosterone system, and how these studies could improve clinical care. Finally, definitive guidelines and best practices for the transition of care for youth with HTN who are entering adulthood is crucially important to answer the above questions.

Pediatric HTN remains a common and important medical condition with long-term health implications. Patients and health care providers alike should be aware of the importance of screening for, diagnosing, and evaluating patients who have HTN and the risk pediatric HTN confers on long-term cardiovascular health across the life course.

References

1. Chen X, Wang Y. Tracking of blood pressure from childhood to adulthood: a systematic review and meta-regression analysis. Circulation. 2008;117(25):3171–80.
2. Flynn JT, Daniels SR, Hayman LL, Maahs DM, McCrindle BW, Mitsnefes M, et al. Update: ambulatory blood pressure monitoring in children and adolescents: a scientific statement from the American Heart Association. Hypertension. 2014;63(5):1116–35.
3. U. S. Preventive Services Task Force. Screening for high blood pressure in children and adolescents: US Preventive Services Task Force Recommendation Statement. J Am Med Assoc. 2020;324(18):1878–83.
4. Flynn JT, Kaelber DC, Baker-Smith CM, Blowey D, Carroll AE, Daniels SR, et al. Clinical practice guideline for screening and management of high blood pressure in children and adolescents. Pediatrics. 2017;140(3):e20171904.
5. Daniels SR, Loggie JM, Khoury P, Kimball TR. Left ventricular geometry and severe left ventricular

6. hypertrophy in children and adolescents with essential hypertension. Circulation. 1998;97(19):1907–11.
6. Assadi F. Effect of microalbuminuria lowering on regression of left ventricular hypertrophy in children and adolescents with essential hypertension. Pediatr Cardiol. 2007;28(1):27–33.
7. Assadi F. Relation of left ventricular hypertrophy to microalbuminuria and C-reactive protein in children and adolescents with essential hypertension. Pediatr Cardiol. 2008;29(3):580–4.
8. Navarini S, Bellsham-Revell H, Chubb H, Gu H, Sinha MD, Simpson JM. Myocardial deformation measured by 3-dimensional speckle tracking in children and adolescents with systemic arterial hypertension. Hypertension. 2017;70(6):1142–7.
9. Berenson GS, Srinivasan SR, Bao W, Newman WP III, Tracy RE, Wattigney WA. Association between multiple cardiovascular risk factors and atherosclerosis in children and young adults. The Bogalusa Heart Study. N Engl J Med. 1998;338(23):1650–6.
10. Wu H-P, Yang W-C, Wu Y-K, Zhao L-L, Chen C-Y, Fu Y-C. Clinical significance of blood pressure ratios in hypertensive crisis in children. Arch Dis Child. 2012;97(3):200–5.
11. Still JL, Cottom D. Severe hypertension in childhood. Arch Dis Child. 1967;42(221):34.
12. Lee GH, Lee IR, Park SJ, Kim JH, Oh JY, Shin JI. Hypertensive crisis in children: an experience in a single tertiary care center in Korea. Clin Hypertens. 2016;22(1):1–6.
13. Seeman T, Hamdani G, Mitsnefes M. Hypertensive crisis in children and adolescents. Pediatr Nephrol. 2019;34(12):2523–37.
14. Jörg R, Milani GP, Simonetti GD, Bianchetti MG, Simonetti BG. Peripheral facial nerve palsy in severe systemic hypertension: a systematic review. Am J Hypertens. 2013;26(3):351–6.
15. Gall E, Chaudhuri A, South AM. Peak blood pressure and prediction of posterior reversible encephalopathy syndrome in children. Pediatr Nephrol. 2020;35(10):1967–75.
16. Deal JE, Barratt TM, Dillon MJ. Management of hypertensive emergencies. Arch Dis Child. 1992;67(9):1089–92.
17. Lande MB, Adams H, Falkner B, Waldstein SR, Schwartz GJ, Szilagyi PG, et al. Parental assessments of internalizing and externalizing behavior and executive function in children with primary hypertension. J Pediatr. 2009;154(2):207–12.e1.
18. Lande MB, Batisky DL, Kupferman JC, Samuels J, Hooper SR, Falkner B, et al. Neurocognitive function in children with primary hypertension. J Pediatr. 2017;180:148–55.e1.
19. Lande MB, Kaczorowski JM, Auinger P, Schwartz GJ, Weitzman M. Elevated blood pressure and decreased cognitive function among school-age children and adolescents in the United States. J Pediatr. 2003;143(6):720–4.
20. Stabouli S, Chrysaidou K, Chainoglou A, Gidaris D, Kotsis V, Zafeiriou D. Uric acid associates

with executive function in children and adolescents with hypertension. Hypertension. 2021;2021:Hypertensionaha12016761.

21. Lande MB, Adams H, Falkner B, Waldstein SR, Schwartz GJ, Szilagyi PG, et al. Parental assessment of executive function and internalizing and externalizing behavior in primary hypertension after antihypertensive therapy. J Pediatr. 2010;157(1):114–9.

22. Lande MB, Batisky DL, Kupferman JC, Samuels J, Hooper SR, Falkner B, et al. Neurocognitive function in children with primary hypertension after initiation of antihypertensive therapy. J Pediatr. 2018;195:85–94.e1.

23. Derhaschnig U, Testori C, Riedmueller E, Hobl EL, Mayr FB, Jilma B. Decreased renal function in hypertensive emergencies. J Hum Hypertens. 2014;28(7):427–31.

24. Mukherjee D, Sinha R, Akhtar MS, Saha AS. Hyponatremic hypertensive syndrome-a retrospective cohort study. World J Nephrol. 2017;6(1):41.

25. Kovalski Y, Cleper R, Krause I, Dekel B, Belenky A, Davidovits M. Hyponatremic hypertensive syndrome in pediatric patients: is it really so rare? Pediatr Nephrol. 2012;27(6):1037–40.

26. Juhola J, Magnussen CG, Viikari JS, Kähönen M, Hutri-Kähönen N, Jula A, et al. Tracking of serum lipid levels, blood pressure, and body mass index from childhood to adulthood: the Cardiovascular Risk in Young Finns Study. J Pediatr. 2011;159(4):584–90.

27. Kelly RK, Thomson R, Smith KJ, Dwyer T, Venn A, Magnussen CG. Factors affecting tracking of blood pressure from childhood to adulthood: the Childhood Determinants of Adult Health Study. J Pediatr. 2015;167(6):1422–8.e2.

28. Sun SS, Grave GD, Siervogel RM, Pickoff AA, Arslanian SS, Daniels SR. Systolic blood pressure in childhood predicts hypertension and metabolic syndrome later in life. Pediatrics. 2007;119(2):237–46.

29. Oikonen M, Nuotio J, Magnussen CG, Viikari JS, Taittonen L, Laitinen T, et al. Repeated blood pressure measurements in childhood in prediction of hypertension in adulthood. Hypertension. 2016;67(1):41–7.

30. Naidoo S, Kagura J, Fabian J, Norris Shane A. Early life factors and longitudinal blood pressure trajectories are associated with elevated blood pressure in early adulthood. Hypertension. 2019;73(2):301–9.

31. Shen W, Zhang T, Li S, Zhang H, Xi B, Shen H, et al. Race and sex differences of long-term blood pressure profiles from childhood and adult hypertension: the Bogalusa Heart Study. Hypertension. 2017;70(1):66–74.

32. Theodore RF, Broadbent J, Nagin D, Ambler A, Hogan S, Ramrakha S, et al. Childhood to early-midlife systolic blood pressure trajectories: early-life predictors, effect modifiers, and adult cardiovascular outcomes. Hypertension. 2015;66(6):1108.

33. Aatola H, Koivistoinen T, Tuominen H, Juonala M, Lehtimäki T, Viikari JSA, et al. Influence of child and adult elevated blood pressure on adult arterial stiffness: the Cardiovascular Risk in Young Finns Study. Hypertension. 2017;70(3):531–6.

34. Raitakari OT, Juonala M, Kähönen M, Taittonen L, Laitinen T, Mäki-Torkko N, et al. Cardiovascular risk factors in childhood and carotid artery intima-media thickness in adulthood: the Cardiovascular Risk in Young Finns Study. J Am Med Assoc. 2003;290(17):2277–83.

35. Ceponiene I, Klumbiene J, Tamuleviciute-Prasciene E, Motiejunaite J, Sakyte E, Ceponis J, et al. Associations between risk factors in childhood (12–13 years) and adulthood (48–49 years) and subclinical atherosclerosis: the Kaunas Cardiovascular Risk Cohort Study. BMC Cardiovasc Disord. 2015;15:89.

36. Hao G, Wang X, Treiber FA, Harshfield G, Kapuku G, Su S. Blood pressure trajectories from childhood to young adulthood associated with cardiovascular risk: results from the 23-year longitudinal Georgia Stress and Heart Study. Hypertension. 2017;69(3):435–42.

37. Davis PH, Dawson JD, Riley WA, Lauer RM. Carotid intimal-medial thickness is related to cardiovascular risk factors measured from childhood through middle age: the Muscatine Study. Circulation. 2001;104(23):2815.

38. Juonala M, Magnussen CG, Venn A, Dwyer T, Burns TL, Davis PH, et al. Influence of age on associations between childhood risk factors and carotid intima-media thickness in adulthood: the Cardiovascular Risk in Young Finns Study, the Childhood Determinants of Adult Health Study, the Bogalusa Heart Study, and the Muscatine Study for the International Childhood Cardiovascular Cohort (i3C) Consortium. Circulation. 2010;122(24):2514–20.

39. Koskinen J, Juonala M, Dwyer T, Venn A, Petkeviciene J, Čeponienė I, et al. Utility of different blood pressure measurement components in childhood to predict adult carotid intima-media thickness. Hypertension. 2019;73(2):335–41.

40. Juhola J, Magnussen CG, Berenson GS, Venn A, Burns TL, Sabin MA, et al. Combined effects of child and adult elevated blood pressure on subclinical atherosclerosis: the International Childhood Cardiovascular Cohort Consortium. Circulation. 2013;128(3):217–24.

41. Aatola H, Hutri-Kähönen N, Juonala M, Viikari JS, Hulkkonen J, Laitinen T, et al. Lifetime risk factors and arterial pulse wave velocity in adulthood: the Cardiovascular Risk in Young Finns Study. Hypertension. 2010;55(3):806–11.

42. Allen NB, Siddique J, Wilkins JT, Shay C, Lewis CE, Goff DC, et al. Blood pressure trajectories in early adulthood and subclinical atherosclerosis in middle age. J Am Med Assoc. 2014;311(5):490–7.

43. Hartiala O, Magnussen CG, Kajander S, Knuuti J, Ukkonen H, Saraste A, et al. Adolescence risk factors are predictive of coronary artery calcification at middle age: the Cardiovascular Risk in Young Finns Study. J Am Coll Cardiol. 2012;60(15):1364–70.

44. Zhang T, Li S, Bazzano L, He J, Whelton P, Chen W. Trajectories of childhood blood pressure and adult left ventricular hypertrophy. Hypertension. 2018;72(1):93–101.

45. Lai CC, Sun D, Cen R, Wang J, Li S, Fernandez-Alonso C, et al. Impact of long-term burden of excessive adiposity and elevated blood pressure from childhood on adulthood left ventricular remodeling patterns: the Bogalusa Heart Study. J Am Coll Cardiol. 2014;64(15):1580–7.

46. Toprak A, Wang H, Chen W, Paul T, Srinivasan S, Berenson G. Relation of childhood risk factors to left ventricular hypertrophy (eccentric or concentric) in relatively young adulthood (from the Bogalusa Heart Study). Am J Cardiol. 2008;101(11):1621–5.

47. Kishi S, Teixido-Tura G, Ning H, Venkatesh BA, Wu C, Almeida A, et al. Cumulative blood pressure in early adulthood and cardiac dysfunction in middle age: the CARDIA study. J Am Coll Cardiol. 2015;65(25):2679–87.

48. Berenson GS, Srinivasan SR, Xu JH, Chen W. Adiposity and cardiovascular risk factor variables in childhood are associated with premature death from coronary heart disease in adults: the Bogalusa Heart Study. Am J Med Sci. 2016;352(5):448–54.

49. Sundström J, Neovius M, Tynelius P, Rasmussen F. Association of blood pressure in late adolescence with subsequent mortality: cohort study of Swedish male conscripts. Br Med J. 2011;342:d643.

50. Falkstedt D, Koupil I, Hemmingsson T. Blood pressure in late adolescence and early incidence of coronary heart disease and stroke in the Swedish 1969 conscription cohort. J Hypertens. 2008;26(7):1313–20.

51. Gray L, Lee IM, Sesso HD, Batty GD. Blood pressure in early adulthood, hypertension in middle age, and future cardiovascular disease mortality: HAHS (Harvard Alumni Health Study). J Am Coll Cardiol. 2011;58(23):2396–403.

52. Miura K, Daviglus ML, Dyer AR, Liu K, Garside DB, Stamler J, et al. Relationship of blood pressure to 25-year mortality due to coronary heart disease, cardiovascular diseases, and all causes in young adult men: the Chicago Heart Association Detection Project in Industry. Arch Intern Med. 2001;161(12):1501–8.

53. Zheng W, Mu J, Chu C, Hu J, Yan Y, Ma Q, et al. Association of blood pressure trajectories in early life with subclinical renal damage in middle age. J Am Soc Nephrol. 2018;29(12):2835–46.

54. Leiba A, Fishman B, Twig G, Gilad D, Derazne E, Shamiss A, et al. Association of adolescent hypertension with future end-stage renal disease. JAMA Intern Med. 2019;179(4):517–23.

55. Leiba A, Twig G, Levine H, Goldberger N, Afek A, Shamiss A, et al. Hypertension in late adolescence and cardiovascular mortality in midlife: a cohort study of 2.3 million 16- to 19-year-old examinees. Pediatr Nephrol. 2016;31(3):485–92.

56. Whelton PK, Carey RM, Aronow WS, Casey DE, Collins KJ, Dennison Himmelfarb C, et al. 2017 ACC/AHA/AAPA/ABC/ACPM/AGS/APhA/ASH/ASPC/NMA/PCNA guideline for the prevention, detection, evaluation, and management of high blood pressure in adults: a report of the American College of Cardiology/American Heart Association Task Force on Clinical Practice Guidelines. J Am Coll Cardiol. 2018;71(19):e127–248.

57. National High Blood Pressure Education Program Working Group on Hypertension Control in Children and Adolescents. Update on the 1987 Task Force Report on high blood pressure in children and adolescents: A Working Group Report from the National High Blood Pressure Education Program. Pediatrics. 1996;98(4):649–58.

58. Dionne JM. Updated guideline may improve the recognition and diagnosis of hypertension in children and adolescents; review of the 2017 AAP blood pressure clinical practice guideline. Curr Hypertens Rep. 2017;19(10):1–14.

59. Bell CS, Samuel JP, Samuels JA. Prevalence of hypertension in children: applying the new American Academy of Pediatrics clinical practice guideline. Hypertension. 2019;73(1):148–52.

60. Blanchette E, Flynn JT. Implications of the 2017 AAP Clinical Practice Guidelines for Management of Hypertension in Children and Adolescents: a review. Curr Hypertens Rep. 2019;21(5):35.

61. Khoury M, Khoury PR, Dolan LM, Kimball TR, Urbina EM. Clinical implications of the revised AAP Pediatric Hypertension Guidelines. Pediatrics. 2018;142(2):e20180245.

62. Dionne JM, Abitbol CL, Flynn JT. Hypertension in infancy: diagnosis, management and outcome. Pediatr Nephrol. 2012;27(1):17–32.

63. Task Force on Blood Pressure Control in Children. Report of the Second Task Force on Blood Pressure Control in Children—1987. Pediatrics. 1987;79(1):1–25.

64. Yang W-C, Zhao L-L, Chen C-Y, Wu Y-K, Chang Y-J, Wu H-P. First-attack pediatric hypertensive crisis presenting to the pediatric emergency department. BMC Pediatr. 2012;12(1):200.

65. Yang WC, Wu HP. Clinical analysis of hypertension in children admitted to the emergency department. Pediatr Neonatol. 2010;51(1):44–51.

66. Redwine KM, Acosta AA, Poffenbarger T, Portman RJ, Samuels J. Development of hypertension in adolescents with pre-hypertension. J Pediatr. 2012;160(1):98–103.

67. Rosner B, Cook NR, Daniels S, Falkner B. Childhood blood pressure trends and risk factors for high blood pressure: the NHANES experience 1988–2008. Hypertension. 2013;62(2):247–54.

68. Din-Dzietham R, Liu Y, Bielo M-V, Shamsa F. High blood pressure trends in children and adolescents in national surveys, 1963 to 2002. Circulation. 2007;116(13):1488–96.

69. Sorof JM, Lai D, Turner J, Poffenbarger T, Portman RJ. Overweight, ethnicity, and the prevalence of hypertension in school-aged children. Pediatrics. 2004;113(3):475–82.

70. Song P, Zhang Y, Yu J, Zha M, Zhu Y, Rahimi K, et al. Global prevalence of hypertension in children: a systematic review and meta-analysis. JAMA Pediatr. 2019;173(12):1154–63.

71. Samuels J, Ng D, Flynn JT, Mitsnefes M, Poffenbarger T, Warady BA, et al. Ambulatory blood pressure patterns in children with chronic kidney disease. Hypertension. 2012;60(1):43–50.

72. Manios Y, Karatzi K, Protogerou AD, Moschonis G, Tsirimiagou C, Androutsos O, et al. Prevalence of childhood hypertension and hypertension phenotypes by weight status and waist circumference: the Healthy Growth Study. Eur J Nutr. 2018;57(3):1147–55.

73. Sharma AK, Metzger DL, Rodd CJ. Prevalence and severity of high blood pressure among children based on the 2017 American Academy of Pediatrics Guidelines. JAMA Pediatr. 2018;172(6):557–65.

74. Dong Y, Song Y, Zou Z, Ma J, Dong B, Prochaska JJ. Updates to pediatric hypertension guidelines: influence on classification of high blood pressure in children and adolescents. J Hypertens. 2019;37(2):297.

75. Luo B, Lin Y, Gao S, Lu Y, Zhao Y, Xie J, et al. Impact of updated pediatric hypertension criteria on prevalence estimates of hypertension among Chinese children. J Hum Hypertens. 2021;35:530–6.

76. Al Kibria GM, Swasey K, Sharmeen A, Day B. Estimated change in prevalence and trends of childhood blood pressure levels in the United States after application of the 2017 AAP guideline. Prev Chronic Dis. 2019;16:E12.

77. Kaelber DC, Localio AR, Ross M, Leon JB, Pace WD, Wasserman RC, et al. Persistent hypertension in children and adolescents: a 6-year cohort study. Pediatrics. 2020;146(4):e20193778.

78. South AM, Palakshappa D, Brown CL. Relationship between food insecurity and high blood pressure in a national sample of children and adolescents. Pediatr Nephrol. 2019;34(9):1583–90.

79. Pickering TG, Hall JE, Appel LJ, Falkner BE, Graves JW, Hill MN, et al. Recommendations for blood pressure measurement in humans: an AHA scientific statement from the Council on High Blood Pressure Research Professional and Public Education Subcommittee. J Clin Hypertens. 2005;7(2):102–9.

80. Expert Panel on Integrated Guidelines for Cardiovascular Health and Risk Reduction in Children and Adolescents, National Heart, Lung, and Blood Institute. Expert Panel on Integrated Guidelines for Cardiovascular Health and Risk Reduction in Children and Adolescents: summary report. Pediatrics. 2011;128(Suppl 5):S213–S56.

81. Nerenberg KA, Zarnke KB, Leung AA, Dasgupta K, Butalia S, McBrien K, et al. Hypertension Canada's 2018 Guidelines for diagnosis, risk assessment, prevention, and treatment of hypertension in adults and children. Can J Cardiol. 2018;34(5):506–25.

82. National High Blood Pressure Education Program Working Group on High Blood Pressure in Children and Adolescents. The Fourth Report on the diagnosis, evaluation, and treatment of high blood pressure in children and adolescents. Pediatrics. 2004;114(2 Suppl 4th Report):555–76.

83. Riley M, Hernandez AK, Kuznia AL. High blood pressure in children and adolescents. Am Fam Physician. 2018;98(8):486–94.

84. Rabi DM, McBrien KA, Sapir-Pichhadze R, Nakhla M, Ahmed SB, Dumanski SM, et al. Hypertension Canada's 2020 Comprehensive Guidelines for the prevention, diagnosis, risk assessment, and treatment of hypertension in adults and children. Can J Cardiol. 2020;36(5):596–624.

85. Muntner P, Shimbo D, Carey RM, Charleston JB, Gaillard T, Misra S, et al. Measurement of blood pressure in humans: a scientific statement from the American Heart Association. Hypertension. 2019;73:e35–66.

86. Lurbe E, Agabiti-Rosei E, Cruickshank JK, Dominiczak A, Erdine S, Hirth A, et al. 2016 European Society of Hypertension Guidelines for the management of high blood pressure in children and adolescents. J Hypertens. 2016;34(10):1887–920.

87. Shah L, Hossain J, Xie S, Zaritsky J. Poor adherence to early childhood blood pressure measurement guidelines in a large pediatric healthcare system. Pediatr Nephrol. 2019;34(4):697–701.

88. de Jong F, Monteaux MC, van Elburg RM, Gillman MW, Belfort MB. Systematic review and meta-analysis of preterm birth and later systolic blood pressure. Hypertension. 2012;59(2):226–34.

89. Juonala M, Cheung MMH, Sabin MA, Burgner D, Skilton MR, Kähönen M, et al. Effect of birth weight on life-course blood pressure levels among children born premature: the Cardiovascular Risk in Young Finns Study. J Hypertens. 2015;33(8):1542–8.

90. Kagura J, Adair LS, Munthali RJ, Pettifor JM, Norris SA. Association between early life growth and blood pressure trajectories in Black South African children. Hypertension. 2016;68(5):1123–31.

91. South AM, Nixon PA, Chappell MC, Diz DI, Russell GB, Jensen ET, et al. Renal function and blood pressure are altered in adolescents born preterm. Pediatr Nephrol. 2019;34(1):137–44.

92. South AM, Shaltout HA, Gwathmey TM, Jensen ET, Nixon PA, Diz DI, et al. Lower urinary α-Klotho is associated with lower angiotensin-(1–7) and higher blood pressure in young adults born preterm with very low birthweight. J Clin Hypertens. 2020;22(6):1033–40.

93. Haikerwal A, Doyle LW, Cheung MM, Wark JD, Opie G, Roberts G, et al. High blood pressure in young adult survivors born extremely preterm or extremely low birthweight in the post surfactant era. Hypertension. 2020;75(1):211–7.

94. Andersen LG, Ängquist L, Eriksson JG, Forsen T, Gamborg M, Osmond C, et al. Birth weight, childhood body mass index and risk of coronary heart disease in adults: combined historical cohort studies. PLoS One. 2010;5(11):e14126.

95. Arnott C, Skilton MR, Ruohonen S, Juonala M, Viikari JSA, Kähönen M, et al. Subtle increases in heart size persist into adulthood in growth restricted babies: the Cardiovascular Risk in Young Finns Study. Open Heart. 2015;2(1) https://doi.org/10.1136/openhrt-2015-000265.

96. Lewandowski AJ, Augustine D, Lamata P, Davis EF, Lazdam M, Francis J, et al. Preterm heart in adult life: cardiovascular magnetic resonance reveals distinct differences in left ventricular mass, geometry, and function. Circulation. 2013;127(2):197–206.

97. Lewandowski AJ, Bradlow WM, Augustine D, Davis EF, Francis J, Singhal A, et al. Right ventricular systolic dysfunction in young adults born preterm. Circulation. 2013;128(7):713–20.

98. Kaijser M, Bonamy Anna-Karin E, Akre O, Cnattingius S, Granath F, Norman M, et al. Perinatal risk factors for ischemic heart disease: disentangling the roles of birth weight and preterm birth. Circulation. 2008;117(3):405–10.

99. Ferreira I, Peeters LL, Stehouwer CD. Preeclampsia and increased blood pressure in the offspring: meta-analysis and critical review of the evidence. J Hypertens. 2009;27(10):1955–9.

100. Kraut EJ, Boohaker LJ, Askenazi DJ, Fletcher J, Kent AL, Selewski DT, et al. Incidence of neonatal hypertension from a large multicenter study [Assessment of Worldwide Acute Kidney Injury Epidemiology in Neonates—AWAKEN]. Pediatr Res. 2018;84(2):279–89.

101. Alagappan A, Malloy MH. Systemic hypertension in very low-birth weight infants with bronchopulmonary dysplasia: incidence and risk factors. Am J Perinatol. 1998;15(1):3–8.

102. Abitbol CL, Bauer CR, Montané B, Chandar J, Duara S, Zilleruelo G. Long-term follow-up of extremely low birth weight infants with neonatal renal failure. Pediatr Nephrol. 2003;18(9):887–93.

103. Sehgal A, Malikiwi A, Paul E, Tan K, Menaham S. Systemic arterial stiffness in infants with bronchopulmonary dysplasia: potential cause of systemic hypertension. J Perinatol. 2016;36(7):564–9.

104. Sehgal A, Morrison J, Alexander B, South AM. Fetal growth restriction and hypertension in the offspring: mechanistic links and therapeutic directions. J Pediatr. 2020;224:115–23.e2.

105. South AM, Nixon PA, Chappell MC, Diz DI, Russell GB, Jensen ET, et al. Association between preterm birth and the renin−angiotensin system in adolescence: influence of sex and obesity. J Hypertens. 2018;36(10):2092–101.

106. South AM, Shaltout HA, Washburn LK, Hendricks AS, Diz DI, Chappell Mark C. Fetal programming and the angiotensin-(1–7) axis: a review

107. Mathewson KJ, Pyhälä R, Hovi P, Räikkönen K, Van Lieshout RJ, Boyle MH, et al. Cardiovascular responses to psychosocial stress reflect motivation state in adults born at extremely low birth weight. Glob Pediatr Health. 2015;2:2333794X15574092.

108. Mathewson KJ, Van Lieshout RJ, Saigal S, Morrison KM, Boyle MH, Schmidt LA. Autonomic functioning in young adults born at extremely low birth weight. Glob Pediatr Health. 2015;2:2333794X15589560.

109. South AM, Shaltout HA, Nixon PA, Diz DI, Jensen ET, O'Shea TM, et al. Association of circulating uric acid and angiotensin-(1–7) in relation to higher blood pressure in adolescents and the influence of preterm birth. J Hum Hypertens. 2020;34(12):818–25.

110. Wegman HL, Stetler C. A meta-analytic review of the effects of childhood abuse on medical outcomes in adulthood. Psychosom Med. 2009;71(8):805–12.

111. Alastalo H, Räikkönen K, Pesonen AK, Osmond C, Barker DJP, Heinonen K, et al. Early life stress and blood pressure levels in late adulthood. J Hum Hypertens. 2013;27(2):90–4.

112. Dong M, Giles Wayne H, Felitti Vincent J, Dube Shanta R, Williams Janice E, Chapman Daniel P, et al. Insights into causal pathways for ischemic heart disease. Circulation. 2004;110(13):1761–6.

113. Danese A, Moffitt TE, Harrington H, Milne BJ, Polanczyk G, Pariante CM, et al. Adverse childhood experiences and adult risk factors for age-related disease: depression, inflammation, and clustering of metabolic risk markers. Arch Pediatr Adolesc Med. 2009;163(12):1135–43.

114. Su S, Wang X, Pollock JS, Treiber FA, Xu X, Snieder H, et al. Adverse childhood experiences and blood pressure trajectories from childhood to young adulthood: the Georgia Stress and Heart study. Circulation. 2015;131(19):1674–81.

115. Lehman BJ, Taylor SE, Kiefe CI, Seeman TE. Relationship of early life stress and psychological functioning to blood pressure in the CARDIA study. Health Psychol. 2009;28(3):338–46.

116. Suglia SF, Koenen KC, Boynton-Jarrett R, Chan PS, Clark CJ, Danese A, et al. Childhood and adolescent adversity and cardiometabolic outcomes: a scientific statement from the American Heart Association. Circulation. 2018;137(5):e15–28.

117. Picone DS, Padwal R, Campbell NRC, Boutouyrie P, Brady TM, Olsen MH, et al. How to check whether a blood pressure monitor has been properly validated for accuracy. J Clin Hypertens. 2020;22(12):2167–74.

118. Johns Hopkins Bloomberg School of Public Health. Selecting blood pressure devices YouTube: Johns Hopkins Bloomberg School of Public Health; 2020 [updated 2020/7/22. YouTube video]. Available from: https://www.youtube.com/watch?v=v_y_JGfYvK8.

119. Duncombe SL, Voss C, Harris KC. Oscillometric and auscultatory blood pressure measurement methods

in children: a systematic review and meta-analysis. J Hypertens. 2017;35(2):213–24.

120. Podoll A, Grenier M, Croix B, Feig DI. Inaccuracy in pediatric outpatient blood pressure measurement. Pediatrics. 2007;119(3):e538–e43.

121. Urbina EM, Khoury PR, McCoy CE, Daniels SR, Dolan LM, Kimball TR. Comparison of mercury blood pressure readings to oscillometric and central blood pressure in predicting target organ damage in youth. Blood Press Monit. 2015;20(3):150.

122. Chiolero A, Paradis G, Lambert M. Accuracy of oscillometric devices in children and adults. Blood Press. 2010;19(4):254–9.

123. Stergiou GS, Alpert B, Mieke S, Asmar R, Atkins N, Eckert S, et al. A universal standard for the validation of blood pressure measuring devices: Association for the Advancement of Medical Instrumentation/European Society of Hypertension/International Organization for Standardization (AAMI/ESH/ISO) Collaboration Statement. J Hypertens. 2018;36(3):472–8.

124. Negroni-Balasquide X, Bell CS, Samuel J, Samuels JA. Is one measurement enough to evaluate blood pressure among adolescents? A blood pressure screening experience in more than 9000 children with a subset comparison of auscultatory to mercury measurements. J Am Soc Hypertens. 2016;10(2):95–100.

125. Sprafka JM, Strickland D, Gómez-Marín O, Prineas RJ. The effect of cuff size on blood pressure measurement in adults. Epidemiology. 1991;2:214–7.

126. Crapanzano MS, Strong WB, Newman IR, Hixon RL, Casal D, Linder CW. Calf blood pressure: clinical implications and correlations with arm blood pressure in infants and young children. Pediatrics. 1996;97(2):220–4.

127. Park MK, Lee DH, Johnson GA. Oscillometric blood pressures in the arm, thigh, and calf in healthy children and those with aortic coarctation. Pediatrics. 1993;91(4):761–5.

128. Schell K, Briening E, Lebet R, Pruden K, Rawheiser S, Jackson B. Comparison of arm and calf automatic noninvasive blood pressures in pediatric intensive care patients. J Pediatr Nurs. 2011;26(1):3–12.

129. Hayes S, Miller R, Patel A, Tumin D, Walia H, Hakim M, et al. Comparison of blood pressure measurements in the upper and lower extremities versus arterial blood pressure readings in children under general anesthesia. Med Devices. 2019;12:297–303.

130. Koebnick C, Mohan Y, Li X, Porter AH, Daley MF, Luo G, et al. Failure to confirm high blood pressures in pediatric care—quantifying the risks of misclassification. J Clin Hypertens. 2018;20(1):174–82.

131. McNiece KL, Poffenbarger TS, Turner JL, Franco KD, Sorof JM, Portman RJ. Prevalence of hypertension and pre-hypertension among adolescents. J Pediatr. 2007;150(6):640–4.e1.

132. Einstadter D, Bolen SD, Misak JE, Bar-Shain DS, Cebul RD. Association of repeated measurements with blood pressure control in primary care. JAMA Intern Med. 2018;178(6):858–60.

133. Daimee UA, Done D, Tang W, Tu XM, Bisognano JD, Bayer WH. The utility of repeating automated blood pressure measurements in the primary care office. J Clin Hypertens. 2016;18(3):250–1.

134. Rhodehouse BC, Fan J, Chen W, McNeal MJ, Durham CG, Erwin JP III. Effect of repeat manual blood pressure measurement on blood pressure and stage of hypertension. In: Baylor University Medical Center Proceedings. Taylor & Francis; 2019.

135. Daley MF, Sinaiko AR, Reifler LM, Tavel HM, Glanz JM, Margolis KL, et al. Patterns of care and persistence after incident elevated blood pressure. Pediatrics. 2013;132(2):e349–e55.

136. Meng L, Liang Y, Liu J, Hu Y, Yan Y, Mi J. Prevalence and risk factors of hypertension based on repeated measurements in Chinese children and adolescents. Blood Press. 2013;22(1):59–64.

137. Johnson PK, Ferguson MA, Zachariah JP. In-clinic blood pressure prediction of normal ambulatory blood pressure monitoring in pediatric hypertension referrals. Congenit Heart Dis. 2016;11(4):309–14.

138. Li Z, Snieder H, Harshfield GA, Treiber FA, Wang X. A 15-year longitudinal study on ambulatory blood pressure tracking from childhood to early adulthood. Hypertens Res. 2009;32(5):404–10.

139. Flynn JT. Differentiation between primary and secondary hypertension in children using ambulatory blood pressure monitoring. Pediatrics. 2002;110(1):89–93.

140. Stergiou GS, Alamara CV, Salgami EV, Vaindirlis IN, Dacou-Voutetakis C, Mountokalakis TD. Reproducibility of home and ambulatory blood pressure in children and adolescents. Blood Press Monit. 2005;10(3):143–7.

141. Stergiou GS, Nasothimiou EG, Giovas PP, Rarra VC. Long-term reproducibility of home vs. office blood pressure in children and adolescents: the Arsakeion school study. Hypertens Res. 2009;32(4):311–5.

142. Urbina E, Alpert B, Flynn J, Hayman L, Harshfield GA, Jacobson M, et al. Ambulatory blood pressure monitoring in children and adolescents: recommendations for standard assessment: a scientific statement from the American Heart Association Atherosclerosis, Hypertension, and Obesity in Youth Committee of the Council on Cardiovascular Disease in the Young and the Council for High Blood Pressure Research. Hypertension. 2008;52(3):433–51.

143. Jones HE, Sinha MD. The definition of daytime and nighttime influences the interpretation of ABPM in children. Pediatr Nephrol. 2011;26(5):775–81.

144. van der Steen MS, Lenders JWM, Thien T. Side effects of ambulatory blood pressure monitoring. Blood Press Monit. 2005;10(3):151–5.

145. Viera AJ, Lingley K, Hinderliter AL. Tolerability of the Oscar 2 ambulatory blood pressure monitor among research participants: a cross-sectional

repeated measures study. BMC Med Res Methodol. 2011;11(1):1–7.

146. Hamdani G, Flynn JT, Daniels S, Falkner B, Hanevold C, Inglefinger J, et al. Ambulatory blood pressure monitoring tolerability and blood pressure status in adolescents: the SHIP AHOY study. Blood Press Monit. 2019;24(1):12.

147. Eissa MAH, Poffenbarger T, Portman RJ. Comparison of the actigraph versus patients' diary information in defining circadian time periods for analyzing ambulatory blood pressure monitoring data. Blood Press Monit. 2001;6(1):21–5.

148. Wühl E, Witte K, Soergel M, Mehls O, Schaefer F. German Working Group on Pediatric Hypertension. Distribution of 24-h ambulatory blood pressure in children: normalized reference values and role of body dimensions. J Hypertens. 2002;20(10):1995–2007.

149. Yip GW, Li AM, So H-K, Choi KC, Leung LC, Fong N-C, et al. Oscillometric 24-h ambulatory blood pressure reference values in Hong Kong Chinese children and adolescents. J Hypertens. 2014;32(3):606–19.

150. Hamdani G, Mitsnefes MM, Flynn JT, Becker RC, Daniels S, Falkner BE, et al. Pediatric and adult ambulatory blood pressure thresholds and blood pressure load as predictors of left ventricular hypertrophy in adolescents. Hypertension. 2021;78(1):30–7.

151. Lee J, McCulloch CE, Flynn JT, Samuels J, Warady BA, Furth SL, et al. Prognostic value of ambulatory blood pressure load in pediatric CKD. Clin J Am Soc Nephrol. 2020;15(4):493–500.

152. Litwin M, Niemirska A, Ruzicka M, Feber J. White coat hypertension in children: not rare and not benign? J Am Soc Hypertens. 2009;3(6):416–23.

153. Kavey R-EW, Kveselis DA, Atallah N, Smith FC. White coat hypertension in childhood: evidence for end-organ effect. J Pediatr. 2007;150(5):491–7.

154. Miyashita Y, Hanevold C, Faino A, Scher J, Lande M, Yamaguchi I, et al. White coat hypertension persistence in children and adolescents: the Pediatric Nephrology Research Consortium study. J Pediatr. 2022;246:154–160.e1.

155. Lurbe E, Invitti C, Torro I, Maronati A, Aguilar F, Sartorio G, et al. The impact of the degree of obesity on the discrepancies between office and ambulatory blood pressure values in youth. J Hypertens. 2006;24(8):1557–64.

156. Stabouli S, Kotsis V, Toumanidis S, Papamichael C, Constantopoulos A, Zakopoulos N. White-coat and masked hypertension in children: association with target-organ damage. Pediatr Nephrol. 2005;20(8):1151–5.

157. Banegas JR, Ruilope LM, de la Sierra A, Vinyoles E, Gorostidi M, de la Cruz JJ, et al. Relationship between clinic and ambulatory blood-pressure measurements and mortality. N Engl J Med. 2018;378(16):1509–20.

158. Cohen JB, Lotito MJ, Trivedi UK, Denker MG, Cohen DL, Townsend RR. Cardiovascular events and mortality in white coat hypertension: a systematic review and meta-analysis. Ann Intern Med. 2019;170(12):853–62.

159. Muntner P, Booth JN III, Shimbo D, Schwartz JE. Is white-coat hypertension associated with increased cardiovascular and mortality risk? J Hypertens. 2016;34(8):1655–8.

160. Fujita H, Matsuoka S, Awazu M. Masked isolated nocturnal hypertension in children and young adults. Pediatr Cardiol. 2018;39(1):66–70.

161. Huang Z, Sharman JE, Fonseca R, Park C, Chaturvedi N, Davey Smith G, et al. Masked hypertension and submaximal exercise blood pressure among adolescents from the Avon Longitudinal Study of Parents and Children (ALSPAC). Scand J Med Sci Sports. 2020;30(1):25–30.

162. Iturzaeta A, Pompozzi L, Casas Rey C, Passarelli I, Torres F. Prevalence of masked hypertension among children with risk factors for arterial hypertension. Arch Argent Pediatr. 2018;116(5):328–32.

163. Hansen TW, Li Y, Boggia J, Thijs L, Richart T, Staessen JA. Predictive role of the nighttime blood pressure. Hypertension. 2011;57(1):3–10.

164. Cuspidi C, Meani S, Salerno M, Valerio C, Fusi V, Severgnini B, et al. Cardiovascular target organ damage in essential hypertensives with or without reproducible nocturnal fall in blood pressure. J Hypertens. 2004;22(2):273–80.

165. Macumber IR, Weiss NS, Halbach SM, Hanevold CD, Flynn JT. The association of pediatric obesity with nocturnal non-dipping on 24-hour ambulatory blood pressure monitoring. Am J Hypertens. 2016;29(5):647–52.

166. Giordano U, Della Corte C, Cafiero G, Liccardo D, Turchetta A, Hoshemand KM, et al. Association between nocturnal blood pressure dipping and insulin resistance in children affected by NAFLD. Eur J Pediatr. 2014;173(11):1511–8.

167. Bakhoum CY, Vuong KT, Carter CE, Gabbai FB, Ix JH, Garimella PS. Proteinuria and nocturnal blood pressure dipping in hypertensive children and adolescents. Pediatr Res. 2021;90(4):876–81.

168. Düzova A, Bayazit AK, Canpolat N, Niemirska A, Bulut IK, Azukaitis K, et al. Isolated nocturnal and isolated daytime hypertension associate with altered cardiovascular morphology and function in children with chronic kidney disease: findings from the Cardiovascular Comorbidity in Children with Chronic Kidney Disease study. J Hypertens. 2019;37(11):2247–55.

169. Thomas J, Stonebrook E, Kallash M. Pediatric hypertension: review of the definition, diagnosis, and initial management. Int J Pediatr Adolesc Med. 2020;9(1):1–6.

170. Yang Q, Zhang Z, Kuklina EV, Fang J, Ayala C, Hong Y, et al. Sodium intake and blood pressure among US children and adolescents. Pediatrics. 2012;130(4):611–9.

171. Cappuccio FP, MacGregor GA. Does potassium supplementation lower blood pressure? A meta-analysis of published trials. J Hypertens. 1991;9(5):465–73.

172. Morris RC Jr, Sebastian A, Forman A, Tanaka M, Schmidlin O. Normotensive salt sensitivity: effects of race and dietary potassium. Hypertension. 1999;33(1):18–23.

173. Sinaiko AR, Gomez-Marin O, Prineas RJ. Effect of low sodium diet or potassium supplementation on adolescent blood pressure. Hypertension. 1993;21(6_pt_2):989–94.

174. Buendia JR, Bradlee ML, Daniels SR, Singer MR, Moore LL. Longitudinal effects of dietary sodium and potassium on blood pressure in adolescent girls. JAMA Pediatr. 2015;169(6):560–8.

175. Al Kibria GM, Nemirovsky A, Sharmeen A, Day B. Age-stratified prevalence, treatment status, and associated factors of hypertension among US adults following application of the 2017 ACC/AHA guideline. Hypertens Res. 2019;42(10):1631–43.

176. Andreoni KA, Forbes R, Andreoni RM, Phillips G, Stewart H, Ferris M. Age-related kidney transplant outcomes: health disparities amplified in adolescence. JAMA Intern Med. 2013;173(16):1524–32.

177. Banerjee T, Crews DC, Wesson DE, Dharmarajan S, Saran R, Ríos Burrows N, et al. Food insecurity, CKD, and subsequent ESRD in US adults. Am J Kidney Dis. 2017;70(1):38–47.

178. Brummett BH, Babyak MA, Siegler IC, Shanahan M, Harris KM, Elder GH, et al. Systolic blood pressure, socioeconomic status, and biobehavioral risk factors in a nationally representative U.S. young adult sample. Hypertension. 2011;58(2):161–6.

179. Drewnowski A, Darmon N. Food choices and diet costs: an economic analysis. J Nutr. 2005;135(4):900–4.

180. Jerrell JM, Sakarcan A. Primary health care access, continuity, and cost among pediatric patients with obesity hypertension. J Natl Med Assoc. 2009;101(3):223–8.

181. Starr MC, Fisher K, Thompson K, Thurber-Smith K, Hingorani S. A pilot investigation of food insecurity among children seen in an outpatient pediatric nephrology clinic. Prev Med Rep. 2018;10:113–6.

182. Starr MC, Wightman A, Munshi R, Li A, Hingorani S. Association of food insecurity and acute health care utilization in children with end-stage kidney disease. JAMA Pediatr. 2019;173(11):1097–9.

183. Davis SK, Liu Y, Quarells RC, Din-Dzietharn R, Metro Atlanta Heart Disease Study Group. Stress-related racial discrimination and hypertension likelihood in a population-based sample of African Americans: the Metro Atlanta Heart Disease Study. Ethn Dis. 2005;15(4):585–93.

184. Brondolo E, Love EE, Pencille M, Schoenthaler A, Ogedegbe G. Racism and hypertension: a review of the empirical evidence and implications for clinical practice. Am J Hypertens. 2011;24(5):518–29.

185. Brickner ME, Hillis LD, Lange RA. Congenital heart disease in adults. First of two parts. N Engl J Med. 2000;342(4):256–63.

186. Simonetti GD, Mohaupt MG, Bianchetti MG. Monogenic forms of hypertension. Eur J Pediatr. 2012;171(10):1433–9.

187. Macumber I, Flynn JT. Does treatment-resistant hypertension exist in children? A review of the evidence. Pediatr Nephrol. 2020;35(6):969–76.

188. Ginsberg JM, Chang BS, Matarese RA, Garella S. Use of single voided urine samples to estimate quantitative proteinuria. N Engl J Med. 1983;309(25):1543–6.

189. Leung AKC, Wong AHC, Barg SSN. Proteinuria in children: evaluation and differential diagnosis. Am Fam Physician. 2017;95(4):248–54.

190. Bigazzi R, Bianchi S, Baldari D, Campese VM. Microalbuminuria predicts cardiovascular events and renal insufficiency in patients with essential hypertension. J Hypertens. 1998;16(9):1325–33.

191. Flynn JT. Microalbuminuria in children with primary hypertension. J Clin Hypertens. 2016;18(10):962–5.

192. Kamrath C, Maser-Gluth C, Haag C, Schulze E. Diagnosis of glucocorticoid-remediable aldosteronism in hypertensive children. Horm Res Paediatr. 2011;76(2):93–8.

193. Stowasser M, Gordon RD, Gunasekera TG, Cowley DC, Ward G, Archibald C, et al. High rate of detection of primary aldosteronism, including surgically treatable forms, after 'non-selective' screening of hypertensive patients. J Hypertens. 2003;21(11):2149–57.

194. Blumenfeld JD, Sealey JE, Schlussel Y, Vaughan ED Jr, Sos TA, Atlas SA, et al. Diagnosis and treatment of primary hyperaldosteronism. Ann Intern Med. 1994;121(11):877–85.

195. Mulatero P, Stowasser M, Loh K-C, Fardella CE, Gordon RD, Mosso L, et al. Increased diagnosis of primary aldosteronism, including surgically correctable forms, in centers from five continents. J Clin Endocrinol Metab. 2004;89(3):1045–50.

196. Fogari R, Preti P, Zoppi A, Rinaldi A, Fogari E, Mugellini A. Prevalence of primary aldosteronism among unselected hypertensive patients: a prospective study based on the use of an aldosterone/renin ratio above 25 as a screening test. Hypertens Res. 2007;30(2):111–7.

197. Funder JW, Carey RM, Mantero F, Murad MH, Reincke M, Shibata H, et al. The management of primary aldosteronism: case detection, diagnosis, and treatment: an Endocrine Society Clinical Practice Guideline. J Clin Endocrinol Metab. 2016;101(5):1889–916.

198. Carss KJ, Stowasser M, Gordon RD, O'Shaughnessy KM. Further study of chromosome 7p22 to identify the molecular basis of familial hyperaldosteronism type II. J Hum Hypertens. 2011;25(9):560–4.

199. South AM, Arguelles L, Finer G, Langman CB. Race, obesity, and the renin-angiotensin-aldosterone system: treatment response in children with primary hypertension. Pediatr Nephrol. 2017;32(9):1585–94.

200. Perrin EC, South AM. Correlation between kidney sodium and potassium handling and the renin-angiotensin-aldosterone system in children with hypertensive disorders. Pediatr Nephrol. 2022;37(3):633–41.

201. South AM, Brady TM, Flynn JT. ACE2 (angiotensin-converting enzyme 2), COVID-19, and ACE inhibitor and Ang II (angiotensin II) receptor blocker use during the pandemic: the pediatric perspective. Hypertension. 2020;76(1):16–22.

202. Ferrario CM, Martell N, Yunis C, Flack JM, Chappell MC, Brosnihan KB, et al. Characterization of angiotensin-(1–7) in the urine of normal and essential hypertensive subjects. Am J Hypertens. 1998;11(2):137–46.

203. Simões e Silva AC, Diniz JS, Regueira Filho A, Santos RA. The renin angiotensin system in childhood hypertension: selective increase of angiotensin-(1–7) in essential hypertension. J Pediatr. 2004;145(1):93–8.

204. South AM, Nixon PA, Chappell MC, Diz DI, Russell GB, Shaltout HA, et al. Obesity is associated with higher blood pressure and higher levels of angiotensin II but lower angiotensin-(1–7) in adolescents born preterm. J Pediatr. 2019;205:55–60.e1.

205. Chappell MC. Biochemical evaluation of the renin-angiotensin system: the good, bad, and absolute? Am J Physiol Heart Circ Physiol. 2016;310(2):H137–H52.

206. Sparks MA, South AM, Badley AD, Baker-Smith CM, Batlle D, Bozkurt B, et al. Severe acute respiratory syndrome coronavirus 2, COVID-19, and the renin-angiotensin system: pressing needs and best research practices. Hypertension. 2020;76(5):1350–67.

207. Viazzi F, Antolini L, Giussani M, Brambilla P, Galbiati S, Mastriani S, et al. Serum uric acid and blood pressure in children at cardiovascular risk. Pediatrics. 2013;132(1):e93–e9.

208. Kanda E, Muneyuki T, Kanno Y, Suwa K, Nakajima K. Uric acid level has a U-shaped association with loss of kidney function in healthy people: a prospective cohort study. PLoS One. 2015;10(2):e0118031.

209. Borghi C, Rosei EA, Bardin T, Dawson J, Dominiczak A, Kielstein JT, et al. Serum uric acid and the risk of cardiovascular and renal disease. J Hypertens. 2015;33(9):1729–41.

210. Cicero AF, Salvi P, D'Addato S, Rosticci M, Borghi C. Association between serum uric acid, hypertension, vascular stiffness and subclinical atherosclerosis: data from the Brisighella Heart Study. J Hypertens. 2014;32(1):57–64.

211. Georgios G, Costas PT, Theodoros K, Nikolaos M, Dimitrios R, Christina C, et al. Serum uric acid is independently associated with diastolic dysfunction in apparently healthy subjects with essential hypertension. Curr Vasc Pharmacol. 2018;16:1–8.

212. Kuwabara M, Hisatome I, Niwa K, Hara S, Roncal-Jimenez CA, Bjornstad P, et al. Uric acid is a strong risk marker for developing hypertension from prehypertension: a 5-year Japanese cohort study. Hypertension. 2018;71(1):78–86.

213. Loeffler LF, Navas-Acien A, Brady TM, Miller ER, Fadrowski JJ. Uric acid level and elevated blood pressure in U.S. adolescents: National Health And Nutrition Examination Survey 1999–2006. Hypertension. 2012;59(4):811–7.

214. Rodrigues TC, Maahs DM, Johnson RJ, Jalal DI, Kinney GL, Rivard C, et al. Serum uric acid predicts progression of subclinical coronary atherosclerosis in individuals without renal disease. Diabetes Care. 2010;33(11):2471–3.

215. Shatat IF, Abdallah RT, Sas DJ, Hailpern SM. Serum uric acid in US adolescents: distribution and relationship to demographic characteristics and cardiovascular risk factors. Pediatr Res. 2012;72(1):95–100.

216. MacIsaac Rachael L, Salatzki J, Higgins P, Walters Matthew R, Padmanabhan S, Dominiczak Anna F, et al. Allopurinol and cardiovascular outcomes in adults with hypertension. Hypertension. 2016;67(3):535–40.

217. Kostka-Jeziorny K, Uruski P, Tykarski A. Effect of allopurinol on blood pressure and aortic compliance in hypertensive patients. Blood Press. 2011;20(2):104–10.

218. Segal MS, Srinivas TR, Mohandas R, Shuster JJ, Wen X, Whidden E, et al. The effect of the addition of allopurinol on blood pressure control in African Americans treated with a thiazide-like diuretic. J Am Soc Hypertens. 2015;9(8):610–9.e1.

219. Feig DI, Soletsky B, Johnson RJ. Effect of allopurinol on blood pressure of adolescents with newly diagnosed essential hypertension: a randomized trial. J Am Med Assoc. 2008;300(8):924–32.

220. Grayson PC, Kim SY, LaValley M, Choi HK. Hyperuricemia and incident hypertension: a systematic review and meta-analysis. Arthritis Care Res (Hoboken). 2010;63(1):102–10.

221. Fabbrini E, Serafini M, Colic Baric I, Hazen SL, Klein S. Effect of plasma uric acid on antioxidant capacity, oxidative stress, and insulin sensitivity in obese subjects. Diabetes. 2014;63(3):976–81.

222. Waring WS, McKnight JA, Webb DJ, Maxwell SR. Uric acid restores endothelial function in patients with type 1 diabetes and regular smokers. Diabetes. 2006;55(11):3127–32.

223. Yu M-A, Sánchez-Lozada LG, Johnson RJ, Kang D-H. Oxidative stress with an activation of the renin-angiotensin system in human vascular endothelial cells as a novel mechanism of uric acid-induced endothelial dysfunction. J Hypertens. 2010;28(6):1234–42.

224. Park YS. Renal scar formation after urinary tract infection in children. Korean J Pediatr. 2012;55(10):367.

225. Stokland E, Hellstrom M, Jakobsson B, Sixt R. Imaging of renal scarring. Acta Paediatr. 1999;88:13–21.

226. Smellie J, Prescod N, Shaw P, Risdon R, Bryant T. Childhood reflux and urinary infection: a follow-up of 10–41 years in 226 adults. Pediatr Nephrol. 1998;12(9):727–36.

227. Castelli PK, Dillman JR, Kershaw DB, Khalatbari S, Stanley JC, Smith EA. Renal sonography with Doppler for detecting suspected pediatric renin-

mediated hypertension–is it adequate? Pediatr Radiol. 2014;44(1):42–9.

228. Chhadia S, Cohn RA, Vural G, Donaldson JS. Renal Doppler evaluation in the child with hypertension: a reasonable screening discriminator? Pediatr Radiol. 2013;43(12):1549–56.

229. Saida K, Kamei K, Hamada R, Yoshikawa T, Kano Y, Nagata H, et al. A simple, refined approach to diagnosing renovascular hypertension in children: a 10-year study. Pediatr Int. 2020;62(8):937–43.

230. Orman G, Masand PM, Kukreja KU, Acosta AA, Guillerman RP, Jadhav SP. Diagnostic sensitivity and specificity of CT angiography for renal artery stenosis in children. Pediatr Radiol. 2021;51(3): 419–26.

231. Trautmann A, Roebuck DJ, McLaren CA, Brennan E, Marks SD, Tullus K. Non-invasive imaging cannot replace formal angiography in the diagnosis of renovascular hypertension. Pediatr Nephrol. 2017;32(3):495–502.

232. Khoury PR, Mitsnefes M, Daniels SR, Kimball TR. Age-specific reference intervals for indexed left ventricular mass in children. J Am Soc Echocardiogr. 2009;22(6):709–14.

233. Killian L, Simpson JM, Savis A, Rawlins D, Sinha MD. Electrocardiography is a poor screening test to detect left ventricular hypertrophy in children. Arch Dis Child. 2010;95(10):832–6.

234. Schwimmer JB, Zepeda A, Newton KP, Xanthakos SA, Behling C, Hallinan EK, et al. Longitudinal assessment of high blood pressure in children with nonalcoholic fatty liver disease. PLoS One. 2014;9(11):e112569.

235. Yoneda M, Yoneda M, Mawatari H, Fujita K, Endo H, Iida H, et al. Noninvasive assessment of liver fibrosis by measurement of stiffness in patients with nonalcoholic fatty liver disease (NAFLD). Dig Liver Dis. 2008;40(5):371–8.

236. Charakida M, Jones A, Falaschetti E, Khan T, Finer N, Sattar N, et al. Childhood obesity and vascular phenotypes: a population study. J Am Coll Cardiol. 2012;60(25):2643–50.

237. Donald AE, Charakida M, Falaschetti E, Lawlor DA, Halcox JP, Golding J, et al. Determinants of vascular phenotype in a large childhood population: the Avon Longitudinal Study of Parents and Children (ALSPAC). Eur Heart J. 2010;31(12):1502–10.

238. Urbina EM. Abnormalities of vascular structure and function in pediatric hypertension. Pediatr Nephrol. 2016;31(7):1061–70.

239. Skrzypczyk P, Pańczyk-Tomaszewska M. Methods to evaluate arterial structure and function in children–state-of-the art knowledge. Adv Med Sci. 2017;62(2):280–94.

240. Urbina EM, Isom S, Bell RA, Bowlby DA, D'Agostino R Jr, Daniels SR, et al. Burden of cardiovascular risk factors over time and arterial stiffness in youth with type 1 diabetes mellitus: the SEARCH for Diabetes in Youth Study. J Am Heart Assoc. 2019;8(13):e010150.

241. Elmenhorst J, Hulpke-Wette M, Barta C, Dalla Pozza R, Springer S, Oberhoffer R. Percentiles for central blood pressure and pulse wave velocity in children and adolescents recorded with an oscillometric device. Atherosclerosis. 2015;238(1):9–16.

242. Hidvégi EV, Illyés M, Benczúr B, Böcskei RM, Rátgéber L, Lenkey Z, et al. Reference values of aortic pulse wave velocity in a large healthy population aged between 3 and 18 years. J Hypertens. 2012;30(12):2314–21.

243. Miyai N, Utsumi M, Gowa Y, Igarashi Y, Miyashita K, Takeda S, et al. Age-specific nomogram of brachial-ankle pulse wave velocity in Japanese adolescents. Clin Exp Hypertens. 2013;35(2):95–101.

244. Thurn D, Doyon A, Sözeri B, Bayazit AK, Canpolat N, Duzova A, et al. Aortic pulse wave velocity in healthy children and adolescents: reference values for the vicorder device and modifying factors. Am J Hypertens. 2015;28(12):1480–8.

245. Urbina EM, Williams RV, Alpert BS, Collins RT, Daniels SR, Hayman L, et al. Noninvasive assessment of subclinical atherosclerosis in children and adolescents: recommendations for standard assessment for clinical research: a scientific statement from the American Heart Association. Hypertension. 2009;54(5):919–50.

246. Doyon A, Kracht D, Bayazit AK, Deveci M, Duzova A, Krmar RT, et al. Carotid artery intima-media thickness and distensibility in children and adolescents: reference values and role of body dimensions. Hypertension. 2013;62(3):550–6.

247. Day TG, Park M, Kinra S. The association between blood pressure and carotid intima-media thickness in children: a systematic review. Cardiol Young. 2017;27(7):1295.

248. Schaefer F, Doyon A, Azukaitis K, Bayazit A, Canpolat N, Duzova A, et al. Cardiovascular phenotypes in children with CKD: the 4C study. Clin J Am Soc Nephrol. 2017;12(1):19–28.

249. Brady TM, Schneider MF, Flynn JT, Cox C, Samuels J, Saland J, et al. Carotid intima-media thickness in children with CKD: results from the CKiD study. Clin J Am Soc Nephrol. 2012;7(12):1930–7.

250. Parati G, Di Rienzo M, Bertinieri G, Pomidossi G, Casadei R, Groppelli A, et al. Evaluation of the baroreceptor-heart rate reflex by 24-hour intra-arterial blood pressure monitoring in humans. Hypertension. 1988;12(2):214–22.

251. Parati G, Saul JP, Di Rienzo M, Mancia G. Spectral analysis of blood pressure and heart rate variability in evaluating cardiovascular regulation: a critical appraisal. Hypertension. 1995;25(6):1276–86.

252. Sorof JM, Poffenbarger T, Franco K, Bernard L, Portman RJ. Isolated systolic hypertension, obesity, and hyperkinetic hemodynamic states in children. J Pediatr. 2002;140(6):660–6.

253. Longin E, Gerstner T, Schaible T, Lenz T, Konig S. Maturation of the autonomic nervous system: differences in heart rate variability in premature vs. term infants. J Perinat Med. 2006;34(4):303–8.

254. De Ferrari GM, Sanzo A, Bertoletti A, Specchia G, Vanoli E, Schwartz PJ. Baroreflex sensitivity predicts long-term cardiovascular mortality after myocardial infarction even in patients with preserved left ventricular function. J Am Coll Cardiol. 2007;50(24):2285–90.

255. Erden M, Kocaman SA, Poyraz F, Topal S, Sahinarslan A, Boyaci B, et al. Incremental effects of serum uric acid levels, autonomic dysfunction, and low-grade inflammation on nocturnal blood pressure in untreated hypertensive patients and normotensive individuals. Arch Turk Soc Cardiol. 2011;39(7):531–9.

256. La Rovere MT, Bigger JT Jr, Marcus FI, Mortara A, Schwartz PJ. Baroreflex sensitivity and heart-rate variability in prediction of total cardiac mortality after myocardial infarction. ATRAMI (Autonomic Tone and Reflexes After Myocardial Infarction) Investigators. Lancet. 1998;351(9101):478–84.

257. Yarows SA, Brook RD. Measurement variation among 12 electronic home blood pressure monitors. Am J Hypertens. 2000;13(3):276–82.

258. White PH, Cooley WC, Transitions Clinical Report Authoring Group, American Academy of Pediatrics, American Academy of Family Physicians, American College of Physicians. Supporting the health care transition from adolescence to adulthood in the medical home. Pediatrics. 2018;142(5):e20182587.

259. O'Brien E, Parati G, Stergiou G, Asmar R, Beilin L, Bilo G, et al. European Society of Hypertension position paper on ambulatory blood pressure monitoring. J Hypertens. 2013;31(9):1731–68.

260. Campbell JF, Shah S, Srivaths P, Acosta AA. Reclassification of adolescent hypertension by ambulatory blood pressure monitoring using adult norms and association with left ventricular hypertrophy. J Clin Hypertens. 2021;23(2):265–71.

261. Mitsnefes M, Flynn JT, Brady T, Baker-Smith C, Daniels SR, Hayman LL, et al. Pediatric ambulatory blood pressure classification: the case for a change. Hypertension. 2021;78(5):1206–10.

262. Haskin O, Wong CJ, McCabe L, Begin B, Sutherland SM, Chaudhuri A. 44-h ambulatory blood pressure monitoring: revealing the true burden of hypertension in pediatric hemodialysis patients. Pediatr Nephrol. 2015;30(4):653–60.

263. Flynn JT. Ambulatory blood pressure monitoring should be routinely performed after pediatric renal transplantation. Pediatr Transplant. 2012;16(6):533–6.

264. Tainio J, Qvist E, Miettinen J, Hölttä T, Pakarinen M, Jahnukainen T, et al. Blood pressure profiles 5 to 10 years after transplant in pediatric solid organ recipients. J Clin Hypertens. 2015;17(2):154–61.

265. Westland R, Schreuder MF, van der Lof DF, Vermeulen A, Dekker-van der Meer IMJ, Bökenkamp A, et al. Ambulatory blood pressure monitoring is recommended in the clinical management of children with a solitary functioning kidney. Pediatr Nephrol. 2014;29(11):2205–11.

266. Dost A, Bechtold-Dalla Pozza S, Bollow E, Kovacic R, Vogel P, Feldhahn L, et al. Blood pressure regulation determined by ambulatory blood pressure profiles in children and adolescents with type 1 diabetes mellitus: impact on diabetic complications. Pediatr Diabetes. 2017;18(8):874–82.

267. Shikha D, Singla M, Walia R, Potter N, Umpaichitra V, Mercado A, et al. Ambulatory blood pressure monitoring in lean, obese and diabetic children and adolescents. Cardiorenal Med. 2015;5(3):183–90.

268. Brown ML, Burkhart HM, Connolly HM, Dearani JA, Cetta F, Li Z, et al. Coarctation of the aorta: lifelong surveillance is mandatory following surgical repair. J Am Coll Cardiol. 2013;62(11):1020–5.

269. Becker AM, Goldberg JH, Henson M, Ahn C, Tong L, Baum M, et al. Blood pressure abnormalities in children with sickle cell anemia. Pediatr Blood Cancer. 2014;61(3):518–22.

270. Bayrakci US, Schaefer F, Duzova A, Yigit S, Bakkaloglu A. Abnormal circadian blood pressure regulation in children born preterm. J Pediatr. 2007;151(4):399–403.

271. Samuel JP, Swinford RD, Portman RJ. Evaluation of hypertension in pediatric patients. In: Pediatric hypertension. New York: Springer; 2013. p. 491–504.

Renovascular Hypertension in Children

49

Agnes Trautmann and Kjell Tullus

Introduction

Renovascular disease is a rare but important cause of childhood hypertension. It accounts for 10% of secondary childhood hypertension [1–3]. Anatomic stenosis of the renal artery results in renal hypoperfusion with consequent release of renin and activation of the renin-angiotensin-aldosterone system (RAAS) developing a renin-mediated hypertension. Renal artery stenosis is important to accurately diagnose, as it is potentially amenable to curative treatment with several endovascular and surgical techniques in more than half of affected children.

Many children with renovascular disease have additional complex abnormalities of other major blood vessels including aorta, cerebral, intestinal or iliac arteries. Usually, children with complex renovascular disease require treatment provided by a specialised multidisciplinary team of paediatric nephrologists, cardiologists, neurologists, interventional radiologists, vascular and neuro-vascular surgeons.

A. Trautmann (✉)
Division of Paediatric Nephrology, Center for Paediatrics and Adolescent Medicine, University of Heidelberg, Heidelberg, Germany
e-mail: agnes.trautmann@med.uni-heidelberg.de

K. Tullus
Division of Paediatric Nephrology, Great Ormond Street Hospital for Children (GOSH), London, UK
e-mail: kjell.tullus@gosh.nhs.uk

Clinical Presentation

Renovascular hypertension is diagnosed at all ages with equally many cases found in all age groups.

Clinical Symptoms

The initial clinical presentation varies from asymptomatic to severe, life threatening symptoms including congestive heart failure or cerebral symptoms. The spectrum of cerebral symptoms is broad with headaches, visual disturbances, signs of acute hypertensive encephalopathy or cerebrovascular incident with convulsions, strokes with focal neurological deficits like facial palsy and hemiplegia. Young infants can also present with more unspecific symptoms and failure to thrive.

At time of diagnosis blood pressure is usually markedly increased, with predominantly stage 2 hypertension (blood pressure > 99th percentile + 5 mmHg). A systolic blood pressure of ≥ 160–180 mmHg is not uncommon. Target organ damage, in particular hypertensive left ventricular hypertrophy, may already be seen at initial presentation, depending on the stage and duration of hypertension.

Renovascular hypertension should also be suspected if there is inadequate blood pressure control with two or more antihypertensive drugs in the absence of any other identifiable cause.

© The Author(s), under exclusive license to Springer Nature Switzerland AG 2023
F. Schaefer, L. A. Greenbaum (eds.), *Pediatric Kidney Disease*,
https://doi.org/10.1007/978-3-031-11665-0_49

Several rare genetic syndromes are associated with childhood renovascular hypertension, with neurofibromatosis type 1 (NF type 1) and Williams' syndrome being the most common. Infants and children with newly diagnosed renovascular hypertension should be carefully examined for syndromal signs (e.g. NF type 1: café au lait macules, axillary/inguinal freckles, neurofibromas, Lisch nodules; Williams' syndrome: facial dysmorphic features like "elfin" faces, cardiovascular disease). Although only a small fraction of children with these genetic syndromes will develop renovascular hypertension, blood pressure should be regularly monitored in these conditions.

Children presenting with non-specific clinical signs of inflammation and suspected large vessel vasculitis, in particular Takayasu's arteritis (TA), are also at risk of developing renovascular hypertension.

Children with new-onset hypertension post-renal transplantation should undergo screening for renovascular disease. An abdominal bruit in transplanted children reflecting the turbulent blood flow at the stenotic anastomosis. A bruit can also be heard over renal arteries in native kidneys especially in slim children. Clinical signs that may point to renovascular hypertension are summarized in Table 49.1.

Laboratory Evaluation

Suspicious, but non-specific laboratory signs for renovascular hypertension include moderate hypokalemia in combination with hypochloremic metabolic alkalosis compatible with secondary hyperaldosteronism and a highly activated renin-angiotensin-aldosterone system. Typically, age-specific plasma renin, aldosterone and plasma-renin-activity (PRA) are increased. However, elevated plasma renin levels and PRA are not specific for renovascular hypertension as they do not allow a differentiation between renovascular and renoparenchymal disease. It is important to note that normal renin levels and PRA values do not exclude renovascular disease.

Table 49.1 Suspicious signs for renovascular hypertension

Suspicious sign	Specification
Blood pressure level	Very high blood pressure (e.g. stage 2 hypertension)
Secondary symptoms of hypertension	Cerebral symptoms
	Cardiac failure
	Facial palsy
Control of hypertension	Difficult, not controlled with ≥ 2 or more drugs
Syndromal disease associated with vascular disease	Neurofibromatosis type 1 (NF 1)
	Williams' syndrome
	Tuberous sclerosis
Signs of vasculitis	Takayasu's vasculitis
Previous vascular insult	Renal artery thrombosis
	Umbilical artery catheterisation
	Previous trauma or radiation
Transplanted kidneys	New onset or worsening of hypertension post-transplant
Clinical examination	Bruit heard over renal artery or arteries
Laboratory diagnostic	Raised peripheral plasma renin
	Moderate hypokalemia

Up to 15% of children with renal artery stenosis, confirmed by DSA, can have normal initial PRA values [4]. Therefore further investigations for renovascular artery stenosis should be performed in case of clinical suspicion (Table 49.1) even in the presence of normal age-specific PRA values.

Laboratory evaluation of renal function is also essential, as renal artery stenosis, especially if bilateral, can compromise renal function due to hypoperfusion.

Vascular Involvement

Renovascular disease in children is often complex with a wide spectrum of renovascular and other vascular involvement. All types of major renal arteries (main, branch and accessory arteries) as well as intrarenal small vessels (segmental, lobar and accessory arteries) can be affected. Bilateral renal artery disease is more common than unilateral disease. Twenty-five to thirty percent of patients are diagnosed with mid aortic syndrome (MAS) combined with bilateral or unilateral disease [5, 6] (Fig. 49.3). MAS is often associated with stenotic lesions in the intestinal arteries, mainly the coeliac trunk and the superior mesenteric artery (SMA) which in many cases both are occluded. The inferior mesenteric artery (IMA) is much less involved and collaterals from the IMA maintain the intestinal blood flow [7]. Importantly, abdominal angina is nearly never seen in children and there is virtually never a need for treatment of the coeliac axis nor the SMA. At least 20% of children also show cerebrovascular involvement, which influences the extent of lowering the blood pressure by treatment without risking cerebral hypoperfusion.

Causes of Renovascular Disease in Childhood

Epidemiology

Renovascular disease is associated with a variety of diseases and pathologies (summarized in Table 49.2). The reported distribution of RVD aetiologies in children varies widely in different parts of the world. However, cross-cohort comparisons are hampered by limited information on the diagnostic criteria used.

In Europe and North America, fibromuscular dysplasia (FMD) accounts for 53–88%, neurofibromatosis type 1 for 10–25%, and Williams' syndrome for 5–10%, of cases (Table 49.2) [8–13]. Whereas Takayasu's arteritis is very rare in Western countries, this disorder has been reported in 73–89% of Indian and South African cohorts [14–18].

Fibromuscular Dysplasia (FMD)

FMD is a non-atherosclerotic, non-inflammatory vascular disorder affecting medium-size arteries. It occurs as unifocal or multifocal disease. The aetiology of FMD is unknown.

FMD can be classified into different types depending on the mainly involved part of the blood vessel (intima, media, adventitia) [19],

Table 49.2 Summary of causes of renovascular hypertension

Cause	Specified diagnoses
Fibromuscular dysplasia	Medial fibroplasia
Syndromal diseases	Neurofibromatosis type 1 (*NF1* gene)
	Williams' syndrome (deletion of chromosome 7q11.23, *Elastin* gene)
	Tuberous sclerosis (*TSC1/TSC2* gene)
	Alagille syndrome (*JAG1* gene)
	Marfan's syndrome (*Fibrillin 1* gene)
	Other syndromes associated with vasculopathies and mid-aortic syndrome
Vasculitis	Takayasu's disease
	Polyarterits nodosa
	Other systemic vasculitides
Extrinsic compression	Neuroblastoma
	Wilms' tumor
	Pheochromocytoma
	Other abdominal and perirenal tumors
Other rare causes	Abdominal radiotherapy
	Previous renal artery thrombosis
	Umbilical artery catheterisation with thrombosis
	Trauma with renal artery disruption
	Congenital rubella syndrome
Renal transplantation	Transplant renal artery stenosis

with medial fibroplasia being the most common type. In childhood, FMD primarily affects the mid and distal renal artery leading to renovascular hypertension [20, 21].

The diagnosis of FMD is based on angiographic appearance and is mainly a diagnosis of exclusion when other conditions have been ruled out. A minority of children display the typical "string of beads" appearance on angiography [22] which is regarded as typical for FMD (Fig. 49.1).

Takayasu Arteritis (TA)

A similar angiographic appearance for renal artery stenosis has been described for vasculiti-

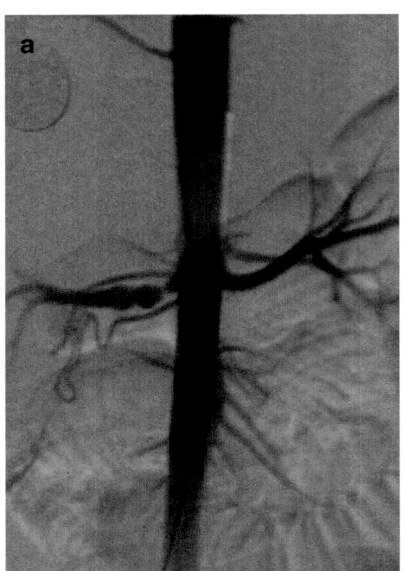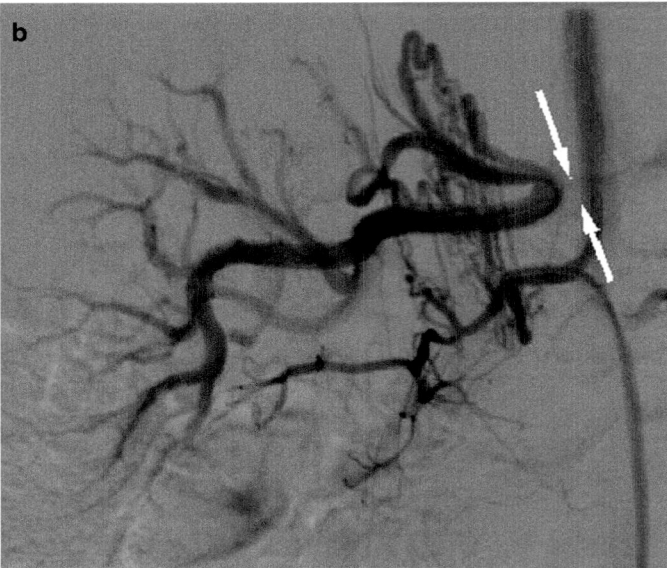

Fig. 49.1 (**a**) Fibromuscular dysplasia: Renal artery stenosis with "string bead" appearance in digital subtraction angiography (DSA) (image kindly provided by Great Ormond Street Hospital, London). (**b**) Obstructed right renal artery in digital subtraction angiography (DSA) (image kindly provided by Great Ormond Street Hospital, London)

des. The by far most frequent vasculitis is Takayasu's arteritis (TA). Rarely, polyarteritis nodosa, and other systemic vasculitides are associated with renovascular hypertension (Table 49.2). TA affects the aorta and its major branches and is mainly a disease of young women in their second and third decades of life. The age of onset is usually between 15 and 30 years [23]. TA has also been reported in young children presenting with malignant hypertension due to renal artery stenosis and cardiac failure [24–27]. However, the rate of misclassification of FMD as TA is suspected to be high in young children.

The aetiology of TA is still undefined. The vascular pathology is characterized by segmental and patchy granulomatous inflammation of all three layers of the aorta and major branches. Finally this inflammation leads to arterial stenosis, thrombosis and aneurysms. Thickened and acutely inflamed vessel walls can be often detected on MRA, CTA and/or PET scan [28] (Fig. 49.2).

The clinical features of TA can be divided into an early, acute and systemic phase, characterized by non-specific clinical features such as low-grade fever, malaise, night sweats, weight loss, arthralgia and fatigue, and a late occlusive phase [29]. Additionally, anaemia and a marked elevation of the erythrocyte sedimentation rate (ESR) can be found in most patients during the systemic phase. The early systemic phase is difficult to diagnose because only half of all patients show these symptoms. The late occlusive phase is characterized by progression from inflammatory into obliterative changes in the aorta and its main branches. In this late occlusive phase, the characteristic features of TA appear, in children predominantly hypertension secondary to renal artery stenosis, cardiac failure and neurological symptoms secondary to hypertension or ischemia [29]. Presentation with vascular bruits, absent or diminished pulses and claudication is less common in children.

The 2006 by EULAR/PRES (European League against Rheumatism/Paediatric Rheumatology European Society) defined consensus criteria for classifying TA are summarized in Table 49.3 [30, 31]. The classification criteria for TA imply that

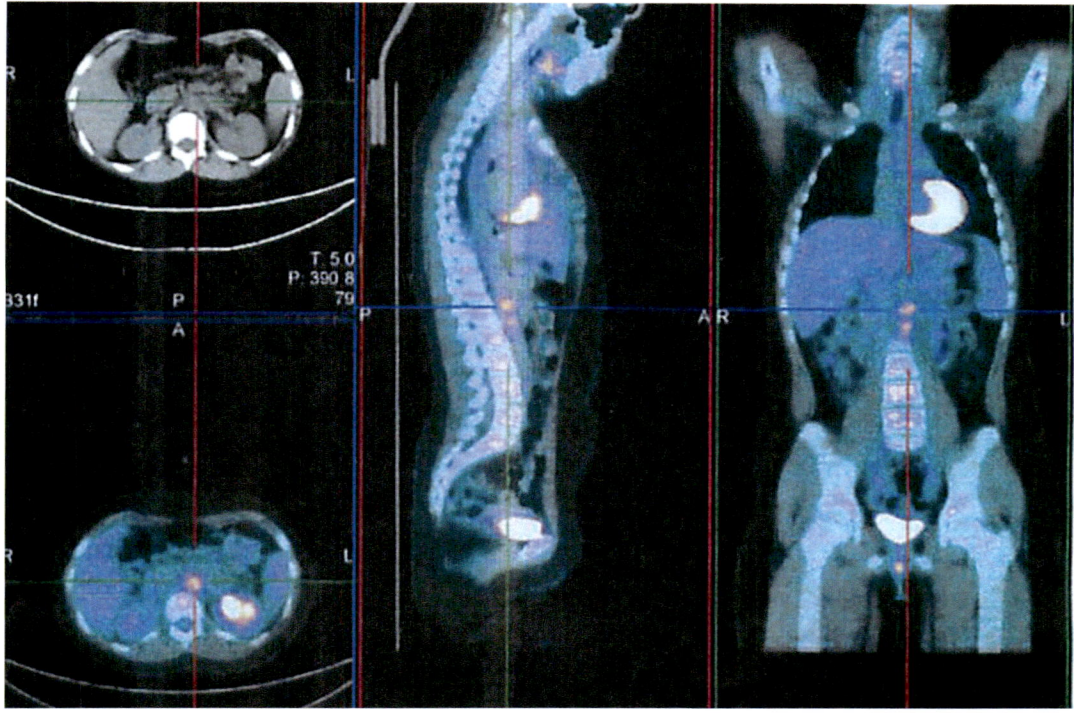

Fig. 49.2 Takayasu's arteritis: PET Scan with lightning of aorta reflecting thickened and inflamed arterial wall (images kindly provided by Great Ormond Street Hospital, London)

Table 49.3 Classification definition for Takayasu's arteritis according to EULAR/PRINTO/PRES (European League against Rheumatism/Paediatric Rheumatology International Trials Organisation/Paediatric Rheumatology European Society) Ankara 2008 consensus criteria (adapted from [31])

Requirement	Criterion	Specification
Mandatory	Angiographic abnormality	Angiographic abnormalities (conventional, CTA or MRA) of the aorta or its main branches and pulmonary arteries showing aneurysm/dilatation
+1 of the 5 following criteria	Hypertension	Systolic/diastolic blood pressure >95th percentile for height
	Pulse deficit or claudication	Lost/decreased/unequal peripheral artery pulse(s) Claudication: focal muscle pain induced by physical activity
	Four limbs blood pressure discrepancy	Discrepancy of four limb systolic blood pressure of >10 mmHg difference in any limb
	Bruits	Audible murmurs or palpable thrills above large arteries
	Acute phase reactant	Erythrocyte sedimentation rate (ESR) >20 mm per first hour or CRP any value above normal (according to local laboratory)

the diagnosis of any vasculitis was already made in the child. In such cases, the classification criteria have shown high sensitivity and specificity when being validated [31].

However, the difficulty is to diagnose vasculitis itself in children, especially if there is a lack of systemic inflammatory signs during the acute systemic phase as well as during the late occlusive phase of TA. Then the criteria are unspecific in diagnosing TA and overlap with features of FMD.

The evaluation of blood vessel wall thickness and inflammation by MR/CT angiography [32] and/or PET scan [28, 33] may help identifying

TA. A markedly thickened blood vessel wall reflecting oedema and inflammation strongly supports the diagnosis of TA (Fig. 49.2).

Differentiation Between Fibromuscular Dysplasia (FMD) and Takayasu's Arteritis (TA)

The differential diagnosis between FMD and TA seems to be difficult in many children. Children with obvious systemic inflammatory symptoms and raised inflammatory parameters (ESR, CRP) are likely to have TA. However, only a minority of children present in the inflammatory early phase of the disease. Inflammatory symptoms are missing during the late occlusive phase of TA. In the late phase of TA the mandatory criteria of angiographic abnormalities with hypertension are the same criteria as used to diagnose FMD. The typical "string of beads" pattern is not regularly seen on angiography in children with FMD.

In that case the evaluation of a thickened, inflamed vessel wall can help in the differential diagnosis, although systematic evaluations of this sign in MRA, CTA or PET scans have not been performed so far.

The ascertainment of the correct differential diagnosis is important for the indication for immunosuppressive treatment in the systemic phase of TA in order to control the active vasculitic process and in view of the timing of interventional or surgical procedures.

Genetic and Syndromic Causes

Several rare genetic syndromes are associated with childhood renovascular disease, with neurofibromatosis type 1 (NF type 1) and Williams syndrome being the most common (Table 49.2). All other associations of syndromes with renovascular disease are rare; these include tuberous sclerosis [34], Alagille syndrome [35, 36] and Marfan's syndrome with predominantly proximal aortic wall abnormalities [37].

To identify new monogenic causes for renovascular hypertension, two studies performed whole-exome sequencing in children with so far unexplained renovascular disease and mid-aortic syndrome [38, 39]. Both studies detected abnormalities in genes causing NF type 1, Williams syndrome, and Alagille syndrome that apparently caused a mild clinical phenotype. However, no new monogenic causes of renovascular disease were identified.

Neurofibromatosis Type 1 (NF Type 1)

The spectrum of NF type 1 associated vasculopathy is broad: Renal arteries are most frequently involved; the stenoses are usually located near the renal ostium. Unilateral and bilateral renal artery stenosis can occur in combination with mid-aortic syndrome by narrowing of the abdominal aorta and stenosis of its major branches (Fig. 49.3). Other common vascular manifestations in NF type 1 are abdominal aortic coarctation, internal carotid aneurysms and cervical vertebral arteriovenous malformations [40–42].

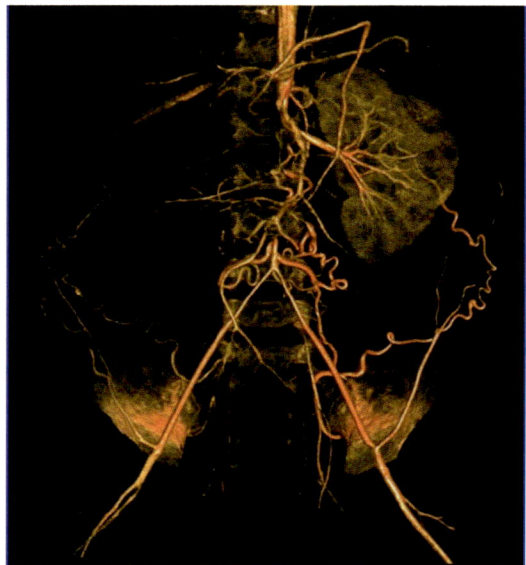

Fig. 49.3 Mid-aortic syndrome with occluded infrarenal aorta and right renal artery stenosis in two-dimensional ('volume-rendered') representation of a three-dimensional computed tomography dataset (image kindly provided by Great Ormond Street Hospital, London)

The real total incidence of secondary hypertension in NF type 1 and age-specific incidences remain unclear [43]; one study reported an incidence of 16%, with most cases involving renal artery stenosis followed by aortic coarctation and pheochromocytoma [44].

In general, blood pressure monitoring every 6–12 months is therefore recommended in all children with NF type 1 [43, 45].

Williams Syndrome

Williams syndrome is associated with cardiovascular abnormalities and a generalized arteriopathy focused on the aorta [46, 47] with consecutive development of mid-aortic syndrome. However, isolated stenoses of the renal and other arteries occur.

Since hypertension is a common feature of Williams syndrome, blood pressure screening is recommended. The reported prevalence ranges between 5% and 70% (summarized in [46]). In most children with Williams syndrome the aetiology of hypertension remains unclear; only in a minority of cases it can be attributed to renal artery stenosis, mid-aortic syndrome or aortic coarctation. It has been argued that arterial vascular stiffness due to defective elastin, resulting in decreased arterial elasticity, vascular smooth muscle cell proliferation and increased intima-media thickness, may contribute to hypertension in this condition [48].

Extrinsic Compression of Renal Artery

Extrinsic compression of the renal artery can mimic renal artery occlusive disease with renal hypoperfusion, activation of the renin-angiotensin-aldosterone-system and development of renin-mediated hypertension. This has been reported in different types of tumours, in particular Wilms tumour [49–51], neuroblastoma [52–54] and pheochromocytoma [55–58]. Mid-aortic syndrome and renal artery stenosis have also been reported after treatment of large tumours (Wilms tumour and neuroblastoma), usually associated with radio- and chemotherapy and postoperative fibrosis causing severe stenosis [59, 60] but also in patients without preceding radiotherapy [61].

Other Rare Causes

Umbilical artery catheterisation during the neonatal period can cause vascular endothelial disruption, thromboembolism with a completely or partially occluded aorta and renal hypoperfusion, renal artery thrombosis, or thromboembolism into the small renal vasculature with renal infarction [62–67].

Renal artery trauma can lead to renovascular hypertension due to surgical injury, disruption of the renal artery or from random accident.

Congenital rubella syndrome can also be associated with renovascular disease [65, 68, 69]. Due to the general recommendation for rubella vaccination, this association is very rarely seen nowadays.

Transplant Renal Artery Stenosis

Data from paediatric cohorts after renal transplantation with newly developed renal artery stenosis are very limited. To date, the prevalence of allograft renal artery stenosis is reported with 4–9% [70, 71]. Clinical presentation usually includes new onset of severe hypertension or significant worsening of pre-existing hypertension during the first few months after renal transplantation.

Imaging

Diagnosing renovascular disease in children is challenging due to the complex anatomical distribution of vascular involvement, the small size of renal arteries affected by age and size of the child and by the degree of arterial branching. Despite the development of non-invasive imaging, selective renal arteriography (digital subtraction angiography, DSA) is still the gold standard imaging method in diagnosing renovascular disease. This might change with further technical developments in the future.

Non-invasive Imaging

For screening, several non-invasive imaging techniques are used in children although its role is still unclear due to the lack of high-quality evidence. The use of non-invasive imaging in children is based on small studies, clinical expert opinion and studies in adults. So far, non-invasive imaging methods cannot reliably diagnose renovascular disease in children, with at least 10–40% false-negative results as well as false-positive results. However, non-invasive imaging can be helpful to rule out extraparenchymal processes, to diagnose renoparenchymal disease, to plan surgery and to follow-up post-surgery.

Kidney Ultrasound and Doppler Studies

Kidney ultrasound combined with renal and abdominal vessel Doppler ultrasound is an important baseline investigation. It can exclude other renal pathologies (renoparenchymal disease, renal scarring), detect extrarenal processes, in particular tumours (e.g. neuroblastoma, Wilms' tumour) and show significant discrepancies of kidney volume and length (≥1 cm) as a possible indirect sign of renovascular hypertension.

Renal Doppler ultrasound can directly visualise a stenosis or be suggestive of renovascular disease when a *parvus et tardus* waveform pattern (Fig. 49.4) or pathologic age-dependent flow parameters (peak systolic flow >2 m/s [72, 73], acceleration time >80 ms, renal artery to aortic flow velocity ratio >3 and difference in resistive index) can be identified. The entire renal artery should be followed when possible from its origin in the abdominal aorta to the renal hilum and a screening for accessory renal arteries and the abdominal aorta is essential [74]. However, renal Doppler ultrasound in children requires advanced

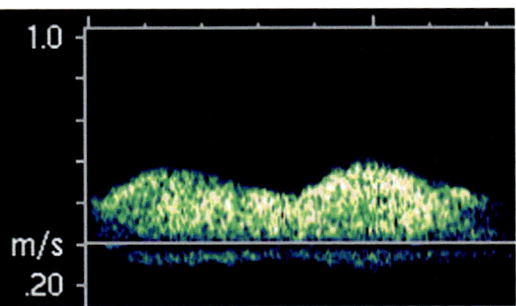

Fig. 49.4 Renal Doppler ultrasound suggestive for renal artery stenosis: *parvus et tardus* waveform pattern (image kindly provided by Great Ormond Street Hospital, London)

technical skills and experience and cooperative children to reliably suspect renovascular disease by Doppler ultrasound.

In general, the experience with renal Doppler ultrasound in children is limited apart from detecting renal artery stenosis in transplanted kidneys [75]. The sensitivity and specificity for Doppler ultrasound was reported in small paediatric cohorts at 63–88% and 73–99% [5, 72, 76–78]—significantly lower than in adult studies. In those small paediatric studies, Doppler ultrasound failed to detect stenoses located in small renal artery branches, segmental renal arteries as well as in main and accessory renal arteries.

CTA and MRA

Magnetic resonance angiography (MRA) or contrast-enhanced multidetector computer tomography angiography (CTA) can be used as next diagnostic steps in diagnosing renovascular disease in children. We do however advocate going directly to DSA in children with a strong suspicion of RAS. With the criteria given in Table 49.1, a majority of children will be shown to have arterial disease and MRA or CTA can never rule out RAS in these cases.

CTA and MRA are able to detect mid-aortic syndrome and sometimes stenosis of intestinal arteries and to assess non-vascular structures like occult renal or suprarenal neoplasms in addition to ultrasound [79].

The advantages of renal CTA versus MRA are a shorter examination time without the need for sedation or general anaesthesia in small children and an easy generation of high-quality 3D images. However, the disadvantage is the significant radiation exposure, even with low-dose protocols [80].

The spatial resolution of MRA has improved significantly with technological advancements and can evaluate renal parenchymal disease with high anatomical detail and improved diagnostic accuracy. However, there is a lack of data in children. To date, only small retrospective studies evaluated whether CTA/MRA can correctly predict renovascular disease, confirmed by DSA [5, 79]. MRA was less sensitive (80%) and specific (62%) than CTA (88% and 81%) and missed renovascular disease mainly in younger children [5]. Lee et al. described a sensitivity of CTA of 90% and MRA of 75% [81].

In summary, CTA and MRA are promising non-invasive imaging methods in diagnosing renovascular disease but currently cannot replace DSA. CTA seems to be more accurate than MRA in diagnosing renovascular hypertension in all age groups, but in particular in young children with small vessel size.

Renal Scintigraphy

Pre- and post-captopril renal scintigraphy with [99mTc] dimercaptosuccinic acid (DMSA) or 99m-Tc-mercaptoacetyltriglycine (MAG3) was initially thought to be a useful screening method for locating renal artery stenosis. However, paediatric studies could not reliably predict renovascular disease and showed low sensitivities of 47–73% [82–84]. Therefore, pre- and post-captopril renal scintigraphy cannot be recommended as a screening method.

DMSA scintigraphy can be informative by evaluating the relative function of each kidney and documenting focal ischemic deficits caused by renal artery stenosis and/or renal scarring. It is important to recognise that kidneys or renal segments with no initial DMSA uptake and suspected no function have the ability to recover after revascularization by angioplasty (Fig. 49.5), especially if the size of the kidney as measured on renal US is still good.

Invasive Imaging

Digital Subtraction Angiography (DSA)

DSA is the diagnostic gold standard in establishing the diagnosis of renovascular disease in children whereas all other non-invasive imaging methods have 10–40% false-negative and false-positive results. DSA provides the best spatial and temporal resolution producing excellent images of the renal arterial lumens and branches, especially if the sizes of the vessels are small.

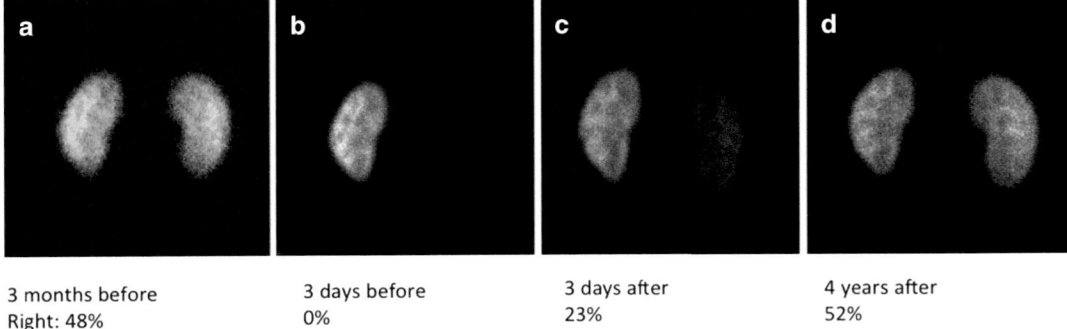

a	**b**	**c**	**d**
3 months before	3 days before	3 days after	4 years after
Right: 48%	0%	23%	52%

Fig. 49.5 DMSA scan with recovery of renal function after percutaneous transluminal angioplasty (PTA). (**a**) Right kidney with normal DMSA uptake 3 months before angioplasty (partial function 48%), (**b**) lacking uptake (0%) 3 days before angioplasty, (**c**) beginning recovery 3 days after angioplasty (23%) and (**d**) stable right partial function 4 years after invention (images kindly provided by Great Ormond Street Hospital, London)

Renal artery stenosis can be defined as a significant reduction of intraluminal diameter (e.g. >60%) and presence of collateral vessels.

DSA is an invasive diagnostic method with a mainly femoral artery approach, requiring general anaesthesia in children, and has a significant ionising radiation exposure. However, the main advantage of DSA is that potentially curative treatment with percutaneous transluminal angioplasty (PTA) can be performed during the same intervention. DSA and angioplasty are recommended to be performed only in clinical centres specialized in paediatric renovascular disease providing a multidisciplinary team including paediatric nephrologists, experienced interventional radiologists and vascular surgeons.

Renal Vein Renin Sampling

In case of bilateral renal artery disease and/or suspected location of stenosis in a segmental artery, renal vein sampling and measurement of plasma renin activity can be useful to identify the more relevant stenotic renal artery or to localize the segmental artery stenosis to a small area of one kidney. Usually, blood samples will be taken from the infrarenal vena cava inferior, the main renal veins and the larger intrarenal branches in order to perform renal vein renin studies during the diagnostic angiography.

Further Imaging

Cranial MR with Angiography

In case of neurological symptoms at initial presentation and suspected cerebrovascular involvement, a cranial MR evaluating cerebral parenchyma and vasculature is recommended.

Echocardiography

To evaluate cardiac function and left ventricular hypertrophy as target organ damage of severe hypertension, echocardiography should be performed in all children at initial presentation and on an annual basis.

Treatment

Treatment of renovascular hypertension is complex and requires input from a multidisciplinary team including interventional radiologists, vascular surgeons and nephrologists. In certain cases input from cardiologists, neurovascular specialists, anaesthetists and other specialists is needed. The goals of treatment are normalization of blood pressure and restoration or preservation of kidney function. Antihypertensive pharmacotherapy will nearly always be the first measure, but is almost never sufficient to control blood pressure. Angioplasty and sometimes open surgery will be needed in nearly all cases.

Pharmacological Treatment

The blood pressure in children with RVH is typically elevated very markedly. Antihypertensive medications usually improve blood pressure somewhat and many children receive combined therapies with multiple drugs [85]. It is however uncommon that blood pressure normalises by pharmacotherapy alone.

While there is no single most effective antihypertensive drug class in children with RVH, RAAS blockers are quite effective in selected individual cases. They do however bear a major chance of harming kidney function as they work by lowering the intra-glomerular pressure. These drugs are therefore contraindicated in children with renal artery stenosis. Selected cases where both angioplasty and surgery are technically unfeasible can benefit from renin-angiotensin blockade. This can often effectively reduce blood pressure but will also impair the function of the whole or part of a kidney (Fig. 49.6).

After successful angioplasty most children will acquire a much improved blood pressure and antihypertensive drugs can be weaned. It is however not uncommon that continued pharmacological treatment is required, albeit with much fewer drugs, to achieve total normalization of blood pressure.

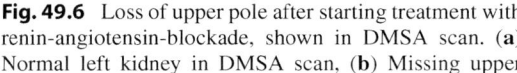

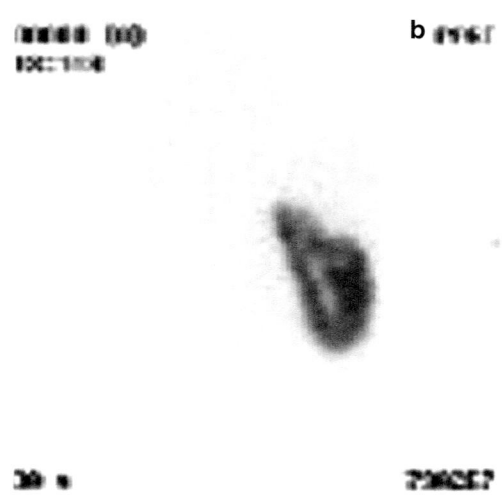

Fig. 49.6 Loss of upper pole after starting treatment with renin-angiotensin-blockade, shown in DMSA scan. (**a**) Normal left kidney in DMSA scan, (**b**) Missing upper pole of left kidney in DMSA scan (images kindly provided by Great Ormond Street Hospital, London)

Angioplasty

The vast majority of children will require interventional treatment. Percutaneous transluminal angioplasty (PTA) is the most commonly used procedure (Fig. 49.7). It is performed under general anaesthesia. The femoral artery is most commonly used for catheterization but in some cases an axillary or and radial approach is needed. The equipment used for adult coronary arteries are generally suitable. Mild to severe stenosis of the main renal arteries and sometimes also the aorta are most amenable to treatment [86]. Even completely occluded arteries can be re-canalized in many cases. Particularly in children with NF type 1 the stenotic tissue may be difficult to open up and a cutting balloon can be needed to reestablish a good-sized vascular lumen (Fig. 49.7).

Unfortunately, the artery can have elastic recoil and cause a residual stenosis after initially successful angioplasty [87]. In some of these cases a stent can be placed to keep the artery open [9, 88–90]. The lumen of the stent can however narrow in size with time. This can be due to intimal hyperplasia within the stent, stent thrombosis, or even stent fracture. Importantly, the fixed diameter of the stent may cause re-stenosis over time as children, and their arteries, grow in size. This is a particular issue in rapidly growing young infants. The use of a stent is therefore generally advised against in children.

A blood vessel that has had successful angioplasty can re-stenose with time and it is therefore not uncommon that a child needs to undergo repeated interventions to achieve optimal results [91].

Children with severe mid aortic syndrome can also benefit from angioplasty. We have seen cases diagnosed with an atretic aorta that have been possible to re-canalize and restore a reasonably wide aorta, normal blood pressure, and normal quality of life [92].

Some children with stenotic vascular lesions that are not amenable to angioplasty due to the small size of the blood vessel can be treated with ethanol ablation of a segment of a kidney [93, 94]. This is particularly useful in polar arteries supplying only a small part of the kidney.

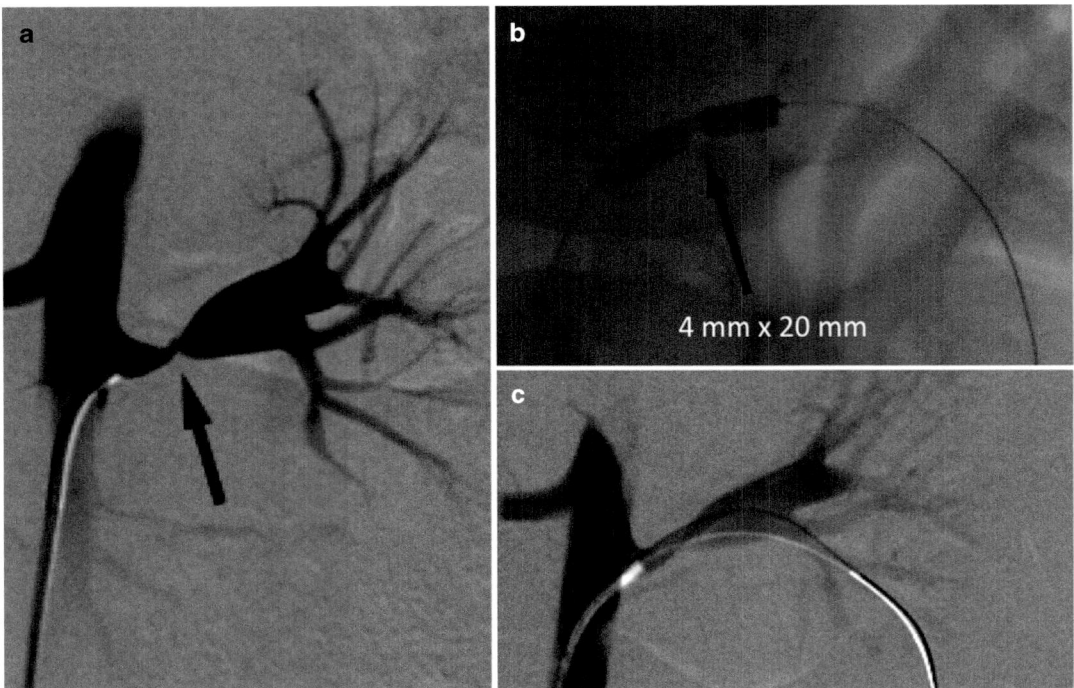

Fig. 49.7 Percutaneous transluminal angioplasty (PTA) of the left renal artery. (**a**) Left renal artery stenosis in angiography, (**b**) Positioning a cutting balloon catheter (4 mm × 20 mm) at the stenotic area, (**c**) improved vascu- lar lumen of left renal artery directly after angioplasty procedure (images kindly provided by Great Ormond Street Hospital, London)

Complications to angioplasty include contrast-induced nephropathy, arterial spasm, thrombosis, arterial dissection and perforation. The risks for these complications vary from 0% to 43% in differ-ent publications [95, 96]. Haemodynamically insig-nificant dissections occur rather often and might be part of the remodelling process after angioplasty. Fatal complications are very uncommon for PTA but we and other centres recommend that vascular surgery should be readily available in case of arte-rial rupture or active extravasation of contrast [97].

Surgery

Surgery should be used in children where angio-plasty has not achieved appropriate blood pressure control, and for aneurysmal disease that is not amenable to endovascular treatment. This assessment needs multi-professional consensus from interventional radiology, vascular surgery and nephrology. A variety of surgical revascular-ization procedures is available, including autolo-gous or synthetic grafts [12, 13, 98, 99]. Autologous grafts can be the splenic or the gastro-duodenal artery that is pulled down to the kidney, or the use of a part of the saphenous vein or internal iliac artery can be used. Dacron is often used for synthetic grafts. Surgery on the renal arteries can be so complicated and time-consuming that it needs to be done outside of the child ("bench surgery", Fig. 49.8), with an ensu-ing auto-transplantation. In children with very complicated pathology, e.g., stenosis of both renal arteries and mid-aortic syndrome, a so-called trouser graft can be used. This extends

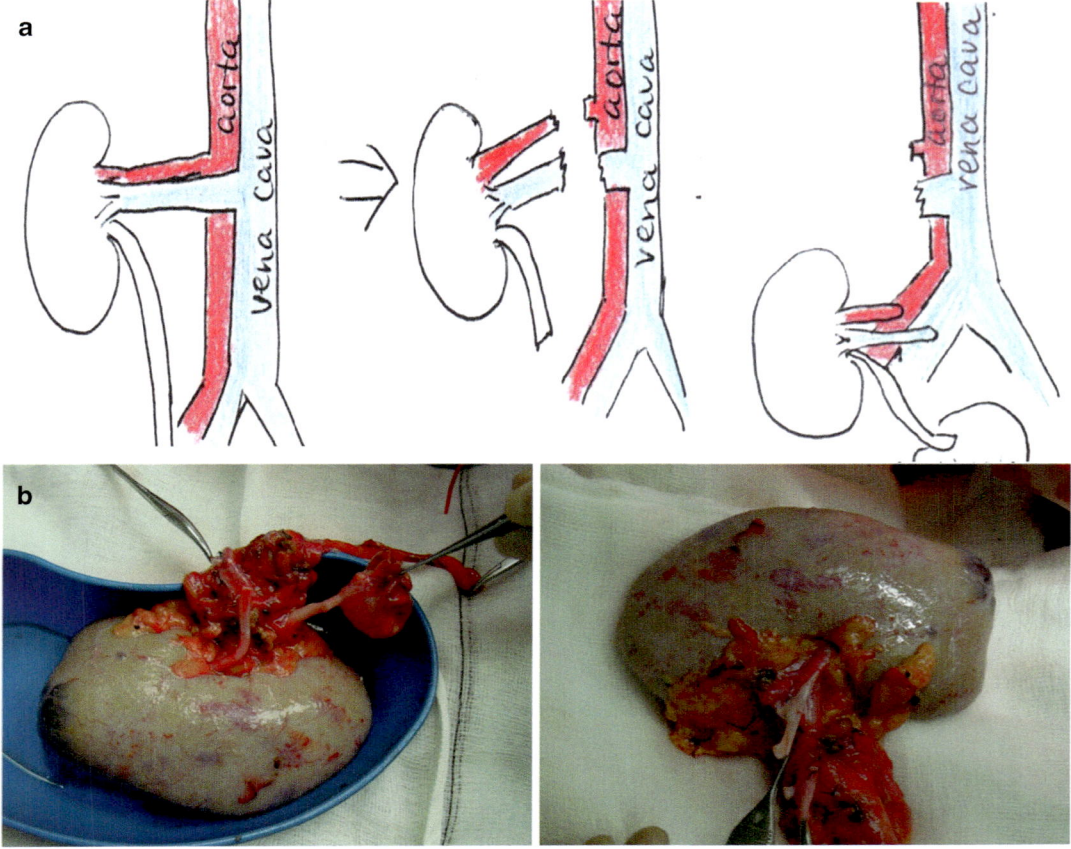

Fig. 49.8 Auto-transplantation: (**a**) Sketch and (**b**) bench surgery (images kindly provided by Great Ormond Street Hospital, London)

from the aorta above the MAS to the aorta below the stenotic lesion and to one or both renal arteries (Fig. 49.9).

In cases where no curative intervention is possible, nephrectomy can be an alternative option. This can be very successful and cure the blood pressure in children with unilateral disease and small non-functioning kidneys [100, 101]. A word of caution is, however, warranted; in some cases kidneys that show less than 10%

function on a pre-treatment DMSA scan recover function after successful angioplasty or revascularization surgery, even up to 50% relative function (Fig. 49.4). These kidneys thus appear to survive on collateral circulation that does not give any relevant kidney function as measured with DMSA. We use the size of the affected kidney measured on ultrasound to decide when to try to recover function or to go directly to nephrectomy.

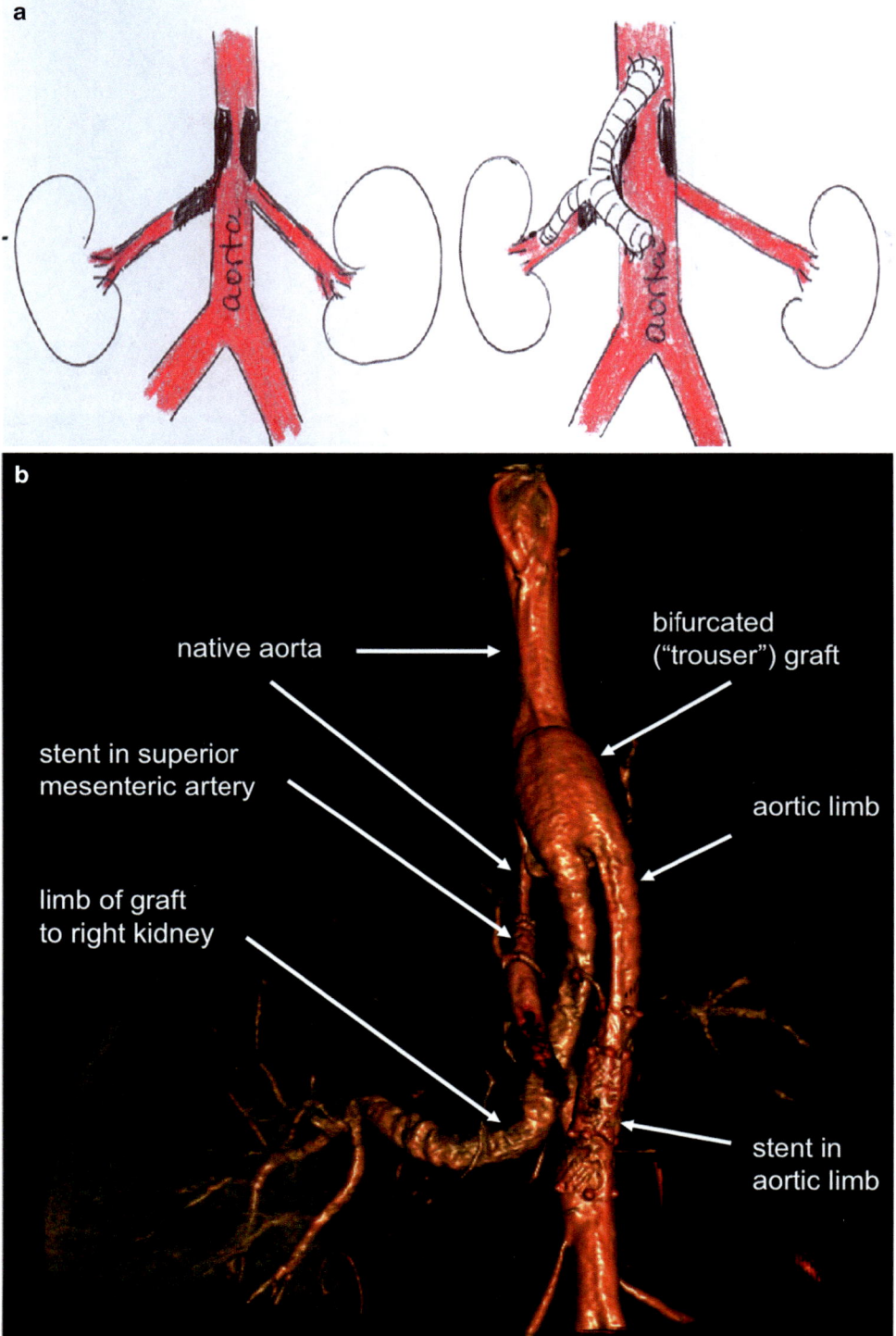

Fig. 49.9 Renal artery trouser graft in mid-aortic syndrome and right renal artery stenosis. (**a**) Sketch of renal artery and mid-aortic stenosis and implementing a renal artery trouser graft in order to plan vascular surgery. (**b**) Complex vascular situation with renal artery trouser graft (images kindly provided by Great Ormond Street Hospital, London)

Outcome

Technical Results

Angioplasty will, in most cases, widen the lumen of the artery. In some cases e.g. with total occlusion of the blood vessel or with a very long and slender renal artery this will however not be possible. In 25–28% of children re-intervention with angioplasty was required [9, 97, 102, 103]. In some children the artery recoils very quickly despite several successful attempts with angioplasty. Some of these children are amenable to surgery. In a recent cohort, 18% of children underwent surgery after initial angioplasty [81].

Blood Pressure

Improvement of blood pressure is the most commonly reported treatment outcome. With the current techniques, PTA normalizes or improves blood pressure in 53–63% of children [9, 97, 103–105]. It typically takes some days before blood pressure settles down and medication can be weaned. Quite often there is a persistent need for one blood pressure drug even after successful intervention.

It is important to analyse the reason when blood pressure improvement is not achieved. Re-stenosis, occurring immediately or with temporal delay, can in many cases explain a failure to improve the blood pressure. In children with widespread renovascular disease, successful treatment of individual stenotic arteries might not be sufficient and the remaining disease continues to drive high blood pressure [9]. Notably, vascular disease in the contralateral kidney and involvement of small intrarenal branches occurs in 50–70% of those children [9, 103] that are not amenable to either PTA or surgery.

Kidney Function

Most studies have not systematically reported the short- and long-term effects of treatment on kidney function. Recovery or stabilization of kidney function is however a very important therapeutic goal. Some kidneys that display no function on DMSA scan regain up to normal function (50% partial function on DMSA) after successful revascularisation. The value of serum creatinine in monitoring kidney function before and after intervention is limited since a major loss of function in one kidney can be "covered up" by a normally functioning contralateral kidney.

Summary

Renovascular stenosis is an unusual but very important cause of severe arterial hypertension in children. It is important to suspect and to diagnose. DSA is the gold standard investigation and angioplasty can be performed at the same time. Surgery is needed in an important minority of cases. Most but not all children will eventually benefit from treatment.

References

1. Bayazit AK, Yalcinkaya F, Cakar N, Duzova A, Bircan Z, Bakkaloglu A, et al. Reno-vascular hypertension in childhood: a nationwide survey. Pediatr Nephrol (Berlin, Germany). 2007;22(9):1327–33.
2. Wyszyńska T, Cichocka E, Wieteska-Klimczak A, Jobs K, Januszewicz P. A single pediatric center experience with 1025 children with hypertension. Acta Paediatr (Oslo, Norway: 1992). 1992;81(3):244–6.
3. Gill DG, Mendes de Costa B, Cameron JS, Joseph MC, Ogg CS, Chantler C. Analysis of 100 children with severe and persistent hypertension. Arch Dis Child. 1976;51(12):951–6.
4. Hiner LB, Falkner B. Renovascular hypertension in children. Pediatr Clin N Am. 1993;40(1):123–40.
5. Trautmann A, Roebuck DJ, McLaren CA, Brennan E, Marks SD, Tullus K. Non-invasive imaging cannot replace formal angiography in the diagnosis of renovascular hypertension. Pediatr Nephrol (Berlin, Germany). 2017;32(3):495–502.
6. Tummolo A, Marks SD, Stadermann M, Roebuck DJ, McLaren CA, Hamilton G, et al. Mid-aortic syndrome: long-term outcome of 36 children. Pediatr Nephrol (Berlin, Germany). 2009;24(11):2225–32.
7. Arslan Z, Patel PAA. Importance of the arc of Riolan in children with severe middle aortic syndrome. Arch Dis Child. 2021;106(12):1190.

8. Deal JE, Snell MF, Barratt TM, Dillon MJ. Renovascular disease in childhood. J Pediatr. 1992;121(3):378–84.

9. Shroff R, Roebuck DJ, Gordon I, Davies R, Stephens S, Marks S, et al. Angioplasty for renovascular hypertension in children: 20-year experience. Pediatrics. 2006;118(1):268–75.

10. Peco-Antić A, Stajić N, Krstić Z, Bogdanović R, Miloševski-Lomić G, Đukić M, et al. Associated extrarenal vascular diseases may complicate the treatment and outcome of renovascular hypertension. Acta Paediatrica (Oslo, Norway: 1992). 2016;105(1):e35–41.

11. Courtel JV, Soto B, Niaudet P, Gagnadoux MF, Carteret M, Quignodon JF, et al. Percutaneous transluminal angioplasty of renal artery stenosis in children. Pediatr Radiol. 1998;28(1):59–63.

12. Stanley JC, Criado E, Upchurch GR Jr, Brophy PD, Cho KJ, Rectenwald JE, et al. Pediatric renovascular hypertension: 132 primary and 30 secondary operations in 97 children. Pediatr Int. 2006;44(6):1219–28. discussion 28–9

13. Stanley JC, Zelenock GB, Messina LM, Wakefield TW. Pediatric renovascular hypertension: a thirty-year experience of operative treatment. J Vasc Surg. 1995;21(2):212–26. discussion 26–7

14. Kumar P, Arora P, Kher V, Rai PK, Gulati S, Baijal SS, et al. Malignant hypertension in children in India. Nephrol Dial Transplant. 1996;11(7):1261–6.

15. Kanitkar M. Renovascular hypertension. Indian Pediatr. 2005;42(1):47–54.

16. McCulloch M, Andronikou S, Goddard E, Sinclair P, Lawrenson J, Mandelstam S, et al. Angiographic features of 26 children with Takayasu's arteritis. Pediatr Radiol. 2003;33(4):230–5.

17. Tyagi S, Kaul UA, Satsangi DK, Arora R. Percutaneous transluminal angioplasty for renovascular hypertension in children: initial and long-term results. Pediatrics. 1997;99(1):44–9.

18. Hari P, Bagga A, Srivastava RN. Sustained hypertension in children. Indian Pediatr. 2000;37(3):268–74.

19. Harrison EG Jr, Hunt JC, Bernatz PE. Morphology of fibromuscular dysplasia of the renal artery in renovascular hypertension. Am J Med. 1967;43(1):97–112.

20. Stanley P, Hieshima G, Mehringer M. Percutaneous transluminal angioplasty for pediatric renovascular hypertension. Radiology. 1984;153(1):101–4.

21. Casalini E, Sfondrini MS, Fossali E. Two-year clinical follow-up of children and adolescents after percutaneous transluminal angioplasty for renovascular hypertension. Investig Radiol. 1995;30(1):40–3.

22. Slovut DP, Olin JW. Fibromuscular dysplasia. N Engl J Med. 2004;350(18):1862–71.

23. Kerr GS, Hallahan CW, Giordano J, Leavitt RY, Fauci AS, Rottem M, et al. Takayasu arteritis. Ann Intern Med. 1994;120(11):919–29.

24. Cilliers AM, Adams PE, Ntsinjana H, Kala U. Review of children with Takayasu's arteritis at a Southern African tertiary care centre. Cardiol Young. 2018;28(9):1129–35.

25. Hahn D, Thomson PD, Kala U, Beale PG, Levin SE. A review of Takayasu's arteritis in children in Gauteng, South Africa. Pediatr Nephrol (Berlin, Germany). 1998;12(8):668–75.

26. Wiggelinkhuizen J, Cremin BJ. Takayasu arteritis and renovascular hypertension in childhood. Pediatrics. 1978;62(2):209–17.

27. Lupi-Herrera E, Sánchez-Torres G, Marcushamer J, Mispireta J, Horwitz S, Vela JE. Takayasu's arteritis. Clinical study of 107 cases. Am Heart J. 1977;93(1):94–103.

28. Blockmans D. PET in vasculitis. Ann N Y Acad Sci. 2011;1228:64–70.

29. Gulati A, Bagga A. Large vessel vasculitis. Pediatr Nephrol (Berlin, Germany). 2010;25(6):1037–48.

30. Ozen S, Ruperto N, Dillon MJ, Bagga A, Barron K, Davin JC, et al. EULAR/PReS endorsed consensus criteria for the classification of childhood vasculitides. Ann Rheum Dis. 2006;65(7):936–41.

31. Ozen S, Pistorio A, Iusan SM, Bakkaloglu A, Herlin T, Brik R, et al. EULAR/PRINTO/PRES criteria for Henoch-Schönlein purpura, childhood polyarteritis nodosa, childhood Wegener granulomatosis and childhood Takayasu arteritis: Ankara 2008. Part II: Final classification criteria. Ann Rheum Dis. 2010;69(5):798–806.

32. Desai MY, Stone JH, Foo TK, Hellmann DB, Lima JA, Bluemke DA. Delayed contrast-enhanced MRI of the aortic wall in Takayasu's arteritis: initial experience. AJR Am J Roentgenol. 2005;184(5):1427–31.

33. Lee SG, Ryu JS, Kim HO, Oh JS, Kim YG, Lee CK, et al. Evaluation of disease activity using F-18 FDG PET-CT in patients with Takayasu arteritis. Clin Nucl Med. 2009;34(11):749–52.

34. Salerno AE, Marsenic O, Meyers KE, Kaplan BS, Hellinger JC. Vascular involvement in tuberous sclerosis. Pediatr Nephrol (Berlin, Germany). 2010;25(8):1555–61.

35. Bérard E, Sarles J, Triolo V, Gagnadoux MF, Wernert F, Hadchouel M, et al. Renovascular hypertension and vascular anomalies in Alagille syndrome. Pediatr Nephrol (Berlin, Germany). 1998;12(2):121–4.

36. Salem JE, Bruguiere E, Iserin L, Guiochon-Mantel A, Plouin PF. Hypertension and aortorenal disease in Alagille syndrome. J Hypertens. 2012;30(7):1300–6.

37. Baum MA, Harris HW Jr, Burrows PE, Schofield DE, Somers MJ. Renovascular hypertension in Marfan syndrome. Pediatr Nephrol (Berlin, Germany). 1997;11(4):499–501.

38. Viering D, Chan MMY, Hoogenboom L, Iancu D, de Baaij JHF, Tullus K, et al. Genetics of renovascular hypertension in children. J Hypertens. 2020;38(10):1964–70.

39. Warejko JK, Tan W, Daga A, Schapiro D, Lawson JA, Shril S, et al. Whole exome sequencing of patients with steroid-resistant nephrotic syndrome. Nat Commun. 2018;13(1):53–62.

40. Oderich GS, Sullivan TM, Bower TC, Gloviczki P, Miller DV, Babovic-Vuksanovic D, et al. Vascular abnormalities in patients with neurofibromatosis

syndrome type I: clinical spectrum, management, and results. J Vasc Surg. 2007;46(3):475–84.

41. Friedman JM, Arbiser J, Epstein JA, Gutmann DH, Huot SJ, Lin AE, et al. Cardiovascular disease in neurofibromatosis 1: report of the NF1 Cardiovascular Task Force. Genet Med. 2002;4(3):105–11.

42. Lin AE, Birch PH, Korf BR, Tenconi R, Niimura M, Poyhonen M, et al. Cardiovascular malformations and other cardiovascular abnormalities in neurofibromatosis 1. Am J Med Genet. 2000;95(2):108–17.

43. Fossali E, Signorini E, Intermite RC, Casalini E, Lovaria A, Maninetti MM, et al. Renovascular disease and hypertension in children with neurofibromatosis. Pediatr Nephrol (Berlin, Germany). 2000;14(8–9):806–10.

44. Tedesco MA, Di Salvo G, Ratti G, Natale F, Calabrese E, Grassia C, et al. Arterial distensibility and ambulatory blood pressure monitoring in young patients with neurofibromatosis type 1. Am J Hypertens. 2001;14(6 Pt 1):559–66.

45. Williams VC, Lucas J, Babcock MA, Gutmann DH, Korf B, Maria BL. Neurofibromatosis type 1 revisited. Pediatrics. 2009;123(1):124–33.

46. Bouchireb K, Boyer O, Bonnet D, Brunelle F, Decramer S, Landthaler G, et al. Clinical features and management of arterial hypertension in children with Williams-Beuren syndrome. Nephrol Dial Transplant. 2010;25(2):434–8.

47. Zalzstein E, Moes CA, Musewe NN, Freedom RM. Spectrum of cardiovascular anomalies in Williams-Beuren syndrome. Curr Hypertens Rep. 1991;12(4):219–23.

48. Pober BR. Williams-Beuren syndrome. N Engl J Med. 2010;362(3):239–52.

49. Friedman AD. Wilms tumor. Pediatr Rev. 2013;34(7):328–30. discussion 30

50. Burnei G, Burnei A, Hodorogea D, Drăghici I, Georgescu I, Vlad C, et al. Diagnosis and complications of renovascular hypertension in children: literature data and clinical observations. J Med Life. 2009;2(1):18–28.

51. D'Angelo P, Catania S, Zirilli G, Collini P, Tropia S, Perotti D, et al. Severe polyuria and polydipsia in hyponatremic-hypertensive syndrome associated with Wilms tumor. Pediatr Blood Cancer. 2010;55(3):566–9.

52. Shinohara M, Shitara T, Hatakeyama SI, Suzuki N, Maruyama K, Kobayashi T, et al. An infant with systemic hypertension, renal artery stenosis, and neuroblastoma. J Pediatr Surg. 2004;39(1):103–6.

53. Marchal AL, Hoeffel JC, Freyd S, Schmitt M, Olive D, Fays J. Arterial hypertension caused by extrinsic compression of the renal artery of tumor origin in a child. Pediatrie. 1986;41(6):475–80.

54. Herman TE. Special imaging casebook. Congenital adrenal neuroblastoma with renovascular hypertension. J Perinatol. 1999;19(6 Pt 1):468–72.

55. Deal JE, Sever PS, Barratt TM, Dillon MJ. Phaeochromocytoma—investigation and management of 10 cases. Arch Dis Child. 1990;65(3):269–74.

56. Gill IS, Meraney AM, Bravo EL, Novick AC. Pheochromocytoma coexisting with renal artery lesions. J Urol. 2000;164(2):296–301.

57. Kuzmanovska D, Sahpazova E, Kocova M, Damjanovski G, Popov Z. Phaeochromocytoma associated with reversible renal artery stenosis. Nephrol Dial Transplant. 2001;16(10):2092–4.

58. Camberos A, Bautista N, Rubenzik M, Applebaum H. Renal artery stenosis and pheochromocytoma: coexistence and treatment. J Pediatr Surg. 2000;35(5):714–6.

59. Koskimies O. Arterial hypertension developing 10 years after radiotherapy for Wilms's tumour. Br Med J (Clin Res Ed). 1982;285(6347):996–8.

60. Wakabayashi S, Takaoka H, Miyauchi H, Sazuka T, Saito Y, Sugimoto K, et al. Usefulness of renal autotransplantation for radiotherapy-induced renovascular hypertension. Intern Med (Tokyo, Japan). 2019;58(13):1897–9.

61. Levin TL, Roebuck D, Berdon WE. Long-segment narrowing of the abdominal aorta and its branches in a survivor of infantile neuroblastoma treated without radiation therapy. Pediatr Radiol. 2011;41(7):933–6.

62. Adelman RD. Long-term follow-up of neonatal renovascular hypertension. Pediatr Nephrol (Berlin, Germany). 1987;1(1):35–41.

63. Adelman RD, Morrell RE. Coarctation of the abdominal aorta and renal artery stenosis related to an umbilical artery catheter placement in a neonate. Pediatrics. 2000;106(3):E36.

64. Merten DF, Vogel JM, Adelman RD, Goetzman BW, Bogren HG. Renovascular hypertension as a complication of umbilical arterial catheterization. Radiology. 1978;126(3):751–7.

65. Starr MC, Flynn JT. Neonatal hypertension: cases, causes, and clinical approach. Pediatr Nephrol (Berlin, Germany). 2019;34(5):787–99.

66. Adelman RD. Neonatal hypertension. Pediatr Clin N Am. 1978;25(1):99–110.

67. Neal WA, Reynolds JW, Jarvis CW, Williams HJ. Umbilical artery catheterization: demonstration of arterial thrombosis by aortography. Pediatrics. 1972;50(1):6–13.

68. Fontaine E, Barthelemy Y, Gagnadoux MF, Cukier J, Broyer M, Beurton D. A review of 72 renal artery stenoses in a series of 715 kidney transplantations in children. Progres en Urologie. 1994;4(2):193–205.

69. Menser MA, Dorman DC, Reye RD, Reid RR. Renal-artery stenosis in the rubella syndrome. Lancet (London, England). 1966;1(7441):790–2.

70. Seeman T. Hypertension after renal transplantation. Pediatr Nephrol (Berlin, Germany). 2009;24(5):959–72.

71. Ghirardo G, De Franceschi M, Vidal E, Vidoni A, Ramondo G, Benetti E, et al. Transplant renal artery stenosis in children: risk factors and outcome after endovascular treatment. Pediatr Nephrol (Berlin, Germany). 2014;29(3):461–7.

72. Brun P, Kchouk H, Mouchet B, Baudouin V, Raynaud A, Loirat C, et al. Value of Doppler ultrasound for the

diagnosis of renal artery stenosis in children. Pediatr Nephrol (Berlin, Germany). 1997;11(1):27–30.

73. Conkbayir I, Yücesoy C, Edgüer T, Yanik B, Yaşar Ayaz U, Hekimoğlu B. Doppler sonography in renal artery stenosis. An evaluation of intrarenal and extrarenal imaging parameters. Clin Imaging. 2003;27(4):256–60.

74. Ilivitzki A, Glozman L, Lopez Alfonso R, Ofer A, Beck Razi N, Rotman Shapira M. Sonographic evaluation of renovascular hypertension in the pediatric population: state-of-the-art. J Clin Ultrasound. 2017;45(5):282–92.

75. Stringer DA, O'Halpin D, Daneman A, Liu P, Geary DF. Duplex Doppler sonography for renal artery stenosis in the post-transplant pediatric patient. Pediatr Radiol. 1989;19(3):187–92.

76. Chhadia S, Cohn RA, Vural G, Donaldson JS. Renal Doppler evaluation in the child with hypertension: a reasonable screening discriminator? Pediatr Radiol. 2013;43(12):1549–56.

77. Castelli PK, Dillman JR, Kershaw DB, Khalatbari S, Stanley JC, Smith EA. Renal sonography with Doppler for detecting suspected pediatric renin-mediated hypertension - is it adequate? Pediatr Radiol. 2014;44(1):42–9.

78. Kchouk H, Brun P, Sentou Y, Raynaud A, Gaux JC, Loirat C. Renal stenosis in hypertensive children. Doppler/arteriographic correlation. Pediatr Nephrol (Berlin, Germany). 1997;22(2):86–90.

79. Vade A, Agrawal R, Lim-Dunham J, Hartoin D. Utility of computed tomographic renal angiogram in the management of childhood hypertension. Pediatr Nephrol (Berlin, Germany). 2002;17(9):741–7.

80. Kurian J, Epelman M, Darge K, Meyers K, Nijs E, Hellinger JC. The role of CT angiography in the evaluation of pediatric renovascular hypertension. Pediatr Radiol. 2013;43(4):490–501. quiz 487–9

81. Lee Y, Lim YS, Lee ST, Cho H. Pediatric renovascular hypertension: treatment outcome according to underlying disease. Pediatr Int. 2018;60(3):264–9.

82. Abdulsamea S, Anderson P, Biassoni L, Brennan E, McLaren CA, Marks SD, et al. Pre- and postcaptopril renal scintigraphy as a screening test for renovascular hypertension in children. Pediatr Nephrol (Berlin, Germany). 2010;25(2):317–22.

83. Minty I, Lythgoe MF, Gordon I. Hypertension in paediatrics: can pre- and post-captopril technetium-99m dimercaptosuccinic acid renal scans exclude renovascular disease? Eur J Nucl Med. 1993;20(8):699–702.

84. Ng CS, de Bruyn R, Gordon I. The investigation of renovascular hypertension in children: the accuracy of radio-isotopes in detecting renovascular disease. Nucl Med Commun. 1997;18(11):1017–28.

85. Tullus K, Brennan E, Hamilton G, Lord R, McLaren CA, Marks SD, et al. Renovascular hypertension in children. Lancet (London, England). 2008;371(9622):1453–63.

86. Agrawal H, Moodie D, Qureshi AM, Acosta AA, Hernandez JA, Braun MC, et al. Interventions in children with renovascular hypertension: a 27-year retrospective single-center experience. Congenit Heart Dis. 2018;13(3):349–56.

87. Eliason JL, Coleman DM, Criado E, Stanley JC. Surgical treatment of abdominal aortic aneurysms in infancy and early childhood. J Vasc Surg. 2016;64(5):1252–61.

88. Imamura H, Isobe M, Takenaka H, Kinoshita O, Sekiguchi M, Ohta M. Successful stenting of bilateral renal artery stenosis due to fibromuscular dysplasia assessed by use of pressure guidewire technique: a case report. Angiology. 1998;49(1):69–74.

89. Ing FF, Goldberg B, Siegel DH, Trachtman H, Bierman FZ. Arterial stents in the management of neurofibromatosis and renovascular hypertension in a pediatric patient: case report of a new treatment modality. Cardiovasc Intervent Radiol. 1995;18(6):414–8.

90. Liang CD, Wu CJ, Fang CY, Ko SF. Endovascular stent placement for management of total renal artery occlusion in a child. J Invasive Cardiol. 2002;14(1):32–5.

91. Humbert J, Roussey-Kesler G, Guerin P, LeFrançois T, Connault J, Chenouard A, et al. Diagnostic and medical strategy for renovascular hypertension: report from a monocentric pediatric cohort. Eur J Pediatr. 2015;174(1):23–32.

92. Minson S, McLaren CA, Roebuck DJ, Tullus K. Infantile midaortic syndrome with aortic occlusion. Pediatr Nephrol. 2012;27(2):321–4. https://doi.org/10.1007/s00467-011-2039-y. Epub 2011 Nov 5. PMID: 22057980.

93. Ishijima H, Ishizaka H, Sakurai M, Ito K, Endo K. Partial renal embolization for pediatric renovascular hypertension secondary to fibromuscular dysplasia. Cardiovasc Intervent Radiol. 1997;20(5):383–6.

94. Teigen CL, Mitchell SE, Venbrux AC, Christenson MJ, McLean RH. Segmental renal artery embolization for treatment of pediatric renovascular hypertension. J Vasc Interv Radiol. 1992;3(1):111–7.

95. Lobeck IN, Alhajjat AM, Dupree P, Racadio JM, Mitsnefes MM, Karns R, et al. The management of pediatric renovascular hypertension: a single center experience and review of the literature. J Pediatr Surg. 2018;53(9):1825–31.

96. Alexander A, Richmond L, Geary D, Salle JL, Amaral J, Connolly B. Outcomes of percutaneous transluminal angioplasty for pediatric renovascular hypertension. J Pediatr Surg. 2017;52(3):395–9.

97. McLaren CA, Roebuck DJ. Interventional radiology for renovascular hypertension in children. Tech Vasc Interv Radiol. 2003;6(4):150–7.

98. O'Neill JA Jr, Berkowitz H, Fellows KJ, Harmon CM. Midaortic syndrome and hypertension in childhood. J Pediatr Surg. 1995;30(2):164–71. discussion 71–2

99. Sandmann W, Dueppers P, Pourhassan S, Voiculescu A, Klee D, Balzer KM. Early and long-term results after reconstructive surgery in 42 children and two young adults with renovascular hypertension due to

fibromuscular dysplasia and middle aortic syndrome. Eur J Vasc Endovasc Surg. 2014;47(5):509–16.

100. Hegde S, Coulthard MG. Follow-up of early unilateral nephrectomy for hypertension. Arch Dis Child Fetal Neonatal Ed. 2007;92(4):F305–6.

101. Tse Y, Marks SD, Brennan E, Hamilton G, McLaren CA, Roebuck DJ, et al. Renal artery revascularisation can restore kidney function with absent radiotracer uptake. Pediatr Nephrol (Berlin, Germany). 2012;27(11):2153–7.

102. Kari JA, Roebuck DJ, Tullus K. Renal artery stenosis in association with congenital anomalies of the kidney and urinary tract. Saudi Med J. 2014;35(10):1264–6.

103. Kari JA, Roebuck DJ, McLaren CA, Davis M, Dillon MJ, Hamilton G, et al. Angioplasty for renovascular hypertension in 78 children. Arch Dis Child. 2015;100(5):474–8.

104. König K, Gellermann J, Querfeld U, Schneider MB. Treatment of severe renal artery stenosis by percutaneous transluminal renal angioplasty and stent implantation: review of the pediatric experience: apropos of two cases. Pediatr Nephrol (Berlin, Germany). 2006;21(5):663–71.

105. Ladapo TA, Gajjar P, McCulloch M, Scott C, Numanoglu A, Nourse P. Impact of revascularization on hypertension in children with Takayasu's arteritis-induced renal artery stenosis: a 21-year review. Pediatr Nephrol (Berlin, Germany). 2015;30(8):1289–95.

Renal Hypertension: Etiology and Management

50

Elke Wühl and Franz Schaefer

Introduction

Blood pressure (BP) is regulated by several setting mechanisms and, apart from the cardiovascular system, the central nervous system and the adrenal glands, the kidneys are key players in BP control.

In 1836 Bright first described the association of a small contracted kidney with left ventricular hypertrophy (LVH) and linked hypertension to kidney disease [1]. In children and adolescents with chronic kidney disease (CKD), arterial hypertension is often the earliest and most prevalent complication of CKD [2]. Large cohort studies in pediatric CKD in Europe [3], Canada [2] and the US [4–6] found controlled or uncontrolled hypertension in more than 40% of children with CKD stage 1 and in up to 90% of those with CKD stage 3 to 5 [2, 6]. Even among patients receiving antihypertensive treatment, BP was uncontrolled in up to 50% of patients [6]. Evaluated by ambulatory BP monitoring (ABPM), the overall prevalence of uncontrolled hypertension ranged between 27% and 48%. The fraction of children with elevated BP not receiving antihypertensive treatment was between 21% and 45% [3, 7–9].

Because untreated or uncontrolled hypertension is an independent risk factor for kidney damage and kidney disease progression as well as for cardiovascular morbidity and mortality, BP control is of utmost importance, especially in patients with prevalent CKD.

This chapter will focus on the pathophysiology of hypertension in pediatric kidney disease and on the indications for antihypertensive treatment, therapeutic options and BP targets in childhood CKD.

The Role of the Kidney in Hypertension

Mechanisms of Blood Pressure Regulation by the Kidneys

The *Pressure-Natriuresis-Diuresis Hypothesis* plays an important role in BP control and the pathophysiology of hypertension. By this mechanism the kidneys regulate arterial pressure by adjusting blood volume. When arterial BP or renal perfusion pressure changes, blood volume is adjusted accordingly by altering the excretion or retention of sodium and water to return arterial BP to normal values [10]. This is accomplished by the interplay of angiotensin II, atrial natriuretic peptide, vasopressin, nitric oxide (NO),

E. Wühl (✉) · F. Schaefer
Division of Pediatric Nephrology, Center for Pediatrics and Adolescent Medicine, Heidelberg University Hospital, Heidelberg, Germany
e-mail: elke.wuehl@med.uni-heidelberg.de; franz.schaefer@med.uni-heidelberg.de

© The Author(s), under exclusive license to Springer Nature Switzerland AG 2023
F. Schaefer, L. A. Greenbaum (eds.), *Pediatric Kidney Disease*,
https://doi.org/10.1007/978-3-031-11665-0_50

kallikrein-kinin, prostaglandins, renal nerves, and other factors. Through this mechanism, the kidneys are even able to override other BP control mechanisms.

To protect the kidneys from BP peaks, transmission of elevated systemic pressure to the glomeruli and to periglomerular capillaries is prevented by preglomerular vasoconstriction [11]. This autoregulation of glomerular filtration rate (GFR) and renal blood flow (RBF) maintains RBF constant within a defined perfusion pressure ranging from approximately 80 to 200 mmHg.

Ideally, higher salt intake leads to an increase in natriuresis and diuresis but almost no change in arterial pressure. However, sensitivity to salt intake varies individually and subjects can be classified according to their arterial pressure response to changes in salt intake.

Subjects in whom arterial pressure is relatively insensitive to changes in sodium intake are so-called *salt-insensitive* individuals while those in whom arterial pressure is related to salt intake are called *salt-sensitive*. In salt-sensitive individuals the pressure-natriuresis relationship is shifted towards higher pressure levels needed to achieve increased sodium excretion; low salt intake results in normal BP but BP steadily increases with increasing salt intake [12].

Subjects with low nephron endowment, e.g., children born small for gestational age or preterm, are especially susceptible to salt sensitivity and increased BP level. Reduced nephron endowment may result in the histopathological finding of 'oligomeganephronia'. In a kidney biopsy study in adult patients with primary hypertension, the total number of glomeruli was reduced by 50%, while the size of the glomeruli was increased 2.3-fold [13].

In a neonate with low nephron number the kidney tries to adapt to the excretory overload by increasing the filtered sodium load per nephron and compensatory growth of the proximal tubule with a consequent increase in sodium reabsorption. A reduced flow at the macula densa induces an increase of glomerular pressure and filtration resulting in restoration of sodium delivery to the macula densa. Thus, extracellular fluid homeostasis is maintained by increased arterial pressure to excrete the sodium load [14]. However, the underlying pathophysiology is not yet fully understood. Pathophysiological mechanisms include genetic predisposition, kidney damage mediated by inflammation, the renin-angiotensin-aldosterone system, and neuronal alterations. After manifestation of salt sensitivity, an individual usually remains salt sensitive [15]. The prevalence of salt-sensitivity increases with age [16] and is associated with an increased risk for cardiovascular events over time [17, 18]. Supported by the observation that 50% of patients with essential hypertension are salt-sensitive, current hypertension guidelines recommend restriction of salt intake [19–21].

Also, dysfunctions of tubular ion transporters have a crucial role in the pathogenesis of hypertension. The Na^+/H^+-exchangers (NHEs), the Na^+-K^+-$2Cl^-$-cotransporter (NKCC), the Na^+-Cl^--cotransporter (NCC), the epithelial sodium cotransporter (ENaC), and the sodium-potassium-ATPase (Na^+/K^+-ATPase) play a major role in sodium homeostasis.

The *renin–angiotensin-aldosterone system* (RAAS) is one of the most powerful regulators of salt homeostasis and BP. The RAAS is activated by either the macula densa, baroreceptor activation, or the sympathetic nervous system. Activation of one of these sensors leads to stimulation of renin release by juxtaglomerular cells. Renin cleaves angiotensinogen to angiotensin I, and angiotensin I is rapidly converted to angiotensin II by the angiotensin-converting enzyme (ACE). Angiotensin II is the most effective component of the RAAS and plays a central role not only in the regulation of fluid volume but also in regulation of vascular resistance. Effects of angiotensin II are mainly mediated via the angiotensin (AT)-1 receptor, i.e., vasoconstriction, aldosterone and vasopressin release, salt and water retention through the kidney, and sympathetic activation, as well as important autocrine and paracrine effects on cell proliferation and migration, and on extracellular matrix formation. The AT-2 receptor-mediated effects of angiotensin II are mainly vasodilatory and antiproliferative and seem to antagonize the effect of angiotensin II at the AT-1 receptor [22]. Additionally, angiotensin II can directly stimulate the activity of ENaC in the collecting duct [23]. This subtle balance between salt homeostasis, BP and the RAAS changes with aging or with decreasing kidney function.

An important role in BP regulation and cardiac function has been ascribed to *renalase*, an amine oxidase mainly expressed by the kidneys [24]. Renalase expression and enzymatic activity are rapidly triggered by modest increases in BP and by brief surges in plasma catecholamines. The active enzyme degrades circulating catecholamines, causing a fall in BP.

Arginine-vasopressin (or *antidiuretic hormone* (ADH)), is a neuropeptide synthesized in the hypothalamus and released in response to increased plasma osmolality, decreased systemic BP, or reduced blood volume. Vasopressin regulates renal water excretion by increasing the osmotic water permeability of the renal collecting duct by activation of the vasopression-2 receptor. In addition, activation of the vasopressin-2 receptor induces NO production, attenuating vasopressin-1 receptor-mediated vasoconstrictor effects [25].

The *kallikrein–kinin system* (KKS) also contributes to the regulation of BP. Kinins, including bradykinin, are formed from kininogen by kininogenase and tissue kallikrein. Bradykinin is mainly degraded by ACE. In the tubular lumen bradykinin causes natriuresis, whereas interstitial bradykinin regulates medullary blood flow [26]. Bradykinin and kallikrein may also act in a paracrine manner on the preglomerular microvessels via release of nitric oxide and prostaglandins [27].

NO, involved in the renal regulation of BP, is produced in the renal medulla and mediates endothelium-dependent vasodilatation. It enhances arterial compliance, reduces vascular resistance and exerts an antiproliferative effect on vascular smooth muscle cells. NO antagonists (e.g. asymmetric dimethylarginine [ADMA]) induce endothelial dysfunction and lead to an increase of BP and decrease in RBF.

Endothelins (ETs) are vasoconstrictor peptides released by endothelial cells. In the kidney, ET-1 is expressed in the glomeruli and medullary collecting ducts. The renal hemodynamic effects are exerted by activation of ET-A and ET-B receptors, located in podocytes, glomeruli, afferent and efferent arterioles, the proximal tubule, the medullary thick ascending limb, and the collecting duct. ET-A is the dominant ET receptor on vascular smooth muscle cells and activation causes vasoconstriction, whereas ET-B receptor activation on endothelial cells results in vasodilation [28].

Atrial natriuretic peptide (ANP), brain natriuretic peptide (BNP), C-type natriuretic peptide (CNP), and urodilatin have been named "*natriuretic peptides*" due to their ability to increase sodium and water excretion, resulting in reduction of intravascular volume and BP [29]. ANP and BNP decrease the secretion of renin and aldosterone, and antagonize the effects of angiotensin II on vascular tone and renal tubular sodium reabsorption. Natriuretic peptides are degraded in the lung and kidney by neutral endopeptidase [30].

Hypertension and the Kidneys

Patients with hypertension are at high risk for progressive kidney damage. The extent of the resulting nephrosclerosis depends on the individual susceptibility, degree of hypertension, the etiology of hypertension and the underlying kidney disease.

The pathogenic factors determining the degree of hypertensive kidney damage can be divided into systemic BP burden, pressure transmission to the kidney vascular bed, and local tissue susceptibility to damage. As long as BP remains within the upper limit of autoregulation, no severe changes occur. However, if this limit is exceeded, acute severe injury may occur. Autoregulatory responses can be compromised by hypertension-induced vascular injury, resulting in amplified kidney damage [31, 32]. Relevant reduction of kidney mass in CKD patients may additionally impair autoregulation [33–35] with consequent enhanced susceptibility to hypertensive injury and accelerated glomerulosclerosis [36, 37].

Pathomechanisms of Hypertension in Chronic Kidney Disease

Sodium retention and consequent *fluid overload* has long been recognized as a critical cause of hypertension in CKD patients. In contrast to patients with essential hypertension, plasma volume is elevated in CKD and correlates with BP. Also, extracellular fluid expansion is consistently found in hypertensive end-stage kidney disease (ESKD) patients. However, the correlation between interdialytic weight gain and BP is weak, suggesting additional volume-independent mechanisms in BP control [38–43]. Furthermore, the high prevalence of arterial hypertension in early CKD, when plasma and extracellular fluid volumes tend to be normal, supports a role of fluid independent mechanisms [44]. This is particularly seen in children with renal hypo/dysplasia, who tend to lose considerable amounts of sodium and water and yet are commonly hypertensive. Additional evidence for volume-independent mechanisms of hypertension in CKD comes from patients undergoing bilateral nephrectomy. In dialyzed children nephrectomy lowers mean BP despite causing anuria [45]. The removal of the native kidneys markedly reduces BP and total peripheral vascular resistance, suggesting an excessive vasopressor function of failing kidneys. Interestingly, previously hypertensive, but not normotensive patients respond to salt and water loading by an increase of BP. Hence, the vascular tone must be affected by kidney-related as well as kidney-unrelated mechanisms.

Activation of the RAAS plays a pivotal role in renal hypertension. Although plasma renin activity is typically significantly elevated in patients with isolated kidney artery stenosis, many patients with CKD have 'inappropriately normal' renin levels considering their degree of hypertension and fluid overload [46, 47]. Enhanced renin secretion by poorly perfused areas such as cysts, scars or due to microangiopathic damage or tubulointerstitial inflammation [48, 49] leads to angiotensin II mediated vaso-constriction and aldosterone-mediated salt retention, increasing both total peripheral resistance and blood volume. In addition, the local angiotensin tone in the diseased kidney is affected by multiple mechanisms, independently of plasma renin activity.

Additionally, *sympathetic overactivity* plays an important role in the pathogenesis of hypertension in CKD. Sympathetic nerve activity is increased in CKD and in dialyzed patients [50, 51], and persists even after kidney transplantation as long as the native kidneys are in place. After bilateral nephrectomy, sympathetic nerve activity and BP normalizes [50]. ACE inhibitor treatment, but not calcium channel blockers, normalizes sympathetic activity, suggesting an effect of renal angiotensin tone on afferent neural signaling [51]. Overactivation of the sympathetic drive is also observed in renovascular and polycystic kidney disease-related hypertension [52].

In addition, renalase expression and blood levels are directly correlated with glomerular filtration rate and are markedly reduced in patients with ESKD. Renalase deficiency may thus contribute to the sympathetic overactivation, hypertension and cardiac disease associated with CKD.

The *vascular endothelium* exerts important endocrine and paracrine functions, including active control of the vascular tone. In CKD, endothelium-dependent vasodilation is impaired [53, 54] and NO production is decreased [55, 56] as a result of impaired biosynthesis and bioavailability of L-arginine, reduced NO synthase (NOS) expression and increased circulating endogenous NOS inhibitors [56]. ADMA, a potent NOS inhibitor, accumulates in CKD due to impaired renal excretion and enzymatic degradation. ADMA independently predicts overall mortality and cardiovascular events in patients with ESKD as well as progression of CKD [57, 58]; however, these findings do not appear to be related to clinical differences in BP [59].

ET-1 is the most potent vasoconstrictor known to date. In ESKD patients, ET-1 plasma levels are increased and correlate with BP level [60]; hence, circulating and possibly renal ET-1 may contribute to hypertension in CKD. With decreasing kidney function, activity of the sympathetic nervous system and oxidative stress are increasingly relevant for the risk of hypertension.

Pressure autoregulation is thought to be impaired in CKD [35], resulting in unrestricted transmission of systemic BP to the glomeruli and subsequent glomerular damage and reduction of renal mass. According to the *Brenner hypothesis*, any critical reduction of functional renal mass leads to *hyperfiltration and intraglomerular hypertension* in the remaining nephrons [61]. The increased filtration pressure causes or aggravates preexisting proteinuria. The exposure of tubular and mesangial structures to macromolecular proteins elicits a marked and persistent tissue response. In addition, proteinuria and enhanced angiotensin II formation stimulate the synthesis and release of several pro-inflammatory cytokines and chemokines, resulting in a local inflammatory and fibrotic tissue response and atrophy of the nephron.

A large body of evidence from epidemiological studies and clinical trials indicates that hypertension is an important driver of *CKD progression*. Numerous interventional trials have demonstrated that lowering BP preserves kidney function in hypertensive patients at risk for progressive kidney disease [62–74]. In addition to hypertension, proteinuria is a major risk factor contributing to CKD progression. Although hypertension aggravates proteinuria and the two risk factors are strongly interrelated, they independently influence kidney survival. Two prospective pediatric trials have demonstrated that hypertension and proteinuria are major independent risk factors for progressive kidney failure in children with CKD [63, 75, 76]. Detailed information on role of hypertension in kidney disease progression is provided in Chap. 55.

Various modifying risk factors, such as low birth weight, high fructose diets or obesity may increase the risk for hypertension [77] in CKD patients.

One potential factor influencing the risk of hypertension is hyperuricemia [78], which is often related to obesity or metabolic syndrome, but also to reduced kidney function. Uric acid levels correlate with endothelial dysfunction and higher BP [79]. Hyperuricemia is involved in the generation of reactive oxygen species (ROS), low NO levels, activation of the RAAS, and endothelial dysfunction. The resulting pro-vasoconstrictive conditions cause ischemia and chemokine release, local inflammation and intrarenal generation of vasoconstrictors that further promote ischemia and block pressure-natriuresis. Sodium retention leads to an increase in serum osmolality, activation of the sympathetic nervous system, constriction of vascular smooth muscle cells, and an increase in systemic vascular resistance. Increasing BP ameliorates tubular ischemia by shifting the pressure-natriuresis curve towards higher pressure and the salt-resistant state [77].

Secondary *hyperparathyroidism*, a complication of CKD, may be another contributor to the high prevalence of hypertension. A retrospective study in adults with CKD demonstrated higher systolic and diastolic BP in patients with elevated parathyroid hormone levels [80]. Since BP correlated highly with serum calcium levels, a mechanistic role of increased cytosolic calcium in patients with severe hyperparathyroidism has been postulated.

BP may also be increased due to *adverse effects of drugs* used in the treatment of CKD. For example, erythropoiesis stimulating agents (ESAs) might increase BP by increasing hematocrit. Hypertension may be secondary to the direct vasoconstrictive actions of steroids, calcineurin inhibitors and other immunosuppressive or anti-inflammatory drugs prescribed in acute or chronic immune-mediated kidney disease or after kidney transplantation.

Factors involved in the pathogenesis of hypertension in CKD are summarized in Fig. 50.1.

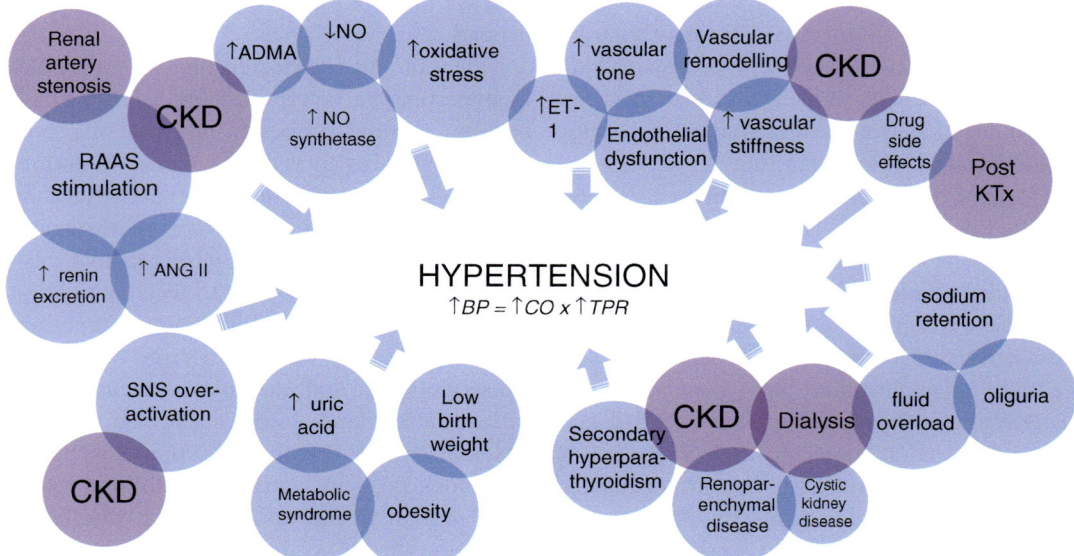

Fig. 50.1 Pathophysiology of hypertension in chronic kidney disease. *RAAS* renin-angiotensin-aldosterone system, *ANG II* angiotensin II, *SNS* sympathetic nervous sys-tem, *CKD* chronic kidney disease, *NO* nitric oxide, *ET-1* endothelin-1, *KTx* kidney transplant, *CO* cardiac output, *TPR* total peripheral resistance, *BP* blood pressure

Hypertension in Specific Renal Conditions

Renoparenchymal hypertension is common in various forms of *acute and chronic glomerulonephritis*. The most common underlying histopathological entities associated with hypertension, even in the absence of kidney failure, are poststreptococcal, focal-segmental, membranoproliferative and crescentic glomerulonephritis. Persistent hypertension is also common in patients with glomerulonephritis secondary to systemic vasculitis, such as systemic lupus erythematosus, and in patients with hemolytic uremic syndrome (HUS).

Hypertension in Acute Kidney Injury

In acute kidney diseases, changes in BP usually mirror changes in disease activity.

In *acute glomerular disease*, e.g., poststreptococcal glomerulonephritis or nephrotic syndrome, patients are often volume expanded due to sodium retention by acute renal impairment

[81]. BP increases due to fluid overload and even in subjects with subclinical volume overload the incidence of hypertension may already be increased. While in these conditions the release of atrial natriuretic peptide is enhanced by sodium retention, the RAAS is often suppressed. In contrast, in patients with acute vasculitis of the kidneys ischemia-induced activation of the RAAS is the main underlying mechanism.

In hypertensive patients with *HUS*, a difference in the pathophysiological mechanisms involved in the origin of hypertension between patients with shiga-toxin associated HUS (STEC-HUS) and patients with atypical, complement-disorder associated HUS (aHUS) is hypothesized. In patients with STEC-HUS, fluid overload and salt retention are supposed to play a major role, but in patients with aHUS complement activation and endothelial dysfunction are probably key players [82, 83]. Of note, while malignant hypertension may indicate aHUS and thrombotic microangiopathy (TMA), in patients with malignant hypertension extremely high BP per se can induce a thrombotic microangiopathy.

Hypertension in Chronic Kidney Disease

Chronic renoparenchymal hypertension is not limited to *glomerular disease*, but is also observed in patients with *congenital anomalies of the kidneys and urinary tract (CAKUT)* or with tubulointerstitial disorders leading to kidney scarring. Recurrent pyelonephritis, reflux nephropathy, obstructive uropathies or polycystic kidney disease, can all lead to activation of the local RAAS, tubulointerstitial fibrosis and tubular atrophy.

The risk of hypertension is more closely associated with the type of underlying kidney disease than with the degree of kidney dysfunction. At any given level of CKD (stage 1–5), children with acquired glomerulopathies or polycystic kidney disease tend to have higher BP than those with renal hypoplasia and/or uropathies. In a survey of the ESCAPE trial group in pediatric CKD patients with CKD 2 to 4, the prevalence of hypertension was 88% in patients with acquired glomerulopathies, 38% in children with hypo-/dysplastic kidney disorders and 57% in other congenital or hereditary kidney diseases [8, 9]. Renoparenchymal disorders are responsible for approximately 75% of cases of secondary hypertension in childhood [84].

A condition that can be associated with malignant hypertension in newborns or in early infancy is autosomal recessive polycystic kidney disease (ARPKD). Children with severe ARPKD may present with episodes of hypertensive crisis associated with high mortality risk, including sudden heart failure, cerebral ischemic or hemorrhagic stroke.

Autosomal dominant polycystic kidney disease (ADPKD), while becoming clinically symptomatic only in adults, has a high prevalence of hypertension in childhood when kidney function is still normal [85].

As described above, the pathophysiological mechanisms in renal parenchymal hypertension encompass an increased activity of the RAAS, sodium and water retention, enhanced activity of the sympathetic nervous system, oxidative stress and endothelial dysfunction.

Renovascular hypertension accounts for about 10% of pediatric patients presenting with secondary hypertension. Renovascular hypertension results from vascular lesions that impair blood flow to one or both kidneys or to kidney segments [86, 87]. Post-stenotic decreased renal perfusion results in stimulation of the RAAS. The most common causes of renovascular hypertension in childhood are idiopathic stenosis of the kidney artery, fibromuscular dysplasia, mid-aortic syndrome, and genetic or syndromic disorders such as neurofibromatosis type 1 (NF1, von Recklinghausen), which can affect not only the renal, but also intrarenal arteries, Williams-Beuren syndrome, and Alagille syndrome.

Kidney artery stenosis should be ruled out in children with very high BP (stage 2 hypertension), hypertensive complications (e.g., hypertensive crisis with cerebral symptoms, heart failure, facial neve palsy), uncontrolled hypertension on more than two antihypertensive drugs, worsening of kidney function after initiation of ACE inhibitor (ACEi) or angiotensin receptor blocker (ARB) therapy, or increased plasma renin activity with hypokalemia.

The preferred therapeutic intervention in childhood renovascular hypertension is revascularization of the stenosis. Detailed information on the management of kidney artery stenosis can be found in Chap. 49.

Hypertension in Pediatric Dialysis Patients

The prevalence of *hypertension in pediatric peritoneal or hemodialysis patients* (CKD stage 5D) is very high. At time of dialysis initiation, up to 80% of patients are hypertensive; out of these 60% are untreated or have uncontrolled hypertension despite antihypertensive drug therapy. After 1 year on dialysis more than 50% of patients remain hypertensive [88–90]. Hypertension may be maintained by the underlying kidney disease, especially in patients with glomerulopathies or PKD, but also by inappropriately high fluid and sodium intake.

In a survey of more than 1300 pediatric dialysis patients in the European ERA/EDTA registry, the overall prevalence of hypertension was similar in hemodialysis (HD; 69.7%) and peritoneal dialysis (PD; 68.2%) patients. However, the percentage of uncontrolled hypertension was higher in HD compared to PD patients (45% vs. 35%) [91]. These epidemiologic data were derived from casual BP measurements, with a single BP recording per patient reported to the registries. For the interpretation of these data, consideration of the time of BP measurement is important because pre-dialysis measurements are usually higher compared with post-dialysis measurements, resulting in a higher probability to be classified as hypertensive when only pre-dialysis measurements are considered.

The dominant factor contributing to hypertension in dialysis patients is volume overload; other contributing factors include, as in non-dialysis CKD patients, activation of the RAAS and the sympathetic nervous system, endothelial dysfunction, increased arterial stiffness, hyperparathyroidism and exposure to BP elevating drugs.

Contrary to the physiologically expected suppression of the RAAS in a state of salt or fluid overload, plasma renin activity was found to be significantly higher in a study comparing hypertensive to normotensive dialysis patients. These findings suggest that in ESKD patients with adequately controlled sodium balance, the RAAS is an important factor involved in the pathogenesis of hypertension [92]. Also, the significant decline in BP observed after bilateral nephrectomy [93] points to volume-independent mechanisms of hypertension in dialysis patients. A further factor contributing to arterial hypertension in ESKD might be the markedly decreased plasma levels of *renalase*. Renalase deficiency and the resulting increase of circulating catecholamine levels may also contribute to the high prevalence of hypertension and cardiovascular disease in ESKD [24, 94].

Hypertension in Pediatric Renal Transplant Recipients

In children and adolescents after kidney transplantation, hypertension is almost as common as

in dialysis patients and constitutes a serious comorbidity [91, 95, 96], not only with respect to cardiovascular morbidity and mortality, but also for kidney transplant survival [97]. Posttransplant hypertension might be caused by the native kidneys, vascular stenosis of the transplant kidney artery, acute or chronic graft dysfunction, and recurrent or de-novo glomerulonephritis in the transplant kidney. In addition, medication side effects of immunosuppressive drugs (steroids, calcineurin inhibitors), including excessive weight gain with steroid treatment, have an important role in posttransplant hypertension.

Hypertension Associated with Disorders of Renal Tubular Sodium Handling

In rare cases, hypertension may be caused by autosomal dominant or recessive single gene mutations (***monogenic hypertension***) [98–100]. Characteristically, all hereditary forms of hypertension lead to suppression of the RAAS with low levels of renin concentration or renin activity ('***low renin hypertension***') due to expansion of plasma volume. In a broader sense, the pathophysiology of these disorders comprises alterations of renal tubular electrolyte handling due to mutations in genes regulating glucocorticoid synthesis or action effecting the mineralocorticoid receptor, or in genes regulating the sodium excretion in the distal tubule.

Apparent mineralocorticoid excess (AME) is an autosomal recessive disorder in which inactivating mutations in the *HSD11B2* gene, encoding the kidney isozyme of 11-β-hydroxysteroid dehydrogenase 2, lead to increased concentrations of cortisol in the kidneys and to activation of the mineralocorticoid receptor due to cross-reaction of cortisol with the non-selective mineralocorticoid receptor. This induces aldosterone-like effects in the tubule, typically causing hypokalemia, metabolic alkalosis, hypernatremia and hypertension.

Glucocorticoid remediable aldosteronism (GRA; familial hyperaldosteronism type 1) is an autosomal dominant disorder due to alterations in the adjacent 11β-hydroxylase and aldosterone synthase genes on chromosome 8q24.3. Unequal cross-over between these genes results in ACTH-stimulated ectopic secretion of aldosterone from the adrenal zona fasciculata. Increased aldosterone secretion stimulates the mineralocorticoid receptor, resulting in suppressed renin levels and hypertension due to upregulation of potassium excretion and sodium reabsorption in the renal tubule.

Hypertension in congenital adrenal hyperplasia (CAH) is caused by autosomal recessive inherited defects in 11β-hydroxylase (Type IV) or 17α-hydroxylase (Type V), leading to overproduction of 21-hydroxylated steroids and overactivation of the mineralocorticoid receptor. The uncontrolled mineralocorticoid activity results in hypertension and hypokalemia. Additionally, in CAH type IV the enzyme block increases the production of sex steroids, with androgenic actions causing virilization in girls and precocious puberty in boys. In CAH type V, the synthesis of sex hormones is compromised, resulting in primary amenorrhea and delayed sexual maturation in girls and in ambiguous genitalia in boys.

Liddle's syndrome is caused by a dominant gain-of-function mutation in the amiloride-sensitive epithelial sodium channel (ENaC) located in the collecting duct. The overactive ENaC causes increased sodium reabsorption and intravascular volume expansion, which leads to hypertension. Moreover, these patients present with hypokalemia, metabolic alkalosis, and occasionally hypercalciuria.

Gordon's syndrome is characterized by familial hyperkalemia with normal kidney function, reduced renal sodium excretion, hypercalciuria and hyperchloremic metabolic acidosis due to dominant mutations in the WNK serine-threonine kinases WNK1 and WNK4 or in *KLHL3* or *CUL3*, associated with loss of inhibitory regulation of the NCC in the thiazide-sensitive distal convoluted tubule.

For accurate assessment of the different forms of low renin hypertension, analysis of serum renin,

aldosterone, serum electrolytes and blood gas analysis, urinary potassium excretion and the urinary steroid profile is required. In addition, further hormonal studies and genetic testing for the disease-causing mutations may be required [98–100].

The etiology of hypertension in pediatric CKD is summarized in Table 50.1. For the diagnostic approach to renal hypertension see Table 50.2. Additional information on the diag-

Table 50.1 Etiology of pediatric renal hypertension

Etiology	Underlying kidney disease/condition
Renoparenchymal	• Acute glomerulonephritis (e.g. post streptococcal glomerulonephritis, Henoch-Schönlein nephritis) • Chronic glomerulonephritis (e.g., FSGS, IgA nephropathy) • Hemolytic uremic syndrome • Interstitial nephritis • Congenital hypo- or dysplasia of the kidneys • Congenital anomalies of the kidneys and urinary tract • Cystic kidney disease (ARPKD, ADPKD) • Recurrent pyelonephritis with scarring • Acute pyelonephritis • Urological interventions • Kidney tumors • Kidney trauma • Chronic kidney failure • Status post kidney transplantation
Renovascular	• Kidney artery stenosis (e.g., fibromuscular dysplasia with neurofibromatosis, Williams-Beuren syndrome) • Vasculitis (e.g., periarteritis nodosa, Takayasu arteritis) • Compression of kidney artery by tumor, bleeding, abscess
Other renal conditions	• Fluid overload in dialysis patients (misjudgment of fluid status) • Side effects of drug treatment in immunosuppressed patients (e.g., steroids, cyclosporine, tacrolimus) • Forms of monogenic ('low-renin') hypertension

FSGS focal-segmental glomerulosclerosis, *ADPKD* autosomal dominant polycystic kidney disease, *ARPKD* autosomal recessive polycystic kidney disease

Table 50.2 Baseline diagnostic measures in suspected renal hypertension

Medical history	
Family history	Hypertension, cardiovascular disease, hereditary kidney disease
Perinatal history	Birth weight, gestational age, oligohydramnios
Current findings	Urinary tract infections, renal or urinary diseases/malformation
Potential renal findings	Dysuria, polydipsia, polyuria, nycturia, hematuria, edema, weight loss, failure to thrive
Indicators for target organ damage	Headache, nose bleeding, vertigo, dizziness, blurred vision, facial palsy, seizures, stroke, dyspnea
Medication	Antihypertensives, steroids, CNI (ciclosporine A, tacrolimus), …
Physical examination	
General	Height, weight, body mass index
Hypertension-associated syndromes	Neurofibromatosis, Williams-Beuren syndrome, …
Cardiovascular exams	Measurements of pulse rate and blood pressure at all 4 extremities Murmur, flow noise at heart, abdomen, flanks, back, neck, head, signs of heart insufficiency
Abdomen	Palpable mass → Wilms tumor, autosomal-dominant or recessive polycystic kidney disease, obstructive uropathy, hepatosplenomegaly → autosomal-recessive polycystic kidney disease
Virilization, ambiguous genitalia	Forms of monogenic hypertension
Basic diagnostics	*Finding → indicating …*
Creatinine, urea (serum)	Creatinine, urea increased → kidney insufficiency
Electrolytes (serum)	Hypokalemia → kidney artery stenosis Hyperkaliemia → kidney insufficiency
Blood gas analysis	Metabolic acidosis → kidney insufficiency
Urinalysis: erythrocytes, leukocytes, glucose, protein, albumin[a]	Hematuria, proteinuria → glomerulonephritis Leukocyturia → pyelonephritis Glucosuria → tubulopathy, diabetes mellitus
Ultrasound of kidneys and urinary tract	Enlarged hyperechogenic kidneys → glomerulonephritis, pyelonephritis Kidney cysts → polycystic kidney disease, cystic dysplastic kidney disease, multicystic dysplastic kidney disease Small, hyperechogenic kidneys → kidney hypoplasia, kidney dysplasia Side differences → unilateral kidney hypo/dysplasia, vesicoureteral reflux with scarring, indicating kidney artery stenosis Tumor
Ophthalmological	Hypertensive retinopathy → end organ damage
Echocardiography	Left ventricular hypertrophy → end organ damage
Further diagnostics	*Finding → indicating…*
Renin, aldosterone levels Renin activity Renin/aldosterone ratio	Hyperreninism → kidney artery stenosis, renoparenchymal hypertension Low-renin hypertension → monogenic hypertension
Urinary steroid profile	→ Forms of monogenic hypertension
Genetic testing	→ Forms of monogenic hypertension
Doppler ultrasound	Flow in kidney arteries, side-different kidney size and resistance indices → kidney artery stenosis
CT or MRI angiography	→ Kidney artery stenosis
Angiography	→ Kidney artery stenosis
Renal scintigraphy	Kidney scars, kidney function
MRI abdomen	Tumor localization and size

[a] Quantitative excretion of protein and albumin in 24 h urine collection or protein/creatinine and albumin/creatinine ratio in morning spot urine samples

nosis of hypertension and BP monitoring in CKD patients is provided in Chap. 49.

Antihypertensive Treatment Strategies in Acute and Chronic Kidney Disease

The main goal of BP control in acute kidney injury is to attain a BP level in the normal range and to avoid acute hypertensive damage to the kidneys and the cardiovascular system.

In CKD-associated hypertension, the growing understanding of the epidemiology, pathophysiology and target organ damage has promoted the search for effective long-term therapeutic strategies (for further information see also Chaps. 49 and 51). These relate to both BP targets and preferred antihypertensive drug choices.

Blood Pressure Target

The therapeutic goal in all CKD children with hypertension is long-term and consistent BP control irrespective of the underlying condition. Hypertension-related cardiovascular end-organ damage such as left ventricular hypertrophy, hypertensive retinopathy, and progressive kidney function deterioration has to be avoided and the risk of long-term cardiovascular sequelae and kidney failure should be minimized. While in children with primary hypertension a BP goal below the 95th BP percentile or below the adult thresholds, whichever is lower, is recommended and this target might be also applicable for hypertension in acute kidney injury, there is ample evidence for beneficial effects of lower BP targets in CKD patients.

In adult CKD patients with diabetic or non-diabetic kidney diseases, meta-analyses of antihypertensive trials showed an almost linear relationship between achieved BP and the annual GFR loss [101]: The better the BP control, the better was kidney survival. As a result, the Seventh Report of the Joint National Committee on Prevention, Detection, Evaluation, and Treatment of High Blood Pressure (JNC7) pub-

lished in 2003 recommended a BP goal of <130/80 mmHg in patients with CKD or diabetes, as compared to <140/90 mmHg in primary hypertension [102]. However, at that point in time the renoprotective superiority of very *strict BP control* had not yet been unequivocally demonstrated in adult nephropathies [103–108]. Thus, the usefulness of lower BP targets in adults with CKD had been questioned. Meanwhile, the findings of the SPRINT trial, published in 2015 [109], gave new impetus to the discussion on BP targets. In this prospective randomized controlled trial including more than 9000 participants aged 50 and older with increased cardiovascular risk (26% in CKD stage 3–4), patients with intensified BP control (systolic BP <120 mmHg) showed 25% lower fatal and nonfatal cardiovascular event rates, 27% lower all-cause mortality, and a 43% reduction of relative risk to die from any cardiovascular cause with the intensive intervention compared to standard treatment (systolic BP <140 mmHg). However, there was no difference in primary cardiovascular outcomes in CKD patients [109] and some methodological aspects of the study are critically discussed [110].

In children with CKD, the Efficacy of Strict Blood Pressure Control and ACE Inhibition on Renal Failure Progression in Pediatric Patients (ESCAPE) Trial has provided evidence for a nephroprotective effect of intensified BP control [63]. CKD children randomized to a target 24-h mean arterial pressure below the 50th percentile for age were 35% less likely to lose 50% GFR or progress to ESKD within 5 years than children with a more conventional BP target between the 50th and 95th BP percentile. The risk to attain the study endpoint was increased by 15% for each mm Hg above the 50th percentile, while a BP below the 50th percentile did not significantly affect renal risk [63]. The protective effect of low normal BP on kidney function seen in the ESCAPE trial was independent of RAAS inhibition since all subjects received the same dose of the ACE inhibitor ramipril. While the benefit was greatest in children with glomerular disorders, it was also significant in children with renal hypoplasia or dysplasia. Survival analysis stratified by the achieved 24-h BP suggested that any BP exceeding the 50th percentile was associated with a compromised kidney outcome [63]. Also in this study, proteinuria was found to be an important modifier of the renoprotective efficacy of intensified BP control. Patients with significant proteinuria had a greater benefit from intensified BP control than non-proteinuric patients.

Based on the findings of the ESCAPE trial [63], the European Society of Hypertension (ESH) pediatric guideline recommends that antihypertensive treatment should be initiated if BP exceeds the 90th percentile and aim for a mean 24-h ambulatory BP target below the 75th percentile in non-proteinuric and below the 50th percentile in proteinuric children and adolescents with CKD [111]. In adolescents aged 16 years and older a BP below 130/80 mmHg should be aimed for in non-proteinuric and below 125/75 mmHg in proteinuric CKD [111]. For young adults with kidney disease, the guideline of the European Societies for Cardiology and Hypertension (ESC/ESH) recommends a BP target of 130–139/70–79 mmHg [21].

The American Academy of Pediatrics Practice Guideline for Management of Hypertension in Children and Adolescents [112] recommends that all children or adolescents with CKD be treated to lower 24-h mean arterial pressure to <50th percentile by ABPM, irrespective of the degree of proteinuria, whereas children with primary hypertension be treated by non-pharmacological or pharmacological intervention to a reduction in systolic and diastolic BP to below the 90th percentile (or below 130/80 mmHg in adolescents ≥13 years old).

Choice of Antihypertensive Drugs

Treatment of Hypertension in Children with Acute Kidney Injury

In view of the different etiologies of acute kidney injury, treatment of hypertension should be individualized. In patients with acute glomerulopathies and edema, such as those presenting with hypertension due to poststreptococcal glomerulonephritis or nephrotic syndrome, where fluid overload and salt retention play a major role, the initial therapy is diuretics. Loop diuretics should be prescribed in patients with severely reduced GFR since thiazides are ineffective when GFR falls below 30. RAAS antagonists can be effective as second line treatment for persistently elevated BP [113], although acute glomerulonephritis typically is a state of low-renin hypertension.

In patients with acute vasculitis, ACE inhibitors are recommended as first line antihypertensive therapy since activation of the RAAS due to renal ischemia is the main pathophysiological mechanism. Since STEC-HUS leads to RAAS activation, ACE inhibitors and angiotensin receptor blockers are the treatment of choice in this condition. In children with hypertension due to atypical HUS mediated by complement activation, treatment of the underlying complement disorder is essential to normalize BP in addition to acute antihypertensive therapy using either RAAS antagonists or calcium channel blockers [83].

Treatment of Hypertension in Children with CKD

The major recommended antihypertensive drug classes (ACEi, ARB, calcium channel blockers (CCB), β-blockers) exert comparable BP lowering effects in CKD patients. A list of antihypertensive drugs used in children with CKD is given in Table 50.3.

In view of the crucial role of the RAAS in kidney failure progression, *RAAS antagonists* (ACEis and ARBs) might confer specific nephroprotective properties beyond their antihypertensive action. RAAS antagonists reduce the intraglomerular pressure, thereby lowering proteinuria and suppressing local inflammatory processes, with subsequent reduction of glomerular hypertrophy and sclerosis, as well as tubulointerstitial inflammation and fibrosis. Most randomized clinical trials have demonstrated superior renoprotective efficacy of RAAS antagonists (ACEis and ARBs) in adults with diabetic and non-diabetic CKD. Several meta-analyses have confirmed the nephroprotective benefit of RAAS antagonists, although the effect size is quite variable [114, 115]. One analysis suggested that the nephroprotection conferred by ACEi might be partially independent of their antihypertensive

Table 50.3 Pharmacological treatment of renal hypertension in children

Class	Drug	Mode of action	Side effects
ACE inhibitors	e. g., Captopril Enalapril Ramipril Fosinopril Benazepril Lisinopril	Inhibition of the conversion of angiotensin I to angiotensin II → vasodilatation, reduction of sympathetic tone, decreased aldosterone dependent salt and water retention, nephroprotection	Cough, hyperkalemia, increase of serum creatinine, hypotension, dizziness, fatigue, headache, laryngioedema, neutropenia *Caveat*: contraindicated in bilateral severe kidney artery stenosis *Caveat*: pre-renal acute kidney failure in dehydration episodes *Caveat*: pregnancy (teratogenic)
Angiotensin-receptor blockers	e. g., Candesartan Valsartan Losartan Irbesartan	Blockade of angiotensin-II-type-1-receptors Nephroprotection (see also ACE inhibitors)	Side effects similar to ACE inhibitors, no cough Rhabdomyolysis, thrombocytopenia
Calcium channel blockers	e. g., Nifedipine Nitrendipine Amlodipine	Reduced influx of calcium into the cells → relaxation of the arterial vascular muscle cells, decrease of peripheral vascular resistance	Headache, flush, tachycardia/palpitations, peripheral edema, fatigue, hypotension, gingival hyperplasia
Diuretics	e. g., Furosemide, Torsemide Hydrochlorothiazide	Increase of renal sodium excretion, decrease of peripheral resistance	Hypokalemia, hyponatremia, alkalosis, extracellular volume depletion, hyperuricemia, diuretics enhance ACE inhibitor effect *Cave* acute kidney failure in dehydration episodes
β-Blockers	e. g., Atenolol Metoprolol Propranolol Carvedilol	Reduction of cardiac output, renin-aldosterone release and of sympathetic activity	Tiredness, dizziness, depression, reduced physical capacity, bradycardia, hypotension, nausea, bronchospasm, *Cave* β-blocker in diabetes mellitus or pulmonary obstruction/asthma
Alpha-blocker	e. g., Doxazosin Phenoxybenzamine	Relaxation of vascular smooth muscle cells, direct vasodilatory effect	Edema, dizziness, fatigue, headache
Centrally acting adrenergic drugs (alpha2-agonists)	e. g., Clonidine	Reduction of sympathetic outflow, decrease in peripheral vascular resistance, decrease of heart rate	Dizziness, headache, fatigue, xerostomia
Vasodilators	e.g. Minoxidil Hydralazine	Activation of gated potassium channels, vasodilatation, lowering of total peripheral resistance	Edema, fluid retention, salt retention, headache, hypertrichosis, leukopenia, nausea, palpitations/tachycardia

Examples of antihypertensives with (some) clinical experience in pediatric hypertension
ACE angiotensin-converting enzyme

and antiproteinuric actions [114]. Thus, RAAS antagonists are considered the first-line pharmacological therapy in hypertensive CKD patients.

For pediatric CKD, the Chronic Kidney Disease in Children (CKiD) Study found an increased prevalence of uncontrolled hypertension in children not receiving ACEi or ARBs, supporting the use of RAAS antagonists as preferred antihypertensive agents in pediatric CKD [5]. Both ACEi and ARBs have been shown to reduce systolic and diastolic BP efficiently [63] in a dose-dependent manner [116]. The drugs were very well tolerated and side effects requiring ACEi or ARB withdrawal due to acute increases of serum creatinine, hyperkalemia or hypotensive episodes were rare [63, 116].

As expected, in patients with underlying CKD the prevalence of reported adverse events is higher, and increases in serum potassium, creatinine and blood urea nitrogen are more commonly reported compared to non-CKD patients. Approximately 25–30% of CKD patients experience an eGFR decline of more than 25% [117]. However, it has been hypothesized that the observed increase in serum creatinine after start of RAAS blockade is due to hemodynamic changes in the glomerulus, which does not reflect kidney injury and should thus be reversible at withdrawal of RAAS blockade [118].

In some patients, the RAAS is incompletely suppressed by ACEi alone, and the possibility of partial secondary resistance due to compensatory upregulation of ACE-independent angiotensin II production ('aldosterone escape') has been suggested [119–121]. Interestingly, in those patients with breakthrough proteinuria followed in the ESCAPE trial [63], BP was still well controlled. Thus, the doses required to achieve the maximal antiproteinuric effect of ARBs may be much higher than the maximally active antihypertensive doses. Significant additional proteinuria lowering was achieved without increased side effects in adults with 64 mg and even 128 mg of candesartan, which has only a minor additional BP lowering effect beyond daily doses of 16–32 mg [122]. Similarly, *dual RAAS blockade* by combined use of an ACEi and an ARB does not exert significant additional antihypertensive effects compared to the maximum recommended dose in monotherapy, but still might improve proteinuria. However, the risk-benefit balance of combining ACEis and ARBs in younger subjects is still debated [123–125].

Other drug classes inhibiting the RAAS exert antihypertensive effects. Aliskiren is a direct *renin antagonist*, blocking the conversion from angiotensinogen to angiotensin I. Its BP lowering effect is comparable to that of ARBs and a combination of aliskiren and valsartan at maximum recommended doses provided significantly greater BP reduction than the respective mono-

therapies [126]. However, combination therapy of aliskiren with ACEi or ARBs significantly increased the risk of cardiovascular events in adults with diabetes or CKD and is therefore not recommended [127, 128].

Mineralocorticoid receptor antagonists (MRA) also lower BP; however, their use is limited by the risk of side effects, including hyperkalemia, gynecomastia, impotence, and amenorrhea. These side effects are more common for the steroidal MRAs spironolactone and eplerenone. Due to the high risk of hyperkalemia, the combination of ACEIs and steroidal MRAs in CKD patients has not been recommended [129]. The novel nonsteroidal MRAs finerenone and esaxerenone have a higher potency and selectivity for the mineralocorticoid receptor and thus seem to have fewer side effects.

Because the antihypertensive effect of MRAs is not superior to ACEis or ARBs, they are not used as first line agents in renal hypertension. However, recent studies support a future role, especially of the nonsteroidal MRAs, in the prevention of cardiovascular disease and CKD progression by reducing oxidative stress, inflammation, fibrosis, endothelial dysfunction and proteinuria [130, 131]. MRAs play an important role in the treatment of some forms of monogenic hypertension (see Table 50.4).

In a substantial number of pediatric CKD patients with hypertension, multidrug antihypertensive therapy is required [3, 63]. The choice of additional antihypertensive drugs in children with CKD is largely arbitrary.

Dihydropyridine *calcium channel blockers* have no antiproteinuric effect and may actually promote proteinuria and more rapid CKD progression [132]. However, their combination with ARBs or ACEis provides powerful BP lowering and even conferred a patient survival advantage as compared to the combination of ARBs or ACEis with thiazide diuretics [133, 134]. Nondihydropyridine calcium channel blockers (diltiazem, verapamil) are antiproteinuric and therefore potentially renoprotective, but have a weaker effect on BP [132].

The use of *β-receptor blockers* appears rational in view of the sympathetic overactivation in

Table 50.4 Dosing of antihypertensive medication in children with CKD (*modified from* [156], *Springer International Publishing*)

Class	Drug	Usual pediatric dosing range[a]	Dosing modifications in CKD stage 3–5 D[a]
Angiotensin receptor blockers	Candesartan	*1–6 years*: 0.2 mg/kg/day up to 0.4 mg/kg/day *6–17 years*: *<50 kg*: 4–16 mg QD *>50 kg*: 8–32 mg QD	No known recommended adjustment but clearance reduced if GFR <30 mL/min; not removed by dialysis; give 50% of usual dose; consider dosing after HD session
	Losartan	0.75 mg/kg/day to 1.4 mg/kg/day; maximum 100 mg daily	Not recommended if GFR <30 mL/min; not removed by dialysis
	Olmesartan	*20–35 kg*: 10–20 mg QD *≥35 kg*: 20–40 mg QD	Clearance reduced if GFR <20 mL/min; do not exceed 20 mg daily in such patients; not removed by dialysis
	Valsartan	*<6 years:* 5–10 mg/day up to 80 mg daily *6–17 years*: 1.3 mg/kg/day up to 2.7 mg/kg/day; maximum 160 mg daily	Clearance reduced if GFR <30 mL/min; not removed by dialysis
Angiotensin converting enzyme inhibitors	Benazepril	0.2 mg/kg/day up to 0.6 mg/kg/day; maximum 40 mg daily	No pediatric data. 20–50% removed by dialysis; give 25–50% of usual dose; consider dosing after HD session
	Captopril	0.3–0.5 mg/kg/dose TID up to 0.6 mg/kg/day; maximum 450 mg daily	No pediatric data. 50% removed by dialysis. Give 25% of usual dose in HD patients; consider dosing after HD session. Give 50% QD of usual daily dose in PD
	Enalapril	0.08 mg/kg/day up to 0.6 mg/kg/day; maximum 40 mg daily	Not studied in children with GFR <30 mL/min. 50% removed by dialysis. Give 50% of usual dose; consider dosing after HD session
	Fosinopril	0.1 mg/kg/day (up to 10 mg/day) up to 0.6 mg/kg/day; maximum 40 mg/day	No known adjustments; not removed by dialysis
	Lisinopril	0.07 mg/kg/day (up to 5 mg/day) up to 0.6 mg/kg/day; maximum 40 mg daily	Not studied in children with GFR <30 mL/min. 50% removed by dialysis. Give 25% of usual dose; consider dosing after HD session
	Quinapril	5–10 mg/day up to 80 mg daily	No pediatric data. For adults with GFR 10–30 mL/min, do not exceed 2.5 mg/day; no data for GFR <10 mL/min
	Ramipril	1.6 mg/m² BSA/day QD up to 6 mg/m²/day; maximum 20 mg daily	No pediatric data. In adults with GFR <40 mL/min, give 25% of usual dose; 20% removal by dialysis. Consider dosing after HD session
α- and β-blocker	Carvedilol	0.1 mg/kg/dose BID (up to 6.25 mg) up to 0.5 mg/kg/dose; maximum 25 mg BID	No adjustment needed; not removed by dialysis
	Labetalol	2–3 mg/kg/day BID up to 10–12 mg/kg/day; maximum 1200 mg daily	No adjustment needed; not removed by dialysis

(continued)

Table 50.4 (continued)

Class	Drug	Usual pediatric dosing range[a]	Dosing modifications in CKD stage 3–5 D[a]
β-Blocker	Atenolol	0.5–1 mg/kg/day up to 100 mg daily	If GFR 15–35 mL/min, do not exceed 50 mg daily (reduction to 50% of usual dose); if GFR <15 mL/min, do not exceed 25 mg daily (reduction to 25% of usual dose). 50% removed by dialysis; consider dosing after HD session
	Metoprolol	Immediate release: 1–2 mg/kg/day BID up to 6 mg/kg/day; maximum 200 mg daily Extended release: 1 mg/kg/day up to 2 mg/kg/day; maximum 200 mg daily	No adjustment needed; not removed by dialysis
	Propranolol	1 mg/kg/day TID-QID up to 8 mg/kg/day; maximum 640 mg daily	No adjustment recommended but can accumulate in kidney impairment; not removed by dialysis
Calcium channel blockers	Amlodipine	0.06 mg/kg/day up to 0.6 mg/kg/day; maximum 10 mg daily	No adjustment needed; not removed by dialysis
	Diltiazem	1.5–2 mg/kg/day up to 6 mg/kg/day; maximum 360 mg daily	No adjustment needed; not removed by dialysis
	Felodipine	2.5–10 mg/day; maximum 10 mg daily	No adjustment needed; not removed by dialysis
	Isradipine	0.05–0.15 mg/kg/dose TID/QID up to 0.8 mg/kg/day; maximum 20 mg daily	No adjustment needed; not removed by dialysis
	Extended-release nifedipine	0.25–0.5 mg/kg/day up to 3 mg/kg/day; maximum 120 mg daily	No adjustment needed; not removed by dialysis
Central α-agonist	Clonidine	5–20 µg/kg/day BID up to 15 µg/kg/day; maximum 0.9 mg daily	No known adjustments; 5% removed on HD
Peripheral α-blockers	Prazosin	0.05–0.1 mg/kg/day TID up to 0.5 mg/kg/day; maximum 20 mg daily	No known adjustments; not removed by dialysis
	Doxazosin	1 mg QD up to 4 mg daily; maximum adult dose is 16 mg daily	No known adjustments; not removed by dialysis
	Terazosin	1 mg QD up to 20 mg daily	No known adjustments; 10% removed on HD
Vasodilators	Hydralazine	0.25 mg/kg/dose TID up to 7.5 mg/kg/day; maximum 200 mg daily	No known adjustments; 25–40% removed by dialysis. Consider dosing after HD session
	Minoxidil	0.1–0.2 mg/kg/day QD-BID up to 1 mg/kg/day; maximum 50 mg daily	No known adjustments
Diuretics	Chlorthalidone	0.3 mg/kg/day up to 2 mg/kg/day; maximum 50 mg daily	Avoid in oligoanuria or with GFR <10 mL/min

Table 50.4 (continued)

Class	Drug	Usual pediatric dosing range[a]	Dosing modifications in CKD stage 3–5 D[a]
	Furosemide	0.5–2 mg/kg/dose QD-QID up to 6 mg/kg/day; maximum 600 mg daily	Avoid in oligoanuria; not removed by dialysis
	Hydroclorothiazide	0.5–1 mg/kg/day; maximum 25 mg daily	Not effective in GFR < 30

BID twice daily, *GFR* glomerular filtration rate, *HD* hemodialysis, *kg* kilogram, *μg* microgram, *mg* milligram, *PD* peritoneal dialysis, *QD* once daily, *QID* four times daily, *TID* three times daily
[a] Recommendations represent the authors' opinions although every effort has been made to confirm by consulting appropriate references. Manufacturers' prescribing information is frequently updated and should be consulted whenever possible

Table 50.5 Advantages of specific antihypertensive combination therapies

Combination	Advantages
ACEi or ARB + diuretic	Enhanced antihypertensive effect of RAAS blockade by diuretic-mediated salt loss
	Decreased risk of RAAS-mediated hyperkalemia by diuretic-mediated potassium excretion
	Reduction of diuretic-mediated increase in plasma renin activity by RAAS blockade
ACEi or ARB + CCB	Attenuated CCB-mediated activation of the sympathetic nervous system by RAAS blockade
	Reduced risk of (dose dependent) CCB-mediated peripheral edema by RAAS blockade
ACEi + ARB[a]	Enhanced RAAS blockade (caveat: increased risk of hyperkalemia, increase in serum creatinine)
	Additional blockade of ACEi-independent pathways in the RAAS → reduced risk of aldosterone rebound phenomenon

ACEi angiotensin converting enzyme inhibitor, *ARB* angiotensin receptor blocker, *CCB* calcium channel blocker, *RAAS* renin-angiotensin-aldosterone system
[a] Combination therapy of ACE + ARB not recommended

CKD. Metoprolol and atenolol were the first antihypertensive drugs used to demonstrate nephroprotective effects by good BP control [135]. Newer β-blockers, such as carvedilol, exert a significantly greater antiproteinuric effect than atenolol at comparable BP reduction [136, 137]. Dosing recommendations for antihypertensive drugs in CKD are given in Table 50.5.

Combination of different drug classes might not only exert additive effects on BP control, but also might counterbalance or increase side effects of antihypertensive agents. Therefore, some antihypertensive drug combinations seem to be more favorable than others (Table 50.6).

In patients with advanced kidney impairment, refractory, multi-drug resistant hypertension usually indicates fluid overload and is an indication to start dialysis therapy.

Because renal hypertension is characterized by the loss of the physiological nocturnal decrease in BP (nocturnal BP dipping) in the majority of patients, the *timing of antihypertensive drug administration* should receive additional attention. For example, bedtime dosing of antihypertensive medication may reconstitute the circadian BP rhythmicity by a more marked effect during the nighttime hours. In a recent study in adult CKD patients randomly assigned to take either all antihypertensive medications in the morning or to take at least one drug in the evening, bedtime dosing improved overall BP control, and reduced significantly the risk for cardiovascular events [138].

In addition to pharmacological treatment, *non-pharmacological interventions* are generally recommended in all children with renal hypertension [21, 111, 139, 140]. These life-style interventions should comprise a reduction of dietary salt intake, high consumption of fruits and vegetables ('DASH' diet), maintenance of a normal body weight, regular physical activity and refraining from smoking. However, it should

Table 50.6 Risk profile and pharmacological treatment[a] of patients with monogenic, 'low renin' hypertension

Form of monogenic hypertension	Age at onset	Cardiovascular symptoms/risks	Recommended therapy	
Apparent mineralocorticoid excess (AME)	Early childhood	Severe hypertension with extensive target organ damage; hypercalciuria, renal failure; low birthweight, failure to thrive	MRA If MRA not effective add dexamethasone K-supplementation Low sodium diet	Spironolactone 1 mg/kg/day in 1–2 doses (max dose 100 mg/day) Eplerenone (adult dosing) 50 mg/day QD or BID Dexamethasone up to 0.01 mg/kg/day
Glucocorticoid remediable aldosteronism (GRA)	Infancy/childhood	Severe hypertension, intracranial aneurysms, cerebral hemorrhage, high associated mortality rate (>50% at age 30)	Physiologic doses of a glucocorticoid (suppression of ACTH secretion) If not effective in reducing BP, then add MRA	Hydrocortisone 10–20 mg/m^2/day Prednisolone 0.1 mg/kg/day Dexamethasone up to 0.01 mg/kg/day Spironolactone 1 mg/kg/day in 1–2 doses (max dose 100 mg/day) Eplerenone (adult dosing) 50 mg/day QD or BID
Congenital adrenal hyperplasia (CAH) (11βhydroxylase deficiency)	Infancy	Hypertension		Hydrocortisone 10–20 mg/m^2/day Prednisolone 0.1 mg/kg/day Dexamethasone up to 0.01 mg/kg/day
Liddle syndrome	Late childhood to adolescence	Hypertension	Direct ENaC inhibition Low sodium diet	Amiloride 0.4–0.625 mg/kg QD (max 20 mg/day) Triamterene 0.5–1 mg/kg/dose BID (max 3–5 mg/kg/day)
Gordon's syndrome	Adolescence to adulthood	Hypertension	Low dose thiazide Low sodium diet	Hydrochlorothiazide 0.5–1 mg/kg QD or BID

ACTH adrenocorticotropic hormone, *BID* twice daily, *BP* blood pressure, *ENaC* epithelial sodium channel, *mg* milligram, *MRA* mineralocorticoid receptor antagonist, *QD* once daily

[a] Recommendations represent the authors' opinions although every effort has been made to confirm by consulting appropriate references. Manufacturers' prescribing information is frequently updated and should be consulted whenever possible

be noted that in children with advanced CKD a high potassium diet might not be feasible. Also, low-salt diets may not be possible in children with renal salt wasting, as often occurs in kidney hypodysplasia.

Treatment of Hypertension in Dialysis Patients

In dialysis patients, where fluid and salt overload play a major role in the pathogenesis of hypertension, *adjustment of dry weight* and *restriction of dietary sodium intake* are the primary measures to correct an elevated BP.

Dry weight is defined as the lowest body weight at the end of a dialysis session at which a patient can remain normotensive without antihypertensive medication until the next dialysis treatment, or the lowest weight a patient can tolerate without exhibiting symptoms of hypotension [141]. However, the determination of dry weight is challenging and often has to be achieved by trial and error. In clinical practice, dry weight is assumed to have been achieved when patients develop signs of intravascular volume depletion, such as drop in BP, cramping, yawning, headache, or abdominal pain (i.e. symptoms often associated with unpleasant and traumatizing experiences for patients). Simple but rather unprecise methods to assess dry weight include monitoring of pre- and post-dialysis weight and clinical assessment of edema, jugular vein distension and crackles on lung auscultation. Bioelectrical impedance analysis, or bioimpedance, is a method that determines the electrical resistance of the body to the flow of an electric current and is correlated with tissue water content. Bioimpedance can be applied to both HD and PD patients and can facilitate the assessment and achievement of dry weight in infants, children and adolescents on dialysis [142]. Further information on the assessment and attainment of dry weight can be found in the chapters on PD, HD and adequacy of dialysis.

To attain dry weight in HD patients, adjusting the duration of dialysis therapy and or the concentration of dialysate sodium are the main strategies to improve fluid removal. There is increasing evidence that matching dialysate sodium with the patient's pre-dialysis serum sodium concentration leads to reduction in thirst, interdialytic weight gain and hypertension [143–145].

In PD patients, optimization of water and sodium removal can be achieved by optimizing osmotic potential (dialysate dextrose concentration, dwell time) and fill volume.

Controlling dietary sodium intake facilitates achievement of dry weight [146], and is associated with decreased thirst, lower interdialytic weight gain, improved BP control, lower left ventricular mass index and decreased mortality in adults [147–149]. Fluid restriction should always be combined with reduction of sodium intake, because increased sodium intake inevitably increases thirst, leading to greater interdialytic weight gain [150]. However, restriction of sodium intake is difficult to achieve given the high sodium intake of most children: while the recommended sodium intake in hypertensive children with CKD is 1500–2300 mg daily (corresponding to 3.8–5.8 g of salt) [151], children with CKD stage 2–4 have been shown to ingest more than 3–5 g of sodium on average [152].

Antihypertensive drugs should only be prescribed if the adjustment of dry weight and sodium restriction do not result in normalization of BP. The preferable drug class in hypertensive pediatric dialysis patients is still unclear. Calcium channel blockers, beta blockers and RAAS antagonists are frequently used; however, RAAS blockade may have an increased risk for hyperkalemia and loss of residual diuresis while calcium channel blockers might complicate fluid removal during dialysis. For dose adjustments of antihypertensive drugs in dialysis patients, see Table 50.5.

Native kidney nephrectomy is typically considered the last resort in the treatment of hypertension in dialysis patients refractory to antihypertensive treatment after optimization of dry weight and salt balance [153].

Treatment of Hypertension in Transplant Patients

Hypertension in *transplant patients* usually requires pharmacological treatment similar to pre-transplant CKD. While CCBs are favorable with respect to counteracting calcineurin inhibitor-induced vasoconstriction, RAAS blockers are also safe and effective and exert antiproteinuric and potentially also renoprotective effects on kidney allograft function. In adult transplant patients, BP control was associated with improved graft survival [154]. However, whether strict BP control is superior to conventional BP control in pediatric kidney transplant patients remains to be shown.

Like in non-transplant CKD patients, non-pharmacological lifestyle measures, including weight reduction in overweight children, a healthy, low-salt, low-sugar, high-fibre diet (DASH-Diet) and physical activity, should be encouraged.

In patients with stable graft function, steroid withdrawal has been shown not only to improve BP, but also to restore nocturnal BP dipping [155]. Treatment options in hypertensive kidney disease are summarized in Fig. 50.2.

Treatment of Patients with Monogenic 'Low-Renin' Hypertension

Because BP elevation in these forms of hypertension is related to functional disturbances of renal tubular sodium handling and to fluid expansion, specific therapies targeting the underlying disease should be prescribed as initial treatment [98–100].

In patients with apparent mineralocorticoid excess (AME), hypertension ameliorates with MRA

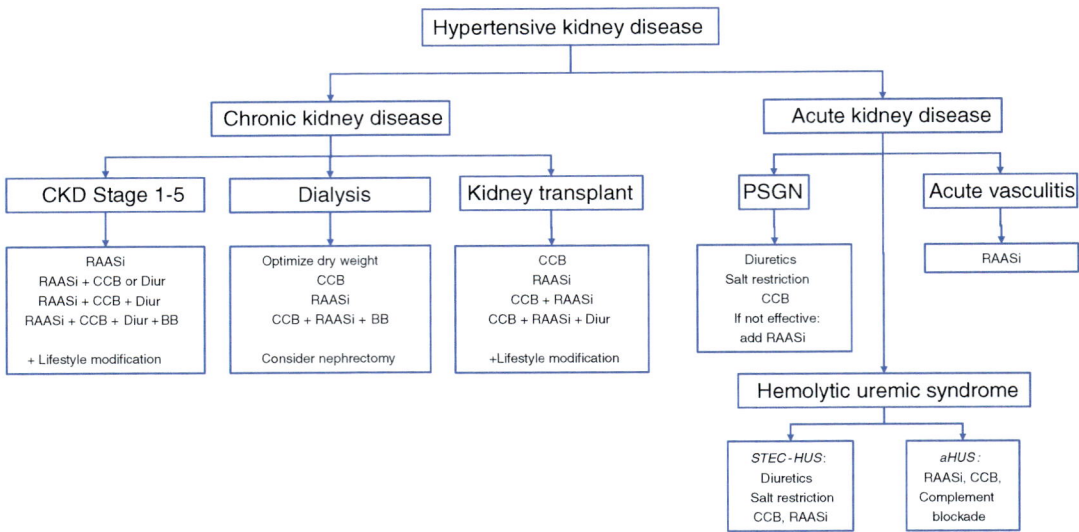

Fig. 50.2 Suggested treatment in hypertensive kidney disease and possible treatment escalation scheme. *CCB* calcium channel blocker, *RAASi* renin angiotensin aldosterone system inhibitor (i.e. ACE inhibitor or angiotensin type I inhibitor), *PSGN* poststreptococcal glomerulonephritis, *aHUS* atypical hemolytic uremic syndrome, *CKD* chronic kidney disease

treatment (spironolactone, eplerenone), along with potential potassium supplements and dietary sodium restriction. Persistently elevated cortisol levels may require glucocorticoid treatment to reduce ACTH-stimulated cortisol production and mineralocorticoid receptor activation.

In patients with *congenital adrenal hyperplasia (CAH type IV or type V)*, treatment consists of glucocorticoids to decrease ACTH secretion. Spironolactone, amiloride, and calcium channel blockers can additionally improve hypertension.

Hypertension in patients with *glucocorticoid remediable aldosteronism* (GRA) responds to treatment with glucocorticoids. If this is not effective to control BP, MRAs, and amiloride or triamterene can be added.

In patients with *Liddle's syndrome*, amiloride or triamterene, targeting the ENaC, are effective in lowering BP. MRAs are not effective in Liddle's syndrome because the ENaC activity is independent of mineralocorticoid regulation.

In Gordon's syndrome, hypertension should be treated with low-dose thiazide, which directly inhibits the underlying NCC overactivity.

Antihypertensive agents are usually of limited efficacy in monogenic forms of hypertension and are not the first-line therapy. For further information on recommended treatment of monogenic hypertension, see Table 50.4.

Monitoring of Patients with Renal Hypertension

Patients with CKD and renoparenchymal hypertension require long-term antihypertensive therapy and life-long monitoring of BP. In patients who recovered from acute kidney injury, BP should be monitored regularly since arterial hypertension and/or proteinuria may manifest years later in patients with subclinical residual kidney damage (e.g., after hemolytic uremic syndrome).

BP should be monitored at each medical appointment in all kidney patients. For further evaluation of BP control and to rule out masked or isolated nocturnal hypertension, conditions that are highly prevalent in CKD, *24-h ABPM* is recommended at least once a year [140]. In patients with insufficiently controlled hypertension at high risk for hypertensive end-organ damage, evaluation should be repeated at even shorter time intervals. Regular *home BP measurements* are recommended for monitoring of BP between outpatient appointments.

Echocardiographic examinations should be performed once yearly for timely diagnosis of left ventricular hypertrophy. If left ventricular hypertrophy is already present, echocardiographic follow-up should be performed every 3–6 months. Additional information on BP monitoring is given in Chap. 49.

Conclusions

Hypertension is a common condition in children with all stages of CKD and contributes to kidney disease progression by a variety of mechanisms, among which the RAAS plays a central role. Thus, RAAS antagonists are the drug class of first choice; other classes of antihypertensive agents should be added as needed until BP is controlled. In pediatric CKD patients, strict BP control is crucial to the preservation of kidney function and cardiovascular health. ABPM-guided treatment to achieve circadian BP control below the 50th to 75th BP percentile for age is the best currently known strategy to achieve maximal nephroprotection.

References

1. Bright R. Morbid appearances in 100 cases connected with albuminous urine. Guys Hosp Rep. 1836;1836:380–402.
2. Wong H, Mylera K, Feber J, Drukker A, Filler G. Prevalence of complications in children with chronic kidney disease according to KDOQI. Kidney Int. 2006;70:585–90.
3. Schaefer F, Doyon A, Azukaitis K, Bayazit A, Canpolat N, Duzova A, et al. Cardiovascular phenotypes in children with CKD: the 4C study. Clin J Am Soc Nephrol. 2017;12(1):19–28.
4. Mitsnefes M, Ho PL, McEnery P. Hypertension and progression of chronic renal insufficiency in children: a report of the North American Pediatric Renal Transplant Cooperative Study (NAPRTCS). J Am Soc Nephrol. 2003;14:2618–22.
5. Flynn JT, Mitsnefes M, Pierce C, Cole SR, Parekh RS, Furth SL, et al. Blood pressure in children with chronic kidney disease: a report form the Chronic Kidney Disease in Children Study. Hypertension. 2008;52:631–7.
6. Halbach S, Flynn J. Treatment of hypertension in children with chronic kidney disease. Curr Hypertens Rep. 2015;17(1):503.
7. Mitsnefes M, Flynn J, Cohn S, Samuels J, Blydt-Hansen T, Saland J, et al. Masked hypertension associates with left ventricular hypertrophy in children with CKD. J Am Soc Nephrol. 2010;21:137–44.
8. Schaefer F, Mehls O. Hypertension in chronic kidney disease. In: Portman RJ, Sorof JM, Ingelfinger JR, editors. Pediatric hypertension. Totowa, NJ: Humana; 2004. p. 371–87.
9. Wühl E, Schaefer F, Mehls O. Prevalence and current treatment policies of hypertension and proteinuria in children with chronic renal failure in Europe. In: Timio M, Wizemann V, Venanzi S, editors. Cardionephrology. Cosenza: Editoriale Bios; 1999. p. 85–8.
10. Guyton AC, Coleman TG, Cowley AV Jr, Scheel KW, Manning RD Jr, Norman RA Jr. Arterial pressure regulation. Overriding dominance of the kidneys in long-term regulation and in hypertension. Am J Med. 1972;52(5):584–94.
11. Romero JC, Ruilope LM, Bentley MD, Fiksen-Olsen MJ, Lahera V, Vidal MJ. Comparison of the effects of calcium antagonists and converting enzyme inhibitors on renal function under normal and hypertensive conditions. Am J Cardiol. 1988;62(11):59G–68G.
12. Ruilope LM. The kidney and control of blood pressure. In: Davison AM, Cameron JS, Grunfeld JP, Ponticelli C, Ritz E, Winearls CG, Van Ypersele C, editors. Oxford textbook of clinical nephrology, vol. 2. Oxford: Oxford University Press; 2008. p. 1321–8.
13. Keller G, Zimmer G, Mall G, Ritz E, Amann K. Nephron number in patients with primary hypertension. N Engl J Med. 2003;348:101–8.
14. Singh RR, Denton KM. Role of the kidney in the fetal programming of adult cardiovascular disease: an update. Curr Opin Pharmacol. 2015;21:53–9.
15. Gu D, Zhao Q, Chen J, Chen JC, Huang J, Bazzano LA, et al. Reproducibility of blood pressure responses to dietary sodium and potassium interventions: the GenSalt study. Hypertension. 2013;62(3):499–505.
16. Weinberger MH, Fineberg NS. Sodium and volume sensitivity of blood pressure. Age and pressure change over time. Hypertension. 1991;18(1):67–71.
17. Morimoto A, Uzu T, Fujii T, Nishimura M, Kuroda S, Nakamura S, et al. Sodium sensitivity and cardiovascular events in patients with essential hypertension. Lancet. 1997;350(9093):1734–7.
18. Luzardo L, Noboa O, Boggia J. Mechanisms of salt-sensitive hypertension. Curr Hypertens Rev. 2015;11(1):14–21.

19. Mancia G, Fagard R, Narkiewicz K, Redon J, Zanchetti A, Bohm M, et al. 2013 ESH/ESC guidelines for the management of arterial hypertension: the task force for the management of arterial hypertension of the European Society of Hypertension (ESH) and of the European Society of Cardiology (ESC). Eur Heart J. 2013;34(28):2159–219.

20. Whelton PK, Carey RM, Aronow WS, Casey DE Jr, Collins KJ, Dennison Himmelfarb C, et al. 2017 ACC/AHA/AAPA/ABC/ACPM/AGS/APhA/ASH/ASPC/NMA/PCNA guideline for the prevention, detection, evaluation, and management of high blood pressure in adults: executive summary: a report of the American College of Cardiology/American Heart Association Task Force on Clinical Practice Guidelines. Hypertension. 2018;71(6):1269–324.

21. Williams B, Mancia G, Spiering W, Agabiti Rosei E, Azizi M, Burnier M, et al. 2018 ESC/ESH guidelines for the management of arterial hypertension. Eur Heart J. 2018;39(33):3021–104.

22. de Gasparo M, Catt KJ, Inagami T, Wright JW, Unger T. International union of pharmacology. XXIII. The angiotensin II receptors. Pharmacol Rev. 2000;52(3):415–72.

23. Mamenko M, Zaika O, Prieto MC, Jensen VB, Doris PA, Navar LG, et al. Chronic angiotensin II infusion drives extensive aldosterone-independent epithelial Na+ channel activation. Hypertension. 2013;62(6):1111–22.

24. Xu J, Li G, Wang P, Velazquez H, Yao X, Li Y, et al. Renalase is a novel, soluble monoamine oxidase that regulates cardiac function and blood pressure. J Clin Invest. 2005;115:1275–80.

25. Birnbaumer M. Vasopressin receptors. Trends Endocrinol Metab. 2000;11(10):406–10.

26. Siragy HM. Evidence that intrarenal bradykinin plays a role in regulation of renal function. Am J Phys. 1993;265(4 Pt 1):E648–54.

27. Beierwaltes WH, Prada J, Carretero OA. Effect of glandular kallikrein on renin release in isolated rat glomeruli. Hypertension. 1985;7(1):27–31.

28. Kohan DE. Endothelin, hypertension and chronic kidney disease: new insights. Curr Opin Nephrol Hypertens. 2010;19(2):134–9.

29. Hunt PJ, Espiner EA, Nicholls MG, Richards AM, Yandle TG. Differing biological effects of equimolar atrial and brain natriuretic peptide infusions in normal man. J Clin Endocrinol Metab. 1996;81(11):3871–6.

30. Roques BP, Noble F, Dauge V, Fournie-Zaluski MC, Beaumont A. Neutral endopeptidase 24.11: structure, inhibition, and experimental and clinical pharmacology. Pharmacol Rev. 1993;45(1):87–146.

31. Karlsen FM, Andersen CB, Leyssac PP, Holstein-Rathlou NH. Dynamic autoregulation and renal injury in Dahl rats. Hypertension. 1997;30(4):975–83.

32. Long DA, Price KL, Herrera-Acosta J, Johnson RJ. How does angiotensin II cause renal injury? Hypertension. 2004;43(4):722–3.

33. Bidani AK, Schwartz MM, Lewis EJ. Renal autoregulation and vulnerability to hypertensive injury in remnant kidney. Am J Phys. 1987;252(6 Pt 2):F1003–10.

34. Griffin KA, Picken M, Bidani AK. Method of renal mass reduction is a critical modulator of subsequent hypertension and glomerular injury. J Am Soc Nephrol. 1994;4(12):2023–31.

35. Christensen PK, Hommel EE, Clausen P, Feldt-Rasmussen B, Parving HH. Impaired autoregulation of the glomerular filtration rate in patients with nondiabetic nephropathies. Kidney Int. 1999;56:1517–21.

36. Bidani AK, Griffin KA. Long-term renal consequences of hypertension for normal and diseased kidneys. Curr Opin Nephrol Hypertens. 2002;11(1):73–80.

37. Bidani AK, Griffin KA. Pathophysiology of hypertensive renal damage: implications for therapy. Hypertension. 2004;44(5):595–601.

38. Sorof JM, Brewer ED, Portmann RJ. Ambulatory blood pressure monitoring and interdialytic weight gain in children receiving chronic hemodialysis. Am J Kidney Dis. 1999;33:667–74.

39. Rahman M, Fu P, Sehgal AR, Smith MC. Interdialytic weight gain, compliance with dialysis regime, and age are independent predictors of blood pressure in hemodialysis patients. Am J Kidney Dis. 2000;35:257–65.

40. Rahman M, Dixit A, Donley V, Gupta S, Hanslik T, Lacson E, et al. Factors associated with inadequate blood pressure control in hypertensive hemodialysis patients. Am J Kidney Dis. 1999;33:498–506.

41. Lingens N, Soergel M, Loirat C, Busch C, Lemmer B, Schärer K. Ambulatory blood pressure monitoring in paediatric patients treated by regular hemodialysis and peritoneal dialysis. Pediatr Nephrol. 1995;9:167–72.

42. Chazot C, Charra B, Laurent G, Didier C, Vo Van C, Terrat JC, et al. Interdialysis blood pressure control by long hemodialysis sessions. Nephrol Dial Transplant. 1995;10:831–7.

43. Savage T, Fabbian F, Giles M, Tomson CRV, Raine AEG. Interdialytic weight gain and 48-hr blood pressure in haemodialysis patients. Nephrol Dial Transplant. 1997;12:2308–11.

44. Blumberg A, Nelp WB, Hegstrîm RM, Scribner BH. Extracellular volume in patients with chronic renal disease treated for hypertension by sodium restriction. Lancet. 1967;2:69–73.

45. Klein IH, Ligtenberg G, Oey PL, Koomans HA, Blankestijn PJ. Sympathetic activity is increased in polycystic kidney disease and is associated with hypertension. J Am Soc Nephrol. 2001;12:2427–33.

46. Brass H, Ochs HG, Armbruster H, Heintz R. Plasma renin activity (PRA) and aldosterone (PA) in patients with chronic glomerulonephritis (GN) and hypertension. Clin Nephrol. 1976;5:57–60.

47. Warren DJ, Ferris TF. Renin secretion in renal hypertension. Lancet. 1970;1(7639):159–62.

48. Loghman-Adham M, Soto CE, Inagami T, Cassis L. The intrarenal renin-angiotensin system in autosomal dominant polycystic kidney disease. Am J Physiol Renal Physiol. 2004;287(4):F775–F88.

49. Ibrahim HN, Hostetter TH. The renin-aldosterone axis in two models of reduced renal mass in the rat. J Am Soc Nephrol. 1998;9:72–6.

50. Converse RL, Jacobsen TN, Toto RD, Jost CMT, Cosentino F, Fouad-Tarazi F, et al. Sympathetic overactivity in patients with chronic renal failure. N Engl J Med. 1992;327:1912–8.

51. Ligtenberg G, Blankenstijn PJ, Oey PL, Klein IH, Dijkhorst-Oei LT, Boomsma F, et al. Reduction of sympathetic hyperactivity by enalapril in patients with chronic renal failure. N Engl J Med. 1999;340(17):1321–8.

52. Miyajima E, Yamada Y, Yoshida Y, Matsukawa T, Shionoiri H, Tochikubo O, et al. Muscle sympathetic nerve activity in renovascular hypertension and primary aldosteronism. Hypertension. 1991;17:1057–62.

53. Thambyrajah J, Landray MJ, McGlynn FJ, Jones HJ, Wheeler DC, Townend JN. Abnormalities of endothelial function in patients with predialysis renal failure. Heart. 2000;83:205–9.

54. Hussein G, Bughdady Y, Kandil ME, Bazaraa HM, Taher H. Doppler assessment of brachial artery flow as a measure of endothelial dysfunction in pediatric chronic renal failure. Pediatr Nephrol. 2008;23:2025–30.

55. Schmidt RJ, Domico J, Samsell LS, Yokota S, Tracy C, Sorkin MI, et al. Indices of activity of the nitric oxide system in hemodialysis patients. Am J Kidney Dis. 1999;34:228–34.

56. Baylis C. Nitric oxide deficiency in chronic kidney disease. Am J Physiol Renal Physiol. 2008;294:F1–9.

57. Zoccali C, Bode-Bîger S, Mallamaci F, Benedetto F, Tripepi G, Malatino L, et al. Plasma concentration of asymmetrical dimethylarginine and mortality in patients with end-stage renal disease: a prospective study. Lancet. 2001;358:2113–7.

58. Fliser D, Kronenberg F, Kielstein JT, Morath C, Bode-Bîger SM, Haller H, et al. Asymmetric dimethylarginine and progression of chronic kidney disease: the mild to moderate kidney disease study. J Am Soc Nephrol. 2005;16:2254–6.

59. Anderstam B, Katzarski K, Bergstrîm J. Serum levels of NO, NG-dimethyl-L-arginine, a potential endogenous nitric oxide inhibitor in dialysis patients. J Am Soc Nephrol. 1997;8:1437–42.

60. Lariviere R, Lebel M. Endothelin-1 in chronic renal failure and hypertension. Can J Physiol Pharmacol. 2003;81(6):607–21.

61. Brenner BM. Nephron adaptation to renal injury or ablation. Am J Phys. 1985;249:F324–7.

62. Peterson JC, Adler S, Burkart JM, Greene T, Hebert LA, Hunsicker LG, et al. Blood pressure control, proteinuria, and the progression of renal disease. The modification of diet in Renal Disease Study. Ann Intern Med. 1995;123:754–62.

63. Wühl E, Trivelli A, Picca S, Litwin M, Peco-Antic A, Zurowska A, et al. Strict blood pressure control and renal failure progression in children. The ESCAPE Trial Group. N Engl J Med. 2009;361:1639–50.

64. Toto RD, Mitchell HC, Smith RD, Lee HC, McIntire D, Pettinger WA. "Strict" blood pressure control and progression of renal disease in hypertensive nephrosclerosis. Kidney Int. 1995;48:851–9.

65. Maschio G, Alberti D, Janin G, Locatelli F, Mann JF, Motolese M, et al. Effect of the angiotensin-converting-enzyme inhibitor benazepril on the progression of chronic renal insufficiency. The angiotensin-converting-enzyme inhibition in Progressive Renal Insufficiency Study Group. N Engl J Med. 1996;334(15):939–45.

66. Lewis EJ, Hunsicker LG, Raymond PB, Rohde RD, for the Collaborative Study Group. The effect of angiotensin-converting-enzyme inhibition on diabetic nephropathy. N Engl J Med. 1993;329:1456–62.

67. Kamper AL, Strandgaard S, Leyssac PP. Effect of enalapril on the progression of chronic renal failure: a randomized controlled trial. Am J Hypertens. 1992;5:423–30.

68. Bantis C, Ivens K, Kreusser W, Koch M, Klein-Vehne N, Grabensee B, et al. Influence of genetic polymorphisms of the renin-angiotensin system on IgA nephropathy. Am J Nephrol. 2004;24:258–67.

69. Zucchelli P, Zuccalà A, Borghi M, Fusaroli M, Sasdelli M, Stallone C, et al. Long-term comparison between captopril and nifidepin in the progression of renal insufficiency. Kidney Int. 1992;42:452–8.

70. Hannedouche T, Landais P, Goldfarb B, elEsper N, Fournier A, Godin M, et al. Randomised controlled trial of enalapril and beta blockers in non-diabetic chronic renal failure. BMJ. 1994;309:833–7.

71. Ihle BU, Whitworth JA, Shahinfar S, Cnaan A, Kincaid-Smith PS, Becker GJ. Angiotensin-converting-enzyme inhibition in non-diabetic progressive renal insufficiency: a controlled double-blind trial. Am J Kidney Dis. 1996;27:489–95.

72. Bakris GL, Copley JB, Vicknair N, Sadler R, Leurgans S. Calcium channel blockers vs. other antihypertensive therapies on progression of NIDDM associated nephropathy. Kidney Int. 1996;50:1641–50.

73. The GISEN Group. Randomised placebo-controlled trial of effect of ramipril on decline in glomerular filtration rate and risk of terminal renal failure in proteinuric, non-diabetic nephropathy. Lancet. 1997;349:1857–63.

74. UK Prospective Diabetes Study (UKPDS). Efficacy of atenolol and captopril in reducing risk of macrovascular and microvascular complications in type-II diabetes. BMJ. 1998;317:713–20.

75. Wingen AM, Fabian-Bach C, Schaefer F, Mehls O. Randomised multicentre study of a low-protein diet on the progression of chronic renal failure in children. European Study Group of Nutritional Treatment of Chronic Renal Failure in Childhood. Lancet. 1997;349(9059):1117–23.

76. van den Belt SM, Heerspink HJL, Gracchi V, de Zeeuw D, Wuhl E, Schaefer F, et al. Early proteinuria lowering by angiotensin-converting enzyme inhibition predicts renal survival in children with CKD. J Am Soc Nephrol. 2018;29(8):2225–33.

77. Johnson RJ, Lanaspa MA, Gabriela Sanchez-Lozada L, Rodriguez-Iturbe B. The discovery of hypertension: evolving views on the role of the kidneys, and current hot topics. Am J Physiol Renal Physiol. 2015;308(3):F167–78.

78. Feig DI, Kang DH, Johnson RJ. Uric acid and cardiovascular risk. N Engl J Med. 2008;359(17):1811–21.

79. Franco MC, Christofalo DM, Sawaya AL, Ajzen SA, Sesso R. Effects of low birth weight in 8- to 13-year-old children: implications in endothelial function and uric acid levels. Hypertension. 2006;48(1):45–50.

80. Raine AE, Bedford L, Simpson AW, Ashley CC, Brown R, Woodhead JS, et al. Hyperparathyroidism, platelet intracellular free calcium and hypertension in chronic renal failure. Kidney Int. 1993;43:700–5.

81. Catapano F, Chiodini P, De Nicola L, Minutolo R, Zamboli P, Gallo C, et al. Antiproteinuric response to dual blockade of the renin-angiotensin system in primary glomerulonephritis: meta-analysis and metaregression. Am J Kidney Dis. 2008;52(3):475–85.

82. Mathew RO, Nayer A, Asif A. The endothelium as the common denominator in malignant hypertension and thrombotic microangiopathy. J Am Soc Hypertens. 2016;10(4):352–9.

83. Cavero T, Arjona E, Soto K, Caravaca-Fontan F, Rabasco C, Bravo L, et al. Severe and malignant hypertension are common in primary atypical hemolytic uremic syndrome. Kidney Int. 2019;96(4):995–1004.

84. Schärer K. Hypertension in children and adolescents. In: Malluche HH, Sawaya BP, Hakim RM, Sayegh MH, editors. Clinical nephrology, dialysis and transplantation: a continuously updated textbook. Deisenhofen: Dustri; 1999. p. 1–28.

85. Massella L, Mekahli D, Paripovic D, Prikhodina L, Godefroid N, Niemirska A, et al. Prevalence of hypertension in children with early-stage ADPKD. Clin J Am Soc Nephrol. 2018;13(6):874–83.

86. Brun P. Hypertension artérielle rénovasculaire. In: Loirat C, Niaudet P, editors. Néphrologie pédiatrique. Paris: Doin; 1993. p. 203–11.

87. Hiner LB, Falkner B. Renovascular hypertension in children. Pediatr Clin N Am. 1993;40:123–40.

88. Mitsnefes M, Stablein D. Hypertension in pediatric patients on long-term dialysis: a report of the North American Pediatric Renal Transplant Cooperataive Study (NAPRTCS). Am J Kidney Dis. 2005;45:309–15.

89. Munshi R, Flynn JT. Hypertension in pediatric dialysis patients: etiology, evaluation, and management. Curr Hypertens Rep. 2018;20(7):61.

90. Halbach SM, Martz K, Mattoo T, Flynn J. Predictors of blood pressure and its control in pediatric patients receiving dialysis. J Pediatr. 2012;160(4):621–5.e1.

91. Kramer AM, van Stralen KJ, Jager KJ, Schaefer F, Verrina E, Seeman T, et al. Demographics of blood pressure and hypertension in children on renal replacement therapy in Europe. Kidney Int. 2011;80:1092–8.

92. Kornerup HJ. Hypertension in end-stage renal disease. The relationship between blood pressure, plasma renin, plasma renin substrate and exchangeable sodium in chronic hemodialysis patients. Acta Med Scand. 1976;200(4):257–61.

93. Zazgornik J, Biesenbach G, Janko O, Gross C, Mair R, Brucke P, et al. Bilateral nephrectomy: the best, but often overlooked, treatment for refractory hypertension in hemodialysis patients. Am J Hypertens. 1998;11(11 Pt 1):1364–70.

94. Desir GV. Renalase deficiency in chronic kidney disease, and its contribution to hypertension and cardiovascular disease. Curr Opin Nephrol Hypertens. 2008;17(2):181–5.

95. Mitsnefes MM, Portman RJ. Ambulatory blood pressure monitoring in pediatric renal transplantation. Pediatr Transplant. 2003;7(2):86–92.

96. Seeman T. Ambulatory blood pressure monitoring in pediatric renal transplantation. Curr Hypertens Rep. 2012;14(6):608–18.

97. Opelz G, Wujciak T, Ritz E. Association of chronic kidney graft failure with recipient blood pressure. Collaborative Transplant Study. Kidney Int. 1998;53(1):217–22.

98. Vehaskari VM. Heritable forms of hypertension. Pediatr Nephrol. 2009;24(10):1929–37.

99. Raina R, Krishnappa V, Das A, Amin H, Radhakrishnan Y, Nair NR, et al. Overview of monogenic or Mendelian forms of hypertension. Front Pediatr. 2019;7:263.

100. Simonetti GD, Mohaupt MG, Bianchetti MG. Monogenic forms of hypertension. Eur J Pediatr. 2012;171(10):1433–9.

101. Bakris GL, Williams M, Dworkin L, Elliot WJ, Epstein M, Toto R, et al. Preserving renal function in adults with hypertension and diabetes: a consensus approach. National Kidney Foundation Hypertension and Diabetes Executive Committees Working Group. Am J Kidney Dis. 2000;36:646–61.

102. Chobanian AV, Bakris GL, Black DL, Cushman WC, Green LA, Izzo JL Jr, et al. The seventh report of the Joint National Committee on Prevention, Detection, Evaluation, and Treatment of High Blood Pressure: the JNC 7 report. JAMA. 2003;289(19):2560–71.

103. Klahr S, Levy AD, Beck GJ. The effects of dietary protein restriction and blood-pressure control on the progression of chronic renal disease. N Engl J Med. 1994;330:877–84.

104. Sarnak MJ, Greene T, Wang X, Beck G, Kusek JW, Collins AJ, et al. The effect of a lower target blood pressure on the progression of kidney disease: long-term follow-up of the modification of diet in renal disease study. Ann Intern Med. 2005;142:342–51.

105. Ruggenenti P, Perna A, Loriga G, Ganeva M, Ene-Iordache B, Turturro M, et al. Blood pressure con-

trol for renoprotection in patients with non-diabetic chronic renal disease (REIN-2): multicenter, randomized controlled trial. Lancet. 2005;365:939–46.

106. Wright JT Jr, Bakris G, Greene T, Agodoa LY, Appel LJ, Charleston J, et al. Effect of blood pressure lowering and antihypertensive drug class on progression of hypertensive kidney disease: results from the AASK trial. JAMA. 2002;288:2421–31.

107. Appel LJ, Wright JT Jr, Greene T, Agodoa LY, Astor BC, Bakris GL, et al. Intensified blood-pressure control in hypertensive chronic kidney disease. N Engl J Med. 2010;363:918–29.

108. Schrier RW, Estacio RO, Mehler PS, Hiatt WR. Appropriate blood pressure control in hypertensive and normotensive type 2 diabetes mellitus: a summary of the ABCD trial. Nat Clin Pract Nephrol. 2008;3:428–38.

109. Group SR, Wright JT Jr, Williamson JD, Whelton PK, Snyder JK, Sink KM, et al. A randomized trial of intensive versus standard blood-pressure control. N Engl J Med. 2015;373(22):2103–16.

110. Kovesdy CP. Hypertension in chronic kidney disease after the Systolic Blood Pressure Intervention Trial: targets, treatment and current uncertainties. Nephrol Dial Transplant. 2017;32(Suppl_2):ii219–i23.

111. Lurbe E, Agabiti-Rosei E, Cruickshank JK, Dominiczak A, Erdine S, Hirth A, et al. 2016 European Society of Hypertension guidelines for the management of high blood pressure in children and adolescents. J Hypertens. 2016;34(10):1887–920.

112. Flynn JT, Falkner BE. New clinical practice guideline for the management of high blood pressure in children and adolescents. Hypertension. 2017;70(4):683–6.

113. Parra G, Rodriguez-Iturbe B, Colina-Chourio J, Garcia R. Short-term treatment with captopril in hypertension due to acute glomerulonephritis. Clin Nephrol. 1988;29(2):58–62.

114. Jafar TH, Schmid CH, Landa M, Giatras I, Toto R, Remuzzi G, et al. Angiotensin-converting enzyme inhibitors and progression of nondiabetic renal disease. A meta-analysis of patient-level data. Ann Intern Med. 2001;135(2):73–87.

115. Casas JP, Weiliang C, Loukogeorgakis S, Vallance P, Smeeth L, Hingorani AD, et al. Effect of inhibitors of the renin-angiotensin system and other antihypertensive drugs on renal outcomes: systematic review and meta-analysis. Lancet. 2005;366:2026–33.

116. Schaefer F, Vande Walle J, Zurowska A, Gimpel C, van Hoeck K, Drozdz D, et al. Efficacy, safety and pharmacokinetics of candesartan cilexetil in hypertensive children from 1 to less than 6 years of age. J Hypertens. 2010;28:1083–90.

117. Lou-Meda R, Stiller B, Antonio ZL, Zielinska E, Yap HK, Kang HG, et al. Long-term safety and tolerability of valsartan in children aged 6 to 17 years with hypertension. Pediatr Nephrol. 2019;34(3):495–506.

118. Bakris GL, Weir MR. Angiotensin-converting enzyme inhibitor-associated elevations in serum creatinine: is this a cause for concern? Arch Intern Med. 2000;160:685–93.

119. Mooser V, Nussberger J, Juillerat L, Burnier M, Waeber B, Bidiville J, et al. Reactive hyperreninemia is a major determinant of plasma angiotensin II during ACE inhibition. J Cardiovasc Pharmacol. 1990;15:276–82.

120. van den Meiracker AH, Man in 't Veld AJ, Admiraal PJ, Ritsema van Eck HJ, Boomsma F, Derkx FH, et al. Partial escape of angiotensin converting enzyme (ACE) inhibition during prolonged ACE inhibitor treatment: does it exist and does it affect the antihypertensive response? J Hypertens. 1992;10:803–12.

121. Shiigai T, Shichiri M. Late escape from the antiproteinuric effect of ACE inhibitors in nondiabetic renal disease. Am J Kidney Dis. 2001;37:477–83.

122. Burgess E, Muirhead N, De Cotret PR, Chiu A, Pichette V, Tobe S, et al. Supramaximal dose of candesartan in proteinuric kidney disease. J Am Soc Nephrol. 2009;20:893–900.

123. ONTARGET Investigators, Yusuf S, Teo KK, Pogue J, Dyal L, Copland I, et al. Telmisartan, ramipril, or both in patients at high risk for vascular events. N Engl J Med. 2008;358(15):1547–59.

124. Mann JF, Schmieder RF, McQueen M, Dyal L, Schumacher H, Pogue J, et al. Renal outcomes with telmisartan, ramipril, or both, in people at high vascular risk (the ONTARGET study): a multicentre, randomised, double-blind, controlled trial. Lancet. 2008;372:547–53.

125. Abutaleb N. ONTARGET should not be over interpreted. Nephrol Dial Transplant. 2010;25(1):44–7.

126. Oparil S, Yarows SA, Patel S, Fang H, Zhang J, Satlin A. Efficacy and safety of combined use of aliskiren and valsartan in patients with hypertension: a randomized, double-blind trial. Lancet. 2007;370:221–9.

127. Parving HH, Brenner BM, McMurray JJ, de Zeeuw D, Haffner SM, Solomon SD, et al. Cardiorenal end points in a trial of aliskiren for type 2 diabetes. N Engl J Med. 2012;367(23):2204–13.

128. European Medicines Agency (2012). http://www.ema.europa.eu/docs/en_GB/document_library/Other/2012/02/WC500122919.pdf.

129. Epstein M, Buckalew V, Altamirano J, Roniker B, Krause S, Kleimann J. Eplerenone reduces proteinuria in type II diabetes mellitus: implications for aldosterone involvement in the pathogenesis of renal dysfunction. J Am Coll Cardiol. 2009;39(Suppl 1):249.

130. Bakris GL, Agarwal R, Anker SD, Pitt B, Ruilope LM, Rossing P, et al. Effect of finerenone on chronic kidney disease outcomes in type 2 diabetes. N Engl J Med. 2020;383(23):2219–29.

131. Wan N, Rahman A, Nishiyama A. Esaxerenone, a novel nonsteroidal mineralocorticoid receptor blocker (MRB) in hypertension and chronic kidney disease. J Hum Hypertens. 2021;35(2):148–56.

132. Remuzzi G, Ruggenenti P, Benigni A. Understanding the nature of renal disease progression. Kidney Int. 1997;51:2–15.

133. Flack JM, Hilkert R. Single-pill combination of amlodipine and valsartan in the management of hypertension. Expert Opin Pharmacother. 2009;10(12):1979–94.

134. Jamerson K, Weber MA, Bakris GL, Dahlöf B, Pitt B, Shi V, et al. Benazepril plus amlodipine or hydrochlorothiazide for hypertension in high risk patients. N Engl J Med. 2008;359:2417–28.

135. Parving HH, Andersen AR, Smidt UM, Svendsen PA. Early aggressive antihypertensive treatment reduces rate of decline in kidney function in diabetic nephropathy. Lancet. 1983;1:1175–9.

136. Marchi F, Ciriello G. Efficacy of carvedilol in mild to moderate essential hypertension and effects on microalbuminuria: a multicenter, randomized open-label, controlled study versus atenolol. Adv Ther. 1995;12:212–21.

137. Fassbinder W, Quarder O, Waltz A. Treatment with carvedilol is associated with a significant reduction in microalbuminuria: a multicenter randomized study. Int J Clin Pract. 1999;53:519–22.

138. Hermida RC, Ayala DE, Mojon A, Fernandez JR. Bedtime dosing of antihypertensive medications reduces cardiovascular risk in CKD. J Am Soc Nephrol. 2011;22:2313–21.

139. Whelton PK, Carey RM, Aronow WS, Casey DE Jr, Collins KJ, Dennison Himmelfarb C, et al. 2017 ACC/AHA/AAPA/ABC/ACPM/AGS/APhA/ASH/ASPC/NMA/PCNA guideline for the prevention, detection, evaluation, and management of high blood pressure in adults: a report of the American College of Cardiology/American Heart Association Task Force on Clinical Practice Guidelines. Hypertension. 2018;71(6):e13–e115.

140. Flynn JT, Kaelber DC, Baker-Smith CM, Blowey D, Carroll AE, Daniels SR, et al. Clinical practice guideline for screening and management of high blood pressure in children and adolescents. Pediatrics. 2017;140(3):e20171904.

141. Jaeger JQ, Mehta RL. Assessment of dry weight in hemodialysis: an overview. J Am Soc Nephrol. 1999;10(2):392–403.

142. Davies SJ, Davenport A. The role of bioimpedance and biomarkers in helping to aid clinical decision-making of volume assessments in dialysis patients. Kidney Int. 2014;86(3):489–96.

143. Munoz Mendoza J, Arramreddy R, Schiller B. Dialysate sodium: choosing the optimal hemodialysis bath. Am J Kidney Dis. 2015;66(4):710–20.

144. Thein H, Haloob I, Marshall MR. Associations of a facility level decrease in dialysate sodium concentration with blood pressure and interdialytic weight gain. Nephrol Dial Transplant. 2007;22(9):2630–9.

145. Basile C, Pisano A, Lisi P, Rossi L, Lomonte C, Bolignano D. High versus low dialysate sodium concentration in chronic haemodialysis patients: a systematic review of 23 studies. Nephrol Dial Transplant. 2016;31(4):548–63.

146. Kooman JP, van der Sande F, Leunissen K, Locatelli F. Sodium balance in hemodialysis therapy. Semin Dial. 2003;16(5):351–5.

147. Kayikcioglu M, Tumuklu M, Ozkahya M, Ozdogan O, Asci G, Duman S, et al. The benefit of salt restriction in the treatment of end-stage renal disease by haemodialysis. Nephrol Dial Transplant. 2009;24(3):956–62.

148. McCausland FR, Waikar SS, Brunelli SM. Increased dietary sodium is independently associated with greater mortality among prevalent hemodialysis patients. Kidney Int. 2012;82(2):204–11.

149. Maduell F, Navarro V. Dietary salt intake and blood pressure control in haemodialysis patients. Nephrol Dial Transplant. 2000;15(12):2063.

150. Lindley EJ. Reducing sodium intake in hemodialysis patients. Semin Dial. 2009;22(3):260–3.

151. K/DOQI clinical practice guidelines on hypertension and antihypertensive agents in chronic kidney disease. Am J Kidney Dis. 2004;43:S1–S290.

152. Hui WF, Betoko A, Savant JD, Abraham AG, Greenbaum LA, Warady B, et al. Assessment of dietary intake of children with chronic kidney disease. Pediatr Nephrol. 2017;32(3):485–94.

153. Baez-Trinidad LG, Lendvay TS, Broecker BH, Smith EA, Warshaw BL, Hymes L, et al. Efficacy of nephrectomy for the treatment of nephrogenic hypertension in a pediatric population. J Urol. 2003;170(4 Pt 2):1655–7. discussion 8

154. Opelz G, Dohler B, Collaborative Transplant Study. Improved long-term outcomes after renal transplantation associated with blood pressure control. Am J Transplant. 2005;5(11):2725–31.

155. Hocker B, Weber LT, John U, Drube J, Fehrenbach H, Klaus G, et al. Steroid withdrawal improves blood pressure control and nocturnal dipping in pediatric renal transplant recipients: analysis of a prospective, randomized, controlled trial. Pediatr Nephrol. 2019;34(2):341–8.

156. Wühl E, Flynn JT. Managment of hypertension in pediatric dialysis patients. In: Warady BA, Alexander SR, Schaefer F, editors. Pediatric dialysis. 3rd ed. Switzerland: Springer Nature; 2021. p. 589–608.

Part XI

Acute Kidney Injury and Neonatal Nephrology

Acute Kidney Injury: Pathophysiology, Diagnosis and Prevention

51

Prasad Devarajan

Introduction

Acute kidney injury (AKI) has been traditionally defined as an abrupt loss of kidney function leading to a rapid decline in glomerular filtration rate (GFR), reduction in urine output, accumulation of waste products such as blood urea nitrogen (BUN) and creatinine, and dysregulation of extracellular volume and electrolyte homeostasis. The term AKI has largely replaced acute renal failure (ARF) since the latter designation over-emphasizes the discrete event of a failed kidney. We now recognize that AKI embodies both the continuum of renal dysfunction that characterizes the clinical spectrum, as well as the diverse molecular, biochemical, and structural injuries to the nephron that occur well before the decline in function. Hence, AKI includes both structural injury and functional impairment. AKI is an increasingly common problem afflicting all ages, occurring in 10–30% of non-critically ill hospitalized children and >30% of children in critical care units. AKI is the leading reason to seek in-patient nephrology consultation and associated with serious short-term and long-term consequences, and therapeutic options are unsatisfactory. The etiology of AKI varies widely according to age, geographical region, and clinical setting [1–7]. Functional AKI induced by dehydration is usually reversible with early fluid therapy. However, the prognosis for patients with structural AKI in the intensive care setting remains guarded. Clinicians now recognize that critically ill patients are dying "of" AKI, and not just simply "with" AKI. Fortunately, the cellular and molecular tools of modern science are providing novel insights into the pathogenetic mechanisms of AKI. Newly discovered pathways are yielding early non-invasive biomarkers for the prediction of AKI and its consequences, as well as innovative strategies for the pro-active treatment and prevention of AKI.

Definitions, Staging, Risk Stratification

Traditionally, AKI has been defined as a rapid decrease in GFR, manifested by an elevated serum creatinine (or a rise from baseline serum creatinine), and/or a reduction in urine output. Based on these criteria, more than 35 different definitions of AKI have plagued the literature, resulting in a wide range of quoted incidence rates, risk factors, and outcomes in the pediatric literature [8]. Essential advances in the field have resulted from consensus AKI definitions, initially in the form of the RIFLE criteria (Risk, Injury, Failure, Loss and End-Stage Kidney Disease) in 2004 with pediatric modifications (pRIFLE) in

P. Devarajan (✉)
Cincinnati Children's Hospital Medical Center,
University of Cincinnati College of Medicine,
Cincinnati, OH, USA
e-mail: prasad.devarajan@cchmc.org

© The Author(s), under exclusive license to Springer Nature Switzerland AG 2023
F. Schaefer, L. A. Greenbaum (eds.), *Pediatric Kidney Disease*,
https://doi.org/10.1007/978-3-031-11665-0_51

2007 [9]. The pRIFLE classification of AKI includes three graded levels of injury (*R*isk, *I*njury, *F*ailure) based upon the severity of reduction in estimated GFR or urine output, as well as two outcome measures (*L*oss of kidney function i.e., persistent failure for >4 weeks, and *E*nd-stage kidney disease i.e., persistent failure for >3 months). Another refinement was the addition of a 0.3 mg/dL serum creatinine rise in less than 48 h, as also embodied in the Acute Kidney Injury Network (AKIN) criteria [10], since studies have shown independent associations with poor outcomes at this creatinine threshold [8]. However, a systematic review of 12 pediatric studies that employed the RIFLE or pRIFLE classification showed continued wide variations in the relationship between RIFLE class and measures of morbidity and mortality [9]. More recently, the above definitions have been harmonized by the Kidney Disease Improving Global Outcomes (KDIGO) AKI Consensus Conference [11, 12] into a single definition of AKI:

- Increase in serum creatinine by ≥0.3 mg/dL [≥26.5 µmol/L] within 48 h, OR
- Increase in serum creatinine to ≥1.5 times baseline within the prior 7 days, OR
- Urine volume ≤0.5 mL/kg/h for 6 h

The KDIGO staging of AKI is shown in Table 51.1. Both the definition and staging include a 0.3 mg/dL serum creatinine increase criterion to specifically be applicable to pediatric

Table 51.1 The Kidney Disease Improving Global Outcomes (KDIGO) AKI criteria (Adapted from Ref. [11])

Stage	Serum creatinine	Urine output
1	1.5–1.9 times baseline, OR ≥0.3 mg/dL (≥26.5 µmol/L) increase	<0.5 mL/kg/h for 6–12 h
2	1.0–2.9 times baseline	<0.5 mL/kg/h for ≥12 h
3	3.0 times baseline, OR SCr ≥4.0 mg/dL (≥353.6 µmol/L), OR Initiation of renal replacement therapy, OR eGFR <35 mL/min per 1.73 m² (<18 years)	<0.3 mL/kg/h for ≥24 h, OR Anuria for ≥12 h

AKI. The staging also allows for a child with eGFR <35 mL/min/1.73 m² to be included in Stage 3, in contrast with the adult criterion of ≥4 mg/dL serum creatinine (which would be unusual in infants and young children). The KDIGO AKI definition has now been extensively validated in both children and adults, and is therefore currently recommended to guide clinical care, and as a standardized inclusion and outcome measure in AKI studies. A neonatal modified KDIGO definition has recently been proposed with slight modifications to the KDIGO criteria, and is the recommended definition for clinical and epidemiological studies in neonates [1]. It is likely that validation and widespread clinical integration of the novel AKI biomarkers discussed later in this chapter will further improve our ability to define and stage AKI.

Some limitations with the KDIGO AKI definition and staging are well recognized, with respect to both the eGFR and the urine output criteria. First, the eGFR measurement is dependent on serum creatinine, which is imprecise for the clinical diagnosis of AKI (as detailed in section "Clinical Presentation"). Second, the definitions outlined above call for an increase in serum creatinine to ≥1.5 times baseline, and the baseline serum creatinine is often unknown. In previously healthy children, it is generally recommended to employ a presumed baseline of 120 mL/min/1.73 m² [13]. In children with available height measurements, the estimated baseline serum creatinine may be imputed by using currently proposed eGFR equations for children [14]. Alternatively, published normative values for serum creatinine based on age and gender can be used. Imputed age- and gender-based serum creatinine norms have been applied to determine baseline serum creatinine and the diagnosis of pediatric AKI in both the hospitalized [15] and the community settings [16]. Third, although a time-dependent reduction in urine output is an important component of AKI diagnosis, most of the published literature is based solely on serum creatinine changes since it is typically more commonly measured and more easily extractable from electronic health records (EHRs). Accurate urine output determination requires an indwelling urinary catheter, which is usually restricted to the critical care setting. In addition, urine output is confounded by hydration status and the clinical use of fluids and diuretics. Finally, the majority of nephrotoxic AKI is non-oliguric. Despite these limitations, recent studies have illustrated that degree of oliguria is strongly associated with poor outcomes in pediatric AKI, and that exclusion of urine output in the definition results in underdiagnosis of AKI, especially in the critical care setting [17, 18].

A new criterion for pediatric AKI was reported, based on a change in reference value of serum creatinine [19]. This study defined pediatric AKI according to pediatric reference change value optimized for AKI in hospitalized children (pROCK) as creatinine increase beyond reference change value of serum creatinine, estimated as the greater of 20 μmol/L or 30% of the initial creatinine level. AKI incidence was lower using the pROCK criteria when compared with the pRIFLE and KDIGO definitions (5.3% versus 15.2% and 10.2%, respectively). In a subsequent study of critically ill children, the pROCK criteria outperformed KDIGO in predicting mortality [20]. However, at the present time, the use of pROCK criteria over the more extensively studied and validated KDIGO criteria is not widely recommended.

The duration of an AKI episode can be used to further refine the diagnosis. For example, transient or reversible AKI (lasting <48 h) portends an improved prognosis when compared to sustained AKI (typically of 2–7 days duration). A new definition of acute kidney disease (AKD) has been proposed for AKI that lasts beyond 7 days and up to 3 months (beyond which the condition is labelled as chronic kidney disease [CKD]). AKD represents a complex syndrome where recurrent bouts of acute injury interact with ongoing regeneration and repair processes. A recent consensus on the evolving definition, management strategies, and research priorities in AKD has been published [21]. AKD is now defined by abnormalities of kidney function and/or structure with implications for health and with a duration of ≤3 months. AKD may include AKI, but also includes abnormalities in kidney function that are not as severe as AKI or that develop over a period of >7 days. The cause(s) of and mechanisms underlying AKD should be actively sought and managed to prevent progression to CKD [21].

In the critical care setting, a simple bedside risk stratification system for AKI has been proposed, which can be incorporated into the real-time EHR for automated alerts. Termed the renal angina index (RAI), it is a composite of known clinical risk factors, including vasopressor use, invasive mechanical ventilation, percent fluid overload, estimated creatinine clearance, and the presence of bone marrow or solid organ transplantation. The RAI has been shown in prospective studies to improve prediction of severe AKI (KDIGO Stage 2 or 3) in critically ill children when compared to an increase in serum creatinine alone [22, 23]. Recent studies have demonstrated the ability of the RAI to predict AKI in children presenting to the emergency department [24] and in children with septic shock [25]. The RAI may be especially useful in identifying children who might benefit best from additional investigative monitoring, including novel biomarkers, and potential early intervention [26–28].

Epidemiology

The precise incidence and prevalence of pediatric AKI are not fully known. However, there is growing evidence to indicate that pediatric AKI is not only common but also rising in incidence globally. While the mounting AKI incidence rate may be attributed in part to increased awareness and better consensus definitions, it is also very likely a consequence of advancements in the non-renal care of otherwise critically ill children. The incidence varies based on the definition used, clinical setting, geographic location, available resources, and the underlying clinical risk factors, as outlined below.

Few data are available to define the incidence of pediatric AKI in the general community setting. In a diverse outpatient cohort of more than 1.5 million children who received care within the Kaiser Permanente Northern California system from 2008 to 2016, the overall incidence of community-based KDIGO-defined pediatric AKI was about 1 per 1000 per year [29]. In contrast, the recent use of EHR systems has provided higher estimates of KDIGO-based AKI in non-critically ill hospitalized children in the 10–30% range. In a retrospective single center study from the United States that utilized EHR to identify AKI in a development and a validation cohort, the incidence of AKI in non-critically ill children was 722/2337 (31%) and 469/1474 (32%), respectively [30]. A prospective cohort study of hospitalized children from Wales used an electronic alert system to identify AKI in 77.3 cases per 1000 person-years [31]. A retrospective multicenter study from China identified AKI in the EHR of 20% among 101,836 hospitalized children [32]. A retrospective analysis from six hospitals in England revealed AKI in 11% of children using the National Health Services AKI e-alert algorithm [33]. In a single center retrospective EHR review in the United States, the incidence of AKI was 10.2% out of 8473 hospitalized children [34]. In the Kaiser Permanente cohort, the incidence of AKI in hospitalized children was 9% [29].

The incidence of AKI in critically ill children and neonates is even higher. In a recent prospective multinational study of 4683 children from 32 ICUs across North America, Europe, Asia, and Australia (AWARE), the overall incidence of AKI was 27% [35]. In a retrospective multicenter analysis of 2022 critically ill neonates from North America, Australia, and India (AWAKEN), the overall incidence of AKI was 30% [36]. This varied with gestational age, with the highest incidence (48%) noted in the 22–29-week gestational age group.

The incidence and etiology of pediatric AKI differs with geographic location and available resources. In resource-rich countries, the etiology has shifted in the past three decades to a hospital-acquired complication of other multisystem illnesses. The AKI is often multifactorial, frequently due to an underlying comorbid condition or its management, and often manifests in the context of multiorgan failure. Primary kidney diseases now account for only 7–10% of AKI in hospitalized children in high-resource settings. Thus, advances in critical care have increasingly rendered pediatric AKI a hospital-acquired disease, especially in developed countries. In contrast, in resource-limited countries, the most common causes of AKI remain in the community-acquired setting and include acute tubular necrosis (ATN) due to gastroenteritis or sepsis, and primary kidney diseases such as acute glomerulonephritis or hemolytic uremic syndrome [37]. In the Global Snapshot conducted by the ISN "0by25" AKI initiative, a prospective observational study of 341 children with AKI from 41 countries identified dehydration, infection, and primary kidney disease as the most common etiologies in low-income countries [38].

The primary risk factors for AKI include critical illness, comorbidities, and nephrotoxin use. The risk of AKI is greatest in critically ill children, in whom the incidence is about 30%. Major contributing factors include sepsis, multiorgan failure, hypotension, shock, congenital heart disease, nephrotoxins, and malignancy [35, 39–41]. Outcomes (including mortality and short- and long-term morbidity) in this population is directly related to AKI severity [42]. Critically ill neonates are also at high risk for AKI, in whom the incidence is also about 30% [36, 43]. Major contributing factors include very low birth weight, low gestational age, sepsis, congenital heart disease, and perinatal asphyxia [44, 45].

Nephrotoxin use is an important risk factor for pediatric AKI worldwide. Non-steroidal anti-inflammatory drugs (NSAIDs) are the most common culprits, accounting for up to 7% of AKI cases in hospitalized children. This risk is further increased in children with dehydration [46]. NSAIDs also cause sub-clinical AKI in children, as signaled by elevation of novel non-invasive biomarkers [47]. Other commonly implicated nephrotoxins include aminoglycosides, vancomycin, piperacillin-tazobactam, antiviral agents, angiotensin converting enzyme (ACE) inhibitors, and loop diuretics. Combinations amplify the risk [48, 49]. The overall risk of radiocontrast agents to cause AKI remains controversial but appears to be low in children with normal kidney function and with the dominant current practice of using low osmolar contrast agents. In a retrospective study of hospitalized children with GFR ≥60 mL/min/1.73 m² who underwent contrast-enhanced CT scanning, the AKI rate was only 2.2% [50].

The global incidence of AKI is higher in pediatric populations with severe chronic illness or underlying comorbid conditions. For example, AKI incidence is high in children with congenital heart disease that requires surgical intervention [51–58], malignancies [59, 60], hematopoietic stem cell transplants [61, 62], liver transplants [63], nephrotic syndrome relapse [64], or sickle cell vaso-occlusive pain crisis [65].

The worldwide COVID-19 pandemic has now added an important new etiology and risk factor for AKI. While this is a rapidly evolving field, recent published data indicate that hospitalized children with COVID-19 infections are at high risk for developing AKI, with an incidence of 20–30% [66–69]. The incidence is even higher—up to 46%—in children with multisystem inflammatory syndrome [70]. The pathogenesis of AKI in COVID-19 infection appears to be multifactorial, including direct viral infection of podocytes and proximal tubular cells, cytokine storm, macrophage activation syndrome, endothelial dysfunction, hypercoagulability, rhabdomyolysis, and complement-mediated injury. AKI in children with COVID-19 infections is directly associated with increased morbidity and mortality, and residual renal impairment at discharge [68, 69].

Clinical Classification

Traditionally, AKI has been classified based on the anatomic location of the initial injury, as prerenal (functional response of structurally normal kidneys to hypoperfusion), intrinsic renal (involving structural damage to the renal parenchyma), or postrenal (congenital or acquired anatomic obstruction to the lower urinary tract). This classification remains convenient for understanding mechanisms as well as the approach to diagnosis and management. With the discovery and validation of novel AKI functional and structural biomarkers discussed below, the terminology is

evolving to include functional, structural and even sub-clinical AKI to better depict the clinical situation and therapeutic response.

AKI may also be classified according to the clinical setting in which it occurs. Community-acquired AKI is more likely to be associated with a single insult, most commonly volume depletion, and is frequently reversible. The medical approach is often conservative, including discontinuing the insult, supportive fluid and electrolyte management, and awaiting spontaneous recovery of renal function. In contrast, hospital-acquired AKI, especially in the critical care setting, is frequently multifactorial, and often part of a more extensive multiorgan dysfunction. Management is more aggressive, with early initiation of renal replacement therapies to optimize the overall care of the patient. Recovery may be partial, and there are significant short- and long-term consequences.

AKI may also be classified according to the urine output, as being non-oliguric (urine output for greater than 6 h of >1 mL/kg/h in infants and >0.5 mL/kg/h in children), oliguric (urine output <1 mL/kg/h in infants, <0.5 mL/kg/h in children, or <400 mL/day in adults), anuric (no urine output), or polyuric (urine output >3 mL/kg/h). Measurement of urine output is especially useful in the critical care setting, since the degree of oliguria reflects the severity of the kidney injury, has important implications for fluid and electrolyte therapy, and provides prognostic information. However, even moderately severe forms of AKI due to nephrotoxins, and the majority of AKI seen in neonatal intensive care, are typically non-oliguric in nature. Furthermore, some children with AKI from ATN may present with polyuria due to a urinary concentrating defect, and polyuria is a characteristic of the recovery (diuretic) phase of AKI.

Functional AKI (Prerenal AKI, Volume-Responsive AKI)

Prerenal AKI is an appropriate functional response of structurally normal kidneys to hypoperfusion. It is the most common form of AKI encountered globally, is often community-acquired, and accounts for 40–55% of all cases. The oliguria in this situation represents a renal mechanism for preserving intravascular volume and has colloquially been termed as "acute renal success". Prerenal AKI is often caused by true volume depletion (e.g., dehydration, bleeding, excessive intestinal or cutaneous losses), early sepsis, or other etiologies leading to effective kidney hypoperfusion (decreased cardiac output, decreased intravascular volume, decreased blood pressure, or "third-spacing"). When prerenal AKI is caused by dehydration, it is usually rapidly reversed by restoration of renal perfusion. However, it is critical to understand that prerenal AKI does not automatically imply fluid responsiveness. AKI due to sepsis or decreased blood pressure often requires the administration of vasoactive agents in addition to fluid resuscitation. In some situations leading to prerenal AKI, such as liver failure, heart failure and nephrotic syndrome, fluid restriction is a mainstay of treatment. The common causes of prerenal AKI are listed in Table 51.2.

Pathophysiology of Prerenal AKI

The kidneys normally receive 25% of the cardiac output, and any decrease in circulatory volume evokes a systemic response leading to the release of potent vasoactive agents (Fig. 51.1). These responses help maintain perfusion to other organs by normalizing circulatory volume and blood pressure, but at the potential expense of GFR. There is an intense baroreceptor-mediated activation of the sympathetic nervous system and renin-angio-

Table 51.2 Common causes of prerenal AKI

Mechanism	Etiology
Volume depletion	Dehydration, hemorrhage, diuretics, burns, shock, nephrotic syndrome, diabetes
Decreased cardiac output	Cardiac failure, arrythmias
Peripheral vasodilatation	Sepsis, anaphylaxis, anti-hypertensive agents
Renal vasoconstriction	Sepsis, non-steroidal anti-inflammatory drugs, angiotensin converting enzyme inhibitors, hepatorenal syndrome

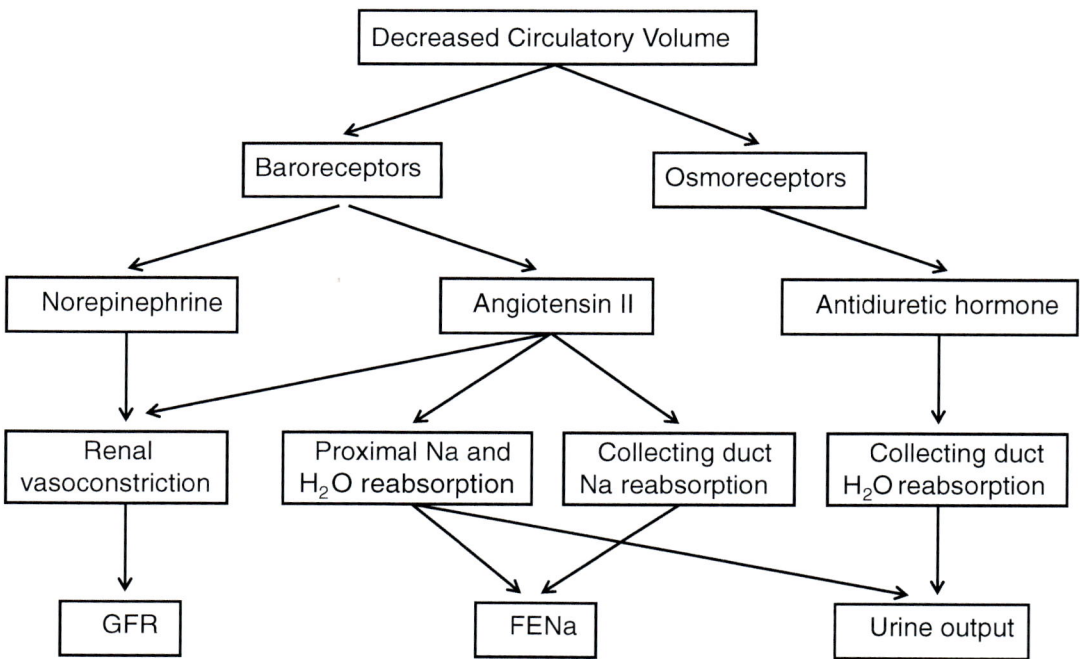

Fig. 51.1 Pathophysiology of prerenal AKI. These neurohormonal mechanisms are physiologically activated in the context of a reduction in effective circulatory volume, and result in an appropriate response by the kidney

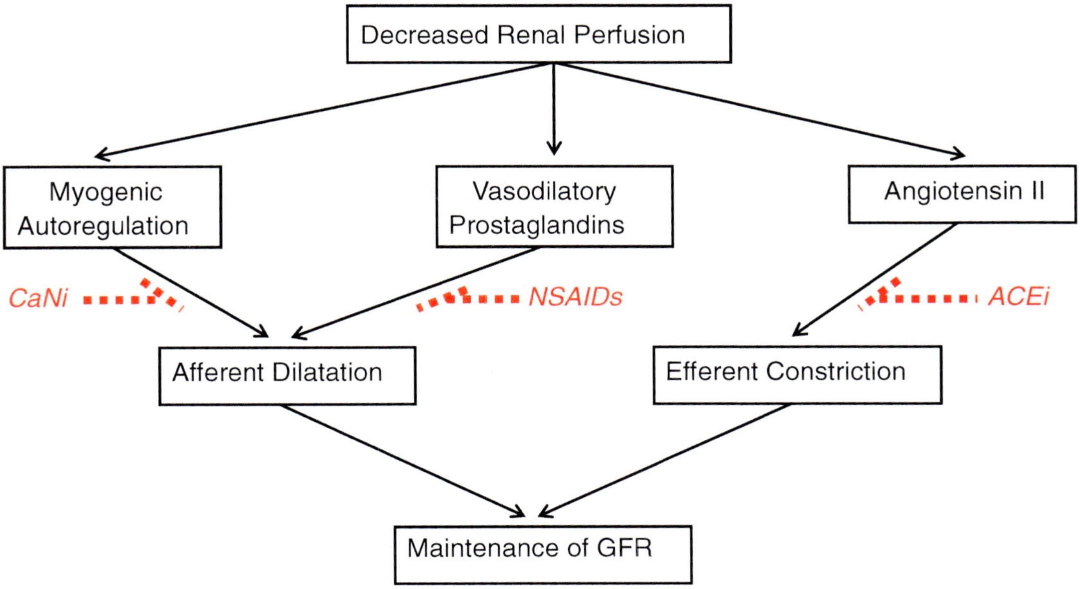

Fig. 51.2 Mechanisms that maintain GFR in prerenal AKI. Iatrogenic interference can precipitate a reduction in GFR. These include the use of calcineurin inhibitors (CaNi), non-steroidal anti-inflammatory drugs (NSAIDs), and angiotensin converting enzyme inhibitors (ACEi)

tensin axis, with resultant renal vasoconstriction mediated by angiotensin II and norepinephrine. Angiotensin II also promotes avid sodium and water reabsorption by the uninjured tubule cells, resulting in oliguria and a decreased fractional excretion of sodium that are the hallmarks of prerenal AKI. In addition, the release of anti-diuretic hormone in response to hypovolemia and a rise in extracellular osmolality results in enhanced water reabsorption by the intact collecting duct, which further contributes to the oliguria.

Concomitantly, at least three distinct intrarenal compensatory mechanisms are brought into play, which help maintain GFR in prerenal states (Fig. 51.2). Myogenic autoregulation refers to the rapid dilatation of the afferent arterioles in physiologic response to a reduction in lateral stretch following hypoperfusion. Calcineurin inhibitors such as tacrolimus and cyclosporine can interfere with the myogenic response and render the transplanted kidney more susceptible to prerenal azotemia. A more effective compensatory mechanism mediating afferent arteriolar dilatation involves the intrare-

nal production of vasodilatory prostaglandins [71]. Under normal physiologic conditions, the cyclooxygenase (constitutional COX-1 and inducible COX-2) enzyme systems catalyze the intrarenal production of prostaglandins that mediate afferent arteriolar dilatation. This system is dramatically upregulated by volume depletion. NSAIDs inhibit this response and can precipitate AKI, especially in the presence of decreased circulatory volume [72, 73]. For example, the use of postnatal indomethacin for patent ductus arteriosus closure in neonates results in AKI in as many as 40% of cases. When indomethacin is used to prevent preterm labor in pregnant women <32 weeks' gestation, the cumulative incidence of AKI within 15 days of life was 43.3% [74]. Another common pediatric scenario in which AKI might occur is the use of NSAIDs in febrile children with a dehydrating illness. In a recent meta-analysis, NSAIDs exposure was associated with an overall 1.6-fold rise in the odds of developing AKI in hospitalized pediatric patients [75]. A third mechanism for maintaining GFR involves the differential effect of angiotensin II on the efferent arteriole. While angiotensin II tends to constrict both the afferent and efferent arteriole, this effect is more marked in the efferent arteriole, leading to increased hydrostatic pressure across the glomerulus and consequent preservation of GFR [76]. Interference with this compensation occurs following ACE inhibitor therapy. In clinical practice, the use of ACE inhibitors appears to increase the incidence of AKI in patients at risk, as has been documented for patients undergoing cardiac surgery, both pre-operatively [77, 78] and post-operatively [79].

It should be noted that compensatory mechanisms that maintain GFR in prerenal AKI are overwhelmed during states of prolonged reduction in renal perfusion pressure, and intrinsic AKI can ensue. Thus, prerenal and intrinsic AKI are along a continuum of renal hypoperfusion states and can co-exist in clinical situations. Furthermore, in some situations, prerenal AKI may be persistent and progressively detrimental, as exemplified by patients with heart failure and liver disease.

Structural AKI (Intrinsic AKI)

Intrinsic AKI is most frequently caused by prolonged ischemia, exogenous nephrotoxins (drugs), endogenous nephrotoxins (myoglobinuria and hemoglobinuria), or sepsis (Table 51.3). Primary kidney etiologies for AKI include vascular disease (e.g., typical and atypical hemolytic uremic syndrome, thrombotic thrombocytopenic purpura, and vasculitides), glomerular disease (e.g., acute glomerulonephritis), and tubulointerstitial disease (e.g., infections and allergic drug reactions). Intrinsic AKI can be associated patho-

Table 51.3 Common causes of intrinsic AKI

Mechanism	Etiology
Acute tubular necrosis	Prolonged ischemia, nephrotoxins
Renal vascular diseases	Hemolytic uremic syndromes, vasculitis
Interstitial diseases	Interstitial nephritis, infections, infiltrations
Glomerulonephritis	Post-infectious, crescentic

logically with ATN. Consequently, it is common clinical practice to use the terms intrinsic AKI and ATN interchangeably. In the clinical setting, intrinsic AKI is frequently multifactorial, with concomitant ischemic, nephrotoxic, and septic components, and with overlapping pathogenetic mechanisms.

Morphology of Intrinsic AKI

ATN is a misnomer since frank tubular cell necrosis is rarely found in human AKI. Even in patients with lethal sepsis and AKI, histopathological findings on post-mortem kidney biopsies taken immediately after death display only limited inflammation, coagulation and cell death. Biopsy findings in other forms of human AKI are also typically paradoxically mild when compared to the severe depression in GFR. There is effacement and loss of proximal tubule apical brush border, disruption of microvilli, patchy loss of tubule cells with exposure of denuded basement membranes, focal proximal tubular dilatation and distal tubular casts, and areas of cellular regeneration. Necrotic cell death is restricted to the outer medullary regions (S3 segment of the proximal tubule and medullary thick ascending limb (mTAL) of Henle's loop). On the other hand, patchy apoptotic cell death has been reported in both distal and proximal tubules, in both ischemic and nephrotoxic forms of human AKI. The relative contribution of damage to the distal tubule adjacent to the S3 segment of the proximal tubule remains controversial. An intense inflammatory response, with peritubular accumulation of leukocytes, is typical in experimental models of AKI but is less prominent in human AKI. In addition, peritubular capillaries in the outer medulla display a striking vascular congestion. The molecular, biochemical, and cellular mechanisms underlying these morphologic changes have uncovered several novel pathways in animal models. This is an extensively studied and rapidly advancing field, and only selected mechanisms that are currently providing promising therapeutic approaches [80] are outlined below.

Alterations in Hemodynamics and Microcirculation

Intrinsic AKI is characterized by persistent hemodynamic abnormalities (Fig. 51.3). Total renal blood flow is reduced to about 50% of normal due to persistent renal vasoconstriction in established AKI, a finding that resulted in the classical term of "vasomotor nephropathy". More importantly, there are regional alterations in renal blood flow, with marked congestion of the outer medullary region. Oxygen tensions are normally lowest in this region that ironically contains tubular segments with the highest energy requirements, namely the S3 segment of the proximal tubule and mTAL. The post-ischemic congestion worsens the relative hypoxia, leading to prolonged injury and necrotic cell death in these segments.

Mechanisms underlying these hemodynamic alterations relate primarily to renal microcirculatory and endothelial damage [81]. The renal microcirculation normally plays a crucial role in maintaining the kidney's functional and structural integrity. However, alterations in microcirculation and oxygenation due to endothelial damage can result in AKI regardless of systemic hemodynamic changes. At the sub-cellular level, AKI-induced mitochondrial damage is a prominent finding in endothelial injury [82]. This leads to a local imbalance of vasoactive substances, including enhanced release of the vasoconstrictor endothelin and reduced release of vasodilatory endothelium-derived nitric oxide (NO). There is substantial evidence from human AKI studies to indicate that endothelial dysfunction results in increased incidence, worsened severity, and prolonged duration of AKI. Plasma levels of endothelin, a potent vasoconstrictor, are increased (and NO levels decreased) in humans with septic AKI. However, while endothelin receptor antagonists ameliorate ischemic AKI in animals, human data are lacking. A human trial of an endothelin receptor antagonist for prevention of contrast-induced AKI resulted in a paradoxical exacerbation of nephrotoxicity. Several newer endothelin receptor blockers have recently been developed for potential use in hypertension and CKD and may hold promise in human AKI.

Similarly, carbon monoxide (CO) and carbon monoxide-releasing molecules have been shown to be protective in animal models of ischemic AKI, likely through vasodilatation and preservation of medullary blood flow as well as cytoprotective and immunomodulatory properties. However, much work is needed in translating these findings to humans, including determination of safe CO dosage, duration of treatment, and frequency of treatment for a given indication. NO, produced in renal endothelial and tubule cells from L-arginine by constitutive and induc-

Fig. 51.3
Pathophysiology of intrinsic AKI—hemodynamic alterations and their consequences

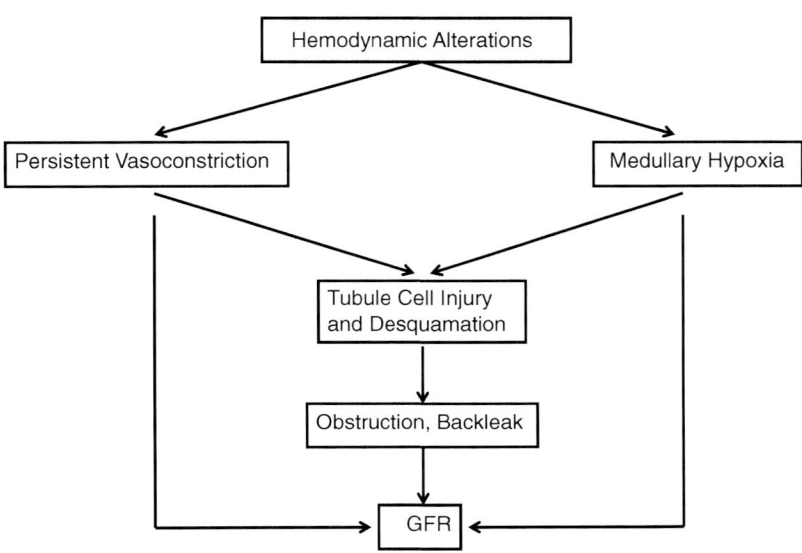

ible NO synthetases (NOS), is also a known renal vasodilator. In a recent meta-analysis of five adult human studies, inhaled NO gas was associated with a reduced risk of AKI after cardiopulmonary bypass surgery with no adverse effects [83]. However, further studies are needed to determine the optimal dosage, timing and duration of NO administration in human AKI.

In the final analysis, it is now apparent that while hemodynamic abnormalities play an important role in the initial phases of AKI, they alone cannot fully account for the profound loss of renal function in established human AKI. Not surprisingly, several human trials of vasodilators have failed to convincingly demonstrate improvement in GFR in established AKI despite augmentation of overall renal blood flow. Persistent renal vasoconstriction may, in fact, represent an adaptive protective mechanism to minimize further cellular injury during the reperfusion period.

Alterations in Tubule Dynamics

Three well known derangements in tubular dynamics in intrinsic AKI include obstruction, back-leak, and activation of tubuloglomerular feedback. The consistent finding of proximal tubular dilatation and distal tubular casts in human AKI are indicative of obstruction to tubular fluid flow. The intraluminal casts stain strongly for Tamm-Horsfall protein, which is normally secreted by the thick ascending limb as a monomer. Conversion into a gel-like polymer is enhanced by the increased luminal sodium concentration typically encountered in the distal tubule in AKI because of impaired proximal tubule sodium reabsorption. This provides an ideal environment for cast formation along with desquamated tubule cells and brush border membranes. Cell death, most prominently noted in the highly susceptible outer medullary regions (S3 segment) of the proximal tubule, provides the sloughed cells and brush borders, with subsequent cellular cast formation and intratubular obstruction. However, it is unlikely that obstruction alone can account for the profound dysfunction in clinical AKI, since human studies using

forced diuresis with furosemide or mannitol did not improve the renal recovery rate of patients with established AKI in most reported studies [84, 85]. Similarly, although movement of the glomerular filtrate back into the circulation has been shown to occur because of intratubular obstruction, this accounts for only a very minor component of the decrease in GFR in human AKI.

A role for activation of tubuloglomerular feedback has been proposed. By physiologic considerations, the increased delivery of sodium chloride to the macula densa due to abnormalities in the injured proximal tubule would be expected to induce afferent arteriolar constriction, mediated by adenosine via A1 adenosine receptor (A1AR) activation, and thereby decrease GFR. Thus, research efforts have focused on specific adenosine receptor antagonists as potential therapeutic agents, since tubuloglomerular feedback activation following ischemic injury may represent a beneficial phenomenon that limits wasteful delivery of ions and solutes to the damaged tubules, thereby reducing the demand for adenosine triphosphate (ATP)-dependent resorptive processes. The protective effects of adenosine inhibition on renal blood flow preservation may be mediated via more selective adenosine receptor activation, and the use of broad-spectrum adenosine receptor antagonists such as theophylline and caffeine is a subject of renewed clinical investigation [86–88].

Alterations in Tubule Cell Metabolism

The various cell types along the nephron display segment-specific susceptibilities to different types of injury, based on their metabolic requirements. The highly active proximal tubule cells need a steady oxygen supply to remain viable, whereas those in the thick ascending limb are relatively resistant to hypoxia. Epithelial cells in the straight segment (S3 segment) of the proximal tubule are most vulnerable to ischemic injury since they are highly dependent on oxidative phosphorylation for energy. The S1 and S2 segments are affected most by toxic nephropathy because of their high rates of endocytosis. The mTAL is particularly vulnerable since it exists in a hypoxic precipice, with low oxygen tension but high oxygen consumption.

A profound reduction in intracellular ATP content is a hallmark of AKI that occurs very early after injury. Approximately 90% of renal intracellular ATP becomes depleted within 10 min of ischemic injury. With reperfusion, ATP levels recover in a bimodal fashion. There is an initial rapid but incomplete (up to 70% of normal) recovery phase, generated by re-phosphorylation of residual adenine nucleotides (ADP and AMP). This is followed by a second slower phase of ATP recovery, which requires resynthesis from purine nucleotide degradation products and salvage pathways. ATP depletion triggers several metabolic consequences in tubule cells. Events that provide insights into potential clinical interventions are detailed below, and their inter-relationship is illustrated in Fig. 51.4.

Alterations in tubule cell adenine nucleotide metabolism have been well documented. Oxygen deprivation leads to a rapid degradation of ATP to

AMP and to hypoxanthine. These metabolites are freely diffusible, and their depletion precludes rapid re-synthesis of ATP during reperfusion. Provision of exogenous adenine nucleotides or thyroxine (which stimulates mitochondrial ATP regeneration) can ameliorate the cellular injury in animal models of ischemic AKI. However, a recent systematic review found a paucity of large, high-quality studies to inform analysis of thyroid hormone interventions for the treatment of humans with AKI. Current evidence suggests that thyroid hormone therapy may be associated with worse outcomes for patients with established AKI; therefore, its use for these patients should be avoided.

ATP depletion leads to impaired calcium sequestration within the endoplasmic reticulum, as well as diminished extrusion of cytosolic calcium into the extracellular space. The resultant increase in free intracellular calcium has been documented following AKI, but its role has remained controversial. Increased intracellular calcium could potentially lead to activation of proteases and phospholipases and cytoskeletal

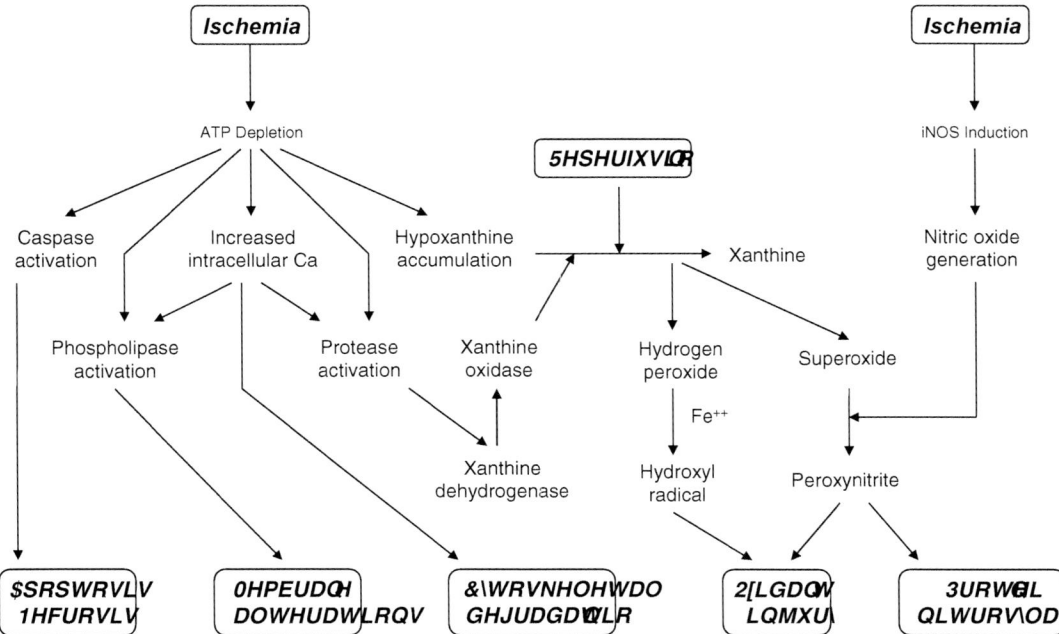

Fig. 51.4 Metabolic consequences of acute ischemia and reperfusion injury to kidney tubule cells. Inhibition of these pathways may provide novel therapeutic approaches to AKI

degradation. A previous meta-analysis suggested that calcium channel blockers may provide some protection from renal injury in the kidney transplant setting, but evidence for their efficacy in other forms of AKI is currently lacking. Any benefit from intracellular calcium blockade may be counterbalanced by the hypotension induced by these agents, with resultant worsening of AKI.

Abundant experimental, and to a lesser extent clinical data, now support a critical role for oxidative stress-related mechanisms in the early injury phase of AKI. Oxidative stress refers to metabolic disturbances, such as increased production of reactive oxygen species (ROS) that leads to the depletion of endogenous antioxidants with resultant cellular damage, dysfunction of proteins, and damage to DNA, lipids, and enzymes. Specifically, there is now substantial evidence for the role of ROS in the pathogenesis of intrinsic AKI. During reperfusion, the conversion of accumulated hypoxanthine to xanthine generates hydrogen peroxide and superoxide (Fig. 51.4). In the presence of iron, hydrogen peroxide forms the highly reactive hydroxyl radical. Concomitantly, ischemia induces NO synthase in tubule cells, and the NO generated interacts with superoxide to form peroxynitrate, which results in cell damage via oxidant injury as well as protein nitrosylation. ROS can cause renal tubule cell injury by oxidation of proteins, peroxidation of lipids, damage to DNA, and induction of apoptosis and autophagy. Studies have documented a dramatic increase in oxidative stress and autophagy, and reduction in antioxidant pathways, in experimental and human AKI. Several scavengers of ROS (such as superoxide dismutase, catalase, and N-acetylcysteine) protect against ischemic AKI in animal models, but human studies have been inconclusive or negative, except for prevention of contrast-induced AKI.

Free iron derived from red cells or other injured cells is one of the most potent factors in the generation of ROS, and the iron scavenger deferoxamine alleviates ischemia-reperfusion injury in animal models and in human clinical trials. However, the systemic toxicity of deferoxamine (hypotension and ocular toxicity) precludes its routine clinical use in human

AKI. Several other molecules are under study for iron chelation [89]. Other potential approaches to minimize the nephrotoxic effects of iron and iron-containing proteins under investigation include administration of haptoglobin to facilitate sequestration of free hemoglobin, administration of hepcidin to prevent iron export from intracellular compartments into the circulation, and pharmacologic upregulation of heme oxygenase-1 (HO1) to accelerate the catabolism of toxic free heme.

Alterations in Tubule, Endothelial, and Glomerular Cell Structure

The cell biologic response of intrinsic kidney cells to ischemic or nephrotoxic AKI is multifaceted, and includes loss of cell polarity and brush borders, cell death, de-differentiation of viable cells, proliferation, and restitution of a normal epithelium, as illustrated in Fig. 51.5. While most prominently described in tubule epithelial cells, structural alterations in the endothelial and glomerular cell cytoskeleton are also of consequence. The major mechanisms underlying this morphologic sequence of events are summarized below.

Cellular ATP depletion results in an early, rapid disruption of the apical actin cytoskeleton and redistribution of actin from the apical domain and microvilli into the cytoplasm. This results in loss of brush border membranes, which contribute to cast formation and obstruction. Intracellular actin released from damaged tubule cells appears in the urine of patients with AKI. Similar changes in endothelial cells may potentiate vascular injury.

Disruption of the apical cytoskeleton also results in loss of tight (zonula occludens) junctions and zonula adherens junctions. Reduced expression, redistribution, and abnormal aggregation of several key proteins that constitute the tight and adherens junctions have been documented after ischemic injury in cell culture, animal models, and human studies. Loss of cadherin staining in the vascular endothelium also suggests that cadherin junctions are altered during injury.

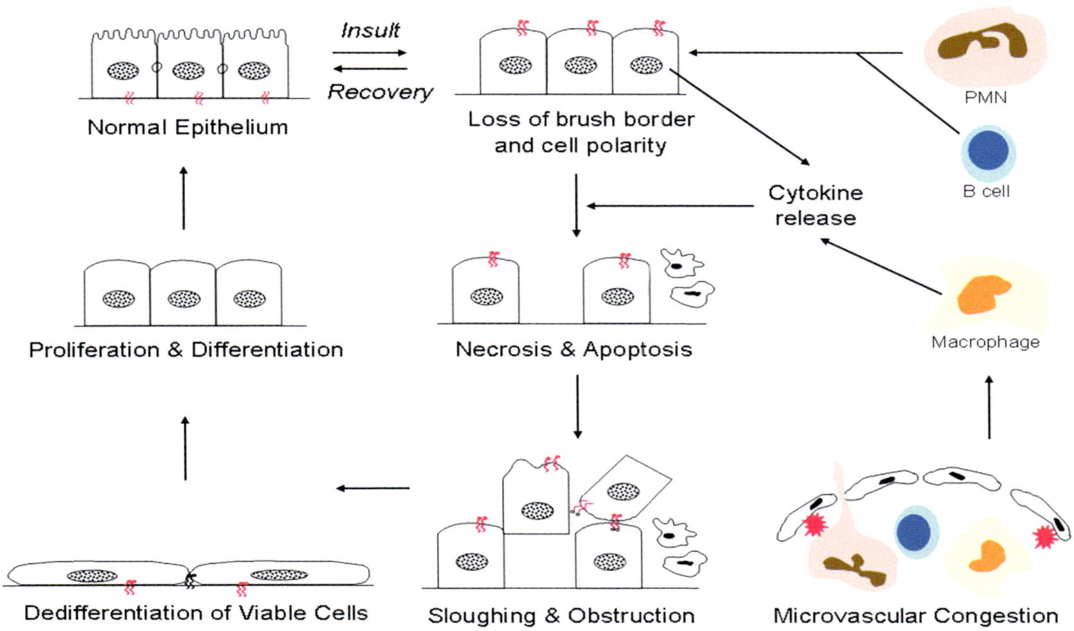

Fig. 51.5 Structural consequences of acute ischemia and reperfusion injury to kidney tubule cells. Novel therapeutic approaches in AKI have targeted prevention of cell death, inhibition of inflammation, and acceleration of the endogenous recovery process

The consequent loss of tight junction barrier function can potentially magnify the transtubular back-leak of glomerular filtrate induced by obstruction. Ischemic injury can also result in podocyte-specific molecular and cellular changes. In healthy podocytes, Neph1 (a component of the podocyte slit diaphragm) complexes with ZO-1 (an actin-related tight junction protein), to link tight junctions to the cortical actin skeleton, thereby providing a structural framework for the slit diaphragm. Slit diaphragms are an important component of the glomerular filtration barrier, and damage to slit diaphragms can lead to impaired filtration. Ischemia induces the dissociation of Neph1 from ZO-1, which results in podocyte effacement and loss of the Neph1-ZO-1 interaction. Although the interaction can be restored after reperfusion, the recovery of podocyte structure is often incomplete.

Other changes occur in the glomerulus during AKI. Podocyte foot processes coarsen during injury, and there is a decrease in heparin sulfate proteoglycan and sialic acid on the endothelial surface layer, which can lead to albuminuria and decrease GFR. Tumour necrosis factor-alpha (TNF-α) has been implicated as a mechanism mediating AKI via glomerular abnormalities. Mice deficient in TNFR1 have normal glomerular morphology and density with minimal cellular detachment, suggesting that TNF-α mediates damage to the glomerular endothelium and is a key determinant of AKI in sepsis.

Ischemic and nephrotoxic insults also result in the early disruption of at least two normally basolaterally polarized proteins, namely Na,K-ATPase and integrins. The Na,K-ATPase is normally tethered to the spectrin-based cytoskeleton at the basolateral domain via the adapter protein ankyrin, where it functions to pump intracellular sodium into the circulation. This provides the driving force for the normal reabsorption of salt and water by the proximal tubule via the apical membrane. A physiologic consequence of the loss of basolateral Na,K-ATPase is impaired proximal tubule sodium reabsorption and a consequent increase in fractional excretion of sodium, which are diagnostic signatures of intrinsic AKI.

The β-1 integrins are normally polarized to the basal domain, where they mediate cell-substratum adhesions. Tubule cell injury leads to a redistribution of integrins to the apical membrane, with consequential detachment of viable cells from the basement membrane. This is followed by abnormal adhesion between these exfoliated cells within the tubular lumen, mediated by an interaction between apical integrin and the Arg-Gly-Asp (i.e., RGD) motif of integrin receptors. Administration of synthetic RGD compounds attenuates tubular obstruction and renal impairment in animal models of ischemic AKI, and the recent availability of orally active integrin antagonists as well as small-molecule peptidomimetics that inhibit RGD-binding integrins holds promise for clinical application in human AKI.

Alterations in Tubule Cell Death

Injured tubule epithelial cells may suffer one of several distinct cellular fates after AKI. Most cells remain viable, suggesting that they either escape injury or are only sub-lethally injured and undergo recovery. A subset of tubule cells displays patchy cell death resulting from at least five pathophysiologic mechanisms: necrosis, apoptosis, necroptosis, ferroptosis, and autophagy. Necrosis is an explosive, unregulated, chaotic process characterized by loss of membrane integrity, cytoplasmic swelling, and cellular fragmentation. Apoptosis is a quiet, regulated, orderly demise typified by cytoplasmic and nuclear shrinkage, DNA fragmentation, and breakdown of the cell into membrane-bound apoptotic bodies that are rapidly cleared by phagocytosis. Clearing dead cells and associated cellular debris is an integral part of tissue homeostasis. While diverse types of phagocytes remove various forms of dying cells during AKI, it remains unknown whether boosting removal of a specific form of dying cell would provide a benefit and which cell type should be targeted for phagocytosis-mediated therapy. Necrosis and apoptosis can coexist and are considered to present two ends of a spectrum. In AKI, the mode of cell death depends primarily on the severity of the insult and the resistance of the cell type. Necrosis occurs after more severe injury and in the more susceptible nephron segments and often is characterized by the activation of phospholipase A2, calpain, and eicosanoids. In contrast, apoptosis predominates after less severe injury, especially in the ischemia-resistant distal nephron segments. Apoptosis can be followed by "secondary necrosis," especially if the apoptotic cells are not removed rapidly.

Apoptosis is a major mechanism of early tubule cell death in contemporary clinical AKI, and considerable attention has been directed toward dissecting the molecular mechanisms involved. Several pathways, including the intrinsic (Bcl-2 family, cytochrome c, caspase 9) extrinsic (Fas, FADD, caspase 8), and regulatory (p53, NF-κB) factors, appear to be activated by ischemic and nephrotoxic AKI, as illustrated in Fig. 51.6. The extrinsic pathway functions by binding death ligands to cell-surface receptor, resulting in procaspase-8 activation, often through mediation with adaptor proteins such as Fas-associated protein with death domain (FADD) or TNF receptor 1-associated death domain. The role of the Fas-FADD pathway in animal models was suggested by demonstration of upregulation of these proteins in apoptotic tubule cells after ischemia and the functional protection afforded by siRNA duplexes targeting the Fas gene. However, convincing human data are lacking. On the other hand, growing evidence implicates an imbalance between the pro-apoptotic (Bax, Bid) and anti-apoptotic (Bcl-2, Bcl-xL) members of the Bcl-2 family in animals and humans so affected. Disequilibrium between Bac/Bcl-2 and Bad/Bid can lead to the formation of mitochondrial pores, which alters cell viability. The proapoptotic transcription factor p53 is activated by HIF-1α and induced at the mRNA and protein levels, and straddles both the intrinsic and extrinsic pathways. Inhibition of p53 by pifithrin-α suppresses ischemia-induced apoptosis by inhibiting transcriptional activation of Bax and mitochondrial translocation of p53. However, pifithrin-α is an unlikely candidate for therapeu-

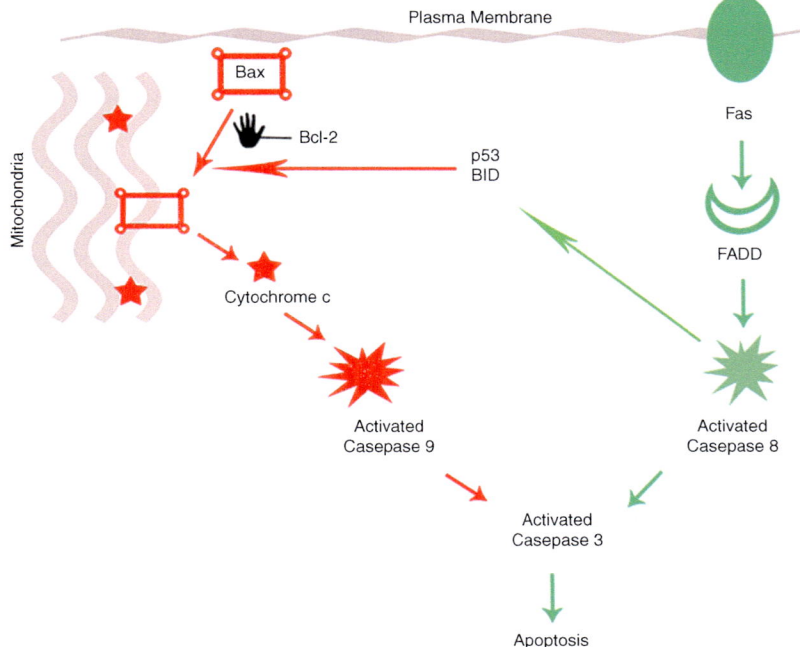

Fig. 51.6 Major tubule cell apoptotic pathways in human AKI. The extrinsic pathway (green) requires activation of Fas and TNF-R1, with subsequent signal transduction and activation of caspase 8. The intrinsic pathway (red) requires translocation of Bax to the mitochondria, thereby releasing cytochrome c and activation of caspase 9. Crosstalk between these pathways is provided largely by the regulatory molecule p53. Inhibition of the central regulatory molecule p53 and the terminal executor caspases hold promise in human AKI

tic consideration in humans because generalized inhibition of p53-dependent apoptosis is likely to promote survival of damaged or mutation-bearing cells in other organ systems. Studies have examined the efficacy of p53 si-RNA as a potential therapeutic agent, as administration of the treatment decreased serum creatinine and tubular necrosis in animal models. Clinical trials examining the effects of p53 si-RNA in human AKI are underway. A recent promising prospective, multicenter, double-blind, randomized, controlled phase 2 trial evaluated the efficacy and safety of a single 10 mg/kg dose of the p53 si-RNA teprasiran in reducing the incidence, severity, and duration of AKI after cardiac surgery in high-risk adult patients [90]. AKI incidence was 37% for teprasiran versus 50% for placebo-treated patients. AKI severity and duration were also improved with teprasiran: 2.5% of teprasiran versus 6.7% of placebo-treated patients had grade 3 AKI; 7% teprasiran versus 13% placebo-treated

patients had AKI lasting for 5 days. No safety issues were identified with teprasiran treatment. Results of larger phase 3 studies, as well as investigations in other forms of AKI, are awaited.

Inhibition of other apoptotic pathways also hold promise for clinical application in human AKI. Caspase activation is by and large the final common "execution" step in apoptosis, and cell-permeant caspase inhibitors have provided particularly attractive targets for study. Currently available caspase inhibitors have largely been investigated only in animals, provide only partial protection, and are most effective when administered before the insult. A vast plethora of other agents, including mesenchymal stem cells, curcumin, erythropoietin (EPO), N-acetyl cysteine, thioredoxin, TNF-α antagonists, A1 adenosine receptor agonists, peroxisome proliferator-activated receptor ligands, NGAL, and poly(ADP-ribose) polymerase inhibitors (to name a few) have all provided encouraging structural and functional protection from experimental AKI, with inhibition of apoptosis and inflammation. Some of these agents are already widely available and have been used safely in other human conditions, and additional results with their use in human AKI should be forthcoming. Challenges for the future clinical use of apoptosis inhibition in AKI include determining the best timing of therapy, optimizing the specificity of inhibitor, minimizing the extrarenal side effects, and tubule-specific targeting of the apoptosis-modulatory maneuvers. The issue of timing is especially important, since inhibiting early cell death may be beneficial but interfering with late onset apoptosis is envisioned to interfere with the removal of dead and unwanted cells.

Necroptosis refers to a programmed cell death that is characterized by caspase-independent regulated necrosis resulting in plasma membrane rupture and subsequent release of damage-associated molecular patterns (DAMPs). Like apoptosis, necroptosis may be induced by multiple extracellular and intracellular stimuli, including tumor necrosis factor (TNF) family members, Fas ligands, interferon, and oxidative stress. However, the downstream mechanisms in necroptosis are distinct, independent of caspase activation, and the resultant cell death is characterized by several necrotic features, including a lack of chromatin condensation or DNA fragmentation. Several novel therapeutic agents that inhibit necroptosis pathways have already shown efficacy in experimental studies, and human translation appears to be promising.

Ferroptosis, a distinct form of iron-dependent cell death now well described in ischemia-reperfusion injuries in organs including the kidney, is characterized primarily by intracellular iron accumulation and lipid peroxidation. Morphologically, ferroptotic cells display mitochondrial changes, including reduced volume, increased membrane density, and decreased mitochondrial cristae and rupture of the outer mitochondrial membrane. The cell nucleus becomes devoid of chromatin condensation. Eventually, the cell membranes rupture and cell death occurs. Targeted regulation of ferroptosis and its signalling pathways are achieving promising results.

The study of autophagy as another mechanism of altered cell viability in AKI has been a topic of considerable recent attention. Autophagy is a physiologic process by which intracellular damaged macromolecules and organelles are degraded and recycled for the synthesis of new cellular components. The process of autophagy involves the formation of a double-membrane structure known as an autophagosome, which first sequesters the cellular constituents and subsequently delivers them to the lysosome for degradation. This results in the recycling of degraded products for the biosynthesis of new cellular components and for meeting the energy needs of the cell. The autophagy process uses lysosomal hydrolases to degrade large intracellular heterogeneous misfolded proteins, protein aggregates, damaged macromolecules, and even entire damaged organelles. Recent progress in identifying the interplay of autophagy, apoptosis, and regulated necrosis has revealed common pathways and molecules in this crosstalk during the pathogenesis of AKI. Autophagy and its associated pathways may pose potentially unique targets for therapeutic interventions in AKI.

The mechanisms whereby most tubule cells escape cell death and either emerge unscathed or recover completely after AKI remain under active investigation. HSPs have surfaced as potential mediators of this cytoprotection. Induction of HSPs is part of a highly conserved innate cellular response that is activated swiftly and robustly after ischemic AKI. The heat shock response is particularly robust in immature kidneys and may form the basis for the common observation that subsequent AKI is less likely to develop in premature infants than adults. Maneuvers that enhance the innate HSP response have potential benefit in human AKI, but clinical evidence is lacking.

Alterations in Tubule Cell Proliferation and Differentiation

Surviving renal tubule cells possess a remarkable ability to regenerate and proliferate after AKI. Morphologically, repair is heralded by the appearance of de-differentiated epithelial cells that express vimentin, a marker for multipotent mesenchymal cells. These cells most likely represent surviving tubule cells that have de-differentiated. In the next phase, the cells upregulate genes encoding a variety of growth factors, such as insulin-like growth factor-1 (IGF-1), hepatocyte growth factor (HGF), and fibroblast growth factor (FGF), and undergo marked proliferation. In the final phase, cells express differentiation factors, such as neural cell adhesion molecule and osteopontin, and undergo re-differentiation until the normal fully polarized epithelium is restored. Thus, during recovery, renal tubule cells recapitulate phases and processes very similar to those during normal kidney development. Emerging data suggest that no pre-existing proximal tubule stem cell population exists, but rather all differentiated proximal tubule cells possess the capacity to proliferate during repair by de-differentiation and self-duplication.

In response to acute injury, animal studies have shown that the surviving, normally quiescent proximal tubule epithelial cells rapidly de-differentiate, proliferate, and enter the S-phase of the cell cycle. Understanding the molecular mechanisms of cell cycle re-entry may provide clues towards accelerating recovery from AKI. With mild injury, these endogenous repair mechanisms can result in the return to a normal structural and functional state. However, when the repair is more severe or dysregulated, the repair process can lead to fibrosis, which can facilitate progression to CKD. Recent experimental data have redefined the role of the surviving epithelial cells in fibrosis. After severe injury, the proximal tubule cell proliferative response is altered due to cell cycle arrest at the G2/M phase, resulting in generation of profibrotic factors including cytokines, growth factors and matrix proteins. Inhibition of the identified profibrotic factors may hold promise in preventing the AKI to CKD transition. For example, HGF is renoprotective and renotrophic in animal models of AKI, because of its proliferative, antiapoptotic, and anti-inflammatory actions. The use of HGF in humans, however, has been hampered at least in part by the widespread expression of its receptor,

raising the possibility of extrarenal side effects. Recent studies have explored the effects of BB3/ANG3777, a small molecule with strong HGF-like activity, which, when first administered at 24 h after renal ischemia in rats, improved survival, augmented urine output, and improved kidney function. BB3/ANG3777 is currently being tested in renal transplant patients. In the case of IGF-1, enthusiasm for its renoprotective effects has been dampened by its exacerbation of inflammation and neutrophil infiltration in the post-ischemic kidney in animals. Human trials with recombinant IGF-1 have not demonstrated a beneficial effect. New growth factors have emerged as potential therapeutic targets that may accelerate renal recovery, including epidermal growth factor and α-melanocyte stimulating hormone (α-MSH), which likely acts via direct hemodynamic effects. α-MSH is an efficacious anti-inflammatory and antiapoptotic cytokine and protects from ischemic, nephrotoxic, and septic AKI in animal models. However, α-MSH therapy was not effective in human AKI trials.

Identification of the source of multipotent mesenchymal cells involved in the regeneration and repair process has been a matter of intense contemporary research. It is now established that renal tubule cells are capable of regeneration, instead of regeneration being driven by an extrarenal progenitor population. Current literature suggests that proximal tubule cells undergo transient de-differentiation after injury and then proliferate to repopulate the tubule. However, mesenchymal stem cells (MSCs) may have important autocrine, paracrine, and growth factor-like effects on kidney regeneration. MSCs are drawn to renal tubules that produce stromal cell-derived factor 1 and remain in the injured kidney for a short period of time. They secrete various growth factors that mediate kidney repair. Administered MSCs clearly enhance recovery from ischemic AKI in animals and recently were tested in clinical settings. Modified MSCs, which were modified to be immune privileged and genetically stable, were tested as a therapy for human AKI. In a cohort of adult patients with AKI after cardiac surgery, administration of allogeneic MSCs did not decrease the time to recovery of kidney function. Endothelial progenitor cells (EPCs) are bone marrow-derived precursors that promote tubular regeneration in the kidney after ischemic injury. Microvesicles from EPCs can protect the kidney from ischemic injury, likely by delivering microRNA that reprograms resident renal cells to a regenerative program. Rats treated with EPC microvesicles had a reduced number of tubular lesions, improved kidney function, reduced apoptosis, and increased tubular proliferation. Six months after ischemic injury, rats showed less fibrosis and glomerulosclerosis, suggesting that EPC vesicles have long-term beneficial renoprotective effects in experimental animals.

Alterations in the Microvasculature

The role of endothelial alterations and endothelial dysfunction in the initiation and extension of AKI has received increasing attention. Morphologically, disruption of the actin cytoskeleton and junctional complexes, like those previously described in tubule epithelial cells, have been documented in endothelial cells in experimental AKI. Consequent endothelial cell swelling, blebbing, and death, with detachment of viable cells, have been observed, and circulating endothelial cells have been demonstrated in humans with septic shock. Sites of endothelial denudation are prone to prolonged vasoconstriction, and systemic or intrarenal administration of fully differentiated endothelial cells into post-ischemic rat kidneys results in functional protection. Furthermore, ischemic injury leads to a marked upregulation of angiostatin, a well-known antiangiogenic factor that induces apoptosis of endothelial cells. Collectively, these findings provide a rationale for the use of pro-angiogenic agents that can increase the pool of or mobilize endothelial progenitor cells. These agents include bone morphogenic protein (BMP), VEGF, statins, and EPO; their putative roles in AKI are currently under investigation. In particular, statins have been shown in pre-clinical studies to ameliorate AKI development via several microvascular mechanisms, including inhibition of vascular superoxide generation and restoration of endothelial derived NO synthase activity. The role of statins in clinical AKI remains controversial. In a recent large retrospective review of adult patients undergoing open cardiac surgery, preoperative statin exposure was a protective factor against all stages of postoperative cardiac surgery associated AKI as well as stage 3 AKI (OR, 0.671, 95% CI, 0.567–0.795), after adjusting for confounding factors [91]. These findings support the need for a larger prospective randomized controlled trial of AKI in adults and children, especially since several commonly available statins are approved for use in children over 8–10 years of age.

EPO is a well-known potent stimulator of erythroid progenitor cells and is commonly used to treat anemia in both children and adults with CKD. In animal models of ischemic AKI, EPO has protective effects via amelioration of microvascular injury as well as additional anti-apoptotic and anti-inflammatory mechanisms. However, several clinical trials in adults with AKI have yielded mixed results. In a meta-analysis of controlled trials in adult patients either at high risk for AKI or following kidney transplant, no reduction of incidence of AKI and no reduction in delayed graft function or improvement in 1-year graft survival after renal transplantation could be documented. Furthermore, in a recent study of extremely low gestational age neonates, EPO did not protect from any AKI or from severe AKI [92].

AKI also leads to increased endothelial expression of a variety of adhesion molecules that promote endothelium-leukocyte interactions. These include intracellular adhesion molecule-1 (ICAM-1), P-selectin, E-selectin, B7-1, vascular adhesion molecule-1 (VCAM-1), and thrombomodulin (TM). Endothelial cells are also involved with coagulation processes via interactions with protein C and TM. Derangements in the coagulation cascade, such as alterations in tissue-type plasminogen activator and plasminogen activator inhibitor-1 in the kidney, may account for the fibrin deposits characteristically found in the renal microvasculature after ischemic injury. The pathways and mechanisms that are involved in formation of interstitial fibrosis after AKI have been examined. Impaired endothelial proliferation and mesenchymal transition processes contribute to vascular dysfunction after AKI. In contrast with tubule epithelial cells, cells of the renal vasculature lack an efficient regenerative capacity, which results in a persistent 30–50% reduction in vascular density after ischemic injury. Vascular dropout likely promotes hypoxia and impairs hemodynamic and sodium regulatory responses in the kidney after AKI and may augment the progression of CKD. Endothelial-to-mesenchymal transition may explain the loss of renal microvessels and the deposition of interstitial fibroblasts, which are seen during ischemic AKI recovery. Numerous genes and molecules have been identified as contributing to kidney fibrosis, including platelet-derived growth factor receptor-β (PDGFR-β), metalloproteinase inhibitor 3 (encoded by the TIMP-3 gene), a disintegrin and metalloproteinase with thrombospondin motifs 1 (encoded by ADAMTS1 gene), transforming growth factor β (TGF-β), and angiotensin II (Ang II).

Alterations in the Inflammatory Response

A growing body of evidence indicates that the inflammatory response plays a major role in ischemic AKI, including particularly in COVID-19 associated AKI [93]. The major components of this response include endothelial injury, leukocyte recruitment, and production of inflammatory mediators by tubule cells. Inflammatory cascades initiated by endothelial dysfunction can be augmented by the generation of several potent mediators by the injured proximal tubule (Fig. 51.5). These include proinflammatory cytokines (TNF-α, IL-6, and IL-1β) and the chemotactic cytokines (MCP-1, IL-8, RANTES). Human studies have shown that the plasma levels of the pro-inflammatory cytokines TNF-α, IL-6 and IL-8 are elevated in AKI and predict mortality. Toll-like receptors (TLRs) represent a major component of this pro-inflammatory response. TLRs are membrane-associated glycoproteins that primarily mediate the function of innate immunity upon induction with pathogen-associated molecular patterns, with resultant production of various pro-inflammatory cytokines and chemokines via intracellular activation of signalling cascades to eliminate the infective agents. TLRs also recognize endogenous host material released during cellular injury, rendering TLRs as crucial surveillance receptors to detect cellular injury. In the kidney, TLRs are expressed primarily in proximal and distal tubule cells. Renal tubular expression of TLR2 is enhanced after ischemic AKI, and TLR2 gene silencing by knockout and antisense treatment prevents ischemia-induced renal dysfunction, neutrophil influx, tubule apoptosis, and induction of MCP-1, TNF-α, IL-6, and IL-1β. Toll-like receptor 4 (TLR4) recently was suggested as another mediator of tubule cell injury. Activation of TLR4 supports the liberation of pro-inflammatory mediators, promotes leukocyte migration and infiltration, and triggers both innate and adaptive immune systems. Mice lacking TLR4 were observed to have reduced tubular damage and fewer proinflammatory cytokines after renal injury. Several compounds have been shown to offer renoprotection via inhibition of TLR4 in experimental animals. Many of these are safe for use in humans, rendering TLR4 inhibition as a novel therapeutic approach in clinical AKI.

Morphologically, several leukocyte subtypes have been shown to aggregate in peritubular capillaries, interstitial space, and even within the tubules after ischemic AKI, and their relative roles remain under investigation. These include neutrophils, macrophages, dendritic cells, B cells and T cells. Neutrophils are the earliest to accumulate in the postischemic kidney and often are found in the peritubular capillary network of the outer medulla, where they adhere to endothelial cells and can cause capillary plugging and congestion. Neutrophils also migrate into the interstitium and increase vascular permeability which aggravates tubular injury. Neutrophil depletion or blockade of neutrophil function provides partial functional protection in some but not all animal models. Furthermore, neutrophils are not a prominent feature of ischemic AKI in humans, casting doubt on the clinical significance of neutrophil infiltration.

Macrophages are the next to accumulate in animal models, classically thought to be largely in response to upregulation of MCP-1 in tubule cells and induction of its cognate receptor CCR2 on macrophages. There is recent evidence for the role of both resident macrophages as well as activated infiltrating macrophages after experimental AKI. Tubule cell injury results in increased expression of damage-associated molecular pattern (DAMP) molecules, Toll-like receptors (TLRs), and pathogen-associated molecular patterns (PAMPs). These signals rapidly recruit neutrophils, natural killer cells, activated macrophages, and resident macrophages to the site of injury. Macrophages recognize the initial damage signals through pattern recognition receptors (PRRs), a family of receptors that recognize DAMPs and PAMPs. This results in downstream stimulation of macrophage phagocytosis, phagolysosomes maturation, antigen presentation, and production of the proinflammatory cytokine, TNFα. Resident macrophages first act to engulf cellular debris as additional bone-marrow derived macrophages and monocytes are recruited. Resident macrophages further prolong inflammation by recruiting other leukocytes to the site of injury. The initial inflammatory macrophage events are subsequently followed by modulation and then inhibition of the inflammatory response. Macrophages have two distinct phenotypes during AKI; the first phenotype contributes to injury, whereas the second promotes kidney repair. Classically activated macrophages, which predominate in early ischemic injury, produce proinflammatory cytokines (such as IL-12). Alternatively activated macrophages, also known as M2 macrophages, are believed to modulate the inflammatory response and promote tissue repair and are prevalent during the recovery and repair phase of AKI.

Dendritic cells (DCs), like macrophages, have pro- and anti-inflammatory functions and work closely with other components of the immune system to respond to kidney injury. Dendritic cells help regulate immune effector cells, and present antigenic material to T cells. Macrophages and DCs share similar functions and have functional plasticity depending on the cues they receive from the microenvironment. There is a contiguous network of DCs, which are identified by presence of the chemokine receptor CX3CR1, in the kidney interstitium and mesangium. DCs are key initiators, potentiators, and effectors in the innate renal immune system. The role of DCs in renal injury is not fully resolved, because some experimental studies suggest that depleting DCs has protective effects while other findings suggest that deleting dendritic cells worsens injury.

CD4+/CD8+ T cells have been identified in animal as well as human models of ischemic AKI and often are observed to increase the production of proinflammatory molecules, such as TNF-α and IFN-γ. T cell depletion is protective in experimental AKI. Inconsistencies exist, however, and recent data suggest that the role of T cells in ischemic AKI may be complex, with the identification of both protective (TH2 phenotype) and deleterious (TH1 phenotype) subtypes of T cells. T helper lymphocytes enhance tissue injury by recruiting neutrophils and other inflammatory cells, while regulatory T cells conversely reduce renal injury and facilitate repair. Moreover, animals deficient in both T and B cells are not protected from ischemic AKI, and depletion of peripheral CD4+ T cells fails to bestow protection from ischemic AKI.

The potential role of B cells in ischemic AKI is intriguing. Compared with wild-type animals, B cell-deficient mice are protected partially from structural and functional ischemic renal injury, despite comparable neutrophil and T cell infiltrations. Wild type serum transfer, but not B cell transfer, into B cell-deficient mice was shown to restore susceptibility to ischemic AKI, implicating a soluble serum factor as a mechanism by which B cell deficiency confers renal protection.

Recent literature has focused on the proximal tubule's role in intra-renal cross talk. Crosstalk between the proximal tubule and the thick ascending limb (TAL) of the loop of Henle recently has been revealed, with TLR4 and Tamm-Horsfall Protein (THP) suggested as likely mediators of the process. THP, also known as uromodulin, is considered a protective molecule, and inhibits proximal tubule production of proinflammatory cytokines and chemokines. Crosstalk between the TAL and proximal tubule suppresses tubular activation of innate immunity and reduces inflammatory injury. During the early phases of AKI, THP production is significantly diminished both at the RNA and protein level, in both experimental and human studies. However, THP is significantly upregulated within 48 h of ischemia in experimental models. The absence of THP in mice resulted in more severe inflammation, increased cast formation, reduced renal function, and diffuse tubular necrosis in the outer medulla. Neutrophil infiltration also was increased in THP-knockout mice, corroborating suggestions that THP functions as an anti-inflammatory and protective molecule during ischemic injury. There is now considerable evidence for a negative association between urinary THP and the development of human AKI [94]. Experimental administration of exogenous THP after AKI mitigates subsequent injury and hastens recovery.

Activation of the complement system in AKI, with resultant amplification of the inflammatory response in the kidney, has received widespread attention in recent years. Whereas ischemia-reperfusion injury in most organs activates the complement cascade along classic pathways, studies in animals and humans have implicated the alternative pathway in AKI. However, other reports have identified a role for the mannose-binding lectin pathway after animal and human ischemic AKI. Also controversial is the identification of the final active complement component. Although earlier studies pointed to the C6b-directed formation of a membrane attack complex, recent observations have identified a predominant role for C5a in ischemic AKI. C5a is a powerful chemoattractant that recruits inflammatory cells such as neutrophils, monocytes, and T cells. The kidney is one of the few organs in which the C5a receptor is normally expressed, in proximal tubule epithelial cells as well as in interstitial macrophages. C5a receptor expression in tubule epithelial cells is upregulated markedly after ischemia-reperfusion injury and sepsis. Inhibition of C5a generation using monoclonal antibodies was found to protect against renal dysfunction induced by ischemia, and in turn to inhibit neutrophil and macrophage influx in experimental models. Pre-treatment with orally active small molecule C5a receptor antagonists substantially reduced the histologic and functional impairment induced by ischemic AKI in animal models. Small molecule antagonists for C5a receptor represent promising agents for the treatment or prevention of ischemic AKI. In addition, the anti-C5 monoclonal antibody (eculizumab) ameliorates experimental ischemic AKI and is widely used in the AKI of atypical hemolytic uremic syndrome. Persistent systemic complement activation is also a hallmark of COVID-19 related AKI in humans, and eculizumab may be beneficial.

Alterations in Gene Expression

Attempts at unraveling the molecular basis of the myriad pathways activated by AKI have been facilitated by advances in functional genomics and transcriptome profiling technologies. Several investigators have used these techniques in human and animal models of AKI to obtain expression profiles of thousands of genes. When combined with bioinformatics tools, these studies have identified novel genes with altered expression, new signal transduction pathways that are activated, and even new drug targets and biomarkers in AKI [95–99]. A few clinically relevant examples are provided here.

One of the first induced molecules to be identified in the postischemic kidney using genomic approaches was kidney injury molecule 1 (KIM-1). KIM-1 protein subsequently was demonstrated to be upregulated in the postischemic animal and human kidney tubules, predominantly on the apical membranes of proximal tubule epithelial cells, where it may play a role in renal regeneration. An ectodomain is shed into the urine, making KIM-1 a promising non-invasive urinary biomarker of ischemic human AKI.

Another example is neutrophil gelatinase-associated lipocalin (NGAL), one of the most highly induced genes in the early postischemic kidney. NGAL protein is markedly upregulated in kidney tubules very early after ischemic AKI in animals and humans and is excreted rapidly in the urine, where it represents a sensitive novel biomarker of early ischemic injury. In the postischemic kidney tubule, NGAL protein is highly expressed in tubule cells that are undergoing proliferation, suggesting its protective or regenerative role after AKI. Exogenous administration of NGAL in experimental models before, during, or even shortly after ischemic or nephrotoxic injury provides remarkable protection at the functional and structural levels, with induction of proliferation and striking inhibition of apoptosis in tubule epithelial cells. In this context, NGAL mitigates iron-mediated toxicity by providing a reservoir for excess iron and may provide a regulated source of intracellular iron to promote regeneration and repair. Exogenously administered NGAL also markedly upregulates HO1, a proven multifunctional protective agent in experimental AKI that works by limiting iron uptake, promoting intracellular iron release, enhancing production of antioxidants such as biliverdin and carbon monoxide, and inducing the cell cycle regulatory protein p21.

Gene expression studies have shown that extracellular signal-regulated kinases (ERK1 and ERK2) are activated 24 h after injury and likely alter cytoskeletal organization and focal complex assembly. ERK 1 and 2 are localized in damaged proximal tubule cells and are activated during renal reperfusion in response to ROS and Ras signaling. ERK1 and 2 have negative downstream effects by phosphorylating proteins that induce the dissolution and restructuring of focal adhesions. Synthetic ERK inhibitors, such as U0126 (already used in humans for chemotherapy), may be relevant in clinical settings as a method that preserves cytoskeletal structure during AKI.

Data mining of gene expression profiles from 150 microarray experiments performed in 21 different models of AKI (including mouse, rat, pig, and human models) identified novel upregulated genes that have now been well characterized—including *LCN2* (*encoding lipocalin 2 or NGAL*), *KIM-1* (kidney injury molecule-1), *CCL2* (*chemokine ligand 2 or MCP-1*), *HMOX1* (*heme oxygenase*), *TNF* (tumor necrosis factor), and *CLU* (Clusterin) [100]. More recent deep sequencing studies have identified significant differences in the responses between AKI subtypes. For exam-

ple, there exists a remarkable diversity of changes in the kidney genomic response to ischemic and septic injuries [101]. In addition, a comparison of ischemic and volume depletion models of AKI, often considered to be a continuum and therefore predicted to have similar gene expression response, unexpectedly showed that less than 10% of expressed genes were differentially regulated in the two models despite identical elevations in the serum creatinine [102]. Volume depletion induced the metabolic pathways and anti-inflammatory molecules. By contrast, ischemic injury activated known and novel inflammatory, coagulation, and epithelial repair pathways, including *LCN2*, *KIM-1*, *CXCL1*, and *IL-6*, all of which were totally unchanged in the volume depletion model. For added complexity, different nephron segments responded with distinct signatures to different injuries. For example, volume depletion predominately affected the inner medulla, whereas ischemic changes were noted primarily in the outer medulla. Ischemic injury induces mRNA expression of *KIM-1* specifically in the proximal tubule and, in contrast, *LCN2* specifically in the distal nephron. Hence, different insults lead to diverse responses reflecting alterations in segment-specific pathophysiology.

Dramatic recent advances in single-cell RNA sequencing (scRNA-seq) and single-nucleus sequencing can now uncover the expression level of every gene in every cell type, enabling the rapid determination of serial gene expression changes in many thousands of cells, identification of previously unknown cell populations, and even novel heterogeneity within a given cell type. For example, scRNA-seq analysis of human kidney transplant biopsies has uncovered 16 distinct cell types and novel cell states within endothelial cells as well as proinflammatory parenchymal responses in the rejecting kidney. Single nuclear approaches have detected unique cell types and cell states within the human kidney, redefined cellular heterogeneity in the proximal tubule and thick ascending limb, and identified novel genomic signatures of fibrosis. Surprising recent data has begun to challenge the dogma that the fibrotic response of the kidney to injury is a late and final common pathway. In a murine bilateral ischemia-reperfusion AKI survival model, early kidney sections at day 1 revealed surprising significant fibrosis adjacent to damaged S3 segments [103]. Single-cell profiling of AKI in mice has also revealed early activation of profibrotic transcriptional signatures [95]. Encouraging new experimental data suggest that this early fibrotic response can be prevented. In murine AKI due to ischemia-reperfusion, intraperitoneal administration of a peptide (pUR4) that binds fibronectin and inhibits fibronectin polymerization (an early event in the fibrotic cascade) soon after injury dramatically attenuated the early fibrotic response [104]. The pUR4 peptide was devoid of any adverse effects, rendering translational application to human AKI a realistic possibility. The NIH-funded Kidney Precision Medicine Project (KPMP) is analyzing human AKI kidney biopsies based on elevations in serum creatinine and a urinary biomarker. These single cell RNA-seq and other advanced deep sequencing studies are expected to yield a detailed molecular atlas of the human kidney, and potentially identify additional new pathways for future therapies.

One of the most remarkable and consistent finding from scRNA-seq studies is the rapid induction of an embryonic phenotype in injured tubule cells [95]. Specifically in injured proximal tubule cells, there is re-expression of genes normally present only in the developing kidney (e.g., *Sox4*, *Cd24a*). This switch to the embryonic state is likely critical for regeneration of tubule cells lost during AKI. The identified candidates that accelerate repair represent new future therapies.

Large-scale genome wide association studies (GWAS) can identify potentially pathogenetic genomic sequences that are statistically enriched in AKI cases compared to controls. A recent GWAS analysis of a discovery cohort of 1400 adults with critical illness (760 with AKI) followed by a separate replication cohort of 200 AKI cases [105] have yielded two single-nucleotide polymorphisms (SNPs) involving the transcription factor interferon regulatory factor 2 (*IRF2*), and an additional two SNPs close to the transcription factor T-box 1 (*TBX1*). The identification of SNPs near IRF2 suggests a potential role for the immune system in AKI, a concept with already strong biologic plausibility. TBX1 is expressed during kidney development, and this finding supports the intriguing concept that ontogeny recapitulates phylogeny after kidney injury, whereby genetic programs involved in nephrogenesis that become dormant after birth are once again reactivated and are essential for the recovery process after injury in post-natal life. Additional GWAS studies with even larger cohorts of control and AKI subjects are under way and may yield new AKI susceptibility genes of critical biological significance.

Alterations in Metabolomics

Recent metabolomic approaches have identified dramatic differences in the response of the kidney to injuries that were previously thought to be closely related. For example, experimental models of ischemia-reperfusion injury display the rapid appearance of alanine, leucine, and glucose in the urine, with a downregulation of urinary creatinine and nicotinamide [106]. In marked contrast, hypoxic injury rapidly induces the urinary excretion of benzoate and fructose, while citrate and isothionate are suppressed [107]. The differential appearance of these metabolites in the urine may hold important clues towards etiology-specific biomarkers and therapeutic targets in humans. Additional recent metabolomic studies in a mouse model of ischemic AKI have identified a deficiency in urinary and intra-renal nicotinamide adenine dinucleotide (NAD), an essential component of energy generation via glycolysis and the Kreb's cycle [108]. In a phase I study of oral NAM supplementation (which generates NAD via a salvage pathway) in adults undergoing cardiac surgery, the rise in serum creatinine was prevented compared to placebo [108]. Additional translational studies are under way.

Unique Aspects of Septic AKI

Although sepsis is one of the most common causes of AKI, the pathogenesis remains incompletely understood. Translational analysis of septic AKI has been limited by the fact that most animal models of this condition do not faithfully mimic the human condition. Kidney biopsies from humans with septic AKI have revealed only mild, nonspecific changes that do not correlate with the profound functional changes. Histological assessment of postmortem kidneys from non-survivors of septic AKI shows mild heterogeneous tubular injury with apical vacuolization, but with an absence of tubular necrosis and only minimal apoptosis. Studies have revealed the surprising finding that unlike in ischemic or nephrotoxic AKI, humans with early septic AKI demonstrate a paradoxical increase in renal blood flow despite a reduction in GFR. Thus, early septic AKI is a hyperemic injury that contrasts with the persistent vasoconstriction characteristic of ischemic and nephrotoxic AKI. In sepsis, at the glomerular level, there is evidence for afferent arteriolar vasoconstriction, efferent arteriolar vasodilatation, and shunting of blood flow via capillaries that bypass the glomerulus, resulting in decreased GFR and oliguria.

Recent evidence shows that microcirculatory dysfunction, inflammation, and metabolic reprogramming are the three fundamental mechanisms that may play a role in the development of septic AKI. Profound heterogeneous changes in microcirculatory flow have been demonstrated, including a decrease in the capillary density, a decrease in the proportion of capillaries with continuous flow and an increase in the proportion of capillaries with intermittent and stop flow. Multiple mechanisms may lead to microcirculatory alterations, including endothelial injury, autonomic nervous system response, shedding of the glycocalyx, and activation of the coagulation cascades.

During sepsis-associated AKI, a reprioritization of energy occurs that seeks to meet metabolic vital needs to ensure survival at the expense of cell function. Functions that consume ATP are downregulated, including protein synthesis and ion transport, especially in the proximal tubular epithelial cells. In addition, experimental studies have suggested that tubular epithelial cells may reprogram their metabolism by switching to aerobic glycolysis and oxidative phosphorylation to fulfill energy requirements during sep-

sis. Furthermore, mitochondria enter a series of quality control processes such as mitophagy and biogenesis to preserve the mitochondrial pool to confer protection and fulfill the necessary energetic requirements. Finally, an early response to septic AKI is cell cycle arrest in tubule cells, which may represent another defense mechanism to preserve energy. Approaches to enhance these survival mechanisms hold promise in human AKI.

AKI and Distant Organ Dysfunction

Substantial experimental and clinical evidence illustrates that AKI leads to dysfunction of other organs, including lung, heart, brain, liver, and intestine via aberrant organ-organ communication. This is clinically important, since the prognosis for patients who have AKI and another organ in a state of dysfunction is especially poor, with a morality rate of 60–80%. Interruption of normal immunological balance and generation of inflammatory mediators are important in AKI-induced distant organ crosstalk. Additional mechanisms include increased endothelial injury, cellular apoptosis, and oxidative stress.

Acute lung injury is a common complication of AKI, and manifests clinically as pulmonary edema and respiratory failure needing mechanical ventilation [109]. Fluid overload from decreased urine output and impaired cardiac function is the major cause of pulmonary edema. In addition, the integrity of alveolar-capillary barrier is impaired by systemic inflammation, oxidative stress, and uremia, causing fluid accumulation in the lung. Increased inflammatory cytokines in the plasma, such as IL-6 and IL-8, have been associated with prolonged ventilator weaning times and increased mortality in AKI patients with acute lung injury.

The term cardiorenal syndrome (CRS) refers to a complex pathophysiological disorder of the heart and kidneys whereby acute or chronic dysfunction in one organ may induce acute or chronic dysfunction in the other organ. In CRS Type 3, also called acute reno-cardiac syndrome, an abrupt worsening of renal function leads to acute cardiac disorder. Cardiovascular failure occurs in about 60% of critically ill adults and is the second most common cause of death (after sepsis). Volume overload decreases myocardial contractility and induces maladaptive myocardial remodeling. Uremic toxin accumulation leads to cardiovascular toxicity and can increase risk for myocardial ischemia by compromising coronary vasoreactivity. Metabolic acidosis also diminishes myocardial contractility. Electrolyte imbalances can trigger arrhythmias.

Liver dysfunction can be observed in critically ill AKI patients and hepatic failure increases the in-hospital mortality in AKI patients. Several clinical studies have found development of hepatic dysfunction in AKI patients leading to alterations in protein synthesis and metabolism of lipid, protein, and drugs. During AKI, there are changes not only in renal drug metabolism, but also in nonrenal metabolism, which can have considerable influence on clinical outcomes due to under- or over-dosing and related toxicity problems. The mechanisms by which AKI impacts liver drug metabolism may be related to uremic toxins, inflammatory cytokines, activated leucocytes, and other neuro-humoral factors. Drug dosing needs to be especially carefully monitored in AKI patients with hepatic dysfunction.

Clinicopathologic Correlations and Therapeutic Implications

The clinical course of AKI can be divided into four phases: initiation, extension, maintenance, and recovery. Clinical recognition of these phases can be facilitated using novel biomarker panels, as described later in this chapter (Fig. 51.7). Advances in our understanding of AKI pathogenesis now allow for postulation of temporal correlations between the clinical and cell biologic alterations. The *initiation phase* is the period during which initial exposure to the ischemic insult occurs, kidney function begins to fall, and parenchymal injury is evolving but not fully entrenched. Intracellular ATP depletion is profound, sublethal injury to the tubule epithelial and endothelial cells predominates, generation of reactive oxygen molecules is initiated, and activation of inflammatory mechanisms commences. Intrarenal protective mechanisms such as induction of HSPs in tubule cells also are brought to play during the initiation phase. If the injury is alleviated at this stage, complete restitution and recovery is very likely. Interventional approaches during this phase might include vasodilators, ATP donors, antioxidants, and iron chelators (Fig. 51.7).

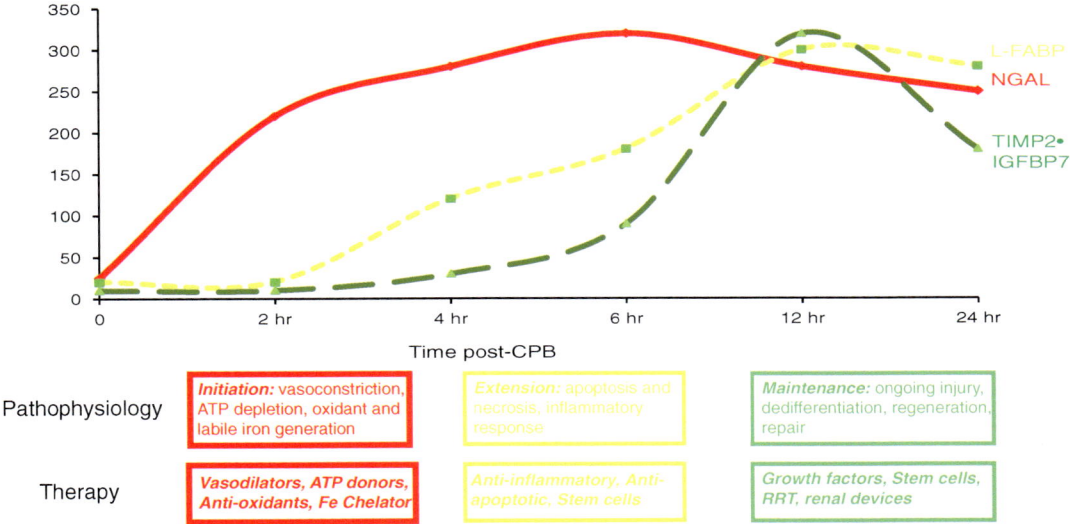

Fig. 51.7 Color coded correlations between time after the initiating insult (in this case, hours after initiation of cardiopulmonary bypass), appearance of non-invasive urinary biomarkers, phase of AKI and the underlying mechanisms, and suggested therapeutic approaches

Prolongation of the initial insult (including reperfusion after ischemia) ushers in the *extension phase*. Blood flow returns to the cortex, and tubules undergo reperfusion-dependent cell death but also commence the regeneration process. By contrast, medullary blood flow remains severely reduced, resulting in more widespread tubule cell death, desquamation, and luminal obstruction. Injured endothelial and epithelial cells amplify the raging inflammatory cascades, and the endothelial denudation potentiates the intense vasoconstriction. The GFR continues to decline. This phase probably represents the optimal window of opportunity for early diagnosis and active therapeutic intervention. Anti-inflammatory agents, anti-apoptotic measures, and stem cells are likely to be particularly efficacious during this phase.

During the *maintenance phase*, parenchymal injury is established, and the GFR is maintained at its nadir even though renal blood flow begins to normalize. Cell injury and regeneration occur simultaneously, and the duration and severity of this phase may be determined by the balance between cell survival and death. Repair of epithelial and endothelial cells appears to be critical to recovery. Measures to accelerate the endogenous regeneration processes may be effective during this phase. These include growth factors, stem cells, and kidney support therapies.

The *recovery phase* is characterized functionally by an improvement in GFR and structurally by reestablishment of tubule integrity, with fully differentiated and polarized epithelial cells. The origin of cells that replenish the damaged epithelial cells has been examined. Fate mapping studies have shown that bone marrow-derived cells do not make a significant contribution. Rather, it is the surviving tubule epithelial cells themselves that dedifferentiate and proliferate to repair the damaged tubule. The normally quiescent surviving proximal tubule cells proliferate by entering the cell cycle and activating cyclin-dependent kinases such as Cdk2 and Cdk4/6, resulting in adaptive repair. Re-expression of kidney developmental genes in injured tubule cells is likely critical for this process. However, the repair process may be incomplete or maladaptive, and AKI can progress to CKD.

Mechanisms Underlying Long-Term Sequelae of AKI

Several studies using large databases in both adults and children have now established the strong correlation between AKI and long-term sequelae, including CKD, hypertension, and end-stage kidney disease (ESKD). The cellular and molecular mechanisms that result in CKD after AKI have been intensely studied in animal models . The three primary morphologic findings include failed tubule recovery/maladaptive tubule repair, capillary rarefaction, and interstitial fibrosis.

The fate of tubule cells that do not regenerate and recover after AKI is variable. In severe AKI, tubule repair may not occur at all, leading to atrophic and fibrotic areas with disconnection of intact glomeruli from surviving tubules and subsequent decline in kidney function. Other surviving cells that undergo dedifferentiation become growth arrested in the G2 phase of the cell cycle and cannot engage proliferative pathways. Such abnormally dedifferentiated "failed-recovery" cells occur in small clusters along entire tubule segments. These senescent tubule epithelial cells acquire the senescence-associated secretory phenotype and actively secrete fibrogenic factors and pro-inflammatory cytokines, thereby creating microenvironments that promote fibrosis and inflammation. Mechanisms underlying this maladaptive repair are emerging.

Capillary rarefaction has been demonstrated after AKI in both animal models and in humans. Persistent hypoxia and resultant endothelial injury results in capillary disintegration. Failure of endothelial cells to regenerate leads to reduced capillary density. In addition, injury to pericytes, which are resident fibroblasts that normally support capillary structure and integrity, results in their detachment from capillaries and worsens capillary disintegration. The consequent persistent local tissue hypoxia drives secretion of pro-fibrotic cytokines, inhibition of vascular repair, and endothelial-mesenchymal transition, all of which promote interstitial fibrosis. Loss of renal vasculature leads to renal VEGF deficiency, and administration of exogenous VEGF or VEGF-derived chimeric molecules preserves capillary density and ameliorates CKD progression in animal models. As a strategy to combat tissue hypoxia, pharmacologic activation of hypoxia-inducible factor (HIF) prevented the development of fibrosis. Pharmacologic activation of Nrf2, a potent antioxidant, has also been effective in ameliorating the sequelae of AKI in animals. All three agents are available for human use and should be tested as ameliorators of the AKI to CKD transition.

The primary cellular drivers of interstitial fibrosis include activated fibroblasts, myofibroblasts derived from activated pericytes and/or endothelial-mesenchymal transition, and persistent influence of inflammatory macrophages and lymphocytes. Fibrosis typically occurs around damaged or atrophic tubules, and is not progressive *per se*. Indeed, the surrounding tubulointerstitium remains normal, and with time, fibrotic tissue shrinks as activated fibroblasts regress. However, fibrosis is progressive in the setting of repeated AKI episodes or if AKI occurs in the setting of previous CKD.

Postrenal AKI

Postrenal AKI is a result of obstruction to the outflow tract on both sides and is uncommon beyond the neonatal period. Postrenal AKI is usually reversed by relief of the obstruction but is accompanied by a very significant post-obstructive diuresis. The common causes of postrenal AKI are listed in Table 51.4. The pathophysiology and management of the obstructive nephropathy syndrome that can result from congenital anomalies are detailed in Chap. 45.

Clinical Presentation

AKI is largely asymptomatic, and its detection must begin with having a high index of suspicion and an awareness of the risk factors. AKI most commonly presents with a progressive accumulation of fluid and/or nitrogenous wastes, in a predisposed patient who has been exposed to one or more of the etiologic factors outlined in Tables 51.2, 51.3 and 51.4. Classic clinical presentations include edema, hypertension, hematuria, and oliguria. Less frequently, one encounters an increase in BUN and creatinine which is not readily explained. In all cases, the evaluation requires a complete history, physical examination, laboratory evaluation, renal imaging, and rarely a kidney biopsy. A diligent search for all drugs and medications ingested is especially important, even when another obvious cause for AKI is evident. The initial approach to a patient with known or suspected AKI should be directed towards (a) identifying the underlying cause, (b) distinguishing between pre-renal and intrinsic AKI, (c) discriminating between AKI and CKD, (d) determining the severity of AKI, and (e) considering a diagnostic fluid challenge.

Identifying the Underlying Cause

The initial history should be directed towards uncovering an obvious risk factor for AKI, such as those listed in Tables 51.2, 51.3 and 51.4. Additional relevant aspects of the AKI history and physical examination are outlined in Tables 51.5 and 51.6, respectively. These, in combination with a careful urinalysis with microscopy, will yield the etiology of AKI in most cases. A short duration of vomiting, diarrhea, or decreased oral intake associated with decreased urine output and typical physical findings of dehydration suggests prerenal volume-responsive functional AKI. Bloody diarrhea with oliguria is consistent with the hemolytic uremic syndrome. A history of pharyngitis or impetigo a few weeks prior to the onset of gross hematuria or edema suggests post-streptococcal glomerulonephritis. The presence of edema should

Table 51.4 Common causes of postrenal AKI

Mechanism	Etiology
Congenital anomalies of the kidney and urinary tract (CAKUT)	Urethral valves, ureteropelvic junction obstruction
Acquired causes	Calculi, clots, neurogenic bladder, drugs that cause urinary retention

Table 51.5 History taking in patients with suspected AKI

- Fluid loss
  - Diarrhea, vomiting
  - Burns
  - Surgery, shock
- Nephrotoxic agents
  - Non-steroidal anti-inflammatory drugs
  - Aminoglycosides
  - Contrast agents
- Glomerular disease
  - Streptococcal infection (Post-streptococcal glomerulonephritis)
  - Bloody diarrhea (Hemolytic-uremic syndrome)
  - Fever, joint complaints, rash (Systemic lupus erythematosus)
- Obstruction
  - Complete anuria
  - Poor urinary stream

Table 51.6 Physical signs in AKI

- Signs of intravascular volume depletion
- Signs of AKI (edema, hypertension)
- Signs of underlying renal disease
  - Butterfly rash, joint swelling (Systemic lupus erythematosus)
  - Purpuric rash (Henoch-Schonlein Purpura)
  - Fever, macular rash (Interstitial nephritis)
  - Palpably enlarged kidneys (Polycystic/ multicystic kidney disease, Renal vein thrombosis)
- Signs of obstruction
  - Poor urinary stream
  - Palpably enlarged bladder
  - Therapeutic catheterization

also prompt a search for nephrotic syndrome, cardiac failure, or liver failure, which would suggest prerenal AKI that should not be treated with fluid resuscitation. Fever, joint complaints, and a malar rash are indicative of systemic lupus erythematosus. In hospitalized patients, nephrotoxic medications or periods of hypotension are commonly associated with intrinsic AKI and should be diligently searched for.

The urinalysis is an important noninvasive test in the diagnostic evaluation. Typically, the urine in conditions that result in prerenal AKI is highly concentrated and contains little protein or blood. In contrast, proteinuria and hematuria are prominent in etiologies leading to intrinsic AKI. A

heme positive urine by dipstick in the absence of RBCs in the sediment on microscopy suggests hemolysis or rhabdomyolysis. Characteristic findings on microscopic examination of the urine sediment can suggest certain diagnoses. Muddy brown granular casts and epithelial cell casts are highly suggestive of intrinsic AKI or ATN. The finding of red cell casts is diagnostic of glomerulonephritis. The concurrent findings of red cell casts, dysmorphic red cells, heavy proteinuria, or lipiduria are referred to as a "nephritic" urinary sediment. This is commonly associated with AKI due to glomerulonephritides. Pyuria with white cell and granular or waxy casts are suggestive of tubular or interstitial disease or urinary tract infection. White cells and white cell casts may also be seen in acute glomerulonephritis. The presence of renal epithelial cells, renal epithelial cell casts and granular casts are characteristic of ATN. In prospective studies of adults with AKI, when a renal epithelial cell, renal epithelial cell cast or granular cast was present, the sensitivity for discriminating no AKI versus AKI was low, but the specificity was very high at 91–95%. In another prospective study of adults with AKI, a urinary sediment scoring system created based on the number of renal tubular epithelial cells and granular casts was significantly associated with severity of AKI and with increased risk of worsening AKI. Urine microscopy is very inexpensive, readily available, noninvasive, and specific for AKI diagnosis and severity, and should therefore be a routine part of evaluating any patient who is suspected to have AKI [110].

Distinguishing Between Functional and Structural AKI

This determination is potentially important because (a) the treatment and prognosis are different, and (b) prompt identification and management of prerenal AKI can prevent the progression to intrinsic AKI. As noted above, the urinalysis with microscopy will often provide an initial differentiation between prerenal and intrinsic AKI. The further distinction is based on the principle that prerenal AKI is associated with maximal reabsorption of solutes and water by the intact proximal tubule, whereas the proximal tubule cell damage typical of intrinsic AKI results in impaired reabsorptive capacity. Urinary indices based on this principle are shown in Table 51.7. The fractional excretion of sodium (FENa) is a convenient bedside screening test for making this distinction. It is calculated from measured concentrations of sodium (Na) and creatinine (Cr) in the urine (U) and plasma (P), as follows:

$$FENa = \left(\left[U/P\right]Na\right)/\left(\left[U/P\right]Cr\right)\times100$$

A FENa below 1% suggests prerenal AKI, in which the reabsorption of almost all the filtered sodium represents an appropriate response to decreased perfusion. A FENa above 2% suggests intrinsic AKI with proximal tubule injury. A FENa between 1% and 2% is non-diagnostic. However, limitations to the utility of FENa should be noted. In neonates, the FENa is generally higher because of their decreased ability to reabsorb sodium resulting from immaturity of proximal tubule function. The FENa can be high following fluid resuscitation, or administration of diuretics.

The fractional excretion of urea (FEUrea) has been proposed as a more accurate determinant of prerenal AKI, especially in patients receiving diuretics and in patients with sepsis. FEUrea is typically <35% in patients with prerenal AKI, and >50% in those with established intrinsic AKI. In the setting of diuretic use, there can be an uncoupling of renal sodium handling from tubular function. FEUrea may represent an alternative diagnostic approach because urea transport is not directly linked to sodium transporters. However, recent studies have revealed that in patients with heart failure receiving intravenous loop diuretic therapy, FEUrea commonly and significantly increased above the pre-diuretic baseline [111].

Multicenter studies in the complex critically ill population have revealed limited utility of both FENa and FEUrea in distinguishing prerenal from intrinsic AKI. These studies raise fundamental questions about the pathophysiologic validity of the prerenal AKI paradigm and suggest that AKI in the critical care setting is a continuum of injury that should likely not be divided into functional (prerenal or transient) or structural (ATN or persistent) sub-types.

By the same principle of increased proximal tubule solute reabsorption, the BUN/creatinine ratio (both expressed as mg/dL) in the serum is often markedly elevated (>20) in prerenal AKI. This is because the intact proximal tubule can avidly reabsorb urea but is impermeable to creatinine. However, increases in BUN without AKI can be encountered in patients receiving steroids or total parenteral nutrition, in catabolic states, and those with gastrointestinal bleeding. In addition, a BUN/creatinine ratio >20 is a poor indicator of prerenal AKI in critically ill patients and should not be used in that setting. This is because of at least two confounding factors. One, critical illness is associated with increased protein catabolism and increased urea generation rate, and a higher severity of illness would be expected to result in a higher BUN and a greater risk for intrinsic AKI. Second, critical illness could result in decreased muscle mass, and a paradoxical reduction in serum creatinine. Indeed, animal studies have demonstrated decreased production of creatinine in sepsis, the most common cause of severe AKI. Thus, in critical illness, both the high BUN and lower serum creatinine are explicable by factors other than a prerenal state.

Distinguishing Between AKI and CKD

A kidney and bladder ultrasound are a sensitive, non-invasive modality that can differentiate not only between AKI and CKD but can also rule out a postrenal etiology. Typically, the kidneys in AKI are normal or enlarged, with increased echogenicity, whereas those in CKD are frequently small and shrunken. Other distinguishing features are shown in Table 51.8.

Table 51.7 Urinary indices in AKI

Measurement	Prerenal AKI	Intrinsic AKI
Urine specific gravity	>1020	<1012
Urine/plasma creatinine	>40	<20
Urine Na (mEq/L)	<20	>40
FENa	<1%	>2%

Determining the Severity of AKI

Estimating the baseline pre-illness serum creatinine can determine the severity of AKI and allow for classification based on the KDIGO criteria. This is best achieved when a previous serum creatinine level is available. If not, the baseline serum creatinine in children can be estimated using the Schwartz formula and a presumed baseline eGFR of 120 mL/min/1.73 m²:

$$\text{Estimated creatinine clearance in mL / min} = 0.413^* L / Pcr$$

Where L = height (cm) and Pcr = plasma creatinine in mg/dL. The constant of 0.413 provides a good approximation of GFR in children of all ages and both genders [14]. However, it should be emphasized that this constant was derived in patients with CKD Stage 2 to 5 and has not been validated for use in AKI.

Another important index of AKI severity is the degree of fluid overload, which is especially useful in the assessment of the critically ill patient. Several recent pediatric AKI studies have demonstrated that increasing degrees of fluid overload are independently associated with mortality and adverse outcomes. Extent of fluid overload during a hospitalization period can be estimated by the following formula:

$$\%\text{Fluid overload} = \left[\text{Total fluid in}\left(L\right) - \text{Total fluid out}\left(L\right)\right] / \text{Admission weight in kg}\right] \times 100$$

The importance of assessing fluid overload was first demonstrated by the Prospective Pediatric Continuous Renal Replacement Therapy (ppCRRT) Registry Group, via analysis of its 340-patient cohort using a tripartite classification for percent fluid overload at CRRT initiation. Patients who developed >20% fluid overload at CRRT initiation had significantly higher mortality (66%) than those who had 10–20% fluid overload (43%) and those with <10% fluid overload (29%). The association between degree of fluid overload and mortality remained after adjusting for intergroup differences and severity of illness. When fluid overload was dichotomized to >20% and <20%, patients with >20% fluid overload had an adjusted mortality OR of 8.5 (95% CI, 2.8–25.7). In addition to impacting mortality, fluid overload can directly worsen kidney function and AKI due to increased renal venous pressure, interstitial edema, and abdominal compartment syndrome. Fluid overload also leads to hemodilution and a falsely reduced serum creatinine concentration, thereby delaying or masking the diagnosis and classification of AKI. Fluid overload at a threshold of 10–20% is independently associated with adverse outcomes in several critically ill pediatric populations [112].

Routine laboratory evaluation for the presence of metabolic complications can also assist in establishing AKI severity. AKI is associated with several life-threatening complications, which require diligent monitoring by the clinician. Fortunately, these complications are uncommon in patients who receive dialytic therapies. Common complications are listed in Table 51.9. Hyponatremia is usually dilutional (secondary to fluid retention and administration of hypotonic fluids). Less common causes

Table 51.8 AKI versus CKD

Acute kidney injury	Chronic kidney disease
Progressive rise in BUN and Cr	Stable elevated BUN and Cr
History of AKI etiology	History of chronic hypertension
Normal growth	Stunted growth
Normal bones	Renal osteodystrophy
No broad urinary casts	Broad waxy urinary casts
Anemia usually mild	Anemia usually severe
Normal or enlarged kidneys	Small shrunken kidneys

Table 51.9 Major complications of AKI

Metabolic	Cardiovascular	Gastrointestinal	Neurologic	Hematologic	Infectious
Hyperkalemia	Pulmonary edema	Nausea, vomiting, anorexia	Altered mental status	Anemia	Pneumonia
Metabolic Acidosis	Arrythmias	Malnutrition	Irritability	Bleeding	Sepsis
Hyponatremia	Pericarditis	Gastritis	Seizures		Infected IV sites
Hypocalcemia	Myocardial infarction	GI Bleeding	Somnolence		
Hyper-phosphatemia	Hypertension	GI ulcers	Coma		

of hyponatremia include sodium depletion (hyponatremic dehydration) and hyperglycemia (serum sodium concentration decreases by 1.6 mEq/L for every 100 mg/dL increase in serum glucose above 100 mg/dL). Hypernatremia in AKI is usually a result of excessive sodium administration (inappropriate fluid therapy or overzealous sodium bicarbonate administration). Hyperkalemia is due to the reduction in GFR, reduction in tubular secretion of potassium, increased catabolism, and metabolic acidosis (each 0.1 unit reduction in arterial pH raises serum potassium by 0.3 mEq/L). Hyperkalemia is most pronounced in patients with excessive endogenous production (rhabdomyolysis, hemolysis, and tumor lysis syndrome). A high anion gap metabolic acidosis is secondary to the impaired renal excretion of acid and the impaired reabsorption and regeneration of bicarbonate. Acidosis is most severe in shock, sepsis, or impaired respiratory compensation. Hypocalcemia is due to increased serum phosphate and impaired renal conversion of vitamin D to the active form. Hypocalcemia is most pronounced in patients with rhabdomyolysis. Metabolic acidosis increases the fraction of ionized calcium (the active form). Therefore, overzealous bicarbonate therapy can decrease the concentration of ionized calcium and precipitate symptoms of hypocalcemia, including tetany, seizures and cardiac arrhythmias. Hyperphosphatemia in AKI is primarily due to impaired renal excretion and can aggravate the hypocalcemia. During recovery from AKI, the vigorous diuretic phase may be accompanied by significant volume depletion, hypernatremia, hypokalemia and hypophosphatemia.

Considering a Diagnostic Fluid Challenge

A common clinical scenario is one where patients present with an increase in BUN and serum creatinine, with a history and physical exam findings consistent with a prerenal etiology, but the duration of the prerenal insult is unknown. Another common diagnostic dilemma occurs when a subject presents with an increase in serum creatinine, but the cause is unclear. In both these cases, a fluid challenge may be diagnostic as well as therapeutic. Typically, fluid challenges in children consist of normal saline in the dose of 10–20 mL/kg repeated once or twice until urine output improves. A reduction in BUN and serum creatinine would suggest a prerenal etiology, whereas an absence of improvement in these parameters (and/or the development of fluid overload) would confirm the diagnosis of intrinsic AKI. Fluid challenges should be avoided in children with pre-renal AKI due to volume-unresponsive states such as liver failure, heart failure and nephrotic syndrome.

Considering a Kidney Biopsy

A renal biopsy is rarely indicated in AKI but should be considered when noninvasive evaluation fails to establish a diagnosis. In pediatric AKI, it is most indicated in patients with suspected acute glomerulonephritis (to identify crescentic forms or specific vasculitides), with suspected lupus nephritis (to classify the disease and establish the activity and chronicity), or with kidney transplant dysfunction.

Problems with Serum Creatinine Measurements in AKI

A progressive increase in serum creatinine (typically 1–2 mg/dL/day) is the hallmark of intrinsic AKI and has served as a biomarker of AKI for several decades. However, serum creatinine concentration is a flawed AKI biomarker for several reasons [113]. Serum creatinine does not differentiate the nature, type and timing of the renal insult. Changes in serum creatinine concentrations often lag changes in GFR until a steady state has been reached, which can take several days. Dialysis readily clears serum creatinine, rendering this marker less useful in the assessment for improving renal function once dialysis has begun. Even normal serum creatinine can vary widely with age, gender, diet, muscle mass, nutritional status, medications, and hydration status. In the acute setting, it is estimated that more than 50% of kidney function must be lost before the serum creatinine even begins to rise because of the concept of renal reserve. However, animal studies have shown that while AKI can be prevented and/or treated by several maneuvers, these measures must be instituted very early after the insult, well before the serum creatinine rises. The lack of early biomarkers of AKI in humans has hitherto impaired our ability to launch potentially effective therapies in a timely manner.

Serum Cystatin C as a Functional Biomarker

The use of cystatin C as an endogenous marker of kidney function in children is well established [114–119]. Cystatin C is a ubiquitous cysteine protease inhibitor protein that is produced by all nucleated cells at a constant rate, freely filtered by the glomerulus, catabolized by the proximal tubule, and does not undergo significant tubular secretion. These qualities make cystatin C a more ideal functional marker of GFR than serum creatinine. Its measurement has been standardized on a clinical laboratory platform. Serum cystatin

C is not affected by gender, diet, hydration, muscle mass, and age (cystatin C levels are nearly identical in adults and children over 12 months of age). Cystatin C outperforms serum creatinine for estimation of GFR in adults and children in the steady state, but its ability to rapidly detect acute changes in GFR is still unclear. Some recent studies have demonstrated that serum cystatin C is an early predictive biomarker of AKI in children [119–121] and adults [122]. However, serum cystatin C measurements are not uniformly available, and the assay is more expensive than serum creatinine. Also, serum cystatin C levels are influenced by steroids and other immunosuppressive therapies, thyroid dysfunction, diabetes, acute inflammation, and high cell turnover. Serum cystatin C remains a functional marker, and not an early marker of structural kidney damage. Additional prospective studies are required to improve our understanding about cystatin C diagnostic cut-off values for prediction of AKI. There remain confounding variables such as method of measurement (standardized clinical laboratory measurements by nephelometry versus turbidimetry, international standardization of reagents) and different reporting equations. The creation of a calibrated reagent (IFCC) has recently allowed for standardization of cystatin C measurements across clinical laboratories and the development of universal GFR estimation equations. New CKD-EPI equations for cystatin C combined with creatinine have now become the preferred method for estimating GFR in adults. For use in children, the Full Age Spectrum (FAS) equations were developed using the assumption that the average GFR of children, adolescents, and young adults is 107.3 mL/min/1.73 m^2. The FAS cystatin C based equations performed as well as or better than the CKD-EPI equations and is currently the preferred mode of reporting eGFR in children and young adults [123].

Novel Early Biomarkers of Kidney Damage in AKI

In the clinical continuum of AKI, we are currently primarily operating in the "established AKI" stage, when the GFR is already reduced and biomarkers of functional injury become apparent, as shown in Fig. 51.8. The genomic and proteomic tools of modern science have identified novel markers for the early stress response of the kidney, which serendipitously appear in the urine or plasma during the "subclinical AKI" phase, well before a change in serum creatinine is detected [124–126]. Thus, they detect structural kidney injury before any functional impairment may be apparent. Many are being developed and validated as early non-invasive structural damage biomarkers for the prediction of AKI and its clinical outcomes in humans. This is a rapidly evolving and expanding field, and the current status of only the most promising examples is summarized in Table 51.10.

The most widely studied and validated early biomarker of AKI in children is neutrophil gelatinase-associated lipocalin (NGAL) [124]. In a prospective study of 71 children undergoing cardiopulmonary bypass, levels of NGAL in the urine and plasma were significantly elevated within 2 h of bypass in those who subsequently developed AKI (defined as a 50% increase in serum creatinine) 1–3 days after surgery [51]. A subsequent prospective study of 374 infants and children undergoing cardiopulmonary bypass confirmed these findings, and additionally established cut-off thresholds as well as a strong association between early NGAL measurements and adverse clinical outcomes, including length of hospital stay and the duration and severity of AKI [54]. A prospective multicenter study of 311 children undergoing cardiac surgery has confirmed the early rise of plasma and urine NGAL concentrations (within 6 h after surgery) in subjects who developed an increase in serum creatinine 2 days later [127]. Early NGAL concentrations were also shown to be associated with longer hospital and ICU stays, and with longer duration of mechanical ventilation. Studies in the heterogeneous pediatric intensive care and emergency department settings have also demonstrated the ability of early NGAL measurements to predict subsequent AKI and its severity [128–130]. Furthermore, urine NGAL levels effectively discriminate between pre-renal AKI and intrinsic AKI [131, 132]. In many reported studies, the addition of NGAL significantly improved the risk prediction for AKI over clinical models alone. Since the widespread

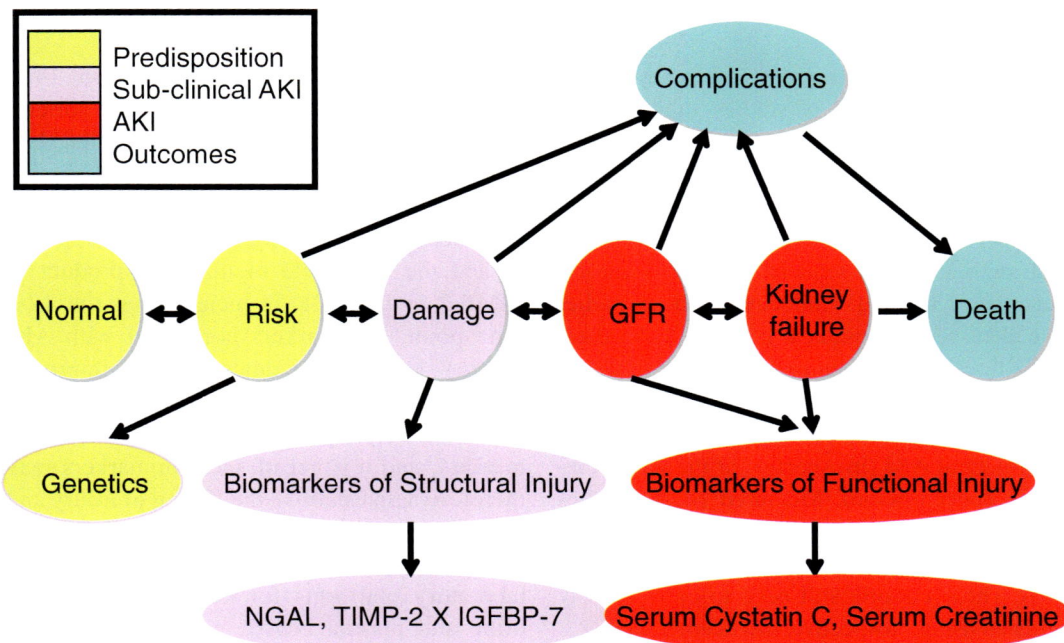

Fig. 51.8 Clinical continuum of AKI, showing the color coded correlations between phases of AKI, and the currently available laboratory methods for their detection

Table 51.10 Novel urinary biomarkers for the prediction of AKI and its outcomes

Biomarker	Source	Function	Cardiac surgery	Kidney transplant	ICU/ED
NGAL	Distal tubule and collecting duct	Regulates iron trafficking, promotes tubule cell survival	2 h post CPB 2 days pre-AKI Predicts AKI severity, dialysis, and death	6 h post-transplant 2–3 days pre DGF Predicts long-term graft loss	On admission 1–2 days pre-AKI Predicts AKI severity, dialysis, and death
IL-18	Proximal tubule	Promotes tubule cell apoptosis and necrosis	6 h post CPB 2 days pre-AKI Predicts AKI severity, dialysis, and death	6 h post-transplant 2–3 days pre DGF Predicts long-term graft loss	On admission 1–2 days pre-AKI Predicts AKI severity, dialysis, and death
L-FABP	Proximal tubule	Antioxidant, suppresses tubule-interstitial damage	6 h post CPB 2 days pre-AKI Not tested for outcomes	Fresh donor urine pre-transplant; predicts DGF	On admission 1–2 days pre-AKI Predicts AKI severity, dialysis, and death
KIM-1	Proximal tubule	Promotes epithelial regeneration, regulates apoptosis	12 h post CPB 1 day pre-AKI Not tested for outcomes	Fresh donor urine pre-transplant; Predicts DGF	On admission 1–2 days pre-AKI Predicts AKI severity, dialysis, and death
TIMP-2 X IGFBP-7	Proximal tubule	Biomarkers of G1 cell cycle arrest	12 h post CPB 1 day pre-AKI Not tested for outcomes	Not tested	12 h after admission; Predicts severe AKI

Times shown (in hours or days) are the earliest time points when the biomarker becomes significantly increased from baseline

AKI acute kidney injury, typically defined as AKIN Stage I or greater, *CPB* cardiopulmonary bypass, *DGF* delayed graft function, *ICU* intensive care unit, *ED* emergency department, *IL-18* interleukin-18, *KIM-1* kidney injury molecule 1, *L-FABP* liver-type fatty acid binding protein, *NGAL* neutrophil gelatinase-associated lipocalin

availability of commercial NGAL assays, there has been an explosion of studies validating the utility of NGAL as an early biomarker. Several multicenter pooled analyses of existing NGAL studies in children and adults have now confirmed the utility of this marker for the early diagnosis of AKI and its clinical sequelae in several clinical scenarios [133–143]. Collectively, these studies have identified proposed cut-offs for NGAL diagnostic thresholds. When urine or plasma NGAL is measured using standardized clinical laboratory platforms, a value of <50 ng/mL effectively rules out structural AKI (irrespective of the serum creatinine concentration). Measured NGAL values of >150 ng/mL are highly predictive of AKI, and values of >500 ng/mL strongly predict severe AKI [143]. These cut-offs still need to be rigorously validated using prospective, multicenter studies.

Studies have examined a combination of urinary biomarkers in children at risk for AKI, including following cardiac surgery [55, 144]. Urinary NGAL was increased in AKI patients within 2 h of bypass initiation, urine interleukin-18 (IL-18) and liver-type fatty acid binding protein (L-FABP) were increased within 6 h, and both urine kidney injury molecule-1 (KIM-1) and the cell cycle biomarkers (product of TIMP-2 and IGFBP-7) increased at the 12-h time point. All markers correlated with AKI severity and clinical outcomes and improved the risk prediction for AKI over clinical models. Thus, they represent temporally sequential markers, and a panel of such biomarkers may therefore help establish the timing of injury and plan appropriate therapies. This concept is illustrated in Fig. 51.7. Standardized clinical laboratory platforms for the measurement of urine and plasma NGAL as well as the cell cycle biomarkers are now available in most countries.

The concept of outcomes in "biomarker-positive, creatinine-negative" patients has been explored. Multicenter studies have enrolled cardiac surgical, critically ill or emergency department patients who were grouped according to their NGAL and serum creatinine status [133]. Studies found that measurement of the levels of NGAL complemented the information obtained by measurement of serum creatinine levels in establishing the diagnosis of AKI and predicting prognosis. A substantial proportion of patients (about 20%) had elevated NGAL levels even in the absence of loss of renal excretory function. This previously undetectable condition (which we now term "subclinical AKI") was associated with a two- to threefold increased risk of death or the need for renal replacement therapy compared to patients without elevations of serum creatinine or tubule damage markers. Notably, even in patients with significant loss of renal function, measurement of tubule damage biomarker levels still added prognostic information, as patients with increased levels of NGAL and serum creatinine levels displayed by far the worst prognosis. Overall, the data support that measurement of tubule damage markers such as NGAL results in a substantial added value to serum creatinine measurements.

Given the above considerations, NGAL and other tubule injury markers may complement a standardized diagnostic approach to AKI, and help clinicians improve their ability to make an early AKI diagnosis. Besides NGAL, other promising biomarkers of tubule damage currently include KIM-1, IL-18, L-FABP, and the cell cycle biomarkers (product of TIMP-2 and IGFBP-7), with additional candidates being continually discovered and verified in this area of intense contemporary research. However, markers of renal function will remain important even after tubule damage markers are fully established. Glomerular filtration markers such as serum creatinine or serum cystatin C are still valuable for the diagnosis and quantification of excretory function loss (e.g., for drug dosing) and prognosis (e.g., for development of CKD). Urine output will still represent a useful criterion for adjustments to fluid balance, and for the commencement or ending of renal replacement therapies. Structural AKI biomarkers may add substantively to our ability to detect AKI early, and to refine our ability to reliably classify AKI, as shown in Table 51.11.

Table 51.11 Biomarkers to refine AKI classification

Functional marker	Structural marker	Classification
–	–	Normal
+	–	Prerenal AKI
–	+	Subclinical AKI
+	+	Intrinsic AKI

Functional markers include serum creatinine, cystatin C, and other markers of GFR. Structural markers include neutrophil gelatinase-associated lipocalin, and others described in the text

Prevention of AKI

Proven measures for prevention of AKI include vigorous fluid administration in patients at high risk for developing AKI, adequate fluid repletion in those with hypovolemia, avoidance of hypotension in critically ill children by providing inotropic support as needed, and close monitoring of renal function and drug levels in children receiving nephrotoxic medications.

Hydration

Vigorous fluid administration (typically with isotonic crystalloid solutions) has been successfully employed to prevent AKI in patients at high risk, including hemoglobinuria, myoglobinuria, early tumor lysis syndrome, renal transplantation, other major surgical procedures, and use of nephrotoxic agents such as radiocontrast, cisplatin, and amphotericin. The efficacy of preoperative hydration strategies was demonstrated by a meta-analysis of 20 randomized controlled trials that investigated the reno-protective effects of perioperative hemodynamic optimization among 4220 adult surgical patients who were undergoing elective or emergent procedures [145]. Postoperative AKI was significantly reduced by perioperative hemodynamic optimization when compared with the control group who did not receive similar goal directed therapy (OR 0.64, 95% CI 0.50–0.83). A more recent meta-analysis with an overall sample of 9308 patients indicated that goal-directed therapy by means of fluids and inotropes improves renal perfusion and oxygenation in high-risk patients undergoing major abdominal and orthopedic surgery [146].

Fluid Resuscitation

A child with a clinical history and physical examination findings consistent with hypovolemia and impending or established prerenal AKI requires immediate vigorous intravenous fluid therapy with normal saline (10–20 mL/kg over 30 min, repeated twice if necessary, until urine output is re-established). Isotonic crystalloids are most used for correcting extracellular volume depletion. Compared to crystalloids, colloids theoretically may result in a greater plasma expansion. However, the difference in required volumes for fluid resuscitation was minimal between crystalloids and colloids. Moreover, colloids carry the risks of hyper-oncotic reduction in glomerular filtration and osmotic tubular damage. It is recommended that serum chloride levels are monitored, since hyperchloremia can cause renal vasoconstriction. If urine output does not improve after restoration of intravascular volume, more invasive monitoring may be required to guide further therapy. In children not responsive to volume repletion alone, preservation of blood pressure and renal perfusion with appropriate inotropic agents is essential to prevent AKI. Patients with established intrinsic AKI require volume restriction to prevent worsening fluid overload. Such patients are best treated by maintaining current volume status by providing for insensible water losses and replacing any ongoing fluid losses.

Nephrotoxin Management

Nephrotoxins are an important risk factor and etiology for pediatric AKI. Monitoring kidney function and drug levels when possible are important for rational adjustment of drug dosing based on known alterations in pharmacokinetics and pharmacodynamics during AKI. It is crucial that clinicians caring for patients requiring potentially nephrotoxic drugs use appropriate drug dosing based on the knowledge of altered clearance rates in early AKI and be vigilant in monitoring for drug efficacy and toxicity. The importance of monitoring serum creatinine levels as a measure of kidney function in children receiving nephrotoxic drugs has been brought into focus in a retrospective single center study of 1660 non-critically ill, hospitalized children [147]. Children who developed AKI as defined by the serum creatinine-based pRIFLE criteria had significantly greater odds of exposure to one or more nephrotoxic medications than patients without AKI (OR 1.7; 95% CI 1.04–2.9). Both increasing dose and duration of nephrotoxin use were associated with increased development of AKI. A recent study demonstrated decreasing AKI duration when a systematic daily serum creatinine monitoring policy was put into practice for children who received multiple nephrotoxic medications. When a systematic daily serum creatinine monitoring program for all non-critically ill children receiving three or more nephrotoxic medications was put in place using an automated EHR-driven protocol in a single center, a 42% reduction in AKI days was observed [148]. This program has now been spread to multiple children's hospitals that could implement a systematic EHR-guided protocol, with excellent published results—follow-up studies have shown a nephrotoxin medication exposure rate decreased by 38% and a reduction in AKI incidence by 64% [149].

Additional quality improvement strategies in the prevention of AKI have been suggested [150]. Briefly, primary prevention at the community level includes raising awareness regarding AKI risk factors among health care professionals and patients by education and establishment of tools that measure these risk profiles. It is suggested that populations and patients at high risk for developing AKI should have a Kidney Health Assessment at least every 12 months to define and modify their AKI risk profile. Primary prevention of AKI in hospitalized patients may be achieved by first screening for AKI risk factors, followed by at least an assessment of serum creatinine, urine dipstick analysis, and urine output. Once AKI has developed, secondary prevention may be directed towards early identification of AKI severity and complications (monitor serum creatinine, urine output, serum electrolytes), minimizing nephrotoxin exposure, ensuring optimal hemodynamic and nutritional status, and treating the underlying cause.

Unproven Pharmacologic Agents for Prevention of AKI

Unproven agents for prevention of AKI include mannitol, loop diuretics, low-dose dopamine, fenoldopam, atrial natriuretic peptide, N-acetylcysteine, and methylxanthines. Their potential use in AKI prevention is briefly discussed here.

Mannitol

Experimental studies suggest that mannitol might be protective by causing a diuresis (which minimizes intratubular cast formation), and by acting as a free radical scavenger (thereby minimizing cell injury). In the clinical setting, the efficacy of mannitol for prevention of AKI in high-risk patients is inconclusive. Indeed, its use may be detrimental, and can result in volume expansion, hyperosmolality, and pulmonary edema. Its use for prevention of AKI is not recommended.

Loop Diuretics

Loop diuretics such as furosemide induce a forced diuresis by reducing active NaCl transport in the thick ascending limb of the loop of Henle. The ensuing decrease in energy requirement may protect the tubule cells in the setting of a decrease in energy delivery. However, the available evidence from clinical studies in adults does not support the routine use of diuretics as prophylaxis for AKI. In some settings, the use of diuretics was harmful. In critically ill children, furosemide was found to be the most common nephrotoxin used and was associated with a twofold greater adjusted risk for developing AKI [151]. Therefore, the use of loop diuretics for prevention of AKI is not recommended. However, in certain select situations, such as contrast induced AKI in susceptible populations, AKI prevention with loop diuretics can be associated with favorable outcomes if euvolemia is carefully maintained.

While controlled studies have demonstrated that the administration of diuretics to patients in the early stages of AKI does not significantly alter the natural history of the disease, furosemide can potentially convert AKI from oliguric to a nonoliguric form and therefore simplify fluid, electrolyte, and nutritional management. The concept here is to use diuretics in well-hydrated, diuretic-responsive patients (primarily furosemide, with sometimes the addition of thiazide diuretics) to maintain urine output, which would prevent fluid overload and allow for nutritional support, both of which would prevent worsening of AKI. In addition, a prospective assessment of a furosemide challenge, or furosemide "stress" test, was able to predict which patients would have worsening AKI based on a lack of response to furosemide within 2 h. In the setting of early AKI, low urine output following the furosemide stress test predicted progressive AKI, need for dialysis, and inpatient mortality [152]. Using a furosemide stress test in patients with increased AKI biomarker levels such as NGAL improves risk stratification and prediction of AKI progression [153].

Dopamine

The use of low "renal-dose" of the inotropic agent dopamine (0.5–3 µg/kg/min) is common in the critical care setting due to its renal vasodilatory and natriuretic effects. However, prospective randomized studies of adult patients at risk for AKI have not shown a beneficial reno-protective effect of "low-dose" dopamine. There are risks associated with even "low-dose" dopamine, including tachycardia, arrhythmias, and myocardial, intestinal and even renal ischemia. Therefore, the routine use of dopamine for prevention of AKI is not recommended.

Fenoldopam

Fenoldopam is a potent, short-acting, selective dopamine A-1 receptor agonist that increases renal blood flow, increases natriuresis, and decreases systemic vascular resistance. Experience with fenoldopam in the pediatric age group is limited. A small, prospective, single center, randomized, double-blind, controlled trial of children undergoing cardiopulmonary bypass revealed a significant reduction in the urinary AKI biomarker NGAL at the end of surgery and 12 h after ICU admission in the group receiving fenoldopam [154]. Confirmation of the benefits of fenoldopam is required in a large, multicenter, randomized, controlled trial prior to routinely recommending this agent for the prevention of AKI.

Natriuretic Peptides

Atrial natriuretic peptide (ANP) and b-type natriuretic peptide (BNP) block tubular reabsorption of sodium and vasodilate the afferent arteriole. The reno-protective effects of these agents have been evaluated primarily in trials of adults undergoing cardiac surgery and with congestive heart failure. While initial data seemed promising, evidence from large, randomized trials have failed to show a conclusive clinic benefit from these agents. Pediatric data for the reno-protective effects of natriuretic peptides is limited. Pending further randomized controlled trial data, the routine use of natriuretic peptides for prophylaxis against AKI is not recommended.

N-Acetylcysteine

N-acetylcysteine (NAC) is a free radical scavenger antioxidant agent that counteracts the deleterious effects of ROS in the generation of tubule cell injury, and also has vasodilatory properties. Several recent meta-analyses have examined the efficacy of N-acetylcysteine in the prevention of AKI following cardiac and other major surgery as well as the prevention of contrast-induced nephropathy in adults. A recent meta-analysis evaluating the preventive effect of NAC on contrast-associated AKI in adults undergoing primary percutaneous coronary intervention suggested that NAC reduces the risk of AKI and all-cause in-hospital mortality [155]. NAC was also shown to prevent postoperative AKI in adults with pre-existing CKD undergoing cardiac surgery [156]. Given that the overall direction of the data is toward benefit and the agent is well tolerated and relatively inexpensive, the use of NAC in high-risk patients is generally recommended. While NAC is commonly used in children for treatment of acetaminophen toxicity and other forms of acute liver failure, data for its reno-protective effects in the pediatric population is limited. The routine use of NAC for AKI prophylaxis in children is not generally recommended, except for judicious use in children with CKD who are at high risk for contrast induced nephropathy. One approach is to use NAC in combination with IV hydration to prevent contrast induced nephropathy in children with CKD stage 3 or greater and a history of contrast-induced AKI in the past, or in children who are already on two nephrotoxins and contrast would be the third nephrotoxin to be used. The efficacy of this approach has not been systematically studied.

Methylxanthines

Methylxanthines are adenosine antagonists that act via A1 and A2A receptors in the kidneys. Previous human clinical trials using caffeine citrate, theophylline or aminophylline have suggested that methylxanthines may prevent AKI or improve renal function in special populations of high-risk neonates and infants, including those with perinatal hypoxia/ischemia or prematurity and undergoing cardiac surgery. In a recent multicenter in preterm neonates, caffeine administration in preterm neonates was associated with reduced incidence and severity of AKI. In this retrospective analysis, for every 4.3 neonates exposed to caffeine, one case of AKI was prevented [86]. In two recent systematic reviews of prophylactic theophylline or aminophylline use for prevention of AKI in highly susceptible neonates with birth asphyxia, the pooled estimate showed a 60% reduction in the incidence of AKI and a significant improvement in fluid balance, with no increase in risk of complications [87, 88]. It should be noted that theophylline has wide variation in metabolism and a narrow therapeutic window, and it is therefore essential to monitor theophylline levels to avoid toxicity.

Prognosis and Outcome

In general, pediatric AKI has serious short- and long-term consequences. The outcome depends upon the etiology, age of the child, and co-morbidities. The short-term outcomes of AKI include mortality and morbidity. Regarding mortality, retrospective analyses of large databases during the past decade in the United States showed that the overall in-hospital mortality rate of hospitalized children with AKI is approximately 15%. Mortality rates have ranged from 9.5% in non-critically ill children to 30% in children requiring intensive care. Even higher in-hospital mortality rates of 35–45% have been reported from other countries. The highest mortality rates are encountered in infants, those who have multiorgan failure, and those requiring renal replacement therapies. Data regarding long-term mortality after pediatric AKI is limited, although small studies have revealed a mortality rate of about 20% during a 2–5 year follow-up period. More recent multinational studies have revealed perhaps an encouraging improvement regarding in-hospital mortality. Both the AWARE study in critically ill children [35] and the AWAKEN study in neonates [36] reported an in-hospital mortality rate of approximately 10%. However, in the Global Snapshot study, children from low-income countries continue to experience a high mortality rate of 20% compared with only 1.2% in those from high-income countries [38].

Regarding short-term morbidity, it is quite clear that AKI is associated with adverse effects, including increased need for and longer duration of ventilatory support, as well as increased length of hospital stay [157]. The AWARE study demonstrated a stepwise increase in mechanical ventilation use as well as ICU lengths of stay (LOS), depending on AKI severity [35]. Critically ill children with stage 1, stage 2, and stage 3 AKI required mechanical ventilation 38.2%, 40.5%, and 50.2% of the time, respectively (vs. no AKI at 29.5%). In the AWARE study, patients with AKI (increase of 1.31 days) and severe AKI (increase of 3 days) had longer ICU LOS after adjusting for severity of illness [35]. These observations confirm previous findings of children who experienced AKI that had longer hospital LOS (36.6 days vs. 20.5 days) than those without AKI [9]. This association is also seen in neonates across all gestational ages. Two single center reports found that AKI increased hospital LOS among neonates by 3.4 days and 11.7 days, respectively. The association between AKI and LOS is evident even in non-critically ill children, including in the settings of nephrotoxin administration and the nephrotic syndrome [64].

Information regarding the long-term outcome of children after an episode of AKI is beginning to accumulate. In a multicenter pooled analysis of 3476 children with hemolytic uremic syndrome followed for a mean of 4.4 years, the combined average death and ESKD rate was 12%, and the combined average renal sequelae rate (CKD, proteinuria, hypertension) was 25%. Thus, long-term follow-up appears to be warranted after an acute episode of hemolytic uremic syndrome. Long-term follow-up of premature infants with neonatal AKI has shown a 45% rate of renal insufficiency. Prominent risk factors for progression include an increased random urine protein/creatinine ratio and a serum creatinine >0.6 mg/dL at 1 year of age. More recent long-term follow-up studies demonstrate that 40–60% of children surviving an AKI episode have a sign of CKD, including proteinuria, hyperfiltration, low eGFR or hypertension In the Translational Research Investigating Biomarker Endpoints in AKI (TRIBE-AKI) prospective study in children after cardiac surgery, hypertension (17%), proteinuria (8%), and a eGFR <90 mL/min/1.73 (13%) were common 5 years later; however, these sequelae were not more common among the children who experienced perioperative AKI [158]. Similarly, the Assessment, Serial Evaluation, and Subsequent Sequelae in Acute Kidney Injury (ASSESS-AKI) prospective study followed children for 4 years after cardiopulmonary bypass [159]. The cohort prevalence of CKD was high (20%); hypertension prevalence was also high (30%). AKI was not significantly associated with the development of CKD or hypertension. However, a subsequently published retrospective study did find that cardiac surgery-associated AKI was associated with a greater risk for CKD stage 2 or greater [160]. The 5-year cumulative incidence of CKD for patients with cardiac surgery-associated AKI was 12%, in comparison with 3% in those without AKI (adjusted HR 3.8). In a longitudinal study of heterogenous critically ill children, AKI was associated with twofold higher odds for CKD or hypertension at 6 years of follow-up [161].

Beyond CKD, AKI episodes are also associated with ESKD. In a retrospective analysis of 1688 surviving children who required dialysis for an acute AKI episode, outcomes after a median of 9.6 years included death (7%), CKD (13%), ESKD (2.6%), and hypertension (12%) [162].

Collectively, these data strongly suggest that long-term follow-up is clearly warranted for children who survive an episode of AKI. Widely available interventions for hypertension and proteinuria hold promise for prevention of CKD progression after AKI, a concept that is especially pertinent to the pediatric population.

Concluding Remarks

AKI represents a very significant and potentially devastating problem in pediatric medicine, with dire immediate and long-term consequences. The incidence appears to be rising globally. Outstanding advances in basic research have illuminated the pathogenesis of AKI and have paved the way for several successful therapeutic approaches in animal models. However, translational research efforts in humans have yielded disappointing results. One reason for this is the lack of early markers for AKI, and hence an unacceptable delay in initiating promising therapies. Fortunately, several potential candidates are currently being developed and tested as sequential non-invasive early biomarkers for the prediction of AKI and its severity. It is likely that not any one biomarker but a collection of strategically selected proteins may provide the "AKI Panel" for the early non-invasive diagnosis of AKI and its consequences. Such a tool of biologically plausible sequential biomarkers would be indispensable for risk stratification, timely institution of potentially effective therapies, monitoring the response to therapies, and for prediction of adverse clinical outcomes. A judicious combination of clinical judgment, established functional markers, novel structural markers based on knowledge of underlying pathophysiology, and technical advances in therapies that counter the complex mechanisms holds the greatest promise for true progress in human intrinsic AKI.

References

1. Starr MC, Charlton JR, Guillet R, Reidy K, Tipple TE, Jetton JG, Kent AL, Abitbol CL, Ambalavanan N, Mhanna MJ, Askenazi DJ, Selewski DT, Harer MW, Neonatal Kidney Collaborative Board. Advances in neonatal acute kidney injury. Pediatrics. 2021;148(5):e2021051220.
2. Hoste EAJ, Kellum JA, Selby NM, et al. Global epidemiology and outcomes of acute kidney injury. Nat Rev Nephrol. 2018;14(10):607–25.
3. Desanti De Oliveira B, Xu K, Shen TH, et al. Molecular nephrology: types of acute tubular injury. Nat Rev Nephrol. 2019;15(10):599–612.
4. Roy J-P, Devarajan P. Acute kidney injury: diagnosis and management. Indian J Pediatr. 2020;87(8):600–7.
5. Devarajan P. The current state of the art in acute kidney injury. Front Pediatr. 2020;9:70.
6. Sandokji I, Greenberg JH. Novel biomarkers of acute kidney injury in children: an update on recent findings. Curr Opin Pediatr. 2020;32(3):354–9.
7. Liu KD, Goldstein SL, Vijayan A, et al. AKI!Now Initiative: recommendations for awareness, recognition, and management of AKI. Clin J Am Soc Nephrol. 2020;15(12):1838–47.
8. Sutherland SM, Byrnes JJ, Kothari M, et al. AKI in hospitalized children: comparing the pRIFLE,

AKIN, and KDIGO definitions. Clin J Am Soc Nephrol. 2015;10(4):554–61.

9. Akcan-Arikan A, Zappitelli M, Loftis LL, Washburn KK, Jefferson LS, Goldstein SL. Modified RIFLE criteria in critically ill children with acute kidney injury. Kidney Int. 2007;71(10):1028–35.

10. Bagga A, Bakkaloglu A, Devarajan P, Mehta RL, Kellum JA, Shah SV, Molitoris BA, Ronco C, Warnock DG, Joannidis M, Levin A, Acute Kidney Injury Network. Improving outcomes from acute kidney injury: report of an initiative. Pediatr Nephrol. 2007;22(10):1655–8.

11. Kidney Disease: Improving Global Outcomes (KDIGO) Acute Kidney Injury Work Group. KDIGO clinical practice guideline for acute kidney injury. Kidney Int Suppl. 2012;2:1–138.

12. Devarajan P. Pediatric acute kidney injury: different from acute renal failure, but how and why? Curr Pediatr Rep. 2013;1(1):34–40.

13. Ciccia E, Devarajan P. Pediatric acute kidney injury: prevalence, impact and management challenges. Int J Nephrol Renovasc Dis. 2017;10:77–84.

14. Schwartz GJ, Munoz A, Schneider MF, Mak RH, Kaskel F, Warady BA, et al. New equations to estimate GFR in children with CKD. J Am Soc Nephrol. 2009;20(3):629–37.

15. Roy J-P, Johnson C, Towne B, et al. Use of height-independent baseline creatinine imputation method with renal angina index. Pediatr Nephrol. 2019;34(10):1777–84.

16. O'Neil ER, Devaraj S, Mayorquin L, et al. Defining pediatric community-acquired acute kidney injury: an observational study. Pediatr Res. 2020;87:564–8.

17. Kaddourah A, Basu RK, Goldstein SL, Sutherland SM, Assessment of Worldwide Acute Kidney Injury, Renal Angina and, Epidemiology (AWARE) Investigators. Oliguria and acute kidney injury in critically ill children: implications for diagnosis and outcomes. Pediatr Crit Care Med. 2019;20(4):332–9.

18. Goldstein SL. Urine output assessment in acute kidney injury: the cheapest and most impactful biomarker. Front Pediatr. 2020;7:565.

19. Xu X, Nie S, Zhang A, Jianhua M, Liu HP, Xia H, Xu H, Liu Z, Feng S, Zhou W, Liu X, Yang Y, Tao Y, Feng Y, Chen C, Wang M, Zha Y, Feng JH, Li Q, Ge S, Chen J, He Y, Teng S, Hao C, Liu BC, Tang Y, Wang LJ, Qi JL, He W, He P, Liu Y, Hou FF. A new criterion for pediatric AKI based on the reference change value of serum creatinine. J Am Soc Nephrol. 2018;29(9):2432–42.

20. Wei C, Hongxia G, Hui F, Danqun J, Haipen L. Impact of and risk factors for pediatric acute kidney injury defined by the pROCK criteria in a Chinese PICU population. Pediatr Res. 2021;89(6):1485–91.

21. Lameire NH, Levin A, Kellum JA, Cheung M, Jadoul M, Winkelmayer WC, Stevens PE, Conference Participants. Harmonizing acute and chronic kidney disease definition and classification: report of a Kidney Disease: Improving Global Outcomes

(KDIGO) Consensus Conference. Kidney Int. 2021;100(3):516–26.

22. Basu RK, Kaddourah A, Goldstein SL, AWARE Study Investigators. Assessment of a renal angina index for prediction of severe acute kidney injury in critically ill children: a multicentre, multinational, prospective observational study. Lancet Child Adolesc Health. 2018;2:112–20.

23. Sethi SK, Raghunathan V, Shah S, Dhaliwal M, Jha P, Kumar M, Paluri S, Bansal S, Mhanna MJ, Raina R. Fluid overload and renal angina index at admission are associated with worse outcomes in critically ill children. Front Pediatr. 2018;6:118.

24. Hanson HR, Carlisle MA, Bensman RS, et al. Early prediction of pediatric acute kidney injury from the emergency department: a pilot study. Am J Emerg Med. 2021;40:138–44.

25. Huang L, Shi T, Quan W, et al. Assessment of early renal anginal index for prediction of subsequent severe acute kidney injury during septic shock in children. BMC Nephrol. 2020;21(1):358.

26. Basu RK, Wang Y, Wong HR, Chawla LS, Wheeler DS, Goldstein SL. Incorporation of biomarkers with the renal angina index for prediction of severe AKI in critically ill children. Clin J Am Soc Nephrol. 2014;9:654–62.

27. Stanski N, Menon S, Goldstein SL, Basu RK. Integration of urinary neutrophil gelatinase-associated lipocalin with serum creatinine delineates acute kidney injury phenotypes in critically ill children. J Crit Care. 2019;53:1–7.

28. Abbasi A, Rabori PM, Farajollahi R, et al. Discriminatory precision of renal angina index in predicting acute kidney injury in children; a systematic review and meta-analysis. Arch Acad Emerg Med. 2020;8(1):e39.

29. Parikh RV, Tan TC, Salyer AS, Auron A, Kim PS, Ku E, Go AS. Community-based epidemiology of hospitalized acute kidney injury. Pediatrics. 2020;146(3):e20192821.

30. Wang L, McGregor TL, Jones DP, Bridges BC, Fleming GM, Shirey-Rice J, McLemore MF, Chen L, Weitkamp A, Byrne DW, Van Driest SL. Electronic health record-based predictive models for acute kidney injury screening in pediatric inpatients. Pediatr Res. 2017;82:465–73.

31. Gubb S, Holmes J, Smith G, et al. Acute kidney injury in children based on electronic alerts. J Pediatr. 2020;220:14–20.

32. Xu X, Nie S, Zhang A, et al. Acute kidney injury among hospitalized children in China. Clin J Am Soc Nephrol. 2018;13:1791–800.

33. Bhojani S, Stojanovic J, Melhem N, et al. The incidence of pediatric acute kidney injury identified using an AKI E-Alert algorithm in six English hospitals. Front Pediatr. 2020;8:29. https://doi.org/10.3389/fped.2020.00029.

34. Sandokji I, Yamamoto Y, Biswas A, et al. A time-updated parsimonious model to predict AKI in hospitalized children. J Am Soc Nephrol. 2020;31(6):1348–57.

35. Kaddourah A, Basu RK, Bagshaw SM, et al. Epidemiology of acute kidney injury in critically ill children and young adults. N Engl J Med. 2017;376:11–20.

36. Jetton JG, Boohaker LJ, Sethi SK, et al. Incidence and outcomes of neonatal acute kidney injury (AWAKEN): a multicenter, multinational, observational cohort study. Lancet Child Adolesc Health. 2017;1(3):184–94.

37. Lameire N, Van Biesen W, Vanholder R. Epidemiology of acute kidney injury in children worldwide, including developing countries. Pediatr Nephrol. 2017;32:1301–14.

38. Macedo E, Cerdá J, Hingorani S, et al. Recognition and management of acute kidney injury in children: the ISN 0by25 Global Snapshot study. PLoS One. 2018;13:e0196586.

39. Chang JW, Jeng MJ, Yang LY, et al. The epidemiology and prognostic factors of mortality in critically ill children with acute kidney injury in Taiwan. Kidney Int. 2015;87:632–9.

40. Fitzgerald JC, Ross ME, Thomas NJ, et al. Risk factors and inpatient outcomes associated with acute kidney injury at pediatric severe sepsis presentation. Pediatr Nephrol. 2018;33:1781–90.

41. Alobaidi R, Morgan C, Goldstein SL, Bagshaw SM. Population-based epidemiology and outcomes of acute kidney injury in critically ill children. Pediatr Crit Care Med. 2020;21:82–91.

42. Fitzgerald JC, Basu RK, Akcan-Arikan A, Izquierdo LM, Piñeres Olave BE, Hassinger AB, Szczepanska M, Deep A, Williams D, Sapru A, Roy JA, Nadkarni VM, Thomas NJ, Weiss SL, Furth S, Sepsis PRevalence, OUtcomes, and Therapies Study Investigators and Pediatric Acute Lung Injury and Sepsis Investigators Network. Acute kidney injury in pediatric severe sepsis: an independent risk factor for death and new disability. Crit Care Med. 2016;44:2241–50.

43. Charlton JR, Boohaker L, Askenazi D, et al. Incidence and risk factors of early onset neonatal AKI. Clin J Am Soc Nephrol. 2019;14(2):184–95.

44. Mwamanenge NA, Assenga E, Furia FF. Acute kidney injury among critically ill neonates in a tertiary hospital in Tanzania; prevalence, risk factors and outcome. PLoS One. 2020;15(2):e0229074. eCollection 2020

45. Askenazi DJ, Heagerty PJ, Schmicker RH, et al. Prevalence of acute kidney injury (AKI) in extremely low gestational age neonates (ELGAN). Pediatr Nephrol. 2020;35(9):1737–48.

46. Balestracci A, Ezquer M, Elmo ME, et al. Ibuprofen-associated acute kidney injury in dehydrated children with acute gastroenteritis. Pediatr Nephrol. 2015;30:1873–8.

47. Nehus E, Kaddourah A, Bennett M, Pyles O, Devarajan P. Subclinical kidney injury in children receiving nonsteroidal anti-inflammatory drugs after cardiac surgery. J Pediatr. 2017;189:175–80.

48. Downes KJ, Cowden C, Laskin BL, et al. Association of acute kidney injury with concomitant vancomycin and piperacillin/tazobactam treatment among hospitalized children. JAMA Pediatr. 2017;171:e173219.

49. Joyce EL, Kane-Gill SL, Priyanka P, et al. Piperacillin/Tazobactam and antibiotic-associated acute kidney injury in critically ill children. J Am Soc Nephrol. 2019;30(11):2243–51.

50. Gilligan LA, Davenport MS, Trout AT, et al. Risk of acute kidney injury following contrast-enhanced CT in hospitalized pediatric patients: a propensity score analysis. Radiology. 2020;294(3):548–56.

51. Mishra J, Dent C, Tarabishi R, Mitsnefes MM, Ma Q, Kelly C, Ruff SM, Zahedi K, Shao M, Bean J, Mori K, Barasch J, Devarajan P. Neutrophil gelatinase-associated lipocalin (NGAL) as a biomarker for acute renal injury after cardiac surgery. Lancet. 2005;365:1231–8.

52. Dent CL, Ma Q, Dastrala S, et al. Plasma neutrophil gelatinase-associated lipocalin predicts acute kidney injury, morbidity and mortality after pediatric cardiac surgery: a prospective uncontrolled cohort study. Crit Care. 2007;11:R127.

53. Bennett M, Dent CL, Ma Q, et al. Urine NGAL predicts severity of acute kidney injury after cardiac surgery: a prospective study. Clin J Am Soc Nephrol. 2008;3:665.

54. Krawczeski CD, Woo JG, Wang Y, et al. Neutrophil gelatinase-associated lipocalin concentrations predict development of acute kidney injury in neonates and children after cardiopulmonary bypass. J Pediatr. 2011;158:1009.

55. Krawczeski CD, Goldstein SL, Woo JG, et al. Temporal relationship and predictive value of urinary acute kidney injury biomarkers after pediatric cardiopulmonary bypass. J Am Coll Cardiol. 2011;58:2301.

56. Li S, Krawczeski CD, Zappitelli M, et al. Incidence, risk factors, and outcomes of acute kidney injury after pediatric cardiac surgery: a prospective multicenter study. Crit Care Med. 2011;39:1493.

57. Jefferies JL, Devarajan P. Early detection of acute kidney injury after pediatric cardiac surgery. Prog Pediatr Cardiol. 2016;41:9.

58. Hirano D, Ito A, Yamada A, et al. Independent risk factors and 2-year outcomes of acute kidney injury after surgery for congenital heart disease. Am J Nephrol. 2017;46:204.

59. Park PG, Hong CR, Kang E, et al. Acute kidney injury in pediatric cancer patients. J Pediatr. 2019;208:243.

60. Xiong M, Wang L, Sue L, et al. Acute kidney injury among hospitalized children with cancer. Pediatr Nephrol. 2021;36:171.

61. Kizilbash SJ, Kashtan CE, Chavers BM, et al. Acute kidney injury and the risk of mortality in children undergoing hematopoietic stem cell transplantation. Biol Blood Marrow Transplant. 2016;22:1264.

62. Koh KN, Sunkara A, Kang G, et al. Acute kidney injury in pediatric patients receiving allogeneic hematopoietic cell transplantation: incidence, risk factors, and outcomes. Biol Blood Marrow Transplant. 2018;24:758.

63. Hamada M, Matsukawa S, Shimizu S, et al. Acute kidney injury after pediatric liver transplantation: incidence, risk factors, and association with outcome. J Anesth. 2017;31:758.

64. Rheault MN, Zhang L, Selewski DT, et al. AKI in children hospitalized with nephrotic syndrome. Clin J Am Soc Nephrol. 2015;10:2110.

65. Baddam S, Aban I, Hilliard L, et al. Acute kidney injury during a pediatric sickle cell vaso-occlusive pain crisis. Pediatr Nephrol. 2017;32(8):1451–6.

66. Wang X, Chen X, Tang F, Luo W, Fang J, Qi C, Sun H, Xiao H, Peng X, Shao J. Be aware of acute kidney injury in critically ill children with COVID-19. Pediatr Nephrol. 2021;36(1):163–9.

67. Chopra S, Saha A, Kumar V, Thakur A, Pemde H, Kapoor D, Ray S, Das A, Pandit K, Gulati A, Sharma AG, Singh P, Sodani R. Acute kidney injury in hospitalized children with COVID19. J Trop Pediatr. 2021;67(2):fmab037.

68. Kari JA, Shalaby MA, Albanna AS, Alahmadi TS, Alherbish A, Alhasan KA. Acute kidney injury in children with COVID-19: a retrospective study. BMC Nephrol. 2021;22(1):202.

69. Raina R, Chakraborty R, Mawby I, Agarwal N, Sethi S, Forbes M. Critical analysis of acute kidney injury in pediatric COVID-19 patients in the intensive care unit. Pediatr Nephrol. 2021;36(9):2627–38.

70. Sethi SK, Rana A, Adnani H, McCulloch M, Alhasan K, Sultana A, Safadi R, Agrawal N, Raina R. Kidney involvement in multisystem inflammatory syndrome in children: a pediatric nephrologist's perspective. Clin Kidney J. 2021;14(9):2000–11.

71. Drożdżal S, Lechowicz K, Szostak B, Rosik J, Kotfis K, Machoy-Mokrzyńska A, Białecka M, Ciechanowski K, Gawrońska-Szklarz B. Kidney damage from nonsteroidal anti-inflammatory drugs-Myth or truth? Review of selected literature. Pharmacol Res Perspect. 2021;9(4):e00817.

72. Misurac JM, Knoderer CA, Leiser JD, Nailescu C, Wilson AC, Andreoli SP. Nonsteroidal anti-inflammatory drugs are an important cause of acute kidney injury in children. J Pediatr. 2013;162(6):1153–9.

73. Clavé S, Rousset-Rouvière C, Daniel L, Tsimaratos M. The invisible threat of non-steroidal anti-inflammatory drugs for kidneys. Front Pediatr. 2019;7:520.

74. Pham JT, Jacobson JL, Ohler KH, Kraus DM, Calip GS. Evaluation of the risk factors for acute kidney injury in neonates exposed to antenatal indomethacin. J Pediatr Pharmacol Ther. 2020;25(7):606–16.

75. Gong J, Ma L, Li M, Ma L, Chen C, Zhao S, Zhou Y, Cui Y. Nonsteroidal anti-inflammatory drugs associated acute kidney injury in hospitalized children: a systematic review and meta-analysis. Pharmacoepidemiol Drug Saf. 2021; https://doi.org/10.1002/pds.5385.

76. Chappell MC. Non-classical renin-angiotensin system and renal function. Compr Physiol. 2012;2(4):2733–52.

77. Arora P, Rajagopalam S, Ranjan R, Kolli H, Singh M, Venuto R, Lohr J. Preoperative use of angiotensin-converting enzyme inhibitors/angiotensin receptor blockers is associated with increased risk for acute kidney injury after cardiovascular surgery. Clin J Am Soc Nephrol. 2008;3(5):1266–73.

78. Terano C, Ishikura K, Miura M, Hamada R, Harada R, Sakai T, Hamasaki Y, Hataya H, Ando T, Honda M. Incidence of and risk factors for severe acute kidney injury in children with heart failure treated with renin-angiotensin system inhibitors. Eur J Pediatr. 2016;175(5):631–7.

79. Moffett BS, Goldstein SL, Adusei M, Kuzin J, Mohan P, Mott AR. Risk factors for postoperative acute kidney injury in pediatric cardiac surgery patients receiving angiotensin-converting enzyme inhibitors. Pediatr Crit Care Med. 2011;12(5):555–9.

80. Benoit SW, Devarajan P. Acute kidney injury: emerging pharmacotherapies in current clinical trials. Pediatr Nephrol. 2018;33(5):779–87.

81. Molema G, Zijlstra JG, van Meurs M, Kamps JAAM. Renal microvascular endothelial cell responses in sepsis-induced acute kidney injury. Nat Rev Nephrol. 2021; https://doi.org/10.1038/s41581-021-00489-1.

82. Sun J, Zhang J, Tian J, Virzì GM, Digvijay K, Cueto L, Yin Y, Rosner MH, Ronco C. Mitochondria in sepsis-induced AKI. J Am Soc Nephrol. 2019;30(7):1151–61.

83. Hu J, Spina S, Zadek F, Kamenshchikov NO, Bittner EA, Pedemonte J, Berra L. Effect of nitric oxide on postoperative acute kidney injury in patients who underwent cardiopulmonary bypass: a systematic review and meta-analysis with trial sequential analysis. Ann Intensive Care. 2019;9(1):129.

84. Waskowski J, Pfortmueller CA, Erdoes G, Buehlmann R, Messmer AS, Luedi MM, Schmidli J, Schefold JC. Mannitol for the prevention of perioperative acute kidney injury: a systematic review. Eur J Vasc Endovasc Surg. 2019;58(1):130–40.

85. Abraham S, Rameshkumar R, Chidambaram M, Soundravally R, Subramani S, Bhowmick R, Sheriff A, Maulik K, Mahadevan S. Trial of furosemide to prevent acute kidney injury in critically ill children: a double-blind, randomized, controlled trial. Indian J Pediatr. 2021;88(11):1099–106.

86. Harer MW, Askenazi DJ, Boohaker LJ, Carmody JB, Griffin RL, Guillet R, Selewski DT, Swanson JR, Charlton JR, Neonatal Kidney Collaborative (NKC). Association between early caffeine citrate administration and risk of acute kidney injury in preterm neonates: results from the AWAKEN study. JAMA Pediatr. 2018;172(6):e180322.

87. Bhatt GC, Gogia P, Bitzan M, Das RR. Theophylline and aminophylline for prevention of acute kidney injury in neonates and children: a systematic review. Arch Dis Child. 2019;104(7):670–9.

88. Bellos I, Pandita A, Yachha M. Effectiveness of theophylline administration in neonates with perinatal asphyxia: a meta-analysis. J Matern Fetal Neonatal Med. 2021;34(18):3080–8.

89. Sharma S, Leaf DE. Iron chelation as a potential therapeutic strategy for AKI prevention. J Am Soc Nephrol. 2019;30(11):2060–71.

90. Thielmann M, Corteville D, Szabo G, Swaminathan M, Lamy A, Lehner LJ, Brown CD, Noiseux N, Atta MG, Squiers EC, Erlich S, Rothenstein D, Molitoris B, Mazer CD. Teprasiran, a small interfering RNA, for the prevention of acute kidney injury in high-risk patients undergoing cardiac surgery: a randomized clinical study. Circulation. 2021;144(14):1133–44.

91. Tian Y, Li X, Wang Y, Zhao W, Wang C, Gao Y, Wang S, Liu J. Association between preoperative statin exposure and acute kidney injury in adult patients undergoing cardiac surgery. J Cardiothorac Vasc Anesth. 2021;36(4):1014–20.

92. Askenazi DJ, Heagerty PJ, Schmicker RH, Brophy P, Juul SE, Goldstein SL, Hingorani S, PENUT Trial Consortium. The impact of erythropoietin on short- and long-term kidney-related outcomes in neonates of extremely low gestational age. Results of a multi-center, double-blind, placebo-controlled randomized clinical trial. J Pediatr. 2021;232:65–72.e7.

93. Legrand M, Bell S, Forni L, Joannidis M, Koyner JL, Liu K, Cantaluppi V. Pathophysiology of COVID-19-associated acute kidney injury. Nat Rev Nephrol. 2021;17(11):751–64.

94. You R, Zheng H, Xu L, Ma T, Chen G, Xia P, Fan X, Ji P, Wang L, Chen L. Decreased urinary uromodulin is potentially associated with acute kidney injury: a systematic review and meta-analysis. J Intensive Care. 2021;9(1):70.

95. Rudman-Melnick V, Adam M, Potter A, Chokshi SM, Ma Q, Drake KA, Schuh MP, Kofron JM, Devarajan P, Potter SS. Single-cell profiling of AKI in a murine model reveals novel transcriptional signatures, pro-fibrotic phenotype, and epithelial-to-stromal crosstalk. J Am Soc Nephrol. 2020;31(12):2793–814.

96. Park J, Shrestha R, Qiu C, Kondo A, Huang S, Werth M, Li M, Barasch J, Suszták K. Single-cell transcriptomics of the mouse kidney reveals potential cellular targets of kidney disease. Science. 2018;360(6390):758–63.

97. Wu H, Malone AF, Donnelly EL, Kirita Y, Uchimura K, Ramakrishnan SM, Gaut JP, Humphreys BD. Single-cell transcriptomics of a human kidney allograft biopsy specimen defines a diverse inflammatory response. J Am Soc Nephrol. 2018;29(8):2069–80.

98. Muto Y, Wilson PC, Ledru N, Wu H, Dimke H, Waikar SS, Humphreys BD. Single cell transcriptional and chromatin accessibility profiling redefine cellular heterogeneity in the adult human kidney. Nat Commun. 2021;12(1):2190.

99. Wu H, Kirita Y, Donnelly EL, Humphreys BD. Advantages of single-nucleus over single-cell RNA sequencing of adult kidney: rare cell types and novel cell states revealed in fibrosis. J Am Soc Nephrol. 2019;30(1):23–32.

100. Devarajan P. Genomic and proteomic characterization of acute kidney injury. Nephron. 2015;131(2):85–91.

101. Mar D, Gharib SA, Zager RA, Johnson A, Denisenko O, Bomsztyk K. Heterogeneity of epigenetic changes at ischemia/reperfusion- and endotoxin-induced acute kidney injury genes. Kidney Int. 2015;88(4):734–44.

102. Xu K, Rosenstiel P, Paragas N, Hinze C, Gao X, Huai Shen T, Werth M, Forster C, Deng R, Bruck E, Boles RW, Tornato A, Gopal T, Jones M, Konig J, Stauber J, D'Agati V, Erdjument-Bromage H, Saggi S, Wagener G, Schmidt-Ott KM, Tatonetti N, Tempst P, Oliver JA, Guarnieri P, Barasch J. Unique transcriptional programs identify subtypes of AKI. J Am Soc Nephrol. 2017;28(6):1729–40.

103. Liu J, Kumar S, Dolzhenko E, Alvarado GF, Guo J, Lu C, Chen Y, Li M, Dessing MC, Parvez RK, Cippà PE, Krautzberger AM, Saribekyan G, Smith AD, McMahon AP. Molecular characterization of the transition from acute to chronic kidney injury following ischemia/reperfusion. JCI Insight. 2017;2(18):e94716.

104. Bowers SLK, Davis-Rodriguez S, Thomas ZM, Rudomanova V, Bacon WC, Beiersdorfer A, Ma Q, Devarajan P, Blaxall BC. Inhibition of fibronectin polymerization alleviates kidney injury due to ischemia-reperfusion. Am J Physiol Renal Physiol. 2019;316(6):F1293–8.

105. Zhao B, Lu Q, Cheng Y, Belcher JM, Siew ED, Leaf DE, Body SC, Fox AA, Waikar SS, Collard CD, Thiessen-Philbrook H, Ikizler TA, Ware LB, Edelstein CL, Garg AX, Choi M, Schaub JA, Zhao H, Lifton RP, Parikh CR, TRIBE-AKI Consortium. A genome-wide association study to identify single-nucleotide polymorphisms for acute kidney injury. Am J Respir Crit Care Med. 2017;195(4):482–90.

106. Chihanga T, Ma Q, Nicholson JD, Ruby HN, Edelmann RE, Devarajan P, Kennedy MA. NMR spectroscopy and electron microscopy identification of metabolic and ultrastructural changes to the kidney following ischemia-reperfusion injury. Am J Physiol Renal Physiol. 2018;314(2):F154–66.

107. Chihanga T, Ruby HN, Ma Q, Bashir S, Devarajan P, Kennedy MA. NMR-based urine metabolic profiling and immunohistochemistry analysis of nephron changes in a mouse model of hypoxia-induced acute kidney injury. Am J Physiol Renal Physiol. 2018;315(4):F1159–73.

108. Poyan Mehr A, Tran MT, Ralto KM, Leaf DE, Washco V, Messmer J, Lerner A, Kher A, Kim SH, Khoury CC, Herzig SJ, Trovato ME, Simon-Tillaux

N, Lynch MR, Thadhani RI, Clish CB, Khabbaz KR, Rhee EP, Waikar SS, Berg AH, Parikh SM. De novo NAD⁺ biosynthetic impairment in acute kidney injury in humans. Nat Med. 2018;24(9):1351–9.

109. Alge J, Dolan K, Angelo J, Thadani S, Virk M, Akcan Arikan A. Two to tango: kidney-lung interaction in acute kidney injury and acute respiratory distress syndrome. Front Pediatr. 2021;18(9):744110.

110. Cavanaugh C, Perazella MA. Urine sediment examination in the diagnosis and management of kidney disease: core curriculum 2019. Am J Kidney Dis. 2019;73(2):258–72.

111. Cox ZL, Sury K, Rao VS, Ivey-Miranda JB, Griffin M, Mahoney D, Gomez N, Fleming JH, Inker LA, Coca SG, Turner J, Wilson FP, Testani JM. Effect of loop diuretics on the fractional excretion of urea in decompensated heart failure. J Card Fail. 2020;26(5):402–9.

112. Selewski DT, Goldstein SL. The role of fluid overload in the prediction of outcome in acute kidney injury. Pediatr Nephrol. 2018;33(1):13–24.

113. Devarajan P. Biomarkers for the early detection of acute kidney injury. Curr Opin Pediatr. 2011;23:194–200.

114. Schwartz GJ, Work DF. Measurement and estimation of GFR in children and adolescents. Clin J Am Soc Nephrol. 2009;4:1832–43.

115. Renganathan A, Warner BB, Tarr PI, Dharnidharka VR. The progression of serum cystatin C concentrations within the first month of life after preterm birth-a worldwide systematic review. Pediatr Nephrol. 2021;36(7):1709–18.

116. Benoit SW, Ciccia EA, Devarajan P. Cystatin C as a biomarker of chronic kidney disease: latest developments. Expert Rev Mol Diagn. 2020;20(10):1019–26.

117. Pottel H, Dubourg L, Goffin K, Delanaye P. Alternatives for the bedside Schwartz equation to estimate glomerular filtration rate in children. Adv Chronic Kidney Dis. 2018;25(1):57–66.

118. Mian AN, Schwartz GJ. Measurement and estimation of glomerular filtration rate in children. Adv Chronic Kidney Dis. 2017;24(6):348–56.

119. Nakhjavan-Shahraki B, Yousefifard M, Ataei N, Baikpour M, Ataei F, Bazargani B, Abbasi A, Ghelichkhani P, Javidilarijani F, Hosseini M. Accuracy of cystatin C in prediction of acute kidney injury in children; serum or urine levels: which one works better? A systematic review and meta-analysis. BMC Nephrol. 2017;18(1):120.

120. Krawczeski CD, Vandevoorde RG, Kathman T, Bennett MR, Woo JG, Wang Y, Griffiths RE, Devarajan P. Serum cystatin C is an early predictive biomarker of acute kidney injury after pediatric cardiopulmonary bypass. Clin J Am Soc Nephrol. 2010;5(9):1552–7.

121. Volpon LC, Sugo EK, Carlotti AP. Diagnostic and prognostic value of serum cystatin C in critically ill children with acute kidney injury. Pediatr Crit Care Med. 2015;16(5):e125–31.

122. Soto K, Coelho S, Rodrigues B, Martins H, Frade F, Lopes S, Cunha L, Papoila AL, Devarajan P. Cystatin C as a marker of acute kidney injury in the emergency department. Clin J Am Soc Nephrol. 2010;5(10):1745–54.

123. Pottel H, Delanaye P, Schaeffner E, Dubourg L, Eriksen BO, Melsom T, Lamb EJ, Rule AD, Turner ST, Glassock RJ, De Souza V, Selistre L, Goffin K, Pauwels S, Mariat C, Flamant M, Ebert N. Estimating glomerular filtration rate for the full age spectrum from serum creatinine and cystatin C. Nephrol Dial Transplant. 2017;32(3):497–507.

124. Devarajan P. Neutrophil gelatinase-associated lipocalin: a promising biomarker for human acute kidney injury. Biomark Med. 2010;4:265–80.

125. Kulvichit W, Kellum JA, Srisawat N. Biomarkers in acute kidney injury. Crit Care Clin. 2021;37(2):385–98.

126. Ostermann M, Zarbock A, Goldstein S, Kashani K, Macedo E, Murugan R, Bell M, Forni L, Guzzi L, Joannidis M, Kane-Gill SL, Legrand M, Mehta R, Murray PT, Pickkers P, Plebani M, Prowle J, Ricci Z, Rimmelé T, Rosner M, Shaw AD, Kellum JA, Ronco C. Recommendations on acute kidney injury biomarkers from the acute disease quality initiative consensus conference: a consensus statement. JAMA Netw Open. 2020;3(10):e2019209.

127. Parikh CR, Devarajan P, Zappitelli M, et al. Postoperative biomarkers predict acute kidney injury and poor outcomes after pediatric cardiac surgery. J Am Soc Nephrol. 2011;22:1737–47.

128. Zappitelli M, Washburn KK, Arikan AA, et al. Urine NGAL is an early marker of acute kidney injury in critically ill children. Crit Care. 2007;11(4):R84.

129. Wheeler DS, Devarajan P, Ma Q, et al. Serum neutrophil gelatinase-associated lipocalin (NGAL) as a marker of acute kidney injury in critically ill children with septic shock. Crit Care Med. 2008;36(4):1297–303.

130. Du Y, Zappitelli M, Mian A, et al. Urinary biomarkers to detect acute kidney injury in the pediatric emergency center. Pediatr Nephrol. 2011;26(2):267–74.

131. Nickolas TL, Schmidt-Ott KM, Canetta P, et al. Diagnostic and prognostic stratification in the emergency department using urinary biomarkers of nephron damage: a multicenter prospective cohort study. J Am Coll Cardiol. 2012;59:246–55.

132. Nickolas TL, O'Rourke MJ, Yang J, Sise ME, Canetta PA, Barasch N, Buchen C, Khan F, Mori K, Giglio J, Devarajan P, Barasch J. Sensitivity and specificity of a single emergency department measurement of urinary neutrophil gelatinase-associated lipocalin for diagnosing acute kidney injury. Ann Intern Med. 2008;148(11):810–9.

133. Haase M, Devarajan P, Haase-Fielitz A, et al. The outcome of neutrophil gelatinase-associated lipocalin-positive subclinical acute kidney injury: a multicenter pooled analysis of prospective studies. J Am Coll Cardiol. 2011;57:1752–61.

134. Haase-Fielitz A, Haase M, Devarajan P. Neutrophil gelatinase-associated lipocalin as a biomarker of acute kidney injury – a critical evaluation of current status. Ann Clin Biochem. 2014;51(Pt 3):335–51.

135. Haase M, Bellomo R, Devarajan P, Schlattmann P, Haase-Fielitz A, NGAL Meta-analysis Investigator Group. Accuracy of neutrophil gelatinase-associated lipocalin (NGAL) in diagnosis and prognosis in acute kidney injury: a systematic review and meta-analysis. Am J Kidney Dis. 2009;54(6):1012–24.

136. Zhou F, Luo Q, Wang L, Han L. Diagnostic value of neutrophil gelatinase-associated lipocalin for early diagnosis of cardiac surgery-associated acute kidney injury: a meta-analysis. Eur J Cardiothorac Surg. 2016;49(3):746–55.

137. Ho J, Tangri N, Komenda P, Kaushal A, Sood M, Brar R, Gill K, Walker S, MacDonald K, Hiebert BM, Arora RC, Rigatto C. Urinary, plasma, and serum biomarkers' utility for predicting acute kidney injury associated with cardiac surgery in adults: a meta-analysis. Am J Kidney Dis. 2015;66(6):993–1005.

138. Wang K, Duan CY, Wu J, Liu Y, Bei WJ, Chen JY, He PC, Liu YH, Tan N. Predictive value of neutrophil gelatinase-associated lipocalin for contrast-induced acute kidney injury after cardiac catheterization: a meta-analysis. Can J Cardiol. 2016;32(8):1033.e19–29.

139. Jiang L, Cui H. Could blood neutrophil gelatinase-associated lipocalin (NGAL) be a diagnostic marker for acute kidney injury in neonates? A systemic review and meta-analysis. Clin Lab. 2015;61(12):1815–20.

140. Kim S, Kim HJ, Ahn HS, Song JY, Um TH, Cho CR, Jung H, Koo HK, Park JH, Lee SS, Park HK. Is plasma neutrophil gelatinase-associated lipocalin a predictive biomarker for acute kidney injury in sepsis patients? A systematic review and meta-analysis. J Crit Care. 2016;33:213–23.

141. Klein SJ, Brandtner AK, Lehner GF, Ulmer H, Bagshaw SM, Wiedermann CJ, Joannidis M. Biomarkers for prediction of renal replacement therapy in acute kidney injury: a systematic review and meta-analysis. Intensive Care Med. 2018;44(3):323–36.

142. Filho LT, Grande AJ, Colonetti T, Della ÉSP, da Rosa MI. Accuracy of neutrophil gelatinase-associated lipocalin for acute kidney injury diagnosis in children: systematic review and meta-analysis. Pediatr Nephrol. 2017;32(10):1979–88.

143. Albert C, Zapf A, Haase M, Röver C, Pickering JW, Albert A, Bellomo R, Breidthardt T, Camou F, Chen Z, Chocron S, Cruz D, de Geus HRH, Devarajan P, Di Somma S, Doi K, Endre ZH, Garcia-Alvarez M, Hjortrup PB, Hur M, Karaolanis G, Kavalci C, Kim H, Lentini P, Liebetrau C, Lipcsey M, Mårtensson J, Müller C, Nanas S, Nickolas TL, Pipili C, Ronco C, Rosa-Diez GJ, Ralib A, Soto K, Braun-Dullaeus RC, Heinz J, Haase-Fielitz A. Neutrophil gelatinase-associated lipocalin measured on clinical laboratory platforms for the prediction of acute kidney injury and the associated need for dialysis therapy: a systematic review and meta-analysis. Am J Kidney Dis. 2020;76(6):826–841.e1.

144. Dong L, Ma Q, Bennett M, Devarajan P. Urinary biomarkers of cell cycle arrest are delayed predictors of acute kidney injury after pediatric cardiopulmonary bypass. Pediatr Nephrol. 2017;32(12):2351–60.

145. Brienza N, Giglio MT, Marucci M, Fiore T. Does perioperative hemodynamic optimization protect renal function in surgical patients? A meta-analytic study. Crit Care Med. 2009;37(6):2079–90.

146. Giglio M, Dalfino L, Puntillo F, Brienza N. Hemodynamic goal-directed therapy and postoperative kidney injury: an updated meta-analysis with trial sequential analysis. Crit Care. 2019;23(1):232.

147. Moffett BS, Goldstein SL. Acute kidney injury and increasing nephrotoxic-medication exposure in noncritically-ill children. Clin J Am Soc Nephrol. 2011;6(4):856–63.

148. Goldstein SL, Kirkendall E, Nguyen H, Schaffzin JK, Bucuvalas J, Bracke T, Seid M, Ashby M, Foertmeyer N, Brunner L, Lesko A, Barclay C, Lannon C, Muething S. Electronic health record identification of nephrotoxin exposure and associated acute kidney injury. Pediatrics. 2013;132(3):e756–67.

149. Goldstein SL, Dahale D, Kirkendall ES, Mottes T, Kaplan H, Muething S, Askenazi DJ, Henderson T, Dill L, Somers MJG, Kerr J, Gilarde J, Zaritsky J, Bica V, Brophy PD, Misurac J, Hackbarth R, Steinke J, Mooney J, Ogrin S, Chadha V, Warady B, Ogden R, Hoebing W, Symons J, Yonekawa K, Menon S, Abrams L, Sutherland S, Weng P, Zhang F, Walsh K. A prospective multi-center quality improvement initiative (NINJA) indicates a reduction in nephrotoxic acute kidney injury in hospitalized children. Kidney Int. 2020;97(3):580–8.

150. Kashani K, Rosner MH, Haase M, Lewington AJP, O'Donoghue DJ, Wilson FP, Nadim MK, Silver SA, Zarbock A, Ostermann M, Mehta RL, Kane-Gill SL, Ding X, Pickkers P, Bihorac A, Siew ED, Barreto EF, Macedo E, Kellum JA, Palevsky PM, Tolwani AJ, Ronco C, Juncos LA, Rewa OG, Bagshaw SM, Mottes TA, Koyner JL, Liu KD, Forni LG, Heung M, Wu VC. Quality improvement goals for acute kidney injury. Clin J Am Soc Nephrol. 2019;14(6):941–53.

151. Slater MB, Gruneir A, Rochon PA, Howard AW, Koren G, Parshuram CS. Risk factors of acute kidney injury in critically ill children. Pediatr Crit Care Med. 2016;17(9):e391–8.

152. Chen JJ, Chang CH, Huang YT, Kuo G. Furosemide stress test as a predictive marker of acute kidney injury progression or renal replacement therapy: a systemic review and meta-analysis. Crit Care. 2020;24(1):202.

153. Matsuura R, Komaru Y, Miyamoto Y, Yoshida T, Yoshimoto K, Isshiki R, Mayumi K, Yamashita T, Hamasaki Y, Nangaku M, Noiri E, Morimura N, Doi K. Response to different furosemide doses

predicts AKI progression in ICU patients with elevated plasma NGAL levels. Ann Intensive Care. 2018;8(1):8.

154. Ricci Z, Luciano R, Favia I, et al. High-dose fenoldopam reduces postoperative neutrophil gelatinase-associated lipocaline and cystatin C levels in pediatric cardiac surgery. Crit Care. 2011;15:R160.

155. Guo Z, Liu J, Lei L, Xue Y, Liu L, Huang H, Chen S, Liu Y, Lin Y, Tao J, Xu Q, Wu K, Zhang L, Chen JY. Effect of N-acetylcysteine on prevention of contrast-associated acute kidney injury in patients with STEMI undergoing primary percutaneous coronary intervention: a systematic review and meta-analysis of randomised controlled trials. BMJ Open. 2020;10(10):e039009.

156. He G, Li Q, Li W, Wang L, Yang J, Zeng F. N-Acetylcysteine for preventing of acute kidney injury in chronic kidney disease patients undergoing cardiac surgery: a meta-analysis. Heart Surg Forum. 2018;21(6):E513–21.

157. Uber AM, Sutherland SM. Acute kidney injury in hospitalized children: consequences and outcomes. Pediatr Nephrol. 2020;35(2):213–20.

158. Greenberg JH, Zappitelli M, Devarajan P, Thiessen-Philbrook HR, Krawczeski C, Li S, Garg AX, Coca S, Parikh CR, Consortium T-A. Kidney outcomes 5 years after pediatric cardiac surgery: the TRIBE-AKI study. JAMA Pediatr. 2016;170:1071–8.

159. Zappitelli M, Parikh CR, Kaufman JS, Go AS, Kimmel PL, Hsu CY, Coca SG, Chinchilli VM, Greenberg JH, Moxey-Mims MM, Ikizler TA, Cockovski V, Dyer AM, Devarajan P, ASsessment, Serial Evaluation, and Subsequent Sequelae in Acute Kidney Injury (ASSESS-AKI) Investigators. Acute kidney injury and risk of CKD and hypertension after pediatric cardiac surgery. Clin J Am Soc Nephrol. 2020;15(10):1403–12.

160. Madsen NL, Goldstein SL, Froslev T, Christiansen CF, Olsen M. Cardiac surgery in patients with congenital heart disease is associated with acute kidney injury and the risk of chronic kidney disease. Kidney Int. 2017;92:751–6.

161. Benisty K, Morgan C, Hessey E, Huynh L, Joffe AR, Garros D, Dancea A, Sauve R, Palijan A, Pizzi M, Bhattacharya S, Doucet JA, Cockovski V, Gottesman RG, Goldstein SL, Zappitelli M. Kidney and blood pressure abnormalities 6 years after acute kidney injury in critically ill children: a prospective cohort study. Pediatr Res. 2020;88(2):271–8.

162. Robinson CH, Jeyakumar N, Luo B, Wald R, Garg AX, Nash DM, McArthur E, Greenberg JH, Askenazi D, Mammen C, Thabane L, Goldstein S, Parekh RS, Zappitelli M, Chanchlani R. Long-term kidney outcomes following dialysis-treated childhood acute kidney injury: a population-based cohort study. J Am Soc Nephrol. 2021;32(8):2005–19.

Management of Pediatric Acute Kidney Injury

Lyndsay A. Harshman, Patrick D. Brophy, and Jordan M. Symons

Introduction

Acute kidney injury (AKI) affects an increasing proportion of critically ill patients who now survive medical and surgical complications that were once often fatal. Despite increased efforts to recognize and prevent AKI, progression to kidney failure continues to occur with alarming frequency. The treatment of AKI in critically ill and injured children requires understanding of medical management of disease with ready availability of renal replacement therapy (RRT) as well as adaptability for use in pediatric patients of all ages and sizes. In this chapter, we review medical management of AKI as well as traditional and emerging RRT modalities.

L. A. Harshman (✉)
Department of Pediatrics, University of Iowa Children's Hospital, Iowa City, IA, USA
e-mail: lyndsay-harshman@uiowa.edu

P. D. Brophy
University of Rochester School of Medicine and Dentistry, Rochester, NY, USA
e-mail: patrick-brophy@uiowa.edu; Patrick_Brophy@URMC.Rochester.edu

J. M. Symons
Department of Pediatrics, University of Washington School of Medicine, Seattle, WA, USA
e-mail: jordan.symons@seattlechildrens.org

Medical Management of AKI

Medical management of AKI includes optimizing renal perfusion, preventing or reducing fluid overload, correcting electrolyte abnormalities and acid-base disturbances, supporting patient nutrition, and closely monitoring administration of nephrotoxic medications all while considering the patient's need for renal replacement if medical management proves ineffective [1–3]. The prevention of AKI is the foremost means of management. The clinician must pay close attention to subtle changes in serum creatinine and corresponding urine output as creatinine increase is a late marker of AKI [4]. Chapter 46 discusses this topic in detail.

Renal Perfusion

Intravenous (IV) fluid is used to treat hypovolemia in an attempt to maintain end organ perfusion, but overly aggressive resuscitation may lead to fluid overload. Both crystalloid and colloid (typically albumin) are utilized in fluid resuscitation; however, two major studies in adults have failed to demonstrate a clear benefit on AKI outcomes or survival difference for colloid versus crystalloid infusions [5, 6]. However, colloid may be advantageous over crystalloid in patients requiring large amounts of fluid resuscitation in the setting of sepsis or burn injury [7].

© The Author(s), under exclusive license to Springer Nature Switzerland AG 2023
F. Schaefer, L. A. Greenbaum (eds.), *Pediatric Kidney Disease*,
https://doi.org/10.1007/978-3-031-11665-0_52

Vasopressors in conjunction with IV fluid resuscitation for vasomotor shock may improve kidney perfusion and are recommended in patients who have or are at risk of AKI [7]. Agents recommended are norepinephrine, vasopressin, and dopamine. Vasopressin and norepinephrine use has increased due to favorable side effect profiles versus the arrhythmic abnormalities noted with dopamine [8, 9].

The use of renal vasodilators to increase renal perfusion does not improve outcomes. Specifically, dopamine has been employed at low dosages in an effort to improve renal perfusion by promoting vasodilatation. Adult studies of "renal dose" dopamine show no benefit and may even suggest harm [10–13]. More recently the selective dopamine agonist fenoldopam has been utilized to augment renal blood flow. Adult literature from single-center studies suggests a decline in both mortality and the need for RRT [14]. Furthermore, meta-analysis of 16 trials of fenoldopam in adults concluded that fenoldopam decreased the incidence of AKI, the need for RRT, intensive care unit (ICU) stay and death from any cause [15]. To date, one available randomized controlled trial has suggested that use of high-dose fenoldopam in pediatric patients on cardiac bypass significantly reduced the use of diuretics and vasodilators during bypass [16]. Current Kidney Disease Improving Global Outcomes (KDIGO) recommendations are against the use of fenoldopam to prevent or treat AKI given the high risk for hypotension associated with its use in ICU patients in comparison to the relatively sparse data available regarding its efficacy [7]. Emerging data from randomized, blinded trials suggest that fenoldopam may be beneficial in complex cardiac surgeries to improve the quality of perfusion during cardiopulmonary bypass and prevent AKI in both adults and children [16, 17]. The role for fenoldopam in AKI requires further clarification.

Volume Status

Awareness of volume status is critical in a patient with AKI since patients may have hypovolemia, euvolemia, or hypervolemia (fluid overload). Volume status should be continually reassessed and correlated with patient intake and output as well as daily weights. Heart rate, blood pressure, capillary refill, and skin turgor are all key components of assessing volume status.

Hypovolemia should be addressed with isotonic fluid to restore intravascular volume, and if necessary, inotropic support. AKI secondary to prerenal azotemia is likely in a severely volume depleted child. Aggressive fluid resuscitation with 10–20 mL/kg normal saline boluses to re-establish intravascular volume is recommended, and if there is no urine output once volume status is restored, a significant dose of furosemide (2 mg/kg IV) may be given. It is important to recognize that administration of furosemide and subsequent diuresis may simply result in conversion of the AKI from oliguric to non-oliguric and will not alter the course of the renal injury itself [18]. If a furosemide trial is used, a single high dose should be administered with observation for response. Furosemide should not be continued if there is ongoing oliguria [19].

Fluid overload has been associated with increased morbidity and mortality in pediatric critical care patients; however, the pathophysiology leading to poor outcome is not fully delineated [20, 21]. Examples of AKI with hypervolemia include following aggressive fluid resuscitation in septic patients and in patients with left ventricular cardiac dysfunction. The use of excessive normal saline for fluid resuscitation is associated with hyperchloremia, which has been demonstrated to diminish renal sodium excretion [22, 23] and impair renal blood flow [24], thus heightening the risk for AKI. Congestive heart failure due to poor left ventricular function can result in poor renal perfusion secondary to deficits in forward flow, which further promotes edema formation through activation of the renin-angiotensin-aldosterone axis and subsequent sodium retention [25]. Diuretic use in the adult ICU patient with AKI is associated with heightened risk of both death and non-recovery of renal function [19]. A trial of high-dose furosemide may be used to relieve hypervolemia given evidence that persistent, positive fluid balance is associated with increasing mortality in adult patients who develop AKI [26]. It is not advisable, however, to rely on diuretic therapy and fluid and nutritional restriction to avoid RRT given that such use of diuretics for either AKI "prophylaxis" or therapy does not improve outcomes [27, 28]. Patients with fluid overload not responsive to diuretics require consideration of RRT.

Cumulative percent fluid overload may be calculated as follows:

```
fluid input (liters) - fluid output
(liters) / ICU admission weight (kg) *
100
```

Evaluation for RRT should occur in the setting of >10% cumulative fluid overload. Initiation of RRT is advised if cumulative fluid overload is >20% [29].

Critically ill pediatric patients presenting with euvolemia but oliguria that is unresponsive to fluid resuscitation may have intrinsic AKI. In this population, continued fluid resuscitation may be detrimental if the patient remains oliguric; thus, guidelines suggest restricting fluid to insensible losses plus replacement of urine output plus extra renal losses [30]. However, nutrition needs may require early RRT to prevent volume overload and electrolyte disturbances.

Electrolyte Abnormalities

Electrolyte abnormalities occur commonly in AKI and may develop rapidly, necessitating vigilant monitoring. Hyperkalemia is common, particularly in oliguric patients, and is potentially life-threatening due to ventricular tachycardia and fibrillation. Medical management of hyperkalemia is directed towards removal of potassium from the body (sodium polystyrene sulfonate, loop diuretic if responsive) and preventing arrhythmias via driving potassium into the cells (albuterol, sodium bicarbonate, insulin + glucose) and stabilizing the cardiac membrane (calcium), as summarized in Table 52.1. Dialysis may be necessary if moderate to severe hyperkalemia is refractory to medical management (Table 52.1).

Hyponatremia occurs more often than hypernatremia in AKI [30]. Hyponatremia is often due to water retention and may be exacerbated by intake of hypotonic fluids. Hyponatremia due to water retention secondary to volume depletion may respond to isotonic fluid. In contrast, fluid

Table 52.1 Medical agents utilized in the management of hyperkalemia

Agent(s)	Mechanism	Dose	Onset	Complications
Sodium bicarbonate	Shifts K+ into cells	1 mEq/kg IV over 10–30 min	15–30 min	Hypernatremia, change in ionized calcium
Albuterol	Shifts K+ into cells	400 µg by nebulizer	30 min	Tachycardia, hypertension
Glucose and insulin	Shifts K+ into cells	Glucose 0.5 g/kg, insulin 0.1 U/kg IV over 30 min	30–120 min	Hypoglycemia
Calcium gluconate 10%	Stabilizes membrane	0.5–1 mL/kg IV over 5–15 min	Immediate	Bradycardia, arrhythmias, hypercalcemia
Calcium chloride	Stabilizes membrane	10 mg/kg IV over 5–15 min	Immediate	Bradycardia, arrhythmias, hypercalcemia
Sodium Polystyrene Sulfonate (Kayexalate®, Concordia Pharmaceuticals, Oakville, Ontario, Canada)	Exchanges Na+ for K+ across the colonic mucosa	1 g/kg orally or PR in sorbitol	30–60 min	Hypernatremia, constipation, colonic membrane irritation if given PR

Used with permission of Elsevier from Andreoli [31]
K^+ potassium, *IV* intravenous, Na^+ sodium, *PR* per rectum

restriction is effective if due to free water excess. RRT may be necessary if renal dysfunction prevents excretion of excess free water. Sodium levels less than <120 mEq/L are associated with a high risk for cerebral edema and seizures. Sodium correction with hypertonic saline solution over several hours should be initiated. Further correction of hyponatremia can be achieved by free water restriction.

Hyperphosphatemia in AKI is secondary to reduction in glomerular filtration rate (GFR). Hyperphosphatemia may be treated with phosphate binders and dietary phosphorus restriction. Selection of a phosphate binder should consider the patient's calcium level. In patients with low ionized calcium, a calcium-containing phosphate binder (e.g. calcium carbonate) should be used; by contrast, in patients with hypercalcemia, a non-calcium phosphate binder, such as sevelamer, is recommended.

Hypocalcemia occurs in AKI secondary to high serum phosphorus. Both total and ionized calcium levels should be monitored since total calcium may be inaccurate due to decreased total calcium secondary to hypoalbuminemia and changes in calcium binding to albumin based on the patient's acid-base status. Initial treatment for mild hypocalcemia in AKI and phosphate retention is correction of hyperphosphatemia, typically using oral phosphate binders. Symptomatic hypocalcemia requires correction with IV calcium. This replacement should be provided with caution in the severely hyperphosphatemic patient given the possibility of systemic calcium phosphate precipitation, potentially worsening existing AKI with calcium phosphate deposition in the renal tubules. Inability to correct hypocalcemia in a symptomatic patient (e.g. tetany and/or seizures) secondary to severe hyperphosphatemia is an indication for dialysis.

For children who are not receiving RRT, several measures can prevent severe metabolic and electrolyte disturbances. First, no supplemental phosphorus or potassium should be provided to the patient unless symptomatic or there is significant hypophosphatemia or hypokalemia. Second, to prevent worsening hypertension and fluid overload, sodium should be restricted to 2–3 mEq/kg/day. Third, parenteral or enteral nutrition should be considered early in the patient's course, as described below, to replete electrolyte abnormalities. If adequate nutrition cannot be provided due to fluid overload, RRT should be initiated. Serum electrolytes, phosphorus, calcium, and albumin should be regularly monitored as dictated by the patient's clinical status.

Acid-Base Disturbances

Metabolic acidosis in AKI is due to renal dysfunction and systemic disease (e.g. sepsis, trauma, burns). Severe acidosis can be treated with IV or oral sodium bicarbonate, with careful monitoring for fluid overload and worsening of hypertension due to the sodium load. Patients with AKI who develop severe, refractory metabolic acidosis may require dialysis therapy, especially in the setting of oligoanuria. It is important to measure the serum total and ionized calcium prior to bicarbonate treatment due to potential for symptomatic hypocalcemia given increased pH-dependent binding of calcium to proteins, which decreases the ionized calcium.

Nutritional Interventions

Patients with AKI are in a hypercatabolic state and should have nutritional support to ensure full calorie, protein, and micronutrient delivery. Nutritional goals include preservation of lean body mass and avoidance of metabolic derangements. Potential benefits include improved wound healing, immune function, and scavenging of oxygen free radicals, with the goal of decreasing patient mortality [32].

Delivery

Adequate nutrition may require supplemental enteral and/or parenteral nutrition if oral intake cannot meet nutritional requirements. Enteral nutrition is preferred if the gastrointestinal tract is functioning given the ease of administration and lower rates of infection. Conversely, parenteral nutrition should be employed when the gastrointestinal tract cannot be utilized and/or enteral feeding cannot provide sufficient nutrition [33]. See Fig. 52.1 for a decision tree illustrating mode of nutritional support in AKI [34].

Protein

Current evidence suggests that patients with AKI require increased protein, particularly when receiving RRT [35]. Protein-energy wasting (PEW) is loss of lean body mass and fat mass and may occur in patients with AKI d [36]. PEW is an independent predictor for patient mortality and is also directly associated with the length of hospital stay and risk of complications [37]. The adult literature recommends an increased protein intake goal of 1.5–2 g/kg per day for hypercatabolic patients or for patients receiving RRT that utilizes high-flux and/or highly efficient filters, which are associated with amino acid losses [38].

Calories and Lipid

General guidelines suggest that critically ill children should receive from 1 to 1.3 times basal metabolic needs in calories [39]; however, additional calories for hypercatabolic states should be provided given the patient's pre-existing state of nutrition. To optimize enteral nutrition, "renal-specific" formulas are an option for patients being medically managed with AKI or on RRT. These formulas may be beneficial given high caloric and protein density with low electrolyte levels [40]. Adequate caloric intake is needed to prevent catabolism, to promote protein synthesis and to offset heat-dependent caloric losses [41]. Parenteral nutrition, including IV lipids, is necessary if enteral nutrition cannot be provided [38, 41].

Nutrients

Levels of vitamin C and water-soluble vitamins, including thiamine and folic acid, may be low in patients with AKI [42]. Use of RRT can exacerbate nutrient and trace element losses due to the very efficient removal of small molecular weight substances [43]. Appropriate replacement is indicated.

Glycemic Control

Stress hyperglycemia is a notable feature of critical illness [44]. Several studies have investigated the impact of conservative versus intensive insulin therapy on patient mortality, with secondary analyses investigating impact of glycemic control on incidence of AKI [45–47]. Tight glycemic control has decreased the incidence of AKI in adults [48]. Insulin is recommended to correct hyperglycemia in AKI, with typical glucose goals between 110 and 150 mg/dL [49].

Avoidance of Nephrotoxins

Many commonly used medications are metabolized and/or excreted by the kidneys. Nephrotoxic medications in the ICU contribute to nearly 25%

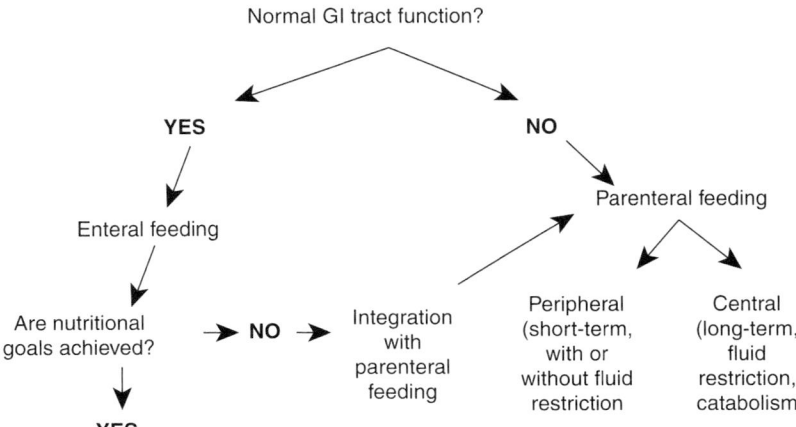

Fig. 52.1 Decision tree for nutritional support in AKI patients with protein energy wasting (PEW) or at risk of PEW. (Used with permission of John Wiley and Sons from Fiaccadori et al. [34])

of AKI cases [50, 51]. Prevention of drug-induced AKI is more effective than any available therapy; recognition of high-risk patients is therefore necessary. The dose and frequency of administration of any potentially nephrotoxic medication should be adjusted (or avoided) based on the patient's GFR.

Common nephrotoxins include aminoglycosides, nonsteroidal anti-inflammatory drugs (NSAIDs), contrast agents, and chemotherapeutic and immunosuppressant medications [52]. AKI induced by drugs occurs by two predominant mechanisms: direct toxicity to renal tubular epithelium, as is seen with aminoglycosides and amphotericin, and interference with autoregulatory mechanisms, leading to unrestricted vasoconstriction and reduced renal blood flow, as is seen with NSAID toxicity. NSAIDs are a common cause of AKI in children, even when ingested at recommended doses; the incidence of AKI may be underestimated both in the inpatient and outpatient settings [53]. Aminoglycosides are widely utilized in pediatric patients. Repeat administration of these agents may lead to renal interstitial and tubular epithelial cell accumulation, and as such, recommendations have been made to administer aminoglycosides every 24 h (or less) to minimize toxicity, with drug levels obtained daily [7].

Contrast-induced AKI (CI-AKI) in adults is associated with an increased risk of mortality in the year following the episode of AKI [54]. The incidence in children is not well-characterized. Patients with chronic kidney disease or diabetes are at increased risk of CI-AKI [54]. Volume and osmolality of contrast administered is directly associated with risk of AKI [55, 56], and non-ionic agents are thought to be safer, especially in patients with chronic kidney disease [57]. The pathophysiology of CI-AKI is still largely unknown. Severe vasoconstriction following contrast administration has been implicated [58, 59], as has direct cytotoxicity via oxygen free radical generation. Serum creatinine rises 1–2 days after the imaging procedure and is usually not accompanied by oligoanuria [60]. Dialysis is required in a minority of patients. No treatment exists other than support if CI-AKI

occurs. However, in recent years, attention has focused on prevention [61, 62]. A meta-analysis of prevention strategies recommends pre- and post-contrast IV volume expansion with bicarbonate-containing fluids and use of low or iso-osmolar contrast agents in the smallest volume possible in patients with pre-existing kidney disease who are at increased risk. N-acetylcysteine and ascorbic acid have also been suggested for use as free radical scavengers in the higher risk populations [57]. N-acetylcysteine is indicated for the prevention of contrast-induced AKI per the 2012 KDIGO guidelines [7]. While older studies have suggested a benefit [63], controversy regarding its use remains as the effect of N-acetylcysteine to prevent AKI can be variable, and several studies have failed to show a significant benefit. There is no significant benefit of either N-acetylcysteine or bicarbonate infusion for prevention of AKI, even among populations at high risk for kidney complications [64]. There have been no randomized trials in children.

Other Medical Therapies

Growth Factors

Renal tubular injury is a major component in the pathogenesis of AKI, and renal tubular repair is a required step for recovery. Growth factors play an important role in the regeneration of epithelial cells. In animal models, several growth factors have been shown to accelerate recovery from renal injury such as erythropoietin, insulin-like growth factor, hepatocyte growth factor, and epidermal growth factor [65]. In cellular and animal models, erythropoietin appears to reduce necrosis and apoptosis in renal epithelial cells while also promoting cell proliferation [66]; however, human studies have failed to yield AKI-related benefit from use of erythropoietin for primary AKI prevention [67]. Similarly, hepatocyte growth factor and insulin-like growth factor-1 appear to limit apoptosis in animal models of renal injury [68, 69], but again, preliminary clinical trials with IGF-1 have not shown benefit to patients. The KDIGO work group recommends against use of IGF-1 to prevent or treat AKI [7].

Adenosine Receptor Antagonists

Theophylline is a non-selective adenosine receptor antagonist that is thought to increase renal blood flow at the level of the afferent arteriole [70]. KDIGO recommendations suggest a single dose of theophylline in high-risk neonates with perinatal asphyxia at risk of AKI [7]. Research to date supports an initial renoprotective effect following theophylline in asphyxiated infants; however, long-term impact on renal function is unclear [71, 72].

Renal Replacement Therapies in AKI

The lack of evidence-based guidelines regarding the definition of pediatric AKI (see Chap. 46) has resulted in much uncertainty and discussion regarding the indications and timing for initiation of RRT as well as the optimal modality to employ. Retrospective reviews in critically ill children demonstrate that those who develop AKI early in a hospital course have greater morbidity and mortality [73, 74]. Use of RRT may prevent and correct life-threatening complications of AKI refractory to medical management. Indications for initiation of RRT in pediatric AKI have traditionally been those used for end-stage renal disease (and are not necessarily easily juxtaposed in the acute setting), including metabolic/electrolyte abnormalities refractory to medical therapy, symptomatic fluid overload, and/or symptomatic uremia; however, metabolic derangement and fluid overload are often late findings in severe renal injury [75]. In the acute setting, consideration of RRT must account for the patient's clinical situation in the context of the aforementioned laboratory abnormalities.

Adult literature suggests that earlier initiation of RRT, for example before the appearance of florid metabolic derangements and symptomatic fluid overload, may yield better patient outcomes, including decreased risk of death, shorter duration of RRT, and shorter hospital stays [76, 77]. For example, volume overload in the setting of AKI refractory to medical management is an indication for RRT even without significant azotemia or elevation in creatinine. Additionally, the presence of multisystem organ dysfunction in the presence of AKI refractory to medical management is a strong indication for initiation of RRT.

More recently, the concept of renal angina [78] has been suggested whereby likelihood of developing AKI is informed by baseline and contextual factors as well as objective evidence to identify those patients at greatest risk for renal injury. Additionally, renal angina criteria stratify patients into moderate-, high-, and very-high risk categories for AKI based on their underlying clinical condition (Table 52.2). Renal angina can be thought of mathematically as "signs of injury" (i.e., fluid overload, estimated creatinine clearance) multiplied by presence of AKI and is comparable to assessment of risk for a myocardial infarction in an adult patient presenting with chest pain. Given that there are currently no reliable biomarkers for establishing the severity or

Table 52.2 Pediatric renal angina criteria

Hazard tranche	Renal angina threshold
Moderate-risk patients Patients admitted to PICU	Doubling of SCr OR eCrCl decrease >50% OR ICU fluid overload >15%
High-risk patients Acute decompensated heart failure Stem-cell-transplant recipient	Serum Cr increase ≥0.3 mg/dL OR eCrCl decrease 25–50% OR ICU fluid overload >10%
Very-high-risk patients Receiving mechanical ventilation and one or more vasoactive medications	Any serum Cr increase OR eCrCl decrease >25% OR ICU fluid overload >5%

Used with permission of Springer Science + Business Media from Basu et al. [78]
PICU pediatric intensive care unit, *SCr* serum creatinine, *OR* odds ratio, *eCrCl* estimated creatinine clearance, *ICU* intensive care unit

prognosis of a patient's AKI, renal angina criteria may help the clinician to predict risk for AKI early in the clinical course and intervene, if needed, with RRT before reaching a state of fluid and metabolic derangement. In one study, the renal angina index obtained on Day 0 of pediatric ICU admission was predictive for progression to AKI on ICU Day 3 [79].

Greater than 20% fluid overload is a significant independent risk factor for increased morbidity and mortality [80]. Other less concrete indications for initiation of RRT include oliguria not responsive to diuretics, escalating ventilatory requirements (especially if pulmonary edema is secondary to fluid overload), need for a large volume of medications/blood products in a currently fluid overloaded patient (>10% overload), and/or when ability to provide adequate nutrition is compromised by fluid restriction secondary to fluid overload and oliguria.

Literature exists regarding when to stop RRT in the patient with AKI. In stopping RRT, the nephrologist may decrease the frequency of therapy from daily to every other day or change modality (e.g. conversion from CRRT to acute hemodialysis [HD]). The decision to stop should be based on evidence for improvement in the underlying disease pathology that led to RRT initiation and improvement in renal function (i.e., increased urine output, diminished azotemia, and decreased fluid overload).

Modality Choice

When initiating RRT for AKI, the clinician should first identify the goals of dialytic therapy. The patient's size, hemodynamic stability, and potential for vascular access also inform modality selection. Choice of therapy will also depend on clinician preference, available resources (e.g. dialysis equipment, nursing staff), and even capabilities for placement of dialysis access.

Acute Peritoneal Dialysis

Acute peritoneal dialysis (PD) provides gradual solute and water clearance through both convec-

tive and diffusion-based mechanisms. Although the use of continuous renal replacement therapy (CRRT) has dramatically increased in the past decade, there remains an important role for acute PD in preterm neonates with limited vascular access and patients admitted to the ICU following surgery for congenital heart defects [81, 82]. Acute PD is still the modality of choice in many countries, especially in the developing world [83–85] as it is a relatively inexpensive form of dialysis that does not require sophisticated technical expertise or equipment. It avoids the risks and complications associated with extracorporeal perfusion, including the possible need for blood-product exposure and systemic anticoagulation. Additionally, large volumes of fluid can be removed slowly over a prolonged period, maintaining hemodynamic stability. Due to the relatively slower solute clearance, including that of nitrogenous waste products, it is not associated with dialysis disequilibrium, which may occur in acute intermittent HD.

Initiation

An in-depth discussion regarding PD access is provided in Chap. 63. In brief, PD does not require vascular access, which can be a challenge in infants and small children, and provides a means for critically ill patients to be dialyzed with preservation of vascular access, thus allowing for rapid institution of therapy even in the less hemodynamically stable patient. Access can be obtained using semi-rigid stylet catheters requiring a trochar and canula method of insertion, the main advantage of which is the ease of bedside insertion by the pediatric nephrologist without surgical intervention and general anesthesia [86]. In patients who can tolerate a surgical procedure, placement of a tunneled permanent catheter is preferred to semi-rigid, temporary catheters to reduce technical complications such as leaks and catheter obstruction [87]. Newer acute placement techniques are performed with soft catheters, often where a Seldinger technique is utilized to insert the catheter over a guidewire (Fig. 52.2). This technique can be well-utilized in infants as it carries a minimal risk of dialysate leakage since no incision is required for the catheter insertion. Consequently, the risk of peritonitis is less, and

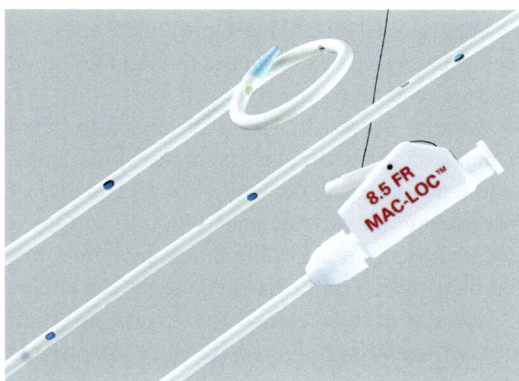

Fig. 52.2 Peritoneal dialysis catheter using Seldinger technique for insertion (8.5FR Mac-Loc™)

these catheters can be kept for up to 5 days without complications [87].

Prescription and Technique

The dialysis prescription for acute PD comprises four major components: the exchange volume, dialysate composition, individual cycle time, consisting of fill, dwell and drain, and total length of the dialysis session. For acute PD, the target exchange fill volume for adequate dialysis in terms of fluid and solute clearance, without the risk of leakage, is 30 mL/kg. However, smaller initial volumes of 10 mL/kg may be used for at least 24–48 h, if there is a risk of leakage from a wide incision site or if a tunneled cuffed catheter is used. Initially, short dwells (e.g. 30 min or hourly exchanges) for 48–72 h are required to remove accumulated solutes and excess fluid. Volume and metabolic control may best be achieved with exchanges performed around-the-clock. Subsequently, in maintenance dialysis, the dwell times can be extended, and total daily therapy time may be reduced, similar to chronic PD, with increasing volumes up to 40–45 mL/kg if a cuffed catheter has been used. PD should be continued until urine output improves, indicating recovering renal function.

Commercial dialysate solutions are available differing in osmolality, osmotic agent, and buffer. The osmotic agent is typically dextrose in a variety of pre-prepared concentrations. The hypertonic dextrose solutions utilized in PD provide a source of additional calories that may be benefi-cial in the critically ill child where IV access for nutrition and maintenance of glycemia may be limited; conversely, hyperglycemia may result from dextrose used in dialysate and insulin therapy may be required [88].

Complications

PD is contraindicated in patients with diaphragmatic defects, omphalocele, gastroschisis, and bladder exstrophy [89]. Complications with PD include catheter malfunction, peritonitis, and poor ultrafiltration. Neonates may have poor drainage due to catheter malposition or kinking, omental wrapping or a fibrin clot, which is exacerbated by the relatively small-bore peritoneal catheters required in the smallest patients. Inadequate drainage may also occur due to constipation. Bedside PD catheter placement with a semi-rigid trochar is associated with a risk of viscus perforation, especially in neonates, both at the time of insertion and with increasing dialysis duration. Severe abdominal pain and shock may occur, and the catheter must be removed for bowel repair and treatment of sepsis. The incidence of peritonitis is highest with the semi-rigid catheter, particularly if it has been kept in place for longer than 72 h [86]. In some cases, patients may develop a diaphragmatic pleuroperitoneal communication following cardiothoracic procedures, which results in a large pleural effusion once PD is initiated. Hypothermia is a complication of PD, particularly in neonates and small children, if dialysate is not warmed prior to infusion into the peritoneal cavity.

Poor ultrafiltration may occur, especially in critically ill infants due to the low fill volume with inadequate fluid reservoir intraperitoneally. Often it is difficult to increase the dwell to the desired volume in the setting of infant acute respiratory distress and low lung volumes as the increasing peritoneal fluid fill volumes results in splinting of the diaphragm. In some cases, during the inflow phase, critically ill infants may desaturate, and require transient compensation in ventilatory pressures. As a result, there is poor ultrafiltration, which increases the fluid retention, thus worsening the respiratory distress. These ill patients are often hypotensive requiring multi-agent inotropic and pressor support. The resultant decrease in bowel perfusion due to vasoconstriction of the mesenteric vessels secondary to pressor support may also contribute to poor ultrafiltration. Additionally, in neonates there is a decrease in the osmotic gradient, because of increased absorption of dextrose from the dialysate, resulting in poor ultrafiltration. With the use of higher dialysate dextrose concentrations to facilitate ultrafiltration, hyperglycemia may occur and necessitate insulin administration.

Electrolyte abnormalities may occur with PD. Hypokalemia may occur, and if noted, potassium should preferably be added to the IV fluid if the patient is not feeding, rather than adding to the dialysate, to avoid frequent bag changes due to changing orders. Potassium can be added to the dialysate if the hypokalemia is severe enough such that the maximum safe concentration of potassium infusion will be exceeded.

Acute Intermittent Hemodialysis

In many countries, acute intermittent HD is the mainstay of dialysis for AKI, particularly in older children. Its main advantage is rapid ultrafiltration and solute removal. It is therefore indicated in AKI that requires rapid fluid removal (acute fluid overload) or rapid solute removal such as hyperkalemia, tumor lysis syndrome, toxic poisonings and other profound metabolic abnormalities. Acute intermittent HD is ideal for hemodynamically stable patients who can tolerate rapid fluid shifts. It is a versatile modality as it allows for ultrafiltration without solute removal, as well as adjustment of the dialysate bath to treat electrolyte abnormalities such as hypernatremia. Moreover, because of the intermittent nature of the dialysis, patients can be mobilized for other procedures. Systematic reviews have suggested that in hemodynamically stable adult patients the continuous forms of RRT do not appear to have a survival advantage over intermittent HD [90–92].

Initiation

When initiating acute HD, one must consider vascular access, HD prescription, and type of dialyzer membrane. Other factors include the patient's ability to tolerate rapid fluid shifts, the need for vasoactive substances to maintain blood pressure, and total fluid removal goals.

Vascular access for HD is discussed in detail in Chap. 65. As with all extracorporeal therapies, treatment success is dependent on the quality of the vascular access. Adequate blood flow (Qb) is essential to providing optimal therapy with minimal interruption. In pediatric patients, the choice of vascular access, catheter size, and insertion site is critical. Short, large bore catheters provide improved performance due to lower resistance to flow [93]; conversely, longer, smaller-bore catheters (e.g. Broviac catheters) are unsuitable due to their high flow resistance.

The HD prescription in AKI must be individualized to provide adequate solute clearance and fluid removal. The prescription for acute intermittent HD is comprised of the dialysis dose delivered per session and the frequency of the sessions. Additional factors affecting the individual HD prescription include the extracorporeal circuit volume, the dialyzer size, blood flow rate, dialysate flow rate, ultrafiltration required, dialysate composition, anticoagulation, and length of session. Blood flow rate is determined by vascular access and determines solute clearance, with higher blood flow increasing solute clearance by optimizing diffusion and convection. Dialysate flow rate is also a determinant of solute clearance [94]. Dialysate flow rate should be at least 1.5 times greater than the blood flow rate to maximize diffusion gradients of solutes. In pediatric patients, HD equipment and prescription require modifications for smaller children (i.e., infants less than 3 kg).

When initiating acute HD for AKI, dialysis dose delivered may change frequently with a need for greater renal support during initial therapy for AKI, as compared to the relatively stable initial dialysis doses provided in initiating chronic HD for end-stage renal disease [95]. Similarly, in patients receiving chronic HD, urea kinetic modeling (Kt/V) is utilized as a measure of dialysis adequacy; however, due to the rapidity of fluid shifts with therapy and frequently changing renal function, Kt/V may not be as reliable in the patient with AKI receiving HD [96]. A review of dialysis dosage in adults concluded that in AKI a Kt/Vurea greater than 1.2 from thrice weekly intermittent HD is associated with improved survival in patients with intermediate severity of illness but does not influence outcomes in more severely ill patients [97]. Increased acute HD treatment frequency may be required despite reaching "adequate" Kt/V to achieve daily fluid removal goals. Although Kt/V recommendations exist, dialysis dosage must be individualized and higher doses of therapy for various metabolic derangements may be required in AKI [97].

The total volume of the extracorporeal circuit includes the volume of the tubing and the dialyzer and should not exceed more than 10% of the patient's blood volume, calculated as 75 mL/kg for older children and 80 mL/kg for infants. If the extracorporeal blood volume exceeds 10–15% of the patient's total blood volume, or the patient has a low hematocrit and/or hemodynamic instability, a blood prime is recommended [98]. When initiating a blood prime, using buffered packed red blood cells (PRBC) or transfusing the PRBC post-membrane in conjunction with a saline prime have been shown to reduce risk of "bradykinin release syndrome" (BRS) [99]. BRS, characterized by a precipitous decline in blood pressure 5–10 min after initiating both acute HD and continuous RRT, has been associated with the use of the AN-69 polyacrylonitrile membrane [99, 100]. Exposure of the primed blood to the negatively charged AN-69 membrane co-activates pre-kallikrein and Hageman factor, resulting in the release of bradykinin, a potent vasodilator. The reaction is potentiated by exposure to blood with an acid pH, which is typical of banked blood used for blood priming the circuit. Thus, the use of a blood prime with an AN-69 membrane can result in profound hypotension. PRBCs to be used in a blood prime should be diluted with normal saline to produce a hematocrit of approximately 35–40%. Buffering the banked blood for priming to physiologic pH prior to priming the circuit or infusing the blood post-filter at the same rate as a saline prime have been shown to be effective in minimizing the BRS, as has avoidance of the AN69 membrane [101, 102].

Dialyzer selection considers the type of membrane desired, the need for a blood prime, the dialyzer membrane surface area, and the ultrafiltration coefficient [103]. The membrane properties of the dialyzer, such as membrane thickness, pore size, and pore density affect dialysis efficiency, with varying clearances for small and middle molecular weight solutes. Dialyzer membrane biocompatibility should be considered when initiating acute HD. See Chap. 66 for additional information on this topic. The use of biocompatible synthetic membranes does not appear to confer any significant clinical advantage either in terms of mortality or AKI recovery when compared to substituted cellulosic membranes [104, 105]. High-flux membranes have larger pores resulting in greater clearances of higher molecular weight solutes but have the risk of back transport from the dialysate of waterborne solute contaminants. In a systematic review comparing the use of high-flux and low-flux membranes in AKI in adults, there was no difference in the risk of mortality or dialysis dependence in survivors [105]. However, in another meta-analysis, there appeared to be a significantly improved renal function recovery with the use of high-flux membranes [104]. High-cut-off-point membranes made from polyamide/polyarylethersulfone, polysulfone, or cellulose triacetate, have greater cytokine clearance and enhanced adsorption properties than conventional high-flux dialyzers [106], and have been developed for use in septic patients with AKI [107, 108]. Treatment using high-cut-off-point membranes has been shown in animal models of sepsis to have beneficial effects on immune cell function and survival [109]. Preliminary clinical studies show that use of these membranes in adult patients with AKI was associated with decreased need for vasopressor therapy, with no reports of serious adverse effects [108].

The smaller blood volumes in infants and young children place them at risk for blood loss due to clotting of the dialyzer; thus, anticoagulation is required with acute intermittent HD for pediatric AKI. Heparin is the most commonly used anticoagulant for intermittent HD. A loading dose of heparin may be given at the start of dialysis followed by intermittent bolus heparin doses. To monitor therapy, the activated partial thromboplastin time (aPTT) or activated clotting time (ACT) may be used. The aPTT should be kept at 1.2–1.5 times the baseline, and the ACT between 120 and 180 s. When heparin is utilized, platelet count should be monitored frequently to assess for development of heparin-induced thrombocytopenia [110]. In coagulopathic patients, heparin-free dialysis can be performed by intermittently flushing the circuit with 0.9% saline; unfortunately, this method increases the ultrafiltration target and decreases dialysis efficiency [111–113]. When using saline anticoagulation, the filter pressure should be monitored, and dialyzer inspected for early clot formation. Regional citrate anticoagulation is also an alternative to systemic heparin anticoagulation in the coagulopathic patient [114] requiring HD for AKI.

Complications

HD in young children can be challenging due to the smaller patient blood volume. This problem is accentuated in the critically ill child, where pressor infusion may be required to support the systemic blood pressure. Moreover, these children may have acute respiratory distress syndrome with hypoxemia or other associated clinical problems such as congestive heart failure or cerebral edema. Therefore, maintenance of an adequate blood pressure in these children is critical to alleviate tissue hypoxia.

Rapid HD using dialyzers with larger surface areas in patients with very high plasma blood urea nitrogen (BUN) concentrations may result in the dialysis disequilibrium syndrome, characterized by neurological symptoms such as fatigue, headache, nausea, vomiting, altered consciousness, convulsions, and coma [115]. Patients with AKI may be at increased risk due to catabolism (high BUN) and pre-existing neurological compromise related to the acute illness. Measures to prevent the disequilibrium syndrome include decreasing the initial dialysis dose, increasing dialysate sodium concentration (143–146 mmol/L), and administration of osmotically active substances such as IV mannitol (0.5–1 g/kg) to prevent rapid osmolar shifts that can cause cerebral edema [116].

Hypotension is one of the most common complications with acute intermittent HD and occurs in part due to rapid fluid and solute removal. Technical advances in the delivery of HD have dramatically reduced the propensity for intradialytic hypotension. The use of volume-controlled dialysis machines and biocompatible synthetic dialysis membranes helped decrease the incidence of intradialytic hypotension. In adult studies, it has been demonstrated that priming the circuit with isotonic saline, discontinuing vasodilator therapy, keeping the dialysate sodium greater than 145 mmol/L and setting the dialysate temperature to below 37 °C result in lesser hemodynamic instability and better outcomes [117]. See Table 52.3 for a summary of recommendations to minimize hemodynamic instability with acute HD. Additionally, use of in-line noninvasive blood volume monitoring to minimize abrupt changes in extracellular volume is useful in young children with hemodynamic instability where large acute changes in extracellular volume are not well tolerated [118]. This method of performing intradialytic noninvasive blood volume monitoring indicates intravascular blood volume change during the dialysis session (Fig. 52.3).

Catheter site complications are possible in acute HD and include infection at the catheter exit site, catheter malfunction, and risk of

Table 52.3 Techniques to improve hemodynamic tolerance of intermittent hemodialysis

All patients:
Use only synthetic or modified cellulose membrane
Connect both lines of the circuit filled with 0.9% saline simultaneously to the central venous catheter
Set dialysate sodium concentration ≥145 mmol/L
Limit maximal blood flow to 150 mL/min with a minimal 4 h session
Set dialysate temperature at ≤37 °C
Advice for hemodynamically unstable patients:
Cool dialysate to 35 °C
Start session with dialysis and continue with ultrafiltration alone
Additional recommendations:
Stop vasodilator therapy

Used with permission of the American Thoracic Society from Schortgen et al. [117]

Fig. 52.3 Intradialytic noninvasive blood volume monitoring: Profile 1: overhydration. Profile 2: euvolemia

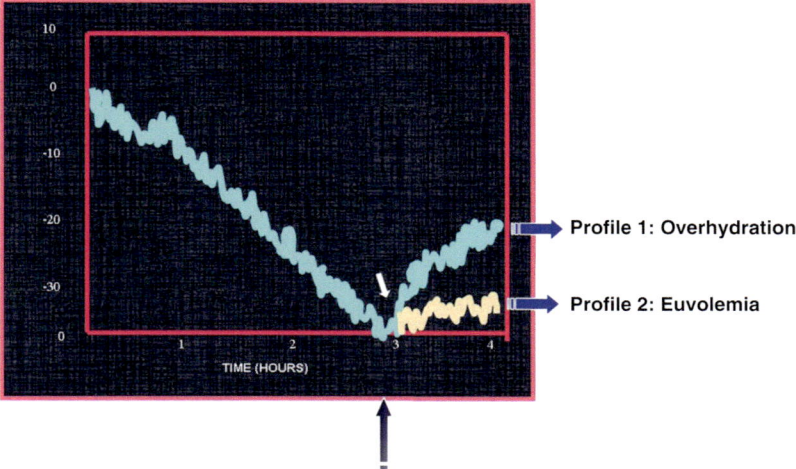

hematologic disturbance (e.g. bleeding, clot). In the event of signs of infection such as fever, line blood cultures should be obtained, and empiric antibiotics started. There is also risk for clotting of the extracorporeal system in acute HD; this can place patients at risk for acute blood loss if the blood is unable to be returned to the patient.

Continuous Renal Replacement Therapies

CRRT is now widely available in pediatric centers throughout the world, and in some has become the preferred method of RRT. CRRT in AKI offers several advantages over traditional dialysis methods when used in critically ill, unstable patients. Because CRRT is continuous, removal of solutes and modification of the volume and composition of the extracellular fluid occur gradually. Unstable patients, who are often intolerant of the abrupt fluid volume and solute concentration changes that accompany standard HD treatments, can be successfully treated with CRRT. The precision and stability with which fluid and electrolyte balance can be maintained using CRRT is unmatched by any currently available dialysis therapies, except perhaps the extended HD techniques mentioned in the following section.

The basic principles of CRRT are similar for adults and children. However, the application of these modalities in children requires attention to several important details unique to therapy in pediatric patients. For example, extracorporeal blood volume may be large compared to the patient blood volume, necessitating blood circuit priming in the very small child as described in the section on acute HD (see "acute intermittent hemodialysis," above). The most demanding considerations arising in pediatric CRRT are related to the need to adapt equipment and prescriptions designed for adult-size patients in order to meet the special needs of the smallest of pediatric patients requiring renal support.

Initiation

The indications for initiating CRRT in children and adults are similar and most often involve the treatment of AKI and fluid overload in a critically ill patient [20, 119]. CRRT may be combined with extracorporeal membrane oxygenation (ECMO) and plasmapheresis circuits.

CRRT refers to a variety of modalities that use one or both solute clearance mechanisms. In continuous venovenous hemofiltration (CVVH), blood flows through the hemofilter, generating large volumes of ultrafiltrate, which is replaced by a physiologic "replacement fluid," either before (pre-dilution) or after (post-dilution) the hemofilter (Fig. 52.4a). Clearance is thus exclusively convective. If a dialysate is infused into the hemofilter, clearance is primarily diffusive, as in HD. Hence, this CRRT modality is called continuous venovenous HD (CVVHD, Fig. 52.4b). When both replacement fluid and dialysate are used, permitting convective and diffusive clearance, the therapy is known as continuous venovenous hemodiafiltration (CVVHDF, Fig. 52.4c).

Initiation of CRRT also requires adequate vascular access, as discussed previously and in Chap. 65.

Fig. 52.4 (**a**) Diagram of a convective based (CVVH) continuous renal replacement therapy (RRT). Note use of either pre- or post-filter replacement fluid rather than dialysate. (**b**) Diagram of diffusion based (CVVHD) continuous RRT. Note use of dialysate rather than replacement fluid. Dialysate flow is countercurrent to blood flow. (**c**) Diagram of combined convective and diffusive based (CVVHDF) continuous RRT. Note use of both dialysate and replacement fluids

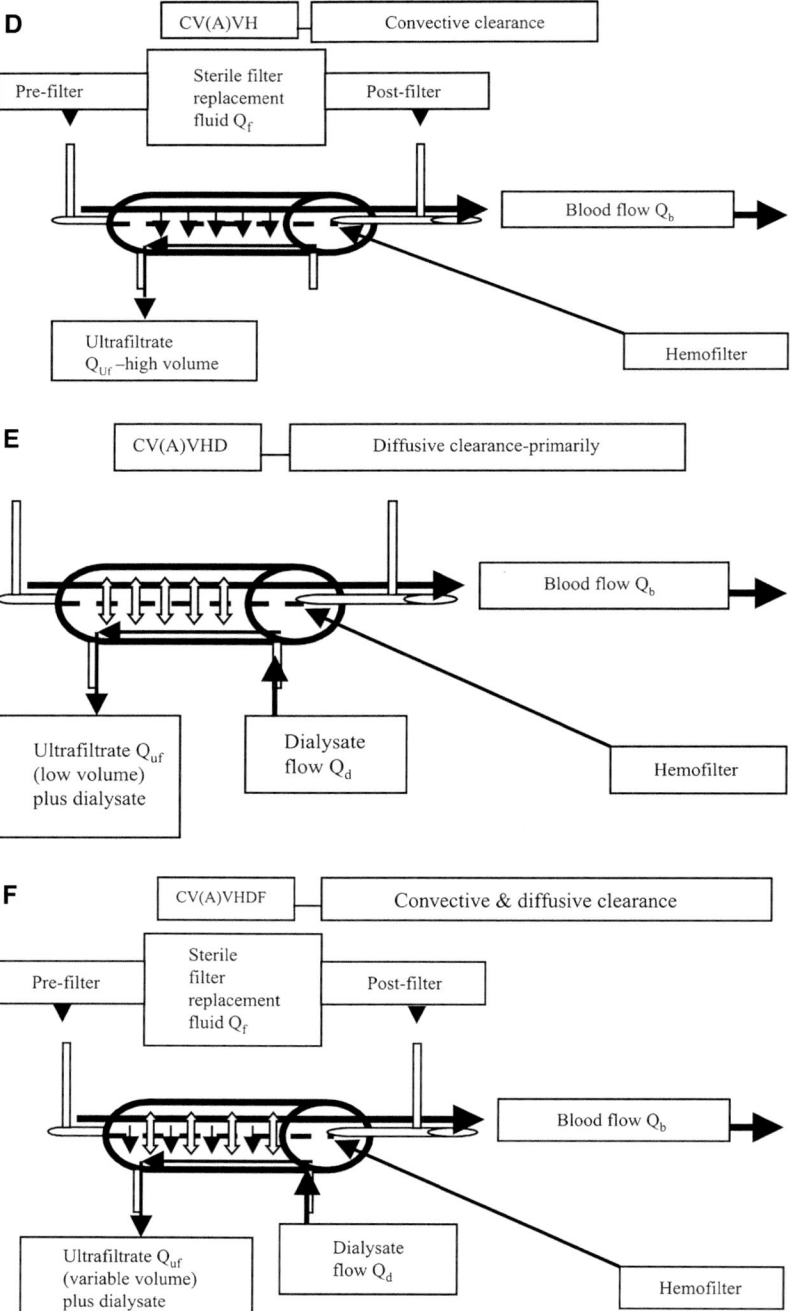

Blood Flow Rates

With a well-functioning vascular access, it is possible to adjust Qb based on to the size of the child and the clinical setting. Higher Qb may support longer filter life by reducing the likelihood of filter fiber clotting. Higher Qb also facilitates increased patient fluid removal by providing greater filter plasma flow rates and reduces the loss of clearance efficiency from pre-dilution mode CVVH or CVVHDF. However, not all patients will tolerate a higher Qb, especially at initiation of CRRT. Hence, we suggest initiating CRRT with lower Qb and advance to the targeted rate over the first 30 min of therapy as tolerated. In contrast to pediatric HD where initial Qb can be readily extrapolated from patient body weight, there are no true "body-weight" recommendations for Qb in any form of pediatric CRRT. The Qb chosen should provide adequate clearance for the size of the patient, with consideration of access limitations and device requirements. Recommendations for Qb range from 4 to 10 mL/kg/min; consequently, Qb may vary widely in CRRT. Depending on the patency of the access, the Qb may need to be higher to maintain flow. For example, 10–12 mL/kg/min may be necessary to accommodate technical requirements (access) and clearance in extremely low birth-weight neonates while 2–4 mL/kg/min may be appropriate in larger adolescents.

Solutions

The tolerability of CRRT has been greatly improved with the introduction of bicarbonate-based CRRT solutions. In the past, with lactate as the buffer, worsening lactic acidosis was common, leading to hypotension and depression of cardiac function [120]. A series of comparative clinical trials of lactate- and bicarbonate-based CRRT fluids in adults [121, 122] and children [123] have demonstrated the superiority of bicarbonate as a buffer; consequently, bicarbonate-based CRRT solutions are now the standard of care, although trace amounts of lactate may be used in solutions to maintain stability.

CRRT solutions also contain sodium, potassium, chloride, glucose, calcium, phosphate, and magnesium. Bicarbonate-based CRRT solutions are available from several manufacturers in a wide array of electrolyte formulations. Most hospital pharmacies stock only a single brand and in only a few formulations. A feature of CRRT, especially in small patients, is the tendency over time for the composition of the CRRT fluids to determine the electrolyte composition of the patient. A fluid low in potassium, phosphorous and magnesium may be appropriate at initiation of CRRT when concentrations of these electrolytes in AKI patients are often elevated. However, depending on the CRRT prescription, within a short time the patient may become deficient in these electrolytes, which can complicate management. Thus, while a "starter" fluid with reduced potassium, phosphorous and magnesium is needed, a fluid that includes these electrolytes in physiologic concentrations should follow. Rather than stocking multiple formulations, some pharmacies may prefer to add potassium, phosphorous, magnesium and even additional bicarbonate to the "starter" solutions as needed, a practice that may add the risk of pharmacy errors and increase costs. Calcium is always left out of solutions when phosphate is present to avoid precipitation. Calcium has usually, but not always, been left out of CRRT solutions used with citrate anticoagulation, as will be discussed below.

Prescription

The optimal "dose" of RRT is not known. Adult AKI studies by Ronco and colleagues using CVVH established a total convective clearance (replacement fluid plus patient fluid removal) target of 35 mL/kg/h as a threshold below which survival was significantly worse [124]. In a subset of these patients with sepsis, there was a trend in favor of improved survival with total convective clearance $\geq$45 mL/kg/h. Despite theoretical considerations that seemed to favor high clearance targets in cytokine-driven illnesses like sepsis [125] and preliminary results in septic adults treated with very high flow CRRT [126], available evidence does not support the use of clearance targets above 20–35 mL/kg/h. For pediatric patients, this translates to 2–3 L/1.73 m^2/h, rates that are reasonably easy to achieve.

Anticoagulation

Effective CRRT requires optimal anticoagulation. Activation of the clotting cascade occurs in CRRT circuits due to contact of the circulating blood with artificial surfaces. Low blood flow rates, turbulent flow, small catheters and high hematocrits hasten clotting. Anticoagulation regimens using mixed molecular weight heparin or sodium citrate are the most commonly used in pediatric CRRT, and either can be effective. An early comparison in pediatric centers showed equal filter life span with heparin and citrate, but more hemorrhagic events in the heparin group [127].

Heparin has been the mainstay of HD anticoagulation for decades. Many pediatric CRRT programs continue to rely on heparin. Heparin is infused in the CRRT circuit pre-filter and titrated to achieve a targeted post-filter activated aPTT 1.5–2 times normal, or an ACT between 180 and 220 s. This is usually accomplished by giving an initial heparin bolus of 20–30 units/kg, followed by a continuous infusion of 10–20 units/kg/h. Alternatively, the circuit may be rinsed and primed with 1–2 L of normal saline to which has been added 2500–5000 units/L of heparin, followed by the pre-filter heparin infusion.

Sodium citrate anticoagulation is widely used in pediatric CRRT programs due to its ease of administration and decreased bleeding risk [128]. By infusing citrate into the arterial limb of the CRRT tubing as it leaves the catheter, calcium ions are bound to the citrate, reducing available calcium and thereby inhibiting coagulation within the circuit, since normal coagulation is calcium-dependent. Systemic hypocalcemia is prevented by infusion of either calcium gluconate or calcium chloride into the patient at a central site. Thus, citrate anticoagulation achieves regional anticoagulation by affecting only the circuit, thereby eliminating the increased risk of bleeding with heparin. Since the original citrate protocol employing 4% trisodium citrate (440 mEq/L sodium), newer modifications utilize anticoagulant citrate dextrose "A" (ACD-A), a less-concentrated formulation, which is also commonly used as the anticoagulant in apheresis procedures.

Adverse effects of citrate anticoagulation include acid-base disturbances, citrate excess and hyperglycemia in infants when ACD-A is used. Patients receiving citrate anticoagulation may develop metabolic alkalosis; fortunately, citrate is readily cleared by dialysis [129]. Citrate excess may be diagnosed by monitoring the ratio of the total calcium to the ionized calcium levels [130]. If hepatic metabolism of citrate is insufficient, citrate accumulates; thus, patients with diminished liver function are at increased risk for citrate excess. Citrate excess can occur when citrate clearance is less than citrate delivery. Citrate is not inherently toxic, but citrate excess causes systemic hypocalcemia. Total calcium levels rise and the ratio of total calcium to systemic ionized calcium levels rises precipitously. As citrate accumulation progresses, it becomes more difficult to maintain the declining systemic ionized calcium levels within normal ranges. Monitoring of ionized calcium is the most sensitive way to detect citrate accumulation [131]. Treatment often requires increasing the removal of citrate by increasing clearance within the circuit (i.e., increased dialysate and/or replacement fluid rate); this assures ongoing anticoagulation while balancing the build-up of citrate in the patient. An initial citrate infusion rate of 50–70% of the usual rate is also recommended in patients with hepatic insufficiency who are at increased risk for citrate toxicity. A pediatric citrate anticoagulation protocol using bicarbonate dialysate has been published [132].

It is also possible in certain situations to use no anticoagulation, relying on periodic saline flushes of the circuit. This approach is typically considered in larger patients with evidence of a sustained coagulopathy due to disseminated intravascular coagulopathy or hepatic failure. However, many of these patients are receiving periodic fresh frozen plasma and platelet infusions to correct the underlying coagulopathy; these infusions will clot a CRRT system when no anticoagulation is used. Moreover, patients with hepatic failure may have a paradoxical hypercoagulable state. An uncontrolled study demonstrated that the no coagulation/saline flushes approach was associated with an inferior circuit life span compared to heparin or citrate anticoagulation [127].

CRRT Use in Combination Therapies

Extra-corporeal Membrane Oxygenation

The widespread use of ECMO in neonatal and pediatric critical care units along with the common occurrence of AKI in these patients with multi-organ dysfunction has led to the need to incorporate CRRT into the ECMO circuit. Fluid overload at CRRT initiation has been shown to be a consistent factor associated negatively with survival in ECMO and preventing the development of significant fluid overload at the outset of ECMO may be more clinically effective than attempting fluid removal later in therapy [133].

The ECMO circuit is fully heparinized, eliminating the need for anticoagulation of the CRRT circuit. Blood flow in the ECMO circuit is often 20–30 times that required for optimal CRRT. Newer ECMO circuits with multiple access phalanges allow the insertion of the CRRT circuit in an entirely pre-oxygenator location, avoiding shunt of oxygenated blood from the patient when the CRRT circuit is placed in a post- to pre-oxygenator position. Close collaboration between CRRT and ECMO teams is required to find the best location for the CRRT circuit and to coordinate therapy goals [134].

Plasma Therapy

Patients with AKI secondary to immune complex–mediated disease and sepsis-associated thrombotic microangiopathy may require both CRRT and plasma therapies (i.e., plasmapheresis, plasma exchange) [135]. CRRT is readily combined concurrently with plasma therapy procedures without interrupting the CRRT circuit. The placement of a three-way stopcock at both arterial and venous limbs of the CRRT circuit at the connection to the double lumen catheter allows diversion of blood through the centrifugation plasmapheresis machine [136].

Plasma exchange removes inflammatory mediators and replaces the volume with fresh frozen plasma in attempt to correct underlying homeostatic abnormalities; conversely, plasmapheresis removes plasma with inflammatory mediators, but replaces the volume with a non-plasma solution (usually albumin) [137].

Additionally, CRRT is believed to have an immunomodulatory effect on inflammatory cytokines in sepsis; however, the impact on patient outcome in sepsis remains unclear and the primary role remains management of fluid overload [138]. CRRT may downregulate the inflammatory response through nonselective extracorporeal removal, mainly by absorption, of cytokines and other mediators, restoring hemodynamic and immunologic homeostasis [139]. One retrospective study demonstrated benefit of isovolemic hemofiltration followed by conventional continuous venovenous hemofiltration in patients with septic shock and oliguric AKI with subsequent improvement in oxygenation and mean arterial pressure as well as significant improvement in survival at 28 days versus those receiving conventional supportive therapy [140].

Complications

CRRT requires the patient to remain relatively immobilized while connected to the CRRT circuit for prolonged periods. As a result, small children typically require sedation and occasionally even pharmacological paralysis to prevent small movements that may disrupt flow in the CRRT circuit. Additionally, a relatively large fraction of total circulating blood volume is in the extracorporeal circuit, placing the child at substantial risk for hypothermia during CRRT. Careful temperature monitoring is required during RRT, particularly when combination therapies are utilized. In-line fluid warmers can be used but increase priming volume. Line warmers that can be applied to the return line offer the best results.

Outcome

The Prospective Pediatric CRRT (ppCRRT) Registry reports an overall pediatric CRRT survival rate of 58% [80]. Survival of pediatric patients treated with CRRT has been reported in single center studies to vary widely by disease and modality [20, 141, 142]. A single center study initially demonstrated that the degree of fluid overload was an independent determinant of outcome in pediatric patients treated with CRRT [20], and that was confirmed by a large multicenter study from the ppCRRT Registry [80].

Patient survival was inversely correlated with percentage fluid overload at initiation of CRRT: survivors had a mean fluid overload of 14.2% while in non-survivors had a mean fluid overload of 25.4%, a difference that was highly significant and independent of diagnosis or severity of illness [20]. Further analysis of the ppCRRT Registry data demonstrated that 20% fluid overload was associated with four times the mortality of pediatric patients receiving CRRT when compared to patients with less than 10% fluid overload at initiation of CRRT [80]. These data suggest that earlier initiation of measures to control fluid accumulation, including CRRT, may improve survival.

Extended Hemodialysis Techniques

Extended hemodialysis techniques, also known as hybrid therapies, utilize intermittent hemodialysis machine technology while providing the slower solute and fluid removal associated with continuous RRT for use in less stable patients with AKI [143, 144]. The terms for these modalities include sustained low-efficiency daily dialysis (SLEDD) or extended daily dialysis (EDD) or slow continuous dialysis (SCD) [145].

SLEDD is a dialytic modality that allows for flexible options in treatment duration, prolonged or even continuous treatments, using conventional dialysis machines with varying pump speeds for 6–18 h daily [146]. Variants such as sustained low-efficiency daily diafiltration (SLEDD-f), aimed at improving clearance of middle molecular inflammatory mediators of the systemic inflammatory response associated with sepsis, have been developed for clinical use [92, 147]. Advantages of SLEDD-f over CVVHDF include faster clearance of small solutes and fluid removal yet maintaining hemodynamic stability [148]. It allows flexible therapeutic schedules so that patients are accessible and can be mobilized for other medical treatments.

Hybrid therapies also have lower heparin requirement than CRRT, but less frequent clotting. The reported incidence of clotting is 17–26% with heparin, while the reported inci-

dence of circuit clotting without anticoagulation is 24–26% using single pass machines and lower using batch systems [149]. Hybrid therapies, with the high diffusive capacity for solutes, are able to correct alkalosis or hypernatremia, while at the same time removing the calcium chelated citrate complexes in citrate anticoagulation, an advantage in patients with liver failure [150]. With hybrid therapies, phosphate removal can be very extensive. Hypophosphatemia and metabolic alkalosis is easily induced in a critically ill patient, especially those on prolonged parenteral nutrition; therefore, preemptive fluid correction with phosphorous and reduction in dialysate bicarbonate are often warranted.

Conclusion

AKI is common in hospitalized children and associated with high risk of mortality and long-term morbidity. Recent advances in the understanding of the pathophysiology of AKI have pointed to newer diagnostic and therapeutic strategies that focus on early recognition and treatment. Exciting developments in technology have made RRT more accessible and more easily applied in the pediatric setting. Yet, despite these advances, mortality rates among children with AKI remain disturbingly high. Hopefully, future developments will improve outcomes for children with AKI.

References

1. Bunchman TE. Treatment of acute kidney injury in children: from conservative management to renal replacement therapy. Nat Clin Pract Nephrol. 2008;4(9):510–4.
2. Himmelfarb J, Joannidis M, Molitoris B, Schietz M, Okusa MD, Warnock D, et al. Evaluation and initial management of acute kidney injury. Clin J Am Soc Nephrol. 2008;3(4):962–7.
3. Andreoli SP. Acute kidney injury in children. Pediatr Nephrol. 2009;24(2):253–63.
4. Zappitelli M, Bernier PL, Saczkowski RS, Tchervenkov CI, Gottesman R, Dancea A, et al. A small post-operative rise in serum creatinine predicts acute kidney injury in children undergoing cardiac surgery. Kidney Int. 2009;76(8):885–92.

5. Finfer S, Bellomo R, Boyce N, French J, Myburgh J, Norton R, et al. A comparison of albumin and saline for fluid resuscitation in the intensive care unit. N Engl J Med. 2004;350(22):2247–56.

6. Vincent JL, Sakr Y, Sprung CL, Ranieri VM, Reinhart K, Gerlach H, et al. Sepsis in European intensive care units: results of the SOAP study. Crit Care Med. 2006;34(2):344–53.

7. Kidney Disease: Improving Global Outcomes (KDIGO) Acute Kidney Injury Work Group. KDIGO clinical practice guideline for acute kidney injury. Kidney Int. 2012;2(Suppl):1–138.

8. De Backer D, Biston P, Devriendt J, Madl C, Chochrad D, Aldecoa C, et al. Comparison of dopamine and norepinephrine in the treatment of shock. N Engl J Med. 2010;362(9):779–89.

9. Delmas A, Leone M, Rousseau S, Albanese J, Martin C. Clinical review: vasopressin and terlipressin in septic shock patients. Crit Care. 2005;9(2):212–22.

10. Venkataraman R, Kellum JA. Prevention of acute renal failure. Chest. 2007;131(1):300–8.

11. Bellomo R, Chapman M, Finfer S, Hickling K, Myburgh J. Low-dose dopamine in patients with early renal dysfunction: a placebo-controlled randomised trial. Australian and New Zealand Intensive Care Society (ANZICS) Clinical Trials Group. Lancet. 2000;356(9248):2139–43.

12. Friedrich JO, Adhikari N, Herridge MS, Beyene J. Meta-analysis: low-dose dopamine increases urine output but does not prevent renal dysfunction or death. Ann Intern Med. 2005;142(7):510–24.

13. Lauschke A, Teichgraber UK, Frei U, Eckardt KU. 'Low-dose' dopamine worsens renal perfusion in patients with acute renal failure. Kidney Int. 2006;69(9):1669–74.

14. Cogliati AA, Vellutini R, Nardini A, Urovi S, Hamdan M, Landoni G, et al. Fenoldopam infusion for renal protection in high-risk cardiac surgery patients: a randomized clinical study. J Cardiothorac Vasc Anesth. 2007;21(6):847–50.

15. Landoni G, Biondi-Zoccai GG, Tumlin JA, Bove T, De Luca M, Calabro MG, et al. Beneficial impact of fenoldopam in critically ill patients with or at risk for acute renal failure: a meta-analysis of randomized clinical trials. Am J Kidney Dis. 2007;49(1):56–68.

16. Ricci Z, Luciano R, Favia I, Garisto C, Muraca M, Morelli S, et al. High-dose fenoldopam reduces postoperative neutrophil gelatinase-associated lipocaline and cystatin C levels in pediatric cardiac surgery. Crit Care. 2011;15(3):R160.

17. Ranucci M, De Benedetti D, Bianchini C, Castelvecchio S, Ballotta A, Frigiola A, et al. Effects of fenoldopam infusion in complex cardiac surgical operations: a prospective, randomized, double-blind, placebo-controlled study. Minerva Anestesiol. 2010;76(4):249–59.

18. Cantarovich F, Rangoonwala B, Lorenz H, Verho M, Esnault VL, High-Dose Flurosemide in Acute Renal Failure Study Group. High-dose furosemide for established ARF: a prospective, randomized, double-blind, placebo-controlled, multicenter trial. Am J Kidney Dis. 2004;44(3):402–9.

19. Mehta RL, Pascual MT, Soroko S, Chertow GM, Group PS. Diuretics, mortality, and nonrecovery of renal function in acute renal failure. JAMA. 2002;288(20):2547–53.

20. Goldstein SL, Currier H, Graf C, Cosio CC, Brewer ED, Sachdeva R. Outcome in children receiving continuous venovenous hemofiltration. Pediatrics. 2001;107(6):1309–12.

21. Askenazi DJ, Koralkar R, Hundley HE, Montesanti A, Patil N, Ambalavanan N. Fluid overload and mortality are associated with acute kidney injury in sick near-term/term neonate. Pediatr Nephrol. 2013;28(4):661–6.

22. Williams EL, Hildebrand KL, McCormick SA, Bedel MJ. The effect of intravenous lactated Ringer's solution versus 0.9% sodium chloride solution on serum osmolality in human volunteers. Anesth Analg. 1999;88(5):999–1003.

23. Reid F, Lobo DN, Williams RN, Rowlands BJ, Allison SP. (Ab)normal saline and physiological Hartmann's solution: a randomized double-blind crossover study. Clin Sci. 2003;104(1):17–24.

24. Wilcox CS. Regulation of renal blood flow by plasma chloride. J Clin Invest. 1983;71(3):726–35.

25. Ronco C, Haapio M, House AA, Anavekar N, Bellomo R. Cardiorenal syndrome. J Am Coll Cardiol. 2008;52(19):1527–39.

26. Grams ME, Estrella MM, Coresh J, Brower RG, Liu KD, National Heart Lung, and Blood Institute Acute Respiratory Distress Syndrome Network, et al. Fluid balance, diuretic use, and mortality in acute kidney injury. Clin J Am Soc Nephrol. 2011;6(5):966–73.

27. Ho KM, Power BM. Benefits and risks of furosemide in acute kidney injury. Anaesthesia. 2010;65(3):283–93.

28. Ho KM, Sheridan DJ. Meta-analysis of frusemide to prevent or treat acute renal failure. BMJ. 2006;333(7565):420.

29. Foland JA, Fortenberry JD, Warshaw BL, Pettignano R, Merritt RK, Heard ML, et al. Fluid overload before continuous hemofiltration and survival in critically ill children: a retrospective analysis. Crit Care Med. 2004;32(8):1771–6.

30. Andreoli SP. Management of acute kidney injury in children: a guide for pediatricians. Paediatr Drugs. 2008;10(6):379–90.

31. Andreoli SP. Acute and chronic renal failure in children. In: Gearhart JP, Rink RC, Mouriquand PDE, editors. Pediatric urology. Philadelphia: Saunders; 2001. p. 777–89.

32. Fiaccadori E, Cremaschi E. Nutritional assessment and support in acute kidney injury. Curr Opin Crit Care. 2009;15(6):474–80.

33. McClave SA, Martindale RG, Vanek VW, McCarthy M, Roberts P, Taylor B, et al. Guidelines for the provision and assessment of nutrition support therapy in the adult critically ill patient: Society of Critical Care Medicine (SCCM) and American Society for

Parenteral and Enteral Nutrition (A.S.P.E.N.). JPEN Parenter Enteral Nutr. 2009;33(3):277–316.

34. Fiaccadori E, Cremaschi E, Regolisti G. Nutritional assessment and delivery in renal replacement therapy patients. Semin Dial. 2011;24(2):169–75.

35. Zappitelli M, Goldstein SL, Symons JM, Somers MJ, Baum MA, Brophy PD, et al. Protein and calorie prescription for children and young adults receiving continuous renal replacement therapy: a report from the Prospective Pediatric Continuous Renal Replacement Therapy Registry Group. Crit Care Med. 2008;36(12):3239–45.

36. Fouque D, Kalantar-Zadeh K, Kopple J, Cano N, Chauveau P, Cuppari L, et al. A proposed nomenclature and diagnostic criteria for protein-energy wasting in acute and chronic kidney disease. Kidney Int. 2008;73(4):391–8.

37. Fiaccadori E, Lombardi M, Leonardi S, Rotelli CF, Tortorella G, Borghetti A. Prevalence and clinical outcome associated with preexisting malnutrition in acute renal failure: a prospective cohort study. J Am Soc Nephrol. 1999;10(3):581–93.

38. Cano NJ, Aparicio M, Brunori G, Carrero JJ, Cianciaruso B, Fiaccadori E, et al. ESPEN guidelines on parenteral nutrition: adult renal failure. Clin Nutr. 2009;28(4):401–14.

39. Briassoulis G, Tsorva A, Zavras N, Hatzis T. Influence of an aggressive early enteral nutrition protocol on nitrogen balance in critically ill children. J Nutr Biochem. 2002;13(9):560.

40. Fiaccadori E, Maggiore U, Giacosa R, Rotelli C, Picetti E, Sagripanti S, et al. Enteral nutrition in patients with acute renal failure. Kidney Int. 2004;65(3):999–1008.

41. Fiaccadori E, Maggiore U, Rotelli C, Giacosa R, Picetti E, Parenti E, et al. Effects of different energy intakes on nitrogen balance in patients with acute renal failure: a pilot study. Nephrol Dial Transplant. 2005;20(9):1976–80.

42. Story DA, Ronco C, Bellomo R. Trace element and vitamin concentrations and losses in critically ill patients treated with continuous venovenous hemofiltration. Crit Care Med. 1999;27(1):220–3.

43. Nakamura AT, Btaiche IF, Pasko DA, Jain JC, Mueller BA. In vitro clearance of trace elements via continuous renal replacement therapy. J Renal Nutr. 2004;14(4):214–9.

44. Van Cromphaut SJ. Hyperglycaemia as part of the stress response: the underlying mechanisms. Best Pract Res Clin Anaesthesiol. 2009;23(4):375–86.

45. Van den Berghe G, Wilmer A, Hermans G, Meersseman W, Wouters PJ, Milants I, et al. Intensive insulin therapy in the medical ICU. N Engl J Med. 2006;354(5):449–61.

46. van den Berghe G, Wouters P, Weekers F, Verwaest C, Bruyninckx F, Schetz M, et al. Intensive insulin therapy in critically ill patients. N Engl J Med. 2001;345(19):1359–67.

47. Hermans G, Wilmer A, Meersseman W, Milants I, Wouters PJ, Bobbaers H, et al. Impact of intensive insulin therapy on neuromuscular complications and ventilator dependency in the medical intensive care unit. Am J Respir Crit Care Med. 2007;175(5):480–9.

48. Schetz M, Vanhorebeek I, Wouters PJ, Wilmer A, Van den Berghe G. Tight blood glucose control is renoprotective in critically ill patients. J Am Soc Nephrol. 2008;19(3):571–8.

49. Kidney Disease: Improving Global Outcomes (KDIGO) Acute Kidney Injury Work Group. KDIGO clinical practice guideline for acute kidney injury. Kidney Int Suppl. 2012;2:S1–138.

50. Mehta RL, Pascual MT, Soroko S, Savage BR, Himmelfarb J, Ikizler TA, et al. Spectrum of acute renal failure in the intensive care unit: the PICARD experience. Kidney Int. 2004;66(4):1613–21.

51. Uchino S, Kellum JA, Bellomo R, Doig GS, Morimatsu H, Morgera S, et al. Acute renal failure in critically ill patients: a multinational, multicenter study. JAMA. 2005;294(7):813–8.

52. Kellum JA, Leblanc M, Venkataraman R. Acute renal failure. Clin Evid. 2008;2008:pii 2001.

53. Misurac JM, Knoderer CA, Leiser JD, Nailescu C, Wilson AC, Andreoli SP. Nonsteroidal anti-inflammatory drugs are an important cause of acute kidney injury in children. J Pediatr. 2013;162(6):1153–9, 9 e1.

54. Rihal CS, Textor SC, Grill DE, Berger PB, Ting HH, Best PJ, et al. Incidence and prognostic importance of acute renal failure after percutaneous coronary intervention. Circulation. 2002;105(19):2259–64.

55. Barrett BJ, Carlisle EJ. Metaanalysis of the relative nephrotoxicity of high- and low-osmolality iodinated contrast media. Radiology. 1993;188(1):171–8.

56. Solomon R. The role of osmolality in the incidence of contrast-induced nephropathy: a systematic review of angiographic contrast media in high risk patients. Kidney Int. 2005;68(5):2256–63.

57. Pannu N, Wiebe N, Tonelli M. Prophylaxis strategies for contrast-induced nephropathy. JAMA. 2006;295(23):2765–79.

58. Cantley LG, Spokes K, Clark B, McMahon EG, Carter J, Epstein FH. Role of endothelin and prostaglandins in radiocontrast-induced renal artery constriction. Kidney Int. 1993;44(6):1217–23.

59. Pflueger A, Larson TS, Nath KA, King BF, Gross JM, Knox FG. Role of adenosine in contrast media-induced acute renal failure in diabetes mellitus. Mayo Clin Proc. 2000;75(12):1275–83.

60. Rudnick MR, Berns JS, Cohen RM, Goldfarb S. Nephrotoxic risks of renal angiography: contrast media-associated nephrotoxicity and atheroembolism – a critical review. Am J Kidney Dis. 1994;24(4):713–27.

61. Taber SS, Mueller BA. Drug-associated renal dysfunction. Crit Care Clin. 2006;22(2):357–74, viii.

62. Peixoto AJ. Critical issues in nephrology. Clin Chest Med. 2003;24(4):561–81.

63. McCullough PA. Contrast-induced acute kidney injury. J Am Coll Cardiol. 2008;51(15):1419–28.

64. Weisbord SD, Gallagher M, Jneid H, et al. Outcomes after angiography with sodium bicarbonate and acetylcysteine. NEJM. 2018;378:603–14.

65. Sharfuddin AA, Molitoris BA. Pathophysiology of ischemic acute kidney injury. Nat Rev Nephrol. 2011;7(4):189–200.

66. Bernhardt WM, Eckardt KU. Physiological basis for the use of erythropoietin in critically ill patients at risk for acute kidney injury. Curr Opin Crit Care. 2008;14(6):621–6.

67. Endre ZH, Walker RJ, Pickering JW, Shaw GM, Frampton CM, Henderson SJ, et al. Early intervention with erythropoietin does not affect the outcome of acute kidney injury (the EARLYARF trial). Kidney Int. 2010;77(11):1020–30.

68. Miller SB, Martin DR, Kissane J, Hammerman MR. Insulin-like growth factor I accelerates recovery from ischemic acute tubular necrosis in the rat. Proc Natl Acad Sci U S A. 1992;89(24):11876–80.

69. Vijayan A, Martin DR, Sadow JL, Kissane J, Miller SB. Hepatocyte growth factor inhibits apoptosis after ischemic renal injury in rats. Am J Kidney Dis. 2001;38(2):274–8.

70. Gouyon JB, Guignard JP. Theophylline prevents the hypoxemia-induced renal hemodynamic changes in rabbits. Kidney Int. 1988;33(6):1078–83.

71. Bhat MA, Shah ZA, Makhdoomi MS, Mufti MH. Theophylline for renal function in term neonates with perinatal asphyxia: a randomized, placebo-controlled trial. J Pediatr. 2006;149(2):180–4.

72. Bakr AF. Prophylactic theophylline to prevent renal dysfunction in newborns exposed to perinatal asphyxia – a study in a developing country. Pediatr Nephrol. 2005;20(9):1249–52.

73. Schneider J, Khemani R, Grushkin C, Bart R. Serum creatinine as stratified in the RIFLE score for acute kidney injury is associated with mortality and length of stay for children in the pediatric intensive care unit. Crit Care Med. 2010;38(3):933–9.

74. Proulx F, Gauthier M, Nadeau D, Lacroix J, Farrell CA. Timing and predictors of death in pediatric patients with multiple organ system failure. Crit Care Med. 1994;22(6):1025–31.

75. Flynn JT. Choice of dialysis modality for management of pediatric acute renal failure. Pediatr Nephrol. 2002;17(1):61–9.

76. Liu KD, Himmelfarb J, Paganini E, Ikizler TA, Soroko SH, Mehta RL, et al. Timing of initiation of dialysis in critically ill patients with acute kidney injury. Clin J Am Soc Nephrol. 2006;1(5):915–9.

77. Bagshaw SM, Uchino S, Bellomo R, Morimatsu H, Morgera S, Schetz M, et al. Timing of renal replacement therapy and clinical outcomes in critically ill patients with severe acute kidney injury. J Crit Care. 2009;24(1):129–40.

78. Basu RK, Chawla LS, Wheeler DS, Goldstein SL. Renal angina: an emerging paradigm to identify children at risk for acute kidney injury. Pediatr Nephrol. 2012;27(7):1067–78.

79. Basu RK, Zappitelli M, Brunner L, Wang Y, Wong HR, Chawla LS, et al. Derivation and validation of the renal angina index to improve the prediction of acute kidney injury in critically ill children. Kidney Int. 2014;85(3):659–67.

80. Sutherland SM, Zappitelli M, Alexander SR, Chua AN, Brophy PD, Bunchman TE, et al. Fluid overload and mortality in children receiving continuous renal replacement therapy: the prospective pediatric continuous renal replacement therapy registry. Am J Kidney Dis. 2010;55(2):316–25.

81. Bonilla-Felix M. Peritoneal dialysis in the pediatric intensive care unit setting: techniques, quantitations and outcomes. Blood Purif. 2013;35(1–3):77–80.

82. Warady BA, Bunchman T. Dialysis therapy for children with acute renal failure: survey results. Pediatr Nephrol. 2000;15(1–2):11–3.

83. Gong WK, Tan TH, Foong PP, Murugasu B, Yap HK. Eighteen years experience in pediatric acute dialysis: analysis of predictors of outcome. Pediatr Nephrol. 2001;16(3):212–5.

84. Anochie IC, Eke FU. Paediatric acute peritoneal dialysis in southern Nigeria. Postgrad Med J. 2006;82(965):228–30.

85. Phadke KD, Dinakar C. The challenges of treating children with renal failure in a developing country. Perit Dial Int. 2001;21(Suppl 3):S326–9.

86. Wong SN, Geary DF. Comparison of temporary and permanent catheters for acute peritoneal dialysis. Arch Dis Child. 1988;63(7):827–31.

87. Chadha V, Warady BA, Blowey DL, Simckes AM, Alon US. Tenckhoff catheters prove superior to cook catheters in pediatric acute peritoneal dialysis. Am J Kidney Dis. 2000;35(6):1111–6.

88. Reznik VM, Griswold WR, Peterson BM, Rodarte A, Ferris ME, Mendoza SA. Peritoneal dialysis for acute renal failure in children. Pediatr Nephrol. 1991;5(6):715–7.

89. Schaefer F, Warady BA. Peritoneal dialysis in children with end-stage renal disease. Nat Rev Nephrol. 2011;7(11):659–68.

90. Rabindranath K, Adams J, Macleod AM, Muirhead N. Intermittent versus continuous renal replacement therapy for acute renal failure in adults. Cochrane Database Syst Rev. 2007;3:CD003773.

91. Bagshaw SM, Berthiaume LR, Delaney A, Bellomo R. Continuous versus intermittent renal replacement therapy for critically ill patients with acute kidney injury: a meta-analysis. Crit Care Med. 2008;36(2):610–7.

92. Abi Antoun T, Palevsky PM. Selection of modality of renal replacement therapy. Semin Dial. 2009;22(2):108–13.

93. Bunchman T, Gardner J, Kershaw D, Maxvold N. Vascular access for hemodialysis or CVVH(D) in infants and children. Nephrol Dial Transplant. 1994;23:314–7.

94. Muller D, Goldstein SL. Hemodialysis in children with end-stage renal disease. Nat Rev Nephrol. 2011;7(11):650–8.

95. Mehta RL. Indications for dialysis in the ICU: renal replacement vs. renal support. Blood Purif. 2001;19(2):227–32.

96. Mehta RL, Bouchard J. Dialysis dosage in acute kidney injury: still a conundrum? J Am Soc Nephrol. 2008;19(6):1046–8.

97. Palevsky PM. Renal replacement therapy in acute kidney injury. Adv Chronic Kidney Dis. 2013;20(1):76–84.

98. Goldstein SL. Overview of pediatric renal replacement therapy in acute renal failure. Artif Organs. 2003;27(9):781–5.

99. Brophy PD, Mottes TA, Kudelka TL, McBryde KD, Gardner JJ, Maxvold NJ, et al. AN-69 membrane reactions are pH-dependent and preventable. Am J Kidney Dis. 2001;38(1):173–8.

100. Parshuram CS, Cox PN. Neonatal hyperkalemic-hypocalcemic cardiac arrest associated with initiation of blood-primed continuous venovenous hemofiltration. Pediatr Crit Care Med. 2002;3(1):67–9.

101. Pasko DA, Mottes TA, Mueller BA. Pre dialysis of blood prime in continuous hemodialysis normalizes pH and electrolytes. Pediatr Nephrol. 2003;18(11):1177–83.

102. Hackbarth RM, Eding D, Gianoli Smith C, Koch A, Sanfilippo DJ, Bunchman TE. Zero balance ultrafiltration (Z-BUF) in blood-primed CRRT circuits achieves electrolyte and acid-base homeostasis prior to patient connection. Pediatr Nephrol. 2005;20(9):1328–33.

103. Fischbach M, Edefonti A, Schroder C, Watson A. Hemodialysis in children: general practical guidelines. Pediatr Nephrol. 2005;20(8):1054–66.

104. Alonso A, Lau J, Jaber BL. Biocompatible hemodialysis membranes for acute renal failure. Cochrane Database Syst Rev. 2008;1:CD005283.

105. Pannu N, Klarenbach S, Wiebe N, Manns B, Tonelli M. Renal replacement therapy in patients with acute renal failure: a systematic review. JAMA. 2008;299(7):793–805.

106. Uchino S, Bellomo R, Morimatsu H, Goldsmith D, Davenport P, Cole L, et al. Cytokine dialysis: an ex vivo study. ASAIO J. 2002;48(6):650–3.

107. Haase M, Bellomo R, Baldwin I, Haase-Fielitz A, Fealy N, Davenport P, et al. Hemodialysis membrane with a high-molecular-weight cutoff and cytokine levels in sepsis complicated by acute renal failure: a phase 1 randomized trial. Am J Kidney Dis. 2007;50(2):296–304.

108. Haase M, Bellomo R, Morgera S, Baldwin I, Boyce N. High cut-off point membranes in septic acute renal failure: a systematic review. Int J Artif Organs. 2007;30(12):1031–41.

109. Rimmele T, Assadi A, Cattenoz M, Desebbe O, Lambert C, Boselli E, et al. High-volume haemofiltration with a new haemofiltration membrane having enhanced adsorption properties in septic pigs. Nephrol Dial Transplant. 2009;24(2):421–7.

110. Warkentin TE, Greinacher A, Koster A, Lincoff AM, American College of Chest Physicians. Treatment and prevention of heparin-induced thrombocytopenia: American College of Chest Physicians Evidence-Based Clinical Practice Guidelines (8th Edition). Chest. 2008;133(6 Suppl):340S–80.

111. Stamatiadis DN, Helioti H, Mansour M, Pappas M, Bokos JG, Stathakis CP. Hemodialysis for patients bleeding or at risk for bleeding, can be simple, safe and efficient. Clin Nephrol. 2004;62(1):29–34.

112. Caruana RJ, Raja RM, Bush JV, Kramer MS, Goldstein SJ. Heparin free dialysis: comparative data and results in high risk patients. Kidney Int. 1987;31(6):1351–5.

113. Sanders PW, Taylor H, Curtis JJ. Hemodialysis without anticoagulation. Am J Kidney Dis. 1985;5(1):32–5.

114. Lohr JW, Slusher S, Diederich D. Safety of regional citrate hemodialysis in acute renal failure. Am J Kidney Dis. 1989;13(2):104–7.

115. Patel N, Dalal P, Panesar M. Dialysis disequilibrium syndrome: a narrative review. Semin Dial. 2008;21(5):493–8.

116. Rees L. Hemodialysis. In: Avner ED, Harmon WE, Niaudet P, editors. Pediatric nephrology. 5th ed. Philadelphia: Lippincott, Williams & Wilkins; 2004.

117. Schortgen F, Soubrier N, Delclaux C, Thuong M, Girou E, Brun-Buisson C, et al. Hemodynamic tolerance of intermittent hemodialysis in critically ill patients: usefulness of practice guidelines. Am J Respir Crit Care Med. 2000;162(1):197–202.

118. Dheu C, Terzic J, Menouer S, Fischbach M. Importance of the curve shape for interpretation of blood volume monitor changes during haemodiafiltration. Pediatr Nephrol. 2009;24(7):1419–23.

119. Bunchman TE, Maxvold NJ, Kershaw DB, Sedman AB, Custer JR. Continuous venovenous hemodiafiltration in infants and children. Am J Kidney Dis. 1995;25(1):17–21.

120. Davenport A, Will EJ, Davison AM. Hyperlactataemia and metabolic acidosis during haemofiltration using lactate-buffered fluids. Nephron. 1991;59(3):461–5.

121. Thomas AN, Guy JM, Kishen R, Geraghty IF, Bowles BJ, Vadgama P. Comparison of lactate and bicarbonate buffered haemofiltration fluids: use in critically ill patients. Nephrol Dial Transplant. 1997;12(6):1212–7.

122. Zimmerman D, Cotman P, Ting R, Karanicolas S, Tobe SW. Continuous veno-venous haemodialysis with a novel bicarbonate dialysis solution: prospective cross-over comparison with a lactate buffered solution. Nephrol Dial Transplant. 1999;14(10):2387–91.

123. Maxvold N, Flynn J, Smoyer W, et al. Prospective crossover comparison of bicarbonate vs lactate-based dialysate for pediatric CVVHD. Blood Purif. 1999;17:27–9.

124. Ronco C, Bellomo R, Homel P, Brendolan A, Dan M, Piccinni P, et al. Effects of different doses in continuous veno-venous haemofiltration on outcomes of acute renal failure: a prospective randomised trial. Lancet. 2000;356(9223):26–30.

125. Di Carlo JV, Alexander SR. Hemofiltration for cytokine-driven illnesses: the mediator delivery hypothesis. Int J Artif Organs. 2005;28(8):777–86.

126. Honore PM, Joannes-Boyau O, Boer W, Collin V. High-volume hemofiltration in sepsis and SIRS: current concepts and future prospects. Blood Purif. 2009;28(1):1–11.

127. Brophy PD, Somers MJ, Baum MA, Symons JM, McAfee N, Fortenberry JD, et al. Multi-centre evaluation of anticoagulation in patients receiving continuous renal replacement therapy (CRRT). Nephrol Dial Transplant. 2005;20(7):1416–21.

128. Mehta RL, McDonald BR, Aguilar MM, Ward DM. Regional citrate anticoagulation for continuous arteriovenous hemodialysis in critically ill patients. Kidney Int. 1990;38(5):976–81.

129. Chadha V, Garg U, Warady BA, Alon US. Citrate clearance in children receiving continuous venovenous renal replacement therapy. Pediatr Nephrol. 2002;17(10):819–24.

130. Meier-Kriesche HU, Gitomer J, Finkel K, DuBose T. Increased total to ionized calcium ratio during continuous venovenous hemodialysis with regional citrate anticoagulation. Crit Care Med. 2001;29(4):748–52.

131. Oudemans-van Straaten HM. Citrate anticoagulation for continuous renal replacement therapy in the critically ill. Blood Purif. 2010;29(2):191–6.

132. Bunchman TE, Maxvold NJ, Barnett J, Hutchings A, Benfield MR. Pediatric hemofiltration: normocarb dialysate solution with citrate anticoagulation. Pediatr Nephrol. 2002;17(3):150–4.

133. Selewski DT, Cornell TT, Blatt NB, Han YY, Mottes T, Kommareddi M, et al. Fluid overload and fluid removal in pediatric patients on extracorporeal membrane oxygenation requiring continuous renal replacement therapy. Crit Care Med. 2012;40(9):2694–9.

134. Ricci Z, Ronco C, Picardo S. CRRT in series with extracorporeal membrane oxygenation in pediatric patients. Kidney Int. 2010;77(5):469–70; author reply 71.

135. Peng ZY, Kiss JE, Cortese-Hasset A, Carcillo JA, Nguyen TC, Kellum JA. Plasma filtration on mediators of thrombotic microangiopathy: an in vitro study. Int J Artif Organs. 2007;30(5):401–6.

136. Yorgin PD, Eklund DK, al-Uzri AA, Whitesell L, Theodorou AA. Concurrent centrifugation plasmapheresis and continuous venovenous hemodiafiltration. Pediatr Nephrol. 2000;14(1):18–21.

137. House AA, Ronco C. Extracorporeal blood purification in sepsis and sepsis-related acute kidney injury. Blood Purif. 2008;26(1):30–5.

138. Servillo G, Vargas M, Pastore A, Procino A, Iannuzzi M, Capuano A, et al. Immunomodulatory effect of continuous venovenous hemofiltration during sepsis: preliminary data. Biomed Res Int. 2013;2013:108951.

139. Grootendorst AF. The potential role of hemofiltration in the treatment of patients with septic shock and multiple organ dysfunction syndrome. Adv Ren Replace Ther. 1994;1(2):176–84.

140. Piccinni P, Dan M, Barbacini S, Carraro R, Lieta E, Marafon S, et al. Early isovolaemic haemofiltration in oliguric patients with septic shock. Intensive Care Med. 2006;32(1):80–6.

141. Symons JM, Brophy PD, Gregory MJ, McAfee N, Somers MJ, Bunchman TE, et al. Continuous renal replacement therapy in children up to 10 kg. Am J Kidney Dis. 2003;41(5):984–9.

142. Flores FX, Brophy PD, Symons JM, Fortenberry JD, Chua AN, Alexander SR, et al. Continuous renal replacement therapy (CRRT) after stem cell transplantation. A report from the prospective pediatric CRRT Registry Group. Pediatr Nephrol. 2008;23(4):625–30.

143. Kudoh Y, Iimura O. Slow continuous hemodialysis – new therapy for acute renal failure in critically ill patients – Part 1. Theoretical consideration and new technique. Jpn Circ J. 1988;52(10):1171–82.

144. Kudoh Y, Shiiki M, Sasa Y, Hotta D, Nozawa A, Iimura O. Slow continuous hemodialysis – new therapy for acute renal failure in critically ill patients – Part 2. Animal experiments and clinical implication. Jpn Circ J. 1988;52(10):1183–90.

145. Tam PY, Huraib S, Mahan B, LeBlanc D, Lunski CA, Holtzer C, et al. Slow continuous hemodialysis for the management of complicated acute renal failure in an intensive care unit. Clin Nephrol. 1988;30(2):79–85.

146. Cruz D, Bobek I, Lentini P, Soni S, Chionh CY, Ronco C. Machines for continuous renal replacement therapy. Semin Dial. 2009;22(2):123–32.

147. Fliser D, Kielstein JT. Technology insight: treatment of renal failure in the intensive care unit with extended dialysis. Nat Clin Pract Nephrol. 2006;2(1):32–9.

148. Marshall MR, Ma T, Galler D, Rankin AP, Williams AB. Sustained low-efficiency daily diafiltration (SLEDD-f) for critically ill patients requiring renal replacement therapy: towards an adequate therapy. Nephrol Dial Transplant. 2004;19(4):877–84.

149. Kumar VA, Craig M, Depner TA, Yeun JY. Extended daily dialysis: a new approach to renal replacement for acute renal failure in the intensive care unit. Am J Kidney Dis. 2000;36(2):294–300.

150. Morath C, Miftari N, Dikow R, Hainer C, Zeier M, Morgera S, et al. Sodium citrate anticoagulation during sustained low efficiency dialysis (SLED) in patients with acute renal failure and severely impaired liver function. Nephrol Dial Transplant. 2008;23(1):421–2.

Neonatal Kidney Dysfunction

53

Isabella Guzzo, Stefano Picca, and David Askenazi

Kidney Function in Neonates

At birth, the kidney replaces the placenta as the major homeostatic organ, maintaining fluid and electrolyte balance and removing harmful waste products. In a healthy term neonate, dynamic changes to renal blood flow occur which lead to alterations in glomerular filtration rate (GFR) over the first few months of life. Tubular development is intact such that conservation or elimination of electrolytes and water are efficient and adequate. Alternatively, the glomerular, tubular and vascular regulation of the kidney in premature infant are abnormal compared to the healthy term counterpart. Describing the "normal" renal physiology in preterm neonates is difficult (as one can argue they are all abnormal); understanding how a term neonate maintains renal blood flow, glomerular filtration and tubular function is critical to extrapolation of how the premature

infant's underdeveloped/immature kidneys function. As we describe neonatal homeostasis, we will contrast the physiology of the "normal" healthy term infant to those of premature infants, understanding that the degree of immaturity and the neonatal course will affect the ability of premature infants "normal" homeostasis.

Healthy term infants are ready to maintain homeostasis of water, electrolytes, and acid/base. In addition, their kidneys function to metabolized drugs/toxins, and eliminate waste products. As the clinician has an integral role in prescribing fluids, electrolytes, and nutrition, proper homeostasis in sick term/near term newborns and premature infants depends on the clinicians' ability to appropriately prescribe fluids, nutrition and electrolytes. Infants who lack ability to remove uremic toxins and maintain appropriate electrolyte/fluid balance with medical management rely on nephrology teams to support the neonate with dialytic therapies designed to maintain homeostasis.

I. Guzzo
Dialysis Unit, Department of Pediatrics, Bambino Gesù Children's Research Hospital IRCCS, Rome, Italy
e-mail: isabella.guzzo@opbg.net

S. Picca
Educational Ambassador of the International Society of Nephrology, Rome, Italy

D. Askenazi (✉)
Department of Pediatrics, University of Alabama at Birmingham, Birmingham, AL, USA
e-mail: daskenazi@peds.uab.edu

Renal Blood Flow in Newborns

Starting with delivery and umbilical cord clamping, major hemodynamic changes occur in renal blood flow which drive changes in neonatal glomerular filtration rate. The proportion of cardiac output distributed to the kidney changes abruptly. Fetal kidneys receive approximately 2.5–5% of cardiac output at birth [1], which increases to 6%

© The Author(s), under exclusive license to Springer Nature Switzerland AG 2023
F. Schaefer, L. A. Greenbaum (eds.), *Pediatric Kidney Disease*,
https://doi.org/10.1007/978-3-031-11665-0_53

by 24 h of life [2, 3], steadily escalates to 10% at 1 week of life, and attains 15–18% at 6 weeks of life [4] as it approaches the fractional cardiac output to the kidneys observed in adults (approximately 20–30%). These dynamic changes in renal blood flow are driven by both increased systemic blood pressure and a substantial decrease in renal vascular resistance. The abrupt and significant drop in renal vascular resistance is due to a redistribution of renal blood flow within the kidney, changes in the number of vascular channels and changes in glomerular arterial resistance [5]. Initially, renal blood flow primarily extends to the outer cortex which gradually distributes to medullary sections over the first few months of life [6].

The auto-regulatory mechanisms which control renal blood flow are driven by both the myogenic reflex of vascular smooth muscles and the tubule-glomerular feedback system. These reflexes aim to maintain constant blood flow by sensing vascular endothelial stretch and distal tubular fluid flow respectively. Nitric oxide, angiotensin II, adenosine, bradykinins, and endothelin play a central role in maintaining adequate blood flow.

The renin angiotensin system is active throughout fetal development and contributes to normal fetal maturation. Congenital abnormalities (i.e., defects to angiotensin II receptors) and secondary abnormalities (i.e., maternal use of angiotensin converting enzyme inhibitor) can significantly affect kidney development. Prostaglandins (potent vasodilators) also serve to increase renal blood flow by active vasodilation of afferent arterioles. These agents are increased in times of stress and help counteract vaso-constrictive effects of angiotensin II and catecholamines. Prostaglandins and inhibitors of prostaglandins are commonly prescribed in neonatal medicine to maintain patency, or electively close patent ductus arteriosus; respectively. Such dynamic changes in renal blood flow, alterations in hemodynamics, and medications to promote vasoconstriction/ vasodilation will greatly affect glomerular filtration rate in neonates.

Glomerulogenesis

Kidney development commences during the 5th week of gestation with partially functional temporary organs (the pronephros and metanephros). The first nephrons are formed by about the 8th week of gestation and increase over time. Four glomerular generations are present after 14 weeks and 12–13 generations of glomeruli after 36 weeks of gestation [7]. The juxtamedullary nephrons develop initially, with superficial ones following. Nephrogenesis continues until 36 weeks of gestation at which time the number of nephrons, 1.6–2.4 million, approximates that of an adult [8]. Autopsy studies suggest that the extra-uterine environment is not amenable to neo-glomerulogenesis, leading to a low nephron number in premature infants [9]. Thus, the premature infant may be programmed for low nephron endowment, and subsequent chronic kidney disease.

In individuals with a lower number of nephrons, single-nephron hyperfiltration can increase total GFR to a similar level as attained by those with normal numbers of glomeruli. However, the impact of low nephron endowment may become problematic over time as single nephron hyperfiltration may cause glomerulosclerosis and ultimately progressive loss of kidney function, especially in the context of other risk factors for CKD such as acute kidney injury, hypertension, diabetes, and other primary kidney diseases.

Glomerular Function Rate (GFR)

GFR is the most useful measurement of kidney function. GFR is measured indirectly through the concept of clearance (the equivalent volume of plasma from which a substance would have to be totally removed to account for its rate of excretion in urine per unit time). Clearance is calculated by dividing the excretion rate of a substance by its plasma concentration ($C_x = U_x \times V$); where U_x and P_x are urine and plasma concentrations of substance x and V is urine flow rate. C_x is expressed as milliliters per minute and is usually normalized to 1.73 m^2, the idealized adult body surface area [10]. GFR is the best clinical test to estimate functional renal mass, which can assist the clinician in prescribing fluids/electrolytes, determine disease progression, and appropriately prescribe medications excreted by the kidney.

The gold standard method for GFR measurement is inulin clearance. Tables 53.1 and 53.2 summarize studies conducted to estimate GFR (measured by inulin clearance) in healthy term and preterm infants, respectively. Dependent on degree of prematurity, GFR steadily improves from 10–20 mL/min/1.73 m² during the first

Table 53.1 Formal GFR measurements for term neonates during the first 2 years of life

Term infants	
Age	mL/min/1.3 m²
1–3 days	21 ± 5
4–14 days	37 ± 7
1–3 months	85 + 35
4–6 months	87 ± 22
7–12 months	96 + 2
1–2 years	105 ± 17

Data from Schwartz and Furth [11]

Table 53.2 Formal GFR measurements for preterm neonates during the first 4 months of life

Premature infants	
Age	mL/min/1.73 m²
1–3 days	14.0 ± 5.0
1–7 days	18.7 ± 5.5
4–8 days	44.3 ± 9.3
3–13 days	47.8 ± 10.7
1.5–4 months	68.4 ± 16.6

Data from Schwartz and Furth [11]

week of life to 30–40 mL/min/1.73 m² by 2 weeks after birth concomitant with alterations in renal blood flow. Thereafter GFR improves steadily over the first few months of life [11, 12]. Serum creatinine (SCr) is the most common method to estimate GFR and monitor kidney function but has significant shortcomings (see Chap. 3).

There are several specific problems with using SCr in neonates: SCr in the first few days of life reflects mother's and not the infant's kidney function. Moreover, GFR in term and preterm infants is generally very low and normal serum creatinine values vary greatly dependent on level of prematurity and age [13] (Fig. 53.1). Finally, bilirubin levels in premature infants rise in the first several days and return to normal after a few weeks. When the colorimetric Jaffe method of SCr is used this may impact SCr interpretation [14].

Attempts to estimate GFR using SCr in neonates have suggested the following formula for children who are <1 year of age [15]: Height (cm) * k/serum creatinine (mg/dL); where $k = 0.33$ for low birth weight and 0.45 for normal birth weight infants. However, caution should be used when applying this equation in clinical practice for several reasons. At best the formula represents a mean estimate and the true GFR may be off in either direction by 20% or more. In addition, the k coefficients were derived using the

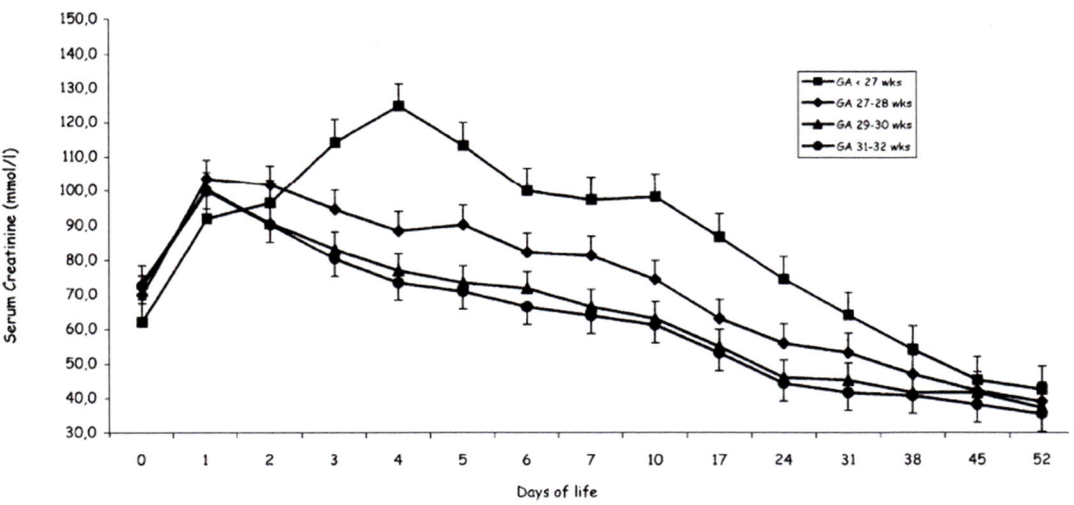

Fig. 53.1 Serum creatinine values over time by gestational age categories. (Used with permission from Gallini et al. [13])

Jaffe calorimetric method to measure SCr. As most hospitals now only use the enzymatic equation, the coefficients may no longer be applicable.

Cystatin C has been extensively studied as a measure of GFR and a marker of acute kidney injury. Since Cystatin C is not influenced by the maternal serum level and is highest at birth, it may be better suited than SCr to monitor kidney function in infants. Cystatin C concentrations significantly decrease during the first three days of life and are independent of gestational age, birth weight and maternal kidney function status in very low birth weight infants [16]. Cystatin C does not differ between males and females and is not influenced by gestational age. Thus, cystatin C seems to have many properties of an ideal marker of kidney function in this age group [17]. However, as only a few studies on this topic have been conducted so far and no studies have linked cystatin C levels with short and long-term outcomes in this population, further research is needed before adopting Cystatin C as a primary marker of kidney function in neonates.

Water, Electrolyte and Acid-Base Disorders in Neonates

Metabolic Acidosis

Neonates typically show a certain degree of acidosis depending on gestational and postnatal age [18]. In full-term neonates, after completion of nephrogenesis at the 34th week of gestation [19], the mechanisms devoted to maintain acid base (AB) equilibrium are still immature. This immaturity concerns both the capacity of H^+ excretion and the HCO_3^- reabsorption threshold [20, 21]. Moreover, the ability of excreting large amounts of acid through ammoniagenesis is impaired in the newborn baby, due to the decreased presence of enzymes necessary for ammoniagenesis, like glutaminase [22]. Finally, neonatal nutrition involves a two to three times higher protein load than older children with consequently higher acid production. In premature infants, this unfavorable condition is even worsened by the inability

to efficiently acidify urine with further acid retention and consequently increased risk of metabolic acidosis. In fact, in preterm infants, plasma bicarbonate levels are lower than in full term neonates for the first 3 weeks of life due to the lower renal threshold for bicarbonate (see Chap. 36). This predisposes preterm neonates to condition known as late metabolic acidosis, which is further promoted by milk formulas containing casein, by parenteral nutrition (especially in TPN containing arginine HCl), and by withdrawal of milk alimentation (and consequently alkali intake), e.g., during episodes of diarrhea.

The acid-base disturbances seen in the NICU occur in an organism with immature homeostatic mechanisms. According to the classic metabolic acidosis classification based on the anion gap, we can take into account a number of clinical situations leading to metabolic acidosis. The anion gap attests the balance (or unbalance) between acid accumulation and loss of base equivalents. It is calculated by: $Na^+ - (Cl^- + HCO_3^-)$ in mEq/L. Metabolic acidosis with a normal anion gap (<16 mEq/L) is seen in neonates with intestinal or renal HCO_3^- losses, which can be due to either proximal or distal renal tubular acidosis (see Chap. 36). Also, the use of the carbonic anhydrase inhibitor acetazolamide in pregnancy has been associated with metabolic acidosis in preterm neonates [23, 24].

The most common conditions causing an anion gap >16 mEq/L in neonates are kidney failure, inborn errors of metabolism (IEM) or lactic acidosis [25]. In kidney failure, the impairment of acid load elimination increases HCO_3^- consumption while in IEM (in particular in organic acidurias [26]. HCO_3^- stores are depleted by the increased production of organic acids. Small bowel drainage following surgical procedures may also induce large HCO_3^- losses. In necrotizing enterocolitis (NEC) acidosis is associated with progressive systemic shock and lactic acidosis [27]. In VLBW infants, metabolic acidosis on the first day of illness is more common in infants with perforated NEC compared to infants without perforation [23].

The treatment of metabolic acidosis in neonates firstly relies on the diagnosis and treatment of the underlying cause. The treatment of renal tubular acidosis with $NaHCO_3$ in critically ill children is controversial [28]. Only one randomized trial examining potential benefits of $NaHCO_3$ in asphyxiated newborn infants is available - it showed no influence on the outcome [29]. No benefit of bicarbonate supplementation has also been found in adult patients. In cardiac arrest, the administration of $NaHCO_3$ has been widely utilized in an attempt to correct acid overproduction caused by decreased tissue oxygenation. There are no available randomized trials demonstrating positive effects of $NaHCO_3$ administration in cardiac arrest in either adult and pediatric patients, including neonates. On the contrary, $NaHCO_3$ may induce CO_2 accumulation in poorly oxygenated districts and hypercarbia [30].

In 2013, a survey in Canadian NICUs showed that $NaHCO_3$ is most frequently administered in septic shock whereas its use is much less frequent in cardiac arrest [31]. With an analogous mechanism, CO_2 accumulation may occur also in ARDS if its elimination by the lungs is insufficient. In this case also, the addition of bicarbonate may induce only a transient rise of pH, usually followed by hypercarbia [32]. A different situation occurs when a net HCO3$^-$ loss or its excessive consumption take place. Examples are gastrointestinal losses and kidney failure. The ability of the neonatal kidney to reabsorb HCO3$^-$ is about one third of that of adult individuals [33] and a mature ammoniagenesis mechanism is lacking [20].

Potential hazards of $NaHCO_3$ supplementation in infants include risk of sodium overload and hypernatremia, hypokalemia and hypocalcemia. Moreover, the use of $NaHCO_3$ in infants has been associated with a number of adverse events like intracranial hemorrhage, deterioration of cardiac function and myocardial injury [34, 35]. In neonates $NaHCO_3$ should be given only after establishment of adequate ventilation and circulation and should be restricted to selected situations like severe acidosis with life-threatening hyperkalemia, massive GI losses, and tubulopathies. In neonatal resuscitation, a dose of 1–2 mmol/kg of a 0.5 mmol/mL solution may be given by slow intravenous push (over at least 2 min) after adequate ventilation and perfusion

have been established [36]. In infants with kidney failure, titration of acid/base balance using sodium citrate is necessary to maintain appropriate metabolic control and growth.

Metabolic Alkalosis

Metabolic alkalosis is almost invariably accompanied by hypokalemia and can be classified on the base of chloride urine concentration. In critical infants, low urinary Cl^- concentration (expressed as Cl^- < 10 mmol/L or, more precisely, as Cl^-/Creatinine ratio < 10 in mol/mol) suggests that the kidneys are avidly holding on to chloride, thus, ruling out chloride loss from the kidneys as the etiology. Low urine chloride metabolic alkalosis may be present as a consequence of loss of gastric secretions (vomiting, nasogastric suction), secretory diarrhea or after rapid correction of hypercapnia, and chronic diuretic which cause low total body chloride). In contrast, metabolic alkalosis with high urine chloride suggests inappropriate losses of chloride from the kidney from primary chloride losing tubulopathies (Bartter syndrome, Gitelman syndrome) and, more frequently, the use of diuretics. If metabolic hypochloruric alkalosis is present in context of systemic hypertension, defects in regulation of aldosterone and renin should be sought (Fig. 53.2).

A peculiar low-chloride associated clinical situation is that of infants after cardiopulmonary bypass surgery. In these patients, metabolic alkalosis is associated with younger age, preoperative ductal dependency and hemodilution [37]. Volume and chloride depletion have been advocated as possible causes [38]. Metabolic alkalosis is also reported in up to 18% of infants referred to surgery for pyloric stenosis [39].

Hyperkalemia

Hyperkalemia may represent a life-threatening condition in the NICU. It is the most common electrolyte disorder associated to heart conduction problems [40]. Non-oliguric hyperkalemia

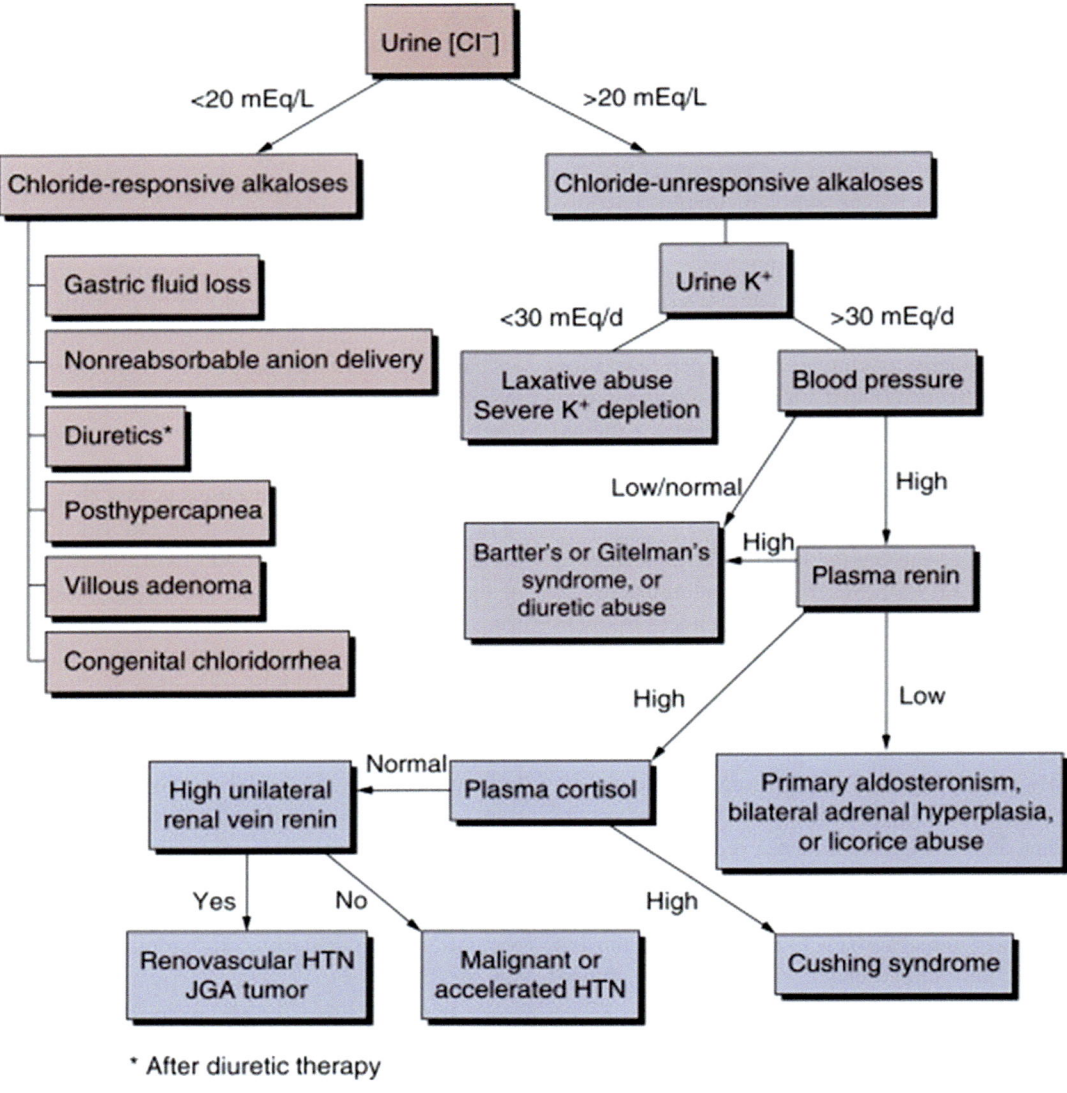

Fig. 53.2 Clinical decision tree diagram for metabolic alkalosis [1] used with permission

of the newborn is defined as a plasma potassium level >6.5 mmol/L in the absence of acute kidney failure [41]. In neonates, spurious hyperkalemia has to be initially excluded since mechanical trauma to red blood cells during venipuncture with consequent release of intracellular potassium is particularly frequent in neonates and prematures. The hemolytic Index is a measure of red color of serum which is due almost exclusively due to hemoglobin. This index (reported as 0 to 4 +) assist in detecting spurious hyperkalemia in infants [42]. Once spurious hyperkalemia is ruled out, a number of causes of true hyperkalemia have to be considered. Hyperkalemia may be induced by increased intake, intra-extracellular potassium redistribution and decreased elimination. Increased intake in critical infants may be seen with acute potassium load and blood transfusion. Acute load is infrequent in non-oliguric infants and it is usually consequent to dosing errors or the administration rate of intravenous potassium containing solutions. Potassium concentration in transfused blood may be as high as 50 mmol/L, so that even small amounts may induce severe hyperkalemia in small infants. This renders the use of fresh blood in newborns mandatory [43]. The most common cause of hyperkalemia due to intra-extracellular potassium redistribution in critically ill infants is metabolic acidosis. In this condition, potassium moves from the intracellular compartment in order to maintain electroneutrality after H^+ ions have accumulated in the intracellular space.

Hyperkalemia is frequent in preterm neonates. It presents as a sudden rise of serum potassium in the first 72 h of life of preterm neonates with a gestational age <28 weeks and may cause heart conduction impairment that may result in sudden death. This condition results from potassium loss from the intracellular space, together with the immature renal excretion of potassium and aldosterone unresponsiveness. Management of hyperkalemia is mandatory when symptoms and/or EKG alterations are present. The latter include tall, peaked T waves with narrow base, prolonged PR interval, decreased or disappearing P wave, widening of QRS, amplified R wave, ventricular fibrillation or asystole. There are three main approaches to the treatment of hyperkalemia: (1) antagonizing the membrane actions of hyperkalemia, (2) driving potassium into cells, and (3) removing potassium from the body. First, stabilization of myocardial function may be obtained by Ca^{2+} infusion. Calcium inactivates sodium channels and increases membrane excitability in 2–3 min. Its effect lasts for 30–60 min, so that an alternative therapy is required after that time. Calcium is given by slow intravenous injection over 5–10 min: 0.11 mmol/kg (0.5 mL/kg of calcium gluconate 10%). Potassium can be driven into intracellular space by insulin in exchange with sodium. I.v. insulin is used with glucose for emergency treatment of hyperkalemia at the dose of intravenous solution of insulin (0.1–0.6 units/kg/h in neonates) with glucose infusion of 0.5–1 g/kg/h (5–10 mL/kg/h of glucose 10%).

The effect starts in 15 min and can last for hours. Blood glucose levels must be carefully monitored to avoid both hypo-and hyperglycemia [43]. Intravenous sodium bicarbonate reverses potassium ions from the extra- to the intracellular compartment to maintain electro-neutrality. A half correction of the base excess (0.3 × weight × BE) over 10–15 min can be administered and the rest given in the next 12–24 h. The main constraint of sodium bicarbonate use is sodium and volume overload, especially when kidney impairment is present. β-2 adrenergic agonists increase sodium-potassium ATPase activity and potassium is driven back into cells. Salbutamol or albuterol can be nebulised or given by intravenous infusions [44, 45]. Finally, removal of potassium is generally obtained by diuretics and cation exchange resins. Furosemide can be administered in 1 mg/kg dosage and repeated in case of need. Since the efficacy of diuretics depends on GFR, higher dosage may be required in kidney failure. Calcium or sodium polystyrene sulfonate (Kayexalate®, Concordia Pharmaceuticals, Oakville, Ontario, Canada) binds potassium by exchanging it with sodium in GI tract so that potassium is eliminated in the stool. In adult patients with life-threatening hyperkalemia, the role of exchange resins has been questioned [46]. In neonates, while potassium elimination can be enhanced by ion resins, gastro-intestinal obstruction and/or perforation can occur following oral or rectal administration of exchange resins [47]. Moreover, in a comparative study in hyperkalemic preterm neonates cation-exchange resin did not lead to a better outcome regarding all-cause mortality than glucose and insulin [48]. Given the above considerations, combined insulin/glucose infusion should be preferred over treatment with rectal cation-resin for acute hyperkalemia in preterm infants [49]. Low potassium formulas are available for children who have poor potassium elimination. In addition, premixing formula with sodium polystyrene sulfonate (Kayexalate®), allowing the resin to settle and providing the supernatant for nutrition, efficiently lowers the oral potassium load without risking bowel obstruction/perforation.

Hypokalemia

True, not alkalosis induced hypokalemia (<3.5 mmol/L) in critically ill infants may develop as a consequence of potassium loss due to intestinal problems (vomiting, nasogastric suction, diarrhea), kidney conditions (diuretic use, recovery from acute kidney injury) or insufficient potassium intake, mainly coming from unbalanced parenteral nutrition. Congenital conditions if untreated can be lethal during the first weeks or months of life. These include congenital chloride diarrhea (a rare autosomal recessive disease characterized by chronic secretory diarrhea), and some inherited conditions like Bartter syndrome, Gitelman syndrome, and related syndromes (see Chap. 33).

In neonates, potassium replacement must be managed with extreme caution, given the rapid change of kalemia induced by small amounts of potassium. Intravenous potassium treatment should only be given for immediately life-threatening emergencies over several minutes while severe hypokalemia may be treated with an infusion of 0.2–0.5 mmol/kg/h to a maximum of 1 mmol/kg. Non-emergencies are best treated using oral supplements if possible, otherwise as small dosages as low as 0.03–0.07 mmol/kg by slow injection. During potassium administration, very frequent monitoring of plasma levels has to be established as well as continuous EKG monitoring while correction occurs [50].

Hypernatremia

Changes in sodium concentration are common in critical neonates, due to the small patient volume and the body fluid changes occurring in the perinatal period. Hypernatremia (>145 mmol/L) must always be considered in relation to the water content and is traditionally classified as hypo-, normo- or hypervolemic. Hypovolemic hypernatremia is often seen when fluid restriction is required and water loss exceeds that of sodium. Other frequent causes of hypovolemic hypernatremia are losses through the gut or the kidney (like watery diarrhea, water loss in post-

obstructive polyuria). Hypernatremia is more frequent in VLBW infants in which water loss through lungs and the immature skin may reach 150 mL/kg/day, thus exposing the preterm to hypernatremia due to free water deficit, especially in the first hours of life. Moreover, renal sodium handling is inversely related to creatinine clearance in the first 2 weeks of life. After 4–5 days from birth sodium balance becomes negative with a sudden decrease of fractional excretion, thus enabling the neonatal kidney to spare sodium. This occurs also in preterm babies [51]. A particular case is that of critically ill infants with severe hypoperfusion and acidosis requiring large amounts of sodium bicarbonate. In this case, often a capillary leak syndrome is present with leak of albumin, sodium and water to the interstitium in a mixed hypovolemic-sodium retaining situation in which sodium is in a third space. Hypervolemic hypernatremia in the NICU is frequently induced by administration of large amounts of sodium with drugs and blood products.

Management of hypernatremia in critically ill infants is usually an urgent treatment. Respiratory distress, necrotizing enterocolitis, and patent ductus arteriosus are associated with hypernatremia and volume expansion [52, 53]. Correction of hypernatremia basically consists in free water administration with correction velocity being the crucial issue. There is evidence that plasma both sodium changes and velocity of these changes are associated with neurological outcome [54]. The rule is to reduce natremia at a speed not >0.5–1.0 mmol/L/h. If plasma sodium is very high (>160 mmol/L), it is advisable to administer a 0.9% saline solution in order to reduce natremia slowly.

Hyponatremia

Hyponatremia (<130 mmol/L) is associated with cerebral edema and permanent neurologic sequelae especially in preterm neonates [55, 56]. In critical neonates, hyponatremia is most frequently seen as a consequence of diuretic use, surgical procedures, diarrhea/vomiting and third space loss. A particular neonatal issue is hyponatremia during therapeutic hypothermia. In these patients, hyponatremia has been related to water loss as a consequence of cooling induced skin vasoconstriction [57]. Total body fluid overload will also cause hyponatremia.

Diuretics are commonly used to treat infants with oxygen-dependent chronic lung disease [58] and congenital heart defect [59]. In acute situations, high-dose diuretics may be required and this may cause hyponatremia which, in turn, hampers the response to the diuretic. Hypokalemia, alkalosis, and calcium wasting can be part of this picture. During surgery, standard neonatal intensive care guidelines recommending hypotonic i.v. infusions containing 20–40 mmol of sodium are often followed [60]. However, these guidelines may not meet metabolic and volume needs in the perioperative period and hyponatremia may result in up to 60% of patients [55, 60, 61]. Careful monitoring of sodium levels and the use of balanced sodium solutions are mandatory in these patients [61]. During neonatal sepsis, capillary leak may take place and large amounts of sodium together with water and albumin are displaced into the interstitium with severe edema poorly responding to diuretics [62].

Replacement of sodium loss in volume depletion must take into account the variation of sodium plasma levels since, if a patient is seizing with a serum sodium <120 mol/L, 3% saline can be given. In patients that are clinically stable, use of isotonic saline can improve sodium concentrations. Like in hypernatremia, correction velocity must not be >1 mmol/kg/h. Careful attention to fluid shifts and serial electrolyte monitoring is essential.

Hypocalcemia

Normal levels of serum calcium are normally achieved during the second week of life when PTH secretion from parathyroid glands can efficiently respond to hypocalcemic stimuli [63]. Before then, normal neonates spontaneously lean towards hypocalcemia. Actually, a physiologic fall in serum calcium concentration, occurs in the first 24 h of life due to the sudden stop of calcium supply from the placenta. PTH is then stimulated but its action becomes valid from 2 to 3 days of life onward [64] . The kidney plays a key role in calcium homeostasis and, although the timing of the action of PTH on renal calcium excretion in neonates is not certain, calciuria increases after the second week of life [65].

NICU infants may develop hypocalcemia (<8.8 mg/dL or ionized calcium <4.9 mg/dL) for a number of reasons. When PTH secretion from immature parathyroid glands is insufficient, a prolongation or a worsening of hypocalcemia occurs (early onset neonatal hypocalcemia) [63]. Under these circumstances, hypocalcemia is rarely symptomatic but EKG alterations (Q-T prolongation) may be present [63]. Preterm infants and children of diabetic mothers [66] are more exposed to the risk of hypocalcemia. Approximately 50% of infants of mothers who have diabetes show hypocalcemia [54].

The etiology of neonatal hypocalcemia is multifactorial. It is probably due to loss of calcium and magnesium with urine, resulting in reduced placental transfer and decreased neonatal secretion of PTH. Another risk factor for early onset hypocalcemia is maternal calcium ingestion during pregnancy, inducing inhibition of the neonate's PTH response and consequent hypocalcemia [67]. Hypocalcemia starting after 5–10 days of age is due to resistance of renal tubule cells to PTH leading to renal retention of phosphorus and hypocalcemia (late onset neonatal hypocalcemia) [63].

Overt hypoparathyroidism in neonates occurs in case of dysgenesis of the parathyroid glands. The most common cause is the DiGeorge syndrome. The phenotype is characterized by hypocalcemia caused by parathyroid gland hypoplasia, defective T-lymphocyte function and impaired cell-mediated immunity caused by impaired thymic differentiation and conotruncal defects of the heart or aortic arch. The syndrome is associated with microdeletions of chromosome 22q11.2. Some neonates may have isolated hypoparathyroidism. Also in the CATCH 22 syndrome (cardiac anomaly, abnormal facies, thymic aplasia, cleft palate, hypocalcemia), haploinsufficiency for genes located in the 22q11 region is associated with contiguous gene deletion syndromes that include not only the DiGeorge syndrome but also the overlapping conotruncal anomaly and velocardiofacial syndromes [63, 68].

In NICU patients, acquired hypocalcemia is frequently drug induced. Aminoglycosides, often used in NICU, can increase renal calcium loss and induce hypocalcemia in neonates [69]. Anticonvulsants such as phenytoin or phenobarbital are potential inducers of cytochrome P450 (CYP450), causing increased vitamin D degradation. Also, the prolonged use of anticonvulsant in the mother during pregnancy can induce hypocalcemia in the newborn [70]. Renal excretion of calcium is notably enhanced during treatment with loop diuretics. This concerns particular populations like infants with heart problems or after cardiosurgery. Ionized calcium also can be reduced in infants treated with sodium bicarbonate, which increases calcium binding to albumin.

Urgent treatment of neonatal hypocalcemia is based on i.v. calcium supply. Calcium gluconate and calcium chloride are both available at 10% concentration. Both preparations have to be administered via a central vein. Although there is no proven superiority of one form over the other for the treatment of ionized hypocalcemia [71], calcium chloride appears to be more irritating for vessels and gluconate should be preferred in neonates. Calcium chloride contains three times more elemental calcium than gluconate (272 vs. 90 mg in 10 mL at 10%, respectively). Serum calcium levels should be corrected by continuous intravenous infusion of calcium (at 1–3 mg of elemental calcium/kg body weight per hour) under strict monitoring of ionized calcium levels, in order to avoid complications as such as bradycardia and arrhythmia or vessel necrosis.

Hypercalcemia

Neonatal hypercalcemia is much less frequent than hypocalcemia. Infants normally show higher total (8.8–11.3 mg/dL) as well as ionized calcium levels (1.19–1.40 mmol/L) than older children or [61]. Hypercalcemia is often asymptomatic.

Hypercalcemic infants can show irritability, dizziness and arterial hypertension. It is not infrequent that hypercalcemia is discovered after diagnosis of nephrocalcinosis or lithiasis.

Hypercalcemia in NICU infants is almost always iatrogenic [63]. Vitamin D and calcium supplementation are a frequent cause of hypercalcemia. Hypophosphatemia is frequently seen in preterm neonates as a consequence of poor intake. Low phosphate levels stimulate PTH secretion which in turn increases intestinal calcium absorption and calcium resorption from the skeleton. Children on Extracorporeal Membrane Oxygenation (ECMO) experience hypercalcemia up to 30% of patients, probably due to aberrant vitamin D-PTH regulation [72].

Rare congenital conditions must be considered in the presence of neonatal hypercalcemia. The calcium-sensing receptor (CASR) is expressed in the PTH producing chief cells of the parathyroid gland and the cells lining the kidney tubule. Inherited abnormalities of the CASR gene can cause either hypercalcemia or hypocalcemia. This autosomal recessive condition affects neonates and induces neonatal severe hyperparathyroidism (NSHPT) [73]. Hypercalcemia is usually severe and can be life-threatening. Typically, PTH levels are normal to high and calcium urinary excretion is low.

Subcutaneous fat necrosis (SFN) can be the consequence of a difficult delivery and is characterized by necrosis of fat and a local macrophagic reaction to the necrotic fat. Hypercalcemia derives from the excess of calcitriol produced by macrophages and is associated with a 15% mortality rate [74]. Of interest, SFN with hypercalcemia has been recently associated with neonatal therapeutic hypothermia [75, 76]. Given the growing use of this therapy, blood calcium levels should be monitored in children undergoing therapeutic hypothermia.

Initial treatment of severe hypercalcemia in critical infants relies on hydration and loop diuretics. Calciuria can rapidly increase, which can worsen kidney function and/or nephrocalcinosis. Withdrawal of hypercalcemic agents such as calcium supplements or vitamin D supplements is mandatory. Treatment of neonatal hyperparathyroidism is an urgent requirement.

Steroids and bisphosphonates have been used with success [77]. More recently, the calcimimetic agent cinacalcet has been used successfully in neonatal hyperparathyroidism in combination with bisphosphonates [78].

Acute Kidney Injury (AKI) in Neonates

Definition and Epidemiology

Previously referred to as acute renal failure, acute kidney injury (AKI) is characterized by a sudden impairment in kidney function, which results in retention of nitrogenous waste products and altered regulation of extracellular fluid volume, electrolytes and acid-base homeostasis. The term "acute kidney injury" has replaced "acute renal failure" by most critical care and nephrology societies, primarily to highlight the importance of recognizing this process at the time of "injury" as opposed to waiting until "failure" has occurred [79].

Despite its limitations (as outlined above and in Chap. 46), SCr is the most commonly used measure to evaluate glomerular filtration in the clinical setting and is more specific than blood urea nitrogen (BUN). BUN is an insensitive measure of glomerular filtration rate (GFR) because it can be increased out of proportion to changes in GFR secondary to high dietary protein intake, gastrointestinal bleed, use of steroids and hypercatabolic states. If the BUN:SCr ratio exceeds 20, increased urea production or increased renal urea reabsorption that occurs in pre-renal azotemia should be suspected [80].

Historically the most common SCr cutpoint used to define neonatal AKI was set at an arbitrary cutoff of 1.5 mg/dL or greater, independent of day of life and regardless of the rate of urine output [81]. In 2009, categorical definition based on a rise in SCr to diagnose and define different stages of AKI [77] was applied to neonates [81]. Since then, we and others have used AKI definitions similar to those published by the 2007 AKIN and 2012 KDIGO guidelines [82–92]. A neonatal AKI definition has been adapted from the KDIGO definition (Table 53.3).

Table 53.3 Neonatal AKI definition

Stage	Serum creatinine (SCr) criteria	Urine output (UOP criteria)
0	No change or rise <0.3 mg/dL	UOP >1 cc/kg/h (over previous 24 h)
1	↑ SCr of ≥0.3 mg/dL or ↑ SCr to 150–199% × baseline	UOP >0.5 cc/kg/h and ≤ 1 cc/kg/h (over previous 24 h)
2	↑ SCr to 200–299% × baseline	UOP >0.1 cc/kg/h and ≤ 0.5 cc/kg/h (over previous 24 h)
3	↑ SCr to ≥300% × baseline or SCr ≥2.5 mg/dL or Receipt of dialysis	UOP ≤0.1 cc/kg/h (over previous 24 h)

Baseline SCr will be defined as the lowest previous SCr value

Table 53.4 Incidence and outcomes of neonates with AKI

Population	Incidence (%)	Mortality AKI v no AKI	Ref.
VLBW[a]	18	55% vs. 5%	[82]
ELBW[b]	12.5	70% vs. 22%	[89]
Sick near-term/term	18	22% vs. 0%	[78]
Sepsis	26	70% vs. 25%	[90]
Asphyxiated Newborn	38	14% vs. 2%	[91]
ECMO[c]	71	72.7% vs. 20%[d]	[92]

[a]Very low birth weight (VLBW) infants <1500 g
[b]Extremely low birth weight (ELBS) infants <1000 g
[c]Extra Corporeal Membrane Oxygenation (ECMO)
[d]In group with highest stage of AKI

The following modifications have been made to account for specific neonatal issues:

- Because SCr normally declines over the first week of life [13], each SCr is compared to lowest previous value.
- As SCr of 2.5 mg/dL represents glomerular filtration rate <10 mL/min/1.73 m^2 in neonates, this cutoff is used to define Stage 3 AKI (as opposed to 4.0 mg/dL in adults).
- UOP criteria have been adapted to levels obtained over 24 h.

Table 53.4 shows the incidence and outcomes of neonatal AKI in different neonatal populations using category AKI definitions similar to that presented here. However, more research is needed to develop, and validate this definition against hard clinical endpoints.

Risk Factors and Etiology

AKI is a common clinical condition in the NICU [93–96]. Up until 2013, limited data coming from small single-center studies identified premature infants, sick near-term or term infants, and infants who undergo cardiopulmonary bypass or ECMO at particular risk for neonatal AKI [88, 97–100]. Also, since there was a wide variation in the incidence of AKI according to the AKI definition used and the number of SCr values measured, a uniform understanding of the risk factors for AKI was difficult to ascertain [101–103]. In 2014, the Neonatal Kidney Collaborative was established and designed a multicenter study to evaluate AKI among critically ill neonates (the Assessment of

Table 53.5 Time to dialysis start, fraction of patients reaching a negative fluid balance and survival rate of infants treated with PD after cardiopulmonary bypass surgery. Only in studies where all patients reached negative fluid balance survival exceeded 50%

Reference	n	Time to PD start	Patients with negative fluid balance (%)	Survivors (%)
Lowrie [179]	17	NA	35	24
Fleming [180]	21	2.5 days (1–6) after surgery	36	38
Golej [181]	116	NA, but 43% of pts. started on PD when CVP >10 mmHg	53	47
Werner [182]	23	2.6 ± 0.6 days	100	53
Dittrich [183]	27	In the OR or first hrs in ICU	100	73
Santos [184]	23	4.8 ± 16.8 h	100	57
Sorof [185]	20	22 h	100	80
Chien [186]	7	1.2 ± 0.4 days after AKI onset	NA	57

Worldwide Acute Kidney Injury Epidemiology in Neonates (AWAKEN)) [104]. In AWAKEN, several risk factors have been evaluated according to gestational age and postnatal age [104]. In particular, perinatal risk factors are associated with early neonatal AKI (first perinatal week) and cardiac and kidney anomalies, surgery and nephrotoxin medications rather than perinatal factors are risk factors of late AKI (after the postnatal week) (Table 53.6) [105, 106]. Furthermore, nearly one third of neonates with late AKI had an episode of early AKI increasing the risk for CKD.

These conditions are important in identifying neonates at risk for development of AKI and because some of them are potentially preventable [107, 108]. The causes of AKI in newborns are typically divided into three groups: pre-renal failure, intrinsic renal failure and post-renal failure with pre-renal and intrinsic being the most frequently reported [109].

Pre-renal and intrinsic renal failure both include congenital and acquired causes of AKI (Table 53.7). The most common form of AKI in neonates is pre-renal failure which accounts for more than 80% of cases.

In numerous studies, **perinatal asphyxia and sepsis** are the most frequent associated conditions [110]. Asphyxia causes renal dysfunction secondary to redistribution of blood flow to more vital organs such as heart and brain at the expense of the others, especially kidneys and gut. The reported incidence of renal failure in asphyxiated neonates varies between 50% and 70% in infants not treated with therapeutic hypothermia [111–113] and 30–40% after introduction of therapeutic hypothermia for the treatment of perinatal asphyxia [114–116]. In asphyxiated newborns, renal outcome correlates with oliguria but also with clinical markers of the severity of asphyxia. In particular, Apgar score at 5 min <6, initial and 12-hour lactate concentrations, and hypoxic ischemic encephalopathy were much better predictors of adverse outcome than kidney function tests [113, 116]. The incidence of AKI among term and near-term neonates with encephalopathy in the AWAKEN cohort was more than 40% and analysis of data including antenatal risk factors selected among factors associated with AKI

Table 53.6 Available filters for neonatal CKRT

Filter	Manufacturer	Surface (m²)	Membrane	Priming (mL)
Miniflow 10	Gambro-Lundia	0.045	AN69	3.5
Minifilter	Minntech	0.07	Polysulfone	6
Carpediem 1	Bellco	0.075	Polysulfone	27.2
Carpediem 3	Bellco	0.245	Polysulfone	41.5
HF20	Gambro-Lundia	0.20	AN69	60
Aquadex UF500	Nuwellis	0.12	Polysulfone	33
FX paed	Fresenius	0.20	Polysulfone	18

Table 53.7 Monitors for pediatric and neonatal CKRT

Monitor	Manufacturer	Pediatric lines	Neonatal lines	Blood pump range (mL/min)	Blood flow steps (mL/min)	Fluid management range (mL/h)
Prismaflex[a]	Gambro-Lundia	Yes	–	20–100	2	50–2500
Multifiltrate	Fresenius	Yes	–	10–100	2	10–7000
Aquarius	Baxter	Yes	–	10–200	2	50–11,000
Plasauto Sigma	Asahi	Yes	Yes	1–400	1	10–12,000
Carpediem	Bellco	–	Yes	2–50	1	10–300
Aqudex	Nuwellis	No	No	5–40	5	10–500

[a]Prismaflex equipped with HF20 circuit

being outborn, low admission temperature, intra-uterine growth restriction and the presence of meconium-stained amniotic fluid (MSAF) [117].

Among the neonatal population, **premature infants and low birth-weight** are particularly sensitive to asphyxia and hypoperfusion [97, 118, 119]. Very low birth weight (VLBW) and extremely low birth weight (ELBW) children are at increased risk for AKI because of prenatal fetal distress secondary to intrauterine growth retardation, placental insufficiency and maternal medications and a postnatal course frequently complicated by hypotension and hypoxia and the need for cardio-pulmonary support [97, 119, 120]. Studies focused on AKI in VLBW/ELBW reported an incidence of 12.5% and 18%, respectively [119, 120]. VLBW infants with AKI were more likely to have low birth weight, low gestational age and low Apgar scores and they frequently required umbilical arterial catheters, assisted ventilation and inotropic support. In another study, infants with AKI had a higher mean airway pressure, a lower mean arterial blood pressure and higher exposure to cefotaxime than non-AKI controls [119].

Given the high vulnerability of the neonatal kidney to the effects of hypoperfusion, **acute tubular necrosis** (ATN) commonly occurs. Pre-renal failure is due to renal hypoperfusion or ischemia in the presence of a normal kidney. Hence, irrespective of whether pre-renal failure is caused by total body volume depletion or decreased effective blood volume, renal function quickly returns to normal if perfusion is rapidly restored. Conversely, if the insult is severe and prolonged, acute tubular necrosis can occur [101]. During renal hypoperfusion many compensatory mechanisms are activated; in particular intrarenal vasodilatory prostaglandins are released. In order to help differentiate pre-renal failure from ATN, urinary indices have been proposed, in particular urine sodium concentration and the fractional excretion of sodium (FENa) [121] (Table 53.7). The assumption is that renal tubules work properly in pre-renal failure and are able to reabsorb solute and water while they are damaged and do not adequately conserve sodium in ATN. The urine samples for measuring indices must be obtained prior to a fluid and diuretic challenge. This could be difficult in oliguric neonates. Urine sodium less than 20 mEq/L and more than 50 mEq/L is suggestive of prerenal and intrinsic renal failure, respectively. FENa is calculated as urine sodium factored by serum sodium divided by urine creatinine factored by serum creatinine:

$$FENa = \text{urine sodium} \times \text{serum creatinine} / \text{serum sodium} \times \text{urine creatinine}$$

In term infants, a FENa above 3% indicates intrinsic renal failure. Preterm babies physiologically lose more sodium than term infants and a FENa of more than 6% can be used to define intrinsic AKI in infants between 29 and 32 weeks of gestation [121, 122].

Sepsis is the second most common condition associated with AKI after perinatal asphyxia [110]. AKI develops in 20–30% of neonates with sepsis [123–126]. In a series of 203 neonates with sepsis, 40 (20%) developed AKI. Increased baseline serum creatinine, vasopressor days, history of necrotizing enterocolitis (NEC) and ECMO requirement were good predictors of AKI in septic neonates. Most AKI episodes were detected within 2 days after sepsis evaluation; 23% of sepsis cases with AKI did not return to their serum creatinine baseline and all of them died [126]. In developing countries with limited resources, sepsis is more common than in developed countries [127, 128] and is the most common cause of AKI in neonates, occurring in 31% of newborns with a mortality rate of 65% [129]. The pathogenesis of AKI in sepsis is multifactorial, including shock, disseminated intravascular coagulation, haemorrhage, cardiac failure, and nephrotoxic drugs. All these conditions cause renal' hypoperfusion with resultant ischemic-reperfusion injury and cytokine- and oxidant-mediated kidney injury.

Administration of **nonsteroidal anti-inflammatory drugs** (NSAID) (for instance, indomethacin for patent ductus arteriosus closure) can inhibit this compensatory mechanism and precipitate AKI during renal hypoperfusion. In a multicenter Italian Study, ibuprofen treatment was identified as a risk factor correlated with impaired kidney function. Interestingly, maternal consumption of NSAID during pregnancy negatively influenced neonatal kidney function as well [130]. The risk of NSAID therapy-associated AKI is even higher when neonates concomitantly receive additional nephrotoxic drugs. Among neonates with patent ductus arteriosus who received gentamicin and NSAID,

the rate of AKI was 14.8% compared to 9.1% for those not exposed to NSAID [131].

Antimicrobial agents are another major class of drugs associated with the development of AKI in preterm infants. Nephrotoxic AKI has been reported in association with aminoglycosides, vancomycin, piperacillin-tazobactam, acyclovir and amphotericin B [132]. In particular, aminoglycosides are widely used in pediatric patients. They accumulate in renal tubular cortical cells and exert nephrotoxicity causing damage to the proximal tubular epithelial cells secondary to lysosomal dysfunction [101, 133, 134]. Several studies have been performed to better understand the risk of nephrotoxicity associated with aminoglycoside therapy. A metanalysis of 16 trials involving 823 neonates comparing once daily aminoglycoside dosing with multiple doses per day found no difference in nephrotoxicity [135]. Similarly, in a Cochrane analysis of 11 studies and 574 neonates once daily dosing did not lead to more nephrotoxicity than twice-daily dosing, at comparable efficacy [136].

In a study that included 281 consecutive cases of AKI in preterm infants in NICU, multivariate logistic regression analysis showed that ceftazidime administration was associated with a greater risk of AKI compared to the other variables selected from univariate analysis including ampicillin, ibuprofen and furosemide [130]. Cephalosporin antibiotics have also been implicated in a case-control study involving 46 matched pairs of infants with and without AKI. Infants who developed AKI had a significantly higher prior exposure to cefotaxime, benzodiazepines, diuretics, and dopamine/dobutamine [119]. Globally, the AKI risk appears to increase with the number of nephrotoxic drugs [137] and the extended use of combination therapies [138].

Conservative Management of Neonatal AKI

Neonatal AKI is associated with a high morbidity and mortality [93]. Unfortunately, very few trials designed to test interventions have been performed in the neonatal population. Management of AKI in newborns is therefore basically supportive and based on maintaining homeostasis until recovery of renal function [110, 122, 139, 140]. The first approach should be to carefully assess risk factors and to precisely define the cause of AKI. In particular, conditions that result in poor renal perfusion such as hypovolemia and sepsis should be promptly recognized and corrected [139, 140].

When and how to implement a fluid challenge continues to be an area of controversy and active investigation. In the resuscitative phase, hypovolemia can be initially corrected by the administration of a **fluid challenge** of 10–20 mL/kg of normal saline in bolus [141]. After active resuscitation has occurred, the goals of therapy should be to limit the degree of fluid overload, meanwhile providing adequate nutrition and medications necessary to promote recovery. Abnormalities in fluid balance are common among neonates and may impact patient outcome even in the absence of AKI. In a cohort of 645 critically ill neonates, a positive fluid balance was reported in more than 60% of patients during the first postnatal week [142]. Furthermore, the degree of fluid overload is an independent predictor of mortality [143, 144]. In a prospective study conducted on 58 neonates, those with AKI had more marked fluid overload and higher mortality rates over the first few days of life [143]. In a study of 154 newborns with AKI, fluid overload in excess of 7% was independently associated with a 13-fold mortality risk [141]. To prevent fluid overload, daily fluid input should not exceed insensible water losses (30 mL/kg/day) plus urinary losses. To guarantee adequate energy and nutrient intake while maintaining restricted fluid intake, concentrated solutions should be used. The volume required to apply drugs should be minimized by administration of pure or highly concentrated infusion volumes [139]. Body weight should be checked twice daily and the estimated fluid overload should be carefully assessed and tracked. Weight monitoring rather than cumulative fluid balance recording is, in fact, considered the most accurate method for measuring fluid balance in neonates and over-

comes the problem of missed in and out measurements [142–145].

In order to maintain fluid balance and allow nutrition and drug infusions, diuretics are commonly used in patients with AKI. Studies in adult patients have not provided any evidence that diuretics improve survival or modify the course of AKI [146]. In young infants with AKI, furosemide use was an independent predictor of poor renal outcome [147] whereas data from AWAKEN suggested that diuretic administration was associated with a decreased risk of early-onset AKI [105]. Although controlled study evidence is lacking, furosemide has been used in neonates with AKI to facilitate clinical management by converting oliguric into non-oliguric AKI. Intravenous furosemide boluses (1 mg/kg) have been adopted for the treatment of oliguria in this setting given the challenges and risks associated with kidney replacement therapies in this difficult group of patients [139]. In addition to furosemide also bumetanide, a potent loop diuretic with similar pharmacologic characteristics as furosemide, was employed to increase urine output in preterm infants with oliguric AKI; while effectively increasing urine output the drug also caused a transient increase in serum creatinine levels, highlighting the nephrotoxic potential of loop diuretics in this vulnerable population [148, 149].

Low-dose **dopamine** has also been utilized to improve urine output in critically ill term and preterm neonates [110]. Dopamine is an endogenous catecholamine that influences different catecholamine receptors in a dose-dependent manner, and, in particular, has been claimed to induce selective renal vasodilation when administered at low dose. Dopamine administration is associated with increased cerebral blood flow and has been shown to be safe and effective for treating hypotension in preterm infants. In oliguric, non-hypotensive neonates, GFR and urine output increased significantly with dopamine infused at a rate of 2.5 µg/kg per min. Moreover, dopamine induced renal and mesenteric vasodilation without an effect on cerebral blood flow when started precociously in preterm neonates treated with indomethacin for the presence of a patent ductus arteriosus. However, an assessment of dopamine use in 19 NICUs and PICUs together with a literature review failed to demonstrate an improvement in renal function and urine output in neonates and pediatric intensive care patients. Moreover, evidence emerged that dopamine may have detrimental effects by worsening renal perfusion in critically ill patients with AKI. More recently, **Fenoldopam**, a selective dopamine A1 receptor agonist that decreases vascular resistance and increases renal blood flow, improved urine output in neonates requiring cardiac surgery with positive fluid balance despite diuretics [150–156]. However, in 40 infants undergoing cardiac surgery with cardiopulmonary bypass, Fenoldopam infused at a low dose (0.1 μg/Kg/min) for 72 h soon after anesthesia did not exert any effects on urine output, fluid balance or AKI incidence [157]. The same authors treated 40 infants undergoing cardiac surgery with a higher dose of Fenoldopam (1 μg/kg/min) during cardiopulmonary bypass. They observed decreased urinary NGAL and cystatin C levels, but no difference in plasma creatinine and urine output between subjects receiving fenoldopam and placebo [158].

Perinatal asphyxia is the primary cause of AKI in neonates. During hypoxia and ischemia, adenosine is released and acts as a vasoconstrictive agent in the kidney contributing to a fall in glomerular filtration rate. In this setting, methylxanthines such as aminophylline and theophylline (non-specific **adenosine receptor antagonists**) can inhibit the vasoconstriction induced by adenosine [159]. Three independent randomized trials in severe asphyxiated term infants and one randomized trial involving preterm neonates have shown that a single dose of theophylline, given early after birth, was associated with decrease in serum creatinine and improved urine output [159–162]. Based on these findings, the KDIGO guidelines recommend a single dose of aminophylline for asphyxiated infants at risk for AKI [163]. More recently, a meta-analysis including 6 randomized trials enrolling 436 neonates treated with prophylactic theophylline as compared to placebo further confirmed the reno-protective

effect of theophylline. A 60% reduction in the incidence of AKI and a decrease in serum creatinine over days 2–5 without significant difference in complications was reported [164]. However, because theophylline has some potentially harmful neurologic effects and because therapeutic hypothermia is now standard of care in these infants, further comparative trials are needed to determine whether these agents improve short-term and long-term renal and neurodevelopmental outcomes [165]. Recently, another methylxanthine, caffeine citrate, administered in the first 7 postnatal days, was associated with a reduced incidence and severity of AKI both in preterm neonates and in premature infants diagnosed with NEC [166, 167].

Few other studies have specifically addressed therapies for AKI in neonates. In an uncontrolled retrospective study of 7 infants with hyperuricemia secondary to AKI treated with intravenous **rasburicase** administration of a single bolus determined a significant decrease of uric acid and creatinine and an increase of urine output within 24 h [168].

As described above, drugs are common causes of AKI in neonates [130–138]. In the setting of AKI, an **evaluation of all medications** should be performed to eliminate nephrotoxic agents and to determine the proper dose of other medications in the context of reduced kidney function and drug clearance. Moreover, whenever possible blood levels should be measured in order to maintain the levels in the therapeutic range and reduce the risk of nephrotoxicity [140]. Involvement of a pharmacist is highly advised especially in those infants receiving nephrotoxic combination therapy for extended periods of time [138–169].

Electrolyte disorders and acidosis are common in neonates with AKI and may complicate the clinical course after AKI. For the management of electrolyte disorders we refer to the above sections of this chapter.

Finally, efforts should be made to provide adequate **nutrition** in NICU patients with AKI [122–170]. Trials in neonates are lacking but extrapolating data from critically ill children, underfeeding is common in AKI and it is important to ensure adequate caloric intake in order to prevent catabolism [171]. Hyperglycemia should be avoided and may require treatment with insulin [137]. Protein intake should be adjusted to meet at least the basal growth requirements (1–2 g/kg/day). These goals could be challenging in oligo/anuric neonates and the risk of fluid overload should be carefully weighed against the risk of malnutrition. If nutrition cannot be provided due to risk of further fluid accumulation, initiation of kidney replacement therapy should be considered.

Dialysis in Newborns

Over the past decades, technological advances and increased expertise have made it possible to support very small infants with dialysis. Nowadays, infants with AKI can receive peritoneal dialysis, hemodialysis or continuous kidney support therapy (CKST) [143, 172, 173]. The **choice of dialysis modality** in critically ill neonates relies on the clinical goals, patient characteristics, and local expertise. Local expertise and facilities affect the dialysis modality choice. Different programs provide neonatal dialysis in one or more location(s) - neonatal ICU, pediatric ICU and/or cardiac ICU.

The **indications** for the different kidney support therapies for neonates and young infants generally resemble those in older children. Whatever the clinical context, general indications for therapy include severe hyperkalemia, intractable acidosis, uremia, fluid overload, prevention of fluid overload, inability to provide adequate nutrition due to concerns of fluid accumulation.

Although most programs that offer dialysis in neonates use peritoneal dialysis, it may not be possible to perform in certain situations; thus HD and/or CKST complements PD. CKST has increased as a form of treatment for children and neonates with AKI in the US [174] and Europe.

In the largest reported multicentric, multinational cohort of neonates with AKI (AWAKEN study), kidney replacement therapy (KRT) was required in 25/605 patients (4.1%). Eleven out of 25 of these patients needed CKRT + ECMO, 9 PD, 4 CKRT and 1 PD + CKRT. No patient was treated with intermittent HD. Although the survival of infants with AKI treated with KRT was higher than that previously reported (76% vs. 44%), the use of KRT was significantly associated with survival (76% vs. 90,9% in AKI patients not treated with KRT; $p < 0.01$) [175].

Peritoneal Dialysis

Peritoneal dialysis (PD) has been extensively used in infants given its simplicity, ability to perform without sophisticated machines, and its slow, continuous action. It is usually well tolerated in small infants [176]. PD has been successfully performed also in very low-birth weight and even extremely low-birth weight neonates, where extracorporeal dialysis faces anatomical barriers.

PD is performed after placement of straight or curled infant catheters. This can happen by percutaneous placement or by surgery. Although surgical implantation is considered the gold standard for PD placement in children, percutaneous placement is a valid alternative and may become essential in low income countries where surgery may not be available. The catheter can be placed by a trocar or, more safely, by Seldinger technique [177].

The most frequent complications include: leakage from catheter entrance, peritonitis, catheter obstruction, bleeding at catheter insertion, exit site infection, hyperglycemia and bowel perforation are the main PD complications [177].

PD prescription in critical neonates is based on frequent, continuous exchanges, with low volumes of dialysate. Regardless whether the catheter is placed percutaneously or surgically, initial loads should be in a low range of 10–20 mL/kg of body weight since larger loads may cause dialysate leakage and diaphragm lifting with respiratory complications [177]. Starting with a standard glucose concentration (1.5 g/dL) is recommended to avoid initial hyperglycemia. Subsequently ultrafiltration rate must be monitored and dialysate glucose concentration adapted according to ultrafiltration needs [177].

Dwell times are usually short, down to 30–40 min in neonates. When large volumes of ultrafiltration are obtained, excessive sodium loss in the ultrafiltrate may occur. This loss is related to patient size and is most marked in neonates. Oral, intravenous or intraperitoneal sodium supplementation may be needed [177].

Outcome data in neonates who undergo PD after cardiopulmonary bypass surgery suggest that early PD improves outcomes. Data on 146 infants who underwent cardiopulmonary bypass surgery, significantly better survival at 30 and 90 days was observed with "early" PD (started at the end of surgery or day after surgery) as compared with controls starting PD after the second day after surgery. The impact of fluid overload on outcome was analyzed in a prospective trial comparing two interventions in infants undergoing cardiac surgery. In the first study period, ascites was passively drained through a PD catheter placed at the time of surgery. In a second series of patients PD was initiated within 2 h of arriving at the cardiac ICU. The infants receiving active PD had significantly more negative net fluid balance, lower mean inotrope score, lower serum cytokine concentrations and earlier sternal closure compared to the infants who had only their peritoneal fluid drained [178].

Further analysis of these and other studies in infants undergoing cardiopulmonary bypass surgery confirmed that attainment of a negative fluid balance is associated with improved survival and other clinical outcomes. Taken together, early start of dialysis, avoidance of fluid overload and its consequent correction appear to favor a good outcome in critically ill infants and may be more important than the choice of treatment modality.

Hemodialysis (HD) can be performed in infants with good results, although poor vascular tolerance and the large extra-corporeal volume provide additional challenges [173].

Hemodialysis

Hemodialysis (HD) can be performed in infants with good results, although poor vascular tolerance and the large extra-corporeal volume provide additional challenges [173]. Although **Extracorporeal Dialysis** has been performed in

neonates in the past five decades the main problems that have been limiting its widespread use are vascular access and cardiovascular tolerance. HD has mainly been used in metabolic crisis and intoxications, when urgent toxic compound removal is needed. There are few reports on the use of *intermittent hemodialysis (HD)* in neonates with AKI. In 1994, Sadowski described 33 acute infants weighing less than 5 kg treated with intermittent HD. A high rate of hypotensive episodes was reported (64%), and a 52% survival rate [173].

Blood flow is mainly dependent on vascular access performance. It is usually prescribed as 5–10 mL/kg body weight; in patients needing a high clearance rate (e.g. hyperammonemic crisis) the maximally achievable flow rate should be used and will be rate limiting for the efficacy of purification. Standard or even lower dialysate flows (300–500 mL/min) combined with low neonatal blood flows usually provide maximal solute extraction. Dialysate warming systems are provided by any HD monitor and preserve neonatal thermoregulation. Vascular access for extracorporeal dialysis is often troublesome in neonates due to the mismatch between vessel size and the diameter of the catheters minimally required to obtain adequate blood flow.

Continuous Kidney Replacement Therapy (CKRT)

Continuous Kidney Replacement Therapy (CKRT) may allow for achievement of the goals of therapy better than HD in neonates. Because it allows for 24 h metabolic and fluid control as opposed to the transient correction and shifts that occur between intermitten HD sessions.

The most commonly used catheters in neonates are dual-lumen, low resistance catheters. 6.5–8 F caliber. The length of the catheter will be depending on whether the catheter is tunneled or not, and whether the catheter is placed in the right internal jugular, left internal jugular, or femoral approach. As an alternative, two smaller single-lumen catheters have been used successfully [187].

Vascular access in children and infants on CKRT can be challenging. Results from the ppCRRT Registry, 5-French catheters showed the poorest function, none of them lasting more than 20 h [188]. Catheterization of the internal jugular vein and the use of CVVHD was found to be associated with the best catheter survival introduction of latest-generation CKRT machines might change the choice of vascular access in neonates (see below).

Until recently, CKRT was performed using tubing, filters and consoles originally conceived for adults [189]. However, problems related to the fluid accuracy and large extracorporeal volumes compared to patient blood volume pose to the smallest neonates. The larger the extracorporeal volume the higher the risk of hemodynamic instability during start, hypocalcemia, acidosis and dilution effect of hemoglobin, platelets and coagulation factors. Blood prime procedures have been reported to minimize the blood exposures.

The creation of monitors and circuits specifically dedicated to neonates has profoundly changed the approach to the extracorporeal treatment of newborns with AKI. In Tables 53.6 and 53.7 list of filters and monitors available for neonates in 2022.

In 2012, Ronco et al. described the creation of the first CKRT monitor for infants <10 kg BW [190] and in 2014 the first patient was treated with this specific device [191]. This machine was approved by the US FDA in April 2020. It provides extraordinary accuracy in blood pump and fluid balance with a blood priming volume ranging 27–42 mL. The machine provides either CVVH and CVVHD (but not both). Blood flow can be set at 1–50 mL/min and dialysis flow from 1 to 10 mL/min, with a maximum effluent flow (net ultrafiltration + dialysate) of 20 mL/min. The maximum fluid removal is 1000 mL per day, with an accuracy of 1 mL per hour. Carpediem® works with such small catheters thanks to a three-roller blood pump that reduces the dead space of the pump tubing segment and the pulsatile profile of the blood flow as compared to conventional two-roller pump systems. This allows continuous aspiration even at very low blood flows through very small catheters [190]. 5F double lumen or combinations of 3.5F and 5F single lumen catheters were used in a series of 26 neonates treated with Carpediem® [192]. 25 of the children survived the CKRT period and 18 survived the NICU stay.

In 2014, Coulthard et al. showed the ability of a syringe-driven machine, the Newcastle Infant Dialysis and Ultrafiltration System (NIDUS®, Allmed, London, UK) to provide better clearance and more accurate ultrafiltration than peritoneal dialysis [193]. The device withdraws 5–12.5 mL aliquots of blood from a single-lumen central venous line, runs it across a dialysis filter and returns it back through a syringe pump. The I-KID study, a randomized clustered wedge study was conducted in England. Study results are expected to be shared in 2022 [194].

Askenazi et al. adapted the Aquadex® (CHF Solutions, Eden Prairie, MN) ultrafiltration system to provide CVVH to neonates [195]. Aquadex® was originally conceived for the treatment of edema in adult cardiac patients but its small priming volume was exploited to create a hemofiltration system in infants. The machine provides a blood flow of 10–40 mL/min; it is equipped with a 0.12 m² polysulfone membrane and a second pump that produces up to 500 mL/h ultrafiltrate in 10 mL/h increments. Reinfusion is provided by an infusion pump external to the circuit. In a 3-center retrospective study among 117 children treated with the Aquadex® system, 72 were under 10 kg body weight and 23 of these survived to discharge. Complications during therapy were seen in 15% of treatments and most were vascular access–related [196].

CKST Prescription for Neonates

No official recommendations for *adequacy* in critically ill infants exist. In neonates with AKI or congenital kidney failure, the daily clearance is potentially much higher than intermitten HD because clearance can occur continuously. The broader aims of metabolic and fluid control, hemodynamic stability, vascular access preservation, nutritional adequacy, and appropriate levels of essential drugs (i.e. anti-microbials) may be more important than waste product removal rates. Some programs aim for filtration rate of 2000 mL/h/1.73 m² others aim for a filtration rate of 20–25 mL/kg/h.

Given the immaturity of neonatal thermoregulation, CKRT induced heat loss could hamper the thermal protection adopted in NICU, especially in low birth weight neonates, with unpredictable consequences on vascular stability. Warming of fluids is needed and different approaches are available. Neonates are at an intrinsically high risk of hemorrhage, and extracorporeal treatment modalities are clearly fraught with an increased risk of hemorrhage. Safe and effective anticoagulation protocols are critical to the success of CKRT.

In the ppCRRT registry, small children <10 kg were more likely to receive heparin anticoagulation compared to citrate regional anticoagulation. In the overall registry, the rates of circuit survival was similar between groups, but the heparin group had higher rates of bleeding than the citrate group [197]. In those receiving heparin anticoagulation, some programs monitor aPTT (goal range 50–70) other target ACT rates of 160–180, while others target anti-Xa levels of 0.3–0.5. The use of citrate regional anticoagulation in smaller children can be more challenging for several reasons. First, traditional CKRT machines require a minimum blood flow, and the blood flow rate per kg is inversely related to body weight. Because the citrate dose depends on blood flow, the amount of citrate used in small children is therefore higher and may require higher clearance rates to achieve target levels. Furthermore, premature infants are born with immature liver function.

In critically ill children with a low body weight.

Management of Hyperammonemia with Kidney Support Therapy

A peculiar indication to KRT in the neonatal age group with metabolic crisis due to Inborn Errors of Metabolism (IEM), most often manifesting as neonatal hyperammonemia or leucinosis. Hyperammonemia is a severe clinical condition characterized by high ammonium levels, excess glutamine accumulation in astrocytes inducing cell swelling and brain edema. In most cases, it presents in full-term neonates with anorexia, seizures, lethargy, coma and death. Most frequently,

it is caused by urea cycle defects (UCD) and organic acidurias (OA). The initial management of an undiagnosed hyperammonemia includes stopping protein intake, intravenous glucose, and initiation of first-line medications including L-arginine, nitrogen scavengers, carbamylglutamate, carnitine, vitamin B12, and biotin. When conservative treatment fails and whenever there is severe symptomatic hyperammonemia, dialysis has to be rapidly established in order to avoid permanent neurological sequelae or death [198]. In leucinosis (maple syrup urine disease; MSUD), deficiency in branched chain ketoacid dehydrogenase leads to the accumulation of branched chains aminoacids (BCAA) leucine, isoleucine, and valine in cells and body fluids. Given the poor renal clearance of BCAA, their accumulation can cause neurologic damage. Medical treatment consists in incorporation of BCAA into protein synthesis with nutritional support but, like in hyperammonemia, it may not be successful and dialysis must be started to clear excess BCAA [199]. In both cases, extracorporeal dialysis provides higher clearances than PD [198, 200]. HD provides highest ammonium clearance and it has been recommended as gold standard of therapy [201], although high volume CKRT (initially at 8 L/h/1.73 m^2) has been proposed as an alternative [198, 200, 202]. The practical application of CKRT in neonatal metabolic decompensation differs from that of AKI since it has been demonstrated in vitro that the clearance of ammonium and leucine achieved with CVVHD depend on dialysate flow rate, being substantially higher with increasing flow rates [200]. However, as in the case of AKI, there is no definite demonstrated association between a specific dialysis modality or of dialysis efficiency with survival. In the study of Schaefer et al. [200], out of nine patients, the five with fastest depuration survived with no or mild neurological impairment while the other four died or survived with severe sequelae. By contrast, in the study of Pela et al. [203], four out of seven neonates with organic acidurias treated with PD survived with no or mild neurological impairment. In a series of 12 neonates with metabolic crises from different IEM, all survivors showed plasma ammonia less than 300 µmol/L after 8 h of KRT and significantly lower ammonia concentration than non-survivors at the same time of treatment. This difference was not related to dialysis modality [180]. In a systematic review of 90 reports on the impact of ammonium levels and dialysis on outcome in 202 infants with UCDs, a higher ammonium level was a determinant for starting dialysis but no significant influence of this treatment on outcome was observed [181]. In a series of 45 hyperammonemic newborns treated with KRT, predialysis ammonium levels were significantly associated with a composite end-point of death or neurological sequelae while the outcome was not related with dialysis modality. Interestingly, while the patients treated with HD had a shorter ammonium decay time compared with all other patients ($p < 0.05$), no significant difference in ammonium reduction rate was observed between patients treated with PD, CAVHD or CVVHD.

The above considerations raise the question if it is correct to evaluate dialysis efficiency by decay time. Under these circumstances, ammonium concentration is strongly dependent on the metabolic state and the majority of patients start dialysis with a medical therapy already under way. Dialysis is part of an overall treatment setting which includes variably efficacious pharmacological support and variably timed initiation of medical treatment and dialysis, with a major modifying influence of the type of underlying metabolic defect on final outcome.

In summary, while ammonium and leucine are small, unbound molecules and behave as such during dialysis (i.e.: best clearance by diffusion, most rapid depuration by HD, less rapid depuration by CKRT and by PD), the dialysis modality does not determine the outcome. A practical approach to the treatment of hyperammonemia in infants has been recently proposed [204].

Outcomes of Neonatal AKI

AKI is associated with significant mortality in critically ill children [205, 206] and adults [207–211], even after controlling for medical co-morbidities, severity of illness scores, and patient demographics. Epidemiological studies in several high-risk groups of neonates have been performed, including very low birth weight infants, near term/term infants with perinatal depression, neonates with severe asphyxia undergoing hypothermia, neonates receiving extra-corporeal membrane oxygenation and infants with cardiopulmonary bypass—associated AKI. Using a categorical AKI frameworks the RIFLE classification systems [205, 207] allow for improved diagnosis and staging of AKI by severity, these studies have provided some evidence that AKI is independently associated with mortality in neonates and young infants even when controlling for potentially confounding demographics, co-morbidities, and interventions.

Critically Ill Neonates

In the multinational retrospective observational Assessment of Worldwide Acute Kidney injury Epidemiology in Neonates (AWAKEN) study using the KDIGO neonatal AKI definition, the incidence of AKI in NICU patients was about 30%, with gestational age following a "U"-shaped distribution (AKI incidence: < 29 week: 45%; ≥29–36 week: 14%; ≥36 week: 41%). Even after controlling for multiple potential confounders, neonates with AKI had 4.6 times higher adjusted odds of death and 8.8 more adjusted hospital days [175]. These associations held true for all gestational age groups [175]. A full account of all studies conducted in this population is beyond the scope of this chapter. Review of outcome studies in premature neonates [212–214], neonates with perinatal asphyxia (REF), those who receive extra-corporeal membrane oxygenation [215] those who undergo cardio-pulmonary bypass surgery have been recently published [216].

Outcomes of Neonates Treated with Kidney Support Therapy (KST) for AKI

The interpretation of outcome of infants treated with dialysis is hampered by several problems. First, the reasons to start KSTt for AKI or not based on AKI diagnosis/criteria. Rather, most pediatric patients initiate kidney support for fluid overload or a combination of fluid overload and AKI. Secondly, the timing of support and the treatment choices are made according to local availability, clinician preference and expertise. Thirdly, the modality, dose and approach are set to institutional practice. Finally, programs will provide kidney support (or choose not to support) neonates based on the severity of illness. Programs that provide kidney support for neonates of higher severity of illness would be expected to have higher mortality rates. Furthermore, most of the studies are retrospective studies at risk for reporting bias.

With this in mind, the overall survival rates of critical ill neonates treated with dialysis are generally poorer than those reported for older children. In the Prospective Pediatric Continuous Renal Replacement Therapy (ppCRRT) Registry, the cohort of children <10 kg (n = 84) had lower survival rates than children >10 kg ($n = 166$) (43% vs 64%). Not differently from older children, fluid overload, high PRISM2 score and urine output at dialysis initiation were found associated with mortality. In particular, patients with fluid overload >20% at the time of CKRT initiation had an almost five times higher odds ratio of death than those who initiated CKRT with <10% fluid excess. Survival was better in neonates who were able to achieve dry weight during CKRT. This suggests that fluid overload predisposes to a poor outcome but its correction may reverse this association [143]. Recent studies using novel and adapted machines with small extra-corporeal volumes suggest better outcomes [196, 217].

Long-term Effects of Prematurity and Neonatal AKI on Chronic Kidney Disease

Links between prematurity/low birth weight and chronic kidney disease in adulthood become increasingly apparent [218]. Figure 53.3 depicts the possible etiology of chronic kidney disease in premature and low birthweight infants. Pre-term delivery disrupts nephrogenesis, which is not complete until around 34–36 weeks gestation. A small number of autopsy studies have suggested that nephrogenesis continues for only a short

time after birth [9, 219, 220]. The remaining nephrons hypertrophy to compensate for decreased nephron mass and, according to Brenner's hypothesis, the resultant "hyperfiltration" eventually becomes deleterious and leads to glomerulosclerosis with sodium retention, systemic hypertension, proteinuria and progressive chronic kidney disease [221]. Thus, premature birth may 'prime' infants for kidney injury and chronic kidney disease. Indeed, premature infants with a birthweight less than 2500 grams have nearly twice the odds of having low glomerular filtration rate, microalbuminuria, end-stage kidney disease and hypertension than their term counterparts [222].

Moreover, the impact of additional AKI events in the NICU on long-term kidney and health outcomes is not yet known. Previously, it was assumed that subjects who survive an episode of AKI would recover kidney function without long-term sequelae; however, recent data from animals [223], critically ill children [224, 225] and adults [226–238] suggest that AKI survivors are indeed at risk for development of CKD. A meta-analysis in adults with AKI showed an

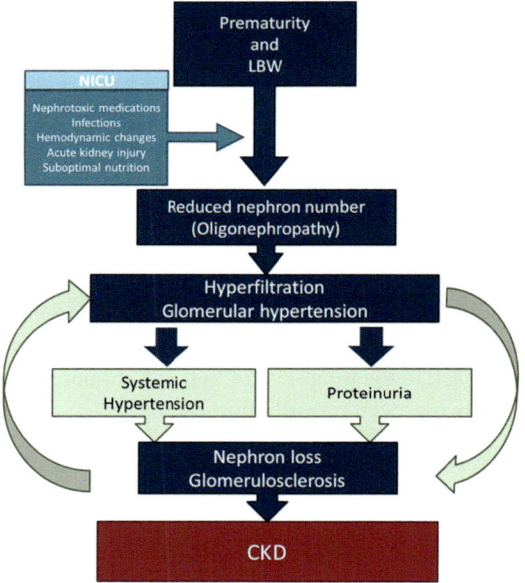

Fig. 53.3 Possible etiology of chronic kidney disease in premature and low birthweight Infants [218] (from Carmody et al. Pediatrics 2013)

almost ninefold risk to develop incident CKD, a threefold risk to progress to end-stage kidney disease and a doubled mortality risk compared to patients without AKI [239].

The role that AKI plays in the development of CKD in the infant population is still unknown. Several small single center retrospective reports have suggested that CKD can develop in infants who had AKI [101, 240]. Human autopsy and animal studies suggest that AKI affects post-natal nephron development. Premature infants who suffer AKI were shown to have fewer layers of nephrons and abnormally configured glomeruli compared to term neonates [9, 220]. Large prospective cohort studies designed to determine risk factors for long-term CKD are needed to define the most appropriate surveillance protocols and identify the subjects at greatest risk.

Future Directions in Neonatal AKI

Our understanding of neonatal AKI has improved and we now have clear epidemiological evidence suggesting that AKI is common and associated with mortality in this age group. New AKI definitions based on SCr, urine output, Cystatin C and emergent urinary biomarkers promise to improve our ability to reliably define neonatal AKI. Studies in VLBW neonates [241, 242], infants undergoing cardiopulmonary bypass surgery [243–251], and other sick NICU patients suggest that these biomarkers can predict a subsequent rise in SCr as well as mortality [84]. However, large comparative studies will be required to determine which functional and kidney injury biomarkers can best predict hard clinical outcomes. Importantly, the normal ranges of urine biomarkers in premature neonates will require careful validation since excretion varies by gestational age, probably due tubular immaturity [241]. With better definitions and earlier indicators of AKI, we will be able to better understand the risk factors, develop preventive strategies, and timely apply appropriate management to improve outcomes in those at risk for AKI.

Another emerging breakthrough regards the provision of extracorporeal treatments for neo-

nates. Thanks to major technological advances, dialysis machines miniaturized for the specific needs of neonates have become available. Machines such as the CARPEDIEM, Aquadex and NIDUS are making important differences in the ability to provide safe and effective therapies in small infants. The main advantage of these machines is the low extra-corporeal volume which drastically lowers the rates of hemodynamic instability at circuit initiation. Furthermore, smaller circuits allow for smaller catheters to be used, enabling extracorporeal therapy even in very small neonates. Maximizing the efficiency and safety of kidney support therapies with these devices will change our approach to the neonate with AKI. One day soon, any infant who could benefit from kidney support therapy will no longer be left without an appropriate and safe treatment option.

References

1. Rudolph AM, Heymann MA, Teramo KA, Barrett CT, Räihä NC. Studies on the circulation of the previable fetus. Pediatr Res. 1971;5:452–65.
2. Jose PA, Fildes RD, Gomez RA, Chevalier RL, Robillard JE. Neonatal renal function and physiology. Curr Opin Pediatr. 1994;6(2):172–7.
3. Yao LP, Jose PA. Developmental renal hemodynamics. Pediatr Nephrol. 1995;9(5):632–7.
4. Paton JB, Fisher DE, DeLannoy CW, Behrman RE. Umbilical blood flow, cardiac output, and organ blood flow in the immature baboon fetus. Am J Obstet Gynecol. 1973;117(4):560–6.
5. Gruskin AB, Edelmann CM Jr, Yuan S. Maturational changes in renal blood flow in piglets. Pediatr Res. 1970;4(1):7–13.
6. Evan AP Jr, Stoeckel JA, Loemker V, Baker JT. Development of the intrarenal vascular system of the puppy kidney. Anat Rec. 1979;194(2):187–99.
7. Chikkannaiah P, Roy M, Kangle R, Patil PV. Glomerulogenesis: can it predict the gestational age? A study of 176 fetuses. Indian J Pathol Microbiol. 2012;55(3):303–7.
8. Abrahamson DR. Glomerulogenesis in the developing kidney. Semin Nephrol. 1991;11(4):375–89.
9. Rodriguez MM, Gomez AH, Abitbol CL, Chandar JJ, Duara S, Zilleruelo GE. Histomorphometric analysis of postnatal glomerulogenesis in extremely preterm infants. Pediatr Dev Pathol. 2004;7(1):17–25.
10. George J, Schwartz M, Alvaro Muñoz, Schneider MF, Mak RH, Kaskel F, Warady BA, Furth S. Formulas

to estimate GFR in children with chronic kidney disease. J Am Soc Nephrol. 2008;

11. Schwartz GJ, Furth SL. Glomerular filtration rate measurement and estimation in chronic kidney disease. Pediatr Nephrol (Berlin, Germany). 2007;22(11):1839–48.

12. Brion LP, Fleischman AR, McCarton C, Schwartz GJ. A simple estimate of glomerular filtration rate in low birth weight infants during the first year of life: noninvasive assessment of body composition and growth. J Pediatr. 1986;109(4):698–707.

13. Gallini F, Maggio L, Romagnoli C, Marrocco G, Tortorolo G. Progression of renal function in preterm neonates with gestational age < or = 32 weeks. Pediatr Nephrol (Berlin, Germany). 2000;15(1–2):119–24.

14. Lolekha PH, Jaruthunyaluck S, Srisawasdi P. Deproteinization of serum: another best approach to eliminate all forms of bilirubin interference on serum creatinine by the kinetic Jaffe reaction. J Clin Lab Anal. 2001;15(3):116–21.

15. Schwartz GJ, Feld LG, Langford DJ. A simple estimate of glomerular filtration rate in full-term infants during the first year of life. J Pediatr. 1984;104(6):849–54.

16. Demirel G, Celik IH, Canpolat FE, Erdeve O, Biyikli Z, Dilmen U. Reference values of serum cystatin C in very low-birthweight premature infants. Acta Paediatr. 2013;102(1):e4–7.

17. Kandasamy Y, Smith R, Wright IM. Measuring cystatin C to determine renal function in neonates. Pediatr Crit Care Med. 2013;14(3):318–22.

18. E. S. Neonates. In: Barrat TM, Avner ED, Harmon WE, editor. Pediatric Nephrol: Lippincott, Williams and Wilins; 1999.

19. Guignard J. Renal morphogenesis and development of renal function. In: Taeusch H, Ballard R, Gleason C, editors. Avery's diseases of the newborn. 8th ed. Philadelphia: Elsevier Saunders; 2005. p. 1257–66.

20. Goldstein L. Renal ammonia and acid excretion in infant rats. Am J Phys. 1970;218(5):1394–8.

21. Quigley R, Baum M. Neonatal acid base balance and disturbances. Semin Perinatol. 2004;28(2):97–102.

22. Day R, Franklin J. Renal carbonic anhydrase in premature and mature infants. Pediatrics. 1951;7(2):182–5.

23. Linder N, Hammel N, Hernandez A, Fridman E, Dlugy E, Herscovici T, et al. Intestinal perforation in very-low-birth-weight infants with necrotizing enterocolitis. J Pediatr Surg. 2013;48(3):562–7.

24. Merlob P, Litwin A, Mor N. Possible association between acetazolamide administration during pregnancy and metabolic disorders in the newborn. Eur J Obstet Gynecol Reprod Biol. 1990;35(1):85–8.

25. Taeusch HW, Ballard RA, Avery ME, Gleason CA. Avery's diseases of the newborn. Elsevier Saunders; 2005.

26. Ozand PT, Gascon GG. Organic acidurias: a review. Part 2. J Child Neurol. 1991;6(4):288–303.

27. Yurdakok M. What next in necrotizing enterocolitis? Turk J Pediatr. 2008;50(1):1–11.

28. Johnson PJ. Sodium bicarbonate use in the treatment of acute neonatal lactic acidosis: benefit or harm? Neonatal Netw. 2011;30(3):199–205.

29. Lokesh L, Kumar P, Murki S, Narang A. A randomized controlled trial of sodium bicarbonate in neonatal resuscitation-effect on immediate outcome. Resuscitation. 2004;60(2):219–23.

30. Ritter JM, Doktor HS, Benjamin N. Paradoxical effect of bicarbonate on cytoplasmic pH. Lancet. 1990;335(8700):1243–6.

31. Parker MJ, Parshuram CS. Sodium bicarbonate use in shock and cardiac arrest: attitudes of pediatric acute care physicians. Crit Care Med. 2013;41(9):2188–95.

32. Baum JD, Robertson NRC. Immediate effects of alkaline infusion in infants with respiratory distress syndrome. J Pediatr. 1975;87:255. e61

33. Schwartz GJ, Evan AP. Development of solute transport in rabbit proximal tubule. I. HCO_3 and glucose absorption. Am J Phys. 1983;245:F382e90.

34. Kette F, Weil MH, Gazmuri RJ. Buffer solutions may compromise cardiac resuscitation by reducing coronary perfusion pressure. JAMA. 1991;266(15):2121–6.

35. Papile LA, Burstein J, Burstein R, Koffler H, Koops B. Relationship of intravenous sodium bicarbonate infusions and cerebral intraventricular hemorrhage. J Pediatr. 1978;93(5):834–6.

36. Niermeyer S, Kattwinkel J, Van Reempts P, Nadkarni V, Phillips B, Zideman D, et al. International Guidelines for Neonatal Resuscitation: An excerpt from the Guidelines 2000 for Cardiopulmonary Resuscitation and Emergency Cardiovascular Care: International Consensus on Science. Contributors and Reviewers for the Neonatal Resuscitation Guidelines. Pediatrics. 2000;106(3):E29.

37. van Thiel RJ, Koopman SR, Takkenberg JJ, Ten Harkel AD, Bogers AJ. Metabolic alkalosis after pediatric cardiac surgery. Eur J Cardiothorac Surg. 2005;28(2):229–33.

38. Wong HR, Chundu KR. Metabolic alkalosis in children undergoing cardiac surgery. Crit Care Med. 1993;21(6):884–7.

39. Tutay GJ, Capraro G, Spirko B, Garb J, Smithline H. Electrolyte profile of pediatric patients with hypertrophic pyloric stenosis. Pediatr Emerg Care. 2013;29(4):465–8.

40. Kundak AA, Dilli D, Karagol B, Karadag N, Zenciroglu A, Okumus N, et al. Non benign neonatal arrhythmias observed in a tertiary neonatal intensive care unit. Indian J Pediatr. 2013;80(7):555–9.

41. Gruskay J, Costarino AT, Polin RA, Baumgart S. Nonoliguric hyperkalemia in the premature infant weighing less than 1000 grams. J Pediatr. 1988;113(2):381–6.

42. Jeffery J, Sharma A, Ayling RM. Detection of haemolysis and reporting of potassium results in samples from neonates. Ann Clin Biochem. 2009;46(Pt 3):222–5.

43. Masilamani K, van der Voort J. The management of acute hyperkalaemia in neonates and children. Arch Dis Child. 2012;97(4):376–80.
44. Greenough A, Emery EF, Brooker R, Gamsu HR. Salbutamol infusion to treat neonatal hyperkalaemia. J Perinat Med. 1992;20(6):437–41.
45. Singh BS, Sadiq HF, Noguchi A, Keenan WJ. Efficacy of albuterol inhalation in treatment of hyperkalemia in premature neonates. J Pediatr. 2002;141:16–20.
46. Gruy-Kapral C, Emmett M, Santa Ana CA, Porter JL, Fordtran JS, Fine KD. Effect of single dose resin-cathartic therapy on serum potassium concentration in patients with end-stage renal disease. J Am Soc Nephrol. 1998;9(10):1924–30.
47. Ohlsson A, Hosking M. Complications following oral administration of exchange resins in extremely low-birth-weight infants. Eur J Pediatr. 1987;146(6):571–4.
48. Malone TA. Glucose and insulin versus cation-exchange resin for the treatment of hyperkalemia in very low birth weight infants. J Pediatr. 1991;118(1):121–3.
49. Vemgal P, Ohlsson A. Interventions for non-oliguric hyperkalaemia in preterm neonates. Cochrane Database Syst Rev. 2012;5:CD005257.
50. Australian Resuscitation C, New Zealand Resuscitation C. Medications and fluids in paediatric advanced life support. ARC and NZRC Guideline 2010. Emerg Med Australasia. 2011;23(4):405–8.
51. Chevalier RL. The moth and the aspen tree: sodium in early postnatal development. Kidney Int. 2001;59(5):1617–25.
52. Hartnoll G, Betremieux P, Modi N. Randomised controlled trial of postnatal sodium supplementation on body composition in 25–30 week gestational age infants. Arch Dis Child Fetal Neonatal Ed. 2000;82(1):F24–8.
53. Modi N. Sodium intake and preterm babies. Arch Dis Child 1993;69(Spec No 1):87–91.
54. Baraton L, Ancel PY, Flamant C, Orsonneau JL, Darmaun D, Roze JC. Impact of changes in serum sodium levels on 2-year neurologic outcomes for very preterm neonates. Pediatrics. 2009;124(4):e655–61.
55. Ertl T, Hadzsiev K, Vincze O, Pytel J, Szabo I, Sulyok E. Hyponatremia and sensorineural hearing loss in preterm infants. Biol Neonate. 2001;79(2):109–12.
56. Moritz ML, Ayus JC. Preventing neurological complications from dysnatremias in children. Pediatr Nephrol (Berlin, Germany). 2005;20(12):1687–700.
57. Prempunpong C, Efanov I, Sant'anna G. The effect of the implementation of therapeutic hypothermia on fluid balance and incidence of hyponatremia in neonates with moderate or severe hypoxic-ischaemic encephalopathy. Acta Paediatr. 2013;102(11):e507–13.
58. Segar JL. Neonatal diuretic therapy: furosemide, thiazides, and spironolactone. Clin Perinatol. 2012;39(1):209–20.
59. Hoch M, Netz H. Heart failure in pediatric patients. Thorac Cardiovasc Surg. 2005;53(Suppl. 2):S129–34.
60. Edjo Nkilly G, Michelet D, Hilly J, Diallo T, Greff B, Mangalsuren N, et al. Postoperative decrease in plasma sodium concentration after infusion of hypotonic intravenous solutions in neonatal surgery. Br J Anaesth. 2013;
61. Sumpelmann R, Mader T, Dennhardt N, Witt L, Eich C, Osthaus WA. A novel isotonic balanced electrolyte solution with 1% glucose for intraoperative fluid therapy in neonates: results of a prospective multicentre observational postauthorisation safety study (PASS). Paediatr Anaesth. 2011;21(11):1114–8.
62. von Rosenstiel N, von Rosenstiel I, Adam D. Management of sepsis and septic shock in infants and children. Paediatr Drugs. 2001;3(1):9–27.
63. Hsu SC, Levine MA. Perinatal calcium metabolism: physiology and pathophysiology. Semin Neonatol. 2004;9(1):23–36.
64. Saggese G, Baroncelli GI, Bertelloni S, Cipolloni C. Intact parathyroid hormone levels during pregnancy, in healthy term neonates and in hypocalcemic preterm infants. Acta Paediatr Scand. 1991;80(1):36–41.
65. Karlen J, Aperia A, Zetterstrom R. Renal excretion of calcium and phosphate in preterm and term infants. J Pediatr. 1985;106(5):814–9.
66. Barnes-Powell LL. Infants of diabetic mothers: the effects of hyperglycemia on the fetus and neonate. Neonatal Netw. 2007;26(5):283–90.
67. Borkenhagen JF, Connor EL, Stafstrom CE. Neonatal hypocalcemic seizures due to excessive maternal calcium ingestion. Pediatr Neurol. 2013;48(6):469–71.
68. Stevens CA, Carey JC, Shigeoka AO. Di George anomaly and velocardiofacial syndrome. Pediatrics. 1990;85(4):526–30.
69. Chiruvolu A, Engle WD, Sendelbach D, Manning MD, Jackson GL. Serum calcium values in term and late-preterm neonates receiving gentamicin. Pediatr Nephrol (Berlin, Germany). 2008;23(4):569–74.
70. Friis B, Sardemann H. Neonatal hypocalcaemia after intrauterine exposure to anticonvulsant drugs. Arch Dis Child. 1977;52(3):239–41.
71. Cote CJ, Drop LJ, Daniels AL, Hoaglin DC. Calcium chloride versus calcium gluconate: comparison of ionization and cardiovascular effects in children and dogs. Anesthesiology. 1987;66(4):465–70.
72. Hak EB, Crill CM, Bugnitz MC, Mouser JF, Chesney RW. Increased parathyroid hormone and decreased calcitriol during neonatal extracorporeal membrane oxygenation. Intensive Care Med. 2005;31(2):264–70.
73. Pacifici GM. Clinical pharmacology of the loop diuretics furosemide and bumetanide in neonates and infants. Paediatr Drugs. 2012;14(4):233–46.
74. Marx SJ, Attie MF, Spiegel AM, Levine MA, Lasker RD, Fox M. An association between neonatal severe primary hyperparathyroidism and familial hypocalciuric hypercalcemia in three kindreds. N Engl J Med. 1982;306(5):257–64.

75. Akcay A, Akar M, Oncel MY, Kizilelma A, Erdeve O, Oguz SS, et al. Hypercalcemia due to subcutaneous fat necrosis in a newborn after total body cooling. Pediatr Dermatol. 2013;30(1):120–3.

76. Strohm B, Hobson A, Brocklehurst P, Edwards AD, Azzopardi D, Register UTC. Subcutaneous fat necrosis after moderate therapeutic hypothermia in neonates. Pediatrics. 2011;128(2):e450–2.

77. Allgrove J. Use of bisphosphonates in children and adolescents. J Pediatr Endocrinol Metab. 2002;15(Suppl. 3):921–8.

78. Wilhelm-Bals A, Parvex P, Magdelaine C, Girardin E. Successful use of bisphosphonate and calcimimetic in neonatal severe primary hyperparathyroidism. Pediatrics. 2012;129(3):e812–6.

79. Mehta RL, Kellum JA, Shah SV, Molitoris BA, Ronco C, Warnock DG, et al. Acute Kidney Injury Network (AKIN): report of an initiative to improve outcomes in acute kidney injury. Crit Care. 2007;11(2):R31.

80. Feld LG, Springate JE, Fildes RD. Acute renal failure. I. Pathophysiology and diagnosis. J Pediatr. 1986;109(3):401–8.

81. Askenazi DJ, Griffin R, McGwin G, Carlo W, Ambalavanan N. Acute kidney injury is independently associated with mortality in very low birthweight infants: a matched case-control analysis. Pediatr Nephrol (Berlin, Germany). 2009;24(5):991–7.

82. Askenazi DJ, Koralkar R, Hundley HE, Montesanti A, Patil N, Ambalavanan N. Fluid overload and mortality are associated with acute kidney injury in sick near-term/term neonate. Pediatr Nephrol (Berlin, Germany). 2012;

83. Selewski DT, Jordan BK, Askenazi DJ, Dechert RE, Sarkar S. Acute kidney injury in asphyxiated newborns treated with therapeutic hypothermia. J Pediatr. 2012;

84. Askenazi DJ, Koralkar R, Hundley HE, Montesanti A, Parwar P, Sonjara S, et al. Urine biomarkers predict acute kidney injury in newborns. J Pediatr. 2012;161(2):270–5 e1.

85. Askenazi DJ, Montesanti A, Hunley H, Koralkar R, Pawar P, Shuaib F, et al. Urine biomarkers predict acute kidney injury and mortality in very low birth weight infants. J Pediatr. 2011;159(6):907–12 e1.

86. Koralkar R, Ambalavanan N, Levitan EB, McGwin G, Goldstein S, Askenazi D. Acute kidney injury reduces survival in very low birth weight infants. Pediatr Res. 2011;69(4):354–8.

87. Phelps CM, Eshelman J, Cruz ED, Pan Z, Kaufman J. Acute kidney injury after cardiac surgery in infants and children: evaluation of the role of angiotensin-converting enzyme inhibitors. Pediatr Cardiol. 2012;33(1):1–7.

88. Aydin SI, Seiden HS, Blaufox AD, Parnell VA, Choudhury T, Punnoose A, et al. Acute kidney injury after surgery for congenital heart disease. Ann Thorac Surg. 2012;94(5):1589–95.

89. Jetton JG, Askenazi DJ. Update on acute kidney injury in the neonate. Curr Opin Pediatr. 2012;24(2):191–6.

90. Li S, Krawczeski CD, Zappitelli M, Devarajan P, Thiessen-Philbrook H, Coca SG, et al. Incidence, risk factors, and outcomes of acute kidney injury after pediatric cardiac surgery: a prospective multicenter study. Crit Care Med. 2011;39(6):1493–9.

91. Bagga A, Bakkaloglu A, Devarajan P, Mehta RL, Kellum JA, Shah SV, et al. Improving outcomes from acute kidney injury: report of an initiative. Pediatr Nephrol (Berlin, Germany). 2007;22(10):1655–8.

92. Khwaja A. KDIGO Clinical practice guidelines for acute kidney injury. Nephron Clin Pract. 2012;120(4):179–84.

93. Jetton JG, Boohaker LJ, Sethi SK, Wazir S, Rohatgi S, Soranno DE, Neonatal Kidney Collaborative (NKC), et al. Incidence and outcomes of neonatal acute kidney injury (AWAKEN): a multicentre, multinational, observational cohort study. Lancet Child Adolesc Health. 2017;1(3):184–94.

94. Shalaby MA, Sawan ZA, Nawawi E, Alsaedi S, Al-Wassia H, Kari JA. Incidence, risk factors, and outcome of neonatal acute kidney injury: a prospective cohort study. Pediatr Nephrol. 2018;33(9):1617–24.

95. Wu Y, Hua X, Yang G, Xiang B, Jiang X. Incidence, risk factors, and outcomes of acute kidney injury in neonates after surgical procedures. Pediatr Nephrol. 2020;35(7):1341–6.

96. Ryan A, Gilhooley M, Patel N, Reynolds BC. Prevalence of acute kidney injury in neonates with congenital diaphragmatic hernia. Neonatology. 2020;117(1):88–94.

97. Carmody JB, Swanson JR, Rhone ET, Charlton JR. Recognition and reporting of AKI in very low birth weight infants. Clin J Am Soc Nephrol. 2014;9:2036–43.

98. Stojanovic V, Barisic N, Milanovic B, Doronjski A. Acute kidney injury in preterm infants admitted to a neonatal intensive care unit. Pediatr Nephrol. 2014;29:2213–20.

99. Alaro D, Bashir A, Musoke R, Wanaiana L. Prevalence and outcomes of acute kidney injury in term neonates with perinatal asphyxia. Afr Health Sci. 2014;14:682–8.

100. Askenazi DJ, Ambalavanan N, Hamilton K, Cutter G, Laney D, Kaslow R, et al. Acute kidney injury and renal replacement therapy independently predict mortality in neonatal and pediatric noncardiac patients on extracorporeal membrane oxygenation. Pediatr Crit Care Med. 2011;12:e1–6.

101. Andreoli SP. Acute renal failure in the newborn. Semin Perinatol. 2004;28(2):112–23.

102. Askenazi DJ, Ambalavanan N, Goldstein SL. Acute kidney injury in critically ill newborns: what do we know? What do we need to learn? Pediatr Nephrol (Berlin, Germany). 2009;24(2):265–74.

103. Agras PI, Tarcan A, Baskin E, Cengiz N, Gurakan B, Saatci U. Acute renal failure in the neonatal period. Ren Fail. 2004;26(3):305–9.

104. Askenazi DJ. AWAKEN-Ing a new frontier in neonatal nephrology. Front Pediatr. 2020;8:21.

105. Charlton JR, Boohaker L, Askenazi D, Brophy PD, D'Angio C, Fuloria M, Neonatal Kidney

Collaborative, et al. Incidence and risk factors of early onset neonatal AKI. Clin J Am Soc Nephrol. 2019;14(2):184–95.

106. Charlton JR, Boohaker L, Askenazi D, Brophy PD, Fuloria M, Gien J, Neonatal Kidney Collaborative (NKC), et al. Late onset neonatal acute kidney injury: results from the AWAKEN Study. Pediatr Res. 2019;85(3):339–48.

107. Hanna MH, Askenazi DJ, Selewski DT. Drug-induced acute kidney injury in neonates. Curr Opin Pediatr. 2016;28(2):180–7.

108. Mah KE, Hao S, Sutherland SM, Kwiatkowski DM, Axelrod DM, Almond CS, et al. Fluid overload independent of acute kidney injury predicts poor outcomes in neonates following congenital heart surgery. Pediatr Nephrol. 2018;33(3):511–20.

109. Gharehbaghi M, Peirovifar A. Evaluating causes of acute renal failure in newborn infants. Pakis J Med Sci. 2007;23(6):877.

110. Selewski DT, Charlton JR, Jetton JG, Guillet R, Mhanna MJ, Askenazi DJ, et al. Neonatal acute kidney injury. Pediatrics. 2015;136(2):e463–73.

111. Karlowicz MG, Adelman RD. Nonoliguric and oliguric acute renal failure in asphyxiated term neonates. Pediatr Nephrol (Berlin, Germany). 1995;9(6):718–22.

112. Gupta BD, Sharma P, Bagla J, Parakh M, Soni JP. Renal failure in asphyxiated neonates. Indian Pediatr. 2005;42(9):928–34.

113. Aggarwal A, Kumar P, Chowdhary G, Majumdar S, Narang A. Evaluation of renal functions in asphyxiated newborns. J Trop Pediatr. 2005;51(5):295–9.

114. Kaur S, Jain S, Saha A, Chawla D, Parmar VR, Basu S, et al. Evaluation of glomerular and tubular renal function in neonates with birth asphyxia. Ann Trop Paediatr. 2011;31(2):129–34.

115. Selewski DT, Jordan BK, Askenazi DJ, Dechert RE, Sarkar S. Acute kidney injury in asphyxiated newborns treated with therapeutic hypothermia. J Pediatr. 2013;162(4):725–729.e1.

116. Bozkurt O, Yucesoy E. Acute kidney injury in neonates with perinatal asphyxia receiving therapeutic hypothermia. Am J Perinatol. 2020; https://doi.org/10.1055/s-0039-1701024.

117. Kirkley MJ, Boohaker L, Griffin R, Soranno DE, Gien J, Askenazi D, Gist KM, Neonatal Kidney Collaborative (NKC). Acute kidney injury in neonatal encephalopathy: an evaluation of the AWAKEN database. Pediatr Nephrol. 2019;34(1):169–76.

118. Perico N, Askenazi D, Cortinovis M, Remuzzi G. Maternal and environmental risk factors for neonatal AKI and its long-term consequences. Nat Rev Nephrol. 2018;14(11):688–703.

119. Viswanathan S, Manyam B, Azhibekov T, Mhanna MJ. Risk factors associated with acute kidney injury in extremely low birth weight (ELBW) infants. Pediatr Nephrol (Berlin, Germany). 2012;27(2):303–11.

120. Koralkar R, Ambalavanan N, Levitan EB, McGwin G, Goldstein S, Askenazi D. Acute kidney injury reduces survival in very low birth weight infant. Pediatr Res. 2011;69(4):354–8.

121. Subramanian S, Agarwal R, Deorari AK, Paul VK, Bagga A. Acute renal failure in neonates. Indian J Pediatr. 2008;75(4):385–91.

122. Gouyon JB, Guignard JP. Management of acute renal failure in newborns. Pediatr Nephrol (Berlin, Germany). 2000;14(10–11):1037–44.

123. Mathur NB, Agarwal HS, Maria A. Acute renal failure in neonatal sepsis. Indian J Pediatr. 2006;73(6):499–502.

124. Burgmaier K, Hackl A, Ehren R, Kribs A, Burgmaier M, Weber LT, Oberthuer A, Habbig S. Peritoneal dialysis in extremely and very low-birth-weight infants. Perit Dial Int. 2020;40(2):233–6.

125. Momtaz HE, Sabzehei MK, Rasuli B, Torabian S. The main etiologies of acute kidney injury in the newborns hospitalized in the neonatal intensive care unit. J Clin Neonatol. 2014;3(2):99–102.

126. Coggins SA, Laskin B, Harris MC, Grundmeier RW, Passarella M, McKenna KJ, et al. Acute kidney injury associated with late-onset neonatal sepsis: a matched cohort study. J Pediatr. 2021;231:185–92 .e4. https://doi.org/10.1016/j.jpeds.2020.12.023.

127. Black RE, Cousens S, Johnson HL, Lawn JE, Rudan I, Bassani DG, et al. Global, regional, and national causes of child mortality in 2008: a systematic analysis. Lancet. 2010;375(9730):1969–87.

128. Mwamanenge NA, Assenga E, Furia FF. Acute kidney injury among critically ill neonates in a tertiary hospital in Tanzania; prevalence, risk factors and outcome. PLoS One. 2020;15(2):e0229074.

129. Vachvanichsanong P, McNeil E, Dissaneevate S, Dissaneewate P, Chanvitan P, Janjindamai W. Neonatal acute kidney injury in a tertiary center in a developing country. Nephrol Dial Transplant. 2012;27(3):973–7.

130. Cuzzolin L, Fanos V, Pinna B, di Marzio M, Perin M, Tramontozzi P, et al. Postnatal renal function in preterm newborns: a role of diseases, drugs and therapeutic interventions. Pediatr Nephrol (Berlin, Germany). 2006;21(7):931–8.

131. Constance JE, Reith D, Ward RM, Balch A, Stockmann C, Korgenski EK, Thorell EA, Sherwin CMT. Risk of nonsteroidal anti-inflammatory drug-associated renal dysfunction among neonates diagnosed with patent ductus arteriosus and treated with gentamicin. J Perinatol. 2017;37(10):1093–102.

132. Hsieh EM, Hornik CP, Clark RH, Laughon MM, Benjamin DK, Smith PB, Best Pharmaceuticals for Children ACT-Pediatric Trials Network. Medication use in the neonatal intensive care unit. Am J Perinatol. 2014;31(9):811–21.

133. Twombley K, Baum M, Gattineni J. Accidental and iatrogenic causes of acute kidney injury. Curr Opin Pediatr. 2011;23(2):208–14.

134. Taber SS, Mueller BA. Drug-associated renal dysfunction. Crit Care Clin. 2006;22(2):357–74. viii

135. Nestaas E, Bangstad HJ, Sandvik L, Wathne KO. Aminoglycoside extended interval dos-

ing in neonates is safe and effective: a meta-analysis. Arch Dis Child Fetal Neonatal Ed. 2005;90(4):F294–300.

136. Rao SC, Srinivasjois R, Hagan R, Ahmed M. One dose per day compared to multiple doses per day of gentamicin for treatment of suspected or proven sepsis in neonates. Cochrane Database Syst Rev. 2011;(11):CD005091.

137. Rhone ET, Carmody JB, Swanson JR, Charlton JR. Nephrotoxic medication exposure in very low birth weight infants. J Matern Fetal Neonatal Med. 2014;27:1485–90.

138. Salerno SN, Liao Y, Jackson W, Greenberg RG, McKinzie CJ, McCallister A, Benjamin DK, Laughon MM, Sanderson K, Clark RH, Gonzalez D. Association between nephrotoxic drug combinations and acute kidney injury in the neonatal intensive care unit. J Pediatr. 2021;228:213–9.

139. Starr MC, Menon S. Neonatal acute kidney injury: a case-based approach. Pediatr Nephrol. 2021; https://doi.org/10.1007/s00467-021-04977-1.

140. Pandey V, Kumar D, Vijayaraghavan P, Chaturvedi T, Raina R. Non-dialytic management of acute kidney injury in newborns. J Renal Inj Prev. 2016;6(1):1–11.

141. Weiss SL, Peters MJ, Alhazzani W, Agus MSD, Flori HR, Inwald DP et al. Surviving Sepsis Campaign International Guidelines for the management of septic shock and sepsis-associated organ dysfunction in children. Pediatr Crit Care Med 2020;21(2):e52-e106.

142. Selewski DT, Akcan-Arikan A, Bonachea EM, Gist KM, Goldstein SL, Hanna M, et al. Neonatal Kidney Collaborative. The impact of fluid balance on outcomes in critically ill near-term/term neonates: a report from the AWAKEN study group. Pediatr Res. 2019;85(1):79–85.

143. Askenazi DJ, Goldstein SL, Koralkar R, Fortenberry J, Baum M, Hackbarth R, et al. Continuous renal replacement therapy for children </=10 kg: a report from the prospective pediatric continuous renal replacement therapy registry. J Pediatr. 2013;162(3):587–92 e3.

144. Duzova A, Bakkaloglu A, Kalyoncu M, Poyrazoglu H, Delibas A, Ozkaya O, et al. Etiology and outcome of acute kidney injury in children. Pediatr Nephrol (Berlin, Germany). 2010;25(8):1453–61.

145. van Asperen Y, Brand PL, Bekhof J. Reliability of the fluid balance in neonates. Acta Paediatr. 2012;101:479–83.

146. Bagshaw SM, Gibney RTN, Kruger P, Hassan I, McAlister FA, Bellomo R. The effect of low-dose furosemide in critically ill patients with early acute kidney injury: a pilot randomized blinded controlled trial (the SPARK study). J Crit Care. 2017;42:138–46.

147. Chiravuri SD, Riegger LQ, Christensen R, Butler RR, Malviya S, Tait AR, et al. Factors associated with acute kidney injury or failure in children undergoing cardiopulmonary bypass: a case-controlled study. Paediatr Anaesth. 2011;21(8):880–6.

148. Oliveros M, Pham JT, John E, Resheidat A, Bhat R. The use of bumetanide for oliguric acute renal failure in preterm infants. Pediatr Crit Care Med. 2011;12(2):210–4.

149. Cotton R, Suarez S, Reese J. Unexpected extra-renal effects of loop diuretics in the preterm neonate. Acta Paediatr. 2012;101(8):835–45.

150. Seri I, Abbasi S, Wood DC, Gerdes JS. Regional hemodynamic effects of dopamine in the sick preterm neonate. J Pediatr. 1998;133(6):728–34.

151. Sassano-Higgins S, Friedlich P, Seri I. A meta-analysis of dopamine use in hypotensive preterm infants: blood pressure and cerebral hemodynamics. J Perinatol. 2011;31:647–55.

152. Lynch SK, Lemley KV, Polak MJ. The effect of dopamine on glomerular filtration rate in normotensive, oliguric premature neonates. Pediatr Nephrol. 2003;18(7):649–52.

153. Seri I, Abbasi S, Wood DC, Gerdes JS. Regional hemodynamic effects of dopamine in the indomethacin-treated preterm infant. J Perinatol. 2002;22(4):300–5.

154. Prins I, Plotz FB, Uiterwaal CS, van Vught HJ. Low-dose dopamine in neonatal and pediatric intensive care: a systematic review. Intensive Care Med. 2001;27(1):206–10.

155. Lauschke A, Teichgraber UK, Frei U, Eckardt KU. 'Low-dose' dopamine worsens renal perfusion in patients with acute renal failure. Kidney Int. 2006;69(9):1669–74.

156. Costello JM, Thiagarajan RR, Dionne RE, Allan CK, Booth KL, Burmester M, et al. Initial experience with fenoldopam after cardiac surgery in neonates with an insufficient response to conventional diuretics. Pediatr Crit Care Med. 2006;7(1):28–33.

157. Ricci Z, Stazi GV, Di Chiara L, Morelli S, Vitale V, Giorni C, et al. Fenoldopam in newborn patients undergoing cardiopulmonary bypass: controlled clinical trial. Interact Cardiovasc Thorac Surg. 2008;7(6):1049–53.

158. Ricci Z, Luciano R, Favia I, Garisto C, Muraca M, Morelli S, et al. High-dose fenoldopam reduces postoperative neutrophil gelatinase-associated lipocaline and cystatin C levels in pediatric cardiac surgery. Crit Care. 2011;15(3):R160.

159. Jenik AG, Ceriani Cernadas JM, Gorenstein A, Ramirez JA, Vain N, Armadans M, et al. A randomized, double-blind, placebo-controlled trial of the effects of prophylactic theophylline on renal function in term neonates with perinatal asphyxia. Pediatrics. 2000;105(4):E45.

160. Bakr AF. Prophylactic theophylline to prevent renal dysfunction in newborns exposed to perinatal asphyxia--a study in a developing country. Pediatr Nephrol. 2005;20(9):1249–52.

161. Eslami Z, Shajari A, Kheirandish M, Heidary A. Theophylline for prevention of kidney dysfunction in neonates with severe asphyxia. Iran J Kidney Dis. 2009;3(4):222–6.

162. Cattarelli D, Spandrio M, Gasparoni A, Bottino R, Offer C, Chirico G. A randomised, double blind, placebo controlled trial of the effect of theophylline in prevention of vasomotor nephropathy in very preterm neonates with respiratory distress syndrome. Arch Dis Child Fetal Neonatal Ed. 2006;91:F80–4.

163. Kidney Disease: Improving Global Outcomes (KDIGO) Acute Kidney Injury Work Group. KDIGO clinical practice guideline for acute kidney injury. Kidney Int Suppl. 2012;2:1–138.

164. Bhatt GC, Gogia P, Bitzan M, Das RR. Theophylline and aminophylline for prevention of acute kidney injury in neonates and children: a systematic review. Arch Dis Child. 2019;104(7):670–9.

165. Askenazi D. Should neonates with perinatal asphyxia receive a single dose of IV theophylline to prevent acute kidney injury? Acta Paediatr. 2016;105(10):1125–6.

166. Harer MW, Askenazi DJ, Boohaker LJ, et al. Association between early caffeine citrate administration and risk of acute kidney injury in preterm neonates: results from the AWAKEN Study. JAMA Pediatr. 2018;172:e180322.

167. Aviles-Otero N, Kumar R, Khalsa DD, Green G, Carmody JB. Caffeine exposure and acute kidney injury in premature infants with necrotizing enterocolitis and spontaneous intestinal perforation. Pediatr Nephrol. 2019;34(4):729–36.

168. Hobbs DJ, Steinke JM, Chung JY, Barletta GM, Bunchman TE. Rasburicase improves hyperuricemia in infants with acute kidney injury. Pediatr Nephrol. 2010;25(2):305–9.

169. Stoops C, Stone S, Evans E, Dill L, Henderson T, Griffin R, et al. Baby NINJA (Nephrotoxic Injury Negated by Just-in-Time Action): reduction of nephrotoxic medication-associated acute kidney injury in the neonatal intensive care unit. J Pediatr. 2019;215:223–8. e6

170. Hay WW Jr, Brown LD, Denne SC. Energy requirements, protein-energy metabolism and balance, and carbohydrates in preterm infants. World Rev Nutr Diet. 2014;110:64–81.

171. Kyle UG, Akcan-Arikan A, Orellana RA, Coss-Bu JA. Nutrition support among critically ill children with AKI. Clin J Am Soc Nephrol. 2013;8(4):568–74.

172. Hakan N, Aydin M, Zenciroglu A, Aydog O, Erdogan D, Karagol BS, et al. Acute peritoneal dialysis in the newborn period: a 7-year single-center experience at tertiary neonatal intensive care unit in Turkey. Am J Perinatol. 2014;31(4):335–8.

173. Sadowski RH, Harmon WE, Jabs K. Acute hemodialysis of infants weighing less than five kilograms. Kidney Int. 1994;45(3):903–6.

174. Warady BA, Bunchman T. Dialysis therapy for children with acute renal failure: survey results. Pediatr Nephrol (Berlin, Germany). 2000;15(1–2):11–3.

175. Jetton JG, Boohaker LJ, Sethi SK, Wazir S, Rohatgi S, Soranno DE, et al. Incidence and outcomes of neonatal acute kidney injury (AWAKEN): a multi-

centre, multinational, observational cohort study. Lancet Child Adolesc Health. 2017;1(3):184–94.

176. Barratt TM. Renal failure in the first year of life. Br Med Bull. 1971;27(2):115–21.

177. Nourse P, Cullis B, Finkelstein F, Numanoglu A, Warady B, Antwi S, et al. ISPD guidelines for peritoneal dialysis in acute kidney injury: 2020 update (paediatrics). Perit Dial Int. 2021;41(2):139–57.

178. Sasser WC, Dabal RJ, Askenazi DJ, Borasino S, Moellinger AB, Kirklin JK, et al. Prophylactic peritoneal dialysis following cardiopulmonary bypass in children is associated with decreased inflammation and improved clinical outcomes. Congenit Heart Dis. 2014;9(2):106–15.

179. Lowrie EG, Huang WH, Lew NL. Death risk predictors among peritoneal dialysis and hemodialysis patients: a preliminary comparison. Am J Kidney Dis. 1995;26(1):220–8.

180. Fleming F, Bohn D, Edwards H, Cox P, Geary D, McCrindle BW, et al. Renal replacement therapy after repair of congenital heart disease in children. A comparison of hemofiltration and peritoneal dialysis. J Thorac Cardiovasc Surg. 1995;109(2):322–31.

181. Golej J, Boigner H, Burda G, Hermon M, Kitzmueller E, Trittenwein G. Peritoneal dialysis for continuing renal support after cardiac ECMO and hemofiltration. Wien Klin Wochenschr. 2002;114(15–16):733–8.

182. Werner HA, Wensley DF, Lirenman DS, LeBlanc JG. Peritoneal dialysis in children after cardiopulmonary bypass. J Thorac Cardiovasc Surg. 1997;113(1):64–8. discussion 8–70

183. Dittrich S, Dahnert I, Vogel M, Stiller B, Haas NA, Alexi-Meskishvili V, et al. Peritoneal dialysis after infant open heart surgery: observations in 27 patients. Ann Thorac Surg. 1999;68(1):160–3.

184. Santos CR, Branco PQ, Gaspar A, Bruges M, Anjos R, Goncalves MS, et al. Use of peritoneal dialysis after surgery for congenital heart disease in children. Perit Dial Int. 2012;32(3):273–9.

185. Sorof JM, Stromberg D, Brewer ED, Feltes TF, Fraser CD Jr. Early initiation of peritoneal dialysis after surgical repair of congenital heart disease. Pediatr Nephrol. 1999;13(8):641–5.

186. Chien JC, Hwang BT, Weng ZC, Meng LC, Lee PC. Peritoneal dialysis in infants and children after open heart surgery. Pediatr Neonatol. 2009;50(6):275–9.

187. El Masri K, Jackson K, Borasino S, Law M, Askenazi D, Alten J. Successful continuous renal replacement therapy using two single-lumen catheters in neonates and infants with cardiac disease. Pediatr Nephrol. 2013;28(12):2383–7.

188. Hackbarth R, Bunchman TE, Chua AN, Somers MJ, Baum M, Symons JM, et al. The effect of vascular access location and size on circuit survival in pediatric continuous renal replacement therapy: a report from the PPCRRT registry. Int J Artif Organs. 2007;30(12):1116–21.

189. Rodl S, Marschitz I, Mache CJ, Koestenberger M, Madler G, Zobel G. Continuous renal replacement

therapy with Prismaflex HF20 disposable set in children from 4 to 15 kg. ASAIO J. 2011;57(5):451–5.

190. Ronco C, Garzotto F, Ricci Z. CA.R.PE.DI.E.M. (Cardio-renal pediatric dialysis emergency machine): evolution of continuous renal replacement therapies in infants. A personal journey. Pediatr Nephrol. 2012;27(8):1203–11.

191. Ronco C, Garzotto F, Brendolan A, Zanella M, Bellettato M, Vedovato S, et al. Continuous renal replacement therapy in neonates and small infants: development and first-in-human use of a miniaturised machine (CARPEDIEM). Lancet. 2014;383(9931):1807–13.

192. Vidal E, Cocchi E, Paglialonga F, Ricci Z, Garzotto F, Peruzzi L, et al. Continuous veno-venous hemodialysis using the cardio-renal pediatric dialysis emergency machineTM: first clinical experiences. Blood Purif. 2019;47(1–3):149–55.

193. Coulthard MG, Crosier J, Griffiths C, Smith J, Drinnan M, Whitaker M, et al. Haemodialysing babies weighing <8 kg with the Newcastle infant dialysis and ultrafiltration system (Nidus): comparison with peritoneal and conventional haemodialysis. Pediatr Nephrol. 2014;29(10):1873–81.

194. Lambert HJ, Sharma S, Matthews JNS. I-KID study protocol: evaluation of efficacy, outcomes and safety of a new infant haemodialysis and ultrafiltration machine in clinical use: a randomised clinical investigation using a cluster stepped-wedge design. BMJ Paediatr Open. 2021;5(1):e001224.

195. Askenazi D, Ingram D, White S, Cramer M, Borasino S, Coghill C, et al. Smaller circuits for smaller patients: improving renal support therapy with Aquadex. Pediatr Nephrol. 2016;31(5):853–60.

196. Menon S, Broderick J, Munshi R, Dill L, DePaoli B, Fathallah-Shaykh S, et al. Kidney support in children using an ultrafiltration device: a multicenter, retrospective study. Clin J Am Soc Nephrol. 2019;14(10):1432–40.

197. Brophy PD, Somers MJ, Baum MA, Symons JM, McAfee N, Fortenberry JD, et al. Multi-centre evaluation of anticoagulation in patients receiving continuous renal replacement therapy (CRRT). Nephrol Dial Transplant. 2005;20(7):1416–21.

198. Picca S, Dionisi-Vici C, Abeni D, Pastore A, Rizzo C, Orzalesi M, et al. Extracorporeal dialysis in neonatal hyperammonemia: modalities and prognostic indicators. Pediatr Nephrol. 2001;16(11):862–7.

199. Jouvet P, Jugie M, Rabier D, Desgres J, Hubert P, Saudubray JM, et al. Combined nutritional support and continuous extracorporeal removal therapy in the severe acute phase of maple syrup urine disease. Intensive Care Med. 2001;27(11):1798–806.

200. Schaefer F, Straube E, Oh J, Mehls O, Mayatepek E. Dialysis in neonates with inborn errors of metabolism. Nephrol Dial Transplant. 1999;14(4):910–8.

201. Summar M. Current strategies for the management of neonatal urea cycle disorders. J Pediatr. 2001;138(Suppl. 1):S30–9.

202. Haberle J, Boddaert N, Burlina A, Chakrapani A, Dixon M, Huemer M, et al. Suggested guidelines for the diagnosis and management of urea cycle disorders. Orphanet J Rare Dis. 2012;7:32.

203. Pela I, Seracini D, Donati MA, Lavoratti G, Pasquini E, Materassi M. Peritoneal dialysis in neonates with inborn errors of metabolism: is it really out of date? Pediatr Nephrol. 2008;23(1):163–8.

204. Raina R, Bedoyan JK, Lichter-Konecki U, Jouvet P, Picca S, Mew NA, et al. Consensus guidelines for management of hyperammonaemia in paediatric patients receiving continuous kidney replacement therapy. Nat Rev Nephrol. 2020;16(8):471–82.

205. Akcan-Arikan A, Zappitelli M, Loftis LL, Washburn KK, Jefferson LS, Goldstein SL. Modified RIFLE criteria in critically ill children with acute kidney injury. Kidney Int. 2007;71(10):1028–35.

206. Zappitelli M, Parikh CR, Akcan-Arikan A, Washburn KK, Moffett BS, Goldstein SL. Ascertainment and epidemiology of acute kidney injury varies with definition interpretation. Clin J Am Soc Nephrol. 2008;3(4):948–54.

207. Ricci Z, Cruz D, Ronco C. The RIFLE criteria and mortality in acute kidney injury: a systematic review. Kidney Int. 2008;73(5):538–46.

208. Cuhaci B. More data on epidemiology and outcome of acute kidney injury with AKIN criteria: benefits of standardized definitions, AKIN and RIFLE classifications. Crit Care Med. 2009;37(9):2659–61.

209. Uchino S. Outcome prediction for patients with acute kidney injury. Nephron Clin Pract. 2008;109(4):c217–23.

210. Macedo E, Castro I, Yu L, Abdulkader RR, Vieira JM Jr. Impact of mild acute kidney injury (AKI) on outcome after open repair of aortic aneurysms. Ren Fail. 2008;30(3):287–96.

211. Bagshaw SM, George C, Bellomo R. Changes in the incidence and outcome for early acute kidney injury in a cohort of Australian intensive care units. Crit Care. 2007;11(3):R68.

212. Wu Y, Wang H, Pei J, Jiang X, Tang J. Acute kidney injury in premature and low birth weight neonates: a systematic review and meta-analysis. Pediatr Nephrol. 2022;37(2):275–87.

213. Coleman C, Tambay Perez A, Selewski DT, Steflik HJ. Neonatal acute kidney injury. Front Pediatr. 2022;10:842544.

214. Starr MC, Charlton JR, Guillet R, Reidy K, Tipple TE, Jetton JG, et al. Advances in neonatal acute kidney injury. Pediatrics. 2021;148(5)

215. Hansrivijit P, Lertjitbanjong P, Thongprayoon C, Cheungpasitporn W, Aeddula NR, Salim SA, et al. Acute kidney injury in pediatric patients on extracorporeal membrane oxygenation: a systematic review and meta-analysis. Medicines (Basel). 2019;6(4):109.

216. Van den Eynde J, Rotbi H, Gewillig M, Kutty S, Allegaert K, Mekahli D. In-hospital outcomes of acute kidney injury after pediatric cardiac surgery: a meta-analysis. Front Pediatr. 2021;9:733744.

217. Goldstein SL, Vidal E, Ricci Z, Paglialonga F, Peruzzi L, Giordano M, et al. Survival of infants treated with CKRT: comparing adapted adult platforms with the Carpediem. Pediatr Nephrol. 2022;37(3):667–75.

218. Carmody JB, Charlton JR. Short-term consequences, long-term risk: prematurity and chronic kidney disease. Pediatrics. 2013;131(6):1168–79.

219. Faa G, Gerosa C, Fanni D, Nemolato S, Locci A, Cabras T, et al. Marked interindividual variability in renal maturation of preterm infants: lessons from autopsy. J Matern Fetal Neonatal Med. 2010;23(Suppl 3):129–33.

220. Sutherland MR, Gubhaju L, Moore L, Kent AL, Dahlstrom JE, Horne RS, et al. Accelerated maturation and abnormal morphology in the preterm neonatal kidney. J Am Soc Nephrol. 2011;22(7):1365–74.

221. Brenner BM, Garcia DL, Anderson S. Glomeruli and blood pressure. Less of one, more the other? Am J Hypertens. 1988;1(4 Pt 1):335–47.

222. White SL, Perkovic V, Cass A, Chang CL, Poulter NR, Spector T, et al. Is low birth weight an antecedent of CKD in later life? A systematic review of observational studies. Am J Kidney Dis. 2009;54(2):248–61.

223. Basile DP. The endothelial cell in ischemic acute kidney injury: implications for acute and chronic function. Kidney Int. 2007;72(2):151–6.

224. Askenazi DJ, Feig DI, Graham NM, Hui-Stickle S, Goldstein SL. 3-5 year longitudinal follow-up of pediatric patients after acute renal failure. Kidney Int. 2006;69(1):184–9.

225. Mammen C, Al Abbas A, Skippen P, Nadel H, Levine D, Collet JP, et al. Long-term risk of CKD in children surviving episodes of acute kidney injury in the intensive care unit: a prospective cohort study. Am J Kidney Dis. 2012;59(4):523–30.

226. Weiss AS, Sandmaier BM, Storer B, Storb R, McSweeney PA, Parikh CR. Chronic kidney disease following non-myeloablative hematopoietic cell transplantation. Am J Transplant. 2006;6(1):89–94.

227. Wald R, Quinn RR, Luo J, Li P, Scales DC, Mamdani MM, et al. Chronic dialysis and death among survivors of acute kidney injury requiring dialysis. JAMA. 2009;302(11):1179–85.

228. Newsome BB, Warnock DG, McClellan WM, Herzog CA, Kiefe CI, Eggers PW, et al. Long-term risk of mortality and end-stage renal disease among the elderly after small increases in serum creatinine level during hospitalization for acute myocardial infarction. Arch Intern Med. 2008;168(6):609–16.

229. Lo LJ, Go AS, Chertow GM, McCulloch CE, Fan D, Ordoñez JD, et al. Dialysis-requiring acute renal failure increases the risk of progressive chronic kidney disease. Kidney Int. 2009;76(8):893–9.

230. Lafrance JP, Djurdjev O, Levin A. Incidence and outcomes of acute kidney injury in a referred chronic kidney disease cohort. Nephrol Dial Transplant. 2010;25(7):2203–9.

231. James MT, Hemmelgarn BR, Wiebe N, Pannu N, Manns BJ, Klarenbach SW, et al. Glomerular filtration rate, proteinuria, and the incidence and consequences of acute kidney injury: a cohort study. Lancet. 2010;376(9758):2096–103.

232. James MT, Ghali WA, Tonelli M, Faris P, Knudtson ML, Pannu N, et al. Acute kidney injury following coronary angiography is associated with a long-term decline in kidney function. Kidney Int. 2010;78(8):803–9.

233. Ishani A, Xue JL, Himmelfarb J, Eggers PW, Kimmel PL, Molitoris BA, et al. Acute kidney injury increases risk of ESRD among elderly. J Am Soc Nephrol. 2009;20(1):223–8.

234. Ishani A, Nelson D, Clothier B, Schult T, Nugent S, Greer N, et al. The magnitude of acute serum creatinine increase after cardiac surgery and the risk of chronic kidney disease, progression of kidney disease, and death. Arch Intern Med. 2011;171(3):226–33.

235. Hsu CY, Chertow GM, McCulloch CE, Fan D, Ordoñez JD, Go AS. Nonrecovery of kidney function and death after acute on chronic renal failure. Clin J Am Soc Nephrol. 2009;4(5):891–8.

236. Choi AI, Li Y, Parikh C, Volberding PA, Shlipak MG. Long-term clinical consequences of acute kidney injury in the HIV-infected. Kidney Int. 2010;78(5):478–85.

237. Ando M, Ohashi K, Akiyama H, Sakamaki H, Morito T, Tsuchiya K, et al. Chronic kidney disease in long-term survivors of myeloablative allogeneic haematopoietic cell transplantation: prevalence and risk factors. Nephrol Dial Transplant. 2010;25(1):278–82.

238. Amdur RL, Chawla LS, Amodeo S, Kimmel PL, Palant CE. Outcomes following diagnosis of acute renal failure in U.S. veterans: focus on acute tubular necrosis. Kidney Int. 2009;76(10):1089–97.

239. Coca SG, Singanamala S, Parikh CR. Chronic kidney disease after acute kidney injury: a systematic review and meta-analysis. Kidney Int. 2011;

240. Abitbol CL, Bauer CR, Montane B, Chandar J, Duara S, Zilleruelo G. Long-term follow-up of extremely low birth weight infants with neonatal renal failure. Pediatr Nephrol. 2003;18(9):887–93.

241. Askenazi D, Koralkar R, Levitan EB, Goldstein SL, Devarajan P, Khandrika S, Mehta R, Ambalavanan N. Baseline values of candidate urine acute kidney injury (AKI) biomarkers vary by gestational age in premature infants. Pediatr Res. 2011;

242. Lavery AP, Meinzen-Derr JK, Anderson E, Ma Q, Bennett MR, Devarajan P, et al. Urinary NGAL in premature infants. Pediatr Res. 2008;64(4):423–8.

243. Bennett M, Dent CL, Ma Q, Dastrala S, Grenier F, Workman R, et al. Urine NGAL predicts severity of acute kidney injury after cardiac surgery: a prospective study. Clin J Am Soc Nephrol. 2008;3(3):665–73.

244. Devarajan P, Krawczeski CD, Nguyen MT, Kathman T, Wang Z, Parikh CR. Proteomic identification of early biomarkers of acute kidney injury after cardiac surgery in children. Am J Kidney Dis. 2010;56(4):632–42.

245. Koyner JL, Garg AX, Shlipak MG, Patel UD, Sint K, Hong K, et al. Urinary cystatin C and acute kidney injury after cardiac surgery. Am J Kidney Dis. 2013;

246. Krawczeski CD, Goldstein SL, Woo JG, Wang Y, Piyaphanee N, Ma Q, et al. Temporal relationship and predictive value of urinary acute kidney injury biomarkers after pediatric cardiopulmonary bypass. J Am Coll Cardiol. 2011;58(22):2301–9.

247. Krawczeski CD, Woo JG, Wang Y, Bennett MR, Ma Q, Devarajan P. Neutrophil gelatinase-associated lipocalin concentrations predict development of acute kidney injury in neonates and children after cardiopulmonary bypass. J Pediatr. 2011;158(6):1009–15 e1.

248. Liangos O, Tighiouart H, Perianayagam MC, Kolyada A, Han WK, Wald R, et al. Comparative analysis of urinary biomarkers for early detection of acute kidney injury following cardiopulmonary bypass. Biomarkers. 2009;14(6):423–31.

249. Mishra J, Dent C, Tarabishi R, Mitsnefes MM, Ma Q, Kelly C, et al. Neutrophil gelatinase-associated lipocalin (NGAL) as a biomarker for acute renal injury after cardiac surgery. Lancet. 2005;365(9466):1231–8.

250. Parikh CR, Mishra J, Thiessen-Philbrook H, Dursun B, Ma Q, Kelly C, et al. Urinary IL-18 is an early predictive biomarker of acute kidney injury after cardiac surgery. Kidney Int. 2006;70(1):199–203.

251. Ramesh G, Krawczeski CD, Woo JG, Wang Y, Devarajan P. Urinary netrin-1 is an early predictive biomarker of acute kidney injury after cardiac surgery. Clin J Am Soc Nephrol. 2010;5(3):395–401.

Part XII

Chronic Kidney Disease

Demographics of CKD and ESRD in Children

54

Julien Hogan and Karlijn J. van Stralen

Introduction

Irreversible kidney damage or so-called chronic kidney disease (CKD) has become a major public health problem worldwide. The adult population has been the subject of extensive epidemiological research [1, 2] but fewer data are available about CKD in children [3]. Despite major scientific advances resulting in substantial improvement in the care of children with CKD, some will still progress and require kidney replacement therapy (KRT). ESKD is a devastating disorder causing substantial mortality and morbidity (most notably cardiovascular, cancer and infection), but this is compounded by specific problems which occur in children such as impaired growth and psychosocial adjustment [4], all of which severely impact upon quality of life [5]. Understanding of the epidemiology of CKD in children is required in order to make a precise and early diagnosis, identify preventable or reversible causes of progression, predict prognosis, and aid the counseling of children and their families.

J. Hogan (✉)
Pediatric Nephrology Unit, Robert Debré University Hospital, Paris, France
e-mail: Julien.hogan2@aphp.fr

K. J. van Stralen
Spaarne Gasthuis Academy, Spaarne Gasthuis Hospital, Hoofddorp, The Netherlands

Part I: CKD (Stages 1–4)

Definition of CKD

Precise data on the epidemiology of CKD in children allowing the evaluation of the incidence and prevalence of CKD and the comparison between countries is lacking. This was in part due to the lack of a universal definition of CKD. For example, the ItalKid Project and North American Pediatric Renal Trials and Collaborative Studies (NAPRTCS) defined CKD as having a glomerular filtration rate (GFR) of below 75 mL/min/1.73 m^2 [6, 7]. Others based their definition on serum creatinine levels themselves or on other thresholds of GFR [8–10]. In 2002, the National Kidney Foundation's Kidney Disease Outcomes Quality Initiative (NKF-K/DOQI) published a classification of CKD applicable to children [11]. CKD was defined by the persistence for more than 3 months of morphological, histological or biological abnormalities of the kidneys and/or a glomerular filtration rate (GFR) below 90 mL/min/1.73 m^2. This classification grades CKD in five stages from stage 1 with normal GFR to end-stage kidney disease (ESKD, stage 5). The K/DOQI classification was revised in 2012 by the KDIGO (Kidney Disease: Improving Global outcomes) to reflect the risk of progression to ESKD and is based on both GFR and albuminuria [12]. Of note, some pediatric specificities need to be considered when using this classification: a) the criteria for duration >3 months does not apply to newborns or infants <3 months of age, (b) the criteria of a GFR <90 mL/min/1.73 m^2 does not apply to children <2 years of age as neonates are born with lower GFR, which increases to normal values in the first 2 years of life, (c) a urinary total protein or albumin excretion rate above the normal value for age may be substituted for albuminuria ≥30 mg/24 h. A similar classification based on the same GFR cut-offs and on the urine protein-creatinine ratio and specifically validated in two large pediatric cohorts (CKID in the USA and ESCAPE in Europe) has been developed recently (Fig. 54.1; Table 54.1) [13].

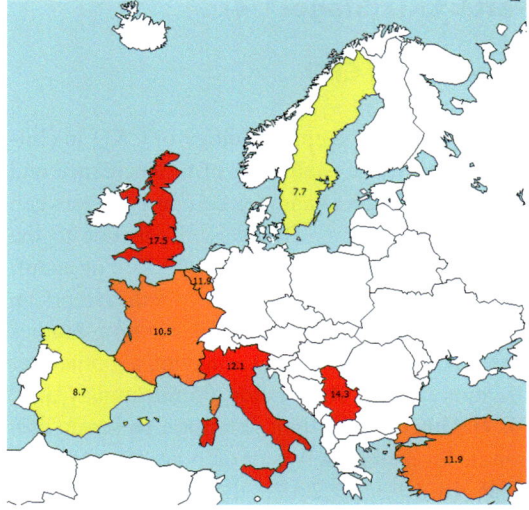

Fig. 54.1 Reported incidence (pmarp) of CKD in children in Europe

The new classification was widely adopted after its introduction; however, its limitations and possible modifications have been a matter of extensive discussions. Moreover, despite efforts to standardize creatinine measurement (by using enzymatic methods instead of colorimetric methods) and GFR estimation, there are still ongoing debates on which eGFR equation should be used in various clinical conditions particularly in early stages of kidney injury [14–17]. In 2009, the bedside Schwartz formula using height and serum creatinine and a unique k coefficient was developed and remains frequently used in clinical practice [18]. Since then many equations have been published using serum creatinine or cystatine C or a combination of both. Recently, papers focused on developing formulas that perform consistently over the whole range of GFR from infants to young adults (FAS [19], CKID U25 [20]).

Screening for CKD

CKD screening and surveillance in adults, either population-based or targeted at risk populations, has become widely advocated and implemented in many countries worldwide, in an attempt to prevent ESKD and the progression of CKD. However, the benefit of screening for early-stage CKD is uncertain [21]. The benefit of such programs in children is even more uncertain [22]. Tests used for CKD screening in children

Table 54.1 CKD classification and estimated risk of progression adapted from (Furth et al. AJKD)

			Baseline UPCR		
			<0.5	[0.5, 2.0]	>2.0
Baseline GFR	I	≥ 90	IR = 2.3 (0.7, 7.0) per 100p-y	–	–
	II	[60–90)	IR = 1.5 (0.8, 2.6) per 100p-y	IR = 8.1 (4.8, 13.8) per 100p-y	IR = 14.2 (6.4, 31.6) per 100p-y
	IIIa	[45–60)	IR = 3.6 (2.5, 5.0) per 100p-y	IR = 6.4 (4.5, 9.1) per 100p-y	IR = 22.8 (13.7, 37.8) per 100p-y
	IIIb	[30–45)	IR = 5.9 (4.4, 7.8) per 100p-y	IR = 10.7 (8.1, 14.1) per 100p-y	IR = 32.0 (23.5, 43.6) per 100p-y
	IV	[15–30)	IR = 17.4 (12.8, 23.6) per 100p-y	IR = 24.8 (19.5, 31.6) per 100p-y	IR = 58.4 (44.5, 76.6) per 100p-y
	V	<15			

Based on baseline GFR and UPCR patients are classified in 6 groups (colors) based on their risk of progression. Incidence rates (IR) of 50% GFR decline or GFR < 15 mL/min/1.73 m^2 are reported

are usually limited to urinary dipstick protein instead of urine albumin/creatinine ratio or on creatinine-based calculation of estimated GFR as recommended for adults. There is also a large variation in the methods used and approaches taken by the different countries, and the findings have shown poor reproducibility [22].

The main studies about screening for CKD in children are summarized in Table 54.2 [23–34]. Mass screening programs to detect CKD in children have been undertaken for many years in several Asian countries such as Japan, Taiwan and Korea [23–25]. Conversely, screening programs have not been adopted in Europe or Australia but screening using urine dipsticks have routinely been performed in healthy children for decades in the United States. In 2000,

the recommendations from the American Academy of Pediatrics were to screen the urine of preschool children and adolescents [35]. This policy has been revised in 2007 and this practice is no longer recommended [36]. Although a decrease in the incidence of ESKD has been observed in Japan and Taiwan, there is only limited evidence that early detection of kidney injury in children may lead to effective interventions to slow progression of CKD and further reduce the risk of developing ESKD [22]. Furthermore, some studies suggest that a urine dipstick is not a cost-effective strategy for screening in children [37] given the high prevalence of transient proteinuria in this population. Although some population-based studies assessing CKD epidemiology by GFR estima-

Table 54.2 Results from studies reporting screening programs from chronic kidney disease in children

Country [Reference]	Study period	Study population	Screening criteria	Main findings
Japan [23]	1974–2002	Population-based 6–14 years old	2 positive urine dipsticks	Prevalence of Pu: 0.07% in 6–11 years 0.35% in 12/14 years old
Taiwan [24]	1992–1996	Population-based 6–15 years old	Pu > 100 mg/dL CKD (SCr >1.7 mg/dL)	Prevalence Pu 0.06% Prevalence CKD 0.002%
Korea [25]	1998–2004	Population-based 6–18 years old	2 positive urine dipsticks	Prevalence Pu 0.2%
Australia [26]	2004–2008	Population-based (57% Arboriginal) 4–14 years old	Single assessment Urine dipsticks uACR≥3.4 mg/mmol	Prevalence of albuminuria at baseline 11.5%
India [27]	2013–2016	Population-based 8–18 years old	Single assessment Urine dipsticks	Prevalence of Pu 1.9% Prevalence of hematuria 5.2%
USA [28]	2009–2014	Population-based 12–18 years old	Albuminuria (uACR) eGFR (bedside Schwartz)	Prevalence of albuminuria: 13.7% Prevalence of persistent albuminuria 3.29% Prevalence of eGFR<60: 0.91%
Singapore [29]	1999–2000	Population-based 12 years old	Urine dipstick	Prevalence of Pu 1.3%
China [30]	2003–2005	Selected population School age children	2 positive urine dipsticks	Prevalence of Pu and/or Hu in 2 specimens: ~1%
Finland [31]	NA	Selected population 8–15 years old	4 urine samples (2 morning, 2 evening. Dipstick and measured Pu	Prevalence of Pu: 10.7% on at least 1 specimen 2.5% on 2 specimens 0.1% on 4 specimens
Iran [32]	NA	Selected population 6–7 years old	Urine dipsticks	Prevalence of Pu: 3.6% Prevalence of persistent Pu: 1.3%
Mexico [33]	2006–2007	Selected population 0–18 years old	Single assessment urine dipstick eGFR (Schwartz)	Prevalence of Pu 16.1% Prevalence of hematuria 17.5% Prevalence of eGFR<60: 1.7%
UK [34]	1967–1969	Selected population 5–16 years old	2 positive urine dipsticks	Prevalence of persistent proteinuria 0.8% on 2 specimens

tion have been performed and indicate that a certain proportion of asymptomatic children have CKD, no systematic national screening program based on GFR assessment in children is currently ongoing.

Demographics of CKD

There is limited information on the epidemiology of early stages of CKD in children. As CKD is usually asymptomatic in its early stages, providing precise epidemiological data is difficult so CKD in children is likely to be underestimated and underreported. Although some pediatric CKD registries using the K/DOQI classification are beginning to emerge, only a few reports on the epidemiology of CKD stages 2–5 in children are available. Due to lack of resources and national renal registries, we know even less about the incidence and prevalence in low income countries. For these countries, data are mostly obtained from reports of major tertiary care referral centers, but the validity of this data is variable.

Europe
The largest population-based study in Europe on the epidemiology of pediatric CKD is the ItalKid project. This study in Italy has been collecting data since 1990 on the epidemiology of childhood CKD, describing the natural history of the disease, and identifying factors that influence its course [6]. So far, nearly 1198 patients have been registered. Other nation-wide European studies are the Serbian CKD registry [38], collecting data on over 336 patients since 2000, the Belgium CKD registry which started in 2001 and has over 143 patients [39], and the data from the Swedish Pediatric Nephrology Association [40]. Also regional studies have taken place in Spain [41], the South-East of the UK [42] and Lorraine in France [8].

Several pediatric nephrology societies from European countries have provided data on the early stages of CKD. Even though age categories and definition of CKD differed between countries, incidence in Europe was consistent, ranging from 8 to 14 per million age-related population

(pmarp) for CKD stages 2–5, and being around 8 pmarp for CKD stage 4–5 (Fig. 54.1). The incidence was highest (17.5 pmarp) in a report from the United Kingdom but the study was hospital-based leading to potential referral filter bias and there may be some uncertainty about the covered geographical area [42].

While an increase in incidence since the 1970s was seen in France [8], this was not seen when comparing two time periods in Sweden [9, 40]. Two studies from Serbia and the UK also suggested an increase in incidence in the past 10 years [38, 42]. Prevalence ranged from about 55–60 to 90–95 pmarp in Spain, Italy, UK and Serbia, depending on the clinical definition of CKD that was used in each study.

In Turkey, the CREDIT study reported a prevalence of CKD stage 3–5 of 2600 pmarp in children aged 5–18 years old in 2007 [43].

North America
In Northern America most of the information on CKD in children derives from two large sources of information namely the North American Pediatric Renal Trials and Collaborative Studies (NAPRTCS) [44] and the Chronic Kidney Disease in Children Prospective Cohort Study (CKiD) [45]. Both studies are collecting data on a voluntary basis and are not population based.

Population-based data are available in adolescents since the NHANES study investigated albuminuria and GFR in a nationally representative sample of the US population including 9225 adolescents aged 12–18 years over 3 study periods. They found a prevalence of 0.91% [95% CI 0.58–1.42%] for CKD stage 3–5 and a prevalence of persistent albuminuria of 3.29% [95% CI 1.94–4.63%] in the 2009–2014 survey [28].

Latin America and the Caribbean
In Chile, a national survey of pediatric nephrologists estimated an incidence of CKD (GFR <30 mL/min/1.73 m^2) in children aged less than 18 years of 5.7 pmarp and a prevalence of 42.5 pmarp in 1996 [46]. Among these patients, half were on conservative treatment and the others were on KRT. Very similar results were found in Argentina, with an incidence of 6.5 pmarp, but with a lower prevalence

(15.4 pmarp) [47]. Fifty-eight percent of this population had ESKD and started with dialysis. In Jamaica, the estimated incidence of CKD was 4.6 pmarp and 28% of them were already in ESKD, without having access to KRT [48].

A study on the epidemiology of CKD conducted in several Latin American countries (Argentina, Brazil, Chile, Colombia, Mexico, Uruguay, and Venezuela) has shown a wide variation in incidence that ranged from 2.8 to 15.8 new cases pmarp [49]. Also an indirect estimation of the incidence of CKD in Mexico suggested a very high incidence, between 24 and 39 per million inhabitants, for which the differences within Mexico were explained by the level of social deprivation [50].

Asia

The estimated prevalence of CKD stage 3–5 among Japanese children in 2010 was 29.8 pmarp [51]. This lower prevalence of pre-dialysis CKD in Japan than in Europe was consistent with the lower prevalence of pediatric ESKD in Japan. Two reports from Vietnam and one from Thailand have suggested an annual incidence of hospitalization for CKD around 5 pmarp, most of patients had already reached ESKD [52–54]. Very little is known about pediatric CKD epidemiology in India and China. A survey conducted in 91 Chinese hospitals found a total of 1658 children aged <15 years with CKD stage 3–5 between 1990 and 2002 which suggests a very low incidence of treated CKD <0.5 pmarp [55]. Patients were referred late with advanced CKD or ESKD in 80% and in-hospital mortality was as high as 72%. Similarly, in India 58% of children had ESKD at the time of CKD diagnosis suggesting that children with CKD are underdiagnosed and referred late [55].

Middle East

The referral center for pediatric kidney diseases in Kuwait provided data on children aged 0–15 years with a GFR <50 mL/min/1.73 m² [10]. The mean incidence was found to be as high as 38 pmarp whereas the prevalence increased from 188 in 1996 to a rate as high as 329 pmarp in 2003. The marked difference in incidence between Kuwaiti children and non-Kuwaiti residents suggested the role of genetic factors. An incidence of 12 pmarp was found in a Turkish survey including children with a GFR <75 mL/min/1.73 m² [56]. An incidence of 11 pmarp and a prevalence of 51 pmarp have been reported in Jordanian children [57].

Africa

Single center studies from sub-Saharan Africa showed very low incidence of CKD estimated at 1–4 pmarp in Nigeria, Sudan, and South Africa [58–61]. Another single center report from Nigeria, however, found an annual incidence of CKD stage 1–5 of 11 pmarp and a prevalence of 48 pmarp [62], which was much higher than the 1.7 pmarp reported in 2004 [63].

Causes of CKD

Type 2 diabetes and hypertension are the leading causes of CKD in adults. The distribution of the causes of CKD in children are very different with major variations between countries. Indeed, congenital abnormalities of the kidney and the urinary tracts (CAKUT) account for 50–60% of CKD cases in children in Europe [6, 38, 39, 42], Japan [51] and the USA [44]. In Turkey and in the Middle East, CAKUT remains the first cause of CKD with often a higher proportion of hereditary nephropathies related to higher rates of consanguinity [10, 56, 57, 64]. Higher proportions of glomerular diseases are found in developing countries such as India, Southeast Asia [52–54], Latin America [48, 49] and Sub-Saharan Africa [58]. The latter may be related to the high prevalence of bacterial, viral and fungal infections in these regions.

Whereas CAKUT predominates in younger patients, glomerulonephritis is the leading cause in children older than 12 years of age. Causes of CKD vary across races, for example, focal segmental glomerulosclerosis, the main cause of glomerular disease, is three times more common in blacks than in whites (19 compared with 6%) and especially among black adolescents (35%) [65].

In general, there is a predominance of male gender (male/female ratio ranging from 1.3 to 3.0). This partly reflects the higher incidence of CAKUT in boys than in girls, but has also been reported in the regions with a high rate of glomerulonephritis.

Part II: KRT (CKD Stage 5D and 5 T)

Epidemiological data on ESKD treated by dialysis or transplantation is more robust thanks to the development of several national and international registries. Unfortunately not every country has such a registry, not all children are reported to the relevant registry, and some countries with registries do not regularly publish reports. Also, as KRT is expensive not all countries are able to offer KRT to children with ESKD. Approximately 80% of the children on KRT live in Europe, Japan or the United States. Dialysis and transplant registries only collect data on treated ESKD; untreated children with ESKD are not captured. However, at least in the developed world, the proportion of children with ESKD who do not receive KRT is likely to be very low [1].

Incidence

The incidence of KRT in children varies greatly between countries but can be estimated between 5 and 10 pmarp [66–70] with extreme values ranging from 0 (Malta) to 17 pmarp (Kuwait)

[71]. However, given that pediatric KRT is extremely rare, numbers in smaller countries are subject to random error. Moreover, variations in incidence may reflect variations in the incidence of CKD, differences in pre-ESKD care or differences in access to KRT. Among large countries with universal access to KRT, the US incidence is consistently high at around 12.9 per million population [72]. In Japan, incidence of pediatric KRT (4.0 pmarp) was consistently much lower than in other high income countries (Table 54.3).

Among lower income countries the incidence is typically lower, as was shown for the Eastern European countries in the ESPN/ERA-EDTA registry [73]. In developing countries where KRT is unaffordable for all but the very wealthy, incidence rates are either not available or were extremely low (<1 pmarp in Bangladesh and Nepal). Some of the variation in incidence may be due to differences in the timing of KRT initiation. In Europe, KRT was generally started at a median GFR of 10.4 mL/min/1.73 m^2 whereas mean GFR ranged from 11.3 to 13.6 mL/min/1.73 m^2 in the United States [72, 74] (Fig. 54.2).

Within-country variations occur by racial group. For example African American in the US, arboriginal children in Australia and New Zealand or children from South Asian origin in the UK [72, 75, 76] have a significantly higher incidence of ESKD than their white counterparts, although differences in the prevalence of other ESKD risk factors such as obesity or disparities in access to medical care may account for at least

Table 54.3 Incidence, prevalence and KRT modality distribution among children with ESKD

	Countries	Year	Age	Incidence/ prevalence	Treatment modality distribution		
					HD	PD	Transplantation
ESPN/ERA-EDTA	36 European countries	2018	0–14	4.9/29.8	43.8	37.9	17.8
					15.9	17.9	66.2
USRDS	USA	2017	0–21	12.9/98.7	51.3	27.8	20.9
					16.6	10	73.4
CORR	Canada	2014	0–19	7.7/65.1	29.5	16.4	54.1
					10	7	83
JSPN Pediatric survey 2012	Japan	2006–2011	0–19	4/–	16	61.7	22.3
					–	–	–
ANZDATA	Australia and New Zealand	2018	0–17	6–9/25–100	25	45	30
					6	12	82

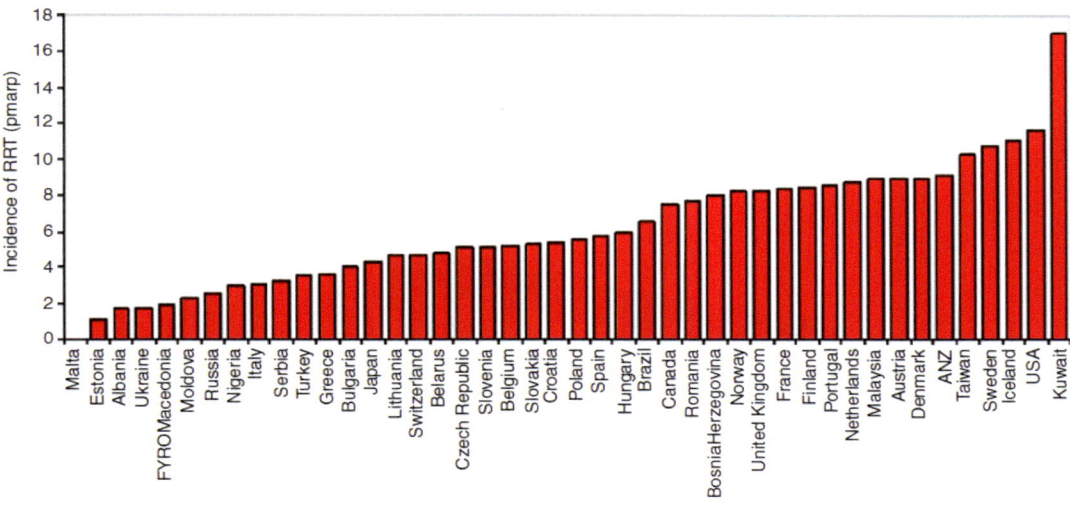

Fig. 54.2 Incidence of KRT in children aged 0–14 between 2008 and 2014

part of these differences. There are also large differences between age groups. The incidence has a typical U-shape distribution, with the highest incidence in the preschool children and in adolescents. Therefore, registries that include patients up to 20 years of age report higher incidence and prevalence data compared with registries excluding those over the age of 15.

Around 20% of patients receive a pre-emptive kidney transplant. In patients starting on dialysis, dialysis modality is strongly dependent on age; while peritoneal dialysis is the treatment of choice in the majority of young children, this pattern decreases with age, with typically higher rates of HD from the age of 10 onwards [75]. Finally, the relative proportion of HD and PD is quite variable between countries and between centers presumably reflecting differences in clinician preference and funding models [77].

Prevalence

The prevalence of treated ESKD is completely dependent on access to KRT in each country. In countries with available data on KRT, the IPNA global registry reports prevalences ranging from less than 1% in some African and Asian countries to 98.7 pmarp in the United States [72, 78]. Indeed, 80% of prevalent ESKD patients live in Europe, North America and Japan, while the prevalence of treated ESKD remains very low in many countries with the highest CKD burden [79]. Within Europe, there are also large differences, with high income countries reporting prevalence rates over 55 pmarp similar to Australia/New Zealand with 56.7 cases per million population [69], while middle income European countries report prevalences around 40 pmarp (Fig. 54.3).

In many countries the prevalence is rising due to the combination of a fairly steady incidence and improved patient survival on KRT. In the United States, the adjusted annual incidence of ESKD in the pediatric population rose slowly during the 1980s then increased marginally from 14 to 15 pmarp between 1990 and 2011 [80]. In contrast, the adjusted prevalence increased from 60 to 85 in between 1990 and 2011. Similar trends were observed in Australia and New Zealand, where the incidence has remained constant at about 8 pmarp over the past 25 years, while the prevalence of KRT increased from approximately 30–50 pmarp [69]. A report from the ERA-EDTA registry on patients aged 0–19 years starting KRT between 1980 and 2000 in 12 Western European countries showed that the incidence of KRT rose from 7 pmarp in 1980–1984 to 10 pmarp in 1985–1989 and remained stable thereafter [81], while the preva-

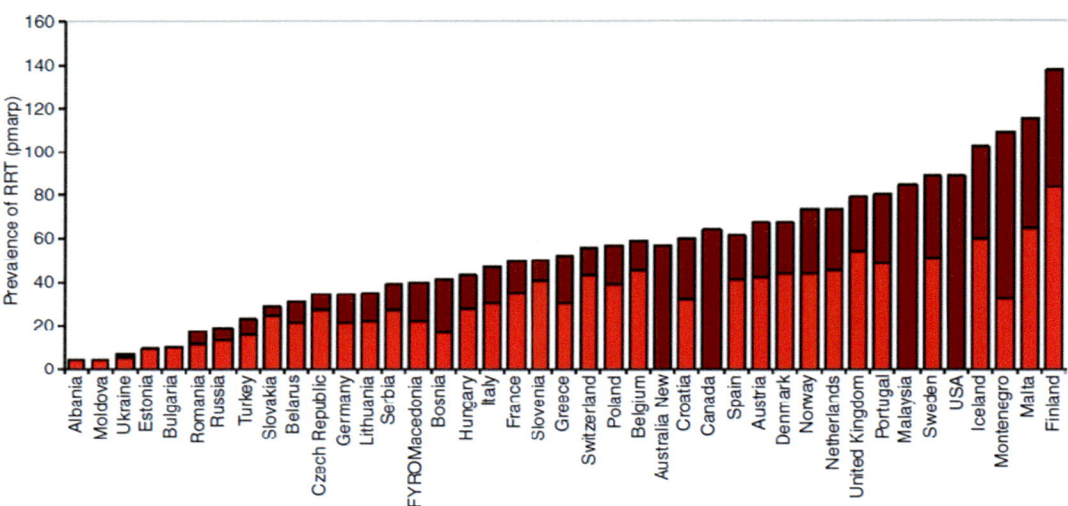

Fig. 54.3 Prevalence of KRT in children on 31st of December 2011 (2012 for Australia and New Zealand and Malaysia). The light bar corresponds to the prevalence in children aged 0–14 years, the sum of the light and the dark bars corresponds to the prevalence in children aged 0–19 years

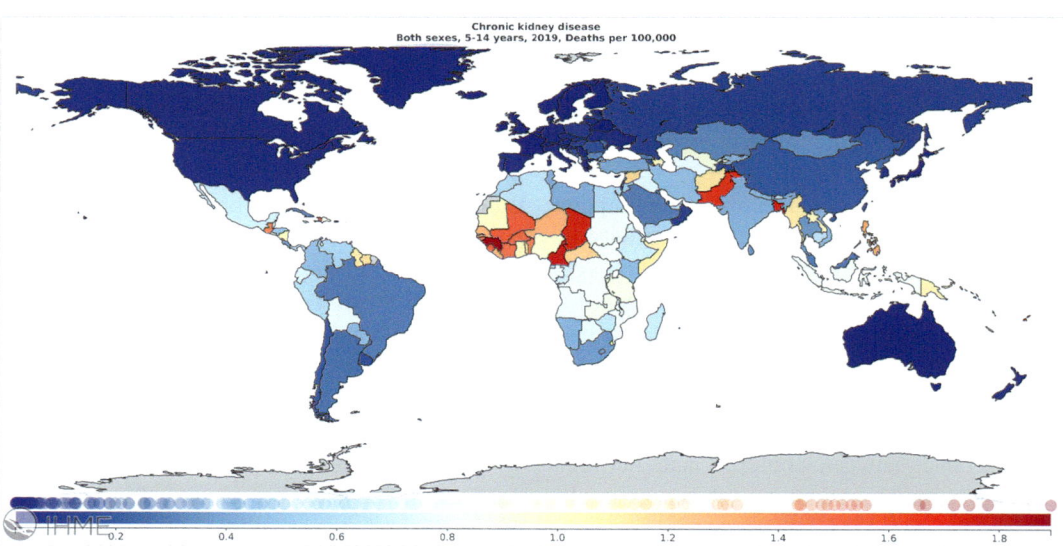

Fig. 54.4 CKD-related death rates in children aged 5–14 years (Global Burden of Disease [83])

lence increased from 22.9 pmarp in 1980 to 62 pmarp in 2000. The increases in prevalence were explained by improved survival and treatment of younger children, while the prevalence was relatively constant for the pubertal age groups.

In developing countries, a lower prevalence of children with ESKD is explained by a low access to KRT [78] and by lower patient survival.

Figure 54.4 presents the death rates per country caused by CKD in children aged 5–14 years old in 2019. As expected, this map perfectly matches maps reporting access to KRT by countries [82].

Transplantation is by far the most common treatment modality in most countries, accounting for 60–80% of patients receiving KRT (Table 54.3). Here again, differences among countries are substantial. For example, fewer than 10% of children on KRT are maintained with a kidney transplant in Belarus, compared with over 90% in Japan and Finland [84]. Recent data show that differences among countries were explained by factors such as the deceased donor rate, the pediatric priority from deceased donor programs, the living donation rate, and healthcare funding models [85]. Compared to adults, children are much more likely to be treated by transplantation due to a combination of fewer comorbidities, higher availability of living donors and, in some cases, preferential allocation of deceased donor kidneys.

Causes of ESKD

the distribution of primary kidney diseases in children reaching ESKD is different than the distribution in children with CKD. Although CAKUT is the most prevalent cause also in children with ESKD, a relatively higher proportion of ESKD cases is caused by glomerular diseases reflecting the faster progression and higher risk of ESKD of this disease group. However, a recent large cohort study from Israel demonstrated that young adults (16–25 years old) with a medical history of kidney disease in childhood but with normal serum creatinine, blood pressure and no proteinuria presented a four-fold increased risk of ESKD over a 30 year follow-up [86]. This underlines the impact of kidney diseases in childhood on ESKD in adulthood and supports long-term follow up of these patients.

There are also very specific local factors. For example, congenital nephrotic syndrome of the Finnish type, explains the very high prevalence of childhood KRT in Finland. Finally, the difference in the distribution of the causes of ESKD in children vs. adults and especially the absence of diabetes or hypertension induced ESKD explains the moderate increase in the prevalence of ESKD in children (+16.6%) in contrast with the major growth experienced by the entire ESKD population (+77%) between 2000 and 2017 in the US [72].

Conclusion

CKD and ESKD in children is a significant public health burden worldwide. Despite significant effort to collect data on children with CKD, the incidence and prevalence of CKD are underestimated in many parts of the world and further studies aiming at improving early CKD diagnosis and at developing effective strategies to slow down CKD progression are needed. For children reaching ESKD, the main challenge is the access to KRT and especially transplantation that remain unavailable to the majority of children with ESKD worldwide.

References

1. Remuzzi G, Benigni A, Finkelstein FO, Grunfeld J-P, Joly D, Katz I, et al. Kidney failure: aims for the next 10 years and barriers to success. Lancet. 2013;382(9889):353–62.
2. Eckardt K-U, Coresh J, Devuyst O, Johnson RJ, Köttgen A, Levey AS, et al. Evolving importance of kidney disease: from subspecialty to global health burden. Lancet. 2013;382(9887):158–69.
3. Harambat J, van Stralen KJ, Kim JJ, Tizard EJ. Epidemiology of chronic kidney disease in children. Pediatr Nephrol. 2012;27(3):363–73.
4. Shroff R, Weaver DJ, Mitsnefes MM. Cardiovascular complications in children with chronic kidney disease. Nat Rev Nephrol. 2011;7(11):642–9.
5. Al-Uzri A, Matheson M, Gipson DS, Mendley SR, Hooper SR, Yadin O, et al. The impact of short stature on health-related quality of life in children with chronic kidney disease. J Pediatr. 2013;163(3):736–41. e1
6. Ardissino G, Daccò V, Testa S, Bonaudo R, Claris-Appiani A, Taioli E, et al. Epidemiology of chronic renal failure in children: data from the ItalKid project. Pediatrics. 2003;111(4 Pt 1):e382–7.
7. Fivush BA, Jabs K, Neu AM, Sullivan EK, Feld L, Kohaut E, et al. Chronic renal insufficiency in children and adolescents: the 1996 annual report of NAPRTCS. North American Pediatric Renal Transplant Cooperative Study. Pediatr Nephrol. 1998;12(4):328–37.
8. Deleau J, Andre JL, Briancon S, Musse JP. Chronic renal failure in children: an epidemiological survey in Lorraine (France) 1975–1990. Pediatr Nephrol. 1994;8(4):472–6.
9. Esbjörner E, Aronson S, Berg U, Jodal U, Linne T. Children with chronic renal failure in Sweden 1978–1985. Pediatr Nephrol. 1990;4(3):249–52. discussion 253-254

10. Al-Eisa A, Naseef M, Al-Hamad N, Pinto R, Al-Shimeri N, Tahmaz M. Chronic renal failure in Kuwaiti children: an eight-year experience. Pediatr Nephrol. 2005;20(12):1781–5.

11. Hogg RJ, Furth S, Lemley KV, Portman R, Schwartz GJ, Coresh J, et al. National Kidney Foundation's Kidney Disease Outcomes Quality Initiative clinical practice guidelines for chronic kidney disease in children and adolescents: evaluation, classification, and stratification. Pediatrics. 2003;111(6 Pt 1):1416–21.

12. Improving Global Outcomes (KDIGO) CKD Work Group. KDIGO 2012 clinical practice guideline for the evaluation and management of chronic kidney disease. Kidney Int Suppl. 2013;(3):1–150.

13. Furth SL, Pierce C, Hui WF, White CA, Wong CS, Schaefer F, et al. Estimating time to ESRD in children with CKD. Am J Kidney Dis. 2018;71(6):783–92.

14. Pottel H, Hoste L, Martens F. A simple height-independent equation for estimating glomerular filtration rate in children. Pediatr Nephrol. 2012;27(6):973–9.

15. Schwartz GJ, Schneider MF, Maier PS, Moxey-Mims M, Dharnidharka VR, Warady BA, et al. Improved equations estimating GFR in children with chronic kidney disease using an immunonephelometric determination of cystatin C. Kidney Int. 2012;82(4):445–53.

16. Sharma AP, Yasin A, Garg AX, Filler G. Diagnostic accuracy of cystatin C-based eGFR equations at different GFR levels in children. Clin J Am Soc Nephrol. 2011;6(7):1599–608.

17. Björk J, Nyman U, Berg U, Delanaye P, Dubourg L, Goffin K, et al. Validation of standardized creatinine and cystatin C GFR estimating equations in a large multicentre European cohort of children. Pediatr Nephrol. 2019;34(6):1087–98.

18. Schwartz GJ, Muñoz A, Schneider MF, Mak RH, Kaskel F, Warady BA, et al. New equations to estimate GFR in children with CKD. J Am Soc Nephrol. 2009;20(3):629–37.

19. Pottel H, Hoste L, Dubourg L, Ebert N, Schaeffner E, Eriksen BO, et al. An estimated glomerular filtration rate equation for the full age spectrum. Nephrol Dial Transplant. 2016;31(5):798–806.

20. Pierce CB, Muñoz A, Ng DK, Warady BA, Furth SL, Schwartz GJ. Age- and sex-dependent clinical equations to estimate glomerular filtration rates in children and young adults with chronic kidney disease. Kidney Int. 2021;99(4):948–56.

21. Qaseem A, Hopkins RH, Sweet DE, Starkey M, Shekelle P, Clinical Guidelines Committee of the American College of Physicians. Screening, monitoring, and treatment of stage 1–3 chronic kidney disease: a clinical practice guideline from the American College of Physicians. Ann Intern Med. 2013;159(12):835–47.

22. Hogg RJ. Screening for CKD in children: a global controversy. Clin J Am Soc Nephrol. 2009;4(2):509–15.

23. Murakami M, Hayakawa M, Yanagihara T, Hukunaga Y. Proteinuria screening for children. Kidney Int Suppl. 2005;94:S23–7.

24. Lin CY, Sheng CC, Chen CH, Lin CC, Chou P. The prevalence of heavy proteinuria and progression risk factors in children undergoing urinary screening. Pediatr Nephrol. 2000;14(10–11):953–9.

25. Cho B-S, Kim S-D. School urinalysis screening in Korea. Nephrology (Carlton). 2007;12(Suppl. 3):S3–7.

26. Kim S, Macaskill P, Hodson EM, Daylight J, Williams R, Kearns R, et al. Beginning the trajectory to ESKD in adult life: albuminuria in Australian aboriginal children and adolescents. Pediatr Nephrol. 2017;32(1):119–29.

27. Chaudhury AR, Reddy TV, Divyaveer SS, Patil K, Bennikal M, Karmakar K, et al. A cross-sectional prospective study of asymptomatic urinary abnormalities, blood pressure, and body mass index in healthy school children. Kidney Int Rep. 2017;2(6):1169–75.

28. Saydah SH, Xie H, Imperatore G, Burrows NR, Pavkov ME. Trends in albuminuria and GFR among adolescents in the United States, 1988–2014. Am J Kidney Dis. 2018;72(5):644–52.

29. Ramirez SP, Hsu SI, McClellan W. Low body weight is a risk factor for proteinuria in multiracial Southeast Asian pediatric population. Am J Kidney Dis. 2001;38(5):1045–54.

30. Zhai Y-H, Xu H, Zhu G-H, Wei M-J, Hua B-C, Shen Q, et al. Efficacy of urine screening at school: experience in Shanghai, China. Pediatr Nephrol. 2007;22(12):2073–9.

31. Vehaskari VM, Rapola J. Isolated proteinuria: analysis of a school-age population. J Pediatr. 1982;101(5):661–8.

32. Shajari A, Shajari H, Zade MHF, Kamali K, Kadivar MR, Nourani F. Benefit of urinalysis. Indian J Pediatr. 2009;76(6):639–41.

33. Koshy SM, Garcia-Garcia G, Pamplona JS, Renoirte-Lopez K, Perez-Cortes G, Gutierrez MLS, et al. Screening for kidney disease in children on World Kidney Day in Jalisco. Mexico Pediatr Nephrol. 2009;24(6):1219–25.

34. Meadow SR, White RH, Johnston NM. Prevalence of symptomless urinary tract disease in Birmingham schoolchildren. I. Pyuria and bacteriuria. Br Med J. 1969;3(5662):81–4.

35. Committee on Practice and Ambulatory Medicine. Recommendations for preventive pediatric health care. Pediatrics. 2000;105(3):645–6.

36. Committee on Practice and Ambulatory Medicine, Bright Futures Steering Committee. Recommendations for preventive pediatric health care. Pediatrics. 2007;120(6):1376.

37. Sekhar DL, Wang L, Hollenbeak CS, Widome MD, Paul IM. A cost-effectiveness analysis of screening urine dipsticks in well-child care. Pediatrics. 2010;125(4):660–3.

38. Peco-Antic A, Bogdanovic R, Paripovic D, Paripovic A, Kocev N, Golubovic E, et al. Epidemiology of chronic kidney disease in children in Serbia. Nephrol Dial Transplant. 2012;27(5):1978–84.

39. Mong Hiep TT, Ismaili K, Collart F, Van Damme-Lombaerts R, Godefroid N, Ghuysen M-S, et al.

Clinical characteristics and outcomes of children with stage 3–5 chronic kidney disease. Pediatr Nephrol. 2010;25(5):935–40.

40. Esbjörner E, Berg U, Hansson S. Epidemiology of chronic renal failure in children: a report from Sweden 1986–1994. Swedish Pediatr Nephrol Assoc Pediatr Nephrol. 1997;11(4):438–42.

41. Areses Trapote R, Sanahuja Ibáñez MJ, Navarro M. Investigadores Centros Participantes en el REPIR II. [Epidemiology of chronic kidney disease in Spanish pediatric population. REPIR II Project]. Nefrologia. 2010;30(5):508–17.

42. Kim JJ, Booth CJ, Waller S, Rasmussen P, Reid CJD, Sinha MD. The demographic characteristics of children with chronic kidney disease stages 3–5 in South East England over a 5-year period. Arch Dis Child. 2013;98(3):189–94.

43. Soylemezoglu O, Duzova A, Yalçinkaya F, Arinsoy T, Süleymanlar G. Chronic renal disease in children aged 5–18 years: a population-based survey in Turkey, the CREDIT-C study. Nephrol Dial Transplant. 2012;27(Suppl. 3):146–51.

44. Seikaly MG, Ho PL, Emmett L, Fine RN, Tejani A. Chronic renal insufficiency in children: the 2001 Annual Report of the NAPRTCS. Pediatr Nephrol. 2003;18(8):796–804.

45. Furth SL, Cole SR, Moxey-Mims M, Kaskel F, Mak R, Schwartz G, et al. Design and methods of the Chronic Kidney Disease in Children (CKiD) prospective cohort study. Clin J Am Soc Nephrol. 2006;1(5):1006–15.

46. Lagomarsimo E, Valenzuela A, Cavagnaro F, Solar E. Chronic renal failure in pediatrics 1996. Chilean survey. Pediatr Nephrol. 1999;13(4):288–91.

47. Grimoldi IA, Briones LM, Ferraris JR, Rodríguez Rilo L, Sojo E, Turconi A, et al. Chronic renal failure, dialysis and transplant: multicentric study: 1996–2003. Arch Argent Pediatr. 2008;106(6):552–9.

48. Miller MEY, Williams JA. Chronic renal failure in Jamaican children—an update (2001–2006). West Indian Med J 2009;58(3):231–234.

49. Orta-Sibu N, Lopez M, Moriyon JC, Chavez JB. Renal diseases in children in Venezuela, South America. Pediatr Nephrol. 2002;17(7):566–9.

50. Franco-Marina F, Tirado-Gómez LL, Estrada AV, Moreno-López JA, Pacheco-Domínguez RL, Durán-Arenas L, et al. An indirect estimation of current and future inequalities in the frequency of end stage renal disease in Mexico. Salud Publica Mex. 2011;53(Suppl. 4):506–15.

51. Ishikura K, Uemura O, Ito S, Wada N, Hattori M, Ohashi Y, et al. Pre-dialysis chronic kidney disease in children: results of a nationwide survey in Japan. Nephrol Dial Transplant. 2013;28(9):2345–55.

52. Huong NTQ, Long TD, Bouissou F, Liem NT, Truong DM, Nga DK, et al. Chronic kidney disease in children: the National Paediatric Hospital experience in Hanoi, Vietnam. Nephrology (Carlton). 2009;14(8):722–7.

53. Mong Hiep TT, Janssen F, Ismaili K, Khai Minh D, Vuong Kiet D, Robert A. Etiology and outcome of chronic renal failure in hospitalized children in Ho Chi Minh City, Vietnam. Pediatr Nephrol. 2008;23(6):965–70.

54. Vachvanichsanong P, Dissaneewate P, McNeil E. Childhood chronic kidney disease in a developing country. Pediatr Nephrol. 2008;23(7):1143–7.

55. Gulati S, Mittal S, Sharma RK, Gupta A. Etiology and outcome of chronic renal failure in Indian children. Pediatr Nephrol. 1999;13(7):594–6.

56. Bek K, Akman S, Bilge I, Topaloğlu R, Calişkan S, Peru H, et al. Chronic kidney disease in children in Turkey. Pediatr Nephrol. 2009;24(4):797–806.

57. Hamed RMA. The spectrum of chronic renal failure among Jordanian children. J Nephrol. 2002;15(2):130–5.

58. Odetunde OI, Okafor HU, Uwaezuoke SN, Ezeonwu BU, Adiele KD, Ukoha OM. Chronic kidney disease in children as seen in a tertiary hospital in Enugu, South-East, Nigeria. Niger J Clin Pract. 2014;17(2):196–200.

59. Anochie I, Eke F. Chronic renal failure in children: a report from Port Harcourt, Nigeria (1985–2000). Pediatr Nephrol. 2003;18(7):692–5.

60. Bhimma R, Adhikari M, Asharam K, Connolly C. The spectrum of chronic kidney disease (stages 2–5) in KwaZulu-Natal, South Africa. Pediatr Nephrol. 2008;23(10):1841–6.

61. Ali E-TMA, Abdelraheem MB, Mohamed RM, Hassan EG, Watson AR. Chronic renal failure in Sudanese children: aetiology and outcomes. Pediatr Nephrol. 2009;24(2):349–53.

62. Olowu WA, Adefehinti O, Aladekomo TA. Epidemiology and clinicopathologic outcome of pediatric chronic kidney disease in Nigeria, a single center study. Arab J Nephrol Transplant. 2013;6(2):105–13.

63. Michael IO, Gabreil OE. Chronic renal failure in children of Benin, Nigeria. Saudi J Kidney Dis Transpl. 2004;15(1):79–83.

64. Madani K, Otoukesh H, Rastegar A, Van Why S. Chronic renal failure in Iranian children. Pediatr Nephrol. 2001;16(2):140–4.

65. Registry Reports | NAPRTCS [Internet]. [cited 2020 Apr 24]. Available from: https://naprtcs.org/registries/annual-report

66. Hattori M. Current trend of pediatric renal replacement therapy in Japan. Contrib Nephrol. 2018;196:223–8.

67. ESPN/ERA-EDTA Registry—Annual reports [Internet]. [cited 2020 Nov 27]. Available from: https://www.espn-reg.org/index.jsp?p=pua

68. Information (CIHI) CI for H. CORR Annual Statistics [Internet]. [cited 2020 Nov 28]. Available from: https://secure.cihi.ca/estore/productSeries.htm?pc=PCC24

69. ANZDATA 42nd Annual Report 2019 (Data to 2018) [Internet]. ANZDATA 42nd Annual Report 2019 (Data to 2018)—ANZDATA. [cited 2020 Jun 12]. Available from: https://www.anzdata.org.au/report/anzdata-42nd-annual-report-2019/

70. Hattori M, Sako M, Kaneko T, Ashida A, Matsunaga A, Igarashi T, et al. End-stage renal disease in Japanese children: a nationwide survey during 2006–2011. Clin Exp Nephrol. 2015;19(5):933–8.

71. Al-Eisa AA, Samhan M, Naseef M. End-stage renal disease in Kuwaiti children: an 8-year experience. Transplant Proc. 2004;36(6):1788–91.

72. USRDS. United States Renal Data System, 2018 Annual Data Report: An overview of the epidemiology of kidney disease in the United States. Bethesda, MD: National Institutes of Health, National Institute of Diabetes and Digestive and Kidney Diseases; 2018.

73. Chesnaye N, Bonthuis M, Schaefer F, Groothoff JW, Verrina E, Heaf JG, et al. Demographics of paediatric renal replacement therapy in Europe: a report of the ESPN/ERA-EDTA registry. Pediatr Nephrol. 2014;29(12):2403–10.

74. van Stralen KJ, Tizard EJ, Jager KJ, Schaefer F, Vondrak K, Groothoff JW, et al. Determinants of eGFR at start of renal replacement therapy in paediatric patients. Nephrol Dial Transplant. 2010;25(10):3325–32.

75. White A, Wong W, Sureshkumar P, Singh G. The burden of kidney disease in indigenous children of Australia and New Zealand, epidemiology, antecedent factors and progression to chronic kidney disease. J Paediatr Child Health. 2010;46(9):504–9.

76. Lewis MA, Shaw J, Sinha MD, Adalat S, Hussain F, Castledine C, et al. UK Renal Registry 12th Annual Report (December 2009): chapter 14: demography of the UK paediatric renal replacement therapy population in 2008. Nephron Clin Pract. 2010;115(Suppl. 1):c279–88.

77. Hogan J, Ranchin B, Fila M, Harambat J, Krid S, Vrillon I, et al. Effect of center practices on the choice of the first dialysis modality for children and young adults. Pediatr Nephrol. 2017;32(4):659–67.

78. IPNA. IPNA Global Registry annual report. 2018. Available from: https://ipna-registry.org/fileadmin/reports/IPNA_Registry_Annual_Report_2018.pdf

79. Harambat J, Ekulu PM. Inequalities in access to pediatric ESRD care: a global health challenge. Pediatr Nephrol. 2016;31(3):353–8.

80. Jafar TH, Stark PC, Schmid CH, Landa M, Maschio G, de Jong PE, et al. Progression of chronic kidney disease: the role of blood pressure control, proteinuria, and angiotensin-converting enzyme inhibition: a patient-level meta-analysis. Ann Intern Med. 2003;139(4):244–52.

81. van der Heijden BJ, van Dijk PCW, Verrier-Jones K, Jager KJ, Briggs JD. Renal replacement therapy in children: data from 12 registries in Europe. Pediatr Nephrol. 2004;19(2):213–21.

82. Liyanage T, Ninomiya T, Jha V, Neal B, Patrice HM, Okpechi I, et al. Worldwide access to treatment for end-stage kidney disease: a systematic review. Lancet. 2015;385(9981):1975–82.

83. Global Burden of Disease. Global Burden of Disease [Internet]Available from: www.healthdata.org/gbd/2019.

84. Harambat J, van Stralen KJ, Schaefer F, Grenda R, Jankauskiene A, Kostic M, et al. Disparities in policies, practices and rates of pediatric kidney transplantation in Europe. Am J Transplant. 2013;13(8):2066–74.

85. Harambat J, van Stralen KJ, Verrina E, Groothoff JW, Schaefer F, Jager KJ, et al. Likelihood of children with end-stage kidney disease in Europe to live with a functioning kidney transplant is mainly explained by nonmedical factors. Pediatr Nephrol. 2014;29(3):453–9.

86. Calderon-Margalit R, Golan E, Twig G, Leiba A, Tzur D, Afek A, et al. History of childhood kidney disease and risk of adult end-stage renal disease. N Engl J Med. 2018;378(5):428–38.

Progression of Chronic Kidney Disease and Nephroprotective Therapy

55

Elke Wühl and Franz Schaefer

Progression of kidney malfunction towards end-stage kidney disease (ESKD) is common in patients with chronic kidney disease (CKD), and once significant impairment of kidney function has occurred CKD tends to progress almost irrespectively of the underlying kidney disorder.

It was first shown in the 1930s that removal of three quarters of the kidney mass in rats leads to progressive glomerulosclerosis and functional deterioration of the remaining nephrons [1]. The glomerular lesions of the remnant kidney were associated with abnormal glomerular permeability and proteinuria. At that time, proteinuria was considered a mere marker of the extent of glomerular damage, despite the findings of Volhard and Fahr in 1914 [2] and von Mollendorf and Stohr [3] in 1924 demonstrating that kidney damage was globally related to pathological amounts of protein excreted in the urine. In 1954 Oliver et al. recognized protein droplets in the cytoplasm of tubular cells. It was proposed that proteinuria could lead to structural and functional nephron damage [4]. In the late 1960s Brenner and coworkers described the pathophysiology of the adaptation processes to nephron loss in the rat remnant kidney model. They found that after removal of nephron mass, arteriolar resistance lowers and plasma flow increases in remnant glomeruli [5]. The tone of afferent arterioles was found to drop by a greater degree than those of the efferent arterioles, increasing glomerular capillary pressure and leading to increased filtration rate per nephron. Brenner also demonstrated that therapies attenuating these changes reduce decline of glomerular function and structural alterations.

Today, there is clear evidence from clinical studies that both hypertension and proteinuria are key players in the pathophysiology of CKD progression in humans [6–8]. The renin-angiotensin system is intrinsically involved in this process, and other potential contributors include genetic background, altered mineral homeostasis, dyslipidemia, renal anemia, inflammation and oxidative stress as well as general cardiovascular risk factors such as obesity, smoking and diabetes. The phenomenon of kidney failure progression following kidney injury or maldevelopment is a current focus of research in adults and children.

This chapter summarizes the current state of knowledge regarding the pathophysiology of kidney disease progression and discusses the evidence base of renoprotective strategies in pediatric CKD.

E. Wühl (✉) · F. Schaefer
Division of Pediatric Nephrology, Center for Pediatrics and Adolescent Medicine, University of Heidelberg, Heidelberg, Germany
e-mail: elke.wuehl@med.uni-heidelberg.de; franz.schaefer@med.uni-heidelberg.de

Natural Course of Chronic Kidney Disease Progression in Children

Information on the natural course of CKD progression in children is still limited. The prospective, population-based ItalKid registry was started in 1990 and over the first 10 years 1197 children with various kidney disorders were registered, including 23% suffering from severe impairment of kidney function [9]. The incidence of kidney replacement therapy (KRT) was 7.3% per year with a 68% cumulative risk of developing CKD Stage 5 by age 20. The decline of kidney function was not linear, but rather characterized by a sharp decline during and after puberty. The probability of kidney survival decreased with lower glomerular filtration rate (GFR) at baseline. This finding supports the general clinical impression that in many children with hypodysplasia of the kidneys, the deterioration of kidney function accelerates around the time of puberty. However, it is still speculative whether this may be due to an increasing discrepancy between body size and functional nephron mass or whether the emerging production of sex steroid hormones at this age may influence kidney survival.

In a retrospective analysis of 176 patients with hypodysplasia of the kidneys, it was suggested that the natural course of kidney function in patients with congenitally reduced renal mass can be divided into three periods: an initial 'hypertrophy' phase characterized by improving kidney function (+6.3 mL/year on average during the first 3 years of life), a subsequent period of stable kidney function attained by 50% of the patients and lasting for a mean of 8 years, and a pattern of kidney function gradually deteriorating towards CKD Stage 5 (Fig. 55.1) [10]. The progression phase started just after infancy in 48% and around puberty in 23%. In 30% of patients kidney function remained stable even beyond puberty. Correlates of deteriorating kidney function were proteinuria, hypertension, past febrile urinary tract infections and lower GFR at onset [10].

An accelerated decline of kidney function was observed during the last 18 months before start of KRT in the Chronic Kidney Disease in Children (CKiD) cohort [11].

In an analysis of 4700 patients with congenital anomalies of the kidneys and the urinary tract followed in the ERA-EDTA Registry, more than two thirds of the patients attained ESKD at adult

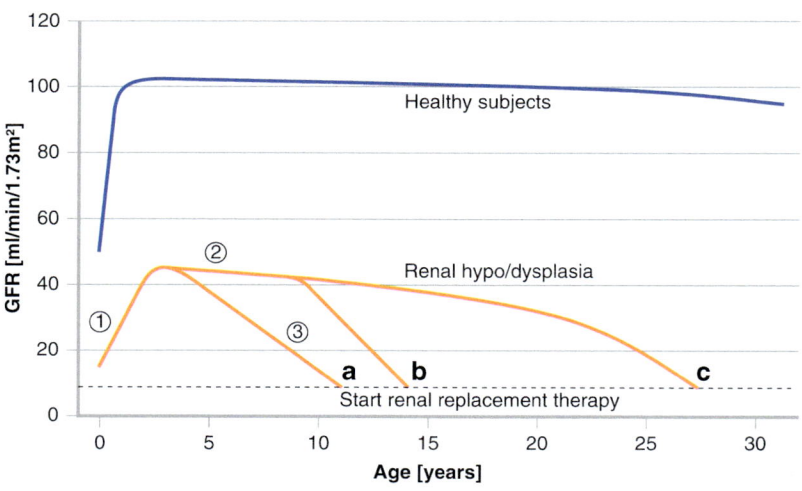

Fig. 55.1 Natural time course of kidney disease progression in children with renal hypodysplasia. ① denotes period of improving kidney function during infancy, ② period of stable kidney function, ③ period of kidney func-

tion deteriorating toward ESKD. Third phase is characterized either by rapid decline soon after infancy (**a**) or at early pubertal age (**b**), or by steady slow decline of renal function (**c**). Modified from Celedon et al. [10]

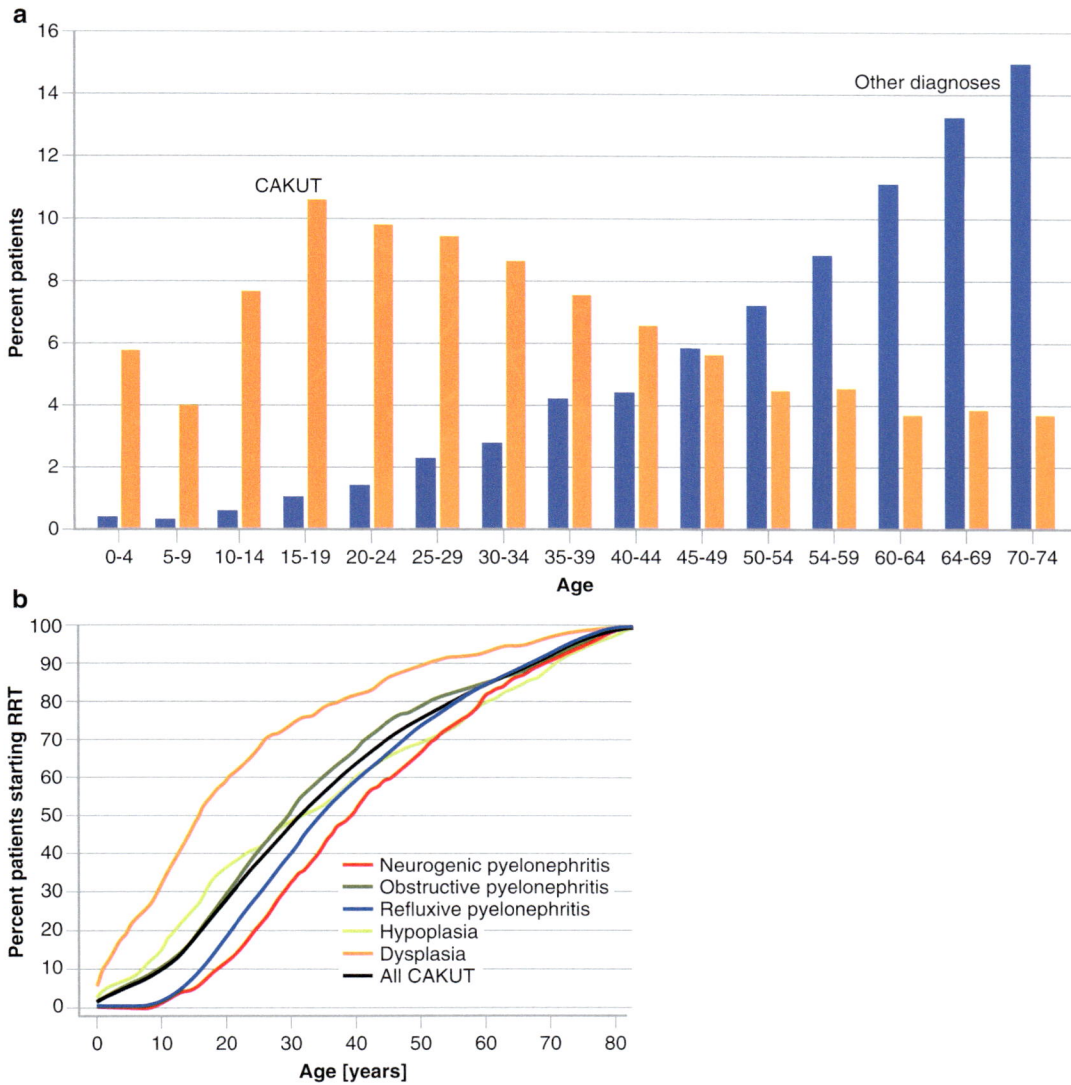

Fig. 55.2 Age distribution at onset of kidney replacement therapy in patients with congenital anomalies of the kidneys and the urinary tract (CAKUT) compared with non-CAKUT patients (**a**) and cumulative percentage of patients starting kidney replacement therapy by CAKUT subcategory (**b**). Data from the European Renal Association – European Dialysis and Transplant Association Registry. Used with permission of American Society of Nephrology from Wühl et al. [12]

age. The mean age at start of kidney replacement therapy was 34 years [12] (Fig. 55.2a, b). These findings support the concept that in patients with a congenital reduction in nephron mass, CKD progression due to ongoing loss of remnant nephrons is a lifelong process.

Mechanisms of Kidney Failure Progression

According to the Brenner hypothesis, any critical loss of functioning kidney mass, irrespective of the nature of the initial injury, leads to glomerular

Fig. 55.3 Mechanisms of kidney disease progression in pediatric nephropathies

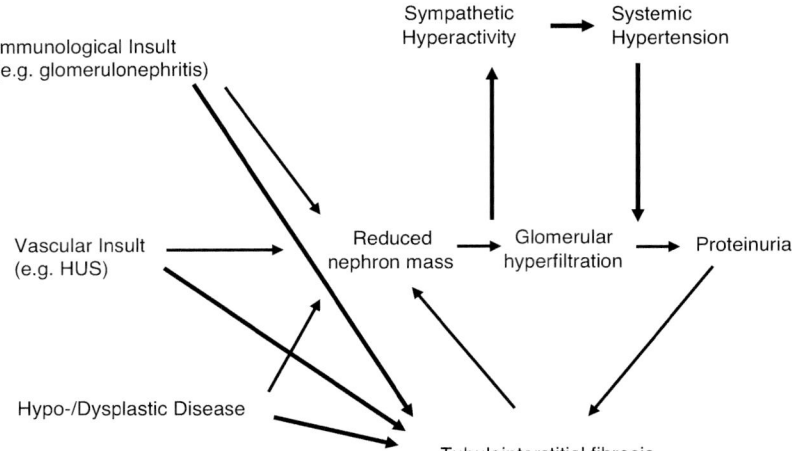

hyperfiltration with an increased single-nephron GFR (Fig. 55.3). The remaining nephrons lose their ability to autoregulate glomerular pressure, resulting in transmission of systemic hypertension to the glomerulus. Increased intraglomerular pressure induces proteinuria, which is the pathophysiological link between glomerular, interstitial [13] and tubular damage [14]. The degree of proteinuria in glomerular diseases correlates with the rate of CKD progression [15].

Recent research has attributed a central role to the podocytes, which are terminally differentiated and unable to respond to injury by proliferation and repair [16]. The key role of this glomerular cell type in the pathophysiology of CKD progression has been demonstrated by a growing number of specific genetic disorders specifically affecting the development, terminal differentiation and postnatal function of the podocytes, which result in congenital or infantile nephrotic syndrome inevitably leading to glomerulosclerosis and progressive kidney failure. The loss of lesioned podocytes may lead to focal and segmental adhesions of the denuded basement membrane to the Bowman capsule, with spreading of the ultrafiltrate into the tubulointerstitial compartment where it causes inflammatory injury ('misdirected filtration').

The formation and maintenance of the glomerular filtration barrier requires a complex interaction between podocytes and glomerular capillary endothelial cells. Vascular endothelial

growth factor (VEGF) overexpression by podocytes has been noted in proteinuric states, and VEGF blocking antibodies prevent glomerular hyperfiltration, hypertrophy and proteinuria. Endothelial cell injury, resulting from disease-specific and/or from non-specific uremia-associated vasculotoxic and inflammatory insults, is frequently involved in progressive glomerular damage [17]. Vascular endothelial cells release endothelin, platelet derived growth factor (PDGF) and fibroblast growth factor (FGF) in response to fluid shear stress [18]. Moreover, injured endothelial cells express increased angiotensinogen and transforming growth factor β (TGFβ) [19], factors causing inflammation and fibrosis. In chronic glomerular injury, endothelial cells lose part of their anti-coagulant properties and intensify their pro-coagulant activity by increased expression of plasminogen activator inhibitor 1 (PAI-1). By release of adhesion molecules such as intracellular adhesion molecule 1 (ICAM-1), endothelial cells facilitate macrophage infiltration and attraction and proliferation of inflammatory cells. In addition, damage to endothelial cells may denude the glomerular basement membrane, all resulting in induction of local platelet aggregation and activation of coagulation with fibrin deposition and microthrombi formation.

Reabsorption of filtered proteins by the tubular epithelial cells can induce direct injury to intracellular lysosomal pathways, oxidative stress and increased local expression of growth factors [20, 21] such as insulin-like growth factor 1 (IGF-1), TGFβ and hepatocyte growth factor (HGF). Moreover, stressed epithelial cells release an array of chemotactic factors including monocyte chemoattractant protein 1 (MCP-1), RANTES, connective tissue growth factor (CTGF), fibronectin and endothelin-1 (ET-1), which promote tubulointerstitial inflammation and fibrosis through recruitment and activation of macrophages [22–28]. Macrophages infiltrating the renal parenchyma in turn perpetuate the production of further cytokines and growth factors. The proteins of the complement system represent another component of proteinuria that may cause tubular damage, and once tubular cells are injured, they may vice versa activate the alternative complement pathway.

Both in the glomerulus and in the tubular apparatus, chronic inflammatory processes promote cell transdifferentiation towards a fibroblast phenotype, driven by a high tone of TGF-ß (epithelial mesenchymal transformation; EMT). Myofibroblastic transformation is characterized by the release of proteinases, cytokines and oxidants [29, 30]. Moreover, myofibroblasts and local fibroblasts begin to deposit fibronectin and laminin, the molecular framework for interstitial collagen deposition [31], and secrete extracellular matrix components including type IV collagen and collagens I, III, and V ('scar' collagens) resulting in scar formation [32]. In addition, the activity of matrix degrading enzymes is inhibited by overproduction of inhibitory peptides (PAI-1, tissue inhibitors of metalloproteinases (TIMPs)) [33, 34]. As a result of increased synthesis and reduced degradation, excessive tubulointerstitial collagen accumulation occurs. The fibrous masses in the tubulointerstitium are believed to compromise oxygen supply to the tubular cells, thereby further contributing to tubular atrophy and nephron loss.

Glomerular sclerosis, tubulointerstitial fibrosis and tubular atrophy result in a further loss of functioning renal mass, closing a vicious circle by further increasing intraglomerular pressure and hypertrophy of the remaining glomeruli (Figs. 55.3 and 55.4).

Angiotensin (Ang) II, the primary effector of the renin angiotensin system, is mechanistically involved in most of the mechanisms described above. Ang II is produced both systemically and locally in the kidney and exerts multiple endocrine, intercrine, autocrine and paracrine effects. Intrarenal Ang II concentrations are a thousand-fold higher than in the circulation. The major source of intrarenal Ang II is auto/paracrine synthesis by tubular, juxtaglomerular and glomerular cells [35–37]. Renin release from the juxtaglomerular apparatus drives systemic Ang II generation and is involved in blood pressure upregulation, but has probably little relevance for intrarenal Ang II action. Most of the intrarenal effects of Ang II are mediated via the Angiotensin II type 1 (AT1) receptor [38]. Ang II is a potent vasoconstrictor that augments intraglomerular pressure by preferentially increasing the efferent arteriolar tone. Ang II also increases intracellular calcium in podocytes [39, 40], inducing cytoskeletal changes and altered podocyte function with resultant protein ultrafiltration even in the absence of structural glomerular damage [41, 42]. Moreover, Ang II increases the proliferation of smooth muscle cells and increases the glomerular and tubular expression of various growth factors, cytokines and chemokines, most importantly of the TGF-β/CTGF system, but also of tumor necrosis factor α (TNFα), PDGF, FGF and vascular cell adhesion molecule 1 (VCAM-1).

Ang II also stimulates oxidative stress, which perpetuates the up-regulation of cytokines, adhesion molecules, and chemoattractants [43, 44]. Finally, intrarenal Ang II stimulates afferent neurons, which are believed to activate central nervous structures regulating sympathetic tone. Hence, Ang II is pathophysiologically involved in the state of sympathetic hyperactivation which is characteristic of CKD and constitutes another important mechanism of renal disease progression and cardiovascular morbidity [45, 46].

In addition, uremia-induced deficiency of nuclear factor erythroid 2-related factor 2 (Nrf2), a transcription factor for the antioxidative stress response and activator of an array of cytoprotective genes, may enhance the susceptibility to kidney injury [47, 48].

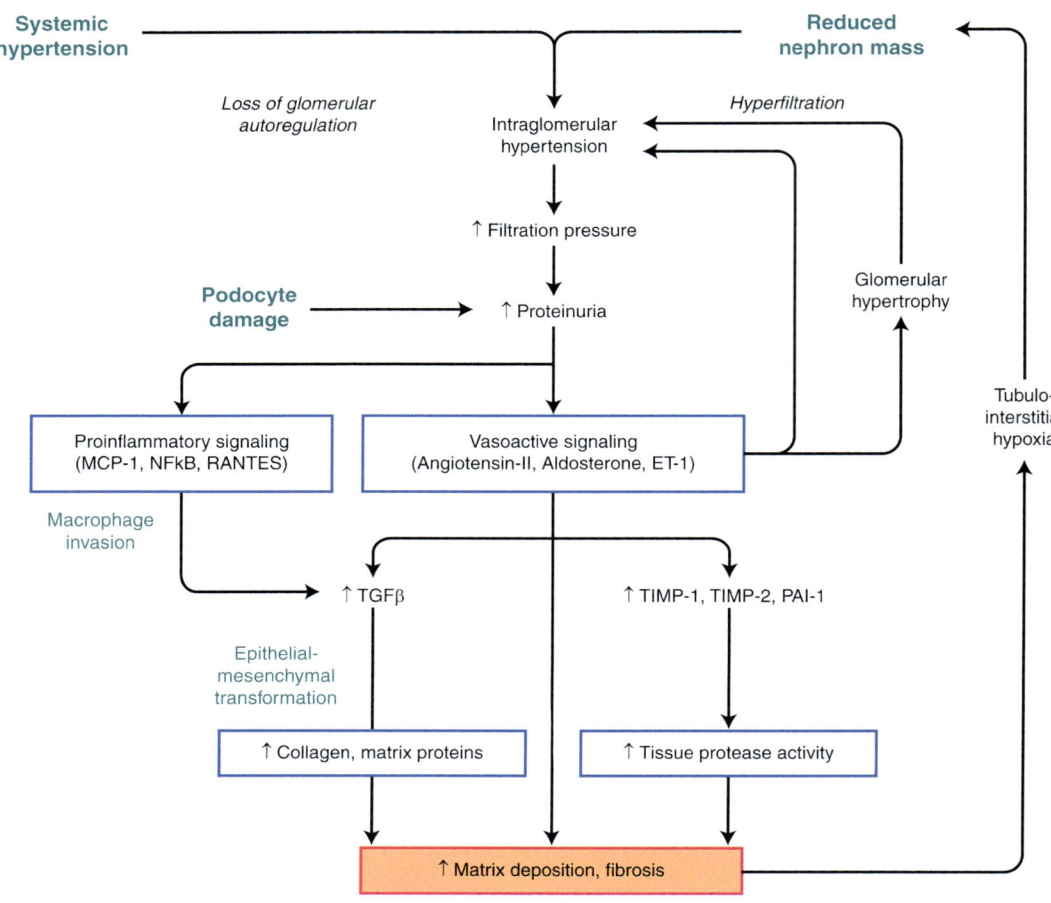

Fig. 55.4 Pathophysiological consequences of hypertension and proteinuria in chronic kidney disease

In patients with reduced nephron mass and anemia, hypoxia of tubular cells may occur due to increased oxygen consumption by tubular cells of the remaining nephrons, a decreased number of interstitial capillaries [49] and accumulation of extracellular matrix between interstitial capillaries and tubular cells, which hampers oxygen diffusion. In turn, hypoxia stimulates the production of profibrotic molecules such as TGFβ and ET-1 by tubular cells, further increasing the synthesis of extracellular matrix by fibroblastic cells and ultimately leads to tubular epithelial cell loss with formation of atubular glomeruli [50, 51].

In addition, hypoxia enhances the local production of reactive oxygen species (ROS). Oxidative stress also induces the release of pro-inflammatory and pro-fibrotic molecules, thereby enhancing the production of extracellular matrix by fibroblasts and favoring cell death.

Factors Modifying the Risk of Kidney Disease Progression

Age at Attainment of Kidney Mass Deficit

The age at which a significant loss of kidney mass occurs may influence the degree of glomerular hypertrophy and the long-term prognosis of kidney function. Patients born with unilateral kidney agenesis are at greater risk for proteinuria, hypertension and CKD than subjects undergoing unilateral nephrectomy by trauma or kidney donation in later life, suggesting that the number of functional nephrons in congenital solitary kidneys might be decreased (possibly by hypogenesis) [52, 53].

Most patients with a solitary functioning kidney experience compensatory kidney growth of the remnant kidney. After unilateral nephrectomy for Wilms' tumor, compensatory renal growth was most marked in patients who underwent surgery at very young age. Marked kidney growth was associated with microalbuminuria in more than 30% of these patients [54]. The possibility that nephrons in infantile solitary kidneys are subject to greater hypertrophic stress is supported by quantitative morphometric studies showing glomerular volumes 5–6 times greater than normal [55].

However, most long-term follow-up studies of congenital solitary kidneys included heterogeneous patient populations. Of note, patients with a congenital solitary kidney due to unilateral multicystic-dysplastic kidney disease (MCDKD) appear to have better functional outcomes over time than patients with unilateral kidney agenesis. In the long-term follow-up study by Sanna-Cherchi, 5% of MCDKD cases but 30% of unilateral kidney agenesis cases required dialysis after their second decade of life (HR 2.43) [53]. In addition, MCDKD patients had a lower prevalence of hypertension (3% vs. 19%) and proteinuria (3% vs. 12%) than patients with unilateral kidney agenesis [56]. It is tempting to speculate that the natural history differences observed with these single-kidney disorders may be related to different underlying pathogenic mechanisms variably affecting the long-term function of the remaining kidney.

Gender

Among adult patients with CKD, women have a higher overall prevalence of pre-dialysis CKD than men, possibly due to the longer life expectancy of women and to CKD overdiagnosis by use of estimated GFR equations. However, decline of kidney function in men is faster, maybe due to unhealthier lifestyles and hormonal differ-

ences, resulting in a higher rate of kidney replacement therapy in men [57].

A kidney survival advantage of females has been suggested by meta-analysis of patient cohorts with autosomal dominant polycystic kidney disease (ADPKD), IgA nephropathy and membranous nephropathy [58]. The advantage seems to be lost in post-menopausal women, suggesting a nephroprotective effect of female sex steroids; however, some confounding by lipid levels or the prevalence of smoking cannot be ruled out. In addition, at all levels of pre-dialysis CKD mortality is higher among men, whereas mortality on KRT is similar for men and women.

Data on a potential sexual dimorphism of kidney survival in children with CKD are scarce. A recent analysis of data from the CKiD Study was able to identify different trajectories of CKD progression in children. However, while females with glomerulopathies showed faster CKD progression than males, no significant sex differences were found in patients with non-glomerular disease. The differences in progression seem likely explained by sex differences in the underlying primary kidney disease and in baseline GFR rather than by a direct effect of sex on progression [59].

Underlying Kidney Disease and Genetic Pathology

Although the pathophysiological principles of CKD progression described above generally apply to all chronic kidney diseases, the time course of deterioration of kidney function for individual disease entities is highly variable. It is evident that patients with aggressive, incompletely controlled immunological nephropathies will have a more rapid progression of CKD than subjects with hypoplasia of the kidneys. However, even within groups of patients suffering from pathogenetically homogeneous hereditary kidney diseases, the rate of CKD progression can vary markedly between individuals. In a growing number of these entities, the progression phenotype can be linked to the underlying genetic defect. In disease entities caused by defects in more than one gene, progression patterns may differ according to the gene involved. For instance, in adults with ADPKD, individuals with mutations in the PKD1 typically have a more severe disease course with earlier need for renal replacement therapy than those with mutations in the PKD2 gene. A gene-phenotype correlation is also obvious in children with the nephronophthisis complex. In children with mutations in the NPHP1 gene, CKD stage 5 is attained at a mean age of 13 years, compared to 8 months in NPHP2 and 19 years in NPHP3 mutation carriers [60]. Even within the same gene, the localization and type of the causative mutations is a key determinant of the renal prognosis. The highly variable times of disease onset and progression to ESKD in steroid resistant nephrotic syndrome caused by different mutations in the NPHS2 gene [61], and in Alport syndrome related to COL4A5 gene mutations [62] are classic examples for genotype-phenotype correlations in recessive and dominant forms of hereditary kidney disorders.

In addition to the causative role of genetic disorders in many if not most pediatric kidney diseases, common polymorphic variants in various genes may determine an individual's susceptibility for kidney injury, kidney disease progression and the response to renoprotective treatment. One of the first common variants studied in the context of CKD progression was the insertion/deletion polymorphism of the angiotensin converting enzyme (ACE) gene. The DD genotype has been shown to predispose for progressive renal failure in IgA nephropathy [63, 64]. Some, though not all studies, found an increased risk for parenchymal damage with the DD genotype in children with congenital urological abnormalities, particularly vesicoureteral reflux [65–67] and an increased risk for poor kidney survival in children with CKD due to kidney hypodysplasia [65].

In adults with non-diabetic proteinuric kidney diseases, the ACE polymorphism has been claimed to predict the nephroprotective efficacy of ACE inhibition. Proteinuria, the rate of GFR decline and progression to CKD stage 5 were lowered by ACE inhibitors in patients with the DD genotype, but not in those with the II or ID genotype [68, 69].

Also, common variants exist in various genes encoding cytokines, growth factors and regulatory peptides involved in CKD progression.

Recent and ongoing meta-analyses of genome-wide association studies (GWAS) are aiming to identify loci associated with incident CKD or the risk of KRT in general population based cohorts [70, 71], as well as in cohorts of adult and pediatric CKD patients [72]. An increasing number of common risk variants in genes related to nephrogenesis (e.g. *ALMS1*, *VEGFA*, *DACH*), glomerular filtration barrier formation and podocytes function (e.g. *DAB2*, *PARD3B*, *VEGFA*), angiogenesis (e.g. *VEGFA*), and renal function (e.g. *UMOD*, *SHROOM3*, *STC1*) have been identified [71]. For example, common variants in the region of the *UMOD* gene encoding uromodulin (Tamm-Horsfall protein) associate with CKD and GFR. Elevated urine uromodulin concentrations, which are associated with a common polymorphism in the *UMOD* region, precede the onset of CKD [73].

Genome-wide association studies may also allow identification of variants related to known CKD risk factors as hypertension or proteinuria in adults [74–76] as well as in children [77].

Epigenetics and Fetal Programming

Fetal programming describes the effect of environmental cues experienced during fetal development on an individual's susceptibility to diseases later in life through epigenetic changes that may be additionally modified postnatally.

Fetal programming may have direct consequences on kidney development and function. Barker and colleagues first demonstrated a correlation of low birth weight with the incidence of cardiovascular disease (CVD) in later adulthood [78]. Subsequent studies suggested that low birth weight is correlated with decreased kidney mass and nephron number, which in turn predisposes to adult hypertension [79]. In line with these findings, a recent study in more than 400 Japanese children born with very low birth weight showed a significant contribution of intrauterine malnutrition to chronic kidney damage [80]. Conversely, higher estimated weights in utero, at birth and at 6 months post-gestational age were found to be associated with higher kidney volume and higher GFR at age 6–7 years [81].

Thus, in interaction with an existing congenital or acquired kidney disease, prenatal programming by epigenetic mechanisms may influence the course of CKD progression [82].

Hypertension

Hypertension is an independent risk factor for renal failure progression in adults [6–8]. While the degree of hypertension is a marker of the underlying renal disease severity, interventional studies have provided evidence that high blood pressure actively contributes to renal failure progression in human CKD. This has been confirmed by hypertension registry data of more than 40,000 adult patients demonstrating an association of systolic blood pressure with incident CKD. Each 10 mmHg increase of baseline or time-varying systolic blood pressure above 120 mmHg was associated with a 6% increase in the risk of developing CKD [83].

In pediatric nephropathies, renal hypertension is common, although typically less severe than in adult kidney disorders. Hypertension prevalence estimates in children with CKD range from 20% to 80%, depending on the degree of renal dysfunction [84]. However, even children with CKD stage 2 or renal hypodysplasia, conditions usually not strongly associated with hypertension, may present with elevated blood pressure [85]. In a large prospective study of children with CKD, systolic blood pressure greater than 120 mmHg has been associated with a faster GFR decline [86] (Fig. 55.5). Among CKD children included in the CKiD Study, time-varying blood pressure $\geq$ 90th percentile (compared to <50th percentile) was associated with an odds ratio of 3.75 in non-glomerular and of 5.96 in glomerular disease for the risk of losing 50% of GFR or progressing to ESKD [87].

Investigations on the physiological diurnal variation of blood pressure by ambulatory blood pressure monitoring have revealed that the integrity of the nocturnal fall of blood pressure ('dipping' pattern) plays a significant role in renal failure progression, in addition to and independent of the absolute blood pressure level.

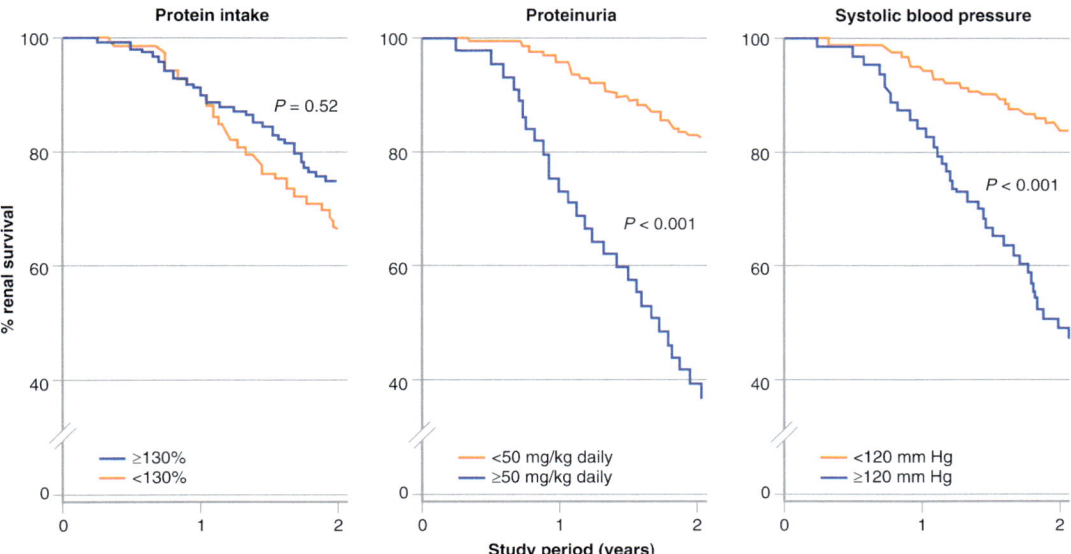

Fig. 55.5 Proteinuria and Hypertension predict the risk of disease progression in children with CKD. Used with permission of Elsevier from Wingen et al. [86]

Non-dipping, a well-known independent cardio-vascular risk factor and common characteristic of renoparenchymal hypertension, is associated with more rapid progression towards kidney failure in adult CKD patients [88–91].

Similarly, elevated night-time blood pressure is correlated with an increased risk of CKD in the general population [92] and with a faster decline of GFR in CKD patients [93]. Overactivation of the sympathetic nervous system and endothelial dysfunction may contribute to the dysregulation of nocturnal blood pressure and circadian pattern [89].

Proteinuria

Population based studies in healthy individuals have demonstrated that proteinuria is an independent risk factor for CKD, KRT and overall mortality [94–96]. In adults with diabetic and non-diabetic kidney disorders, proteinuria is clearly predictive of the renal prognosis [15, 97, 98]. In the Ramipril Efficacy in Nephropathy (REIN) trial [99], urinary protein excretion was the only baseline variable correlated with GFR decline and progression to KRT.

In children, the spectrum of underlying kidney disorders markedly differs from adults. Congenital renal hypodysplasia with or without urinary tract abnormalities is the leading underlying pediatric kidney disorder, accounting for more than 60% of CKD cases. The European Study Group for Nutritional Treatment of Chronic Renal Failure in Childhood first demonstrated in 200 children with CKD stages 3–4 that proteinuria and hypertension are also major predictors of GFR decline in pediatric kidney disease [86] (Fig. 55.5). The ItalKid Project confirmed that proteinuria predicts renal disease progression in children with renal hypodysplasia [100]. In the ESCAPE (Effect of Strict Blood Pressure Control and ACE Inhibition on Progression of Chronic Renal Failure in Pediatric Patients) trial, baseline proteinuria and residual proteinuria during ACE inhibition were quantitatively associated with CKD progression [101, 102].

In a joint analysis of 1200 children with CKD stages 2–4 from the CKiD Study and the ESCAPE Trial, patients with glomerular disease showed a 43% shorter time to ESKD or 50% GFR loss than children with non-glomerular disease [103]. The average time to reach this endpoint was more than 10 years in non-proteinuric children with mild to moderate CKD as compared to 1.3 years in those with CKD stage 4 and nephrotic range proteinuria [103] (Fig. 55.6).

Metabolic Acidosis

In the Cardiovascular Comorbidity in Children with CKD Study (4C Study), pediatric patients with CKD stage 3–5 with time-averaged serum bicarbonate below 18 mmol/l had a significantly higher risk of CKD progression compared to those with a serum bicarbonate of 22 mmol/L or more [104]. These findings are in keeping with findings in interventional trials in adult CKD patients suggesting that *metabolic acidosis* is associated with faster decline in eGFR [105–107] (Table 55.1).

Dyslipidemia and Insulin Resistance

Abnormalities of lipid metabolism are a common complication in CKD. In the CKiD Study, 45% of children had *dyslipidemia*, with an increased risk in children with GFR < 30. Obese and overweight children in the cohort had significantly higher odds ratios of having dyslipidemia, with the highest risk in the most obese subjects. Dyslipidemia was also independently associated with nephrotic–range proteinuria. [108].

Epidemiological studies give some evidence that dyslipidemia is an independent risk factor not only for CVD but also for progressive chronic renal failure [109]. The dyslipidemic pattern differs between the major renal disease entities [110] and the degree of dyslipidemia parallels the degree of renal function impairment. Underlying mechanisms of uremic dyslipidemia include insulin resistance [111], obesity, hyperparathyroidism [112], malnutrition, acidosis [113] and impaired catabolism of triglyceride-rich lipoproteins by decreased activity of lipoprotein lipase and hepatic triglyceride lipase.

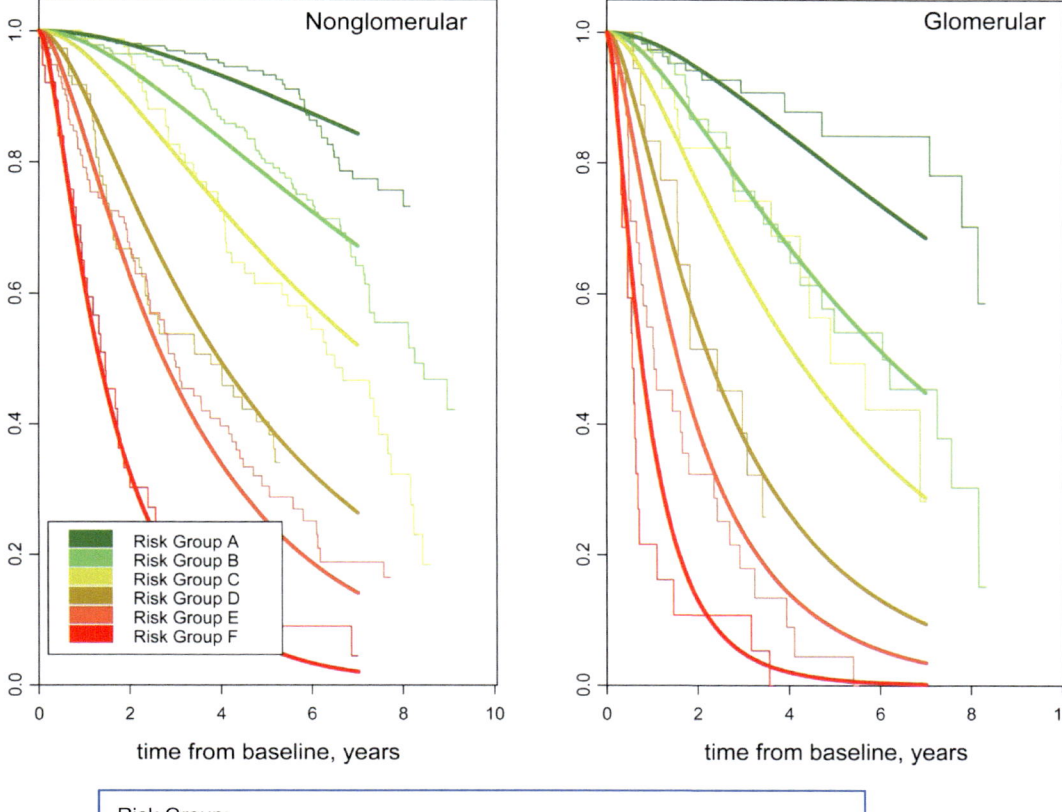

Risk Group:

A – CKD stage I to IIIa and UPCR < 0.5;

B – CKD stage IIIb and UPCR < 0.5 *or* CKD stage II to IIIa and UPCR 0.5 to 2;

C – CKD stage IIIb and UPCR 0.5 to 2 *or* CKD stage II and UPCR > 2;

D – CKD stage IV and UPCR < 0.5 *or* CKD stage IIIa and UPCR > 2;

E - CKD stage IV and UPCR 0.5 to 2 *or* CKD stage IIIb and UPCR > 2;

F - CKD stage IV and UPCR > 2.

Fig. 55.6 Survival curves for the time from assessment of CKD (baseline) to a composite clinical event (50% GFR decline, kidney replacement therapy, or GFR less than 15 mL/min/1.73 m^2) stratified by CKD diagnosis and risk group. Used with permission of Elsevier from Furth [103])

In animal models, hypercholesterolemia accelerates the rate of progression of kidney disease [114]. A link between dyslipidemia and oxidative stress in the pathogenesis of renal damage was shown in unilaterally nephrectomized rats, in which hyperlipidemia increased glomerular and tubulointerstitial infiltration and aggravated glomerulosclerosis [115].

There are also observations in humans that the *insulin resistance syndrome* may underlie or mediate the association between lipids and loss of renal function. A strong relationship between the *metabolic syndrome* and the risk for CKD and microalbuminuria was found in a large, adult, non-diabetic general population [116]. A relationship between serum cholesterol and GFR decline was also shown in adult patients with type 1 diabetes and overt nephropathy [117]; patients with a total cholesterol level > 7 mmol/L showed an at least three times faster decline in GFR than subjects with lower cholesterol levels.

Table 55.1 Potential therapeutic strategies for prevention of kidney disease progression

Therapeutic target	Agents	Action	Treatment aim
Renin-angiotensin-aldosterone system	ACE inhibitors Angiotensin receptor blockers Aldosterone antagonists Renin inhibitors	RAAS blockade: antiproteinuric, antihypertensive, anti-fibrotic, and anti-inflammatory effects	Blood pressure control Reduction of proteinuria Attenuation of glomerular sclerosis and tubulointerstitial fibrosis
Hypertension	All antihypertensive drug classes	Antihypertensive Additional antiproteinuric effect by blood pressure control	Strict blood pressure control [101, 135, 136, 239, 240]: – BP target <75th Pct in non-proteinuric children – BP target <50th Pct in proteinuric children
Proteinuria	ACE inhibitors, some CCBs (non-dihydropyridines) and ß-blockers (e.g., carvedilol)	Antiproteinuric	Minimization of proteinuria: urinary protein excretion <300 mg/m^2/d [143, 144]
Metabolic acidosis	Bicarbonate	Renoprotective	Serum bicarbonate level > 22 mmol/L [107]
Inflammation	e.g., Endothelin A receptor antagonist, Pentoxifylline, Neprilysin, bardoxolone	Anti-inflammatory and antifibrotic action	Reduction of inflammation and fibrosis, attenuation of glomerular sclerosis and tubulointerstitial fibrosis
Dyslipidemia	Statins	Lipid lowering	Normalization of lipid profile
Anemia	Erythropoietin	Improved oxygen supply, reduced oxidative stress, direct protective effects	Normalization of hemoglobin levels
Mineral metabolism, Hyperparathyroidism	Phosphate binders (Calcium-free) Vitamin D Calcimimetics	Renoprotective Anti-fibrotic (vitamin D) Reduction of proteinuria, blood pressure, glomerular sclerosis (calcimimetics)	Calcium, phosphate, PTH and vitamin D levels within target range for CKD patients [241]
Hyperuricemia	Allopurinol	Renoprotective	Normalization of serum uric acid levels [229]
Renal disease progression	Low Protein Diet (0.8–1.1 g/kg/d)	Reduction of serum urea levels	Reduction of serum urea levels, delay of end-stage renal disease

RAAS renin-angiotensin-aldosterone-system, *ACE* angiotensin converting enzyme, *ACEi* ACE inhibitor, *ARBs* angiotensin receptor blockers, *CCBs* Calcium channel blockers, *BP* blood pressure, *Pct* percentile, *CKD* chronic kidney disease

Additionally, *obesity* appears to be a negative prognostic factor for both diabetic and non-diabetic nephropathies and an independent risk factor for accelerated progression [118, 119]. As adipose tissue generates high levels of circulating free fatty acids (FFA) and FFA uptake and oxidation in CKD are reduced by hypoadiponectinemia, leptin resistance, and increased cytokine release from adipose tissue and macrophages, intracellular FFA accumulate [120]. This may cause renal mesangial and epithelial cell injury and renal disease progression as a consequence of FFA-induced lipotoxicity.

However, the evidence for dyslipidemia as an independent risk factor for renal disease development and/or progression is not as strong in clinical studies as it is in experimental settings. It is unclear whether dyslipidemia independently increases the renal risk in those without other risk factors for kidney disease because most studies have been performed in patients with pre-existing renal disease or patients with associated renal risk factors such as hypertension or diabetes.

Hyperuricemia

Data regarding the role of hyperuricemia in the progression of CKD are conflicting. While in the Modification of Diet in Renal Disease (MDRD) study [121] a single elevated uric acid level was not predictive of future kidney failure in adults, a retrospective cohort study from Taiwan suggested that higher uric acid levels are associated with a more rapid eGFR decline and higher risk of kidney failure, particularly in patients without proteinuria [122]. In line with the latter findings, data from the CKiD Study indicated that hyperuricemia may also be an independent risk factor for faster CKD progression in children and adolescents [123].

Bone Metabolism

Disturbances of the *bone mineral metabolism* also may influence CKD progression. Phosphorus accumulation [124], elevated serum alkaline phosphatase [125] and low 25-hydroxyvitamin D levels are associated with progression, potentially via their relation to fibroblast growth factor 23 (FGF23), which has been identified as an independent risk factor for CKD progression in adults and children [126].

Environmental Factors

Additionally, environmental effects may affect progression of CKD, such as exposure to *smoking*. Smoking has been associated with an increased risk of renal disease progression in adults [127]. In the CKiD cohort, second hand smoking exposure was independently associated with nephrotic range proteinuria [128].

Treatment Strategies in Kidney Disease Progression

Based on the current understanding of the mechanisms of kidney disease progression, several principal nephroprotective strategies have emerged in recent years. These are based mainly on clinical evidence established in adult patients, but growing evidence also supports their efficacy in children. Efficient control of blood pressure and minimization of proteinuria are the two most important measures to preserve residual kidney function. Other approaches, such as the prevention and treatment of CKD-associated anemia, dyslipidemia and mineral metabolism disorder, have an experimental basis whereas their clinical importance is still less clear. The level of clinical evidence in support of the various nephroprotective strategies will be discussed below and is summarized in Table 55.2.

Blood Pressure Control

Numerous studies in adults have shown that antihypertensive therapy slows the rate of kidney failure progression [129]. There seems to be a linear relationship between the blood pressure level achieved by antihypertensive treatment and the rate of annualized GFR decline in CKD patients [129]. This relationship appears to persist well into the normal range of blood pressure [15, 130], although interventional trials comparing different blood pressure targets yielded somewhat conflicting results.

In children with CKD, the ESCAPE Trial provided evidence that intensified blood pressure control targeting for a 24-h mean arterial pressure below the 50th percentile provides superior long-term nephroprotection compared to a higher target range (50th to 95th percentile) [101]. In this randomized clinical trial, the ACE inhibitor ramipril was administered at a fixed dose in 385 children with CKD. Subsequently, the patients were randomized for conventional or intensified blood pressure control to be achieved by administration of additional antihypertensive drugs not affecting the renin-angiotensin-aldosterone system (RAAS). Within 5 years of observation, the risk of losing 50% of eGFR or progressing to KRT was reduced by 35% (from 42.7 to 29.9%) in the strict blood pressure control arm [101] (Fig. 55.7).

Intensified blood pressure control effectively improved kidney survival in children with an

Table 55.2 Evidence levels for efficacy of nephroprotective treatment strategies in adults and children with CKD

Renoprotective treatment	Evidence in adults	Evidence in children	Effect of Intervention	Drugs licensed for … in ….
Antihypertensive treatment (RAAS blockade/CCBs/ß-Blockers)/Strict BP control	Multiple RCTS, meta-analyses	One RCT; few observational studies	+ BP control reduces risk of CKD; evidence for beneficial effect of strict BP control especially in proteinuric CKD	Hypertension in adults and children
RAAS blockade – antihypertensive + antiproteinuric treatment				
ACEi/ARBs	RCTs	RCTs	++ Antihypertensive + antiproteinuric	Hypertension in adults and children
Aldosterone antagonists	RCTs	RCT underway (finerenone)	+ Antihypertensive + antiproteinuric, reduced risk of CKD (finerenone)	Spironolactone: hyperaldosteronism in adults and children; eplerenone: left ventricular dysfunction in adults; Finerenone: diabetic and non-diabetic CKD in adults
Renin antagonists	RCT	None	+ Antihypertensive + antiproteinuric	Hypertension in adults
Combined RAAS blockade (ACEi + ARB or ACEi/ARB + aldosterone / renin antagonist)	RCTs	None	+ Antihypertensive + antiproteinuric; increased risk of side effects, combined RAAS blockade not recommended	NA
SGLT2 inhibitors	RCTs	None	++ Antihypertensive, antiproteinuric, anti-inflammatory, reduction of CKD progression rate	Diabetic / non-diabetic CKD in adults
Bicarbonate	RCTs	Observational studies	+ Reduced risk of CKD progression	Metabolic acidosis
Tolvaptan (in ADPKD)	RCTs	RCT	+ Retardation of cyst growth and CKD progression	Progressive ADPKD in adults
Antihypertensive chronotherapy	RCTs	None	+? Nephroprotective effects reported, but quality of studies questioned	NA
Anti-inflammatory agents				
Endothelin receptor antagonists	RCTs	RCT underway (sparsentan)	+? Antihypertensive + antiproteinuric, but unfavourable side effect profile for some compounds	Sparsentan: FSGS in adults

(continued)

Therapy					
Bardoxolone	RCTs	None	+?	Inconclusive findings	Not licensed
Pentoxifylline	RCTs	None	?	Inconclusive findings	Peripheral arterial disease in adults
Neprilysin	RCTs	None	?	Inconclusive findings	Heart failure in adults
Statins	RCTs	None	+?	Reduced risk of CKD progression in some studies	Dyslipidemia
Allopurinol, Febuxostat	RCTs	None	+?	Inconclusive findings	Hyperuricemia
Vitamin D	Observational studies	Observational studies	+	Inconclusive findings	Vitamin D deficiency, rickets, CKD
Erythropoiesis stimulating agents	Observational studies	None	?	Inconclusive findings	Anemia
Low protein diet	RCTs	One RCT	+?	Inconclusive findings	NA

RCT randomized, controlled trial; + positive effect; ++ strong positive effect; +? Positive effects reported, but findings still inconclusive;? effect unknown; *NA* not applicable, *ADPKD* autosomal dominant polycystic kidney disease, *FSGS* focal segmental glomerulosclerosis, *BP* blood pressure, *ACEI* angiotensin converting enzyme inhibitor, *ARB* angiotensin receptor blocker, *CCB* calcium channel blocker

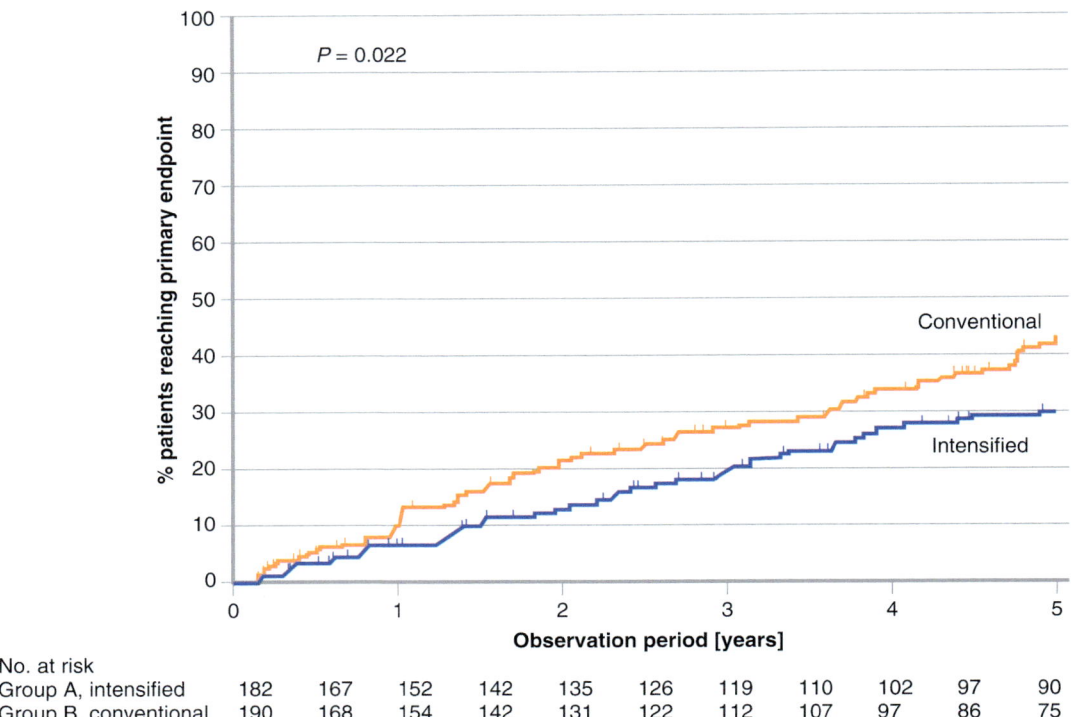

No. at risk
Group A, intensified	182	167	152	142	135	126	119	110	102	97	90
Group B, conventional	190	168	154	142	131	122	112	107	97	86	75

Fig. 55.7 Progression of chronic renal disease in children with CKD according to blood pressure control. The cumulative probability of reaching the primary composite end point of a 50% decline in the GFR or progression to end-stage renal disease is shown for patients randomized to either conventional or intensified blood pressure control in the ESCAPE Trial Used with permission of Massachusetts Medical Society from Wühl et al. [101]

underlying glomerulopathy as well as renal dysplasia or hypo-dysplasia, albeit not in other congenital or hereditary nephropathies [101].

The kidney survival benefit of intensified blood pressure control demonstrated by the ESCAPE Trial is in partial contrast to findings in other studies in adult CKD populations (MDRD Trial, ABCD Trial, AASK Trial, REIN-2 extension trial [131–133] in which no significant benefit was demonstrated for the cohorts as a whole. These partially discrepant findings may be explained by methodological and population differences. Patient age, ethnicity, pharmacological treatment protocols, duration of follow-up and dropout rates varied markedly between the mentioned studies. Furthermore, the use of ambulatory blood pressure monitoring may have enabled more sensitive monitoring of achieved blood pressure level in the pediatric ESCAPE Trial than in the adult trials, in which casual blood pressure

readings were exclusively used. Remarkably, for all adult CKD studies mentioned above, patients with proteinuria were more likely to benefit from intensified blood pressure control. This is consistent with the results of a meta-analysis of nearly 10,000 CKD patients in which intensified blood pressure control in patients with proteinuria appeared to protect against renal failure [134].

In the ESCAPE trial [101], strict blood pressure control was tolerated very well in the vast majority of children. Since the absolute risk of cardiovascular events in children is very low, the "J curve" phenomenon, i.e., an increase of cardiovascular events in patients achieving a very low blood pressure level, seems to be largely confined to elderly patients with advanced atherosclerosis.

The findings of the ESCAPE Trial [101] have been adopted by the most recent pediatric guideline published by the European Society of

Hypertension, which recommends a blood pressure target (for casual blood pressure and for ambulatory blood pressure monitoring) below the 75th percentile in non-proteinuric children with CKD, and below the 50th percentile in those with proteinuria [135]. The AAP Clinical Practice Guideline for Screening and Management of High Blood Pressure in Children and Adolescents, published in 2017, recommends a blood pressure goal below the 50th percentile for all children with CKD [136].

For adults and adolescents above age 15, the latest European hypertension guideline recommends a systolic target blood pressure of 130–140 mmHg [137], while the US guideline recommends a target blood pressure of <130/80 mmHg for adults with CKD [138] and the most recent KDIGO guideline suggests a systolic target blood pressure of <120 mmHg by standardized office readings [139]. For further information, please see also Chap. 50.

Proteinuria Control

In line with the experimental evidence given above, multiple clinical studies have confirmed that proteinuria is not only a marker, but also an important mechanism of kidney disease progression. Its reduction is associated with a slowing of GFR loss in the long term [15, 140–142].

In the ESCAPE trial, the level of residual proteinuria during antiproteinuric treatment was negatively associated with kidney survival in children with CKD [101, 102]. In a post-hoc analysis of the trial data, the initial antiproteinuric effect of the pharmacological intervention predicted the long-term preservation of kidney function [102]. The maximal effect was observed in children who achieved a proteinuria reduction of more than 60%. In the MDRD and REIN trials in adults with CKD, each 1 g/d reduction in proteinuria achieved within 3–4 months of antiproteinuric therapy slowed the subsequent GFR decline by 1–2 mL/min per year [15, 143]. Hence, the goal of antiproteinuric treatment is to reduce proteinuria as much as possible, ideally to <300 mg/m^2/day [144, 145].

Pharmacological Treatment Options

Antihypertensive and Antiproteinuric Pharmacotherapy

While the different classes of *antihypertensive agents* are comparable with respect to their blood pressure lowering efficacy, they differ markedly regarding their effects on proteinuria and CKD progression [141, 142, 146, 147].

By virtue of their pharmacological properties, *ACE inhibitors* (ACEis) and *angiotensin II type I receptor blockers* (ARBs) are the first options in both adults and children with CKD. These RAAS antagonists have an excellent safety profile, which is almost indistinguishable from placebo. In adults with essential hypertension, treatment with RAAS antagonists has been associated with the best quality of life among all antihypertensive agents.

RAAS antagonists suppress the local angiotensin II tone (ACEis) or action (ARBs). This results in a reduction of intraglomerular pressure and proteinuria, diminished local release of TGF-ß and other growth factors, cytokines and chemokines, with consequently attenuated glomerular hypertrophy and sclerosis, tubulointerstitial inflammation and fibrosis [85]. They also normalize central nervous sympathetic tone by reduced renal afferent nerve stimulation.

Several randomized trials in adults with diabetic or non-diabetic kidney disease have demonstrated a more effective reduction of proteinuria, usually by 30–40%, by ACEis as compared to placebo and/or other antihypertensive agents [144]. In the long term, this is associated with a reduced rate of renal failure progression [140, 144, 148–156].

Very similar results were obtained in randomized comparisons of ARBs with placebo or conventional antihypertensive agents in diabetic nephropathy [147, 157, 158]. It has been reasoned that ACEis might have a specific renoprotective advantage by inducing accumulation of vasodilatory and antifibrotic bradykinins, but the course of GFR was similar in clinical trials comparing ACEi and ARB therapy [159, 160]. However, a recent network meta-analysis suggested that ACEis are superior to ARBs and other antihypertensive agents in reducing adverse renal events in patients with non-dialysis CKD 3–5, but are not superior to ARBs in lowering odds of kidney events in patients with advanced CKD [161].

Prescription of RAAS antagonists typically reduces the risk of doubling serum creatinine or attaining ESRD by 30–40%, but the superiority of RAAS antagonists is related to the prevailing degree of proteinuria. In adults, the superior nephroprotection of ACEis over other antihypertensive agents has been most clearly shown in patients with proteinuria exceeding 500 mg/day.

While the maximal antiproteinuric effects of RAAS antagonists occur at doses exceeding those providing maximal antihypertensive action [162], regulatory authority approval is usually available only for the doses used to treat hypertension. Therefore, it is generally recommended to administer these drugs, after confirming tolerability in a short run-in period, at their highest approved doses [141, 163].

Early pediatric studies showed stable longterm renal function with ACE inhibition in children following hemolytic uremic syndrome [164], stable GFR during 2.5 years of losartan treatment in children with proteinuric CKD [165], and attenuated histopathological progression in children with IgA nephropathy receiving combined RAAS blockade [166]. The ESCAPE trial demonstrated efficient blood pressure control and proteinuria reduction by the ACE inhibitor ramipril [101, 167]. Subsequently, several randomized clinical trials demonstrated efficient, dose-dependent antihypertensive and antiproteinuric efficacy of ARBs in children [168–171]. One comparative trial suggested superior 24-h blood pressure lowering with the ARB valsartan relative to the ACEi enalapril, without any difference in antiproteinuric efficacy [168].

In the EARLY PRO-TECT Alport study, ramipril treatment significantly reduced the risk of disease progression in children and young adolescents with Alport syndrome by almost half and diminished the slope of albuminuria progression and the decline in GFR [172]. Early ACEi treatment is not curative, but may delay, or even prevent, the need for dialysis and kidney trans-

plantation until relatively late in life for substantial numbers of patients with Alport syndrome due to hemizygous missense variants and even truncating variants [173].

The CKiD study has provided observational evidence that children with moderate to severe CKD benefit from ACEi and ARB use by a KRT risk reduction of 21–37% [174].

The antiproteinuric response within in the first 2–3 months of administration is predictive of the long term renoprotective effect [102, 143] and may be utilized to individualize the appropriate drug dose. The specific glomerulodynamic effects of RAAS antagonists induce an immediate drop of the GFR, usually by approximately 10–15%, when these drugs are first administered. In patients with CKD, this may cause a significant increase in serum creatinine. It is important to know that a marked initial GFR decline is actually a positive predictor of the long-term nephroprotective effect [175]. Rapid acute renal failure soon after administration of a RAAS antagonist is a very rare event and usually related to concomitant volume depletion or previously unidentified bilateral renal artery stenoses.

Notably, a gradual rebound of proteinuria after the second treatment year during ongoing ACE inhibition was observed in the ESCAPE trial [101]. This effect was dissociated from a persistently good blood pressure control (Fig. 55.8), and may limit the long-term renoprotective efficacy of ACEi monotherapy in pediatric CKD. In several adult studies, subsets of patients developed partial secondary resistance to ACE inhibitors ('aldosterone escape' by compensatory upregulation of ACE-independent angiotensin II production) [176–179]. Such patients might benefit from the use of ARBs, which should not be affected by aldosterone escape.

Combined RAAS blockade using ACEi and ARB concomitantly has only a minor effect on blood pressure (3–4 mmHg vs. monotherapy), but increases the antiproteinuric effect of ACEi or ARB monotherapy by 30–40% [180, 181]. However, the findings of the ONTARGET in adult populations with high cardiovascular risk (CKD and diabetes) do not support the concept of

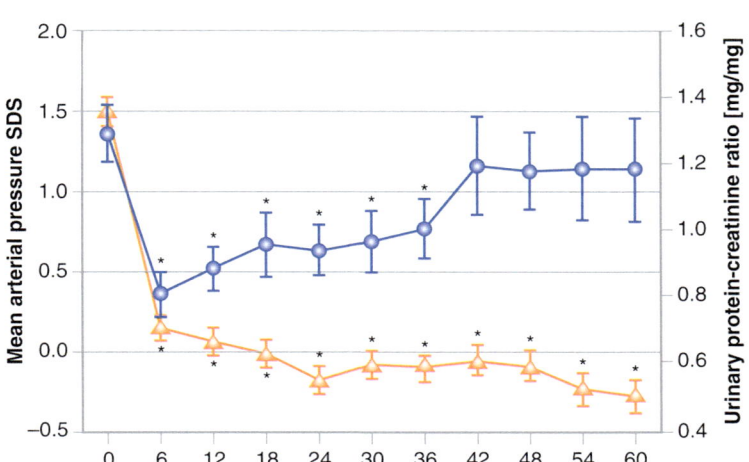

Fig. 55.8 Dissociation of antihypertensive and antiproteinuric effects of ACE-inhibition in children with CKD and fixed ramipril treatment (6 mg/m²/day) participating in the ESCAPE Trial. Used with permission of Massachusetts Medical Society from Wühl et al. [101]

dual RAAS blockade in patients with low GFR or albuminuria [182, 183]. However, it is questionable whether these findings in a high-risk adult population with diabetes and established CVD can be extrapolated to pediatric CKD patients [184].

Aldosterone antagonists also act by RAAS suppression resulting in reduced blood pressure. While the use of spironolactone is limited by its endocrine side effects, the newer aldosterone antagonist eplerenone has minimal affinity for progesterone and androgen receptors; apart from the risk of hyperkalemia, reported side effects were similar to placebo [185]. Combined therapy of eplerenone and an ACEi increased patient survival in adults with congestive heart failure. However, the combination therapy of both compounds is limited in CKD patients by the potentiated risk of hyperkalemia. A Cochrane review analyzing the results of 44 studies on the use of aldosterone antagonists in combination with ACEi or ARB found uncertain effects of aldosterone antagonists when added to ACEi or ARB (or both) on the risk of death, major cardiovascular events, and kidney failure in patients with proteinuric CKD [186]. Aldosterone antagonists may reduce proteinuria, eGFR, and systolic blood pressure in patients who have mild to moderate CKD but may increase the risk of hyperka-

lemia, acute kidney injury and gynecomastia when added to ACEi and/or ARB.

In contrast, finerenone, a novel nonsteroidal selective mineralocorticoid receptor antagonist, has been shown in animal studies to block inflammation and fibrosis in both the heart and kidneys with only minor effects on serum potassium. In the placebo-controlled Fidelio-DKD trial involving >5700 adults with CKD and type 2 diabetes, finerenone significantly lowered the risk of CKD progression and cardiovascular events [187]. A clinical trial assessing the antiproteinuric efficacy of finerenone in pediatric CKD is currently underway.

The simultaneous use of novel, well-tolerated oral potassium binders may improve the tolerability of combined RAAS blockade, including aldosterone antagonists, in patients with increased risk for hyperkalemia [188].

The *renin-antagonist* aliskiren, which blocks the conversion from angiotensinogen to angiotensin I, has been shown to effectively reduce blood pressure. Preliminary data showed a blood pressure lowering effect comparable to that of ARBs and the combination therapy of aliskiren and valsartan at maximum recommended doses provided significantly higher reductions in blood pressure than did monotherapy [189]. However, due to the higher risk of cardiovascular complications found in the ALTITUDE study, the combination therapy of aliskiren with ACEis or ARBs in patients with CKD is not recommended [190].

Calcium channel blockers (CCBs) are safe and can achieve blood pressure goals in patients with CKD. However, CCBs of the dihydropyridine type (amlodipine, nifedipine) fail to reduce progression of CKD. Although being excellent antihypertensive agents, dihydropyridine calcium channel blockers have no antiproteinuric effect and may actually promote proteinuria and more rapid CKD progression [142]. This is in contrast to non-dihydropyridine calcium channel blockers (diltiazem, verapamil), which have some antiproteinuric effect [142]. Therefore dihydropyridine CCBs should be avoided in proteinuric patients unless administered in combination with RAAS antagonists to improve blood pressure control [163], and may be acceptable as first-line antihypertensive monotherapy only in non-proteinuric patients.

CKD is often a state of overactivation of the sympathetic nervous system, and antiadrenergic drugs play an important role in its management. *β-blockers* are effective in lowering blood pressure in CKD patients; metoprolol and atenolol were the first antihypertensive agents for which beneficial effects on the decline of kidney function in CKD patients were demonstrated [149]. In the AASK trial, the beta-blocker metoprolol had an antiproteinuric effect almost comparable to ramipril, in marked contrast to amlodipine [141]. The antiproteinuric action may be due to sympatholytic effects. Newer β-blockers such as carvedilol have even better antiproteinuric effects compared to atenolol [191, 192].

Antihypertensive Combination Therapies

Because hypertension is a multifactorial disorder, monotherapy is often not effective in lowering blood pressure to the target range. Treatment with a single antihypertensive agent typically controls blood pressure in less than half of the patients.

Although most patients can be started on a single-drug regimen, consideration should be given to starting with two drugs of different classes for those with stage 2 hypertension. In addition, other patient-specific factors, such as age, concurrent medications, drug adherence, drug interactions, the overall treatment regimen, and comorbidities, should be considered. However, of those patients started on a single agent, many will subsequently require ≥2 drugs from different pharmacological classes to reach blood pressure goals. Drug regimens with complementary activity should be considered to maximize lowering of blood pressure. In addition, use of combination therapy may also improve adherence [137, 138].

In the ESCAPE trial [101], one third of patients required combination therapy to attain a blood pressure level in the normal range (<95th percentile), and 40% to reach a blood pressure in the lower normal range (<50th percentile). Likewise, 41% of the more than 700 patients participating in the European Cardiovascular Comorbidities in Children with CKD (4C) study were on two or more antihypertensive drugs [193], and 35% of the CKiD Study participants received combination therapy at baseline [194].

In CKD patients, RAAS antagonists are most commonly combined with a diuretic or with a calcium channel blocker, whereas their combination with a β-blocker usually does not exert an additive effect on blood pressure control. Fixed-dose combinations ('single pill') preparations are becoming increasingly popular in antihypertensive therapy, and may help maximize treatment adherence and efficacy [137, 138].

Antihypertensive Chronotherapy

In view of the fact that nocturnal blood pressure non-dipping is an independent risk factor for CKD progression, the timing of antihypertensive drugs may be relevant. Even with long-acting agents with recommended once daily administration, evening dosing lowers night-time blood pressure more efficiently, thereby partially restoring the physiologic nocturnal dipping pattern. However, these effects seem to differ for individual antihypertensive drug classes. Whereas bedtime administration of calcium channel blockers and ACE inhibitors tends to restore the dipping pattern, evening dosing of β-blockers has no effect on the circadian blood pressure rhythm [195].

While antihypertensive 'chronotherapy' has not yet been demonstrated to affect CKD progression, in a study randomly assigning hypertensive CKD patients to either take all prescribed hypertension medications in the morning or at least one of them at bedtime, bedtime dosing was associated with improved blood pressure control and significant reduction of cardiovascular risk [196].

SGLT-2 Inhibition

Several drugs developed to enhance glucose control in patients with diabetes mellitus type 2, such as metformin, glucagon-like peptide 1 (GLP-1) agonists, dipeptidyl peptide 4 (DPP-4) antagonists, and specific *sodium-glucose cotransporter 2 (SGLT2) inhibitors*, have recently been demonstrated to not only improve metabolic control but to exert additional beneficial effects on the cardiovascular system and the kidneys. Among these medications, SGLT2 inhibitors (gliflozins) have emerged as a particularly promising novel drug class. Apart from their glucose lowering effect, SGLT2 inhibitors decrease blood pressure, body weight, and albuminuria. The nephroprotective effects are based on a decrease of sodium delivery to the distal tubule and reduced glomerular blood flow leading to reversal of glomerular hypertension and hyperfiltration [197]. Large clinical outcome trials with the SGLT2 inhibitors dapagliflozin, canagliflozin, and empagliflozin in adult CKD patients with diabetic nephropathy have demonstrated a potent long-term nephroprotective effect of SGLT2 inhibition, with proteinuria reduction by 30–50% and impressive beneficial effects on hard renal outcomes such as doubling of serum creatinine, eGFR decline, need for KRT, and death from renal disease [198–200]. These nephroprotective effects have been

confirmed in non-diabetic CKD patients [201]. To date, based on the results of the clinical trial programs, the SGLT2 inhibitors have been approved for the treatment of diabetic nephropathy. Unfortunately, pediatric trials with these novel compounds are currently not planned.

Due to the complementary effects of SGLT2 inhibitors and RAAS antagonists on glomerular perfusion and intraglomerular pressure (vasoconstriction of the afferent vessel by the SGLT2 inhibitor and vasodilatation of the efferent vessel by RAAS inhibition), combined therapy with these two drug classes might further reduce intraglomerular pressure and exert additive nephroprotective effects [202].

Anti-inflammatory Drugs

While RAAS antagonists exert indirect anti-inflammatory and antifibrotic properties via blockade of RAAS-dependent profibrotic and inflammatory pathways as outlined above, other non-specific *anti-inflammatory and antifibrotic drugs* may decrease fibrogenesis by reducing macrophage infiltration and subsequent recruitment of fibroblasts or generation of ROS. For example, pirfenidone, exerting anti-fibrotic, anti-oxidant, and anti-inflammatory properties, interfering with the expression, secretion and the effect of TGF-β, improved kidney function and proteinuria and reduced kidney scarring in animal models; however, in clinical trials in FSGS or diabetic nephropathy patients, pirfenidone showed conflicting results, failing to prevent proteinuria or GFR decline particularly in patients with renal dysfunction [203, 204].

Endothelin$_A$ (ET$_A$) receptor mediated inflammation, fibrosis and proteinuria can be reduced by *endothelin A receptor antagonists* (ERAs). ERAs have been shown to reduce albuminuria and blood pressure, but also cause sodium and fluid retention and anemia. A large randomized controlled trial in patients with diabetes mellitus type 2 and CKD using the relatively unselective ERA avosentan was terminated early because of an increased frequency of heart failure [205]. Atrasentan, a more selective endothelin receptor antagonist, reduced the risk of renal events compared with placebo in pre-selected patients with diabetes and CKD [206]. Combined ET_A and angiotensin II blockade by sparsentan, a drug comprising moieties of irbesartan and atrasentan, achieved significantly greater reductions in proteinuria compared to irbesartan in patients with primary FSGS [207].

Despite their relevant side effect profile, the large body of pre-clinical data supporting a beneficial effect of ERAs, as well as encouraging results from clinical trials in IgA nephropathy, FSGS, Alport syndrome, sickle cell nephropathy, and resistant hypertension, hold promise that ET_A receptor antagonists may ultimately have a beneficial effect on a wide range of kidney disorders [208].

It has been shown that Nrf2 expression is consistently downregulated in CKD [209] and that activation of Nrf2 may prevent or attenuate fibrosis. Interventions that increase Nrf2 system components have been already described, but their effectiveness and clinical relevance require further clinical studies [209]. One pharmacological promotor of Nrf2 activity is *bardoxolone*. Initial phase 1 studies showed that bardoxolone increased GFR; however, subsequent phase 3 studies in patients with CKD and diabetes type 2 were prematurely terminated due to an increased risk of heart failure, elevation of transaminases, hypomagnesemia and muscle cramps. Worryingly, bardoxolone seems to increase urinary albumin excretion, indicating ongoing or even worsening glomerular damage. This might explain why after an initial increase GFR declined over 24 weeks in patients allocated to bardoxolone in the BEAM study [210]. Studies to further elaborate whether bardoxolone effectively retards kidney fibrosis and progression in specific kidney diseases such as Alport syndrome (CARDINAL trial) or ADPKD are underway.

Pentoxifylline (PTF), a non-specific phosphodiesterase inhibitor, has anti-inflammatory, antiproliferative, and anti-fibrotic properties. So far, the small clinical trials evaluating PTF in patients with CKD yielded conflicting data. A meta-analysis of 11 studies on PTF in combination with ACEi or ARB treatment including 705 adult

patients suggested that combination therapy may lead to a greater reduction in proteinuria and attenuate the decline in eGFR in patients with CKD stages 3–5 [211].

Neprilysin (neutral endopeptidase or membrane metallo-endopeptidase) degrades numerous peptide hormones, including bradykinin, endothelin, and atrial and brain natriuretic peptides (ANP, BNP). Thus, *neprilysin inhibition* (NEPi) may be a therapeutic strategy enhancing the activity of the natriuretic peptide system, inducing natriuresis, diuresis and inhibition of the RAAS and the sympathetic nervous system. Sacubitril/valsartan, the first *angiotensin receptor-neprilysin inhibitor* (ARNI), has been shown to substantially improve not only cardiovascular outcomes in adults with heart failure, but also to delay CKD progression in this population. However, ARNIs have not shown similar effects on kidney function in the short-to-medium term in CKD patients [212].

In patients with ADPKD, *tolvaptan*, an oral selective antagonist of the vasopressin V2 receptor, has demonstrated beneficial disease-modifying properties in adults. Tolvaptan reduced total kidney volume and the decline of kidney function in adults with relatively early-stage ADPKD and high likelihood of rapid disease progression [213, 214] and also in those with more advanced disease [215]. Preliminary results of a placebo-controlled trial in pediatric ADPKD patients have shown efficient lowering of urine osmolality and a nominal reduction of total kidney volume after one-year of exposure to the drug [216].

Other Supportive Treatment Strategies

Metabolic acidosis is common in patients with CKD and may contribute to the development and worsening of proteinuria and tubulointerstitial fibrosis, accelerating the rate of decline in renal function. In a randomized controlled trial evaluating the renoprotective potential of oral bicarbonate supplementation in adult patients with CKD, only 4 of 67 patients receiving bicarbonate progressed to dialysis as compared to 22 of 67 patients in the untreated control group [107]. CKD progression rate was reduced to 1 mL/min/year in patients with serum bicarbonate levels ≥22 mmol/L compared to >2.5 mL/min/year in patients with uncorrected low bicarbonate levels [107]. In adults with hypertensive nephropathy and relatively preserved GFR (mean GFR 75 mL/min/1.73 m^2), 5 years of oral sodium bicarbonate substitution (0.5 mEq/kg lean body weight daily) provided effective kidney protection when added to blood pressure reduction and ACE-inhibition [106]. Therefore, tight control of metabolic acidosis may become an important component of renoprotective therapy in patients with progressive CKD.

Treatment of uremic *dyslipidemia* is another component of renoprotective therapy. General measures to prevent dyslipidemia in CKD patients include prevention or treatment of malnutrition and correction of metabolic acidosis, hyperparathyroidism and anemia, all of which may contribute to dyslipidemia [112, 217, 218]. In addition, based on evidence from the general population, therapeutic life style modification (diet, exercise, weight reduction) is recommended for adults and children with CKD related dyslipidemia by the KDIGO Clinical Practice Guideline for Lipid Management in Chronic Kidney Disease [219]. Experimental evidence suggests that statins may retard kidney disease progression not only by their lipid lowering, but also by lipid-independent pleiotropic effects, inhibiting signalling molecules at several points in inflammatory pathways. Anti-inflammatory effects and improved endothelial function are thought to be partially responsible both for CVD risk reduction and improved kidney function [220]. Lipid lowering pharmacological treatment is common in adults with CKD, based on the benefit of this approach for primary and secondary prevention of CVD in the general adult population. However, in children with CKD, treatment of hypercholesterolemia is not recommended and treatment for hypertriglyceridemia should focus on severe cases due to lack of clear benefits coupled with safety concerns related to long-term use in children [219].

A meta-analysis including 10 studies on the impact of statin therapy on CKD progression suggested that high-dose, but not low-dose statin use, may be nephroprotective in CKD patients [221]. In addition, the degree of CKD and proteinuria may influence the effect of statin therapy on CKD progression. A study in almost 3500 adults with CKD demonstrated significant effects on GFR decline in patients with CKD stages 3b to 5 or proteinuria >1000 mg/d, whereas no significant effects were seen in mild to moderate CKD and non-proteinuric patients [222].

Several studies in adults with CKD suggested that dietary phosphorus restriction may stabilize kidney function [223]. However, no conclusions were possible from studies in children [224]. Experimental studies have suggested a PTH-independent beneficial effect of *phosphate restriction* on CKD progression. A high calcium phosphorus product may be detrimental to renal survival by aggravating intrarenal vasculopathy as well as by causing tubulointerstitial calcifications, which may stimulate tubulointerstitial inflammation and fibrosis. In view of these pathophysiological associations, it is currently discussed whether calcium-free phosphate binders may have some renoprotective potential in patients with CKD.

Sevelamer or colestilan may prove beneficial beyond phosphate lowering due to their pleiotropic effects, which include lipid lowering and anti-inflammatory properties. A lower all-cause mortality was found in patients with CKD stage 3–5D treated with sevelamer compared to patients on calcium-based phosphate binders [225].

Treatment with non-hypercalcemic doses of active *vitamin D* attenuates renal failure progression in uremic rats. This effect may be due to the immune modulatory and antifibrotic properties of vitamin D in combination with inhibitory actions on the RAAS [226]. In children with CKD, 25(OH)D levels >50 nmol/L were associated with better preservation of renal function, even in the presence of concomitant ACEi therapy [227].

In addition, there is increasing evidence for interactions between vitamin D, FGF23, and klotho regulating calcium phosphate homeostasis. Alterations of this endocrine axis may contribute to kidney disease progression by activation of the RAAS, vitamin D deficiency, reduced renal production of klotho and reduced FGF23 signaling [228]. FGF23 levels are independently associated with progression of CKD and may serve as a biomarker and mechanism of CVD [126]. These findings provide further arguments for close monitoring and early intervention to maintain mineral, vitamin D and PTH homeostasis in CKD.

Another biomarker of progressive CKD is serum uric acid. While allopurinol treatment improved renal outcome in CKD patients compared to placebo without a change in blood pressure level [229], and febuxostat treatment slowed down kidney disease progression [230], the CKD-FIX Trial could not demonstrate a beneficial effect of *uric acid lowering treatment* on kidney disease progression in stage 3–4 CKD patients [231].

Historically, *low protein diet* was prescribed for prevention of renal progression. However, the effects and consequences of this diet on CKD progression and delay of ESKD are inconclusive. A large randomized trial in adults failed to demonstrate efficacy of a low protein diet on the progression of non-diabetic kidney disease [232], whereas, in a recent review, protein restriction was associated with a risk reduction of kidney death [233]. Thus, though the progression rate was not significantly influenced by protein restriction, kidney replacement therapy could be postponed.

In children reduced protein intake to the minimal acceptable lower limit did not slow CKD progression [86, 234]. Further reductions may be effective but not acceptable for patients. Furthermore, a low protein diet may increase the risk of low-calorie intake, which may jeopardize the preservation of adequate statural growth. Therefore, it does not seem to be justified to prescribe a low protein diet in children with CKD.

Recently, studies in ADPKD patients have identified a chronic shift in energy production from mitochondrial oxidative phosphorylation to aerobic glycolysis as a contributor to cyst growth, making the cyst cells particularly sensitive to the availability of glucose. Therefore, low calorie or ketogenic diets may be a potential intervention to delay ADPKD progression [235]. A clinical trial evaluating the effect of a ketogenic diet on cyst growth and CKD progression in adult ADPKD patients is underway (NCT04680780).

Erythropoiesis stimulating agents (ESA) have emerged as a tissue-protective survival factor in various non-hematopoietic organs [236]. It has been suggested that normalizing hemoglobin in CKD patients might attenuate renal disease progression by increasing oxygen supply to the kidneys, preventing tubular atrophy and interstitial fibrosis. In addition, erythropoietin might counteract oxidative stress and apoptosis and may have direct protective effects on tubular cells [237] and podocytes [238]. However, this concept has not been substantiated in clinical trials on CKD progression to date.

Conclusions

Progression of childhood CKD towards kidney failure is common and once a significant impairment of kidney function has occurred it progresses irrespectively of the underlying kidney disease. Onset of CKD and progression rate in defined disease entities may be influenced by genetic factors. Hypertension and proteinuria are the most important independent risk factors for CKD progression. RAAS antagonists preserve kidney function, not only by lowering blood pressure, but also by their antiproteinuric and anti-inflammatory properties. Intensified blood pressure control exerts additional renoprotective effects in pediatric CKD; therefore, therapeutic strategies to prevent progression should comprise blood pressure control aiming for a target blood pressure below the 50th to 75th percentile. Furthermore, there is increasing evidence that treatment with SGLT2 inhibitors contributes to preservation of kidney function in adults with CKD. Other factors contributing in a multifactorial manner to CKD progression include anemia, metabolic acidosis, dyslipidemia and disorders of mineral metabolism. Measures to preserve renal function should therefore also comprise the maintenance of hemoglobin, serum bicarbonate, lipids and mineral metabolism in the normal range.

References

1. Chanutin A, Ferris EB. Experimental renal insufficiency produced by partial nephrectomy 1. Control diet. Arch Int Med. 1932;49:767–87.
2. Volhard F, Fahr TH. Die Bright'sche Nierenkrankheit. Berlin: Julius Springer; 1914. p. 232.
3. von Mollendorf W, Stohr P. Lehrbuch der histologie. Jena: Fischer; 1924. p. 343.
4. Oliver J, Macdowell M, Lee YC. Cellular mechanisms of protein metabolism in the nephron. I. The structural aspects of proteinuria, tubular absorption, droplet formation, and the disposal of proteins. J Exp Med. 1954;99:589–604.
5. Hostetter TH, Olson JL, Rennke HG, Venkatachalam MA, Brenner BM. Hyperfiltration in remnant nephrons: a potentially adverse response to renal ablation. Am J Phys. 1981;241(1):F85–93.
6. Klag MJ, Whelton PK, Randall BL, Neaton JD, Brancati FL, Ford CE, et al. Blood pressure and end-stage renal disease in men. N Engl J Med. 1996;334(1):13–8.
7. Iseki K, Ikemiya Y, Iseki C, Takishita S. Proteinuria and the risk of developing end-stage renal disease. Kidney Int. 2003;63(4):1468–74.
8. Locatelli F, Marcelli D, Comelli M, Alberti D, Graziani G, Buccianti G, et al. Proteinuria and blood pressure as causal components of progression to end-stage renal failure. Northern Italian Cooperative Study Group. Nephrol Dial Transplant. 1996;11(3):461–7.
9. Ardissino G, Dacco V, Testa S, Bonaudo R, Claris-Appiani A, Taioli E, et al. Epidemiology of chronic renal failure in children: data from the ItalKid project. Pediatrics. 2003;111:e382–e7.
10. Gonzalez Celedon C, Bitsori M, Tullus K. Progression of chronic renal failure in children with dysplastic kidneys. Pediatr Nephrol. 2007;22(7):1014–20.
11. Zhong Y, Munoz A, Schwartz GJ, Warady BA, Furth SL, Abraham AG. Nonlinear trajectory of GFR in children before RRT. J Am Soc Nephrol. 2014;25(5):913–7.
12. Wuhl E, van Stralen KJ, Verrina E, Bjerre A, Wanner C, Heaf JG, et al. Timing and outcome of renal replacement therapy in patients with congenital malformations of the kidney and urinary tract. Clin J Am Soc Nephrol. 2013;8(1):67–74.
13. Remuzzi G, Bertani T. Pathophysiology of progressive nephropathies. N Engl J Med. 1998;339:1448–56.
14. Olbricht CJ, Cannon LK, Garg LC, Tisher CC. Activities of cathepsins B and L in isolated nephron segments from proteinuric and nonproteinuric rats. Am J Phys. 1986;250:F1055–62.
15. Peterson JC, Adler S, Burkart JM, Greene T, Hebert LA, Hunsicker LG, et al. Blood pressure control, proteinuria, and the progression of renal disease. The Modification of Diet in Renal Disease Study. Ann Intern Med. 1995;123:754–62.
16. Kriz W. Progressive renal failure—inability of podocytes to replicate and the consequences for development of glomerulosclerosis. Nephrol Dial Transplant. 1996;11:1738–42.
17. Takano T, Brady HR. The endothelium in glomerular inflammation. Curr Opin Nephrol Hypertens. 1995;4:277–86.
18. Malek AM, Greene AL, Izumo S. Regulation of endothelin 1 gene by fluid shear stress is transcriptionally mediated and independent of protein kinase C and cAMP. Proc Natl Acad Sci U S A. 1993;90:5999–6003.
19. Lee LK, Meyer TW, Pollock AS, Lovett DH. Endothelial cell injury initiates glomerular sclerosis in the rat remnant kidney. J Clin Invest. 1995;96:953–64.
20. Hirschberg R, Wang S. Proteinuria and growth factors in the development of tubulointerstitial injury and scarring in kidney disease. Curr Opin Nephrol Hypertens. 2005;14:43–52.
21. Wang SN, Lapage J, Hirschberg R. Glomerular ultrafiltration and apical tubular action of IGF-1, TGF-beta, and HGF in nephrotic syndrome. Kidney Int. 1999;56:1247–51.
22. Wang SN, Hirschberg R. Growth factor ultrafiltration in experimental diabetic nephropathy contributes to interstitial fibrosis. Am J Physiol Renal Physiol. 2000;278:F554–60.
23. Wang SN, Lapage J, Hirschberg R. Loss of tubular bone morphogenetic protein-7 in diabetic nephropathy. J Am Soc Nephrol. 2001;12:2392–9.
24. Donadelli R, Abbate M, Zanchi C, Corna D, Tomasone S, Benigni A, et al. Protein traffic activates NF-kB gene signaling and promotes MCP-1-dependent interstitial inflammation. Am J Kidney Dis. 2000;36:1226–41.
25. Morigi M, Macconi D, Zoja C, Donadelli R, Buelli S, Zanchi G, et al. Protein overload-induced NF-kappB activation in proximal tubular cells requires H2O2 through a PKC-dependent pathway. J Am Soc Nephrol. 2002;13:1179–89.
26. Zoja C, Donadelli R, Colleoni S, Figliuzzi M, Bonazzola S, Morigi M, et al. Protein overload stimulates RANTES production by proximal tubular cells depending on NF-kappaB activation. Kidney Int. 1998;53:1608–15.
27. Zoja C, Morigi M, Figliuzzi M, Bruzzi I, Oldroyd S, Benigni A, et al. Proximal tubular cell synthesis and secretion of endothelin-1 on challenge with albumin and other proteins. Am J Kidney Dis. 1995;26:934–41.
28. Kees-Folts D, Sadow JL, Schreiner GF. Catabolism of albumin is associated with the release of an inflammatory lipid. Kidney Int. 1994;45:1697–709.
29. Floege J, Burns MW, Alpers CE, Yoshimura A, Pritzl P, Gordon K, et al. Glomerular cell proliferation and PDGF expression precede glomerulosclerosis in the remnant kidney model. Kidney Int. 1992;41:297–309.

30. Couser WG. Pathogenesis of glomerular damage in glomerulonephritis. Nephrol Dial Transplant. 1998;13:10–5.

31. Strutz F, Neilson EG. New insights into mechanisms of fibrosis in immune renal injury. Springer Semin Immunopathol. 2003;24:459–79.

32. Kelly CJ, Neilson EG. Tubulointerstitital diseases. In: Brenner BM, editor. The kidney. Philadelphia: Saunders; 2004. p. 1483–512.

33. Eddy AA, Fogo A. Plasminogen activator inhibitor-1 in chronic kidney disease: evidence and mechanisms of action. J Am Soc Nephrol. 2006;17:2999–3012.

34. Catania JM, Chen G, Parrish AR. Role of matrix metalloproteinases in renal pathophysiologies. Am J Physiol Renal Physiol. 2007;292:F905–F11.

35. Schalenkamp MA, Danser AH. Angiotensin II production and distribution in the kidney-II. Model based analysis of experimental data. Kidney Int. 2006;69:1553–7.

36. Schalenkamp MA, Danser AH. Angiotensin II production and distribution in the kidney: I. A kinetic model. Kidney Int. 2006;69:1543–52.

37. Navar LG, Nishiyama A. Why are angiotensin concentrations so high in the kidney? Curr Opin Nephrol Hypertens. 2004;13:107–15.

38. Schmitz D, Berk BC. Angiotensin II signal transduction stimulation of multiple mitogen activated protein kinase pathways. Trends Endocrinol Metab. 1997;8:261–6.

39. Nitschke R, Henger A, Ricken S, Gloy J, Muller V, Greger R, et al. Angiotensin II increases the intracellular calcium activity in podocytes of the intact glomerulus. Kidney Int. 2000;57:41–9.

40. Henger A, Huber T, Fischer KG, Nitschke R, Mundel P, Schollmeyer P, et al. Angiotensin II increases the cytosolic calcium activity in rat podocytes in culture. Kidney Int. 1997;52:687–93.

41. Yoshioka T, Mitarai R, Kon V, Deen WM, Rennke HG, Ishikawa I. Role of antiotensin II in overt functional proteinuria. Kidney Int. 1997;52:687–93.

42. Bohrer MP, Deen WM, Robertson CR, Brenner BM. Mechanism of the angiotensin II-induced proteinuria in the rat. Am J Phys. 1977;233:F13–21.

43. Taal MW, Chertow GM, Rennke HG, Gurnani A, Jiang T, Shasafaei A, et al. Mechanisms underlying renoprotection during renin-angiotensin system blockade. Am J Physiol Renal Physiol. 2001;280:F343–55.

44. Taal MW, Omer SA, Nadim MK, Mackenzie HS. Cellular and molecular mediators in common pathway mechanisms of chronic renal disease progression. Curr Opin Nephrol Hypertens. 2000;9:323–31.

45. Converse RL, Jacobsen TN, Toto RD, Jost CM, Consentino F, Fouad-Tarazi F, et al. Sympathetic overactivity in patients with chronic renal failure. N Engl J Med. 1992;327:1912–8.

46. Hausberg M, Kosch M, Harmelink P, Barenbrock M, Hohage H, Kisters K, et al. Sympathetic nerve activity in end-stage renal disease. Circulation. 2002;165:1974–9.

47. Nezu M, Suzuki N, Yamamoto M. Targeting the KEAP1-NRF2 system to prevent kidney disease progression. Am J Nephrol. 2017;45(6):473–83.

48. Stenvinkel P, Chertow GM, Devarajan P, Levin A, Andreoli SP, Bangalore S, et al. Chronic inflammation in chronic kidney disease progression: role of Nrf2. Kidney Int Rep. 2021;6(7):1775–87.

49. Kang DH, Kanellis J, Hugo C, Truong L, Anderson S, Kerjaschki D, et al. Role of the microvascular endothelium in progressive renal disease. J Am Soc Nephrol. 2002;13:806–16.

50. Orphanides C, Fine LG, Norman JT. Hypoxia stimulates proximal tubular cell matrix production via a TGF-1-independent mechanism. Kidney Int. 1997;52:637–47.

51. Fine LG, Orphanides C, Norman JT. Progressive renal disease: the chronic hypoxia hypothesis. Kidney Int Suppl. 1998;65:S74–8.

52. Argueso L, Ritchey ML, Boyle ET Jr, Milliner DS, Bergstralh EL, Kramer SA. Prognosis of patients with unilateral renal agenesis. Pediatr Nephrol. 1992;6:412–6.

53. Sanna-Cherchi S, Ravani P, Corbani V, Parodi S, Haupt R, Piaggio G, et al. Renal outcome in patients with congenital abnormalities of the kidney and urinay tract. Kidney Int. 2009;76:528–33.

54. Di Tullio MT, Casale F, Indolfe P, Polito C, Guliano M, Martini A, et al. Compensatory hypertrophy and progressive renal damage in children nephrectomized for Wilms' tumor. Med Pediatr Oncol. 1996;26:325–8.

55. Bhathena DB, Julian BA, McMorrow RG, Baehler RW. Focal sclerosis of hypertrophic glomeruli in solitary funtioning kidneys of humans. Am J Kidney Dis. 1985;5:226–32.

56. Matsell DG, Bao C, Po White T, Chan E, Matsell E, Cojocaru D, et al. Outcomes of solitary functioning kidneys-renal agenesis is different than multicystic dysplastic kidney disease. Pediatr Nephrol. 2021;

57. Carrero JJ, Hecking M, Chesnaye NC, Jager KJ. Sex and gender disparities in the epidemiology and outcomes of chronic kidney disease. Nat Rev Nephrol. 2018;14(3):151–64.

58. Neugarten J, Acharya A, Silbiger SR. Effect of gender on the progression of nondiabetic renal diseas: a meta-analysis. J Am Soc Nephrol. 2000;11:319–29.

59. Bonneric S, Karadkhele G, Couchoud C, Patzer RE, Greenbaum LA, Hogan J. Sex and glomerular filtration rate trajectories in children. Clin J Am Soc Nephrol. 2020;15(3):320–9.

60. Hildebrandt F, Otto E, Omran H. Nephronophthise und verwandte Krankheiten. Med Genet. 2000;12:225–31.

61. Hinkes B, Vlangos C, Heeringa S, Mucha B, Gbadegesin R, Liu J, et al. Specific podocin mutations correlate with age of onset in steroid-resistant nephrotic syndrome. J Am Soc Nephrol. 2008;19(2):365–71.

62. Bekheirnia MR, Reed B, Gregory MC, McFann K, Shamshirsaz AA, Masoumi A, et al. Genotype-phenotype correlation in X-linked Alport syndrome. J Am Soc Nephrol. 2010;21(5):876–83.

63. Bantis C, Ivens K, Kreusser W, Koch M, Klein-Vehne N, Grabensee B, et al. Influence of genetic polymorphisms of the renin-angiotensin system on IgA nephropathy. Am J Nephrol. 2004;24:258–67.

64. Maruyama K, Yoshida M, Nishio H, Shirakawa T, Kawamura T, Tanaka R, et al. Polymorphisms of renin-angiotensin system genes in childhood IgA nephropathy. Pediatr Nephrol. 2001;16:350–5.

65. Hohenfellner K, Hunley TE, Brezinska R, Brodhag P, Shyr Y, Brenner W, et al. ACE I/D gene polymorphism predicts renal damage in congenital uropathies. Pediatr Nephrol. 1999;13:514–8.

66. Erdogan H, Mir S, Serdaroglu E, Berdeli A, Aksu N. Is ACE gene polymorphism a risk factor for renal scarring with low grade reflux? Pediatr Nephrol. 2004;19:734–7.

67. Dudley J, Johnston A, Gardner A, McGraw M. The deletion polymorphism of the ACE gene is not an independent risk factor for renal scarring in children with vesico-ureteric reflux. Nephrol Dial Transplant. 2002;17:652–4.

68. Perna A, Ruggenenti P, Testa A, Spoto B, Benini R, Misefari V, et al. ACE genotype and ACE inhibitors induced renoprotection in chronic proteinuric nephropathies1. Kidney Int. 2000;57:274–81.

69. Ruggenenti P, Perna A, Zoccali C, Gherardi G, Benini R, Testa A, et al. Chronic proteinuric nephropathies. II. Outcomes and response to treatment in a prospective cohort of 352 patients: differences between women and men in relation to the ACE gene polymorphism. Gruppo Italiano di Studi Epidemologici in Nefrologia (Gisen). J Am Soc Nephrol. 2000;11(1):88–96.

70. Boger CA, Gorski M, Li M, Hoffmann MM, Huang C, Yang Q, et al. Association of eGFR-related loci identified by GWAS with incident CKD and ESRD. PLoS Genet. 2011;7(9):e1002292.

71. Kottgen A, Pattaro C, Boger CA, Fuchsberger C, Olden M, Glazer NL, et al. New loci associated with kidney function and chronic kidney disease. Nat Genet. 2010;42(5):376–84.

72. Pediatric Investigation of Genetic Factors Linked with Renal Progression (PediGFR): Chronic Kidney Disease in Children Cohort (CKiD) [Internet]. Available from: http://www.ncbi.nlm.nih.gov/projects/gap/cgi-bin/study.cgi?study_id=phs000650.v1.p1.

73. Kottgen A, Hwang SJ, Larson MG, Van Eyk JE, Fu Q, Benjamin EJ, et al. Uromodulin levels associate with a common UMOD variant and risk for incident CKD. J Am Soc Nephrol. 2010;21(2):337–44.

74. Kottgen A, Albrecht E, Teumer A, Vitart V, Krumsiek J, Hundertmark C, et al. Genome-wide association analyses identify 18 new loci associated with serum urate concentrations. Nat Genet. 2013;45(2):145–54.

75. Pattaro C, Kottgen A, Teumer A, Garnaas M, Boger CA, Fuchsberger C, et al. Genome-wide association and functional follow-up reveals new loci for kidney function. PLoS Genet. 2012;8(3):e1002584.

76. Eckardt KU, Barthlein B, Baid-Agrawal S, Beck A, Busch M, Eitner F, et al. The German Chronic Kidney Disease (GCKD) study: design and methods. Nephrol Dial Transplant. 2012;27(4):1454–60.

77. Wuttke M, Wong CS, Wuhl E, Epting D, Luo L, Hoppmann A, et al. Genetic loci associated with renal function measures and chronic kidney disease in children: the Pediatric Investigation for Genetic Factors Linked with Renal Progression Consortium. Nephrol Dial Transplant. 2016;31(2):262–9.

78. Barker DJ, Osmond C, Golding J, Kuh D, Wadsworth ME. Growth in utero, blood pressure in childhood and adult life, and mortality from cardiovascular disease. BMJ. 1989;298(6673):564–7.

79. Dotsch J, Plank C, Amann K. Fetal programming of renal function. Pediatr Nephrol. 2012;27(4):513–20.

80. Uemura O, Ishikura K, Kaneko T, Hirano D, Hamasaki Y, Ogura M, et al. Perinatal factors contributing to chronic kidney disease in a cohort of Japanese children with very low birth weight. Pediatr Nephrol. 2021;36(4):953–60.

81. Bakker H, Gaillard R, Franco OH, Hofman A, van der Heijden AJ, Steegers EA, et al. Fetal and infant growth patterns and kidney function at school age. J Am Soc Nephrol. 2014;25(11):2607–15.

82. Reddy MA, Natarajan R. Recent developments in epigenetics of acute and chronic kidney diseases. Kidney Int. 2015;88(2):250–61.

83. Hanratty R, Chonchol M, Havranek EP, Powers JD, Dickinson LM, Ho PM, et al. Relationship between blood pressure and incident chronic kidney disease in hypertensive patients. Clin J Am Soc Nephrol. 2011;6(11):2605–11.

84. Halbach S, Flynn J. Treatment of hypertension in children with chronic kidney disease. Curr Hypertens Rep. 2015;17(1):503.

85. Schaefer F, Mehls O. Hypertension in chronic kidney disease. In: Portman RJ, Sorof JM, Ingelfinger JR, editors. Pediatric hypertension. Totowa, NJ: Humana Press; 2004. p. 371–87.

86. Wingen AM, Fabian-Bach C, Schaefer F, Mehls O. Randomised multicentre study of a low-protein diet on the progression of chronic renal failure in children. European Study Group of Nutritional Treatment of Chronic Renal Failure in Childhood. Lancet. 1997;349(9059):1117–23.

87. Reynolds BC, Roem JL, Ng DKS, Matsuda-Abedini M, Flynn JT, Furth SL, et al. Association of time-varying blood pressure with chronic kidney disease progression in children. JAMA Netw Open. 2020;3(2):e1921213.

88. Ohkubo T, Hozawa A, Yamaguchi J, Kikuya M, Ohmori K, Michima M, et al. Prognostic significance of the nocturnal decline in blood pressure in individuals with and without high 24-h blood pressure: the Ohasama study. J Hypertens. 2002;20(11):2183–9.

89. Jeong JH, Fonkoue IT, Quyyumi AA, DaCosta D, Park J. Nocturnal blood pressure is associated with sympathetic nerve activity in patients with chronic kidney disease. Physiol Rep. 2020;8(20):e14602.

90. Ida T, Kusaba T, Kado H, Taniguchi T, Hatta T, Matoba S, et al. Ambulatory blood pressure monitoring-based analysis of long-term outcomes for kidney disease progression. Sci Rep. 2019;9(1):19296.

91. Timio M, Venanzi S, Lolli S, Lippi G, Verdura C, Monarca C, et al. 'Non-dipper' hypertensive patients and progressive renal insufficiency: a 3-year longitudinal study. Clin Nephrol. 1995;43:382–7.

92. Kanno A, Kikuya M, Asayama K, Satoh M, Inoue R, Hosaka M, et al. Night-time blood pressure is associated with the development of chronic kidney disease in a general population: the Ohasama Study. J Hypertens. 2013;31(12):2410–7.

93. Redon J, Plancha E, Swift PA, Pons S, Munoz J, Martinez F. Nocturnal blood pressure and progression to end-stage renal disease or death in non-diabetic chronic kidney disease stages 3 and 4. J Hypertens. 2010;28(3):602–7.

94. Tarver-Carr M, Brancati F, Eberhardt M, Powe N. Proteinuria and the risk of chronic kidney disease (CKD) in the United States. J Am Soc Nephrol. 2000;11:168A.

95. Hoy WE, Wang Z, vanBuynder P, Baker PR, Mathews JD. The natural history of renal disease in Autralian Aborigines. Part I. Changes in albuminuria and glomerular filtration rate over time. Kidney Int. 2001;60:243–8.

96. Iseki K, Kinjo K, Iseki C, Takishita S. Relationship between predicted creatinine clearance and proteinuria and the risk of developing ESRD in Okinawa. Japan Am J Kidney Dis. 2004;44(5):806–14.

97. Risdon RA, Sloper JC, de Wardener HE. Relationship between renal functionand histological changes found in renal biopsy specimens from patients with persistant glomerular nephritis. Lancet. 1968;2:363–6.

98. Remuzzi G, Ruggenenti P, Perico N. Chronic renal disease: renoprotective benefits of renin-angiotensin system inhibition. Ann Intern Med. 2002;136:604–15.

99. Ruggenenti P, Perna A, Mosconi L, Matalone M, Pisoni R, Gaspari F, et al. Proteinuria predicts end-stage renal failure in non-diabetic chronic nephropathies. The "Gruppo Italiano di Studi Epidemiologici in Nefrologia" (GISEN). Kidney Int Suppl. 1997;63:S54–S7.

100. Ardissino G, Testa S, Dacco V, Vigano S, Taioli E, Claris-Appiani A, et al. Proteinuria as a predictor of disease progression in children with hypodysplastic nephropathy. Pediatr Nephrol. 2004;19:172–7.

101. Wühl E, Trivelli A, Picca S, Litwin M, Peco-Antic A, Zurowska A, et al. Strict blood pressure control and renal failure progression in children. The ESCAPE Trial Group. N Engl J Med. 2009;361:1639–50.

102. van den Belt SM, Heerspink HJL, Gracchi V, de Zeeuw D, Wuhl E, Schaefer F, et al. Early proteinuria lowering by angiotensin-converting enzyme inhibition predicts renal survival in children with CKD. J Am Soc Nephrol. 2018;29(8):2225–33.

103. Furth SL, Pierce C, Hui WF, White CA, Wong CS, Schaefer F, et al. Estimating time to ESRD in children with CKD. Am J Kidney Dis. 2018;71(6):783–92.

104. Harambat J, Kunzmann K, Azukaitis K, Bayazit AK, Canpolat N, Doyon A, et al. Metabolic acidosis is common and associates with disease progression in children with chronic kidney disease. Kidney Int. 2017;92(6):1507–14.

105. Dobre M, Yang W, Chen J, Drawz P, Hamm LL, Horwitz E, et al. Association of serum bicarbonate with risk of renal and cardiovascular outcomes in CKD: a report from the Chronic Renal Insufficiency Cohort (CRIC) study. Am J Kidney Dis. 2013;62(4):670–8.

106. Mahajan A, Simoni J, Sheather SJ, Broglio KR, Rajab MH, Wesson DE. Daily oral sodium bicarbonate preserves glomerular filtration rate by slowing its decline in early hypertensive nephropathy. Kidney Int. 2010;78(3):303–9.

107. de Brito-Ashurst I, Varagunam M, Raftery MJ, Yaqoob MM. Bicarbonate supplementation slows progression of CKD and improves nutritional status. J Am Soc Nephrol. 2009;20:2075–84.

108. Gunta SS, Mak RH. Is obesity a risk factor for chronic kidney disease in children? Pediatr Nephrol. 2013;28(10):1949–56.

109. Muntner P, Coresh J, Clinton Smith J, Eckfeldt J, Klag MJ. Plasma lipids and risk of developing renal dysfunction: the Atherosclerosis Risk in Communities Study. Kidney Int. 2000;58:293–301.

110. Saland MJ, Ginsberg H, Fisher EA. Dyslipidemia in pediatric renal disease: epidemiology, pathophysiology, and management. Curr Opin Pediatr. 2002;14:197–204.

111. Cheng SC, Chu TS, Huang KY, Chen YM, Chang WK, Tsai TJ, et al. Association of hypertriglyceridemia and insulin resistance in uremic patients undergoing CAPD. Perit Dial Int. 2001;21:282–9.

112. Mak RH. 1,25-Dihydroxyvitamin D3 corrects insulin and lipid abnormalities in uremia. Kidney Int. 1998;53:1353–7.

113. Mak RH. Effect of metabolic acidosis on hyperlipidemia in uremia. Pediatr Nephrol. 1999;13:891–3.

114. Abrass CK. Cellular lipid metabolism and the role of lipids in progressive renal disease. Am J Nephrol. 2004;24:46–53.

115. Scheuer H, Gwinner W, Hohbach J, Grone EF, Brandes RP, Malle E, et al. Oxidant stress in hyperlipidemia-induced renal damage. Am J Physiol Renal Physiol. 2000;278:F63–74.

116. Chen J, Muntner P, Hamm LL, Jones DW, Batuman V, Fonseca V, et al. The metabolic syndrome and chronic kidney disease in US adults. Ann Int Med. 2004;140:167–74.

117. Zhou M, Sevilla L, Vallega G, Chen P, Palacin M, Zorzano A, et al. Insulin-dependent protein trafficking in skeletal muscle cells. Am J Phys. 1998;275:E187–E96.

118. Herget-Rosenthal S, Dehnen D, Kribben A, Quellmann T. Progressive chronic kidney disease in primary care: modifiable risk factors and predictive model. Prev Med. 2013;57(4):357–62.

119. Wang Y, Chen X, Song Y, Caballero B, Cheskin LJ. Association between obesity and kidney disease: a systematic review and meta-analysis. Kidney Int. 2008;73(1):19–33.

120. Bagby SP. Obesity-initiated metabolic syndrome and the kidney: a recipe for chronic kidney disease? J Am Soc Nephrol. 2004;15(11):2775–91.

121. Madero M, Sarnak MJ, Wang X, Greene T, Beck GJ, Kusek JW, et al. Uric acid and long-term outcomes in CKD. Am J Kidney Dis. 2009;53(5):796–803.

122. Tsai CW, Lin SY, Kuo CC, Huang CC. Serum uric acid and progression of kidney disease: a longitudinal analysis and mini-review. PLoS One. 2017;12(1):e0170393.

123. Rodenbach KE, Schneider MF, Furth SL, Moxey-Mims MM, Mitsnefes MM, Weaver DJ, et al. Hyperuricemia and progression of CKD in children and adolescents: the Chronic Kidney Disease in Children (CKiD) cohort study. Am J Kidney Dis. 2015;66(6):984–92.

124. Staples AO, Greenbaum LA, Smith JM, Gipson DS, Filler G, Warady BA, et al. Association between clinical risk factors and progression of chronic kidney disease in children. Clin J Am Soc Nephrol. 2010;5(12):2172–9.

125. Taliercio JJ, Schold JD, Simon JF, Arrigain S, Tang A, Saab G, et al. Prognostic importance of serum alkaline phosphatase in CKD stages 3–4 in a clinical population. Am J Kidney Dis. 2013;62(4):703–10.

126. Wolf M. Update on fibroblast growth factor 23 in chronic kidney disease. Kidney Int. 2012;82(7):737–47.

127. Lee S, Kang S, Joo YS, Lee C, Nam KH, Yun HR, et al. Smoking, smoking cessation, and progression of chronic kidney disease: results from KNOW-CKD Study. Nicotine Tob Res. 2021;23(1):92–8.

128. Omoloja A, Jerry-Fluker J, Ng DK, Abraham AG, Furth S, Warady BA, et al. Secondhand smoke exposure is associated with proteinuria in children with chronic kidney disease. Pediatr Nephrol. 2013;28(8):1243–51.

129. Bakris GL, Williams M, Dworkin L, Elliot WJ, Epstein M, Toto R, et al. Preserving renal function in adults with hypertension and diabetes: a consensus approach. National Kidney Foundation Hypertension and Diabetes Executive Committees Working Group. Am J Kidney Dis. 2000;36:646–61.

130. Sarnak MJ, Greene T, Wang X, Beck G, Kusek JW, Collins AJ, et al. The effect of a lower target blood pressure on the progression of kidney disease: long-term follow-up of the modification of diet in renal disease study. Ann Intern Med. 2005;142:342–51.

131. Schrier RW, Estacio RO, Mehler PS, Hiatt WR. Appropriate blood pressure control in hypertensive and normotensive type 2 diabetes mellitus: a summary of the ABCD trial. Nat Clin Pract Nephrol. 2008;3:428–38.

132. Ruggenenti P, Perna A, Loriga G, Ganeva M, Ene-Iordache B, Turturro M, et al. Blood pressure control for renoprotection in patients with non-diabetic chronic renal disease (REIN-2): multicenter, randomized controlled trial. Lancet. 2005;365: 939–46.

133. Wright JT Jr, Bakris G, Greene T, Agodoa LY, Appel LJ, Charleston J, et al. Effect of blood pressure lowering and antihypertensive drug class on progression of hypertensive kidney disease: results from the AASK trial. JAMA. 2002;288:2421–31.

134. Lv J, Ehteshami P, Sarnak MJ, Tighiouart H, Jun M, Ninomiya T, et al. Effects of intensive blood pressure lowering on the progression of chronic kidney disease: a systematic review and meta-analysis. CMAJ. 2013;185(11):949–57.

135. Lurbe E, Agabiti-Rosei E, Cruickshank JK, Dominiczak A, Erdine S, Hirth A, et al. 2016 European Society of Hypertension guidelines for the management of high blood pressure in children and adolescents. J Hypertens. 2016;34(10):1887–920.

136. Flynn JT, Kaelber DC, Baker-Smith CM, Blowey D, Carroll AE, Daniels SR, et al. Clinical practice guideline for screening and management of high blood pressure in children and adolescents. Pediatrics. 2017;140(3)

137. Williams B, Mancia G, Spiering W, Agabiti Rosei E, Azizi M, Burnier M, et al. 2018 ESC/ESH Guidelines for the management of arterial hypertension. Eur Heart J. 2018;

138. Whelton PK, Carey RM, Aronow WS, Casey DE Jr, Collins KJ, Dennison Himmelfarb C, et al. 2017 ACC/AHA/AAPA/ABC/ACPM/AGS/APhA/ASH/ASPC/NMA/PCNA Guideline for the Prevention, Detection, Evaluation, and Management of High Blood Pressure in Adults: Executive Summary: A Report of the American College of Cardiology/American Heart Association Task Force on Clinical Practice Guidelines. Hypertension. 2018;71(6):1269–324.

139. Cheung AK, Chang TI, Cushman WC, Furth SL, Hou FF, Ix JH, et al. Executive summary of the KDIGO 2021 clinical practice guideline for the management of blood pressure in chronic kidney disease. Kidney Int. 2021;99(3):559–69.

140. The GISEN Group (Gruppo Italiano di Studi Epidemiologici in Nephrologia). Randomized placebo-controlled trial of effect of ramipril on decline in glomerular filtration rate and risk of terminal renal failure in proteinuric, non-diabetic nephropathy. Lancet. 1997;349:1857–63.

141. Wright JT Jr, Bakris G, Greene T, Agodoa LY, Appel LJ, Charleston J, African American Study of Kidney Disease and Hypertension, et al. Effect of blood pressure lowering and antihypertensive drug class on progression of hypertensive kidney disease: Results from the AASK trial. JAMA. 2003;288:2421–31.

142. Remuzzi G, Ruggenenti P, Benigni A. Understanding the nature of renal disease progression. Kidney Int. 1997;51:2–15.

143. Ruggenenti P, Perna A, Remuzzi G. Retarding progression of chronic renal disease: the neglected issue of residual proteinuria. Kidney Int. 2003;63:2254–61.

144. Jafar TH, Schmid CH, Landa M, Giatras I, Toto R, Remuzzi G, et al. Angiotensin-converting enzyme inhibitors and progression of nondiabetic renal disease. A meta-analysis of patient-level data. Ann Intern Med. 2001;135(2):73–87.

145. Ruggenenti P, Schieppati A, Remuzzi G. Progression, remission, regression of chronic renal diseases. Lancet. 2001;357:1601–8.

146. Brenner BM, Cooper ME, DeZeeuw D, Keane WF, Mitch WE, Parving HH, et al. Effects of losartan on renal and cardiovascular outcomes in patients with type 2 diabetes and nephropathy. N Engl J Med. 2001;345:861–9.

147. Lewis EJ, Hunsicker LG, Raymond PB, Rohde RD, for the Collaborative Study G. The effect of angiotensin-converting-enzyme inhibition on diabetic nephropathy. N Engl J Med. 1993;329:1456–62.

148. Maschio G, Alberti D, Janin G, Locatelli F, Mann JF, Motolese M, et al. Effect of the angiotensin-converting-enzyme inhibitor benazepril on the progression of chronic renal insufficiency. The Angiotensin-Converting-Enzyme Inhibition in Progressive Renal Insufficiency Study Group. N Engl J Med. 1996;334(15):939–45.

149. Parving HH, Andersen AR, Smidt UM, Svendsen PA. Early aggressive antihypertensive treatment reduces rate of decline in kidney function in diabetic nephropathy. Lancet. 1983;1:1175–9.

150. Zucchelli P, Zuccalö A, Borghi M, Fusaroli M, Sasdelli M, Stallone C, et al. Long-term comparison between captopril and nifidepin in the progression of renal insufficiency. Kidney Int. 1992;42:452–8.

151. Kamper AL, Strandgaard S, Leyssac PP. Effect of enalapril on the progression of chronic renal failure: a randomized controlled trial. Am J Hypertens 1992;5:423–430.

152. van Essen GG, Apperloo AJ, Rensma PL, Stegeman CA, Sluiter WJ, de Zeeuw D. Are angiotensin converting enzyme inhibitors superior to beta blockers in retarding progressive renal function decline? Kidney Int Suppl. 1997;63:S58–62.

153. Hannedouche T, Landais P, Goldfarb B, elEsper N, Fournier A, Godin M, et al. Randomised controlled trial of enalapril and beta blockers in non-diabetic chronic renal failure. BMJ. 1994;309:833–7.

154. Bannister KM, Weaver A, Clarkson AR, Woodroffe AJ. Effect of angiotensin converting enzyme and calcium channel inhibition on progression of IgA nephropathy. Contrib Nephrol. 1995;111:184–92.

155. Ihle BU, Whitworth JA, Shahinfar S, Cnaan A, Kincaid-Smith PS, Becker GJ. Angiotensin-converting-enzyme inhibition in non-diabetic progresive renal insufficiency: a controlled double-blind trial. Am J Kidney Dis. 1996;27:489–95.

156. Ruggenenti P, Perna A, Gherardi G, Garini G, Zocalli C, Salvadori M, et al. Renoprotective properties of ACE-inhibition in non-diabetic nephropathies with non-nephrotic proteinuria. Lancet. 1999;354:359–64.

157. Viberti G, Mogensen CE, Groop LC, Pauls JF, European Microalbuminuria Captopril Study Group. Effect of captopril on progression to clinical proteinuria in patients with insulin-dependent diabetes mellitus and microalbuminuria. JAMA. 1994;271:275–9.

158. Parving HH, Hommel E, Smidt UM. Protection of kidney function and decrease in albuminuria by captopril in insulin-dependent diabetics with nephropathy. BMJ. 1988;297:1086–91.

159. Nakao N, Yoshimura A, Morita H, Takada M, Kayano T, Ideura T. Combination treatment of angiotensin-II receptor blocker and angiotensin-converting-enzyme inhibitor in non-diabetic renal disease (COOPERATE): a randomised controlled trial. Lancet. 2003;361:117–24.

160. Barnett AH, Bain SC, Bouter P, Karlberg B, Madsbad S, Jervell J, et al. Angiotensin-receptor blockade versus converting-enzyme inhibition in type 2 diabetes and nephropathy. N Engl J Med. 2004;351:1952–61.

161. Zhang Y, He D, Zhang W, Xing Y, Guo Y, Wang F, et al. ACE inhibitor benefit to kidney and cardiovascular outcomes for patients with non-dialysis chronic kidney disease stages 3–5: a network meta-analysis of randomised clinical trials. Drugs. 2020;80(8):797–811.

162. Burgess E, Muirhead N, De Cotret PR, Chiu A, Pichette V, Tobe S, et al. Supramaximal dose of candesartan in proteinuric kidney disease. J Am Soc Nephrol. 2009;20:893–900.

163. Wilmer WA, Rovin BH, Hebert CJ, Rao SV, Kumor K, Hebert LA. Management of glomerular proteinuria: a commentary. J Am Soc Nephrol. 2003;14:3217–32.

164. Van Dyck M, Proesmans W. Renoprotection by ACE inhibitors after severe hemolytic uremic syndrome. Pediatr Nephrol. 2004;19:688–90.

165. Ellis D, Vats A, Moritz ML, Reitz S, Grosso MJ, Janosky JE. Long-term antiproteinuric and renoprotective efficacy and safety of losartan in children with proteinuria. J Pediatr. 2003;143:89–97.

166. Tanaka H, Suzuki K, Nakahata T, Tsugawa K, Konno Y, Tsuruga K, et al. Combined therapy of enalapril and losartan attenuates histologic progression in immunoglobulin A nephropathy. Pediatr Int. 2004;46:576–9.

167. Wühl E, Mehls O, Schaefer F, Group ET. Antihypertensive and antiproteinuric efficacy of

ramipril in children with chronic renal failure. Kidney Int. 2004;66(2):768–76.

168. Schaefer F, Litwin M, Zachwieja J, Zurowska A, Turi S, Grosso A, et al. Efficacy and safety of valsartan compared to enalapril in hypertensive children: a 12-week, randomized, double-blind, parallel-group study. J Hypertens. 2011;29(12): 2484–90.

169. Schaefer F, Coppo R, Bagga A, Senguttuvan P, Schlosshauer R, Zhang Y, et al. Efficacy and safety of valsartan in hypertensive children 6 months to 5 years of age. J Hypertens. 2013;31(5):993–1000.

170. Schaefer F, van de Walle J, Zurowska A, Gimpel C, van Hoeck K, Drozdz D, et al. Efficacy and safety of candesartan cilexetil suspension in hypertensive infants: the CINCH trial. Pediatr Nephrol. 2009;24:OC044. (Abstract)

171. Trachtman H, Hainer JW, Sugg J, Teng R, Sorof JM, Radcliffe J, et al. Efficacy, safety and pharmacokinetics of candesartan cilexetil in hypertensive children aged 6 to 17 years. J Clin Hypertens (Greenwich). 2008;10:743–50.

172. Gross O, Tonshoff B, Weber LT, Pape L, Latta K, Fehrenbach H, et al. A multicenter, randomized, placebo-controlled, double-blind phase 3 trial with open-arm comparison indicates safety and efficacy of nephroprotective therapy with ramipril in children with Alport's syndrome. Kidney Int. 2020;97(6):1275–86.

173. Kashtan CE, Gross O. Clinical practice recommendations for the diagnosis and management of Alport syndrome in children, adolescents, and young adults-an update for 2020. Pediatr Nephrol. 2021;36(3):711–9.

174. Abraham AG, Betoko A, Fadrowski JJ, Pierce C, Furth SL, Warady BA, et al. Renin-angiotensin II-aldosterone system blockers and time to renal replacement therapy in children with CKD. Pediatr Nephrol. 2017;32(4):643–9.

175. Bakris GL, Weir MR. Angiotensin-converting enzyme inhibitor-associated elevations in serum creatinine: is this a cause for concern? Arch Int Med. 2000;160:685–93.

176. Mooser V, Nussberger J, Juillerat L, Burnier M, Waeber B, Bidiville J, et al. Reactive hyperreninemia is a major determinant of plasma angiotensin II during ACE inhibition. J Cardiovasc Pharmacol. 1990;15:276–82.

177. van den Meiracker AH, Manin't Veld AJ, Admiraal PJ, Ritsema van Eck HJ, Boomsma F, Derkx FH, et al. Partial escape of angiotensin converting enzyme (ACE) inhibition during prolonged ACE inhibitor treatment: does it exist and does it affect the antihypertensive response? J Hypertens. 1992;10:803–12.

178. Shiigai T, Shichiri M. Late escape from the antiproteinuric effect of ACE inhibitors in nondiabetic renal disease. Am J Kid Dis. 2001;37:477–83.

179. Bomback AS, Klemmer PJ. The incidence and implications of aldosterone breakthrough. Nat Clin Pract Nephrol. 2007;3:486–92.

180. Doulton TW, He FJ, MacGregor FA. Systemic review of combined angiotensin-converting enzyme inhibition and angiotensin receptor blockade in hypertension. Hypertension. 2005;45:880–6.

181. MacKinnon M, Shurraw S, Akbari A, Knoll GA, Jaffey J, Clark HD. Combination therapy with an angiotensin receptor blocker and an ACE inhibitor in proteinuric renal disease: a systematic review of the efficacy and safety data. Am J Kidney Dis. 2006;48:8–20.

182. Investigators O, Yusuf S, Teo KK, Pogue J, Dyal L, Copland I, et al. Renal outcomes with telmisartan, ramipril, or both, in patients at high vascular risk (The ONTARGET Study): a multicenter, randomized, double-blind, controlled trial. N Engl J Med. 2008;358:1547–59.

183. Mann JF, Schmieder RF, McQueen M, Dyal L, Schumacher H, Pogue J, et al. Renal outcomes with telmisartan, ramipril, or both, in people at high vascular risk (the ONTARGET study): a multicentre, randomised, double-blind, controlled trial. Lancet. 2008;372:547–53.

184. Abutaleb N. ONTARGET should not be over interpreted. Nephrol Dial Transplant. 2010;25(1):44–7.

185. White WB, Carr AA, Krause S, Jordan R, Roniker B, Oigman W. Assessment of the novel selective aldosterone blocker eplerenone using ambulatory and clinical blood pressure in patients with systemic hypertension. Am J Cardiol. 2003;92:38–42.

186. Chung EY, Ruospo M, Natale P, Bolignano D, Navaneethan SD, Palmer SC, et al. Aldosterone antagonists in addition to renin angiotensin system antagonists for preventing the progression of chronic kidney disease. Cochrane Database Syst Rev. 2020;10:CD007004.

187. Bakris GL, Agarwal R, Anker SD, Pitt B, Ruilope LM, Rossing P, et al. Effect of finerenone on chronic kidney disease outcomes in type 2 diabetes. N Engl J Med. 2020;383(23):2219–29.

188. Weir MR, Bakris GL, Bushinsky DA, Mayo MR, Garza D, Stasiv Y, et al. Patiromer in patients with kidney disease and hyperkalemia receiving RAAS inhibitors. N Engl J Med. 2015;372(3):211–21.

189. Oparil S, Yarows SA, Patel S, Fang H, Zhang J, Satlin A. Efficacy and safety of combined use of aliskiren and valsartan in patients with hypertension: a randomized, double-blind trial. Lancet. 2007;370:221–9.

190. European Medicines A. http://www.ema.europa.eu/docs/en_GB/document_library/Other/2012/02/WC500122919.pdf. 2012.

191. Marchi F, Ciriello G. Efficacy of carvedilol in mild to moderate essential hypertension and effects on microalbuminuria: a multicenter, randomized. open-label, controlled study versus atenolol. Adv Ther. 1995;12:212–21.

192. Fassbinder W, Quarder O, Waltz A. Treatment with carvedilol is associated with a significant reduction in microalbuminuria: a multicenter randomized study. Int J Clin Pract. 1999;53:519–22.

193. Schaefer F, Doyon A, Azukaitis K, Bayazit A, Canpolat N, Duzova A, et al. Cardiovascular phenotypes in children with CKD: the 4C study. Clin J Am Soc Nephrol. 2017;12(1):19–28.

194. Flynn JT, Mitsnefes M, Pierce C, Cole SR, Parekh RS, Furth SL, et al. Blood pressure in children with chronic kidney disease: a report from the Chronic Kidney Disease in Children study. Hypertension. 2008;52(4):631–7.

195. Hermida RC, Diana EA, Calvo C. Administration-time-dependent effects of antihypertensive treatment on the circadian pattern of blood pressure. Curr Opin Nephrol Hypertens. 2005;14:453–9.

196. Hermida RC, Ayala DE, Mojón A, Fernández JR. Bedtime dosing of antihypertensive medications reduces cardiovascular risk in CKD. J Am Soc Nephrol. 2011;22:2313–21.

197. Piperidou A, Loutradis C, Sarafidis P. SGLT-2 inhibitors and nephroprotection: current evidence and future perspectives. J Hum Hypertens. 2020;

198. Heerspink HJL, Kosiborod M, Inzucchi SE, Cherney DZI. Renoprotective effects of sodium-glucose cotransporter-2 inhibitors. Kidney Int. 2018;94(1):26–39.

199. Piperidou A, Sarafidis P, Boutou A, Thomopoulos C, Loutradis C, Alexandrou ME, et al. The effect of SGLT-2 inhibitors on albuminuria and proteinuria in diabetes mellitus: a systematic review and meta-analysis of randomized controlled trials. J Hypertens. 2019;37(7):1334–43.

200. Sarraju A, Li J, Cannon CP, Chang TI, Agarwal R, Bakris G, et al. Effects of canagliflozin on cardiovascular, renal, and safety outcomes in participants with type 2 diabetes and chronic kidney disease according to history of heart failure: Results from the CREDENCE trial. Am Heart J. 2021;233:141–8.

201. Heerspink HJL, Stefansson BV, Correa-Rotter R, Chertow GM, Greene T, Hou FF, et al. Dapagliflozin in patients with chronic kidney disease. N Engl J Med. 2020;383(15):1436–46.

202. Herrington WG, Preiss D, Haynes R, von Eynatten M, Staplin N, Hauske SJ, et al. The potential for improving cardio-renal outcomes by sodium-glucose co-transporter-2 inhibition in people with chronic kidney disease: a rationale for the EMPA-KIDNEY study. Clin Kidney J. 2018;11(6):749–61.

203. Cho ME, Kopp JB. Pirfenidone: an anti-fibrotic therapy for progressive kidney disease. Expert Opin Investig Drugs. 2010;19(2):275–83.

204. Allinovi M, De Chiara L, Angelotti ML, Becherucci F, Romagnani P. Anti-fibrotic treatments: a review of clinical evidence. Matrix Biol. 2018;68–69:333–54.

205. Mann JF, Green D, Jamerson K, Ruilope LM, Kuranoff SJ, Littke T, et al. Avosentan for overt diabetic nephropathy. J Am Soc Nephrol. 2010;21:527–35.

206. Heerspink HJL, Parving HH, Andress DL, Bakris G, Correa-Rotter R, Hou FF, et al. Atrasentan and renal events in patients with type 2 diabetes and chronic kidney disease (SONAR): a double-blind, randomised, placebo-controlled trial. Lancet. 2019;393(10184):1937–47.

207. Trachtman H, Nelson P, Adler S, Campbell KN, Chaudhuri A, Derebail VK, et al. DUET: a phase 2 study evaluating the efficacy and safety of sparsentan in patients with FSGS. J Am Soc Nephrol. 2018;29(11):2745–54.

208. Benigni A, Buelli S, Kohan DE. Endothelin-targeted new treatments for proteinuric and inflammatory glomerular diseases: focus on the added value to anti-renin-angiotensin system inhibition. Pediatr Nephrol. 2021;36(4):763–75.

209. Juul-Nielsen C, Shen J, Stenvinkel P, Scholze A. Systematic review of the nuclear factor erythroid 2-related factor 2 (NRF2) system in human chronic kidney disease: alterations, interventions, and relation to morbidity. Nephrol Dial Transplant. 2021;

210. Pergola PE, Raskin P, Toto RD, Meyer CJ, Huff JW, Grossman EB, et al. Bardoxolone methyl and kidney function in CKD with type 2 diabetes. N Engl J Med. 2011;365(4):327–36.

211. Liu D, Wang LN, Li HX, Huang P, Qu LB, Chen FY. Pentoxifylline plus ACEIs/ARBs for proteinuria and kidney function in chronic kidney disease: a meta-analysis. J Int Med Res. 2017;45(2):383–98.

212. Judge PK, Haynes R. TaleNeprilysin and Neprilysin inhibition in chronic kidney disease. Curr Opin Nephrol Hypertens. 2021;30(1):123–30.

213. Torres VE, Chapman AB, Devuyst O, Gansevoort RT, Grantham JJ, Higashihara E, et al. Tolvaptan in patients with autosomal dominant polycystic kidney disease. N Engl J Med. 2012;367(25):2407–18.

214. Torres VE, Higashihara E, Devuyst O, Chapman AB, Gansevoort RT, Grantham JJ, et al. Effect of Tolvaptan in autosomal dominant polycystic kidney disease by CKD stage: results from the TEMPO 3:4 trial. Clin J Am Soc Nephrol. 2016;11(5):803–11.

215. Torres VE, Gansevoort RT, Czerwiec FS. Tolvaptan in later-stage polycystic kidney disease. N Engl J Med. 2018;378(5):489–90.

216. Mekahli D, Guay-Woodford L, Cadnaparphornchai M, Greenbaum LA, Litwin M, Seeman T, et al. Randomized, placebo-controlled, phase 3b trial of tolvaptan in the treatment of children and adolescents with autosomal dominant polycystic kidney disease (ADPKD): 1-year data. Abstract FC130. Nephrol Dial Transplant. 2021;36. https://academic.oup.com/ndt/article/36/Supplement_1/gfab134.001/6289663

217. Mak RH. Metabolic effects of erythropoietin in patients on peritoneal dialysis. Pediatr Nephrol. 1998;12:660–5.

218. Mak RH. Effect of metabolic acidosis on insulin action and secretion in uremia. Kidney Int. 1998;54(2):603–7.

219. Wanner C, Tonelli M, Kidney Disease: Improving Global Outcomes Lipid Guideline Development Work Group M. KDIGO Clinical Practice Guideline for Lipid Management in CKD: summary of recommendation statements and clinical approach to the patient. Kidney Int. 2014;85(6):1303–9.

220. Epstein M, Campese VM. Pleiotropic effects of 3-hydroxy-3-methylglutaryl coenzyme a reductase inhibitors on renal function. Am J Kidney Dis. 2005;45:2–14.

221. Sanguankeo A, Upala S, Cheungpasitporn W, Ungprasert P, Knight EL. Effects of statins on renal outcome in chronic kidney disease patients: a systematic review and meta-analysis. PLoS One. 2015;10(7):e0132970.

222. Hu PJ, Wu MY, Lin TC, Chen TT, Wu YC, Su SL, et al. Effect of statins on renal function in chronic kidney disease patients. Sci Rep. 2018;8(1):16276.

223. Klahr S, Levy AD, Beck GJ. The effects of dietary protein restriction and blood-pressure control on the progression of chronic renal disease. N Engl J Med. 1994;330:877–84.

224. K/DOQI Clinical practice guidelines for bone metabolism and disease in children with chronic kidney disease. Am J Kidney Dis. 2005;46(Suppl. 1):S12–S100.

225. Patel L, Bernard LM, Elder GJ. Sevelamer versus calcium-based binders for treatment of hyperphosphatemia in CKD: a meta-analysis of randomized controlled trials. Clin J Am Soc Nephrol. 2016;11(2):232–44.

226. Martinez-Arias L, Panizo S, Alonso-Montes C, Martin-Virgala J, Martin-Carro B, Fernandez-Villabrille S, et al. Effects of calcitriol and paricalcitol on renal fibrosis in CKD. Nephrol Dial Transplant. 2021;

227. Shroff R, Aitkenhead H, Costa N, Trivelli A, Litwin M, Picca S, et al. Normal 25-Hydroxyvitamin D levels are associated with less proteinuria and attenuate renal failure progression in children with CKD. J Am Soc Nephrol. 2016;27(1):314–22.

228. de Borst MH, Vervloet MG, ter Wee PM, Navis G. Cross talk between the renin-angiotensin-aldosterone system and vitamin D-FGF-23-klotho in chronic kidney disease. J Am Soc Nephrol. 2011;22(9):1603–9.

229. Siu YP, Leung KT, Tong MK, Kwan TH. Use of allopurinol in slowing the progression of renal disease through its ability to lower serum uric acid level. Am J Kidney Dis. 2006;47:51–9.

230. Whelton A, Macdonald PA, Zhao L, Hunt B, Gunawardhana L. Renal function in gout: long-term treatment effects of febuxostat. J Clin Rheumatol. 2011;17(1):7–13.

231. Badve SV, Pascoe EM, Tiku A, Boudville N, Brown FG, Cass A, et al. Effects of allopurinol on the progression of chronic kidney disease. N Engl J Med. 2020;382(26):2504–13.

232. Levey AS, Greene T, Sarnak MJ, Wang X, Beck GJ, Kusek JW, et al. Effect of dietary protein restriction on the progression of kidney disease: long-term follow-up of the Modification of Diet in Renal Disease (MDRD) Study. Am J Kidney Dis. 2006;48:876–88.

233. Fouque D, Laville M, Boissel JP. Low-protein diets for chronic kidney disease in non diabetic adults (Cochrane review). In: The renal health library. Oxford: Update Software Ltd.; 2005.

234. Chaturvedi S, Jones C. Protein restriction for children with chronic renal failure. Cochrane Database Syst Rev. 2007;17:CD006863.

235. Carriazo S, Perez-Gomez MV, Cordido A, Garcia-Gonzalez MA, Sanz AB, Ortiz A, et al. Dietary care for ADPKD patients: current status and future directions. Nutrients. 2019;11(7)

236. Bahlmann FH, Fliser D. Erythropoietin and renoprotection. Curr Opin Nephrol Hypertens. 2009;18(1):15–20.

237. Sharples EJ, Patel N, Brown P, Stewart K, Mota-Philipe H, Shaeff M, et al. Erythropoietin protects the kidney against the injury and dysfunction caused by ischemia-reperfusion. J Am Soc Nephrol. 2004;15:2115–24.

238. Eto N, Wada T, Inagi R, Takano H, Shimizu A, Kato H, et al. Podocyte protection by darbepoetin: preservation of the cytoskeleton and nephrin expression. Kidney Int. 2007;72:455–63.

239. Lurbe E, Cifkova R, Cruickshank JK, Dillon MJ, Ferreira I, Invitti C, et al. Management of high blood pressure in children and adolescents: recommendations of the European Society of Hypertension. J Hypertens. 2009;27(9):1719–42.

240. National High Blood Pressure Education Program Working Group on High Blood Pressure in Children and Adolescents. The fourth report on the diagnosis, evaluation, and treatment of high blood pressure in children and adolescents. Pediatrics. 2004;114:555–76.

241. KDIGO 2017 Clinical Practice Guideline Update for the Diagnosis, Evaluation, Prevention, and Treatment of Chronic Kidney Disease–Mineral and Bone Disorder (CKD-MBD). Kidney Int Suppl. 2017;7:1–59.

Growth and Puberty in Chronic Kidney Disease

56

Dieter Haffner and Lesley Rees

Introduction

Maintaining optimum growth is one of the most challenging problems in the management of children with chronic kidney disease (CKD): reports published in 2013 showed that approximately 50% of children requiring kidney replacement therapy (KRT) before their 13th birthday had a final height below the normal range [1–4]. Short stature is a marker for increased mortality and hampers the psychosocial integration of pediatric CKD patients [5–7]. There is, however, evidence that, alongside advancements in the medical and technical management of CKD and kidney replacement therapy (KRT), height prognosis has substantially improved over the past decades [1, 2, 4, 8–11]. In 799 pre-dialysis children with mostly mild to moderate CKD (median age 11 years, estimated glomerular filtration rate (eGFR) 50 mL/min/1.73 m^2) followed in the Chronic Kidney Disease in Children (CKiD) Study, the median height standard deviation score (SDS) was −0.55. Among 594 patients from 12 European countries with CKD stage 3–5 (median eGFR 30 mL/min/1.73 m^2) who were followed prospectively in the 4C Study, mean height SDS was −1.57, with 36% of patients having a height below the third percentile. In 1001 children in the International Pediatric Peritoneal Dialysis Network (IPPN), the mean height SDS at initiation of dialysis was −1.97 [10]. Hence, these data from contemporaneous large cohort studies demonstrate that growth failure progressively occurs with decreasing eGFR. In the 2020 USRDS report the percentage of incident end-stage kidney disease (ESKD) patients with short stature was lowest in the oldest patients age groups, being 20.3% at 18–19.9 years, 25.8% at 14–17, 20.1% at 10–13, 38.8% at 5–9 and 51.9% at 0–4 years of age [11, 12].

There appears to be a positive trend over time: e.g. in Germany, the mean standardized height in children on KRT has increased over the past 20 years from −3.0 SDS to −1.8 SDS [1]. Yet this is not the case in all parts of the world, particularly in those with inadequate local resources, where height prognosis remains dismally low [2, 13]. Even across Europe, the 4C Study observed growth failure to vary widely between countries, from 7% to 44% [9].

There is no single cause of failing growth in children with CKD (Fig. 56.1). The two most important influences are the severity of CKD and young age at its onset, so that children with CKD due to congenital kidney abnormalities manifest-

D. Haffner (✉) · L. Rees
Department of Paediatric Kidney, Liver and Metabolic Diseases, Hannover Medical School, Hannover, Germany

Department of Paediatric Nephrology, Gt Ormond St Hospital for Children NHS Foundation Trust, London, UK
e-mail: Haffner.dieter@mh-hannover.de;
Lesley.Rees@gosh.nhs.uk

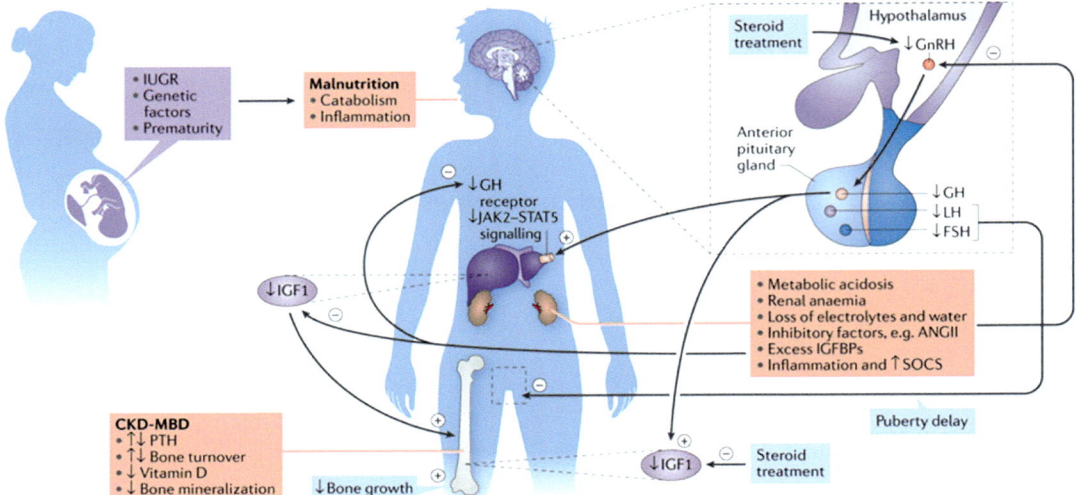

Fig. 56.1 The etiology of growth failure in CKD is multifactorial and includes intrauterine growth restriction (IUGR), genetic factors such as parental height and primary renal disease, prematurity, and malnutrition which especially limits growth in children with congenital CKD. Mineral and bone disorder (CKD-MBD), metabolic acidosis, anemia, loss of electrolytes and water, and disturbances of the somatotropic and gonadotropic hormone axes are additional factors. CKD is a state of growth hormone (GH) insensitivity, characterized by deficiency of functional insulin-like growth factor I (IGF-I), to reduced GH receptor expression in target organs like the liver, disturbed GH receptor signaling via the Janus kinase - signal transducers, activators of transcription (JAK2-STAT5) due to inflammation induced SOCS (suppressor of cytokine signalling), and increased IGF-binding capacity due to excess of IGFBPs. Finally, reduced release of hypothalamic gonadotropin-releasing hormone (GnRH), due to uremia-related inhibitory factors such as angiotensin II (AngII), and steroid treatment may result in decreased circulating levels of bioactive luteinizing hormone (LH), hypogonadism and reduced pubertal growth spurt. PTH, parathyroid hormone; FSH, follicle stimulating hormone; IGFBP, insulin-like growth factor binding proteins. [Reproduced with permission of [30]]

ing in infancy are usually more severely affected than those with acquired conditions developing in later childhood. This review summarizes the current knowledge of the phenotype, pathophysiology and therapeutic options for children with failing growth resulting from CKD.

Normal Growth

The physiological growth pattern can be divided into fetal, infantile, mid-childhood and pubertal phases (Fig. 56.2) [14]. During fetal life, nearly 30% of final height has already been achieved, so low birth weight and prematurity can substantially influence subsequent growth and final height attainment: although many otherwise normal infants born prematurely grow normally, and those who are small for gestational age (SGA) catch up in the first 6 months of life, around 10%, particularly if SGA, remain below the normal range for height into adulthood. A further one third to one half of total postnatal growth occurs during the first 2 years of life, and 20% during the pubertal phase. Throughout each postnatal phase the predominant influences on growth are different. Whereas in infancy, growth mainly depends on nutritional intake, growth in mid-childhood is driven by the somatotropic hormone axis. During puberty, the gonadotropic hormone axis stimulates growth via increased proliferation of growth plate chondrocytes and modulation of growth hormone (GH) secretion from the pituitary gland, resulting in the pubertal growth spurt (Fig. 56.2) [14].

Fig. 56.2 Typical growth pattern in congenital chronic kidney disease. Relative loss in the nutrient-dependent infantile and gonadal hormone-dependent puberty phases, and percentile-parallel growth in the mainly GH-dependent growth period in mid-childhood are shown. The shaded area represents the normal range, third to 97th centiles. (Reproduced with permission of [14])

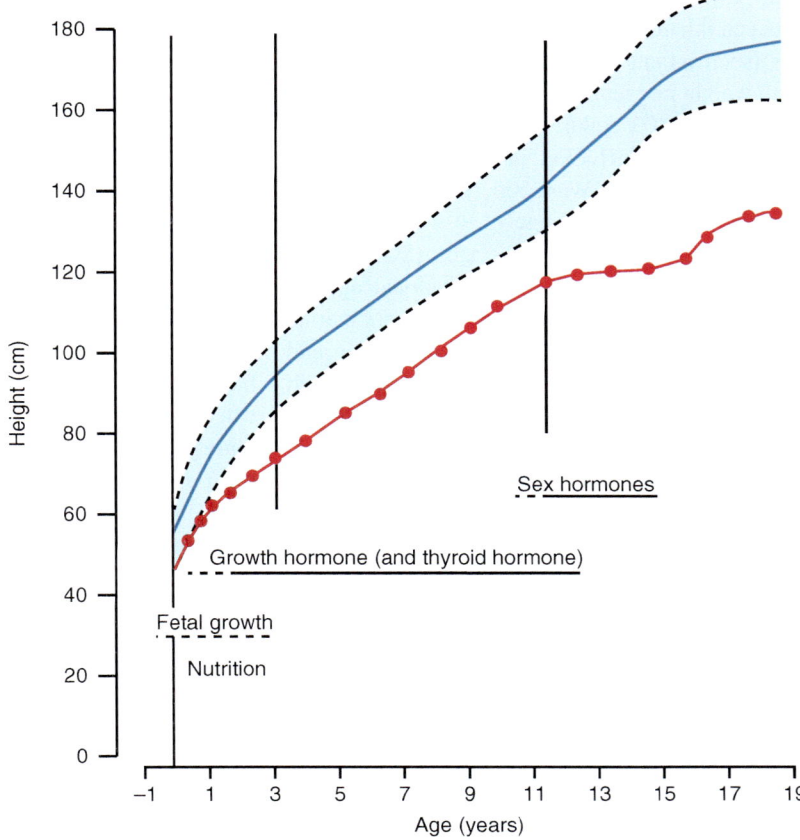

Effect of CKD on the Phases of Growth

The classical growth pattern for a child born with CKD was described in 1974 [15]. Length at birth is usually already below the mean (Fig. 56.2) [16]. As with any chronic disease, height velocity is most affected during periods of rapid growth. Marked growth retardation occurs during the first 2 years of life, followed by percentile parallel growth in mid-childhood, but catch-up growth is unusual. In the pre-pubertal years, the appearance of secondary sexual characteristics is delayed and the growth rate again decreases disproportionately [17, 18]. The pubertal growth spurt is later than normal and its magnitude impaired, resulting in further loss of growth

potential and reduced final height (Fig. 56.2) [14]. Over the last 20 years, although these basic principles remain, this classic description has been reassessed as there have been new concepts and treatments for most patients in all postnatal phases of growth.

The Fetal Phase

Reduced fetal growth was described as a feature of the classic growth pattern of the child with CKD in 1994, and has been demonstrated in several studies since [16, 19–22]. Both prematurity and low birth weights are common. The incidence is particularly high in infants on dialysis but perhaps more surprisingly is high in children with less severe CKD as well [23]. Registry data do not always distinguish between infants who do or do not have co morbidities (such infants often have below normal mean birth weight and length) but it has been shown that of just over 400 children with a mean eGFR of around 40 mL/min/1.73 m^2 in the US CKD registry, low birth weight (LBW, <2500 g) occurred in 17%, prematurity (gestational age < 36 weeks) in 12% and small for gestational age (SGA, birth weight < tenth percentile for gestational age) in 14%. It has been hypothesized that poor intrauterine growth conditions, e.g. maternal malnutrition and smoking, could cause both intrauterine growth retardation and kidney dysplasia [24, 25]. Likewise genetic abnormalities, e.g. dysregulation of Wilms' tumor suppressor gene, could cause both short stature and renal hypodysplasia [26]. Interestingly, in the US CKD registry 40% of patients had needed intensive care (ICU) at birth. The comparable overall incidence of abnormal birth history in the US population is 7–8%. Low birth weight, prematurity, SGA and requirement for ICU were all risk factors for poor growth outcomes, independent of renal function [21]. Likewise, intrauterine growth retardation, neonatal distress and parental height were shown to be important independent predictors of poor growth outcome in a cohort of 509 German children with CKD stage 3–5 [27].

The Infantile Phase

It is not surprising that adverse effects on growth are most intense during the infantile phase, and in particular the first 6 months of life, as the rate of growth is as high as 25 cm per year at birth, 18 cm per year at 6 months of age, and still 12 cm per year at 12 months of age. These figures are higher than at any other time during childhood and adolescence. Such growth challenges require nutrient intakes that are relatively higher than at any other age. As the infantile phase is predominantly dependent on nutrition, inadequate intake at this time can have a dramatic influence on growth. Indeed, any circumstances leading to decreased growth rates in this phase result in severe growth retardation and a potentially irreversible loss of growth potential [28, 29]. The decrease in mean standardized height can amount

to 0.6 SD per month in infants with CKD stage 5. In recent years the increasing acceptance of KRT for all infants, including those with associated comorbidities, has increased the challenge to achieve normal growth in this age group [20]. Malnutrition in young children with CKD is due to inadequate nutritional intake and frequently recurrent vomiting as well. In addition, catabolic episodes due to infections, loss of water and electrolytes, and CKD-mineral and bone disorder (CKD-MBD) are major contributing factors to growth impairment in this period. If these disturbances are adequately controlled, severe stunting can be avoided in the majority of patients without untreatable comorbidities [19, 20, 30]. However, most infants suffering from severe CKD need supplementary feeding in order to provide adequate nutrient, water and electrolyte intake [31].

The Childhood Phase

During this phase, the somatotropic hormone axis becomes the most important influence on growth. Growth is closely correlated with the degree of kidney dysfunction in this period. Although there is no critical threshold, growth patterns are typically stable if the GFR remains above 25 mL/min/1.73 m^2 and tend to diverge from the percentiles below this level [23]. Sequels of CKD such as anemia, metabolic acidosis and malnutrition seem to be less important in midchildhood. However, even a growth rate that parallels the centiles may not be 'normal', as children with good renal function and steroid-free immunosuppression following transplantation exhibit significant catch-up, compatible with the concept of continued suppression of an intrinsic catch-up growth potential in the uremic state [32, 33].

The Pubertal Phase

Pubertal Development
Delayed onset and progression of pubertal development was a common feature when KRT programs for children started [17]. Studies of the timing of pubertal onset have been hampered by the fact that bone age is only a crude marker for

assessment in CKD. Indeed, the distribution of bone age at pubertal onset varies at least as much as the distribution of chronological age in these patients. However, data from the late eighties demonstrated a delay of pubertal onset by 2–2.5 years in children with ESKD [17]. Menarche occurred after the upper limit of the normal age range (i.e. 15 years) in almost half of the girls treated by dialysis or transplantation [34]. Moreover, despite the achievement of pubertal stage IV or V, a substantial proportion of dialysis patients presented with permanently impaired reproductive function [35]. Fortunately, in the last twenty years most children requiring KRT before pubertal age present with normal or only slightly delayed pubertal onset. In two recent studies, mean age at pubertal onset as well as age at menarche did not differ between children on KRT and healthy children; and the serum levels of pubertal reproductive hormones were normal in the great majority of patients [1, 36]. Bone maturation in patients on KRT continues to be delayed by approximately 1.4 years compared to healthy children, although this does not negatively impact on pubertal development [1]. The age at onset of puberty has been positively correlated with the age at transplantation. Thus, early renal transplantation is a prerequisite for prevention of pubertal delay in children with stage 5 CKD [18, 36]. A recent analysis of the CKiD cohort including children with CKD stage 3–5 revealed delayed menarche in 10% of adolescent patients which was associated with African American race, lower eGFR, ever corticosteroid use, and longer duration of CKD [18, 37]. Delayed menarche was strongly associated with reduced height (<−2.0 SDS). Thus, delayed puberty is an important contributor to short stature in female patients even prior to dialysis. Patients who show delayed puberty—defined in boys by a testicular volume < 4 mL at the age of 14 years and in girls by a breast stage <B2 at age 13.5 years—should undergo work up by a pediatric endocrinologist including potential induction of puberty [30].

Pubertal Growth

During the last two decades in parallel with the improvement in sexual maturation has been an improvement in pubertal height gain [1, 2, 17, 18]. Longitudinal growth in 384 German

children on KRT who were followed between 1998 and 2009 was compared with 732 children enrolled in the European Dialysis and Transplant Association (EDTA) Registry between 1985 and 1988 (Fig. 56.3) [1]. In line with previous

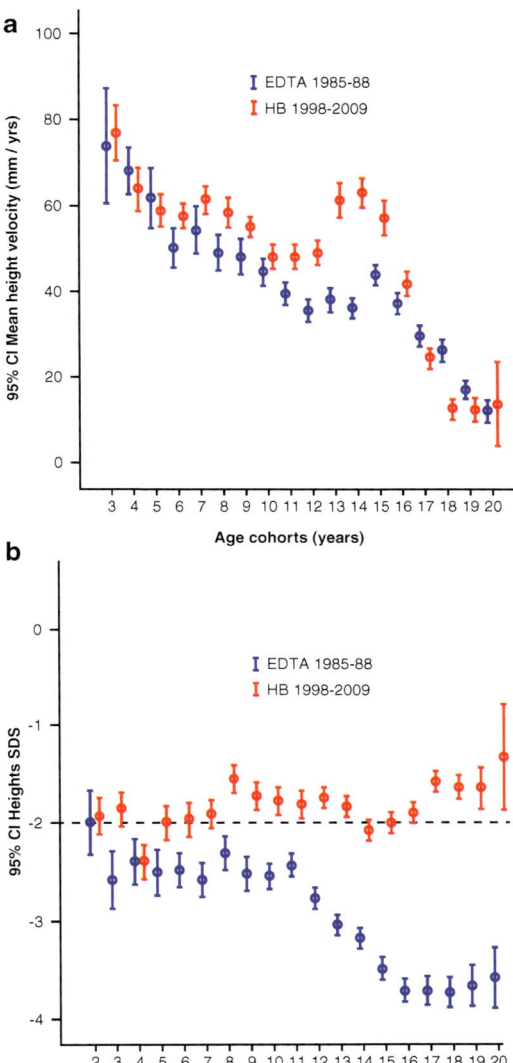

Fig. 56.3 (**a**) Mean height velocity of European children with renal replacement therapy in the EDTA study 1985–1988 (blue lines) versus the Hannover/Berlin (H/B) pediatric population cohort 1998–2009 (red lines) in different age cohorts. (**b**) Age-dependent height standard deviation score of European children on kidney replacement therapy 1985–1988 (EDTA study, n = 732, blue error bars) and in the HB group (n = 384, red error bars). EDTA European Dialysis and Transplant Association, CI Confidence interval. Reproduced with permission of [1]

studies, the pubertal growth spurt in the EDTA patients was delayed by approximately 2.5 years. In many patients no clear pubertal growth spurt was present, and consequently standardized height decreased during pubertal age. In contrast, a clear pubertal growth spurt was present and the onset of the pubertal growth spurt was within the normal range in the majority of the patients followed-up more recently. Consequently, standardized height even improved during puberty and until adult height. A strong negative correlation between total pubertal height gain and age at transplantation was reported in two studies a [18, 36]. Thus, whereas 20 years ago a loss of about 1.0 SD was expected during puberty, nowadays normal or only slightly reduced pubertal growth spurt can be expected if long-term dialysis is avoided.

Segmental Growth

It has been postulated that during malnutrition there is preferential preservation of growth of vital organs at the expense of less vital tissues such as the limbs, so that malnutrition during childhood results in disproportionate stunting with impairment of leg growth, and preserved trunk and head growth [38]. Consequently, relative leg length is increasingly used as a biomarker of childhood nutrition in epidemiological studies [39, 40]. Information pertaining to segmental growth has been collected in the CKD Growth and Development Study, in which more than 800 pediatric CKD patients before and after transplantation have been enrolled since 1998 [41–43]. Patients with a long-term history of CKD and KRT showed an age related disproportionate growth pattern [41–43]. Growth impairment and disproportionality was most obvious in early childhood. Sitting height was mostly preserved, whereas growth of the legs and arms was most severely affected. This resulted in a markedly elevated sitting height index (ratio of sitting height to total body height). Leg length was more affected in prepubertal patients. Consequently, body disproportion was less pronounced in pubertal patients. In addition to transplant func-

tion and steroid exposure, congenital CKD, smallness for gestational age, young age, and use of recombinant human growth hormone (rhGH) in the pre-transplant period were significantly associated with growth outcome (stature and degree of body disproportion. Catch-up growth after kidney transplantation is mainly related to improved trunk growth in children aged less than 4 years and stimulated leg growth in older children resulting in complete normalization of body proportions until attainment of adult height in the vast majority of patients [42, 44].

Adult Height and Height Prediction

When interpreting the adult heights of patients treated for CKD in childhood, it has to be remembered that the data obtained at any time will reflect treatment practices spanning the previous two decades. Furthermore, most reports of adult heights do not or incompletely discriminate according to patient characteristics (e.g. diagnoses, ages of onset of CKD, types and durations of KRT), and in particular registries do not separate out children with co morbidities that affect growth in their own right. With that in mind, reduced adult heights have been reported in up to 50% of CKD patients, although there has been a trend for improvement over the past decade [1–4, 17, 18, 45]. Mean adult heights vary from 148–158 cm for females and 162–168 cm for males (second centiles 151 and 163 cm respectively).

The ESPN/EDTA registry has shown that, after adjustment for age and period of start of KRT, final height increased significantly from -1.93 SDS in children who started KRT before 1990, to -1.78 in children in 1990–1999, and to -1.61 in those starting KRT after 1999 ($p < 0.001$). While 55% of patients attained an adult height within the normal range between 1990 and 19,995, this figure had risen to 62% between 2006–2011 [2]. The improvement in adult height over time was independent of age at the start of KRT (Fig. 56.4). Poorest growth outcomes were associated with earlier start and longer duration of dialysis or a diagnosis of a metabolic disorder such as cystinosis and hyper-

Fig. 56.4 Changes in final height SDS over time according to age and period of start of KRT (n = 981). The horizontal line in the middle of the box represents the median, the bottom and top of the box represent the lower and upper quartiles, respectively, and the ends of the whiskers represent the tenth and the 90th percentiles. (Reproduced with permission of [2])

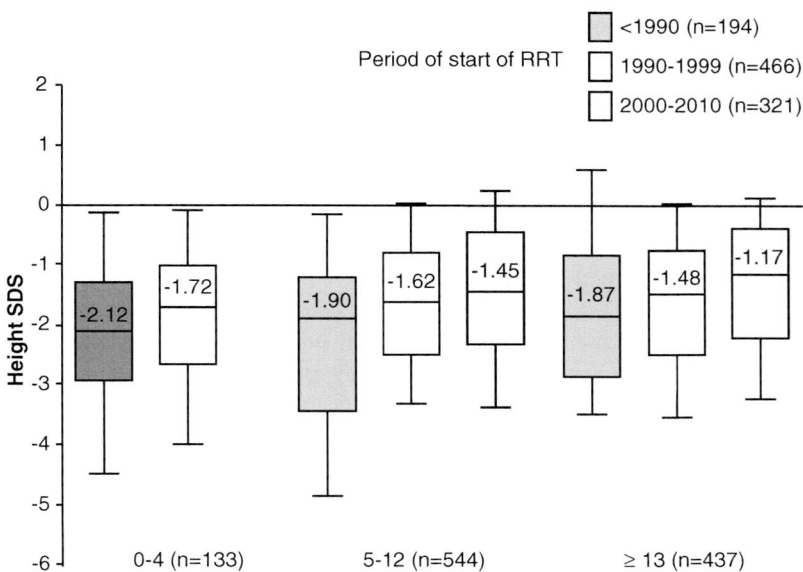

oxaluria; whereas those with a longer time spent with a renal transplant and those treated with rhGH did the best [2–4, 46–49].

There is evidence that over the years, final height post transplantation is improving [3]. This is likely to be due to a combination of factors such as better growth attained pre transplant, e.g. by adequate nutrition and rhGH therapy, pre-emptive transplantation thus avoiding dialysis, and to the development of protocols that mini-mize the use of corticosteroids. European data show an improvement in final height from −2.06 SDS in children who reached adulthood in 1990–1995 to −1.33 SDS in 2006–2011[2]. In the 2014 NAPRTCS report, the mean height SDS of those >19 years of age was −1.37. Twenty-five percent of these patients had a height SDS of −2.2 or worse, and 10% were more than 3.2 SD below the mean. This has improved considerably as adult height SDS was −1.93 with the 1987–1991 cohort, −1.51 for 1992–1996 cohort; −1.06 for the 1997–2001 cohort, −0.98 for the 2002–2006 cohort and −0.89 for the most recent cohort (https://naprtcs.org/system/files/2014_Annual_Transplant_Report.pdf).

Older age at start of KRT, starting KRT more recently, cumulative time with a transplant, and greater height SDS at initiation of KRT were independently associated with a higher adult height SDS. Most impressively, recent results of the avoidance of steroids post transplant alto-gether are excellent, with mean final heights of 177 cm and 175 cm in males transplanted prepu-bertally and postpubertally respectively, with sim-ilar figures of 165 cm and 162 cm for females [4].

The application of adult height prediction methods in children suffering from CKD is not recommended. In several validation studies final height was overpredicted by 3–10 cm [17, 18, 46]. Most likely this reflects the complexity and thus unpredictability of growth and development under the conditions of chronic uremia, with highly variable and dynamic impacts of disease progression, medications, bone disease, KRT modalities, skeletal maturation, and pubertal tim-ing [18, 46].

Causes of Growth Failure in CKD

Growth failure in CKD is due to a complex inter-play of many different factors, with varying effects at different ages and stages of CKD (Fig. 56.1). While some factors, such as nutritional and hormonal abnormalities, and hemato-logical and metabolic derangements such as acidosis, electrolyte imbalance, and CKD-MBD are potentially correctable, the effects of others, such as birth parameters, associated syndromes, race and parental heights, are not [27]. There is a substantial global variation of the degree of growth failure in children on KRT which is at least partly explained by differences in economics. In a recent survey of the IPPN network gross national income was a strong independent predictor of standardized height, adding to the impact of other well-known factors, e.g. congenital CKD, anuria, and dialysis vintage as outlined below [50]. Likewise the country of residence was an independent predictor of growth outcome in a large European cohort of children with CKD stage 3–5, which may be related to differences in the timing of diagnosis and/or referral to a center specialized for children with CKD—which in turn may have economic causes [9].

Cause of Renal Disease

Congenital Abnormalities of the Kidneys and Urinary Tract (CAKUT)

Renal tubular sodium and bicarbonate losses are common in children with CAKUT, and can cause salt depletion and acidosis both of which can contribute to growth failure [51]. Supplementation with salt and bicarbonate may be necessary, along with free access to water.

Glomerulopathies

Growth may be affected in children with glomer-ulopathies, even in early CKD [52]. The nephrotic state per se and glucocorticoid treatment are known risk factors. Prolonged high corticosteroid doses lead to severe growth failure. Although partial catch-up growth can be seen after cessation of glucocorticoid treatment, this is usually restricted to young (prepubertal) patients [53]. Congenital nephrotic syndrome is often associated with severe growth retardation during the first months of life, even in patients with pre-served kidney function, and seems to be secondary to persistent edema, recurrent infections, losses of peptide and protein-bound hormones in the urine, and/or protein-calorie malnutrition [54, 55]. In the Finnish-type nephrotic syndrome adequate nutritional support is vital and bilateral nephrectomies and initiation of dialysis may be necessary to stabilize growth. In less severe types of congenital nephrotic syndrome, unilateral nephrectomy and/or treatment with prostaglandin synthesis inhibitors and RAS antagonists can reduce proteinuria and thereby stabilize growth and the overall clinical condition [54–56].

Tubular and Interstitial Nephropathies

Tubular dysfunction characterized by losses of electrolytes, bicarbonate, and water can lead to severe growth failure even in the presence of normal glomerular function. The growth suppressive effects of isolated tubular defects are illustrated by the severe growth failure typically seen in patients suffering from renal tubular acidosis, Bartter syndrome, and nephrogenic diabetes insipidus [57]. Supplementation with electrolytes, water and bicarbonate may be able to prevent growth failure or even induce catch-up growth [58].

The most severe growth failure, which may be very difficult to treat, occurs in patients suffering from complex tubular disorders such as Fanconi syndrome [58–61]. In these patients, only partial catch-up growth can usually be achieved even with vigorous water and electrolyte supplementation. Systemic metabolic disorders (such as cystinosis, primary hyperoxaluria and mitochondrial cytopathies) resulting in complex tubular dysfunction, progressive loss of kidney function, and involvement of other vital organs (e.g. liver, bone, and brain) also lead to severe growth failure [61–63]. In children with nephropathic cystinosis, growth failure occurs already in infancy when glomerular function is typically not yet compromised. Progressive growth failure is further sustained by generalized deposition of cystine crystals altering the function of the growth plate, bone marrow, hypothalamus, and pituitary and thyroid glands. Early initiation of treatment with cystine depleting agents (cysteamine) results in an improvement of growth rates and substantial delay in the development of ESKD [61, 64]. Nevertheless, in a recent European study mean standardized height in children suffering from nephropathic cystinosis with CKD 2–5 was 1.0 SDS lower compared to that in children with other causes of CKD at comparable age and degree of CKD, compatible with an additional impact of an underlying osteoblast defect in this disease [65, 66]. In patients with primary hyperoxaluria, supplementary treatment with citrate and pyridoxine can delay the progression of CKD in some patients, and possibly improve longitudinal growth [62]. However real catch-up growth after combined liver-kidney transplantation is rarely observed even in prepubertal oxalosis patients [48]. New ribonucleic acid interference (RNAi) therapies are expected to become the standard of treatment in these children, so that end-stage kidney disease, KRT and consecutive growth failure may be avoidable in the vast majority of cases in the future [67].

Stage of CKD and Dialysis

Even moderate reduction of GFR has been reported to result in impaired growth. The principal registry providing data on the epidemiology of growth in conservatively managed CKD is the North American Pediatric Renal Trials and Collaborative Studies (NAPRTCS). The 2006 report covers the 10 years between 1994–2004 and includes a very large cohort of over 5000 children with GFRs of up to 75 mL/min/1.73 m². As expected, the most growth retarded were the youngest children, with a mean standardized height for under 2 years of age of −2.3 SD, but mean height SDS was reduced at all ages (−1.7, −1.4, −1.0 at 2–6, 6–12 and > 12 years respectively), with over one third overall being below the third centile for height. Standardized height worsened with progression of CKD, so that there was a strong correlation between creatinine clearance and height SDS (−3.2, −1.9, −1.5, and −0.9 for GFR <10, 10–25, 25–50 and > 50 mL/min/1.73 m² respectively) [68]. This means that many children, and particularly the very young,

are already short at the time of entry to KRT programmes [69]. This has been confirmed more recently in a cohort of 42 children followed during the first 6 years of life, when the mean height SDS was normal at CKD stage 1–2, approximately −0.5 at CKD stage 3–5 and much less, at −1.5 SDS, for those on dialysis [70].

That short stature becomes more common in children on dialysis has been confirmed by the United States Renal Data System (USRDS), a registry collecting data on patients on KRT programs in the US. The 2007 report shows that the height and weight of approximately half of children on dialysis were below the 20th centile for the normal population [71]. Comparison of 2007 and 2016 data demonstrates that the prevalence of short stature in the incident pediatric ESKD population has not improved over the past 10 years [12]. The British Association for Paediatric Nephrology (BAPN) report for height SDS of prevalent patients on dialysis at the end of 2017 was −2 with interquartile range of −1 to −3, having been −1.3 (−0.3 to −2.4) SDS at the start of KRT (UK Renal Registry (2021) UK Renal Registry 23rd Annual Report – data to 31/12/2019, Bristol, UK. Available from renal. org/audit-research/annual-report). Children on dialysis were shorter than their transplanted peers whose mean Height SDS was −1.0 (−0.2 to −2), although both groups are below the heights of the normal age matched population. The International Pediatric Dialysis Registry collects data from more than 3000 children on peritoneal dialysis (PD) from around the world, and is, therefore, able to provide comparisons of all aspects of PD according to region in the largest cohort of children on PD to date. Currently, the mean standardized height on commencing PD is −2.35 SDS, and is below normal worldwide, but there is a large variation, ranging in 21 countries from −1.3 in the UK, to −3.5 in Brazil. Regional variations in resources are likely to contribute to these differences [31]. Given our knowledge that in the majority of reports standardized height declines with increasing time on dialysis, the obvious key to prevention of growth deterioration is pre-emptive transplantation [72].

Protein-Calorie Malnutrition

Anorexia is a common symptom of CKD, due to a combination of altered taste sensation, decreased clearance of cytokines that affect appetite and satiety, obligatory losses of salt and water leading to a preference for salty foods and large volumes of water, and the need for multiple medications. Vomiting is also common, particularly in infants, whose diet is liquid and therefore high volume, and because gastro-esophageal reflux is frequent and elevated polypeptide hormones result in abnormal gastrointestinal motility. PD results in raised intra-abdominal pressure, which may affect both appetite and cause vomiting and constipation, and dietary and fluid restrictions may result in an inadequate diet. Peritoneal dialysate losses of protein and sodium may be high. Finally, co-morbidities may cause poor feeding in their own right [31, 73]. Nutritional deficiency is, therefore, one of the most frequent and important factors contributing to growth failure. The Pediatric Renal Nutrition Taskforce has produced guidelines for the nutritional management of children with CKD stages 2–5 and on dialysis (*vide infra*) [74, 75].

Protein-Energy Wasting

Protein-energy wasting (PEW) is characterized by maladaptive responses including anorexia, elevated basic metabolic rate, wasting of lean body tissue, and under-utilization of fat tissue for energy [76]. It differs from malnutrition in which appetite is maintained, and weight loss is associated with protective metabolic responses such as a decreased basic metabolic rate and preservation of lean body mass at the expense of fat mass. Malnutrition can usually be overcome by nutritional supplementation or changes in the composition of the diet, whereas PEW can only be partially reversed by increased nutrition. Why some children develop PEW is unknown, but inflammation is likely to play a role [77]. However, growth failure is one of the main manifestations of PEW in children with CKD. New understandings of the pathophysiology of PEW in CKD have the potential for novel therapeutic strategies such as ghrelin agonists and melanocortin antagonists [31].

Obesity

At this stage it is important to mention obesity, which is emerging as a growing problem for children with CKD. In the ESPN/ERA-EDTA registry including 25 countries, of 5199 patients below the age of 18 years the prevalence of underweight was 4.3%, while 19.6% and 11.2% were overweight or obese respectively [78]. Receiving steroid therapy and living with a kidney transplant were independent risk factors for overweight. The incidence of obesity parallels that around the world in the normal population. The IPPN database demonstrates this regional variation, with BMI-SDS ranging from a mean of 0.8 in the US to −1.4 in India in children of all ages [31]. Twenty six percent of infants were obese in the US and 50% malnourished in Turkey [31, 58]. In North America, the frequency of obesity is increasing in the CKD population both before as well as at CKD stage 5 [79]. Obesity is a particularly a problem after kidney transplantation. This has been studied in the NAPRTCS database in a retrospective cohort study of 4326 children transplanted between 1995 and 2006, and followed up to 2007. Median BMI increased by 11% at 6 months but with no substantial changes thereafter [80]. In Europe, children with the lowest BMI and those over 5 years of age at transplant showed the greatest increases in BMI post-transplant [78]. UK 2017 data shows that the mean BMI of transplanted children was 1 SDS (0–1.8), whereas it was 0 (−0.8–1.1) for children on dialysis (UK Renal Registry (2021) UK Renal Registry 23rd Annual Report—data to 31/12/2019, Bristol, UK. Available from renal.org/audit-research/annual-report). The use of steroid sparing regimens may mitigate post transplant obesity [4]. Important to note, among transplanted recipients, a very short stature (OR: 1.64, 95% CI: 1.40–1.92) and glucocorticoid treatment (OR: 1.23, 95% CI: 1.03–1.47) were associated with a higher risk of being overweight/obese. Hence, at least in post-transplant patients, obesity is also a risk factor for poor growth.

Metabolic Acidosis

Metabolic acidosis (serum bicarbonate <22 mEq/L) usually begins when the GFR falls below 50% of normal, and is associated with decreased longitudinal growth and increased protein breakdown [81, 82]. Metabolic acidosis is also associated with endocrine consequences: in experimental uremia there is increased glucocorticoid production, increased protein degradation, and profound effects on the somatotropic hormone axis. The latter is characterized by down regulation of spontaneous GH secretion by the pituitary gland, decreased expression of the GH-receptor and insulin like growth factor I (IGF-I) receptor in target organs, and decreased IGF I serum concentrations [83]. Hence, metabolic acidosis induces a state of GH insensitivity, which is likely to contribute to impaired longitudinal growth in CKD patients.

Disturbances of Water and Electrolyte Balance

Although the relationship between salt loss and growth failure has not been formally proven in CKD, children with isolated tubular disorders resulting in urinary salt and water losses show severe growth retardation which can be at least partly resolved by adequate salt and water supplementation. The same applies to patients with a reduced chloride diet or with familial chloride diarrhea [84]. Growth impairment in diabetes insipidus supports the concept that polyuria may also contribute to growth failure in CKD patients [85].

CKD-Mineral and Bone Disorder (CKD-MBD)

It is widely accepted that skeletal deformities due to CKD-MBD contribute to uremic growth failure [86, 87]. Pronounced secondary hyperparathyroidism can interfere with longitudinal growth by destruction of the growth plate architecture, epiphyseal displacement and metaphyseal fractures. Severe destruction of the metaphyseal bone architecture may result in complete growth arrest.

Treatment with 1,25-dihydroxyvitamin D_3 $(1,25(OH)_2D_3)$ improves growth in uremic rats, but this not been demonstrated in children with CKD [88, 89].

PTH levels primarily reflect osteoblast activity. Therefore, it has been speculated that low PTH levels may be associated with poor bone and statural growth, and conversely high PTH levels might be expected in well growing children; and similarly, that poor growth might be expected with adynamic bone disease and better growth in its absence. Information on this issue is conflicting. Diminished growth rates have been shown in four dialyzed patients who had adynamic bone disease on bone biopsy, and PTH levels were positively correlated with the annual change in standardized height [90]. However, the proportion of patients showing adynamic bone disease in this population, where all subjects received high-dose intermittent calcitriol treatment, was rather high (25%). Therefore, this does not represent patients treated nowadays [91]. Indeed, low bone turnover was noted in only 4% of pediatric patients on dialysis in a recent study. In addition, there was no relationship between PTH levels and growth rates in 35 prepubertal children on dialysis for more than one year. Moreover, stable growth was seen with PTH levels only slightly above the normal range, and even catch-up growth occurred in children younger than 2 years [92]. In addition, one well-designed direct histomorphometric assessment in children on dialysis revealed no association between low bone turnover and body growth [93]. The IPPN offers the most up to date information from the largest cohort of PD patients: the annual prospective change in standardized height tended to correlate inversely with time-integrated mean PTH levels: patients with mean PTH levels >500 pg/mL (i.e. > 9 times upper limit of normal (ULN)) showed a significant loss in height SDS as compared to children with lower PTH levels (−0.28 versus −0.05 SDS per year; p < 0.05) [94]. Thus, dialyzed children with normal or only slightly elevated PTH levels have the potential for normal growth, whereas patients with high PTH levels (>500 pg/mL) are at increased risk of growth failure.

Anemia

Longstanding anemia in CKD patients has profound systemic consequences including anorexia and catabolism due to altered energy turnover, and multiple dysfunctions of organ systems. Retardation of growth and development is a hallmark of untreated chronic anemias of non-renal origin, such as thalassemia major. Theoretically, anemia may interfere with growth via mechanisms such as poor appetite, undercurrent infections, cardiac complications and reduced oxygen supply to cartilage. The advent of recombinant human erythropoietin in the late 1980s permitted study of the effects of anemia correction on longitudinal growth in CKD. Although short-term stimulatory effects of erythropoietin on longitudinal growth have been reported anecdotally, no persistent catch-up growth could be demonstrated in several multicenter clinical trials [95, 96] Partial correction of anemia has, though, improved exercise capacity and decreased heart rate and resting oxygen consumption [95, 97].

Endocrine Changes

Uremia interferes with the metabolism and regulation of various peptide hormones. This leads to inappropriate concentrations of circulating hormones and/or altered hormone action on target tissues (Fig. 56.1). Distinct alterations of the somatotropic and gonadotropic hormone axes have been identified, which are believed to play an important role in uremic growth failure [98].

Gonadotropic Hormone Axis

Gonadal Hormones

Low or low normal total and free testosterone (T) as well as dihydrotestosterone (DHT) plasma concentrations due to decreased synthesis and/or increased metabolic clearance have been reported in adolescents and adults with longstanding uremia [99]. The reduced conversion of T to DHT secondary to diminished 5α-reductase activity might contribute to the delayed pubertal development seen in some boys on dialysis [100]. Likewise, plasma estradiol levels in women tend to decrease in parallel with GFR reduction, and some adolescent girls show low-normal or decreased estradiol levels in relation to pubertal age [100, 101]. However, these observations were all made more than 20 years ago. At least in transplanted children this issue seems to be resolved nowadays. In a recent study, the majority of transplanted children without prior long-term dialysis had normal estradiol and testosterone levels [36]. This may at least partly explain the improvement of pubertal development in patients on KRT during the last decades [1].

Gonadotropins

Increased plasma concentrations of LH and FSH in combination with decreased or low-normal gonadal hormones suggest a state of compensated hypergonadotropic hypogonadism in patients with CKD stage 5 [102]. However, in patients on dialysis, gonadotrophin secretion may be inadequate relative to the degree of hypogonadism. This is compatible with an additional defect of pituitary gonadotropin release and the analysis of spontaneous pulsatile LH secretion has provided insights into the underlying pathophysiology [103, 104]. In dialyzed patients mean LH plasma levels are elevated despite significantly reduced pituitary LH secretion, due to the markedly impaired kidney metabolic clearance of LH. When kidney function is restored by kidney transplantation, pulsatile LH secretion normalizes and hypergonadotropic FSH and/or LH levels are only rarely observed [36, 103]. Animal studies suggest that a primary hypothalamic defect may contribute to the delayed onset of puberty in patients with uremia. The observed reduced release of hypothalamic gonadotropin-releasing hormone (GnRH) is due to uremia-related inhibitory factors and/or to an increased tone of the inhibitory neurotransmitter gamma-aminobutyric acid [105, 106].

Beyond the quantitative alterations of gonadotropin release, uremia also affects the biological quality of circulating gonadotropins. In pubertal and adult dialysis patients the proportion of bioactive LH in relation to the total immunochemically measurable amount of LH is reduced. This might be due to altered glycosylation and/or accumulation of less active isoforms [105–107].

In summary, insufficient activation of the hypothalamic GnRH pulse generator, likely mediated via circulating inhibitors, appears to be the key abnormality underlying delayed puberty and altered sexual functions in patients with CKD stage 5. However, kidney transplantation is able to completely normalize all these alterations in the majority of patients if long periods on dialysis treatment are avoided.

Somatotropic Hormone Axis

Growth Hormone Secretion and Metabolism

In both pediatric and adult CKD patients fasting GH concentrations are normal or even increased, depending on the stage of CKD. GH, a 22-kilodalton protein, is almost freely filtered by the glomerulus (sieving coefficient ~0.82) and thereby ultimately cleared from the circulation [108]. Indeed, a linear relationship between GFR and the metabolic clearance rate of GH has been shown; GH clearance is reduced by approximately 50% in patients with CKD stage 5 [108, 109]. The prolonged plasma half-life of GH, rather than increased endogenous secretion, explains the increased circulating GH concentrations in uremia. Pituitary GH secretion is unaltered in prepubertal patients but decreased in adolescents with CKD, suggesting insufficient stimulation by gonadal steroids during puberty [110, 111]. In addition, malnutrition and metabolic acidosis negatively impact GH secretion rates in children with CKD [112].

Growth Hormone Receptor and GH Signaling

Experimental studies have advanced our understanding of uremic GH resistance. Both, the GH-induced hepatic as well as the growth plate cartilage IGF-I synthesis is diminished, due to either decreased expression of the GH receptor (GH-R) and/or a postreceptor signaling defect [113, 114]. Whereas reduced expression of the GH-R encoding mRNA in liver and growth plate chondrocytes was seen, hepatic and growth plate cartilage GH-R protein levels were comparable in uremic and non-uremic animals when corrected for uremia-associated anorexia by pair feeding [113–115]. Thus, whereas a decreased GH-R abundance in the liver and the growth plate cartilage is questionable, a postreceptor GH signaling defect was identified as cause of the diminished hepatic IGF-I secretion upon GH stimulation. In fact, aberrant GH-dependent JAK-STAT signaling has been noted in experimental animals [116]. Binding of GH to its receptor leads to activation of the JAK-STAT cascade by tyrosine phosphorylation, and transcriptional activation of IGF-I synthesis and proteins of the suppressor of cytokine signaling (SOCS) family. The latter are responsible for dephosphorylation of the GH-activated cascade and as such provide a GH-regulated negative feedback loop. However, under the conditions of chronic uremia the equilibrium between GH-induced transcriptional activation of IGF-I and SOCS is shifted towards SOCS overstimulation. Recent studies suggest that the chronic inflammatory state associated with CKD contributes to GH resistance, as SOCS are also induced by inflammatory cytokines [117, 118].

In humans, GH binding protein (GHBP), which enters the circulation by proteolytic cleavage of the extracellular receptor domain, is taken as a measure of GH receptor expression. In line with animal experiments, GHBP plasma levels in CKD patients are decreased and are related to residual kidney function [119].

Insulin-Like Growth Factor Plasma Binding and Tissue Action

Apart from GH resistance, insensitivity to IGF-I is also found in patients with advanced CKD [120–122]. While serum concentrations of IGF-I and IGF-II are usually within the normal range in children with CKD stage 1–4, IGF-I levels are slightly reduced and those of IGF-II mildly increased in dialyzed patients [123]. In contrast to the unchanged total amount of circulating immunoreactive IGF, somatomedin bioavailability is reduced in advanced CKD pointing to the existence of circulating inhibitors [124]. A low-molecular weight somatomedin inhibitor (~1 kDa) was reported to circulate in uremic serum in an early study, but this has not been characterized further. Later studies focused on the accumulation of the specific high-affinity IGF-binding proteins (IGFBP1–6), which are normally cleared by the kidneys and are considered the main cause of diminished somatomedin bioactivity in uremia. In particular, the concentrations of IGFBP-1, −2, −3, −4 and − 6 increase as kidney function declines and IGFBP-1, -2 and -6 have been shown to inhibit IGF I bioactivity in-vitro [125, 126]. In contrast, the serum concentration of IGFBP-5 is normal and IGFBP-5 proteins undergo intense proteolytic cleavage in chronic uremia [126]. Likewise, the elevated level of IGFBP-3 is mostly due to the accumulation of proteolytic fragments whereas intact IGFBP-3 is markedly diminished [127]. The molar excess of IGFBPs over IGFs is approximately 150% in children with CKD and 200% in children on dialysis as compared to 25% in children without CKD. An inverse correlation between growth retardation and IGFBP-1, -2, and -4 serum concentrations has been described [128]. Reduced IGF bioactivity can be normalized by removing unsaturated IGFBP [124]. These data are in favor of the concept that serum IGFBPs increase with progression of CKD, and that the greater excess of IGFBPs by CKD stage 5 contributes to the more severe growth failure and reduced response to rhGH therapy in these children. In addition, cellular IGF signaling is impaired in the uremic state; it remains to be elucidated whether a postreceptor mechanism similar to the one observed for GH signaling is responsible for this phenomenon [118, 122, 124].

In summary, the marked deficiency of IGF-I synthesis, the modest elevation of GH levels due to decreased metabolic clearance, and increased IGF plasma binding capacity, strongly support the concept of a multilevel homeostatic failure of the GH-IGF-I system.

Corticosteroid Treatment

Long-term glucocorticoid treatment in patients after transplantation leads to diminished longitudinal growth by impairment of the somatotropic hormone axis. High-dose glucocorticoid treatment suppresses pulsatile GH release from the pituitary gland mainly by reduction of pulse amplitude [129]. The physiologic increase in GH secretion during puberty is reduced in allograft recipients receiving glucocorticoid treatment (≥ 4 mg/m² per day) and the association between sex steroid plasma concentrations and GH release observed in healthy adolescents is blunted [129]. These changes are mainly due to increased hypothalamic somatostatin release.

In addition to reduced GH release, corticosteroids suppress GH-R mRNA and protein in animals and most likely also in humans [130]. Consequently, hepatic IGF-I mRNA levels are reduced in animals receiving glucocorticoids. However, plasma concentrations of IGF-I in patients treated by glucocorticoids are normal or only slightly reduced. In individual children on corticosteroid treatment impaired longitudinal growth occurs despite normal GH secretion and plasma IGF-I levels, suggesting insensitivity to GH and IGF-I at the level of the growth plate. Indeed, a direct growth inhibiting effect of dexamethasone on the growth plate was shown by local injection in rabbits [131]. In cultured growth plate chondrocytes glucocorticoids decreased DNA synthesis and cell proliferation in a dose-dependent fashion, associated with reduced expression of the GH receptor and diminished paracrine IGF-I synthesis [132]. In addition, pharmacological doses of glucocorticoids also impaired the proliferative response to the calciotropic hormones calcitriol and PTH [132]. This is at least partly related to a diminished release of paracrine IGF-I secretion by these hormones. IGF-I modulates its own activity in cultured rat growth plate chondrocytes by the synthesis of both inhibitory (IGFBP-3) and stimulatory (IGFBP-5) binding proteins. This is modified by glucocorticoid treatment. Therefore, glucocorticoid treatment not only interferes with the somatotropic hormone axis with respect to GH secretion and GH / IGF-I receptor signaling, but also by modulation of paracrine IGF-I synthesis and binding by IGF binding proteins. Even more important, based on *in vivo* studies in rabbits catch-up growth after glucocorticoid exposure may remain incomplete in general [131]. Consequently, all efforts must be undertaken to reduce steroid exposure in children with CKD before and after kidney transplantation [133].

Treatment of Growth Failure in Chronic Kidney Disease

General Measures

The main measures for prevention and treatment of growth failure in children with CKD are summarized in Table 56.1. Close growth monitoring with intervals depending on previous growth, age and stage of CKD is essential. Early referral to a pediatric nephrology center followed by careful nutritional and metabolic management is vital in the prevention of growth retardation [134]. Growth retardation is clearly correlated to the degree of CKD. Therefore, adequate measures should be undertaken to preserve GFR, and to provide adequate dialysis in those children who require maintenance dialysis [72]. Preservation of kidney function requires treatment of elevated blood pressure, aiming for blood pressure values below the 50th and 75th percentile in proteinuric and non-proteinuric children, respectively [135]. Renin-angiotensin aldosterone system inhibitors, preferentially angiotensin-converting enzyme inhibitors or angiotensin receptor inhibitors, should be used to treat high blood pressure and ameliorate proteinuria in children with CKD [136]. Nephrotoxic medication should be avoided, and urinary tract infections in children with congenital abnormalities of the kidneys and urinary tract (CAKUT) should be treated. Finally,

Table 56.1 Main measures for prevention and treatment of growth failure in pediatric CKD

Prevention:
- Close growth monitoring with intervals depending on previous growth, age and stage of CKD
- Preserve kidney function by:
  - treating elevated blood pressure and reducing proteinuria, preferably using RAAS inhibitors
  - avoiding nephrotoxic medication
  - prompt treatment of urinary tract infections
- Provide adequate energy and protein intake and consultation with a renal dietician.
  - Consider enteral feeding by gastrostomy or nasogastric tube in cases of persistent insufficient oral intake
- Substitute water and electrolyte losses and correct metabolic acidosis
- Keep PTH levels in the recommended CKD stage-dependent target range and substitute native vitamin D in cases of low vitamin D levels
- Aim for early (preemptive) kidney transplantation with minimal steroid exposure in patients with end-stage CKD
- Provide adequate dialysis in patients requiring maintenance dialysis

Treatment:
- Consider use of growth hormone treatment in cases of persistent growth failure, i.e. height < third percentile and height velocity < 25th percentile, excluding patients who have received a transplant within the last 12 months
- Consider intensified dialysis or hemodiafiltration in in patients requiring maintenance dialysis presenting with persistent growth failure
- Consider use of rhGH therapy in pediatric kidney transplant recipients for whom expected catch-up growth cannot be achieved by steroid minimization, or for patients where steroid withdrawal is not feasible due to high immunological risks, particularly in children with suboptimal graft function (eGFR <50 mL/min/1.73 m^2)

CKD chronic kidney disease, *RAAS* renin-angiotensin aldosterone system, *PTH* parathyroid hormone, *eGFR* estimated glomerular filtration rate

disease specific treatment, e.g. treatment with cysteamine in patients with nephropathic cystinosuis, may be required.

Adequate **nutritional management** is crucial in infants and young children, who frequently need supplementary feeding via nasogastric tube or, preferably, gastrostomy [75, 137]. In a retrospective analysis of growth in 101 infants and young children with severe CKD it could be demonstrated that persistent catch-up growth can be achieved in the majority of patients when there is good metabolic control and enteral feeding is commenced at the first sign of growth delay (Fig. 56.5) [20]. However, spontaneous growth as well as catch-up growth after initiation of enteral feeding is limited in patients with comorbidities [20, 138]. The use of enteral feeding varies around the world, as has been clearly demonstrated by the IPPN report of 153 infants on PD: gastrostomies are most commonly used in the US, where 80% of infants on PD are gastrostomy fed; 20% have gastrostomies in Europe, but there are very small numbers or none in the rest of the world [13]. Nasogastric feeding is commonest in Europe and Latin America. Gastrostomy feeding, rather than demand or nasogastric tube feeding, is associated with better preservation of linear growth in the infants in the IPPN database (Fig. 56.6)) [13]. This may be related to decreased vomiting with gastrostomies as compared to nasogastric tubes. Catch-up growth in children started on enteral feeding after the age of 2 years may be substantial but is markedly reduced in those on dialysis and strongly negatively correlated with age [139]. The assurance of adequate caloric and energy intake requires the patient and families to be advised by a kidney dietician, especially when supplementary feeding via nasogastric or gastrostomy tube is required [74, 137] In general, the initial prescription for energy intake in children with CKD should approximate that of healthy children of the same age (suggested dietary intake, SDI) [74]. To optimize growth in children with suboptimal weight gain and linear growth, energy intake should be adjusted towards the higher end of the SDI [74]. Caloric intake should account for growth failure and be related to "height age" rather than to chronological age if the child's height is below the normal range. Calorie intake in excess of 100% of SDI may not improve catch-up growth but rather results in

obesity and may thereby negatively contribute to long-term cardiovascular morbidity in CKD patients [140, 141]. If there is excessive weight gain dietary energy intake should be reduced for children on PD to compensate for the energy derived from dialysate glucose, estimated at 8–12 kcal/kg per day. In addition; to promote optimal growth, target protein intake in children with CKD should be at the upper end of the SDI [74]. In patients on PD, a slightly higher intake (+0.2 g/kg/day) is recommended to compensate for dialytic protein losses. The aim is to maintain a normal serum albumin and a urea below 20 mmol/L as far as possible. High protein intakes should be avoided since, despite many attempts, anabolizing or growth promoting effects of high-protein diets have neither been demonstrated in animal models nor in children with CKD. On the contrary, high protein diets may be detrimental by aggravating metabolic acidosis and augmenting the dietary phosphorus load.

Metabolic acidosis should be vigorously treated by alkali supplementation aiming for serum bicarbonate levels equal or above 22 mEq/L. This can be assured by treatment with sodium bicarbonate and/or the use of HCO_3-based or lactate based dialysis solutions in patients on dialysis [11]. In addition, supplementation of water and electrolytes is essential in patients presenting with polyuria and/or salt losing nephropathies. Supplementation of sodium chloride is also important in young children on PD, since significant amounts of sodium chloride (i.e. 2–5 mmol/kg body weight) may be eliminated via ultrafiltration.

Dialysis and Intensified Dialysis

Although dialysis attenuates the uremic state, longitudinal growth is not usually improved and long-term PD or HD are associated with a gradual loss of standardized height in children and adolescents, and can be as high as 1 SD per year in infants [9, 142–144]. Children on dialysis who maintain some residual kidney function have the best growth; indeed residual kidney function may be a better predictor of longitudinal growth than dialytic clearance [145, 146]. However, a recent

Fig. 56.5 Course of mean standardized height and body mass index (BMI) of children presenting within the first 6 months of life with a glomerular filtration rate less than 20 mL/min/1.73 m^2 receiving tube feeding in order to provide at least 100% of the recommended daily allowance (RDA) of healthy children. (**a**) Height SDS and BMI values for all patients. (**b**) Height SDS and BMI values for patients without comorbidites. (**c**) Height SDS and BMI values for patients with comorbidities. (Reproduced with permission of [20])

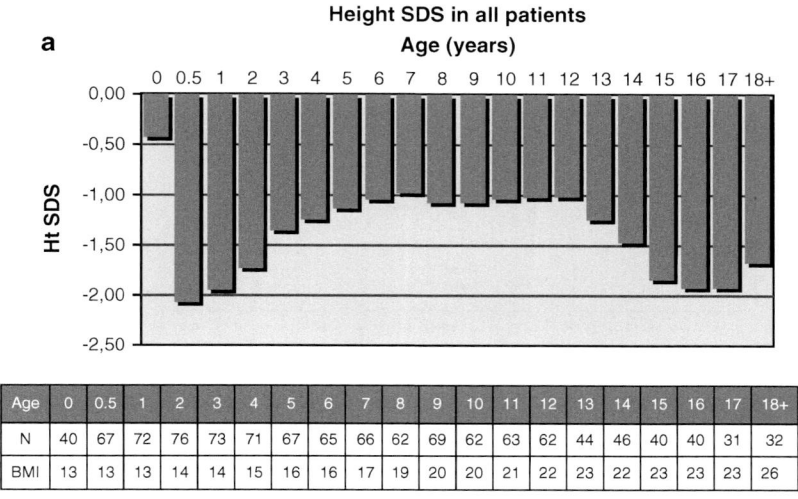

Height SDS in all patients

Age	0	0.5	1	2	3	4	5	6	7	8	9	10	11	12	13	14	15	16	17	18+
N	40	67	72	76	73	71	67	65	66	62	69	62	63	62	44	46	40	40	31	32
BMI	13	13	13	14	14	15	16	16	17	19	20	20	21	22	23	22	23	23	23	26

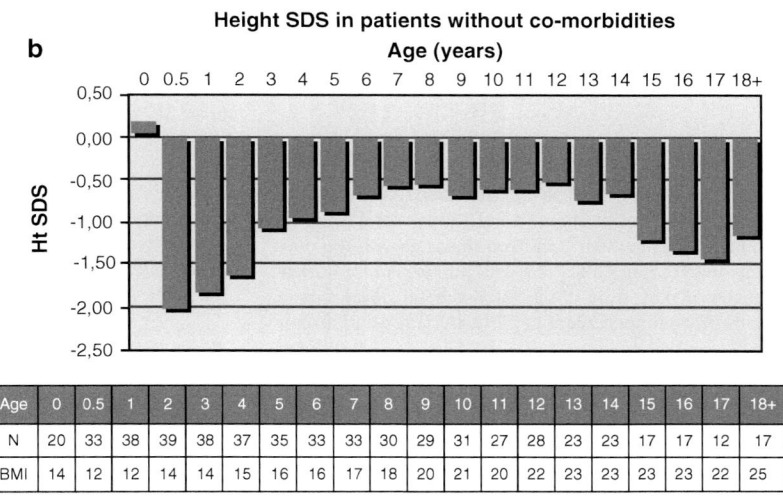

Height SDS in patients without co-morbidities

Age	0	0.5	1	2	3	4	5	6	7	8	9	10	11	12	13	14	15	16	17	18+
N	20	33	38	39	38	37	35	33	33	30	29	31	27	28	23	23	17	17	12	17
BMI	14	12	12	14	14	15	16	16	17	18	20	21	20	22	23	23	23	23	22	25

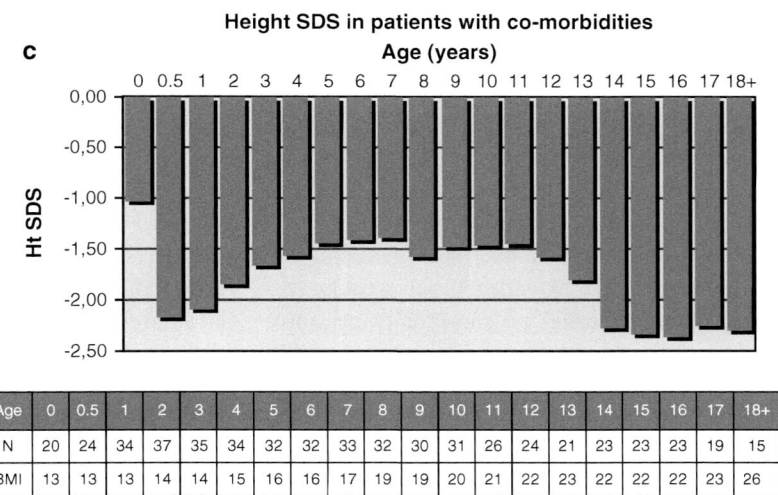

Height SDS in patients with co-morbidities

Age	0	0.5	1	2	3	4	5	6	7	8	9	10	11	12	13	14	15	16	17	18+
N	20	24	34	37	35	34	32	32	33	32	30	31	26	24	21	23	23	23	19	15
BMI	13	13	13	14	14	15	16	16	17	19	19	20	21	22	23	22	22	22	23	26

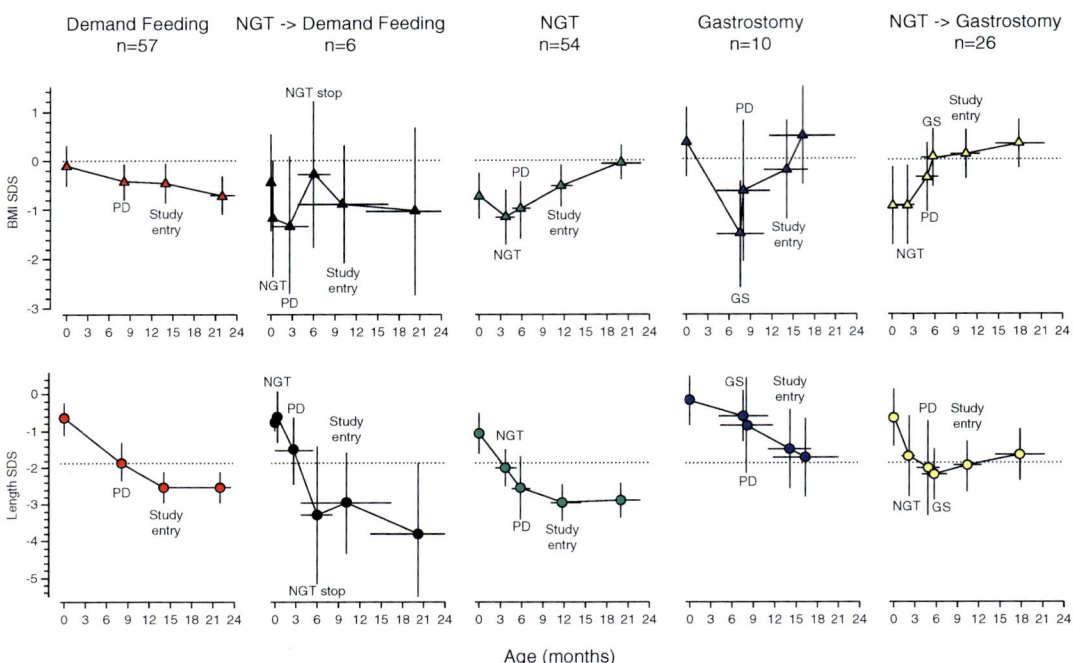

Fig. 56.6 Whereas both nasogastric tube (NGT) and gastrostomy (GS) feeding improve nutritional status, only GS feeding associates with stabilized linear growth in young infants undergoing CPD. The data points represent mean estimates at key time points of postnatal development, (i.e., birth, commencement of CPD, initiation and discontinuation of nasogastric tube or gastrostomy feeding, enrollment to IPPN [study entry], and last available observation). Two-dimensional error bars denote the 95% confidence intervals to mean age and SDS at the respective time point. [Reproduced with permission of [13]]

Italian study in infants on chronic PD reported catch-up growth in 50% of patients [147]. High peritoneal transporter status, a condition associated with increased morbidity and mortality in adults, is associated with poor longitudinal growth in children on chronic PD [148]. This might be due to the putative association of high peritoneal transport with inflammation, which can suppress statural growth by interference with GH signaling (*vide supra*), or excessive losses of proteins and amino acids important to growth.

It has been suggested that intensified dialysis, achieved by either extended thrice-weekly sessions, daily nocturnal or short daily sessions, might be able to induce catch-up growth [148–150]. According to a French study, catch-up growth can be maximized when intensified hemodiafiltration (3 h, 6 times a week) and rhGH therapy are combined [148, 149, 151–154]. Using this approach in 15 mainly prepubertal children for an average observation time of 21 months, there was an average increase in growth velocity from 3.8 cm/year at baseline to 8.9 cm/year (Fig. 56.7). This resulted in a mean of 1.7 SDS gain of standardized height, representing complete catch-up growth according to the attainment of the target height SDS [153]. A recent non-randomized study demonstrated superior growth in children treated with hemodiafiltration compared to those with conventional hemodialysis (HD) (Fig. 56.8) [155]. From a pathophysiological point of view, intensified hemodiafiltration (HDF) is a better substitute for physiological kidney function and may allow substantially better clearance of uremic toxins, e.g. middle-molecular weight compounds [155]. As a result, microinflammation and metabolic acidosis may be abolished, leading to improved appetite and tissue anabolism. The improved removal of inflammatory cytokines might reverse

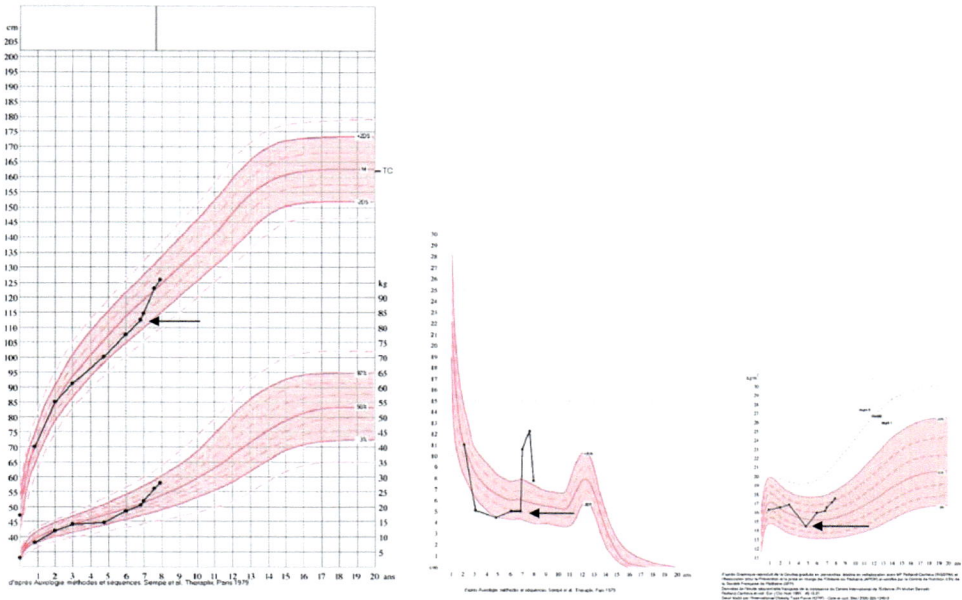

Patient 14, a girl on daily on line hemodiafiltration
Protein diet intake(g/kg/d) : 2.4±0.4 ; protein nitrogen appearance(g/kg/d) : 1.3 ±0.14
Mean growth velocity (cm/year) : 9.6
Achieved height versus mid parental target height (SDS) : +0.3

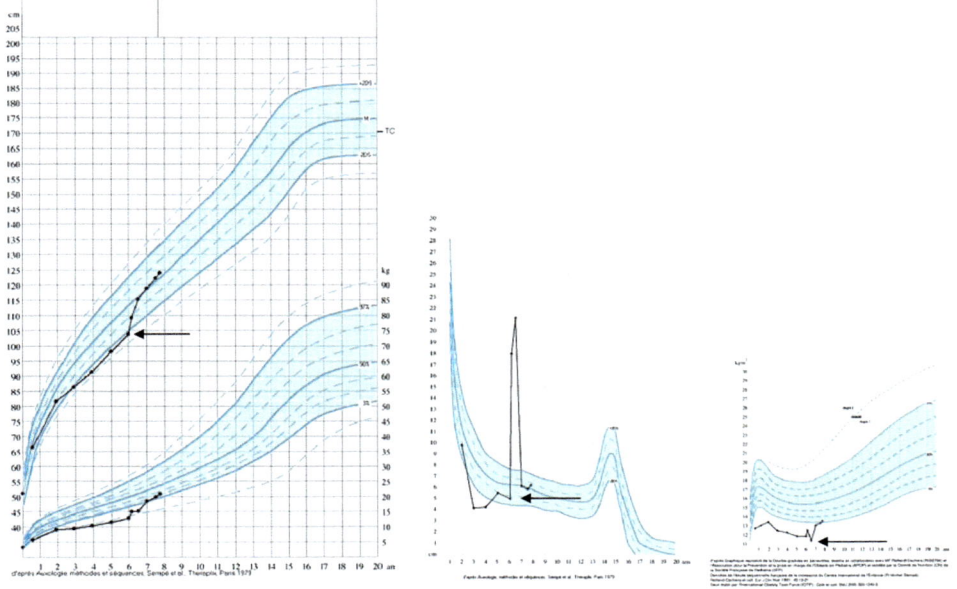

Patient 1, a boy on daily on line hemodiafiltration.
Protein diet intake(g/kg/d) : 2.7±0.2 ; protein nitrogen appearance(g/kg/d) : 1.44 ±0.15
Mean growth velocity (cm/year) : 10.4
Achieved height versus mid parental target height (SDS) : +0.2

Fig. 56.7 Examples of growth charts (height and weight chart; growth velocity chart in centimeters per year; body mass under chart) of two patients on daily online hemodi- afiltration (start indicated by bars) in addition to rhGH treatment . TC on height chart is the familial target height in (centimeters). [Reproduced with permission of [153]]

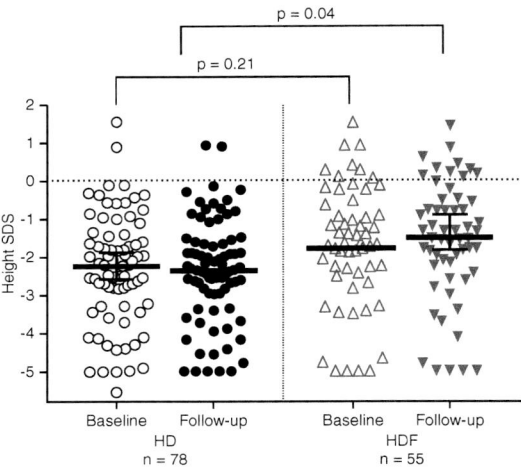

Fig. 56.8 Improved height SDS in children on hemodi-afiltration (HDF) compared to hemodialysis (HD). The figure shows change in height SDS in the HD and HDF arms at baseline and 1-year follow-up. Data are shown as median and interquartile range. Within-group analyses performed by Wilcoxon matched-pairs signed-rank test and HD versus HDF cohorts compared by Mann–Whitney U test. At 12 months the height SDS in the HDF group was higher than in the HD group (P = 0.04). (Reproduced with permission of [155])

GH resistance enabling the full therapeutic potential of rhGH [152]. The positive effects of intensified dialysis, particularly home HD, usually outweigh the potential impact on psychosocial integration and treatment costs. Prospective randomized trials appear required to provide definite proof to this promising concept. In particular, the relative contribution of concomitant rhGH therapy to the growth improvement observed with intensified dialysis remains to be defined.

Transplantation

Although many of the metabolic and endocrine disorders contributing to uremic growth failure are resolved by kidney transplantation, post-transplant catch-up growth is usually restricted to young children and occurs far from regularly [3, 156]. As well as transplant function, age, severity of stunting at time of transplantation and gluco-corticoid dosage are inversely associated with longitudinal growth. One retrospective study found that while standardized height was comparable at time of transplantation, it was significantly higher among living-related donor (LRD) than deceased donor transplant (DDT) recipients 5 years later [157]. This benefit of LRD grafts was independent of GFR arguing for preferential LRD in children with respect to post-transplant growth.

It must be stressed that even low-dose glu-cocorticoid treatment (<4 mg/m^2/day) results in growth suppression in children after transplantation. While complete steroid withdrawal has been associated with unacceptably high rejection rates in children with azathioprine and/ or cyclosporine A medication, withdrawal or even complete steroid avoidance appears much safer with the currently preferred immu-nosuppressants [158]. In a randomized trial of late steroid withdrawal in patients on treatment with cyclosporine A, mycophenolate mofetil steroid-free patients showed improved growth compared to controls (i.e. change in height SDS; 0.6 ± 0.1 versus −0.2 ± 0.1) within 27 months [159]. However, catch-up growth in pubertal patients was rather limited compared to that in prepubertal patients. It seems logical

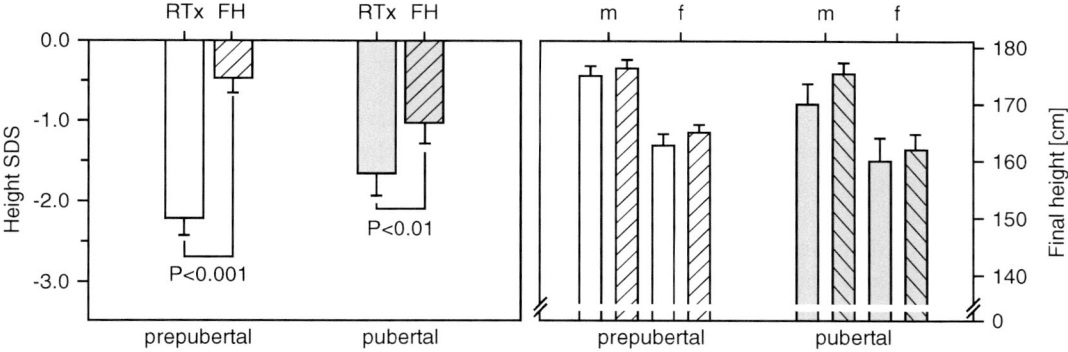

Fig. 56.9 Mean standardized height at time of renal transplantation compared to adult height and comparison of adult height with genetic target height in patients with steroid-withdrawal during month 4–6 after transplantation Mean standardized height at the time of transplantation and final height in prepubertal (n = 36) and pubertal (n = 24) patients. (d) Mean adult height (open bars) and genetic target height (hatched bars) in boys (n = 25) and girls (n = 17). Data in (c) and (d) are given as mean ± SEM. (Reproduced with permission of [4])

that if steroids are withdrawn at an early stage, or even completely avoided, a better growth outcome will be observed. Indeed, a retrospective analysis of longitudinal growth in a cohort of 74 children who had been weaned off steroids within 6 months of transplantation showed remarkable results [4, 159]. Mean adult height was -0.5 ± 1.1 SDS and -1.0 ± 1.3 SDS in prepubertal and pubertal patients and was within the normal range (>-2 SD) in 94% and 80% of them respectively (Fig. 56.9). Likewise, early steroid-withdrawal (< 6 weeks) and complete steroid avoidance improved standardized height by approximately 1.0 SDS within 3–5 years post-transplantation [32, 33, 160, 161]. Although experimental data indicate that mTOR inhibitors may interfere with chondrocyte proliferation and/or gonadal hormone synthesis, recent case control studies in transplanted children revealed similar growth rates in patients with and without mTOR inhibitor treatment [162].

In summary, efforts to avoid a height deficit before transplantation, early (preemptive) kidney transplantation, and immunosuppressive strategies characterized by the early withdrawal or even complete avoidance of steroids can improve adult height and normalize body proportions in children after successful transplantation.

Endocrine Therapies

Vitamin D

Calcitriol deficiency is a major cause of secondary hyperparathyroidism and CKD-MBD. Although calcitriol supplementation reverses the biochemical, radiographic, and histological signs of high turnover bone disease, neither experimental nor clinical studies demonstrate consistent improvement in longitudinal growth [89, 162–164]. These conflicting results might be due to differences in the mode of administration and to the pleiotropic calcitriol-specific effects on growth plate chondrocytes. In addition, only a week association between parathyroid hormone (PTH) levels and linear growth was reported in children with advanced CKD [94]. In general, minimal PTH suppressive active vitamin D analogues dosages should be used in order to keep PTH levels in the desired target range [165]. Finally, supplementation with cholecalciferol or ergocalciferol should be initiated in children with serum 25-hydroxyvitamin D concentrations below 75 nmol/L (<30 ng/mL) [166].

Calcimimetics

Uncontrolled and controlled studies provide evidence that calcimimetics are an effective therapy for secondary hyperparathyroidism in pediatric dialysis patients [167]. Calcimimetics suppress PTH secretion by activating the calcium-sensing receptor (CaR). The CaR is expressed by epiphyseal chondrocytes; its stimulation stimulates chondrocytic proliferation and differentiation. Thus, calcimimetics may affect longitudinal growth in uremia as well. In fact, the calcimimetic cinacalcet improved food efficiency and body weight gain in uremic rats, but no effects on growth plate morphology and/or longitudinal growth were seen [168]. Likewise, no beneficial or adverse effect on longitudinal growth was noted during calcimimetic treatment periods of up-to three years in children on dialysis [167]. A comprehensive European guideline on the use of cinacalcet in children on dialysis was published recently [169].

Growth Hormone

Pharmacological treatment of children with CKD and growth delay with rhGH actually predated the elucidation of the pathomechanisms that underlie chronic uremic alterations of the GH-IGF-1 axis [114, 169–171]. Administration of rhGH markedly stimulates IGF-I synthesis with only a modest effect on IGFBPs, thereby normalizing somatomedin bioactivity and promoting longitudinal growth [172]. The efficacy and safety of long-term treatment with rhGH in children with CKD before and after kidney transplantation is well established and clinical practice recommendations on this topic were recently published in 2019 [30].

Efficacy of rhGH in Prepubertal Children

In prepubertal children with pre-dialysis CKD, rhGH therapy typically doubles height velocity during the first treatment year [173]. Catch-up growth continues asymptotically during extended treatment [174–176]. In dialyzed children, the treatment response is significantly attenuated compared to children with pre-dialysis CKD (0.8 SD vs. 1.3 SD) [177]. RhGH responsiveness is similarly poor in children on peritoneal dialysis and standard hemodialysis, but as noted previously, can be markedly improved when dialytic clearance is augmented by daily HDF [153].

Based on the current experience with rhGH in pediatric CKD patients, a model to predict growth response was developed [178]. The prediction model was developed using a cohort of 208 prepubertal children with CKD stage 3-5D followed in a pharmaco-epidemiological survey (KIGS), and validated in an independent group of 67 CKD patients registered at the Dutch Growth Research Foundation. The height velocity during the first rhGH treatment year (PHV) was predicted by the following equation: PHV (centimeters per year) = 13.3 − [age (years) × 0.38 + (weight SDS × 0.39)] − [hereditary renal disorder (0 when absent or 1 when present) × 1.16] + [Ln rhGH dose (milligrams per kilogram per week) × 1.04] + [GFR (milliliters per minute × 1.73 m^2) × 0.023]. This equation explains 37% of the overall variability of the growth response. The SE of the estimate or error SD of the prediction model was 1.6 cm and nonresponders in the validation group were correctly identified. This model may help in predicting non-responders and in tailoring treatment strategies for growth retarded children with CKD.

Several RCTs have shown the benefit of rhGH therapy in short prepubertal renal transplant recipients. A meta-analysis of five prospective RCTs involving a total of 401 patients showed that patients receiving rhGH therapy had a significantly higher growth velocity 1 year after the initiation of therapy than the control group, with a mean height SDS difference of 0.68 (95% CI 0.25–1.11) [173].

Effects of rhGH on Pubertal Growth and Adult Height

In a study following patients with CKD and ESKD from late prepubertal age to final height, the average height increment in rhGH treated patients was twice that seen in a matched control group [46]. The main benefit for total growth and final height was achieved before the onset of the pubertal growth spurt, whereas no overall effect on pubertal height gain was observed (Fig. 56.10).

Data on adult height are available from 11 non-randomized trials in which rhGH was administered for at least 2 years, comprising a total of 836 patients on various modes of KRT [30]. In

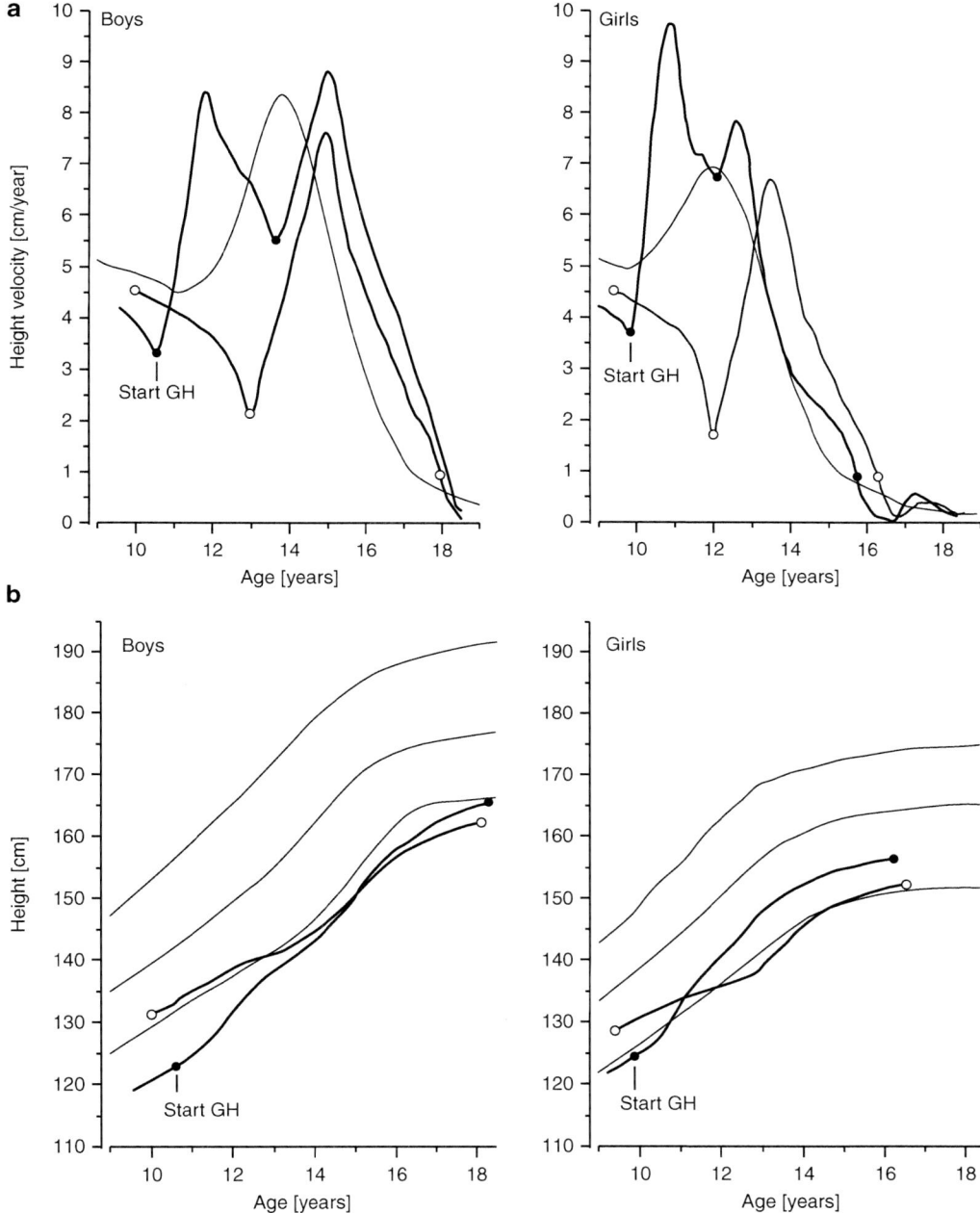

Fig. 56.10 (**a**) Synchronized mean height velocity curves of 32 boys (left panel) and 6 girls (right panel) with CKD during rhGH Treatment (closed circles), as compared with 50 children with CKD not treated with rhGH (open circles) and 232 normal children (thin lines). The dots indicate the time of the first observation, which corresponds to the start of rhGH treatment in the growth hormone-treated children, minimal prespurt height velocity, and the time of the end of the pubertal growth spurt. (Reproduced with permission of [46]). (**b**) Synchronized mean height curves of 32 boys (left panel) and 6 girls (right panel) with CKD during rhGH treatment (closed circles), as compared with 50 children with CKD not treated with rhGH (open circles). Normal values are indicated by the third, 50th, and 97th percentile. The dots indicate the time of the first observation, which corresponds to the start of rhGH treatment in the growth hormone-treated children, and the time of the end of the pubertal growth spurt. (Reproduced with permission of [46])

five studies a matched historical control group was included. The median change in standardized height until attainment of adult height amounted to 1.1 SDS (range 0.2–1.6 SDS) in rhGH treated patients (p < 0.05 for each final height measurement versus initial height measurement). This change corresponded to a median absolute increase in rhGH treated patients by 7.4 cm (range 1.4–10.8 cm) in boys and 7.0 cm (range 1.3–10.1 cm) in girls, based on European reference values. However, this calculation may underestimate the rhGH effect since in the non-rhGH treated controls adult height was significantly below the initial standardized height indices in all except one study. Height attained at the start of rhGH and throughout the duration of rhGH treatment were positively associated with final height, whereas time spent on dialysis, age at puberty onset, and age of start of rhGH were negatively associated with final height [46, 47]. Taken together, the available studies suggest that rhGH improves adult height in short prepubertal and pubertal CKD patients prior to and after kidney transplantation.

Efficacy of rhGH in Infants

According to standard concepts of the pathophysiology of uremic growth failure, malnutrition and fluid and electrolyte imbalances have a much greater impact on infant growth than alterations of somatotropic hormones. Consequently, correction of the nutritional status has been considered the primary measure to restore normal growth in growth retarded infants, postponing the option of endocrine therapeutic intervention to beyond the second year of life. This concept has been challenged by several reports of initiating rhGH in growth retarded infants with CKD [179–181]. A randomized controlled study involving 30 growth retarded infants (mean age: 16 months) with moderate CKD (mean eGFR: 25 mL/min/1.73 m^2) revealed excellent catch-up growth from from −3.0 to −1.1 SDS within 24 months of treatment, in contrast to no significant change in controls [179]. Another study reported an increase in height SDS from −3.3 to −2.2 within 12 months in 8 infants with a mean age of 22 months and CKD stage 3–4 [180]. In a ran-

domized study of 16 infants with stage 3–4 CKD who were receiving at least 80% of the recommended daily allowence for calories and of whom seven were enterally fed, those randomized to rhGH showed significantly higher length gains (14.5 versus 9.5 cm/year; delta height SDS +1.43 versus −0.11) [181]. Hence, the results of these studies lend further support to the previous observation that the relative efficacy and cost efficiency of rhGH is actually best when initiated at young age, i.e. during infancy and early childhood [30]. While the provision of adequate nutrition is certainly vital to growth and development of infants with CKD, some children show growth failure despite adequate nutrition. In these patients, any further increases of energy intake typically lead to fat deposition, but not catch-up growth. Early rhGH therapy appears to be an attractive option to accelerate length and weight gain in such infants. The fact that the enhanced growth also helps the infant achieve the body size required for kidney transplantation more expeditiously is another substantial benefit [30].

General rhGH Treatment Strategies

Children from 6 months of age with stage 3–5 CKD or on dialysis should be candidates for rhGH therapy if they have persistent growth failure, defined as a height below the third percentile for age and sex and a height velocity below the 25th percentile, once other potentially treatable risk factors for growth failure have been adequately addressed, and provided the child has growth potential (open epiphysis on X-ray of the wrist) [30]. RhGH therapy should also be considered for children older than 6 months with stage 3–5 CKD or on dialysis who present with a height between the third and tenth percentile but persistent low height velocity (<25th percentile), once other potentially treatable risk factors for growth failure have been adequately addressed. Such early, preventive therapy is probably more cost-effective than starting at a more advanced age when growth retardation has become more evident and higher absolute rhGH doses are required.

Children suffering from nephropathic cystinosis often show severe growth retardation despite somewhat mild reductions in GFR, which is thought to be related to the deleterious effects of Fanconi syndrome, resulting in hypophosphatemic rickets and malnutrition and/or an underlying obstoblast/osteoclast defect [61]. Therefore, rhGH treatment is recommended in short children with nephropathic cystinosis at all stages of CKD [30].

The growth response to rhGH treatment is positively associated with residual kidney function, target height, initial target height deficit and duration of rhGH treatment, and inversely correlated with the age at start of treatment [46, 47, 174, 177, 178]. Daily dosing is more effective than three doses per week and the optimal dose is 0.045–0.05 mg/kg body weight per day by subcutaneous injections in the evening [30]. Parents and physicians should encourage children from about 8 to 10 years of age to do the rhGH injections on their own if adequate training and adherence can be assured, because this may ultimately improve patient adherence and self-esteem [30]. Whereas discontinuation of rhGH results in catch-down growth in approximately 75% of CKD patients this phenomenon is rarely observed when rhGH treatment is discontinued after kidney transplantation, highlighting the close relationship between kidney function and growth [182]. Furthermore, although the absolute height gain achieved by rhGH is independent of age, the reference range increases with age. Thus, rhGH treatment should be started as early as growth retardation becomes evident (i.e. height below third percentile) [30]. If height velocity in the first year of rhGH treatment is less than 2 cm per year over baseline, it is recommended to assess patient adherence to rhGH therapy through the measurement of serum IGF-I levels and/or the use of an injection pen with downloadable memory function, ensuring administration of the correct weight-adjusted GH dose, and addressing any, possibly subclinical, nutritional and metabolic issues [30].

The primary treatment target should be to return the child's height into her/his individual genetic percentile channel. Treatment may be suspended once this target is reached, but growth should be monitored closely as outlined above. In patients receiving rhGH while on conservative treatment rhGH should be continued after the initiation of dialysis, but stopped at the time of kidney transplantation. RhGH therapy should, however, subsequently also be considered for pediatric kidney transplant recipients for whom expected catch-up growth cannot be achieved by steroid minimization or for patients in whom steroid withdrawal is not feasible due to high immunological risk, particularly in children with suboptimal graft function (eGFR <50 mL/min/1.73 m^2). Growth should be monitored for at least 1 year post-transplantation before rhGH therapy is considered, in order to allow for spontaneous catch-up growth without need for rhGH therapy [30].

Potential Adverse Events Associated with rhGH Therapy

The safety of long-term rhGH treatment in CKD has been evaluated in several clinical studies and registries [30]. RhGH therapy in short children with CKD stage 3–5D and after kidney transplantation was not associated with an increased incidence of malignancy, slipped capital femoral epiphysis, avascular necrosis, glucose intolerance, pancreatitis, CKD progression, acute allograft rejection or fluid retention. Intracranial hypertension (ICH), manifesting in 3 out of 1376 CKD patients, was the only adverse event significantly associated with rhGH therapy [183]. However, in all three instances ICH occurred after discontinuation of rhGH. Due to the potentially increased risk of ICH in CKD, baseline fundoscopy is recommended prior to therapy initiation [30]. Furthermore, hydration should be carefully monitored in CKD patients receiving rhGH since overhydration may be a predisposing factor for ICH. In the presence of symptoms like headache or vomiting, an immediate workup for ICH including fundoscopy should be performed.

Although insulin secretion increases during the first year of rhGH treatment and hyperinsulinemia persists during long-term therapy, normal glucose tolerance is preserved during up to 5 years of rhGH administration in CKD patients on conservative treatment, dialysis, and after kidney tansplantation. Hyperinsulinemia is most pronounced in transplanted patients on concomitant glucocorticoid therapy. Hyperinsulinemia may, at least in theory, contribute to the development of atherosclerosis or induce diabetes mellitus by exhaustion of ß-cells. However, up to now this has not been observed in CKD patients receiving rhGH [183].

Aggravation of secondary hyperparathyroidism has rarely been reported in CKD patients on rhGH treatment, and the underlying pathomechanisms remain to be elucidated [184]. RhGH might have a direct stimulatory effect on the parathyroid gland and/or might have subtle effects on calcium homeostasis which in turn stimulate PTH secretion. Finally, increased longitudinal bone growth by rhGH treatment may unmask preexisting renal osteodystrophy. Therefore, bone metabolism should be evaluated carefully in candidates for rhGH therapy and severe hyperparathyroidism and renal osteodystrophy should be adequately treated before initiation of such therapy in CKD patients. Likewise, rhGH therapy should be stopped in patients with persistent severe secondary hyperparathyroidism (PTH > 500 pg/mL). RhGH may be reinstituted when PTH levels return to the desired PTH target range [30].

Future Perspectives

Despite attention to nutrition and the availability of rhGH therapy, the problem of CKD associated growth failure has not been resolved in the majority of dialysis patients. If early kidney transplantation is not possible, the concept of intensified hemodiafiltration combined with rhGH may be a promising option for patients suffering from growth retardation and GH insensitivity on conventional dialysis therapy. Independent of concomitant rhGH therapy, hemodiafiltration appears to allow improved growth rates than conventional hemodialysis and, if available, should be the preferred extracorporeal dialysis modality in all growing children.

Self-reported nonadherence to rhGH is associated with poorer growth velocity in children with CKD. Therefore, monitoring and optimizing adherence to rhGH therapy is key to satisfactory

growth outcomes [185]. Another promising avenue of clinical research may be the provision of recombinant IGF-I administered as monotherapy or in combination with rhGH, as well as targeting of the SOCS2 signaling pathway [186].

A particular challenge is the management of severely diminished pubertal height gain seen in some adolescents with CKD. In such adolescents, pharmacological inhibition of epiphyseal closure may allow an extended duration of the remaining growth period. Since the closure of the epiphyseal growth plate is induced by local estrogen action, inhibition of estrogen synthesis is a principal therapeutic option. Whereas gonadotropin-releasing hormone analogues arrest pubertal progress, the potential growth benefit would come at the psychological disadvantage of delayed sexual maturation. In boys, aromatase inhibitors, which suppress local conversion of testosterone to estradiol, might extend the growth phase without affecting pubertal development and thereby increase the time window for the use of rhGH therapy. Indeed, the combined use of armomatase inhibitors and rhGH was associated with modest increases in adult height in boys with idiopathic short stature.

[187, 188]. However, some important questions about their long-term safety exist which at the moment prevent this from being generally recommended [189]. It would be fascinating to study its efficacy in adolescents on long-term dialysis. Nevertheless, successful early (preemptive) kidney transplantation with minimal steroid exposure is ultimately the best current measure to improve growth and final height in children with CKD stage 5.

References

1. Franke D, Winkel S, Gellermann J, Querfeld U, Pape L, Ehrich JH, Haffner D, Pavicic L, Zivicnjak M. Growth and maturation improvement in children on renal replacement therapy over the past 20 years. Pediatr Nephrol. 2013;28:2043–51.
2. Harambat J, Bonthuis M, van Stralen KJ, Ariceta G, Battelino N, Bjerre A, Jahnukainen T, Leroy V, Reusz G, Sandes AR, Sinha MD, Groothoff JW, Combe C, Jager KJ, Verrina E, Schaefer F, for the ESPN/ERA-EDTA Registry. Adult height in patients

with advanced CKD requiring renal replacement therapy during childhood. Clin J Am Soc Nephrol. 2013;

3. Fine RN, Martz K, Stablein D. What have 20 years of data from the north american pediatric renal transplant cooperative study taught us about growth following renal transplantation in infants, children, and adolescents with end-stage renal disease? Pediatr Nephrol. 2010;25:739–46.

4. Klare B, Montoya CR, Fischer DC, Stangl MJ, Haffner D. Normal adult height after steroid-withdrawal within 6 months of pediatric kidney transplantation: a 20 years single center experience. Transpl Int. 2012;25:276–82.

5. Wong CS, Gipson DS, Gillen DL, Emerson S, Koepsell T, Sherrard DJ, Watkins SL, Stehman-Breen C. Anthropometric measures and risk of death in children with end-stage renal disease. Am J Kidney Dis. 2000;36:811–9.

6. Furth SL, Stablein D, Fine RN, Powe NR, Fivush BA. Adverse clinical outcomes associated with short stature at dialysis initiation: a report of the north american pediatric renal transplant cooperative study. Pediatrics. 2002;109:909–13.

7. Ku E, Fine RN, Hsu CY, McCulloch C, Glidden DV, Grimes B, Johansen KL. Height at first RRT and mortality in children. Clin J Am Soc Nephrol. 2016;11:832–9.

8. Hartung EA, Furth SL. Growth in children on renal replacement therapy: a shrinking problem? Pediatr Nephrol. 2013;28:1905–8.

9. Behnisch R, Kirchner M, Anarat A, Bacchetta J, Shroff R, Bilginer Y, Mir S, Caliskan S, Paripovic D, Harambat J, Mencarelli F, Büscher R, Arbeiter K, Soylemezoglu O, Zaloszyc A, Zurowska A, Melk A, Querfeld U, Schaefer F, and the 4C Study Consortium. Determinants of statural growth in european children with chronic kidney disease: findings from the cardiovascular comorbidity in children with chronic kidney disease (4C) study. Front Pediatr. 2019;7:278.

10. Schaefer F, Benner L, Borzych-Dużałka D, Zaritsky J, Xu H, Rees L, Antonio ZL, Serdaroglu E, Hooman N, Patel H, Sever L, Vondrak K, Flynn J, Rébori A, Wong W, Hölttä T, Yildirim ZY, Ranchin B, Grenda R, Testa S, Drożdż D, Szabo AJ, Eid L, Basu B, Vitkevic R, Wong C, Pottoore SJ, Müller D, Dusunsel R, Celedon CG, Fila M, Sartz L, Sander A, Warady BA, International Pediatric Peritoneal Dialysis Network (IPPN) Registry. Global variation of nutritional status in children undergoing chronic peritoneal dialysis: a longitudinal study of the international pediatric peritoneal dialysis network. Sci Rep. 2019;9:4886-z.

11. Rodig NM, McDermott KC, Schneider MF, Hotchkiss HM, Yadin O, Seikaly MG, Furth SL, Warady BA. Growth in children with chronic kidney disease: a report from the chronic kidney disease in children study. Pediatr Nephrol. 2014;29:1987–95.

12. United States Renal Data System. USRDS annual data report: Epidemiology of kidney disease in the United States, vol. 2020. Bethesda, MD: National Institutes of Health, National Institute of Diabetes and Digestive and Kidney Diseases; 2020. p. 2021.

13. Rees L, Azocar M, Borzych D, Watson AR, Buscher A, Edefonti A, Bilge I, Askenazi D, Leozappa G, Gonzales C, van Hoeck K, Secker D, Zurowska A, Ronnholm K, Bouts AH, Stewart H, Ariceta G, Ranchin B, Warady BA, Schaefer F, International Pediatric Peritoneal Dialysis Network (IPPN) Registry. Growth in very young children undergoing chronic peritoneal dialysis. J Am Soc Nephrol. 2011;22:2303–12.

14. Schaefer F, Mehls O. Endocrine, metabolic and growth disorders. In: Holliday MA, Barrat TM, Avner ED, editors. Pediatric nephrology. 3rd ed. Baltimore: Williams & Wilkins; 1994. p. 1241–86.

15. Downie AB, Mulligan J, Stratford RJ, Betts PR, Voss LD. Are short normal children at a disadvantage? the wessex growth study. BMJ. 1997;314:97–100.

16. Karlberg J, Schaefer F, Hennicke M, Wingen AM, Rigden S, Mehls O. Early age-dependent growth impairment in chronic renal failure. european study group for nutritional treatment of chronic renal failure in childhood. Pediatr Nephrol. 1996;10:283–7.

17. Schaefer F, Seidel C, Binding A, Gasser T, Largo RH, Prader A, Scharer K. Pubertal growth in chronic renal failure. Pediatr Res. 1990;28:5–10.

18. Nissel R, Brazda I, Feneberg R, Wigger M, Greiner C, Querfeld U, Haffner D. Effect of renal transplantation in childhood on longitudinal growth and adult height. Kidney Int. 2004;66:792–800.

19. Kari JA, Gonzalez C, Ledermann SE, Shaw V, Rees L. Outcome and growth of infants with severe chronic renal failure. Kidney Int. 2000;57:1681–7.

20. Mekahli D, Shaw V, Ledermann SE, Rees L. Long-term outcome of infants with severe chronic kidney disease. Clin J Am Soc Nephrol. 2010;5:10–7.

21. Greenbaum LA, Munoz A, Schneider MF, Kaskel FJ, Askenazi DJ, Jenkins R, Hotchkiss H, Moxey-Mims M, Furth SL, Warady BA. The association between abnormal birth history and growth in children with CKD. Clin J Am Soc Nephrol. 2011;6:14–21.

22. Franke D, Volker S, Haase S, Pavicic L, Querfeld U, Ehrich JH, Zivicnjak M. Prematurity, small for gestational age and perinatal parameters in children with congenital, hereditary and acquired chronic kidney disease. Nephrol Dial Transplant. 2010;25:3918–24.

23. Schaefer F, Wingen AM, Hennicke M, Rigden S, Mehls O. Growth charts for prepubertal children with chronic renal failure due to congenital renal disorders. european study group for nutritional treatment of chronic renal failure in childhood. Pediatr Nephrol. 1996;10:288–93.

24. Cetin I, Mando C, Calabrese S. Maternal predictors of intrauterine growth restriction. Curr Opin Clin Nutr Metab Care. 2013;16:310–9.

25. Jagadapillai R, Chen J, Canales L, Birtles T, Pisano MM, Neal RE. Developmental cigarette smoke exposure: kidney proteome profile alterations in low birth weight pups. Toxicology. 2012;299:80–9.

26. Menendez-Castro C, Hilgers KF, Amann K, Daniel C, Cordasic N, Wachtveitl R, Fahlbusch F, Plank C, Dotsch J, Rascher W, Hartner A. Intrauterine growth restriction leads to a dysregulation of wilms' tumour supressor gene 1 (WT1) and to early podocyte alterations. Nephrol Dial Transplant. 2013;28:1407–17.

27. Franke D, Alakan H, Pavicic L, Gellermann J, Muller D, Querfeld U, Haffner D, Zivicnjak M. Birth parameters and parental height predict growth outcome in children with chronic kidney disease. Pediatr Nephrol. 2013;28:2335–41.

28. Jones RW, Rigden SP, Barratt TM, Chantler C. The effects of chronic renal failure in infancy on growth, nutritional status and body composition. Pediatr Res. 1982;16:784–91.

29. Kleinknecht C, Broyer M, Huot D, Marti-Henneberg C, Dartois AM. Growth and development of nondialyzed children with chronic renal failure. Kidney Int Suppl. 1983;15:40.

30. Drube J, Wan M, Bonthuis M, Wühl E, Bacchetta J, Santos F, Grenda R, Edefonti A, Harambat J, Shroff R, Tönshoff B, Haffner D, European Society for Paediatric Nephrology Chronic Kidney Disease Mineral and Bone Disorders, Dialysis, and Transplantation Working Groups. Clinical practice recommendations for growth hormone treatment in children with chronic kidney disease. Nat Rev Nephrol. 2019;15:577–89.

31. Rees L, Mak RH. Nutrition and growth in children with chronic kidney disease. Nat Rev Nephrol. 2011;7:615–23.

32. Sarwal MM, Ettenger RB, Dharnidharka V, Benfield M, Mathias R, Portale A, McDonald R, Harmon W, Kershaw D, Vehaskari VM, Kamil E, Baluarte HJ, Warady B, Tang L, Liu J, Li L, Naesens M, Sigdel T, Waskerwitz J, Salvatierra O. Complete steroid avoidance is effective and safe in children with renal transplants: a multicenter randomized trial with three-year follow-up. Am J Transplant. 2012;12:2719–29.

33. Delucchi A, Valenzuela M, Lillo AM, Guerrero JL, Cano F, Azocar M, Zambrano P, Salas P, Pinto V, Ferrario M, Rodriguez J, Cavada G. Early steroid withdrawal in pediatric renal transplant: five years of follow-up. Pediatr Nephrol. 2011;26:2235–44.

34. Rizzoni G, Broyer M, Brunner FP, Brynger H, Challah S, Kramer P, Oules R, Selwood NH, Wing AJ, Balas EA. Combined report on regular dialysis and transplantation of children in europe, XIII, 1983. Proc Eur Dial Transplant Assoc Eur Ren Assoc. 1985;21:66–95.

35. Burke BA, Lindgren B, Wick M, Holley K, Manivel C. Testicular germ cell loss in children with renal failure. Pediatr Pathol. 1989;9:433–44.

36. Tainio J, Qvist E, Vehmas R, Jahnukainen K, Holtta T, Valta H, Jahnukainen T, Jalanko H. Pubertal development is normal in adolescents after renal transplantation in childhood. Transplantation. 2011;92:404–9.

37. Kim HS, Ng DK, Matheson MB, Atkinson MA, Warady BA, Furth SL, Ruebner RL. Delayed menarche in girls with chronic kidney disease and the association with short stature. Pediatr Nephrol. 2020;35:1471–5.

38. Zivicnjak M, Franke D, Ehrich JH, Filler G. Does growth hormone therapy harmonize distorted morphology and body composition in chronic renal failure? Pediatr Nephrol. 2000;15:229–35.

39. Gunnell D, Whitley E, Upton MN, McConnachie A, Smith GD, Watt GC. Associations of height, leg length, and lung function with cardiovascular risk factors in the midspan family study. J Epidemiol Community Health. 2003;57:141–6.

40. Kinra S, Sarma KV, Hards M, Smith GD, Ben-Shlomo Y. Is relative leg length a biomarker of childhood nutrition? long-term follow-up of the hyderabad nutrition trial. Int J Epidemiol. 2011;40:1022–9.

41. Zivicnjak M, Franke D, Filler G, Haffner D, Froede K, Nissel R, Haase S, Offner G, Ehrich JH, Querfeld U. Growth impairment shows an age-dependent pattern in boys with chronic kidney disease. Pediatr Nephrol. 2007;22:420–9.

42. Franke D, Thomas L, Steffens R, Pavicic L, Gellermann J, Froede K, Querfeld U, Haffner D, Zivicnjak M. Patterns of growth after kidney transplantation among children with ESRD. Clin J Am Soc Nephrol. 2015;10:127–34.

43. Franke D, Steffens R, Thomas L, Pavicic L, Ahlenstiel T, Pape L, Gellermann J, Muller D, Querfeld U, Haffner D, Zivicnjak M. Kidney transplantation fails to provide adequate growth in children with chronic kidney disease born small for gestational age. Pediatr Nephrol. 2017;32:511–9.

44. Grohs J, Rebling RM, Froede K, Hmeidi K, Pavičić L, Gellermann J, Müller D, Querfeld U, Haffner D, Živičnjak M. Determinants of growth after kidney transplantation in prepubertal children. Pediatr Nephrol. 2021;36:1871–80.

45. Offner G, Latta K, Hoyer PF, Baum HJ, Ehrich JH, Pichlmayr R, Brodehl J. Kidney transplanted children come of age. Kidney Int. 1999;55:1509–17.

46. Haffner D, Schaefer F, Nissel R, Wuhl E, Tonshoff B, Mehls O. Effect of growth hormone treatment on the adult height of children with chronic renal failure. german study group for growth hormone treatment in chronic renal failure. N Engl J Med. 2000;343:923–30.

47. Nissel R, Lindberg A, Mehls O, Haffner D, Pfizer International Growth Database (KIGS) International Board. Factors predicting the near-final height in growth hormone-treated children and adolescents with chronic kidney disease. J Clin Endocrinol Metab. 2008;93:1359–65.

48. Nissel R, Latta K, Gagnadoux MF, Kelly D, Hulton S, Kemper MJ, Ruder H, Soderdahl G, Otte JB, Cochat P, Roquet O, Jamieson NV, Haffner D. Body

growth after combined liver-kidney transplantation in children with primary hyperoxaluria type 1. Transplantation. 2006;82:48–54.

49. Brinkert F, Lehnhardt A, Montoya C, Helmke K, Schaefer H, Fischer L, Nashan B, Bergmann C, Ganschow R, Kemper MJ. Combined liver-kidney transplantation for children with autosomal recessive polycystic kidney disease (ARPKD): Indication and outcome. Transpl Int. 2013;26:640–50.

50. Schaefer F, Borzych-Duzalka D, Azocar M, Munarriz RL, Sever L, Aksu N, Barbosa LS, Galan YS, Xu H, Coccia PA, Szabo A, Wong W, Salim R, Vidal E, Pottoore S, Warady BA, & IPPN investigators (2012) Impact of global economic disparities on practices and outcomes of chronic peritoneal dialysis in children: Insights from the international pediatric peritoneal dialysis network registry. Perit Dial Int 32: 399–409.

51. Hiraoka M. Medical management of congenital anomalies of the kidney and urinary tract. Pediatr Int. 2003;45:624–33.

52. Tullus K, Webb H, Bagga A. Management of steroid-resistant nephrotic syndrome in children and adolescents. Lancet Child Adolesc Health. 2018;2:880–90.

53. Rees L, Greene SA, Adlard P, Jones J, Haycock GB, Rigden SP, Preece M, Chantler C. Growth and endocrine function in steroid sensitive nephrotic syndrome. Arch Dis Child. 1988;63:484–90.

54. Dufek S, Holtta T, Trautmann A, Ylinen E, Alpay H, Ariceta G, Aufricht C, Bacchetta J, Bakkaloglu SA, Bayazit A, Cicek RY, Dursun I, Duzova A, Ekim M, Iancu D, Jankauskiene A, Klaus G, Paglialonga F, Pasini A, Printza N, Said Conti V, do Sameiro Faria M, Schmitt CP, Stefanidis CJ, Verrina E, Vidal E, Vondrak K, Webb H, Zampetoglou A, Bockenhauer D, Edefonti A, Shroff R. Management of children with congenital nephrotic syndrome: Challenging treatment paradigms. Nephrol Dial Transplant. 2018;

55. Dufek S, Ylinen E, Trautmann A, Alpay H, Ariceta G, Aufricht C, Bacchetta J, Bakkaloglu S, Bayazit A, Caliskan S, do Sameiro Faria M, Dursun I, Ekim M, Jankauskiene A, Klaus G, Paglialonga F, Pasini A, Printza N, Conti VS, Schmitt CP, Stefanidis C, Verrina E, Vidal E, Webb H, Zampetoglou A, Edefonti A, Holtta T, Shroff R, ESPN Dialysis Working Group. Infants with congenital nephrotic syndrome have comparable outcomes to infants with other renal diseases. Pediatr Nephrol. 2019;34:649–55.

56. Boyer O, Schaefer F, Haffner D, Bockenhauer D, Hölttä T, Bérody S, Webb H, Heselden M, Lipska-Zie Tkiewicz BS, Ozaltin F, Levtchenko E, Vivarelli M. Management of congenital nephrotic syndrome: consensus recommendations of the ERKNet-ESPN working group. Nat Rev Nephrol. 2021;17:277–89.

57. Haffner D, Weinfurth A, Manz F, Schmidt H, Bremer HJ, Mehls O, Scharer K. Long-term outcome of paediatric patients with hereditary tubular disorders. Nephron. 1999;83:250–60.

58. Lopez-Garcia SC, Emma F, Walsh SB, Fila M, Hooman N, Zaniew M, Bertholet-Thomas A, Colussi G, Burgmaier K, Levtchenko E, Sharma J, Singhal J, Soliman NA, Ariceta G, Basu B, Murer L, Tasic V, Tsygin A, Decramer S, Gil-Pena H, Koster-Kamphuis L, La Scola C, Gellermann J, Konrad M, Lilien M, Francisco T, Tramma D, Trnka P, Yuksel S, Caruso MR, Chromek M, Ekinci Z, Gambaro G, Kari JA, Konig J, Taroni F, Thumfart J, Trepiccione F, Winding L, Wuhl E, Agbas A, Belkevich A, Vargas-Poussou R, Blanchard A, Conti G, Boyer O, Dursun I, Pinarbasi AS, Melek E, Miglinas M, Novo R, Mallett A, Milosevic D, Szczepanska M, Wente S, Cheong HI, Sinha R, Gucev Z, Dufek S, Iancu D, Kleta R, Schaefer F, Bockenhauer D, European dRTA Consortium. Treatment and long-term outcome in primary distal renal tubular acidosis. Nephrol Dial Transplant. 2019;

59. Greco M, Brugnara M, Zaffanello M, Taranta A, Pastore A, Emma F. Long-term outcome of nephropathic cystinosis: a 20-year single-center experience. Pediatr Nephrol. 2010;25:2459–67.

60. Haffner D, Weinfurth A, Seidel C, Manz F, Schmidt H, Waldherr R, Bremer HJ, Mehls O, Scharer K. Body growth in primary de toni-debre-fanconi syndrome. Pediatr Nephrol. 1997;11:40–5.

61. Hohenfellner K, Rauch F, Ariceta G, Awan A, Bacchetta J, Bergmann C, Bechtold S, Cassidy N, Deschenes G, Elenberg E, Gahl WA, Greil O, Harms E, Herzig N, Hoppe B, Koeppl C, Lewis MA, Levtchenko E, Nesterova G, Santos F, Schlingmann KP, Servais A, Soliman NA, Steidle G, Sweeney C, Treikauskas U, Topaloglu R, Tsygin A, Veys K, Vigier VR, Zustin J, Haffner D. Management of bone disease in cystinosis: Statement from an international conference. J Inherit Metab Dis. 2019;42:1019–29.

62. Rumsby G, Cochat P. Primary hyperoxaluria. N Engl J Med. 2013;369:2163.

63. Emma F, Salviati L. Mitochondrial cytopathies and the kidney. Nephrol Ther. 2017;13(Suppl. 1):S23–8.

64. Kimonis VE, Troendle J, Rose SR, Yang ML, Markello TC, Gahl WA. Effects of early cysteamine therapy on thyroid function and growth in nephropathic cystinosis. J Clin Endocrinol Metab. 1995;80:3257–61.

65. Ewert A, Leifheit-Nestler M, Hohenfellner K, Büscher A, Kemper MJ, Oh J, Billing H, Thumfart J, Stangl G, Baur AC, Föller M, Feger M, Weber LT, Acham-Roschitz B, Arbeiter K, Tönshoff B, Zivicnjak M, Haffner D. Bone and mineral metabolism in children with nephropathic cystinosis compared with other CKD entities. J Clin Endocrinol Metab. 2020;105:dgaa267. https://doi.org/10.1210/clinem/dgaa267.

66. Battafarano G, Rossi M, Rega LR, Di Giovamberardino G, Pastore A, D'Agostini M, Porzio O, Nevo N, Emma F, Taranta A, Del Fattore A. Intrinsic bone defects in cystinotic mice. Am J Pathol. 2019;189:1053–64.

67. Weigert A, Martin-Higueras C, Hoppe B. Novel therapeutic approaches in primary hyperoxaluria. Expert Opin Emerg Drugs. 2018;23:349–57.

68. Seikaly MG, Salhab N, Gipson D, Yiu V, Stablein D. Stature in children with chronic kidney disease: analysis of NAPRTCS database. Pediatr Nephrol. 2006;21:793–9.

69. North american pediatric renal trials and collaborative studies. (2005). NAPRTCS annual report 2005. available at: https://Web.emmes.com/study/ped/annlrept/annlrept2005.pdf.

70. Katsoufis CP, DeFreitas MJ, Infante JC, Castellan M, Cano T, Safina Vaccaro D, Seeherunvong W, Chandar JJ, Abitbol CL. Risk assessment of severe congenital anomalies of the kidney and urinary tract (CAKUT): A birth cohort. Front Pediatr. 2019;7:182.

71. United states renal data system (USRDS). 2008 report. USRDS coordinating center, minneapolis, pp. 296–297.

72. Haffner D. Strategies for optimizing growth in children with chronic kidney disease. Front Pediatr. 2020;8:399.

73. Rees L, Brandt ML. Tube feeding in children with chronic kidney disease: technical and practical issues. Pediatr Nephrol. 2010;25:699–704.

74. Shaw V, Polderman N, Renken-Terhaerdt J, Paglialonga F, Oosterveld M, Tuokkola J, Anderson C, Desloovere A, Greenbaum L, Haffner D, Nelms C, Qizalbash L, Vande Walle J, Warady B, Shroff R, Rees L. Energy and protein requirements for children with CKD stages 2–5 and on dialysis-clinical practice recommendations from the pediatric renal nutrition taskforce. Pediatr Nephrol. 2020;35:519–31.

75. Rees L, Shaw V, Qizalbash L, Anderson C, Desloovere A, Greenbaum L, Haffner D, Nelms C, Oosterveld M, Paglialonga F, Polderman N, Renken-Terhaerdt J, Tuokkola J, Warady B, Walle JV, Shroff R, Pediatric Renal Nutrition Taskforce. Delivery of a nutritional prescription by enteral tube feeding in children with chronic kidney disease stages 2–5 and on dialysis-clinical practice recommendations from the pediatric renal nutrition taskforce. Pediatr Nephrol. 2021;36:187–204.

76. Mak RH, Cheung WW, Zhan JY, Shen Q, Foster BJ. Cachexia and protein-energy wasting in children with chronic kidney disease. Pediatr Nephrol. 2012;27:173–81.

77. Rees L. Protein energy wasting; what is it and what can we do to prevent it? Pediatr Nephrol. 2019;

78. Bonthuis M, van Stralen KJ, Verrina E, Groothoff JW, Alonso Melgar A, Edefonti A, Fischbach M, Mendes P, Molchanova EA, Paripovic D, Peco-Antic A, Printza N, Rees L, Rubik J, Stefanidis CJ, Sinha MD, Zagozdzon I, Jager KJ, Schaefer F. Underweight, overweight and obesity in paediatric dialysis and renal transplant patients. Nephrol Dial Transplant. 2013;28(Suppl. 4):iv195–204.

79. Rees L, Jones H. Nutritional management and growth in children with chronic kidney disease. Pediatr Nephrol. 2013;28:527–36.

80. Foster BJ, Martz K, Gowrishankar M, Stablein D, Al-Uzri A. Weight and height changes and factors associated with greater weight and height gains after pediatric renal transplantation: a NAPRTCS study. Transplantation. 2010;89:1103–12.

81. Bailey JL, Wang X, England BK, Price SR, Ding X, Mitch WE. The acidosis of chronic renal failure activates muscle proteolysis in rats by augmenting transcription of genes encoding proteins of the ATP-dependent ubiquitin-proteasome pathway. J Clin Invest. 1996;97:1447–53.

82. Boirie Y, Broyer M, Gagnadoux MF, Niaudet P, Bresson JL. Alterations of protein metabolism by metabolic acidosis in children with chronic renal failure. Kidney Int. 2000;58:236–41.

83. Brungger M, Hulter HN, Krapf R. Effect of chronic metabolic acidosis on the growth hormone/IGF-1 endocrine axis: new cause of growth hormone insensitivity in humans. Kidney Int. 1997;51:216–21.

84. Grossman H, Duggan E, McCamman S, Welchert E, Hellerstein S. The dietary chloride deficiency syndrome. Pediatrics. 1980;66:366–74.

85. Sharma S, Ashton E, Iancu D, Arthus MF, Hayes W, Van't Hoff W, Kleta R, Bichet DG, Bockenhauer D. Long-term outcome in inherited nephrogenic diabetes insipidus. Clin Kidney J. 2018;12:180–7.

86. Schmitt CP, Mehls O. Mineral and bone disorders in children with chronic kidney disease. Nat Rev Nephrol. 2011;7:624–34.

87. Haffner D, Fischer DC. Bone cell biology and pediatric renal osteodystrophy. Minerva Pediatr. 2010;62:273–84.

88. Mehls O, Ritz E, Gilli G, Wangdak T, Krempien B. Effect of vitamin D on growth in experimental uremia. Am J Clin Nutr. 1978;31:1927–31.

89. Mehls O, Knoller N, Oh J, Wesch H, Wunsche B, Schmitt CP. Daily but not pulse calcitriol therapy improves growth in experimental uremia. Pediatr Nephrol. 2000;14:658–63.

90. Kuizon BD, Goodman WG, Juppner H, Boechat I, Nelson P, Gales B, Salusky IB. Diminished linear growth during intermittent calcitriol therapy in children undergoing CCPD. Kidney Int. 1998;53:205–11.

91. Bakkaloglu SA, Wesseling-Perry K, Pereira RC, Gales B, Wang HJ, Elashoff RM, Salusky IB. Value of the new bone classification system in pediatric renal osteodystrophy. Clin J Am Soc Nephrol. 2010;5:1860–6.

92. Cansick J, Waller S, Ridout D, Rees L. Growth and PTH in prepubertal children on long-term dialysis. Pediatr Nephrol. 2007;22:1349–54.

93. Waller S, Shroff R, Freemont AJ, Rees L. Bone histomorphometry in children prior to commencing renal replacement therapy. Pediatr Nephrol. 2008;23:1523–9.

94. Borzych D, Rees L, Ha IS, Chua A, Valles PG, Lipka M, Zambrano P, Ahlenstiel T, Bakkaloglu SA, Spizzirri AP, Lopez L, Ozaltin F, Printza N, Hari P, Klaus G, Bak M, Vogel A, Ariceta G, Yap HK, Warady BA, Schaefer F, International Pediatric PD Network (IPPN). The bone and mineral disorder of children undergoing chronic peritoneal dialysis. Kidney Int. 2010;78:1295–304.

95. Morris KP, Sharp J, Watson S, Coulthard MG. Non-cardiac benefits of human recombinant erythropoietin in end stage renal failure and anaemia. Arch Dis Child. 1993;69:580–6.

96. Jabs K. The effects of recombinant human erythropoietin on growth and nutritional status. Pediatr Nephrol. 1996;10:324–7.

97. Martin GR, Ongkingo JR, Turner ME, Skurow ES, Ruley EJ. Recombinant erythropoietin (epogen) improves cardiac exercise performance in children with end-stage renal disease. Pediatr Nephrol. 1993;7:276–80.

98. Haffner D, Zivicnjak M. Pubertal development in children with chronic kidney disease. Pediatr Nephrol. 2017;32:949–64.

99. Belgorosky A, Ferraris JR, Ramirez JA, Jasper H, Rivarola MA. Serum sex hormone-binding globulin and serum nonsex hormone-binding globulin-bound testosterone fractions in prepubertal boys with chronic renal failure. J Clin Endocrinol Metab. 1991;73:107–10.

100. Van Kammen E, Thijssen JH, Schwarz F. Sex hormones in male patients with chronic renal failure. I. the production of testosterone and of androstenedione. Clin Endocrinol. 1978;8:7–14.

101. Ferraris JR, Domene HM, Escobar ME, Caletti MG, Ramirez JA, Rivarola MA. Hormonal profile in pubertal females with chronic renal failure: before and under haemodialysis and after renal transplantation. Acta Endocrinol. 1987;115:289–96.

102. Schaefer F, Seidel C, Mitchell R, Scharer K, Robertson WR. Pulsatile immunoreactive and bioactive luteinizing hormone secretion in adolescents with chronic renal failure. the cooperative study group on pubertal development in chronic renal failure (CSPCRF). Pediatr Nephrol. 1991;5:566–71.

103. Schaefer F, Veldhuis JD, Robertson WR, Dunger D, Scharer K. Immunoreactive and bioactive luteinizing hormone in pubertal patients with chronic renal failure. cooperative study group on pubertal development in chronic renal failure. Kidney Int. 1994;45:1465–76.

104. Schaefer F, Daschner M, Veldhuis JD, Oh J, Qadri F, Scharer K. In vivo alterations in the gonadotropin-releasing hormone pulse generator and the secretion and clearance of luteinizing hormone in the uremic castrate rat. Neuroendocrinology. 1994;59:285–96.

105. Daschner M, Philippin B, Nguyen T, Wiesner RJ, Walz C, Oh J, Sandow J, Mehls O, Schaefer F. Circulating inhibitor of gonadotropin releasing hormone secretion by hypothalamic neurons in uremia. Kidney Int. 2002;62:1582–90.

106. Schaefer F, Vogel M, Kerkhoff G, Woitzik J, Daschner M, Mehls O. Experimental uremia affects hypothalamic amino acid neurotransmitter milieu. J Am Soc Nephrol. 2001;12:1218–27.

107. Mitchell R, Bauerfeld C, Schaefer F, Scharer K, Robertson WR. Less acidic forms of luteinizing hormone are associated with lower testosterone secretion in men on haemodialysis treatment. Clin Endocrinol. 1994;41:65–73.

108. Haffner D, Schaefer F, Girard J, Ritz E, Mehls O. Metabolic clearance of recombinant human growth hormone in health and chronic renal failure. J Clin Invest. 1994;93:1163–71.

109. Schaefer F, Baumann G, Haffner D, Faunt LM, Johnson ML, Mercado M, Ritz E, Mehls O, Veldhuis JD. Multifactorial control of the elimination kinetics of unbound (free) growth hormone (GH) in the human: regulation by age, adiposity, renal function, and steady state concentrations of GH in plasma. J Clin Endocrinol Metab. 1996;81:22–31.

110. Tonshoff B, Veldhuis JD, Heinrich U, Mehls O. Deconvolution analysis of spontaneous nocturnal growth hormone secretion in prepubertal children with preterminal chronic renal failure and with end-stage renal disease. Pediatr Res. 1995;37:86–93.

111. Schaefer F, Veldhuis JD, Stanhope R, Jones J, Scharer K. Alterations in growth hormone secretion and clearance in peripubertal boys with chronic renal failure and after renal transplantation. cooperative study group of pubertal development in chronic renal failure. J Clin Endocrinol Metab. 1994;78:1298–306.

112. Challa A, Chan W, Krieg RJ Jr, Thabet MA, Liu F, Hintz RL, Chan JC. Effect of metabolic acidosis on the expression of insulin-like growth factor and growth hormone receptor. Kidney Int. 1993;44:1224–7.

113. Troib A, Landau D, Kachko L, Rabkin R, Segev Y. Epiphyseal growth plate growth hormone receptor signaling is decreased in chronic kidney disease-related growth retardation. Kidney Int. 2013;84:940–9.

114. Schaefer F, Chen Y, Tsao T, Nouri P, Rabkin R. Impaired JAK-STAT signal transduction contributes to growth hormone resistance in chronic uremia. J Clin Invest. 2001;108:467–75.

115. Edmondson SR, Baker NL, Oh J, Kovacs G, Werther GA, Mehls O. Growth hormone receptor abundance in tibial growth plates of uremic rats: GH/IGF-I treatment. Kidney Int. 2000;58:62–70.

116. Rabkin R, Sun DF, Chen Y, Tan J, Schaefer F. Growth hormone resistance in uremia, a role for impaired JAK/STAT signaling. Pediatr Nephrol. 2005;20:313–8.

117. Wiezel D, Assadi MH, Landau D, Troib A, Kachko L, Rabkin R, Segev Y. Impaired renal growth hormone JAK/STAT5 signaling in chronic kidney disease. Nephrol Dial Transplant. 2014;29:791–9.

118. Tsao T, Fervenza F, Friedlaender M, Chen Y, Rabkin R. Effect of prolonged uremia on insulin-like growth factor-I receptor autophosphorylation and tyrosine kinase activity in kidney and muscle. Exp Nephrol. 2002;10:285–92.

119. Tonshoff B, Cronin MJ, Reichert M, Haffner D, Wingen AM, Blum WF, Mehls O. Reduced concentration of serum growth hormone (GH)-binding protein in children with chronic renal failure: Correlation with GH insensitivity. the european study group for nutritional treatment of chronic renal failure in child-

hood. the german study group for growth hormone treatment in chronic renal failure. J Clin Endocrinol Metab. 1997;82:1007–13.

120. Fouque D. Insulin-like growth factor 1 resistance in chronic renal failure. Miner Electrolyte Metab. 1996;22:133–7.

121. Powell DR, Liu F, Baker BK, Hintz RL, Lee PD, Durham SK, Brewer ED, Frane JW, Watkins SL, Hogg RJ. Modulation of growth factors by growth hormone in children with chronic renal failure. the southwest pediatric nephrology study group. Kidney Int. 1997;51:1970–9.

122. Ding H, Gao XL, Hirschberg R, Vadgama JV, Kopple JD. Impaired actions of insulin-like growth factor 1 on protein synthesis and degradation in skeletal muscle of rats with chronic renal failure. evidence for a postreceptor defect. J Clin Invest. 1996;97:1064–75.

123. Tonshoff B, Blum WF, Wingen AM, Mehls O. Serum insulin-like growth factors (IGFs) and IGF binding proteins 1, 2, and 3 in children with chronic renal failure: Relationship to height and glomerular filtration rate. the european study group for nutritional treatment of chronic renal failure in childhood. J Clin Endocrinol Metab. 1995;80:2684–91.

124. Blum WF, Ranke MB, Kietzmann K, Tonshoff B, Mehls O. Growth hormone resistance and inhibition of somatomedin activity by excess of insulin-like growth factor binding protein in uraemia. Pediatr Nephrol. 1991;5:539–44.

125. Powell DR, Liu F, Baker BK, Hinzt RL, Kale A, Suwanichkul A, Durham SK. Effect of chronic renal failure and growth hormone therapy on the insulin-like growth factors and their binding proteins. Pediatr Nephrol. 2000;14:579–83.

126. Ulinski T, Mohan S, Kiepe D, Blum WF, Wingen AM, Mehls O, Tonshoff B. Serum insulin-like growth factor binding protein (IGFBP)-4 and IGFBP-5 in children with chronic renal failure: Relationship to growth and glomerular filtration rate. the european study group for nutritional treatment of chronic renal failure in childhood. german study group for growth hormone treatment in chronic renal failure. Pediatr Nephrol. 2000;14:589–97.

127. Lee DY, Park SK, Yorgin PD, Cohen P, Oh Y, Rosenfeld RG. Alteration in insulin-like growth factor-binding proteins (IGFBPs) and IGFBP-3 protease activity in serum and urine from acute and chronic renal failure. J Clin Endocrinol Metab. 1994;79:1376–82.

128. Tonshoff B, Kiepe D, Ciarmatori S. Growth hormone/insulin-like growth factor system in children with chronic renal failure. Pediatr Nephrol. 2005;20:279–89.

129. Schaefer F, Hamill G, Stanhope R, Preece MA, Scharer K. Pulsatile growth hormone secretion in peripubertal patients with chronic renal failure. cooperative study group on pubertal development in chronic renal failure. J Pediatr. 1991;119:568–77.

130. Olney RC. Mechanisms of impaired growth: effect of steroids on bone and cartilage. Horm Res. 2009;72(Suppl. 1):30–5.

131. Baron J, Klein KO, Colli MJ, Yanovski JA, Novosad JA, Bacher JD, Cutler GB Jr. Catch-up growth after glucocorticoid excess: a mechanism intrinsic to the growth plate. Endocrinology. 1994;135:1367–71.

132. Klaus G, Jux C, Fernandez P, Rodriguez J, Himmele R, Mehls O. Suppression of growth plate chondrocyte proliferation by corticosteroids. Pediatr Nephrol. 2000;14:612–5.

133. Haffner D, Leifheit-Nestler M. CKD-MBD post kidney transplantation. Pediatr Nephrol. 2021;36:41–50.

134. Bertram JF, Goldstein SL, Pape L, Schaefer F, Shroff RC, Warady BA. Kidney disease in children: latest advances and remaining challenges. Nat Rev Nephrol. 2016;12:182–91.

135. Lurbe E, Agabiti-Rosei E, Cruickshank JK, Dominiczak A, Erdine S, Hirth A, Invitti C, Litwin M, Mancia G, Pall D, Rascher W, Redon J, Schaefer F, Seeman T, Sinha M, Stabouli S, Webb NJ, Wuhl E, Zanchetti A. 2016 European society of hypertension guidelines for the management of high blood pressure in children and adolescents. J Hypertens. 2016;34:1887–920.

136. van den Belt SM, HJL H, Gracchi V, de Zeeuw D, Wuhl E, Schaefer F, ESCAPE Trial Group. Early proteinuria lowering by angiotensin-converting enzyme inhibition predicts renal survival in children with CKD. J Am Soc Nephrol. 2018;29:2225–33.

137. Rees L, Shaw V, Qizalbash L, Anderson C, Desloovere A, Greenbaum L, Haffner D, Nelms C, Oosterveld M, Paglialonga F, Polderman N, Renken-Terhaerdt J, Tuokkola J, Warady B, Walle JV, Shroff R, Pediatric Renal Nutrition Taskforce. Delivery of a nutritional prescription by enteral tube feeding in children with chronic kidney disease stages 2–5 and on dialysis-clinical practice recommendations from the pediatric renal nutrition taskforce. Pediatr Nephrol. 2020;

138. Behnisch R, Kirchner M, Anarat A, Bacchetta J, Shroff R, Bilginer Y, Mir S, Caliskan S, Paripovic D, Harambat J, Mencarelli F, Buscher R, Arbeiter K, Soylemezoglu O, Zaloszyc A, Zurowska A, Melk A, Querfeld U, Schaefer F, and the 4C Study Consortium. Determinants of statural growth in european children with chronic kidney disease: findings from the cardiovascular comorbidity in children with chronic kidney disease (4C) study. Front Pediatr. 2019;7:278.

139. Marlais M, Stojanovic J, Jones H, Cleghorn S, Rees L. Catch-up growth in children with chronic kidney disease started on enteral feeding after 2 years of age. Pediatr Nephrol. 2020;35:113–8.

140. Coleman JE, Watson AR. Gastrostomy buttons for nutritional support in children with cystinosis. Pediatr Nephrol. 2000;14:833–6.

141. Ledermann SE, Shaw V, Trompeter RS. Long-term enteral nutrition in infants and young chil-

dren with chronic renal failure. Pediatr Nephrol. 1999;13:870–5.

142. Neu AM, Bedinger M, Fivush BA, Warady BA, Watkins SL, Friedman AL, Brem AS, Goldstein SL, Frankenfield DL. Growth in adolescent hemodialysis patients: data from the centers for medicare & medicaid services ESRD clinical performance measures project. Pediatr Nephrol. 2005;20:1156–60.

143. Quinlan C, Bates M, Sheils A, Dolan N, Riordan M, Awan A. Chronic hemodialysis in children weighing less than 10 kg. Pediatr Nephrol. 2013;28:803–9.

144. Rees L, Schaefer F, Schmitt CP, Shroff R, Warady BA. Chronic dialysis in children and adolescents: challenges and outcomes. Lancet Child Adolesc Health. 2017;1:68–77.

145. Shroff R, Wright E, Ledermann S, Hutchinson C, Rees L. Chronic hemodialysis in infants and children under 2 years of age. Pediatr Nephrol. 2003;18:378–83.

146. Chadha V, Blowey DL, Warady BA. Is growth a valid outcome measure of dialysis clearance in children undergoing peritoneal dialysis? Perit Dial Int. 2001;21(Suppl. 3):179.

147. Vidal E, Edefonti A, Murer L, Gianoglio B, Maringhini S, Pecoraro C, Sorino P, Leozappa G, Lavoratti G, Ratsch IM, Chimenz R, Verrina E, Italian Registry of Paediatric Chronic Dialysis. Peritoneal dialysis in infants: the experience of the italian registry of paediatric chronic dialysis. Nephrol Dial Transplant. 2012;27:388–95.

148. Schaefer F, Klaus G, Mehls O. Peritoneal transport properties and dialysis dose affect growth and nutritional status in children on chronic peritoneal dialysis. mid-european pediatric peritoneal dialysis study group. J Am Soc Nephrol. 1999;10:1786–92.

149. Tom A, McCauley L, Bell L, Rodd C, Espinosa P, Yu G, Yu J, Girardin C, Sharma A. Growth during maintenance hemodialysis: impact of enhanced nutrition and clearance. J Pediatr. 1999;134:464–71.

150. Katz A, Bock GH, Mauer M. Improved growth velocity with intensive dialysis. consequence or coincidence? Pediatr Nephrol. 2000;14:710–2.

151. Fischbach M, Zaloszyc A, Laetitia H, Menouer S, Terzic J. Why does three times per week hemodialysis provide inadequate dialysis for children? Hemodial Int. 2014;18(Suppl 1):39.

152. Fischbach M, Fothergill H, Seuge L, Zaloszyc A. Dialysis strategies to improve growth in children with chronic kidney disease. J Ren Nutr. 2011;21:43–6.

153. Fischbach M, Terzic J, Menouer S, Dheu C, Seuge L, Zalosczic A. Daily on line haemodiafiltration promotes catch-up growth in children on chronic dialysis. Nephrol Dial Transplant. 2010;25:867–73.

154. Fischbach M, Fothergill H, Zaloszyc A, Menouer S, Terzic J. Intensified daily dialysis: the best chronic dialysis option for children? Semin Dial. 2011;24:640–4.

155. Shroff R, Smith C, Ranchin B, Bayazit AK, Stefanidis CJ, Askiti V, Azukaitis K, Canpolat N, Agbas A, Aitkenhead H, Anarat A, Aoun B, Aofolaju D, Bakkaloglu SA, Bhowruth D, Borzych-Duzalka D, Bulut IK, Buscher R, Deanfield J, Dempster C, Duzova A, Habbig S, Hayes W, Hegde S, Krid S, Licht C, Litwin M, Mayes M, Mir S, Nemec R, Obrycki L, Paglialonga F, Picca S, Samaille C, Shenoy M, Sinha MD, Spasojevic B, Stronach L, Vidal E, Vondrak K, Yilmaz A, Zaloszyc A, Fischbach M, Schmitt CP, Schaefer F. Effects of hemodiafiltration versus conventional hemodialysis in children with ESKD: The HDF, heart and height study. J Am Soc Nephrol. 2019;30:678–91.

156. Laster ML, Fine RN. Growth following solid organ transplantation in childhood. Pediatr Transplant. 2014;18:134–41.

157. Pape L, Ehrich JH, Zivicnjak M, Offner G. Growth in children after kidney transplantation with living related donor graft or cadaveric graft. Lancet. 2005;366:151–3.

158. Grenda R. Steroid withdrawal in renal transplantation. Pediatr Nephrol. 2013;28:2107–12.

159. Hocker B, Weber LT, Feneberg R, Drube J, John U, Fehrenbach H, Pohl M, Zimmering M, Frund S, Klaus G, Wuhl E, Tonshoff B. Improved growth and cardiovascular risk after late steroid withdrawal: 2-year results of a prospective, randomised trial in paediatric renal transplantation. Nephrol Dial Transplant. 2010;25:617–24.

160. Webb NJ, Douglas SE, Rajai A, Roberts SA, Grenda R, Marks SD, Watson AR, Fitzpatrick M, Vondrak K, Maxwell H, Jaray J, Van Damme-Lombaerts R, Milford DV, Godefroid N, Cochat P, Ognjanovic M, Murer L, McCulloch M, Tonshoff B. Corticosteroid-free kidney transplantation improves growth: 2-year follow-up of the TWIST randomized controlled trial. Transplantation. 2015;99:1178–85.

161. Grenda R, Watson A, Trompeter R, Tonshoff B, Jaray J, Fitzpatrick M, Murer L, Vondrak K, Maxwell H, van Damme-Lombaerts R, Loirat C, Mor E, Cochat P, Milford DV, Brown M, Webb NJ. A randomized trial to assess the impact of early steroid withdrawal on growth in pediatric renal transplantation: the TWIST study. Am J Transplant. 2010;10:828–36.

162. Billing H, Burmeister G, Plotnicki L, Ahlenstiel T, Fichtner A, Sander A, Hocker B, Tonshoff B, Pape L. Longitudinal growth on an everolimus- versus an MMF-based steroid-free immunosuppressive regimen in paediatric renal transplant recipients. Transpl Int. 2013;26:903–9.

163. Schmitt CP, Ardissino G, Testa S, Claris-Appiani A, Mehls O. Growth in children with chronic renal failure on intermittent versus daily calcitriol. Pediatr Nephrol. 2003;18:440–4.

164. Sanchez CP, He YZ. Bone growth during daily or intermittent calcitriol treatment during renal failure with advanced secondary hyperparathyroidism. Kidney Int. 2007;72:582–91.

165. Shroff R, Wan M, Nagler EV, Bakkaloglu S, Cozzolino M, Bacchetta J, Edefonti A, Stefanidis CJ, Vande Walle J, Ariceta G, Klaus G, Haffner D, Schmitt CP, European Society for Paediatric Nephrology Chronic Kidney Disease Mineral and Bone Disorders and Dialysis Working Groups. Clinical practice recommendations for treatment with active vitamin D analogues in children with chronic kidney disease stages 2–5 and on dialysis. Nephrol Dial Transplant. 2017;32:1114–27.

166. Shroff R, Wan M, Nagler EV, Bakkaloglu S, Fischer DC, Bishop N, Cozzolino M, Bacchetta J, Edefonti A, Stefanidis CJ, Vande Walle J, Haffner D, Klaus G, Schmitt CP, European Society for Paediatric Nephrology Chronic Kidney Disease Mineral and Bone Disorders and Dialysis Working Groups. Clinical practice recommendations for native vitamin D therapy in children with chronic kidney disease stages 2–5 and on dialysis. Nephrol Dial Transplant. 2017;32:1098–113.

167. Warady BA, Ng E, Bloss L, Mo M, Schaefer F, Bacchetta J. Cinacalcet studies in pediatric subjects with secondary hyperparathyroidism receiving dialysis. Pediatr Nephrol. 2020;35:1679–97.

168. Nakagawa K, Perez EC, Oh J, Santos F, Geldyyev A, Gross ML, Schaefer F, Schmitt CP. Cinacalcet does not affect longitudinal growth but increases body weight gain in experimental uraemia. Nephrol Dial Transplant. 2008;23:2761–7.

169. Bacchetta J, Schmitt CP, Ariceta G, Bakkaloglu SA, Groothoff J, Wan M, Vervloet M, Shroff R, Haffner D, European Society for Paediatric Nephrology and the Chronic Kidney Disease-Mineral and Bone Disorders and Dialysis Working Group of the, ERA-EDTA. Cinacalcet use in paediatric dialysis: a position statement from the european society for paediatric nephrology and the chronic kidney disease-mineral and bone disorders working group of the ERA-EDTA. Nephrol Dial Transplant. 2020;35:47–64.

170. Mehls O, Ritz E, Hunziker EB, Eggli P, Heinrich U, Zapf J. Improvement of growth and food utilization by human recombinant growth hormone in uremia. Kidney Int. 1988;33:45–52.

171. Kovacs G, Fine RN, Worgall S, Schaefer F, Hunziker EB, Skottner-Lindun A, Mehls O. Growth hormone prevents steroid-induced growth depression in health and uremia. Kidney Int. 1991;40:1032–40.

172. Powell DR, Durham SK, Liu F, Baker BK, Lee PD, Watkins SL, Campbell PG, Brewer ED, Hintz RL, Hogg RJ. The insulin-like growth factor axis and growth in children with chronic renal failure: a report of the southwest pediatric nephrology study group. J Clin Endocrinol Metab. 1998;83:1654–61.

173. Hodson EM, Willis NS, Craig JC. Growth hormone for children with chronic kidney disease. Cochrane Database Syst Rev. 2012;(2):CD003264.

174. Haffner D, Wuhl E, Schaefer F, Nissel R, Tonshoff B, Mehls O. Factors predictive of the short- and

175. Fine RN, Kohaut E, Brown D, Kuntze J, Attie KM. Long-term treatment of growth retarded children with chronic renal insufficiency, with recombinant human growth hormone. Kidney Int. 1996;49:781–5.

176. Hokken-Koelega A, Mulder P, De Jong R, Lilien M, Donckerwolcke R, Groothof J. Long-term effects of growth hormone treatment on growth and puberty in patients with chronic renal insufficiency. Pediatr Nephrol. 2000;14:701–6.

177. Wuhl E, Haffner D, Nissel R, Schaefer F, Mehls O. Short dialyzed children respond less to growth hormone than patients prior to dialysis. german study group for growth hormone treatment in chronic renal failure. Pediatr Nephrol. 1996;10:294–8.

178. Mehls O, Lindberg A, Nissel R, Haffner D, Hokken-Koelega A, Ranke MB. Predicting the response to growth hormone treatment in short children with chronic kidney disease. J Clin Endocrinol Metab. 2010;95:686–92.

179. Fine RN, Attie KM, Kuntze J, Brown DF, Kohaut EC. Recombinant human growth hormone in infants and young children with chronic renal insufficiency. genentech collaborative study group. Pediatr Nephrol. 1995;9:451–7.

180. Maxwell H, Rees L. Recombinant human growth hormone treatment in infants with chronic renal failure. Arch Dis Child. 1996;74:40–3.

181. Santos F, Moreno ML, Neto A, Ariceta G, Vara J, Alonso A, Bueno A, Afonso AC, Correia AJ, Muley R, Barrios V, Gomez C, Argente J. Improvement in growth after 1 year of growth hormone therapy in well-nourished infants with growth retardation secondary to chronic renal failure: Results of a multicenter, controlled, randomized, open clinical trial. Clin J Am Soc Nephrol. 2010;5:1190–7.

182. Fine RN, Brown DF, Kuntze J, Wooster P, & Kohau7t EE (1996) Growth after discontinuation of recombinant human growth hormone therapy in children with chronic renal insufficiency. the genentech cooperative study group. J Pediatr 129: 883–891.

183. Fine RN, Ho M, Tejani A, Blethen S. Adverse events with rhGH treatment of patients with chronic renal insufficiency and end-stage renal disease. J Pediatr. 2003;142:539–45.

184. Picca S, Cappa M, Martinez C, Moges SI, Osborn J, Perfumo F, Ardissino G, Bonaudo R, Montini G, Rizzoni G. Parathyroid hormone levels in pubertal uremic adolescents treated with growth hormone. Pediatr Nephrol. 2004;19:71–6.

185. Akchurin OM, Schneider MF, Mulqueen L, Brooks ER, Langman CB, Greenbaum LA, Furth SL, Moxey-Mims M, Warady BA, Kaskel FJ,

Skversky AL. Medication adherence and growth in children with CKD. Clin J Am Soc Nephrol. 2014;9:1519–25.

186. Kovacs GT, Oh J, Kovacs J, Tonshoff B, Hunziker EB, Zapf J, Mehls O. Growth promoting effects of growth hormone and IGF-I are additive in experimental uremia. Kidney Int. 1996;49:1413–21.

187. Mauras N, Gonzalez de Pijem L, Hsiang HY, Desrosiers P, Rapaport R, Schwartz ID, Klein KO, Singh RJ, Miyamoto A, Bishop K. Anastrozole increases predicted adult height of short adolescent males treated with growth hormone: a randomized, placebo-controlled, multicenter trial for one to three years. J Clin Endocrinol Metab. 2008;93:823–31.

188. Miller BS, Ross J, Ostrow V. Height outcomes in children with growth hormone deficiency and idiopathic short stature treated concomitantly with growth hormone and aromatase inhibitor therapy: data from the ANSWER program. Int J Pediatr Endocrinol. 2020, 2020:19-z. Epub 2020 Oct 6

189. Saroufim R, Eugster EA. Non-GH agents and novel therapeutics in the management of short stature. Indian J Pediatr. 2021; https://doi.org/10.1007/s12098-021-03824-3. Online ahead of print

Neurodevelopment in Chronic Kidney Disease

57

Rebecca J. Johnson and Lyndsay A. Harshman

Introduction

Neurodevelopmental outcomes for young children with end-stage kidney disease (ESKD) historically were poor [1, 2]. As medical and surgical management of the disease have improved, cognitive and developmental outcomes have improved as well [3, 4]. However, our understanding of how the biochemical and hormonal milieu of kidney failure affects the growing brain remains incomplete. We also recognize that the treatments for kidney failure and their complications affect neurodevelopment, although the full effects may not be recognized for years.

Critical brain growth occurs *in utero* and throughout infancy [5], and it continues into young adulthood as well [6]. Early experiences and environment can affect vision, hearing, language, and responses to social cues [5, 7]. Structural maturation of specific neural pathways occurs throughout childhood and adolescence, which presumably corresponds to maturation of cognitive abilities and suggests that sensitive periods for neuronal architecture and function of discrete regions of the brain occur throughout these stages of life [8]. Thus, infancy, childhood, and adolescence are characterized by growth in cognition, memory and comprehension, and the long duration of childhood chronic kidney disease (CKD) has the potential to influence or interrupt brain development over an extended span of time.

The psychology literature is concordant with the observations of neuroscientists. Armstrong and Horn [9] presented a model of late effects that outlines how childhood chronic illness can impact neurodevelopment and neurocognitive function. They noted that most childhood chronic health conditions and their treatments affect the growth and development of children's brains. Brain structures, processes, and functions that develop prior to onset of disease are likely to be less affected, although exceptions such as toxic exposures or cerebral infarction may still have an impact. Secondly, the age of the child over the course of the disease determines the scope and severity of neurocognitive effects. Brain structures, functions, and processes that develop after the age of disease onset are likely to be most affected; thus, the younger the child is at onset of disease and treatment, the more global and severe the effects on development may be. We can synthesize this into a model for a given child who is treated for a chronic illness: the course will be an interaction between the age at diagnosis, the extent of disease

R. J. Johnson (✉)
Division of Developmental and Behavioral Health, Children's Mercy Kansas City and the University of Missouri—Kansas City School of Medicine, Kansas City, MO, USA
e-mail: rejohnson@cmh.edu

L. A. Harshman
University of Iowa Stead Family Children's Hospital, Iowa City, IA, USA

© The Author(s), under exclusive license to Springer Nature Switzerland AG 2023
F. Schaefer, L. A. Greenbaum (eds.), *Pediatric Kidney Disease*,
https://doi.org/10.1007/978-3-031-11665-0_57

and treatment intensity, whether the disease is successfully managed, the time since the treatment, and the age of the child when neurodevelopmental function is assessed [10–12].

This model of disrupted neurocognitive development is particularly relevant to childhood CKD and offers a useful paradigm for understanding the range of possible consequences on cognition [13]. CKD is a lifelong condition that differs from some insults originally envisioned by Armstrong and colleagues [11, 12]. Approximately 50% of all pediatric CKD diagnoses are due to congenital, non-glomerular anomalies [14] and *half* of all CKD patients with congenital disease will progress to kidney transplantation [15]. Some of these children will have a history of preterm birth and a complicated neonatal course with early hypoxia and mechanical ventilation, hypotension or hypertension, anemia, potential stroke, multiple surgical procedures with general anesthesia, and exposure to a wide range of drugs. Any of these exposures can adversely affect neurodevelopment.

Even children who develop kidney disease at a later stage of life may experience a prolonged course of disease with comorbidities. A large proportion of children with CKD will require chronic dialysis therapy prior to receiving a kidney transplant. While such treatment is lifesaving and more refined than decades ago, it provides far less clearance than normal kidney function and does not fully normalize the biochemical and hormonal milieu. In this chapter, we will review the effects of dialysis on brain structure and function.

Patients, families, and the nephrology team often expect a great deal from kidney transplantation, including dramatic amelioration of the metabolic abnormalities associated with advanced CKD/dialysis. Yet transplantation requires exposure to a range of drugs known to have neurologic effects, including glucocorticoids, calcineurin inhibitors, cytotoxic agents, and monoclonal/polyclonal antibodies. These effects will be discussed at greater length later in the chapter.

Children with CKD experience frequent interruptions in schooling and may have a consequent lack of engagement in their education. School absences may have a higher than anticipated impact on future educational attainment, employment, and social adjustment. In fact, the social and emotional cost of chronic disease has a substantial impact on children with CKD, draining energy from the important work of cognitive and social growth and development. This is discussed in detail in Chap. 63.

This chapter will provide readers with both a summary of literature and an in-depth analysis of current knowledge. Tables 57.1, 57.2, and 57.3 provide a comprehensive listing of publications of cognitive and developmental testing in children with CKD: assessments of children diagnosed before 24 months of age (Table 57.1), assessments of children diagnosed after 24 months of age (Table 57.2), and comparisons of different treatment groups (e.g., pre- vs. post-transplant and dialysis vs. transplant) (Table 57.3). We have highlighted selected findings from these core studies in the sections below.

Table 57.1 Assessments of children diagnosed with CKD at less than 24 months of age

Study	CKD *n*	Treatment group[a]	Age at diagnosis[b]	Mean age at assessment (range)	Skills assessed	Tests	Control group
Popel et al. [24]	15	Transplant	<24 mos.	56 mos.	IQ/Cognitive Visual-Motor Integration	WPPSI-III VMI Fifth Edition	No
Hartmann et al. [25]	15	Transplant	<2.3 yrs.	8.3 yrs.	IQ/Cognitive Neuromotor	HAWK-III Zurcher Neuromotorik	No
Johnson & Warady [22]	12	Transplant	<16 mos.	11 yrs. (no range)	IQ/Cognitive Academic Memory/ Learning Executive Functions	WISC-IV WIAT-II-A WRAML2 BRIEF	Siblings

Table 57.1 (continued)

Study	CKD n	Treatment group[a]	Age at diagnosis[b]	Mean age at assessment (range)	Skills assessed	Tests	Control group
Laakkonen et al. [19]	21	PD	<24 mos.	16 mos. and 5+ yrs.	Infant (Broad Dev.) IQ/Cognitive Memory/ Learning Sensorimotor	AIMS MFED WPPSI NEPSY VMI DMA	No
Hijazi et al. [91]	31	Mixed	<18 mos.	8.4 years (no range)	Broad Development	Chart review	No
Madden et al. [21]	16	Mixed	<12 mos.	5.8 yrs. (1.6–12.1 yrs.)	Infant (Broad Dev.) IQ/Cognitive	Griffiths MDS WISC-III	No
Shroff et al. [18]	11	Mixed	<24 mos.	0–6 yrs.	Infant (Broad Dev.)	Griffiths MDS BSID	No
Ledermann et al. [92]	16	Mixed	<12 mos.	Half ≥5 yrs., half <5 yrs.	Infant (Broad Dev.) IQ/Cognitive	Griffiths MDS WISC	No
Warady, Belden, & Kohaut [4]	28	Mixed	<3 mos.	1 yr. and 4–7 yrs.	Infant (Broad Dev.) IQ/Cognitive	MDAT BSID WISC-III SB	No
Elzouki et al. [3]	15	Mixed	<16 mos.	14 mos. to 10.4 yrs.	Infant (Screen)	DDST	No
Honda et al. [93]	15	Mixed	<24 mos.	Every 6 mos., then 5–6 yrs.	Infant (Broad Dev.) IQ/Cognitive	Enjoji Method Tanaka-Binet	No
Bock et al. [94]	15	Mixed	<6 mos.	7.1 mos. (2–16 mos.); at Time 1; repeated	Infant (Broad Dev.)	BSID	No
McGraw & Haka-Ikse [1]	10	Transplant	<1 month	13 mos. to 4.5 yrs.	Infant (Broad Dev.)	Revised Yale Developmental Schedules	No
Rotundo et al. [2]	23	Mixed	<12 mos.	0.5–14 yrs. (n = 20)	Infant (Screen) Infant (Broad Dev.) IQ/Cognitive	DDST BSID SB	No

Att. attention; *CKD* chronic kidney disease; *Dev.* DEVELOPMENT; *ESKD* end stage kidney disease; *IQ* intelligence quotient; *Mod.* moderate; *PD* peritoneal dialysis

TESTS (alphabetical by abbreviation): *AIMS* Alberta Infant Motor Scale; *BRIEF* Behavior Rating Inventory of Executive Function; *BSID* Bayley Scales of Infant Development; *DDST* Denver Developmental Screening Test; *DMA* Direct Memory Access; *Griffiths MDS* Griffiths Mental Development Scales; *HAWK-III* Hamburg-Wechsler-Intelligence Scale for Children, Third Edition; *MDAT* Modified Developmental Assessment Test; *MFED* Munich Functional Developmental Diagnostic; *NEPSY* NEPSY: A Developmental Neuropsychological Assessment; *SB* Stanford-Binet Intelligence Scales; *WIAT-II-A* Wechsler Individual Achievement Test, Second Edition Abbreviated; *WRAML2* Wide Range Assessment of Memory and Learning, Second Edition; *VMI* Beery Buktenica Test of Visual Motor Integration; *WISC (III, IV)* Wechsler Intelligence Scale for Children, Third or Fourth Edition; *WPPSI (III)* Wechsler Preschool and Primary Scale of Intelligence

[a]Mixed: participant group that includes some combination of patients on conservative therapy, undergoing dialysis, or post-transplant

[b]Age at diagnosis presented as Mean (Range) unless otherwise indicated

Table 57.2 Assessments of children diagnosed with CKD at greater than 24 months of age

Study	CKD n	Treatment group[a]	Age at diagnosis[b]	Mean age at assessment (range)	Skills assessed	Tests	Control group
Hooper et al. [32]	368	Mild to mod. CKD	8 yrs. since diagnosis	6–16 yrs.	IQ/cognitive Academic Att./ Concentration Executive functions	WASI WIAT-II-A CPT-II BRIEF	No
Falger et al. [47]	27	Transplant	7.7 yrs. (0.25–15 yrs. dialysis onset)	14.1 yrs. (6.5–17 yrs.)	IQ/cognitive Sensorimotor	WISC-III KABC Zurich NMA	No
Slickers et al. [95]	29	Mixed	4.4 (0–16 yrs.)	12.5 (7–19 yrs.)	IQ/Cognitive Memory / Learning Att./ Concentration	WASI WRAML GDS	No
Duquette et al. [33]	30	Mixed	5.1 yrs.	12. 7 yrs. (6–18 yrs.)	IQ/Cognitive Academic	WASI WIAT-II	Healthy
Gipson et al. [35]	20	Mixed	7.2 yrs.	13.4 yrs. (17.5–19 yrs.)	IQ/Cognitive Memory / Learning Att./ Concentration Sensorimotor Language Executive functions	WASI WRAML GDS RFFT COWAT Tower of London WJ-III Numbers Reversed	Healthy
Bawden et al. [30]	22	Mixed	Unknown	11.8 yrs. (no range)	IQ/Cognitive Academic Memory / Learning Att./ Concentration Sensorimotor	WISC-III WRAT-3 WRMT-R Word Attack WIAT Reading Comprehension WRAML NVSRT EOWPVT VMI Grooved Pegboard Finger-Tapping Test	Siblings
Qvist et al. [31]	33	Transplant	<5 yrs.	8 yrs. (7–12 yrs.)	IQ/Cognitive	WISC-R NEPSY	No
Groothoff et al.	126	Mixed	0–14 yrs.	29.4 yrs. (21–42 yrs.)	IQ/Cognitive	WAIS (Dutch)	Normative comparison
Crocker et al. [96]	24	Mixed	Unknown	6–16 yrs.	IQ/Cognitive Academic Memory/ Learning Sensorimotor Language	WISC-III WRAT-3 WRAML WRMT Word Attack WIAT Reading Comprehension NVSRT EOWPVT VMI Grooved Pegboard Finger-Tapping Test	No

Table 57.2 (continued)

Study	CKD n	Treatment group[a]	Age at diagnosis[b]	Mean age at assessment (range)	Skills assessed	Tests	Control group
Hulstijn-Dirkmaat et al. [17]	31	Mixed	<5 yrs.	Repeated	Infant (Broad Dev.) IQ/Cognitive	BSID McCarthy Scales of Children's Abilities	No
Fennell et al. [26–28]	56	Mixed	6.1 yrs. (no range)	13.6 yrs. (6–18 yrs.)	IQ/Cognitive Memory/ Learning Att./ Concentration Sensorimotor Visuospatial	WISC-R WAIS-R RPM VMI SRT CPT Brown-Peterson Tasks Other	Healthy

Att. Attention; *CKD* chronic kidney disease; *Dev.* development; *ESKD* end stage kidney disease; *IQ* intelligence quotient; *Mod.* moderate; *PD* peritoneal dialysis
TESTS (alphabetical by abbreviation): *BRIEF* Behavior Rating Inventory of Executive Function; *BSID* Bayley Scales of Infant Development; *COWAT* Controlled Oral Word Association Test; *CPT, CPT-II* Conners' Continuous Performance Test, First or Second Edition; *EOWPVT* Expressive One-Word Picture Vocabulary Test; *GDS* Gordon Diagnostic System; *KABC* Kaufman Assessment Battery for Children; *NEPSY* NEPSY: A Developmental Neuropsychological Assessment; *NVSRT* Nonverbal Selective Reminding Test; *RFFT* Ruff Figural Fluency Test; *RPM* Raven's Progressive Matrices; *SRT* Buschke Selective Reminding Test; *WIAT, WIAT-II, WIAT-II-A* Wechsler Individual Achievement Test, First or Second Edition, Second Edition Abbreviated; *WJ-III* Woodcock-Johnson III, Tests of Cognitive Abilities; *WRAML* Wide Range Assessment of Memory and Learning; *WRAT-3* Wide Range Achievement Test, Third Edition; *WRMT, WRMT-R* Woodcock Reading Mastery Tests, First Edition or Revised; *VMI* Beery Buktenica Test of Visual Motor Integration; *WAIS, WAIS-R* Wechsler Adult Intelligence Scale, First Edition or Revised; *WASI* Wechsler Abbreviated Scale of Intelligence; *WISC (R, III)* Wechsler Intelligence Scale for Children, Revised or Third Edition; *Zurich NMA* Zurich Neuromotor Assessment
[a]Mixed: participant group that includes some combination of patients on conservative therapy, undergoing dialysis, or post-transplant
[b]Age at diagnosis presented as Mean (Range) unless otherwise indicated

Table 57.3 Comparisons of different treatment groups

Study	CKD n	Treatment group	Age at diagnosis[a]	Mean age at assessment (range)	Skills assessed	Tests	Control group
Icard et al. [44]	26	Pre-/Post Transplant CKD vs. Transplant	Unknown	Transplant group 10.7 yrs. (5.3–17.9) and 12.8 mos. later CKD Group: 7.8 yrs. (0.2–16.2) and 10.9 mos. later	IQ/Cognitive	Mullen Scales of Early Learning WASI	Healthy
Brouhard et al. [23]	62	Dialysis vs. Transplant	n = 34 < 10 yrs.; n = 28 > 10 yrs.	13.7 yrs.	IQ/Cognitive Academic	TONI-2 WRAT	Siblings
Lawry, Brouhard, & Cunningham [97]	24	Dialysis vs. Transplant	Duration CKD 2.8–4 yrs.	14.9 yrs. dialysis; 13.7 yrs. transplant; (6–18 yrs.)	IQ/Cognitive Academic	WISC-R WAIS-R WJ-R	No

(continued)

Table 57.3 (continued)

Study	CKD n	Treatment group	Age at diagnosis[a]	Mean age at assessment (range)	Skills assessed	Tests	Control group
Mendley & Zelko [45]	9	Pre-/Post Transplant	11.7 yrs.	14.2 yrs. and 15.8 yrs.	IQ/Cognitive Memory/ Learning Att./ Concentration Sensorimotor Visuospatial	WISC-III WAIS-R PASAT CHIPASAT SRT MVDT Grooved Pegboard Trail-Making Test CAT CPT	No
Davis et al. [16]	37	Pre-/Post Transplant	<30 mos.	14 months post-transplant	Infant (Broad Dev.) IQ/Cognitive	BSID SB	No
So et al. [46]	9	Pre-/Post Transplant	<7 mos.	<12 mos. and 3–22 mos. post-tansplant	Infant (Screen) Infant (Broad Dev.)	DDST BSID	No
Rasbury et al. [98]	18	Pre-/Post Dialysis	10.6 yrs. (ESKD)	12.8 yrs.	IQ/Cognitive Memory/ Learning	CFIT Learning Task	Healthy
Fennell et al. [99]	20	Pre-/Post Transplant	Unknown	11.7 yrs. and 1 mo. and 1 yr. post-transplant	IQ/Cognitive Academic Memory/ Learning Att./ Concentration Executive Functions	WISC PIAT HRCT Auditory Vigilance Task Free Recall Task	Healthy
Rasbury et al. [100]	14	Pre-/Post Transplant	Unknown	11.2 yrs. (no range) and 6 mos. post-transplant	IQ/Cognitive Academic Memory/ Learning Att./ Concentration	WISC-R PIAT CPT HRCT Auditory Vigilance Task Free Recall Task	Healthy

Att. Attention; *CKD* chronic kidney disease; *Dev.* development; *ESKD* end stage kidney disease; *IQ* intelligence quotient; *Mod.* moderate; *PD* peritoneal dialysis

TESTS (alphabetical by abbreviation): *BSID* Bayley Scales of Infant Development; *CAT* Cognitive Abilities Test; *CFIT* Culture Fair Intelligence Test; *CHIPASAT* Children's Paced Auditory Serial Addition Test; *CPT* Conners' Continuous Performance Test; *DDST* Denver Developmental Screening Test; *HRCT* Halstead-Reitan Category Test; *MVDT* Meier Visual Discrimination Test; *PASAT* Paced Auditory Serial Addition Test; *PIAT* Peabody Individual Achievement Test; *SB* Stanford-Binet Intelligence Scales; *SRT* Buschke Selective Reminding Test; *TONI-2* Test of Nonverbal Intelligence, Second Edition; *WJ-R* Woodcock-Johnson Revised, Tests of Achievement; *WRAT* Wide Range Achievement Test; *WAIS-R* Wechsler Adult Intelligence Scale, Revised; *WASI* Wechsler Abbreviated Scale of Intelligence; *WISC (R, III)* Wechsler Intelligence Scale for Children, Revised or Third Edition

[a]Age at diagnosis presented as mean (range) unless otherwise indicated

Early Development

Several studies have described developmental outcomes for children who were diagnosed with CKD during infancy. These studies have either assessed children shortly after their diagnosis or have reported developmental progress during the period of early childhood using broad measures (cognitive, motor, language) such as the Bayley Scales of Infant Development (BSID) or the Griffiths Mental Development Scale. Davis et al. [16] assessed 37 children younger than 30 months of age who were undergoing kidney transplant, and again an average of 14 months post-transplant, utilizing either the BSID or the Stanford-Binet Intelligence Scales (SB), depending on the child's age. Prior to transplant, most patients had significantly delayed psychomotor development and 18 patients had mental development scores classified as delayed. Post-transplant psychomotor performance improved, with the group mean reaching the low average range, and many of the patients with cognitive delay (12 of 18) improving their scores to the average range. Persistently abnormal cognitive function was associated with the earliest onset of kidney failure. In a similar study, 28 patients diagnosed with ESKD before three months of age [4] were assessed at a mean age of 5.9 years (the majority post-transplant), using a range of instruments, including the Modified Developmental Assessment Test (MDAT) and the Wechsler Intelligence Scale for Children, Third edition, (WISC-III) as well as the BSID and SB. Overall, 22 of the 28 children (79%) had general mental development that placed within the broad range of average.

Hulstijn-Dirkmaat et al. [17] prospectively evaluated 31 young children (mean age of 2.5 years) with a broad range of CKD, using the BSID and the McCarthy Scales of Children's Abilities. In this sample, 32% of patients had comorbid conditions or disease (cerebral complications or unexplained neurological impairment, visual/hearing disorder, congenital heart disease); children with comorbid conditions were evenly distributed between dialysis and non-dialysis groups. Overall, the patients had significantly delayed cognitive development, with a mean developmental index of 78.5 (SD 19.5), and a distribution of scores skewed below that of the normal population. Children _without_ comorbidities who did not yet require dialysis had a group mean in the average range, compared to those on dialysis, whose group mean placed in the borderline range for cognitive functioning. Among children _with_ comorbidities, those with CKD who did not yet require dialysis scored in the borderline range for cognitive development, while those on dialysis had a mean score in the impaired range. Thus, comorbid disease and more advanced CKD (i.e., need for dialysis) were independently associated with lower neurodevelopmental scores.

Other studies have found the developmental outcomes of very young children with CKD to be linked to comorbid medical conditions or risk factors. Shroff et al. [18] evaluated a group of 11 children who began kidney replacement therapy between 0 and 24 months of age; six achieved age-appropriate developmental milestones. The remaining five had significant special education needs, with developmental outcomes linked to medical co-morbidities including VACTERL association (e.g., vertebral defects, anal atresia, Cardiac defects, tracheoesophageal fistula, renal anomalies, and limb abnormalities), infantile hemiplegia, deafness, congenital hypothyroidism, transposition of the great vessels, and an undiagnosed syndrome that included dysmorphism, developmental delay, and non-functioning kidneys. Laakkonen et al. [19] examined neurodevelopmental outcomes for 21 patients who began kidney replacement therapy with peritoneal dialysis (PD) before 24 months of age and were at least 5 years of age. A comprehensive battery of tests was used (see Table 57.1) which targeted development, cognition, sensory and motor function, memory and learning. Six of these patients were considered to have normal neurodevelopment; the remaining 15 had some degree of neurodevelopmental impairment, ranging from minor (n = 9) to major (n = 6). Those with major impairment all had documented pre-dialysis risk factors (e.g., perinatal asphyxia, severe hypotension, alcohol exposure, severe neonatal respiratory distress).

In contrast to studies that have evaluated young children with more advanced stages of CKD, Hooper et al. [20] reported on preschool children with mild to moderate CKD. Measures of developmental level/IQ were administered to 124 children 12–68 months who had a mean estimate glomerular filtration rate (eGFR) of 50 ml/min per 1.73 m². While all mean scores placed in the average range in this group with mild disease, the authors noted that an unexpectedly high percentage (27%) had developmental/IQ scores that placed in the at-risk range, defined as scores more than 1 SD below the mean of a normal distribution.

To summarize, children diagnosed with CKD in infancy are at risk for delayed neurodevelopment; the magnitude of the delay is influenced by medical and neurological comorbidities, as well as the age of onset and severity of disease. There is some evidence that transplant early in life benefits neurodevelopmental catch-up.

Intellectual Function (IQ)

ESKD Onset in Infancy and Early Childhood

Many studies in pediatric CKD have specifically examined intellectual function (IQ). The most used measure to assess IQ is the Wechsler Intelligence Scale for Children (WISC); its most current version is the Fifth Edition (WISC-V). The WISC includes a Full-Scale IQ (FSIQ) and five index scores: Verbal Comprehension (VCI), Visual Spatial (VSI), Fluid Reasoning (FRI), Processing Speed (PSI), and Working Memory (WMI).

A few studies have looked at long-term intellectual functioning of children diagnosed with ESKD as infants or early in life. The previously noted study by Warady et al. [4] assessed IQ in 28 patients who were diagnosed with ESKD before 3 months of age. Using the WISC-III, they showed a divergence in verbal (acquired knowledge and verbal reasoning) and nonverbal (ability to understand and manipulate nonverbal stimuli such as colors, patterns, and shapes) performance at a mean age of 5.9 years: 72% of the children had average verbal scores, whereas only 56% reached average nonverbal scores. In a similar study, Madden et al. [21] assessed the IQ of 16 patients with ESKD who initiated dialysis during the first year of life. These subjects were also studied at a mean age of 5.8 years. The IQ range for the sample was 50–102 with an average IQ of 87 for the ESKD group (approximately 1 standard deviation below the mean). Ten children had IQ scores within one standard deviation of the mean. This average and distribution of scores were clearly abnormal (i.e., average IQ = 100) with a distribution that skewed lower.

Johnson and Warady [22] built on the above studies by adding a sibling control group. They assessed late neurocognitive outcomes for 12 patients diagnosed with ESKD as infants (mean age at testing: 10 years). All but one had functioning transplants, and for those with transplants mean eGFR was consistent with mild to moderate CKD. Mean WISC-IV index scores ranged from 80 to 82 (borderline to low average) and the mean FSIQ score was 76.8. The distribution of FSIQ scores ranged from 55–102 and are strikingly similar to those reported by Madden et al. [21] noted above. Nine of the patients were compared to their healthy siblings and these participants had FSIQ, Processing Speed Index (PSI), and Working Memory Index scores significantly lower than siblings. For example, only one-third of patients had an FSIQ in the average range or above, in contrast to 6 of 9 siblings. For the patient group, higher FSIQ and the VCI were associated with older age at start of dialysis; higher FSIQ and the PSI were associated with fewer months on dialysis, and higher PSI was associated with younger age at transplant. The Test of Nonverbal Intelligence (TONI-2), a test of intellectual functioning that does not require verbal responses, was utilized in another study of 62 children with CKD that included sibling controls [23]. While these subjects were diagnosed later in life, the pattern of intellectual functioning was very similar: patients' mean percentile ranks for nonverbal intelligence ranged from the 27th to the 35th percentile, regardless of whether they were on dialysis or post-transplant, while siblings' mean percentile ranks ranged from the 32nd to the 56th percentile.

Popel et al. [24] found similar results using data from a longitudinal, prospective study to evaluate predictors of developmental outcomes for children who received a transplant before the age of 5 years. These patients started dialysis in the first 2 years of life (73% initiating dialysis in the first year of life), with a mean age of 30 months at transplant. At a mean age of 56 months (all post-transplant), mean scores on FSIQ, visual-motor integration, and adaptive skills were approximately one SD below the population normative mean. Hartmann et al. [25] assessed the neurocognitive and neuromotor outcomes of 15 patients with severe congenital CKD who received a kidney transplant at a mean age of 2.8 years and were evaluated a mean age of 8.3 years. Six of these patients received a pre-emptive kidney transplant and the other nine underwent dialysis for a mean of 11 months (±8.6 months). Neuromotor function was assessed as abnormal for eight patients. Performance IQ (PIQ) was lower (m = 89) than the normative mean of 100, and lower PIQ was associated with abnormal neuromotor function. Time on dialysis was inversely correlated with verbal IQ. Pre-emptive kidney transplant and duration of dialysis less than 3 months were protective; participants meeting these criteria demonstrated better neurocognitive outcomes.

Existing data indicate that children diagnosed with ESKD as infants or very early in childhood achieve intellectual outcomes which vary depending on comorbidities. Many achieve normal or near normal intellectual function, but with a distribution that is skewed below normal. Patients tend to perform less well than their unaffected siblings. Younger age at transplant and shorter duration of dialysis appear to benefit neurocognitive outcomes. These are impressive outcomes given the complexity of ESKD with onset in infancy, yet they indicate a substantial risk for learning impairment and academic difficulties.

Mixed Age Groups Including Mild to Moderate CKD

Children with onset of ESKD before school-age and those with mild-to-moderate CKD demonstrate IQ impairment that is similarly skewed below the population mean, although the effect is less striking than those diagnosed with ESKD as infants or in early childhood, and more children perform in the average to above average range. Fennell et al. [26–28] published some of the earliest data regarding associations between standardized neuropsychological tests and CKD. Compared to a healthy control group matched for age, sex, and ethnicity, a group of children with a range of eGFR, from moderate CKD to post-transplant, performed more poorly on selected indices of non-verbal IQ (Wechsler subtests Similarities, Digits Forward, and Digits Backward).

Gipson et al. [29] studied children and adolescents with advanced CKD (a mix of dialysis-dependent patients and patients being treated conservatively) and included a comparison group of healthy children. This sample of 20 children with CKD had an average age at diagnosis of 7 years and an age range of 7.5–19 years at the time of assessment. Patients with CKD scored significantly lower than the healthy controls on a measure of intelligence (Wechsler Abbreviated Scale of Intelligence [WASI] Full Scale IQ).

Using a sibling control group, Bawden et al. [30] evaluated 22 patients who were listed for transplant and either receiving dialysis or approaching dialysis. Intelligence was assessed via the WISC-III. Those with CKD/ESKD had a group mean score that was average to low average. Overall, the group scored significantly lower than the sibling group on measures of VIQ, PIQ, and FSIQ.

Qvist et al. [31] assessed children diagnosed in early childhood with ESKD secondary to congenital nephrotic syndrome. At a mean age of 8 years, this group had an average IQ of 87 (low average range) on the WISC-Revised, and 6–24% of patients were characterized as impaired based on the results of neuropsychological tests (NEPSY).

Hooper et al. [32] used a cross-sectional analysis of the Chronic Kidney Disease in Children (CKiD) study to describe cognitive function in 368 school-age children with mild to moderate CKD. While the group had mean IQ scores in the average range, the number of subjects whose scores placed one or more SDs below the mean on a measure of nonverbal ability (WASI block design) was more than twice that of the normative group. Several risk factors for low scores were identified in this study, including proteinuria, low birth weight (LBW), and history of seizures.

Duquette et al. [33] examined 30 patients (mean age = 12.7 years) with childhood-onset CKD, half on dialysis and half with pre-dialysis CKD, and compared them to a healthy control group. The two groups differed significantly on some key variables: the control group had higher maternal education and a larger proportion of children who identified as Caucasian. Nonetheless, after controlling for maternal education and race, the control group scored significantly higher on measures of VIQ, PIQ, and FSIQ than patients with CKD. Fifty-seven percent of the CKD group had FSIQ scores below the 25th percentile, compared to only 15% of the control group. Kidney function (eGFR) was a significant predictor of intellectual functioning, while age of CKD onset and duration of CKD were not associated with IQ in this study.

Groothoff et al. [34] obtained estimates of cognitive functioning in a group of 126 adults (mean age = 29.4 years) who began kidney replacement therapy between the ages of 1.9 and 14.9 years. The majority had a functioning transplant; 16 and 12 were on hemodialysis (HD) and PD, respectively. Groups mean scores for Verbal, Performance, and FSIQ placed in the average range. Compared to a matched control group, however, IQ scores and educational attainment were significantly lower for the CKD group.

Executive Function

Executive functioning (EF) is a term used in the field of psychology that refers to the management of complex cognitive processes, including planning, organization, problem solving, working memory, and attention. These skills are required for optimal performance on tests of intellectual functioning (IQ), but are assessed more directly with EF-specific cognitive tasks. A number of researchers have examined attention and memory abilities in children with CKD, believing these abilities may be particularly susceptible to effects of the disease. The early work of Fennell et al. [26–28] sought to examine the relationship between EF and CKD. Their subjects, a group of children receiving a range of kidney replacement therapies (HD, PD, transplant), scored worse than healthy controls on a variety of measures of EF (e.g., working memory, attention). The NEPSY was administered by Qvist et al. [31] to children with congenital nephrotic syndrome to assess attention, concentration, and memory skills. Results indicated that impairment was more frequent in children with a history of major central nervous system (CNS) infarcts, hemiplegia, and/or those with a seizure disorder or an abnormal EEG.

Gipson et al. [35] included measures of memory and executive function in their study of children and adolescents with CKD and compared them to healthy controls. Patients scored significantly lower on all of the memory indices and on the "initiation" and "sustaining" EF domains, which assess task initiation and ability to sustain attention. Memory and EF findings persisted even after the authors controlled for IQ and age. Of note, the severity of memory deficits was positively related to the age at onset of CKD.

In Johnson and Warady's (2013) long-term follow-up of patients who had been diagnosed with ESKD as infants, EF findings were similar to those for IQ: better verbal ability and memory were associated with older age at start of dialysis and fewer months on dialysis, and younger age at transplant was associated with higher overall memory scores. Shorter time on dialysis and younger age at transplant were also associated with better scores on the Metacognitive Index of the parent-report BRIEF. When compared to their healthy siblings, the patients scored significantly worse on the Wide Range Assessment of Memory and Learning, Second Edition Verbal Memory Index (but not the Visual Memory

Index), the BRIEF Metacognition Index, and the BRIEF Global Executive Composite score.

The CKiD study is the largest study to examine EF, but unlike many of the other studies discussed, included only children with mild to moderate CKD and without history of kidney transplant [32]. Mean scores were in the average range for a variety of attention-related measures (Conners' Continuous Performance Test, Second Edition) and parent ratings of executive functioning (BRIEF). However, on several of the BRIEF measures (Metacognition Index, Working Memory and Planning subscales, and the Global Executive Composite score) a larger than expected proportion of patients scored one or more SD below the mean ("at risk" for lower EF). If we consider these results broadly, 33–40% of children with early-stage CKD would be considered at risk for some impairment in EF. CKD-associated risk factors including low birth weight, proteinuria, hypertension, and history of seizures were associated with slightly worse scores on several measures. Conversely, higher eGFR appeared protective, as it was associated with a lesser chance of scoring in the "at risk" range. Older subjects had slightly worse scores, suggesting that EF growth was diverging from their peers. It is important to emphasize that overall mean scores were average and group findings were statistically, but not necessarily clinically, significant. In another study of CKiD participants, Johnson et al. [36]examined parent ratings of attention problems using the Behavior Assessment System for Children, Second Edition (BASC-2) Parent Rating Scales. Parents rated 28% of the sample as at risk for attention problems. Persistent hypertension and unresolved proteinuria predicted rating of attention problems. Taken together, these findings suggest that even mild to moderate CKD is associated with increased risk for sub-optimal neurocognitive functioning, which may be relevant for some patients. The CKiD study also collected parent ratings of attention and executive functioning for preschool participants with mild to moderate CKD. Thirty percent of the participants had parent ratings that placed in the "at-risk" range (ratings higher than 1 SD above the mean [worse]) for overall executive functioning [20].

Executive functioning was examined by the Neurocognitive Assessment and Magnetic Resonance Imaging Analysis of Children and Young Adults with Chronic Kidney Disease (NiCK) Study, a cross-sectional study of youth with CKD stages 2–5 [37]. This study compared 90 participants with CKD to 70 controls. Those with CKD scored significantly worse than controls in several areas of executive functioning, including attention, memory, and inhibitory control. In addition, performance was associated with eGFR: participants with CKD exhibited lower performance on tests of executive functioning as eGFR declined. Using ambulatory blood pressure monitoring, the authors also found that blood pressure abnormalities, including increased diastolic load and decreased diastolic dipping, were associated with neurocognitive impairment.

Lande et al. [38] also found an association between blood pressure variability (BPV) and executive functioning. They assessed 650 children 6+ years old with mild to moderate CKD enrolled in the CKiD study and had a mean follow-up period of 4 years. Children with systolic visit-to-visit BPV in the upper tertile obtained lower scores on a measure of executive functioning (D-KEFS Category Switching) than those with BPV in the lower tertile. This association remained significant in multivariate analyses that controlled for mean BP, demographic characteristics, and CKD-related variables.

Academic Achievement and Educational/Vocational Outcomes

There are limited data to describe academic achievement outcomes for children with mild to moderate pediatric CKD. An initial evaluation of academic achievement data collected as part of the Chronic Kidney Disease in Children (CKiD) multicenter prospective cohort study [39] suggested that general academic achievement scores were skewed toward the lower end of the normal range in CKD. The group's mean performance on the Wechsler Individual Achievement Test, Second Edition, Abbreviated (WIAT-II-A) was in the average range, but across all academic domains more patients were "at risk" (scoring one or more SDs below the normative mean for age) than would be expected given a normal distribution. One third of subjects scored "at risk" on the WIAT-II-A Numerical Operations subtest, which is more than twice the expected rate. CKD-related characteristics including eGFR, proteinuria, hypertension, and anemia were not associated with low achievement. Among children evaluated in the CKiD cohort, ADD/ADHD was self-reported for 9% of the sample; however, this was not significantly associated with risk for academic underachievement. Children displaying lower total achievement scores had significantly more school absence (5.5 days versus 3 days). Use of an IEP or 504 plan was reported by 29% of the CKiD sample and children with lower total achievement scores had a higher rate of IEP or 504 plan usage (51% versus 17%).

When we consider the study by Duquette et al. [33], which compared 30 patients with CKD or ESKD to a group of 41 age and gender-matched healthy controls, we must keep in mind differences in key variables: the control group had higher maternal education and a larger proportion of children who identified as Caucasian. In addition, the CKD participants had more previous grade retentions, use of specialized educational plans, and more school absences. Allowing for these caveats, the patients scored significantly lower than the controls on the WIAT-II Word Reading and Math Reasoning domains. Higher eGFR was positively correlated with all academic scores, suggesting that less advanced disease causes fewer adverse educational consequences. The authors also examined whether children in either group met criteria for a learning disorder, using three different formulas: an ability-achievement discrepancy formula, which requires an academic standard score to be at least 15 points lower than FSIQ; a regression formula, which statistically adapts the discrepancy formula using achievement scores predicted by FSIQ; and a low achievement formula, which defines learning disability as a standard score below the 25th percentile for age. The two groups differed significantly only when the low achieve-

ment formula was used. Using this approach, 43%, 37%, and 40% of the CKD group met criteria for a learning disorder in reading, math, and spelling, respectively, compared to 7%, 2%, and 5% of the control group. Thus, for children with CKD, for whom the disease process may depress both cognitive performance and academic achievement, discrepancy formulas (which require a significant discrepancy between cognitive and achievement scores) may be of limited use. The authors also noted that children with CKD had a 40% rate of grade retention, compared to 2.4% of the control group, suggesting that current educational services are not meeting the needs of these patients.

Brouhard et al. [23] compared 62 dialysis and transplant patients (average age 13.7 years, roughly half with disease onset prior to 10 years) to a healthy sibling control group, using the Wide Range Achievement Test (WRAT), a brief measure of academic achievement that assesses three areas: spelling, arithmetic, and reading. There were no significant differences between the dialysis and transplant groups. When compared to siblings, the combined patient group scored significantly lower across all domains, with sibling mean scores placing in the average range and patient mean scores placing in the low average range. Using available data for approximately half the study sample, 85% percent of sibling participants were in regular education classes full-time while only 64% of patients were in a regular setting. Over half (56%) of the patients had missed 21 or more days of school in the last semester, compared to only one sibling (4%). The percentage of a patient's life with ESKD was negatively correlated with the WRAT Arithmetic score.

Early onset of disease, type of disease (e.g., congenital nephrotic syndrome), and associated comorbidities confer risk to academic achievement. Studies have historically varied in terms of whether those with significant CNS risk factors are included in analyses. When Johnson and Warady [22] compared the performance of nine children diagnosed with ESKD in infancy to that of their healthy siblings, patients with major neurological risk factors, including stroke or asphyxia, Galloway Mowat syndrome, and Joubert syndrome, were excluded. Healthy siblings outperformed patients across all domains of the WIAT-II-A, including Word Reading, Spelling, and Numerical Operations, as well as the Total Achievement score. Mean scores for siblings placed in the average range; in contrast, all patient mean scores placed in the low average range. Based on parent report, only one of the siblings had ever been diagnosed with a learning or attention disorder, while three patients (33%) had been diagnosed with a learning disorder, and one with an attention disorder (11%). In another study that excluded patients with syndromes known to influence neuropsychological functioning, and that also included a sibling control group [30], 22 patient-sibling pairs participated in academic assessment and no significant differences were found on measures of achievement. These patients ranged in age from 6 to 16 years, were on a transplant waiting list, and were approaching or receiving dialysis. The average age of onset of ESKD was not reported. These results are more consistent with those from the CKiD study and suggest better academic achievement outcomes for children diagnosed later in childhood compared to those diagnosed in infancy.

In a more severely affected cohort, Qvist et al. [31] examined educational outcomes for children diagnosed with ESKD early in life. In this sample, a large proportion (88%) of children had a diagnosis of congenital nephrotic syndrome (severe Finnish type), many with comorbid events in early infancy including history of stroke. Thirty-three children who underwent transplant before 5 years of age were followed prospectively. The authors reported outcomes an average of 6 years post-transplant, when the patients were 7–12 years of age. Twenty-six patients (79%) attended a regular school, although six of these children required remedial education services. The remaining seven children attended a specialized school, two of them to accommodate hearing impairment rather than intellectual impairment. Risk factors for requiring a specialized educational setting included: longer time on dialysis, more hypertensive crises (the majority of which occurred during dialysis),

more seizures (which occurred for some patients during dialysis and for others post-transplant), and major infarcts/hemiplegia. While major cerebral infarcts were more common in those requiring special education (3/7), watershed infarcts and abnormal EEGs were also seen among those in remedial and regular classes.

A small number of studies have examined much longer-term educational and vocational outcomes for patients who had ESKD as children. Having ESKD as a child appears to be associated with lower educational attainment, lower socioeconomic class, and higher rates of unemployment [34, 40], although at least one study reported more positive outcomes [40]. Offner et al. [41] described 124 adults with a mean age of 25 years who had received a kidney transplant between 1970 and 1993, when they were a mean age of 12.1 years. Mean eGFR had declined over the years, from 76 to 45 ml/min/1.73 m^2, and 80% of the sample had maintained or developed hypertension. Education and employment levels were roughly the same as the general German population at that time (9% unemployed in general population, versus 14% in the sample), although 45% lived with their parents. In contrast, a large study of 126 Dutch adults by Groothoff et al. [34] reported that only 42.2% of patients completed intermediate or advanced vocational training compared to 72.2% of the general population. Reynolds et al. [40] examined long-term outcomes for patients who underwent dialysis or transplant during adolescence (at a mean age of 14.4 years) and found that (1) the social distribution of kidney patients was lower than that of a healthy comparison group; (2) kidney patients had lower educational achievement; (3) significantly fewer were employed full-time, although two-thirds were employed in some capacity; and (4) that more kidney patients were receiving social security benefits compared to the control group (42% vs. 15%). Seventy-one percent of patients in this study reported that their disease and its treatment had significantly affected their education. The authors reported that onset of illness before 11 years of age and current self-reported low energy were associated with unemployment.

Qualitative research exploring educational and vocational outcomes have produced similar themes. Kerklaan et al. [42] interviewed 30 young adults 18–35 years of age who were diagnosed with CKD during childhood. These participants described long-term impact of school absences and reduced participation in social activities, including social anxiety, feelings of inferiority, and falling behind peers with activities and accomplishments. Longer duration of dialysis during childhood seemed to be related to more negative impact on friendships and participation in recreational activities. Participants described limitations to school, work, and social/leisure activities secondary to treatment burden; challenges with independence (e.g., moving out of parents' home); and difficulty forming adult relationships. Some described reorienting their plans and goals, being inspired to pursue certain professions (e.g., nursing, counseling), and unique, positive opportunities that arose secondary to the diagnosis of CKD.

The available data examining academic and vocational outcomes are consistent with what we know about the impact of CKD on cognitive and intellectual functioning. Children with CKD are at risk for lower academic achievement and poorer educational and vocational outcomes. The age of onset of CKD, disease severity, and comorbid conditions all influence the degree to which academic achievement is affected. The available evidence suggests that the academic achievement of children with CKD will be significantly below that of their siblings if kidney replacement therapy is required early in life. It is important to consider that in addition to the medical effects of CKD (such as uremia, acidosis, hypertension, and fatigue), children with CKD miss more academic instruction, and often have less time and energy to complete homework. The emotional and financial strain of kidney replacement therapy, as well as the time commitment, may also result in fewer opportunities for enrichment activities (music lessons, field trips) all of which also may impact a child's learning and achievement.

Pediatric nephrologists and allied health professionals have an opportunity to reduce the impact of CKD on academic achievement, particularly for children receiving chronic outpatient dialysis. This might include provision of school services in the dialysis unit, adjusting dialysis schedules to accommodate the school day, and working with families and schools to develop individualized education or remediation plans. Children who are struggling academically should be referred early for cognitive and psychoeducational evaluation.

Cognitive Outcomes and Kidney Transplantation

Kidney transplantation is a central goal in the management of children with advanced CKD, promising improved survival and quality of life. A substantial body of literature indicates that both cognitive performance and academic achievement are improved among children with kidney transplant when compared to those receiving dialysis. The available literature indicates that, in general, children with kidney transplant have improved performance on a range of tests of cognitive abilities and achievement post-transplant, although not full normalization. This is supported by more recent meta-analytic data from over thirty pediatric studies demonstrating that, in general, children with kidney transplant have intelligence equivalent to children with mild/moderate CKD and significantly better intelligence assessment than children receiving dialysis [43].

Icard et al. [44] reported results for six patients with advanced CKD who received a transplant. Compared to a control group of children with CKD being treated conservatively, children who received a transplant demonstrated a meaningful increase in their intellectual and developmental functioning. In fact, children receiving a transplant had, on average, a 12-point increase in their standard intelligence scores from pre- to post-transplant. Mendley and Zelko [45] obtained baseline intellectual assessment (WISC-III or WAIS-R) and performed within-subject comparisons of nine patients just prior to and 1 year after kidney transplant, using a wide range of neuropsychological tests. At baseline, intelligence scores placed within the broad range of average, although skewed slightly lower than a normal distribution. All were attending regular education classes full-time with excellent attendance. After transplant, there was significant improvement in specific aspects of neurocognitive performance. Mental processing speed and decision-making speed (as assessed by the computerized Cognitive Abilities Test) improved from pre- to post transplant and subjects showed more consistent performance after transplant. Sustained attention (assessed by the Connors' Continuous Performance Test Signal Detection Index) and working memory (assessed by the Paced Auditory Serial Addition Test) also improved after transplant.

A study of an early cohort of infants (diagnosed and treated between 1978 and 1985) demonstrated how successful kidney transplantation has the potential to ameliorate developmental deficits [46]. All nine children had significant improvement in head circumference Z-score after transplant even as linear growth lagged. Performance on developmental assessment improved in most infants, with post-transplant Bayley cognitive and motor development scores placing within the broad range of average for most children. Seizures noted while children were on dialysis were not present after transplant.

Falger et al. [47] evaluated the intellectual functioning of 27 patients who had transplants in childhood (mean age at transplant was 9 years); evaluations took place an average of 6 years post-transplant (average age at assessment was 14 years). Median FSIQ was 97, but the range was wide (49–133). Five patients had neurological comorbidities, and their mean FSIQ score was 81, with a range of 49–101 (encompassing severe impairment to normal function). Twenty-one subjects had an FSIQ score > 85, and two were in the high average range (>115). The VIQ was significantly higher than the PIQ, which was significantly lower than a control population. The patients also scored significantly lower than a control group on 5 of 11 WISC-III subtests, even when excluding subjects with neurologic morbidity.

The assessment of long-term intellectual and metacognitive functioning and academic achievement for a group of 12 children transplanted in early life is described previously in this chapter [22]. Performance on some indices was related to younger age at transplant and fewer months on dialysis; however, post-transplant evaluation showed persistence of IQ and achievement gaps when a subgroup of patients was compared to their unaffected siblings. Molnar-Varga et al. [48] also examined how age and duration of dialysis impact later cognitive functioning. They compared 35 kidney transplant recipients who were a median of 28 months post-transplant to 35 healthy controls on a measure of intelligence (Woodcock-Johnson International Edition). The mean FSIQ score placed in the broad range of average, but greater than 1 SD lower than control participants (mean score 85 versus 107). Earlier age at onset of dialysis and longer time on dialysis were associated with lower scores in the transplant group, as was cumulative days hospitalized (standardized for age).

We must also consider how the introduction of a range of new medications at the time of transplantation has the potential to affect the CNS. While high dose glucocorticoid therapy is almost always of short duration, many children continue to receive lower dose glucocorticoids for years or even decades. The hippocampus has high concentrations of glucocorticoid receptors and neurochemical and electrophysiologic changes occur in the presence of these hormones [49]. Prolonged supraphysiologic exposure can accelerate neuronal loss in the hippocampus and increase the severity of other neurologic insults. Cellular toxicity, dendritic atrophy, and damage to hippocampal structure have been shown in a primate model of chronic exposure [50]. The effects of low doses over longer duration are unknown [51].

Calcineurin inhibitors are a mainstay of lifelong immunosuppression, but our knowledge of the neurocognitive effects of chronic use of this class of medications in children is limited. Acute neurotoxicity has been described in a subset of patients and can include headache, tremor, insomnia, paresthesia, mental status changes, visual and auditory hallucinations, cortical blindness, seizures and memory loss [52, 53]. These side effects are more often observed in patients undergoing bone marrow or liver transplant, likely because of the greater intensity of immunosuppression required. In a study of 14 pediatric kidney recipients receiving calcineurin inhibitors, 86% reported myalgias, tremor, fatigue and headache, and half of the group had symptoms most of the time [54]. Acute, reversible encephalopathy with MRI findings was reported in two children, ages 7 and 17 years, after kidney transplant who were treated with tacrolimus at levels of 10–11 ng/ml [55]. Both subjects recovered completely and tolerated lower tacrolimus levels of 6–7 ng/ml.

Many potential mechanisms have been proposed to explain calcineurin inhibitor neurotoxicity, and these hypotheses are relevant to our concerns regarding brain development in young children with CKD. Calcineurin represents >1% of total brain protein, and intracellular binding proteins for cyclosporine and tacrolimus are found throughout the CNS. Both drugs may interfere with the activity of excitatory (N-methyl-D-aspartic acid [NMDA]) and inhibitory (γ-aminobutyric acid [GABA]) amino acid receptors through calcineurin, which may impact memory formation [52]. Intra-cranial injection of cyclosporine to day-old chicks disrupts memory formation [56]. Further, cyclosporine is toxic to glial cells in culture in a manner that appears to correlate with the white matter changes which are seen by CT and MRI in affected transplant recipients [52]. Cyclosporine has also been shown to induce apoptosis of oligodendrocytes and neurons in culture [57]. It is only possible to speculate to what degree these observed changes affect the normal dendritic pruning, myelination, and formation of complex connections which characterize infant and early childhood brain development.

Clinical observations suggest that sirolimus may not have independent neurologic toxicity [58]. However, it appeared to enhance the toxic effects of cyclosporine on brain mitochondrial glucose metabolism in a rat model [59]. In contrast, mycophenolate mofetil is not thought to have a neurotoxic profile.

Genetics of Neurodevelopment and Kidney Development

While only a fraction of adult CKD is caused by genetic disorders, genetic forms of kidney disease are common in pediatric CKD, representing approximately 40% of all cases. Single gene mutations explain an array of kidney diseases [60], yet there can be no doubt that there is much more to learn about genetic etiologies. A few genetic disorders are known to be associated with both CKD and mental retardation, but the full spectrum of neurodevelopmental abnormalities associated with genetic CKD has not been clearly defined. Causative genes have been identified in approximately half of kidney diseases with classic Mendelian inheritance [60], but we recognize other organ systems are affected in addition to the kidneys and urinary tract.

We now know that copy number variants (CNVs) are common in the human genome and can be identified and analyzed using array-based technologies [61]. Certain rare CNVs appear etiologic in developmental disorders, including schizophrenia, attention deficit disorder, developmental delay, behavior abnormalities and learning disability [62–64]. In a study of 522 patients with congenital kidney malformations, including kidney aplasia, agenesis, hypoplasia and dysplasia, rare CNVs were more likely in cases than controls, and large CNVs and gene-disrupting events were strikingly more frequent [65]. Among the genomic disorders associated with kidney developmental disturbance were those previously recognized to be associated with neuropsychiatric traits (e.g., DiGeorge, Wolf-Hirschhorn, Kallman, Potocki-Lupinski syndromes). Further, there were novel CNVs spanning genes having murine orthologs associated with kidney and neurodevelopmental defects.

These findings may change our understanding of the relationship between developmental and neurocognitive abnormalities and childhood CKD. Rather than attributing neurodevelopmental delay exclusively to uremic metabolic disturbance, we must consider that defects in pleiotropic genes involved in the morphology of brain and kidney may play a causative role in neurodevelopmental delays.

Neuroimaging

Neuroimaging provides a noninvasive opportunity to examine brain structure and function. Given the observed neurocognitive findings in the pediatric CKD population, research has more recently moved to defining the neural mechanisms for cognitive dysfunction. Neuroimaging studies in children with CKD and ESKD are few and are limited by broadly defined inclusion criteria including age at the time of evaluation, age at diagnosis, type of therapy, and underlying disease. In seeking a deeper understanding of the documented cognitive deficits in CKD, it is critical to ask: (1) is there a structural or functional brain basis for the observed neurocognitive deficits in this population; and (2) are there specific regions of the brain that are most associated with these deficits?

Imaging data can largely be reviewed by modality: computerized tomography (CT), structural magnetic resonance imaging (sMRI), and functional magnetic resonance imaging (fMRI). Twenty neuroimaging studies that include pediatric CKD patients have been published in the literature between 1977 and the present. Of these studies, 13 utilized CT-based neuroimaging and 7 utilized MRI. Most early studies on the topic of neuroimaging in pediatric CKD used CT. Within the more modern pediatric MRI subset, six have evaluated structural MRI and only one has examined brain function through use of regional cerebral blood flow. Study populations in the published literature vary widely in sample size, age, and primary disease etiology.

Contemporary neuroimaging data available from CT are available from 1997 to 2006. Nine of the thirteen published studies in the pediatric CKD literature using CT as a neuroimaging modality were case-control or prospective in nature. CT-based studies focused on pediatric populations with ESKD or post-transplantation without inclusion of less severe disease CKD phenotypes. In general, CT data from these studies demonstrate higher risk for global cerebral atrophy, silent white matter infarcts, and ventriculomegaly [3, 66, 67]. Cerebral atrophy is well-described in pediatric nephrology literature dating prior to 1990, with reports of up to 60% of patients having atrophy that was not associated with type of renal disease, hypertension severity, or corticosteroid therapy [68]. Cerebral atrophy in ESKD, however, has been correlated with age of onset of renal disease [66] and dialytic modality [69, 70]. Qualitative imaging also shows that lower cerebral density [69, 71] and ventriculomegaly secondary to brain atrophy [72] are more often associated with requirement for and duration of pediatric HD compared with receipt of PD [70].

The use of MRI can provide high-resolution qualitative and quantitative assessment of the brain. sMRI provides information related to volumes within and between regions of the brain. Additionally, if the MRI is performed in a research-based scan sequence, it is often possible to obtain sequences that evaluate white and gray matter as well as blood flow within the brain—the former representing sMRI and latter representing functional fMRI.

Data from the Neurocognitive Assessment and Magnetic Resonance Imaging Analysis of Children and Young Adults with Chronic Kidney Disease (NiCK) Study performed volumetric brain assessment using sMRI in youth with CKD compared to normal controls [73]. Although the sample size was adequately powered to detect a statistical difference between populations (N = 90), the CKD sample was very heterogenous with regard to chronological age, stage of disease, disease etiology, and inclusion of dialysis/transplant patients. Statistical analyses, including corrections for multiple comparisons and adjustments for age and sex, did not support any specific brain regional differences between CKD patients and controls. Furthermore, there were no CKD-related clinical predictors to link differences in brain regions of interest to neurocognitive performance. Single-center data by Solomon et al. [74] evaluated 18 males with mild to moderate CKD due to congenital anomalies of the kidney and urinary tract in comparison to matched, healthy peers. Cerebellar gray matter volume was significantly smaller in children with CKD compared to peers (Fig. 57.1). In contrast, cerebral gray matter volume was increased in CKD participants. Reduced

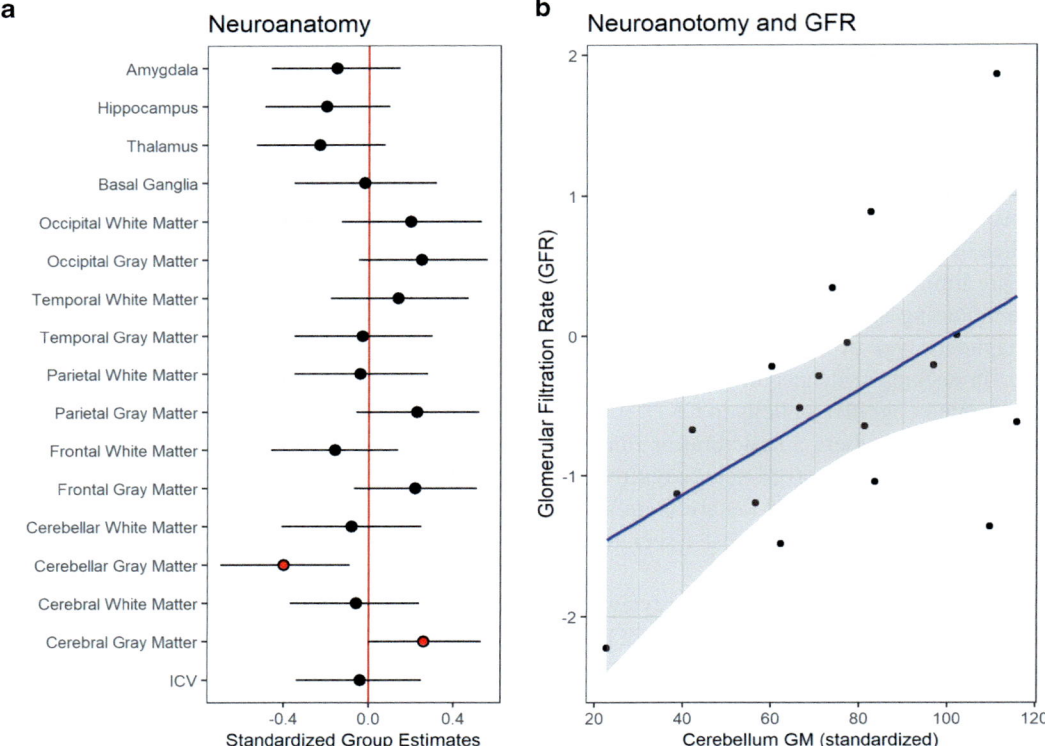

Fig. 57.1 Neuroanatomical differences between controls and pediatric chronic kidney disease [74]. Panel A shows the standardized group estimates (x-axis) and 95% confidence limits of the estimates for each of the regions of interest (ROI) included in the analysis (y-axis). Estimates are adjusted for age, socioeconomic status, and maternal education. The red (vertical) line marks 0, or no significant effect of group on ROI. Red circles mark significant group estimates. Panel B shows the relationship between estimated glomerular filtration rate, eGFR, (x-axis) and standardized cerebellum gray matter volume (y-axis) in the CKD group

cerebellum gray matter volume was associated with disease severity, operationalized as eGFR and predicted lower verbal fluency scores in the CKD sample. Enlarged cerebral gray matter in the CKD sample predicted lower scores on mathematics assessment.

sMRI also serves to inform the microstructural white matter integrity of the brain via diffusion tensor imaging (DTI). DTI is an MRI modality that allows for examination of white matter integrity—i.e., axonal or white matter microstructural changes that disrupt the diffusive property of water in the axon. These microstructural changes have been shown in diseases such as hypertension, diabetes mellitus, and atherosclerosis [75, 76]. The result of this microstructural disruption is a change in a physical diffusive property of the axon called decreased fractional anisotropy. Matsuda-Abedini et al. [77] conducted a quantitative white matter analysis utilizing a heterogenous sample of patients with varying CKD etiologies (including patients on PD and post-transplant) and control patients. This demonstrated the presence of decreased white matter integrity, specifically decreased fractional anisotropy, within the anterior limb of the internal capsule. It is possible that the entirety of the white matter integrity difference within the sample was not captured given the multisite nature of the study; specifically, MRI sequences are highly scanner dependent and statistically significant differences can emerge (or be lost) due to differences in magnet strength or brand of scanner utilized. Lastly, the sample did not have parallel neurocognitive data to further inform the significance of white matter changes within the anterior limb of the internal capsule finding.

fMRI studies examine the use of oxygen within the brain or rate of arterial cerebral blood flow with specialized scan sequences called 'resting state' or 'arterial spin labeling,' respectively. Additional analysis of data from the NiCK Study lends evidence for regional cerebral blood flow abnormalities that may underlie cognitive changes in pediatric CKD [78]. In a study by Liu et al. [78], patients with CKD, including dialysis and transplant patients, showed higher global cerebral blood flow compared to control subjects. Perhaps of most interest, one area showed regional cerebral blood flow differences between patients and control subjects—including a region called the "default mode" network (Fig. 57.2). Neuroscience literature supports that the brain is organized into functional networks, and the

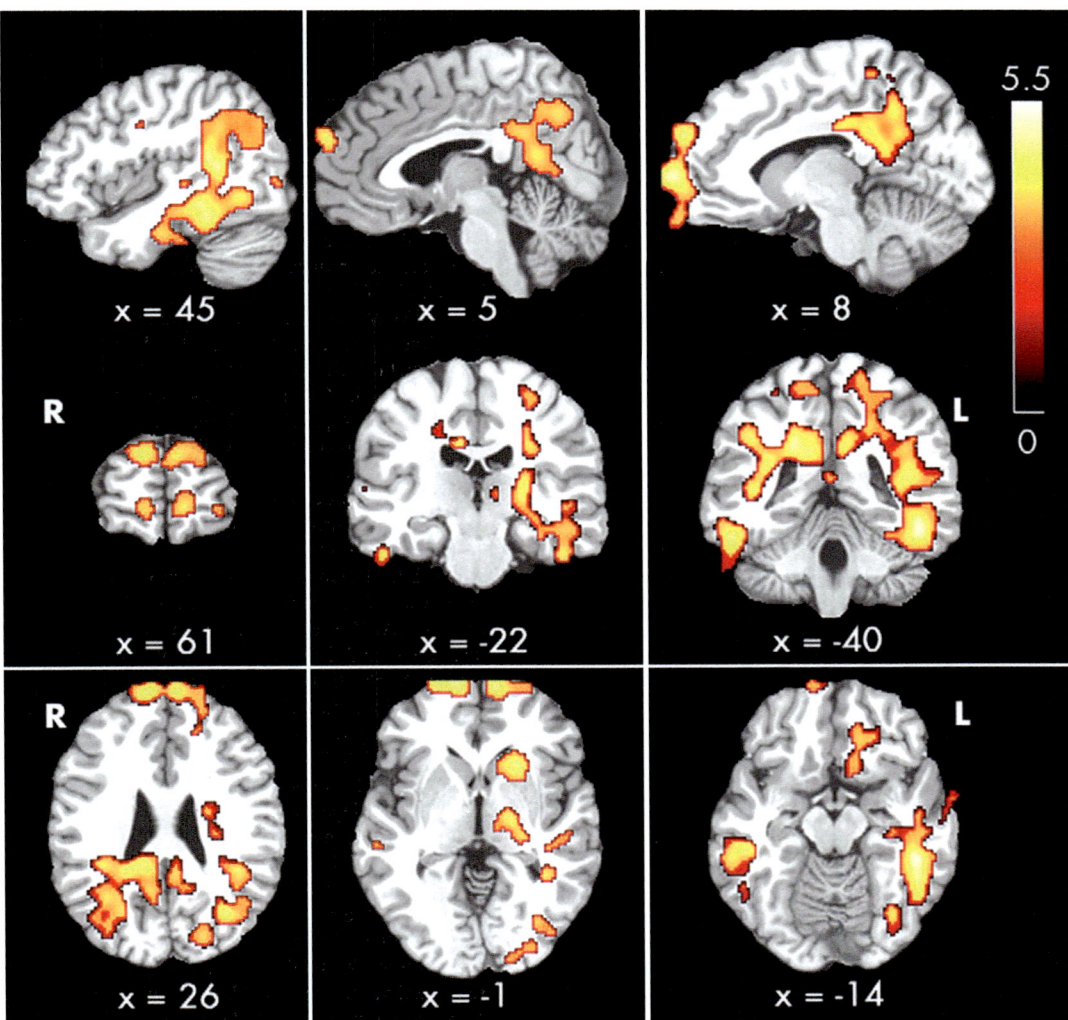

Fig. 57.2 From Liu et al. [78], reprinted with permission: demonstration of voxel-wise group comparison of cerebral blood flow after removal of effects of hematocrit level, age, and sex. Contrast shown here demonstrates the regions where those with CKD have greater cerebral blood flow than controls. Of note, there were no regions in this analysis where controls had greater regions than those with CKD. Color bar indicates *t* scores. *x, y, z* = coordinates in Montreal Neurological Institute (MNI) space

default mode network is a critical loop for attention regulation and, perhaps, EF processes [79–82]. Hematocrit-related effects explained most of the observed group differences in cerebral blood flow. Thus, Liu et al. hypothesized that chronic anemia experienced in pediatric CKD could be a potential cause of vascular endothelial damage due to increased compensatory blood flow to meet demands for deficits in tissue oxygen delivery.

More Frequent Hemodialysis and Neurocognitive Functioning

There were improvements in blood pressure, phosphate control and health-related quality of life in a prospective controlled trial of daily or nocturnal HD in adults [83, 84]. One cohort was studied with an expanded battery of cognitive tests; executive function and global cognition were not affected, but memory and verbal fluency were improved [85]. The subjects who received daily HD saw improvement on the Rey Auditory Verbal Learning Test Immediate Recall and the Controlled Oral Word Association Test after 12 months. The frequent nocturnal HD group did not see a benefit in cognition and had poorer performance on one test of attention. A smaller longitudinal study of 14 adults showed benefits to attention and working memory, psychomotor efficiency and processing speed, and learning efficiency when subjects were converted from thrice weekly HD to nocturnal treatments 5–7 times per week [86].

Reports of frequent HD and nocturnal dialysis in children have focused on improvements in growth and metabolic control, rather than on cognition. There remains interest in expanding these treatment choices to more children. Improvement in blood pressure control and middle molecule clearance coupled with reduction or removal of dietary restrictions could benefit both cognition and quality of life. Nonetheless, it is recognized that these treatment schedules are burdensome. In one of the largest series reporting patient outcomes for more frequent dialysis, daily in-center hemodiafiltration required 3-hour treatments six

times per week [87]. Home nocturnal HD performed 6–7 nights per week provides improved metabolic control and elimination of dietary restrictions [88] but increased perceived treatment burden for the family. The NxStage System is most often used for home HD but is only appropriate for those over 30 kg; we do not have an alternative to PD for the smallest patients. These preliminary observations in selected dialysis programs have engendered enthusiasm for alternative regimens for HD in children and it has been recommended that pediatric nephrologists consider ways to implement more frequent HD and strategies for supporting families who wish to pursue it [89, 90].

Conclusion

The cognitive deficits observed in pediatric CKD patients represent a potentially under-recognized consequence of pediatric CKD in day-to-day clinical practice. The findings presented in this chapter demonstrate that our pediatric CKD patients are most at risk for cognitive dysfunction in the domain of executive functions; specifically, attention and working memory. Cognitive and academic performance may be associated with features on neuroimaging including differences in gray matter volume. These cognitive, academic, and neuroimaging differences likely emerge in early childhood and can be detected during the early stages of CKD. This signals a need for greater attention to the developing brain in the midst of a life-long, chronic disease process. Current data represent a limited understanding of the medical determinants of cognitive dysfunction in CKD and an even more minimal understanding of the genetic and epigenetic drivers of cognitive development and performance in CKD. Certainly, research efforts to understand cognition in CKD may be better served through parallel inclusion of a chronic disease control model that includes healthy controls. Nephrologists should remain aware of the burden of managing chronic disease at a young age and how that differs from the experience of adults who develop CKD later in life.

When treating children with CKD, it is important that nephrology care incorporate a psychologist as part of the treatment team to provide understanding for families and patients regarding the impact of CKD progression on neurodevelopment and neurocognitive performance and available academic accommodations and interventions. This will allow patients and caregivers to obtain more comprehensive information about the potential for cognitive rehabilitation and learn how best to support children and adolescents with CKD as they navigate educational and vocational endeavors.

Acknowledgments The authors wish to acknowledge Susan R. Mendley, MD for her contributions to the previous edition of this chapter.

References

1. McGraw ME, Haka-Ikse K. Neurologic-developmental sequelae of chronic renal failure in infancy. J Pediatr. 1985;106(4):579–83.
2. Rotundo A, Nevins TE, Lipton M, Lockman LA, Mauer SM, Michael AF. Progressive encephalopathy in children with chronic renal insufficiency in infancy. Kidney Int. 1982;21(3):486–91.
3. Elzouki A, Carroll J, Butinar D, Moosa A. Improved neurological outcome in children with chronic renal disease from infancy. Pediatr Nephrol. 1994;8(2):205–10.
4. Warady BA, Belden B, Kohaut E. Neurodevelopmental outcome of children initiating peritoneal dialysis in early infancy. Pediatr Nephrol. 1999;13(9):759–65.
5. Levitt P. Structural and functional maturation of the developing primate brain. J Pediatr. 2003;143(4 Suppl):S35–45.
6. Brain Development Cooperative G. Total and regional brain volumes in a population-based normative sample from 4 to 18 years: the NIH MRI Study of Normal Brain Development. Cereb Cortex. 2012;22(1):1–12.
7. Sabatini MJ, Ebert P, Lewis DA, Levitt P, Cameron JL, Mirnics K. Amygdala gene expression correlates of social behavior in monkeys experiencing maternal separation. J Neurosci. 2007;27(12):3295–304.
8. Paus T, Zijdenbos A, Worsley K, Collins DL, Blumenthal J, Giedd JN, et al. Structural maturation of neural pathways in children and adolescents: in vivo study. Science. 1999;283(5409):1908–11.
9. Armstrong FD, Horn M. Educational issues in childhood cancer. Sch Psychol Q. 1995;10:292–304.
10. Armstrong FD. Neurodevelopment and chronic illness: mechanisms of disease and treatment. Ment Retard Dev Disabil Res Rev. 2006;12:168–73.
11. Armstrong FD, Mulhern RK. Acute lymphoblastic leukemia and brain tumors. In: Brown RT, editor. Cognitive aspects of chronic illness in children. New York: The Guilford Press; 1999. p. 1–14.
12. Mulhern RK, Merchant TE, Gajjar A, Reddick WE, Kun LE. Late neurocognitive sequelae in survivors of brain tumours in childhood. Lancet Oncol. 2004;5(7):399–408.
13. Gerson AC, Butler R, Moxey-Mims M, Wentz A, Shinnar S, Lande MB, et al. Neurocognitive outcomes in children with chronic kidney disease: Current findings and contemporary endeavors. Ment Retard Dev Disabil Res Rev. 2006;12(3):208–15.
14. North American Pediatric Renal Trials and Collaborative Studies—NAPRTCS 2014 Annual Transplant Report. Rockville, MD; 2014.
15. Seikaly MG, Ho PL, Emmett L, Fine RN, Tejani A. Chronic renal insufficiency in children: the 2001 Annual Report of the NAPRTCS. Pediatr Nephrol. 2003;18(8):796–804.
16. Davis ID, Chang PN, Nevins TE. Successful renal transplantation accelerates development in young uremic children. Pediatrics. 1990;86(4):594–600.
17. Hulstijn-Dirkmaat GM, Damhuis IH, Jetten ML, Koster AM, Schroder CH. The cognitive development of pre-school children treated for chronic renal failure. Pediatr Nephrol. 1995;9(4):464–9.
18. Shroff R, Wright E, Ledermann S, Hutchinson C, Rees L. Chronic hemodialysis in infants and children under 2 years of age. Pediatr Nephrol. 2003;18(4):378–83.
19. Laakkonen H, Lonnqvist T, Valanne L, Karikoski J, Holmberg C, Ronnholm K. Neurological development in 21 children on peritoneal dialysis in infancy. Pediatr Nephrol. 2011;26(10):1863–71.
20. Hooper SR, Gerson AC, Johnson RJ, Mendley SR, Shinnar S, Lande MB, et al. Neurocognitive, social-behavioral, and adaptive functioning in preschool children with mild to moderate kidney disease. J Dev Behav Pediatr. 2016;37(3):231–8.
21. Madden SJ, Ledermann SE, Guerrero-Blanco M, Bruce M, Trompeter RS. Cognitive and psychosocial outcome of infants dialysed in infancy. Child Care Health Dev. 2003;29(1):55–61.
22. Johnson RJ, Warady BA. Long-term neurocognitive outcomes of patients with end-stage renal disease during infancy. Pediatr Nephrol. 2013;28(8):1283–91.
23. Brouhard BH, Donaldson LA, Lawry KW, McGowan KR, Drotar D, Davis I, et al. Cognitive functioning in children on dialysis and post-transplantation. Pediatr Transplant. 2000;4(4):261–7.
24. Popel J, Joffe R, Acton BV, Bond GY, Joffe AR, Midgley J, et al. Neurocognitive and functional outcomes at 5 years of age after renal transplant in early childhood. Pediatr Nephrol. 2019;34(5):889–95.

25. Hartmann H, Hawellek N, Wedekin M, Vogel C, Das AM, Balonwu K, et al. Early kidney transplantation improves neurocognitive outcome in patients with severe congenital chronic kidney disease. Transpl Int. 2015;28(4):429–36.

26. Fennell RS, Fennell EB, Carter RL, Mings EL, Klausner AB, Hurst JR. Association between renal-function and cognition in childhood chronic-renal-failure. Pediatr Nephrol. 1990;4(1):16–20.

27. Fennell RS, Fennell EB, Carter RL, Mings EL, Klausner AB, Hurst JR. A longitudinal-study of the cognitive function of children with renal-failure. Pediatr Nephrol. 1990;4(1):11–5.

28. Fennell RS, Fennell EB, Carter RL, Mings EL, Klausner AB, Hurst JR. Correlations between performance on neuropsychological tests in children with chronic renal failure. Child Nephrol Urol. 1990;10(4):199–204.

29. Gipson DS, Duquette PJ, Icard PF, Hooper SR. The central nervous system in childhood chronic kidney disease. Pediatr Nephrol. 2007;22(10):1703–10.

30. Bawden HN, Acott P, Carter J, Lirenman D, MacDonald GW, McAllister M, et al. Neuropsychological functioning in end-stage renal disease. Arch Dis Child. 2004;89(7):644–7.

31. Qvist E, Pihko H, Fagerudd P, Valanne L, Lamminranta S, Karikoski J, et al. Neurodevelopmental outcome in high-risk patients after renal transplantation in early childhood. Pediatr Transplant. 2002;6(1):53–62.

32. Hooper SR, Gerson AC, Butler RW, Gipson DS, Mendley SR, Lande MB, et al. Neurocognitive functioning of children and adolescents with mild-to-moderate chronic kidney disease. Clin J Am Soc Nephrol. 2011;6(8):1824–30.

33. Duquette PJ, Hooper SR, Wetherington CE, Icard PF, Gipson DS. Brief report: intellectual and academic functioning in pediatric chronic kidney disease. J Pediatr Psychol. 2007;32(8):1011–7.

34. Groothoff JW, Grootenhuis M, Dommerholt A, Gruppen MP, Offringa M, Heymans HS. Impaired cognition and schooling in adults with end stage renal disease since childhood. Arch Dis Child. 2002;87(5):380–5.

35. Gipson DS, Hooper SR, Duquette PJ, Wetherington CE, Stellwagen KK, Jenkins TL, et al. Memory and executive functions in pediatric chronic kidney disease. Child Neuropsychol. 2006;12(6):391–405.

36. Johnson RJ, Gerson AC, Harshman LA, Matheson MB, Shinnar S, Lande MB, et al. A longitudinal examination of parent-reported emotional-behavioral functioning of children with mild to moderate chronic kidney disease. Pediatr Nephrol. 2020;35(7):1287–95.

37. Ruebner RL, Laney N, Kim JY, Hartung EA, Hooper SR, Radcliffe J, et al. Neurocognitive dysfunction in children, adolescents, and young adults with CKD. Am J Kidney Dis. 2016;67(4):567–75.

38. Lande MB, Mendley SR, Matheson MB, Shinnar S, Gerson AC, Samuels JA, et al. Association of blood pressure variability and neurocognition in chil-dren with chronic kidney disease. Pediatr Nephrol. 2016;31(11):2137–44.

39. Harshman LA, Johnson RJ, Matheson MB, Kogon AJ, Shinnar S, Gerson AC, et al. Academic achievement in children with chronic kidney disease: a report from the CKiD cohort. Pediatr Nephrol. 2019;34(4):689–96.

40. Reynolds JM, Morton MJ, Garralda ME, Postlethwaite RJ, Goh D. Psychosocial adjustment of adult survivors of a paediatric dialysis and transplant programme. Arch Dis Child. 1993;68(1):104–10.

41. Offner G, Latta K, Hoyer PF, Baum HJ, Ehrich JH, Pichlmayr R, et al. Kidney transplanted children come of age. Kidney Int. 1999;55(4):1509–17.

42. Kerklaan J, Hannan E, Hanson C, Guha C, Cho Y, Christian M, et al. Perspectives on life participation by young adults with chronic kidney disease: an interview study. BMJ Open. 2020;10(10):e037840.

43. Chen K, Didsbury M, van Zwieten A, Howell M, Kim S, Tong A, et al. Neurocognitive and educational outcomes in children and adolescents with CKD: a systematic review and meta-analysis. Clin J Am Soc Nephrol. 2018;13(3):387–97.

44. Icard P, Hooper SR, Gipson DS, Ferris ME. Cognitive improvement in children with CKD after transplant. Pediatr Transplant. 2010;14(7):887–90.

45. Mendley SR, Zelko FA. Improvement in specific aspects of neurocognitive performance in children after renal transplantation. Kidney Int. 1999;56(1):318–23.

46. So SK, Chang PN, Najarian JS, Mauer SM, Simmons RL, Nevins TE. Growth and development in infants after renal transplantation. J Pediatr. 1987;110(3):343–50.

47. Falger J, Latal B, Landolt MA, Lehmann P, Neuhaus TJ, Laube GF. Outcome after renal transplantation. Part I: intellectual and motor performance. Pediatr Nephrol. 2008;23(8):1339–45.

48. Molnar-Varga M, Novak M, Szabo AJ, Kelen K, Streja E, Remport A, et al. Neurocognitive functions of pediatric kidney transplant recipients. Pediatr Nephrol. 2016;31(9):1531–8.

49. Suri D, Vaidya VA. Glucocorticoid regulation of brain-derived neurotrophic factor: relevance to hippocampal structural and functional plasticity. Neuroscience. 2013;239:196–213.

50. Sapolsky RM, Uno H, Rebert CS, Finch CE. Hippocampal damage associated with prolonged glucocorticoid exposure in primates. J Neurosci. 1990;10(9):2897–902.

51. Antonow-Schlorke I, Schwab M, Li C, Nathanielsz PW. Glucocorticoid exposure at the dose used clinically alters cytoskeletal proteins and presynaptic terminals in the fetal baboon brain. J Physiol. 2003;547(Pt 1):117–23.

52. Bechstein WO. Neurotoxicity of calcineurin inhibitors: impact and clinical management. Transpl Int. 2000;13(5):313–26.

53. Veroux P, Veroux M, Puliatti C, Morale W, Cappello D, Valvo M, et al. Tacrolimus-induced neurotoxic-

ity in kidney transplant recipients. Transplant Proc. 2002;34(8):3188–90.

54. Neu AM, Furth SL, Case BW, Wise B, Colombani PM, Fivush BA. Evaluation of neurotoxicity in pediatric renal transplant recipients treated with tacrolimus (FK506). Clin Transpl. 1997;11(5 Pt 1):412–4.

55. Parvex P, Pinsk M, Bell LE, O'Gorman AM, Patenaude YG, Gupta IR. Reversible encephalopathy associated with tacrolimus in pediatric renal transplants. Pediatr Nephrol. 2001;16(7):537–42.

56. Bennett PC, Zhao W, Lawen A, Ng KT. Cyclosporin A, an inhibitor of calcineurin, impairs memory formation in day-old chicks. Brain Res. 1996;730(1–2):107–17.

57. McDonald JW, Goldberg MP, Gwag BJ, Chi SI, Choi DW. Cyclosporine induces neuronal apoptosis and selective oligodendrocyte death in cortical cultures. Ann Neurol. 1996;40(5):750–8.

58. Maramattom BV, Wijdicks EFM. Sirolimus may not cause neurotoxicity in kidney and liver transplant recipients. Neurology. 2004;63:1958–9.

59. Serkova N, Jacobsen W, Niemann CU, Litt L, Benet LZ, Leibfritz D, et al. Sirolimus, but not the structurally related RAD (everolimus), enhances the negative effects of cyclosporine on mitochondrial metabolism in the rat brain. Br J Pharmacol. 2001;133(6):875–85.

60. Hildebrandt F. Genetic kidney diseases. Lancet. 2010;375(9722):1287–95.

61. Purcell S, Neale B, Todd-Brown K, Thomas L, Ferreira MA, Bender D, et al. PLINK: a tool set for whole-genome association and population-based linkage analyses. Am J Hum Genet. 2007;81(3):559–75.

62. Stefansson H, Rujescu D, Cichon S, Pietilainen OP, Ingason A, Steinberg S, et al. Large recurrent microdeletions associated with schizophrenia. Nature. 2008;455(7210):232–6.

63. Elia J, Glessner JT, Wang K, Takahashi N, Shtir CJ, Hadley D, et al. Genome-wide copy number variation study associates metabotropic glutamate receptor gene networks with attention deficit hyperactivity disorder. Nat Genet. 2011;44(1):78–84.

64. Shaw-Smith C, Pittman AM, Willatt L, Martin H, Rickman L, Gribble S, et al. Microdeletion encompassing MAPT at chromosome 17q21.3 is associated with developmental delay and learning disability. Nat Genet. 2006;38(9):1032–7.

65. Sanna-Cherchi S, Kiryluk K, Burgess KE, Bodria M, Sampson MG, Hadley D, et al. Copy-number disorders are a common cause of congenital kidney malformations. Am J Hum Genet. 2012;91(6):987–97.

66. Passer JA. Cerebral atrophy in end-stage uremia. Proc Clin Dial Transplant Forum. 1977;7:91–4.

67. Papageorgiou C, Ziroyannis P, Vathylakis J, Grigoriadis A, Hatzikonstantinou V, Capsalakis Z. A comparative study of brain atrophy by computerized tomography in chronic renal failure and chronic hemodialysis. Acta Neurol Scand. 1982;66(3):378–85.

68. Steinberg A, Efrat R, Pomeranz A, Drukker A. Computerized tomography of the brain in children with chronic renal failure. Int J Pediatr Nephrol. 1985;6(2):121–6.

69. Schnaper HW, Cole BR, Hodges FJ, Robson AM. Cerebral cortical atrophy in pediatric patients with end-stage renal disease. Am J Kidney Dis. 1983;2(6):645–50.

70. La Greca G, Biasioli S, Chiaramonte S, Dettori P, Fabris A, Feriani M, et al. Studies on brain density in hemodialysis and peritoneal dialysis. Nephron. 1982;31(2):146–50.

71. Dettori P, La Greca G, Biasioli S, Chiaramonte S, Fabris A, Feriani M, et al. Changes of cerebral density in dialyzed patients. Neuroradiology. 1982;23(2):95–9.

72. Kretzschmar K, Nix W, Zschiedrich H, Philipp T. Morphologic cerebral changes in patients undergoing dialysis for renal failure. AJNR Am J Neuroradiol. 1983;4(3):439–41.

73. Hartung EA, Erus G, Jawad AF, Laney N, Doshi JJ, Hooper SR, et al. Brain magnetic resonance imaging findings in children and young adults with CKD. Am J Kidney Dis. 2018;72(3):349–59.

74. Solomon MA, van der Plas E, Langbehn KE, Novak M, Schultz JL, Koscik TR, et al. Early pediatric chronic kidney disease is associated with brain volumetric gray matter abnormalities. Pediatr Res. 2020;

75. Kodl CT, Franc DT, Rao JP, Anderson FS, Thomas W, Mueller BA, et al. Diffusion tensor imaging identifies deficits in white matter microstructure in subjects with type 1 diabetes that correlate with reduced neurocognitive function. Diabetes. 2008;57(11):3083–9.

76. Kozera GM, Dubaniewicz M, Zdrojewski T, Madej-Dmochowska A, Mielczarek M, Wojczal J, et al. Cerebral vasomotor reactivity and extent of white matter lesions in middle-aged men with arterial hypertension: a pilot study. Am J Hypertens. 2010;23(11):1198–203.

77. Matsuda-Abedini M, Fitzpatrick K, Harrell WR, Gipson DS, Hooper SR, Belger A, et al. Brain abnormalities in children and adolescents with chronic kidney disease. Pediatr Res. 2018;84(3):387–92.

78. Liu HS, Hartung EA, Jawad AF, Ware JB, Laney N, Port AM, et al. Regional cerebral blood flow in children and young adults with chronic kidney disease. Radiology. 2018;288(3):849–58.

79. Gusnard DA, Akbudak E, Shulman GL, Raichle ME. Medial prefrontal cortex and self-referential mental activity: relation to a default mode of brain function. Proc Natl Acad Sci U S A. 2001;98(7):4259–64.

80. Raichle ME, MacLeod AM, Snyder AZ, Powers WJ, Gusnard DA, Shulman GL. A default mode of brain function. Proc Natl Acad Sci U S A. 2001;98(2):676–82.

81. Simpson JR Jr, Snyder AZ, Gusnard DA, Raichle ME. Emotion-induced changes in human medial prefrontal cortex: I. During cognitive task performance. Proc Natl Acad Sci U S A. 2001;98(2):683–7.

82. Raichle ME. The brain's default mode network. Annu Rev Neurosci. 2015;38:433–47.

83. Group FHNT, Chertow GM, Levin NW, Beck GJ, Depner TA, Eggers PW, et al. In-center hemodialysis six times per week versus three times per week. N Engl J Med. 2010;363(24):2287–300.

84. Rocco MV, Lockridge RS Jr, Beck GJ, Eggers PW, Gassman JJ, Greene T, et al. The effects of frequent nocturnal home hemodialysis: the Frequent Hemodialysis Network Nocturnal Trial. Kidney Int. 2011;80(10):1080–91.

85. Kurella Tamura M, Unruh ML, Nissenson AR, Larive B, Eggers PW, Gassman J, et al. Effect of more frequent hemodialysis on cognitive function in the frequent hemodialysis network trials. Am J Kidney Dis. 2013;61(2):228–37.

86. Jassal SV, Devins GM, Chan CT, Bozanovic R, Rourke S. Improvements in cognition in patients converting from thrice weekly hemodialysis to nocturnal hemodialysis: a longitudinal pilot study. Kidney Int. 2006;70(5):956–62.

87. Fischbach M, Fothergill H, Zaloszyc A, Menouer S, Terzic J. Intensified daily dialysis: the best chronic dialysis option for children? Semin Dial. 2011;24(6):640–4.

88. Geary DF, Piva E, Tyrrell J, Gajaria MJ, Picone G, Keating LE, et al. Home nocturnal hemodialysis in children. J Pediatr. 2005;147(3):383–7.

89. Muller D, Zimmering M, Chan CT, McFarlane PA, Pierratos A, Querfeld U. Intensified hemodialysis regimens: neglected treatment options for children and adolescents. Pediatr Nephrol. 2008;23(10):1729–36.

90. Warady BA, Chadha V. Chronic kidney disease in children: the global perspective. Pediatr Nephrol. 2007;22(12):1999–2009.

91. Hijazi R, Abitbol CL, Chandar J, Seeherunvong W, Freundlich M, Zilleruelo G. Twenty-five years of infant dialysis: a single center experience. J Pediatr. 2009;155(1):111–7.

92. Ledermann SE, Scanes ME, Fernando ON, Duffy PG, Madden SJ, Trompeter RS. Long-term outcome of peritoneal dialysis in infants. J Pediatr. 2000;136(1):24–9.

93. Honda M, Kamiyama Y, Kawamura K, Kawahara K, Shishido S, Nakai H, et al. Growth, development and nutritional status in Japanese children under 2 years on continuous ambulatory peritoneal dialysis. Pediatr Nephrol. 1995;9(5):543–8.

94. Bock GH, Conners CK, Ruley J, Samango-Sprouse CA, Conry JA, Weiss I, et al. Disturbances of brain maturation and neurodevelopment during chronic renal failure in infancy. J Pediatr. 1989;114(2):231–8.

95. Slickers J, Duquette P, Hooper S, Gipson D. Clinical predictors of neurocognitive deficits in children with chronic kidney disease. Pediatr Nephrol. 2007;22(4):565–72.

96. Crocker JF, Acott PD, Carter JE, Lirenman DS, MacDonald GW, McAllister M, et al. Neuropsychological outcome in children with acquired or congenital renal disease. Pediatr Nephrol. 2002;17(11):908–12.

97. Lawry KW, Brouhard BH, Cunningham RJ. Cognitive functioning and school performance in children with renal failure. Pediatr Nephrol. 1994;8(3):326–9.

98. Rasbury WC, Fennell RS 3rd, Fennell EB, Morris MK. Cognitive functioning in children with end stage renal disease pre- and post-dialysis session. Int J Pediatr Nephrol. 1986;7(1):45–50.

99. Fennell RS 3rd, Rasbury WC, Fennell EB, Morris MK. Effects of kidney transplantation on cognitive performance in a pediatric population. Pediatrics. 1984;74(2):273–8.

100. Rasbury WC, Fennell RS 3rd, Morris MK. Cognitive functioning of children with end-stage renal disease before and after successful transplantation. J Pediatr. 1983;102(4):589–92.

Nutritional Challenges in Pediatric Kidney Disease

58

Rayna Levitt and Caitlin E. Carter

Introduction

Provision of adequate nutrition is a cornerstone of optimal management and improvement of outcomes for children with chronic kidney disease (CKD). Nutrition impacts short-term outcomes, including renal disease progression, growth, and development as well as long-term outcomes, including cardiovascular risk. Presently, the majority of guidelines for the nutritional management of children with CKD are based on consensus opinions and practice-based evidence.

Important considerations include the provision of adequate energy and macronutrients, the achievement of fluid and electrolyte balance, the provision of adequate micronutrients, and the prevention of metabolic bone disease. Extremes of body mass index, representing under-nutrition and over-nutrition are associated with poor outcomes and should be addressed when designing nutritional care plans for children with CKD. Promoting optimal nutrition for children with CKD necessitates multidisciplinary collaboration, including input from registered dietitians, physicians, nurses, and social workers.

R. Levitt · C. E. Carter (✉)
Division of Nephrology, Rady Children's Hospital,
University of California San Diego,
San Diego, CA, USA
e-mail: rlevitt@rchsd.org; cecarter@health.ucsd.edu

Nutrition Assessment

In 2009, in recognition of the growing population of children with CKD, the National Kidney Foundation published the Kidney Disease Outcomes Quality Initiative's (KDOQI) Clinical Practice Guidelines for Nutrition in Children with CKD [1]. These practice guidelines expanded upon guidelines that were published by KDOQI in 2000 by setting out evidenced based nutrition recommendations for pediatric patients with CKD, including patients receiving dialysis and those who have received kidney transplants. The guidelines were recommended as a starting point for those providing medical nutrition therapy to this complex patient population [2]. In 2019, the Pediatric Renal Nutrition Task Force, a team of pediatric nephrologists and pediatric renal dietitians from eight countries in Europe and North America, was established to develop clinical practice recommendations (CPRs) to update the 2009 KDOQI guidelines in areas where new evidence has become available [3]. This group conducted an in-depth review of evidence for current practices along with consensus opinion to establish updated practice guidelines.

The primary goal of evaluating nutrition status of children with CKD is to support growth and development, while preventing protein-energy wasting (PEW) and its well documented negative effects on patient outcomes [4, 5]. Provision of medical nutrition therapy in this population also aims to ensure that vitamin and mineral needs are met. There is a risk posed by over-nutrition as well, illustrated by obesity resulting from factors such as overzealous tube-feeding and the frequent use of corticosteroid therapy. Nutrition assessment in this patient population should involve the use of multiple measures of nutrition status as no single measure can provide an accurate picture. Children with CKD require more frequent monitoring of their nutrition status than their healthy counterparts, and the collection and comparison of measures over time can be used to form a more complete picture. The recommended components of assessment include anthropometric measures, evaluation of dietary intake, and review of biochemical data.

Anthropometric Measures

Height, weight and head circumference are the most easily attained measures used in nutrition assessment. They should be accurately measured using calibrated equipment and standardized techniques [1].

- Weight should be assessed at every clinic visit and weight gain or loss trends should be noted.
- Height should be evaluated in order to give context to the weight assessment. For children under 2 years of age, recumbent length should be measured. Standing height can be measured for those over 2 years who are able to stand. In order to determine if the height achieved is appropriate given a child's genetic potential, mid-parental height should be assessed. While anecdotal data can be used for this, it is best if the heights of both biological parents can be measured [6].

Mid-Parental Height Calculation:	
Boys:	[(mother's height + 13 cm) + father's height]/2
Girls:	[mother's height + (father's height-13 cm)]/2

(chart adapted from KDOQI 2009)

- Head circumference should be measured for children under 2 years of age.

These measures are plotted on percentile charts. In the U.S., the recommendations of the Centers for Disease Control and Prevention (CDC) are to use the World Health Organization growth charts to monitor growth for infants and children ages 0–<2 years of age and to use the CDC growth charts to monitor growth for children ages 2 years and older [7]. These values can also be expressed as standard deviation scores (number of standard deviations from the mean for a normal population of the same age). If an applicable underlying genetic disorder is present, it is appropriate to utilize a disease specific growth charts to assess growth parameters.

- Weight for length (for children <2 years) or BMI (for children ages 2–20 years) should be calculated every time weight and height are measured and plotted on percentile charts.

When evaluating BMI in children with CKD, it may be preferable to express their BMI relative to height age (the age at which the child's height would be at the 50th percentile). Children with CKD commonly experience poor linear growth and delayed skeletal maturation. Comparison of BMI to other children with the same chronological age may result in an underestimation of that child's BMI percentile. It is therefore more appropriate to compare BMI to those of children with similar height and maturation [1, 4, 5]. When evaluating weight or using weight to calculate BMI, it is important to first evaluate whether edema is present. For dialysis patients, estimated dry weight should be used when calculating weight for length or BMI.

In addition to anthropometric measurements, nutrition-focused physical exam (NFPE) can be included as part of the patient assessment as it can identify muscle wasting, subcutaneous fat loss, edema and macronutrient deficiencies [8]. The value of NFPE has been noted in the general pediatric population as it can identify malnutrition that has a negative impact on growth and development. Since children with CKD are known to be at risk of poor growth, it may add value to the assessment of this patient population as well.

Dietary Assessment

It is recommended that dietary intakes of children with CKD be assessed with a minimum frequency of annually, or as often as every 2 weeks depending on the age of the child and stage of disease. More frequent assessments are recommended for younger children and children with advanced stages of CKD. Children who depend solely on enteral feeding should have more frequent monitoring. This is especially true of enterally fed infants who may benefit from feeding adjustments as often as weekly [6, 9]. The dietary intake assessment should either take the form of a prospective 3-day diet diary or a 24-h diet recall. A 3-day diary should include one weekend day to represent variation in the diet due to change in schedules on weekends. The 24-h diet recall may be better suited to adolescents who, may not be compliant with completion of a food diary. Either technique can be utilized by a registered dietitian to estimate daily intake of energy, macronutrients, vitamins and minerals. They can provide information about diet adequacy and, over time, can highlight changes in appetite that may lead to weight loss or increased risk of malnutrition. If dietary assessment reveals that the diet is inadequate, in addition to other considerations, the dietitian should evaluate whether food insecurity is a contributing factor. In 2018, one in seven U.S. households with children was affected by food insecurity, which can be exacerbated by families facing increased medical expenses [10].

Assessing Protein Status: Normalized Protein Catabolic Rate vs. Serum Albumin

Lower serum albumin is associated with increased morbidity and mortality [11]. The 2000 KDOQI Nutrition Guidelines recommended albumin be used as a marker of nutritional status in pediatric dialysis patients [2]. There are several shortfalls, however, in the use of albumin levels as a measure of nutritional status in children with CKD. Serum albumin concentrations decrease for various non-nutritional reasons, such as the presence of fluid overload, urinary and dialysate protein losses, inflammation, infection and liver disease [4]. In addition, it is possible for serum albumin to be normal in patients who are known to have a poor oral intake and who appear malnourished with a decrease in lean body or fat mass. Despite these limitations, hypoalbuminemia has been associated with mortality in children initiating dialysis therapy and albumin levels above 4 g/dL in adolescent patients on hemodialysis (HD) have been associated with a reduced risk of death and decreased hospitalizations [6]. For this reason, serum albumin levels continue to be monitored and are interpreted in the context of other assessment data.

Normalized protein catabolic rate (nPCR) has been validated as an objective tool that may assist in the nutritional assessment of adolescent HD patients. The calculation of nPCR is based on the increase in the level of blood urea nitrogen between the end of one HD treatment and the beginning of the subsequent treatment and it is theoretically more accurate than food diaries or diet recalls. Calculations using BUN values from the end of one dialysis treatment and BUN values at the start of a subsequent treatment may more accurately reflect protein intake than calculations using BUN values from the start and end of a same day HD treatment [12]. Higher nPCR in adolescents has been found to be a good predictor of weight gain, whereas lower nPCR has been shown to predict weight loss.

Normalized protein nitrogen appearance (nPNA) is a similar measure of estimated protein intake that can be calculated for patients on peritoneal dialysis (PD). It is calculated by determining the total daily excretion of urea in the dialysate and urine, as well as the daily dialysate protein losses. These values are entered into an estimating equation and are normalized for body size.

Equations for Calculation of Normalized Protein Catabolic Rate (nPCR) and Normalized Protein Equivalent of Nitrogen Appearance (nPNA)

nPCR

1. **Calculate urea generation rate (G, mg/min):**
   $G = [(C2 \times V2) - (C1 \times V1)]/t$
   C1 = post-dialysis BUN (mg/dL)
   C2 = pre-dialysis BUN (mg/dL)
   V1 = post-dialysis total body water (dL;
   V1 = 5.8 dL/kg × post dialysis weight in kg)
   V2 = pre-dialysis total body water (dL;
   V2 = 5.8 dL/kg × predialysis weight in kg)
   t = time (minutes) from the end of one dialysis treatment to the start of the next dialysis treatment

2. **Calculate nPCR:**
   5.43 × estG/V1 + 0.17

nPNA

1. **Calculate total nitrogen appearance (TNA, g/day):**
   0.03 + 1.138 urea-Nurine +0.99 urea-Ndialysate +1.18 BSA + 0.965 protein-Ndialysate

2. **Calculate protein equivalent of nitrogen appearance (PNA, g/day):**
   TNA × 6.25

3. **Normalize PNA to body weight (nPNA):**
   PNA/weight (kg)

N = nitrogen, BSA = body surface area, BUN = blood urea nitrogen
Adapted from: National Kidney Foundation KDOQI Clinical Practice Guideline for Nutrition in Children with CKD: 2008 Update. Am J Kidney Dis. 2009; 53(3 Suppl 2):S1-S123 [1] and from Roman B. Nutrition Management of Pediatric Chronic Kidney Disease. Support Line. 2013 April;35(2):12–21 [4]

nPCR and nPNA are expressed in grams of protein per kilogram body weight per day (g/kg/day). The target nPCR or nPNA should be equivalent to the protein goal for age, which is based on the dietary reference intake (DRI) plus an allowance for dialytic protein and amino acid losses. Because nPCR fluctuates on a daily basis depending upon what is eaten, a single nPCR value does not give a good picture of protein intake; the observation of trends from month to month provides more information [1]. Among the shortfalls of nPCR are that it may overestimate protein intake in severely catabolic patients and underestimate protein intake in growing children, and has not been shown to have predictive value in infants and young children. For these reasons, like other assessment tools, it should be used in conjunction with other data to provide a complete picture of nutritional status.

Nutrition Management

Health care teams have moved away from prescribing "renal diets" as the standard diet for all children with CKD. Dietary modifications should be individualized based upon disease state and biochemical data as well as factors such as the child's age, development and food preferences. Children with CKD may require modifications to their intake of calories, protein, fat, phosphorus, calcium, sodium, potassium and fluid. In order to promote growth and development and facilitate adherence to diet recommendations, restrictions should be kept as liberal as possible. The diet can then be liberalized or tightened depending on the response in the relevant parameter. The nutrition care plan should be monitored frequently. Adjustments should be made over time in response to changes in the child's nutritional status, age, development, anthropometrics, food preferences, renal function, biochemistries, need for and mode of renal replacement therapy, medications and psychosocial status. Diet instructions should begin with a simple explanation of the role of the nutrient in the body, the rationale for the diet modification, the desired outcomes to be achieved (e.g., specific amount of weight gain, normalize serum phosphorus levels) and what happens if the modifications are not made. Guidelines for change should be practical, individualized to the patient's and the family's lifestyle, cultural food preferences and eating habits, and should be positive in that they emphasize the foods that the child can eat to replace those that need to be limited or avoided. Food models, pictures of foods from supermarket advertisements, and food containers with labels and ingredient lists can be used to make teaching sessions more interesting and relatable. During follow up, food records and diet histories can be used to assess the child's and family's understanding of and adherence to the diet to identify problems that may exist with modifying dietary intake. Nutritional counseling is recommended on an ongoing basis in order to address the dynamic nature of a child's development, food preferences, residual renal function and medical condition. Caregivers outside of the family (grandparents, school staff, daycare providers, and babysitters) should be aware of diet modifications and should be provided with copies of teaching materials to use as reference guides to ensure consistent adherence to diet modifications. Adolescents should receive sufficient education to allow them to independently make appropriate choices when they are at restaurants, with friends, or at school.

Energy

Energy Requirements

Adequate energy intake can lead to increases in body weight and improvement in linear growth. Meeting caloric requirements is important to avoid using protein as an energy source through gluconeogenesis. There is no evidence that children with CKD have different energy requirements than their same-aged healthy counterparts. For this reason, the KDOQI 2009 guidelines and the Pediatric Renal Nutrition Task Force (PRNT) agree that initial energy goals for children with CKD 2–5D be the same as those for healthy children of the same chronological age [1, 3]. The PRNT utilizes the terminology suggested dietary intake (SDI) (see Table 58.1 from PRNT paper) as the guideline rather than estimated energy requirements used by KDOQI. The SDI provides a range of values. These SDI for energy can be adjusted for physical activity level and BMI [1, 3]. If weight gain and linear growth are poor, energy intake should be adjusted towards the higher end of the SDI. Weight and linear growth

Table 58.1 Energy and protein requirements for infants, children and adolescents with CKD2–5D aged 0–18 years

SDI for energy and protein: birth[a] to 18 years			
Month	SDI[b] energy (kcal/kg/day)	SDI protein (g/kg/day)	SDI protein (g/day)
0	93–107	1.52–2.5	8–12
1	93–120	1.52–1.8	8–12
2	93–120	1.4–1.52	8–12
3	82–98	1.4–1.52	8–12
4	82–98	1.3–1.52	9–13
5	72–82	1.3–1.52	9–13
6–9	72–82	1.1–1.3	9–14
10–11	72–82	1.1–1.3	9–15
12	72–120	0.9–1.14	11–14
Year	**SDI energy (kcal/kg/day)**		**SDI protein (g/kg/day)**	**SDI protein (g/day)**
–	Male	Female		
2	81–95[c]	79–92[c]	0.9–1.05	11–15
3	80–82	76–77	0.9–1.05	13–15
4–6	67–93	64–90	0.85–0.95	16–22
7–8	60–77	56–75	0.9–0.95	19–28
9–10	55–69	49–63	0.9–0.95	26–40
11–12	48–63	43–57	0.9–0.95	34–42
13–14	44–63	39–50	0.8–0.9	34–50
15–17	40–55	36–46	0.8–0.9	Male: 52–65 Female: 45–49

For children with poor growth, reference to the SDI for height age may be appropriate. Height age is the age that corresponds to an individual's height when plotted on the 50th centile on a growth chart

[a]Thirty-seven/40 weeks gestation. Premature infants have higher energy and protein requirements. The increased need for these and other nutrients (sodium, potassium, calcium, and phosphorus) must be balanced against the nutritional interventions to control the effects of CKD. This is outside the scope of this CPR

[b]Suggested Dietary Intake (SDI) is based on the Physical Activity Level (PAL) used by the international bodies: 1–3 year PAL 1.4; 4–9 year PAL 1.6; and 10–17 year PAL 1.8. Where guidelines have given a range of energy requirements for different levels of PAL, the lowest PAL has been taken for SDI energy in consideration that children with CKD are likely to have low activity levels

[c]Scientific Advisory Committee on Nutrition [13] reports energy requirements as kcal/day: male 1040 kcal/day; female 932 kcal/day

should be monitored over time and calorie goals should be adjusted according to the child's weight gain or loss and needs for catch-up growth.

There are many factors that can contribute to inadequate caloric intake in children with CKD. Decreased appetite is common. This may be related to alterations in taste perception that can decrease spontaneous intake of food [14]. High fluid intake requirements in polyuric patients or the requirement to take multiple medications can also diminish appetite. Other factors impacting intake include vomiting and gastro-esophageal reflux, delayed gastric emptying and elevation of cytokine levels, including tumor necrosis factor [15]. Changes in hormones that regulate appetite such as leptin and ghrelin can also contribute to decreased intake. Frequent hospitalizations, multiple surgeries, nasogastric tube use and developmental delays impacting feeding with or without the factors previously listed can lead to oral aversion or delayed development of oral feeding skills. Nutrition supplementation should be initiated promptly if a downward trend in weight percentile is noted [3].

Obesity is increasing both in the population of healthy children around the world as well as in the population of children with CKD. In 2015–2016, the prevalence of obesity in the U.S. was 13.9% among preschool-aged children (2–5 years of age), 18.4% among school-aged children (6–11 years of age) and 20.6% among adolescents (12–19 years of age) [3, 16].

The International Pediatric PD Network (IPPN) registry found that children starting chronic peritoneal dialysis (PD) therapy had an overweight/obesity prevalence as high as 19.7% [3, 16, 17]. Nasogastric and gastric tube feeds have been found to be an independent predictor of overweight/obesity, which suggests that there may be over-utilization of supplemental feeds through NG/GT tubes in some patients, leading to an imbalance between caloric intake and energy expenditure [18]. The Chronic Kidney Disease in Children (CKiD) study found the median energy consumption of children with CKD to be higher than recommended in all age groups [19, 20]. With recognition that the epidemic of obesity in the general pediatric population has been linked to increased rates of hypertension, hypercholesterolemia, impaired glucose tolerance, insulin resistance, type 2 diabetes, sleep apnea and asthma, the potential adverse impact of these co-morbidities on children with CKD should be investigated. Future prospective studies should examine any potential link between obesity and poor outcomes, especially with respect to cardiovascular events, so that appropriate dietary and lifestyle modifications can be defined.

Appetite Stimulants

When patients are not meeting nutritional needs, nutrition counseling and calorie supplementation provide the first line of defense; however, complementary strategies for improving appetite and treating or preventing malnutrition have been examined. Megestrol acetate (MA), a synthetic progesterone derivative with appetite stimulating properties, has been studied in the pediatric CKD population. In a retrospective cohort study, Hobbs et al. followed 25 patients with a mean age of 8.9 ± 5.4 years who had demonstrated decreases in BMI and poor weight gain [21]. The mean duration of therapy was 5.4 ± 6.3 months. During treatment, there was a significant increases in BMI ($P < 0.0001$) and weight ($P < 0.0001$). Linear growth continued to improve. MA was well tolerated with the exception of one patient who experienced a side effect of cushingoid features. The authors conclude that MA may provide a safe short-term strategy to improve nutritional status in children with CKD. Possible side effects of MA such as diarrhea, headaches, dizziness, hyperglycemia, hypertension, adrenal suppression, adrenal insufficiency and thromboembolic events have been cited as causes for taking caution in its use in infants with CKD [22]. Cyproheptadine is an antihistamine that increases appetite by exerting an anti-serotoninergic effect on the brain. It has been studied as a potential appetite stimulant in underweight children who are otherwise healthy, children with cystic fibrosis and those with cancer-related cachexia, and has been found to significantly increase caloric intake and height velocity [23, 24]. The appetite stimulating effects of the gut hormone ghrelin suggest that it could be an effective treatment for anorexia in adult CKD patients. This hormone is felt to potentially play a key role in the pathogenesis of protein-energy wasting, inflammation and cardiovascular complications in CKD [25–27]. Ghrelin has been found to acutely induce lipolysis and insulin resistance and could potentially increase the risk of diabetes [28]. Though further studies demonstrating the long-term efficacy of ghrelin are needed, along with evaluation of its use in children, it appears possible that administration of long-acting ghrelin mimetics holds the promise of improving appetite and nutrition in patients with CKD.

Nutritional Supplementation

When voluntary oral intake is low, calories can be maximized by adding concentrated sources of carbohydrate and fat to the diet, choosing calorie dense foods, and limiting calorie-free foods and fluids such as water. Calories can be added to foods using heart-healthy margarines or oils, cream and other fats, sugars, syrups, or commercial carbohydrate modules. Commercial calorie supplements such as milkshakes or energy bars may be useful; however, their phosphorus and potassium content should be taken into consideration. Standard pediatric enteral supplements have fairly high calcium and phosphorus content to support bone growth. These products are contraindicated in children with hyperphosphatemia and/or hyperkalemia. Standard products may be used in combination with low mineral and electrolyte pediatric renal products for these patients. Adult renal products can be used for older children and teens.

For infants with CKD, breastfeeding is the preferred method of feeding. If breastfeeding is not possible or breastmilk is not available, whey-based infant formulas are recommended. If a low potassium, low phosphorus formula option is needed, a low renal solute load infant formula such as Similac PM 60/40®(Abbott Laboratories, Chicago, IL, USA) can be used either to fortify or supplement breastfeeding or on its own. Breastmilk and infant formula should be fortified for infants who require fluid restriction or for those who require more energy or nutrient dense feeds.

To meet requirements, commercial glucose polymer powders, liquid fat products or powdered fat and carbohydrate combination products can be added to infant feedings to increase their standard energy density (20 kcal/oz., 0.67 kcal/mL) as high as 60 kcal/oz. (2 kcal/mL) without significantly increasing electrolyte and mineral content. The choice to add a carbohydrate module, fat, or a combination of both should be made after considering serum glucose and lipid profiles, the presence of malabsorption or chronic respiratory disease (carbohydrate metabolism increases carbon dioxide production), and the cost to the caregivers. When making more than two or three increases in energy density, the distribution of calories from carbohydrate and fat should be kept similar to the base feeding. Unless fat malabsorption is present, "heart-healthy" oils such as corn or canola oil can provide a low-cost option, especially for infants on PD who have hypertriglyceridemia as a consequence of absorbing excess glucose from the dialysate. Powdered products may be preferred over oils, however, due to the difficulty of blending oil with formula and the tendency of the oil to adhere to feeding bottles and feeding tubes. Increasing the caloric density of powdered formulas by concentration (i.e., adding more formula powder or liquid concentrate and less water) is typically not recommended because of the accompanying increase in sodium, potassium, and phosphorus concentrations. If concentration of feeds or if dietary supplements are required, they should be introduced in a gradual manner to optimize acceptance and tolerance. Increases in energy density of 2–4 kcal/oz. are generally better tolerated than larger increases.

If using adult formulas, clinicians should evaluate the protein and electrolyte content of the formula to ensure its safety and appropriateness based on the child's age and weight. Serum magnesium levels require monitoring when using adult renal formulas because their magnesium content is significantly higher than breast milk, infant and pediatric formulas. The acceptance of these products can be improved by mixing them with fruit, and/or ice to make shakes or slush-type drinks.

For children undergoing PD, energy contribution resulting from glucose absorption from peritoneal dialysate solutions may provide an additional 8–26 kcal/kg [2]. The amount of glucose absorbed can vary depending on the mode of dialysis (time on dialysis, cycles and dwell times), the glucose concentration of the dialysate and the characteristics of the peritoneal membrane [3, 5] For underweight children on PD therapy, clinicians need not calculate the calories absorbed from dialysate as this might compromise the nutritional quality of the diet. These calories should be considered as "bonus" calories to help promote weight gain. However, for children on PD who are exceeding weight gain goals, it may be important to take the estimated calorie contribution from PD fluid into account.

Infant, Pediatric and Adult Renal Formula Options

Formula	Distributed by	Used for
Similac PM 60/40®	Abbott Laboratories, Chicago, IL, USA	Infant formula for infants requiring low renal solute load, low electrolyte formula Can be used alone or to supplement breast milk Can be used in combination with other formulas to achieve desired mineral and electrolyte balance
RenaStart®	Vitaflo, USA	Intended for children ages 1 and up For children requiring formula low in protein, calcium, chloride, potassium, phosphorus and vitamin A Can be used in combination with other formulas to achieve desired mineral and electrolyte balance Not intended for use as a sole source of nutrition
Suplena®	Abbott Nutrition	Calorie dense adult nutrition supplement for patients with potassium and phosphorus restrictions
Nepro®	Abbott nutrition	Calorie dense adult nutrition supplement for patients with potassium and phosphorus restrictions who require additional protein

Formula	Distributed by	Used for
NovaSource Renal®	Nestle nutrition	Calorie dense adult nutrition supplement for patients with potassium and phosphorus restrictions
Renalcal®	Nestle nutrition	Calorie dense adult nutrition supplement for patients requiring minimal additional electrolytes and minerals. Can be used in combination with other formulas to achieve desired mineral and electrolyte balance Not intended for use as a soul source of nutrition

Despite efforts to provide adequate calories through oral nutrition supplementation and formula concentration, many factors such as gastroesophageal reflux, vomiting, medication taste, uremia and thirst for large volumes of water due to polyuria can contribute to inadequate oral intake and poor weight gain. For children who are not able to meet their nutrition requirements orally, enteral feeding is recommended.

Enteral Feeding

Nasogastric, gastrostomy, gastrojejunostomy, and jejunostomy tubes have all been used successfully to provide additional nutrition, fluids and/or medications by intermittent bolus or continuous infusion. Nasogastric tubes are a good option for short-term enteral feeding or may be used as a bridge until a long-term tube can be placed, but they are not recommended for long-term use as they are associated with an increase in emesis. Although oral feeding is preferred when possible, tube feeding should be considered for children who are unable to meet their energy needs despite dietary intervention and who are underweight and/or growth delayed. In addition to the benefits of promoting weight gain and growth, enteral feeding can help relieve the stress that many caregivers experience when efforts to provide adequate oral nutrition are failing. If oral intake is limited or absent and enteral feeding is provided, oral stimulation is encouraged in order to promote development of feeding skills and prevent the development of food aversion [1]. Oral stimulation and nonnutritive sucking opportunities should be provided to infants who are completely dependent on tube feeding to help smooth their transition to oral feeding after successful transplantation. Limiting practice with oral feeding can have a significant negative impact on oral motor skill development. Occupational therapists or speech therapists are central in facilitating the development and strengthening of oral feeding skills and preventing or extinguishing oral aversion. Using a multidisciplinary approach, the prospects for a transition to oral feeding post-transplant are good. Even if oral intake improves after transplant, some children will benefit from retaining the G-tube to help ensure adequate hydration and adherence to recommended medications.

The choices of formula and feeding plan are guided by age, serum chemistries, gastrointestinal function, and fluid allowance. In addition, caregiver related factors, including the ability of caregivers to mix and measure formula recipes and financial barriers to accessing ingredients, must be considered. Feedings are initiated and advanced according to pediatric guidelines and tolerance [29]. Volumes and rates that are based on body weight help to avoid intolerance in patients who are underweight or small for their age. Whenever possible, the volume of feeds should be minimized to optimize tol-erance and keep the hours of feeding manageable within the child's daily schedule. Infants should be given intermittent bolus feeds to maintain normal blood sugars. Continuous overnight feeds are generally avoided for infants due to an increased risk of aspiration resulting from vomiting and gastroesophageal reflux associated with uremia. Continuous feedings may be required if the patient's tolerance of bolus feedings is poor. Continuous overnight feeds are generally preferred for children and adolescents to facilitate daytime hunger and optimize oral intake. Reported complications of enteral feeding include tube blockage, tube displacement emesis, leakage around the gastrostomy exit site, skin irritation and itching, exit site infection, hemorrhage and peritonitis [30], When vomiting and gastroesophageal reflux are not responsive to medical therapy, jejunal feeding or a fundoplication may be warranted. To decrease the risk of peritonitis, the placement of gastrostomy, gastrojejunostomy, and jejunostomy tubes should occur before or concomitant with insertion of a PD catheter, whenever possible [31–33]. In particular, percutaneous endoscopic gastrostomy insertion after PD initiation carries a high risk for fungal peritonitis and potential PD failure. Suggested precautions for lowering the risk of peritonitis include antibiotic and antifungal prophylaxis, withholding PD for 2–3 days, and gastrostomy placement by an experienced endoscopy team [9, 33].

Age	Initial hourly infusion	Daily increases	Goal
Continuous feedings			
0–1 year	10–20 mL/h or 1–2 mL/kg/h	5–10 mL/8 h or 1 mL/kg/h	21–54 mL/h or 6 mL/kg/h
1–6 years	20–30 mL/h or 2–3 mL/kg/h	10–15 mL/8 h or 1 mL/kg/h	71–92 mL/h or 4–5 mL/kg/h
6–14 years	30–40 mL/h or 1 mL/kg/h	15–20 mL/8 h or 0.5 mL/kg/h	108–130 mL/h or 3–4 mL/kg/h
>14 years	50 mL/h or 0.5–1 mL/kg/h	25 mL/8 h or 0.4–0.5 mL/kg/h	125 mL/h
Bolus feedings			
0–1 year	60–80 mL every 4 h or 10–15 mL/kg/feed	20–40 mL every 4 h	80–240 mL every 4 h or 20–30 mL/kg/feed
1–6 years	80–120 mL every 4 h or 5–10 mL/kg/feed	40–60 mL every 4 h	280–375 mL every 4 h or 15–20 mL/kg/feed
6–14 years	120–160 mL every 4 h or 3–5 mL/kg/feed	60–80 mL every 4 h	430–520 mL every 4 h or 10–20 mL/kg/feed
>14 years	200 mL every 4 h or 3 mL/kg/feed	100 mL every 4 h	500 mL every 4 h or 10 mL/kg/feed

Parenteral Nutrition

When oral and/or enteral nutrition intake is not sufficient or not tolerated, parenteral nutrition (PN) may be necessary to provide adequate nutrition. When delivering PN in fluid restricted patients, concentrated solutions of amino acids, dextrose, and lipids are required. Energy requirements during PN are 10% lower than enteral requirements because there is no thermal effect of feeding. Standard amino acid solutions (i.e., both essential and nonessential amino acids) are generally used and provided according to daily enteral protein recommendations specific to the child's age and renal replacement therapy. Amino acids, dextrose, and lipids can be advanced according to normal pediatric PN guidelines and serum urea, glucose, and triglyceride concentrations should be monitored. Mineral and electrolyte content should be adjusted to maintain acceptable serum concentrations, and acetate and chloride content should be adjusted to maintain normal acid-base balance. Standard pediatric dosages of parenteral multivitamins and trace elements can be used; the risk of toxicity, especially for vitamin A, is minimal with a daily injectable multivitamin provided that the child has no other exogenous source of vitamin A (i.e., oral diet is minimal).

Intradialytic Parenteral Nutrition (IDPN)

Intradialytic PN (IDPN) is a non-invasive method of delivering supplemental nutrition to malnourished patients on HD. It can be delivered using the HD access during treatments, allowing the volume of fluid to be removed through ultrafiltration. The KDOQI guidelines recommend a trial of IDPN for children receiving maintenance HD who are unable to meet their nutritional requirements through oral or enteral feeding [1]. IDPN is only supplemental and cannot be used as a sole source of nutrition, but it can be used to augment inadequate oral and/or enteral intake in malnourished children. It can provide a significant amount of protein, but will only meet a small percentage of overall caloric needs [34].

There have been several studies of IDPN use in children. Goldstein et al. demonstrated that IDPN could reverse weight loss and promote weight gain within 6 weeks of its initiation in three teenage patients who had experienced a ≥ 10% weight loss over a 3 month period [35]. In this study, IDPN provided 40% of the weekly prescribed protein intake. Orellana et al. examined IDPN in teenaged patients who had lost 10% of their body weight in a 3 month period and were below 90% of their ideal body weight [36]. Of the nine patients studied, seven patients who had organic illness demonstrated an improvement of weight or BMI during the first 5 months of IDPN therapy. The other two patients had psychosocial associated malnutrition and did not demonstrate similar improvement of weight or BMI. The lack of weight gain in these patients was postulated to be due to issues such as depression or inadequate access to food after initiation of IDPN, which may have limited their ability to improve their oral or enteral intake [37].

The optimal composition of IDPN has not been defined, but it is typically designed to provide amino acids in amounts to meet the estimated daily protein needs along with dextrose and 20% or 30% lipid components to increase calorie provision [1]. The goal infusion rate provides optimal caloric intake while avoiding hyperglycemia and hyperlipidemia. It is important to monitor for hyperglycemia, hypokalemia, hypophosphatemia and hyperlipidemia. It has been suggested to limit the glucose infusion rate to ≤9 mg/kg/min. This can help minimize hyperglycemia and prevent refeeding syndrome. Lipid infusions should be limited to no more than 1–2 g/kg/day, starting as low as 0.5 g/kg/day. It is recommended to hold or reduce intralipid (IL) infusions if triglycerides exceed 250 mg/dL [34]. It is also important to be aware of the additional fluid contribution in patients who routinely present with fluid overload between dialysis treatments. As critics of PN, Dudley et al. point to potential problems such as disorders of glucose homeostasis, acid-base, fluid and electrolyte disturbances, impaired renal function, metabolic bone disease and nephrolithiasis. They state that IDPN is not more beneficial than enteral supplements in patients who are compliant with supplementation and have adequate intestinal function.

They do, however, recommend a minimum 3 month trial of IDPN for malnourished children on HD in whom enteral support has not demonstrated benefits or is not viable [38]. Although IDPN is costly, it is recommended for patients who have experienced a weight loss of >10% for three consecutive months and who are below 90% of their ideal body weight (or who have a BMI for height age that is below the fifth percentile) and who have not responded to oral and/or enteral supplementation [1, 34, 37].

The use of IL infusion alone has been studied in children receiving HD as a method of sparing protein degradation and supporting positive nitrogen balance. Hasken et al. found that the provision of 0.5–1 gram/kg IL therapy during each dialysis session could contribute to improvements in serum albumin, predialysis BUN, and nPCR in malnourished pediatric HD patients [39]. The cohort exhibited a 5% weight gain without any changes in cholesterol or triglyceride levels. One benefit from this approach is a reduction in cost compared to delivering full IDPN.

Limiting Energy Intake

Increased appetite and excessive energy intake are common in children treated with high-dose corticosteroid therapy for conditions such as nephrotic syndrome, vasculitis, and renal transplantation. Children and caregivers should receive early education about the potential for overweight and obesity and be provided with strategies for controlling caloric intake, optimizing dietary balance and increasing physical activity to maintain a healthy weight. Overweight is sometimes seen in infants and children on PD as a result of significant dialysate glucose absorption, which is usually greater in young infants because of the enhanced permeability of their peritoneal membrane for small molecules. To help control weight gain in these patients, dialysate calories should be considered when estimating energy intake. Icodextrin dialysate, which contains a poorly absorbed, high-molecular-weight, starch-derived glucose polymer to provide the osmotic force for ultrafiltration, can be used to lower the caloric load without sacrificing clearance of metabolic waste or fluid removal.

Protein

Protein Requirements

Children need to be in positive nitrogen balance to support growth. Along with providing adequate protein, the diet must also provide adequate non-protein calories from fats and carbohydrates in order to prevent protein from being utilized to meet energy needs. It is also critical that the correct balance of amino acids be provided. The PRNT suggests a range for the SDI for protein that is designed to represent the daily amount of protein considered to meet the needs for 97.5% of the population (see Table 58.1) [3]. They suggest that the target for protein intake should be at the upper end of the SDI in order to support optimal growth. The lower end of the SDI is considered to be the minimum safe intake. Children treated with HD or PD may need to have protein intakes above the SDI in order to compensate for protein losses into the dialysate. During periods of peritonitis, there may be an increase in peritoneal protein losses that necessitates a further increase in protein intake. Protein needs may increase due to proteinuria, glucocorticoids, acidosis, other infections and catabolism. In contrast, children who have a persistently high BUN level that is believed to be associated with dietary intake may need their protein intake adjusted towards the lower end of the SDI. If protein intake is excessive, patients may experience increased accumulation of nitrogenous waste products and increased symptoms of uremia. For children following a lacto-ovo vegetarian or vegan diet, it is recommended that the SDI be increased by a factor of 1.2 (lacto-ovo vegetarian) to 1.3 (vegan) to compensate for the lower bioavailability of non-animal protein. The restriction of dietary protein in the early stages of CKD is not recommended as it may increase the risk of malnutrition, protein-energy wasting and poor growth. A high intake of protein may also be detrimental to health as it may negatively impact acid-base balance and urea levels as well as increase phosphorus intake [3]. During the immediate post-transplant period, protein needs are increased by approximately 50% in association with surgical stress and the catabolic effects of steroids. Needs are decreased back to normal recommendations approximately 3 months after transplantation [1].

Modifying Dietary Protein Intake

Despite anorexia and decreased appetite, voluntary protein intake usually exceeds recommendations, which can be acceptable as long as serum urea and phosphate levels are within acceptable limits. Occasionally, protein intake may be inadequate as a result of anorexia, oral-motor problems, low meat intake, or a low phosphorus diet that limits protein-rich dairy foods. Persistently low urea levels (i.e., <50 mg/dL or <18 mmol/L) may be a sign of overall inadequate protein and caloric intake in children receiving dialysis. KDOQI guidelines recommend the use of protein supplements to augment poor oral and/or enteral protein intake [1]. Powdered protein modules (see Table 58.2) can be added to expressed breast milk, infant formula, beverages, pureed foods, cereals, or other moist foods to boost their protein content. Minced or chopped meat, chicken, fish, egg, tofu, or skim milk powder can be added to soups, pasta, or casseroles. High levels of phosphorus often accompany high protein diets and this should be considered when making efforts to increase dietary protein content. Renal nutrition supplements that are rich in protein can also be given orally or enterally to increase protein intake.

Carbohydrates

Prescribed oral, enteral and/or parenteral diets for children with CKD should include a balance of calories from carbohydrates and unsaturated fats within the physiological ranges recommended as the acceptable macronutrient distribution ranges of the DRI [5]. Recommended carbohydrate intake should account for 45–65% of total daily caloric intake, with less than 10% coming from added sugars. In addition, children on PD may receive up to an additional 8 ± 2.8 calories/kg/day from absorption of intraperitoneal dextrose [40, 41]. Diets with excess simple carbohydrates or fats may lead to potential increased risk of chronic diseases such as coronary heart disease, obesity and diabetes. Cardiovascular disease (CVD) is the leading cause of morbidity and death in children with CKD. After transplantation, glucocorticosteroids and immunosuppressive agents such as tacrolimus may cause impaired glucose tolerance, glycosuria, and a relative resistance to insulin that may lead to diabetes. The management of children who have or who develop diabetes should follow the recommendations of the American Diabetes Association, including the avoidance of simple carbohydrates, weight control, and physical activity [42].

Fiber

Obtaining an adequate intake of dietary fiber has traditionally been difficult for patients following a renal diet, but with a shift towards recommending fewer processed and packaged foods, and more whole and plant-based foods, it is easier to include fiber in the diet of children with CKD. Among the benefits of consuming adequate dietary fiber are the reduction of constipation and improvement of hypercholesterolemia with a reduction in total and LDL cholesterol levels as well as a decrease in overall risk of CVD. Recent literature has promoted the benefits of dietary fiber in improving the composition and metabolism of gut microbiota, which has been linked in adults with reducing obesity, diabetes and dyslipidemia [43]. An increased intake of high fiber foods may require an increase in the use of phosphate or potassium binders or an adjustment of the potassium content of the dialysate, but it is important to avoid restricting fiber for the sole purpose of controlling labs. For children who have difficulty meeting their fiber needs from food, fiber supplements can be used to increase fiber intake; however, care should be

Table 58.2 Examples of modular protein additives

Beneprotein powder	Nestle nutrition	Contains 6 g of protein, 25 kcal per 7 g scoop
Complete amino acid mix	Nutricia	Contains 7.8 g protein, 31 kcal per TBSP
Liquid protein fortifier	Abbott nutrition	Contains 1 g protein, 4 kcal per 6 mL

taken to ensure that these supplements do not contain potassium. For patients following a fluid restriction, fiber intake may need to be limited to prevent the hardening of stools and subsequent constipation.

Fat

Dietary fat is an important source of calories for growing children, but high fat diets are also associated with an increased risk of CVD events, a major contributor to morbidity and mortality in patients with kidney disease. The KDOQI guidelines recommended that fat intake account for 25–35% of caloric intake in children above age 4, with slightly higher intake of 30–40% in younger children. [1] Less than 10% of fat intake should come from saturated fats. In the CKiD cohort, while overall energy intake was higher than recommended, the median percentage of caloric intake from fat was within this range [19]. Supplemental fats can be used for children with poor weight gain and fat intake can be safely restricted to the lower end of this range in circumstances of excessive weight gain of dyslipidemia.

CVD is the leading cause of death in adults with childhood onset CKD [44, 45] and dyslipidemia is one of many factors that increase the risk of CVD. Lipid metabolism is disrupted in CKD, with up to 45% of children with in the CKiD cohort having dyslipidemia and dyslipidemia is more prevalent and more severe in children with lower glomerular filtration rate (GFR) and nephrotic range proteinuria [46]. Dyslipidemia in children with CKD has not been directly associated with increased CVD events; however, higher triglyceride levels and lower LDL have been associated with increased carotid artery intima-media thickness and reduced brachial artery flow-mediated dilation, both of which are associated with atherosclerosis [47]. There is consensus that lipid profiles should be monitored annually in children with CKD and that diet and lifestyle modification is warranted for children with dyslipidemia. These modifications include increased physical activity to achieve 5 h of moderate to vigorous physical activity and increasing dietary fiber, fruit, and vegetable intake while decreasing intake of saturated and trans fats. Increased intake of monounsaturated and polyunsaturated fatty acids (e.g. oils from canola, corn, flaxseed, safflower, soy, olives, and peanuts) should be encouraged as total and LDL cholesterol are decreased with increased intake.

Because CVD events are rare, even in high-risk children, there have not been sufficient data to show a decrease in CVD risk with statin therapy in children. However, while KDOQI/KDIGO guidelines do not recommend lipid lowering pharmacotherapy for children with CKD [48], the American Heart Association (AHA) [49] recommends that children with increased risk of CVD have target triglyceride level <150 mg/dL and LDL <100 mg/dL for highest risk, which includes end-stage renal disease (ESRD), and <130 mg/dL for moderate risk, which includes CKD. The AHA recommends initiation of lipid lowering therapy if these targets cannot be achieved with 3 months of diet and lifestyle modification.

Consumption of omega-3 fatty acids (ALA, EPA, and DHA) can have beneficial effects on cardiovascular risk factors including inflammation, thrombosis, triglycerides, vascular and cardiac hemodynamics and arrhythmias [50]. Omega-3 fatty acids can be found in fatty fish such as tuna mackerel, trout, salmon, herring, sardines, and anchovies. Adequate intake of omega-3 fatty acids is 0.5 gm for children less than 1 year and rises to 1.6 g for males and 1.1 gm for non-pregnant females by age 14. Most individuals meet this level of intake through dietary ingestion, and there has not been sufficient evidence to recommend supplementation in treatment of hypertriglyceridemia.

Omega-3 fatty acid supplementation has been shown to result in modest improvement in lipid profile in children on dialysis, but there has not been convincing evidence that supplementation mitigates CV risk in adults or children with CKD [51, 52]. A recent meta-analysis of studies evaluating the effects of omega-3 polyunsaturated fats in adult patients with CKD showed a modestly reduced risk of CV events in patients on dialysis, but no benefit in regards to reduction of CV events, progression to ESRD, mortality, or graft rejection in patients with pre-dialysis CKD [53].

Potassium

The PRNT recently provided updated recommendations for management of potassium intake in children with CKD 2–5 [54], recognizing that there are limited data to support many of the recommendations. Maintenance of normal serum potassium levels depends on potassium intake, urinary potassium excretion and transcellular shifts of potassium, which can happen rapidly in response to increased potassium intake, acid-base disturbances, and insulin. Because 98% of total body potassium is intracellular, even small transcellular shifts can result in significant changes in serum potassium levels. Dyskalemias are associated with cardiac arrhythmias and muscle dysfunction and can be fatal if severe and not treated emergently. Urinary potassium excretion decreases as GFR decreases, and with the use of medications such as calcineurin inhibitors and renin-angiotensin-aldosterone inhibitors. Daily dialysis (either HD or PD) will typically provide sufficient potassium clearance to permit a diet without potassium restriction; however, children with more standard HD prescriptions or with CKD 4–5 not yet on dialysis often require dietary potassium restriction. High dietary potassium has been associated with increased mortality in adult patients on dialysis [55]. Recommendations for dietary potassium intake should target normal serum potassium levels and must account for all of these contributing factors. The KDIGO recommended potassium restriction is 30–40 mg/kg/day for older children and 40–120 mg/kg/day for younger children, but there are minimal data to support this recommendation [1].

Sources of dietary potassium intake can be difficult to identify on dietary history and bioavailability of ingested potassium varies widely. Most dietary potassium comes from breast milk, infant formula, milk, potatoes, tomatoes and other fruits and vegetables. Providers must also ask about salt substitutes, which are commonly used to avoid high sodium intake. A food is considered to have high potassium content if it contains >200 mg/serving. Restricting high potassium foods or soaking high potassium foods and rinsing them prior to ingestion reduces potassium intake. For infants or children on enteral

formula, specific renal formulas with low potassium formulas can substitute for standard formula. In older children, high potassium foods such as oranges, bananas, potatoes and potato products, tomatoes and tomato products, legumes, lentils, yogurt and chocolate should be limited. Additional carbohydrate or fat additive may be required to achieve adequate caloric intake while limiting potassium intake [21]. If dietary restriction is insufficient to control elevated serum potassium levels, potassium binders such as sodium polystyrene sulfonate or patiromer can be used to prevent hyperkalemia; however, both binders have gastrointestinal side effects that must be monitored. These binders can be given orally or enterally. Alternately, fluids such as nutritional supplements and formulas can be pre-treated with the binder to reduce their potassium content. The insoluble resin is allowed to sit in the formula for 30 min and potassium is exchanged for sodium (SPS) or calcium (patiromer). The potassium-depleted formula can then be decanted from the sediment at the bottom of the container. Along with the decrease in potassium content, the decanted portion of formula may also affect concentration of other electrolytes and minerals [56, 57].

Hypokalemia occurs in children who have excessive potassium losses due to frequent dialysis or high urinary potassium excretion due to renal tubular dysfunction. Severe hypokalemia requires emergent intravenous (IV) supplementation to avoid cardiac arrhythmia. Dietary increases in potassium intake and cessation of binders is usually sufficient to correct the hypokalemia chronically.

Sodium

Recommendations for sodium intake depend on the specific cause and severity of CKD. Serum sodium cannot be used to differentiate between sodium excess and sodium depletion because it reflects water balance rather than total body sodium. For children with salt-wasting syndromes and associated polyuria, including obstructive uropathy, renal dysplasia, tubular disease, and polycystic kidney disease, urinary sodium losses commonly exceed dietary sodium intake, resulting in need for sodium supplementation. Conversely, for children with glomerular disease or oliguria/anuria, high sodium intake is associated with fluid overload and hypertension.

Salt restriction in adults with CKD is associated with lower blood pressure and proteinuria, both risk factors for CKD progression and CV mortality, but studies evaluating the relationship between sodium intake and those outcomes have been variable [58]. For children who are pre-hypertensive, hypertensive or edematous, restriction of daily sodium intake to 1500 mg/day for children aged 2–3 years, 1900 mg/day for children aged 4–8 years, 2200 mg/day for children aged 9–13 years and 2300 mg/day for adolescents aged ≥14 years is recommended [1]. This can be difficult to achieve, but families can start by limiting processed foods, canned foods, and fast foods, which are all high in sodium. Families should be taught to read nutritional labels and strategies to increase consumption of fresh foods that are flavorful and appealing to the child.

For children with excessive sodium losses in the urine or through PD, sodium supplementation is required to prevent sodium depletion, volume depletion, and impaired growth. Supplementation should begin with a goal of providing at least the age related DRI of sodium and chloride and can be adjusted as needed [1]. Supplements can be given separately or added to breast milk or infant formula, provided that the infant reliably receives the full volume of breast milk of formula. As infants transition to table food, dietary sodium intake increases and adjustments to sodium chloride supplementation should be made accordingly.

For patients with calcium-based kidney stone formation, decreased sodium intake has been shown to decrease urinary calcium excretion, but has not definitively been proven to reduce the risk of calcium-based stones [59].

Salt and Sugar in Hypertension

Regulation of total body sodium content is an important homeostatic mechanism for maintaining normal blood pressure—as blood pressure rises, urinary sodium excretion increases. The underlying mechanisms resulting in the pre-

sumed causal relationship between higher dietary sodium intake and higher blood pressure have not been fully described. In studies in adults, lower dietary sodium intake is associated with lower blood pressure and lower CVD risk. Higher sodium intake is associated with higher systolic blood pressure and risk for pre-hypertension and hypertension in U.S. children and adolescents [60] and reduction in sodium intake over time was temporally associated with a decreased incidence of hypertension among children participating in the NHANES study [61]. A meta-analysis of studies assessing the effect of sodium restriction for 2 weeks or longer on children with elevated blood pressure showed reduction in blood pressure on a lower sodium diet [62]. Based on these data and consistent data from adult studies [63] indicating improved outcomes at lower sodium intake, the CDC recommends that dietary intake of sodium should be restricted to 2300 mg for adults and 1500 mg for children with hypertension. Epidemiologic studies have linked fructose intake with hypertension and elevated uric acid [64]. Reduction in sugar-added beverages consumption is strongly associated with reduction in blood pressure [65]. Indeed, an important component of the DASH (dietary approaches to stop hypertension) diet is limitation of added sugar (fructose).

Fluid Intake

Similar to sodium intake, recommendations for target daily fluid intake should be adjusted based on the child's clinical condition, taking into account the underlying cause of CKD, the volume of urine output, the GFR, and the presence of edema and hypertension. Infants and children with polyuria due to nephrogenic diabetes insipidus or salt losing nephropathy, typically have high obligatory fluid output and require high fluid intake to prevent chronic dehydration, malaise, and poor growth. High fluid intake may also be recommended for children with nephrolithiasis or urinary tract infections to prevent recurrence. There is currently a study underway to evaluate the potential benefit of prescribed increase in fluid intake on progression of renal disease in adult patients with autosomal dominant polycystic kidney disease [66]. After kidney transplantation, high fluid intake is prescribed to maintain adequate perfusion of the transplanted kidney, to replace high urine volume, and regulate intravascular volume. For all of these conditions, water and calorie free fluids are encouraged to prevent excessive weight gain and hyperglycemia.

Once CKD progresses to oliguria or anuria, fluid limitation is often required to avoid fluid overload, hypertension, and subsequent cardiac, cerebrovascular, renal and respiratory complications. Children on PD may not need fluid restriction because higher glucose concentration dialysates can increase ultrafiltration to maintain euvolemia. Fluid limits are more often needed for patients on HD to limit interdialytic fluid gain to less than 5% of dry weight between dialysis sessions. The prescribed total fluid intake is based on insensible fluid losses, urine output, ultrafiltration capacity, other losses, and current amount of fluid overload. Insensible water losses for children and adolescents are 20 mL/kg/day or 400 mL/m^2 with maximum estimates of 800 mL/ day in adults [1], and can be 1.5–2 times higher in neonates and preterm infants. In anuric children, fluid intake above this threshold can lead to hypervolemia. Higher interdialytic weight gain is associated with higher blood pressure and left ventricular mass index in children on dialysis [67] and higher ultrafiltration rates is associated with increased mortality for adults on HD [68]. These data emphasize the importance of fluid restriction between dialysis treatments.

Limiting fluid intake can be difficult for children and their families and requires careful education about reducing sodium intake and about the water content of many fruits and vegetables.

Calcium and Phosphorous

Calcium and Phosphorous Intake

Appropriate calcium and phosphorous management is critical to maintaining normal bone health and growth while reducing the risk of extraosseous calcification in the kidneys and vascular system. Elevated serum phosphorus levels occur early in CKD and can lead to elevated levels of parathyroid hormone (PTH) and FGF23, which are associated

with high bone turnover calcium deposition in organs and arteries. The PNRT and KDOQI recommend daily intake of calcium and phosphorous within age adjusted ranges for healthy children, with a goal of maintaining normal serum calcium and phosphorous levels [68]. Periodic food frequency questionnaires and/or a 3-day food diary can be used to assess dietary phosphorous intake in children with CKD. Absorption of calcium and phosphate varies by food source and vitamin D status.

Calcium

Children have higher calcium requirements than adults due to increasing skeletal mass, particularly during the periods of most rapid growth including infancy and puberty. Suggested dietary intake of calcium, including from dietary and calcium based phosphate binders, should be 1–2 times the standard daily intaking, ranging from 220 mg/day in infancy to 1300 mg/day in adolescence [69]. Most dietary calcium comes from breast milk, formula, cow's milk, other dairy products and cereals. Absorption of calcium is affected by bioavailability. Abnormal bone mineralization is seen at all stages of CKD, with increasing frequency at lower GFR [70, 71]. Increased calcium intake in childhood is associated with increased bone density [72–74] and phosphate binder usage (primarily calcium containing), was found to be protective for incident fracture in the CKiD cohort [71].

Patients with insufficient calcium intake should be encouraged to consume food with high endogenous calcium content (such as dairy products) as well as calcium-fortified foods. This must be balanced with the goal of limiting phosphorous intake, which is also high in many dairy products. If dietary intake alone cannot meet the SDI, calcium supplementation should be recommended, and should be taken between meals to maximize absorption. Salts of calcium such as calcium gluconate, lactate, acetate, or carbonate are usually well tolerated by children and can be given in doses of less than 500 mg at a time to optimize absorption. Calcium chloride should not be used to supplement patients with CKD as it may cause metabolic acidosis, and calcium citrate should be avoided due to concerns for increased aluminum absorption [1].

Serum calcium should be maintained in the normal range for age. When hypocalcemia is present, vitamin D supplementation should also be considered to increase intestinal calcium absorption, as low vitamin D levels impair calcium absorption [75]. Patients with hypocalcemia and persistently elevated PTH levels may require calcium intake above the 200% SDI upper limit, and this should be monitored closely to avoid hypercalcemia. Hypercalcemia should also be avoided as it can lead to extraosseous calcification. In general, mild to moderate hypercalcemia can be treated with serial reduction in calcium supplementation, calcium-based phosphate binders, and vitamin D supplements. A variety of calcium-free phosphorous binders (i.e. sevelamer) are available as substitutes. In addition, synthetic vitamin D analogues such as paricalcitol and doxercalciferol may have less hypercalcemic effect. For patients on HD or PD, dialysate calcium content can be decreased.

After transplantation, glucocorticoid therapy can induce osteoporosis; therefore, calcium supplementation may be needed for children who are unable to meet the SDI for calcium through dietary intake alone.

Phosphorous

Elevated serum phosphorous levels occur relatively early in CKD progression due to decreased urinary phosphorous excretion. This stimulates higher levels of the phosphaturic hormones PTH and FGF-23, which results in high bone turnover with bone calcium loss. This leads to calcium deposition in organs and small vessels.

Targeting a normal serum phosphorous for age and decreasing dietary phosphorous intake, even prior to onset of hyperphosphatemia, can help prevent both elevated serum phosphorous and PTH levels. Dietary phosphorous intake should be limited to the SDI for age starting early in CKD, with more strict limitations to the lower limit of SDI as CKD progresses, or in the setting of ongoing hyperphosphatemia or hyperparathyroidism [69]. For infants and formula fed children, whey based infant formulas and specific renal formulas with low phosphorous content can be used to reduce phosphorous intake. For children who are not formula fed, attention to sources of dietary phosphorous is particularly important, as intestinal phosphate absorption is affected by the source of phosphorous. Inorganic dietary phosphorous, found in processed foods, has much higher absorption (up to 100%) compared to phosphorous found in meats, fish, dairy, vegetables, and other plant-based foods.

For many children, dietary restriction is insufficient to control serum phosphate levels, and mealtime phosphate binders are required to impair intestinal phosphorous absorption to achieve normal serum phosphorous levels. Calcium-based binders (calcium carbonate and calcium acetate) are preferred in infants and young children due to their higher calcium requirements. Non-calcium based binders (e.g. sevelamer carbonate) can be added if calcium based binders are insufficient to achieve normal phosphorous levels. Sevelamer carbonate may also be used to pre-treat breast milk, infant formula or cow's milk in order to reduce phosphate content [76].

Despite the importance of normalization of serum phosphorous, achieving control of serum phosphorous levels is particularly challenging. For example, the majority of subjects in the CKiD study ingest more phosphorous than recommended, especially in the younger age group [19].

For children with renal tubular disorders and associated urinary phosphorous wasting or those with intensified dialysis regimens resulting in hypophosphatemia, phosphorous supplementation is often required as hypophosphatemia is associated with morbidity, mortality, and poor growth.

Acid Load

Progressive renal dysfunction resulting in decreased urinary ammonia excretion despite stable acid generation leads to increased prevalence of acidosis in children with impaired renal function. In the CkiD cohort, 25% of children with CKD had serum bicarbonate <22 mEq/L [77]. Children with tubular dysfunction from dysplasia or inherited tubular defects are at higher risk for acidosis. In the 4C cohort, 43–60% of children had serum bicarbonate <22 mmol/L [78]. Normalization of acid-base status in children with glomerular disease has been associated with reduced progression of kidney disease [79]. While dietary acid load is more difficult to quantify, increased urinary acid excretion, a correlate of dietary acid intake, has been associated with CKD progression and hypertension in small pediatric studies [80, 81]. Reducing dietary acid load by increasing intake of fruits and vegetables may improve acidosis, minimize requirement for alkali supplementation, and slow kidney disease progression.

Vitamins, Minerals and Trace Elements

Children with CKD and ESRD are at increased risk for vitamin and mineral deficiencies due to multiple nutritional factors, including anorexia, poor intake, dietary restrictions, abnormal renal metabolism, drug-nutrient interactions, and poor intestinal absorption. In addition, there are concerns about potential losses of water-soluble vitamins during dialysis. Thiamine (B1), pyridoxine (B6), folate (B9), and vitamin C are all small to middle-sized molecules that are easily cleared on HD. PD is thought to result in less diffusive clearance of these molecules, but higher protein losses may result in greater losses of protein bound vitamins and trace elements [82]. A recent study of adults on thrice weekly HD and typical doses of vitamin B and C supplementation (given after dialysis), showed that almost all patients had high vitamin B levels at baseline, while over 80% of patients had normal vitamin C levels. When the dose of supplementation was reduced by 50%, vitamin B levels generally stayed normal; however, there were significant losses of B vitamins into the dialysate effluent [83]. While vitamin C clearance during dialysis is hypothesized, no difference in vitamin C levels over time were seen in adult patients receiving three times weekly versus six times weekly in the Frequent Hemodialysis Network Study [84]. Children with protein energy malnutrition may be particularly susceptible to thiamine deficiency because it is extensively protein bound.

Current practice, consistent with KDOQI guidelines, is to provide vitamin and trace element supplementation for children on dialysis to achieve DRI for healthy children, with the goal of avoiding complications of vitamin insufficiencies. There are minimal pediatric data available to support this recommendation [82]. Thiamine deficiency is rare in children, but can lead to severe lactic acidosis and neurologic complications in the acute phase; therefore, supplementation to avoid deficiency is recommended [82]. Folate (B9), pyridoxine (B6), and cobalamin (B12) supplementation may mitigate hyperhomocysteinemia, which potentially reduces cardiovascular risk [85]. In addition, folate deficiency can result in erythropoietin resistant anemia that can be corrected with supplementation [86].

Vitamin C is thought to be low in patients with CKD due to decreased intake to accommodate low potassium and low oxalate diets, low dose vitamin C supplementation due to concern for conversion to oxalate, and clearance of vitamin C during dialysis. Scurvy has been reported in a pediatric PD patient.

There are no pediatric renal vitamins available in the US. Adult B and C vitamin formulations can be used in older children and adolescent patients. Younger children can be prescribed liquid adult vitamins or can be offered split doses of adult renal vitamins or every other day dosing. These preparations contain no more that 6–100 mg of vitamin C to avoid oxalate retention.

Trace Elements

Trace elements are important components of many enzymatic pathways and proteins. Deficiencies of these micronutrients may have major adverse effects in growing children. Dialysis can lead to the accumulation of trace elements either because of insufficient elimination or because of contamination. It can alternately lead to excessive removal of trace elements. Zinc and selenium contents vary by formula type and, for breast-fed infants, are largely determined by maternal diet [82].

Low dietary intake of copper has been noted in children receiving dialysis and the KDOQI guidelines recommend monitoring intake every 4–6 months [1]. Copper deficiency can cause anemia and neutropenia. Clinical signs of copper overload should also be assessed, as excess copper is associated with CKD [1].

Selenium acts as a cofactor for oxidation and reduction enzymes such as glutathione peroxidase. Low serum selenium levels have been found in patients with CKD and those receiving dialysis, although it is not removed by dialysis. Selenium depletion appears most likely in critically ill patients on continuous renal replacement therapy.

Zinc deficiency is relatively common in adult dialysis patients, resulting from poor dietary intake and removal by HD because it is not protein bound [82]. Zinc deficiency can present as failure to thrive, dermatitis, and inflammatory disease in children. Monitoring of trace elements in dialysis may be warranted, but there are no specific recommendations for children.

Supplemental oral or IV iron is usually required by all children on erythropoietin-stimulating agents to avoid depletion of iron stores and to maintain target hemoglobin concentrations. Current KDIGO guidelines recommend iron administration during erythropoietin therapy to maintain transferrin saturation greater than 20% and serum ferritin greater than 100 ng/mL to ensure adequate iron stores [87]. Iron stores in patients with kidney disease may be depleted by frequent blood draws and chronic blood loss in the gastrointestinal tract and HD circuit. In addition, iron metabolism is disrupted in patients with advanced CKD and other chronic inflammatory conditions due to increased levels of the regulatory protein hepcidin. Hepcidin prevents duodenal iron absorption and movement of iron into the circulation, making iron unavailable for erythropoiesis. This is thought to explain resistance to enteral iron supplementation for patients with CKD.

Enteral or parenteral iron supplementation are options. Oral supplementation at a dose of 3–6 mg/kg of elemental iron daily is often successful, particularly for patients with lower serum ferritin levels and who are earlier in their CKD course. For patients with significant iron losses on dialysis and with hepcidin mediated iron deficiency (i.e. those with normal or high ferritin levels), IV iron supplementation is preferred. There are several formulations of intravenous iron available, with the more recently developed formulations less likely to result in hypotension [88]. IV iron can be given as a loading dose with serial infusions or as maintenance therapy on a weekly to monthly basis depending on patient need. There are limited data on the use of IV iron in children with CKD and ESRD. Studies including adults on HD, demonstrated higher dose IV iron supplementation was non-inferior, with a statistical trend towards superiority for a composite endpoint of mortality and cardiovascular morbidity ascribed to lower exogenous erythropoietin dose [89]. In this population, higher dose IV iron supplementation was also found to be safe, without an increased risk of infection [90].

Vitamin D

Vitamin D is obtained from the diet (D2, ergocalciferol) and exposure to ultraviolet light (D3, cholecalciferol). The liver hydroxylates the vitamin D precursors to form 25-hydroxy vitamin D (25[OH]D). A second hydroxylation occurs in the kidney, leading to the formation of 1,25 dihydroxyvitamin D (1,25(OH)2D), calcitriol). Calcitriol regulates intestinal calcium absorption, bone resorption and renal excretion of phosphate and calcium. As GFR declines, plasma concentrations of calcitriol decrease. This leads to a decrease in intestinal calcium absorption and reduced renal phosphate excretion. The result is hypocalcemia and hyperphosphatemia, which stimulate PTH and FGF-23 secretion, leading to mineral bone disorder.

Clinical practice guidelines focused on optimizing bone health in children with CKD recommend defining sufficient 25[OH]D levels as >75 nmol/L (>30 ng/mL) and supplementation with vitamin D (cholecalciferol or ergocalciferol) for children with CKD who have levels below this threshold [90]. This is based on data demonstrating that children with CKD who were treated with ergocalciferol have longer time prior to developing hyperparathyroidism [91]. In addition, Stein et al. [92] reported 100 pediatric CKD patients and found a high prevalence of hyperparathyroidism early in CKD which was associated with lower 25[OH]D levels, independent of calcitriol level. There may also be a relationship between vitamin D deficiency in CKD and CVD as measured by arterial stiffness and LVMI [93, 94].

Low 25[OH]D levels have been documented in patients with nephrotic syndrome and can be at least partially attributed to loss of vitamin D binding proteins in the urine. Supplementation with vitamin D3 in 43 children with nephrotic syndrome showed improved 25[OH]D vitamin D level. There was no change in bone mineral content or bone mineral density at 6 months [95]. There is a risk of nephrocalcinosis and urolithiasis with excess vitamin D supplementation, so levels should be monitored periodically.

For children with PTH elevated above target range for CKD stage, treatment with vitamin D analogs such as calcitriol [96] reduce PTH levels; however, the effect on bone outcomes including, fracture and growth is less clear. Daily calcitriol, at the lowest effective dose, with monitoring for hypercalcemia, is recommended.

Other Fat-Soluble Vitamins

Vitamin A is best known for its effects on vision. Vitamin A toxicity can cause dry skin, pruritus, weight loss, anorexia, taste disturbances, bone and joint pain, hypercalcemia, and neuropsychiatric symptoms [97]. Vitamin A is not removed by dialysis and patients with CKD and ESRD have been found to exhibit elevated serum levels without supplementation [1]. The total intake for vitamin A should be limited to the DRI and supplementation should only be used in patients with very low dietary intake. Vitamin K and E, the other primary fat soluble vitamins, are not removed by dialysis and intake should be limited to the DRI to avoid toxicity, which is less common for these fat soluble vitamins than for vitamin A.

Transplantation

When caring for children after kidney transplantation, it is important to view the post-transplant period as a dynamic phase of CKD. Factors such as electrolyte balance, linear growth, and weight gain remain important components of nutrition assessment. The primary goal of medical nutrition therapy post kidney transplant is to promote optimal nutrition status while helping patients offset or minimize the side effects of immunosuppressive medications. These side effects may include protein catabolism, hypertension, hyperglycemia, hyperkalemia, dyslipidemias, hypophosphatemia, hypomagnesemia, osteoporosis, increased infection risk and gastrointestinal disturbances. Patients should be closely monitored for changes in kidney function resulting from recurrence of disease, rejection episodes, lapses in taking medication, and gradual decline in graft function.

Immediately post-transplant, patients may require restrictions of sodium, potassium, phosphorus and/or fluid until full graft function is established. Assuming the kidney is functioning well, a balanced, heart healthy diet is recommended. Intake of saturated, trans-fats and sodium should be limited, although some toddlers may require sodium supplementation. For children receiving tube feeds, formula can typically be changed to a standard pediatric variety. Energy needs should be established based on age and gender, starting at 100% estimated energy requirement and adjusting for activity and body size [1]. Protein needs are increased for the first 3 months post-transplant to allow for healing of the surgical site. Subsequently, needs should be based on DRI or recommended daily allowance for age and gender.

Hydration is critical after transplant to ensure adequate perfusion of the graft. For infants and toddlers, 2500 mL/ 1.0 m^2 body surface area is recommended. For older children and adolescents, 1.5–4 L/day may be required [98]. Sugar-free, caffeine-free beverages should be encouraged. It is important to educate patients and families on strategies for ensuring that fluid goals are met. Cell phone apps, water bottles, watch alarms or incentive charts may all be helpful in reminding patients to drink throughout the day. Tube fed patients who are able to transition successfully to taking nutrition orally may continue to require the g-tube in order to meet fluid goals.

Children will benefit from a nutrition assessment to evaluate if their diets are balanced. Children who lack variety in their diets should be encouraged to take a daily multivitamin. Phosphorus and magnesium supplementation are often required immediately post-transplant as these minerals are often wasted in the urine. Calcium intake should be evaluated, and supplements should be encouraged if dietary intake is poor, particularly for children taking corticosteroids as part of their immunosuppressive protocol. Vitamin D levels should be evaluated routinely as supplementation should be provided if insufficiency or deficiency is present.

Weight management can be particularly difficult for children who are taking steroids as part of their post-transplant immunosuppressive regimen. The steroid-induced increase in appetite along with the liberalization of diet restrictions that may have been present prior to transplant can lead to rapid weight gain and obesity. Education on diet and lifestyle modification should be provided and repeated in order to help prevent this outcome.

Food safety and hygiene are important in order to prevent food borne illness in this immunosuppressed population. Families should be specifically instructed about washing hands and food preparation surfaces, separating foods to avoid cross-contamination, prompt refrigeration of foods and heating foods to the proper temperatures to kill pathogens. Additionally, foods such as grapefruit and pomegranate should be avoided because they can alter the absorption of certain medications, including some immunosuppressants and calcium-channel blockers.

Potential side effects of common transplant medications	Nutrition therapy
HTN/edema	Low-sodium diet
Hypotension	Encourage increased fluid intake, sodium if appropriate
Hyperkalemia/ hypomagnesemia/ hypophosphatemia	Adjust mineral intake with diet and/or with supplementation
Hyperglycemia	Carbohydrate control/ Insulin

Potential side effects of common transplant medications	Nutrition therapy
Diarrhea/constipation	Add fiber/fluid/physical activity Polyethylene glycol/Docusate Sodium prescribed when needed
Nausea/vomiting	Small frequent meals/ medication if needed
Anemia	Supplement with iron
Growth suppression	Ensure adequate intake of protein, calories Growth hormone may be warranted but is typically note used within the first year post transplant
Osteoporosis	Calcium/Vitamin D, weight bearing exercise
Increased appetite	Calorie control, exercise
Hyperlipidemia	Low fat diet, exercise, Omega-3 supplementation
Anorexia	Small frequent meals

References

1. National Kidney Foundation Kidney Disease Outcomes Quality Initiative. K/DOQI clinical proactive guideline for nutrition in children with CKD: 2008 update. Am J Kindey Dis. 2009;53(3):S1–S124.
2. National Kidney Foundation Dialysis Outcome Qualtiy Initiative. Clinical practice guidelines for nutrition in chronic renal failure. K/DOQI Am J Kidney Dis. 2000;35(6 Suppl 2):S1–140.
3. Shaw V, Polderman N, Renken-Terhaerdt J, Paglialonga F, Oosterveld M, Tuokkola J, et al. Energy and protein requirements for children with CKD stages 2–5 and on dialysis-clinical practice recommendations from the Pediatric Renal Nutrition Taskforce. Pediatr Nephrol. 2020;35(3):519–31.
4. Roman B. Nutrition management of pediatric chornic kidney disease. Support Line. 2013;35(2):12–21.
5. Mak RH, Cheung WW, Zhan JY, Shen Q, Foster BJ. Cachexia and protein-energy wasting in children with chronic kidney disease. Pediatr Nephrol. 2012;27(2):173–81.
6. Rees L, Jones H. Nutritional management and growth in children with chronic kidney disease. Pediatr Nephrol. 2013;28(4):527–36.
7. Prevention CDC. Growth Charts—WHO Child Growth Standards 2010 [updated 2010/09/09. Available from: https://www.cdc.gov/growthcharts/ who_charts.htm.
8. Corkins KG. Nutrition-focused physical examination in pediatric patients. Nutr Clin Pract. 2015;30(2):203–9.

9. Nelms CL, Shaw V, Greenbaum LA, Anderson C, Desloovere A, Haffner D, Oosterveld MJS, Paglianlonga F, Polderman N, Qizalbash RL, Renken-Terhaerdt J, Tuokkola J, Walle JV, Shroff R, Warady BA. Assessment of nutritional status in chidlren with chronic kidney diseases—clinical practice recommendations from the Pediatric Rneal Nutrition Taskforce. Pediatrc Nephrol. 2021;36(4):995–1010.

10. Service USDoAER. USDA ERS—Food Security and Nutrition Assistance 2020 [updated 2020/12/16. Available from: https://www.ers.usda.gov/data-products/ag-and-food-statistics-charting-the-essentials/food-security-and-nutrition-assistance.

11. Rees L, Mak RH. Nutrition and growth in children with chronic kidney disease. Nat Rev Nephrol. 2011;7(11):615–23.

12. Srivaths PR, Sutherland S, Alexander S, Goldstein SL. Two-point normalized protein catabolic rate overestimates nPCR in pediatric hemodialysis patients. Pediatr Nephrol. 2013;28(5):797–801.

13. Scientific Advisory Committee on Nutrition (2011) Dietary reference values for energy https://assets.publishing.service.gov.uk/government/uploads/system/uploads/attachment_data/file/339317/SACN_Dietary_Reference_Values_for_Energy.pdf. Accessed February 8, 2022.

14. Armstrong JE, Laing DG, Wilkes FJ, Kainer G. Smell and taste function in children with chronic kidney disease. Pediatr Nephrol. 2010;25(8):1497–504.

15. Foster BJ, McCauley L, Mak RH. Nutrition in infants and very young children with chronic kidney disease. Pediatr Nephrol. 2012;27(9):1427–39.

16. Hales CM, Carroll MD, Fryar CD, Ogden CL. Prevalence of obesity among adults and youth: United States, 2015–2016. NCHS Data Brief. 2017;288:1–8.

17. Schaefer F, Benner L, Borzych-Duzalka D, Zaritsky J, Xu H, Rees L, et al. Global variation of nutritional status in children undergoing chronic peritoneal dialysis: a longitudinal study of the International Pediatric Peritoneal Dialysis Network. Sci Rep. 2019;9(1):4886.

18. Rees L, Azocar M, Borzych D, Watson AR, Buscher A, Edefonti A, et al. Growth in very young children undergoing chronic peritoneal dialysis. J Am Soc Nephrol. 2011;22(12):2303–12.

19. Hui WF, Betoko A, Savant JD, Abraham AG, Greenbaum LA, Warady B, et al. Assessment of dietary intake of children with chronic kidney disease. Pediatr Nephrol. 2017;32(3):485–94.

20. Chen W, Ducharme-Smith K, Davis L, Hui WF, Warady BA, Furth SL, et al. Dietary sources of energy and nutrient intake among children and adolescents with chronic kidney disease. Pediatr Nephrol. 2017;32(7):1233–41.

21. Hobbs DJ, Bunchman TE, Weismantel DP, Cole MR, Ferguson KB, Gast TR, et al. Megestrol acetate improves weight gain in pediatric patients with chronic kidney disease. J Ren Nutr. 2010;20(6):408–13.

22. Williams JL, Perius M, Humble A, Sigler D, Urbanes A, Shapiro HS. Effect of megestrol acetate on the nutritional status of malnourished hemodialysis patients. J Ren Nutr. 1997;7(4):231.

23. Mahachoklertwattana P, Wanasuwankul S, Poomthavorn P, Choubtum L, Sriprapradang A. Short-term cyproheptadine therapy in underweight children: effects on growth and serum insulin-like growth factor-I. J Pediatr Endocrinol Metab. 2009;22(5):425–32.

24. Sant'Anna AMGA, Hammes PS, Porporino M, Martel C, Zygmuntowiez C, Ramsay M. Use of cyproheptadine in young children with feeding difficulties and poor growth in a pediatric feeding program. J Pediatr Gastr Nutr. 2014;59(5):674–8.

25. Gunta SS, Mak RH. Ghrelin and leptin pathophysiology in chronic kidney disease. Pediatr Nephrol. 2013;28(4):611–6.

26. Wynne K, Giannitsopoulou K, Small CJ, Patterson M, Frost G, Ghatei MA, et al. Subcutaneous ghrelin enhances acute food intake in malnourished patients who receive maintenance peritoneal dialysis: a randomized, placebo-controlled trial. J Am Soc Nephrol. 2005;16(7):2111–8.

27. Ashby DR, Ford HE, Wynne KJ, Wren AM, Murphy KG, Busbridge M, et al. Sustained appetite improvement in malnourished dialysis patients by daily ghrelin treatment. Kidney Int. 2009;76(2):199–206.

28. Mak RH, Ikizler AT, Kovesdy CP, Raj DS, Stenvinkel P, Kalantar-Zadeh K. Wasting in chronic kidney disease. J Cachexia Sarcopenia Muscle. 2011;2(1):9–25.

29. Pediatric Nutrition Care Manual: Academy of Nutrition and Dietetics; 2017. Available from: https://www.eatrightstore.org/product-type/subscriptions/pediatric-nutrition-care-manual.

30. Rees L, Brandt ML. Tube feeding in children with chronic kidney disease: technical and practical issues. Pediatr Nephrol. 2010;25(4):699–704.

31. Rees L, Shaw V, Qizalbash L, Anderson C, Desloovere A, Greenbaum L, et al. Delivery of a nutritional prescription by enteral tube feeding in children with chronic kidney disease stages 2–5 and on dialysis-clinical practice recommendations from the Pediatric Renal Nutrition Taskforce. Pediatr Nephrol. 2021;36(1):187–204.

32. Ledermann SE, Spitz L, Moloney J, Rees L, Trompeter RS. Gastrostomy feeding in infants and children on peritoneal dialysis. Pediatr Nephrol. 2002;17(4):246–50.

33. von Schnakenburg C, Feneberg R, Plank C, Zimmering M, Arbeiter K, Bald M, et al. Percutaneous endoscopic gastrostomy in children on peritoneal dialysis. Perit Dial Int. 2006;26(1):69–77.

34. Juarez MD. Intradialytic parenteral nutrition in pediatrics. Front Pediatr. 2018;6:267.

35. Goldstein SL, Baronette S, Gambrell TV, Currier H, Brewer ED. nPCR assessment and IDPN treatment of malnutrition in pediatric hemodialysis patients. Pediatr Nephrol. 2002;17(7):531–4.

36. Orellana P, Juarez-Congelosi M, Goldstein SL. Intradialytic parenteral nutrition treatment and biochemical marker assessment for malnutrition in adolescent maintenance hemodialysis patients. J Ren Nutr. 2005;15(3):312–7.

37. Srivaths PR, Wong C, Goldstein SL. Nutrition aspects in children receiving maintenance hemodialysis: impact on outcome. Pediatr Nephrol. 2009;24(5):951–7.

38. Dudley J, Rogers R, Sealy L. Renal consequences of parenteral nutrition. Pediatr Nephrol. 2014;29(3):375–85.

39. Haskin O, Sutherland SM, Wong CJ. The effect of intradialytic intralipid therapy in pediatric hemodialysis patients. J Ren Nutr. 2017;27(2):132–7.

40. Grodstein GP, Blumenkrantz MJ, Kopple JD, Moran JK, Coburn JW. Glucose absoprtio during continous ambulatory peritoneal dialysis. Kidney Int. 1981;19:564–7.

41. Bodnar DM, Busch S, Fuchs J, Piedmonte M, Schreiber M. Estimating glucose absorption in peritoneal dialysis using peritoneal equilibration tests. Adv Perit Dial. 1993;9:114–8.

42. American Diabetes Association. Children and Adolescents: Standard of Medical Care in Diabetes—2019. Diabetes Care. 2019;42(Suppl. 1):S129–47.

43. Camerotto C, Cupisti A, D'Alessandro C, Muzio F, Gallieni M. Dietary fiber and gut microbiota in renal diets. Nutrients. 2019;11(9)

44. Okuda Y, Soohoo M, Ishikura K, Tang Y, Obi Y, Laster M, Rhee CM, Streja E, Kalantar-Zadeh K. Primary causes of kidney disease and mortality in dialysis-dependent children. Pediatr Nephrol. 2020;35(5):851–60.

45. Mitsnefes MM. Cardiovascular disease in children with chronic kidney disease. J Am Soc Nephrol. 2012;23(4):578–85.

46. Saland JM, Pierce CB, Mitsnefes MM, Flynn JT, Goebel J, Kupferman JC, et al. Dyslipidemia in children with chronic kidney disease. Kidney Int. 2010;78(11):1154–63.

47. Khandelwal P, Murugan V, Hari S, Lakshmy R, Sinha A, Hari P, et al. Dyslipidemia, carotid intima-media thickness and endothelial dysfunction in children with chronic kidney disease. Pediatr Nephrol. 2016;31(8):1313–20.

48. Sarnak MJ, Bloom R, Muntner P, Rahman M, Saland JM, Wilson PW, et al. KDOQI US commentary on the 2013 KDIGO Clinical Practice Guideline for Lipid Management in CKD. Am J Kidney Dis. 2015;65(3):354–66.

49. de Ferranti SD, Steinberger J, Ameduri R, Baker A, Gooding H, Kelly AS, et al. Cardiovascular risk reduction in high-risk pediatric patients: a scientific statement from the American Heart Association. Circulation. 2019;139(13):e603–e34.

50. Mozaffarian D, Wu JHY. Omega-3 fatty acids and cardiovasular disease: effects on risk factors, molecular pathways, and clinical events. J Am Coll Card. 2011;58(20):2047–67.

51. Ateya AM, Sabri NA, El Hakim I, Shaheen SM. Effect of Omega-3 fatty acids on serum lipid profile and oxidative stress in pediatric patients on regular hemodialysis: a randomized placebo-controlled study. J Ren Nutr. 2017;27(3):169–74.

52. Omar ZA, Montser BA, Farahat MAR. Effect of high-dose omega 3 on lipid profile and inflammatory markers in chronic hemodialysis children. Saudi J Kidney Dis Transpl. 2019;30(3):634–9.

53. Saglimbene VM, Wong G, van Zwieten A, Palmer SC, Ruospo M, Natale P, Campbell K, Teixeira-Pinto A, Craig JC, Strippoli GFM. Effects of omega-3 polyunsaturated fatty acid intake in patients with chronic kidney disease: systematic review and meta-analysis of randomized controlled trials. Clin Nutr. 2020;39(2):358–68.

54. Desloovere A, Renken-Terhaerdt J, Tuokkola J, Shaw V, Greenbaum LA, Haffner D, et al. The dietary management of potassium in children with CKD stages 2–5 and on dialysis-clinical practice recommendations from the Pediatric Renal Nutrition Taskforce. Pediatr Nephrol. 2021;

55. Noori N, Kalantar-Zadeh K, Kovesdy CP, Murali SB, Bross R, Nissenson AR, et al. Dietary potassium intake and mortality in long-term hemodialysis patients. Am J Kidney Dis. 2010;56(2):338–47.

56. Taylor JM, Oladitan L, Carlson S, Hamilton-Reeves JM. Renal formulas pretreated with medications alters the nutrient profile. Pediatr Nephrol. 2015;30(10):1815–23.

57. Paloian NJ, Bowman B, Bartosh SM. Treatment of infant formula with patiromer dose dependently decreases potassium concentration. Pediatr Nephrol. 2019;34(8):1395–401.

58. McMahon EJ, Campbell KL, Bauer JD, Mudge DW. Altered dietary salt intake for people with chronic kidney disease. Cochrane Database Syst Rev. 2015;(2):CD010070.

59. Zisman AL. Effectiveness of treatment modalities on kidney stone recurrence. Clin J Am Soc Nephrol. 2017;12(10):1699–708.

60. Yang Q, Zhang Z, Kuklina EV, Fang J, Ayala C, Hong Y, Loustalot F, Dai S, Gunn JP, Tian N, Cogswell M, Merritt R. Sodium intake and blood pressure among US children and adolescents. Pediatrics. 2012;130(4):611–9.

61. Overwyk KJ, Zhao L, Zhang Z, Wiltz J, Dunford EK, Cogswell ME. Trends in blood pressure and usual dietary sodium intake among children and adolescents, National Health and Nutrition Examination Survey 2003 to 2016. Hypertension. 2019;74(2):260–6.

62. He FJ, MacGregor GA. Importance of slat in determine blood pressure in children: meta-analysis of controlled trials. Hypertension. 2006;48(5):861.

63. Adler AJ, Taylor F, Martin N, Gottlieb S, Taylor RS, Ebrahim S. Reduced dietary salt for the prevention of cardiovascular disease. Cochrane Database Syst Rev. 2014;(12):CD009217.

64. Nguyen S, Choi HK, Lustig RH, Hsu CY. Sugar-sweetened beverages, serum uric acid and blood pressure in adolescents. J Pediatr. 2009;154:807–13.

65. Chen L, Caballero MDC, et al. Reducing comsumption of sugar-sweetened beverages is associated with reduction: a prospective study among United States adults. Circulation. 2010;121:2398–406.

66. Wong ATY, Mannix C, Grantham JJ, Allman-Farinelli M, Badve SV, Boudville N, et al. Randomised controlled trial to determine the efficacy and safety of prescribed water intake to prevent kidney failure due to autosomal dominant polycystic kidney disease (PREVENT-ADPKD). BMJ Open. 2018;8(1):e018794.

67. Paglialonga F, Consolo S, Galli MA, Testa S, Edefonti A. Interdialytic weight gain in oligoanuric children and adolescents on chronic hemodialysis. Pediatr Nephrol. 2015;30(6):999–1005.

68. Kalantar-Zadeh K, Regidor DL, Kovesdy CP, Van Wyck D, Bunnapradist S, Horwich TB, Fonarow GC. Fluid retention is associated with cardiovascular mortality in patients undergoing long-term hemodialysis. Circulation. 2009;119(5):671–9.

69. McAlister L, Pugh P, Greenbaum L, Haffner D, Rees L, Anderson C, Desloovere A, Nelms C, Oosterveld M, Paglialonga F, Polderman N, Qizalbash L, Renken-Terhaerdt J, Tuokkola J, Warady B, Walle JV, Shaw V, Shroff R. The dietary management of calcium and phosphate in children with CKD stages 2–5 and on dialysis-clinical practice recommendation from the Pediatric Renal Nutrition Taskforce. Pediatr Nephrol. 2020;35(3):501–18.

70. Wesseling-Perry K, Pereira RC, Tseng CH, Elashoff R, Zaritsky JJ, Yadin O, Sahney S, Gales B, Jüppner H, Salusky IB. Early skeletal and biochemical alterations in pediatric chronic kidney disease. Clin J Am Soc Nephrol. 2012;7(1):146–52.

71. Denburg MR, Kumar J, Jemielita T, Brooks ER, Skversky A, Portale AA, Salusky IB, Warady BA, Furth SL, Leonard MB. Fracture Burden and risk factors in childhood CKD: results from the CKiD cohort study. J Am Soc Nephrol. 2016;27(2):543–50.

72. Bonjour JP, Carrie AL, Ferrari S, Clavien H, Slosman D, Theintz G, et al. Calcium-enriched foods and bone mass growth in prepubertal girls: a randomized, double-blind, placebo-controlled trial. J Clin Invest. 1997;99(6):1287–94.

73. Cadogan J, Eastell R, Jones N, Barker ME. Milk intake and bone mineral acquisition in adolescent girls: randomised, controlled intervention trial. BMJ. 1997;315(7118):1255–60.

74. Matkovic V, Goel PK, Badenhop-Stevens NE, Landoll JD, Li B, Ilich JZ, et al. Calcium supplementation and bone mineral density in females from childhood to young adulthood: a randomized controlled trial. Am J Clin Nutr. 2005;81(1):175–88.

75. Shroff R, Wan M, Nagler EV, Bakkaloglu S, Fischer DC, Bishop N, et al. Clinical practice recommendations for native vitamin D therapy in children with chronic kidney disease stages 2–5 and on dialysis. Nephrol Dial Transplant. 2017;32(7):1098–113.

76. Raaijmakers R, Houkes LM, Schroder CH, Willems JL, Monnens LA. Pre-treatment of dairy and breast milk with sevelamer hydrochloride and sevelamer carbonate to reduce phosphate. Perit Dial Int. 2013;33(5):565–72.

77. Rodig NM, McDermott KC, Schneider MF, Htochkiss HM, Yadin O, Seikaly MG, Furth SL, Warady BA. Growth in children with chronic kidney disease: a report from the Chronic Kidney Disease in Children Study. Pediatr Nephrol. 2014;29(10):1987–95.

78. Harambat J, Kunzmann K, Azukaitis K, Bayazit AK, Canpolat N, Doyon A, et al. Metabolic acidosis is common and associates with disease progression in children with chronic kidney disease. Kidney Int. 2017;92(6):1507–14.

79. Brown DD, Roem J, Ng DK, Reidy KJ, Kumar J, Abramowitz MK, Mak RH, Furth SL, Schwartz GJ, Warady BA, Kaskel FJ, Melamed ML. Low serum bicarbonate and CKD progression in children. Clin J Am Soc Nephrol. 2020;15(6):755–65.

80. López M, Moreno G, Lugo G, Marcano G. Dietary acid load in children with chronic kidney disease. Eur J Clin Nutr. 2020;74(Suppl 1):57–62.

81. Krupp D, Shi L, Remer T. Longitudinal relationships between diet-dependent renal acid load and blood pressure development in healthy children. Kidney Int. 2014;85(1):204–10.

82. Harshman LA, Lee-Son K, Jetton JG. Vitamin and trace element deficiencies in the pediatric dialysis patient. Pediatr Nephrol. 2018;33(7):1133–43.

83. Schwotzer N, Kanemitsu M, Kissling S, Darioli R, Benghezal M, Rezzi S, et al. Water-soluble vitamin levels and supplementation in chronic online hemodiafiltration patients. Kidney Int Rep. 2020;5(12):2160–7.

84. Raimann JG, Abbas SR, Liu L, Larive B, Beck G, Kotanko P, et al. The effect of increased frequency of hemodialysis on vitamin C concentrations: an ancillary study of the randomized Frequent Hemodialysis Network (FHN) daily trial. BMC Nephrol. 2019;20(1):179.

85. Clase CM, Ki V, Holden RM. Water-soluble vitamins in people with low glomerular filtration rate or on dialysis: a review. Semin Dial. 2013;26(5):546–67.

86. Bamgbola OF, Kaskel F. Role of folate deficiency on erythropoietin resistance in pediatric and adolescent patients on chronic dialysis. Pediatr Nephrol. 2005;20(11):1622–9.

87. KDIGO clinical practice guidelines for anemia in chronic kidney disease. Kindeny Int Suppl. 2012;2:279–325.

88. Atkinson MA, Warady BA. Anemia in Chronic Kidney Disease. Pediatr Nephrol. 2018;33:227–38.

89. Macdougall IC, White C, Anker SD, Bhandari S, Farrington K, Kalra P, McMurray JJV, Murray H, Tomson CRV, Wheeler DC, Winerals CG, Ford I. Intravenous iron in patients undergoing maintenance hemodialysis. NEJM. 2019;380(5):447–58.

90. Macdougall IC, Bhandari S, White C, Anker SD, Farrington K, Karla PA, Mark PB, McMurray JJV, Reid C, Robertson M, Tomson CRV, Wheeler DC, Winerals CG, Ford I. Intravenous iron dosing and infection risk in patients on hemodialysis: a prespecified secondary analysis of the PIVOTAL trial. JASN. 2020;31:1118–27.

91. Shroff R, Wan M, Gullett A, Ledermann S, Shute R, Knott C, Wells D, Aitkenhead H, Manickavasagar B, van't Hoff W, Rees L. Ergocalciferol supplementation in children with CKD delays the onset of secondary hyperparathyroidism: a randomized trial. Clin J Am Soc Nephrol. 2012;7(2):216–23.

92. Stein DR, Feldman HA, Gordon CM. Vitamin D status in children with chronic kidney disease. Pediatr Nephrol. 2012;27(8):1341–50.

93. Patange AR, Valentini RP, Gothe MP, Du W, Pettersen MD. Vitamin D deficiency is associated with increased left ventricular mass and diastolic dysfunction in children with chronic kidney disease. Pediatr Cardiol. 2013;34(3):536–42.

94. Patange AR, Valentini RP, Du W, Pettersen MD. Vitamin D deficiency and arterial wall stiffness in children with chronic kidney disease. Pediatr Cardiol. 2012;33(1):122–8.

95. Banerjee S, Basu S, Sen A, Sengupta J. The effect of vitamin D and calcium supplementation in pediatric steroid-sensitive nephrotic syndrome. Pediatr Nephrol. 2017;32(11):2063–70.

96. Shroff R, Wan M, Nagler EV, Bakkaloglu S, Cozzolino M, Bacchetta J, Edefonti A, Stefanidis CJ, Vande Walle J, Ariceta G, Klaus G, Haffner D, Schmitt CP, European Society for Paediatric Nephrology Chronic Kidney Disease Mineral and Bone Disorders and Dialysis Working Groups. Clinical Practice Recommendations for treatment with active vitamin D analogues in children with chronic kidney disease stages 2-5 and on dialysis. Nephrol Dial Transplant. 2017;32(7):1114–27.

97. Holden RM, Ki V, Morton AR, Clase C. Fat-soluble vitamins in advanced CKD/ESKD: a review. Semin Dial. 2012;25(3):334–43.

98. Asfaw M, Mingle J, Hendricks J, Pharis M, Nucci AM. Nutrition management after pediatric solid organ transplantation. Nutr Clin Pract. 2014;29(2):192–200.

Anemia in Chronic Renal Disease

59

Larry A. Greenbaum

Abbreviations

CKD	Chronic kidney disease
CRP	C-reactive protein
DA	Darbepoetin alpha
ESA	Erythropoiesis stimulating agent
FDA	Food and Drug Administration
GFR	Glomerular filtration rate
Hb	Hemoglobin
HD	Hemodialysis
HIF	Hypoxia inducible factor
IL-6	Interleukin-6
IV	Intravenous
KDIGO	Kidney Disease: Improving Global Outcomes
Kg	Kilogram
LVH	Left ventricular hypertrophy
MCV	Mean corpuscular volume
PD	Peritoneal dialysis
PEG	Polyethylene glycol
PHD	Propyl hydroxylase domain
PHIs	Prolyl hydroxylase inhibitors
PTH	Parathyroid hormone
rHuEPO	Recombinant human erythropoietin
SLE	Systemic lupus erythematosus
TIBC	Total iron binding capacity
TSAT	Transferrin saturation

L. A. Greenbaum (✉)
Pediatric Nephrology, Emory University and
Children's Healthcare of Atlanta, Atlanta, GA, USA
e-mail: lgreen6@emory.edu

Introduction

Anemia is one of the most common problems in children with chronic kidney disease (CKD); it is almost universal in children with stage 5 CKD. The development of recombinant human erythropoietin (rHuEPO) revolutionized the treatment of anemia in CKD, but anemia management remains challenging. Many management issues remain uncertain, including the ideal target hemoglobin (Hb). There are guidelines for the management of anemia in CKD [1–3].

Pathophysiology of Anemia

A variety of factors contribute to anemia in CKD (Table 59.1). The principal etiology is decreased production of EPO by the kidneys. However, many children are still anemic despite administration of erythropoiesis stimulating agents (ESAs) [4, 5], emphasizing the multifactorial etiology of anemia in children with CKD.

Erythropoietin Deficiency

The kidneys produce EPO and kidney damage leads to decreased EPO production. In children with CKD, EPO levels are inappropriately low for the degree of anemia [6]. The degree of EPO deficiency generally worsens as the glomerular

Table 59.1 Causes of anemia in CKD

Erythropoietin deficiency.
Blood loss
Hemolysis
Bone marrow suppression
Iron deficiency
Inadequate dialysis
Malnutrition
Chronic or acute inflammation
Infection
Hyperparathyroidism
B12 or folate deficiency
Aluminum toxicity
Carnitine deficiency
Medications (e.g. ACE inhibitors)
Systemic disease
   Hemoglobinopathy
   Hypothyroidism
   Systemic lupus erythematosus
   Malignancy

ACE angiotensin-converting enzyme

filtration rate (GFR) decreases, but the level of GFR at which inadequate EPO causes anemia varies between patients, partially due to the nature of the underlying kidney disease [7]. On average, a GFR below 43 mL/min/1.73 m^2 is associated with a decline in Hb in children with CKD [8].

Blood Loss

Excessive blood loss may directly cause anemia, or it may lead to iron deficiency (see below). Causes of blood loss in children with CKD include phlebotomy, blood lost in the dialyzer and tubing during hemodialysis (HD) [9], gastrointestinal losses [9], and increased menstrual bleeding due to the acquired platelet function defect of CKD. Children receiving HD have increased intestinal blood loss when compared to other children with CKD [9] and have lower Hb values than children receiving peritoneal dialysis (PD) [5]. Increased blood loss is associated with rHuEPO resistance in pediatric HD patients [10].

Decreased Red Blood Cell Survival

Red blood cells in children with CKD have a decreased lifespan [9]. This may be partially due to carnitine deficiency (see below) [11], and a direct consequence of EPO deficiency, since red cell survival increases in CKD patients after starting rHuEPO [12]. Red blood cells in patients receiving HD have an increased osmotic fragility. Hemolytic anemia may occur due to a child's primary disease [e.g. systemic lupus erythematosus (SLE)].

Bone Marrow Suppression

In an in vitro assay, serum from children with CKD directly suppressed red blood cell production [6]. The specific inhibitory substances have not been identified, but dialysis appears to effectively remove some of these molecules, allowing for decreased doses of rHuEPO [13]. In a study of teenagers receiving HD, the children with Hb less than 11 g/dL had a slightly lower Kt/V$_{urea}$ (1.46 v.s 1.53), but dialysis adequacy did not predict anemia in the multiple regression analysis, perhaps due to the high overall Kt/V in this patient population [14]. Severe bone marrow suppression may occur in children after renal transplantation due to medications [15] or infections, especially parvovirus B19 [16].

Iron Deficiency

Iron deficiency is a significant cause of anemia in patients with CKD; it is multifactorial (Table 59.2). In a study of older children, a serum transferrin saturation (TSAT) less than 20% was an independent predictor of anemia [14]. However, serum ferritin was not predictive of anemia, perhaps because ferritin is often elevated in CKD patients with concurrent inflammation, which may inhibit red cell synthesis (see below). This is supported by a study of children receiving PD where Hb was inversely related to serum ferritin [17].

Table 59.2 Causes of iron deficiency in children with CKD

Blood loss
  Phlebotomy
  Hemodialysis
  Menses
  Gastrointestinal
  Surgical procedures
Dietary iron deficiency
Poor absorption of enteral iron
  Inflammation
  Medications (phosphate binders, gastric acid inhibitors)
Iron depletion during ESA therapy

ESA erythropoiesis-stimulating agent

Iron deficiency often develops after initiation of an ESA because the increase in red blood cell synthesis depletes iron stores. In some patients, there is a functional iron deficiency following ESA treatment; there are adequate supplies of iron, but the transfer of iron from ferritin is not fast enough to meet the high demand for red blood cell synthesis.

Inadequate Dialysis

In adults receiving dialysis, there is evidence that anemia is associated with inadequate dialysis. An increase in dialysis dose leads to an improvement in Hb. In addition, there is an inverse relationship between Kt/V and ESA dose. Resistance to ESAs was associated with a lower Kt/V in a study of pediatric HD patients [10]. Dialysis is effective at removing hepcidin (see below) [18], suggesting a possible mechanism for the relationship between dialysis dose and anemia.

Malnutrition

Malnutrition may be another factor contributing to anemia in CKD. In one pediatric study, low albumin was one predictor of anemia [14]. There are many possible explanations for the relationship between malnutrition and anemia. Generalized malnutrition may be a marker for nutritional iron deficiency or for deficiency of other nutrients that influence red cell production or survival. Another possible explanation for this observation is the relationship between markers of malnutrition and markers of inflammation [19]. As described below, inflammation is another mechanism of resistance to rHuEPO. It is possible that inflammation causes malnutrition, and this directly causes resistance to ESAs. An alternative explanation is that inflammation directly causes rHuEPO resistance, and that malnutrition is a surrogate marker of inflammation. A malnutrition inflammation score predicted ESA resistance in a study of pediatric HD patients [10].

Inflammation

Acute and chronic inflammation are well-known causes of decreased red blood cell synthesis. Inflammation is one of the mechanisms of the anemia of chronic disease and of the decreased erythropoiesis that occurs during infections. Markers of inflammation are commonly increased in CKD patients. There are a variety of putative mechanisms. Surgical procedures and acute infections are more common in CKD patients, especially those who are receiving dialysis or have a kidney transplant. The impaired immune system in uremia may lead to an increase in non-specific inflammation [20]. CKD patients may have underlying systemic diseases, such as SLE or granulomatosis with polyangiitis. HD may induce inflammation via complement activation, direct activation of inflammatory cells by the dialysis membrane, and diffusion of endotoxin into the patient from the dialysate. Use of ultra-pure dialysis in HD patients decreases inflammatory markers, increases Hb levels, and decreases ESA use [21].

Hepcidin is an important mediator of ESA resistance [22]. Hepcidin, which is produced in the liver, inhibits intestinal absorption of iron and release of iron stores from the reticuloendothelial system. This is accomplished through down-regulation of ferroprotein, the principal transmembrane transporter of iron. Hepcidin is normally down-regulated in anemia, increasing absorption of iron and release of iron stores. In contrast, hepcidin increases when iron stores are adequate. Hepcidin is also up-regulated by inflammation. Interleukin 6 (IL-6) induces production of hepcidin and is risk factor for ESA resistance [23, 24]. Hepcidin's effect on release of iron stores explains inflammatory block, a condition where body stores of iron are adequate, but there is ineffective delivery of iron to the bone marrow. Findings in patients with inflammatory blockade may include elevated C-reactive protein (CRP) levels, resistance to ESAs, high serum ferritin levels, and low levels of serum iron and TSAT [25]. This mechanism is common to the anemia of many chronic diseases.

Hyperparathyroidism

Hyperparathyroidism may decrease bone marrow production of red blood cells [26] and rarely causes pancytopenia [27]. Elevated parathyroid hormone (PTH) levels are associated with ESA resistance in pediatric HD patients [10] and PTH is inversely related to Hb in pediatric dialysis patients [5]. Treatment of hyperparathyroidism via parathyroidectomy may lead to an increase in Hb.

B12 or Folate Deficiency

Patients with CKD may rarely develop a megaloblastic anemia due to folate or vitamin B12 deficiency. Poor nutritional intake combined with dialytic losses may predispose CKD patients to deficiencies of these water-soluble vitamins. There is some evidence that routine folate supplementation improves the response to rHuEPO, even in the absence of low serum levels of folic acid [28].

Aluminum Toxicity

Aluminum overload may cause a microcytic anemia in patients with CKD [29]. Currently, aluminum overload is an uncommon cause of anemia due to the recognition of the dangers of aluminum-containing phosphate binders.

Carnitine Deficiency

Carnitine deficiency may occur in CKD, principally due to removal of carnitine by dialysis, although decreased dietary intake and endogenous synthesis may also contribute [11]. Renal losses of carnitine are significant in children with Fanconi syndrome. Carnitine deficiency may decrease red blood cell survival by reducing the strength of the red cell membrane [11]. Intravenous (IV) carnitine may reduce rHuEPO dose requirements in adults receiving HD, but there is disagreement regarding the strength of the evidence; carnitine should not be used routinely in children, if at all, outside of a research setting [1, 11, 30–32]. Oral carnitine should not be used in patients receiving HD [11].

Medications

A variety of medications can inhibit erythropoiesis, especially certain medications used in renal transplant recipients [15, 33]. Angiotensin-converting enzyme inhibitors and angiotensin receptor blockers are especially pertinent in CKD patients because of their widespread use [34].

Summary

Erythropoietin deficiency and iron deficiency are the most common causes of anemia in children with CKD. Inflammation and hyperparathyroidism are important mediators of ESA resistance.

Epidemiology of Anemia in Pediatric CKD

Anemia is common in children with CKD, even in patients with stage 3 CKD [5, 35]. In one study, anemia was more common in children greater than 2 years old, males, and patients receiving antihypertensive medications [35]. In another cohort, African American race was associated with an increased risk of anemia in children with CKD [4].

In children receiving PD, anemia is quite common and varies by region [17]. Risk factors for anemia include inflammation, decreased residual urine output and hyperparathyroidism [17].

Anemia is common in children after kidney transplantation [36]. The principal cause of anemia is allograft dysfunction, although current immunosuppressive medications appear to be responsible for the increased prevalence of anemia in these patients. Iron deficiency is common in children who are anemic after renal transplantation.

Clinical Effects of Anemia

There are a variety of clinical effects of anemia (Table 59.3). The clinical consequences of anemia in patients with CKD are difficult to discern because anemia identifies patients with co-morbidities such as inflammation and malnutrition. A variety of studies demonstrated an association between anemia and morbidity and mortality, but these conclusions may be biased by co-morbidities.

Studies in adult CKD patients have shown an association between anemia and increased mortality and hospitalization rates [37–40]. In a pediatric analysis, anemia 30 days after initiation of dialysis was associated with a significant increase in mortality and hospitalization rate

Table 59.3 Clinical effects of anemia

Cardiovascular
  Left ventricular hypertrophy
Systemic
  Fatigue
  Depression
  Decreased quality of life
  Sleep disturbances
  Decreased exercise tolerance
  Impaired cognitive function
  Loss of appetite

[41]. In analysis of children receiving PD, anemia was associated with increased mortality, hypertension, and left ventricular hypertrophy (LVH) [17], suggesting that in patients with ESKD low Hb may partially reflect fluid overload ("dilutional anemia"). In children with CKD, anemia was associated with an increased risk of hospitalization [42].

In a group of children receiving dialysis, treatment of anemia with rHuEPO was associated with an elevated cardiac index in 6 months and a significant reduction in left ventricular mass index by 12 months [43]. In one study [44], children with severe LVH had significantly lower Hb values than children without LVH. However, anemia did not predict LVH in the final multiple regression model.

There is uncertainty regarding the direct deleterious consequences of a lower Hb in adults with CKD. These include observational studies that have corrected for a variety of co-morbidities [45]. More importantly, randomized studies using ESAs to target different Hb levels have failed to demonstrate a benefit of higher Hb targets on morbidity or mortality [46, 47]. In fact, a higher Hb target has resulted in a significant increase in morbidity and mortality in randomized studies [48, 49].

In randomized studies in adults, a higher Hb improves quality of life [47], although this is not a consistent finding [48, 50]. In a placebo-controlled trial, randomization to rHuEPO resulted in less fatigue, improved exercise tolerance and improved scores of physical symptoms and depression [51]. There is evidence of the deleterious effects of anemia on child development. There is an association in children with CKD between anemia and lower scores of health-related quality of life [52]. Studies of the effect of rHuEPO in children with CKD have shown improvement in quality of life, exercise tolerance, appetite, peak oxygen consumption and treadmill time during exercise testing, Wechsler intelligence score, and ventilatory aerobic threshold [53–55]. There does not appear to be a beneficial effect of anemia correction on the growth retardation associated with CKD [56].

Clinical Evaluation of Anemia

Initial Evaluation

Alternative causes of anemia should be evaluated prior to treating patients with an ESA (Table 59.4). The diagnosis of anemia in children should be based on age and gender specific normal ranges.

The initial evaluation of children with CKD and anemia should include a complete blood count, reticulocyte count, ferritin, iron, total iron binding capacity (TIBC) and a TSAT. The TSAT is calculated by dividing the serum iron by the TIBC. Measurement of EPO levels generally does not have clinical utility. A cost-effectiveness analysis in adults argues against routine screening for aluminum overload or deficiencies of folate or B12 [57]. EPO deficiency causes a normocytic anemia; macrocytosis or microcytosis should lead to consideration of other etiologies (Table 59.4).

Table 59.4 Indications for additional evaluation in children with chronic kidney disease and anemia

Indication	Response
Macrocytosis	Consider B12 or folate deficiency, unless due to brisk reticulocytosis
Decreased platelets and/or white blood cells	Consider malignancy, acute infection, SLE, severe hyperparathyroidism or medications
History of using aluminum-containing phosphate binders or other symptoms of aluminum overload	Consider aluminum toxicity
Anemia despite adequate reticulocytosis	Consider excessive blood loss or hemolysis
Microcytosis	Consider iron deficiency, hemoglobinopathy, or inflammation
Iron deficiency prior to starting an ESA	Evaluate for causes of iron deficiency (see Table 59.2)
Low reticulocyte count and falling hemoglobin in a patient being treated with an ESA	Consider non-adherence, anti-erythropoietin antibodies, parvovirus B19 infection

ESA human erythropoiesis stimulating agent, *SLE* systemic lupus erythematosus

A low mean corpuscular volume (MCV) occurs with iron deficiency, thalassemia and in up to 50% of patients with anemia of chronic disease. A high MCV suggests the possibility of B12 or folate deficiency. Measurement of serum levels of B12 and folate is indicated if there is an elevated MCV or if there is anemia without an alternative explanation. RBC folate is useful when a serum folate level is inconclusive or if recent intake of folate may lead to a falsely normal serum folate level.

Concomitant depression of white cells or platelets raises the specter of malignancy, although an isolated low white blood cell count may be due to a transient viral infection or a medication. SLE may cause depression of the white blood cell count, platelet count and an autoimmune Coombs positive hemolytic anemia. EPO deficiency causes an inappropriately low reticulocyte count, and the presence of an adequate reticulocytosis suggests alternative explanations, such as blood loss or hemolysis. An elevated CRP, indicating inflammation, may provide an explanation for anemia refractory to ESAs.

Iron deficiency is common in children with CKD, even prior to starting an ESA. There are a variety of explanations for iron deficiency in children with CKD (Table 59.2). All children with CKD should be queried about gastrointestinal blood loss and, when appropriate, menstrual losses. A more aggressive work-up (e.g. testing stool for occult blood or endoscopy) is appropriate in children with significant, unexplained iron deficiency prior to receiving ESA therapy. Along with low serum ferritin and TSAT, children with iron deficiency typically have a low MCV. Because it is a marker of inflammation, serum ferritin may be misleadingly normal in children with CKD despite iron deficiency.

Evaluation of the ferritin and TSAT establishes a baseline, since iron deficiency is likely to develop during ESA treatment. In addition, while all patients starting an ESA should receive oral iron supplementation unless iron overload is present, iron deficiency prior to starting ESA therapy may significantly attenuate the response to therapy. Such patients are candidates for IV iron.

Chronic Monitoring

Routine monitoring in children with anemia due to CKD includes periodic assessment of Hb, MCV, and iron stores. The development of macrocytosis in a patient after starting an ESA is usually due to the expected reticulocytosis; an increasing Hb, arguing against a nutritional deficiency anemia, supports this explanation. Iron overload may also cause an increased MCV [58]. Microcytosis is usually due to iron deficiency.

A decrease in Hb is expected during acute infections [59] or after surgical procedures [60]. ESA dose requirements increase following blood loss that causes a fall in Hb; this persists until the Hb returns to the target range. Depleted iron stores are the usual explanation for a poor response to ESA therapy. Some children have a functional iron deficiency, and may respond to IV iron, even though the ferritin levels are adequate. Additional evaluation is indicated in children who have an unexplained increase in ESA dose requirement, need unexpectedly large doses of ESA, or have a decreasing Hb (Table 59.4).

A reticulocyte count is the usual first step in evaluating unexplained anemia or an excessive ESA requirement. An appropriately elevated reticulocyte count (corrected for the degree of anemia) argues that the patient is anemic due to blood loss or hemolysis. Blood loss is also suggested by a minimal increase in ferritin and TSAT despite the use of multiple doses of IV iron. The child should then have stool tested for occult blood; an evaluation for hemolysis may also be appropriate. Inadequate reticulocytosis suggests that there is a defect in red cell production. This may be due to poor adherence or technique failure in a patient receiving home ESA. There may be a readily identifiable explanation, such as severe secondary hyperparathyroidism. Alternatively, additional testing may be necessary. A serum aluminum level is an appropriate test in the child with a history of using aluminum-containing phosphate binders. One of the most common causes of a poor response to ESA is an inflammatory block due to acute or chronic inflammation. An elevated CRP supports this diagnosis [20]. Other testing, depending on the patient, may include screening for anti-EPO antibodies (see below), and serum levels of folate and B12. A hematologist should evaluate refractory anemia with no identifiable explanation [31, 61].

Treatment of Anemia

Treatment with an ESA is necessary in many children with CKD, including children with chronic allograft dysfunction [62]. Almost all children receiving dialysis are treated with an ESA. In addition, almost all treated patients require oral or IV iron. Other underlying causes of anemia should be corrected (Table 59.1). Blood transfusions should be reserved for children with symptomatic anemia or with worsening anemia due to blood loss, hemolysis, or unresponsiveness to ESAs [1].

Target Hemoglobin

A number of randomized studies in adult patients with CKD have demonstrated that targeting higher Hb levels leads to increased morbidity and mortality [46, 48, 49, 63]. In one study, targeting a higher Hb led to a decrease in dialysis adequacy and a higher use of IV iron [46]. The TREAT trial compared placebo and darbepoetin alpha (DA) in adults with CKD. The risk of stroke was almost doubled in the patients randomized to receive DA to achieve a Hb of 13 g/dL, although there was a modest improvement in fatigue in the DA group [49]. Stroke was also increased when adult HD patients were randomized to a higher Hb target [63]. In the CREATE trial, the group randomized to a higher Hb had more episodes of hypertension and headache [47]. In the CHOIR trial, the group randomized to a higher Hb had an increased risk of death or cardiovascular event and there was no difference in quality of life between the groups [48]. In a retrospective cohort study of adult kidney transplant recipients, patients receiving an ESA with a Hb level above 12.5 g/dL had an increase in mortality [64].

The reason for the increased morbidity and mortality associated with a higher Hb target is unresolved. It could be attributed to a higher Hb level or to the need for higher doses of ESAs, which have been postulated to have untoward effects beyond increasing the Hb. High ESA dose is associated with increased morbidity and mortality, but this appears to be partially related to resistance to ESAs due to co-morbidities [65–67]. However, in studies that randomized CKD patients to ESA or placebo, the groups receiving ESAs had an increased risk of stroke [49] and access clotting [51]. Moreover, in a randomized study of rHuEPO in patients with ischemic stroke, the group receiving rHuEPO had significantly increased mortality [68]. Dialysis patients who have high Hb levels without the use of ESAs do not have increased mortality [69]. A higher Hb target could lead to more variation in Hb levels, which has been associated with increased mortality [70].

The negative consequences of targeting higher Hb concentrations in the trials of ESAs has led the US Food and Drug Administration (FDA) to recommend that ESAs be given at the lowest dose possible to avoid blood transfusions and that ESAs should be reduced or withheld if the Hb exceeds 11 g/dL and withheld if the Hb exceeds 12 g/dL. Moreover, all ESAs have a black box warning and patients must receive education regarding the possible adverse effects of ESAs. A combination of these concerns, and possibly a change in the payment structure for ESAs, has led to a decrease in the dose of ESAs and Hb levels in US dialysis patients [71].

There are no data on the ideal target Hb in children or whether the target should be adjusted based on age and gender. Kidney Disease: Improving Global Outcomes (KDIGO) recommends an upper limit Hb of 11.5 g/dL in adults, but recommends targeting pediatric CKD patients between 11–12 g/dL. The British NICE guidelines recommend a target of 10–12 g/dL for all patient 2 years and older, with a target of 9.5–11.5 g/dL in children less than 2 years [2, 3]. The Canadian Society of Nephrology recommends a target of 10–11 g/dL for adults, but considers 9.5–11.5 g/dL an acceptable range [72]. The US KDOQI commentary on KDIGO advocates the FDA-recommended upper cutoff of 11 g/dL for adults, but a range of 11–13 g/dL for children

[73]. There are clearly clinical situations that require different target Hb values. For example, specific children may require a higher target Hb (e.g. a child with underlying cyanotic heart disease) or a lower target (e.g. a child with sickle cell disease).

Some patients remain anemic or develop refractory anemia despite ESA therapy and correction of other etiologies of anemia. This is especially common in patients who have inflammation. Ongoing escalation of ESA dose in these patients has been associated with adverse outcomes in adults [49], suggesting that ESA dose should not be increased without limit in patients who are hyporesponsive. Patients who do not respond to an ESA or stop responding to an ESA should have an evaluation of possible etiologies of anemia (Tables 56.1 and 56.4).

Hemoglobin Monitoring

Hb monitoring is preferred over hematocrit because Hb measurements are more standardized and consistent. For patients receiving HD, blood samples should be taken immediately prior to dialysis. This may lead to a falsely low Hb value due to hemodilution from fluid gain between dialysis sessions. Hence, this should be considered in children with significant interdialytic weight gain. It is reasonable to measure Hb prior to a HD session after a short interdialytic period (2 days) since the effect of hemodilution on Hb is generally less significant [31].

The frequency of monitoring varies depending on the patient. Children who are being given a stable dose of ESA and within their target Hb can have a Hb level performed as infrequently as monthly in a dialysis patient, and even less often in a predialysis patient (minimum of every 3 months). After the initiation of ESA or after a dosing change, a Hb should generally be obtained at least monthly until the Hb has stabilized within the target range. Protocols that use less frequent monitoring and dose adjustments may reduce costs and minimize Hb cycling, large variations in Hb values that are associated with increased morbidity in adults [74, 75].

Erythropoiesis Stimulating Agents

rHuEPO was the first ESA, but a number of other preparations are now available. Two preparations, DA and methoxy polyethylene glycol (PEG)-epoetin beta, are modified forms of EPO. The main advantage of other preparations is a longer half-life, which permits less frequent dosing. This is especially advantageous in children who require subcutaneous dosing given the discomfort and fear associated with injections. Less frequent dosing may also decrease provider burden in a dialysis unit and provide cost savings [76]. Hypoxia-inducible factor (HIF) prolyl hydroxylase inhibitors (PHIs) have a different mechanism of action than the other ESAs, including both stimulation of EPO production and increasing iron bioavailability. HIH-PHIs have the advantage of oral administration, but regulatory approval has been slow due to safety concerns; they have not been systematically studied in children.

There are no studies directly comparing different ESAs in children, and limited studies in adults except for comparisons of the HIF-PHIs with other ESAs. Availability of the different preparations varies by country.

Recombinant Human Erythropoietin

Multiple studies in adult patients demonstrated the efficacy of IV and subcutaneously administered rHuEPO for correcting the anemia of CKD. A placebo controlled trial demonstrated that rHuEPO is effective in children with CKD [55], and studies in adults demonstrate that use of ESAs decreases the need for transfusions [49, 51, 77].

Pharmacokinetics

The pharmacokinetics of rHuEPO in CKD has been studied in children and adults. There are clear differences based on the route of administration, with less complete absorption of subcutaneous rHuEPO, but a significantly longer half-life when compared to IV administration. In studies of children with CKD, the measured mean half-life of rHuEPO is 5.6–7.5 h for IV dosing and 14.2–25.2 h for subcutaneous dosing. For IV dosing, there is evidence in adults that the half-life of rHuEPO increases as the dose increases.

Dosing

There are dramatic differences in the dosing needs of children with CKD who are receiving rHuEPO, even when adjusted for patient size [78, 79]. Some have recommended dosing children independent of weight and utilizing "adult" dosing [80]. A variety of variables influence the dosing needs of patients (Table 59.5), but it remains difficult to predict the dosing needs of an individual patient. Factors affecting the necessary dose per kilogram (kg) of rHuEPO in children with CKD include the stage of CKD (higher in stage 5), the mode of dialysis (higher in HD due to increased blood loss) [81, 82], the age of the patient (higher in younger patients) [78, 79, 82], the route of administration (higher with IV versus subcutaneous) [79], and the dosing frequency (higher with less frequent dosing regimens). Concurrent causes of poor response to rHuEPO, such as iron deficiency, inflammation, or hyperparathyroidism, often result in higher doses. Blood loss, due to HD, blood draws, and other sources, increase the need for rHuEPO. Blood draws can be especially problematic in the youngest patients, because they often need more frequent monitoring and the relative losses per kg of body weight tend to be higher. Finally, residual renal production of EPO can decrease the need for rHuEPO.

In children receiving PD or predialysis patients, an appropriate starting dose for subcutaneous rHuEPO is 100 units/kg/week divided into two doses, although once weekly dosing may be appropriate in a child with mild anemia. Children less than 5 years are likely to need a higher dose,

Table 59.5 Factors influencing erythropoietin dosing

Route of administration
Mode of dialysis
Initial and target hemoglobin
Endogenous erythropoietin
Patient age
Dosing frequency
Presence of other causes of anemia (see Table 59.1)

and a starting dose of 150 units/kg/week may be appropriate in such patients, especially if severe anemia (Hb < 8 g/dL) is present. Alternatively, a study of children receiving PD demonstrated that the average weekly dose of EPO was 4300 IU/m² independent of age [17], suggesting that body surface area can be used to dose EPO in children independent of age or weight. For children receiving HD and IV rHuEPO dosing, a starting dose of 150 units/kg/week divided into three doses is reasonable, again with the caveat that higher doses are likely necessary in children less than 5 years. A starting dose of 200–300 units/kg/week may be more appropriate in such patients, especially if there is concomitant severe anemia.

In children receiving chronic subcutaneous dosing of rHuEPO, the majority can be maintained on weekly dosing to minimize the number of painful injections. However, some patients require more frequent injections. Less frequent dosing regimens of rHuEPO are effective in adults with pre-dialysis CKD [83].

When children receive IV dosing during HD, it is important to inject rHuEPO via the bloodlines. Use of the venous drip chamber may result in reduced drug delivery due to "trapping" of rHuEPO, although this appears to be somewhat machine dependent.

For children receiving subcutaneous dosing, the site of injection should be rotated. The discomfort of subcutaneous dosing can be reduced by utilizing the multidose vial, which contains the local anesthetic benzyl alcohol as a preservative.

Frequent dose adjustments are typically necessary in patients receiving rHuEPO. This is probably due to variations in the factors that cause anemia (Table 59.1) and that influence rHuEPO dosing (Table 59.5). In addition, more active erythropoiesis is needed to increase a patient's Hb. Hence, the dose that patients need to increase their Hb level into the target range is often more than the dose needed to maintain a stable Hb. Patients may need higher doses of rHuEPO at the start of therapy or after a decrease in Hb due to blood loss or a transient illness.

Most children, when they initiate HD, are converted to IV dosing of rHuEPO, which should then almost always be given thrice weekly. Based on adult studies, the total weekly dose of rHuEPO should be increased by 50% when a patient changes from subcutaneous to IV dosing. Similarly, patients changing from IV dosing to subcutaneous dosing should have their weekly dose decreased by 33%. However, most pediatric patients who convert between IV and subcutaneous dosing are also changing dialysis modality. Given the higher needs for rHuEPO in children on HD [78], patients changing to IV dosing because they are initiating HD may need an additional increase in their dose. In children less than 10 years and certainly those less than 5 years, rHuEPO dosing requirements during HD are very high [79]. This suggests that these patients may need an increase in their rHuEPO dose after beginning HD, irrespective of any change in route of administration. Young children should have careful monitoring of the Hb when initiating HD, increasing the dose of rHuEPO further if necessary. Even in older children, there is extreme variability in the dose requirements when converting to IV dosing; dose requirements may increase or decrease. The ability to more aggressively treat iron deficiency in children receiving HD (see below) may result in a decrease in rHuEPO requirements.

The goal of rHuEPO therapy is to maintain patient Hb within a desired target range. Overly rapid increases in Hb can be associated with hypertension, and should be avoided. In patients with a Hb below the target, the goal is to increase the Hb by 1–2 g/dL per month. The dose of rHuEPO should be increased by 25% if the patient is below the target Hb and has not increased at least 1 g/dL over the last month. The dose should be reduced by 25% if the Hb is greater than the target Hb or the Hb has increased by more than 2 g/dL over the last month. The rHuEPO should be temporarily held if the Hb is more than 1 g/dL over the target Hb or the Hb has increased by more than 2 g/dL over the last month and is above the target Hb.

Complications

An increase in blood pressure after starting rHuEPO therapy may occur in children [55, 84].

This appears to be more common in children who receive higher doses of rHuEPO, and have a consequent more rapid increase in Hb [85]. Hence, rapid increases in Hb should be avoided. While the increase in red cell mass appears to be one mechanism of the hypertension, there also appears to be a direct effect of rHuEPO on the vasculature.

An increase in vascular access clotting following rHuEPO treatment has been attributed to the increase in Hb. There may also be a small negative effect on dialytic clearance, but this is not clinically significant.

Iron deficiency may develop in children treated with rHuEPO [55, 84]. This is secondary to iron utilization for red blood cell synthesis. Consequently, unless iron overload is present, all patients treated with rHuEPO should receive iron supplementation and be screened for iron deficiency before and during therapy.

A rare complication of rHuEPO is the development of anti-EPO antibodies [86]. These antibodies neutralize both endogenous EPO and rHuEPO, resulting in red cell aplasia. Immunosuppressive therapy, including after renal transplantation, results in hematologic recovery in many patients [87]. Patients with undetectable anti-EPO antibodies may subsequently respond to rHuEPO [87].

Darbepoetin Alpha

DA (Aranesp™) is a genetically engineered molecule with a longer half-life than rHuEPO, permitting less frequent administration. The longer half-life of DA is due two additional N-glycosylation sites.

Efficacy

Studies in adults demonstrate comparable efficacy of rHuEPO and DA, despite less frequent dosing of DA [88, 89]. One study demonstrated that many CKD patients do well when receiving DA subcutaneously as infrequently as once every 3–4 weeks [90].

In a prospective study, children receiving rHuEPO were randomized to rHuEPO or DA at a less frequent dosing interval (0.42 µg of DA per week for each 100 units/week of rHuEPO). There was no significant difference in Hb or side effects between the groups at the end of the 20-week study; the median weekly dose of DA was 0.41 mcg/kg, with 25th and 75th percentiles of 0.25 and 0.82 mcg/kg, respectively [91]. A small prospective study evaluated the response to converting seven children receiving HD from thrice weekly rHuEPO to weekly DA (1 mcg of DA per week for each 200 units/week of rHuEPO). Especially in the younger children who were receiving high doses of rHuEPO, there were problems initially with elevated Hb levels and associated hypertension. This was corrected by reducing the dose of DA, suggesting that this dose conversion ratio may be inappropriate in younger children, and that careful monitoring of the initial response is necessary when converting to DA. The mean steady-state dose of DA after 3 months was 0.51 mcg/kg/week [92].

In a large prospective study, children with CKD and anemia were given DA at a starting dose of 0.45 µg/kg/week. There was a significant improvement in Hb and it was sustained during the 28 weeks of the study. By the end of the study, slightly more than half the patients were receiving DA at dosing intervals of at least 2 weeks [93]. A small study has described the successful use of DA in infants, with a starting dose of 0.5 µg/kg/week [94]. The dose was able to be reduced and the dosing interval was increased to 3–4 weeks in some of the infants [94]. In another study in children, the initial dose in naïve patients was 0.45 mcg/kg and patients previously treated with rHuEPO were converted using a dose of 1 mcg of DA per 200 IU of rHuEPO [95]. The final dose was higher in the patients converted from rHuEPO, perhaps because most of these patients were receiving dialysis and none of the naïve patients were dialysis patients [95]. In a prospective registry study in children, including dialysis and pre-dialysis patients, the geometric mean dose range was 1.4–2.0 mcg/kg/month (0.3–0.5 mcg/kg/week) [96].

Pharmacokinetics

One study evaluated the half-life of DA in pediatric patients with CKD [97]. Each patient received one dose of DA (0.5 mcg/kg) intravenously and subcutaneously. The half-life of DA with IV administration was 22.1 h (SD = 4.5 h). The half-life was 42.8 h (SD = 4.8 h) with subcutaneous administration. The pharmacokinetics were comparable to a similarly designed study in adults except for increased bioavailability (54% vs. 37%) and an earlier T_{max} (36 h vs. 54 h) in the pediatric patients when DA was administered subcutaneously [97, 98]. Hence, DA may be absorbed more rapidly in pediatric patients [97]. More rapid absorption was also seen in pediatric studies of rHuEPO [99].

Dosing

Based on protein mass, 1 mcg of DA is equivalent to 200 units of rHuEPO. Nevertheless, the recommended DA dose by the manufacturer when converting patients from rHuEPO to DA is not a direct conversion based on the 1 mcg of DA to 200 units rHuEPO ratio (Table 59.6). The recommended conversion ratios are based on an analysis of the dose conversion clinical trials [100]. This analysis indicates that proportionally less DA was needed in patients who began the trial on higher doses of rHuEPO

[100]. The explanation for this observation is unclear. It is possible that the efficacy of DA increases at higher doses. Alternatively, there may simply be a "regression to the mean" in those patients who were on very high doses of rHuEPO. These patients may have had a transient reason (e.g. inflammation) that led to high ESA dose requirements that subsequently resolved, allowing lowering of the DA dose during the study.

One challenge with DA administration in children is the lack of a multidose vial. First, many small pediatric patients are likely to need less than 25 μg, the smallest available single-dose vial. This results in wasting of the unused medication. Second, pediatric patients may not tolerate the discomfort of 1 mL injections or may require multiple injections in order to tolerate the full 1 mL volume of the single-dose vials. A useful alternative is to utilize DA in more concentrated single-dose prefilled syringes. Thus, dosing of DA necessitates knowledge of the available preparations (Table 59.7), and requires creative adjustments of doses and dosing intervals to minimize wasting of medication.

Recommendations for converting patients from rHuEPO to DA based on adult data are available (Table 59.6). Patients who are receiving rHuEPO twice or thrice weekly should receive DA weekly, and patients who are receiving weekly rHuEPO should receive DA every other week.

Based on the pediatric literature, a reasonable starting dose of DA in ESA naïve patients is approximately 0.5 mcg/kg given weekly. Alternatively, the same total dose could be given every 2 weeks (i.e. 1 mcg/kg every 2 weeks). Every 2-week dosing at initiation should be

Table 59.6 Starting dose of darbepoetin alpha based on previous dosing of rHuEPO

Previous weekly rHuEPO dose (units/week)	Weekly darbepoetin alpha dose (mcg/week)
<2500	6.25
2500–4999	12.5
5000–10,999	25
11,000–17,999	40
18,000–33,999	60
34,000–89,999	100
≥90,000	200

Table based on manufacturer's recommendations
rHuEPO recombinant human erythropoietin

Table 59.7 Available preparations of darbepoetin alpha (single use vials)

*25 mcg	*40 mcg	[a]60 mcg	[a]100 mcg	[a]150 mcg	[a]200 mcg	[a]300 mcg	500 mcg

[a]Preparations that are available in low volume prefilled syringes (0.3–0.6 mL, depending on the dose)

Table 59.8 Dose adjustment table for darbepoetin alpha

6.25.	10	15	20	30	40	50	60	80	100	130	150	200

Doses are in micrograms. The dose to the left of the current dose should be used for dose decreases and the dose to the right of the current dose for dose increases reserved for patients with a Hb that is only mildly below target. Close monitoring of the Hb is essential for all patients due to the variable response to DA.

As occurs with rHuEPO, frequent dose adjustments of DA are often necessary [88]. Since DA has a long half-life, it is important not to increase the dose too quickly to avoid overshooting the target Hb. Many patients require lower doses after their Hb reaches the target range. When adjusting DA dosing, it is desirable to round doses based on the available preparations (Table 59.7) to avoid excessive wasting of the medication. Nevertheless, excessive rounding is not appropriate; some patients will need to discard some of their medication. Table 59–8 presents one system for dose adjustment. It is unclear whether the DA is evenly distributed in the prefilled syringes. Hence, gentle mixing of the medication and transfer to a 1 mL syringe has been recommended for patients who do not need a full dose [94].

Dose frequency of DA can be gradually reduced from weekly to every other week to every 3 weeks to every 4 weeks [101]. Not all patients will tolerate decreased dose frequency, especially beyond every 3 weeks. The dose frequency can be reduced whenever the patient has a Hb level that would normally mandate decreasing the dose. Alternatively, the dose frequency can be reduced in patients who are on a stable DA dose and have a Hb in the target range. The total weekly dose should remain the same. For patients receiving DA less often than weekly, consideration should be given to increasing the dose frequency if a patient requires more than 1 dose increase, especially if the total weekly dose is relatively high.

Complications

Side effect profiles have been similar in studies comparing IV DA with IV rHuEPO [88, 89]. In one study, there was a statistically significant increase in pruritus in the DA group [89]. Injection site pain is more severe in children with subcutaneous DA than with rHuEPO [102].

There have been cases of antibodies developing to DA leading to pure red cell aplasia [103].

Methoxy Polyethylene Glycol-Epoetin Beta

Methoxy PEG-epoetin beta is made by linking EPO with a large polymer chain via amide bonds between amino acids and methoxy PEG butanoic acid. Methoxy PEG-epoetin beta is also called Continuous Erythropoietin Receptor Activator (C.E.R.A.). A long half-life permits less frequent dosing [104].

Efficacy

A number of studies have demonstrated the effectiveness of methoxy PEG-epoetin beta in adult patients with CKD [105–111]. In a direct comparison with DA in adult HD patients, methoxy PEG-epoetin beta was superior at maintaining Hb at the prescribed target [112]. Methoxy PEG-epoetin beta given either every 2 weeks or every 4 weeks was comparable to rHuEPO in adult dialysis patients [107, 109].

Methoxy PEG-epoetin beta is effective in adult kidney transplant recipients [113, 114]. In a randomized study, once-monthly methoxy PEG-epoetin beta was compared with every 1–2 weeks DA, with similar efficacy and side effect profiles [115].

Two clinical trials have demonstrated that methoxy PEG-epoetin beta is effective in children with CKD [116, 117]. Children with stable anemia undergoing HD were converted from EPO or DA to methoxy PEG-epoetin beta, and Hb remained stable [116]. Similar efficacy was seen in a clinical trial that included children with pre-dialysis CKD and children receiving PD or HD [117].

Pharmacokinetics

The half-life of methoxy PEG-epoetin beta was 134 h and 139 h in adult PD patients following IV and subcutaneous dosing, respectively [118]. The peak reticulocyte count occurred at a mean of

occur with an inflammatory block, a condition where inflammation prevents effective delivery of iron for erythropoiesis. Clinical signs of infection, a low serum iron, an elevated CRP, and an increasing ferritin support a diagnosis of an inflammatory block.

KDIGO recommends treating adult CKD patients with IV iron when the TSAT is <30% and the ferritin is <500 ng/mL, assuming there is an indication (desire to increase the Hb or decrease the ESA dose). It is clear that some patients respond to IV iron despite an elevated ferritin [130]. This has led to controversy regarding the upper limit of ferritin in the KDIGO guidelines, with some suggesting that there is no evidence base for an upper limit for ferritin of 500 ng/mL [72, 73]. There has been an increase in the use of IV iron worldwide [131], and in the US the mean serum ferritin in HD patients increased to close to 800 ng/ml [71].

The KDIGO cutoffs for initiating IV iron in pediatric patients are a TSAT <20% and a ferritin <100 ng/ml. This is quite conservative and many pediatric nephrologists treat patients with TSATs <20–30% despite ferritin values >100 ng/ml. The upper limit of ferritin for holding IV iron for pediatric patients varies among clinicians, with some practitioners using cutoffs of 500–800 ng/ml. This variation is due to the lack of evidence supporting a specific cutoff.

Iron Therapy

After EPO deficiency, iron deficiency is the leading cause of anemia in children with CKD. Treatment of iron deficiency often allows achievement of the target Hb with a lower dose of ESA. Iron therapy should not be given to patients who have iron overload, which is commonly defined as a ferritin greater than 800 ng/mL or a TSAT>50%.

Oral Iron

Only a small percentage of oral iron is absorbed, limiting its efficacy in patients who have high iron requirements due to blood loss, such as children receiving HD [9]. Adherence to therapy may be problematic due to problems with gastrointestinal side effects, including abdominal discomfort and constipation [132]. In HD patients, oral iron appears to be of limited benefit and is poorly tolerated [133].

There is an up-regulation in oral iron absorption in patients who have a low serum ferritin or decreased marrow iron stores. However, HD patients have decreased absorption of oral iron when compared to normal controls; inflammation, which is common in HD patients, decreases iron absorption. This is partially mediated by hepcidin, which inhibits iron absorption from the intestines, and is increased by inflammation [22].

Oral iron absorption is decreased when given with food; hence, iron should be given either 1 h before or 2 h after a meal. Calcium carbonate and calcium acetate decrease iron absorption; oral iron should not be given at the same time as these phosphate binders. Sevelamer seems to have little effect on oral iron absorption [134]. H2-receptor antagonists and proton pump inhibitors may also adversely affect iron absorption.

Oral iron may be adequate therapy in children who are not receiving HD. In children receiving HD, oral iron is often not sufficient to correct absolute or functional iron deficiency [135, 136]. Children receiving chronic IV iron should not receive oral iron given the limited benefits and high rate of side effects of oral iron.

Ferrous sulfate, an iron salt, is the most commonly prescribed oral iron preparation; other iron salts include ferrous fumarate, ferrous gluconate and polysaccharide iron complex. Iron salts rapidly release iron ions, which increases the risk of gastrointestinal side effects. The iron salts are inexpensive options. Children should receive a dose of 3–6 mg/kg/day of elemental iron (maximum dose: 150–300 mg/day).

There are a variety of alternative options to iron salts, but many are expensive, with prices that range from 20 to more than 500 times the cost of ferrous sulfate. The possible advantages include increased effectiveness due to increased bioavailability, and improved tolerability with some preparations.

Ferric citrate was originally approved as a phosphate binder, but has been shown to be effective in treating iron deficiency, though gastrointestinal side effects are common [137–139]. In a randomized study in adults with CKD, ferric citrate was superior to ferrous sulfate for correcting iron deficiency [140]. There is limited pediatric experience with ferric citrate as a phosphate binder [141].

Ferric maltol is an oral iron preparation that was approved by the FDA and European Medical Agency for iron deficiency based on studies of patients with inflammatory bowel disease and CKD [142, 143]. It is better tolerated than iron salts [142]. Because of its improved bioavailability, doses of 30 mg twice daily are effective in adults. A randomized study in adult inflammatory bowel disease patients showed comparable 26 and 52 week efficacy when compared to IV ferric carboxymaltose [144]. There is no published pediatric experience.

Sucrosomial® iron has improved bioavailability and gastrointestinal tolerance compared to iron salts [144]. It is effective in adults with CKD at a dose of 30 mg daily, and had comparative long-term efficacy in increasing hemoglobin in adult CKD patients not on dialysis when compared to 125 mg of IV iron gluconate given weekly, though iron stores improved more with IV iron gluconate [145]. It is much less expensive than the other alternatives to iron salts (ferric citrate and ferric maltol) and is cost-effective when compared to IV iron preparations [146]. It is available over the counter in the US, though only via on-line sources. There is no published pediatric experience.

Intravenous Iron

IV iron is more effective than oral iron in correcting anemia in adult patients with CKD, although the benefit is relatively small in pre-dialysis patients [132, 147, 148]. IV iron is believed to be cost effective in HD patients due to decrease ESA utilization [149, 150]. Studies in children, including a meta-analysis [151], have shown the efficacy of IV iron in correcting iron deficiency,

improving Hb levels, and reducing rHuEPO dose requirements [135, 136, 152–155]. There is limited experience using IV iron in pediatric kidney transplant recipients [156].

Acute dosing of IV iron is used for patients who have evidence of iron deficiency, which is most commonly defined based on measures of iron stores. The dose given is relatively large. Chronic dosing utilizes smaller doses to maintain iron stores and provide a regular source of iron for erythropoiesis. Acute dosing results in a more significant change in Hb and iron stores [157]. For children receiving PD or who are predialysis, the goal is usually to minimize the need for IV line placement by maximizing the dose given during a single infusion. A chronic dosing strategy is generally only utilized in patients receiving HD due to the burden of IV placement.

Preparations

There are a variety of IV iron preparations available (Table 59.9). The European Pediatric PD Working Group recommended not using iron dextran due to concerns about life-threatening anaphylactic reactions [30]. These preparations have different side effect profiles. In addition, there is no preparation that is ideal in every situation. Iron sucrose and ferric gluconate have limitations on individual doses and must be given over an extended period when higher doses are utilized. This somewhat limits their utility in patients who are not receiving HD. In contrast, ferric carboxymaltose, ferric derisomaltose and ferumoxytol can be given more rapidly at higher doses. However, ferric carboxymaltose, ferric derisomaltose and ferumoxytol are not designed to be given in a chronic dosing strategy due to product packaging in very high doses.

Ferric gluconate is generally well-tolerated [158, 159], and an effective treatment for CKD patients with iron deficiency [130, 160–163]. Ferric gluconate is available in 62.5 mg vials. Acute dosing in adult HD patients is typically 125 mg administered over 10 min given over 8 consecutive HD sessions (total dose = 1000 mg). The recommended acute dose in children receiving HD is a maximum of 1.5 mg/kg over 10 min. In adults, ferric gluconate doses of 250 mg, over

Table 59.9 Intravenous iron preparations[a]

Compound	Adult dosing	Adult administration
LMW Iron dextran[b]	500–1000 mg	Test dose (25 mg) needed; Remainder of dose over >60 min
Ferric gluconate	125 mg	Diluted infusion over 1 h Undiluted up to 12.5 mg/min
Iron sucrose	100 mg	Injection: 2–5 min (≤200 mg) Infusion: ≤200 mg: 15 min; 300 mg: 1.5 h; 400 mg: 2.5 h; 500 mg: 3.5–4 h
Ferric carboxymaltose	≥50 kg: 750 mg × 2 (≥1 week apart) or 15 mg/kg (max 1 g) × 1 dose <50 kg: 15 mg/kg (once or twice ≥1 week apart)	Injection: 100 mg/min (≤750 mg) or over 15 min (1 g dose); infusion (diluted) over ≥15 min
Ferric derisomaltose	≥ 50 kg: 1 g <50 kg: 2 mg/kg	Infusion: ≥30 min
Ferumoxytol	1020 mg (one dose) or 510 mg (2 doses) ≥ 3 days apart	Infusion: 510 mg: ≥ 15 min; 1020 mg ≥ 30 min

LMW low molecular weight

[a]Dosing and administration recommendations may vary by country and change over time. Review current, local recommendations prior to using

[b]Smaller doses may be used for maintenance therapy, typically in hemodialysis patients

60 or 90 min, were well tolerated [164], as were infusions over 1–4 h) [165]. In children, one study reported administration of doses ranging from 1.5 to 8.8 mg/kg, with the child receiving the highest dose having a significant adverse event [152]. Thus, acute doses of ferric gluconate in patients not receiving HD should not exceed 4 mg/kg (250 mg if >60 kg), which should be given over at least 90 min.

Iron sucrose is generally well-tolerated [166, 167] and effective in correcting iron deficiency in patients with CKD [168–170]. Iron sucrose is available in 50 mg vials. Adult HD patients are usually given 50 or 100 mg over 5 min [166]. Infusions of 100 mg over 10 consecutive dialysis sessions is used for acute dosing to provide a total of 1000 mg. For chronic dosing in adult HD patients, doses of 50 or 100 mg avoids wasting medication and can be given weekly or every other week [166].

In adult PD or predialysis pat over 1.5–2 h, appear to be well tolerated. Doses of iron sucrose as high as 500 mg have been given, but the infusion time must be extended to avoid side effects, and this dose may not be tolerated in smaller adults [169, 171, 172]. In children, a dose of 2 mg/kg (maximum 100 mg) over 3 min or 5 mg/kg (maximum 300 mg) over 90 min is well-tolerated [173]. The 5 mg/kg dose can be repeated the next day [173].

Ferric carboxymaltose is effective in treating iron deficiency and is approved for use in non-dialysis CKD patients [174–178]. When ferric carboxymaltose was directly compared to iron sucrose, there was more hypertension in the ferric carboxymaltose group and more hypotension in the iron sucrose group [177]. There are recommendations for acute dosing in adults: 15 mg/kg (maximum 750 mg) with a second dose at least 1 week later. It is administered over 15 min. There is substantial pediatric experience with ferric carboxymaltose, but limited experience in children with CKD [179–183]. In one study, the usual dose was 15 mg/kg, with a maximum dose of 750 mg [179]. In another study, the usual dose was 20 mg/kg, with a maximum dose of 1000 mg in children >35 kg and 500 mg in children <35 kg [183]. Ferric carboxymaltose is available in 750 mg vials, precluding its use in a chronic dosing strategy (see below) or in small children without wasting medication. Hypophosphatemia is a complication in adults with CKD and children who receive ferric carboxymaltose for other indications [177, 184–187].

Ferumoxytol, approved for CKD patients, is effective when given to adults at a dose of 510 mg, followed by a second dose 3–8 days later, though single doses of 1020 mg also appear safe [188–191]. The infusion rate should not exceed 30 mg of iron/second. The large vial size (510 mg) limits

its utility in small children or for use in a chronic dosing strategy. There is limited pediatric experience, albeit not in children with CKD [192, 193]. In one study, ferumoxytol at a dose of 10 mg/kg (maximum 510 mg) was administered over 60 min and 15 min for the first infusion and subsequent infusions, respectively [193].

Ferric derisomaltose is approved and marketed in more than 30 countries worldwide, including the US, the EU, Canada, and Australia for treating iron deficiency. It has comparative efficacy to iron sucrose in patients without CKD and patients with pre-dialysis CKD. There is no published pediatric experience [194, 195].

Acute Dosing

Acute doses of IV iron are given when the patient has evidence of iron deficiency (see criteria above). The goal of acute IV iron dosing is to normalize the serum ferritin and the TSAT. In some cases, an acute dose may be used as a trial of IV iron in a patient with normal iron studies, but a poor response to an ESA. In these patients, the goal of acute IV iron is a reduction in ESA dose or correction of resistant anemia.

In adult HD patients, studies suggest that a total dose of 1000 mg of iron, divided over multiple consecutive dialysis sessions, is appropriate, since smaller doses are not as effective [162]. A total dose of 1000 mg has been used in older children with good results [136]. A randomized study of children receiving HD compared 2 acute dosing regimens of ferric gluconate (1.5 mg/kg/dose and 3.0 mg/kg/dose; maximum dose, 125 mg/dose) given during 8 consecutive HD sessions. The patients had a TSAT <20% and/or a ferritin less than 100 ng/mL at baseline. Both doses led to an increase in Hb and normalization of iron indices. Since there was no difference in the response, the authors recommended a dose of 1.5 mg/kg/dose (maximum of 125 mg/dose) for 8 consecutive HD sessions [196]. This provides a total dose of 12 mg/kg (maximum dose of 1000 mg). Based on the available evidence, the total dose for acute pediatric dosing should be between 12 and 25 mg/kg (1000 mg maximum) divided over up to 12 HD sessions, depending on the dose and iron preparation (see above discussion of specific preparations).

Chronic Dosing

Acute dosing is effective in correcting iron deficiency, but especially in HD patients there is a risk of ongoing episodes of iron deficiency due to continued blood loss. Transient iron deficiency may lead to decreased red blood cell synthesis. This has led to more frequent chronic IV iron use. Observational studies in adults suggests that maintenance therapy may be associated with better outcomes than an acute dosing strategy [197, 198].

In one pediatric study, 1 mg/kg of ferric gluconate for 12 weeks led to a significant increase in Hb [135]. In another pediatric study, chronic IV iron sucrose (2 mg/kg [max = 200 mg] weekly) produced a reduction in rHuEPO dose [153]. A randomized 16-week study in children receiving HD compared maintenance IV iron dextran (doses of 25, 50 or 100 mg/week based on weight; doses therefore ranged from 1.25–2.5 mg/kg/week) with oral iron (4–6 mg/kg/day). The patients receiving IV iron had a significant increase in ferritin when compared to the oral iron group. There was a trend toward a reduction in rHuEPO dose in the IV iron group when compared to the oral iron group [155].

Another study randomized children receiving HD to intermittent IV iron versus maintenance IV iron. There was a higher rate of iron overload in the children receiving intermittent IV iron [199]. This observation may be secondary to a decreased ability to utilize stored iron in children receiving HD due to an inflammatory block. The low doses of maintenance IV iron are immediately employed for red cell synthesis, avoiding an excessive accumulation of stored iron. This contrasts with intermittent IV iron; the high doses cannot all be utilized immediately, increasing the risk of eventual iron overload.

One pediatric study prospectively followed children who were started on a maintenance dose of 1 mg/kg/week of ferric gluconate and then adjusted the dose of ferric gluconate based on iron studies. The majority of the patients completing the study required a dose of 1.5 mg/kg to maintain adequate iron stores [200].

Maintenance IV iron in children receiving HD should be started at about 1 mg/kg/week, usually given as a once/week dose. The maintenance dose is titrated to keep the TSAT above 20% and the ferritin above 100 ng/mL; IV iron should be held if the TSAT is greater than 50% or the ferritin is greater than 500 ng/mL.

Complications

There are some complications of IV iron that are specific to the particular preparation. Iron dextran may cause an acute anaphylactic reaction, which is potentially fatal [201]. Iron sucrose [159] and ferric gluconate [162] have a safer side effect profile, although all IV iron preparations have the potential to cause serious adverse reactions. Children and adults who have had anaphylactic reactions to iron dextran have tolerated other iron preparations [152, 202, 203]. High doses of iron dextran may cause patients to develop arthralgias and myalgias [204].

There are reports of laboratory findings and clinical symptoms that may be due to acute iron toxicity during the use of iron sucrose and ferric gluconate. This effect is related to the dose and infusion rate and is presumably secondary to rapid release of free iron. Symptoms with ferric gluconate have included loin pain, hypotension, emesis and paresthesias [205]. Iron sucrose side effects have included rash, flushing, and hypotension, which were rapidly reversible [206]. These side effects limit the maximum single dose of these compounds when compared to iron dextran, which releases free iron at a slower rate.

Use of IV iron may increase generation of reactive oxidative species, which has the potential to impair endothelial cell function, promote atherosclerosis, cause inflammation, and decrease immune function [207–210]. There is evidence of an association between higher iron dose and increased adverse outcomes, recognizing a variety of potential confounders [211]. These adverse events may be less likely with iron preparations that release iron more gradually (e.g. ferric carboxymaltose, ferumoxytol and ferric derisomaltose) than iron sucrose or ferric gluconate. This was seen in a randomized study comparing iron sucrose with ferumoxytol [177]. Yet, there is not yet enough evidence to reach a conclusion on this issue given the limitations with the extant literature [212].

Ferumoxytol is associated with higher rates of adverse events than iron sucrose or ferric gluconate [167]. Adverse reactions include injection site reactions, hypersensitivity reactions and hypotension that can be severe [213]. Patients should be observed for at least 30 min after receiving ferumoxytol. Its use may also transiently affect MRI interpretation since it is also used as a contrast agent for MRIs [213].

Iron overload is a potential complication of IV iron therapy, and may occur in CKD patients receiving IV iron [214–216]. There is concern that current IV iron protocols may lead to more problems with iron overload, which has been seen in children receiving acute or maintenance IV iron [153, 199].

IV iron may cause hypophosphatemia, which appears to be mediated by increased levels of FGF-23 and urinary phosphate wasting [217, 218]. Clinically significant, sustained hypophosphatemia is associated with ferric carboxymaltose [186, 187, 219].

IV iron may increase the risk of infection [220]. A multivariate analysis did not find a relationship between IV iron and infection, although there was a trend toward more infections among those patients who received large amounts of IV iron versus those who received lower doses [221]. Given this potential complication, IV iron should be held in patients with acute infections.

References

1. Kidney Disease: Improving Global Outcomes (KDIGO) Anemia Work Group. KDIGO Clinical Practice Guideline for Anemia in Chronic Kidney Disease. Kidney Int. 2012;2:279–335.
2. Mikhail A, Brown C, Williams JA, et al. Renal association clinical practice guideline on Anaemia of Chronic Kidney Disease. BMC Nephrol. 2017;18:345.
3. Chronic kidney disease: assessment and management. 2021. (Accessed August 30, 2021, 2021, at https://www.nice.org.uk/guidance/ng203/chapter/Recommendations#managing-anaemia)
4. Atkinson MA, Pierce CB, Zack RM, et al. Hemoglobin differences by race in children with CKD. Am J Kidney Dis. 2010;55:1009–17.
5. van Stralen KJ, Krischock L, Schaefer F, et al. Prevalence and predictors of the sub-target Hb level

in children on dialysis. Nephrol Dial Transplant. 2012;27:3950–7.

6. McGonigle RJ, Boineau FG, Beckman B, et al. Erythropoietin and inhibitors of in vitro erythropoiesis in the development of anemia in children with renal disease. J Lab Clin Med. 1985;105:449–58.

7. Mercadal L, Metzger M, Casadevall N, et al. Timing and determinants of erythropoietin deficiency in chronic kidney disease. Clin J Am Soc Nephrol. 2012;7:35–42.

8. Fadrowski JJ, Pierce CB, Cole SR, Moxey-Mims M, Warady BA, Furth SL. Hemoglobin decline in children with chronic kidney disease: baseline results from the chronic kidney disease in children prospective cohort study. Clin J Am Soc Nephrol. 2008;3:457–62.

9. Muller-Wiefel DE, Sinn H, Gilli G, Scharer K. Hemolysis and blood loss in children with chronic renal failure. Clin Nephrol. 1977;8:481–6.

10. Bamgbola OF, Kaskel FJ, Coco M. Analyses of age, gender and other risk factors of erythropoietin resistance in pediatric and adult dialysis cohorts. Pediatr Nephrol. 2009;24:571–9.

11. Eknoyan G, Latos D, Lindberg J. Practice recommendations for the use of L-Carnitine in dialysis-related carnitine disorder National Kidney Foundation Carnitine Consensus Conference. Am J Kidney Dis. 2003;41:868–76.

12. Polenakovic M, Sikole A. Is erythropoietin a survival factor for red blood cells? J Am Soc Nephrol. 1996;7:1178–82.

13. Richardson D, Lindley E, Bartlett C, Will E. A randomized, controlled study of the consequences of hemodialysis membrane composition on erythropoietic response. Am J Kidney Dis. 2003;42:551–60.

14. Frankenfield DL, Neu AM, Warady BA, Fivush BA, Johnson CA, Brem AS. Anemia in pediatric hemodialysis patients: results from the 2001 ESRD Clinical Performance Measures Project. Kidney Int. 2003;64:1120–4.

15. Arbeiter K, Greenbaum L, Balzar E, et al. Reproducible erythroid aplasia caused by mycophenolate mofetil. Pediatr Nephrol. 2000;14:195–7.

16. Subtirelu MM, Flynn JT, Schechner RS, Pullman JM, Feuerstein D, Del Rio M. Acute renal failure in a pediatric kidney allograft recipient treated with intravenous immunoglobulin for parvovirus B19 induced pure red cell aplasia. Pediatr Transplant. 2005;9:801–4.

17. Borzych-Duzalka D, Bilginer Y, Ha IS, et al. Management of anemia in children receiving chronic peritoneal dialysis. J Am Soc Nephrol. 2013;24:665–76.

18. Zaritsky J, Young B, Gales B, et al. Reduction of serum hepcidin by hemodialysis in pediatric and adult patients. Clin J Am Soc Nephrol. 2010;5:1010–4.

19. Kalantar-Zadeh K, Ikizler TA, Block G, Avram M, Kopple J. Malnutrition-inflammation complex syndrome in dialysis patients: causes and consequences. Am J Kidney Dis. 2003;42:864–81.

20. Barany P. Inflammation, serum C-reactive protein, and erythropoietin resistance. Nephrol Dial Transplant. 2001;16:224–7.

21. Susantitaphong P, Riella C, Jaber BL. Effect of ultrapure dialysate on markers of inflammation, oxidative stress, nutrition and anemia parameters: a meta-analysis. Nephrol Dial Transplant. 2013;28:438–46.

22. Atkinson MA, White CT. Hepcidin in anemia of chronic kidney disease: review for the pediatric nephrologist. Pediatr Nephrol. 2012;27:33–40.

23. Ganz T. Molecular pathogenesis of anemia of chronic disease. Pediatr Blood Cancer. 2006;46:554–7.

24. Won HS, Kim HG, Yun YS, et al. IL-6 is an independent risk factor for resistance to erythropoiesis-stimulating agents in hemodialysis patients without iron deficiency. Hemodial Int. 2012;16:31–7.

25. Barany P, Divino Filho JC, Bergstrom J. High C-reactive protein is a strong predictor of resistance to erythropoietin in hemodialysis patients. Am J Kidney Dis. 1997;29:565–8.

26. Rao DS, Shih MS, Mohini R. Effect of serum parathyroid hormone and bone marrow fibrosis on the response to erythropoietin in uremia. N Engl J Med. 1993;328:171–5.

27. Nomura S, Ogawa Y, Osawa G, Katagiri M, Harada T, Nagahana H. Myelofibrosis secondary to renal osteodystrophy. Nephron. 1996;72:683–7.

28. Pronai W, Riegler-Keil M, Silberbauer K, Stockenhuber F. Folic acid supplementation improves erythropoietin response. Nephron. 1995;71:395–400.

29. Kaiser L, Schwartz KA. Aluminum-induced anemia. Am J Kidney Dis. 1985;6:348–52.

30. Schroder CH, European Pediatric Peritoneal Dialysis Working Group. The management of anemia in pediatric peritoneal dialysis patients. Guidelines by an ad hoc European committee. Pediatr Nephrol 2003;18:805–809.

31. Locatelli F, Aljama P, Barany P, et al. Revised European best practice guidelines for the management of anaemia in patients with chronic renal failure. Nephrol Dial Transplant. 2004;19(Suppl. 2):ii1–47.

32. Morgans HA, Chadha V, Warady BA. The role of carnitine in maintenance dialysis therapy. Pediatr Nephrol. 2021;36:2545–51.

33. Malyszko J, Glowinska I, Mysliwiec M. Treatment of anemia with erythropoietin-stimulating agents in kidney transplant recipients and chronic kidney disease-another drawback of immunosuppression? Transplant Proc. 2012;44:3013–6.

34. Erturk S, Nergizoglu G, Ates K, et al. The impact of withdrawing ACE inhibitors on erythropoietin responsiveness and left ventricular hypertrophy in haemodialysis patients. Nephrol Dial Transplant. 1999;14:1912–6.

35. Atkinson MA, Martz K, Warady BA, Neu AM. Risk for anemia in pediatric chronic kidney disease patients: a report of NAPRTCS. Pediatr Nephrol. 2010;25:1699–706.

36. Mitsnefes MM, Subat-Dezulovic M, Khoury PR, Goebel J, Strife CF. Increasing incidence of post-kidney transplant anemia in children. Am J Transplant. 2005;5:1713–8.

37. Foley RN, Parfrey PS, Harnett JD, Kent GM, Murray DC, Barre PE. The impact of anemia on cardiomyopathy, morbidity, and and mortality in end-stage renal disease. Am J Kidney Dis. 1996;28:53–61.

38. Collins AJ, Li S, St Peter W, et al. Death, hospitalization, and economic associations among incident hemodialysis patients with hematocrit values of 36 to 39%. J Am Soc Nephrol. 2001;12:2465–73.

39. Locatelli F, Pisoni RL, Combe C, et al. Anaemia in haemodialysis patients of five European countries: association with morbidity and mortality in the Dialysis Outcomes and Practice Patterns Study (DOPPS). Nephrol Dial Transplant. 2004;19:121–32.

40. Fort J, Cuevas X, Garcia F, et al. Mortality in incident haemodialysis patients: time-dependent haemoglobin levels and erythropoiesis-stimulating agent dose are independent predictive factors in the ANSWER study. Nephrol Dial Transplant. 2010;25:2702–10.

41. Warady BA, Ho M. Morbidity and mortality in children with anemia at initiation of dialysis. Pediatr Nephrol. 2003;18:1055–62.

42. Staples AO, Wong CS, Smith JM, et al. Anemia and risk of hospitalization in pediatric chronic kidney disease. Clin J Am Soc Nephrol. 2009;4:48–56.

43. Morris KP, Skinner JR, Hunter S, Coulthard MG. Cardiovascular abnormalities in end stage renal failure: the effect of anaemia or uraemia? Arch Dis Child. 1994;71:119–22.

44. Mitsnefes MM, Daniels SR, Schwartz SM, Meyer RA, Khoury P, Strife CF. Severe left ventricular hypertrophy in pediatric dialysis: prevalence and predictors. Pediatr Nephrol. 2000;14:898–902.

45. McMahon LP, Cai MX, Baweja S, et al. Mortality in dialysis patients may not be associated with ESA dose: a 2-year prospective observational study. BMC Nephrol. 2012;13:40.

46. Besarab A, Bolton WK, Browne JK, et al. The effects of normal as compared with low hematocrit values in patients with cardiac disease who are receiving hemodialysis and epoetin. N Engl J Med. 1998;339:584–90.

47. Drueke TB, Locatelli F, Clyne N, et al. Normalization of hemoglobin level in patients with chronic kidney disease and anemia. N Engl J Med. 2006;355:2071–84.

48. Singh AK, Szczech L, Tang KL, et al. Correction of anemia with epoetin alfa in chronic kidney disease. N Engl J Med. 2006;355:2085–98.

49. Pfeffer MA, Burdmann EA, Chen CY, et al. A trial of darbepoetin alfa in type 2 diabetes and chronic kidney disease. N Engl J Med. 2009;361:2019–32.

50. Finkelstein FO, Finkelstein SH. The impact of anemia treatment on health-related quality of life in patients with chronic kidney disease in the contemporary era. Adv Chronic Kidney Dis. 2019;26:250–2.

51. Canadian Erythropoietin Study Group. Association between recombinant human erythropoietin and quality of life and exercise capacity of patients receiving haemodialysis. Canadian Erythropoietin Study Group. BMJ. 1990;300:573–8.

52. Gerson A, Hwang W, Fiorenza J, et al. Anemia and health-related quality of life in adolescents with chronic kidney disease. Am J Kidney Dis. 2004;44:1017–23.

53. Montini G, Zacchello G, Baraldi E, et al. Benefits and risks of anemia correction with recombinant human erythropoietin in children maintained by hemodialysis. J Pediatr. 1990;117:556–60.

54. Burke JR. Low-dose subcutaneous recombinant erythropoietin in children with chronic renal failure. Australian and New Zealand Paediatric Nephrology Association. Pediatr Nephrol. 1995;9:558–61.

55. Jabs K, Alexander S, McCabe D, Lerner G, Harmon W. Primary results from the U.S. multicenter pediatric recombinant erythropoietin (EPO) study. J Am Soc Nephrol. 1994;5:546.

56. Jabs K. The effects of recombinant human erythropoietin on growth and nutritional status. Pediatr Nephrol. 1996;10:324–7.

57. Hutchinson FN, Jones WJ. A cost-effectiveness analysis of anemia screening before erythropoietin in patients with end-stage renal disease. Am J Kidney Dis. 1997;29:651–7.

58. Gokal R, Weatherall DJ, Bunch C. Iron induced increase in red cell size in haemodialysis patients. Q J Med. 1979;48:393–401.

59. Hymes LC, Hawthorne SM, Clowers BM. Impaired response to recombinant erythropoietin therapy in children with peritonitis. Dial Transplant. 1994;23:462–3.

60. van Iperen CE, Kraaijenhagen RJ, Biesma DH, Beguin Y, Marx JJ, van de Wiel A. Iron metabolism and erythropoiesis after surgery. Br J Surg. 1998;85:41–5.

61. National Kidney Foundation. KDOQI clinical practice guidelines and clinical practice recommendations for anemia in chronic kidney disease. Am J Kidney Dis. 2006;47:S1–S145.

62. Aufricht C, Balzar E, Steger H, et al. Subcutaneous recombinant human erythropoietin in children with renal anemia on continuous ambulatory peritoneal dialysis. Acta Paediatr. 1993;82:959–62.

63. Parfrey PS, Foley RN, Wittreich BH, Sullivan DJ, Zagari MJ, Frei D. Double-blind comparison of full and partial anemia correction in incident hemodialysis patients without symptomatic heart disease. J Am Soc Nephrol. 2005;16:2180–9.

64. Heinze G, Kainz A, Horl WH, Oberbauer R. Mortality in renal transplant recipients given erythropoietins to increase haemoglobin concentration: cohort study. BMJ. 2009;339:b4018.

65. Kausz AT, Solid C, Pereira BJ, Collins AJ, St PW. Intractable anemia among hemodialysis patients: a sign of suboptimal management or a marker of disease? Am J Kidney Dis. 2005;45:136–47.

66. Solomon SD, Uno H, Lewis EF, et al. Erythropoietic response and outcomes in kidney disease and type 2 diabetes. N Engl J Med. 2010;363:1146–55.

67. Zhang Y, Thamer M, Stefanik K, Kaufman J, Cotter DJ. Epoetin requirements predict mortality in hemodialysis patients. Am J Kidney Dis. 2004;44:866–76.

68. Ehrenreich H, Weissenborn K, Prange H, et al. Recombinant human erythropoietin in the treatment of acute ischemic stroke. Stroke. 2009;40:e647–56.

69. Goodkin DA, Fuller DS, Robinson BM, et al. Naturally occurring higher hemoglobin concentration does not increase mortality among hemodialysis patients. J Am Soc Nephrol. 2011;22:358–65.

70. Regidor DL, Kopple JD, Kovesdy CP, et al. Associations between changes in hemoglobin and administered erythropoiesis-stimulating agent and survival in hemodialysis patients. J Am Soc Nephrol. 2006;17:1181–91.

71. Fuller DS, Pisoni RL, Bieber BA, Port FK, Robinson BM. The DOPPS practice monitor for U.S. dialysis care: update on trends in anemia management 2 years into the bundle. Am J Kidney Dis. 2013;62:1213–6.

72. Moist LM, Troyanov S, White CT, et al. Canadian Society of Nephrology commentary on the 2012 KDIGO Clinical Practice Guideline for Anemia in CKD. Am J Kidney Dis. 2013;62:860–73.

73. Kliger AS, Foley RN, Goldfarb DS, et al. KDOQI US commentary on the 2012 KDIGO Clinical Practice Guideline for Anemia in CKD. Am J Kidney Dis. 2013;62:849–59.

74. Lines SW, Lindley EJ, Tattersall JE, Wright MJ. A predictive algorithm for the management of anaemia in haemodialysis patients based on ESA pharmacodynamics: better results for less work. Nephrol Dial Transplant. 2012;27:2425–9.

75. Gilbertson DT, Ebben JP, Foley RN, Weinhandl ED, Bradbury BD, Collins AJ. Hemoglobin level variability: associations with mortality. Clin J Am Soc Nephrol. 2008;3:133–8.

76. Schiller B, Doss S, De Cock E, Del Aguila MA, Nissenson AR. Costs of managing anemia with erythropoiesis-stimulating agents during hemodialysis: a time and motion study. Hemodial Int. 2008;12:441–9.

77. Eschbach JW, Abdulhadi MH, Browne JK, et al. Recombinant human erythropoietin in anemic patients with end-stage renal disease. Results of a phase III multicenter clinical trial. Ann Intern Med. 1989;111:992–1000.

78. Ho M, Stablein DM. North American Pediatric Renal Transplant Cooperative Study (NAPRTCS) Annual Report. Rockville, Maryland, 2003.

79. Centers for Medicare & Medicaid Services. 2002 annual report, end stage renal disease clinical performance measures project. Am J Kidney Dis. 2003;42:S1–S96.

80. Port RE, Mehls O. Erythropoietin dosing in children with chronic kidney disease: based on body size or on hemoglobin deficit? Pediatr Nephrol. 2009;24:435–7.

81. Sieniawska M, Roszkowska-Blaim M. Recombinant human erythropoietin dosage in children undergoing hemodialysis and continuous ambulatory peritoneal dialysis. Pediatr Nephrol. 1997;11:628–30.

82. Jander A, Wiercinski R, Balasz-Chmielewska I, et al. Anaemia treatment in chronically dialysed children: a multicentre nationwide observational study. Scand J Urol Nephrol. 2012;46:375–80.

83. Spinowitz B, Germain M, Benz R, et al. A randomized study of extended dosing regimens for initiation of epoetin alfa treatment for anemia of chronic kidney disease. Clin J Am Soc Nephrol. 2008;3:1015–21.

84. Brandt JR, Avner ED, Hickman RO, Watkins SL. Safety and efficacy of erythropoietin in children with chronic renal failure. Pediatr Nephrol. 1999;13:143–7.

85. Yalcinkaya F, Tumer N, Cakar N, Ozkaya N. Low-dose erythropoietin is effective and safe in children on continuous ambulatory peritoneal dialysis. Pediatr Nephrol. 1997;11:350–2.

86. Casadevall N, Nataf J, Viron B, et al. Pure red-cell aplasia and antierythropoietin antibodies in patients treated with recombinant erythropoietin. N Engl J Med. 2002;346:469–75.

87. Bennett CL, Cournoyer D, Carson KR, et al. Long-term outcome of individuals with pure red cell aplasia and antierythropoietin antibodies in patients treated with recombinant epoetin: a follow-up report from the Research on Adverse Drug Events and Reports (RADAR) Project. Blood. 2005;106:3343–7.

88. Nissenson AR, Swan SK, Lindberg JS, et al. Randomized, controlled trial of darbepoetin alfa for the treatment of anemia in hemodialysis patients. Am J Kidney Dis. 2002;40:110–8.

89. Vanrenterghem Y, Barany P, Mann JF, et al. Randomized trial of darbepoetin alfa for treatment of renal anemia at a reduced dose frequency compared with rHuEPO in dialysis patients. Kidney Int. 2002;62:2167–75.

90. Walker R. Aranesp (darbepoetin alfa) administered at a reduced frequency of once every 4 weeks (Q4W) maintains hemoglobin levels in patients with chronic kidney disease (CKD) receiving dialysis. National Kidney Foundation Clinical Nephrology Meeting; 2002.

91. Warady BA, Arar MY, Lerner G, Nakanishi AM, Stehman-Breen C. Darbepoetin alfa for the treatment of anemia in pediatric patients with chronic kidney disease. Pediatr Nephrol. 2006;21:1144–52.

92. De Palo T, Giordano M, Palumbo F, et al. Clinical experience with darbepoietin alfa (NESP) in children undergoing hemodialysis. Pediatr Nephrol. 2004;19:337–40.

93. Geary DF, Keating LE, Vigneux A, Stephens D, Hebert D, Harvey EA. Darbepoetin alfa (Aranesp) in children with chronic renal failure. Kidney Int. 2005;68:1759–65.

94. Durkan AM, Keating LE, Vigneux A, Geary DF. The use of darbepoetin in infants with chronic renal impairment. Pediatr Nephrol. 2006;21:694–7.

95. Andre JL, Deschenes G, Boudailliez B, et al. Darbepoetin, effective treatment of anaemia in paediatric patients with chronic renal failure. Pediatr Nephrol. 2007;22:708–14.

96. Schaefer F, Hoppe B, Jungraithmayr T, et al. Safety and usage of darbepoetin alfa in children with chronic kidney disease: prospective registry study. Pediatr Nephrol. 2016;31:443–53.

97. Lerner G, Kale AS, Warady BA, et al. Pharmacokinetics of darbepoetin alfa in pediatric patients with chronic kidney disease. Pediatr Nephrol. 2002;17:933–7.

98. Macdougall IC, Gray SJ, Elston O, et al. Pharmacokinetics of novel erythropoiesis stimulating protein compared with epoetin alfa in dialysis patients. J Am Soc Nephrol. 1999;10:2392–5.

99. Evans JH, Brocklebank JT, Bowmer CJ, Ng PC. Pharmacokinetics of recombinant human erythropoietin in children with renal failure. Nephrol Dial Transplant. 1991;6:709–14.

100. Scott SD. Dose conversion from recombinant human erythropoietin to darbepoetin alfa: recommendations from clinical studies. Pharmacotherapy. 2002;22:160S–5S.

101. Disney A, Jersey PD, Kirkland G, et al. Darbepoetin alfa administered monthly maintains haemoglobin concentrations in patients with chronic kidney disease not receiving dialysis: a multicentre, open-label, Australian study. Nephrology. 2007;12:95–101.

102. Schmitt CP, Nau B, Brummer C, Rosenkranz J, Schaefer F. Increased injection pain with darbepoetin-alpha compared to epoetin-beta in paediatric dialysis patients. Nephrol Dial Transplant. 2006;21:3520–4.

103. Macdougall IC, Casadevall N, Locatelli F, et al. Incidence of erythropoietin antibody-mediated pure red cell aplasia: the Prospective Immunogenicity Surveillance Registry (PRIMS). Nephrol Dial Transplant. 2015;30:451–60.

104. Fishbane S, Pannier A, Liogier X, Jordan P, Dougherty FC, Reigner B. Pharmacokinetic and pharmacodynamic properties of methoxy polyethylene glycol-epoetin beta are unaffected by the site of subcutaneous administration. J Clin Pharmacol. 2007;47:1390–7.

105. Macdougall IC, Walker R, Provenzano R, et al. C.E.R.A. corrects anemia in patients with chronic kidney disease not on dialysis: results of a randomized clinical trial. Clin J Am Soc Nephrol. 2008;3:337–47.

106. Canaud B, Mingardi G, Braun J, et al. Intravenous C.E.R.A. maintains stable haemoglobin levels in patients on dialysis previously treated with darbepoetin alfa: results from STRIATA, a randomized phase III study. Nephrol Dial Transplant. 2008;23:3654–61.

107. Levin NW, Fishbane S, Canedo FV, et al. Intravenous methoxy polyethylene glycol-epoetin beta for haemoglobin control in patients with chronic kidney disease who are on dialysis: a randomised non-inferiority trial (MAXIMA). Lancet. 2007;370:1415–21.

108. Klinger M, Arias M, Vargemezis V, et al. Efficacy of intravenous methoxy polyethylene glycol-epoetin beta administered every 2 weeks compared with epoetin administered 3 times weekly in patients treated by hemodialysis or peritoneal dialysis: a randomized trial. Am J Kidney Dis. 2007;50:989–1000.

109. Sulowicz W, Locatelli F, Ryckelynck JP, et al. Once-monthly subcutaneous C.E.R.A. maintains stable hemoglobin control in patients with chronic kidney disease on dialysis and converted directly from epoetin one to three times weekly. Clin J Am Soc Nephrol. 2007;2:637–46.

110. Roger SD, Locatelli F, Woitas RP, et al. C.E.R.A. once every 4 weeks corrects anaemia and maintains haemoglobin in patients with chronic kidney disease not on dialysis. Nephrol Dial Transplant. 2011;26:3980–6.

111. Frimat L, Mariat C, Landais P, Kone S, Commenges B, Choukroun G. Anaemia management with C.E.R.A. in routine clinical practice: OCEANE (Cohorte Mircera patients non-dialyses), a national, multicenter, longitudinal, observational prospective study, in patients with chronic kidney disease not on dialysis. BMJ Open. 2013;3

112. Carrera F, Lok CE, de Francisco A, et al. Maintenance treatment of renal anaemia in haemodialysis patients with methoxy polyethylene glycol-epoetin beta versus darbepoetin alfa administered monthly: a randomized comparative trial. Nephrol Dial Transplant. 2010;25:4009–17.

113. Sanchez-Fructuoso A, Guirado L, Ruiz JC, et al. Anemia control in kidney transplant patients treated with methoxy polyethylene glycol-epoetin beta (mircera): the Anemiatrans Group. Transplant Proc. 2010;42:2931–4.

114. Esposito C, Abelli M, Sileno G, et al. Effects of continuous erythropoietin receptor activator (CERA) in kidney transplant recipients. Transplant Proc. 2012;44:1916–7.

115. Campistol JM, Carreno A, Morales JM, et al. Once-monthly pegylated epoetin Beta versus darbepoetin alfa every two weeks in renal transplant recipients: a randomized trial. Transplantation. 2013;95:e6–e10.

116. Fischbach M, Wühl E, Reigner SCM, Morgan Z, Schaefer F. Efficacy and long-term safety of C.E.R.A. maintenance in pediatric hemodialysis patients with anemia of CKD. Clin J Am Soc Nephrol. 2018;13:81–90.

117. Warady BA, Reigner SM, Tirodkar C, Drozdz D. A study to ascertain the optimum starting dose of subcutaneous (SC) C.E.R.A. for maintenance treatment of anaemia in paediatric patients with chronic kidney disease (CKD) on dialysis or not yet on dialysis. Eur Renal Assoc. 2022;

118. Macdougall IC, Robson R, Opatrna S, et al. Pharmacokinetics and pharmacodynamics of intravenous and subcutaneous continuous erythropoietin receptor activator (C.E.R.A.) in patients with

chronic kidney disease. Clin J Ame Soc Nephrol. 2006;1:1211–5.

119. Choi P, Farouk M, Manamley N, Addison J. Dose conversion ratio in hemodialysis patients switched from darbepoetin alfa to PEG-epoetin beta: AFFIRM study. Adv Ther. 2013;30:1007–17.

120. Wedekin M, Ehrich JH, Pape L. Effective treatment of anemia in pediatric kidney transplant recipients with methoxy polyethylene glycol-epoetin beta. Pediatr Transplant. 2011;15:329–33.

121. Schaefer F. C.E.R.A. (continuous erythropoietin receptor activator—methoxy polyethylene glycol epoetin beta) in paediatric dialysis patients with anaemia of chronic kidney disease: real-world evidence from the ipdn and iphn registries. Eur Renal Assoc. 2022;

122. Locatelli F, Del Vecchio L. Are prolyl-hydroxylase inhibitors potential alternative treatments for anaemia in patients with chronic kidney disease? Nephrol Dial Transplant. 2020;35:926–32.

123. Haase VH. Hypoxia-inducible factor-prolyl hydroxylase inhibitors in the treatment of anemia of chronic kidney disease. Kidney Int Suppl. 2011;2021(11):8–25.

124. Chertow GM, Pergola PE, Farag YMK, et al. Vadadustat in patients with anemia and non-dialysis-dependent CKD. N Engl J Med. 2021;384:1589–600.

125. Mikhail AI, Schön S, Simon S, et al. A prospective observational study of iron isomaltoside in haemodialysis patients with chronic kidney disease treated for iron deficiency (DINO). BMC Nephrol. 2019;20:13.

126. López-Ruzafa E, Vázquez-López MA, Lendinez-Molinos F, et al. Reference values of reticulocyte hemoglobin content and their relation with other indicators of iron status in healthy children. J Pediatr Hematol Oncol. 2016;38:e207–12.

127. Teixeira C, Barbot J, Freitas MI. Reference values for reticulocyte parameters and hypochromic RBC in healthy children. Int J Lab Hematol. 2015;37:626–30.

128. Davidkova S, Prestidge TD, Reed PW, Kara T, Wong W, Prestidge C. Comparison of reticulocyte hemoglobin equivalent with traditional markers of iron and erythropoiesis in pediatric dialysis. Pediatr Nephrol. 2016;31:819–26.

129. Hayes W. Measurement of iron status in chronic kidney disease. Pediatr Nephrol. 2019;34:605–13.

130. Coyne DW, Kapoian T, Suki W, et al. Ferric gluconate is highly efficacious in anemic hemodialysis patients with high serum ferritin and low transferrin saturation: results of the Dialysis Patients' Response to IV Iron with Elevated Ferritin (DRIVE) Study. J Am Soc Nephrol. 2007;18:975–84.

131. Bailie GR, Larkina M, Goodkin DA, et al. Variation in intravenous iron use internationally and over time: the Dialysis Outcomes and Practice Patterns Study (DOPPS). Nephrol Dial Transplant. 2013;28:2570–9.

132. Shepshelovich D, Rozen-Zvi B, Avni T, Gafter U, Gafter-Gvili A. Intravenous versus oral iron supplementation for the treatment of anemia in CKD: an updated systematic review and meta-analysis. Am J Kidney Dis. 2016;68:677–90.

133. Hodson EM, Craig JC. Oral iron for patients receiving dialysis: what is the evidence? Semin Dial. 2014;27:8–10.

134. Pruchnicki MC, Coyle JD, Hoshaw-Woodard S, Bay WH. Effect of phosphate binders on supplemental iron absorption in healthy subjects. J Clin Pharmacol. 2002;42:1171–6.

135. Tenbrock K, Muller-Berghaus J, Michalk D, Querfeld U. Intravenous iron treatment of renal anemia in children on hemodialysis. Pediatr Nephrol. 1999;13:580–2.

136. Greenbaum LA, Pan CG, Caley C, Nelson T, Sheth KJ. Intravenous iron dextran and erythropoietin use in pediatric hemodialysis patients. Pediatr Nephrol. 2000;14:908–11.

137. Fishbane S, Block GA, Loram L, et al. Effects of ferric citrate in patients with nondialysis-dependent CKD and iron deficiency anemia. J Am Soc Nephrol. 2017;28:1851–8.

138. Ganz T, Bino A, Salusky IB. Mechanism of action and clinical attributes of Auryxia(®) (ferric citrate). Drugs. 2019;79:957–68.

139. Choi YJ, Noh Y, Shin S. Ferric citrate in the management of hyperphosphataemia and iron deficiency anaemia: a meta-analysis in patients with chronic kidney disease. Br J Clin Pharmacol. 2021;87:414–26.

140. Womack R, Berru F, Panwar B, Gutiérrez OM. Effect of ferric citrate versus ferrous sulfate on iron and phosphate parameters in patients with iron deficiency and CKD: a randomized trial. Clin J Am Soc Nephrol. 2020;15:1251–8.

141. Hanudel MR, Laster M, Ramos G, Gales B, Salusky IB. Clinical experience with the use of ferric citrate as a phosphate binder in pediatric dialysis patients. Pediatr Nephrol. 2018;33:2137–42.

142. Khoury A, Pagan KA, Farland MZ. Ferric Maltol: A New Oral Iron Formulation for the Treatment of Iron Deficiency in Adults. Ann Pharmacother. 2021;55:222–9.

143. Pergola PE, Kopyt NP. Oral Ferric Maltol for the Treatment of Iron-Deficiency Anemia in Patients With CKD: A Randomized Trial and Open-Label Extension. Am J Kidney Dis. 2021;78:846–56.e1.

144. Howaldt S, Domènech E, Martinez N, Schmidt C, Bokemeyer B. Long-Term Effectiveness of Oral Ferric Maltol vs Intravenous Ferric Carboxymaltose for the Treatment of Iron-Deficiency Anemia in Patients With Inflammatory Bowel Disease: A Randomized Controlled Noninferiority Trial. Inflamm Bowel Dis. 2021;

145. Pisani A, Riccio E, Sabbatini M, Andreucci M, Del Rio A, Visciano B. Effect of oral liposomal iron versus intravenous iron for treatment of iron deficiency anaemia in CKD patients: a randomized trial. Nephrol Dial Transplant. 2015;30:645–52.

146. Riccio E, Sabbatini M, Capuano I, Pellegrino AM, Petruzzelli LA, Pisani A. Oral Sucrosomial® iron

versus intravenous iron for recovering iron deficiency anaemia in ND-CKD patients: a cost- minimization analysis. BMC Nephrol. 2020;21:57.

147. Albaramki J, Hodson EM, Craig JC, Webster AC. Parenteral versus oral iron therapy for adults and children with chronic kidney disease. Cochrane Database Syst Rev. 2012;1:CD007857.

148. Rozen-Zvi B, Gafter-Gvili A, Paul M, Leibovici L, Shpilberg O, Gafter U. Intravenous versus oral iron supplementation for the treatment of anemia in CKD: systematic review and meta-analysis. Am J Kidney Dis. 2008;52:897–906.

149. Pizzi LT, Bunz TJ, Coyne DW, Goldfarb DS, Singh AK. Ferric gluconate treatment provides cost savings in patients with high ferritin and low transferrin saturation. Kidney Int. 2008;74:1588–95.

150. Wong G, Howard K, Hodson E, Irving M, Craig JC. An economic evaluation of intravenous versus oral iron supplementation in people on haemodialysis. Nephrol Dial Transplant. 2013;28:413–20.

151. Gillespie RS, Wolf FM. Intravenous iron therapy in pediatric hemodialysis patients: a meta-analysis. Pediatr Nephrol. 2004;19:662–6.

152. Yorgin PD, Belson A, Sarwal M, Alexander SR. Sodium ferric gluconate therapy in renal transplant and renal failure patients. Pediatr Nephrol. 2000;15:171–5.

153. Morgan HE, Gautam M, Geary DF. Maintenance intravenous iron therapy in pediatric hemodialysis patients. Pediatr Nephrol. 2001;16:779–83.

154. Warady BA, Zobrist RH, Wu J, Finan E. Efficacy and safety of sodium ferric gluconate complex in anemic children on hemodialysis. Pediatr Nephrol. 2005; In press

155. Warady BA, Kausz A, Lerner G, et al. Iron therapy in the pediatric hemodialysis population. Pediatr Nephrol. 2004;19:655–61.

156. Gillespie RS, Symons JM. Sodium ferric gluconate for post-transplant anemia in pediatric and young adult renal transplant recipients. Pediatr Transplant. 2005;9:43–6.

157. Kshirsagar AV, Freburger JK, Ellis AR, Wang L, Winkelmayer WC, Brookhart MA. The comparative short-term effectiveness of iron dosing and formulations in US hemodialysis patients. Am J Med 2013;126:541.e1-.e14.

158. Michael B, Coyne DW, Fishbane S, et al. Sodium ferric gluconate complex in hemodialysis patients: adverse reactions compared to placebo and iron dextran. Kidney Int. 2002;61:1830–9.

159. Coyne DW, Adkinson NF, Nissenson AR, et al. Sodium ferric gluconate complex in hemodialysis patients. II. Adverse reactions in iron dextran-sensitive and dextran-tolerant patients. Kidney Int. 2003;63:217–24.

160. Javier AM. Weekly administration of high-dose sodium ferric gluconate is safe and effective in peritoneal dialysis patients. Nephrology Nursing Journal: Journal of the American Nephrology Nurses' Association. 2002;29:183–6.

161. Giordano A, Arrigo G, Lavarda F, Colasanti G, Petrini C. Comparison of two iron gluconate treatment modalities in chronic hemodialysis patients: results of a randomized trial. J Nephrol. 2005;18:181–7.

162. Nissenson AR, Lindsay RM, Swan S, Seligman P, Strobos J. Sodium ferric gluconate complex in sucrose is safe and effective in hemodialysis patients: North American Clinical Trial. Am J Kidney Dis. 1999;33:471–82.

163. Panesar A, Agarwal R. Safety and efficacy of sodium ferric gluconate complex in patients with chronic kidney disease. Am J Kidney Dis. 2002;40:924–31.

164. Folkert VW, Michael B, Agarwal R, et al. Chronic use of sodium ferric gluconate complex in hemodialysis patients: safety of higher-dose (> or =250 mg) administration. Am J Kidney Dis. 2003;41:651–7.

165. Jain AK, Bastani B. Safety profile of a high dose ferric gluconate in patients with severe chronic renal insufficiency. J Nephrol. 2002;15:681–3.

166. Aronoff GR, Bennett WM, Blumenthal S, et al. Iron sucrose in hemodialysis patients: safety of replacement and maintenance regimens. Kidney Int. 2004;66:1193–8.

167. Bailie GR. Comparison of rates of reported adverse events associated with i.v. iron products in the United States. Am J Health Syst Pharm. 2012;69:310–20.

168. Charytan C, Levin N, Al-Saloum M, Hafeez T, Gagnon S, Van Wyck DB. Efficacy and safety of iron sucrose for iron deficiency in patients with dialysis-associated anemia: North American clinical trial. Am J Kidney Dis. 2001;37:300–7.

169. Van Wyck DB, Roppolo M, Martinez CO, Mazey RM, McMurray S. for the United States Iron Sucrose Clinical Trials G. A randomized, controlled trial comparing IV iron sucrose to oral iron in anemic patients with nondialysis-dependent CKD. Kidney Int. 2005;68:2846–56.

170. Goldstein SL, Morris D, Warady BA. Comparison of the safety and efficacy of 3 iron sucrose iron maintenance regimens in children, adolescents, and young adults with CKD: a randomized controlled trial. Am J Kidney Dis. 2013;61:588–97.

171. Chandler G, Harchowal J, Macdougall IC. Intravenous iron sucrose: establishing a safe dose. Am J Kidney Dis. 2001;38:988–91.

172. Blaustein DA, Schwenk MH, Chattopadhyay J, et al. The safety and efficacy of an accelerated iron sucrose dosing regimen in patients with chronic kidney disease. Kidney International - Supplement. 2003:S72–7.

173. Anbu AT, Kemp T, O'Donnell K, Smith PA, Bradbury MG. Low incidence of adverse events following 90-minute and 3-minute infusions of intravenous iron sucrose in children on erythropoietin. Acta Paediatr. 2005;94:1738–41.

174. Covic A, Mircescu G. The safety and efficacy of intravenous ferric carboxymaltose in anaemic patients undergoing haemodialysis: a multi-centre, open-label, clinical study. Nephrol Dial Transplant. 2010;25:2722–30.

175. Charytan C, Bernardo MV, Koch TA, Butcher A, Morris D, Bregman DB. Intravenous ferric carboxymaltose versus standard medical care in the treatment of iron deficiency anemia in patients with chronic kidney disease: a randomized, active-controlled, multi-center study. Nephrol Dial Transplant. 2013;28:953–64.

176. Onken JE, Bregman DB, Harrington RA, et al. A multicenter, randomized, active-controlled study to investigate the efficacy and safety of intravenous ferric carboxymaltose in patients with iron deficiency anemia. Transfusion (Paris). 2014;54:306–15.

177. Macdougall IC, Bock AH, Carrera F, et al. FIND-CKD: a randomized trial of intravenous ferric carboxymaltose versus oral iron in patients with chronic kidney disease and iron deficiency anaemia. Nephrol Dial Transplant. 2014;29:2075–84.

178. Onken JE, Bregman DB, Harrington RA, et al. Ferric carboxymaltose in patients with iron-deficiency anemia and impaired renal function: the REPAIR-IDA trial. Nephrol Dial Transplant. 2014;29:833–42.

179. Powers JM, Shamoun M, McCavit TL, Adix L, Buchanan GR. Intravenous Ferric Carboxymaltose in Children with Iron Deficiency Anemia Who Respond Poorly to Oral Iron. J Pediatr. 2017;180:212–6.

180. Mantadakis E, Roganovic J. Safety and efficacy of ferric carboxymaltose in children and adolescents with iron deficiency anemia. J Pediatr. 2017;184:241.

181. Tan MLN, Windscheif PM, Thornton G, Gaynor E, Rodrigues A, Howarth L. Retrospective review of effectiveness and safety of intravenous ferric carboxymaltose given to children with iron deficiency anaemia in one UK tertiary centre. Eur J Pediatr. 2017;176:1419–23.

182. DelRosso LM, Picchietti DL, Ferri R. Comparison between oral ferrous sulfate and intravenous ferric carboxymaltose in children with restless sleep disorder. Sleep. 2021;44

183. Sasankan N, Duncan H, Curtis L, et al. Ferric Carboxymaltose Across All Ages in Paediatric Gastroenterology Shows Efficacy Without Increased Safety Concerns. J Pediatr Gastroenterol Nutr. 2021;72:506–10.

184. Posod A, Schaefer B, Mueller T, Zoller H, Kiechl-Kohlendorfer U. Hypophosphatemia in children treated with ferric carboxymaltose. Acta Paediatr. 2020;109:1491–2.

185. Kirk SE, Scheurer ME, Bernhardt MB, Mahoney DH, Powers JM. Phosphorus levels in children treated with intravenous ferric carboxymaltose. Am J Hematol. 2021;96:E215–e8.

186. Schaefer B, Tobiasch M, Viveiros A, et al. Hypophosphataemia after treatment of iron deficiency with intravenous ferric carboxymaltose or iron isomaltoside-a systematic review and meta-analysis. Br J Clin Pharmacol. 2021;87:2256–73.

187. Schaefer B, Zoller H, Wolf M. Risk factors for and effects of persistent and severe hypophosphatemia following ferric carboxymaltose. J Clin Endocrinol Metab. 2021;

188. Khan H, May P, Kuo E, et al. Safety and efficacy of a single total dose infusion (1020 mg) of ferumoxytol. Ther Adv Hematol. 2021;12:20406207211006022.

189. Auerbach M, Strauss W, Auerbach S, Rineer S, Bahrain H. Safety and efficacy of total dose infusion of 1,020 mg of ferumoxytol administered over 15 min. Am J Hematol. 2013;88:944–7.

190. Spinowitz BS, Kausz AT, Baptista J, et al. Ferumoxytol for treating iron deficiency anemia in CKD. J Am Soc Nephrol. 2008;19:1599–605.

191. Provenzano R, Schiller B, Rao M, Coyne D, Brenner L, Pereira BJ. Ferumoxytol as an intravenous iron replacement therapy in hemodialysis patients. Clinical Journal of The American Society of Nephrology: CJASN. 2009;4:386–93.

192. Hassan N, Cahill J, Rajasekaran S, Kovey K. Ferumoxytol infusion in pediatric patients with gastrointestinal disorders: first case series. Ann Pharmacother. 2011;45:e63.

193. Hassan N, Boville B, Reischmann D, Ndika A, Sterken D, Kovey K. Intravenous Ferumoxytol in Pediatric Patients With Iron Deficiency Anemia. Ann Pharmacother. 2017;51:548–54.

194. Wolf M, Auerbach M, Kalra PA, Glaspy J, Thomsen LL, Bhandari S. Safety of ferric derisomaltose and iron sucrose in patients with iron deficiency anemia: The FERWON-IDA/NEPHRO trials. Am J Hematol. 2021;96:E11–e5.

195. Bhandari S, Kalra PA, Berkowitz M, Belo D, Thomsen LL, Wolf M. Safety and efficacy of iron isomaltoside 1000/ferric derisomaltose versus iron sucrose in patients with chronic kidney disease: the FERWON-NEPHRO randomized, open-label, comparative trial. Nephrol Dial Transplant. 2021;36:111–20.

196. Warady BA, Zobrist RH, Wu J, Finan E. Sodium ferric gluconate complex therapy in anemic children on hemodialysis. Pediatr Nephrol. 2005;20:1320–7.

197. Besarab A, Kaiser JW, Frinak S. A study of parenteral iron regimens in hemodialysis patients. Am J Kidney Dis. 1999;34:21–8.

198. Brookhart MA, Freburger JK, Ellis AR, Wang L, Winkelmayer WC, Kshirsagar AV. Infection risk with bolus versus maintenance iron supplementation in hemodialysis patients. J Am Soc Nephrol. 2013;24:1151–8.

199. Ruiz-Jaramillo Mde L, Guizar-Mendoza JM, Gutierrez-Navarro Mde J, Dubey-Ortega LA, Amador-Licona N. Intermittent versus maintenance iron therapy in children on hemodialysis: a randomized study. Pediatr Nephrol. 2004;19:77–81.

200. Warady BA, Zobrist RH, Finan E. Ferrlecit Pediatric Study Group. Sodium ferric gluconate complex maintenance therapy in children on hemodialysis. Pediatr Nephrol. 2006;21:553–60.

201. Fletes R, Lazarus JM, Gage J, Chertow GM. Suspected iron dextran-related adverse drug events in hemodialysis patients. Am J Kidney Dis. 2001;37:743–9.

202. Van Wyck DB, Cavallo G, Spinowitz BS, et al. Safety and efficacy of iron sucrose in patients sensitive to iron dextran: North American clinical trial. Am J Kidney Dis. 2000;36:88–97.

203. Bastani B, Rahman S, Gellens M. Lack of reaction to ferric gluconate in hemodialysis patients with a history of severe reaction to iron dextran. ASAIO J. 2002;48:404–6.

204. Auerbach M, Chaudhry M, Goldman H, Ballard H. Value of methylprednisolone in prevention of the arthralgia-myalgia syndrome associated with the total dose infusion of iron dextran: a double blind randomized trial. J Lab Clin Med. 1998;131:257–60.

205. Pascual J, Teruel JL, Liano F, Sureda A, Ortuno J. Serious adverse reactions after intravenous ferric gluconate. Nephrol Dial Transplant. 1992;7:271–2.

206. Hoigne R, Breymann C, Kunzi UP, Brunner F. Parenteral iron therapy: problems and possible solutions. Schweiz Med Wochenschr. 1998;128:528–35.

207. Fishbane S, Mathew A, Vaziri ND. Iron toxicity: relevance for dialysis patients. Nephrol Dial Transplant. 2014;29:255–9.

208. Drueke T, Witko-Sarsat V, Massy Z, et al. Iron therapy, advanced oxidation protein products, and carotid artery intima-media thickness in end-stage renal disease. Circulation. 2002;106:2212–7.

209. Reis KA, Guz G, Ozdemir H, et al. Intravenous iron therapy as a possible risk factor for atherosclerosis in end-stage renal disease. Int Heart J. 2005;46:255–64.

210. Vaziri ND. Understanding iron: promoting its safe use in patients with chronic kidney failure treated by hemodialysis. Am J Kidney Dis. 2013;61:992–1000.

211. Bailie GR, Larkina M, Goodkin DA, et al. Data from the Dialysis Outcomes and Practice Patterns Study validate an association between high intravenous iron doses and mortality. Kidney Int. 2015;87:162–8.

212. Blumenstein I, Shanbhag S, Langguth P, Kalra PA, Zoller H, Lim W. Newer formulations of intravenous iron: a review of their chemistry and key safety aspects - hypersensitivity, hypophosphatemia, and cardiovascular safety. Expert Opin Drug Saf. 2021;20:757–69.

213. Lu M, Cohen MH, Rieves D, Pazdur R. FDA report: Ferumoxytol for intravenous iron therapy in adult patients with chronic kidney disease. Am J Hematol. 2010;85:315–9.

214. Canavese C, Bergamo D, Ciccone G, et al. Validation of serum ferritin values by magnetic susceptometry in predicting iron overload in dialysis patients. Kidney Int. 2004;65:1091–8.

215. Ferrari P, Kulkarni H, Dheda S, et al. Serum iron markers are inadequate for guiding iron repletion in chronic kidney disease. Clinical Journal of The American Society of Nephrology: CJASN. 2011;6:77–83.

216. Rostoker G, Griuncelli M, Loridon C, et al. Hemodialysis-associated hemosiderosis in the era of erythropoiesis-stimulating agents: a MRI study. Am J Med. 2012;125:991–9.e1.

217. Schouten BJ, Hunt PJ, Livesey JH, Frampton CM, Soule SG. FGF23 elevation and hypophosphatemia after intravenous iron polymaltose: a prospective study. Journal of Clinical Endocrinology & Metabolism. 2009;94:2332–7.

218. Schaefer B, Tobiasch M, Wagner S, et al. Hypophosphatemia after intravenous iron therapy: Comprehensive review of clinical findings and recommendations for management. Bone. 2022;154:116202.

219. Wolf M, Rubin J, Achebe M, et al. Effects of Iron Isomaltoside vs Ferric Carboxymaltose on Hypophosphatemia in Iron-Deficiency Anemia: Two Randomized Clinical Trials. JAMA. 2020;323:432–43.

220. Ishida JH, Johansen KL. Iron and infection in hemodialysis patients. Semin Dial. 2014;27:26–36.

221. Hoen B, Paul-Dauphin A, Kessler M. Intravenous iron administration does not significantly increase the risk of bacteremia in chronic hemodialysis patients. Clin Nephrol. 2002;57:457–61.

Disorders of Bone Mineral Metabolism in Chronic Kidney Disease

60

Claus Peter Schmitt and Rukshana C. Shroff

Introduction

Disturbances of bone and mineral metabolism almost inevitably develop in the course of chronic kidney disease (CKD). These comprise altered calcium and phosphate homeostasis, abnormal synthesis and secretion of parathyroid hormone (PTH) and vitamin D, and alterations in bone metabolism and function. If not treated appropriately, severe and sometimes disabling complications may occur. Alterations of bone and mineral metabolism originating in childhood contribute not only to degenerative bone disease, but also to vascular morbidity and mortality in young adult life. Hence, adequate control of bone and mineral metabolism is one of the major challenges in the treatment of pediatric patients with chronic renal failure.

With the growing awareness that mineral dysregulation in CKD is closely linked to abnormal bone pathology, and that these in turn lead to extra-skeletal calcification, Kidney Disease Improving Global Outcomes (KDIGO) have proposed a broad and encompassing term chronic kidney disease - mineral and bone disorder (CKD-MBD) to describe this clinical entity [1]. CKD-MBD is defined as a systemic disorder of mineral and bone metabolism that is manifested by either one or a combination of the following:

- Abnormalities of calcium, phosphorus, PTH, or vitamin D metabolism
- Abnormalities in bone turnover, mineralization, linear growth, or strength
- Vascular or other soft tissue calcification

A proposed framework for classifying CKD-MBD divides patients into four types based on the presence or absence of abnormalities in the three primary components used in the definition of the disorder: laboratory abnormalities, bone disease, and calcification of extraskeletal tissue. In this chapter we discuss the pathophysiology, clinical presentation and treatment of CKD-MBD in children.

Epidemiology

Metabolic derangements begin as early as in CKD stage II (glomerular filtration rate [GFR] of 60–90 ml/min/1.73 m^2), plasma levels of active 1,25-dihydroxyvitamin D [1,25(OH)$_2$D$_3$] decline and parathyroid hormone [PTH] and fibroblast growth factor-23 [FGF23] levels start to increase [2] (Fig. 60.1), with Fibroblast growth factor 23 (FGF-23), a phosphaturic hormone, being the earliest marker of disrupted mineral homeostasis

C. P. Schmitt (✉)
Division of Pediatric Nephrology, Center for Pediatric and Adolescent Medicine, Heidelberg, Germany
e-mail: clauspeter.schmitt@med.uniheidelberg.de

R. C. Shroff
Renal Unit, UCL Great Ormond Street Hospital and Institute of Child Health, London, UK
e-mail: Rukshana.Shroff@gosh.nhs.uk

© The Author(s), under exclusive license to Springer Nature Switzerland AG 2023
F. Schaefer, L. A. Greenbaum (eds.), *Pediatric Kidney Disease*,
https://doi.org/10.1007/978-3-031-11665-0_60

[3]. Mineralization defects have been demonstrated in 29% of children with CKD stage 2 [4]. When end stage renal disease (ESRD) is reached, most patients have abnormal bone histology. The specific features of bone disease depend on the degree of hyperparathyroidism and the therapeutic measures taken to control the disease, whereas the mode of dialysis therapy, PD or HD, does not appear to play a major role [5]. Adynamic bone disease has a high prevalence, being observed in 40–50% of adult and almost 30% of pediatric

ESRD patients (Fig. 60.2) [5–7]. Amongst children, CKD related bone disease can manifest as bone pain and deformities, growth retardation and fractures and have long-term consequences. In a cohort of 249 young Dutch adults with onset of end-stage renal failure before the age of 14 years 61% had severe growth retardation, 37% bone disease (defined by at least one of the following conditions: deforming bone abnormalities, chronic pain related to the skeletal system, disabling bone abnormalities, aseptic bone necrosis and atraumatic fractures and 18% disabilities resulting from bone impairment [8].

There is a complex interplay between CKD-related bone disease and cardiovascular disease that begins early in the course of CKD, is seen even in children [9], and leads to a significant decrease in life expectancy [10, 11]. Several large national registries have published similar findings for pediatric dialysis recipients. The United States Renal Data Systems (USRDS) has reported that 23% of all deaths in dialysis patients were from cardiovascular causes [12], and 50% of all deaths in young adults who received dialysis as children were from cardiovascular or cerebrovascular causes [10]. Encouragingly, recent reports suggest that there is a substantial decrease in mortality rates over time among US patients [13]. Cardiovascular disease in CKD is discussed in greater detail in Chap. 61.

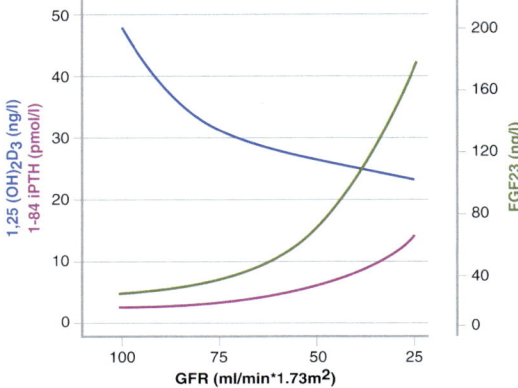

Fig. 60.1 Mean plasma intact PTH, 1,25(OH)₂D₃ (left y-axis) and FGF23 concentrations (right y-axis) in patients with different degree of CKD. Individual values may vary considerably especially in patients with advanced renal failure

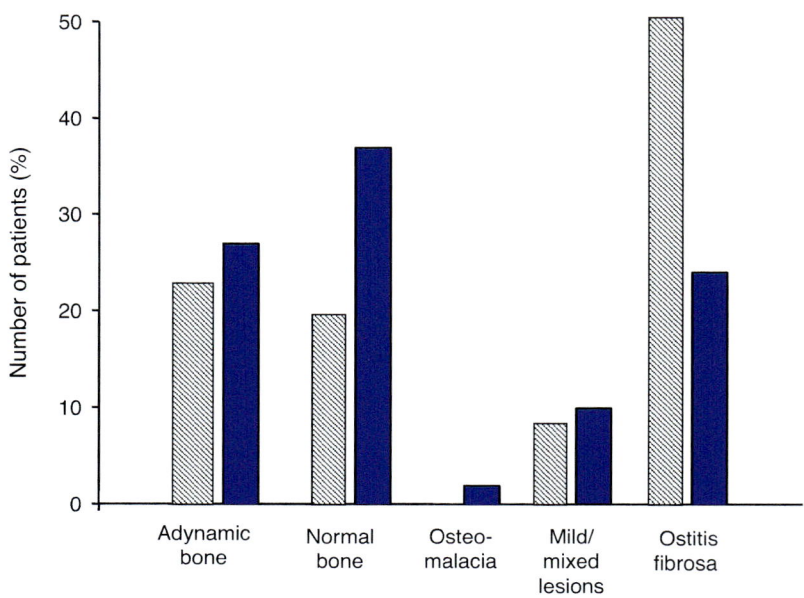

Fig. 60.2 Spectrum of renal osteodystrophy in children with CKD stage 5 diagnosed in the USA in the early 1990s (hatched bars, adapted from [6]) and in Poland in the late 1990s (filled bars, adapted from [5])

Pathogenesis

Bone and mineral homeostasis are regulated in a complex network of local and systemic factors. Patients with CKD develop major disturbances in calcium, $1,25(OH)_2D$ and phosphate homeostasis and subsequently abnormal parathyroid gland function, which ultimately drives the course of the disease (Fig. 60.3). FGF23 has added a new dimension to the Ca-P-PTH axis and advanced our understanding of mineral dysregulation in CKD [3]. FGF23, along with its membrane receptor klotho, acts through an intricate negative feedback system involving PTH and vitamin D to regulate serum calcium and phosphate levels.

Disorders of Calcium Homeostasis

In healthy individuals 99% of total body calcium is stored in the bone, 0.975% in soft tissues and only 0.025% is circulating in blood. Plasma ionized calcium levels are tightly controlled by PTH and $1,25(OH)_2D$. The parathyroid gland senses changes in ionized calcium by a G-protein coupled membrane receptor. Acute hypocalcemia is counteracted by an instantaneous and marked increase in PTH release from storage vesicles, rapidly normalizing plasma calcium levels, and by an increased PTH gene transcription and synthesis rate, an adaptive response which takes several hours to occur. In addition, hypocalcemia stabilizes PTH mRNA by increased binding of a cytosolic adenosine-uridine-rich protein (AUF1) in the 3′ untranslated region of the PTH mRNA [14]. A subsequent increase in $1,25(OH)_2D$ synthesis further stabilizes plasma calcium levels via stimulation of gastrointestinal calcium absorption. A recent study has shown that 76% of children with CKD4-5D had a dietary Ca intake <100% Reference Nutrient Intake, largely because a restriction of dairy foods as part of a P controlled diet limits Ca intake, and additional Ca from medications is required to meet the KDOQI guideline of 100–200% normal recommended Ca intake [15].

In CKD, reduced $1,25(OH)_2D$ synthesis impairs intestinal calcium resorption, resulting in an activation of the regulatory circuits described above and a resetting of ionized calcium at low or low-normal levels. The calcemic response of bone to PTH is reduced and higher PTH levels are required to maintain calcium homeostasis and bone turnover. Uremic toxins, low levels of $1,25(OH)_2D$, accumulation of inactive PTH fragments and osteoprotegerin, and altered PTH receptor expression have been implicated in the skeletal resistance to PTH, providing yet another

Fig. 60.3
Pathophysiology of secondary hyperparathyroidism

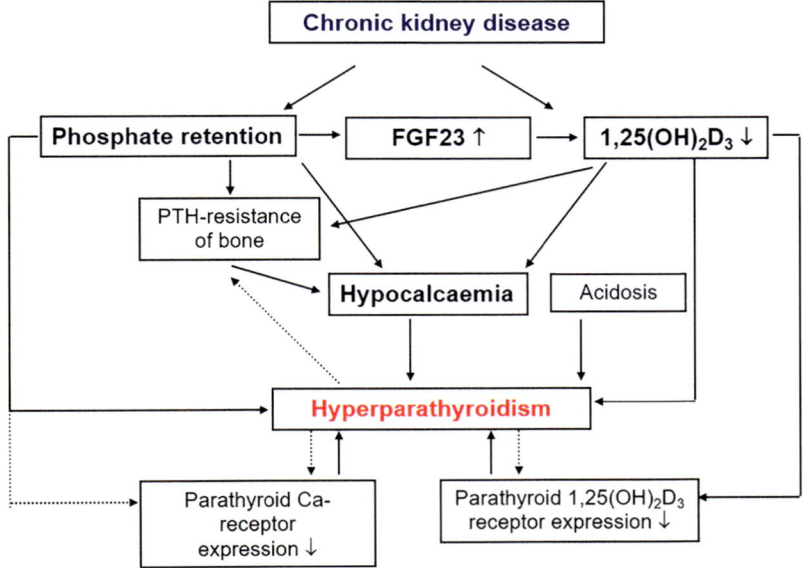

mechanism contributing to the development of hyperparathyroidism (Fig. 60.3) [16].

Plasma ionized calcium is the major regulator of the parathyroids at the level of gene expression, secretion and cell proliferation. Induction of hypocalcemia stimulates PTH release, PTH peptide synthesis via stabilization of PTH mRNA and, if sustained, induces profound parathyroid cell proliferation [17]. Hypocalcemia appears to be a more important regulator of the parathyroid than vitamin D, as suggested by the efficient control of hyperparathyroidism in vitamin D-receptor knock-out mice by a selective increase of dietary calcium content [18]. Moreover, calcimimetic agents suppress PTH by up to 80%, independent of plasma phosphate and $1,25(OH)_2D$ levels.

Abnormalities of $1,25(OH)_2D$ Metabolism in CKD

$25(OH)D$ is converted to the systemically active $1,25(OH)_2D$ by the enzyme 1-alpha hydroxylase. Progressive loss of intact renal parenchyma, low $25(OH)D$ levels and increased FGF-23 release from the bone result in low circulating $1,25(OH)_2D$ levels. This in turn leads to reduced intestinal calcium absorption and hypocalcemia; it is estimated that the intestinal calcium absorption increases from ~45% to 65% in the presence of adequate vitamin D. Hypocalcaemia triggers PTH release in order to maintain calcium homeostasis and to stimulate 1-alpha hydroxylase.

$1,25(OH)_2D$ controls parathyroid gland function not only via modulating plasma ionized calcium, but also directly by suppressing PTH gene transcription [19] and by upregulating its own receptor in parathyroid cells. Moreover $1,25(OH)_2D$ binds to a response element in the promoter region of the calcium receptor, resulting in increased calcium receptor abundance, thereby increasing the sensitivity of the parathyroid gland to ionized calcium [20]. Hypocalcemia on the other hand compromises vitamin D action by upregulating calreticulin, a repressor of the vitamin response element in the parathyroid glands [21]. In addition, $1,25(OH)_2D$ regulates parathyroid cell prolifera-

tion, with low levels promoting parathyroid gland hyperplasia.

FGF23 controls $1,25(OH)_2D$ production through a complex feedback mechanism [22]. FGF23 suppresses the renal 1-alpha-hydroxylase and thereby reduces conversion of $25(OH)D$ to $1,25(OH)_2D$. In addition, FGF23 increases the activity of 24,25 hydroxylase to degrade $1,25(OH)_2D$.

$1,25(OH)_2D$ has numerous additional important functions outside the bone and parathyroid. The hormone is an important regulator of the immune system and affects the contractility, growth and migration of vascular smooth muscle cells (VSMCs) as well as the evolution of vascular calcifications. Both endothelial and VSMCs express high-affinity Vitamin D3 receptors. $1,25(OH)_2D$ deficiency may contribute to cardiovascular disease by unrepressed production of proteins involved in arterial calcification such as bone morphogenetic protein-2 [23, 24] or by suppressed production of local inhibitors of mineralization, e.g. matrix GLA protein [25]. High doses of $1,25(OH)_2D$ on the other hand promote vascular calcification via an increased calcium phosphate product and transition of vascular smooth muscle cells to an osteoblast like phenotype. Of note in this context, $1,25(OH)_2D$ is not only an endocrine factor exclusively secreted by the kidney. Extrarenal 1-α-hydroxylase expression has been demonstrated in various tissues such as bone, smooth muscle cells and parathyroid glands [26, 27], suggesting an additional paracrine mode of action independent of renal conversion.

25-Hydroxy Vitamin D Deficiency

The widespread deficiency of $25(OH)D$ is even more pronounced in CKD patients than in the general population, related to multiple potential causes [28]: (1) Patients with CKD may be less active and have less sunlight exposure; (2) The endogenous synthesis of vitamin D in the skin is reduced in CKD; (3) Ingestion of foods that are natural sources of vitamin D may be diminished; (4) Proteinuria may be accompanied by high urinary losses of vitamin D binding protein (VDBP), leading to increased renal losses of all vitamin D metabolites; (5) 25(OH)D and VDBP may be lost in peritoneal dialysis fluid. There is debate about what levels of vitamin D can be considered adequate. Current clinical practice recommendations for children with CKD suggest a target level of 30–48 ng/ml (75–120 nmol/L) [29].

Low 25(OH)D levels result in muscle weakness [30] and bone pain and aggravate renal bone disease [31, 32]. Bone histomorphological changes are correlated with plasma 25(OH)D levels [31, 33]. *In vitro*, a concentration of 40 ng/ml 25(OH)D is as efficient in suppressing PTH as calcitriol at a maximally PTH suppressive dose. A randomized trial in 47 children with CKD2–4 demonstrated a longer time to development of secondary hyperparathyroidism with vit. D supplementation as compared to those children on placebo [34].

Abnormalities of Phosphate Metabolism and Phosphaturic Hormone FGF23

Phosphate excretion declines early with failing renal function and this is a driving force of CKD-MBD. When the GFR falls to <50 ml/min/1.73 m^2, phosphate accumulates [2]. In early stages, the decline in renal phosphate excretion is counteracted by the phosphaturic hormones Fibroblast Growth Factor 23 (FGF23) and PTH. Clinical studies have identified increased FGF23 levels as the earliest biological marker of deranged calcium - phosphate homeostasis in CKD, even before PTH levels start to rise [3, 35, 36] (Fig. 60.2). FGF23 is mainly secreted by osteocytes and acts on the type IIa and IIc sodium-phosphate co-transporters (NaPi) in the apical membrane of proximal tubular cells to increase urinary phosphate excretion. It suppresses 1,25(OH)$_2$D synthesis by suppressing 1-α hydroxylase (CYP27B1) and increasing 1,25(OH)$_2$D degradation to 24,25(OH)2D by promoting CYP24A1 [37]. Thus, by reducing circulating 1,25(OH)$_2$D levels, FGF23 reduces phosphate absorption from the gut. Also, FGF23 suppresses PTH mRNA and decreases serum PTH [38]. In

turn, FGF23 secretion is stimulated by phosphorus, 1,25(OH)$_2$D and PTH. Mutations in the FGF23 gene result in severe hypo- and hyperphosphatemic disorders (see Chap. 34). Recent data suggests that FGF23 may in fact play a key role in calcium homeostasis and increased FGF23 is associated with higher calcium levels [39].

FGF23 signaling requires the presence of the transmembrane protein klotho on its target cells. Klotho is highly expressed in the kidneys where it serves as a high-affinity receptor for FGF23 [40]. When its extracellular domain is shed from the cell surface, it enters the circulation as soluble klotho and functions as a humoral factor that regulates ion channels and transporters (including NaPi and the calcium channel TRPV5 in the gut). Klotho deficiency develops with declining GFR and leads to a state of relative FGF23 resistance. However, FGF23 may be a 'double edged sword': although elevated FGF23 levels increase phosphate excretion in early stages of CKD, they have been associated with increased cardiovascular mortality both in CKD patients [41] and the general population. FGF23 exerts a direct toxic effect on the myocardium and is associated with left ventricular hypertrophy [42, 43].

A decline in circulating P concentrations can be observed in very early CKD when circulating FGF23 levels and bone FGF23 expression are increased. In contrast, in advanced stages of CKD hyperphosphatemia does contribute to increased FGF23 and treatment with active vitamin D analogs further contributes to increasing FGF23 levels. In all CKD stages, non-mineral metabolism factors such as iron status, erythropoietin and inflammation may also contribute to increased FGF23 production. In murine models, both absolute and "functional" iron deficiency increase bone FGF23 expression [44]. Erythropoietin can also stimulate FGF23 production and, conversely, FGF23 may suppress erythropoiesis [45]. FGF23 levels are higher in patients with glomerular diseases when compared to those with congenital anomalies of the kidneys and urinary tract (CAKUT) [46]; inflammation increases bone and circulating FGF23 levels [44].

Hyperphosphatemia has multiple deleterious effects. It contributes to hyperparathyroidism independently of plasma calcium and 1,25(OH)₂D [47, 48] via increasing PTH gene transcription, PTH peptide secretion and parathyroid cell proliferation. Furthermore, hyperphosphatemia reduces renal 1,25(OH)₂D synthesis, inhibits the suppressive action of 1,25(OH)₂D on the parathyroid glands and promotes resistance of bone to PTH. Another indirect mechanism by which high phosphate drives hyperparathyroidism is via physicochemical precipitation of calcium-phosphate salts, a process aggravating hypocalcemia. High phosphate levels are very difficult to control as phosphate binders are one of the most difficult medications to comply with. The International Pediatric Peritoneal Dialysis Network has shown that 45% of all children have hyperphosphataemia, with the prevalence increasing to >80% amongst adolescents [49].

Secondary Hyperparathyroidism

The multiple effects of 1,25(OH)₂D deficiency, hypocalcemia and hyperphosphatemia in CKD lead to the development of secondary hyperparathyroidism, with a progressive demineralisation of the bone. Pre-pro PTH gene transcription rate, mRNA stability, protein synthesis and secretion of the mature protein are increased. Persistent hyperparathyroidism induces distinct changes in parathyroid gland morphology and function. Parathyroid cell proliferation results in diffuse and polyclonal and eventually monoclonal cell growth, associated with the formation of adenoma. Regulatory systems include endothelin, TGF-alpha, epidermal growth factor receptor and the cell cycle inhibitor p21 [50–53]. Monoclonal parathyroid cell growth is the result of an array of possible genetic aberrations such as gene deletions, loss of heterozygosity, clonal rearrangement and /or oncogene overexpression and tumor suppressor gene inactivation. Polymorphisms in the PTH, Vitamin D receptor and calcium receptor genes may also be involved and explain some of the clinical variability of the disease [54]. Reduced expression of the parathyroid calcium sensing receptor and of the vitamin D receptor

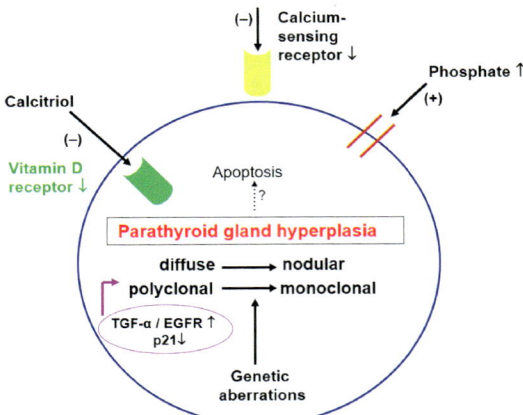

Fig. 60.4 Cellular alterations of parathyroid gland function in CKD

leads to a progressive escape from the two key physiological control mechanisms and ultimately to parathyroid gland autonomy (Fig. 60.4).

Minute to minute analyses of PTH secretion have revealed distinct alterations of the dynamics of oscillatory PTH release in uremic patients, including a markedly reduced secretory capacity to counteract changes in ionized calcium by modulation of the frequency and mass of PTH secretory bursts [55, 56].

Apoptosis is a rare event in normal parathyroid tissue; parathyroid cells can survive for >25 years, so, although uremia is associated with increased apoptosis of parathyroid cells, this mechanism is insufficient to counterbalance enhanced proliferation [57]. Whether an inversion of this imbalance, i.e. regression of parathyroid hyperplasia, occurs in uremic patients, or after correction of uremia, remains controversial [58].

In uremia, *fragments of the intact 1–84 PTH* peptide accumulate in the circulation and exert distinct biological activity, most notable 7–84 PTH fragments that are thought to be biologically inactive are present in the circulation and offset the classic biological actions of PTH [59–61]. 7–84 PTH internalizes the PTH type-1 receptor without prior activation. This may be one explanation for the reduced PTH1R level in uremia, the resistance of bone to PTH and the dissociation of phosphorus and calcium homeostasis in CKD patients. Interindividual variation of 7–84 PTH /1–84 PTH ratios is high. Alternatively, PTH fragments may also signal via receptors distinct from the PTH1R, e.g. through a C-terminal PTH receptor [62] and by this impact on bone. Up to now, there is only limited evidence that the differentiation of PTH fragments is clinically helpful for defining low and high turnover bone disease. The use of PTH assays measuring 7–84 in addition to 1–84, intact-PTH is therefore currently not recommended for routine clinical practice.

Oxidative stress is increased in CKD, and the amino acid methionine at two positions in the PTH peptide is prone to oxidation. A large proportion of circulating PTH measured by standard assay systems is oxidized and may thus not be biologically active. Non-oxidized PTH concentrations are 1.5–2.25 fold higher in patients in renal failure as compared to health controls [63]. Oxidation blunts the biological activity of the peptide. Oxidized PTH (oxPTH) loses its PTH receptor-stimulating properties, whereas non-oxidized PTH is a full agonist of the receptor [63]. Measurements of non-oxidized PTH should reflect the hormone status more precisely, but a recent bone biopsy study in 31 patients with CKD suggests no additional benefit [64]. Non-oxidized PTH measurements are currently not recommended for routine clinical practice.

The Impact of Metabolic Acidosis

Metabolic acidosis, an almost inevitable covariate in patients with failing renal function, has a number of untoward effects on bone. These include physicochemical dissolution of bone with inhibition of osteoblast and activation of osteoclast activity leading to a net calcium efflux from the bone. This is associated with impaired bone mineralization and an increased incidence of osteomalacia, which can be improved by correction of metabolic acidosis [65]. Moreover some evidence suggests that metabolic acidosis increases PTH levels in CKD patients and enhances the peripheral actions of PTH on bone

by increasing the expression and ligand affinity of the PTH receptor [66]. The relative quantitative contribution of metabolic acidosis to bone disease in CKD patients remains uncertain.

Further Mediators of CKD Bone Disease

The kidney-bone-vessel interaction is not confined to the homeostasis of calcium-phosphate and $1,25(OH)_2D$ synthesis, but a number of other key molecules are involved.

Bone morphogenetic protein-7 (BMP-7) is produced and secreted in postnatal life mainly by renal collecting tubule cells. CKD is associated with a marked deficiency of circulating BMP-7, most likely due to reduced renal synthesis. In the uremic rat model, adynamic bone disease develops if serum calcium, phosphate, vitamin D and PTH levels are maintained in the normal range. This observation has led to the hypothesis that the variable histopathological appearance of uremic bone may reflect the net balance of hyperparathyroidism inducing a high-turnover and BMP-7 deficiency causing a low-turnover state. At least in the uremic rat, exogenous administration of BMP-7 can reverse both adynamic and high turnover bone disease by improving osteoblast number and bone formation activity [67] . Moreover, BMP-7 reduces vascular calcifications in uremic animals, possibly by increasing the skeletal deposition of phosphorus and calcium [68] . The Diabetes Heart Study showed that single nucleotide polymorphisms in the BMP-7 gene have significant and reciprocal effects on vascular calcification and bone density [69]. Despite these notable discoveries BMP-7 has not entered the clinical arena so far; neither have circulating BMP-7 measurements been established as a biomarker of bone health nor have therapeutic studies progressed beyond the preclinical phase to date.

Osteoprotegerin (OPG) is a soluble protein of the tumor necrosis factor (TNF) receptor superfamily and a decoy receptor for the *receptor activator of nuclear factor kappa B ligand (RANKL)*. By binding RANKL, OPG inhibits nuclear kappa

B, which is an essential transcription factor for immune and inflammation related genes, cell survival and differentiation. OPG inhibits the differentiation of osteoclast precursors into mature osteoclasts and regulates the resorptive action. OPG-deficient mice exhibit media calcifications. In humans, circulating OPG levels associate with vascular calcifications and in CKD patients in particular with aortic and coronary calcifications [70, 71]. Low levels of soluble RANKL indicate a higher risk for cardiovascular events [72] and predict CV mortality in patients with CKD [73]. Prospective clinical trials with the OPG analogue, RANKL inhibitor denosumab suggest improved bone mineral density in early stages of CKD [74], the impact on vascular calcifications is yet uncertain.

Sclerostin is a glycoprotein secreted by osteocytes. It binds to a transmembrane complex (consisting of the frizzled receptor and the low-density lipoprotein receptor-related protein 5 or 6 coreceptor) and inhibits the Wingless-type mouse mammary tumor virus integration site (Wnt) pathway. The Wnt pathway stimulates stem cell and pre-osteoblast proliferation, induces osteoblastogenesis, inhibits osteoblast and osteocyte apoptosis and attenuates osteoclastogenesis. Sclerostin is produced by osteocytes and has an anti-anabolic effect on bone. Ageing, mechanical unloading of the skeleton, low PTH levels and progression of CKD have been associated with high circulating sclerostin levels. In HD patients, sclerostin levels correlate negatively with histomorphometric parameters of bone turnover, osteoblast number and function [75]. Sclerostin expression is increased during vascular smooth muscle cell calcification, where it potentially inhibits local arterial Wnt signalling and thus may represent a defense response against calcification. High circulating sclerostin levels have been associated with improved survival in hemodialysis patients [76].

Bone Histology in CKD-MBD

The term "renal osteodystrophy" is reserved for the spectrum of histological changes in CKD-associated bone disease, including changes in bone turn-over, mineralization and volume (TMV). The type of renal osteodystrophy in an individual patient depends on the therapeutic interventions taken to counteract an otherwise progressive disease (Fig. 60.5). Changes in bone turnover develop early in the course of CKD, prior to measurable changes in mineral homeostasis, possibly effected by osteocyte cytokines such as sclerostin [77]. In untreated children with CKD histological signs of fibrosis and demineralization prevail, whereas aggressive long-term treatment with calcium and vitamin D is associated with low bone turn over. At present, an adequate balance with normal or mild alterations in bone morphology is achieved only in a minority of the children [1]. A histological classification of renal osteodystrophy is given in Table 60.1, and respective histopathological illustrations are given in Fig. 60.6.

Children with some forms of rare inherited kidney diseases may have an element of bone disease independent of the degree of kidney failure and CKD-MBD, due to potential functions of the mutated genes in bone homeostasis. Exacerbated skeletal disease is prevalent in patients with cystinosis, primary hyperoxaluria and some primary ciliopathies [78–80]. Understanding the impact

Fig. 60.5 The type of renal bone disease depends on therapeutic interventions

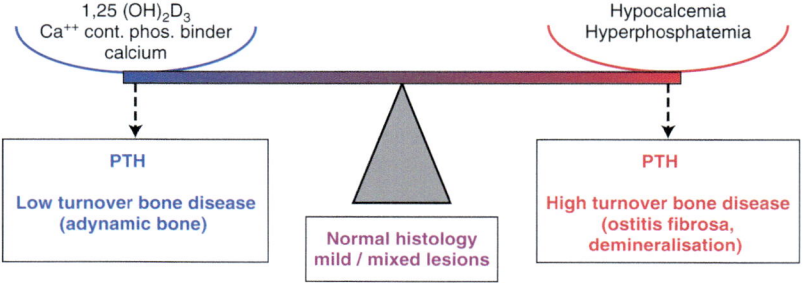

1,25 $(OH)_2D_3$
Ca^{++} cont. phos. binder
calcium

Hypocalcemia
Hyperphosphatemia

PTH
Low turnover bone disease (adynamic bone)

Normal histology
mild / mixed lesions

PTH
High turnover bone disease (ostitis fibrosa, demineralisation)

Table 60.1 Histological classification of renal osteodystrophy

Type	Etiology	Description	Comments
High turnover bone disease (Ostitis fibrosa)	Hyperparathyroidism	– Increased bone formation, resorption and osteoid deposition/seams – Disorganized collagen (woven bone), marrow fibrosis	– Frequent in untreated patients – Skeletal deformities, bone pain, epiphysiolysis
Low turnover: I Adynamic bone	– Relatively low PTH – Ca++ load, vit. D metabolites – Uremic toxins – Altered cytokines/growth factors	– Low bone formation and resorption rate – Decreased osteoid deposition	– Most common type – Increased fracture risk (?) – Extraosseus calcifications (?)
II Osteomalacia	– Aluminium – Unknown factors	– Accumulation of osteoid – Inhibition of the mineralization process	– Incidence ↓ with adequate dialysate purification and withdrawal of aluminium cont. Phosphate binders
Mixed disease	– Hyperparathyroidism – Aluminium – Unknown factors	– Increased remodelling, resorption and osteoid, – Areas of low bone formation	

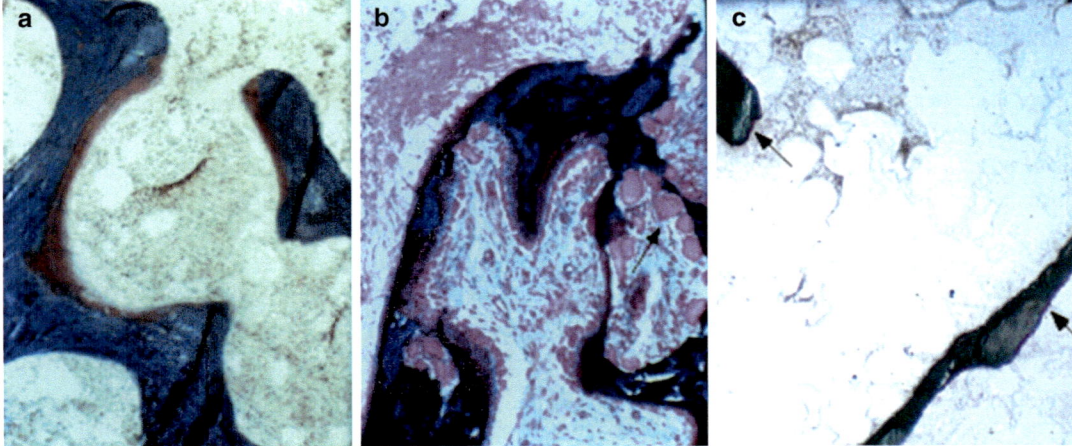

Fig. 60.6 Representative examples of different types of bone histology in patients with CKD (courtesy of LD Quarles, Department of Nephrology and Hypertension, University of Kansas Medical Center, Kansas City, Kansas, USA). (**a**) Histologic appearance of normal bone. Goldner Masson trichrome staining shows mineralized lamellar bone in blue and adjacent nonmineralized osteoid in red-brown. Osteoid comprises less than 25% of bone surfaces. The cellular area between the osseous structures is the marrow space. (**b**) Goldner Masson trichrome staining showing osteitis fibrosa due to second-ary hyperparathyroidism with increased number of osteoclasts (arrow) and extensive bone marrow fibrosis (as shown by the light blue staining of the marrow). The increased resorption results in a thin and scalloped appearance of mineralized trabecular bone. Osteoid and bone formation are relatively increased, too. (**c**) Adynamic bone disease, characterized by reduction in bone formation and resorption. The osteoid seams are thin (red lines at the bone surface; arrows), and there is little evidence of cellular activity

of the different genetic defects on the growing skeleton will likely lead to targeted therapeutic strategies.

Bone Mineral Accrual and Peak Bone Mass

Bone mass is mainly genetically determined [81], but exogenous factors also play a major role. Bone mass markedly increases during childhood, reaching a peak at 25–30 years of age [82]. The growing skeleton of children is uniquely vulnerable to factors that can impair bone accrual including poor growth, delayed maturation, muscle deficits, decreased physical activity, abnormal mineral metabolism, and secondary hyperparathyroidism. Skeletal calcium increases from 25 g in newborns to 900 and 1200 g in adult females and males, respectively. Increased $1,25(OH)_2D$ levels coincide with an increased rate of skeletal calcium accumulation during puberty [83]. In healthy adolescents approximately 25% of total skeletal mass is laid down during the 2-year interval of peak height velocity. This gives rise to an increased calcium and phosphate requirement in children, especially during periods of rapid growth, and the enormous buffering capacity of the growing skeleton. Calcium balance studies have shown that in healthy children on a high calcium diet the amount of calcium incorporated into the skeleton increases up to a threshold dietary intake above which no further bone accumulation occurs [84]. Calcium requirements are highest in the first year of life (503 ± 91 mg/day) and during pubertal growth (396 ± 164 mg/day), dropping thereafter to normal adult requirements (114 ± 133 mg/day) [84].

The mineral requirements of the growing skeleton have two important consequences: the normal range for Ca and P varies substantially with age (Fig. 60.10), and secondly, the high Ca and P requirements of the bones can 'buffer' increased dietetic calcium and phosphate loads, preventing extra-skeletal mineralization and ectopic calcification. Normal serum calcium and phosphate

levels fall steeply from birth until the age of 1–2 years and then gradually reduce up to the age of 7 years when they reach adult levels. Children with CKD are highly prone to develop mineralization defects. Almost one third of children with CKD stage 2 and more than of 90% of children on dialysis have deficient mineralisation [4], while this is the case in only 3% of adult dialysis patients [85]. Hence, calcium balance studies are urgently required in children with CKD to determine balance at different levels of calcium intake and at different stages of puberty, ideally correlating this data with bone histology.

Osteomalacia in animals with FGF23 deficiency suggests that FGF23 may play a direct role in skeletal mineralization; both overexpression [86] and ablation of FGF23 [87] in mice with normal renal function is associated with abnormal mineralization of osteoid, although by different mechanisms. The phosphaturic effect of increased FGF23 may cause rickets and osteomalacia through an insufficiency of mineral substrate.

Both, bone mass and bone geometry are altered in children with uremic bone disease, depending on the degree of hyperparathyroidism, disturbed vitamin D metabolism and therapeutic counteractions taken to control the disease. In CKD patients DXA (dual energy x-ray absorptiometry) scans are not a reliable measure of bone mineral density (BMD), but peripheral quantitative CT (pQCT) scans provide a useful measure [88]. In children with CKD low calcium and high PTH levels have been associated with a decrease in tibial BMD on pQCT [89]; this study also showed that a 1 SD decrease in BMD was associated with a twofold increase in fracture risk.

Linear Growth

Longitudinal growth is a unique feature of childhood. Growth occurs through the modelling of new bone by skeletal accretion and longitudinal growth in the growth plate. Bone formation in children occurs by two distinct mechanisms: skeletal remodelling of existing mineralized tissue that is controlled by osteoclasts and osteoblasts and modelling of new bone by skeletal accretion and longitudinal growth from the growth plate, through the action of chondrocytes [4, 90]. The growth plate is an avascular tissue between the epiphyses and metaphyses of long bones. During endochondral bone formation it is progressively replaced by bone. Bone formation in the endochondral growth plate is regulated by growth hormone (GH) and the PTH/PTH-related protein-receptor axis that together promote chondrocyte proliferation, matrix synthesis and chondrocyte differentiation into osteogenic cells [91].

Clinical Manifestations

Symptoms of renal osteodystrophy can develop early, especially in children with CKD from infancy. Initial signs are often vague and nonspecific and may not come to the attention of the caregivers. Especially young infants require meticulous monitoring, since the high growth velocity, the high mineral demand and the enhanced pressure load to joints with increasing mobility can rapidly lead to severe deformations.

Bone Pain

Bone pain is a common manifestation in children with CKD. Initial symptoms may be difficult to distinguish from other causes of pain, but become more specific with progressive disease and localize to the weight bearing joints. Since symptoms vary considerably among individual patients, they do not allow for conclusions regarding the type and severity of the underlying bone disease. Limping, bone deformities and axial displacement require a prompt and thorough diagnostic process, including biochemical and radiographic studies. A recent study reported that significant bone pain hindered the daily

activities of 58% of children with advanced (i.e. stages 4–5) CKD [88].

Myopathy

Patients with severe bone disease may also show muscular symptoms such as muscle weakness and wasting, exercise limitation, and waddling gait. The pathogenesis seems to be complex. One major reason is vitamin D deficiency, but inefficient clearance of uremic toxins, insulin resistance, carnitine deficiency, malnutrition and anemia may also contribute [92]. Muscle fat mass is increased in CKD children and negatively correlated with physical performance [93]. Some studies indicate an abnormal oxygen conductance from the muscular microcirculation to the normal functioning mitochondria [94]. Myopathy may further reduce bone strength 96).

Skeletal Deformities

Bone deformities include bowing of the weight bearing bones, with genua valga being most frequent. Genua vara, coxa vara, ulnar deviation and ankle deformations may also be seen, whereas avascular necrosis rarely occurs unless glucocorticoids are given. In infants, skeletal abnormalities often resemble vitamin D deficient rickets. Widening of the metaphyseal regions may develop in all long bones. The degree is dependent on the severity of metabolic bone disease and metaphyseal growth which varies with age. Particular attention has to be paid to deformities in small children when they start to bear weight. Physical examination should always include a detailed bone status and in case of suspicious findings be followed by radiological studies. According to the International Pediatric Peritoneal Dialysis Network clinical symptoms and/or radiological signs of bone disease are seen in about 15% of children on PD including 5% with limb deformities, with the latter possibly necessitating corrective orthopedic procedures [49].

Slipped Epiphyses

Pronounced secondary hyperparathyroidism, hypocalcemia and severe osteitis fibrosa cause disintegration of the growth plate and increase the risk of epiphysiolysis. Fibrotic alterations develop in the region connecting the epiphysis and the metaphysis. The growth cartilage columns are disorganized and partly substituted by fibrous tissue predisposing to local displacement with shear stress. Slipped epiphyses are more common in children with severe hyperparathyroidism, especially when insufficiently controlled for an extended period of time. The most frequently affected site is the proximal femur, followed by distal radius, ulna, distal femur, humerus, tibia and fibula, often depending on the mechanical stress put on the joints. Virtually any epiphysis may be involved (Figs. 60.7 and 60.8). Since epiphyseal slipping is a potentially severe and eventually incapacitating complication

resulting in osteonecrosis, severe deformities, and degenerative joint disease, one should always be aware of the characteristic clinical symptoms. These include pain, limping, waddling gait, inability to walk and limited range of motion on examination. In infants the deformities may develop within few weeks. Diagnosis is established by radiography, treatment includes correction of factors involved in the metabolic bone disease, in particular control of secondary hyperparathyroidism, reduced weight bearing and conservative orthopedic measures. If these measures are not successful, surgical intervention for stabilization may be required. Surgery should only be performed after control of secondary hyperparathyroidism has been achieved, if necessary by cinacalcet therapy or even parathyroidectomy. Even though prospective studies are missing, a failure of orthopaedic corrective measures has been documented in patients with uncontrolled high turnover bone disease.

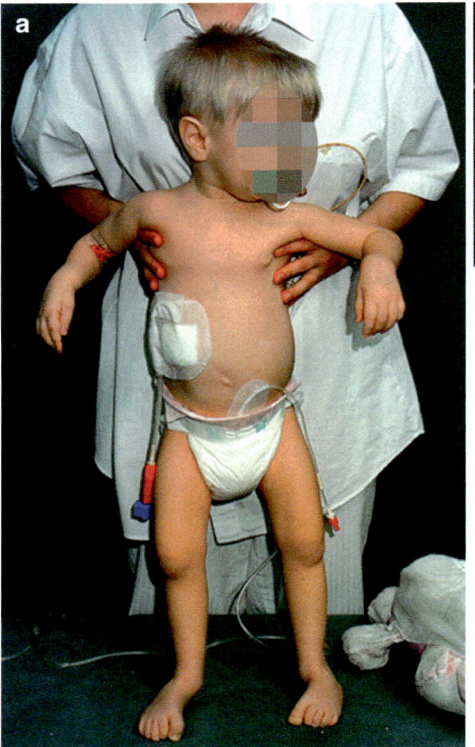
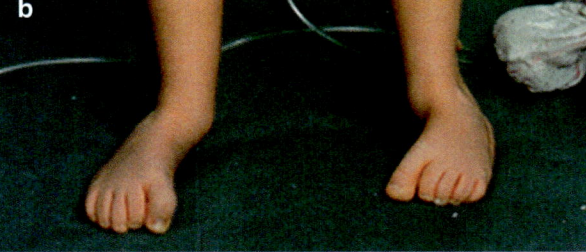

Fig. 60.7 3-year-old boy with ESRD at age 1 year due to prune belly syndrome. He rapidly developed severe renal osteodystrophy with epiphyseal slipping of multiple joints after non-adherence to calcitriol therapy

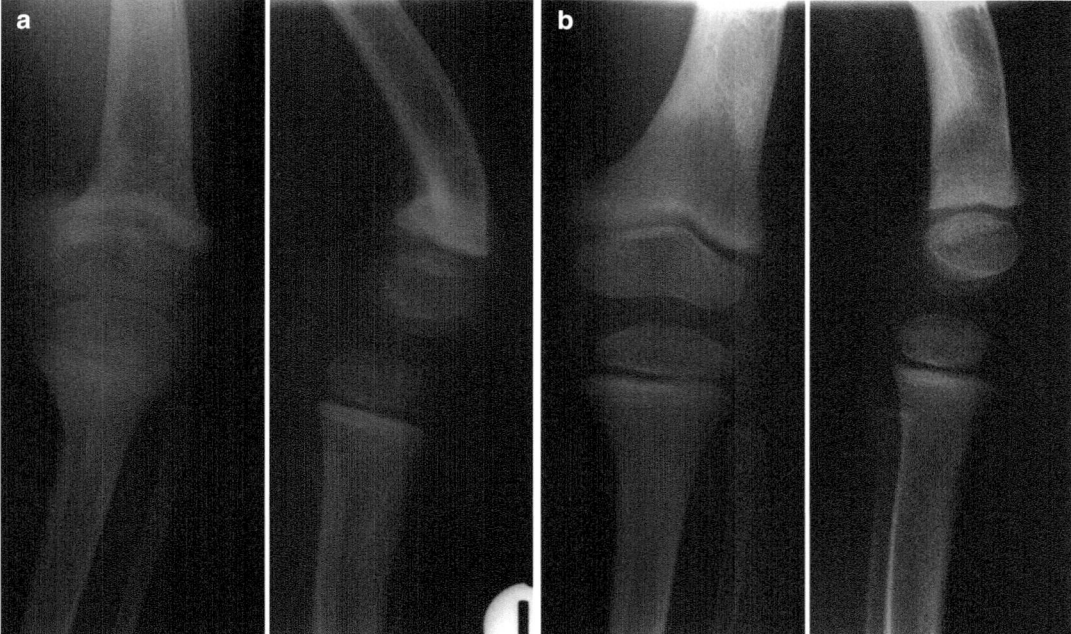

Fig. 60.8 X-rays of the left knee of the same boy as in Fig. 60.7. (**a**) Prior to therapy. (**b**) After 1 year of treatment with calcitriol and calcium i.v. and i.p. and parathy- roidectomy with autotransplantation of parathyroid tissue. The severe deformities have substantially improved, sur- gical intervention was not required

Fractures

Healthy children have an incidence of 14 fractures per 1000 person years, mainly localized to the limbs [95]. In children with CKD fracture risk is increased [96]. Besides complete fractures, bone deformities, slipped epiphyses and microfractures are common. While microfractures may occur and be rapidly repaired at high bone turnover, subjects with low bone turnover may be at increased risk of macrofractures; however this concept has not been proven consistently [97]. In large prospective studies of children with CKD, including the North-American Chronic Kidney Disease in Childhood (CKiD) cohort, a 2.4- and three-fold higher rate of fractures have been reported in boys and girls, respectively, with pre- dialysis CKD as compared to healthy children [98]. Fracture risk in pediatric CKD is associated with baseline-walking difficulty, Tanner stages 4–5 pubertal development, lower height Z-score, higher parathyroid hormone (PTH) levels, lower Ca and 25-hydroxyvitamin D (25D) levels and

team sports participation [98]. Phosphate binder use, and particularly Ca-based phosphate binder use has been associated with decreased fracture risk in children with pre-dialysis CKD, suggest- ing that improved phosphate control and/or increased calcium intake may exert some protec- tive action [98].

Studies using peripheral quantitative CT scans have demonstrated that children with CKD have significant deficits in cortical volumetric bone mineral density. A reduction in tibial cortical BMD z-score over 1 year follow-up was associ- ated with low serum calcium and high PTH levels [89] as well as uremic myopathy [96]. Growth hormone appears to have a protective effect [96].

Bone biopsies in adults demonstrate that both low and high bone turnover are associated with distinct abnormalities contributing to the dimin- ished mechanical competence of bone in CKD. Low turnover bone is characterized by lower cancellous bone volume and reduced tra- becular thickness, high turnover bone by a reduced mineral to matrix ratio and lower stiffness [85]. The fracture risk of adult dialysis patients correlates with plasma iPTH in a U-shaped manner, with the lowest risk observed at average PTH levels around 300 pg/ml [99]. After pediatric kidney transplantation the incidence of fractures is increased five-fold as compared to healthy children, i.e. to 76 fractures per 1000 patient years, two thirds of which affect the vertebrae [95].

Growth Retardation

Growth failure, a regular feature of children with CKD, is mainly due to endogenous growth hormone and IGF1 resistance, malnutrition (especially in infants) and metabolic acidosis. The effects of altered Vitamin D and PTH metabolism on growth are not entirely clear.

In children with CKD a short-term improvement of growth rate has been reported with 1,25-OH$_2$-D treatment [100]; this however was not confirmed in long-term observations. Excessive vitamin D treatment may even result in adynamic bone disease and growth retardation [91]. *In vitro*, calcitropic and somatotropic hormones interact with the proliferation of growth plate chondrocytes [101]. PTH-rP, which acts via the type I PTH receptor, is an important local inhibitor of growth plate chondrocyte maturation [102]. In rats, intermittent bolus injection of PTH increases growth rate whereas this is not seen with continuous PTH infusion, indicating that fluctuations in the level and not the PTH plasma concentration alone impact on bone [103].

From clinical observation it is not clear which PTH range is optimal for growth. In two studies a positive correlation between mean plasma PTH levels and growth was observed, suggesting that higher PTH levels promote growth [91, 104]. Others reported a normal growth rate in children with CKD stage II-IV with PTH levels in the normal range, as well as in CKD stage V with mean plasma PTH concentrations only 50% above the upper limit of normal. In these children particular attention was paid to adequate nutritional support and a strict control of serum phosphate levels within the normal range [105]. Whether normal

bone turnover was maintained in these children is unclear since bone biopsies were not performed [104–106]. In 214 children followed prospectively in the International Pediatric PD Network (IPPN) Registry, the annual change in height SDS tended to be inversely correlated with mean plasma PTH levels. Patients with mean PTH > 500 ng/ml exhibited a significant loss in height SDS [43].

Cardiovascular Calcifications

Cardiovascular mortality is markedly increased in uremic patients. Vascular calcification is one of the main mechanisms underlying this most important long-term complication of renal replacement therapy. In a study published in 2000 36 of 39 young adults with childhood onset of CKD already had significant coronary artery calcifications [10]. Alterations of the morphological and functional properties of arteries have been reported as early as in the second decade of life in children on dialysis [9, 10, 107, 108]. The presence of vascular calcification on CT scan is directly related to hyperphosphatemia, the average calcium x phosphate product over time, intake of calcium containing phosphate binders and plasma PTH levels [9, 10]. In a post mortem analysis of 120 children with CKD, soft tissue and vascular calcification was associated with the use of active vitamin D and calcium containing phosphate binders [109]. Both low and high levels of 1,25(OH)2D have been associated with coronary artery calcification: very low 1,25(OH)2D levels were associated with high turnover bone disease as well as with greater inflammation whereas very high 1,25(OH)2D increase gut calcium absorption and suppress bone calcium and phosphate uptake with adynamic bone disease [110]. Although calcium balance studies have not been performed in children with CKD. Calcium supply should be higher with rapid growth, but it is suspected that the calcium load is often too high in children with advanced CKD treated with active vitamin D, calcium containing phosphate binders and dialysis solutions containing unphysiologically high calcium lev-

Fig. 60.9 Bone disease and soft tissue calcification. Low PTH levels (low turnover bone disease) prevent mineral deposition into bone, high PTH levels result in mineral release from bone. Excessive minerals precipitate in soft tissues

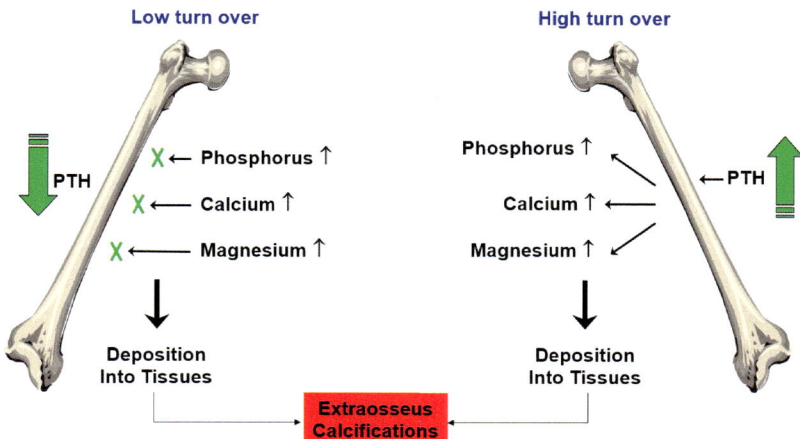

els. On the other hand, the calcium buffering capacity of bone is reduced in patients with low- and high-turn-over bone disease (Fig. 60.9). Noteworthy, calcifications are not merely a passive process of precipitation but triggered by oxidative stress, advanced glycation endproducts and regulated by locally and systemically acting proteins [71]. The plasma protein fetuin is significantly reduced in CKD patients and correlates with cardiovascular mortality [111] and vascular calcification even in children on dialysis [112].

Calcifications may also occur in other sites than the vascular wall, such as the lung or and in periarticular areas. Calciphylaxis, a severe form of extra-skeletal calcifications, has been described in children with tertiary hyperparathyroidism [113]. It is characterized by painful nodules that become mottled or violaceous, indurated and ultimately ulcerated. Accurate diagnosis and optimal treatment of disturbance in bone and mineral metabolism may be crucial in preventing these life-limiting sequelae in children with CKD. Vascular calcification is discussed in detail in chap. 58.

Post-transplant Bone Disease

Successful renal transplantation should reverse all pathologic conditions that lead to CKD-associated mineral and bone disease. In both adult and pediatric kidney recipients, bone histologic changes associated with secondary hyper-

parathyroidism resolve within 6 months after kidney transplantation; bone mineral content Z-scores, however, remain significantly reduced, especially in cortical bone [114]. Interestingly, a disconnect is observed between circulating PTH levels and bone turnover post transplantation; some patients have persistently elevated rates of bone turnover while others develop adynamic lesions, despite moderately elevated serum PTH levels [115].

Immunosuppressive treatment, in particular glucocorticoids, and any degree of CKD developing in the post-transplant course interferes with bone metabolism. Persistent hypophosphatemia is a common finding in renal allograft recipients, especially within the first months post-surgery. Tubular dysfunction secondary to any toxicity, persistent HPT and increased plasma FGF23 levels are considered the main causes of exaggerated renal phosphate secretion after transplantation. Of note, plasma phosphate levels can be normal despite reduced total body phosphate content. In these patients increased skeletal phosphate removal due to increased PTH and inappropriately low calcitriol levels may counterbalance the phosphatonin (FGF23)-induced persistent renal phosphate loss [116]. Likewise, magnesium, an integral part of the hydroxyapatite structure of the bone and essential for osteoblast and osteoclast function, is wasted secondary to calcineurin inhibitor use.

According to bone biopsy studies in adults, loss of bone volume and mineralization leading to low turn-over bone disease is frequent in adults after successful transplantation [117, 118]. The risk of fracture is particularly high the first several months following transplantation. Skeletal lesions may improve subsequently, depending on renal function and pharmacological treatment, but do not resolve completely in the majority of patients [115]. Assessment of BMD by means of DXA shows conflicting results, possibly due to the inadequate standardization and the failure to correct for height and muscular mass. PQCT results demonstrate nearly normal BMD for height and muscle mass, while cortical thickness is reduced [119]. The fracture risk is increased (see above). Avascular necrosis is reported to develop in 4% of children after organ transplantation, most often in the femoral head, but it may also develop in the talus, the humeral neck and other skeletal sites [120]. Avascular necrosis has become less common in recent years, due to steroid sparing with newer immunosuppressive protocols.

Assessment of Renal Bone Disease

Apart from thorough physical examination, the diagnosis of the uremic bone mineral metabolic disorder is mainly based on repeated biochemical analyses (Table 60.2). Even though no single biochemical marker is able to provide a complete assessment of renal osteodystrophy, bone biopsies are rarely performed for the clinical management of patients. In a study of 161 children undergoing chronic PD, high PTH and low serum calcium levels were seen in those with defective mineralization, irrespective of their bone turnover rate [122]. As recommended by KDIGO

guidelines, a thorough assessment of CKD-MBD parameters requires serial assessment of phosphate, calcium and PTH levels, considered together, with trends in levels being most useful in guiding clinical decision making [123]. The 2010 Cochrane review on 'Interventions for Bone Disease in Children with CKD' [124] and the 2013 NICE guideline on hyperphosphataemia management in adults and children with CKD and on dialysis [125, 126] emphasize the lack of pediatric information and the need for more research in children with CKD.

Biochemistry

Serum Calcium

Measurement of total calcium is the mostly used method to assess serum calcium levels. Normal serum concentrations depend on age (Fig. 60.10). Of note, normal total serum calcium may not indicate normal serum ionized calcium levels, and should be corrected for serum albumin concentration if this is low. pH corrected ionized calcium levels are the best reflection of free (biologically available) calcium. Importantly, serum calcium levels are not a reflection of the total body calcium stores, since calcium levels are tightly regulated by multiple negative feedback systems as described above.

Serum calcium is usually normal or low in untreated patients with advanced CKD, with the maintenance of calcium homeostasis being exerted mainly by a compensatory increase in PTH. Once treatment with active vitamin D and calcium containing phosphate binders is initiated, serum calcium levels increase and PTH

Table 60.2 Suggested monthly intervals for the frequency of measurements for biochemical markers of renal osteodystrophy [121]. More frequent measurements may be required in young children, in patients treated with severe renal osteodystrophy, non-compliant patients, and after renal transplantation

CKD stage	GFR (ml/min*1.73 m^2)	Calcium/Ca^{++}, phosphate, AP, PTH	Total ALP	PTH	Serum 25(OH)$_2$D$_3$	Bicarbonate
2	60–89	6	12	12	12	6
3	30–59	6	6	6	6–12	6
4	15–29	3	3	3	3–12	3
5	<15, dialysis	1	1–3	1–3	3–12	1

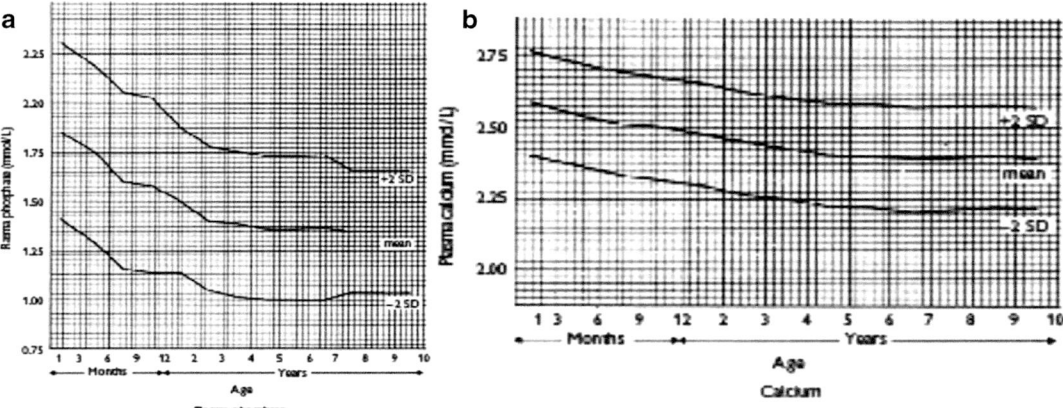

Fig. 60.10 Age-dependent calcium and phosphate percentiles in the plasma of healthy children. (**a**) Calcium, (**b**) Phosphate. *SD* standard deviation. Permission obtained from Blackwell Scientific © Claytob B.E. et al. Pediatric chemical pathology; clinical tests and reference ranges (1980)

declines. Hypercalcemia is still rare in calcitriol treated children with stage IV CKD [104], but seen in about 6% of measurements in children on peritoneal dialysis treated with calcitriol, calcium containing phosphate binders and PD solutions with calcium concentrations of 1.75 mmol/L [127]. Children with low turn-over bone disease and children with tertiary hyperparathyroidism treated with calcitriol are particularly prone to hypercalcemia, because the calcium buffering capacity of bone is reduced. An important differential diagnosis of hypercalcemia in children on dialysis is volume depletion. This condition is usually characterized by a high total but normal ionized calcium concentration. Alternative causes of hypercalcemia to consider include immobilization and, rarely, paraneoplastic release of PTHrP and extrarenal calcitriol production in granulomatous diseases such as tuberculosis and sarcoidosis.

Serum Phosphate

Dietary phosphate intake usually exceeds renal phosphate removal if GFR drops below 40 ml/min/1.73 m^2 but may be noted earlier if phosphate intake is high. The serum concentration of phosphate should be kept in the normal range. Of note, the renal phosphate threshold and serum phosphate concentrations are age-dependent with an upper limit of normal of 2.4 mmol/L in small infants, 2.1 and 1.9 in preschool and school children, and 1.44–1.9 mmol/L in adolescents according to different reference tables [128]; (Fig. 60.10). The physiological range depends on whether a child is growing or postpubertal. In non-fasting adolescents serum phosphate is subject to significant circadian variations following an M-shaped curve with peaks at 4 PM and 3:30 AM and a maximal diurnal amplitude of 1 mmol/L [129]. These fluctuations are not related to food intake and largely disappear with advancing CKD [130].

Parathyroid Hormone

Plasma PTH levels are a key element in the diagnosis and therapeutic monitoring of renal osteodystrophy and should be measured together with calcium, phosphate, alkaline phosphatase and blood bicarbonate at least every 6 months when GFR drops below 60, every 3 months at a GFR below 30 ml/min/1.73 m^2 and every month when end stage renal disease is reached (Table 60.2).

However, the interpretation of PTH measurements is compromised by significant variation between PTH assays and the variable presence of biologically inactive PTH fragments and oxidized

PTH as discussed above. The target range for PTH which allows for normal bone turnover and growth and which is not associated with increased vascular calcifications is not clear. In children with CKD stage 5, values of iPTH below 200 pg/ml have been suggested to indicate adynamic bone disease whereas values above 500 pg/ml are associated with osteitis fibrosa; however, considerable overlap exists [6]. A study of the IPPN registry found a markedly increasing risk of symptomatic bone disease with PTH exceeding 300 pg/ml and impaired longitudinal growth at mean PTH concentrations above 500 pg/ml, whereas the risk of hypercalcemia increased at levels below 100 pg/ml [49]. These findings support a PTH target range of 100–300 pg/ml in the pediatric age group (Table 60.3). In another study, children with PTH levels below twice the upper limit of normal had less vascular calcification compared to those with PTH levels above twice the upper limit of normal [9].

Alkaline Phosphatase

Measurements of serum total alkaline phosphatases, a marker of osteoblast activity, can be helpful in predicting bone turnover in conjunction with PTH [131]. Values are strongly age dependent with higher activity present during periods of rapid growth. Bone specific alkaline phosphatase may further increase predictability of bone turnover and may be advantageous in subgroups of patients, e.g. with hepatic diseases, to exclude measurement of non-skeletal enzyme. The potential benefits have to be weighed against the considerably higher costs.

Table 60.3 Target iPTH range in children with CKD 2–5 (adapted from 133;135). Recommendations for CKD stage 2–4 are opinion based; stage 5 recommendations are evidence based but still debated. Whole-PTH assays provide values which are only 50–60% values obtained with iPTH assays; this however may vary considerably

CKD stage	GFR (ml/min*1.73 m²)	Target iPTH range (pg/ml)
2	60–89	35–70
3	30–59	35–70
4	15–29	70–110
5	<15, dialysis	100–300

25(OH)D and 1,25(OH)₂D

Serum levels of 25(OH)D give an estimate of vitamin D body stores; it's serum half-life is 3 weeks. There is debate about what levels of vitamin D can be considered adequate, but most authorities agree that a level of 20–30 ng/ml is sufficient to maintain normal serum calcium levels and prevent hyperparathyroidism. Recently published ESPN guidelines suggest that serum 25D levels be maintained above 75 nmol/L (30 ng/ml), and below 120 nmol/L (48 ng/ml) [29]. These levels maintain optimal gut Ca absorption and prevent seasonal fluctuations that can predispose even healthy children to nutritional rickets [28]. Serum levels <5 ng/ml have been categorized as severe deficiency, 5–15 ng/ml as mild deficiency and serum levels of 16–30 ng/ml as vitamin D insufficiency. Since 25(OH)D may have numerous physiological functions, vitamin D deficiency must be avoided at all stages of CKD. 25(OH)D serum levels should be measured 6–12 monthly depending on CKD stage in children not on vitamin D treatment. In case vitamin D supplementation is required, levels should be measured again after 3 months [29] (Table 60.2). Oral 1,25(OH)2D is rapidly absorbed and peak plasma levels are reached within 3 h in children with CKD [89]. Due to the short plasma half-life of 1,25(OH)₂D (4–6 h), the clinical usefulness of 1,25(OH)₂D measurements in plasma is limited. However, plasma 1,25(OH)₂D levels have been correlated with the presence of vascular calcification in children on dialysis [110].

Additional Serum Markers of Bone Turn Over

Biomarkers of bone formation, e.g. osteocalcin and procollagen type I carboxyl terminal peptides, and of bone resorption, e.g. type I collagen cross linked telopeptide and pyridinoline, have not been studied widely to date in children with CKD. Most of them are eliminated via the kidney and accumulate with reduced renal function. TRAP-5b and osteoprotegerin may prove as useful indicators of bone metabolism, based on the central role of RANK ligand/osteoprotegerin in bone metabolism [71]. FGF23 has been correlated with indices of bone mineralization in children [4] and sclerostin, an inhibitor of bone formation, with bone turn-over rates [75]. Further studies correlating the circulating levels of these potential biomarkers to bone histology, growth and established biochemical markers will be required to determine their added value in the monitoring of uremic bone disease.

Aluminum

Aluminum containing phosphate binders are not recommended in children and dialysis water purification has generally improved. Therefore, aluminum related bone disease and encephalopathy should not develop anymore, and plasma aluminum levels do not need to be determined on a regular base. Exposure to aluminum, however, may still occur in some countries.

Imaging

Radiography of the Skeleton

Conventional radiographs of the skeleton are relatively insensitive in detecting renal bone disease, and only grossly evaluate bone structure and mineralization. They should be performed in patients if results are expected to impact on treatment, in case of bone pain and suspicion of fracture and in children with genetic diseases with specific bone involvement [121]. Hand and wrist X-rays can demonstrate severe hyperparathyroidism induced hyperosteoclasia and osteitis fibrosa as subperiostal resorption zones (Fig. 60.11), subperiostal erosions of the phalanges, and acroosteolyses at the end phalanges and at sites of ligament endings. In the skull, hyperparathyroidism results in ground-glass- or granular appearance, focal radiolucencies and sclerotic areas. In children with CKD widened radiolucent areas of the growth zones also indicate accumulation of fibrous tissue, in contrast to nutritional rickets where the radiolucent areas are mainly due to accumulation of unmineralized growth cartilage. Brown tumours

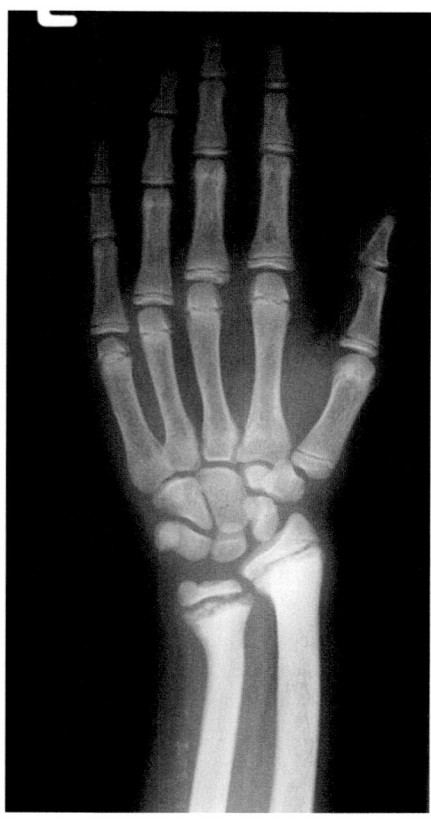

Fig. 60.11 Left hand X-ray in 18-year-old boy with signs of severe renal bone disease: subperiostal erosions, especially of the middle phalanges, brown tumor in the second digit, "ricket-like" lesions and vascular calcifications at the forearm (Courtesy of J. Troeger, University Hospital for Pediatric and Adolescent Medicine, Heidelberg, Germany)

also present accumulation of hyperosteoclastic tissue. They can typically be seen at the metaphyses of long bones but also at other skeletal sites such as the jaw. In contrast to hyperosteoclastic patients, there are no specific signs of osteomalacia. Even Looser zones, straight wide radiolucent bands within the cortex, can represent osteomalacia lesions but also fibrous tissue.

Measurements of Bone Mineral Density

Measurements of bone mineral density are not routinely used in the monitoring of CKD-associated bone disease. Prospective interventional studies are lacking and problems in interpreting results are common. Dual-energy X-ray absorptiometry (DXA) is the most widely used method for measuring bone mineral content and bone mineral density (BMD). BMD (g/cm^2) is often falsely taken as a surrogate parameter of bone strength and fracture risk. BMD increases physiologically in childhood with age and, more closely, with measures of body size such as height and weight. As a consequence, measurements should not be normalized to age but to body height, bone size or muscle function [132]. The interpretation of DEXA measurements is further complicated by the lacking distinction between cortical and cancellous bone. The ISCD 2007, the KDIGO 2017 guideline update and the European Pediatric Clinical Practice Points [121] recommend against routine DXA BMD testing in CKD3–5 since BMD does not predict the type of renal osteodystrophy. This is because PTH excess has generally catabolic effects on cortical bone with decrease in cortical volumetric BMD and cortical thickness whereas it exerts anabolic effects on trabecular bone. A recent study showed that combination of routine biomarkers were better predictors of cortical BMD evaluated by pQCT, and BMD measurement by DXA did not correlate with biochemical data or pQCT measures [88]. Thus, these imaging techniques are not recommended for routine screening tools of bone health or fracture risk prediction in pediatric CKD patients [121].

Peripheral Quantitative Computer Tomography (pQCT)

Peripheral Quantitative Computer Tomography (pQCT) is an alternative technology which permits resolution of cancellous and cortical bone. pQCT of the tibia provides a detailed picture of bone health, including volumetric bone density, separate evaluation of cortical and trabecular components, and measurement of bone dimensions, parameters of bone strength and muscle mass. The reported measurement error in children and adolescents is <2%. pQCT has been widely used in children with CKD and is a good predictor of future fracture risk [89]. In children with CKD, pQCT revealed reduced cortical area and a decline in cortical BMD with time, in association with high PTH plasma levels [96]. pQCT also unmasks differences in total bone density between patients with high turnover and adynamic bone disease [118]. Despite these promising findings, routine application of pQCT has not yet been recommended due to a lack of prospective information regarding an impact of pQCT monitoring on treatment outcomes.

Bone Biopsy

Micromorphometric analysis of the bone is the gold standard for characterization and quantification of renal bone disease. The biopsy procedure is safe and well tolerated by most children. It provides information on the current histologic status and, if double tetracycline staining is performed, the dynamics of bone formation and mineralization can be assessed. Bone biopsies are not needed for routine diagnosis and treatment of renal osteodystrophy, but may be considered if the clinical and biochemical findings do not explain underlying bone disease, e.g. severe bone deformity or pain, low-energy fracture, persistent hypercalcemia or hypophosphatemia, despite optimized treatment [121]. Since few bone biopsies have been performed in children with CKD in the last 20 years, cooperation with the few remaining centres with respective experience regarding the technical procedure and histomorphometric analyses is recommended. Bone biopsies may have a role in clinical trials in which the effect of therapeutic interventions require histological verification.

Imaging of the Parathyroid Glands

In children with severe secondary hyperparathyroidism, sonography of the parathyroid glands should be performed. Parathyroid glands usually cannot be detected by ultrasound unless they are enlarged. The indication of advanced imaging procedures in patients with refractory hyperparathyroidism is controversial. MIBI scan and MRI may give additional information in cases where parathyroidectomy is considered, e.g. an ectopic gland, especially prior to re-exploration of unsuccessful parathyroidectomy. Preoperative imaging by ultrasound, and even by MIBI scan or MRI, may fail to detect adenomas. Therefore, a negative result should not prevent thorough surgical exploration if clinically indicated.

Imaging of Vascular Alterations

The intima media thickness (IMT) of the common carotid artery as assessed by high resolution sonography is a sensitive marker of early vascular lesions, and in adults with CKD it is a strong predictor of future cardiovascular events and death [133]. In children with CKD, carotid IMT has been correlated with the time averaged serum Ca x P product, the cumulative dose of calcium-based phosphate binders, and the mean calcitriol dose [9, 107, 108]. In experienced hands, sequential sonographic IMT assessments can be a valuable diagnostic tool of vasculopathy secondary to altered bone and mineral metabolism.

In cases of severely disturbed bone and mineral metabolism, plain x-rays may be performed to screen for vascular and soft tissue calcifications (Fig. 60.11).

Coronary artery calcifications can be assessed quantitatively by electron-beam or ECG-gated computer tomography, and vessel stiffness by applanation tonometry, ultrasound based or newer oscillometric techniques. These are discussed in detail in Chap. 58.

Treatment

CKD-MBD management in children needs to focus on three key areas. First, to maintain normal calcium - phosphate homeostasis so as to obtain acceptable bone quality and cardiovascular status, second to provide optimal growth in order to maximize the final height and third, to correct all metabolic and clinical abnormalities that can worsen bone disease, growth and cardio-vascular disease, i.e. metabolic acidosis, anaemia, malnutrition and 25(OH)vitamin D deficiency.

Many of the factors contributing to the development of secondary hyperparathyroidism and renal osteodystrophy are present early in the course of renal disease (Fig. 60.1). Since patients are usually asymptomatic, insufficient attention is often paid to progressive alterations in bone and mineral homeostasis. With advancing renal failure, parathyroid glands become hyperplastic and less sensitive to therapeutic interventions. Therefore, **prevention** should always be the primary objective in children with CKD in order to delay the development and its osseous and cardio-vascular sequelae. An overview of key preventative strategies is given in Table 60.6. A scheme summarizing the treatment in patients with established hyperparathyroidism is given in Fig. 60.12.

Optimal control of serum **phosphate** levels is probably the crucial element of preventive management. Hyperphosphatemia is an independent risk factor for secondary hyperparathyroidism, renal osteodystrophy and vascular calcifications. As early as in CKD stage II, regular dietary counseling should be performed and drug therapy may already be considered. On the other hand, hypophosphatemia, as commonly seen in children with associated tubulopathies even in CKD stage II–IV or after renal transplantation, may induce hypophosphatemic osteomalacia and should also be avoided.

Serum **calcium** must be maintained in the normal range, taking care of maintaining a normal serum calcium phosphorus ion product. The upper limit for the serum calcium × phosphorus ion product recommended for adults (55 mg^2/dl^2) is applicable in adolescents, whereas the upper normal limit is higher in children below 12 years of age (65 mg^2/dl^2) and even higher in infants. The calcium × phosphate product is rarely used in clinical practice now since it is not a 'biological' value and does not represent the true physic-chemical coupling in hydroxyapatite crystals (chemical formula $Ca_{10}(PO_4)_6(OH)_2$). Clinicians are advised to follow serum calcium and serum phosphate levels, particularly trends in both of these, rather than the calcium × phosphate product.

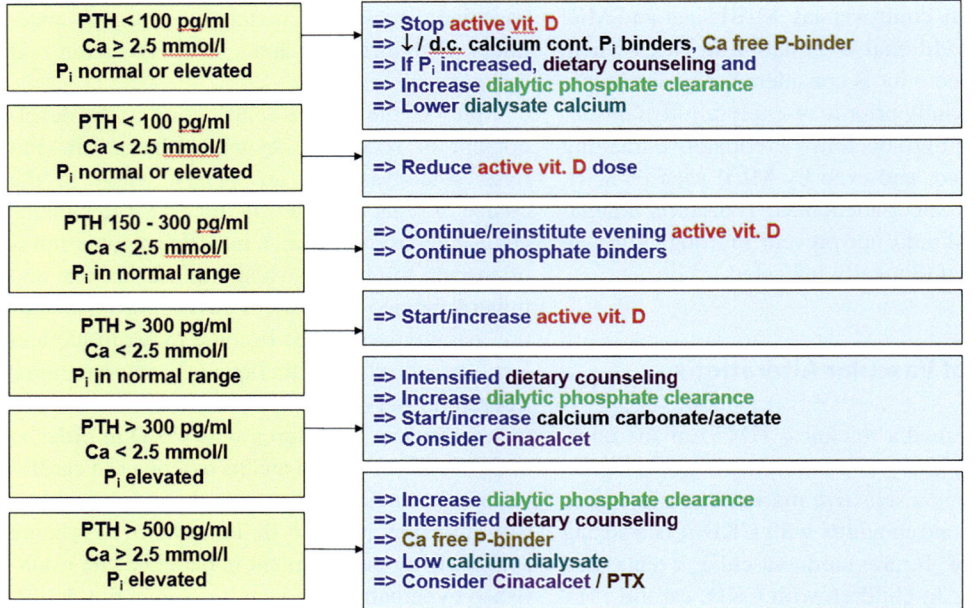

Fig. 60.12 Therapeutic algorithm for treatment of hyperparathyroidism in children with CKD

In CKD stage 5, serum calcium levels in the upper normal range should be avoided [128, 134] and hypercalcemia must be prevented. In case of hypercalcemia, all calcium containing phosphate binders must be withheld, vitamin D therapy be stopped and, if hypercalcemia persists, PD fluid with 1.25 mMol/L calcium be administered. Even lower dialysate calcium concentrations may be used in HD patients. On the other hand, pediatricians must keep in mind that growing infants and children need a positive calcium balance. In growing children hyperparathyroidism may often be triggered insufficient calcium supply. The routine use of dialysate calcium concentrations of 1.25 mmol/L may be inadequate in patients with major UF associated calcium losses. Thus 1.5 and 1.75 mMol/L dialysate calcium concentrations are often needed, depending on the oral calcium load and active vitamin D treatment.

The sensitivity of the skeleton to **PTH** effects decreases with declining renal function. Therefore, an increasing PTH target level has been suggested. These target levels are given in Table 60.3. For CKD stage II–IV target PTH recommendations only reflect expert opinion. For patients with CKD stage V there is some biopsy-derived evidence for the indicated target ranges, which, however, is challenged by recent studies [105, 135]. If plasma PTH levels are below the target range and serum calcium levels are increased vitamin D therapy and calcium containing phosphate binders should be reduced or even discontinued, a reduction in dialysate calcium concentration may be justified. Of note, growth hormone should not be given to patients with uncontrolled hyperparathyroidism, symptomatic high turn-over bone disease or slipped epiphysis.

Diet

Regular dietary counseling is an essential part of CKD-MBD management. Optimal control of serum P concentration is a crucial element of preventative management, starting early in the course of CKD. K/DOQI and the Pediatric Renal Nutrition Taskforce [136] have published guidelines on the dietary management of Ca and P in children with CKD2–5D. They recommend regular dietary counseling from early CKD and limiting dietary P intake to within the age-appropriate normal ranges for children in the mild-moderate stages of CKD and to the lower limit of the normal range in patients with advanced CKD who have persistent hyperphosphatemia or hyperparathyroidism [128, 136, 137]. For detailed dietary recommendations regarding dietary calcium and phosphorus intake, please refer to Chap. 55.

Importantly, processed foods are likely to contain inorganic P additives (such as phosphoric acid and sodium phosphate), which are almost completely absorbed, unlike organic phosphates that have a lower bioavailability. Aggressive dietary P restriction is difficult since it may compromise adequate intake of other nutrients, especially protein and Ca [15]. P intake is directly linked to protein intake, with 10–12 mg of P accompanying each gram of protein; any reduction in P intake should not compromise protein intake. In a recent study 67% of children with CKD stages 4–5 had a dietary Ca intake below the recommended nutrient intake, and additional Ca from medications, mainly in the form of P binders, was required to maintain nutritional Ca requirements [15].

Dialysis

The efficacy of dialysis in removing excess phosphate is modifiable to some extent but overall limited [138]. E.g., an anuric child of 20 kg body weight and a daily protein intake of 1.4 g/kg ingests 430 mg phosphate per day. Concomitant intake of calcitriol and phosphate binders will result in absorption of roughly 50% of phosphate (215 mg/d). This amount of phosphate is the maximum that can be eliminated by conventional dialysis. At a protein intake of 2 g/kg*d, the phosphate balance will be positive by more than 60 mg per day on a conventional PD or hemodialysis schedule. A weekly creatinine clearance of more than 80 L/1.73m^2 would be required to compensate the dietary phosphate load. This efficacy can only be achieved by frequent [139] or long nocturnal hemodialysis [140]. Slow-flow nocturnal hemodialysis performed over 6–9 h per night five to six times per week dramatically improves phosphate clearance and may even require phosphate supple-

mentation p.o. or in the dialysis bath to prevent phosphate depletion and aggravation of bone disease [141, 142]. If such intensified hemodialysis is not available or not feasible, repeated dietary counseling and optimized oral phosphate binder management are essential (see below). In children receiving automated peritoneal dialysis, total PD fluid turnover should be maximized using maximally tolerable fill volumes, maximally acceptable cycler times and additional day time exchanges [138]. In a prospective multi-centre study serum phosphate levels were similar between HD and HDF patients but PTH levels declined in the HDF cohort over 12 months while remaining static in those on HD [143]. A further study has shown that FGF23, a middle molecular weight substance, if cleared more efficiently on HDF, with 30% lower levels than conventional HD [144].

Phosphate Binders

Restriction of dietary phosphorus intake may be sufficient in early stages of CKD. However, even with some dietary restriction of phosphate intake, normophosphatemia may only be maintained at the expense of increased PTH and FGF 23 plasma levels, both of which decrease tubular phosphate reabsorption. As renal function deteriorates, dietary control of phosphate becomes more difficult and overt hyperphosphatemia usually develops. Oral phosphate binding agents should be added. Calcium salts are used as first line phosphate binders. They have limited phosphate binding capacity (Table 60.4). The dose required depends on the oral phosphorus intake, and often reaches several grams per day. While in hypocalcemic and rapidly growing children the additional calcium load still is beneficial, many patients tend to develop hypercalcemia with prolonged administration. Significantly more calcium is absorbed and little phosphorus retained when calcium containing phosphate binders are not given with meals. Calcium acetate contains 25% of elemental calcium, calcium carbonate 40%. Calcium acetate binds more phosphorus per unit of calcium content and thus allows for higher doses and improved phosphate

Table 60.4 Phosphate binding agents

Compound	Calcium content (%)	Calcium absorbed (%)	Phosphate bound per g compound	Phosphate bound per Ca^{++} absorbed	Comment
Calcium Carbonate	40	20–30	39 mg / g	≈ 1 mg/8 mg	High Ca^{++} load, inexpensive, GI side effects
Calcium Acetate	25	22 (between meals 40)	45 mg / g	≈ 1 mg/3 mg	GI side effects, less Ca^{++} load than CaCO$_3$, inexpensive
Mg + Ca carbonate	Variable	20–30% of Ca	NA	≈ 1 mg/2.3 mg	Less Ca^{++} load, GI side effects, long term effects?
Sevelamer HCl/– Carbonate	0	0	Similar to calcium acetate[a]	NA	Ca^{++} and Al^{+++} free, cholesterol ↓, costs ↑, acidosis ↑ (in case of HCl)
Aluminum cont. Binders	0	0	Similar to calcium acetate	NA	Effective but toxic, not recommended

NA not applicable or no data
[a]See Ref. [145]

Table 60.5 Suggested treatment for vitamin D supplementation in children with CKD and on dialysis. With permission from [29]

Age	25(OH) D serum (nmol/L)[a]	Vitamin D supplementation dose (daily)	Monitoring
Intensive replacement phase			
<1 year		600 IU/day[b]	– Serum calcium and urinary calcium levels 1–3 monthly based on CKD stage
>1 year[b]	<12	8000 IU/day	– 25(OH)D levels: after 3 months
	12–50	4000 IU/day	
	50–75	2000 IU/day	
Maintenance phase			
<1 year	>75[d]	400 IU/day	– 25(OH)D levels: after 6–12 monthly
>1 year[c]		1000–2000 IU/ day based on CKD stage	

[a]To convert nmol/L to ng/ml divide by 2.5
[b]In infants <1 year, a fixed dose is recommended irrespective of the level of 25(OH)D
[c]Consider adjusting dose by body size (weight or body surface area)
[d]If levels remain <75 nmol/L, then give doses as per the 'intensive replacement' schedule for a further course of intensive replacement and recheck levels

control. If given at similar doses, calcium acetate results in a reduced incidence of hypercalcemia as compared to calcium carbonate (Table 60.4).

On the other hand, less gastrointestinal side effects have been reported with calcium carbonate. An individual choice is required to assure optimal patient compliance and control of calcium and phosphate uptake.

Calcium citrate is also effective, but citrate increases aluminum resorption and should therefore be avoided (Table 60.5).

Magnesium Salts

Magnesium salts have a relatively weak intestinal phosphate binding activity and require higher dosing, but avoid calcium exposure. An inverse relationship between serum Mg, hyperparathyroidism and vascular calcification has been demonstrated in adult dialysis patients and thus potential benefits have been attributed to magnesium salts [146]. Interestingly, in addition to the beneficial effects of intestinal phosphate binding of magnesium, experimental studies suggest inhibition of vascular smooth muscle cell transition into an osteoblast like phenotype, and inhibition of nanocrystal formation from calcium and phosphate ions, a key mechanism in the formation of ectopic calcification in CKD [147]. Diarrhea, hyperkalemia and hypermagnesemia are their main side effects. The long-term effects of an increased magnesium load are not clear. At present, magnesium containing phosphate binders may be given as adjuncts to calcium containing binders.

Table 60.6 Measures for prevention of MBD in children with CKD

- Active screening for hyperparathyroidism—measurement of PTH begins when the GFR falls to <90 ml/min/1.73 m²
- Control of hyperphosphataemia
  - Diet
  - Phosphate binders:
    first line—calcium-based phosphate binders
    second line or if hypercalcaemia—calcium-free phosphate binders
    (in addition to calcium-based binders or as a substitute)
- Control of hypocalcaemia using lowest possible dose of vitamin D
  - native vitamin D in CKD 1–3
  - active vitamin D analogues in CKD 4–5 and 5D
- Improve dialysis efficiency for phosphate removal
- Pre-emptive renal transplantation where possible
- Avoid vitamin K antagonists like warfarin to prevent inactivation of calcification antagonist MGP
- Cinacalcet, especially in case of high doses of active vitamin D and high serum calcium concentrations
- Parathyroidectomy—in case of hyperparathyroidism refractory to all therapeutic measures including cinacalcet

Calcium Free Phosphate Binders

Growing evidence for a role of the oral calcium load in the progression of cardiovascular calcifications urged the development of calcium free phosphate binders. They are especially indicated in patients with a calcium intake exceeding twice the recommended daily intake (which increases from 210 mg elemental calcium per day in the first 6 months of life to 1250 mg/d in adolescents), reduced PTH levels (with likely adynamic bone disease), hypercalcemia or even emerging soft tissue calcifications.

Sevelamer hydrochloride is a hydrogel of polyallylamine, which is resistant to digestive degradation and therefore not absorbed. It binds dietary phosphate and releases hydrochloric acid. This may reduce plasma bicarbonate levels [145], a problem which can be circumvented by the use of sevelamer carbonate [148]. Intestinal binding of bile acids significantly lowers LDL cholesterol. The major advantage of sevelamer is that in contrast to calcium containing phosphate binders, sevelamer reduces serum phosphate without increasing serum calcium levels. Hypercalcemia occurs less frequently: in an 8-week cross-over study in children, sevelamer and calcium acetate were equally effective at reducing serum phosphate levels, but significantly less hypercalcaemia occurred in the sevelamer group [145].

Aluminum Containing Phosphate Binders

Aluminum containing phosphate binders are efficient phosphate absorbers but may result in aluminum intoxication. Their administration is not recommended in children. If their use cannot be avoided, e.g. in case of a severely increased calcium phosphate product not manageable otherwise, dosage should be limited to 30 mg/kg*d. Aluminum containing binders should only be given if other calcium free alternatives (see below) are not available. Regular monitoring of aluminum blood levels is needed. In case of persistent hyperparathyroidism cinacalcet and even parathyroidectomy should be considered (see below) to avoid extended exposure to aluminum containing binders.

Lanthanum carbonate binds intestinal phosphate more effectively than calcium carbonate and sevelamer. However, patients on extended treatment show increased lanthanum serum levels. Significant tissue accumulation has been demonstrated in rats. In light of the past experience with aluminum toxicity, lanthanum containing phosphate binders are currently not recommended in children with CKD. Nonetheless, according to the International Pediatric PD Network 1.6% of all children monitored worldwide until 2020 have been receiving lanthanum containing phosphate binders.

Iron-Based Phosphate Binders

Iron-based phosphate binders reduce serum phosphate and FGF 23 concentrations while simultaneously increasing serum iron stores in patients with CKD and on dialysis [149, 150]. A recent randomized open-label study has shown that sucroferric oxyhydroxde is as effective as Ca acetate in controlling serum P levels in children with CKD [151]. Similar to other P-binders, adverse events are primarily GI-related.

Newer P-Binders

Intestinal P absorption is regulated by sodium-dependent P co-transporter type 2b (NPT2b). Treatment with niacin (vitamin B3) or its metabolite nicotinamide/niacinamide, both of which modulate NPT2b expression, result in a sustained reduction in serum P concentrations in adult dialysis patients [152]. However, in a randomized trial of adult HD patients, NPT2b inhibition was not effective in reducing serum P concentrations [153]. Targeting salivary P using P-binding chewing gum has also been proposed [154]. These agents have not yet been studied in children.

Long-term Safety of Phosphate Binder Therapy

The long-term cardiovascular safety of phosphate binder therapy is still controversial. A randomized clinical trial in adults with a GFR of 20–45 ml/min/1.73 m^2 demonstrated an increase in arterial calcification with calcium, lanthanum and sevelamer binder therapy, but not in placebo treated patients [155]. Others showed progressive arterial calcification in predialysis patients on low-phosphorus diet alone. Progression was less in calcium carbonate-treated patients, and absent in sevelamer-treated patients [156]. The Independent trial demonstrated improved survival in predialysis patients randomized to sevelamer as compared to those treated with calcium carbonate [157, 158]. A recent meta-analysis comprising 104 studies involving 13,744 adults concluded that sevelamer may lower death (all causes) compared to calcium-based binders in patients on dialysis and incur less treatment-related hypercalcaemia, but demonstrated no clinically important benefits of any phosphate binder on cardiovascular endpoints or fracture risk. Likewise no such beneficial effects could be demonstrated in patients with CKD2–5 [159]. Respective data in children is scant. Still, in view of the key pathophysiological role of phosphate in CKD MBD cardiovascular disease, most children with hyperphosphatemia are treated with phosphate binders, considering the calcium demand of the growing bone and the treatment associated calcium load.

Vitamin D

Oral treatment with ergocalciferol or cholecalciferol is suggested when serum 25(OH)D concentrations are below 30–40 ng/ml in order to prevent muscular weakness, secondary hyperparathyroidism and osteomalacia. At least in early stages of CKD, supplementation of cholecalciferol can prevent or reduce hyperparathyroidism and should be prescribed before calcitriol is considered. In an RCT of 25(OH)D therapy in children with CKD stages 2–4, children on ergocalciferol who achieved 25D levels >75 nMol/L had a significantly longer time to development of secondary hyperparathyroidism compared to those on placebo [34].

No clear consensus exists on the preferable type of native vitamin D supplement (ergo vs cholecalciferol), its dosage, frequency of administration or duration of treatment in healthy children or children with CKD. The KDIGO and ESPN guidelines recommend a loading regimen or intensive replacement period for a variable duration of 4–12 weeks followed by a maintenance regimen [29, 128]. Both guidelines further recommend escalating doses for intensive replacement depending on the baseline 25(OH)D level; cholecalciferol doses range from 2000 to 8000 IU/day for intensive phase replacement and 1000–2000 IU/day for maintenance therapy. The therapeutic window is wide; hypercalcemia, hypercalciuria, and symptomatic toxicity have been reported only when serum 25(OH)D levels exceed 250 nmol/L. Current clinical practice recommendations for children with CKD suggest a target level of 75–120 nmol/L (30–48 ng/ml).

Vitamin D repletion strategies include daily, weekly, monthly and even 3-monthly dosing regimens. Several trials have evaluated the short-term safety, efficacy and tolerability of these protocols. A recent randomized trial compared cholecalciferol dosing regimens for achieving and maintaining 25OHD concentrations ≥30 ng/ml in children with CKD stages 2–4, and showed that cholecalciferol as daily, weekly or monthly administration yielded similar 25OHD concentrations without toxicity [160]. Children with glomerular disease required higher doses of cholecalciferol compared to those with non-glomerular disease.

Active Vitamin D Sterols

Recent ESPN guidelines have addressed treatment with active vitamin D sterols [161]. These are indicated in pediatric CKD patients whose serum PTH levels remain elevated despite normal serum 25D and P levels. Alfacalcidol (1-α hydroxyvitamin D_2) or calcitriol (1,25-dihydroxyvitamin D_3) are most commonly used. The dose of calcitriol depends on initial PTH, Ca and phosphate values. An initial dose of 5–10 ng/kg*d is effective and safe in most children with CKD [128, 161]. Alfacalcidol is often used in infants and small children since a liquid formula is available, and the dose can be carefully titrated. Higher doses relative to calcitriol may be required due to the requisite hepatic metabolism to 1,25 vitamin D. The frequency of calcium, phosphate and PTH monitoring should be adapted to the dose of vitamin D administered. All vitamin D analogues can get adsorbed to plastic tubing to varying degrees, and therefore should not be administered via feeding tubes.

Calcitriol efficiently controls secondary hyperparathyroidism. With prolonged treatment a substantial number of children, however, develop adynamic bone disease, which has been associated with a reduced growth rate and frequent episodes of hypercalcemia [58, 63].

A second consequence to consider with active vitamin D treatment is the increase not only of intestinal absorption of calcium [162] but also of phosphate. Calcitriol increases intestinal phosphate absorption from around 60% to 90% [163] (Fig. 60.13). Calcitriol use often is limited by aggravated hyperphosphatemia and hypercalcemia. Calcitriol, hypercalcemia and hyperphosphatemia contribute to extraosseus tissue calcifications and decreased survival in children with end stage renal disease [67, 68]. Deterioration of renal function is not accelerated by calcitriol [164], at least if administered at moderate doses not resulting in increased serum calcium and phosphate concentrations.

All activated vitamin D analogs increase FGF23 secretion. Although the consequences of these increased FGF23 levels in dialyzed patients remain to be completely determined, current evidence suggests that excessive circulating FGF23 is associated with increased mortality rates and cardiovascular disease [41]. Two randomized trials have demonstrated that vitamin D analogs do not improve cardiac function for patients with CKD stages 3–5 during one year of treatment [165, 166].

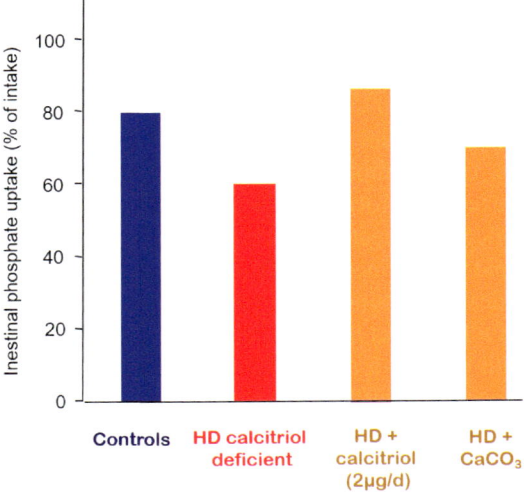

Fig. 60.13 Effect of calcitriol and oral phosphate binder on intestinal phosphate uptake. Calcitriol significantly increases phosphate uptake in hemodialysis patients (HD). $CaCO_3$, given at a dose of 75 mEq prior to a standardized meal, reduces phosphate uptake but increases oral calcium intake by 1.4 g compared to placebo, the intestinal calcium uptake increases to 28% of the ingested amount as compared to 14% with placebo

The Mode of Calcitriol Administration

The mode of calcitriol administration is of minor importance. Some studies including bone biopsies suggested a strong effect of calcitriol on bone metabolism with intermittent oral, intravenous and intraperitoneal administration. These studies, however, were not controlled against a daily administration mode [127]. Prospective randomized studies comparing daily versus intermittent oral calcitriol in healthy children and children with CKD stages 2–4 revealed no differences in PTH suppression, intestinal calcium absorption, the incidence of hypercalcemia and hyperphosphatemia or longitudinal growth rates [167, 168]. Overall, the response to calcitriol depends less on the mode of administration than on the degree of secondary hyperparathyroidism, hyperphosphatemia and the degree of parathyroid gland autonomy.

Synthetic Vitamin D Analogues

Synthetic vitamin D analogues have been developed to reduce intestinal calcium and phosphorus absorption at equipotent PTH suppressive action. Three sterols have been approved, i.e. 22-oxacalcitriol, 19-nor-1,25 dihydroxy vitamin D2 (paricalcitol) and 1α-hydroxyvitamin D2 (doxercalciferol). In adult hemodialysis patients, paricalcitol treatment is associated with a more rapid achievement of PTH control and fewer episodes of sustained hypercalcemia and increased $Ca \times P$ product than calcitriol therapy In children with CKD 3–5 and on hemodialysis paricalcitol appears to be efficacious and safe [169, 170]. The still limited evidence for a superior efficacy-safety profile of the synthetic vitamin D analogues must be balanced against their high costs.

There is also observational evidence for a survival benefit associated with the use of vitamin D sterols in general, which awaits confirmation in prospective trials. It may reflect a plethora of beneficial immunological and cardiovascular effects of active vitamin D compounds. In summary, active vitamin D sterols are indispensable therapeutic agents in the management of CKD but should always be used with caution and in awareness of their limited therapeutic window, beyond which major untoward effects to the bone, cardiovascular and potentially other systems may occur.

Calcimimetic Agents

Calcimimetics are a new class of compounds that bind to the parathyroid calcium sensing receptor, increase its sensitivity to ionized calcium by allosteric modification, and dose dependently decrease plasma PTH levels by up to 80%. The effect is largely independent of baseline PTH and phosphate levels and thus allows for control of parathyroid gland function even in patients with otherwise refractory hyperparathyroidism. **Cinacalcet** is the only currently approved calcimimetic agent. Cinacalcet also reduces serum calcium and phosphate levels, possibly via increased mineral deposition into bone. A randomized clinical trial in adult dialysis patients suggested attenuation of vascular and cardiac valve calcification with cinacalcet plus low-dose vitamin D sterols [171]. However, in a large placebo-controlled trial only a non-significant 7% reduction in death or first cardiovascular event was observed. A nominally significant 12% reduction in the risk of death was observed after adjustment for the unevenly distributed baseline characteristics [172].

Observational studies, industry sponsored phase 2 and 3 randomized studies, and one single arm extension study in pediatric dialysis patients demonstrated good efficiency of cinacalcet, i.e. suppression of PTH, and good tolerability [173]. Cinacalcet has therefore been licensed for children on dialysis above 3 years of age. According to a recent position statement of the respective European Working groups, the starting dose of cinacalcet should be about 0.2 mg/kg/day based on dry weight [174]. The dose may be increased at 4-week intervals by about 0.2 mg/kg/day to a maximum daily dose of 2.5 mg/kg (and not exceeding 180 mg), based on serum PTH levels and albumin corrected calcium levels >2.2 mmol/L. The cinacalcet dose should be decreased in case of PTH levels between 100 and 150 pg/ml, and lower serum calcium, and withheld if PTH levels fall <100 pg/ml and if albumin-corrected serum calcium levels are <2 mmol/L and/or ionized calcium levels <1.0 mmol/L. About 10–20% of the children on cinacalcet developed episodes of hypocalcemia in clinical trials. A fatality reported together with diarrhea-associated hypocalcemia and long QT time demonstrates the need of careful serum monitoring, i.e. within one week after initiation of cinacalcet and up-titration, and monthly with stable cinacalcet dose. Next to hypocalcemia, the main side effects of cinacalcet are nausea and vomiting, which can be attenuated by evening administration. Prior to start of cinacalcet a normal corrected QT (cQT) time should be verified by ECG. Concomitant medications with the potential to increase the QTc or to interfere with cinacalcet metabolism need to be carefully considered [174]. At present, it is recommended to initiate cinacalcet in children in whom SHPT cannot adequately be controlled with standard of care therapy. Whether cinacalcet is useful earlier in the course of treatment, i.e. to prevent high dose active vit. D analogues is yet unknown. The calcium sensing receptor is expressed on epiphyseal chondrocytes and calcimimetics have been shown to reduce serum testosterone levels in HD patients by 30%. Hence, an impact on longitudinal growth and pubertal development cannot be ruled out. Reassuringly, animal studies and the clinical data obtained thus far do not suggest an impact of cinacalcet on pubertal development and longitudinal growth [174, 175].

Etelcalcetide is a novel calcium receptor sensitizing, calcimimetic compound with a prolonged half-life, administered intravenously. It has been licensed for adult patients on hemodialysis and has the potential to improve treatment adherence since it is administered during hemodialysis sessions. A recent phase 1, single dose clinical trial in 11 children on hemodialysis demonstrated similar pharmacokinetics and pharmacodynamics as in adults [176]. A pediatric single arm study over 6 months is currently under way.

Whether the different pharmacodynamics with three-times-weekly i.v. dosing as compared to daily oral cinacalcet administration is of clinical relevance is currently unclear.

Parathyroidectomy

Despite intensive vitamin D and phosphate binder treatment, some children with CKD may develop refractory hyperparathyroidism, in particular if renal transplantation cannot be performed for an extended period of time. In young adult CKD patients, the incidence of parathyroidectomy is more than 2 per 100 patient years. In our experience the incidence of parathyroidectomy in children has been at least similar to adults. Indications for parathyroidectomy are persistent and recurrent hypercalcemia and hyperphosphatemia despite optimized dietary efforts and medication including cinacalcet, progressive and debilitating bone disease and progressive extraosseus calcifications. Latest findings in adults indicate a more than 50% reduction in the incidence of unremitting hyperparathyroidism and thus the need of parathyroidectomy, possibly related to the use of cinacalcet [177].

Total parathyroidectomy and autotransplantation of tissue fragments in the abdominal subcutaneous layer is preferred to subtotal parathyroidectomy, since the remaining tissue tends to grow again and the transplant is easier to access for diagnostic and curative purposes. Total parathyroidectomy without autotransplantation may result in difficulties to control calcium homeostasis, in particular after kidney transplantation. Ablation of parathyroid tissue by ethanol injection has been suggested as an alternative to surgery; published pediatric experience is limited to a 15 year boy successfully treated 2 months after renal transplantation [178]. Some centers give active vitamin D 72 h prior to surgery to lessen postoperative hypocalcemia; this, however, is not indicated if calcium and phosphate values are markedly increased.

Postoperatively serum ionized calcium needs to be monitored closely, because most of the children develop "hungry bone" syndrome. Due to the rapid decline of PTH, skeletal calcium uptake increases markedly. In most of the children calcium infusions are required within few hours after operation, especially in children with high preoperative PTH and alkaline phosphatase levels. Calcium infusion can be started at a rate of 0.05 mmol/kg*h (2 mg/kg*h) of elemental calcium, but must continuously be adapted according to the changes in serum ionized calcium levels. Calcium infusion is often required for several days, subsequent oral calcium administration for many weeks. In addition, patients should be given high doses of calcitriol (up to 2 µg/d) and dialyzed with a high dialysate calcium concentration. Serum phosphate levels also decline; however, phosphorus supplementation may aggravate hypocalcemia and should only be initiated in case of significant hypophosphatemia.

Success rate is high in children. Parathyroid tissue fragments autotransplanted subcutaneously, usually start to secret PTH soon. Symptomatic hypocalcemia may develop in children not adhering to the medication; irreversible recurrent nerve palsy is rare. PTH and calcium x phosphate product remain within in the target range for many years [179].

Treatment After Renal Transplantation

Children receiving a renal allograft are at risk for multifactorial, progressive bone disease. Persistent hyperparathyroidism, hypophosphatemia and glucocorticoid use require close monitoring of bone metabolism, even if transplant function is normal. Serum calcium, phosphate and bicarbonate should be measured weekly within the first 2 months and at least monthly during the following months. Subsequent determinations also have to be adapted to renal function. PTH should be checked initially and 1 month post transplantation. If plasma PTH remains elevated further controls and therapeutic measures are required. If renal function is reduced, the frequency of determinations should be according to the stage of CKD (Table 60.2) and subsequent treatment strategies follow the guidelines for CKD (Table 60.3). Hypophosphatemia should be corrected. Glucocorticoids should be given at the lowest dose possible and may be withdrawn in patients with stable transplant function. Calcium and active vitamin D therapy lessen glucocorticoid induced bone loss in adults and have been recommended, however no pediatric data have been provided to date. Likewise, next to a case report only one observational study on the off-label use of cinacalcet in 20 children after kidney transplantation has been published [180]. It suggests efficient PTH suppression, and acceptable tolerability despite relatively high cinacalcet doses. The effect of cinacalcet on urine calcium excretion and allograft function is uncertain; some adult studies highlighted the potential risk of nephrocalcinosis. In case cinacalcet is used in children after transplantation, e.g. in order to circumvent parathyroidectomy, careful monitoring is required.

Future Therapeutic Perspectives

Bisphosphonates, selectively blocking osteoclasts and thus bone resorption, appear to be safe at all stages of CKD. Dose reduction is probably required in CKD stage 5, at least based on pharmacokinetic studies. These agents have been recommended for high-risk adult transplant patients on glucocorticoid treatment, although according to a recent meta-analysis the evidence for a reduction in fracture risk and bone pain is low [153]. Important concerns regard their long-lasting action and the risk of hypocalcemia associated with overdosing. Likewise, the effects of bisphosphonates on vascular calcifications need further study, because low bone turnover might exacerbate vascular calcifications. Even if bisphosphonates prove safe, their efficacy in CKD is uncertain. More clinical research data are mandatory before their use in growing children with CKD or glucocorticoid-induced osteoporosis can be considered.

BMP-7 has been used successfully in animal models of renal osteodystrophy and vascular calcification. Human data are currently limited to orthopedic interventions, where it has been employed successfully to induce healing of pathologic fractures. **Blockade of** the Wnt pathway inhibitor **sclerostin** is currently investigated in patients with osteoporosis. Whether sclerostin is a simple marker or an active mediator of bone and cardiovascular disease in CKD and whether sclerostin blockade mitigates these essential comorbidities is currently unknown.

Prognosis

Despite an increasing number of therapeutic options, the management of mineral metabolism remains difficult. More than one third of adults with pediatric-onset CKD have clinical symptoms of bone disease and almost one out of five patients is disabled by bone disease [8]. The CKD-associated alterations of bone mineral metabolism disorders and their treatment during childhood years substantially contribute to the development of uremic arteriopathy, and probably to the excessive cardiovascular mortality in early adult life [10]. Barriers to success are limited patient compliance, the limited efficacy of prescribed measures, the prohibitive costs of novel, more efficacious therapies, and the progressive development of parathyroid autonomy.

Still, there is hope that prevention of mineral dysregulation with early and appropriate use of phosphate binders, prevention of 25(OH)D deficiency, new vitamin D analogues and calcimimetics may reduce the prevalence of mineral disorder and prevent bone disease and vasculopathy in children with CKD. Moreover, the attention to the various clinical practice guidelines available now for pediatric patients with CKD, the establishment of patient registries monitoring achievement of targets and prospective, randomized trials evaluating clinical outcome parameters should result in more favorable long-term outcomes of children with CKD.

References

1. Moe S, Drueke T, Cunningham J, Goodman W, Martin K, Olgaard K, et al. Definition, evaluation, and classification of renal osteodystrophy: a position statement from Kidney Disease: Improving Global Outcomes (KDIGO). Kidney Int. 2006;69(11):1945–53.
2. Levin A, Bakris GL, Molitch M, Smulders M, Tian J, Williams LA, et al. Prevalence of abnormal serum vitamin D, PTH, calcium, and phosphorus in patients with chronic kidney disease: results of the study to evaluate early kidney disease. Kidney Int. 2007;71(1):31–8.
3. Isakova T, Wolf MS. FGF23 or PTH: which comes first in CKD? Kidney Int. 2010;78(10):947–9.
4. Wesseling-Perry K, Pereira RC, Wang H, Elashoff RM, Sahney S, Gales B, et al. Relationship between plasma fibroblast growth factor-23 concentration and bone mineralization in children with renal failure on peritoneal dialysis. J Clin Endocrinol Metab. 2009;94(2):511–7.
5. Ziólkowska H, Pańiczyk-Tomaszewska M, Debiński A, Polowiec Z, Sawicki A, Sieniawska M. Bone biopsy results and serum bone turnover parameters in uremic children. Acta Paediatr. 2000;89(6):666–71.
6. Salusky IB, Ramirez JA, Oppenheim W, Gales B, Segre GV, Goodman WG. Biochemical markers of renal osteodystrophy in pediatric patients undergoing CAPD/CCPD. Kidney Int. 1994;45(1):253–8.
7. Spasovski GB, Bervoets AR, Behets GJ, Ivanovski N, Sikole A, Dams G, et al. Spectrum of renal bone disease in end-stage renal failure patients not yet on dialysis. Nephrol Dial Transplant. 2003;18(6):1159–66.
8. Groothoff JW, Offringa M, Van Eck-Smit BL, Gruppen MP, Van De Kar NJ, Wolff ED, et al. Severe bone disease and low bone mineral density after juvenile renal failure. Kidney Int. 2003;63(1):266–75.
9. Shroff RC, Donald AE, Hiorns MP, Watson A, Feather S, Milford D, et al. Mineral metabolism and vascular damage in children on dialysis. J Am Soc Nephrol. 2007;18(11):2996–3003.
10. Oh J, Wunsch R, Turzer M, Bahner M, Raggi P, Querfeld U, et al. Advanced coronary and carotid arteriopathy in young adults with childhood-onset chronic renal failure. Circulation. 2002;106(1):100–5.
11. Parekh RS, Carroll CE, Wolfe RA, Port FK. Cardiovascular mortality in children and young adults with end-stage kidney disease. J Pediatr. 2002;141(2):191–7.
12. US Renal Data System. USRDS 2002 Annual Data Report: Atlas of End-Stage Renal Disease in the United States, Bethesda, MD, National Institutes of Health, National Institutes of Digestive and Kidney Diseases, 2002. 2007. Ref Type: Generic.

13. Mitsnefes MM, Laskin BL, Dahhou M, Zhang X, Foster BJ. Mortality risk among children initially treated with dialysis for end-stage kidney disease, 1990–2010. JAMA. 2013;309(18):1921–9.

14. Moallem E, Kilav R, Silver J, Naveh-Many T. RNA-Protein binding and post-transcriptional regulation of parathyroid hormone gene expression by calcium and phosphate. J Biol Chem. 1998;273(9):5253–9.

15. McAlister L, Silva S, Shaw V, Shroff R. Dietary calcium intake does not meet the nutritional requirements of children with chronic kidney disease and on dialysis. Pediatr Nephrol. 2020;35(10):1915–23.

16. Iwasaki Y, Yamato H, Nii-Kono T, Fujieda A, Uchida M, Hosokawa A, et al. Insufficiency of PTH action on bone in uremia. Kidney Int Suppl. 2006;102:S34–6.

17. Naveh-Many T, Rahamimov R, Livni N, Silver J. Parathyroid cell proliferation in normal and chronic renal failure rats. The effects of calcium, phosphate, and vitamin D. J Clin Invest. 1995;96(4):1786–93.

18. Li YC, Amling M, Pirro AE, Priemel M, Meuse J, Baron R, et al. Normalization of mineral ion homeostasis by dietary means prevents hyperparathyroidism, rickets, and osteomalacia, but not alopecia in vitamin D receptor-ablated mice. Endocrinology. 1998;139(10):4391–6.

19. Silver J, Moallem E, Kilav R, Sela A, Naveh-Many T. Regulation of the parathyroid hormone gene by calcium, phosphate and 1,25-dihydroxyvitamin D. Nephrol Dial Transplant. 1998;13(Suppl. 1):40–4.

20. Canaff L, Hendy GN. Human calcium-sensing receptor gene. Vitamin D response elements in promoters P1 and P2 confer transcriptional responsiveness to 1,25-dihydroxyvitamin D. J Biol Chem. 2002;277(33):30337–50.

21. Sela-Brown A, Russell J, Koszewski NJ, Michalak M, Naveh-Many T, Silver J. Calreticulin inhibits vitamin D's action on the PTH gene in vitro and may prevent vitamin D's effect in vivo in hypocalcemic rats. Mol Endocrinol. 1998;12(8):1193–200.

22. Juppner H, Wolf M, Salusky IB. FGF-23: More than a regulator of renal phosphate handling? J Bone Miner Res. 2010;25(10):2091–7.

23. Drissi H, Pouliot A, Koolloos C, Stein JL, Lian JB, Stein GS, et al. 1,25-(OH)2-vitamin D3 suppresses the bone-related Runx2/Cbfa1 gene promoter. Exp Cell Res. 2002;274(2):323–33.

24. Virdi AS, Cook LJ, Oreffo RO, Triffitt JT. Modulation of bone morphogenetic protein-2 and bone morphogenetic protein-4 gene expression in osteoblastic cell lines. Cell Mol Biol (Noisy -legrand). 1998;44(8):1237–46.

25. Fraser JD, Otawara Y, Price PA. 1,25-Dihydroxyvitamin D3 stimulates the synthesis of matrix gamma-carboxyglutamic acid protein by osteosarcoma cells. Mutually exclusive expression of vitamin K-dependent bone proteins by clonal osteoblastic cell lines. J Biol Chem. 1988;263(2):911–6.

26. Segersten U, Correa P, Hewison M, Hellman P, Dralle H, Carling T, et al. 25-hydroxyvitamin D(3)-1alpha-hydroxylase expression in normal and pathological parathyroid glands. J Clin Endocrinol Metab. 2002;87(6):2967–72.

27. Somjen D, Weisman Y, Kohen F, Gayer B, Limor R, Sharon O, et al. 25-hydroxyvitamin D3-1alpha-hydroxylase is expressed in human vascular smooth muscle cells and is upregulated by parathyroid hormone and estrogenic compounds. Circulation. 2005;111(13):1666–71.

28. Shroff R, Knott C, Rees L. The virtues of vitamin D--but how much is too much? Pediatr Nephrol. 2010;25(9):1607–20.

29. Shroff R, Wan M, Nagler EV, Bakkaloglu S, Fischer DC, Bishop N, et al. Clinical practice recommendations for native vitamin D therapy in children with chronic kidney disease stages 2–5 and on dialysis. Nephrol Dial Transplant. 2017;32(7):1098–113.

30. Schott GD, Wills MR. Muscle weakness in osteomalacia. Lancet. 1976;1(7960):626–9.

31. Mucsi I, Almasi C, Deak G, Marton A, Ambrus C, Berta K, et al. Serum 25(OH)-vitamin D levels and bone metabolism in patients on maintenance hemodialysis. Clin Nephrol. 2005;64(4):288–94.

32. Shah N, Bernardini J, Piraino B. Prevalence and correction of 25(OH) vitamin D deficiency in peritoneal dialysis patients. Perit Dial Int. 2005;25(4):362–6.

33. Coen G, Mantella D, Manni M, Balducci A, Nofroni I, Sardella D, et al. 25-hydroxyvitamin D levels and bone histomorphometry in hemodialysis renal osteodystrophy. Kidney Int. 2005;68(4):1840–8.

34. Shroff R, Wan M, Gullett A, Ledermann S, Shute R, Knott C, et al. Ergocalciferol supplementation in children with CKD delays the onset of secondary hyperparathyroidism: a randomized trial. Clin J Am Soc Nephrol. 2012;7(2):216–23.

35. Larsson T, Nisbeth U, Ljunggren O, Juppner H, Jonsson KB. Circulating concentration of FGF-23 increases as renal function declines in patients with chronic kidney disease, but does not change in response to variation in phosphate intake in healthy volunteers. Kidney Int. 2003;64(6):2272–9.

36. Shigematsu T, Kazama JJ, Yamashita T, Fukumoto S, Hosoya T, Gejyo F, et al. Possible involvement of circulating fibroblast growth factor 23 in the development of secondary hyperparathyroidism associated with renal insufficiency. Am J Kidney Dis. 2004;44(2):250–6.

37. Holick MF. Vitamin D deficiency. N Engl J Med. 2007;357(3):266–81.

38. Ben-Dov IZ, Galitzer H, Lavi-Moshayoff V, Goetz R, Kuro-o M, Mohammadi M, et al. The parathyroid is a target organ for FGF23 in rats. J Clin Invest. 2007;117(12):4003–8.

39. Wan M, Smith C, Shah V, Gullet A, Wells D, Rees L, et al. Fibroblast growth factor 23 and soluble klotho in children with chronic kidney disease. Nephrol Dial Transplant. 2013;28(1):153–61.

40. Kuro-o M. Overview of the FGF23-Klotho axis. Pediatr Nephrol. 2010;25(4):583–90.

41. Gutierrez OM, Mannstadt M, Isakova T, Rauh-Hain JA, Tamez H, Shah A, et al. Fibroblast growth factor

23 and mortality among patients undergoing hemodialysis. N Engl J Med. 2008;359(6):584–92.

42. Faul C, Amaral AP, Oskouei B, Hu MC, Sloan A, Isakova T, et al. FGF23 induces left ventricular hypertrophy. J Clin Invest. 2011;121(11):4393–408.

43. Gutierrez OM, Januzzi JL, Isakova T, Laliberte K, Smith K, Collerone G, et al. Fibroblast growth factor 23 and left ventricular hypertrophy in chronic kidney disease. Circulation. 2009;119(19):2545–52.

44. David V, Martin A, Isakova T, Spaulding C, Qi L, Ramirez V, et al. Inflammation and functional iron deficiency regulate fibroblast growth factor 23 production. Kidney Int. 2016;89(1):135–46.

45. Coe LM, Madathil SV, Casu C, Lanske B, Rivella S, Sitara D. FGF-23 is a negative regulator of prenatal and postnatal erythropoiesis. J Biol Chem. 2014;289(14):9795–810.

46. Denburg MR, Kalkwarf HJ, de Boer IH, Hewison M, Shults J, Zemel BS, et al. Vitamin D bioavailability and catabolism in pediatric chronic kidney disease. Pediatr Nephrol. 2013;28(9):1843–53.

47. Almaden Y, Canalejo A, Hernandez A, Ballesteros E, Garcia-Navarro S, Torres A, et al. Direct effect of phosphorus on PTH secretion from whole rat parathyroid glands in vitro. J Bone Miner Res. 1996;11(7):970–6.

48. Slatopolsky E, Finch J, Denda M, Ritter C, Zhong M, Dusso A, et al. Phosphorus restriction prevents parathyroid gland growth. High phosphorus directly stimulates PTH secretion in vitro. J Clin Invest. 1996;97(11):2534–40.

49. Borzych D, Rees L, Ha IS, Chua A, Valles PG, Lipka M, et al. The bone and mineral disorder of children undergoing chronic peritoneal dialysis. Kidney Int. 2010;78(12):1295–304.

50. Cozzolino M, Lu Y, Finch J, Slatopolsky E, Dusso AS. p21WAF1 and TGF-alpha mediate parathyroid growth arrest by vitamin D and high calcium. Kidney Int. 2001;60(6):2109–17.

51. Cozzolino M, Lu Y, Sato T, Yang J, Suarez IG, Brancaccio D, et al. A critical role for enhanced TGF-alpha and EGFR expression in the initiation of parathyroid hyperplasia in experimental kidney disease. Am J Physiol Renal Physiol. 2005;289(5):F1096–102.

52. Gogusev J, Duchambon P, Stoermann-Chopard C, Giovannini M, Sarfati E, Drueke TB. De novo expression of transforming growth factor-alpha in parathyroid gland tissue of patients with primary or secondary uraemic hyperparathyroidism. Nephrol Dial Transplant. 1996;11(11):2155–62.

53. Kanesaka Y, Tokunaga H, Iwashita K, Fujimura S, Naomi S, Tomita K. Endothelin receptor antagonist prevents parathyroid cell proliferation of low calcium diet-induced hyperparathyroidism in rats. Endocrinology. 2001;142(1):407–13.

54. Aucella F, Morrone L, Stallone C, Gesualdo L. The genetic background of uremic secondary hyperparathyroidism. J Nephrol. 2005;18(5):537–47.

55. Schmitt CP, Schaefer F. Calcium sensitivity of the parathyroid in renal failure: another look with new methodology. Nephrol Dial Transplant. 1999;14(12):2815–8.

56. Schmitt CP, Huber D, Mehls O, Maiwald J, Stein G, Veldhuis JD, et al. Altered instantaneous and calcium-modulated oscillatory PTH secretion patterns in patients with secondary hyperparathyroidism. J Am Soc Nephrol. 1998;9(10):1832–44.

57. Zhang P, Duchambon P, Gogusev J, Nabarra B, Sarfati E, Bourdeau A, et al. Apoptosis in parathyroid hyperplasia of patients with primary or secondary uremic hyperparathyroidism. Kidney Int. 2000;57(2):437–45.

58. Bonarek H, Merville P, Bonarek M, Moreau K, Morel D, Aparicio M, et al. Reduced parathyroid functional mass after successful kidney transplantation. Kidney Int. 1999;56(2):642–9.

59. Lepage R, Roy L, Brossard JH, Rousseau L, Dorais C, Lazure C, et al. A non-(1-84) circulating parathyroid hormone (PTH) fragment interferes significantly with intact PTH commercial assay measurements in uremic samples. Clin Chem. 1998;44(4):805–9.

60. Slatopolsky E, Finch J, Clay P, Martin D, Sicard G, Singer G, et al. A novel mechanism for skeletal resistance in uremia. Kidney Int. 2000;58(2):753–61.

61. Waller S, Ridout D, Cantor T, Rees L. Differences between "intact" PTH and 1-84 PTH assays in chronic renal failure and dialysis. Pediatr Nephrol. 2005;20(2):197–9.

62. Divieti P, Geller AI, Suliman G, Juppner H, Bringhurst FR. Receptors specific for the carboxyl-terminal region of parathyroid hormone on bone-derived cells: determinants of ligand binding and bioactivity. Endocrinology. 2005;146(4):1863–70.

63. Hocher B, Oberthur D, Slowinski T, Querfeld U, Schaefer F, Doyon A, et al. Modeling of oxidized PTH (oxPTH) and non-oxidized PTH (n-oxPTH) receptor binding and relationship of oxidized to non-oxidized PTH in children with chronic renal failure, adult patients on hemodialysis and kidney transplant recipients. Kidney Blood Press Res. 2013;37(4–5):240–51.

64. Ursem SR, Heijboer AC, D'Haese PC, Behets GJ, Cavalier E, Vervloet MG, Evenepoel P. Non-oxidized parathyroid hormone (PTH) measured by current method is not superior to total PTH in assessing bone turnover in chronic kidney disease. Kidney Int. 2021;99(5):1173–8.

65. Cochran M, Wilkinson R. Effect of correction of metabolic acidosis on bone mineralisation rates in patients with renal osteomalacia. Nephron. 1975;15(2):98–110.

66. Disthabanchong S, Martin KJ, McConkey CL, Gonzalez EA. Metabolic acidosis up-regulates PTH/PTHrP receptors in UMR 106-01 osteoblast-like cells. Kidney Int. 2002;62(4):1171–7.

67. Davies MR, Lund RJ, Mathew S, Hruska KA. Low turnover osteodystrophy and vascular calcification are amenable to skeletal anabolism in an animal

model of chronic kidney disease and the metabolic syndrome. J Am Soc Nephrol. 2005;16(4):917–28.

68. Davies MR, Lund RJ, Hruska KA. BMP-7 is an efficacious treatment of vascular calcification in a murine model of atherosclerosis and chronic renal failure. J Am Soc Nephrol. 2003;14(6):1559–67.

69. Freedman BI, Bowden DW, Ziegler JT, Langefeld CD, Lehtinen AB, Rudock ME, et al. Bone morphogenetic protein 7 (BMP7) gene polymorphisms are associated with inverse relationships between vascular calcification and BMD: the Diabetes Heart Study. J Bone Miner Res. 2009;24(10):1719–27.

70. Ozkok A, Caliskan Y, Sakaci T, Erten G, Karahan G, Ozel A, et al. Osteoprotegerin/RANKL axis and progression of coronary artery calcification in hemodialysis patients. Clin J Am Soc Nephrol. 2012;7(6):965–73.

71. Schoppet M, Shroff RC, Hofbauer LC, Shanahan CM. Exploring the biology of vascular calcification in chronic kidney disease: what's circulating? Kidney Int. 2008;73(4):384–90.

72. Wei T, Wang M, Wang M, Gan LY, Li X. Relationship of sRANKL level and vascular calcification score to cardiovascular events in maintenance hemodialysis patients. Blood Purif. 2009;28(4):342–5.

73. Huang QX, Li JB, Huang N, Huang XW, Li YL, Huang FX. Elevated osteoprotegerin concentration predicts increased risk of cardiovascular mortality in patients with chronic kidney disease: a systematic review and meta-Analysis. Kidney Blood Press Res. 2020;45(4):565–75.

74. Broadwell A, Chines A, Ebeling PR, Franek E, Huang S, Smith S, et al. Denosumab safety and efficacy among subjects in the FREEDOM extension study with mild-to-moderate chronic kidney disease. J Clin Endocrinol Metab. 2020; dgaa851. Online ahead of print

75. Cejka D, Herberth J, Branscum AJ, Fardo DW, Monier-Faugere MC, Diarra D, et al. Sclerostin and Dickkopf-1 in renal osteodystrophy. Clin J Am Soc Nephrol. 2011;6(4):877–82.

76. Viaene L, Behets GJ, Claes K, Meijers B, Blocki F, Brandenburg V, et al. Sclerostin: another bone-related protein related to all-cause mortality in haemodialysis? Nephrol Dial Transplant. 2013;28(12):3024–30.

77. Sabbagh Y, Graciolli FG, O'Brien S, Tang W, Dos Reis LM, Ryan S, et al. Repression of osteocyte Wnt/beta-catenin signaling is an early event in the progression of renal osteodystrophy. J Bone Miner Res. 2012;27(8):1757–72.

78. Hruska KA, Mahjoub MR. New pathogenic insights inform therapeutic target development for renal osteodystrophy. Kidney Int. 2019;95(2):261–3.

79. Bacchetta J, Farlay D, Abelin-Genevois K, Lebourg L, Cochat P, Boivin G. Bone impairment in oxalosis: an ultrastructural bone analysis. Bone. 2015;81:161–7.

80. Claramunt-Taberner D, Flammier S, Gaillard S, Cochat P, Peyruchaud O, Machuca-Gayet I, et al. Bone disease in nephropathic cystinosis is related to cystinosin-induced osteoclastic dysfunction. Nephrol Dial Transplant. 2018;33(9):1525–32.

81. Langman CB. Genetic regulation of bone mass: from bone density to bone strength. Pediatr Nephrol. 2005;20(3):352–5.

82. Baxter-Jones AD, Faulkner RA, Forwood MR, Mirwald RL, Bailey DA. Bone mineral accrual from 8 to 30 years of age: an estimation of peak bone mass. J Bone Miner Res. 2011;26(8):1729–39.

83. Aksnes L, Aarskog D. Plasma concentrations of vitamin D metabolites in puberty: effect of sexual maturation and implications for growth. J Clin Endocrinol Metab. 1982;55(1):94–101.

84. Matkovic V, Heaney RP. Calcium balance during human growth: evidence for threshold behavior. Am J Clin Nutr. 1992;55(5):992–6.

85. Malluche HH, Mawad HW, Monier-Faugere MC. Renal osteodystrophy in the first decade of the new millennium: analysis of 630 bone biopsies in black and white patients. J Bone Miner Res. 2011;26(6):1368–76.

86. Jonsson KB, Zahradnik R, Larsson T, White KE, Sugimoto T, Imanishi Y, et al. Fibroblast growth factor 23 in oncogenic osteomalacia and X-linked hypophosphatemia. N Engl J Med. 2003;348(17):1656–63.

87. Shimada T, Kakitani M, Yamazaki Y, Hasegawa H, Takeuchi Y, Fujita T, et al. Targeted ablation of Fgf23 demonstrates an essential physiological role of FGF23 in phosphate and vitamin D metabolism. J Clin Invest. 2004;113(4):561–8.

88. Lalayiannis AD, Crabtree NJ, Ferro CJ, Askiti V, Mitsioni A, Biassoni L, et al. Routine serum biomarkers, but not dual-energy X-ray absorptiometry, correlate with cortical bone mineral density in children and young adults with chronic kidney disease. Nephrol Dial Transplant. 2020; ahead of print

89. Denburg MR, Tsampalieros AK, de Boer IH, Shults J, Kalkwarf HJ, Zemel BS, et al. Mineral metabolism and cortical volumetric bone mineral density in childhood chronic kidney disease. J Clin Endocrinol Metab. 2013;98(5):1930–8.

90. Bacchetta J, Harambat J, Cochat P, Salusky IB, Wesseling-Perry K. The consequences of chronic kidney disease on bone metabolism and growth in children. Nephrol Dial Transplant. 2012;27(8):3063–71.

91. Kuizon BD, Salusky IB. Growth retardation in children with chronic renal failure. J Bone Miner Res. 1999;14(10):1680–90.

92. Marrades RM, Roca J, Campistol JM, Diaz O, Barbera JA, Torregrosa JV, et al. Effects of erythropoietin on muscle O2 transport during exercise in patients with chronic renal failure. J Clin Invest. 1996;97(9):2092–100.

93. Alayli G, Ozkaya O, Bek K, Calmasur A, Diren B, Bek Y, et al. Physical function, muscle strength and muscle mass in children on peritoneal dialysis. Pediatr Nephrol. 2008;23(4):639–44.

94. Sala E, Noyszewski EA, Campistol JM, Marrades RM, Dreha S, Torregrossa JV, et al. Impaired muscle oxygen transfer in patients with chronic renal failure. Am J Physiol Regul Integr Comp Physiol. 2001;280(4):R1240–8.

95. Helenius I, Remes V, Salminen S, Valta H, Makitie O, Holmberg C, et al. Incidence and predictors of fractures in children after solid organ transplantation: a 5-year prospective, population-based study. J Bone Miner Res. 2006;21(3):380–7.

96. Tsampalieros A, Kalkwarf HJ, Wetzsteon RJ, Shults J, Zemel BS, Foster BJ, et al. Changes in bone structure and the muscle-bone unit in children with chronic kidney disease. Kidney Int. 2013;83(3):495–502.

97. Parfitt AM. Renal bone disease: a new conceptual framework for the interpretation of bone histomorphometry. Curr Opin Nephrol Hypertens. 2003;12(4):387–403.

98. Denburg MR, Kumar J, Jemielita T, Brooks ER, Skversky A, Portale AA, Salusky IB, Warady BA, Furth SL, Leonard MB. Fracture burden and risk factors in childhood CKD: results from the CKiD Cohort Study. J Am Soc Nephrol. 2016;27(2):543–50.

99. Danese MD, Kim J, Doan QV, Dylan M, Griffiths R, Chertow GM. PTH and the risks for hip, vertebral, and pelvic fractures among patients on dialysis. Am J Kidney Dis. 2006;47(1):149–56.

100. Chesney RW, Moorthy AV, Eisman JA, Jax DK, Mazess RB, Deluca HF. Increased growth after long-term oral 1alpha,25-vitamin D3 in childhood renal osteodystrophy. N Engl J Med. 1978;298(5):238–42.

101. Klaus G, Weber L, Rodriguez J, Fernandez P, Klein T, Grulich-Henn J, et al. Interaction of IGF-I and 1 alpha, 25(OH)2D3 on receptor expression and growth stimulation in rat growth plate chondrocytes. Kidney Int. 1998;53(5):1152–61.

102. Vortkamp A, Lee K, Lanske B, Segre GV, Kronenberg HM, Tabin CJ. Regulation of rate of cartilage differentiation by Indian hedgehog and PTH-related protein. Science. 1996;273(5275):613–22.

103. Schmitt CP, Hessing S, Oh J, Weber L, Ochlich P, Mehls O. Intermittent administration of parathyroid hormone (1-37) improves growth and bone mineral density in uremic rats. Kidney Int. 2000;57(4):1484–92.

104. Schmitt CP, Ardissino G, Testa S, Claris-Appiani A, Mehls O. Growth in children with chronic renal failure on intermittent versus daily calcitriol. Pediatr Nephrol. 2003;18(5):440–4.

105. Cansick J, Waller S, Ridout D, Rees L. Growth and PTH in prepubertal children on long-term dialysis. Pediatr Nephrol. 2007;22(9):1349–54.

106. Waller S, Reynolds A, Ridout D, Cantor T, Gao P, Rees L. Parathyroid hormone and its fragments in children with chronic renal failure. Pediatr Nephrol. 2003;18(12):1242–8.

107. Goodman WG, Goldin J, Kuizon BD, Yoon C, Gales B, Sider D, et al. Coronary-artery calcification in young adults with end-stage renal disease who are undergoing dialysis. N Engl J Med. 2000;342(20):1478–83.

108. Litwin M, Wuhl E, Jourdan C, Trelewicz J, Niemirska A, Fahr K, et al. Altered morphologic properties of large arteries in children with chronic renal failure and after renal transplantation. J Am Soc Nephrol. 2005;16(5):1494–500.

109. Milliner DS, Zinsmeister AR, Lieberman E, Landing B. Soft tissue calcification in pediatric patients with end-stage renal disease. Kidney Int. 1990;38(5):931–6.

110. Shroff R, Egerton M, Bridel M, Shah V, Donald AE, Cole TJ, et al. A bimodal association of vitamin D levels and vascular disease in children on dialysis. J Am Soc Nephrol. 2008;19(6):1239–46.

111. Ketteler M, Bongartz P, Westenfeld R, Wildberger JE, Mahnken AH, Bohm R, et al. Association of low fetuin-A (AHSG) concentrations in serum with cardiovascular mortality in patients on dialysis: a cross-sectional study. Lancet. 2003;361(9360):827–33.

112. Shroff RC, Shah V, Hiorns MP, Schoppet M, Hofbauer LC, Hawa G, et al. The circulating calcification inhibitors, fetuin-A and osteoprotegerin, but not Matrix Gla protein, are associated with vascular stiffness and calcification in children on dialysis. Nephrol Dial Transplant. 2008;

113. Brandenburg VM, Sinha S, Specht P, Ketteler M. Calcific uraemic arteriolopathy: a rare disease with a potentially high impact on chronic kidney disease-mineral and bone disorder. Pediatr Nephrol. 2014;

114. Tsampalieros A, Griffin L, Terpstra AM, Kalkwarf HJ, Shults J, Foster BJ, et al. Changes in DXA and quantitative CT measures of musculoskeletal outcomes following pediatric renal transplantation. Am J Transplant. 2014;14(1):124–32.

115. Sanchez CP, Salusky IB, Kuizon BD, Ramirez JA, Gales B, Ettenger RB, et al. Bone disease in children and adolescents undergoing successful renal transplantation. Kidney Int. 1998;53(5):1358–64.

116. Bhan I, Shah A, Holmes J, Isakova T, Gutierrez O, Burnett SM, et al. Post-transplant hypophosphatemia: tertiary 'Hyper-Phosphatoninism'? Kidney Int. 2006;70(8):1486–94.

117. Cruz EA, Lugon JR, Jorgetti V, Draibe SA, Carvalho AB. Histologic evolution of bone disease 6 months after successful kidney transplantation. Am J Kidney Dis. 2004;44(4):747–56.

118. Monier-Faugere MC, Mawad H, Qi Q, Friedler RM, Malluche HH. High prevalence of low bone turnover and occurrence of osteomalacia after kidney transplantation. J Am Soc Nephrol. 2000;11(6):1093–9.

119. Ruth EM, Weber LT, Schoenau E, Wunsch R, Seibel MJ, Feneberg R, et al. Analysis of the functional muscle-bone unit of the forearm in pediatric renal transplant recipients. Kidney Int. 2004;66(4):1694–706.

120. Helenius I, Jalanko H, Remes V, Tervahartiala P, Salminen S, Sairanen H, et al. Avascular bone necrosis of the hip joint after solid organ transplan-

tation in childhood: a clinical and MRI analysis. Transplantation. 2006;81(12):1621–7.

121. Bakkaloglu SA, Bacchetta J, Lalayiannis AD, Leifheit-Nestler M, Stabouli S, Haarhaus M, et al. Bone evaluation in paediatric chronic kidney disease: clinical practice points from the European Society for Paediatric Nephrology CKD-MBD and Dialysis working groups and CKD-MBD working group of the ERA-EDTA. Nephrol Dial Transplant. 2021;36(3):413–25.

122. Bakkaloglu SA, Wesseling-Perry K, Pereira RC, Gales B, Wang HJ, Elashoff RM, et al. Value of the new bone classification system in pediatric renal osteodystrophy. Clin J Am Soc Nephrol. 2010;5(10):1860–6.

123. Ketteler M, Block GA, Evenepoel P, Fukagawa M, Herzog CA, McCann L, et al. Executive summary of the 2017 KDIGO Chronic Kidney Disease-Mineral and Bone Disorder (CKD-MBD) Guideline Update: what's changed and why it matters. Kidney Int. 2017;92(1):26–36.

124. Geary DF, Hodson EM, Craig JC. Interventions for bone disease in children with chronic kidney disease. Cochrane Database Syst Rev. 2010;(1):CD008327.

125. NICE clinical guideline 157. www.nice.org.uk/guidance/CG157 2013.

126. Dasgupta I, Shroff R, nett-Jones D, McVeigh G. Management of hyperphosphataemia in chronic kidney disease: summary of National Institute for Health and Clinical Excellence (NICE) guideline. Nephron Clin Pract. 2013;124(1–2):1–9.

127. Salusky IB, Kuizon BD, Belin TR, Ramirez JA, Gales B, Segre GV, et al. Intermittent calcitriol therapy in secondary hyperparathyroidism: a comparison between oral and intraperitoneal administration. Kidney Int. 1998;54(3):907–14.

128. Massry SG, Coburn JW, Chertow GM, Hruska K, Langman C, Malluche H, Martin K, McCann LM, McCarthy JT, Moe S, Salusky IB. K/DOQI clinical practice guidelines for bone metabolism and disease in chronic kidney disease. Am J Kidney Dis. 2003;42(4 Suppl. 3):S1–201.

129. Markowitz ME, Rosen JF, Laxminarayan S, Mizruchi M. Circadian rhythms of blood minerals during adolescence. Pediatr Res. 1984;18(5):456–62.

130. Trivedi H, Moore H, Atalla J. Lack of significant circadian and post-prandial variation in phosphate levels in subjects receiving chronic hemodialysis therapy. J Nephrol. 2005;18(4):417–22.

131. Urena P, Hruby M, Ferreira A, Ang KS, de Vernejoul MC. Plasma total versus bone alkaline phosphatase as markers of bone turnover in hemodialysis patients. J Am Soc Nephrol. 1996;7(3):506–12.

132. Schonau E. The peak bone mass concept: is it still relevant? Pediatr Nephrol. 2004;19(8):825–31.

133. London GM, Guerin AP, Marchais SJ, Metivier F, Pannier B, Adda H. Arterial media calcification in end-stage renal disease: impact on all-cause and cardiovascular mortality. Nephrol Dial Transplant. 2003;18(9):1731–40.

134. Klaus G, Watson A, Edefonti A, Fischbach M, Ronnholm K, Schaefer F, et al. Prevention and treatment of renal osteodystrophy in children on chronic renal failure: European guidelines. Pediatr Nephrol. 2006;21(2):151–9.

135. Waller S, Ledermann S, Trompeter R, van't Hoff W, Ridout D, Rees L. Catch-up growth with normal parathyroid hormone levels in chronic renal failure. Pediatr Nephrol. 2003;18(12):1236–41.

136. McAlister L, Pugh P, Greenbaum L, Haffner D, Rees L, Anderson C, et al. The dietary management of calcium and phosphate in children with CKD stages 2-5 and on dialysis-clinical practice recommendation from the Pediatric Renal Nutrition Taskforce. Pediatr Nephrol. 2020;35(3):501–18.

137. Initiative NKFDOQ. KDOQI clinical practice guideline for nutrition in children with CKD: 2008 update. Executive summary. Am J Kidney Dis. 2009;53:S11–S104. https://www.kidney.org/sites/default/files/docs/cpgpednutr2008.pdf

138. Schmitt CP, Borzych D, Nau B, Wühl E, Zurowska A, Schaefer F. Dialytic phosphate removal: a modifiable measure of dialysis efficacy in automated peritoneal dialysis. Perit Dial Int. 2009;29(4):465–71.

139. Fischbach M, Terzic J, Menouer S, Dheu C, Seuge L, Zalosczic A. Daily on line haemodiafiltration promotes catch-up growth in children in chronic dialysis. Nephrol Dial Transplant 2009.; epub ahead of print.

140. Thumfart J, Puttkamer CV, Wagner S, Querfeld U, Muller D. Hemodiafiltration in a pediatric nocturnal dialysis program. Pediatr Nephrol. 2014;29(8):1411–6.

141. Geary DF, Piva E, Tyrrell J, Gajaria MJ, Picone G, Keating LE, et al. Home nocturnal hemodialysis in children. J Pediatr. 2005;147(3):383–7.

142. Hothi DK, Harvey E, Piva E, Keating L, Secker D, Geary DF. Calcium and phosphate balance in adolescents on home nocturnal haemodialysis. Pediatr Nephrol. 2006;21(6):835–41.

143. Shroff R, Smith C, Ranchin B, Bayazit AK, Stefanidis CJ, Askiti V, et al. Effects of hemodiafiltration versus conventional hemodialysis in children with ESKD: the HDF, heart and height study. J Am Soc Nephrol. 2019;30(4):678–91.

144. Perouse de MT, Ranchin B, Leclerc AL, Bertholet-Thomas A, Belot A, Cochat P, et al. Online hemodiafiltration in children and hypoparathyroidism: a single-centre series of cases. Nephrol Ther. 2014;10:35–8.

145. Pieper AK, Haffner D, Hoppe B, Dittrich K, Offner G, Bonzel KE, et al. A randomized crossover trial comparing sevelamer with calcium acetate in children with CKD. Am J Kidney Dis. 2006;47(4):625–35.

146. Wei M, Esbaei K, Bargman J, Oreopoulos DG. Relationship between serum magnesium, parathyroid hormone, and vascular calcification in patients on dialysis: a literature review. Perit Dial Int. 2006;26(3):366–73.

147. Vervloet M. Modifying phosphate toxicity in chronic kidney disease. Toxins (Basel). 2019;11(9):522.

148. Gonzalez E, Schomberg J, Amin N, Salusky IB, Zaritsky J. Sevelamer carbonate increases serum bicarbonate in pediatric dialysis patients. Pediatr Nephrol. 2010;25(2):373–5.

149. Yokoyama K, Hirakata H, Akiba T, Fukagawa M, Nakayama M, Sawada K, et al. Ferric citrate hydrate for the treatment of hyperphosphatemia in nondialysis-dependent CKD. Clin J Am Soc Nephrol. 2014;9(3):543–52.

150. Floege J, Covic AC, Ketteler M, Rastogi A, Chong EM, Gaillard S, et al. A phase III study of the efficacy and safety of a novel iron-based phosphate binder in dialysis patients. Kidney Int. 2014;

151. Greenbaum LA, Jeck N, Klaus G, Fila M, Stoica C, Fathallah-Shaykh S, et al. Safety and efficacy of sucroferric oxyhydroxide in pediatric patients with chronic kidney disease. Pediatr Nephrol. 2020; ahead of print

152. Bostom AG. New evidence for the phosphorus-lowering effects of niacin. Am J Kidney Dis. 2010;56(1):185.

153. Palmer SC, Chung EYM, McGregor DO, Bachmann F, Strippoli G. Interventions for preventing bone disease in kidney transplant recipients. Rev Cochrane Database Syst Rev. 2019;10(10):CD005015.

154. Savica V, Calo LA, Monardo P, Davis PA, Granata A, Santoro D, et al. Salivary phosphate-binding chewing gum reduces hyperphosphatemia in dialysis patients. J Am Soc Nephrol. 2009;20(3):639–44.

155. Block GA, Wheeler DC, Persky MS, Kestenbaum B, Ketteler M, Spiegel DM, et al. Effects of phosphate binders in moderate CKD. J Am Soc Nephrol. 2012;23(8):1407–15.

156. Russo D, Miranda I, Ruocco C, Battaglia Y, Buonanno E, Manzi S, et al. The progression of coronary artery calcification in predialysis patients on calcium carbonate or sevelamer. Kidney Int. 2007;72(10):1255–61.

157. Di IB, Bellasi A, Russo D. Mortality in kidney disease patients treated with phosphate binders: a randomized study. Clin J Am Soc Nephrol. 2012;7(3):487–93.

158. Di IB, Molony D, Bell C, Cucciniello E, Bellizzi V, Russo D, et al. Sevelamer versus calcium carbonate in incident hemodialysis patients: results of an open-label 24-month randomized clinical trial. Am J Kidney Dis. 2013;62(4):771–8.

159. Ruospo M, Palmer SC, Natale P, Craig JC, Vecchio M, Elder GJ, Strippoli GF. Phosphate binders for preventing and treating chronic kidney disease-mineral and bone disorder (CKD-MBD). Cochrane Database Syst Rev. 2018;8(8):CD006023.

160. Iyengar A, Kamath N, Reddy HV, Sharma J, Singhal J, Uthup S, et al. Determining the optimal cholecalciferol dosing regimen in children with CKD: a randomized controlled trial. Nephrol Dial Transplant. 2020; Epub ahead of print

161. Shroff R, Wan M, Nagler EV, Bakkaloglu S, Cozzolino M, Bacchetta J, et al. Clinical practice recommendations for treatment with active vitamin D analogues in children with chronic kidney disease stages 2-5 and on dialysis. Nephrol Dial Transplant. 2017;32(7):1114–27.

162. Brickman AS, Coburn JW, Friedman GR, Okamura WH, Massry SG, Norman AW. Comparison of effects of 1 alpha-hydroxy-vitamin D3 and 1,25-dihydroxy-vitamin D3 in man. J Clin Invest. 1976;57(6):1540–7.

163. Ramirez JA, Emmett M, White MG, Fathi N, Santa Ana CA, Morawski SG, Fordtran JS. The absorption of dietary phosphorus and calcium in hemodialysis patients. Kidney Int. 1986;30(5):753–9.

164. Palmer SC, McGregor DO, Craig JC, Elder G, Macaskill P, Strippoli GF. Vitamin D compounds for people with chronic kidney disease not requiring dialysis. Cochrane Database Syst Rev. 2009;(4):CD008175.

165. Wang AY, Fang F, Chan J, Wen YY, Qing S, Chan IH, et al. Effect of paricalcitol on left ventricular mass and function in CKD--the OPERA trial. J Am Soc Nephrol. 2014;25(1):175–86.

166. Thadhani R, Appelbaum E, Pritchett Y, Chang Y, Wenger J, Tamez H, et al. Vitamin D therapy and cardiac structure and function in patients with chronic kidney disease: the PRIMO randomized controlled trial. JAMA. 2012;307(7):674–84.

167. Ardissino G, Schmitt CP, Testa S, Claris-Appiani A, Mehls O. Calcitriol pulse therapy is not more effective than daily calcitriol therapy in controlling secondary hyperparathyroidism in children with chronic renal failure. European Study Group on Vitamin D in Children with Renal Failure. Pediatr Nephrol. 2000;14(7):664–8.

168. Ardissino G, Schmitt CP, Bianchi ML, Dacco V, Claris-Appiani A, Mehls O. No difference in intestinal strontium absorption after oral or IV calcitriol in children with secondary hyperparathyroidism. The European Study Group on Vitamin D in Children with Renal Failure. Kidney Int. 2000;58(3):981–8.

169. Webb NJA, Lerner G, Warady BA, Dell KM, Greenbaum LA, Ariceta G, Hoppe B, Linde P, Lee HJ, Eldred A, Dufek MB. Efficacy and safety of paricalcitol in children with stages 3 to 5 chronic kidney disease. Pediatr Nephrol. 2017;32(7):1221–32.

170. Greenbaum LA, Benador N, Goldstein SL, Paredes A, Melnick JZ, Mattingly S, et al. Intravenous paricalcitol for treatment of secondary hyperparathyroidism in children on hemodialysis. Am J Kidney Dis. 2007;49(6):814–23.

171. Raggi P, Chertow GM, Torres PU, Csiky B, Naso A, Nossuli K, et al. The ADVANCE study: a randomized study to evaluate the effects of cinacalcet plus low-dose vitamin D on vascular calcification in patients on hemodialysis. Nephrol Dial Transplant. 2011;26(4):1327–39.

172. Chertow GM, Block GA, Correa-Rotter R, Drueke TB, Floege J, Goodman WG, et al. Effect of cinacalcet on cardiovascular disease in patients undergoing dialysis. N Engl J Med. 2012;367(26):2482–94.

173. Warady BA, Ng E, Bloss L, Mo M, Schaefer F, Bacchetta J. Cinacalcet studies in pediatric subjects with secondary hyperparathyroidism receiving dialysis. Pediatr Nephrol. 2020;35(9):1679–97.

174. Bacchetta J, Schmitt CP, Ariceta G, Bakkaloglu SA, Groothoff J, Wan M, et al. Cinacalcet use in paediatric dialysis: a position statement from the European Society for Paediatric Nephrology and the Chronic Kidney Disease-Mineral and Bone Disorders Working Group of the ERA-EDTA. Nephrol Dial Transplant. 2020;35(1):47–64.

175. Nakagawa K, Pérez EC, Oh J, Santos F, Geldyyev A, Gross ML, Schaefer F, Schmitt CP. Cinacalcet does not affect longitudinal growth but increases body weight gain in experimental uraemia. Nephrol Dial Transplant. 2008;23(9):2761–7.

176. Sohn W, Salusky IB, Schmitt CP, Taylan C, Walle JV, Ngang J, et al. Phase 1, single-dose study to assess the safety, tolerability, pharmacokinetics, and pharmacodynamics of etelcalcetide in pediatric patients with secondary hyperparathyroidism receiving hemodialysis. Pediatr Nephrol. 2021;36(1):133–42.

177. Parfrey PS, Chertow GM, Block GA, Correa-Rotter R, Drueke TB, Floege J, et al. The clinical course of treated hyperparathyroidism among patients receiving hemodialysis and the effect of cinacalcet: the EVOLVE trial. J Clin Endocrinol Metab. 2013;98(12):4834–44.

178. Ohta T, Sakano T, Fuchinoue S, Tsuji T, Tanabe K, Hattori M, et al. A case of post-transplant hyperparathyroidism treated with ethanol injection. Pediatr Nephrol. 2002;17(4):236–8.

179. Schaefer B, Schlosser K, Wuhl E, Schall P, Klaus G, Schaefer F, et al. Long-term control of parathyroid hormone and calcium-phosphate metabolism after parathyroidectomy in children with chronic kidney disease. Nephrol Dial Transplant. 2010;25(8):2590–5.

180. Bernardor J, Schmitt CP, Oh J, Sellier-Leclerc AL, Büscher A, Dello Strologo L, et al. The use of cinacalcet after pediatric renal transplantation: an international CERTAIN Registry analysis. Pediatr Nephrol. 2020;35(9):1707–18.

Cardiovascular Disease in Pediatric Chronic Kidney Disease

61

Anke Doyon and Mark Mitsnefes

Epidemiology

Cardiovascular Mortality: Leading Cause of Death in Children with CKD

In 1998, the National Kidney Foundation Task Force on cardiovascular disease (CVD) declared an epidemic of cardiac disease in end-stage kidney disease (ESKD) patients [1]. This report however provided no information on CVD in children. Over the next two decades, there have been important studies around the world addressing CVD in children with ESKD.

In 2002, as a follow up on a Task Force, Parekh et al. [2], using the United States Renal Data System (USRDS) database, performed the first analysis to evaluate the risk of a cardiac death in children and young adults (age 0–30 years) and to identify factors potentially associated with CVD mortality. A total of 1380

deaths between 1990 and 1996 were analyzed. There were 311 cardiac deaths (23% of the total). These data were in great contrast to the general pediatric population where CVD mortality was low and accounted for less than 3% of all causes of death [3]. The analysis also showed that the rates of cardiac deaths in this age group were approximately 1000 times higher than in the general pediatric population. Subsequent reports from international registries over the next few years have confirmed that CVD is the leading cause of death in children with ESKD and in adults with childhood onset of CKD. The Australia and New Zealand Dialysis and Transplant (ANZDATA) [4], Dutch national cohort study (LERIC) [5] and a large German study [6] report that 40–50% of all deaths are from cardiovascular or cerebrovascular causes. Cross-sectional studies of young adults with childhood-onset ESKD have found a cardiac death rate of 35% in U.S. children transplanted at age 0–19 years [7]; 23% in 150 German patients transplanted as children between 1970 and 1993 (almost ten times higher than the occurrence of malignancies [8]), and 32% in another series of dialyzed or transplanted young adults from Germany [9].

Foster et al. analyzed the long-term survival of 18,911 patients who received a first kidney transplant during childhood (at <21 years old, 1983–2006) and confirmed that the majority of deaths

A. Doyon
Division of Pediatric Nephrology, Center for Pediatric and Adolescent Medicine, Heidelberg, Germany
e-mail: anke.doyon@med.uni-heidelberg.de

M. Mitsnefes (✉)
Division of Nephrology and Hypertension, Cincinnati Children's Hospital Medical Center, Cincinnati, OH, USA
e-mail: mark.mitsnefes@cchmc.org

F. Schaefer, L. A. Greenbaum (eds.), *Pediatric Kidney Disease*,
https://doi.org/10.1007/978-3-031-11665-0_61

were from cardiovascular causes especially after graft failure (45%) versus those with a functioning graft (25%) [10]. The hazard ratios (HR) for cardiovascular mortality associated with dialysis after graft failure was 7.8 as compared to those with functioning graft. As other studies, this study also observed an improvement in cardiovascular mortality in transplant recipients. However, even in these patients, the mortality rates were still significantly higher (approximately 10 times) than in the general pediatric population. Mitsnefes et al. [11] analyzed data from more than 20,000 pediatric ESKD patients followed over two decades, with follow-up to 2010. The authors demonstrated that mortality rates for children and adolescents being treated with dialysis have improved dramatically between 1990 and 2010.

While most published studies analyzing mortality in young adults have focused on patients who developed ESKD during childhood, there have been very few studies examining cardiovascular morbidity and mortality specifically in patients who developed ESKD during young adulthood (21–29 years). Using USRDS data collected in 2003–2013, Modi et al. [12] showed that the risk for cardiovascular mortality in these young adults was 143–500 times higher compared to age-matched young adults in the general population. During the study follow-up period, 16.2% of the cohort died, and CVD accounted for 38% of all deaths. The risk of death among those with onset of disease during young adulthood was similar to that of young adults with childhood-onset ESKD (1–11 years or 12–21 years). Presence of diabetes, coronary artery disease, and heart failure were notable risk factors for cardiovascular-related mortality.

Modi et al. also compared the risk of cardiovascular-related hospitalizations. Not surprisingly, the rates of cardiovascular hospitalization during the five-year follow-up period were highest for those 22–29 years and lowest for those 1–11 years, with risk remaining stable in children but increasing over time in the adolescent group until reaching the hospitalization rate of young adults. As expected, patients receiving hemodialysis and peritoneal dialysis were at higher risk for cardiovascular-related hospitalizations compared to patients receiving preemptive transplantation.

Ku et al. [13] compared trends over time in mortality from CVD-related causes of death among more than 80,000 children and young adults <30 years of age starting dialysis in 1995–2015. Overall, 40% of deaths were cardiovascular-related causes. The risk of cardiovascular-related death was stable initially, began improving after the early 2000s, and became significantly lower after 2006 in those starting dialysis as either children or young adults (Fig. 61.1).

Taken together, these data show that despite significant improvement in patient survival, mostly due to decrease in cardiovascular (especially in those after kidney transplantation) and infectious disease mortality, CVD remains the world-wide biggest obstacle to long-term survival of children and adolescents with ESKD, especially those on maintenance dialysis [14] (Fig. 61.2). Not surprisingly, the American Heart Association guidelines for cardiovascular risk reduction in high-risk pediatric patients continue to stratify pediatric CKD patients in the "highest risk" category for the development of CVD [15, 16].

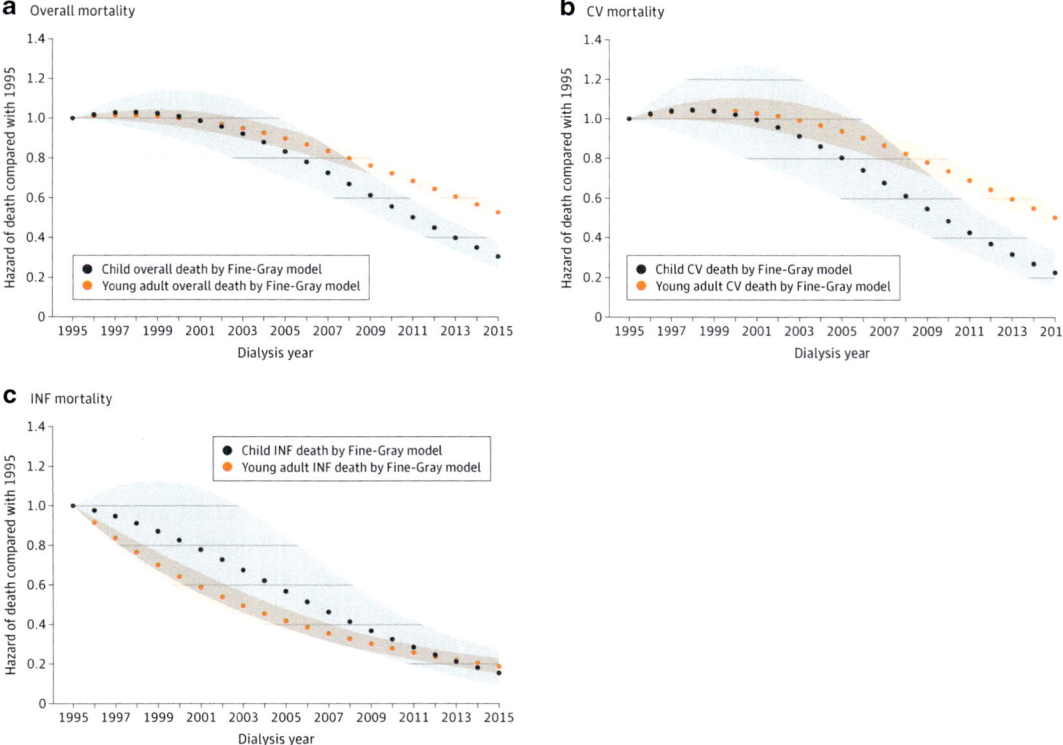

Fig. 61.1 Trend in cause-specific deaths among children and young adults by calendar year of dialysis initiation using fine-Gray models. Shaded areas represent 95%CIs for the point estimates in young adults and children. *CV* indicates cardiovascular, *INF* infection. From Ku et al. [13]

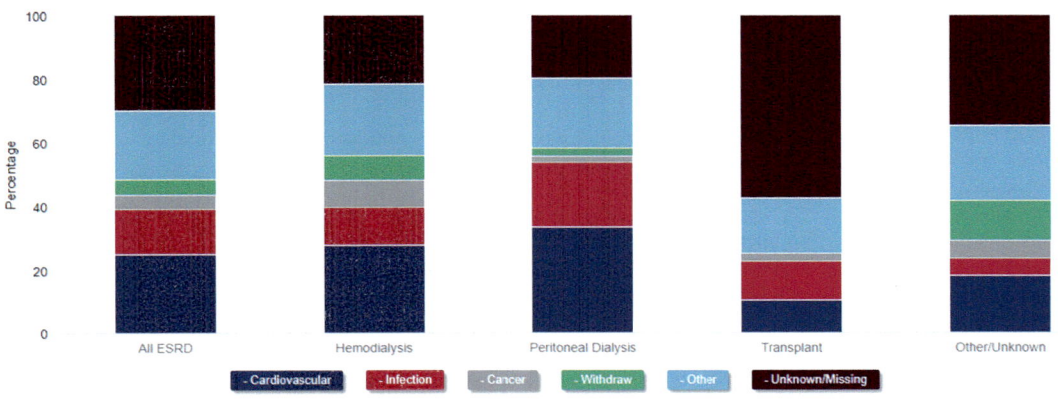

Fig. 61.2 Cause of death in children with ESKD, by treatment modality, 2010–2019. The most common cause of death in children with ESRD was a cardiovascular cause, followed by an infectious cause, but the causes of death differed by treatment modality. For example, children receiving PD died more commonly of infections than children receiving HD. A large proportion of the causes of death in children were of unknown cause (30%), and the cause was particularly likely to be unknown for children with a kidney transplant. *US Renal Data System: USRDS 2020 Annual Data Report: ESRD among Children and Adolescents.* https://adr.usrds.org/2020/end-stage-renal-disease/7-%20esrd-among-children-and-adolescents

Specific Causes of Cardiac Death

The term "cardiac death" may include several diagnostic categories, such as cardiac arrest, arrhythmia, myocardial infarction, valvular heart disease, cardiomyopathy, etc. (Table 61.1).

Although it is common to group these diagnoses together, this may obscure the issue; the diagnosis of arrhythmia could be due to hyperkalemia (possibly due to noncompliance, dietary mistakes, acidosis, insufficient dialysis, etc.) or due to coronary artery disease or other causes. Therefore, diagnostic categories do not necessarily permit conclusions regarding the pathogenesis of CVD events.

In the initial USRDS study almost 20 years ago of Parekh et al., cardiac arrest was the most common cause in each of the age groups, followed by arrhythmia and cardiomyopathy [2]. The incidence of cardiac arrest in the youngest age group (0–4 years) was 5–10 times higher

Table 61.1 Most common cardiovascular risks, abnormalities and cardiac causes of death

Cardiovascular risks and abnormalities[a]	Cardiac causes of death
CV Risks	*Dialysis*
Hypertension	Cardiac arrest/arrhythmias
Dyslipidemia	Cerebrovascular disease
Hyperphosphatemia	Congestive heart failure/pulmonary edema
Increased Ca × P product	Cardiomyopathy
Anemia	Acute myocardial infarction
Early CV abnormalities	Pericarditis
Left Ventricular hypertrophy	*Transplant*
LV Systolic and diastolic dysfunction	Cardiac arrhythmias
Increased cIMT	Cerebrovascular disease
Increased PWV	Acute myocardial infarction
Coronary artery calcification	Cardiomyopathy

[a]The frequency of cardiovascular risks and abnormalities increases with advancing of CKD with the greatest prevalence during maintenance dialysis. Despite some improvement, many of these factors persist after transplantation

than in other age groups, perhaps, as noted by the authors, a reflection of the difficulty of ascertaining the true cause of death in young children. Some of these young children might have died from other co-morbid conditions such as congenital disorders which are not included in the USRDS database.

The most recent study by Ku et al. [13] also using the USRDS indicated that while sudden cardiac death remained the leading cause of death, its risk has improved steadily but to a greater degree in children versus young adults comparing 2015 versus 1995. In contrast, trends differed for heart failure-related mortality: while the risk of dying from heart failure did not change over time in children, it began to decline in those starting dialysis as young adults after 2008. The risk of dying from a myocardial infarction was significantly lower after 2005 compared to 1995 in young adults, but was not different during most of the follow-up time in children although the event rate was very low. The risk of dying of a stroke began to improve after 2009–2010 in both those starting dialysis as children and young adults.

The high rate of sudden cardiac death in children, especially in infants with ESKD, is poorly understood and warrants further investigation. In adults, sudden cardiac death is often a result of fatal arrhythmias due to acute ischemia of preexisting atherosclerotic disease. It is believed that arrhythmias are also the likely cause of most cases of sudden cardiac death in children. However, the origin of acquired malignant arrhythmias in children is unlikely to be an atherosclerotic lesion. Instead, dilated, especially hypertrophic cardiomyopathies are a leading cause of sudden cardiac death in children [17]. The macroscopic and microscopic structural abnormalities in cardiomyopathies involve fibrosis and cellular hypertrophy that predispose to an electrical instability with resultant arrhythmias. Ischemia of small coronary vessels secondary to medial hypertrophy might result in dispersion of repolarization properties and arrhythmia from re-entrant or autonomic mechanisms. As we discuss in more detail below in this chapter, many children with CKD develop left ventricular hypertrophy (LVH), which is frequently severe, especially in children on prolonged dialysis therapy [18, 19]. It is currently unknown if LVH in young patients with CKD is characterized by structural abnormalities similar to familial or idiopathic hypertrophic cardiomyopathies associated with sudden cardiac death. To what extent LVH can contribute to an increased risk for sudden cardiac death in children with CKD is also not known. Deadly arrhythmias in children with ESKD could also be evoked by acute changes in the cardiac extra- or intracellular ionic milieu, especially involving abnormalities of sodium- and potassium-based repolarization currents.

Symptomatic ischemic heart disease and myocardial infarction are typical complications of CVD in older patients with CKD and account for more than 50% of death in these patients [20]. In contrast, young patients as a rule have no symptoms of ischemic heart disease such as angina pectoris and no myocardial infarction but remain asymptomatic. Could this imply that ischemic heart disease is silent and therefore underdiagnosed? Silent myocardial ischemia is frequently found in patients with CKD, especially during dialysis [21]. Myocardial infarction may also be disguised, as has been noted in younger women who may have significantly different symptoms at initial presentation [22]. There is a paucity of studies regarding EKG monitoring in children with CKD, but circadian rhythms of blood pressure (BP) and heart rate are altered in children with CKD [23]. There are no systematic autopsy studies in young patients with CKD focusing on vascular and coronary pathology. Therefore, the lack of symptomatic ischemic heart disease in young patients and paucity of cardiac deaths due to confirmed myocardial infarction remains an important observation; however, it is presently unknown whether absence of symptoms truly implies absence of advanced vascular and cardiac disease.

Risk Factors

In the general population, CVD in most patients is the result of atherosclerosis. Atherosclerosis is a multifactorial disease affecting the heart and large and medium-sized arteries, with a focal distribution, and with the characteristic appearance of lipid-rich plaques in the intima of the arterial wall. Clinical manifestations include coronary heart disease, cerebrovascular disease, aortic aneurysm, and peripheral arterial occlusive disease. This disease is slowly progressive over several decades. Atherosclerosis has a multifactorial pathogenesis, but the occurrence of the disease is associated with typical risk factors: dyslipidemia, hypertension, smoking, male gender, diabetes, abdominal obesity, lack of physical activity. In the INTERHEART study, a case-control study of acute myocardial infarction performed in 52 countries more than 15 years ago, these traditional risk factors (in combination with psychosocial factors, consumption of fruits, vegetables, and alcohol) accounted for 90% of the attributable risk in men and 94% in women, indicating their worldwide predictive value irrespective of gender, race, or region [24].

CKD has been appropriately described as a "vasculopathic state" because of the extraordinary risk indicated by the accumulation of numerous risk factors [25]. The occurrence and prevalence of these risk factors have been exhaustively described [26–28]. Traditional risk factors (for atherosclerosis), non-traditional (uremic) risk factors and cardiomyopathy (a risk factor in itself) most likely act synergistically, resulting in altered vascular and cardiac structure and function in CKD [29].

What makes children with CKD so highly predisposed to the development of accelerated atherosclerosis/arteriosclerosis and premature CVD during young adulthood is likely a unique combination of extremely highly prevalent traditional and CKD-related risk factors (Table 61.1).

Traditional Risk Factors

The high prevalence of traditional cardiovascular risk factors is already evident in children with early stages of CKD. Many publications from the Chronic Kidney Disease in Children (CKiD) study, an observational cohort study of more than one thousand children (aged 1–16 years) with CKD stages 2–4 initiated in the early 2000s, provided contemporary data on the prevalence of cardiovascular risk factors over the last decade. An initial cross-sectional study showed that 54% of participants had **hypertension**; among children receiving antihypertensive medication, 48% still had elevated blood pressures [30]. Ambulatory blood pressure monitoring (ABPM) demonstrated a high frequency of masked hypertension (38%) [31]. During a 4-year follow up, only 46% of hypertensive patients achieved controlled clinic BP [32]. In a study comparing ambulatory BP control over two time periods (2005–2008 and 2010–2013), there was a significantly higher prevalence of masked hypertension and a lower prevalence of normotension in the more recent period [33]. Recent data indicate that unrecognized and untreated hypertension is more prevalent and persistent in younger children [34]. Thus, despite publication of the initial CKiD hypertension data in 2008–2010, plus published recommendations and guidelines for stricter BP control in patients with CKD, hypertension has remained under-recognized and under-treated in children with CKD.

Dyslipidemia was initially found in 43% of the CKiD cohort: 32% had triglycerides levels >130 mg/dL; 21% had HDL-cholesterol levels <40 mg/dL and 21% had total cholesterol >200 mg/dL [35]. Dyslipidemia persisted (51%) 6.5 years later in the CKiD participants [36]. Likewise, the prevalence of dyslipidemia was 61.5% in children with CKD enrolled in KNOW-PedCKD, the KoreaN cohort study for Outcomes in patients With Pediatric Chronic Kidney Disease [37].

Among the CKiD participants, about 30% were either **overweight or obese** [38]. Although diabetes is very rare in children with CKD, hyperinsulinemia and insulin resistance was present in 9% and 19% respectively of the CKiD cohort [38]. Importantly, almost one half of the CKiD cohort had a combination of traditional cardiovascular risk factors [38]. Even lean patients had a high prevalence of multiple traditional cardiovascular risks, with nearly one-quarter having two or three cardiovascular risk factors. Overweight or obese study participants had a very high prevalence of multiple risk factors, similar to rates in severely obese

(BMI > 40 kg/m²) children without kidney disease. This pattern differentiates the population of children with CKD from healthy children, in whom the coexistence of multiple cardiovascular risk factors is extremely infrequent, and restricted to those who are obese (metabolic syndrome). However, classical **metabolic syndrome** is also very frequent in the CKiD cohort with a prevalence of 40% in overweight patients and 60% in the obese children [39]. In this study, those with persistent metabolic syndrome had approximately twice the odds of kidney function decline (>10% per year) compared to those without multiple cardiometabolic risk factors and normal BMI.

The frequency of traditional risk factors is highest in children on maintenance dialysis (Table 61.1). Successful kidney transplantation leads to elimination of many uremia-related risk factors for atherosclerotic CVD. However, transplant recipients are not free from multiple complications and transplantation frequently amplifies many of the traditional risk factors (Table 61.1). One multicenter study determined that 38% of kidney transplant recipients had a coexistence of at least three traditional cardiovascular risk factors [40].

CKD-Related Risk Factors

While the high prevalence of traditional risk factors might explain a higher prevalence of accelerated CAD and premature cardiac death in young adults, it cannot explain the high rates of cardiac death in 0–19 year olds on maintenance dialysis or after transplant. To understand the risk of cardiac disease in these children, the focus has been on evaluation of uremia-related risk factors. As in adults, abnormal mineral metabolism is frequent in children with CKD. The role of mineral and bone disorder (MBD) in development of vascular disease in CKD will be discussed extensively later in this chapter. As with traditional risks, the rates of abnormalities are higher in dialysis patients versus those with pre-ESKD (Table 61.1).

Despite widely spread use of erythropoietin and iron therapy, **anemia** is still frequently poorly controlled, especially in children with advanced CKD [41] or on maintenance dialysis [42]. Data from the CKiD study indicate that 26% of children with non-glomerular and 43% of children with glomerular CKD had hemoglobin levels less than the fifth percentile using age- and sex-specific norms [43]. Data from the Korean cohort (KNOW-PedCKD) demonstrated 40% prevalence of anemia [44].

One of the largest studies to date from the international Pediatric Peritoneal Dialysis Network (IPPN) (1394 pediatric patients aged 1 month to 20 years from 81 pediatric dialysis centers in 30 countries) showed that 25% of patients had a hemoglobin level < 10 g/dL despite more than 95% of participants received erythropoietin therapy [45]. In an early USRDS study, severe anemia has been linked to overall mortality in these children but not to cardiac death [46]. Similarly, in the IPPN study overall death occurred more frequently in those with hemoglobin <11 g/dL (4.2%) versus those with hemoglobin >11 g/dL (2.6%) [45].

Inflammation is also mainly evident in chronically dialyzed children. However, there have been no studies examining the role of inflammation in cardiac death of children with ESKD. Even though there have been no studies of a direct link between specific traditional and uremia-related risks and CVD mortality, epidemiological data presented above showing remarkable decrease in mortality post-transplant versus dialysis, clearly point out to dialysis vintage as a major cause of cardiac death in children and young adults with childhood onset of ESKD.

In summary, children and adolescents with CKD harbor a multitude of risk factors for CVD that at this age seems without parallel [47]. The overall effect of these risk factors and their relative contribution to morbidity and mortality in young patients is yet unknown. While studies in adult CKD patients predominantly focus on symptomatic cardiovascular events and all-cause mortality to identify risk factors, these end-points fortunately are rare in the pediatric setting. Studies in this age group therefore have to rely on surrogate endpoints such as the identification and progression rate of subtle cardiovascular changes (Table 61.1). The scarce knowledge about the extent of the progression of cardiovascular altera-

tions and promoting factors is often a result of relative small patient numbers in individual pediatric nephrology centers. For this reason, multicenter studies are a logic and reasonable consequence to advance cardiovascular research in children with CKD. In this regard, two large consortiums in Europe and the United States have formed more than a decade ago to monitor and evaluate the children with CKD with a special emphasis on the cardiovascular status. In addition to the CKiD study that was introduced earlier in the chapter [48], the European consortium has initiated the Cardiovascular Comorbidity in Children with Chronic Kidney Disease Study (4C Study) which prospectively follows more than 700 children with more advanced CKD all over Europe [49]. In both studies, yearly exams evaluate the cardiovascular status in these patients by vascular ultrasound, BP measurement, other traditional and CKD related CVD risk factors, echocardiography and assessment of arterial stiffness. It has provided important insight about who is or will be at a particularly high risk to suffer from cardiovascular complications. In this chapter, we describe the current findings from the above multicenter observational studies.

Vascular Disease in Pediatric CKD

Non-invasive Studies of Vascular Abnormalities

Coronary Artery Calcification

CT scans were the earliest imaging modalities to detect vascular abnormalities such as coronary artery calcifications (CAC) in young adults with ESKD. Braun et al. [50] were the first to describe increased calcium scores in young dialysis patients when compared with non-dialysis patients with known or suspected coronary artery disease and a number of studies confirmed this finding for young patients with ESKD starting in childhood or adolescents [6, 51–58]. Also, coronary calcium scores increased significantly in dialysis patients even over short time periods [52, 57]. Two studies reported the occurrence of CAC only starting at the age of 20 or 31 years in their patient cohorts respectively [53, 57] whereas others detected them already during adolescence [51, 58]. The percentage of patients with proven CAC was highly variable between studies and ranged between 10% and 92%, possibly reflecting the wide age range, differences in cumulative time on dialysis or after transplantation, and variation in medical treatment policies. Recent studies of CAC in children with ESKD have been performed by Srivaths et al. [54–56]. In their initial study, 5 of 16 patients (31%) had CAC. In a follow up study, the CT was repeated 1 year after the initial evaluation. Three patients with initial CAC progressed based on increased Agaston score; one patient developed new and none of the patients resolved CAC.

Although heterogeneous in age, duration and mode of renal replacement therapy, several risk factors for the presence and severity of CAC were consistently identified in the majority of studies. Among them are the patients' age, cumulative time on dialysis, CRP, PTH, FGF23, mean serum phosphorus and calcium-phosphorus product levels, and cumulative exposure to active vitamin D.

Carotid Intima-Media Thickness

In adults, carotid intima-media thickness consensus (cIMT) measurement is considered a valid and reliable assessment of atherosclerotic burden [59–62] that can predict coronary atherosclerosis and its clinical sequelae, such as myocardial infarction and stroke [60, 62]. Measurement of cIMT is recommended by the American Heart Association for risk stratification in adults whose CV risk is not clear or is intermediate [61] and as a standard non-invasive assessment of subclinical atherosclerosis in children and adolescents [61].

Briefly, cIMT is measured at the far wall of an ultrasound image recorded with a high-frequency probe. Normal values were first developed for children between 10 and 20 years based on measurements in 241 healthy children [63] and later on for children between 6 and 18 years in a cohort of 1155 healthy non-obese and non-hypertensive children [64]. The study demonstrated low inter- and intraobserver variation,

confirming the suitability of cIMT measurements as a surrogate marker of the vascular health status in multicenter trials.

Ultrasound studies in pediatric predialysis, dialysis and transplanted patients revealed significant alterations of the vessel wall compared to healthy controls, which start well before attainment of ESKD. This was first shown in smaller studies [65, 66] and confirmed in the large observational multicenter studies of CKiD and 4C.

CKD patients of the CKiD study showed increased cIMT which was correlated with hypertension and dyslipidemia [67]. The baseline evaluation of the 4C Study cohort revealed elevated cIMT in 42% of patients (Fig. 61.3) [68]. cIMT was higher in girls and associated with higher systolic blood pressure SDS, BMI SDS, physical activity and serum phosphorus [68].

Oxidative stress has been suspected as a potential factor involved in the pathogenesis of large vessel arteriopathy, but so far, few associations to the clinical vascular status have been reported in pediatric CKD. In 134 predialysis and dialysis patients aged 2–16 years, reduced glutathione levels but not other oxidative stress markers such as malondialdehyde, nitric oxide and homocysteine were found to be associated with cIMT [69].

In children with ESKD receiving **dialysis**, cIMT is more markedly increased than in the predialytic CKD population [58, 65, 69]. In these children cIMT is consistently linked to abnormal mineral metabolism and associated medications, as indicated by associations with serum phosphorus, calcium-phosphorus product, iPTH levels, and calcium based phosphate binder therapy. In addition, a strong association between active vitamin D dosage and cIMT was noted in the largest study of cIMT to date in pediatric dialysis patients [58]. Notably, not only an excess of active vitamin D but also 1.25 Vitamin D deficiency is a risk factor for increased cIMT in dialyzed children, constituting a U-shaped relationship of serum 1.25-vitamin D levels and cIMT [70].

Increased cIMT in pediatric **kidney transplant recipients** has consistently been demon-

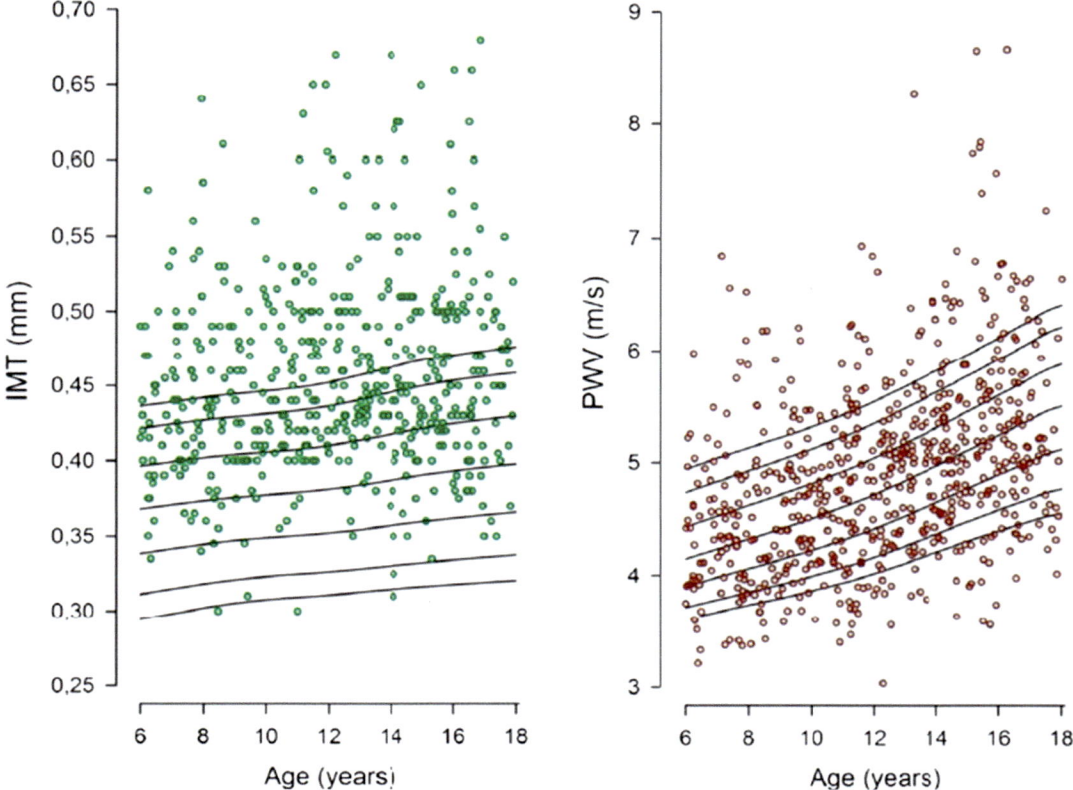

Fig. 61.3 Surrogate marker measurements. Distribution of carotid intima-media thickness (IMT; left panel) and pulse wave velocity (PWV; right panel). Curves represent 5th, 10th, 25th, 50th, 75th, 90th, and 95th reference percentiles. From Schaefer et al. [69]

strated. A meta-analysis of 2016 estimated that cIMT was about 0.05 mm higher in these patients than in healthy controls [71]. It included 9 studies and a total of 259 mostly kidney and few liver transplant patients. In a study of 109 children in three German centers, cIMT was elevated in 43% of patients with a kidney transplant [72].

There is scarce information about the progression of cIMT over time in children with CKD. Time on dialysis is associated with higher cIMT levels, as reported by Chavarria et al. in 60 dialyzed children [73] and by Oh et al. in 39 young adults with childhood-onset ESKD [6]. In a prospective study following 24 children with CKD stage 3–5 and 32 patients on dialysis, cIMT values increased both in the predialysis and the dialysis patients. By contrast, among patients

who were transplanted during the observation period, those with elevated cIMT at baseline showed significant regression after transplantation [74]. In children of the 4C cohort who underwent pre-emptive kidney transplantation when reaching ESKD, cIMT did not regress but increased significantly less than in children who started dialysis [75].

Importantly, clinical morphologic measures appear to reflect structural changes even on the molecular level. In patients of the 4C Study, cIMT measured by ultrasound was correlated with arterial calcium content in arterial biopsies and corresponding transcriptional alterations regarding pro-calcifying factors, calcification inhibitors and extracellular matrix components were demonstrated [75].

Pulse Wave Velocity

In recent years, research has focused not only on morphological but also on functional measures of the vascular status. A variety of technologies to non-invasively assess arterial properties *in vivo* have been introduced. Among different techniques, pulse wave velocity (PWV) is one of the most studied in children with CKD. PWV is a measure of arterial stiffness derived from the propagation of the pulse wave along the vessel wall between two defined points of the arterial tree. Similarly to normal values of blood pressure, PWV is strongly age- and height-dependent and considerably lower in children and young adolescents than in adults. Therefore, age- or height normalized values should be used for the interpretation of PWV. The European Heart Association rates PWV as "gold-standard" to assess arterial stiffness and recommends its measurement for the evaluation of cardiovascular risk. In adults, a relationship to mortality independent of blood pressure and other confounding factors was demonstrated in 241 patients with ESKD and 439 patients with CKD stage 2–5 [76, 77]. Savant et al. reported PWV comparable to healthy children in a group of patients from the CKiD study with more than 50% of patients in CKD stage 1 or 2 [78]. The baseline assessment of children with **pre-dialytic CKD** of the 4C study (CKD stage 3–5) showed elevated PWV in 20% of patients (Fig. 61.3) [68]. PWV in these patients was associated with higher systolic blood pressure, albuminuria and iPTH and with lower vitamin D levels [68]. While slightly different methods were used in both studies (applanation tonometry vs. oscillometric recording) a turning point towards increasing arterial stiffness at CKD stage 3 might be implied.

Considerably increased PWV has been reported in several smaller studies in pediatric **dialysis** patients [58, 77, 79]. The 3H study found higher PWV in patients on conventional hemodialysis than in patients receiving hemodiafiltration [80]. PWV decreased over time in both groups.

Increased PWV has also been detected in a cross-sectional analysis of pediatric **transplant recipients** [81]. In a longitudinal analysis of 4C Study patients who started renal replacement therapy, PWV decreased after pre-emptive kidney transplantation but increased after the start of dialysis treatment [75]. The 4C study recently analyzed changes in PWV in children with ESKD who underwent kidney transplantation [82]. In their analysis, PWV significantly increased after transplantation and was significantly higher in girls compared to boys. PWV was positively associated with time on dialysis and diastolic blood pressure in both sexes. Authors concluded that girls with CKD are more susceptible to develop arterial stiffness compared to boys and that this difference persist after transplantation and might contribute to higher mortality rates seen in girls with kidney failure.

Blood pressure has been identified as the most important predictor for PWV in all CKD stages. In addition, associations to markers of CKD-MBD and uremic toxins have been described in pediatric cohorts [83–86]. There is also evidence that the NO pathway is altered in CKD which associates with measurements of arterial structure and function. Shroff et al. showed that HDL derived from pediatric CKD patients inhibited NO production in vitro, which was correlated inversely to measures of PWV and cIMT in these subjects [87].

ABPM and Ambulatory Arterial Stiffness Index (AASI)

Ambulatory Blood Pressure Monitoring (ABPM) does not only characterize BP status, rhythm and daily variability but can also provide information about vascular stiffness. The Ambulatory Arterial Stiffness Index (AASI) is computed as 1 minus the diastolic-on-systolic blood pressure slope of the linear regression line between 24-h ambulatory diastolic and systolic blood pressure readings. It was found highly correlated with PWV and the central and peripheral augmentation index. In children with hypertension, AASI is increased and associated with the duration and origin of hypertension [88]. In a study of 51 kidney transplant recipients, AASI was increased in hypertensive subjects and the main determinants were dipping time, volume overload and time on dialysis, while PWV was increased also in normotensive patients and predicted by a dialysis vintage of more than 1 year. This observation led to the interpretation that PWV might represent structural long-term changes of the vessels, while AASI rather demonstrates the volume- and pressure-associated arterial stiffness [89]. While further evaluation of AASI as a cardiovascular marker is desirable, it could be a useful tool to monitor volume status and to adjust diuretic therapy [90].

Flow-Mediated Dilation, Postischemic Reactive Hyperemia

Endothelial-dependent flow-mediated dilation (FMD) measures the dilation of an artery after a short occlusion of the subjacent arteries. It depends on the potential of the vessel endothelium to produce nitric oxide (NO) or prostanoids to trigger vasodilatation and thereby characterizes endothelial reactivity and function [91]. Practically, the dilation of the brachial artery is measured by ultrasound at baseline and after the release of a BP cuff which has been placed on the upper arm or the forearm and has been inflated to approximately 50 mmHg above the systolic BP for several minutes. Despite a high interobserver and within-subject variability [92], a multitude of studies in adults have used FMD as surrogate marker for endothelial dysfunction. Several recent studies in adult CKD patients have demonstrated a reduction of FMD in both predialysis and dialysis patients [93]. Moreover, reduced FMD was predictive of fatal and non-fatal cardiovascular events in a prospective study of 304 adult predialysis patients [94]. The applicability of FMD in children is compromised by the limited tolerance to a BP cuff inflated over several minutes, and the unpleasant phase of hyperemia often prevents repeated measurements. Nevertheless a few small studies have been performed in children with CKD, two of which found decreased FMD in 23% and 71% of children with CKD stage 2–4 and 4, respectively [95, 96]. In another study which included predialysis, dialysis and transplanted patients, 60% had impaired FMD, which was significantly associated with cIMT [97]. A study of 44 pediatric patients after kidney transplantation found that treatment including everolimus resulted in reduced FMD compared to standard calcineurin inhibitor treatment [98]. While this study was cross-sectional only, it indicated that implications of different treatment regimens may become apparent by comparing surrogate endpoints, making them a feasible option also for prospective clinical trials.

Mechanisms of Vascular Calcification in CKD

Patients with CKD develop different types of vascular pathology. The predominant alteration consists of progressive calcification of the tunica media (Fig. 61.4). Additionally, calcification of

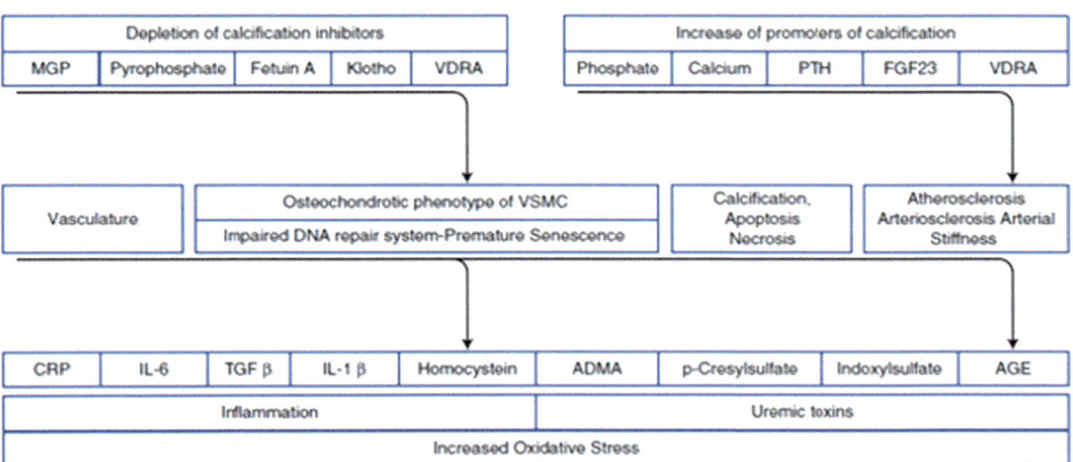

Fig. 61.4 Pathophysiologic mechanisms of vascular calcification. *MGP* Matrix Gla protein, *VDRA* vitamin D receptor agonist, *AGE* advanced glycosylation products, *ADMA* asymmetric dimethylarginin

the intima can occur and further deteriorate the vascular phenotype. Vascular smooth muscle cells (VSMC) play a key role in medial calcification. They are actively involved in calcification processes and undergo alterations including premature senescence and apoptosis, loss of calcification inhibitory capacities, osteogenic transformation and deposition of hydroxyapatite [99]. As a dysregulated mineral metabolism in CKD plays a key role in this process KDIGO explicitly includes "vascular or other soft-tissue calcification" in the definition of CKD-MBD [100]. The so-called kidney-vascular-bone axis reflects the direct and deleterious consequences of an unbalanced mineral metabolism on the vascular system.

The Kidney-Vascular-Bone Axis

In addition to hypertension and dyslipidemia, mineral metabolism plays a crucial role for vascular alterations in CKD. Among the directly or indirectly involved factors are serum levels of calcium, phosphate, vitamin D, PTH, FGF23 and Klotho.

Although serum calcium levels are usually low in untreated CKD patients, medications such as calcitriol and calcium-based phosphate binders can significantly increase serum calcium, especially in the presence of low-bone turnover disease. High calcium uptake by VSMC can induce matrix vesicle calcification similar to processes in the bone [101] and promote apoptosis of the cells leading to release of calcium in the extracellular matrix and formation of calcification "nidus" [102]. High phosphate levels are frequent in advanced CKD and might even occur at milder stages depending on phosphate intake. Phosphate is a key mediator of medial calcification. In vitro experiments have demonstrated that phosphate can induce an osteochondrogenic state in VSMC [103].

Given the outlined consequences of an altered mineral metabolism, a linear association of arterial deterioration and calcification with failing kidney function would seem logical. However, vessels of dialysis patients seem to be substantially more prone to calcification from hypercalcemia and hyperphosphatemia than vessels of

healthy individuals, as demonstrated in both in vitro and in vivo models of human vessels. In a model of intact human vessels, Shroff et al. showed that calcium accumulation already started during pre-dialysis CKD while the number of VSMC and vessel architecture was normal. In dialysis vessels however, calcification was significantly accelerated and vessels showed deranged architecture, increased VSMC death and deposition of hydroxyapatite laden vesicles. In addition to high serum calcium levels, it is likely that reduced concentration or activity of calcification inhibitors such as Fetuin-A and MGP contribute to the calcification process [104, 105].

Calcium and phosphate levels are subject to tight regulatory circles. An important mechanism of phosphate homeostasis includes FGF23 and Klotho. FGF23 is induced by high phosphate levels, it increases urinary phosphate excretion and inhibits 1.25 vitamin D synthesis [106]. Klotho is a coreceptor for FGF23 and is involved in the regulation of phosphaturia and 1.25 vitamin D production [107]. There is a free soluble form, but it is also expressed in arteries and VSMC [108]. FGF23 is upregulated and vascular Klotho downregulated early in the course of CKD [109] and several studies have linked increased calcification to reduced vascular Klotho expression in CKD [108, 109]. Reversal of Klotho insufficiency by transgenic overexpression in mice with CKD ameliorated phosphate extretion, preserved renal function and decreased calcification, potentially identifying a new therapeutic option [110]. Increases in FGF23 have been linked to increased mortality independently of phosphate levels [111]. *In vitro*, FGF23 enhances phosphate-induced calcification [112] and *in vivo*, the severity of calcification in patients with a nonzero Agatston score is associated with FGF23 in CKD patients [113]. In children on dialysis with coronary artery calcification, Srivath et al. found significantly increased FGF23 levels compared to those without calcification [55]. In adults however, there are conflicting results about the role of FGF23 for vascular calcification, endothelial dysfunction and arterial elasticity [114, 115].

Regarding phosphate binders, there seem to be different effects on aortic calcification depending on the type of phosphate binder [116]. As there are no data about the effect of phosphate binders on arterial calcification and Klotho or FGF23 in children, future studies are recommendable to improve therapeutic approaches.

Calcium levels are controlled by vitamin D levels, which themselves play a role in vascular calcification. Besides increasing calcium levels, vitamin D receptor agonists themselves can induce calcification by induction of an osteoblast phenotype of VSMC [117]. They also increase the secretion of alkaline phosphatase, which can worsen the calcification inhibitory capacity of VSMC by degrading pyrophosphate, a potent calcification inhibitor [118]. However, there is also evidence from a mouse model that vitamin D receptor agonists induce Klotho and lower FGF23, thereby exerting a beneficial effect on medial calcification [119]. These contradictory observations may help to explain the bimodal relation between vitamin D levels and calcification in clinical studies [70].

Calcification Inhibitors

Evidently, additional or permissive factors contribute to the disposition of a vessel for calcification particularly in dialysis. In fact, healthy individuals benefit from strong inhibitors of calcification such as pyrophosphate, Fetuin A and MGP. These inhibitors are loaded in vesicles of VSMCs and are released in the presence of increased serum calcium scores. Under normal conditions these vesicles can prevent calcification, but if the inhibitory contents are compromised or if their capacity is overrun by extreme dysbalance of mineral homeostasis, hydroxyapatite crystals can form from these calcium-rich vesicles. Uptake of hydroxyapatite crystals in turn can lead to apoptosis and necrosis of VSMCs, further diminishing the calcification inhibitory capacity of the vessel [99]. This is the initiation of a vicious cycle as a consequence of the disturbed mineral metabolism in CKD and aggravated by abnormalities of mechanisms protective of calcification. Inhibitors of calcification have been studied extensively in adults and to a lesser extent in children with CKD.

The active form of **MGP** is y-carboxylated and antagonizes BMP signaling, which is involved in endothelial dysfunction, formation of vascular lesions calcification and neoangiogenesis [120]. Vitamin K deficiency, as it occurs e.g. with warfarin treatment or in CKD, therefore leads to reduced levels of active MGP and a disposition to increased calcification. But serum levels of MGP alone have no protective effect on calcification, instead MGP therefore has to be expressed in VSMC [121]. Accordingly, no associations of serum levels of undercarboxylated or y-carboxylated MGP to vascular measures have been identified in two studies with dialyzed and transplanted children [85, 122]. Nevertheless, histologically, pediatric dialysis patients showed deposition of undercarboxylated MGP in calcified vessels [104].

Fetuin A is a circulating calcification inhibitor and also a content of VSMC vesicles. In the presence of fetuin A, calcium and phosphate form soluble calciprotein particles instead of hydroxyapatite crystals and thereby prevent ectopic calcification [123]. In children, there are conflicting results of fetuin A levels in dialysis patients. One study found reduced fetuin levels in pediatric dialysis patients compared to healthy controls and children with mild CKD or after transplantation [124]. They were positively correlated with 25OHD dosage and calcium, but not with 25OHD serum levels. Another study found higher fetuin A serum levels in dialysis patients and an inverse correlation with time on dialysis. Vascular calcification was associated with lower fetuin A levels and vascular measures were inversely correlated to aoPWV and augmentation index [85]. Histologically, increased fetuin-A staining was demonstrated in calcified vessels of dialysis patients [105].

Promoters of Calcification and Premature Aging in CKD

There is evidence that the balance of vascular homeostasis shifts towards calcification not only by the loss of inhibitors but also by promoting factors. Uremic toxins induce oxidative stress which in turn hampers the ability of VSMC to regenerate. Instead, a disabled DNA damage repair system leads to senescence of the cells. An important marker in this process is prelaminin A. Nuclear laminas are of essential significance for the nuclear integrity of cells, and prelamin A normally is converted to laminin A over several steps including farnesylation and subsequental cleavage by the metalloproteinase FACE1/Zmpste24. Oxidative stress induces a down-regulation of FACE1/Zmpste24 and thereby inhibits the completion of functional laminin A [125]. Other than being a biomarker for premature cell senescence, farnesylated prelamin A is possibly actively involved in cell damage, specifically to the nuclear structure. In vessels of pediatric dialysis patients, there was a high prelamin A deposition in calcified arteries which provoked a osteogenic differentiation of VSMC and a senescence-associated secretory phenotype with increased expression of bone morphogenetic protein 2, osteoprotegerin and interleukin 6 [126]. These factors in turn can induce osteogenic differentiation in endothelial and mesenchymal progenitor cells, hereby involving also the vessel endothelium and initiating yet another vicious cycle in the calcification process [127].

Uremic Toxins and Endothelial Dysfunction

Another important pathway of vascular damage is endothelial dysfunction, triggered by the uremic milieu and accumulating toxins. Uremic toxins can be either water-soluble or protein-bound, accumulating either by reduced excretion or alterations of metabolic pathways in uremia. Besides well-studied factors such as homocystein, recently discovered toxins include *p*-cresylsulfate, indoxylsulfate, aysmmetric dimethylarginin (ADMA), advanced glycation endproducts and many more.

Hyperhomocysteinemia is a well-known risk factor for ischemic heart disease and stroke [128]. Homocysteine impairs endothelial function and inhibits endothelium-dependent vasodilatation. It also inhibits angiogenesis and endothelial repair [129]. Plenty of studies have linked homocysteine levels to increased mortality in adults. The highest homocysteine levels in this regard are found in patients with mutations in enzymes or cofactors of the homocysteine metabolism. Also in dialysis patients, homocystein is significantly increased compared to the normal population and high values are associated with an elevated risk for vascular complications [130]. According to a meta-analysis of Wald et al. [131] the risk for ischaemic heart disease, pulmonary embolism and stroke increases with homocysteine levels as identified by comparing individuals with genetically caused higher homocysteine levels to controls without the mutation. However, several controlled clinical trials including trials with CKD patients have failed to show a beneficial outcome when homocystein levels were reduced by substituting folic acid together with either vitamin B6, vitamin B12 or both [132–134]. Several explanations have been proposed to explain this, for example the fact that most studies treated patients with only mildly elevated homocysteine, which might not lead to a measurable effect. Also, homocysteine might be not the real culprit but only a measurable effect of yet another toxic agent. Finally, folic acid, the treatment for hyperhomocysteinemia, increases levels of S-adenosylmethionin, which in turn can increase ADMA levels by providing a methyl donor group to N-methyltransferases. By increasing another uremic toxin, this might partly explain the failure of folic acid to prevent cardiovascular disease by reducing homocysteine [135]. Data about homocysteine and the vascular status in children with CKD is scarce; one small study showed no associations of homocysteine to the cardiovascular status as assessed by flow-mediated dilation of the brachial artery and cIMT [97].

ADMA is a methylated L-arginine derivative which accumulates in chronic kidney disease [136]. It is protein-bound and therefore poorly dialzed. *In vitro* ADMA production is increased by activation of the NADPH oxidase and *in vivo* by angiotensin II infusion [137]. ADMA inhibits NO production, which leads to an increase of systemic vascular resistance, blood pressure and sodium retention [138]. Furthermore, it promotes an inflammatory phenotype and premature senescence of endothelial cells [129]. In children with

CKD stage 1 to 4, increased systolic BP and non-dipping nocturnal BP in 24 h BP measurements were found associated with increased ADMA relative to arginine and symmetric dimethyl-arginine levels in the urine [139].

p-cresylsulfate and **indoxylsulfate** are produced by intestinal bacterial from *p*-cresol and tryptophan respectively. The EUTox working group analyzed *p*-cresylsulfate and indoxylsulfate in 139 adult patients and both were inversely correlated with renal function and mortality [140, 141]. *p*-Cresyl sulfate was also positively correlated with vascular calcification and mortality [140]. Indoxyl sulfate was associated with vascular calcification and pulse wave velocity [141]. In 609 children with CKD from the 4C Study cohort, serum levels of indoxyl sulfate and *p*-cresylsulfate at the baseline visit were inversely correlated with eGFR. Serum indoxyl sulfate levels were associated with higher cIMT and progression of PWV within 12 months of follow-up [86]. Indoxyl sulfate, but not *p*-cresyl sulfate levels were also independently associated with the prospective loss of kidney function in the same study cohort [142].

The Heart in Pediatric CKD

Cardiac Remodeling

Cardiac remodeling is a chronic and progressive process resulting in genome expression, molecular, cellular, and interstitial transformations that manifest as changes in the size, shape, and function of the heart after cardiac injury [143]. The triggers that initiate cardiac injury are diverse. In case of CKD, mechanical or hemodynamic overload is the initial stimulus, although hormones and cytokines may play an important role in its maintenance. The first response to imposed pressure or volume overload is the hypertrophy of cardiomyocytes (Fig. 61.5). The patterns of sarcomere formation induced by pressure or volume overload are distinct. Pressure-induced hypertrophy, concentric LVH, is characterized by a parallel addition of sarcomeres resulting in the increase of cross-sectional area and diameter of the myocytes. Concentric LVH is closely associated with

systolic or pulse pressure. From a physiological view, increased systolic BP and pulse pressure due to increased peripheral resistance and arterial stiffness are the principal factors opposing LV ejection and leading to increased LV workload. With volume-induced hypertrophy, eccentric LVH, addition of sarcomeres occurs in series resulting in longitudinal cell growth with secondary addition of new sarcomeres in parallel. Both myocyte diameter and length are proportionally increased, resulting in a balanced increase in overall wall thickness and LV volume. In the transition to maladaptive LVH, LV dilatation becomes disproportional to wall thickness with myocytes elongated without an increase in diameter.

In patients with CKD, the principal features of volume-induced LV enlargement include volume and sodium retention, anemia, and arteriovenous shunt.

Experimental models of cardiac hypertrophy developed over the last two decades support the theory that mechanical stress due to either pressure or volume overload is a trigger for activation of multiple other mechanisms leading to myocardial remodeling [144, 145]. These factors include metabolic defects in fuel utilization and efficiency, inflammatory responses, lipotoxicity, pathological growth of myocytes and loss of cytoprotective signaling [145]. In patients with CKD, these mechanisms might be activated independently of hemodynamic overload since uremia *per se* is associated with alteration in multiple factors [146–148].

Studies over the last decade have identified fibroblast growth factor 23 (**FGF23**), a bone-derived circulating peptide, as a novel CKD-related risk factor in the development of LVH. Plasma concentrations of FGF23 increase early and progressively in both children [149] and adults [150] with advancing CKD. High FGF23 is associated with premature death [111, 151], cardiovascular events [152], and LVH [153, 154], with experimental data favoring a direct pathophysiologic role of FGF23 in promoting LVH via an FGF receptor 4-dependent pathway [155, 156]. The CKiD study determined that among children and adolescents with GFR

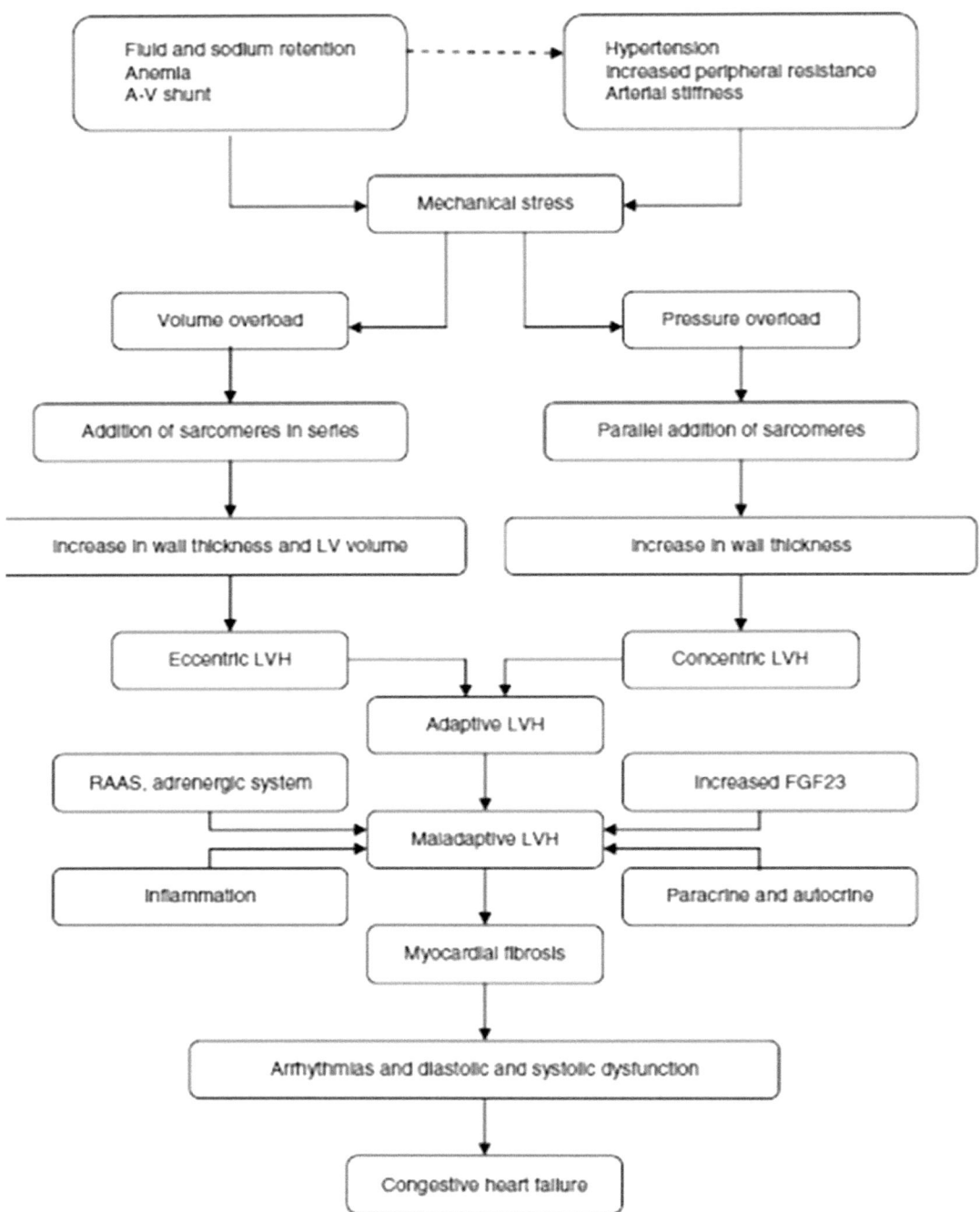

Fig. 61.5 Pathophysiologic mechanisms of LVH. Myocyte hypertrophy is likely an adaptive mechanism designed to improve pump function by expanding the number of contractile units in the myocardium while simultaneously reducing wall stress by increasing wall thickness. The transduction of mechanical stress occurs through the integrin proteins, transmembrane receptors that couple extra cellular matrix components directly to the intracellular cytoskeleton and nucleus. A signal for hypertrophy is mediated by a complex cascade of signaling systems within cardiomyocytes resulting in gene reprogramming. Activated hypertrophy-related genes induce the synthesis of new contractile proteins that are organized into new sarcomeres

$\geq$45 mL/min per 1.73 m^2, higher plasma FGF23 concentrations were independently associated with a higher prevalence of LVH [157]. This association was strongest in participants with FGF23 levels $\geq$170 RU/mL in whom the odds of LVH was three times higher than in those with FGF23 levels <100 RU/mL.

One of the possible mechanisms of LVH and LV dysfunction is abnormal sphingolipid metabolism leading to **cardiac lipotoxicity**. This condition leading to dilated cardiomyopathy has been described in congenitally obese Zucker diabetic fatty (ZDF) rats [158] and in adults with obesity and diabetes [159]. This is especially relevant to CKD patients, a population with a high prevalence of obesity, metabolic syndrome, and diabetes. In adult incident hemodialysis patients, Mitsnefes et al. [160] demonstrated that high plasma glucosylceramides were consistently and independently associated with CVD outcomes including uncontrolled hypertension, LVH, and decreased ejection fraction. The authors also reported that higher levels of glucosylceramide, C16GC, were associated with increased risk of CVD and all-cause mortality independent of diabetes, comorbidity index, and lipid levels.

A recent study demonstrated that mice with CKD had **T cells** infiltrating the heart and T cell depletion significantly improved both diastolic function and myocardial strain [161]. In the same study, children with CKD had increasing frequency of T cells bearing activation markers PD-1 and/or CD57 that was associated with worsening diastolic function on echocardiogram.

The association of different biomarkers with abnormal cardiac structure and function was examined in the Chronic Renal Insufficiency Cohort (CRIC) Study [162]. The researchers found that the novel biomarker growth differentiation factor 15 (**GDF-15**), a marker of inflammation and tissue injury, and clinical biomarkers N-terminal pro-B-type natriuretic peptide (**NT-proBNP**) and high-sensitivity troponin T (**hsTnT**), were associated with increased LVM and systolic dysfunction.

Initially, LVH is beneficial. It optimizes ejection performance by normalizing systolic wall stress and reducing tension among greater number of sarcomeres. Maladaptive cardiac hypertrophy which develops secondary to prolonged and proportionally increased pressure and volume overload (see above) with declined renal function is a proposed mechanism of congestive heart failure. This in turn results in excessive cardiac myocyte work relative to the supply of oxygen. As a consequence, myocyte death and fibrosis develops, with chamber dilatation and systolic dysfunction. However, the specific mechanisms of *cardiac myocyte death* are not well-determined. Unlike in direct cardiac injury (e.g. acute ischemia) where both necrosis and apoptosis produce cell death, chronic remodeling and transition to overt heart failure have been associated primarily with an elevated degree of apoptosis. However, it is not clear whether apoptosis is a cause or consequence of heart failure. With time, capillary density, coronary reserve and subendocardial perfusion decrease resulting in myocardial fibrosis [163]. *Intermyocardiocyte fibrosis* is a unique feature of uremic heart disease. Experimental uremic models showed selective increase in cardiac interstitial cells and nuclear volume but not in endothelial cell volume [164]. During this phase, patients present with arrhythmias and diastolic and systolic dysfunction, ultimately transitioning to overt heart failure.

Early Markers of Cardiomyopathy

Since symptomatic CVD is very rare in children, the focus of research has been on identifying in children with CKD early markers or intermediate CV outcomes. Over the last two decades, echocardiographically detected abnormalities of the LV such as LVH and LV dysfunction have been accepted as early markers of cardiomyopathy. In adults, the CRIC study demonstrated that the prevalence of LVH was 32%, 48%, 57%, and 75% for eGFR categories $\geq$60, 45–59, 30–44, and <30 mL/min per 1.73 m^2, respectively [165]. These abnormalities historically have been considered as strong independent predictors of coronary artery disease, heart failure and cardiac mortality both in the general population and in adults with hypertension and CKD. As early as in 1989, Silberberg et al. [166] showed that adult patients on maintenance dialysis who were diagnosed with LVH had a 52% higher 5-year mortality rate than patients without LVH. A few years later, Foley et al. [167] determined that LV dilatation and systolic dysfunction at start of dialysis were independently associated with mortality. The results of these studies triggered an investigation of cardiac structure and function in pediatric patients with CKD. Studies over last two decades have proven that abnormalities of LV are also present in children with CKD.

Evaluation of LVM in Children

M mode echocardiographic measurement is currently the most commonly clinically used imaging modality to assess LVM. The LVM is calculated according to recommendations from the American Society of Echocardiography [168]. This method applies measurements of LV end-diastolic diameter (LVED) and septal (IVS) and posterior wall (PW) thicknesses and accurately predicts LVM through the equation: $0.8[1.04\{[LVED +PW + IVS]^3 - LVED^3\}.] + 0.6$. Adjusting the calculated LVM to account for differences in age, height and weight is the next step to establish uniform reference values and criteria for LVH. Unfortunately, there is no uniform definition of LVH in children. The most ideal *indexing* parameter is lean body mass (LBM), but this is difficult to measure. Indexing LVM by patient height raised to approximately cubic exponential power has been shown to produce the greatest reduction in LVM variability in normal subjects, most correctly to detect differences between normal and obese subjects [169], and, importantly, correlates most closely to indexing by lean body mass [170]. However, in children, dispersion of residual variation of $LVM/height^{2.7}$ increases with either increasing height or age suggesting that other variables effect ventricular growth in children. Though further investigation is needed to determine the most ideal indexing parameter, dividing LVM by $height^{2.7}$ ($g/m^{2.7}$) seems to work well for older children and adolescents [171]. For children older than 9 years, the value of LVM index 95th percentile is relatively stable and is $38-42$ $g/m^{2.7}$. The most recent American Academy of Pediatrics Clinical Practice

Guidelines (CPG) published in 2017 for screening and management of high BP in children and adolescents formally recommend LVM index value of 51 $g/m^{2.7}$ as a conservative cut point to define LVH in children >8 years of age [172]. This value is above 99th percentile for children and adolescents and associated with up to a fourfold increase in cardiovascular morbidity in adults with hypertension [171]. The use of this value to define LVH in young children is problematic since the normative values for LVM index ($g/m^{2.7}$) are significantly higher than in older children as can be seen in study by Khoury et who published pediatric reference values for LVM index ($g/m^{2.7}$) based on the analysis of 2273 non-obese, healthy children and adolescents (0–18 years) [173] (Table 61.2. The data indicate that indexing of LVM to a power of $height^{2.7}$ is age and gender specific. For example, the 95th percentile for LVM index varies from 40 to 45 $g/m^{2.7}$ in adolescent girls and boys to about 70 $g/m^{2.7}$ in one-year old children; boys have a slightly larger LVM for a given height throughout childhood and adolescence (Fig. 61.6).

One of the potential pitfalls in using age-dependent LVM indexing in children with CKD is related to short stature. Foster et al. [174] demonstrated that LVMI ($g/m^{2.7}$) varies not only according to age but also according to absolute height with higher values in children with shorter height, especially in those with height < 110 cm. Given that the CKD patients have significantly reduced height relative to age, poor growth may result in some miss-classification of diagnosis of LVH in very young children. To account for short stature, Borzych et al. [175] suggested substituting chronological age by height age (*i.e.*, the age of a child of the same height growing at the 50th height percentile) using Khoury et al. [173] references. Chinali et al. studied 400 healthy children and proposed to use a single value of 45 $g/m^{2.16}$ across the whole pediatric age range to diagnose LVH, arguing that the allometric exponent 2.16 fully normalizes the LVMI in children of all ages and both sexes and removes the need to calculate specific percentiles for height and sex (Fig. 61.7) [176]. This alternative method of indexing LVM is promising and potentially, if validated in larger

Table 61.2 LVM (g) and LVMI (g/m$^{2.7}$) percentile values

Age	Gender	N	Variable	Percentile						Minimum	Maximum
				10th	25th	50th	75th	90th	95th		
<6 months	Boys	62	LVM	7.22	9.04	10.94	14.16	16.28	17.6	6.27	21.18
			LVMI	40.19	46.92	56.44	66.41	75.72	80.1	32.41	83
	Girls	43	LVM	7.59	9.27	11.15	13.76	16.05	16.5	5.49	28.74
			LVMI	39.05	48.62	55.38	65.98	73.47	85.6	21.22	109.2
6 months ≤2 years	Boys	73	LVM	16.95	20.25	23.88	27.84	32.47	33.7	9.43	36.32
			LVMI	36.17	40.66	44.95	53.29	61.27	68.6	26.71	74.75
	Girls	53	LVM	15.39	17.45	22.25	26.46	31.98	34.6	12.22	35.98
			LVMI	32.91	38.67	42.04	49.85	52.86	57.1	24.18	61.06
2 ≤4 years	Boys	124	LVM	24.37	28.52	33.31	38.79	45.48	48.4	13.27	58.13
			LVMI	28.44	33.88	39.5	45.19	48.74	52.4	21.25	77.07
	Girls	84	LVM	24.7	28.4	33.34	38.15	43.88	46.1	17.9	50.98
			LVMI	28.87	31.85	37.88	43.11	47.65	55.3	20.63	66.58
4 ≤6 years	Boys	133	LVM	34.36	39.13	45.49	52.62	59.26	63.2	22.92	83.51
			LVMI	27.68	30.68	36.96	40.2	45.12	48.1	18.76	57.25
	Girls	111	LVM	29.24	34.57	39.67	46.59	50.38	57.3	17.68	76.64
			LVMI	25.85	28.06	32.29	36.43	43.47	44.3	18.17	59.25
6 ≤8 years	Boys	117	LVM	40.23	45.14	51.73	62.06	70.48	77.4	25.95	97.29
			LVMI	24.47	28.56	31.79	36.28	40.18	44.6	20.27	59.47
	Girls	110	LVM	36.88	40.6	48.38	55.84	65.54	72.1	25.29	89.3
			LVMI	23.15	25.77	29.71	33.15	37.73	43.5	20.11	54.76
8 ≤10 years	Boys	111	LVM	45.32	51.49	62.09	73.42	84.61	91.1	32.35	122
			LVMI	22.45	24.85	29.11	34.57	38.25	41	15.24	53.19
	Girls	99	LVM	39.22	48.08	54.76	70.87	75.49	83.6	31.6	91.82
			LVMI	19.07	22.12	26.63	30.37	34.3	36	13.46	44.35

LVM left ventricular mass, *LVMI* left ventricular mass index (with permission of Elsevier from Khoury et al. [173])

studies, could replace currently utilized normative data.

Cardiac MRI is considered to be the most accurate imaging modality to measure LVM. While the normative pediatric percentile values have been developed [177], this modality has limited availability and still remains too expansive to recommend it for routine use. In addition to measurement of LVM, M mode echocardiography can be used to define *LV geometric pattern* (Fig. 61.8).

LV geometry is evaluated based on the 95th percentiles for LVM index and relative wall thickness. Relative wall thickness (RWT) is calculated from measurements made at end diastole as the ratio of the PW thickness plus IVS thickness over the LVED. Normal geometry is defined as LVM index and RWT below the 95th percentile. Concentric remodeling is defined as LVM index below the 95th percentile with RWT greater than the 95th percentile. Eccentric LVH is defined as LVM index greater than the 95th percentile and RWT below the 95th percentile. Concentric LVH is defined as both LVM index and RWT greater than the 95th percentile. As in case of LVM index, the 95th percentile values for RWT are not uniform and vary from 0.375 to 0.41.

Thus, the frequencies of different geometric patterns may differ depending on the cut off points used in the study.

Studies of LVH in Children with CKD

As in adults, LVH develops when **CKD** is mild or moderate in children and progresses as kidney function deteriorates. The baseline data on LVH from the CKiD cohort indicated a prevalence of 17% [31]. In this study, in addition to confirmed hypertension (elevated casual and ambulatory BP) and lower hemoglobin, masked hypertension (normal casual BP and elevated ambulatory BP) and female gender were independently associated with LVH. The likelihood of having LVH was four times higher in children having masked hypertension compared to children with normal clinic and ambulatory BP. The follow up study determined that over 4 years, the prevalence of LVH diminished from 16% to 11% [178]. Decrease in BP corresponded to regression of LVH in these children. As in the cross-sectional baseline analysis, the likelihood of developing of LVH was four times higher in females. The 4C study reported an increase in the prevalence of LVH from 10.6% in CKD stage 3a to 48% in CKD stage 5 [68].

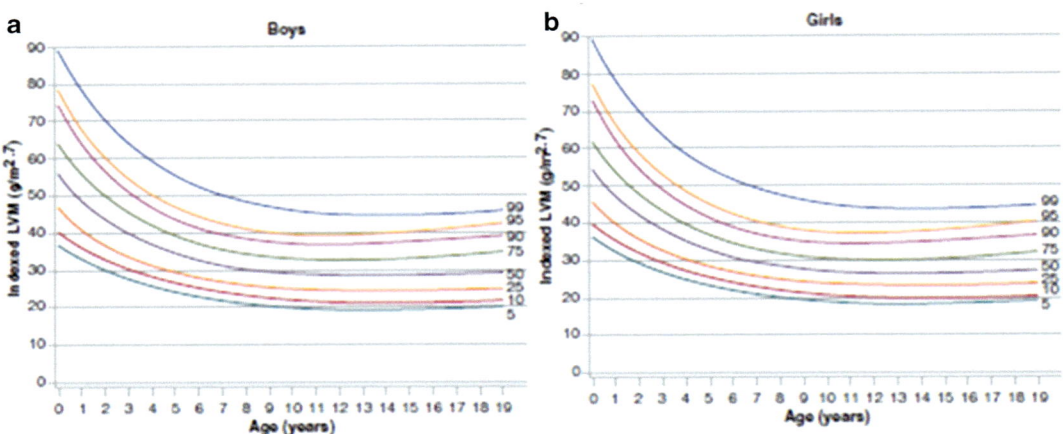

Fig. 61.6 The estimates of the 5th, 10th, 25th, 50th, 75th, 90th, and 95th quantiles of LVM indexed to height$^{2.7}$ for ages 0 through 18 years. Values displayed separately for boys (**a**) and girls (**b**) (used with permission of Elsevier from Khoury et al [173])

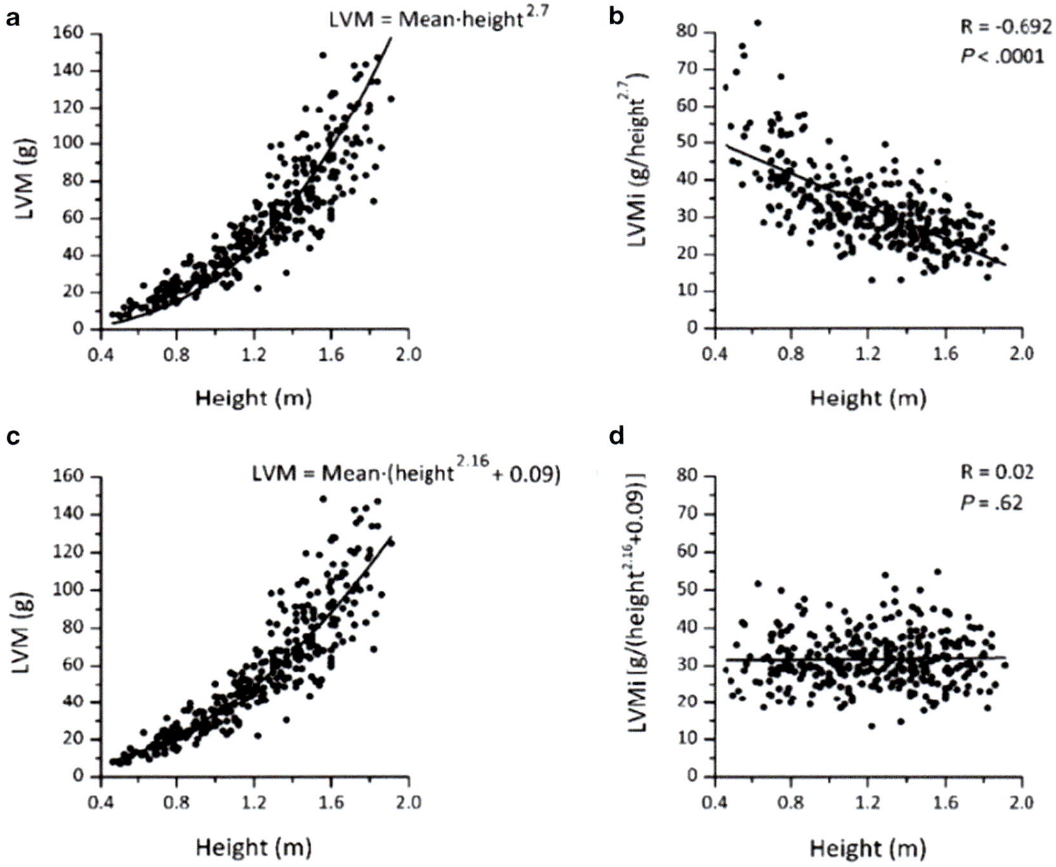

Fig. 61.7 (**a**) Regression of LVM with height 2.7; (**b**) distribution of residuals for height 2.7; (**c**) regression of LVM with height2.16; (**d**) distribution of residuals for height2.16; and. *LVMi* LVM index (adapted and used with permission of Elsevier from Chinali et al [176])

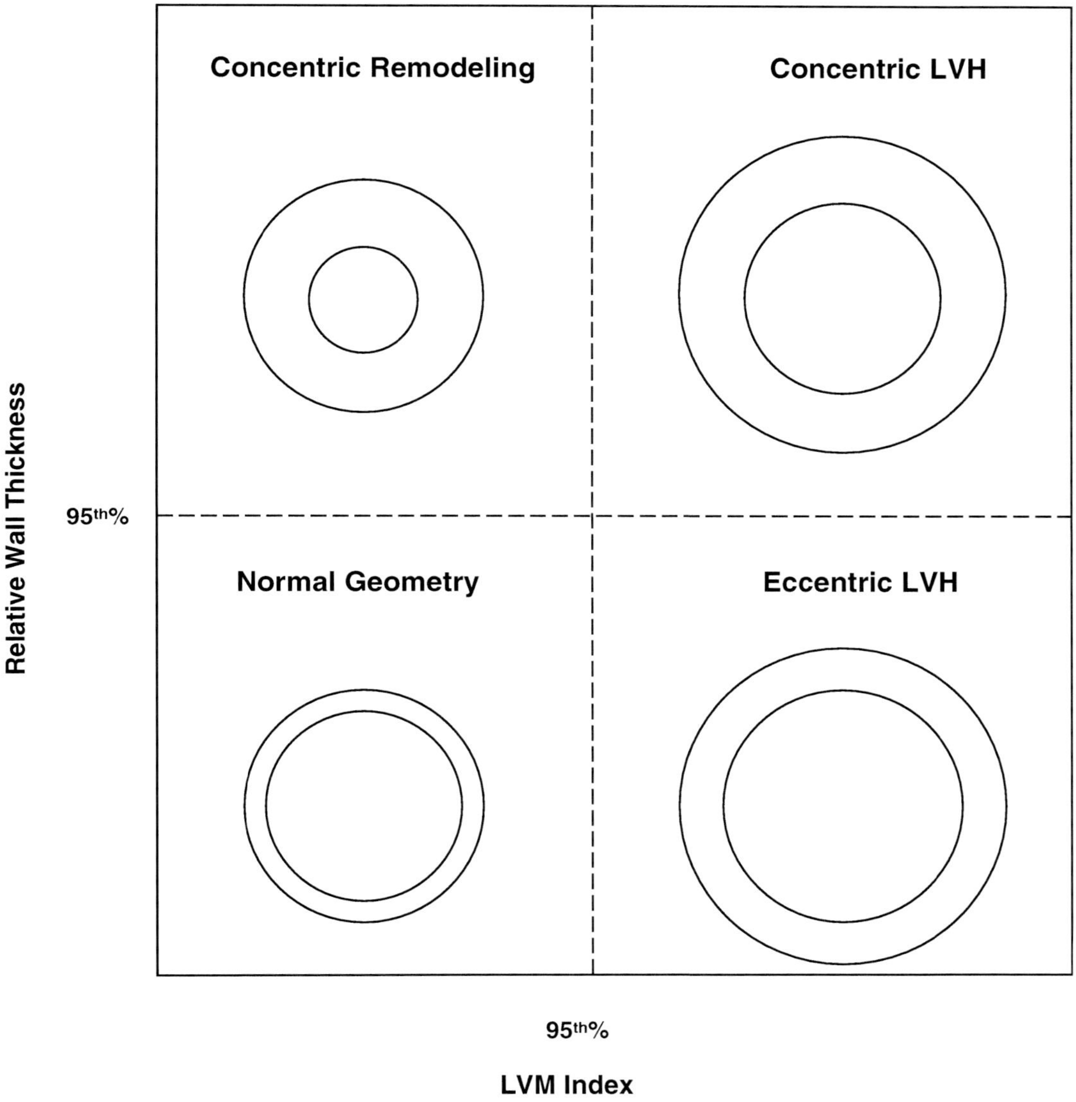

Fig. 61.8 LV geometry

Since the early 2000s there have been many studies around the world evaluating LVH in patients on maintenance **dialysis** and all indicated a much higher prevalence of LVH (40–80%) [18, 179–185] than in children prior to dialysis or after kidney transplantation. Small retrospective studies also suggest that with a better BP and volume control LVH regression might be achieved in young patients on dialysis [179, 180, 186]. The largest retrospective analysis from the International Pediatric Peritoneal Dialysis Network (IPPN), using height-age adjusted normative values for LVMI [175], demonstrated an overall LVH prevalence of 48.1% [187]. In the prospective analysis, the incidence of LVH developing *de novo* in patients with normal baseline LVM was 29%, and the incidence of regression from LVH to normal LVM 40% per year on PD. Transformation to and regression from concentric LV geometry occurred in 36% and 28% of the patients, respectively. Hypertension, high body mass index, use of continuous ambulatory peritoneal dialysis, renal disease other than hypo/dysplasia, and hyperparathyroidism were identified as independent predictors of LVH.

As in children prior to transplantation, most single-center pediatric studies indicate that LVH remains common (30–50%) **post-transplant** and relates to not adequately controlled blood pressure [181, 188–193]. A study from the Midwest Pediatric Nephrology Consortium (MWPNC) showed that LVH was significantly more common in those with metabolic syndrome (55%) than in those without (32%) [40]. In contrast to the above studies, some studies showed a significantly lower frequency of LVH. Englund et al. [194] reported the results of a longitudinal analysis of children who received renal transplants 10–20 years ago. Of 53 children who received a renal transplant between 1981 and 1991, 47 survived and were observed for 10 to 20 years. Before primary transplant, 51% of the 53 children were prescribed antihypertensive treatment. At the 10-year follow-up, echocardiography showed minor LVH in only two children with hypertension. No child without hypertension at 10 years showed LVH. Progressive aortic insufficiency was discovered in two children, one of whom had a supravalvular aortic aneurysm requiring surgical repair 10 years after transplant. Low prevalence of LVH post-transplant (4.5%) attributed to well-controlled ambulatory blood pressure was observed in a study by Balzano et al. [195].

There are have been few small studies assessing LVH status in children with CKD using cardiac MRI. In a study by Schaefer et al. [196], LVH has been demonstrated in 12 of 15 (80%) patients with CKD, while the prevalence of LVH was seven of 18 (39%) in the transplant patient group. Avendt et al. [197] found only 3 of 20 patients on maintenance dialysis and 1 of 18 patients post kidney transplant to have LVH. In the largest study to date (n = 120) utilizing cardiac MRI, Cheang et al. [198] demonstrated increased LV mass to volume ratio (MVR) in children with severe CKD suggesting LV concentric remodeling.

Left Ventricular Function and Pediatric CKD

In contrast to adults, in whom *systolic dysfunction* is frequently associated with early cardiac failure and decreased survival, in children with CKD systolic LV function is usually preserved [181, 199, 200]. The majority of pediatric studies have examined LV systolic performance using indices of performance which are dependent on loading conditions. This presents a major problem in patients with CKD or on dialysis because they may have substantial alteration of preload and afterload. A load independent index of contractility can be determined based on the relation between heart rate-corrected velocity of circumferential fiber shortening (VCF) and end-systolic wall stress (WS) by calculation of the difference between measured and predicted VCF for the calculated WS [201]. Using this index, Mitsnefes et al. [202] showed that children with CKD or on maintenance dialysis had increased LV contractility at rest. However, patients on dialysis had decreased contractile reserve during exercise, which might herald the development of a maladaptive stage of LVH. The mechanism of increased contractility in pediatric patients with CKD is not clear. The combination of increased heart rate, cardiac output and hypertension in these patients is consistent with a hyperdynamic circulation and suggests the possible role of sympathetic overactivity. Similar results were demonstrated in a more recent study by Gu et al. [203].

A study from the ESCAPE trial argues that subclinical systolic dysfunction is already present in predialysis children [204]. The authors analyzed LV shortening at the midwall level (midwall shortening [mS]), which more accurately reflects the contractile force independent of pathologic changes in LV geometry [205, 206]. Using this index, the study determined that the prevalence of subclinical systolic dysfunction as defined by impaired mS was more than fivefold higher in patients with CKD compared with control subjects (24.6 *versus* 4.5%; $P < 0.001$). Systolic dysfunction was most common (48%) in patients with concentric hypertrophy and associated with lower hemoglobin levels. The authors concluded that the combination of concentric LV geometry with midwall dysfunction might represent a cardiac phenotype designating an increased risk for development of overt CVD.

Additional, more novel and sensitive, assessments of cardiac systolic function, including strain and strain rate, have been shown to detect differences in function prior to ejection or shortening fraction in a variety of populations, such as Duchenne muscular dystrophy [207], sickle cell disease [208] and survivors of childhood acute leukemia [209]. An analysis of the 4C study showed a high prevalence of subclinical systolic dysfunction in children with CKD characterized by lower radial and circumferential LV strain paired with a mild cardiac systolic dyssynchrony [210].

Relatively few studies have assessed *LV diastolic function* in pediatric patients with CKD [181, 200, 211–214]. Doppler measurement of mitral inflow velocity has been the most widely used method to assess LV diastolic function. Unfortunately, the transmitral Doppler velocities and, therefore the E/A ratio, are affected by several factors, including left atrial pressure and preload. This is particularly important for patients with advanced CKD, since many of them are hypervolemic. Tissue Doppler Imaging (TDI) is a more reliable method to assess diastolic function in CKD patients since it is less load dependent and provides a more accurate measure of diastolic function. Studies employing TDI determined that children with CKD have abnormal diastolic function [211, 212]. In these studies, children on maintenance dialysis had significantly worse diastolic function than children with mild-to-moderate CKD or post-transplant. Poor diastolic function in patients on dialysis was associated with anemia, hyperphosphatemia, increased calcium-phosphorus ion product and LVH. Data from the 4C study demonstrated an independent association of worse E/e', a marker of LV compliance, with higher systolic BP and a

better E/e' z-score with RAS inhibition [214]. Recent data from the CKID study showed that 15% of participants had abnormally high E/e' ratio [215]. In adjusted analysis, a higher E/e' ratio was independently associated with ambulatory (sustained) hypertension, higher LVM index Z score, increased BMI Z score, lower hemoglobin, higher phosphorus level, and younger age. Casual blood pressure was not significantly associated with higher E/e'. These data indicated that ambulatory blood pressure might better identify children with CKD at risk for subclinical cardiac dysfunction than clinic blood pressure alone. Long-term significance of diastolic dysfunction in pediatric patients with CKD is not known. Longitudinal studies are necessary to determine if abnormal diastolic function predicts the development of systolic dysfunction and congestive heart failure in these patients.

Hothi et al. [216]. measured myocardial stunning as a marker of cardiac function in children on maintanence hemodialysis. Eleven of 12 patients developed myocardial stunning with varying degrees of compensatory hyperkinesis in unaffected segments, maintaining left ventricular ejection fraction throughout treatment. Recently, these authors evaluated regional LV function and mechanical synchronicity echographically by two-dimensional segmental longitudinal, circumferential and radial myocardial strain [217]. All patients were assessed pre-dialysis and at the end of dialysis. Radial strain was lower in uremic patients and increased during HD. Circumferential strain was preserved in uremic patients and fell during HD. Intrasegmental deformation synchronicity was progressively worse pre-dialysis and end of dialysis compared with controls. Some observations suggest that cardiac MRI and MR Spectroscopy could play a potentially useful role in the early detection and monitoring of cardiac dysfunction in children with CKD. Malatesta-Munter et al. [218] studied the biomarkers of cardiac function that included peak LV myocardial circumferential strain (Ecc) to assess regional LV function, T2 relaxation time to quantify myocardial structural composition, and phosphocreatinine/ATP (PCr/ATP) ratio from phosphorus-31 Magnetic Resonance Spectroscopy (^{31}P MRS) to assess muscle energy metabolism. This report demonstrated decreased Ecc (45%), decreased energy metabolism and abnormal myocardial micro-composition. These abnormalities were detected despite uniformly normal ejection fractions.

Clinical Approach to CVD in Children with CKD

The primary goal to prevent and minimize development of CVD in children with CKD is avoidance of long-term dialysis and preemptive transplantation if feasible. For those children who must have long-term dialysis, the strategy is directly linked to achievement of adequate dialysis outcomes, including aggressive monitoring and management of hypertension, dyslipidemia, mineral metabolism, anemia, nutrition, inflammation, and other dialysis complications. Unfortunately, achieving recommended Kt/V urea does not necessarily lead to control of the above problems. Epidemiologic data on cardiac death in both peritoneal dialysis and hemodialysis clearly indicate that current dialysis adequacy recommendations based on Kt/V are not adequate to decrease CVD morbidity in children with ESKD. Unlike in adults, there have been no randomized pediatric studies examining the role of more frequent or nocturnal hemodialysis in cardiac outcomes. However, small single-center studies of frequent or nocturnal dialysis indicate clinically important improvement in children' health including growth, hypertension, cardiac hypertrophy and function [219–222]. Hemodiafiltration (HDF) is also advocated as a preferred dialysis modality that might improve cardiovascular health in children with ESKD. Results from the HDF, Heart and Height (3H) study, a nonrandomized observational study comparing outcomes on conventional hemodialysis (HD) versus postdilution online HDF in children showed that HDF was associated with a lack

of progression in vascular measures versus progression with HD, as well as an increase in height not seen in the HD cohort [223]. The study also indicated improved patient-related outcomes among children on HDF correlating with improved BP control and clearances. Taking the potential for a longer and possibly more productive life, the benefits of HDF, more frequent and longer dialysis treatment might be more far reaching in children than in older adults [224].

Otherwise, management strategies should be specific to the stage of CKD (predialysis, dialysis, or transplant) as each has a unique subset of common risk factors. KDOQI and/or KDIGO recommendations for the management of most common individual CV risk factors are relatively recent but overall these guidelines are not based on strong evidence, especially when applied to children. For these reasons, the recommendations should always be tailored to the specific patient. Typically, separate recommendations are provided for advanced and end-stage kidney disease.

As in the general pediatric population, traditional risk factors like hypertension, dyslipidemia, and obesity should be a primary focus in CV risk reduction in children with CKD. In addition, evaluation and treatment of mineral metabolism abnormalities should be a prioritized focus of management.

Hypertension

The most recent 2012 KDIGO recommendations on BP control are restricted to non-dialysis (CKD and transplant) patients only [225]. These guidelines do not focus on methodological or diagnostic issues or lifestyle modification options to treat hypertension and are restricted to pharmacological treatment only. The recommendations are based on renal outcomes; however, because of the association of hypertension with LVH and increased cIMT, they can be reasonably applied to prevent and minimize CV outcomes. The BP targets refer to manual auscultatory BP. However, some of the recommendations are based on the results of studies utilizing ambulatory blood pressure monitoring. Since the publication of the 2012 KDIGO recommendations, there have been updated guidelines on management of BP in children from USA, Europe and Canada. While these updated guidelines are generally consistent with KDIGO recommendations, they are not identical. There are three main recommendations. First, KDIGO recommends initiation of BP lowering treatment when BP is consistently above the 90th percentile for age, sex, and height (1C level of evidence). This recommendation is consistent with the Canadian guidelines [226] but not with that of the 2017 AAP [172] or 2016 European Society of Hypertension (ESH) guidelines [227], which recommend starting BP medications if BP is consistently above the 95th percentile in the general pediatric population. The AAP 2017 also recommends using adult guidelines for initiating treatment (BP is >130/80 mmHg) for children aged 13 years and older. However, some of these patients might have small stature and may require a lower BP threshold to initiate treatment.

The second recommendation is to lower manually obtained clinic BP below 50th percentile for age, sex, and height, particularly for those children who have proteinuria (2D level of evidence). However, this recommendation is based on the results of the ESCAPE study even though the ESCAPE trial used mean arterial pressure from ABPM to classify BP [228]. A 2017 KDIGO controversy conference report on BP in kidney disease advised to revise this recommendation accordingly [229]. However, because ABPM is not widely available, the conference also recommended using oscillometric devices as an alternative.

The third recommendation is the use of ACEI or ARB irrespective of the level of proteinuria. Despite only 2D level of evidence, this recommendation is relatively well accepted by the pediatric nephrology community. The KDIGO guidelines are slightly different from the 2016 ESH guidelines [227]. Based largely on the ESCAPE trial results, ESH guidelines recommend that in children with CKD, BP targets

should be below the 50th percentile in the presence of proteinuria (the same as KDIGO) and below the 75th percentile (versus 90th percentile KDIGO) in the absence of proteinuria.

In the child on dialysis the presence of hypertension is mostly related to fluid overload, and attainment of dry weight will result in lowering of BP in the majority of patients. Dry weight and dialysis prescription need to be frequently adapted to avoid fluid overload induced hypertension. Thus, more frequent or prolonged dialysis sessions are the primary intervention to control hypertension. In addition, supportive measures aiming for a low extracellular volume as dietary salt restriction, low dialysate sodium content and restriction of fluid intake are important to complement an adequate dialysis prescription. The BP targets for dialysis patients are not as strict as for non-dialysis patients. The KDOQI guidelines recommend the BP target to be below the 95th percentile for age, sex, and height [230]. The KDIGO 2019 Controversy Conference on BP and volume management in dialysis addresses four major topics including BP measurement and targets, pharmacologic management, dialysis prescriptions as they relate to BP and volume and extracellular volume assessment and management with a focus on technology-based solutions; and volume-related patient symptoms and experiences [231].

Dyslipidemia

The latest guidelines for lipid screening and treatment in children with CKD by KDIGO published in 2013 recommend evaluation with a lipid profile (total cholesterol, LDL cholesterol, HDL cholesterol, triglycerides) in newly diagnosed CKD (including those treated with chronic dialysis or kidney transplantation) [232]. Management of dyslipidemia should include therapeutic lifestyle changes including dietary modification, weight reduction, increased physical activity, reducing alcohol intake, and treatment of hyperglycemia (if present), especially in overweight/obese children. In case of significant hypertriglyceridemia, dietary changes include a very low-fat diet (15% total calories), medium-chain triglycerides, and fish oils to replace some long-chain triglycerides. The initiation of statin therapy is based on a risk assessment and LDL-cholesterol level. Because children with CKD belong to a high level risk factor group, the statins are recommended at LDL-cholesterol level > 160 mg/dL. However, if there are additional moderate risks (e.g., hypertension, obesity, nephrotic syndrome as a cause of CKD), statins should be started at LDL-cholesterol >130 mg/dL. Given the lack of evidence for the benefit and safety of combination therapy with bile acid resins, colestipol and ezetimibe in pediatric CKD populations, the KDIGO Work Group does not recommend the use of such multi-drug regimens even in children with severely elevated LDL-C. Pharmacological treatment of hypertriglyceridemia with fibrates is not recommended in children with CKD because of concerns of developing pancreatitis.

Obesity and Physical Inactivity

Evidence from adult maintenance dialysis populations suggests a survival advantage conferred by higher BMI [233]; however, this appears to be limited to those with low body fat and high muscle mass [234]. Per KDOQI, "the safety and efficacy of weight loss in the overweight dialysis patient is unknown. Therefore, weight loss in the dialysis patients should be approached with close monitoring by a registered dietician and physician" [230]. However, increased levels of physical activity are encouraged to improve exercise capacity [235]. It is unknown whether obesity in children with ESKD confers survival benefits while on maintenance dialysis. For children with CKD prior to dialysis or post-transplant, treatment of obesity and maintenance of normal body habitus (BMI between fifth and 85th percentile for age, sex) is advisable. This recommendation is based on the evidence that obesity is associated with worse long-term outcomes. For example, it has been long known that severe childhood obesity is a significant risk factor for CKD in children and adults [237–239]. After pediatric renal

transplantation obesity is associated with higher rates of graft dysfunction and graft loss [239, 240]. Recommendations on management of obesity in CKD children should be individualized according to their age, physical tolerance, CKD stage, dialysis and co-morbidities and, as in the general pediatric population, include dietary modification, behavior modification and physical activity. Older adolescents with CKD, extreme obesity (BMI ≥ 40) and other comorbidities associated with long-term risks who failed to respond to dietary or behavior modifications may consider weight loss surgery.

Left Ventricular Hypertrophy

Overall, based on data that LVH is more frequent in children diagnosed with hypertension, it seems appropriate to perform echocardiography in children with CKD and in renal transplant recipients who have elevated casual BP and/or masked hypertension on ABPM. Echocardiography also should be considered in children with severe anemia. If LVH is diagnosed, periodic follow-up echocardiographic monitoring is suggested. Although not perfect, we suggest using the 2017 AAP CPG recommendations to diagnose LVH. Specifically, one can use the references of Khoury et al. [173] for children ≤8 years of age and a single cut off point of 51 $g/m^{2.7}$ for older children. If the child has a short stature, height age adjustment is warranted as described by Borzych et al. [175]. As we mentioned above in this chapter, alternative approach using a single cut off point of 45 $g/m^{2.16}$ to define LVH has recently been introduced and used in Europe [176].

Mineral and Bone Disorder

In clinical practice, the focus should be on maintaining serum phosphorus and calcium levels at age-appropriate normal range and on prevention of significant hyperparathyroidism and low vitamin D levels. The most recent KDIGO Clinical Practice Guideline Update for the Diagnosis,

Evaluation, Prevention, and Treatment of Chronic Kidney Disease–Mineral and Bone Disorder (CKD-MBD) [241] provides specific recommendations on timing of assessment and treatment options if abnormal markers of MBD are found (discussed in details in chap. 58). The dietary management of calcium and phosphate in children with CKD stages 2–5 and on dialysis is updated by recommendations from the Pediatric Renal Nutrition Taskforce [242].

Future

Since the first description of increased cardiovascular risk in children with CKD more than two decades ago, significant improvements have been achieved and guidelines have been developed to address individual cardiovascular risk factors. However, many recommendations are still based on opinion rather than on clear clinical evidence. Current and future longitudinal multicenter studies have the potential not only to monitor the implementation of treatment goals, but also to analyze the success in improving cardiovascular outcome in pediatric patients with CKD. Insights from these studies will also pose new questions which have to be brought from bedside to bench and vice versa, ultimately helping to continuously improve recommendations for each individual patient.

Acknowledgments We thank Dr. Uwe Querfeld for his contribution to this chapter in the first edition of the textbook.

References

1. Levey AS, et al. Controlling the epidemic of cardiovascular disease in chronic renal disease: what do we know? What do we need to learn? Where do we go from here? National Kidney Foundation Task Force on Cardiovascular Disease. Am J Kidney Dis. 1998;32(5):853–906.
2. Parekh RS, et al. Cardiovascular mortality in children and young adults with end-stage kidney disease. J Pediatr. 2002;141(2):191–7.
3. Mathews TJ, et al. Annual summary of vital statistics: 2008. Pediatrics. 2011;127(1):146–57.
4. McDonald SP, Craig JC. Long-term survival of children with end-stage renal disease. N Engl J Med. 2004;350(26):2654–62.
5. Groothoff JW, et al. Mortality and causes of death of end-stage renal disease in children: a Dutch cohort study. Kidney Int. 2002;61(2):621–9.
6. Oh J, et al. Advanced coronary and carotid arteriopathy in young adults with childhood-onset chronic renal failure. Circulation. 2002;106(1):100–5.
7. U.S.Renal Data System. USRDS 2000 Annual Data Report. Bethesda: The National Institutes of Health, National Institute of Diabetes and Digestive and Kindney Diseases; 2000.
8. Offner G, et al. Kidney transplanted children come of age. Kidney Int. 1999;55(4):1509–17.
9. Briese S, et al. Arterial and cardiac disease in young adults with childhood-onset end-stage renal disease-impact of calcium and vitamin D therapy. Nephrol Dial Transplant. 2006;21(7):1906–14.
10. Foster BJ, et al. Change in mortality risk over time in young kidney transplant recipients. Am J Transplant. 2011;11(11):2432–42.
11. Mitsnefes MM, et al. Mortality risk among children initially treated with dialysis for end-stage kidney disease, 1990–2010. JAMA. 2013;309(18):1921–9.
12. Modi ZJ, et al. Risk of cardiovascular disease and mortality in young adults with end-stage renal disease: an analysis of the US Renal Data System. JAMA Cardiol. 2019;4(4):353–62.
13. Ku E, et al. Trends in cardiovascular mortality among a cohort of children and young adults starting dialysis in 1995 to 2015. JAMA Netw Open. 2020;3(9):e2016197.
14. US Renal Data System: USRDS 2020 annual data report:ESRDamongchildrenandadolescents.https://adr.usrds.org/2020/end-stage-renal-disease/7-%20esrd-among-children-and-adolescents.
15. Kavey RE, et al. Cardiovascular risk reduction in high-risk pediatric patients: a scientific statement from the American Heart Association Expert Panel on Population and Prevention Science; the Councils on Cardiovascular Disease in the Young, Epidemiology and Prevention, Nutrition, Physical Activity and Metabolism, High Blood Pressure Research, Cardiovascular Nursing, and the Kidney in Heart Disease; and the Interdisciplinary Working Group on Quality of Care and Outcomes Research: endorsed by the American Academy of Pediatrics. Circulation. 2006;114(24):2710–38.
16. de Ferranti SD, et al. Cardiovascular risk reduction in high-risk pediatric patients: a scientific statement from the American Heart Association. Circulation. 2019;139(13):e603–34.
17. Maron BJ. Sudden death in young athletes. N Engl J Med. 2003;349(11):1064–75.
18. Mitsnefes MM, et al. Severe left ventricular hypertrophy in pediatric dialysis: prevalence and predictors. Pediatr Nephrol. 2000;14(10–11):898–902.
19. Mitsnefes MM, et al. Severe cardiac hypertrophy and long-term dialysis: the Midwest Pediatric

Nephrology Consortium study. Pediatr Nephrol. 2006;21(8):1167–70.

20. US Renal Data System: USRDS 2020 Annual Data Report: Mortality and causes of death. https://adr. usrds.org/2020/end-stage-renal-disease/5-mortality.

21. Nakamura S, et al. Prediction of coronary artery disease and cardiac events using electrocardiographic changes during hemodialysis. Am J Kidney Dis. 2000;36(3):592–9.

22. Shaw LJ, et al. Insights from the NHLBI-Sponsored Women's Ischemia Syndrome Evaluation (WISE) Study: Part I: gender differences in traditional and novel risk factors, symptom evaluation, and gender-optimized diagnostic strategies. J Am Coll Cardiol. 2006;47(Suppl. 3):S4–S20.

23. Barletta GM, et al. Heart rate and blood pressure variability in children with chronic kidney disease: a report from the CKiD study. Pediatr Nephrol. 2014;29(6):1059–65.

24. Yusuf S, et al. Effect of potentially modifiable risk factors associated with myocardial infarction in 52 countries (the INTERHEART study): case-control study. Lancet. 2004;364(9438):937–52.

25. Luke RG. Chronic renal failure--a vasculopathic state. N Engl J Med. 1998;339(12):841–3.

26. Muntner P, et al. Traditional and nontraditional risk factors predict coronary heart disease in chronic kidney disease: results from the atherosclerosis risk in communities study. J Am Soc Nephrol. 2005;16(2):529–38.

27. Zoccali C. Traditional and emerging cardiovascular and renal risk factors: an epidemiologic perspective. Kidney Int. 2006;70(1):26–33.

28. Zoccali C, et al. Adipose tissue cytokines, insulin sensitivity, inflammation, and cardiovascular outcomes in end-stage renal disease patients. J Ren Nutr. 2005;15(1):125–30.

29. Querfeld U. The clinical significance of vascular calcification in young patients with end-stage renal disease. Pediatr Nephrol. 2004;19(5):478–84.

30. Flynn JT, et al. Blood pressure in children with chronic kidney disease: a report from the Chronic Kidney Disease in Children study. Hypertension. 2008;52(4):631–7.

31. Mitsnefes M, et al. Masked hypertension associates with left ventricular hypertrophy in children with CKD. J Am Soc Nephrol. 2010;21(1):137–44.

32. Kogon AJ, et al. Nephrotic-range proteinuria is strongly associated with poor blood pressure control in pediatric chronic kidney disease. Kidney Int. 2014;85(4):938–44.

33. Barletta G, Pierce C, Mitsnefes M, Samuels J, Warady B, Furth S, Flynn J. Are blood pressure indices improving in children with chronic kidney disease? A period analysis. ASN Kidney Week. 2016;

34. Reynolds BC, et al. Association of time-varying blood pressure with chronic kidney disease progression in children. JAMA Netw Open. 2020;3(2):e1921213.

35. Saland JM, et al. Dyslipidemia in children with chronic kidney disease. Kidney Int. 2010;78(11):1154–63.

36. Saland JM, et al. Change in dyslipidemia with declining glomerular filtration rate and increasing proteinuria in children with CKD. Clin J Am Soc Nephrol. 2019;14(12):1711–8.

37. Baek HS, et al. Dyslipidemia in pediatric CKD patients: results from KNOW-PedCKD (KoreaN cohort study for Outcomes in patients With Pediatric CKD). Pediatr Nephrol. 2020;35(8):1455–61.

38. Wilson AC, et al. Prevalence and correlates of multiple cardiovascular risk factors in children with chronic kidney disease. Clin J Am Soc Nephrol. 2011;6(12):2759–65.

39. Lalan S, et al. Cardiometabolic risk factors, metabolic syndrome, and chronic kidney disease progression in children. J Pediatr. 2018;202:163–70.

40. Wilson AC, et al. High prevalence of the metabolic syndrome and associated left ventricular hypertrophy in pediatric renal transplant recipients. Pediatr Transplant. 2010;14(1):52–60.

41. Furth SL, et al. Metabolic abnormalities, cardiovascular disease risk factors, and GFR decline in children with chronic kidney disease. Clin J Am Soc Nephrol. 2011;6(9):2132–40.

42. Atkinson MA, et al. Risk for anemia in pediatric chronic kidney disease patients: a report of NAPRTCS. Pediatr Nephrol. 2010;25(9):1699–706.

43. Furth SL, et al. Estimating time to ESRD in children with CKD. Am J Kidney Dis. 2018;71(6):783–92.

44. Lee KH, et al. Anemia and iron deficiency in children with Chronic Kidney Disease (CKD): data from the know-ped CKD study. J Clin Med. 2019;8(2)

45. Borzych-Duzalka D, et al. Management of anemia in children receiving chronic peritoneal dialysis. J Am Soc Nephrol. 2013;24(4):665–76.

46. Warady BA, Ho M. Morbidity and mortality in children with anemia at initiation of dialysis. Pediatr Nephrol. 2003;18(10):1055–62.

47. Querfeld U. Cardiovascular considerations of pediatric ESRD. In: Warady B, Schaefer F, Fine R, Alexander S, editors. Pediatric dialysis. Dordrecht/Boston/London: Kluwer Academic Publishers; 2004. p. 353–67.

48. Furth SL, et al. Design and methods of the Chronic Kidney Disease in Children (CKiD) prospective cohort study. Clin J Am Soc Nephrol. 2006;1(5):1006–15.

49. Querfeld U, et al. The Cardiovascular Comorbidity in Children with Chronic Kidney Disease (4C) study: objectives, design, and methodology. Clin J Am Soc Nephrol. 2010;5(9):1642–8.

50. Braun J, et al. Electron beam computed tomography in the evaluation of cardiac calcification in chronic dialysis patients. Am J Kidney Dis. 1996;27(3):394–401.

51. Civilibal M, et al. Coronary artery calcifications in children with end-stage renal disease. Pediatr Nephrol. 2006;21(10):1426–33.

52. Civilibal M, et al. Progression of coronary calcification in pediatric chronic kidney disease stage 5. Pediatr Nephrol. 2009;24(3):555–63.

53. Ishitani MB, et al. Early subclinical coronary artery calcification in young adults who were pediatric kidney transplant recipients. Am J Transplant. 2005;5(7):1689–93.

54. Srivaths PR, et al. Malnutrition-inflammation-coronary calcification in pediatric patients receiving chronic hemodialysis. Hemodial Int. 2010;14(3):263–9.

55. Srivaths PR, et al. Elevated FGF 23 and phosphorus are associated with coronary calcification in hemodialysis patients. Pediatr Nephrol. 2011;26(6):945–51.

56. Srivaths PR, et al. High serum phosphorus and FGF 23 levels are associated with progression of coronary calcifications. Pediatr Nephrol. 2014;29(1):103–9.

57. Goodman WG, et al. Coronary-artery calcification in young adults with end-stage renal disease who are undergoing dialysis. N Engl J Med. 2000;342(20):1478–83.

58. Shroff RC, et al. Mineral metabolism and vascular damage in children on dialysis. J Am Soc Nephrol. 2007;18(11):2996–3003.

59. Touboul PJ, et al. Mannheim carotid intima-media thickness consensus (2004–2006). An update on behalf of the Advisory Board of the 3rd and 4th Watching the Risk Symposium, 13th and 15th European Stroke Conferences, Mannheim, Germany, 2004, and Brussels, Belgium, 2006. Cerebrovasc Dis. 2007;23(1):75–80.

60. Lorenz MW, et al. Prediction of clinical cardiovascular events with carotid intima-media thickness: a systematic review and meta-analysis. Circulation. 2007;115(4):459–67.

61. Urbina EM, et al. Noninvasive assessment of subclinical atherosclerosis in children and adolescents: recommendations for standard assessment for clinical research: a scientific statement from the American Heart Association. Hypertension. 2009;54(5):919–50.

62. Greenland P, et al. Prevention Conference V: Beyond secondary prevention: identifying the high-risk patient for primary prevention: noninvasive tests of atherosclerotic burden: Writing Group III. Circulation. 2000;101(1):E16–22.

63. Jourdan C, et al. Normative values for intima-media thickness and distensibility of large arteries in healthy adolescents. J Hypertens. 2005;23(9):1707–15.

64. Doyon A, et al. Carotid artery intima-media thickness and distensibility in children and adolescents: reference values and role of body dimensions. Hypertension. 2013;62(3):550–6.

65. Mitsnefes MM, et al. Cardiac and vascular adaptation in pediatric patients with chronic kidney disease: role of calcium-phosphorus metabolism. J Am Soc Nephrol. 2005;16(9):2796–803.

66. Litwin M, et al. Altered morphologic properties of large arteries in children with chronic renal failure and after renal transplantation. J Am Soc Nephrol. 2005;16(5):1494–500.

67. Brady TM, et al. Carotid intima-media thickness in children with CKD: results from the CKiD study. Clin J Am Soc Nephrol. 2012;7(12):1930–7.

68. Schaefer F, et al. Cardiovascular phenotypes in children with CKD: the 4C study. Clin J Am Soc Nephrol. 2017;12(1):19–28.

69. Garcia-Bello JA, et al. Carotid intima media thickness, oxidative stress, and inflammation in children with chronic kidney disease. Pediatr Nephrol. 2013;

70. Shroff R, et al. A bimodal association of vitamin D levels and vascular disease in children on dialysis. J Am Soc Nephrol. 2008;19(6):1239–46.

71. Al Nasser Y, et al. Subclinical cardiovascular changes in pediatric solid organ transplant recipients: a systematic review and meta-analysis. Pediatr Transplant. 2016;20(4):530–9.

72. Borchert-Morlins B, et al. Factors associated with cardiovascular target organ damage in children after renal transplantation. Pediatr Nephrol. 2017;32(11):2143–54.

73. Chavarria LA, et al. Intima media thickness in children undergoing dialysis. Pediatr Nephrol. 2012;27(9):1557–64.

74. Litwin M, et al. Evolution of large-vessel arteriopathy in paediatric patients with chronic kidney disease. Nephrol Dial Transplant. 2008;23(8):2552–7.

75. Schmidt BMW, et al. Early effects of renal replacement therapy on cardiovascular comorbidity in children with end-stage kidney disease: findings from the 4C-T study. Transplantation. 2018;102(3):484–92.

76. Blacher J, et al. Impact of aortic stiffness on survival in end-stage renal disease. Circulation. 1999;99(18):2434–9.

77. Covic A, et al. Increased arterial stiffness in children on haemodialysis. Nephrol Dial Transplant. 2006;21(3):729–35.

78. Savant JD, et al. Vascular stiffness in children with chronic kidney disease. Hypertension. 2017;69(5):863–9.

79. Kis E, et al. Pulse wave velocity in end-stage renal disease: influence of age and body dimensions. Pediatr Res. 2008;63(1):95–8.

80. Shroff R, et al. Effect of haemodiafiltration vs conventional haemodialysis on growth and cardiovascular outcomes in children—the HDF, heart and height (3H) study. BMC Nephrol. 2018;19(1):199.

81. Azukaitis K, et al. Pathophysiology and consequences of arterial stiffness in children with chronic kidney disease. Pediatr Nephrol. 2021;36(7):1683–95.

82. Sugianto RI, et al. Insights from the 4C-T study suggest increased cardiovascular burden in girls with end stage kidney disease before and after kidney transplantation. Kidney Int. 2021; https://doi.org/10.1016/j.kint.2021.11.032. Epub ahead of print. , 2021. S0085–2538(21)01163–7. Epub ahead of print

83. Makulska I, et al. The importance of fetuin-A in vascular calcification in children with chronic kidney disease. Adv Clin Exp Med. 2019;28(4):499–505.

84. Kis E, et al. Effects of bone and mineral metabolism on arterial elasticity in chronic renal failure. Pediatr Nephrol. 2009;24(12):2413–20.

85. Shroff RC, et al. The circulating calcification inhibitors, fetuin-A and osteoprotegerin, but not matrix Gla protein, are associated with vascular stiffness and calcification in children on dialysis. Nephrol Dial Transplant. 2008;23(10):3263–71.

86. Holle J, et al. Indoxyl sulfate associates with cardiovascular phenotype in children with chronic kidney disease. Pediatr Nephrol. 2019;34(12):2571–82.

87. Shroff R, et al. HDL in children with CKD promotes endothelial dysfunction and an abnormal vascular phenotype. J Am Soc Nephrol. 2014;25(11):2658–68.

88. Simonetti GD, et al. Ambulatory arterial stiffness index is increased in hypertensive childhood disease. Pediatr Res. 2008;64(3):303–7.

89. Degi A, et al. Ambulatory arterial stiffness index in children after kidney transplantation. Pediatr Transplant. 2013;17(7):598–604.

90. Mitsnefes MM. Ambulatory arterial stiffness index: Is there an additional value to characterize cardiovascular risk in children with kidney transplant? Pediatr Transplant. 2013;17(7):595–7.

91. Corretti MC, et al. Guidelines for the ultrasound assessment of endothelial-dependent flow-mediated vasodilation of the brachial artery: a report of the International Brachial Artery Reactivity Task Force. J Am Coll Cardiol. 2002;39(2):257–65.

92. De Roos NM, et al. Within-subject variability of flow-mediated vasodilation of the brachial artery in healthy men and women: implications for experimental studies. Ultrasound Med Biol. 2003;29(3):401–6.

93. Moody WE, et al. Endothelial dysfunction and cardiovascular disease in early-stage chronic kidney disease: cause or association? Atherosclerosis. 2012;223(1):86–94.

94. Yilmaz MI, et al. Vascular health, systemic inflammation and progressive reduction in kidney function; clinical determinants and impact on cardiovascular outcomes. Nephrol Dial Transplant. 2011;26(11):3537–43.

95. Wilson AC, et al. Flow-mediated vasodilatation of the brachial artery in children with chronic kidney disease. Pediatr Nephrol. 2008;23(8):1297–302.

96. Hussein G, et al. Doppler assessment of brachial artery flow as a measure of endothelial dysfunction in pediatric chronic renal failure. Pediatr Nephrol. 2008;23(11):2025–30.

97. Muscheites J, et al. Assessment of the cardiovascular system in pediatric chronic kidney disease: a pilot study. Pediatr Nephrol. 2008;23(12):2233–9.

98. Ruben S, et al. Impaired microcirculation in children after kidney transplantation: everolimus versus mycophenolate based immunosuppression regimen. Kidney Blood Press Res. 2018;43(3):793–806.

99. Shanahan CM. Mechanisms of vascular calcification in CKD-evidence for premature ageing? Nat Rev Nephrol. 2013;9(11):661–70.

100. Kidney disease: improving global outcomes (KDIGO) CKD-MBD Work Group. KDIGO clinical practice guideline for the diagnosis, evaluation, prevention, and treatment of Chronic Kidney Disease-Mineral and Bone Disorder (CKD-MBD). Kidney Int Suppl. 2009;S1–130.

101. Reynolds JL, et al. Human vascular smooth muscle cells undergo vesicle-mediated calcification in response to changes in extracellular calcium and phosphate concentrations: a potential mechanism for accelerated vascular calcification in ESRD. J Am Soc Nephrol. 2004;15(11):2857–67.

102. Shroff R, Long DA, Shanahan C. Mechanistic insights into vascular calcification in CKD. J Am Soc Nephrol. 2013;24(2):179–89.

103. Speer MY, et al. Runx2/Cbfa1, but not loss of myocardin, is required for smooth muscle cell lineage reprogramming toward osteochondrogenesis. J Cell Biochem. 2010;110(4):935–47.

104. Shroff RC, et al. Chronic mineral dysregulation promotes vascular smooth muscle cell adaptation and extracellular matrix calcification. J Am Soc Nephrol. 2010;21(1):103–12.

105. Shroff RC, et al. Dialysis accelerates medial vascular calcification in part by triggering smooth muscle cell apoptosis. Circulation. 2008;118(17):1748–57.

106. Siomou E, Stefanidis CJ. FGF-23 in children with CKD: a new player in the development of CKD-mineral and bone disorder. Nephrol Dial Transplant. 2012;27(12):4259–62.

107. Hu MC, Kuro-o M, Moe OW. Klotho and chronic kidney disease. Contrib Nephrol. 2013;180:47–63.

108. Lim K, et al. Vascular Klotho deficiency potentiates the development of human artery calcification and mediates resistance to fibroblast growth factor 23. Circulation. 2012;125(18):2243–55.

109. Fang Y, et al. Early chronic kidney disease-mineral bone disorder stimulates vascular calcification. Kidney Int. 2014;85(1):142–50.

110. Hu MC, et al. Klotho deficiency causes vascular calcification in chronic kidney disease. J Am Soc Nephrol. 2011;22(1):124–36.

111. Gutierrez OM, et al. Fibroblast growth factor 23 and mortality among patients undergoing hemodialysis. N Engl J Med. 2008;359(6):584–92.

112. Jimbo R, et al. Fibroblast growth factor 23 accelerates phosphate-induced vascular calcification in the absence of Klotho deficiency. Kidney Int. 2013;

113. Scialla JJ, et al. Fibroblast growth factor 23 is not associated with and does not induce arterial calcification. Kidney Int. 2013;83(6):1159–68.

114. Sarmento-Dias M, et al. Fibroblast growth factor 23 is associated with left ventricular hypertrophy, not with uremic vasculopathy in peritoneal dialysis patients. Clin Nephrol. 2016;85(3):135–41.

115. Yilmaz MI, et al. FGF-23 and vascular dysfunction in patients with stage 3 and 4 chronic kidney disease. Kidney Int. 2010;78(7):679–85.

116. Block GA, et al. Effects of phosphate binders in moderate CKD. J Am Soc Nephrol. 2012;23(8): 1407–15.

117. Zebger-Gong H, et al. 1,25-Dihydroxyvitamin D3-induced aortic calcifications in experimental uremia: up-regulation of osteoblast markers, calcium-transporting proteins and osterix. J Hypertens. 2011;29(2):339–48.

118. O'Neill WC. Pyrophosphate, alkaline phosphatase, and vascular calcification. Circ Res. 2006;99(2):e2.

119. Lau WL, et al. Vitamin D receptor agonists increase klotho and osteopontin while decreasing aortic calcification in mice with chronic kidney disease fed a high phosphate diet. Kidney Int. 2012;82(12):1261–70.

120. Yao Y, et al. Inhibition of bone morphogenetic proteins protects against atherosclerosis and vascular calcification. Circ Res. 2010;107(4):485–94.

121. Schoppet M, et al. Exploring the biology of vascular calcification in chronic kidney disease: what's circulating? Kidney Int. 2008;73(4):384–90.

122. van Summeren MJ, et al. Circulating calcification inhibitors and vascular properties in children after renal transplantation. Pediatr Nephrol. 2008;23(6):985–93.

123. Heiss A, et al. Hierarchical role of fetuin-A and acidic serum proteins in the formation and stabilization of calcium phosphate particles. J Biol Chem. 2008;283(21):14815–25.

124. Schaible J, et al. Serum fetuin-A and vitamin D in children with mild-to-severe chronic kidney disease: a cross-sectional study. Nephrol Dial Transplant. 2012;27(3):1107–13.

125. Muteliefu G, et al. Indoxyl sulfate promotes vascular smooth muscle cell senescence with upregulation of p53, p21, and prelamin A through oxidative stress. Am J Physiol Cell Physiol. 2012;303(2):C126–34.

126. Liu Y, et al. Prelamin A accelerates vascular calcification via activation of the DNA damage response and senescence-associated secretory phenotype in vascular smooth muscle cells. Circ Res. 2013;112(10):e99–109.

127. Yao Y, et al. A role for the endothelium in vascular calcification. Circ Res. 2013;113(5):495–504.

128. Homocysteine Studies Collaboration. Homocysteine and risk of ischemic heart disease and stroke: a meta-analysis. JAMA. 2002;288:2015–22.

129. Jourde-Chiche, N., et al., Vascular incompetence in dialysis patients--protein-bound uremic toxins and endothelial dysfunction. Semin Dial, 2011. 24(3): p. 327–337.

130. Robinson K, et al. Hyperhomocysteinemia confers an independent increased risk of atherosclerosis in end-stage renal disease and is closely linked to plasma folate and pyridoxine concentrations. Circulation. 1996;94(11):2743–8.

131. Wald DS, Law M, Morris JK. Homocysteine and cardiovascular disease: evidence on causality from a meta-analysis. BMJ. 2002;325(7374):1202.

132. Jamison RL, et al. Effect of homocysteine lowering on mortality and vascular disease in advanced chronic kidney disease and end-stage renal disease: a randomized controlled trial. JAMA. 2007;298(10):1163–70.

133. Toole JF, et al. Lowering homocysteine in patients with ischemic stroke to prevent recurrent stroke, myocardial infarction, and death: the Vitamin Intervention for Stroke Prevention (VISP) randomized controlled trial. JAMA. 2004;291(5):565–75.

134. Bazzano LA, et al. Effect of folic acid supplementation on risk of cardiovascular diseases: a meta-analysis of randomized controlled trials. JAMA. 2006;296(22):2720–6.

135. Maron BA, Loscalzo J. The treatment of hyperhomocysteinemia. Annu Rev Med. 2009;60:39–54.

136. Vallance P, et al. Accumulation of an endogenous inhibitor of nitric oxide synthesis in chronic renal failure. Lancet. 1992;339(8793):572–5.

137. Wilcox CS. Asymmetric dimethylarginine and reactive oxygen species: unwelcome twin visitors to the cardiovascular and kidney disease tables. Hypertension. 2012;59(2):375–81.

138. Kielstein JT, et al. Cardiovascular effects of systemic nitric oxide synthase inhibition with asymmetrical dimethylarginine in humans. Circulation. 2004;109(2):172–7.

139. Kuo HC, Hsu CN, Huang CF, Lo MH, Chien SJ, Tain YL. Urinary arginine methylation index associated with ambulatory blood pressure abnormalities in children with chronic kidney disease. J Am Soc Hypertens. 2012;6:385–92.

140. Liabeuf S, et al. Free p-cresylsulphate is a predictor of mortality in patients at different stages of chronic kidney disease. Nephrol Dial Transplant. 2010;25(4):1183–91.

141. Barreto FC, et al. Serum indoxyl sulfate is associated with vascular disease and mortality in chronic kidney disease patients. Clin J Am Soc Nephrol. 2009;4(10):1551–8.

142. Holle J, et al. Serum indoxyl sulfate concentrations associate with progression of chronic kidney disease in children. PLoS One. 2020;15(10):e0240446.

143. Cohn JN, Ferrari R, Sharpe N. Cardiac remodeling-concepts and clinical implications: a consensus paper from an international forum on cardiac remodeling. Behalf of an International Forum on Cardiac Remodeling. J Am Coll Cardiol. 2000;35(3):569–82.

144. Swynghedauw B. Molecular mechanisms of myocardial remodeling. Physiol Rev. 1999;79(1):215–62.

145. Mishra S, Kass DA. Cellular and molecular pathobiology of heart failure with preserved ejection fraction. Nat Rev Cardiol. 2021;18(6):400–23. Online ahead of print

146. London GM, Parfrey PS. Cardiac disease in chronic uremia: pathogenesis. Adv Ren Replace Ther. 1997;4(3):194–211.

147. Guerin AP, et al. Cardiovascular disease in renal failure. Minerva Urol Nefrol. 2004;56(3):279–88.

148. Wang X, Shapiro JI. Evolving concepts in the pathogenesis of uraemic cardiomyopathy. Nat Rev Nephrol. 2019;15(3):159–75.

149. Portale AA, et al. Disordered FGF23 and mineral metabolism in children with CKD. Clin J Am Soc Nephrol. 2014;9(2):344–53.

150. Isakova T, et al. Fibroblast growth factor 23 is elevated before parathyroid hormone and phosphate in chronic kidney disease. Kidney Int. 2011;79(12):1370–8.

151. Isakova T, et al. Fibroblast growth factor 23 and risks of mortality and end-stage renal disease in patients with chronic kidney disease. JAMA. 2011;305(23):2432–9.

152. Scialla JJ, et al. Fibroblast growth factor-23 and cardiovascular events in CKD. J Am Soc Nephrol. 2014;25(2):349–60.

153. Gutierrez OM, et al. Fibroblast growth factor 23 and left ventricular hypertrophy in chronic kidney disease. Circulation. 2009;119(19):2545–52.

154. Faul C, et al. FGF23 induces left ventricular hypertrophy. J Clin Invest. 2011;121(11):4393–408.

155. Grabner A, et al. Activation of cardiac fibroblast growth factor receptor 4 causes left ventricular hypertrophy. Cell Metab. 2015;22(6):1020–32.

156. Leifheit-Nestler M, et al. Induction of cardiac FGF23/FGFR4 expression is associated with left ventricular hypertrophy in patients with chronic kidney disease. Nephrol Dial Transplant. 2016;31(7): 1088–99.

157. Mitsnefes MM, et al. FGF23 and left ventricular hypertrophy in children with CKD. Clin J Am Soc Nephrol. 2018;13(1):45–52.

158. Zhou YT, et al. Lipotoxic heart disease in obese rats: implications for human obesity. Proc Natl Acad Sci U S A. 2000;97(4):1784–9.

159. Sharma S, et al. Intramyocardial lipid accumulation in the failing human heart resembles the lipotoxic rat heart. FASEB J. 2004;18(14):1692–700.

160. Mitsnefes MM, et al. Plasma glucosylceramides and cardiovascular risk in incident hemodialysis patients. J Clin Lipidol. 2018;12(6):1513–1522 e4.

161. Winterberg PD, et al. T Cells play a causal role in diastolic dysfunction during uremic cardiomyopathy. J Am Soc Nephrol. 2019;

162. Stein NR, et al. Associations between cardiac biomarkers and cardiac structure and function in CKD. Kidney Int Rep. 2020;5(7):1052–60.

163. Amann K, et al. Reduced capillary density in the myocardium of uremic rats--a stereological study. Kidney Int. 1992;42(5):1079–85.

164. Tyralla K, Amann K. Morphology of the heart and arteries in renal failure. Kidney Int Suppl. 2003;84:S80–3.

165. Park M, et al. Associations between kidney function and subclinical cardiac abnormalities in CKD. J Am Soc Nephrol. 2012;23(10):1725–34.

166. Silberberg JS, et al. Impact of left ventricular hypertrophy on survival in end-stage renal disease. Kidney Int. 1989;36(2):286–90.

167. Foley RN, et al. The prognostic importance of left ventricular geometry in uremic cardiomyopathy. J Am Soc Nephrol. 1995;5(12):2024–31.

168. Devereux RB, Reichek N. Echocardiographic determination of left ventricular mass in man. Anatomic validation of the method. Circulation. 1977;55(4):613–8.

169. de Simone G, et al. Left ventricular mass and body size in normotensive children and adults: assessment of allometric relations and impact of overweight. J Am Coll Cardiol. 1992;20(5):1251–60.

170. Daniels SR, et al. Echocardiographically determined left ventricular mass index in normal children, adolescents and young adults. J Am Coll Cardiol. 1988;12(3):703–8.

171. de Simone G, et al. Effect of growth on variability of left ventricular mass: assessment of allometric signals in adults and children and their capacity to predict cardiovascular risk. J Am Coll Cardiol. 1995;25(5):1056–62.

172. Flynn JT, et al. Clinical practice guideline for screening and management of high blood pressure in children and adolescents. Pediatrics. 2017;140(3)

173. Khoury PR, et al. Age-specific reference intervals for indexed left ventricular mass in children. J Am Soc Echocardiogr. 2009;22(6):709–14.

174. Foster BJ, et al. A novel method of expressing left ventricular mass relative to body size in children. Circulation. 2008;117(21):2769–75.

175. Borzych D, et al. Defining left ventricular hypertrophy in children on peritoneal dialysis. Clin J Am Soc Nephrol. 2011;6(8):1934–43.

176. Chinali M, et al. Left ventricular mass indexing in infants, children, and adolescents: a simplified approach for the identification of left ventricular hypertrophy in clinical practice. J Pediatr. 2016;170:193–8.

177. Sarikouch S, et al. Sex-specific pediatric percentiles for ventricular size and mass as reference values for cardiac MRI: assessment by steady-state free-precession and phase-contrast MRI flow. Circ Cardiovasc Imaging. 2010;3(1):65–76.

178. Kupferman JC, et al. BP Control and left ventricular hypertrophy regression in children with CKD. J Am Soc Nephrol. 2013;

179. Mitsnefes MM, et al. Changes in left ventricular mass in children and adolescents during chronic dialysis. Pediatr Nephrol. 2001;16(4):318–23.

180. Ulinski T, et al. Reduction of left ventricular hypertrophy in children undergoing hemodialysis. Pediatr Nephrol. 2006;21(8):1171–8.

181. Johnstone LM, et al. Left ventricular abnormalities in children, adolescents and young adults with renal disease. Kidney Int. 1996;50(3):998–1006.

182. Morris KP, et al. Cardiac abnormalities in end stage renal failure and anaemia. Arch Dis Child. 1993;68(5):637–43.

183. O'Regan S, et al. Echocardiographic assessment of cardiac function in children with chronic renal failure. Kidney Int Suppl. 1983;15:S77–82.

184. Palcoux JB, et al. Echocardiographic patterns in infants and children with chronic renal failure. Int J Pediatr Nephrol. 1982;3(4):311–4.

185. Drukker A, Urbach J, Glaser J. Hypertrophic cardiomyopathy in children with end-stage renal disease and hypertension. Proc Eur Dial Transplant Assoc. 1981;18:542–7.
186. Melhem N, et al. Improved blood pressure and left ventricular remodelling in children on chronic intermittent haemodialysis: a longitudinal study. Pediatr Nephrol. 2019;34(10):1811–20.
187. Bakkaloglu SA, et al. Cardiac geometry in children receiving chronic peritoneal dialysis: findings from the international pediatric peritoneal dialysis network (IPPN) registry. Clin J Am Soc Nephrol. 2011;6(8):1926–33.
188. Matteucci MC, et al. Left ventricular hypertrophy, treadmill tests, and 24-hour blood pressure in pediatric transplant patients. Kidney Int. 1999;56(4):1566–70.
189. Morgan H, et al. Ambulatory blood pressure monitoring after renal transplantation in children. Pediatr Nephrol. 2001;16(11):843–7.
190. Mitsnefes MM, et al. Changes in left ventricular mass index in children and adolescents after renal transplantation. Pediatr Transplant. 2001;5(4):279–84.
191. El-Husseini AA, et al. Echocardiographic changes and risk factors for left ventricular hypertrophy in children and adolescents after renal transplantation. Pediatr Transplant. 2004;8(3):249–54.
192. Kitzmueller E, et al. Changes of blood pressure and left ventricular mass in pediatric renal transplantation. Pediatr Nephrol. 2004;19(12):1385–9.
193. Pais P, et al. Nocturnal hypertension and left ventricular hypertrophy in pediatric renal transplant recipients in South India. Pediatr Transplant. 2020;24(4):e13710.
194. Englund M, Berg U, Tyden G. A longitudinal study of children who received renal transplants 10–20 years ago. Transplantation. 2003;76(2):311–8.
195. Balzano R, et al. Use of annual ABPM, and repeated carotid scan and echocardiography to monitor cardiovascular health over nine yr in pediatric and young adult renal transplant recipients. Pediatr Transplant. 2011;15(6):635–41.
196. Schaefer B, et al. Cardiac magnetic resonance imaging in children with chronic kidney disease and renal transplantation. Pediatr Transplant. 2012;16(4):350–6.
197. Avendt MB, Taylor MD, Mitsnefes MM. Cardiac MRI assessment in children and young adults with end-stage renal disease. Clin Nephrol. 2018;90(3):172–9.
198. Cheang MH, et al. A comprehensive characterization of myocardial and vascular phenotype in pediatric chronic kidney disease using cardiovascular magnetic resonance imaging. J Cardiovasc Magn Reson. 2018;20(1):24.
199. Colan SD, et al. Left ventricular mechanics and contractile state in children and young adults with end-stage renal disease: effect of dialysis and renal transplantation. J Am Coll Cardiol. 1987;10(5):1085–94.
200. Goren A, Glaser J, Drukker A. Diastolic function in children and adolescents on dialysis and after kidney transplantation: an echocardiographic assessment. Pediatr Nephrol. 1993;7(6):725–8.
201. Colan SD, Borow KM, Neumann A. Left ventricular end-systolic wall stress-velocity of fiber shortening relation: a load-independent index of myocardial contractility. J Am Coll Cardiol. 1984;4(4):715–24.
202. Mitsnefes MM, et al. Left ventricular mass and systolic performance in pediatric patients with chronic renal failure. Circulation. 2003;107(6):864–8.
203. Gu H, et al. Elevated ejection-phase myocardial wall stress in children with chronic kidney disease. Hypertension. 2015;66(4):823–9.
204. Chinali M, et al. Reduced systolic myocardial function in children with chronic renal insufficiency. J Am Soc Nephrol. 2007;18(2):593–8.
205. de Simone G, et al. Assessment of left ventricular function by the midwall fractional shortening/end-systolic stress relation in human hypertension. J Am Coll Cardiol. 1994;23(6):1444–51.
206. de Simone G, et al. Left ventricular chamber and wall mechanics in the presence of concentric geometry. J Hypertens. 1999;17(7):1001–6.
207. Amedro P, et al. Speckle-tracking echocardiography in children with duchenne muscular dystrophy: a prospective multicenter controlled cross-sectional study. J Am Soc Echocardiogr. 2019;32(3):412–22.
208. Whipple NS, et al. Ventricular global longitudinal strain is altered in children with sickle cell disease. Br J Haematol. 2018;183(5):796–806.
209. Corella Aznar EG, et al. Use of speckle tracking in the evaluation of late subclinical myocardial damage in survivors of childhood acute leukaemia. Int J Cardiovasc Imaging. 2018;34(9):1373–81.
210. Chinali M, et al. Advanced parameters of cardiac mechanics in children with CKD: the 4C study. Clin J Am Soc Nephrol. 2015;10(8):1357–63.
211. Mitsnefes MM, et al. Impaired left ventricular diastolic function in children with chronic renal failure. Kidney Int. 2004;65(4):1461–6.
212. Mitsnefes MM, et al. Abnormal cardiac function in children after renal transplantation. Am J Kidney Dis. 2004;43(4):721–6.
213. Simpson JM, et al. Systolic and diastolic ventricular function assessed by tissue Doppler imaging in children with chronic kidney disease. Echocardiography. 2013;30(3):331–7.
214. Doyon A, et al. impaired systolic and diastolic left ventricular function in children with chronic kidney disease: results from the 4C study. Sci Rep. 2019;9(1):11462.
215. Mitsnefes MM, et al. Diastolic function and ambulatory hypertension in children with chronic kidney disease. Hypertension. 2021;78(5):1347–54.
216. Hothi DK, et al. Pediatric myocardial stunning underscores the cardiac toxicity of conventional hemodialysis treatments. Clin J Am Soc Nephrol. 2009;4(4):790–7.

217. Hothi DK, et al. Hemodialysis-induced acute myo-cardial dyssynchronous impairment in children. Nephron Clin Pract. 2013;123(1–2):83–92.

218. Malatesta-Muncher R, et al. Early cardiac dysfunction in pediatric patients on maintenance dialysis and post kidney transplant. Pediatr Nephrol. 2012;27(7):1157–64.

219. Fischbach M, et al. Daily on-line haemodiafiltration: a pilot trial in children. Nephrol Dial Transplant. 2004;19(9):2360–7.

220. Hoppe, A., et al., A hospital-based intermittent nocturnal hemodialysis program for children and adolescents. J Pediatr, 2011. 158(1): p. 95–9, 99 e1.

221. Fischbach M, et al. Daily on line haemodiafiltration promotes catch-up growth in children on chronic dialysis. Nephrol Dial Transplant. 2010;25(3):867–73.

222. Laskin BL, et al. Short, frequent, 5-days-per-week, in-center hemodialysis versus 3-days-per week treatment: a randomized crossover pilot trial through the Midwest Pediatric Nephrology Consortium. Pediatr Nephrol. 2017;32(8):1423–32.

223. Shroff R, et al. Effects of hemodiafiltration versus conventional hemodialysis in children with ESKD: the HDF, heart and height study. J Am Soc Nephrol. 2019;30(4):678–91.

224. Lacson E Jr, Lazarus M. Dialysis time: does it matter? A reappraisal of existing literature. Curr Opin Nephrol Hypertens. 2011;20(2):189–94.

225. Taler SJ, et al. KDOQI US commentary on the 2012 KDIGO clinical practice guideline for management of blood pressure in CKD. Am J Kidney Dis. 2013;62(2):201–13.

226. Nerenberg KA, et al. 1. Can J Cardiol. 2018;34(5):506–25.

227. Lurbe E, et al. 2016 European Society of Hypertension guidelines for the management of high blood pressure in children and adolescents. J Hypertens. 2016;34(10):1887–920.

228. Wuhl E, et al. Strict blood-pressure control and progression of renal failure in children. N Engl J Med. 2009;361(17):1639–50.

229. Cheung AK, et al. Blood pressure in chronic kidney disease: conclusions from a Kidney Disease: Improving Global Outcomes (KDIGO) Controversies Conference. Kidney Int. 2019;95(5):1027–36.

230. K/DOQI clinical practice guidelines for cardiovascular disease in dialysis patients. Am J Kidney Dis. 2005;45(4 Suppl 3):S1–153.

231. Flythe JE, et al. Blood pressure and volume management in dialysis: conclusions from a Kidney Disease: Improving Global Outcomes (KDIGO) Controversies Conference. Kidney Int. 2020;97(5):861–76.

232. KDIGO clinical practice guideline for lipid management in chronic kidney disease. Kidney Int Suppl. 2013;3(3):259–305.

233. Hakim RM, Lowrie E. Obesity and mortality in ESRD: is it good to be fat? Kidney Int. 1999;55(4):1580–1.

234. Nishizawa Y, Shoji T, Ishimura E. Body composition and cardiovascular risk in hemodialysis patients. J Ren Nutr. 2006;16(3):241–4.

235. Goldstein SL, Montgomery LR. A pilot study of twice-weekly exercise during hemodialysis in children. Pediatr Nephrol. 2009;24(4):833–9.

236. Gunta SS, Mak RH. Is obesity a risk factor for chronic kidney disease in children? Pediatr Nephrol. 2013;28(10):1949–56.

237. Inge TH, et al. perioperative outcomes of adolescents undergoing bariatric surgery: the Teen-Longitudinal Assessment of Bariatric Surgery (Teen-LABS) Study. JAMA Pediatr. 2013;

238. Vivante A, et al. Body mass index in 1.2 million adolescents and risk for end-stage renal disease. Arch Intern Med. 2012;172(21):1644–50.

239. Mitsnefes MM, Khoury P, McEnery PT. Body mass index and allograft function in pediatric renal transplantation. Pediatr Nephrol. 2002;17(7):535–9.

240. Hanevold CD, et al. Obesity and renal transplant outcome: a report of the North American Pediatric Renal Transplant Cooperative Study. Pediatrics. 2005;115(2):352–6.

241. KDIGO. Clinical practice guideline update for the diagnosis, evaluation, prevention, and treatment of chronic kidney disease–mineral and bone disorder (CKD-MBD). Kidney Int Suppl. 2017;2017(7):1–59.

242. McAlister L, et al. The dietary management of calcium and phosphate in children with CKD stages 2-5 and on dialysis-clinical practice recommendation from the Pediatric Renal Nutrition Taskforce. Pediatr Nephrol. 2020;35(3):501–18.

Ethical Issues in End Stage Kidney Disease

62

Aaron Wightman and Michael Freeman

Introduction

Since the development of pediatric nephrology as a discipline in the twentieth century, we have experienced a progressive expansion of our capabilities in caring for children with significant kidney disease. As treatments improved, patients and their families have been asked to choose from a wider array of treatments, and decisions to pursue or forgo those interventions have acquired greater ethical weight. Moreover, as care of children with kidney disease is provided within the context of health care systems and policies on a regional, national, and international level, the ethics of medical care must be considered with a broader lens than simply doing "what is best" for our individual patients. In this chapter we will review both the structures of contemporary bioethics as it applies to decisions made by patients and their families, as well as some of the current areas of ethical concern within pediatric nephrology.

A. Wightman (✉)
Department of Pediatrics, University of Washington School of Medicine, Seattle Children's Hospital, Seattle, WA, USA
e-mail: Aaron.Wightman@seattlechildrens.org

M. Freeman
Departments of Pediatrics and Humanities, Penn State College of Medicine, Penn State Hershey Children's Hospital, Hershey, PA, USA
e-mail: mfreeman3@pennstatehealth.psu.edu

Contemporary Bioethics and the Limits of Parental Decision-Making

When providing care to a competent adult, there is a strong presumption that the decisions made by the patient should direct care. While it is true that factors such as the clinician's assessment of what might be beneficial or harmful to the patient, as well as broader system issues regarding resource availability may also play a role, the wishes of the patient are generally paramount. This framework of medical decision-making is derived from an understanding that individual adults have both a right to dictate the care that they receive based on a fundamental respect for bodily integrity and are in the best position to assess how a given treatment course will support their own goals and values [1]. In contrast, by nature of the fact that they are continuing to grow and develop, children are assumed to lack a long-standing system of values or the appropriate understanding of the implications of a given treatment decision. As such, there is a long-standing tradition of deference to parental decisions in pediatric care.

Although parents are generally considered the primary decision-makers in the pediatric setting, their authority is not absolute. Both the child, as well as society more broadly, have an interest in the child's well-being. This is reflected across laws in numerous countries that place limits on parental activities such as corporal punishment, and mandate that parents provide for children's basic needs, including nutrition, education, and health care [2, 3]. While the details of these laws are shaped by local custom and other social aspects, they reflect an acknowledgement that the community has an obligation to provide for children given their vulnerable state. Within the context of healthcare, this raises the possibility of significant conflict when a decision made by a patient and their family is incompatible with what the clinician thinks would be most beneficial to the patient.

Historically, when these conflicts have arisen, they have been resolved by an assessment of what would broadly be considered in the child's best interest [4]. Within bioethics, the best interest standard requires a decision-maker to consider the child's present and future self-regarding interests alone and select the treatment that maximizes benefit and minimizes harms [4]. While the best interests standard is well suited to conflicts when the risks and benefits of each treatment course are clearly disproportionate (such as a decision to forgo antibiotic therapy for bacterial pyelonephritis), there are other instances in which the determination of what is "best" is dependent on highly personalized assessment of the relative value of different factors. In a more complicated case, such as dialysis for a preterm infant, it is entirely possible that parents and clinicians may consider the same risks and benefits of treatment and reach different conclusions on what is "best." Additionally, children have a variety of physical, intellectual, social and emotional interests and a precise determining what actions "best" support these interests may not be possible. Finally, the best interest standard fails to acknowledge that we do not typically require that parents do what is absolutely "best" for children in all circumstances. Given the varied obligations that parents have to themselves, their children, and their community this would be impossible.

Instead of seeking to overrule parental authority for decisions that are not in the best interests of the child, Diekema argues such actions should be reserved for parental choices, generally refus-

als, that place a child at clear risk of significant harm [5]. The harm principle allows for the differing values that parents may place on benefits and burdens of treatment options when compared to the opinions of medical professionals, but does not allow for parents to refuse a treatment in which serious, imminent harm is expected to occur and where there is a reasonable intervention that could avoid that harm [5]. The best interest standard and harm principle were further operationalized through the concept of the zone of parental discretion, which sought to highlight the range of choices parents may make so long as they do not exceed a harm threshold [6]. Although the concept of "best-interest" is frequently referenced in the clinical setting, there is broad consensus within the field of pediatric ethics that in complex medical decision-making, such as the care of children with chronic kidney disease (CKD), the best interests standard is better considered aspirational to guide decision-making and the harm principle is better reserved for situations where clinicians must consider overruling parental authority [7].

Ethical Issues in Dialysis and ESRD

Withholding, Withdrawal, and Forgoing Dialysis Treatment

There is no universally accepted criterion for forgoing life-sustaining treatments such as dialysis. Decisions concerning withholding or withdrawing dialysis remain a source of controversy and distress for children, their families, and nephrologists. Withdrawal of dialysis is common among adults on dialysis, accounting for approximately one quarter of deaths among dialysis patients in the United States. Withdrawal of life-sustaining treatments is also a leading cause of death in neonatal and pediatric intensive care units [8, 9]. Less is known about withholding or withdrawal of dialysis treatment for children, although one analysis of French-speaking pediatric nephrology centers from 1995–2001 found 50 cases where dialysis was withheld or withdrawn among

440 children with end-stage kidney disease (11.5%) [10]. The most common reasons for withdrawal included concerns of subsequent quality of life, severe neurological handicap, and consequences of the disease on the family [10].

Decisions made to forgo dialysis should be individualized, shared, and consistent with the interests of the child and the benefits and burdens resulting from renal replacement therapy or compassionate conservative treatment [11]. Choices should reflect the patient and family's goals of care that are achievable and be centered upon the patient's quality of life [11–13]. Four concepts that may influence decisions to forgo dialysis treatment include: perception of moral difference between withholding and withdrawing treatment, the technological imperative, futility, and time-limited trials of therapy.

Withholding, Withdrawal, Equivalence

Withholding dialysis is defined as foregoing dialysis in a patient for whom dialysis has yet to be initiated (i.e. never starting). Withdrawal of dialysis means the discontinuation and forgoing of ongoing dialysis therapy (i.e. stopping after dialysis has been started or attempted). Both situations are similar in that life-sustaining treatments are possible but are not provided.

A series of surveys of pediatric specialists, intensivists, neonatologists, general practitioners, intensivists, and palliative care specialists have shown that many clinicians do not feel that decisions to withhold and withdraw life-sustaining treatments are morally the same [14–18]. Clinicians may sense that withdrawing dialysis or other life sustaining-treatments feels more distressing than never starting. This may reflect a perception of greater moral agency, responsibility, and culpability on the part of the healthcare provider for a patient's death associated with withdrawal of treatment (commission) vs. never initiating treatment (omission). There is a tendency to describe a situation in which treatment has begun as "the train has left the station" and

cannot be stopped [19]. Other clinicians may sense it is more problematic to withhold rather than to withdraw a life-sustaining treatment like dialysis. For example, Ladin and colleagues found that many adult nephrologists do not routinely discuss withholding dialysis treatment with elderly patients for fear of missing out on potentially beneficial therapy, being perceived as abandoning the patient or not providing care, and concern that withholding dialysis did not represent an "active" option [20]. Others have argued that withholding a life-sustaining treatment like dialysis precludes the possibility of an unexpected recovery and denies an opportunity to learn more about the benefits and burdens of therapy and the patient's prognosis. If dialysis is initiated and later withdrawn, the treatment is forgone only after its lack of utility has been confirmed [21].

Nephrologists' perceptions of a moral difference between withholding and withdrawing dialysis may result in negative consequences for patients. Implicit belief that withholding is preferable to withdrawing can create an "up front barrier" to appropriate treatment which may result in both inappropriate under treatment (reticence to begin therapy due to concerns of being trapped by biomedical technology that once begun cannot be stopped) and overtreatment (failure to withdraw harmful treatment once started) [22, 23]. Overtreatment may result in waste of limited medical and financial resources by insisting on a therapy that is no longer beneficial or desirable for the patient [22–24]. Others who feel withholding dialysis is more problematic than withdrawal may require all patients to undergo dialysis treatment, as withholding precludes a dying patient of a chance, even if extremely limited, of benefitting from dialysis treatment. While this approach offers the opportunity for unlikely patients to benefit, it would result in suffering for the majority who will not benefit and significant waste of resources by providing treatment unlikely to be beneficial [21, 25, 26].

It is generally accepted that there is no ethical distinction between withholding and withdrawing life-sustaining treatments, even if there may be an emotional distinction for patient, family and the medical team [1, 11, 19, 23]. The equivalence thesis is an important concept in understanding these difficult cases. The equivalence thesis holds that all other things being equal, if it is permissible to withhold a medical treatment for a patient, it is also permissible to withdraw the same treatment and vice versa [27, 28]. Both not initiating and stopping life-sustaining therapy can be justified, depending upon the circumstances. Both can be instances of allowing to die, and both can be instances of killing [27, 28]. In situations where the physician has a clear duty to treat, omission of treatment by withholding or withdrawing violates that duty. Conversely, if there is no a clear duty to treat, then both withholding and withdrawing could be considered to be permissible [27, 29]. Given the consequences that arise from implicit beliefs of moral differences between withholding and withdrawing, nephrologists would be better served to combine the concepts into a single term, foregoing.

Technological Imperative

The technological imperative may influence pediatric nephrologists reluctance to forgo dialysis treatment [30]. The technological imperative has been suggested as something which is imprinted on physicians early in training: the drive to use the best, most modern and most high-tech interventions because they are available [31]. It may be best understood at its core as "That which is possible to do must be done" [32]. Pediatric nephrologists are well trained in the technical aspects of dialysis, but are less well trained in holding back, declining to offer therapy when the burdens outweigh the benefits or when a patient or family does not want the treatment. Recognizing that the technological imperative that is a natural part of pediatric nephrology may help clinicians when faced with a patient or family who desire to forgo medically available treatment. The technological imperative should not be allowed to stand in the way of shared decision-making, as it sometimes is just as powerful to leave a tool unused.

Futility

When considering life-sustaining treatments such as dialysis, nephrologists may be tempted to claim that treatment should not be provide because it is futile. Futility is a tool used by clinicians to make a unilateral decision to forgo a treatment because the treatment cannot produce the benefit that the patient or family seek [33]. In this sense a claim of futility is extremely powerful because if a treatment is futile not only is there no duty for clinicians to perform it, but there may also be a duty not to perform it. In spite of this, futility has important limitations that generally preclude its use in pediatric nephrology. The greatest limitation of futility is that it has many different meanings to clinicians, families, patients, and society [33]. Generally, three definitions of futility are most often utilized [34]. First, physiologic futility is a claim that the treatment cannot produce the benefit sought. A classic example is treating a viral infection with antibiotics. Antibiotics cannot accomplish the goal of treating viral infection. In contrast the goal of dialysis treatment is to improve fluid and metabolic balance. If access can be obtained and BP is sufficient, dialysis will almost always improve fluid and metabolic balance. Therefore, dialysis is unlikely to be physiologically futile. Second, quantitative futility is a claim that, while it is possible the treatment may produce the benefit sought, it is so unlikely as to not be worth it. In proposing this definition, Schneiderman and colleagues ask clinicians to reflect on the last 100 similar patients or the published literature [35]. If chance of failure is >99%, then the treatment is futile. For dialysis, if access can be obtained and blood pressure managed this threshold is very rarely achieved. Third, qualitative futility is a judgement that while a treatment has a reasonable prospect of producing the benefit sought it isn't worthwhile all things considered. This judgement does not reflect clinical expertise or medical judgement and instead is a cost/benefit analysis informed by the goals of care which are typically determined by the patient or their parents with the input of clinicians rather by clinicians alone.

The purpose of this discussion is not to claim that in every instance dialysis should be pursued; rather, that futility is an inappropriate reason not to do so. The assessment of benefit in such cases goes beyond whether dialysis will provide metabolic clearance and ultrafiltration to more global questions focused on quality of life for the patient. These considerations are inherently value-based and should be determined by the child's informed parents except when there is reason to believe that the parents are not acting as appropriate decision makers for the child [12, 33, 36].

Time-Limited Trial of Therapy

In the setting of uncertainty or discordance between a treating team or between treating team and family, a time-limited trial is sometimes considered as a third option in addition to initiating or forgoing life-sustaining treatments like dialysis [24, 37, 38]. A time-limited trial is an agreement between care providers and surrogate decision-makers to provide a medical therapy over a defined period of time to determine if the patient improves or deteriorates according to agreed-upon objective clinical outcomes [37]. Time-limited trials offer potential benefits of alleviating the burden of decision-making in the setting of uncertainty, avoiding interprofessional conflict, and providing support for patients, their families, and clinicians. A trial of dialysis therapy may allow for further information to be gathered about the benefits and burdens of dialysis without committing the child to a lifetime of renal replacement therapy [11, 38, 39]. Yet, when considering life-sustaining treatments such as dialysis unlikely to meet a physiologic definition of futility, time-limited trials have important limitations. These include the arbitrary duration of a trial, use of value-laden considerations as "objective" outcomes, and concern that parents may have a different understanding of a "trial" than clinicians. With the exception of some neonates, most children with chronic kidney failure will require some form of renal replacement therapy for the remainder of their lives. As the treatment is life-long, any time duration of a trial is arbitrary. Seemingly objective outcome often considered in a time-limited trial of dialysis include factors such as dialysis catheter failure, peritonitis, extubation, or neural imaging findings. Catheter failure and peritonitis are relatively common and treatable complications of dialysis treatment and thus do not seem to describe failure of dialysis treatment. Rather than being objective, outcomes such as extubation or neuroimaging findings instead reflect implicit assessments of the quality of a life on chronic mechanical ventilation or with a neurodevelopmental disability. This is an example of a technical criteria fallacy in which inherently value based decisions are medicalized without engagement in the key ethical arguments that would justify their use [40]. Finally, parents may have a different conception of a trial of a life-sustaining treatment like dialysis. Parents have described a "trial" of therapy as treatment until a complication arose where it was clear that the burdens of continued treatment (generally pain) outweighed the benefits of continued treatment; otherwise, treatment continues indefinitely [24, 41]. This is a reasonable assessment, but is a description of initiating treatment, not a trial. Treating teams and families should continually reassess whether the benefits of any treatment outweigh its burdens and whether the treatment continues to support the patient's goals of care. For an efficacious life-sustaining treatment like dialysis, nephrologists are better suited to avoid discussion of time-limited trials and instead focus on initiation or forgoing treatment with the understanding that such a decision should be continually revisited in light of the benefits and burdens experienced by the child [10, 24].

Palliative Care

Discussion about initiation or forgoing life-sustaining treatments like dialysis and transplant can feel dichotomous in nature. It is important to recognize that relationships between patients, families, and clinicians are not. This means duties to care and support patients, families, and colleagues persist regardless of any decision made about life-sustaining treatments and intensification of palliative treatments should occur in conjunction with any decision to forgo life-sustaining treatments [42]. This highlights the importance of continued care including palliative care.

Pediatric palliative care strives to (1) relieve physical, psychological, social, practical, and existential suffering, (2) improve quality of life, (3) facilitate decision-making, and (4) assist with care coordination for children with life-threatening or life-shortening conditions [43–47]. Even in resource-limited health system settings, the Worldwide Palliative Care Alliance identifies early integration of palliative care as a human right for children [48]. While initially limited to patients with terminal illnesses such as children with kidney failure where renal replacement treatments were forgone, pediatric societies increasingly recommend PPC for all children with a "life-threatening" condition [43, 44, 45, 47, 49] This encompasses children with life-limiting conditions, where cure is not possible, and children with life-threatening conditions, where cure is possible and disease-directed treatments are ongoing [43–45, 47, 49] Importantly, most, if not all, children with advanced CKD fall into one of those two groups [47, 50].

CKD is an incurable, life-long and life-shortening condition which imposes significant burdens on children and their families. Children with kidney failure receiving dialysis treatment or who received a kidney transplant experience poorer health-related quality of life (HRQoL) compared to healthy peers and peers with other chronic illnesses [51–57]. CKD negatively affects mental health and well-being including high rates of depression and anxiety [58–60]. Further, pain needs of children with CKD may go under recognized. For example a multicenter study utilizing the Patient Reported Outcomes Measurement Information System (PROMIS) demonstrated that about half of children with CKD, regardless of stage or transplant history, experienced pain within the last week interfering with daily activities [61]. Children with CKD also experience impaired sleep, with studies showing high rates of sleep disturbances in children with non-

dialysis dependent (37%) and dialysis dependent CKD (86%) [62, 63]. The importance of recognizing and developing strategies to address these burdens was highlighted by a recent qualitative study in which adolescents with CKD shared their desire that outcomes such as fatigue, lifestyle restrictions, and physical activity be prioritized [64].

To date, utilization of pediatric palliative care for children with CKD and their families has been limited [27, 65, 66]. This calls for future clinical and research efforts to integrate palliative care into the care of children with CKD similar to the evolution in practice in adult nephrology and other pediatric chronic diseases [47, 67, 68–70].

Ethical Issues in Kidney Transplantation

Consideration of Quality of Life in Transplant Decisions

Some have argued that transplant listing decisions should consider degree of improvement in quality of life that can be expected from transplant rather than expected graft and patient survival [71]. The net effect would be to prioritize children without intellectual disabilities as transplant candidates. Indeed, survey data suggests many pediatric kidney transplant programs do consider cognition as criterion for kidney transplant and may utilize different considerations for potential candidates with intellectual disabilities [72, 73]. These approaches appear to lack empiric support. Graft and recipient survival following kidney transplant do not appear to be notably different between recipients with and without intellectual disability [74]. Further, a successful kidney transplant improves the quality of life for children with kidney failure regardless of level of cognition [75, 76]. Rather than focusing on relative degree of improvement in quality of life that can be expected from a transplant, nephrologists are better suited to reflect on whether of whether the potential recipient would benefit sufficiently relative to the burdens that transplantation would pose.

Assessment of Adherence

Transplant organs remain an inherently scarce resource. As such, within the transplant system there is a strong emphasis on avoiding circumstances expected to result in premature graft loss. Assessment of a potential recipient's adherence to treatment recommendations is part of that process and referral to transplantation may be delayed or denied due to concerns of non-adherence [77]. There is evidence that non-adherence is common in the pediatric kidney disease population, particularly among adolescents [78–80]. Potentially as a result of this phenomenon, older adolescents and young adults demonstrate a markedly increased rate of graft failure as compared to both younger children and older adults [81].

While adherence is a critical for a transplant recipient to be successful, there are important limitations in applying concerns about non-adherence to clinical practice. Physicians' ability to predict the future adherence of their patients are quite limited [82, 83]. Further, patients who are members of minority population are more likely to be judged to be non-adherent [84, 85]. This is of particular significance, as many of the studies that have sought to describe factors that might predict non-adherence rely, at least in part, on healthcare provider's assessment of non-adherence [80, 86]. These same studies have frequently identified psychosocial risk factors as predictive of non-adherence, including gender, ethnic background, being a member of a single parent household, and socio-economic status [86, 87]. Given the subjectivity of many assessments of non-adherence, particularly in disease states where more 'objective' markers of adherence such as drug levels are not routinely followed, it becomes readily apparent how this can represent a vicious cycle. Patients who are socially disadvantaged by these psycho-social criteria may be more likely to experience delays or denial in transplant due to concerns regarding adherence or be judged to be non-adherent following transplant. This in turn has the potential to reinforce existing biases and disparities in care.

Acknowledgement of these concerns is not meant to be an argument against the inclusion of assessments of adherence and social support within the transplant process. Instead, nephrologists should be aware of the limitations of their ability to assess these factors and incorporate this uncertainty into the relative weight placed on these factors in decisions.

Assessments of Alcohol and Other Substance Use

A recent study of pediatric transplant programs suggest that substance use by potential pediatric transplant recipients remains a concern for clinicians and in some cases sobriety or cessation therapy is a requirement for listing a patient for organ transplantation [88]. Unfortunately, substance use is very common among adolescents with chronic illness. In a recent study of youth in the US with a variety of chronic illnesses, 36.5% of high school students reported alcohol use and 20% reported marijuana use [89]. Similar to studies of the broader adolescent population in the US [90]. Population level studies in a variety of other countries demonstrate prevalent adolescent substance use as well [91, 92].

In pediatric populations, studies suggest a correlation between substance use behaviors and non-adherence to medical regiments [89, 93]. Studies assessing the influence of alcohol and other substance use on post-transplant outcomes among adults have been mixed, but are broadly indicative of worse outcomes, at least among heavy substance users [94–98]. As such, consideration of substance use among potential pediatric transplant recipients is a valid concern in considering post-transplant outcomes. Unfortunately, many pediatric transplant programs lack clear policies regarding substance use in transplant referral and listing decisions [88]. In a recent study of transplant center practices, the majority of programs did not routinely or universally use urine or blood toxicology screening to assess for substance use, instead utilizing this testing only in circumstances of clinician suspicion of substance use or in the setting of patient self-report [88]. This approach is not reliable due to the limitations of self-report of substance use by adolescents in the clinical setting [99, 100] and pediatric clinician's limited ability to assess substance use by clinical impression alone [100].

From an ethical standpoint, the use of screening approaches that are neither standardized nor universal increases the risk of clinician bias influencing the selection of patients that require more intensive screening. While research suggests that substance use in pediatrics may increase the risk of a poor transplant outcome as compared to a control population, it is important to acknowledge that many transplant candidates may be at greater risk of poorer transplant outcome than their peers due to a variety of factors such as their underlying disease [101], concurrent illnesses [81], and age at transplantation [81]. Undue emphasis on "risk" arising from substance use (as opposed to other categories) may perpetuate existing racial, ethnic and psychosocial biases in transplant care.

Justice and Broader Social Concerns in Pediatric Kidney Care

Caregiver Burden

Pediatric CKD affects not only the child, but their family and community. Caregiver burden is a multidimensional construct reflecting an individual's perception of overload during the caregiving process in one or more of four perspectives: physical, psychological, social, and financial [102]. While caregiver burdens may be greatest for younger children and those with more advanced kidney disease, they are experienced caring for all children at all levels of CKD [64, 103–108, 109]. At its most significant, caregivers (particularly mothers) experience extraordinary burdens which, in some circumstances exceed their available physical, financial, or psychological resources so they are unable to meet their duties to themselves or to others for whom they are responsible [64, 103–105, 110, 111]. This experience has been reported by caregivers throughout the world and is influenced by the available social resources within each country [105]. Patients also express concern over caregiver burden. In a recent study, adolescents and young adults with kidney disease expressed guilt over the stress and burdens that their treatment imposed upon their families [64].

In light of the severity of the burdens experienced by at least some caregivers and the concern for caregiving demands voiced by adolescents and young adults, it seems cruel and unjust for nephrologists not to discuss expected burdens with parents. This raises challenging ethical questions, including how clinicians and parents could or should incorporate considerations of caregiver burden into medical decision-making for a child with kidney disease. Where caregiving burden is significant, it is possible a treatment choice may be in the best interest of a child, but not in the best interest of other children in the family, the family as a whole, or the community. Yet, the dominant frameworks of pediatric medical decision-making utilize the best interest standard, which focuses exclusively on the self-regarding interests of the child when weighing treatment options. Such frameworks seek to highlight the primacy of the needs of the child, protect the child from exploitation by those more powerful, and hold that a child's basic needs must always be met [5, 112, 113]. While intuitively appealing, such a stance overlooks that parents, siblings, and other caregivers are also moral agents with finite resources and pragmatically that even in the wealthiest countries public resources may be insufficient to meet the needs of children with kidney disease and their families [105]. Yet it seems unfair for societal failures to support children and families to fall exclusively on the vulnerable child with kidney disease. The ethical tension between the needs of the child, other members of the family, and community in a setting of constrained resources does not offer a ready solution. It highlights a gap in the current ethical framework of pediatric medical decision-making. Recognition of caregiver burden calls for advocacy from the pediatric nephrology community to appeal for greater supports for children and their families, but also for nephrologists to recognize the situation their patient and their patient's families find themselves.

Racism, Disparities and Structural Injustices

Social determinants play a dramatic role in shaping health outcomes for children with CKD and their families [114]. Healthy People 2020 organizes social determinants of health around 5 key domains: (1) economic stability, (2) education, (3) neighborhood and built environment, (4) social and community context, and (5) health and healthcare [115]. These are influenced by societal problems of structural racism, sexism, ableism, classism and the biases associated with them which are experienced differently by particular individuals and groups within populations [116–120]. In addition, adverse environmental conditions and differences in access to healthcare, housing, clean water, healthy food, and opportunities for exercise experienced by particular groups can influence both the emergence and the progression of kidney disease [116, 119]. This insight supports the need for critical reflection in nephrology clinical practice and research. For example, the use of race as a prognostic factor or association with an outcome of interest may overlook the impact of racism rather than race in influencing clinical outcomes [121–124]. The intersection between kidney disease and racial, ethnic, gender, and socioeconomic disparities further highlights how particular groups are disadvantaged [125, 126]. One notable example is the intersection between race, socioeconomic deprivation and access to kidney transplant [127–130]. Nephrologists should seek to become aware of the impact of social determinants of health, systemic inequities, and implicit biases and work to dismantle structural causes of inequity that impact the health and well-being of patients, families, and colleagues [118, 119, 131]. Additionally, nephrologists should seek to engage with the communities they serve to promote partnerships and build trust and be trustworthy to the underserved populations that historically have been victimized by acts of injustice [119, 131–133].

Further, it is incumbent upon nephrologists to recognize how historic injustices, including colonialism and racism, contribute to the inequities resulting in high rates of acquired kidney disease in children in low- and middle-income countries. These impacts include high prevalence of bacterial, viral, and parasitic infections, limited access to reproductive care, low birth weight, malnutrition, food insecurity, poor sanitation, unsafe water supply, and pollution, all of which contribute to the development of kidney disease [116, 134–137]. These injustices highlight the need for increased and sustained efforts to support children with kidney disease and those caring for them throughout the world as an integral part of pediatric nephrologists' roles as advocates and global citizens.

Ethical Care in the Setting of Resource Limitations

It is important to acknowledge that all health care environments have limited resources. In the setting of national or other public health systems, these limitations may be dictated by realities of budgeting and health care prioritization. In the setting of private insurance, these limitations may be enacted by the policies of individual insurance programs. Institutions may vary in their ability to provide ancillary support services to the populations they serve, and families may be limited in the financial or psychosocial burdens that they can assume when caring for a child with kidney disease.

Given this reality, it is evident that there are inequities in the healthcare provided and received in different clinical settings. This is a challenge to the notion of fairness, which suggests that differential treatment of individuals is only justified if there is a morally significant difference between them [1]. Considerations such as wealth are not thought to be morally significant. Yet, resource limitations in a given practice environment may force nephrologists to deviate from what they consider optimal kidney care [138–140]. This in turn induces moral distress, a term that describes the distress that occurs not because of uncertainty regarding the most ethical course of action, but because the most appropriate ethical course is known but cannot be pursued [138, 139, 141].

Resource constraints and the lack of equity in resources for pediatric kidney care are likely beyond the efforts of individual clinicians to address. Given these constraints, however, one can consider three general guidelines in the provision of care that is limited by resource availability:

1. *In the face of resource limitations, ethically optimal care is contextual*: Different practice environments may have different prevailing standards of nephrologic care. While it is incumbent upon healthcare providers to provide the optimal care their treatment environment allows, they cannot be considered ethically required to provide care for which there is insufficient resource support. If better care could be provided in another practically accessible care setting (for example, transfer to another institution with increased resource availability or placement of the child in a different home environment to allow the provision of outpatient dialysis services), these interventions should be considered. However, it is important to recognize that these transitions may themselves be restricted due to a lack of resources and may be associated with other significant burdens that make this approach untenable.

2. *In the face of resource limitations, ethically optimal care is holistic*: It is important to recognize that a given treatment course may result in benefits and burdens beyond simple medical efficacy. The impact of treatment recommendations on patients and their family should be assessed with this in mind. For example, if the medial costs associated with the "standard of care" in a given setting might be financially ruinous to a family, deviation from this standard of care may be ethically permissible or even necessary. If the harm experienced by the child and their family from a treatment course exceeds the value of the health benefits gained, an alternative treatment course should be considered.

   It is important to note that this concept may be applied more broadly on a systems

level. As an example, while the overall benefits of the use of phosphate binders as a whole are at times called into question [142], meta-analyses have suggested that the use of sevelamer results in a reduction in all-cause mortality as compared to calcium containing phosphate binders [143]. However, sevelamer based phosphate binders are substantially more expensive than calcium-containing phosphate binders and as such wholesale transition away from calcium containing binders may place a substantially increased burden on patients, dialysis units and healthcare systems [144–146]. The relative utility of making changes of this type depend on the resources available and the alternative use to which those resources might be applied.

3. *In the face of resource limitations, ethically optimal care requires advocacy*: While it is true that resource constraints may be beyond the ability for individual medical practitioners to control, our obligations to our patients require us to serve as an advocate to ensure that their health care needs can be addressed appropriately. At its core, advocacy involves attempting to address the factors that constrain healthcare providers from providing the highest quality care possible. On an individual patient level, advocacy often takes the form of seeking to secure resources that have, in the view of the healthcare provider, been misallocated or circumstances in which the patient may experience a disproportionate benefit from receiving those resources. This may be as simple as obtaining additional financial support for patients facing significant transportation barriers, or as complex as petitioning private or national formularies to consider an exception to provide a therapy that is typically not available. More expansively, advocacy on the local, regional, national and international level seeks to alleviate those resource limitations that adversely and unjustly affect the populations that we care for and about.

References

1. Beauchamp TL, Childress JF. Principles of biomedical ethics. 8th ed. New York City: Oxford University Press; 2012.
2. Kobulsky JM, Dubowitz H, Xu Y. The global challenge of the neglect of children. Child Abuse Negl. 2020;110:104296. https://doi.org/10.1016/j.chiabu.2019.104296.
3. Assembly UG. Convention on the rights of the child. United Nations, Treaty Series. 1989;1577(3): 1–23.
4. Buchanan AE, Brock DW. Deciding for others: the ethics of surrogate decision making. 1989.
5. Diekema DS. Parental refusals of medical treatment: the harm principle as threshold for state intervention. Theor Med Bioethics. 2004;25(4):243–64.
6. Gillam L. The zone of parental discretion: an ethical tool for dealing with disagreement between parents and doctors about medical treatment for a child. Clin Ethics 2016;11(1):1-8.
7. McDougall RJ, Notini L. Overriding parents' medical decisions for their children: a systematic review of normative literature. J Med Ethics. 2014;40(7):448–52.
8. Vernon DD, Dean JM, Timmons OD, Banner W Jr, Allen-Webb EM. Modes of death in the pediatric intensive care unit: withdrawal and limitation of supportive care. Crit Care Med. 1993;21(11):1798–802.
9. Carter BS, Howenstein M, Gilmer MJ, Throop P, France D, Whitlock JA. Circumstances surrounding the deaths of hospitalized children: opportunities for pediatric palliative care. Pediatrics. 2004;114(3):e361–6. https://doi.org/10.1542/peds.2003-0654-F.
10. Fauriel I, Moutel G, Moutard ML, Montuclard L, Duchange N, Callies I, et al. Decisions concerning potentially life-sustaining treatments in paediatric nephrology: a multicentre study in French-speaking countries. Nephrol Dial Transplant. 2004;19(5):1252–7. https://doi.org/10.1093/ndt/gfh100.
11. Renal Physicians Association. Shared decision making in the appropriate initiation of and withdrawal from dialysis. 2nd ed. Rockville, MD: RPA; 2010.
12. American Academy of Pediatrics Committee on Bioethics. Guidelines on foregoing life-sustaining medical treatment. Pediatrics. 1994;93(3):532–6.
13. Committee on Hospital Care and Institute for Patient-and Family-Centered Care. Patient- and family-centered care and the pediatrician's role. Pediatrics. 2012;129(2):394–404. https://doi.org/10.1542/peds.2011-3084.
14. Sprung CL, Paruk F, Kissoon N, Hartog CS, Lipman J, Du B, et al. The Durban World Congress Ethics Round Table Conference Report: I. Differences between withholding and withdrawing life-sustaining treatments. J Crit Care. 2014;29(6):890–5. https://doi.org/10.1016/j.jcrc.2014.06.022.
15. Chung GS, Yoon JD, Rasinski KA, Curlin FA. US Physicians' Opinions about distinctions between withdrawing and withholding life-sustaining treatment. J Relig Health. 2016;55(5):1596–606. https://doi.org/10.1007/s10943-015-0171-x.
16. Rebagliato M, Cuttini M, Broggin L, Berbik I, de Vonderweid U, Hansen G, et al. Neonatal end-of-life decision making: Physicians' attitudes and relationship with self-reported practices in 10 European countries. JAMA. 2000;284(19):2451–9. https://doi.org/10.1001/jama.284.19.2451.
17. Feltman DM, Du H, Leuthner SR. Survey of neonatologists' attitudes toward limiting life-sustaining treatments in the neonatal intensive care unit. J Perinatol. 2012;32(11):886–92. https://doi.org/10.1038/jp.2011.186.
18. Solomon MZ, Sellers DE, Heller KS, Dokken DL, Levetown M, Rushton C, et al. New and lingering controversies in pediatric end-of-life care. Pediatrics. 2005;116(4):872–83. https://doi.org/10.1542/peds.2004-0905.
19. Fox RRC, Swazey JP. The courage to fail : a social view of organ transplants and dialysis. Chicago: University of Chicago Press; 1974.
20. Ladin K, Pandya R, Perrone RD, Meyer KB, Kannam A, Loke R, et al. Characterizing approaches to dialysis decision making with older adults: a qualitative study of nephrologists. Clin J Am Soc Nephrol. 2018;13(8):1188–96. https://doi.org/10.2215/CJN.01740218.
21. Orentlicher D. Matters of life and death: making moral theory work in medical ethics and the law. Princeton, NJ: Princeton University Press; 2001.
22. Derse AR. Limitation of treatment at the end-of-life: withholding and withdrawal. Clin Geriatr Med. 2005;21(1):223–38., xi. https://doi.org/10.1016/j.cger.2004.08.007.
23. Wilkinson D, Savulescu J. A costly separation between withdrawing and withholding treatment in intensive care. Bioethics. 2014;28(3):127–37. https://doi.org/10.1111/j.1467-8519.2012.01981.x.
24. Wightman A. Management dilemmas in pediatric nephrology: time-limited trials of dialysis therapy. Pediatric Nephrol. 2017;32(4):615–20. https://doi.org/10.1007/s00467-016-3545-8.
25. Ladin K, Pandya R, Kannam A, Loke R, Oskoui T, Perrone RD, et al. Discussing conservative management with older patients with CKD: an interview study of nephrologists. Am J Kidney Dis. 2018;71(5):627–35. https://doi.org/10.1053/j.ajkd.2017.11.011.
26. Buchak L. Why high-risk, non-expected-utility-maximising gambles can be rational and beneficial: the case of HIV cure studies. J Med Ethics. 2017;43(2):90–5. https://doi.org/10.1136/medethics-2015-103118.
27. Levine DZ, Truog RD. Discontinuing immunosuppression in a child with a renal transplant: are there limits to withdrawing life support? Am J Kidney Dis. 2001;38(4):901–15.

28. Rachels J. Active and passive euthanasia. N Engl J Med. 1975;292(2):78–80. https://doi.org/10.1056/NEJM197501092920206.

29. Wilkinson D, Butcherine E, Savulescu J. Withdrawal aversion and the equivalence test. Am J Bioeth. 2019;19(3):21–8. https://doi.org/10.1080/15265161.2019.1574465.

30. Ying I, Levitt Z, Jassal SV. Should an elderly patient with stage V CKD and dementia be started on dialysis? Clin J Am Soc Nephrol. 2014;9(5):971–7. https://doi.org/10.2215/CJN.05870513.

31. VR F. Who shall live? Health, economics and social choice. Singapore: World Scientific Publishing 2011.

32. Hofmann B. Is there a technological imperative in health care? Int J Technol Assess Health Care. 2002;18(3):675–89.

33. Helft PR, Siegler M, Lantos J. The rise and fall of the futility movement. N Engl J Med. 2000;343(4):293–6. https://doi.org/10.1056/NEJM200007273430411.

34. Beauchamp TL, Childress JF. Principles of biomedical ethics. 6th ed. New York: Oxford University Press; 2009.

35. Schneiderman LJ, Jecker NS, Jonsen AR. Medical futility: its meaning and ethical implications. Ann Internal Med. 1990;112(12):949–54.

36. Committee on Fetus and Newborn, 1994 to 1995. The Initiation or withdrawal of treatment for high-risk newborns. Pediatrics. 1995;96(2):362–3.

37. Quill TE, Holloway R. Time-limited trials near the end of life. JAMA. 2011;306(13):1483–4. https://doi.org/10.1001/jama.2011.1413.

38. Scherer JS, Holley JL. The role of time-limited trials in dialysis decision making in critically ill patients. Clin J Am Soc Nephrol. 2016;11(2):344–53. https://doi.org/10.2215/CJN.03550315.

39. Dionne JM, d'Agincourt-Canning L. Sustaining life or prolonging dying? Appropriate choice of conservative care for children in end-stage renal disease: an ethical framework. Pediatric Nephrol (Berlin, Germany). 2015;30(10):1761–9. https://doi.org/10.1007/s00467-014-2977-2.

40. Veatch RM. The technical criteria fallacy. Hastings Center Rep. 1977;7(4):15–6.

41. Wightman A, Zimmerman CT, Neul S, Lepere K, Cedars K, Opel D. Caregiver experience in pediatric dialysis. Pediatrics. 2019; https://doi.org/10.1542/peds.2018-2102.

42. Feudtner C, Mott AR. Expanding the envelope of care. Arch Pediatr Adoles Med. 2012;166(8):772–3. https://doi.org/10.1001/archpediatrics.2012.150.

43. Liben S, Papadatou D, Wolfe J. Paediatric palliative care: challenges and emerging ideas. Lancet. 2008;371(9615):852–64. https://doi.org/10.1016/S0140-6736(07)61203-3.

44. Kang TI, Munson D, Hwang J, Feudtner C. Integration of palliative care into the care of children with serious illness. Pediatr Rev. 2014;35(8):318–25.; quiz 26. https://doi.org/10.1542/pir.35-8-318.

45. Hospice SO, Medicine P, Care CO. Pediatric palliative care and hospice care commitments, guidelines, and recommendations. Pediatrics. 2013;132(5):966–72. https://doi.org/10.1542/peds.2013-2731.

46. Organization WH. Palliative care. 2020. https://www.who.int/news-room/fact-sheets/detail/palliative-care. Accessed Accessed Feb. 20, 2021.

47. House TR, Wightman A. Adding life to their years: the current state of pediatric palliative care in chronic kidney disease. Kidney360 2021;2(6): 1063.

48. Ezer T, Lohman D, de Luca GB. Palliative care and human rights: a decade of evolution in standards. J Pain Symptom Manag. 2018;55(2S):S163–S9. https://doi.org/10.1016/j.jpainsymman.2017.03.027.

49. Network ICsPC. What is children's palliative care? 2015. http://www.icpcn.org/about-icpcn/what-is-childrens-palliative-care/ Accessed Feb. 20, 2021.

50. Thumfart J, Reindl T, Rheinlaender C, Muller D. Supportive palliative care should be integrated into routine care for paediatric patients with life-limiting kidney disease. Acta Paediatr. 2018;107(3):403–7. https://doi.org/10.1111/apa.14182.

51. Goldstein SL, Graham N, Burwinkle T, Warady B, Farrah R, Varni JW. Health-related quality of life in pediatric patients with ESRD. Pediatric Nephrol. 2006;21(6):846–50. https://doi.org/10.1007/s00467-006-0081-y.

52. Buyan N, Turkmen MA, Bilge I, Baskin E, Haberal M, Bilginer Y, et al. Quality of life in children with chronic kidney disease (with child and parent assessments). Pediatric Nephrol. 2010;25(8):1487–96. https://doi.org/10.1007/s00467-010-1486-1.

53. Splinter A, Tjaden LA, Haverman L, Adams B, Collard L, Cransberg K, et al. Children on dialysis as well as renal transplanted children report severely impaired health-related quality of life. Qual Life Res. 2018;27(6):1445–54. https://doi.org/10.1007/s11136-018-1789-4.

54. Tjaden LA, Vogelzang J, Jager KJ, van Stralen KJ, Maurice-Stam H, Grootenhuis MA, et al. Long-term quality of life and social outcome of childhood end-stage renal disease. J Pediatr. 2014;165(2):336–42 e1. https://doi.org/10.1016/j.jpeds.2014.04.013.

55. Tong A, Tjaden L, Howard K, Wong G, Morton R, Craig JC. Quality of life of adolescent kidney transplant recipients. J Pediatr. 2011;159(4):670–5 e2. https://doi.org/10.1016/j.jpeds.2011.04.007.

56. Lopes MT, Ferraro AA, Koch VHK. Confiabilidade da tradução da versão brasileira do questionário PedsQL—DREA para avaliação da qualidade de vida de crianças e adolescentes. Braz J Nephrol. 2015;37:158–65.

57. Varni JW, Limbers CA, Burwinkle TM. Impaired health-related quality of life in children and adolescents with chronic conditions: a comparative analysis of 10 disease clusters and 33 disease categories/severities utilizing the PedsQL 4.0 Generic Core Scales. Health Qual Life Outcomes. 2007;5:43. https://doi.org/10.1186/1477-7525-5-43.

58. Moreira JM, Bouissou Morais Soares CM, Teixeira AL, Simoes ESAC, Kummer AM. Anxiety, depression, resilience and quality of life in children and

adolescents with pre-dialysis chronic kidney disease. Pediatric Nephrol. 2015;30(12):2153–62. https://doi.org/10.1007/s00467-015-3159-6.

59. Bailey PK, Hamilton AJ, Clissold RL, Inward CD, Caskey FJ, Ben-Shlomo Y, et al. Young adults' perspectives on living with kidney failure: a systematic review and thematic synthesis of qualitative studies. BMJ Open. 2018;8(1):e019926. https://doi.org/10.1136/bmjopen-2017-019926.

60. Kogon AJ, Matheson MB, Flynn JT, Gerson AC, Warady BA, Furth SL, et al. Depressive symptoms in children with chronic kidney disease. J Pediatr. 2016;168(164-70):e1. https://doi.org/10.1016/j.jpeds.2015.09.040.

61. Selewski DT, Massengill SF, Troost JP, Wickman L, Messer KL, Herreshoff E, et al. Gaining the patient reported outcomes measurement information system (PROMIS) perspective in chronic kidney disease: a Midwest Pediatric Nephrology Consortium study. Pediatric Nephrol. 2014;29(12):2347–56. https://doi.org/10.1007/s00467-014-2858-8.

62. Sinha R, Davis ID, Matsuda-Abedini M. Sleep disturbances in children and adolescents with non-dialysis-dependent chronic kidney disease. Arch Pediatr Adolesc Med. 2009;163(9):850–5. https://doi.org/10.1001/archpediatrics.2009.149.

63. Davis ID, Baron J, O'Riordan MA, Rosen CL. Sleep disturbances in pediatric dialysis patients. Pediatric Nephrol. 2005;20(1):69–75. https://doi.org/10.1007/s00467-004-1700-0.

64. Hanson CS, Gutman T, Craig JC, Bernays S, Raman G, Zhang Y, et al. Identifying important outcomes for young people with CKD and their caregivers: a nominal group technique study. Am J Kidney Dis. 2019;74(1):82–94. https://doi.org/10.1053/j.ajkd.2018.12.040.

65. Thumfart J, Bethe D, Wagner S, Pommer W, Rheinlander C, Muller D. A survey demonstrates limited palliative care structures in paediatric nephrology from the perspective of a multidisciplinary healthcare team. Acta Paediatr. 2018; https://doi.org/10.1111/apa.14688.

66. Keefer P, Lehmann K, Shanley M, Woloszyk T, Khang E, Luckritz K, et al. Single-center experience providing palliative care to pediatric patients with end-stage renal disease. J Palliat Med. 2017;20(8):845–9. https://doi.org/10.1089/jpm.2016.0353.

67. Lam DY, Scherer JS, Brown M, Grubbs V, Schell JO. A conceptual framework of palliative care across the continuum of advanced kidney disease. Clin J Am Soc Nephrol. 2019; https://doi.org/10.2215/CJN.09330818.

68. Davison SN, Levin A, Moss AH, Jha V, Brown EA, Brennan F, et al. Executive summary of the KDIGO controversies conference on supportive care in chronic kidney disease: developing a roadmap to improving quality care. Kidney Int. 2015;88(3):447–59. https://doi.org/10.1038/ki.2015.110.

69. Weaver MS, Heinze KE, Kelly KP, Wiener L, Casey RL, Bell CJ, et al. Palliative care as a standard of care in pediatric oncology. Pediatr Blood Cancer. 2015;62(Suppl 5):S829–33. https://doi.org/10.1002/pbc.25695.

70. Hancock HS, Pituch K, Uzark K, Bhat P, Fifer C, Silveira M, et al. A randomised trial of early palliative care for maternal stress in infants prenatally diagnosed with single-ventricle heart disease. Cardiol Young. 2018;28(4):561–70. https://doi.org/10.1017/S1047951117002761.

71. Savulescu J. Resources, Down's syndrome, and cardiac surgery. BMJ. 2001;322(7291):875–6.

72. Wall A, Lee GH, Maldonado J, Magnus D. Genetic disease and intellectual disability as contraindications to transplant listing in the United States: a survey of heart, kidney, liver, and lung transplant programs. Pediatr Transplant. 2020;24(7):e13837. https://doi.org/10.1111/petr.13837.

73. Willem L, Knops N, Mekahli D, Cochat P, Edefonti A, Verrina E, et al. Renal replacement therapy in children with severe developmental disability: guiding questions for decision-making. Eur J Pediatr. 2018; https://doi.org/10.1007/s00431-018-3238-3.

74. Wightman A, Diekema D, Goldberg A. Consideration of children with intellectual disability as candidates for solid organ transplantation: a practice in evolution. Pediatr Transplant. 2018;22(1) https://doi.org/10.1111/petr.13091.

75. Ohta T, Motoyama O, Takahashi K, Hattori M, Shishido S, Wada N, et al. Kidney transplantation in pediatric recipients with mental retardation: clinical results of a multicenter experience in Japan. Am J Kidney Dis. 2006;47(3):518–27. https://doi.org/10.1053/j.ajkd.2005.11.015.

76. Wightman A, Bradford MC, Smith J. Health-related quality of life changes following renal transplantation in children. Pediatr Transplant. 2019;23(2):e13333. https://doi.org/10.1111/petr.13333.

77. Furth SL, Hwang W, Neu AM, Fivush BA, Powe NR. Effects of patient compliance, parental education and race on nephrologists' recommendations for kidney transplantation in children. Am J Transplant. 2003;3(1):28–34. https://doi.org/10.1034/j.1600-6143.2003.30106.x.

78. Dobbels F, Ruppar T, De Geest S, Decorte A, Van Damme-Lombaerts R, Fine RN. Adherence to the immunosuppressive regimen in pediatric kidney transplant recipients: a systematic review. Pediatr Transplant. 2010;14(5):603–13.

79. Chua AN, Warady BA. Adherence of pediatric patients to automated peritoneal dialysis. Pediatric Nephrol. 2011;26(5):789–93.

80. Hoegy D, Bleyzac N, Robinson P, Bertrand Y, Dussart C, Janoly-Dumenil A. Medication adherence in pediatric transplantation and assessment methods: a systematic review. Patient Prefer Adherence. 2019;13:705–19. https://doi.org/10.2147/PPA.S200209.

81. Foster BJ, Dahhou M, Zhang X, Platt RW, Samuel SM, Hanley JA. Association between age and graft failure rates in young kidney transplant recipients.

Transplantation. 2011;92(11):1237–43. https://doi.org/10.1097/TP.0b013e31823411d7.

82. Burgess SW, Sly PD, Morawska A, Devadason SG. Assessing adherence and factors associated with adherence in young children with asthma. Respirology. 2008;13(4):559–63.

83. Finney JW, Hook RJ, Friman PC, Rapoff MA, Christophersen ER. The overestimation of adherence to pediatric medical regimens. Child Health Care. 1993;22(4):297–304.

84. Phillips LA, Leventhal EA, Leventhal H. Factors associated with the accuracy of physicians' predictions of patient adherence. Patient Educ Couns. 2011;85(3):461–7. https://doi.org/10.1016/j.pec.2011.03.012.

85. Bogart LM, Catz SL, Kelly JA, Benotsch EG. Factors influencing physicians' judgments of adherence and treatment decisions for patients with HIV disease. Med Decis Mak. 2001;21(1):28–36.

86. Connelly J, Pilch N, Oliver M, Jordan C, Fleming J, Meadows H, et al. Prediction of medication nonadherence and associated outcomes in pediatric kidney transplant recipients. Pediatr Transplant. 2015;19(5):555–62. https://doi.org/10.1111/petr.12479.

87. Killian MO, Schuman DL, Mayersohn GS, Triplett KN. Psychosocial predictors of medication nonadherence in pediatric organ transplantation: a systematic review. Pediatr Transplant. 2018;22(4):e13188. https://doi.org/10.1111/petr.13188.

88. Monnin K, Lofton AM, Naclerio C, Buchanan CL, Campbell K, Tenenbaum RB, et al. Understanding substance use policies and associated ethical concerns: a survey of pediatric transplant centers. Pediatr Transplant. 2021:e13984. https://doi.org/10.1111/petr.13984.

89. Weitzman ER, Ziemnik RE, Huang Q, Levy S. Alcohol and marijuana use and treatment nonadherence among medically vulnerable youth. Pediatrics. 2015.:peds.2015-0722; https://doi.org/10.1542/peds.2015-0722.

90. Johnson RM, Fleming CB, Cambron C, Dean LT, Brighthaupt S-C, Guttmannova K. Race/ethnicity differences in trends of Marijuana, cigarette, and alcohol use among 8th, 10th, and 12th graders in Washington State, 2004–2016. Prev Sci. 2019;20(2):194–204. https://doi.org/10.1007/s11121-018-0899-0.

91. Pilatti A, Read JP, Pautassi RM. ELSA 2016 Cohort: alcohol, tobacco, and marijuana use and their association with age of drug use onset, risk perception, and social norms in Argentinean College Freshmen. Front Psychol. 2017;8:1452.

92. Kraus L, Seitz NN, Piontek D, Molinaro S, Siciliano V, Guttormsson U, et al. 'Are the times a-changin'? Trends in adolescent substance use in Europe. Addiction. 2018;113(7):1317–32.

93. Wray J, Waters S, Radley-Smith R, Sensky T. Adherence in adolescents and young adults following heart or heart-lung transplantation. Pediatr

Transplant. 2006;10(6):694–700. https://doi.org/10.1111/j.1399-3046.2006.00554.x.

94. Alhamad T, Koraishy FM, Lam NN, Katari S, Naik AS, Schnitzler MA, et al. Cannabis dependence or abuse in kidney transplantation: implications for posttransplant outcomes. Transplantation. 2019;103(11):2373–82. https://doi.org/10.1097/TP.0000000000002599.

95. Greenan G, Ahmad SB, Anders MG, Leeser A, Bromberg JS, Niederhaus SV. Recreational marijuana use is not associated with worse outcomes after renal transplantation. Clin Transplant. 2016;30(10):1340–6.

96. Dobbels F, Denhaerynck K, Klem ML, Sereika SM, De Geest S, De Simone P, et al. Correlates and outcomes of alcohol use after single solid organ transplantation: a systematic review and meta-analysis. Transplant Rev. 2019;33(1):17–28.

97. Hurst FP, Altieri M, Patel PP, Jindal TR, Guy SR, Sidawy AN, et al. Effect of smoking on kidney transplant outcomes: analysis of the United States renal data system. Transplantation. 2011;92(10)

98. Lentine KL, Lam NN, Naik AS, Axelrod DA, Zhang Z, Dharnidharka VR, et al. Prescription opioid use before and after kidney transplant: implications for posttransplant outcomes. Am J Transplant. 2018;18(12):2987–99. https://doi.org/10.1111/ajt.14714.

99. Williams RJ, Nowatzki N. Validity of adolescent self-report of substance use. Subst Use Misuse. 2005;40(3):299–311. https://doi.org/10.1081/JA-200049327.

100. Delaney-Black V, Chiodo LM, Hannigan JH, Greenwald MK, Janisse J, Patterson G, et al. Just say "I don't": lack of concordance between teen report and biological measures of drug use. Pediatrics. 2010;126(5):887–93.

101. Chinnakotla S, Verghese P, Chavers B, Rheault MN, Kirchner V, Dunn T, et al. Outcomes and risk factors for graft loss: lessons learned from 1056 pediatric kidney transplants at the University of Minnesota. J Am College Surg. 2017;224(4):473–86. https://doi.org/10.1016/j.jamcollsurg.2016.12.027.

102. Chou KR. Caregiver burden: a concept analysis. J Pediatric Nurs. 2000;15(6):398–407. https://doi.org/10.1053/jpdn.2000.16709.

103. Tong A, Lowe A, Sainsbury P, Craig JC. Experiences of parents who have children with chronic kidney disease: a systematic review of qualitative studies. Pediatrics. 2008;121(2):349–60. https://doi.org/10.1542/peds.2006-3470.

104. Aldridge MD. How do families adjust to having a child with chronic kidney failure? A systematic review. Nephrol Nurs J. 2008;35(2):157–62.

105. Wightman A. Caregiver burden in pediatric dialysis. Pediatric Nephrol. 2019; https://doi.org/10.1007/s00467-019-04332-5.

106. Geense WW, van Gaal BGI, Knoll JL, Cornelissen EAM, van Achterberg T. The support needs of parents having a child with a chronic kidney disease:

a focus group study. Child: Care Health Develop. 2017;43(6):831–8. https://doi.org/10.1111/cch.12476.

107. Parham R, Jacyna N, Hothi D, Marks SD, Holttum S, Camic P. Development of a measure of caregiver burden in paediatric chronic kidney disease: the paediatric renal caregiver burden scale. J Health Psychol. 2014; https://doi.org/10.1177/1359105314524971.

108. Wong G, Medway M, Didsbury M, Tong A, Turner R, Mackie F, et al. Health and wealth in children and adolescents with chronic kidney disease (K-CAD study). BMC Public Health. 2014;14:307. https://doi.org/10.1186/1471-2458-14-307.

109. Bignall ON 2nd, Goldstein SL. Childhood CKD affects the entire family. Am J Kidney Dis. 2015;65(3):367–8. https://doi.org/10.1053/j.ajkd.2014.11.013.

110. Murray TH. The worth of a child. Berkeley: University of California Press; 1996.

111. Ong ZH, Ng CH, Tok PL, Kiew MJX, Huso Y, Shorey S, et al. Sources of distress experienced by parents of children with chronic kidney disease on dialysis: a qualitative systematic review. J Pediatric Nurs. 2020;57:11–7. https://doi.org/10.1016/j.pedn.2020.10.018.

112. Ross LF. Children, families, and health care decision making. Issues in biomedical ethics. Oxford, New York: Clarendon Press; 1998.

113. Kopelman LM. Using the best interests standard to generate actual duties. AJOB Primary Res. 2013;4(2):11–4. https://doi.org/10.1080/21507716.2013.782371.

114. Hall YN. Social determinants of health: addressing unmet needs in nephrology. Am J Kidney Dis. 2018;72(4):582–91. https://doi.org/10.1053/j.ajkd.2017.12.016.

115. Promotion OoDPaH. Social determinants of health. 2010. https://www.healthypeople.gov/2020/topics-objectives/topic/social-determinants-of-health. Accessed 25 Feb. 2021.

116. Krissberg JR, Sutherland SM, Chamberlain LJ, Wise PH. Policy in pediatric nephrology: successes, failures, and the impact on disparities. Pediatric Nephrol. 2020; https://doi.org/10.1007/s00467-020-04755-5.

117. Freeman MA, Myaskovsky L. An overview of disparities and interventions in pediatric kidney transplantation worldwide. Pediatric Nephrol. 2015;30(7):1077–86. https://doi.org/10.1007/s00467-014-2879-3.

118. Bignall O, Raglin Bignall W. Silence is not an option: the time is now to become antiracist pediatric nephrologists. Kidney Notes. 2020:4.

119. Bignall ONR 2nd, Crews DC. Stony the road we trod: towards racial justice in kidney care. Nat Rev Nephrol. 2021;17(2):79–80. https://doi.org/10.1038/s41581-020-00389-w.

120. Longino K, Kramer H. Racial and ethnic disparities, kidney disease, and COVID-19: a call to action. Kidney Med. 2020;2(5):509–10. https://doi.org/10.1016/j.xkme.2020.07.001.

121. Boyd R, Lindo E, Weeks L, McLemore M. On racism: a new standard for publishing on racial health inequities. Health Affairs Blog. 2020;

122. Dharnidharka VR, Seifert ME. Kidney transplant results in children: progress made, but blacks lag behind. Kidney Int. 2015;87(3):492–4. https://doi.org/10.1038/ki.2014.366.

123. Patzer RE, Mohan S, Kutner N, McClellan WM, Amaral S. Racial and ethnic disparities in pediatric renal allograft survival in the United States. Kidney Int. 2015;87(3):584–92. https://doi.org/10.1038/ki.2014.345.

124. Rao S, Segar MW, Bress AP, Arora P, Vongpatanasin W, Agusala V, et al. Association of genetic west african ancestry, blood pressure response to therapy, and cardiovascular risk among self-reported black individuals in the Systolic Blood Pressure Reduction Intervention Trial (SPRINT). JAMA Cardiol. 2020; https://doi.org/10.1001/jamacardio.2020.6566.

125. Wilson Y, White A, Jefferson A, Danis M. Intersectionality in clinical medicine: the need for a conceptual framework. Am J Bioeth. 2019;19(2):8–19. https://doi.org/10.1080/15265161.2018.1557275.

126. Wesselman H, Ford CG, Leyva Y, Li X, Chang CH, Dew MA, et al. Social determinants of health and race disparities in kidney transplant. Clin J Am Soc Nephrol. 2021;16(2):262–74. https://doi.org/10.2215/CJN.04860420.

127. Plumb LA, Sinha MD, Casula A, Inward CD, Marks SD, Caskey FJ, et al. Associations between deprivation, geographic location, and access to pediatric kidney care in the United Kingdom. Clin J Am Soc Nephrol. 2021;16(2):194–203. https://doi.org/10.2215/CJN.11020720.

128. Samuel SM, Foster BJ, Tonelli MA, Nettel-Aguirre A, Soo A, Alexander RT, et al. Dialysis and transplantation among Aboriginal children with kidney failure. Can Med Assoc J. 2011;183(10):E665–72. https://doi.org/10.1503/cmaj.101840.

129. Patzer RE, Amaral S, Klein M, Kutner N, Perryman JP, Gazmararian JA, et al. Racial disparities in pediatric access to kidney transplantation: does socioeconomic status play a role? Am J Transplant. 2012;12(2):369–78. https://doi.org/10.1111/j.1600-6143.2011.03888.x.

130. Kucirka LM, Grams ME, Balhara KS, Jaar BG, Segev DL. Disparities in provision of transplant information affect access to kidney transplantation. Am J Transplant. 2012;12(2):351–7. https://doi.org/10.1111/j.1600-6143.2011.03865.x.

131. Goldberg AM, Bignall ONR 2nd. Mind the Gap: acknowledging deprivation is key to narrowing kidney health disparities in both children and adults. Clin J Am Soc Nephrol. 2021;16(2):185–7. https://doi.org/10.2215/CJN.19321220.

132. Manning KD. More than medical mistrust. Lancet. 2020;396(10261):1481–2. https://doi.org/10.1016/S0140-6736(20)32286-8.

133. Wilkins CH. Effective engagement requires trust and being trustworthy. Med Care. 2018;56(10 Suppl. 1):S6–8. https://doi.org/10.1097/MLR.0000000000000953.

134. Garcia-Garcia G, Jha V. World Kidney Day 2015: CKD in disadvantaged populations. Am J Kidney Dis. 2015;65(3):349–53. https://doi.org/10.1053/j.ajkd.2014.12.001.

135. Harambat J, Ekulu PM. Inequalities in access to pediatric ESRD care: a global health challenge. Pediatric Nephrol. 2016;31(3):353–8. https://doi.org/10.1007/s00467-015-3263-7.

136. Kayange NM, Smart LR, Tallman JE, Chu EY, Fitzgerald DW, Pain KJ, et al. Kidney disease among children in sub-Saharan Africa: systematic review. Pediatr Res. 2015;77(2):272–81. https://doi.org/10.1038/pr.2014.189.

137. Jha V, Arici M, Collins AJ, Garcia-Garcia G, Hemmelgarn BR, Jafar TH, et al. Understanding kidney care needs and implementation strategies in low- and middle-income countries: conclusions from a "Kidney Disease: Improving Global Outcomes" (KDIGO) controversies conference. Kidney Int. 2016;90(6):1164–74. https://doi.org/10.1016/j.kint.2016.09.009.

138. Ducharlet K, Philip J, Gock H, Brown M, Gelfand SL, Josland EA, et al. Moral distress in nephrology: perceived barriers to ethical clinical care. Am J Kidney Dis. 2020;76(2):248–54.

139. Flood D, Wilcox K, Ferro AA, Montano CM, Barnoya J, Garcia P, et al. Challenges in the provision of kidney care at the largest public nephrology center in Guatemala: a qualitative study with health professionals. BMC Nephrol. 2020;21(1):1–10.

140. Luyckx VA, Miljeteig I, Ejigu AM, Moosa MR, editors. Ethical challenges in the provision of dialysis in resource-constrained environments. Elsevier; 2017.

141. Lamiani G, Borghi L, Argentero P. When healthcare professionals cannot do the right thing: A systematic review of moral distress and its correlates. J Health Psychol. 2017;22(1):51–67.

142. Kestenbaum BR, de Boer IH. Comparative safety of phosphate binders without proven efficacy—how did we get here? JAMA Internal Med. 2019;179(6):749–50.

143. Spoendlin J, Paik JM, Tsacogianis T, Kim SC, Schneeweiss S, Desai RJ. Cardiovascular outcomes of calcium-free vs calcium-based phosphate binders in patients 65 years or older with end-stage renal disease requiring hemodialysis. JAMA Internal Med. 2019;179(6):741–9.

144. Peter WLS, Wazny LD, Weinhandl ED. Phosphate-binder use in US dialysis patients: prevalence, costs, evidence, and policies. Am J Kidney Dis. 2018;71(2):246–53.

145. Bajait CS, Pimpalkhute SA, Sontakke SD, Jaiswal KM, Dawri AV. Prescribing pattern of medicines in chronic kidney disease with emphasis on phosphate binders. Indian J Pharmacol. 2014;46(1):35.

146. Rizk R, Hiligsmann M, Karavetian M, Evers SMAA. Economic evaluations of interventions to manage hyperphosphataemia in adult haemodialysis patients: a systematic review. Nephrology. 2016;21(3):178–87. https://doi.org/10.1111/nep.12584.

Psychosocial Issues in Children with Chronic Kidney Disease

63

Amy J. Kogon and Stephen R. Hooper

Introduction

The psychosocial functioning of children and adolescents with chronic kidney disease (CKD) typically receives little attention in the busy pediatric nephrology clinic, but there is a growing literature to suggest that it should play a critical role in the overall care of this population. It is important for the quality of care received by the child and their family, the impact that psychiatric difficulties can exert on that quality of care, the interaction of such problems with other neurodevelopmental functions such as cognitive functioning and social development, and the economics of care as related to poor adherence to and the risk of adverse events. Psychosocial issues have been shown to have an adverse impact on disease progression and health care costs [1–4].

This chapter provides a comprehensive overview of what is known about the broad area of psychosocial issues in children with CKD going back approximately three decades. Couched within the context of the epidemiology of childhood psychiatric disorders, this chapter discusses many of the available studies addressing (1) psychiatric disorders and symptoms, (2) social functioning, (3) quality of life, and (4) long-term functional outcomes. Additionally, guidance for measuring psychosocial issues in the clinical setting and associated management strategies will be reviewed. The chapter concludes with a brief discussion of gaps in the literature and future clinical research suggestions for the future.

Psychiatric and Psychosocial Challenges

In general, the psychiatric and psychosocial challenges faced by all children and adolescents is staggering. Based on data from the National Survey of Children's Health [5], approximately 7.7 million children and adolescents in the United States have at least one mental health disorder. These disorders included depression, anxiety, attention deficit-hyperactivity disorder, and a variety of other conditions. With rates of identification ranging from 7.6% to over 27%, this equates to about 1 in 7 children and teenagers (14.3%) who have a condition that could be treated; however, nearly half of these individuals do not receive treatment to address their mental health needs. Left untreated, these conditions can impact neurodevelopment, general health, and wellbeing. These rates coincide with rates of psychiatric disorders

A. J. Kogon (✉)
Department of Pediatrics, Children's Hospital of Philadelphia, University of Pennsylvania, Philadelphia, PA, USA
e-mail: kogona@chop.edu

S. R. Hooper
Department of Allied Health Sciences, School of Medicine, University of North Carolina-Chapel Hill, Chapel Hill, NC, USA
e-mail: stephen_hooper@med.unc.edu

© The Author(s), under exclusive license to Springer Nature Switzerland AG 2023
F. Schaefer, L. A. Greenbaum (eds.), *Pediatric Kidney Disease*,
https://doi.org/10.1007/978-3-031-11665-0_63

from large epidemiological studies in the United States (e.g., The Smokey Mountain Study = 13.3% [6]), although some have been alarmingly higher (e.g., National Comorbidity Survey = 40.3%) [7], and with rates across the globe (13.4%) [8]. These rates are lower than those for children with various disabilities, such as cerebral palsy, with rates as high as 57% [9]. Additionally, these rates do not include those children and adolescents who may be experiencing significant psychological stress/distress or those who may have subthreshold psychiatric symptoms.

Further, studies of children with pediatric chronic illnesses have clearly demonstrated the consequences of co-morbid psychiatric disease on the primary medical disease, with higher health care utilization and costs [10], worse medical adherence [11], and worse control of the underlying medical condition [10, 11]. These outcomes are less rigorously studied in children and adolescents with CKD, but a study of pediatric hemodialysis (HD) patients and a study that included renal transplant patients identified a relationship between adherence and depressive

and/or anxiety symptoms [12, 13]. Accordingly, a complete understanding of the psychiatric and psychosocial challenges of CKD is critically important to optimal clinical management and care across the lifespan.

Psychiatric Disorders and Symptoms

Life with CKD is difficult, and as a child the multiple adversities related to living with such a complex disease can predispose to psychiatric complications (see Fig. 63.1). Children with CKD experience higher rates of psychiatric illness when compared to their healthy peers. Although there are many reports on the prevalence of psychiatric disease, estimates vary depending on the specific population evaluated and the tools used for diagnosis. The difficulties surrounding psychiatric complications in pediatric CKD exist universally, with studies documenting the morbidity of psychiatric complications extending from North and South America to Asia (see Table 63.1).

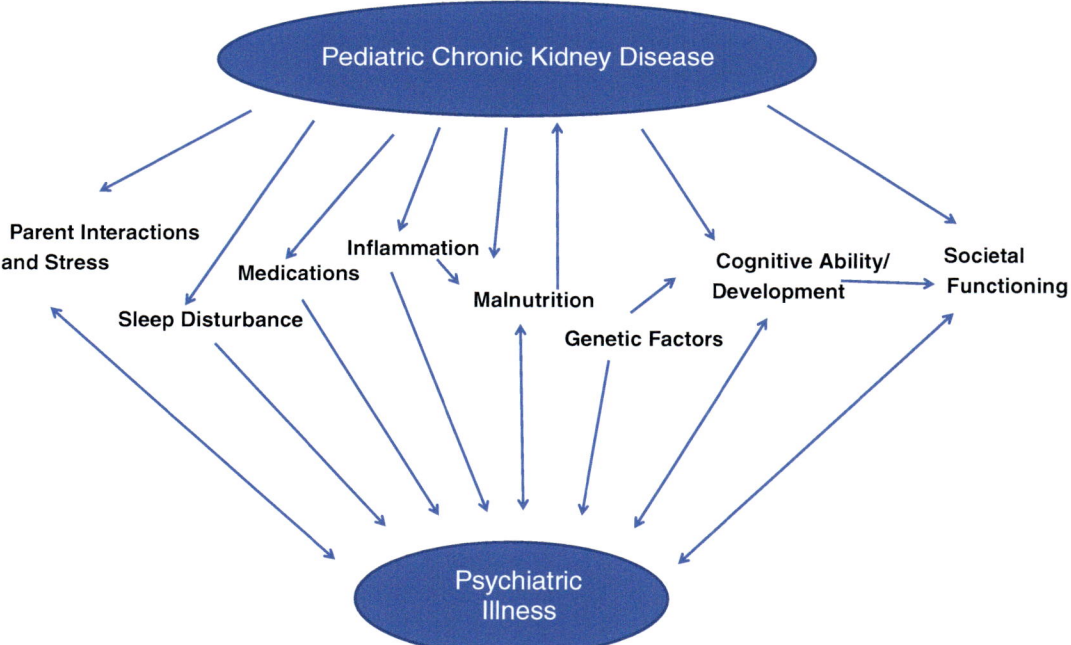

Fig. 63.1 The multiple factors that contribute to psychiatric illness and symptoms in pediatric patients with chronic kidney disease

Table 63.1 Studies examining the psychiatric and social functioning and quality of life functioning in pediatric chronic kidney disease

Study	Sample	Measures	Findings
Psychiatric disorders and symptoms			
Garralda et al. 1988 [14]	22 children on dialysis, 22 children with CKD not on dialysis; 31 controls matched to age and sex with dialysis patients; 2–18 years	Patients: Full psychiatric interview with a doctor, The Birleson Depression inventory, Lipsitt self-concept scale for self-esteem, General health questionnaire if they left school, Denver developmental screening test Teachers: Rutter Child Scale Parents: Modified psychiatric interview with parents, Rutter parental screening, Behavior check list, Highlands Dependency questionnaire or Vinelands Social Maturity scale, Modified social stress and supports interview, General health Questionnaire to assess mental distress in parents	Excess psychiatric adjustment noted in ill children with marked disturbance more common in dialysis group. By composite report, a definite psychiatric disorder noted in 32% dialysis, 23% CKD and 21% of controls. Marked worrying/anxiety identified in 30% of dialysis, 40% of CKD and 14% of control participants
Eisenhauer et al. 1988 [23]	15 children with CKD: 8 ESKD and 7 mild CKD 8–16 years old	DICA	Depression was most common psychiatric disorder diagnosed in those with ESKD at 63% and anxiety the most common disorder diagnosed in those with mild disease at 57%
Reynolds et al. 1991 [32]	29 functioning renal transplant recipients, 22 on HD, 22 CKD and 31 healthy controls 1–18 years of age	Rutter A and B, Birleson and Lipsitt questionnaires	92% of parents reported improvements in their child's health after transplant and none of parents felt that their child had serious behavioral or emotional difficulty as compared to 1/3 of those with CKD and dialysis. Parents also described their child as happier and less irritable than before transplant. Behavioral problems in the Rutter A questionnaire were more than twice as common in the group who had transplants than in the HD or healthy group. Behavior at school of transplanted patients as assessed by Rutter B did not differ from controls but showed worse scores than HD
Brownbridge et al. 1991 [33]	73 ESKD, 32 HD, 28 CAPD, 13 transplant recipients; 2–21 years of age	Study specific questionnaires completed by patients and parents for measures of health status; Structured family interviews; CDI STAIC Rutter A scale Leeds scale for the self-assessment of anxiety and depression	Transplant recipients had less functional impairment and less social impairment, but groups did not differ on levels of anxiety, depression or behavioral disturbance. Patients on CAPD had less social impairment, lower depression scores, and less behavioral disturbance than HD patients. Parents of children on CAPD had less depression and anxiety then the parents with children on HD

(continued)

Table 63.1 (continued)

Study	Sample	Measures	Findings
Fukunishi et al. 1993 [27]	23 children on CAPD, 23 healthy controls; 4–18 years if age	DICA obtained monthly for 3 months followed by 9 months psychiatric interview	69.6% of dialysis patients had an anxiety disorder vs 8.7% of controls. 65.2% of dialysis patients experienced separation anxiety
Fukunishi et al. 1995 [28]	26 patients on CAPD, 27 transplant recipients, 27 controls; 6–15 years old	DICA –administered at least 3 times over 3 months Interviewed parents regarding school maladjustment	65% of dialysis patients had separation anxiety which associated with the family psychological environment. After receiving a transplant, school maladjustment remained and adjustment disorder was in 27% which was related to poor relationship with peers. For those on CAPD, 68% had separation anxiety, along with 18.5% of transplant recipients and 3.7% of controls
Brownbridge et al. 1999 [90]	60 dialysis patients 2–21 years of age	Structured family interview	Low adherence associated with self-ratings of anxiety and depression
Fielding et al. 1999 [90]	60 patients on dialysis; 2–21 years of age	Patient: CDI, STAIC Parents: Rutter A scale, Leeds Scale for the self-assessment of anxiety and depression	Poorer socioeconomic status associated with more behavioral disturbances in children and increased depression and anxiety in parents. Children who suffered greater functional impairment as a result of illness were more likely to be depressed, anxious, and show behavioral disturbance. Children's scores on social impairment scale correlated with parents' depression and anxiety scores
Soliday et al. 2000	41 parents of children with kidney disease:15 with SSNS, 12 with CKD, 14 transplant recipients compared to 34 controls; 1–18 years	CBCL PSI-SF FES	Mean scores on CBCL and parenting stress scores were within normal limits. 28.6% of transplant patients had clinically significant levels of internalizing symptoms and 20% of children with SSNS had clinically significant externalizing symptoms
Penkower et al. 2003 [91]	22 renal transplant recipients; 13–18 years	Face to face interviews BDI state anxiety, state-trait anxiety and state anger subscales of Spielberger	36.4% demonstrated symptoms of depression, 36.4% anxiety and 18.2% excessive state anger. Adolescents with excessive anger were at greatest risk for missing medications
Wallace et al. 2004 [30]	64 renal transplants recipients; 6–21 years old	FEATS CDI Davidson Trauma Scale	36% had results consistent with depression and/or PTSD; FEATS identified a subset of patients who were not identified using the self-report measures. Davidson scores correlated with hospital days and FEATS correlated with height Z score and donor type. Depression wad identified by CDI in 19% and PTSD by Davidson scores in 42%

Table 63.1 (continued)

Study	Sample	Measures	Findings
Bakr et al. 2007 [16]	9–15 years, 19 children on HD, 19 children CKD	Semi-structured clinical interview for children and adolescents on structured observation and self-report	Prevalence of psychiatric disorders 52.6%: 68.4% HD, 36.8% CKD. Adjustment disorder 18.4%, Depression 10.3%, NC 7.7%, Anxiety 5.1%
Berney-Martinet et al. 2009 [29]	Matched 20 CKD, 40 transplant recipients and 40 controls; 12–18 years	K-SADS-PL CBCL	Lifetime depressive disorder in of 35% transplant recipients, 35% CKD, and 15.2% of controls. Anxiety disorders seen in 22.5% of transplant recipients, 35% of CKD, and 5% of controls. Behavioral disorder seen in 30% transplant recipients, 15% of CKD, 20% of controls
Amr et al. 2009 [34]	19 patients on HD, 19 CKD and 19 controls	CBCL SCICA	Mean internalizing score was significantly higher in dialysis than in CKD and controls. No difference in externalizing scales. Mean scores of SCICA observed problems and total self-reports higher in the control group than CKD groups. Positive correlation between SCICA self-report and CBCL
Dobbels et al. 2010 [26]	23 kidney transplant recipients; 10–18 years old	BDI KIDSCREEN-27	Depressive symptoms occurred in 17.4% and 75% of those with depressive symptoms were non-adherent to medications. Parents rated their adolescents to be significantly lower on psychological well-being, autonomy, and school functioning
Hernandez et al. 2011 [36]	67 patients on dialysis: 43 PD, 24 HD; 4–18 years old	Birleson Scale	10% with high occurrence of depressive symptoms and 42% without any symptoms-all of those with high depressive symptoms were female and none had a friend to confide in. For those on PD, depressive symptoms associated with lower Kt/v
Kogon et al. 2013 [25]	44 children: 20 pre-ESKD, 15 dialysis, 9 transplant recipients; 9–18 years	CDI-II	30% of cohort had depression: 25% of those pre-ESKD, 13% of those on dialysis, 67% of the transplant recipients
Selewski et al. 2014 [92]	233 children with CKD III-V including ESKD; 8–17 years old	PROMIS	Recent hospitalizations and edema predicted worse depression and anxiety scores. Those with 2 or more co-existing medical conditions had worse score in depression, anxiety, social-peer relationships
Moreira et al. 2015 [93]	28 pre-ESKD CKD, 28 controls; 9–18 years old	CDI self-report for childhood anxiety related disorder scales	Higher clinically significant depressive symptoms and higher scores for separation anxiety in those with CKD. Less resilience in those with depression

(continued)

Table 63.1 (continued)

Study	Sample	Measures	Findings
Yousefichaijan et al. 2016 [31]	80 children stage 1–3 CKD and 80 controls; 7–17 years old	Obsessive compulsive inventory-child	Mean scores for doubting/checking, ordering, and total scores significantly higher in CKD
Kogon et al. 2016 [38]	420 children CKD; Median age 11.45 years	BASC	Genomic disorders associated with more internalizing problems
Kogon et al. 2016 [24]	344 CKD subjects; 6–17 years	CDI	7% diagnosed with depression. Higher scores associated with less maternal education and lower HRQOL
Kogon et al. 2019 [37]	71 CKD stage II & higher (including ESKD) and 64 controls; 8–25 years old	CDI-II or BDI	Depression in 17% of those with CKD and 12.5% controls. Obesity associated with depression
Cueller et al. 2019 [40]	47 patients with ESKD: 12 PD, 17 HD, 18 renal transplant recipients; 7–18 years old	CDI	64% with symptoms of depression: 61% of transplant recipients, 65% of HD patients, and 66% of those on PD. More depression associated with shorter duration of ESKD and older age. Less depression in transplant recipients from a living donor
Dinc et al. 2019 [15]	66 CKD subjects: 21 transplant recipients, 27 dialysis, 18 CKD and 37 controls	Parent: Parental Attitude Scale, Symptom Checklist-90 by mothers Self: CDI, STAIC, K-SADS	Higher median CDI score for CKD group but no difference in STAIC scores. 41% of children in CKD group diagnosed with current psychiatric disorder vs 16% in control group: 43% of those with transplant, 33% of those on dialysis,50% of those with CKD. A past psychiatric disorder was identified in 52% of those CKD vs 22% of controls: 71% of those with renal transplant, 30% of those on dialysis, 61% of controls. Major depression identified in 9% of CKD overall vs 0% controls: 9.5% of those with a transplant, 15% of those on dialysis, 0% of those with pre-ESKD CKD. No differences found within CKD modalities. No difference in STAIC scores versus controls
Kang et al. 2019 [21]	166 participants with CKD stage 1–4; <18 years old	Korea-CBCL	20.5% had significant mental health problems, 22.3% had psychosocial adjustment problems. 12.7% had clinically significant internalizing problem and 9% had clinically significant externalizing problem. Those with short stature and with multiple comorbidities were more likely to score within the clinical range
Johnson et al. 2020 [20]	845 CKD patients	BASC	On depression scale, higher income and IQ associated with fewer symptoms. Time in study associated with lower depression scores

Table 63.1 (continued)

Study	Sample	Measures	Findings
Social functioning			
Fukunishi et al. 1995 [41]	30 CAPD, 35 transplant recipients, 33 controls; 6–15 years old		No difference between CAPD and transplant patients for school maladjustment with academic problems. CAPD endorsed significantly worse school absenteeism than controls and CAPD and transplant patients had worse and relationships with peers than controls
Qvist et al. 2004 [39]	32 children with renal transplant; under the age of 5	CBCL, CBCL-TRF, HRQOL	Total scores on CBCL did not differ from normative sample. Somatic complains and social problems more frequent in boys. Patients with low scores had more comorbidity and were more likely to attend a special school. Girls had less externalizing problems as rated by teacher than reference. Scores on attention scales were higher in boys and girls as rated by parents and teachers. HRQOL scores differed significantly
Gerson et al. 2004 [94]	13 pediatric renal transplant patients 2–21 years old	BASC Children's Health Questionnaire Young Adolescent Body Image Scale PSI-SF FES	More attention problems associated with worse adherence and better child behavior associated with better medication adherence
Berney-Martinet et al. 2009 [29]	Matched 20 CKD, 40 transplant recipients, 40 controls; 12–18 years old	CBCL	Transplant scored lower than CKD in social competence score; no difference between groups in activities score. Social issues related to psychiatric problems
Hooper et al. 2009 [19]	26 children with CKD: 13 on dialysis, 13 CKD and 33 controls 7–19 years old	BASC	More internalizing problems and behavior symptoms index score in CKD group, although scores fell within the average range. No group differences on adaptive skills or externalizing problems. On parent ratings, CKD participants scored worse on anxiety and depression
Hooper et al. 2016 [22]	124 preschool children mild to moderate CKD	BASC-2, ABAS-II	Parent rating of social-behavioral functioning were in the average range. No problems noted for internalizing, externalizing, or overall behavioral symptoms. On ABAS-II, scores were in the low average to average range in particular for the Practical Composite Score-reflecting capabilities in age-appropriate social functioning. 32–51% of preschoolers were at risk for not developing age-appropriate activities of daily living. No CKD related variables were risk factors

(continued)

Table 63.1 (continued)

Study	Sample	Measures	Findings
Xiao et al. 2019 [35]	318 patients and reference population, CKD stage II or higher including ESKD 13–19 years old	National Youth Risk Behavior Survey	Children with CKD reported significantly lower prevalence of risk behaviors
Johnson et al. 2020 (repeated from above) [20]	845 CKD patients	BASC-2 Parent Rating Scale	Average BASC scores for the group, with ratings improving over time. Male was risk factor for poorer scores. Persistent hypertension was associated with worse scores on the Behavioral Symptoms Index
Quality of life			
Fadrowski et al. 2006 [58]	78 adolescents with CKD, including ESKD; 11–18 years old	CHQ	Increasing height associated with positive change in physical and psychosocial summary score. Increasing age associated with decreasing psychosocial score
Sundaram et al. 2007 [52]	51 liver transplant and 26 kidney transplant recipients; 11–18 years old	CHQ-PF and CF	Caregivers reported lower physical functioning and general health than the normative population, but similar psychological health. All caregivers shared a negative emotional impact on them and their families. Parent-youth concordance was highest for physical functioning, pain, behavior problems, and self-esteem, but lowest for mental health and family cohesion
Falger et al. 2008 [44]	37 children renal transplant recipients; 5–17 years old	Child Quality of Life Questionnaire & CBCL completed by parents and youth.	Parents and youth reported impaired emotional functioning, which was correlated with adverse family relationships and maternal distress. No differences between parent and child quality of life ratings, but ratings were correlated with maternal distress
Gerson et al. 2010 [61]	402 children with mild to moderate CKD 2–16 years old	PedsQL completed by parents and youth	Patients had significantly lower physical, school, emotional and social domain scores than healthy youth. Longer disease duration and older age were associated with higher quality of life. Short stature associated with lower physical functioning scores
Diseth et al. 2011 [53]	28 transplant recipients and 40 cancer survivors and 42 controls; 12–19 years old	Strengths & Difficulties Questionnaire & PedsQL completed by parents and youth; General Health Questionnaire & Quality of Life Scales for parents	PedsQL emotional functioning of the transplant group was lower than the health controls, but similar to that of the cancer group. Parents from both transplant and cancer groups reported similar levels of negative impact of their child's illness on their functioning and on family functioning

Table 63.1 (continued)

Study	Sample	Measures	Findings
Heath et al. 2011 [50]	225 patients with CKD stages 3–5: 47 dialysis, 128 transplant recipients, 49 pre-ESKD; 6–18 years old	Generic Children's Quality of Life Measure Questionnaire completed by child	No significant differences between scores when compared to normative group, and no differences seen across various treatment modalities
Marciano et al. 2011 [48]	136 CKD patients: 39 dialysis, 29 transplant recipients 75 ore-ESKD	Strengths & Difficulties Questionnaire; PedsQL rated by parents & youth	Parents of CKD patients reported the rate of emotional & disruptive disorders to be about 50% higher than in normative group. In contrast, about 1/3 of children reported emotional problems. There was a large negative correlation between the presence of behavior and emotional disorders and the PedsQL total score
Park et al. 2012 [51]	92 children with ESKD: 11 HD, 44 PD = 44, 37 transplant recipients; 2–18 years old	PedsQL ESKD Module	Children with kidney transplant or on dialysis did not differ on perceptions of family and peer interactions, worry, physical appearance, or communication. Parents reported communication problems were worse for children on dialysis than transplant recipients
Neul et al. 2013 [55]	53 dialysis patients and their parents	PedsQL & PedsQL ESKD Module administered at 6-month intervals over a 2-yr. period completed by both patients and parents.	Parent Global PedsQL ratings did not change over time, but ratings were lower in girls and in those with longer dialysis vintage. Emotional and school domains decreased over time. Patient reported scores were higher compared to the parent ratings
Al-Uzri et al. 2013 [57]	483 children with mild to moderate CKD; 2–17 years old	PedsQL completed by parents and youth over two visits.	Significant association between catch-up growth and growth hormone use on parent reports of child physical and social functioning domains. Older children had higher ratings than their parents on all PedsQL scales.
Haavisto et al. 2013 [45]	77 transplant patients: 16 heart, 44 kidney, 14 liver; 6–16 years old	HRQOL & CBCL completed by parents, patients, & teachers.	No differences in HRQOL scores between transplant recipients, but younger participants had lower scores compared to norms. When compared to normative data, the adolescent transplant group reported less distress and more vitality, but more problems attending school and being with friends. Parents and teachers reported more internalizing problems than the normative group, but scores were in the average range. Parents reported more problems with health and physical functioning than patients

(continued)

Table 63.1 (continued)

Study	Sample	Measures	Findings
Killis-Pstrusinska et al. 2013 [46]	203 children with CKD: 25 HD, 41 PD and 137 pre-ESKD and 388 parent proxies; 2–18 years old	PedsQL Inventory completed by patients & parents	Lower HRQOL scores in all CKD groups compared to norms, and HD patients had the lowest scores. There was significant discordance between parents and patients on emotional functioning in the PD group, but not in the HD or conservative treatment groups
Baek HS et al. 2017 [54]	376 parents and 305 children; <18 years of age	PedsQL	Lower HRQOL identified in female patients and those with more co-morbidities and by parent report in those with lower kidney function and anemia. Growth and bone mineral density were positively correlated with QOL. There was no relationship between HRQOL and age or duration of disease
Splinter et al. 2018 [47]	192 ESKD patients 8–18 years in Europe	PedsQL	Patients reported significantly lower scores compared to the healthy norms and other chronic health conditions. Those who had undergone a preemptive transplant reported better physical health scores that were similar to other chronic conditions
Francis A et al. 2018 [49]	375 children 6–18 years with CKD stages I-5 including dialysis and transplant recipients	Health Utilities Index (HUI)	The lowest scores were for those on dialysis, followed by transplant recipients, then CKD stages 3–5 with the highest scores seen in those with CKD stages 1–2
Pardede SO et al. 2019 [56]	112 children including hemodialysis; 2–18 years of age	PedsQL	The lowest scores were seen in the school and emotional domains. HRQOL was lowest in those with CKD diagnosis >60 months, female and in middle school.
Carlson et al. 2020 [60]	733 children and adolescents with mild to moderate CKD; Median age 11 years	PedsQL completed by parents and children over multiple visits.	Presence of anemia was associated with significantly lower overall HRQOL and physical functioning as per child ratings. On parent ratings, anemia was associated with lower emotional functioning scores. Caregivers did not observe declines in their children's other PedsQL subscales in the presence of anemia
Díaz-González de Ferris ME et all 2021 [59]	734 children median age of 11 years	PedsQL	Average HRQOL scores were higher in younger children, but were more highly related to number of medications, with lower HRQOL associated with the number of unique medications

Long-term functional outcomes

Roscoe et al. 1991 [95]	118 adolescents treated between 1966 and 1986	Functional status obtained by structured telephone interview	80% survival after 15 years for transplanted patients. 29% were living on their own or with a spouse, the rest mostly living with a family member.14% were neither enrolled in an educational program nor employed

Table 63.1 (continued)

Study	Sample	Measures	Findings
Mellerio et al. 2014 [96]	374 adult aged patients transplanted as children; Median age 27 and 12.3 years since first transplant	Questionnaire with data compared to French general population using indirect standardization matched for gender, age, period	Compared to the general population 31% versus 52.2% lived with partner, 36% v 21% lived with parents and 19% v 10% were unemployment. Factors predictive of poor outcome were primary disease severity, presence of comorbidities or disabilities, being on dialysis, and female gender
Lewis et al. 2014 [64]	236 young adults with ESKD presenting as children compared to those presenting as adults.	Questionnaires	30% of those with a pediatric and 20% of those with an adult presentation were labeled disabled. There was lower educational attainment in pediatric presentation and those with pediatric presentation less likely to have full or part-time paid work (57% v 76%) and less likely to be living with a partner
Murray et al. 2014 [65]	57 young adults:5 CKD, 8 dialysis, 45 TX; 27 were pediatric presentation	Semi-structured interview	Median age leaving school was 16 year: 17.5% still studying, 75% completed education, 60% employed, and 33% unemployed. For those with pediatric presentation: 7% were in special ed. and 26% earned a general certificate of secondary education. 75% felt that their employment or work was negatively affected by ESKD. 33% unemployed and not in school vs 22% in general population. 8.5% were receiving welfare vs 4% in general population
Enden et al. 2018 [97]	29 young adult men who underwent renal transplantation in childhood and 56 matched survivors of childhood acute lymphoblastic leukemia and 52 controls with other childhood illness	RAND-36 BDI	Compared to leukemia survivors and controls transplant recipients had higher BDI scores and reported more bodily pain and worse general health which associated with older age, longer duration of dialysis, multiple transplantations and lower graft function. Transplant recipients were less likely to be in permanent relationship (40% v 8-% controls and 50% leukemia survivors). Transplant recipients reported lower HRQOL. 10% of transplant recipients had at least one child compared to 21% of leukemia survivors, and 43% of controls. 4% transplant recipients graduated from university compared to 14% of leukemia survivors and 18% of controls. 67% of transplant recipients were employed compared to 90% leukemia survivors and 100% of controls

(continued)

Table 63.1 (continued)

Study	Sample	Measures	Findings
Groothoff et al. 2018 [42]	144 patients with onset of ESKD before 14 years of age born before 1979		67.4% of ESKD patients were employed with 19.1% involuntarily unemployed vs 6.4% of general population. 53% had low skill occupation and 10% had high skilled-significantly different than general population. Being on dialysis, motor disabilities and chronic fatigue most important predictors of unemployment. Average income was significantly lower than general population. 21% felt that disease has significant negative influence on professional achievement and career. 34% lived with their parents but 10 years later 67.4% were married or lived with a partner. 31.5% had offspring compared to 74.4%, and 65% of ESKD children scored lower in all domains of developmental milestones than healthy peers
Hamilton et al. 2019 [43]	417 transplant recipients and 173 dialysis patients; 16–30 year old	Study developed survey	Compared to the general population those with ESKD were less likely to live with partner or have children, more likely to live with parents, had poorer quality of life and were twice the likely to have a psychological problem. They were also less likely to have drunk alcohol, 1.6 years older at first alcohol consumption, less likely to have tried cannabis or street drugs, spent money gambling or been in trouble with the law, and twice as likely to have never had sex
Kerklaan et al. 2020 [98]	30 patients diagnosed with non-ESKD CKD during childhood; 18–35 years old	Semi-structured interview	Struggled with daily restrictions, felt defeated hopeless and lagging behind studies and life goals. 20% worked full time, 23% part-time, and 13% unemployed. 43% were students, 26% married or living together, 60% single, 63% living with parents/families, 23% living with partner, and 7% had 1 child

CKD chronic kidney disease, *ESKD* end stage kidney disease, *DICA* diagnostic interview for children and adolescents, *CAPD* continuous ambulatory peritoneal dialysis, *CDI* children's depression inventory, *STAIC* state-trait anxiety inventory for children, *CBCL* child behavior checklist, *PSI-SF* parenting stress index-short form, *FES* family environment scale, *SSNS* steroid-sensitive nephrotic syndrome, *BDI* beck depression index, *FEATS* formal elements of art therapy scale, *PTSD* post-traumatic stress disorder, *K-SADS-PL* Kiddie Schedule for Affective Disorders and Schizophrenia Present and Lifetime Version, *SCICA* semi-structured clinical interview for children and adolescents, *HRQOL* health related quality of life, *PROMIS* The Patient-Reported Outcomes Measurement Information System, *BASC* Behavior Assessment System for Children, *ABAS* Adaptive Behavior Assessment System, *CHQ-PF/CF* Child health questionnaire-Parent form/child form

With respect to general rates of psychiatric disorders in pediatric CKD, Garralda et al. completed modified psychiatric interviews with parents and determined that psychiatric disorders were more common in dialysis patients and CKD patients than in healthy controls [14]. More recently, a study from Turkey also found a high prevalence of psychiatric disorders in children with CKD, including those with a transplant and on dialysis, when compared to the control group. Specifically, they found that 41% of children with CKD were diagnosed with a current psychiatric disorder, compared to 16% in the control group, and that 52% of those with CKD reported a prior psychiatric diagnosis as compared to 7% in the control group [15]. A study from Egypt of children on dialysis and with pre-dialysis CKD evaluated for the presence of a psychiatric disorder using a semi-structured clinical interview. The overall prevalence of psychiatric disorders was 53%, including 68% of patients on HD and 37% of CKD patients without end-stage kidney disease (ESKD) [16].

Emotional-behavioral functioning more broadly has often been assessed through the use of the omnibus ratings scales, such as the Child Behavioral Checklist (CBCL)[17] and Behavior Assessment System for Children (BASC) [18]. A study compared ESKD, CKD, and controls and found that behavior ratings on the BASC by parents and children fell within the average range. Parent ratings showed increased number of internalizing symptoms, but otherwise did not show concerns for social-behavior functioning [19]. Likewise, the Chronic Kidney Disease in Children (CKiD) cohort study investigated emotional-behavioral functioning in children using the BASC-2 completed by parents and found that, on average, children with CKD scored in the typical range, although more children than expected scored >1 standard deviation towards a score of impairment [20]. This was also shown in a study of children with CKD stage I–IV in Korea, which found that based on the parent-proxy CBCL 20.5% and 22.3% of children had scores consistent with clinically significant mental health and psychosocial adjustment problems,

respectively [21]. Similar to the findings in older children, this pattern has been demonstrated in preschool children with CKD. The median parent scores on the BASC-2 were consistently within the average range, although 37% of children scored >1 standard deviation above the mean on adaptive behavior problems [22].

In addition to the general prevalence rates of psychiatric disorders and emotional-behavioral functioning in pediatric CKD, there also have been studies that have focused on the prevalence of depression and anxiety. The prevalence of depression or elevated depressive symptoms identified in studies of children with CKD ranges from 7% to 67% (see Fig. 63.2) [23]. The most commonly used instrument to document these findings is the Children's Depression Inventory (CDI). In CKiD, one of the largest studies to date to evaluate depressive symptoms, 7% of 344 children with CKD had a diagnosis of depression or elevated depressive symptoms [24]. This study, which is part of a multi-year, prospective, observational cohort design, identified a lower prevalence than described in other studies, which have primarily been single-center studies. This may be due to selection bias since participants in the CKiD study may be self-selected and have a lower likelihood of psychiatric comorbidity. A single-center study that used the CDI to evaluate for depression in children and adolescents with CKD found that 30% of the participants scored within the clinical range. The most likely to be depressed were the transplant patients (67%) followed by the pre-ESKD patients (25%) and the dialysis patients (13%). This pattern persisted even after adjustment for age and gender [25]. Similarly, Berney-Martinet et al. evaluated CKD patients, healthy controls and transplant recipients for the lifetime prevalence of depression with the Kiddie Schedule for Affective Disorders and Schizophrenia (K-SADS). They found that 35% of transplant recipients and 35% of pre-ESKD recipients have been depressed, compared to 15% of controls. Another study of adolescent transplant patients identified that 17.4% were depressed based on the Beck Depression Inventory [26].

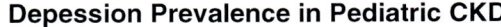

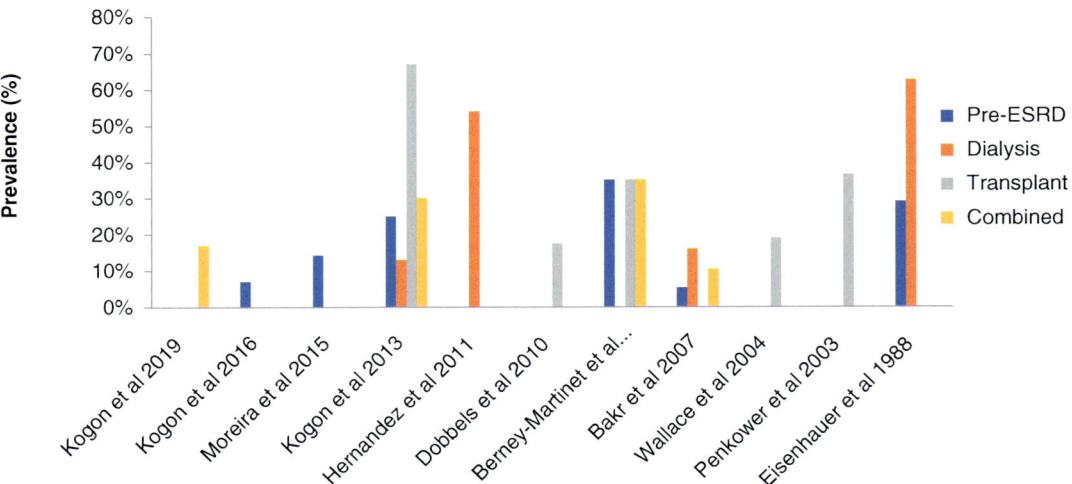

Fig. 63.2 Studies depicting depression prevalence in pediatric chronic kidney disease: prior to end-stage kidney disease (pre-ESRD), dialysis, and transplant

Although less studied than depression, anxiety disorders are also common in children with CKD compared to controls. A study in Japan from 1993 found that 69.6% of children on peritoneal dialysis (PD) experienced an anxiety disorder as compared to only 8.7% of controls, with separation anxiety disorder being the most common in both groups [27]. A subsequent study by the same group also found anxiety to be more common in renal transplant recipients, though not as common as in dialysis patients, than in controls [28]. In another study, the prevalence of an anxiety disorder was 22.5% kidney transplant recipients, 35% in those with pre-ESKD CKD and only 5% in healthy controls [29]. Post-traumatic stress is also of concern, particularly for those with more morbid disease. In a study of renal transplant recipients, 6–21 years of age, 42% of participants had Davidson Trauma Scale scores consistent with post-traumatic stress disorder (PTSD), and the scores correlated with the number of hospital days in the previous year [30] One study from Iran evaluated 80 children with CKD stages 1–3 and 80 healthy children for the presence of obsessive compulsive disorder (OCD) using the Obsessive Compulsive Inventory-Child Version. The mean total scores of children with CKD were signifi-

cantly higher than for the healthy children, with higher scores being noted particularly in the symptom of doubting/checking and ordering [31].

Renal transplantation remains the optimal therapy for ESKD and is highly advocated for patients on dialysis. Despite receiving a renal transplant, the challenges of living with CKD remain, and as noted above, renal transplant recipients may still suffer from psychiatric and emotional distress. Many studies have compared the burden of psychosocial disease of living with a transplant to pre-ESKD and dialysis. One study clearly demonstrated that families report considerable improvements in a child's physical health. Yet, behavioral problems were twice as common in children who had received a transplant than in the healthy and pre-ESKD groups. Additionally school behavior in the transplant group, as rated by teachers, was similar to the healthy group and overall families reported an improvement in their children's behavior and quality of life [32]. Berney-Martinet et al. likewise did not find that transplantation associated with a lower prevalence of depression when compared to those who were pre-ESKD [29]. Another study also showed similar scores on the CDI and the State-trait anxiety inventory for children (STAIC) between the transplant and dialysis groups [33]. Other studies even document that the prevalence of psychiatric disorders in renal transplant recipients exceeds those with pre-ESKD CKD [25].

Studies have attempted to identify the risk factors for psychiatric morbidity in children with CKD. Although limited by sample size, most studies have not found disease-related variables to be significantly associated with psychiatric functioning [14, 24, 25, 34, 35], although one study reported higher parent-rated internalizing problems scores in children with non-glomerular disease than glomerular disease [20]. When comparing psychiatric morbidity by dialysis modalities, children undergoing PD appear to fare better than those undergoing in-center HD [33]. A study in Peru showed that 10% of children and adolescents with CKD reported high depressive symptomatology based on the Birleson Scale, and for children on PD the presence of depressive symptoms was significantly associated with Kt/V [36]. Additionally, as in the general population, obesity may play a role in increasing the risk for symptoms of depression [24, 37]. There is also evidence of a genetic role for depression. A CKiD study found that children with CKD who also had a pathogenic genomic copy number variation were more likely to endorse increased internalizing symptoms [38]. An increase in comorbidities, including preterm birth and developmental delay, also likely predisposes an individual with CKD to worse psychiatric functioning [21, 39].

Overall, psychiatric disorders and symptoms appear to be more common in pediatric CKD than in the general pediatric population, and the complications do not fully resolve with transplant. However, longitudinal studies of psychiatric functioning have found that instead of worsening with progression or duration of disease, there are fewer psychiatric complications in those with longer duration of disease and over time [40]. This can be seen in a CKiD study of parent-completed BASC-2 scores that identified improved scores over time [20]. These findings suggest that some children with CKD adapt to their circumstances; however, the examination for the presence of psychiatric disorders and emotional distress remain a critical area.

Social Functioning

The research on social functioning of children and adolescents with CKD is more limited than that of psychiatric functioning (see Table 63.1). Unlike other illnesses, such as childhood cancer, there are no studies directly comparing the classroom and extracurricular behaviors of children with CKD to healthy peers. Much of the available literature is embedded within studies that investigate psychosocial functioning more broadly. For example, the opportunities to make friends is likely impacted by CKD, but there are few studies examining this important social function. One study found that only 30% of children on dialysis, 55% of children with CKD not on dialysis and 83% of control participants reported having a special friend [14]. Similarly, the children with CKD also reported more loneliness than the control participants. Interestingly, in this study, those with CKD not on dialysis reported double the prevalence of being lonely (10%) than those on dialysis. In Japan, a study used the Diagnostic Interviews for Children and Adolescents monthly for 3 months in order to assess school adjustment of children with a renal transplant, children on PD, and control participants [41]. They found the children on dialysis had the most indicators of school maladjustment and that even children in the transplant group indicated significantly more school maladjustment than the control participants.

Evidence for the impact of social functioning and psychosocial development in CKD is also found in studies that compare risky behaviors in adolescents with CKD to control participants. In a multicenter study of North American adolescents with CKD stage II or higher, including ESKD, completed the National Youth Risk Behavior Survey [35]. Compared to a reference group, adolescents with CKD reported significantly fewer high-risk behaviors, including smoking, sexual activity, and unsafe driving, than the reference group. Although it is reassuring that adolescents with CKD appear to be participating in less high-risk behavior than their peers, there is concern that this indicates a delay in developmental milestones since engaging in risky behavior is part of normal adolescent behavior.

Additionally, children with CKD report a delay in the ages of first sexual intercourse and first alcoholic beverage [42, 43]. These delays may indicate a break with typical development that could negatively impact adult outcomes.

Quality of Life

As seen in Table 63.1, quality of life is heavily studied in pediatric CKD. The bulk of these studies have been cross-sectional, with only a few longitudinal studies. Most of the literature has focused on quality of life in patients receiving renal replacement therapies, while other studies have focused on group comparisons across different chronic health conditions and specific CKD groupings. The measure of quality of life usually includes multiple domains (i.e. physical, school, emotional and social) that reveal particular aspects of health related quality of life (HRQOL) that may be affected more than other aspects in particular settings.

There have been a number of studies examining quality of life in kidney transplant recipients. Falger et al. looked at the psychosocial adjustment post-transplant using the Netherlands-based Quality of Life Questionnaire and the CBCL [44]. They found that the dimension measuring emotional functioning was rated as impaired according to both parent and youth report. There were no statistical differences between parent and child ratings with regard to quality of life. Maternal distress showed a negative correlation with most dimensions of the quality of life scale. In Belgium, Dobbels et al. conducted a cross-sectional study with adolescent kidney transplant patients [26]. They assessed HRQOL using the short form of the KIDSCREEN and depression using the BDI. Adolescent transplant patients perceived their physical and psychological functioning about the same as healthy controls. However, parent's ratings of their adolescent's psychological well-being, level of perceived autonomy, and school functioning were significantly lower when compared to healthy controls. Finally, Haavisto et al. examined the quality of life in kidney transplant patients [45]. Data were collected from patients, caregivers and teachers. Using a Finnish HRQOL Questionnaire and U.S. normative date, the adolescent transplant group had significantly less self-reported feelings of distress and experienced more vitality than the controls; but, they described more problems attending school and being with friends. Additionally, parents described the transplant group as experiencing more problems in health and physical functioning than the transplant patients themselves. Taken together, while a transplant clearly contributes to improved health for children and adolescents with CKD, quality of life ratings remain significantly lower.

With respect to renal replacement therapies, a number of studies also have compared quality of life findings across different treatment modalities. Killis-Pstrusinska et al. administered the PedsQL (Pediatric Quality of Life Inventory) to Polish children with CKD and to their parents [46]. The sample included children on HD and PD and pre-ESKD patients. Children on PD reported significantly better quality of life compared to those on HD, and there was significant disagreement between parents and children, with parents reporting worse quality of life. Another study from Europe also demonstrated significantly lower HRQOL across all domains of ESKD (dialysis and transplant) when compared to healthy norms and other chronic conditions, with those who had received a preemptive transplant reporting higher scores on physical health [47]. They also identified that comorbidities was the most important determinant associated with lower HRQOL. Marciano et al. investigated the prevalence of behavior disorders (measured using the Strengths and Difficulties Questionnaire) and the relationship to HRQOL (measured using the PedsQL Global score) in children from Brazil with CKD, including pre-ESKD and dialysis patients and kidney transplant recipients [48]. Parents reported a negative correlation between the presence of behavior and emotional disorders and the HRQOL score. A large study from Australia and New Zealand used the Health Utilities Index (HUI) to show that children on dialysis had the lowest HRQOL, followed by transplant recipients, children with CKD stages 3–5 and children with CKD stages 1–2 [49].

In contrast, several studies have not demonstrated significant concerns for quality of life in children and adolescents with CKD receiving renal replacement therapies. Specifically, Heath et al. evaluated dialysis and kidney transplant patients in the United Kingdom using the Generic Children's Quality of Life Measure (GCQ) and compared their results with normative data [50]. The GCQ questionnaire assesses how the child views his or her life and how they would like it to be. Quality of life is measured as the discrepancy between the two viewpoints. No significant differences between the mean GCQ scores of the participants in various treatment modalities or from the mean of the normative group were observed. Similarly, Park et al. examined the quality of life in Korean children on HD or PD and transplant recipients using the PedsQL End-Stage Renal Disease Module [51]. There were no significant group differences on perceptions regarding family and peer interactions and communication. However, parent reports suggested that communication problems were worse in children on dialysis than in transplant recipients.

A few studies have compared quality of life in children with CKD and other medical conditions. Sundaram et al. evaluated a cohort of liver and kidney transplant patients using the Child Health Questionnaire (CHQ) completed by both parent and child [52]. Caregivers reported lower physical functioning and general health, but similar psychological health to the normative population. Caregivers expressed a negative emotional impact of their child's health on themselves and the family. Diseth et al. evaluated the mental health and quality of life of 28 transplanted youth and compared them to healthy controls and children who had survived acute lymphoblastic leukemia in Norway [53]. In addition to the Strength and Difficulties Questionnaire, the PedsQL was administered to youth and their parents. Similar to previous reports, emotional functioning of the transplant group was poorer than the healthy group, but similar to the cancer group. With regard to maternal mental health and maternal quality of life, parents of the transplant and the cancer groups reported similar degrees of impact of the child's illness on their functioning and on family functioning.

One of the challenges with examining the CKD population is that most studies enroll small numbers, with heterogeneity of age and CKD severity. These challenges likely explain some of the inconsistencies between reports. However, there are several consistent risk factors for lower HRQOL. Repeatedly, females have reported lower HRQOL than males [54–56] and those with short stature suffer lower HRQOL, particularly in the physical functioning domains [54, 57, 58]. Expectedly, maternal distress and adverse family relationships has also repeatedly been identified as associating with poorer HRQOL [44]. Similarly, emotional and behavioral disorders also associate with poorer HRQOL [48]. Other factors identified as associating with HRQOL include number of medications prescribed and the presence of anemia [59, 60]. The relationships between duration of disease and age with HRQOL are more mixed [54, 56, 59, 61].

Lastly, there are only a few longitudinal studies examining quality of life in CKD Neul et al. used a longitudinal case control method to track changes in physical, emotional, social, and educational functioning in dialysis patients and parents over 2 years [55]. The PedsQL and the End-Stage Module of the PedsQL were administered at approximately 6-month intervals. Parent-reported Global PedsQL scores did not change over time; however, global scores assessed by parents were significantly lower in females than males. After adjusting for a number of variables (e.g. dialysis), parents rating of school functioning declined significantly over the 2 years. Further, patients on dialysis had significantly lower emotional functioning. In contrast, patients reported more positive functioning compared to their parent's perceptions. Fadrowski et al. conducted a longitudinal study of physical and psychosocial functioning [58]. In this multicenter study, adolescents and their parents completed the CHQ over 4 years. After adjusting for targeted covariates, the Physical Summary score declined as glomerular filtration rate declined. Additionally, annualized height gains were associated with a improvements in Physical and Psychosocial summary scores, as seen in other studies [49, 57]. Finally, the effect of anemia on

HRQOL using the PedsQL was investigated in 773 children with mild to moderate CKD, with approximately 30% having anemia at the index visit [60]. The presence of anemia was associated with significantly lower overall HRQOL and physical functioning as reported by the children. For the parent ratings, the development of anemia was associated with lower emotional functioning and decreased physical functioning over time compared to those who remained anemia-free. No other findings on the PedsQL were noted.

Long-Term Functional Outcomes

As can be seen in Table 63.1, there is a paucity of scientific exploration into the long-term functional outcomes of childhood CKD. In a study from the United Kingdom that compared 976 young adults with ESKD to the general population, ESKD patients were more likely to live at home with parents and to be unemployed. Further, those who were employed were more likely to participate in low-skill occupations and have significantly lower incomes [43, 62]. Similar findings have been reported in young adults with ESKD in France, the United Kingdom and the United States [63–66].

Fortunately, there is some evidence that socio-professional outcomes are improving for young adults with ESKD. A study from the Netherlands compared the socio-professional achievements of adults with ESKD in 2010 and 2000. In 2010, they were more likely to live with a partner and to have completed a high level educational degree [67]. Clearly, this is an area of interest from a psychosocial perspective, and there is a need for more evidence-based interventions.

Identification and Measurement of Psychosocial Issues in the Clinical Setting

The identification of psychosocial issues may be straight forward. A patient may present with somatic complaints that are not compatible with their medical condition; they may appear withdrawn, with blunted affect; or demonstrate concerning grooming or social habits. A family member or member of the treatment team may raise concern. There are several methods for making a formal diagnosis, including standardized inventories, clinical or structured interviews or direct observation. Interpretation of data gathered from these methods requires consideration of the type of measurement being employed (e.g., is it a rating scale, a clinical interview, an observation?), its psychometric properties (i.e., is it reliable and valid?), who is providing the information (i.e., parents, teachers, the child or adolescent?) including their honesty, forthrightness and insightfulness, and the clinical utility of the obtained information (i.e., how will the information be used and what resources are available to address the chronicity and/or severity of the concerns?).

Clinical interview is a long-held approach to obtaining patient information [68]. When systematic and structured, this approach can provide substantial information about the psychosocial functioning of a child or adolescent. Children can be interviewed alone or with their parent or caregiver. Adolescents typically are interviewed alone. The challenge with clinical interviews is that they tend not to be systematic and there is no assurance that all diagnostic questions will be asked of each patient. This can be addressed by using a structure interview that addresses all necessary questions based on the clinical situation. Examples of structured interviews include the Diagnostic Interview of Children and Adolescents (DICA) [69], the Kiddie Schedule for Affective Disorders and Schizophrenia (K-SADS) [70], the Child and Adolescent Psychiatric Assessment (CAPA) [71], and the Preschool Age Psychiatric Assessment (PAPA) [72], for preschoolers and early elementary age children. The primary advantages of a structured interview is that it increases the probability that necessary questions will be asked, particularly with respect to diagnostic criteria; however, it can be time consuming, limiting its application in a rapid-paced clinical setting. Nonetheless, structured interviews are usually considered the gold standard in clinical research for psychiatric conditions, and several studies have employed these scales with pediatric CKD.

Another approach to psychosocial assessment is behavioral rating scales. These scales are standardized, normed across a wide age range, typically have strong psychometric properties, and are cost and time efficient, with many now being computer administered and scored. They require some level of literacy on the part of the respondent, but can be completed by a child, adolescent, parent, teacher, or other caregiver. Further, rating scales have been developed to assess a wide variety of psychosocial issues as well as to assess specific concerns. For example, omnibus rating scales that utilize a multi-rater, multi-setting, multi-instrument assessment design include the Child Behavior Checklist (CBCL) [17], Behavior Assessment Scale for Children (BASC) [18], and the Conners' Rating Scale-3 (Conners) [73]. These scales provide a vast amount of information, as informed by the rater, and can assist in identifying psychosocial difficulties as well as screening for psychiatric diagnoses. All of these measures have been used in the assessment of psychosocial functioning in pediatric CKD.

Similarly, rating scales have been developed to identify symptoms and behaviors associated with specific disorders. For example, the Child Depression Inventory-2 (CDI-2) [74] assess for depression or depression symptoms and has been commonly used to identify depression in pediatric CKD. There are also specific rating scales for anxiety (e.g., Multidimensional Anxiety Scale for Children-2 [75]), anger [76], attention deficit hyperactivity disorder (Vanderbilt ADHD Diagnostic Rating Scale [77]), self-esteem (Multidimensional Self-Concept Scale [78]), OCD (Yale-Brown Obsessive-Compulsive Survey [79]), quality of life (PedsQL [80]) and other conditions [81]

While most assessments of psychosocial functioning typically use some combination of clinical interviews and rating scales, the applicability and utility of any of these approaches are determined by the nature of the clinic and the type of services that can be offered. Additionally, the use of multi-rater, multi-setting, multi-instrument assessment models, while providing a wide array of data on the social and emotional functioning of the patient, can present discrepancies in the data across different instruments and different raters. In fact, discrepancies between child and parent perceptions regarding the presence and the severity of psychosocial issues should be expected as they are consistently observed in nearly all of the studies cited in this chapter. For this reason, obtaining information from multiple informants is advisable [82]. Additionally, it is important to note that perceptual discordance is particularly pronounced during adolescence [57] and it is important to consider this discordance in the interpretation of psychosocial measures. Working with a pediatric psychologist or other mental health professional (e.g., social worker, counselor, child psychiatrist) can assist in the interpretation of these assessments.

Management of Psychosocial Issues in the Clinical Setting

Addressing the psychosocial needs of children and adolescents with CKD is important but can present challenges. Nephrology providers manage the medical complexity of CKD and may have limited time to address psychosocial issues, especially given limited knowledge in this area. In addition, families may be reluctant to raise yet another problem that may need to be addressed by adding more providers, appointments, or medications to their already complicated regimens. Moreover, there are no data specific to treating psychosocial issues in the context of pediatric CKD.

To address the psychiatric challenges, a medical social worker is often already part of the team in many pediatric nephrology programs and can be a good resource for families. The social worker can address any background stressors and can provide coping strategies to the patients. Community mental health provides also may be an option, although in the United States access can be limited by insurance constraints and community providers may feel more comfortable partnering with the medical team given the complexity of CKD. Referral to pediatric psychologists can be helpful for administration of evidence-based therapies, such as cognitive-behavioral therapy, to address psychiatric issues. In the United States, access to pediatric psychologists can also be a barrier. For adolescents, referral to an adolescent medicine specialist can be helpful for strategies to manage living with a chronic condition. Lastly, pharmacotherapy for treatment of anxiety, depression, ADHD, and other psychiatric conditions can be useful. Although not specifically studied in children and adolescents with CKD, the selective serotonin uptake inhibitors have been studied in adults with CKD and ESKD and therefore should be considered first-line agents for managing depression and anxiety. Fluoxetine and citalopram do not require dosage adjustments in CKD, while the maximum dosage of sertraline may need to be reduced [83].

There are additional options to support the social and behavioral health of children and adolescents with CKD. Families can be supported by connecting them with other families of children with CKD, which can include connections through social media or kidney camps. Attending kidney camps has been shown to be beneficial for both patients and their families [84–86]. Pediatric psychologists and medical social workers can provide parenting tools and stress management techniques. In addition, child life providers can help manage the anxiety and psychological trauma that may come from repeated invasive medical procedures and encounters. To reduce stress in the school setting, medical social workers can advocate for a patient's needs and accommodations.

While a discussion of school-related functions is beyond the scope of this chapter, there is a longstanding recognition of the negative impact of physical illness on educational and eventual occupational functioning as these disruptions can affect psychosocial functioning. Educational and occupational problems appear to be major areas of concern for children and their parents; chronic school absenteeism is alarmingly common in children with CKD [87]. Not only do school absences have a direct impact on gaining fundamental academic proficiencies, but missed school also interferes with children acquiring essential social competencies and developing social support networks. Even with the relatively reassuring educational and occupational assessments of children with CKD [88], continued efforts need to be made to allow for school-based accommodations as well as work-based accommodations for absences due to medical appointments and sporadic exacerbations of kidney disease.

Finally, the type of mental health treatment and/or social supports for children and adolescents with CKD may vary by developmental level. For example, adolescents with CKD may face barriers during their transition to early adulthood, particularly with respect to their healthcare. The transition to adulthood is an important period in human development that requires an individual to increase autonomy, find gainful employment, and build social relationships. Pediatric CKD and the medical complications that can be associated with CKD can prevent many adolescents from making this transition and facing these developmental challenges successfully. To date, intervention research geared toward the medical and psychosocial barriers that impede transition to adulthood is emergent and several possibilities exist that might prove instrumental in smoothing the transition for adolescents with CKD. The issue of transition is critical to the psychosocial health of this population, particularly given the medical needs that will continue into adulthood and the concomitant psychosocial burden that many of these youth will experience as they move into the adult world [89].

Gaps in the Literature and Future Directions

It is clear that children and adolescents with CKD experience psychosocial challenges and that these challenges should be addressed. More research is needed to provide evidence-based literature to define appropriate interventions. In addition, more interdisciplinary support, such as therapists, psychologists and psychiatrists, would enable better care for pediatric CKD patients. Research that clearly establishes the relationships between psychosocial distress and outcomes, such as healthcare costs and utilization and educational and professional attainment, and demonstrates improvement in outcomes with appropriate interventions would be helpful to justify increased psychosocial support.

Conclusions

Children with CKD have many challenges, including short stature, chronic school absenteeism and reduced social opportunities. Consequently, children and adolescents with CKD at all stages of disease may experience mental health and adjustment problems that extend into adulthood and affect quality of life. Although renal transplant is the optimal therapy for ESKD, it is not curative, and children and adolescent renal transplant recipients have psychosocial issues, and some may even be exacerbated. Disease related variables have not consistently been shown to associate with psychiatric functioning, but obesity, genetics, comorbidities and preterm birth may predispose a child with CKD to impaired psychosocial health. There are many tools to measure psychosocial performance to aid in identification of impairment. Although medical social workers, community mental health providers and adolescent medicine doctors may offer support and strategies to struggling patients, more research is needed to define the interventions that will improve the psychosocial health, and ultimately improve the long-term outcomes of children with CKD.

References

1. Bruce MA, Beech BM, Sims M, et al. Social environmental stressors, psychological factors, and kidney disease. J Investig Med. 2009;57(4):583–9. https://doi.org/10.2310/JIM.0b013e31819dbb91.
2. Cukor D, Cohen SD, Peterson RA, Kimmen PL. Psychosocial aspects of chronic disease: ESRD as a paradigmatic illness. J Am Soc Nephrol. 2007;18(12):3042–55. https://doi.org/10.1681/ASN.2007030345.
3. Gerson AC, Riley A, Fivush BA, et al. Assessing health status and health care utilization in adolescents with chronic kidney disease. J Am Soc Nephrol. 2005;16(5):1427–32. https://doi.org/10.1681/ASN.2004040258.
4. Spiegel BMR, Melmed G, Robbins S, Esrailian E. Biomarkers and health-related quality of life in end-stage renal disease: a systematic review. Clin J Am Soc Nephrol. 2008;3(6):1759–68. https://doi.org/10.2215/CJN.00820208.
5. Whitney DG, Peterson MD. US National and State-Level Prevalence of Mental Health Disorders and Disparities of Mental Health Care Use in Children. JAMA Pediatr. 2019;173(4):389–91. https://doi.org/10.1001/jamapediatrics.2018.5399.
6. Costello EJ, Mustillo S, Erkanli A, Keeler G, Angold A. Prevalence and development of psychiatric disorders in childhood and adolescence. Arch Gen Psychiatry. 2003;60(8):837–44. https://doi.org/10.1001/archpsyc.60.8.837.
7. Kessler RC, Avenevoli S, Costello EJ, et al. Prevalence, persistence, and sociodemographic correlates of DSM-IV disorders in the National Comorbidity Survey Replication Adolescent Supplement. Arch Gen Psychiatry. 2012;69(4):372–80. https://doi.org/10.1001/archgenpsychiatry.2011.160.
8. Polanczyk GV, Salum GA, Sugaya LS, Caye A, Rohde LA. Annual research review: a meta-analysis of the worldwide prevalence of mental disorders in children and adolescents. J Child Psychol Psychiatry Allied Discip. 2015;56(3):345–65. https://doi.org/10.1111/jcpp.12381.
9. Downs J, Blackmore AM, Epstein A, et al. The prevalence of mental health disorders and symptoms in children and adolescents with cerebral palsy: a systematic review and meta-analysis. Dev Med Child Neurol. 2018;60(1):30–8. https://doi.org/10.1111/dmcn.13555.
10. Richardson LP, Russo JE, Lozano P, McCauley E, Katon W. The effect of comorbid anxiety and depressive disorders on health care utilization and costs among adolescents with asthma. Gen Hosp Psychiatry. 2008;30(5):398–406. https://doi.org/10.1016/j.genhosppsych.2008.06.004.
11. Smith BA, Modi AC, Quittner AL, Wood BL. Depressive symptoms in children with cystic fibrosis and parents and its effects on adherence to airway clearance. Pediatr Pulmonol. 2010;45(8):756–63. https://doi.org/10.1002/ppul.21238.
12. Brownbridge G, Fielding DM. Psychosocial adjustment and adherence to dialysis treatment regimes. Pediatr Nephrol. 1994;8(6):744–9. https://doi.org/10.1007/BF00869109.
13. Maikranz JM, Steele RG, Dreyer ML, Stratman AC, Bovaird JA. The relationship of hope and illness-related uncertainty to emotional adjustment and adherence among pediatric renal and liver transplant recipients. J Pediatr Psychol. 2007;32(5):571–81. https://doi.org/10.1093/jpepsy/jsl046.

14. Garralda ME, Jameson RA, Reynolds JM, Postlethwaite RJ. Psychiatric adjustment in children with chronic renal failure. J Child Psychol Psychiatry. 1988;29(1):79–90. https://doi.org/10.1111/j.1469-7610.1988.tb00691.x.

15. Senses Dinc G, Cak T, Cengel Kultur E, Bilginer Y, Kul M, Topaloglu R. Psychiatric morbidity and different treatment modalities in children with chronic kidney disease. Arch Pediatr. 2019;26(5):263–7. https://doi.org/10.1016/j.arcped.2019.05.013.

16. Bakr A, Amr M, Sarhan A, et al. Psychiatric disorders in children with chronic renal failure. Pediatr Nephrol. 2007;22(1):128–31. https://doi.org/10.1007/s00467-006-0298-9.

17. Achenbach TM, Rescorla L. Manual for the ASEBA school-age forms and profiles. Burlington, VT: University of Vermont, Research Center for Children, Youth and Families; 2001.

18. Reynolds C, Kamphaus R. Behavior assessment system for children. 2nd ed. Circle Pines, MN: American Guidance Service, Inc.; 2004.

19. Hooper SR, Duquette PJ, Icard P, Wetherington CE, Harrell W, Gipson DS. Social-behavioural functioning in paediatric chronic kidney disease. Child Care Health Dev. 2009;35(6):832–40. https://doi.org/10.1111/j.1365-2214.2009.00992.x.

20. Johnson RJ, Gerson AC, Harshman LA, et al. A longitudinal examination of parent-reported emotional-behavioral functioning of children with mild to moderate chronic kidney disease. Pediatr Nephrol. 2020;35(7):1287–95. https://doi.org/10.1007/s00467-020-04511-9.

21. Kang NR, Ahn YH, Park E, et al. Mental health and psychosocial adjustment in pediatric chronic kidney disease derived from the KNOW-Ped CKD study. Pediatr Nephrol. 2019;34(10):1753–64. https://doi.org/10.1007/s00467-019-04292-w.

22. Hooper SR, Gerson AC, Johnson JR, et al. Neurocognitive, social-behavioral, and adaptive functioning in preschool children with mild to moderate kidney disease. J Dev Behav Pediatr. 2016;37(3):231–8. https://doi.org/10.1097/DBP.0000000000000267.

23. Eisenhauer GL, Arnold WC, Livingston RL. Identifying psychiatric disorders in children with renal disease. South Med J. 1988;81(5):572–6. https://doi.org/10.1097/00007611-198805000-00008.

24. Kogon AJ, Matheson MB, Flynn JT, et al. Depressive symptoms in children with chronic kidney disease. J Pediatr. 2016;168:164–170.e1. https://doi.org/10.1016/j.jpeds.2015.09.040.

25. Kogon AJ, Vander Stoep A, Weiss NS, Smith J, Flynn JT, McCauley E. Depression and its associated factors in pediatric chronic kidney disease. Pediatr Nephrol. 2013;28(9) https://doi.org/10.1007/s00467-013-2497-5.

26. Dobbels F, Decorte A, Roskams A, Van Damme-Lombaerts R. Health-related quality of life, treatment adherence, symptom experience and depression in adolescent renal transplant patients.

Pediatr Transplant. 2010;14(2):216–23. https://doi.org/10.1111/j.1399-3046.2009.01197.x.

27. Fukunishi I, Honda M, Kamiyama Y, Ito H. Anxiety disorders and pediatric continuous ambulatory peritoneal dialysis. Child Psychiatry Hum Dev. 1993;24(1):59–64. https://doi.org/10.1007/BF02353719.

28. Fukunishi I, Kudo H. Psychiatric problems of pediatric end-stage renal failure. Gen Hosp Psychiatry. 1995;17(1):32–6. https://doi.org/10.1016/0163-8343(94)00060-Q.

29. Berney-Martinet S, Key F, Bell L, Lépine S, Clermont M-J, Fombonne E. Psychological profile of adolescents with a kidney transplant. Pediatr Transplant. 2009;13(6):701–10. https://doi.org/10.1111/j.1399-3046.2008.01053.x.

30. Wallace J, Yorgin PD, Carolan R, et al. The use of art therapy to detect depression and post-traumatic stress disorder in pediatric and young adult renal transplant recipients. Pediatr Transplant. 2004;8(1):52–9. https://doi.org/10.1046/j.1397-3142.2003.00124.x.

31. Yousefichaijan P, Sharafkhah M, Rafeie M, Salehi B. Obsessive Compulsive Inventory-Child Version (OCV-CI) to evaluate obsessive compulsive disorder in children with early stages of chronic kidney disease: a case control study. Nephrourol Mon. 2016;8(1):e34017. https://doi.org/10.5812/numonthly.34017.

32. Reynolds JM, Garralda ME, Postlethwaite RJ, Goh D. Changes in psychosocial adjustment after renal transplantation. Arch Dis Child. 1991;66(4):508–13. https://doi.org/10.1136/adc.66.4.508.

33. Brownbridge G, Fielding DM. Psychosocial adjustment to end-stage renal failure: comparing haemodialysis, continuous ambulatory peritoneal dialysis and transplantation. Pediatr Nephrol. 1991;5(5):612–6. https://doi.org/10.1007/BF00856653.

34. Amr M, Bakr A, Gilany AH, Hammad A, El-Refaey A, El-Mougy A. Multi-method assessment of behavior adjustment in children with chronic kidney disease. Pediatr Nephrol. 2009;24(2):341–7. https://doi.org/10.1007/s00467-008-1012-x.

35. Xiao N, Stolfi A, Malatesta-Muncher R, et al. Risk behaviors in teens with chronic kidney disease: a study from the midwest pediatric nephrology consortium. Int J Nephrol. 2019;2019 https://doi.org/10.1155/2019/7828406.

36. Hernandez EG, Loza R, Vargas H, Jara MF. Depressive symptomatology in children and adolescents with chronic renal insufficiency undergoing chronic dialysis. Int J Nephrol. 2011;2011:1–7. https://doi.org/10.4061/2011/798692.

37. Kogon AJ, Kim JY, Laney N, et al. Depression and neurocognitive dysfunction in pediatric and young adult chronic kidney disease. Pediatr Nephrol May 2019. doi:https://doi.org/10.1007/s00467-019-04265-z.

38. Verbitsky M, Kogon AJ, Matheson M, et al. Genomic disorders and neurocognitive impairment in pediatric CKD. J Am Soc Nephrol. 2017;28(8) https://doi.org/10.1681/ASN.2016101108.

39. Qvist E, Närhi V, Apajasalo M, et al. Psychosocial adjustment and quality of life after renal transplantation in early childhood. Pediatr Transplant. 2004;8(2):120–5. https://doi.org/10.1046/j.1399-3046.2003.00121.x.

40. Rodriguez Cuellar CI, García de la Puente S, Hernández Moraria J, Bojórquez Ochoa A, Filler G, Zaltzman GS. High depression rates among pediatric renal replacement therapy patients: a cross-sectional study. Pediatr Transplant. 2019;23(8) https://doi.org/10.1111/petr.13591.

41. Fukunishi I, Honda M. School adjustment of children with end-stage renal disease. Pediatr Nephrol. 1995;9(5):553–7. https://doi.org/10.1007/BF00860928.

42. Groothoff JW, Offringa M, Grootenhuis M, Jager KJ. Long-term consequences of renal insufficiency in children: lessons learned from the Dutch LERIC study. Nephrol Dial Transplant. 2018;33(4):552–60. https://doi.org/10.1093/ndt/gfx190.

43. Hamilton AJ, Caskey FJ, Casula A, Ben-Shlomo Y, Inward CD. Psychosocial health and lifestyle behaviors in young adults receiving renal replacement therapy compared to the general population: findings from the SPEAK Study. Am J Kidney Dis. 2019;73(2):194–205. https://doi.org/10.1053/j.ajkd.2018.08.006.

44. Falger J, Landolt MA, Latal B, Rüth EM, Neuhaus TJ, Laube GF. Outcome after renal transplantation. Part II: quality of life and psychosocial adjustment. Pediatr Nephrol. 2008;23(8):1347–54. https://doi.org/10.1007/s00467-008-0798-x.

45. Haavisto A, Korkman M, Sintonen H, et al. Risk factors for impaired quality of life and psychosocial adjustment after pediatric heart, kidney, and liver transplantation. Pediatr Transplant. 2013;17(3):256–65. https://doi.org/10.1111/petr.12054.

46. Kiliś-Pstrusińska K, Medyńska A, Chmielewska IB, et al. Perception of health-related quality of life in children with chronic kidney disease by the patients and their caregivers: Multicentre national study results. Qual Life Res. 2013;22(10):2889–97. https://doi.org/10.1007/s11136-013-0416-7.

47. Splinter A, Tjaden LA, Haverman L, et al. Children on dialysis as well as renal transplanted children report severely impaired health-related quality of life. Qual Life Res. 2018;27(6):1445–54. https://doi.org/10.1007/s11136-018-1789-4.

48. Marciano RC, Bouissou Soares CM, Diniz JSS, et al. Behavioral disorders and low quality of life in children and adolescents with chronic kidney disease. Pediatr Nephrol. 2011;26(2):281–90. https://doi.org/10.1007/s00467-010-1683-y.

49. Francis A, Didsbury MS, Van Zwieten A, et al. Quality of life of children and adolescents with chronic kidney disease: a cross-sectional study. Arch Dis Child. 2019;104(2):134–40. https://doi.org/10.1136/archdischild-2018-314934.

50. Heath J, MacKinlay D, Watson AR, et al. Self-reported quality of life in children and young people with chronic kidney disease. Pediatr Nephrol. 2011;26(5):767–73. https://doi.org/10.1007/s00467-011-1784-2.

51. Park KS, Hwang YJ, Cho MH, et al. Quality of life in children with end-stage renal disease based on a PedsQL ESRD module. Pediatr Nephrol. 2012;27(12):2293–300. https://doi.org/10.1007/s00467-012-2262-1.

52. Sundaram SS, Landgraf JM, Neighbors K, Cohn RA, Alonso EM. Adolescent health-related quality of life following liver and kidney transplantation. Am J Transplant. 2007;7(4):982–9. https://doi.org/10.1111/j.1600-6143.2006.01722.x.

53. Diseth TH, Tangeraas T, Reinfjell T, Bjerre A. Kidney transplantation in childhood: mental health and quality of life of children and caregivers. Pediatr Nephrol. 2011;26(10):1881–92. https://doi.org/10.1007/s00467-011-1887-9.

54. Baek HS, Kang HG, Choi HJ, et al. Health-related quality of life of children with pre-dialysis chronic kidney disease. Pediatr Nephrol. 2017;32(11):2097–105. https://doi.org/10.1007/s00467-017-3721-5.

55. Neul SK, Minard CG, Currier H, Goldstein SL. Health-related quality of life functioning over a 2-year period in children with end-stage renal disease. Pediatr Nephrol. 2013;28(2):285–93. https://doi.org/10.1007/s00467-012-2313-7.

56. Pardede SO, Rafli A, Gunardi H. Quality of life in chronic kidney disease children using assessment Pediatric Quality Of Life Inventory™. Saudi J Kidney Dis Transpl. 2019;30(4):812–8. https://doi.org/10.4103/1319-2442.265456.

57. Al-Uzri A, Matheson M, Gipson DS, et al. The impact of short stature on health-related quality of life in children with chronic kidney disease. J Pediatr. 2013;163(3):736–741.e1. https://doi.org/10.1016/j.jpeds.2013.03.016.

58. Fadrowski J, Cole SR, Hwang W, et al. Changes in physical and psychosocial functioning among adolescents with chronic kidney disease. Pediatr Nephrol. 2006;21(3):394–9. https://doi.org/10.1007/s00467-005-2122-3.

59. Díaz-González de Ferris ME, Pierce CB, Gipson DS, et al. Health-related quality of life in children with chronic kidney disease is affected by the number of medications. Pediatr Nephrol. 2021;36(5):1307–10. https://doi.org/10.1007/s00467-021-04919-x.

60. Carlson J, Gerson AC, Matheson MB, et al. A longitudinal analysis of the effect of anemia on health-related quality of life in children with mild-to-moderate chronic kidney disease. Pediatr Nephrol. 2020;35(9):1659–67. https://doi.org/10.1007/s00467-020-04569-5.

61. Gerson AC, Wentz A, Abraham AG, et al. Health-related quality of life of children with mild to moderate chronic kidney disease. Pediatrics. 2010;125(2):e349–57. https://doi.org/10.1542/peds.2009-0085.

62. Tjaden LA, Grootenhuis MA, Noordzij M, Groothoff JW. Health-related quality of life in patients with pediatric onset of end-stage renal disease: state of the art and recommendations for clinical practice. Pediatr Nephrol. 2016;31(10):1579–91. https://doi.org/10.1007/s00467-015-3186-3.

63. Mellerio H, Alberti C, Labèguerie M, et al. Adult social and professional outcomes of pediatric renal transplant recipients. Transplantation. 2014;97(2):196–205. https://doi.org/10.1097/TP.0b013e3182a74de2.

64. Lewis H, Marks SD. Differences between paediatric and adult presentation of ESKD in attainment of adult social goals. Pediatr Nephrol. 2014;29(12):2379–85. https://doi.org/10.1007/s00467-014-2864-x.

65. Murray PD, Dobbels F, Lonsdale DC, Harden PN. Impact of end-stage kidney disease on academic achievement and employment in young adults: a mixed methods study. J Adolesc Health. 2014;55(4):505–12. https://doi.org/10.1016/j.jadohealth.2014.03.017.

66. Murray PD, Brodermann MH, Gralla J, Wiseman AC, Harden PN. Academic achievement and employment in young adults with end-stage kidney disease. J Ren Care. 2019;45(1):29–40. https://doi.org/10.1111/jorc.12261.

67. Tjaden LA, Maurice-Stam H, Grootenhuis MA, Jager KJ, Groothoff JW. Impact of renal replacement therapy in childhood on long-term socioprofessional outcomes: a 30-year follow-up study. J Pediatr. 2016;171:189–195.e2. https://doi.org/10.1016/j.jpeds.2015.12.017.

68. MacKinnon RA, Michels R, Buckley P. The psychiatric interview in clinical practice. 3rd ed. Washington, D.C.: American Psychiatric Association; 2016.

69. Herjanic B, Reich W, Welner Z. Diagnostic interview for Children and Adolescents-Fourth Edcition (DICA-IV). North Tonawonda, NY: Multi-Health Systems Incorporated; 1997.

70. Kaufman J, Birmaher B, Brent D, et al. Schedule for affective disorders and schizophrenia for school-age children-present and lifetime version (K-SADS-PL): initial reliability and validity data. J Am Acad Child Adolesc Psychiatry. 1997;36(7):980–8. https://doi.org/10.1097/00004583-199707000-00021.

71. Angold A, Jane CE. The Child and Adolescent Psychiatric Assessment (CAPA). J Am Acad Child Adolesc Psychiatry. 2000;39(1):39–48. https://doi.org/10.1097/00004583-200001000-00015.

72. Egger HL, Erkanli A, Keeler G, Potts E, Walter BK, Angold A. Test-retest reliability of the Preschool Age Psychiatric Assessment (PAPA). J Am Acad Child Adolesc Psychiatry. 2006;45(5):538–49. https://doi.org/10.1097/01.chi.0000205705.71194.b8.

73. Conners K. Conners' behavior rating scale-3. North Tonawanda, NY: Multi-Health Systems Incorporated; 2008.

74. Kovacs M. CDI-2: Children's depression inventory 2nd edition technical manual. 2nd ed. Toronto: Multi-Health Systems Incorporated; 2011.

75. J M. Multidimensional anxiety scale for children-2. San Antonio, TX: Pearson; 2012.

76. Speilberger C. State-trait anger expression inventory-2. Odessa, FL: Psychological Assessment Resources, Inc.; 1999.

77. Wolraich ML, Lambert W, Doffing MA, Bickman L, Simmons T, Worley K. Psychometric properties of the vanderbilt ADHD diagnostic parent rating scale in a referred population. J Pediatr Psychol. 2003;28(8):559–67. https://doi.org/10.1093/jpepsy/jsg046.

78. Bracken B. Multidimensional self-concept scale. Austin, TX: Pro-Ed; 1993.

79. Goodman WK, Price LH, Rasmussen SA, et al. The Yale-Brown obsessive compulsive scale: I. Development, use, and reliability. Arch Gen Psychiatry. 1989;46(11):1006–11. https://doi.org/10.1001/archpsyc.1989.01810110048007.

80. Varni JW. The PedsQL measurement model for the pediatric quality of life inventory. Chicago: PedsMetrics; 2021.

81. Frankel KA, Harrison JN, Njoroge WFM, editors. Clinical guide to psychiatric assessment of infants and young children. New York: Springer; 2019.

82. Cremeens J, Eiser C, Blades M. Factors influencing agreement between child self-report and parent proxy-reports on the Pediatric Quality of Life Inventory™ 4.0 (PedsQL™) generic core scales. Health Qual Life Outcomes. 2006;4 https://doi.org/10.1186/1477-7525-4-58.

83. Nagler EV, Webster AC, Vanholder R, Zoccali C. Antidepressants for depression in stage 3–5 chronic kidney disease: a systematic review of pharmacokinetics, efficacy and safety with recommendations by European Renal Best Practice (ERBP). Nephrol Dial Transplant. 2012;27(10):3736–45. https://doi.org/10.1093/ndt/gfs295.

84. Klee KM. Benefits of a mainstreamed summer camp experience for teens with ESRD. Adv Perit Dial. 1992;8:423–5.

85. Warady BA. Therapeutic camping for children with end-stage renal disease. Pediatr Nephrol. 1994;8(3):387–90. https://doi.org/10.1007/BF00866373.

86. Klee K, Greenleaf K, Watkins S. Summer camps for children and adolescents with kidney disease. ANNA J. 1997;24(1)

87. Richardson KL, Weiss NS, Halbach S. Chronic school absenteeism of children with chronic kidney disease. J Pediatr. 2018;199:267–71. https://doi.org/10.1016/j.jpeds.2018.03.031.

88. Harshman LA, Johnson RJ, Matheson MB, et al. Academic achievement in children with chronic kidney disease: a report from the CKiD cohort. Pediatr Nephrol. 2019;34(4):689–96. https://doi.org/10.1007/s00467-018-4144-7.

89. Icard PF, Hower SJ, Kuchenreuther AR, Hooper SR, Gipson DS. The transition from childhood to adulthood with ESRD: educational and social challenges. Clin Nephrol. 2008;69(1):1–7. https://doi.org/10.5414/CNP69001.

90. Fielding D, Brownbridge G. Factors related to psychosocial adjustment in children with end-stage renal failure. Pediatr Nephrol. 1999;13(9):766–70. https://doi.org/10.1007/s004670050695.

91. Penkower L, Dew MA, Ellis D, Sereika SM, Kitutu JMM, Shapiro R. Psychological distress and adherence to the medical regimen among

adolescent renal transplant recipients. Am J Transplant. 2003;3(11):1418–25. https://doi.org/10.1046/j.1600-6135.2003.00226.x.

92. Selewski DT, Massengill SF, Troost JP, et al. Gaining the Patient Reported Outcomes Measurement Information System (PROMIS) perspective in chronic kidney disease: a Midwest Pediatric Nephrology Consortium study. Pediatr Nephrol. 2014;29(12):2347–56. https://doi.org/10.1007/s00467-014-2858-8.

93. Moreira JM, Bouissou Morais Soares CM, Teixeira AL, Silva ACSE, Kummer AM. Anxiety, depression, resilience and quality of life in children and adolescents with pre-dialysis chronic kidney disease. Pediatr Nephrol. 2015;30(12):2153–62. https://doi.org/10.1007/s00467-015-3159-6.

94. Gerson AC, Furth SL, Neu AM, Fivush BA. Assessing associations between medication adherence and potentially modifiable psychosocial variables in pediatric kidney transplant recipients and their families. Pediatr Transplant. 2004;8(6):543–50. https://doi.org/10.1111/j.1399-3046.2004.00215.x.

95. Roscoe JM, Smith LF, Williams EA, et al. Medical and social outcome in adolescents with end-stage renal failure. Kidney Int. 1991;40(5):948–53. https://doi.org/10.1038/ki.1991.299.

96. Mellerio H, Alberti C, Labèguerie M, et al. Adult social and professional outcomes of pediatric renal transplant recipients. Transp J. 2014;97(2):196–205. https://doi.org/10.1097/TP.0b013e3182a74de2.

97. Endén K, Tainio J, Jalanko H, Jahnukainen K, Jahnukainen T. Lower quality of life in young men after pediatric kidney transplantation when compared to healthy controls and survivors of childhood leukemia—a cross-sectional study. Transpl Int. 2018;31(2):157–64. https://doi.org/10.1111/tri.13040.

98. Kerklaan J, Hannan E, Hanson C, et al. Perspectives on life participation by young adults with chronic kidney disease: an interview study. BMJ Open. 2020;10(10) https://doi.org/10.1136/bmjopen-2020-037840.

Part XIII

Kidney Replacement Therapy

Initiation of Kidney Replacement Therapy: Strategic Choices and Preparation

64

Jérôme Harambat and Iona Madden

Introduction

During the past three decades, the management of children with chronic kidney disease (CKD) and end-stage kidney disease (ESKD) has improved dramatically. In high-income regions, though the financial cost is important, provision of kidney replacement therapy (KRT) by dialysis or pre-emptive transplantation is considered standard care for the great majority of children for whom this therapy is indicated. However, in lower income countries, the economic, human, and technical resources required for the treatment of childhood ESKD make it a major health challenge.

Children with CKD and their families/caregivers experience a complex decision on KRT initiation and treatment modality choice for a lifelong condition. The timing and circumstances of KRT initiation, and the choice of KRT modality can significantly impact clinical outcomes as well as the child's and caregivers' mental health and social life. The chosen KRT modality for children should ensure the lowest risk of mortality and morbidity and provide the best quality of life. In this regard, (living donor) pre-emptive kidney transplantation, when feasible, is considered the best choice of KRT in children. However, the majority of pediatric patients with ESKD will require dialysis. Chronic peritoneal dialysis (PD) can offer several advantages over hemodialysis (HD) for children.

This chapter outlines the current distribution of KRT modalities among incident and prevalent pediatric patients worldwide, the main outcomes according to KRT modality, the optimal timing of KRT initiation (dialysis initiation, preemptive kidney transplantation), the dialysis preparation and transplant workup. In addition, the chapter explores the pros and cons of each KRT modality taking into consideration the widely variable access to KRT around the world, and the lifetime perspectives of the choice to be made. Topic reviews that include more comprehensive management, complications and outcomes of the different modalities of KRT are discussed in separate chapters.

Current Distribution of Initial KRT Modalities Among Pediatric Patients Worldwide

The incidence, prevalence, and treatment modalities of pediatric ESKD worldwide are only partially known because of differences in pediatric patient definitions, disease classification, and lack of national registries and health information systems, especially in low- and middle-income

J. Harambat (✉) · I. Madden
Pediatric Nephrology Unit, Department of Pediatrics, University of Bordeaux, University Children's Hospital, Bordeaux, France
e-mail: jerome.harambat@chu-bordeaux.fr; iona.madden@chu-bordeaux.fr

countries [1, 2]. Most of the epidemiological data on pediatric ESKD requiring KRT (dialysis or kidney transplantation) is derived from high-income countries due to the availability of robust national or international registries mainly in Europe, Australia and New Zealand, and the United States [1].

The incidence of ESKD in children varies widely across different countries but ranges from 5–15 per million children per year among patients under 20 years. The number of children starting KRT has decreased in the United States where the incidence rate was the highest worldwide, remained stable in other high-income countries [3, 4], and may have increased in some lower income countries. The prevalence of ESKD in children varies between 40–60 per million children in Western Europe and Australia, with the prevalence being higher in the US (around 100 per million children) and lower in South America and Eastern Europe. Globally the prevalence of children undergoing KRT (functioning transplant or maintenance dialysis) may be increasing, yet there is considerable variation in access to and practices of initiating KRT worldwide. Several factors may have contributed to the increase: improved survival of ESKD children, broadening pediatric KRT acceptance criteria, and better access to pediatric KRT (especially dialysis) in low- and middle-income countries.

However, major disparities currently exist in access to kidney care services for children, particularly in low- and middle-income countries so that most pediatric patients with ESKD in these countries have no or limited options for KRT and the vast majority of children receiving KRT worldwide reside in high-income countries [1, 5, 6]. A wide variation in the initial KRT modalities exists across the world.

Kidney transplantation is the preferred KRT option in children and adults with CKD, conferring significant survival advantage, improved quality of life, and health system cost savings. According to the Global kidney Health Atlas,

kidney transplantation is not available in more than 20% of countries worldwide (>60% of African countries) and the proportion of countries that cannot provide pediatric kidney transplantation is expected to be much higher [7]. In Europe and the United States, approximately 20% of children start KRT with pre-emptive kidney transplantation [3, 4]. The access to pediatric kidney transplantation is influenced by ethnic, economic and geographic disparities [8–10]. For example, across 32 countries in Europe, a strong association was found between country income based on the GDP per capita and the country-specific rate of pediatric kidney transplantation [11]. In some countries, kidney transplantation is not available as an option for initial KRT in children.

Children who do not receive pre-emptive kidney transplantation may receive PD or HD, but the prevalence of the use of each of these modalities varies substantially depending on the center, country, reimbursement system for ESKD care, and public policies [5, 12]. In Europe and the UK, there is an almost equal distribution between HD and PD as initial modality. HD is the most common initial dialysis modality in the US and Brazil, while PD is more frequently chosen as first modality in Australia/New Zealand and Japan (Fig. 64.1). There seems to be trend towards a decrease in PD use versus HD as first KRT modality, particularly in the UK and the US [3, 13]. PD may be the preferred chronic dialysis modality in low-resource settings although HD in adult dialysis facilities is often the only option because of the cost and logistical challenges associated with PD in children [14, 15]. Globally, PD, most commonly provided with an automated cycling device (CCPD), is usually the first dialysis modality for infants and young children, while HD predominates among children above 10 years and adolescents. Home hemodialysis (HHD) is offered to a small number of selected children by a few centers [16].

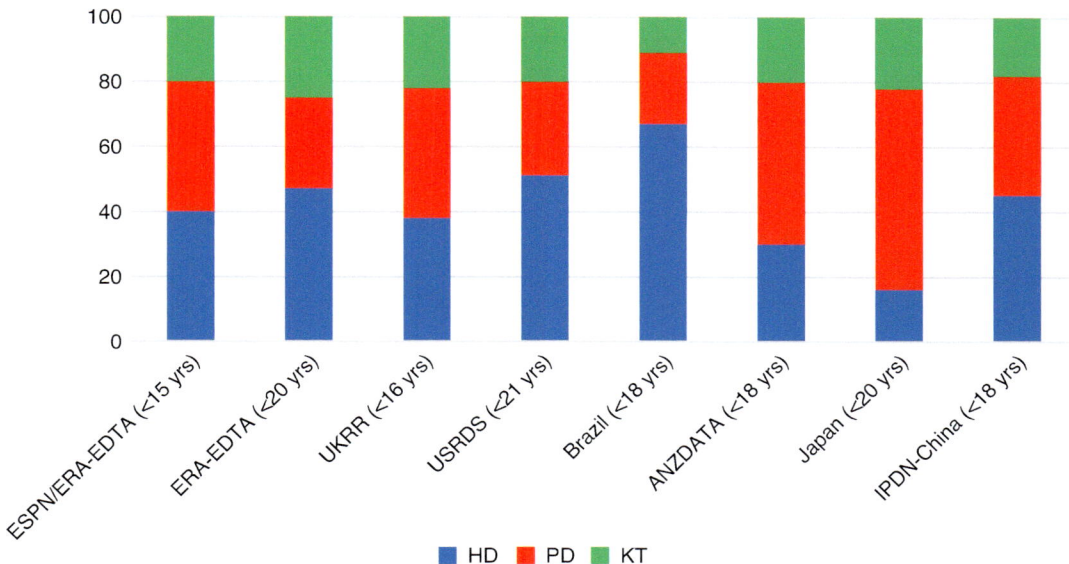

Fig. 64.1 Distribution of initial kidney replacement therapy modality in children according to various registries
ANZDATA Australia and New Zealand Dialysis and Transplant Registry, ESPN/ERA-EDTA European Society for Paediatric Nephrology/European Renal Association- European Dialysis and Transplant Association, IPDN-China International Pediatric Dialysis Network-China, UKRR United Kingdom Renal Registry, USRDS United States Renal Data System, HD hemodialysis, PD peritoneal dialysis, KT kidney transplantation

Main Outcomes According to KRT Modality

It has been established that (pre-emptive) kidney transplantation offers better patient survival than dialysis [17–19]. In the US, children treated with HD or PD have a five and two times higher 1-year mortality rate after initiation of KRT than those receiving a preemptive transplantation [3]. In Europe, starting KRT with dialysis is associated with a two-fold higher hazard of death as compared to preemptive kidney transplantation [20]. Children and adolescents <21 years of age initiating KRT with preemptive transplantation have a higher 5-year survival of 96–97% in the US and Europe as compared to ~86% (US) and ~ 90–92% (Europe) with dialysis [3, 21]. Mortality on dialysis is particularly high in infants and children younger than 5 years of age. In the very long-term, both European and US data suggest that children treated with dialysis would have a deficit in their expected remaining lifetime of 40–50 years vs. 12–20 years for

transplanted patients [3, 22]. Nonetheless, about 80% of pediatric patients are either started on dialysis to bridge the preparation time needed for transplantation or will require dialysis after graft loss [3, 4].

Survival comparisons by dialysis modality in a randomized clinical trial setting proved extremely difficult [23]. Consequently, survival comparisons rely on registry data [24, 25]. In the pediatric dialysis population, there seems to be a consistent trend showing survival advantage in patients on PD with a 20–30% reduced mortality risk as compared to those who start KRT on HD [24–26] (Fig. 64.2). In the USA, this better survival on PD was only present in children <5 years, whereas in Europe, the effect size was smaller in children <5 years and no difference was observed in infants <12 months [26]. Furthermore, European data show that this PD treatment effect was stronger during the first year of dialysis, in older children, and in children late referred to pediatric nephrology care [25]. However, despite adjusted or stratified analyses, the risk of indica-

Fig. 64.2 Cumulative incidence of mortality in European children on hemodialysis and peritoneal dialysis at start of kidney replacement therapy (used with permission from [25])

HD hemodialysis, *PD* peritoneal dialysis

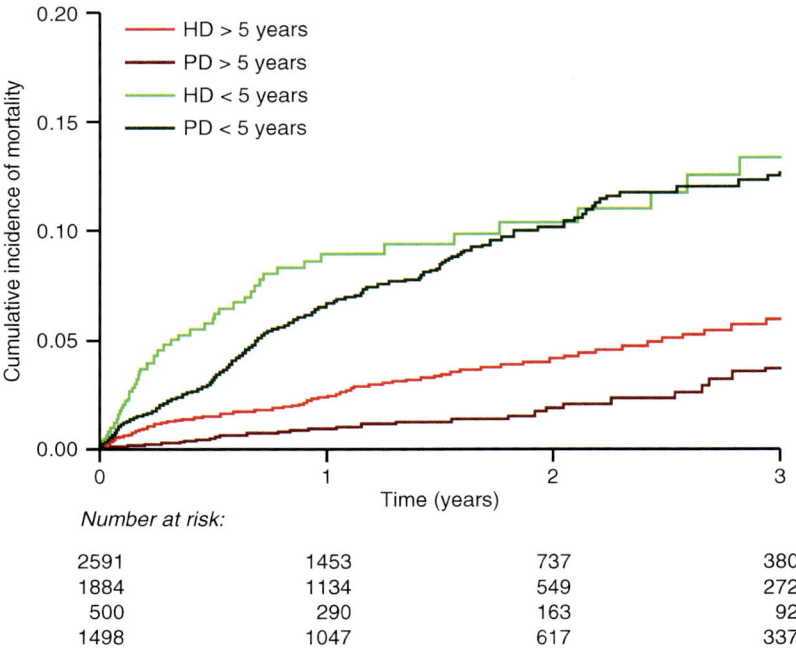

Optimal Timing of KRT Initiation

Current Recommendations and Guidelines

tion bias inherent to observational studies remains, as sicker patients are more likely to be started with HD. Dialysis in neonates is challenging but technically feasible. Data on 264 patients from 4 international registries who commenced chronic dialysis in the first month of life showed a 3- and 5-year survival rates of 80 and 76%, respectively [27].

Children and adolescents undergoing dialysis report severely decreased health-related quality of life (QoL) compared to those with a functioning transplant but, surprisingly, most studies did not find significant differences between patients on HD and those on PD [28, 29]. However, PD has been associated with more dietary and fluid freedom, and less disruption in children's schooling and social life compared with HD [30].

Moreover, preemptive kidney transplantation has been associated with improved post-transplant outcomes such as significantly reduced risk of graft loss [19, 31, 32], reduced risk of acute rejection [33], and better health-related QoL in the domain of physical health [34].

In 2020, a position statement from an expert group recommended dialysis initiation when the eGFR drops below 10 mL/min/1.73 m^2 or when the child has uremic symptoms refractory to medication or dietary management [35]. All other recommendations come from adult guidelines. The Kidney Disease Outcomes Quality Initiative (KDOQI) suggested in 2006 that dialysis should be considered when eGFR is <14 mL/min/1.73 m^2 and recommended when eGFR falls to <8 mL/min/1.73 m^2 [36]. The updated 2015 KDOQI (for HD) stated that symptoms and signs associated with CKD complications, rather than a specific eGFR, should guide the decision to initiate dialysis [37]. The KDIGO conference report in 2018 confirmed that there is no specific eGFR threshold for dialysis initiation in the absence of symptoms, and that current data do not support pre-emptive dialysis initiation [38].

Regarding transplantation as an initial KRT modality, the European Renal Best Practice (ERBP) recommended to develop programs for preemptive living donor kidney transplantation [39]. There is no guidance for the timing of preemptive transplantation but a statement that the optimal timing should be to avoid dialysis in a patient who otherwise would need to start it according to current guidelines i.e., shortly or a few months before the need to initiate dialysis [39]. Indeed, in adults, neither patient nor graft survival was influenced by the level of pretransplant eGFR [40]. A recent KDIGO clinical practice guideline also recommended that patients should be referred for evaluation 6–12 months before anticipated dialysis to facilitate preemptive kidney transplantation [41]. The KDIGO guideline specifically recommends preemptive kidney transplantation (living or deceased donor) in children when the eGFR is <15 mL/min/1.73 m^2 or earlier with symptoms [41].

Pre-ESKD Care and Referral for KRT Initiation

Optimal CKD care should include timely referral and frequent visits with a multidisciplinary team of physicians, nurses, dieticians, social workers and pharmacists. This integrated model of CKD care has been associated with improvement in measurable outcomes [42, 43]. Recommendations for "timely referral" to a pediatric nephrologist should allow access to multidisciplinary care for CKD, patient and family education and support, and considering a preemptive kidney transplantation.

Delayed referral, lack of patient preparedness and urgent-start of dialysis have been associated with higher morbidity on dialysis, lower access to kidney transplantation, and worse kidney graft survival [44–46]. Late referral has been defined as starting dialysis between 1 and 3 months after the first appointment with a pediatric nephrologist. Late referral in adults has been associated with limited choice of dialysis modality and worse clinical outcomes, including more hospitalizations and deaths [47]. Similar findings have

been reported in children. In the UK, 25% of children with ESKD were referred late (defined as having <3 months between first visit with a pediatric nephrologist and commencement of KRT). These patients were less likely to receive a kidney transplant after 1 year of dialysis (21% vs. 61% for early referral) without difference in mortality [45]. In a study from Poland, children with a late referral had more metabolic and clinical complications, more admissions to ICU, and a lower chance to receive a kidney transplant within 3 years [48]. Of 1527 children in the ESPN/ERA-EDTA registry whose first appointment with a pediatric nephrologist was known, late starters (45%, defined as eGFR <8 mL/min/1.73 m^2 at start of KRT) were significantly more likely to be late referrals [49]. However, the access to kidney transplantation at 1, 2, and 5 years was similar regardless of the timing of referral [49].

Urgent Versus Non-urgent and Planned Versus Unplanned Start of KRT

In 2018, a KDIGO Consensus Conference defined urgent-start dialysis by the need to initiate dialysis imminently or in less than 48 h after presentation in order to correct life-threatening manifestations [38]. An unplanned start is defined as dialysis initiation when access is not ready for use or when dialysis is initiated with a modality that is not the patient and family's choice. HD and PD are possible in both planned or unplanned and urgent or non-urgent start of dialysis. However, children requiring KRT in the setting of hyperkalemia, volume overload or critical illness may not be good candidates for urgent start with PD. The risk factors for urgent and unplanned start of dialysis include late referral, lower socio-economic background, lower health literacy, acute illness, rapid (and often unpredictable) loss of kidney function, and severe symptoms [50–52]. When urgent or unplanned start dialysis limit the initial modality choice, patients and families need to subsequently be provided with education and support to allow them choosing their preferred modality when feasible. Conversely, a planned initiation of dialysis is performed when the modality has been chosen prior to the need for dialysis and the access is ready for use. A preemptive kidney transplantation is by definition a planned modality of KRT.

Outcome According to the Timing of KRT Initiation

There is a large variation around the world in the threshold of eGFR for the initiation of dialysis in children. There is variation in approach both between and within countries. The median eGFR at dialysis initiation in pediatric patients in Europe and the USA is around 8 mL/min/1.73 m² but the range is wide, from less than 5 to over 10 mL/min/1.73 m² [49, 53, 54]. In the Japanese registry, the median eGFR at KRT initiation (including kidney transplant) was 12 mL/min/1.73 m² [55]. There is a trend towards earlier start of dialysis: a USRDS registry study including more than 15,000 children found that the proportion of children starting dialysis with an eGFR >10 mL/min/1.73 m² increased from 16% in 1995 to 40% in 2015 [54]. In Canada, there has been a change over the past 20 years with dialysis currently being initiated at an eGFR ≥10.5 mL/min/1.73 m² in one-third of children, a higher rate than previously reported [56]. The reasons for this trend are unclear. Possible reasons could be the adoption of changing trends in the clinical practice guidelines, starting from KDOQI 2006 in which the recommendations were to consider dialysis if eGFR was below 14 and start when eGFR was below 8 mL/min/1.73 m² [36]. However, updates from KDOQI 2015 and KDIGO 2019 recommend commencement of dialysis when the patient becomes symptomatic [37, 38].

A specific eGFR value for initiating dialysis in the absence of symptomatic kidney failure has not been established in adults. The IDEAL trial could not demonstrate a benefit of commencing dialysis at higher levels of eGFR [57]. Recently, there have been three large pediatric registry studies from USRDS and ESPN/ERA-EDTA examining the association between eGFR at ini-

tiation of chronic dialysis and clinical outcomes [49, 53, 54]. Of nearly 10,000 incident dialysis patients aged 1–17 years in the USRDS registry (1995–2016), higher eGFR at dialysis start was associated with a higher mortality risk. Specifically, compared with eGFR of 7 to <9 mL/min/1.73 m², eGFR <5 and ≥12 mL/min/1.73 m² were associated with lower and higher mortality, with adjusted HR of 0.57 and 1.31, respectively [53]. In stratified analyses, mortality risk was associated with higher eGFR in children ≥6 years, whereas the association was attenuated among those younger than 6 years. Although this study suggests that initiating dialysis at eGFR >12 mL/min/1.73 m² is associated with increased mortality, there seems to be a similar outcome across the range of 5–12 mL/min/1.73 m² in which the majority of ESKD patients will start KRT [53]. Another study from the USRDS assessed the association between eGFR at dialysis initiation and hazard of death in a total of 15,000 children aged 1–18 years in the period 1995–2015 [54]. Mortality risk was 36% higher among those with higher (> 10 mL/min/1.73 m²) versus lower (≤ 10 mL/min/1.73 m²) eGFR at dialysis initiation. The mortality associated with higher eGFR risk was more pronounced among children receiving HD (HR 1.56) while the association with eGFR was no longer significant among those treated by PD [54]. In Europe, a retrospective ESPN/ERA-EDTA Registry study of ~3000 children aged <18 years from 21 countries found no difference in mortality risk and access to transplantation between children who started dialysis at eGFR ≥8 mL/min/1.73 m² vs. < 8 mL/min/1.73 m² [49] (Fig. 64.3).

Notably, the ESPN/ERA-EDTA Registry study found no significant difference in other outcomes such as anemia, hyperphosphatemia, growth, and access to transplantation between late starters at eGFR <8 mL/min/1.73 m² (median 6) and early starters at eGFR ≥8 mL/min/1.73 m² (median 10.5) [49]. However, the prevalence of hypertension was higher in late starters (61%) than in early starters (54%) [49]. In a Turkish study of 245 children, patients with early-start dialysis at eGFR >10 mL/min/1.73 m² (mean 13.5) and late-starters at eGFR <7 mL/

Fig. 64.3 Cumulative incidence of death and kidney transplantation within 5 years of dialysis initiation for European children starting dialysis early (eGFR ≥8 mL/min/1.73 m²) (A) and children starting dialysis late (eGFR <8 mL/min/1.73 m²) (B). Used with permission from [49]

Tx kidney transplantation, *eGFR* estimated glomerular filtration rate, *RRT* renal replacement therapy

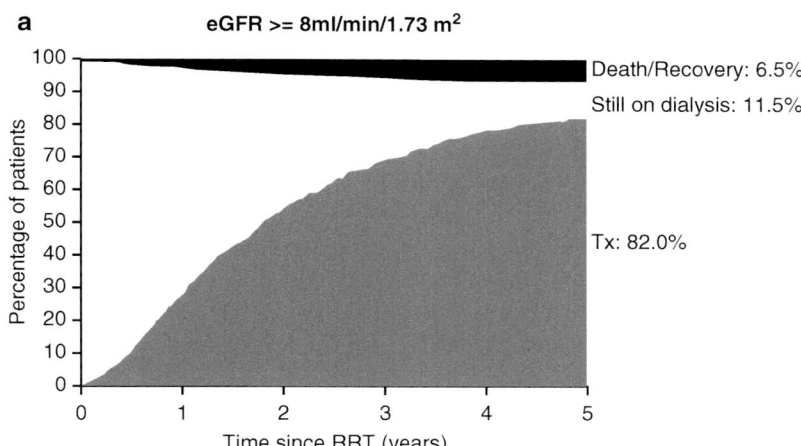

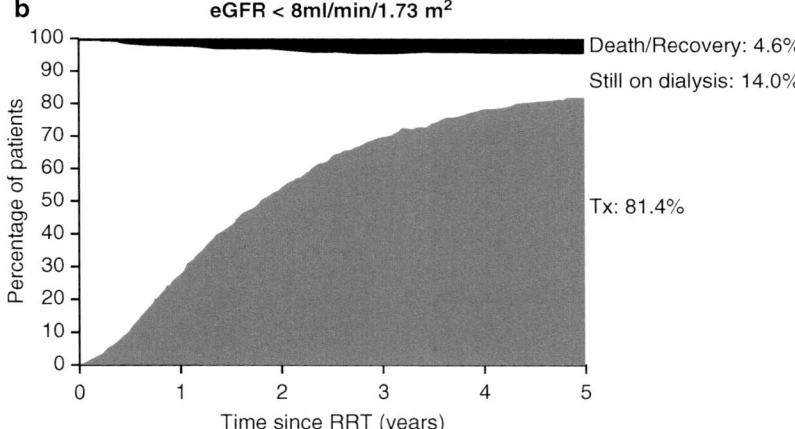

min/1.73 m² (mean 5.5) did not significantly differ in left ventricular mass index (LVMI) and left ventricular hypertrophy (LVH) [58].

Regarding nutrition and growth, the ESPN/ERA-EDTA study showed that height SDS was not different at start of dialysis with an eGFR above or below 8 mL/min/1.73 m² (−1.79 vs. −1.76), and the drop in height SDS after 1 year of dialysis was similar in both groups (−0.22 vs. −0.24) [49]. The distribution of BMI was also comparable between the two groups. However, in a cohort study of the International Pediatric Peritoneal Dialysis Network (IPDN) (1000 PD children from 35 countries), an underweight status was twice more common in children starting PD at eGFR <6 mL/min/1.73 m² (11%) compared to those starting PD at eGFR 9–12 mL/min/1.73 m² (5%) [59].

There is no pediatric data to suggest that patient or graft survival could be influenced by the level of eGFR at time of preemptive kidney transplantation.

KRT Initiation

The timing of KRT initiation is a complex decision that needs to take into account the eGFR and the rate of its loss, the treatment modalities available, and symptoms or signs attributable to kidney failure. Initiation of KRT is usually considered in case of inability to control volume status or blood pressure, deterioration in nutritional status or growth failure, severe biochemical abnormalities such as hyperkalemia, hyperphosphatemia or metabolic acidosis, and patient reported outcome measures such as fatigue, nausea and loss of appetite, declining cognitive performance, or poor QoL [30, 35].

While the optimal timing for starting KRT is unknown and the reasons for initiating dialysis are highly variable, risk equations may be potentially helpful to predict the time when KRT will be necessary although validation studies are limited in children [60, 61]. This may be combined with, and not replace, clinical judgement. The decision to start KRT should ideally always be reached by discussions between the child when appropriate, caregivers, and the CKD multidisciplinary care team.

Once maintenance dialysis has been initiated in pediatric patients there is a recovery rate of 2% within 2 years after the start of dialysis [62]. There is a particularly high chance of recovery (>10%) in children starting dialysis for vasculitis, ischemic kidney failure, and hemolytic uremic syndrome, which should be considered when planning expedited kidney transplantation [62].

Dialysis Availability and Choice of Modality

Dialysis modalities include in-center and, rarely, home HD, as well as continuous ambulatory and automated PD. Prescription patterns can be categorized as conventional, intensive (short daily or nocturnal), or exceptionally palliative in children [63, 64]. Availability of modalities and prescription patterns usually depends more on local resources and infrastructures, reimbursement policies, center practices and expertise, than patient and family preferences. In most high-income countries, in-center hemodialysis is the predominant modality whereas PD is the first option in some areas. In high-income countries, PD may be more cost effective than HD, yet the opposite might be true in low- and middle-income countries where KRT is offered to children but manufacturing or importing PD fluids could be more expensive [38].

The selection of dialysis modality is based on the patient's age and comorbidity, family support and psychosocial conditions, local resources,

Table 64.1 Issues to be considered in the selection of kidney replacement therapy modality in children

Factors to be considered
Patient and family preference
Patient age and size
Medical/surgical comorbidities, contraindications
Geographic location, distance to the center
Local nephrology/surgical expertise
Family burden
Psychosocial support
School attendance
Growth
Lifelong morbidity and mortality
Healthcare system, out-of-pocket costs

modality contraindications, healthcare team expertise, and child and family choice (Table 64.1). The only absolute contraindication for maintenance HD is the absence of possible vascular access or prohibitive cardiovascular instability (Table 64.2). PD is contraindicated if the peritoneal membrane is not functional or PD catheter is not possible (Table 64.2). All other conditions are relative contraindications.

There is no study to suggest that either PD or HD is superior in children with ESKD. PD is often preferred and widely used in infants and small children for whom the creation and maintenance of a suitable vascular access can be challenging. Home dialysis modalities such as automated PD using a cycling device (CAPD) and rarely home HD (HHD) can improve patient autonomy, flexibility and QoL, and facilitate regular school attendance [35, 63]. PD is also preferred over HD in children with cardiovascular instability, and some reports have suggested benefits of HHD in children with cardiac failure [65]. Preserving residual kidney function is important in the choice of KRT modality and should be a goal for pediatric nephrologists. Although PD may be associated with a slower decline in residual kidney function than HD, the evidence regarding the effect of initial dialysis modality and therapeutic strategy is limited in children [66, 67].

In addition to medical factors, the proximity to a pediatric HD center and the heavy burden of home dialysis care for families should be considered when choosing a dialysis modality. In some countries, it has been reported that children with

Table 64.2 Contraindications to the different kidney replacement therapy modalities in children

	Preemptive kidney transplantation	Peritoneal dialysis	Hemodialysis
Absolute contraindications	• Active infection • Severe irreversible multisystem organ failure • Severe pulmonary or cardiac dysfunction in a child not suitable for multiorgan transplant • Life-threatening extrarenal disorder not correctable by kidney transplant • Uncontrolled malignancy	• Abdominal wall defects • Diaphragmatic hernia • Bladder exstrophy • Obliterated peritoneal cavity • Peritoneal membrane failure	• No vascular access • Severe cardiovascular instability • Unavailability of facilities
Relative contraindications	• Active systemic disease (lupus, vasculitis, antiglomerular basement membrane disease) • Unstable psychiatric disorder • Ongoing, health-compromising nonadherent behavior	• Ileo/colostomies • Recent major abdominal surgery • Infant with organomegaly • Inadequate living situation for home dialysis, lack of caregiver support	• Difficult vascular access • Coagulopathy • Unstable psychiatric disorder

social disadvantage tend to receive more commonly HD than PD compared to those from wealthier families and have less access to preemptive kidney transplantation [46, 68]. This suggests delayed referral as well as concerns by healthcare providers and/or caregivers themselves about their ability to safely provide dialysis at home. Further investigation is needed to clarify whether social inequities exist in the provision of KRT in children. Although the published data is limited in pediatric nephrology, there has been growing recognition of the importance of patient and caregiver involvement in planning CKD care and shared decision-making regarding KRT modality [68–70]. The modality selection should therefore reflect informed child and family choice adapted to their health and social conditions and appropriate to the healthcare system and local resources.

Dialysis Preparation and Transplant Workup

Dialysis Preparation

Many children, for various reasons, require a variable period of dialysis before transplantation is possible. Dialysis is considered a bridge to kidney transplantation and should be as short as possible to improve outcomes [19, 31]. Adequate dialysis preparation enables better understanding of the dialysis process, reduces fear and anxiety regarding long-term dialysis, thus ensuring improved therapy adherence and better overall outcomes.

Before starting dialysis, patients and their caregivers should meet the following criteria: (i) they need to have a good understanding of the different treatment options available, (ii) they should have a functioning permanent access for the dialysis modality of their choice, and (iii) they should not require hospitalization for untreated complications of acute or chronic uremia [30, 35, 38, 71].

1. Education

   Patient education and decision support are essential in helping patients and families to better understand ESKD and available KRT options, improve literacy and possibly outcomes. In adults, early education has been associated with better survival after dialysis initiation [72]. Effective education programs should be offered to the child if appropriate, and the family or caregivers when the eGFR is <30 mL/min/1.73 m^2 (CKD stage 4). Comprehensive education material should provide information related to all forms of dialysis. In addition, a thorough psychological, social and economic evaluation of the family or caregivers is required to determine their ability to cope with the burden of care associated with the provision of home KRT (PD or HHD) [63]. The multidisciplinary care team can therefore individualize the training plan to meet the needs of the parents or caregiver.

2. Dialysis access

PD access should be prepared whenever possible at least 2 weeks before starting KRT. For late-referred patients, this might imply switching to HD temporarily or definitively. However, urgent-start PD has been proven safe in adults, and early catheter use feasible in children. Gastrostomy tube feeding in children already receiving PD is not contraindicated but a gastrostomy tube should be ideally inserted prior to the placement of a PD catheter [73]. There are guidelines regarding optimal timing and placement technique for PD catheters, access type, PD training, and prevention of complications in the pediatric population [74–76]. Constipation has been associated with increased risk of post placement PD catheter migration and should be addressed preoperatively. The use of a double-cuff Tenckhoff catheter has been recommended [75], and omentectomy to prevent PD catheter occlusion should be considered at the time of catheter insertion.

Among children receiving HD, central venous catheter (CVC) is the predominant vascular access choice. The International Pediatric HD Network reported the use of an arteriovenous fistula (AVF) in 26% of children initiating HD; this rate was higher in an ESPN/ERA-EDTA study (45%), and much lower (< 15%) in a recent USRDS report [3, 77, 78]. A vascular access with an AVF has been associated with better dialysis efficacy, fewer medical complications, less vascular access procedures, lower costs, and higher deceased donor transplantation rate than an access with a CVC [77, 78]. It is therefore recommended that children start HD with a functioning AVF which should be created at least 3 months before anticipated use [79]. However, in some circumstances such as in infants and young children depending on size and surgical expertise, those requiring unplanned HD, those with an anticipated short period of dialysis before (living donor) kidney transplantation, or patient choice, a cuffed CVC is preferred [79]. The choice for access thus requires individualization for each patient and a dedicated vascular access clinic may optimize the timing and quality of vascular access in this setting [79–81].

Kidney Transplant Workup

1. General principles

The pre-transplant evaluation (Table 64.3) is an essential part of the kidney transplant process and aims to reduce complications and increase graft and patient survival [41, 82]. The transplant workup should be started 6 to 12 months before the patient is likely to require KRT in known CKD patients, but should start as soon as possible in patients with a late referral. It includes a medical and psychosocial evaluation, and patient/caregiver education. The initial phase is to rule out any contraindications (Table 64.2). The medical evaluation also includes the detection of anti-Human Leukocyte Antigen (HLA) antibodies to the donor, the detection and treatment of any infection prior to transplantation, the completion of immunizations, screening for coagulation and thrombosis abnormalities, and the correction of any significant urinary tract abnormality. In certain cases, the indication for native nephrectomy should be discussed. Patients and their families or caregivers should be provided with sufficient information regarding patient survival, transplant complications and immunosuppressive drugs used and their side effects.

2. Blood group

The majority of kidney transplantations are ABO compatible and most allocation schemes allocate donor kidneys on the basis of blood

Table 64.3   Proposed pre-transplant assessment check list

	Relevant workup		Date/frequency
Planned transplant type	Living or deceased donor		
Chronic kidney disease evaluation	Diagnosis (± genetic testing when relevant)		
	Dialysis history		
	Previous transplants (living donor – deceased donor)		
	Creatinine		
	eGFR		
	PTH, calcium and phosphorus levels		
Immunology	Blood group		
	Tissue typing		
	Cross match		
	HLA antibodies		/3 months
Infectious disease workup	Serologies/PCR	CMV	/3 months if negative
		EBV	/3 months if negative
		Hepatitis B	
		Hepatitis C	
		Hepatitis A	
		Varicella	
		Measles/mumps/rubella	
		Toxoplasmosis	
		HIV	
		Syphilis (VDRL/TPHA)	
	Immunization history		
	Interferon gamma release assay (Quantiferon)	All patients who have not had BCG	
	Chest X-ray for latent TB if required	All patients who have not had BCG	
	Urine culture		
Metabolic workup	Liver function		
	Fasting glucose level		
	CYP3A5/TPMT	If azathioprine used	
Coagulation	Family/patient history – bleeding and clotting		
	Protein C		
	Protein S		
	Anti-thrombin functional		
	Lupus anticoagulant (DRVVT)		
	Anti-cardiolipin IgG - B2GP1 (if required)		
	Factor VIII		
	Factor XII		
	Activated Protein C Resistance		
	Factor V Leiden mutation		
	Prothrombin		
	Factor II mutation		
	G6PD deficiency screen		
Imaging	Ultrasound of aorta, inferior vena cava and iliac vessels		
	Magnetic resonance angiography/venography	Under 20 kg / previous transplants	
	Angiography/Venography (if required)		
	Bladder ultrasound scan	Pre/Post micturition	
	Voiding cystourethrogram	Patients with urinary tract abnormalities	
	Urodynamics (If required)		
	Cardiac ultrasound and electrocardiogram		/6–12 months

(continued)

Table 64.3 (continued)

	Relevant workup		Date/frequency
Reviews/ Referrals	Detailed interview with nephrology consultant		
	Detailed interview with transplant surgeon	Including transplant plan (anatomical position, transplant ureter…)	
	Urology review if required	Bladder plan	/12 months
	Detailed interview with anaesthetist	Access plan for transplant	/6 months
	Ear Nose and Throat (ENT) review		
	Dental review		
	Dermatology review		
	Ophthalmology review if required		
	Other if required (neurology, liver)		
Psychosocial assessment	Psychologist		
	Pediatric psychiatrist		
	Social worker		

BCG Bacille Calmette-Guerin, *CMV* cytomegalovirus, *CYP3A5* cytochrome P450 3A5, *EBV* Epstein-Barr virus, *eGFR* estimated glomerular filtration rate, *G6PD* glucose-6-phosphate dehydrogenase; *HIV* human immunodeficiency virus, *HLA* human leukocyte antigen, *PCR* polymerase chain reaction, *PTH* Parathormone, *TB* tuberculosis, *TPMT* Thiopurine methyltransferase

group identity. However, given donor shortages, an increasing number of centers provide living donor blood group incompatible transplantation. Recipient anti-B or anti-A titers are measured and depending on the level, the decision is made regarding the kidney transplantation feasibility and the treatment required to prevent a reaction (rituximab, plasmapheresis, immunoadsorption) [83].

3. Histocompatibility and immunogenetics

HLA typing is performed for all patients undergoing kidney transplantation and refers to the characterization of the individual's HLA genes and the identification of the HLA molecules expressed on the surface of their cells. DNA technology has led to the identification of many more alleles and is the gold standard for HLA typing. Sensitization is the development of antibodies to HLA antigens and their presence is likely to result in antibody mediated rejection and early graft loss. Sensitization can happen in the following main situations: previous transplant, blood, platelet or fresh frozen plasma transfusions, and pregnancy. It can also happen spontaneously through cross-sensitization from infection and pro-inflammatory events [84]. Several different assays are available to determine the sensitivity of a potential transplant recipient to donor HLA antigens. Microbead array and ELISA techniques have been proven to be more sensitive than cytotoxicity. Pre-transplant cross-matching is mandatory and aims to confirm the absence of donor-directed HLA antibodies. A positive cross-match is a potential contraindication for kidney transplantation.

Assays for Cross-match Testing

– The complement-dependent **cytotoxic crossmatch** is the most common test where donor lymphocytes are incubated with recipient serum in the presence of complement. If donor specific antibodies are present, cell lysis is observed, and the crossmatch is deemed positive.

– The **flow cytometry cross-match** is a more sensitive cross-match. Recipient serum is added to the donor lymphocytes, followed by the addition of a secondary fluorochrome-conjugated antibody that detects human IgG. Samples with the patient's serum incubated with the donor cells are compared with a negative control containing pooled sera from normal, healthy, unsensitized individuals. It is particularly useful in sensitized patients and can be performed with peripheral blood cells.

- **Virtual cross-matching** involves reviewing the donor HLA profile against the patient's HLA antibody profile to determine whether the patient has donor-directed antibodies that would cause a positive cross-match test result. This technique can be performed in a certain number of patients with a low immunological risk and reduces the cold ischemia time. A further cross-match test must be performed retrospectively to confirm the negative virtual cross-match.

4. Infectious Disease Issues

Infections are an important cause of morbidity and mortality post-transplant. As such, pre-transplant infectious screening is an essential step in preparing for kidney transplantation [85]. The urinary tract, skin, teeth, and sinuses should be carefully examined for signs of infection or site of chronic infection. Lack of prior exposure to certain pre-transplant viruses may affect transplantation outcomes. Post-transplant viral disease may be more severe (CMV, influenza), increase the risk of chronic allograft dysfunction (CMV, BK virus) and can increase the risk of post-transplant lymphoproliferative disease (EBV) [86].

Routine childhood immunizations should be completed prior to kidney transplantation according to age-appropriate guidelines and should be updated using expedited regimens where necessary [86, 87]. Live vaccines, such as varicella, tuberculosis and measles, should be administered at least two months prior to transplantation. Live vaccines are contraindicated after transplantation [87].

5. Coagulation and thrombosis screening

The patient's history of bleeding and/or clotting is an important aspect. All patients should have a pre-transplant coagulation and thrombophilia screen to avoid bleeding/clotting complications.

6. Urinary tract abnormalities

The lower urinary tract should be evaluated using a voiding cystourethrogram to detect any abnormality that should be corrected prior to transplantation in patients with history of congenital abnormalities of the urinary tract or infection. Bladder and urethra abnormalities may be responsible for ureterohydronephrosis of the transplant, thereby increasing the risk of graft loss. These and other abnormalities may increase the risk of urinary tract infection. Patients with lower urinary tract obstruction are at the highest risk of post-transplant bladder dysfunction. These patients should be assessed carefully with urodynamic studies. It may be necessary to create an appendicovesicostomy in patients that require clean intermittent catheterization and/or to enlarge the bladder with an intestinal segment in patients with a small pathologic bladder [85, 86].

7. Native nephrectomy

The need for native nephrectomy is controversial. The benefits of retaining native kidneys may include preservation of residual urine output, production of native erythropoietin and better vitamin D/calcium homeostasis. However, in certain cases, native nephrectomy may be beneficial, although data are limited and no guidelines exist. Native nephrectomy prior to transplant may be considered in patients with glomerular disease with significant proteinuria (to reduce risk of thrombosis due to low albumin), autosomal dominant polycystic kidney disease (to avoid symptoms secondary to extremely large polycystic kidneys such as pain, hematuria and pressure effects causing gastrointestinal or respiratory symptoms), high-grade vesicoureteral reflux (to reduce post-transplant infection/bladder dysfunction), severe uncontrollable hypertension, and malignancy or malignant predisposition (WT1 gene variants) [88–90]. These indications are center-dependent and no clear guidelines detailing for example proteinuria/polyuria cut-offs or the degree of hypertension exist.

8. Donor options

Access to kidney transplantation is highly variable globally and even regionally, with a limited number of low-middle and low-income countries offering pediatric kidney transplantation [3, 5–8, 11]. While well-established national policies and organizations for organ procurement and allocation account for higher deceased donor (DD) transplantation rates in high-income countries, most low-middle and low-income countries initiate pediatric kidney transplantation through a living related donor (LD) program [3, 7, 11]. The transplanted kidney has a limited survival and most children with ESKD will require two, three or even more kidney transplants in their lifetime. In this regard, a LD transplant provides a better long-term graft survival and is a better option for children [86]. Even in LD kidney transplant recipients, there is a benefit in graft survival for preemptive transplantation (vs. non preemptive) [19, 31]. When there is no LD identified or available, the choice of accepting or declining a DD kidney is a difficult decision-making process involving recipient's age and size, current morbidity, time spent on dialysis and sensitization, as well as donor history, age and size, kidney risk profile, HLA matching and expected cold ischemia time [91].

An important dilemma for pediatric nephrologists is, if there is only one possible living donor, should the first kidney transplant be from a LD or a DD. The pros for receiving a DD kidney first are that children have access to good-quality donors in a relatively short period of time. Therefore, the LD could be saved for a later time after first transplant failure when the waiting time may become longer. An argument against this would be that later, the potential donor will be older and may have health issues preventing re-transplantation with a LD [91]. This question has been addressed in the US by data from the Scientific Registry of Transplant Recipients (SRTR) showing in almost 15,000 pediatric kidney transplant recipients that the cumulative graft life was similar with both strategies,

i.e. living first-deceased second and deceased first-living second [92]. The same authors examined this question of optimal timing regarding the order of DD and LD kidney transplantation using a Markov decision process model to compare the relative survival benefit of each strategy over a time horizon of 20 years [93]. It was shown that for the most highly sensitized patients (PRA > 80%), a DD-first strategy was associated with a survival advantage, but for all other patients (with PRA < 80%), a LD-first strategy conferred a better patient survival [93].

Although the choice of donor should be made on an individual basis, we, and others, feel that the best treatment should be proposed for children with ESKD and recommend that a preemptive living donor kidney transplantation should always be considered as the first option.

Summary: Lifetime Perspectives

The initiation of KRT and subsequent changes of modality are intrinsic processes in the life of a child with ESKD and should be planned and reflect patients' life goals and preferences when possible. There are pros and cons of each KRT modality (CAPD/CCPD, in-center HD, home HD, preemptive/post-dialysis transplantation, living/deceased donor) to be considered in order to provide personalized care for a child with ESKD (Table 64.4). Both the short- and long-term benefits and risks of each KRT modality across the entire patient's lifespan should be carefully evaluated, considering the widely variable practice patterns and access to KRT around the world. From a lifetime perspective, it is essential for pediatric nephrologists not only to provide the best initial KRT modality available but also to keep in mind the subsequent best treatment modality and access for an individual patient.

We suggest that an integrated life plan approach for pediatric KRT should take into account the long-term consequences of the decisions and choices to be made such as dialysis

Table 64.4 Advantages and disadvantages of different kidney replacement therapy modalities in children

Modality		Advantages	Disadvantages
Kidney transplantation (KT)	KT (compared to dialysis)	Avoids dialysis morbidity and mortality	Variable access to transplantation
		Better patient survival	Not suitable for smaller children (< 10 kg)
		Better psychosocial outcome	Surgical complications
		Better quality of life	Infections
		Fewer restrictions (dietary, time, medications)	Malignancy
		Better growth	Burden of graft failure/repeated KRT modalities
		More cost-effective	
	Preemptive (compared to non-preemptive) KT	Better graft survival	Psychosocial difficulties
	Non-preemptive KT		Increased risk of graft failure
	Living donor (compared to deceased donor) KT	Better long-term graft survival	Kidney health risk for the donor
		Shorter waiting time	Psychological and socioeconomic issues for the donor
		Better graft quality	Possibility of poorer HLA matching
		Reduced delayed graft function	
		Reduced hospital costs	
	Deceased donor (compared to living donor) KT	Priority in allocation schemes	Increased risk of graft failure
Peritoneal dialysis (PD)		Increased patient freedom	Dependent on parental/caregiver participation
		Longer preservation of residual kidney function	Caregiver burden
		Avoidance of vascular access	Medicalization of the home
		Improved school attendance	Infections
		Fewer dietary restrictions	Risk of peritoneal membrane failure if on PD for years
		Technically more feasible in smaller children	
		Possible for patients who live far away from HD centre	
		Lower cost compared to HD	
Hemodialysis (HD)	In-centre HD (ICHD)	Long-term technique survival	Limited by availability of vascular access
		Suitable if patients/parents/caregivers unable to perform dialysis at home	Availability dependent on local resources
		Decreased treatment duration	Increased cost when compared to other modalities
	Home hemodialysis (HHD)	Increased flexibility with dialysis times	Dependent on parental/caregiver participation
		Improved school attendance compared to ICHD	Caregiver burden
		Reduced intradialytic symptoms and hypotensive episodes	More rapid loss of residual kidney function
		Improved cardiovascular outcomes compared to ICHD	Medicalization of the home
		More cost-effective compared to ICHD	Increased AVF complications
		Improved nutrition and growth compared to ICHD	Increased home utility bills (water, electricity)

AVF arteriovenous fistula, *HD* hemodialysis, *HHD* home hemodialysis, *HLA* human leukocyte antigen, *ICHD* in-center hemodialysis, *KRT* kidney replacement therapy, *KT* kidney transplantation, *PD* peritoneal dialysis

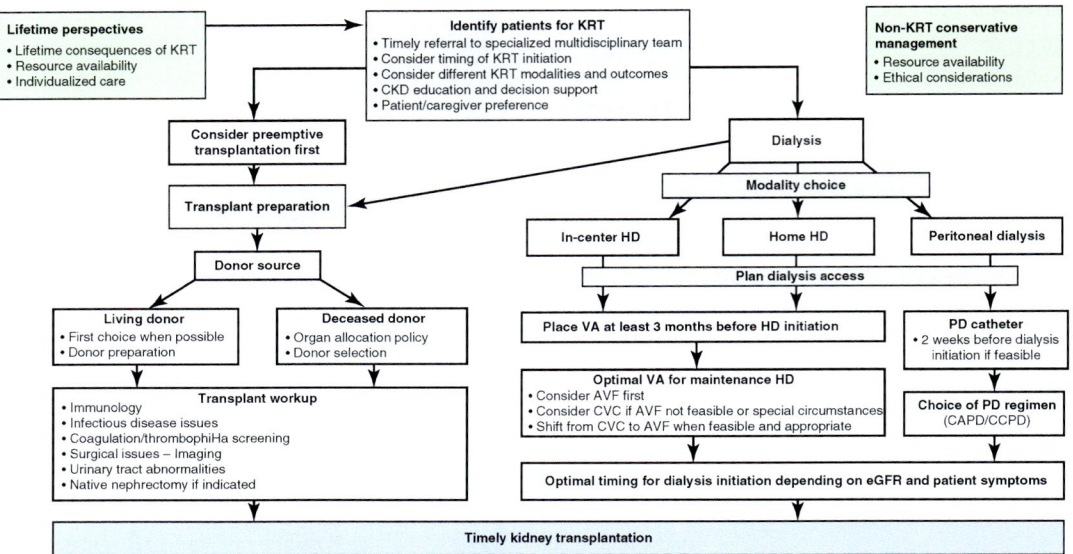

Abbreviations: AVF, Arteriovenous Fistula; CAPD, Continuous Ambulatory Peritoneal Dialysis; CCPD, Continuous Cyclic Peritoneal Dialysis; CKD, Chronic Kidney Disease; eGFR, Estimated Glomerular Filtration Rate; CVC, Central Venous Catheter; HD, Hemodialysis; KRT, Kidney Replacement Therapy; PD, Peritoneal dialysis; VA, Vascular access

Fig. 64.4 Integrated ESKD life plan approach for kidney replacement therapy modalities in children

AVF arteriovenous fistula, *CAPD* continuous ambulatory peritoneal dialysis, *CCPD* continuous cyclic perito-

neal dialysis, *CKD* chronic kidney disease, *eGFR* estimated glomerular filtration rate, *CVC* central venous catheter, *HD* hemodialysis, *KRT* kidney replacement therapy, *PD* peritoneal dialysis, *VA* vascular access

access sustainability, cardiovascular morbidity and mortality associated with prolonged dialysis, cumulative functioning graft survival according to the order of donor type, long-term morbidity of cumulative immunosuppressive load post-transplant, family/caregiver burden, interference of modalities with social life and relationships, growth and cognitive outcomes, QoL, and patient-centered outcomes (Fig. 64.4).

The (very) long-term outcome studies clearly favor early (living donor) kidney transplantation in children with ESKD, which appears to have a beneficial effect on overall mortality, morbidity, and psychosocial maturation. The cumulative duration of dialysis in relation to years with a functioning kidney graft has been strongly associated with many adverse outcomes, especially with cardiovascular mortality, but also short stature, impaired cognitive performance, locomotor disorders, social dependence and depression [94–99]. The impact of dialysis on physical condition is also reflected by the sharp difference in physical health perception of dialysis and transplanted patients. On the other hand, some registry data

(ANZDATA, ERA-EDTA) suggested that a short period of dialysis (up to 1 year) did not affect overall mortality [17, 100]. A longer period of dialysis has been associated with a higher risk of death regardless of donor source [19]. Although PD patients may have short-term survival advantage compared to HD, no studies showed significant differences in long-term outcome of PD and HD. However, PD may certainly be favorable over HD to achieve the longest and most feasible dialysis access life plan for the individual patient.

Although dialysis is the most unfavorable mode of KRT, kidney transplantation is associated with considerable late morbidity. Disabling co-morbidity was reported by 40% of all kidney transplant recipients in the Dutch late outcomes study (LERIC) [98]. Apart from clinical bone disease, the most frequently reported disabling problems were daily headaches, tremors and severe itching, most of them appearing in transplanted patients. Malignancies, infection, cumulative cardiovascular burden (hypertension-related LVH and arterial wall stiffening) are the most life-threatening problems after kidney transplantation [99, 101]. Although current data shows a much lower mortality in pediatric kidney transplant recipients than in those remaining on dialysis, the need for many decades of kidney graft function will expose more patients to risk of life-threatening infections and malignancies at relatively young adult age.

The approaches to optimize long-term outcomes and QoL in pediatric patients with ESKD include timely referral for multidisciplinary CKD care, education and support for patients and caregivers, promotion of pre-emptive and living-related transplantation, reduction of KRT time on dialysis to the minimum, favor home dialysis therapies, consider intensive dialysis, individualization of the subsequent KRT modality and dialysis access plan in a lifespan perspective. There is general consensus that providing personalized care which incorporates patient goals and preferences has become a priority.

References

1. Harambat J, van Stralen KJ, Kim JJ, Tizard EJ. Epidemiology of chronic kidney disease in children. Pediatr Nephrol. 2012;27(3):363–73.
2. Ploos van Amstel S, Noordzij M, Warady BA, Cano F, Craig JC, Groothoff JW, Ishikura K, Neu A, Safouh H, Xu H, Jager KJ, Schaefer F. Renal replacement therapy for children throughout the world: the need for a global registry. Pediatr Nephrol. 2018;33(5):863–71.
3. United States Renal Data System. USRDS 2018 Annual Data Report: Epidemiology of kidney disease in the United States. Chapter 7: ESRD among children, adolescents, and young adults. Bethesda, MD: National Institutes of Health, National Institute of Diabetes and Digestive and Kidney Diseases; 2018.
4. Bonthuis M, Vidal E, Bjerre A, Aydoğ Ö, Baiko S, Garneata L, Guzzo I, Heaf JG, Jahnukainen T, Lilien M, Mallett T, Mirescu G, Mochanova EA, Nüsken E, Rascher K, Roussinov D, Szczepanska M, Tsimaratos M, Varvara A, Verrina E, Veselinović B, Jager KJ, Harambat J. Ten-year trends in epidemiology and outcomes of pediatric kidney replacement therapy in Europe: data from the ESPN/ERA-EDTA Registry. Pediatr Nephrol. 2021;36(8):2337–48.
5. Lalji R, Francis A, Wong G, Viecelli AK, Tong A, Teixeira-Pinto A, McCulloch M, Bello AK, Levin A, Lunney M, Osman MA, Ye F, Jha V, Feehally J, Harris DC, Johnson DW. Disparities in end-stage

kidney disease care for children: a global survey. Kidney Int. 2020;98(3):527–32.
6. McCulloch M, Luyckx VA, Cullis B, Davies SJ, Finkelstein FO, Yap HK, Feehally J, Smoyer WE. Challenges of access to kidney care for children in low-resource settings. Nat Rev Nephrol. 2021;17(1):33–45.
7. Iyengar A, McCulloch MI. Paediatric kidney transplantation in under-resourced regions-a panoramic view. Pediatr Nephrol. 2021; https://doi.org/10.1007/s00467-021-05070-3.
8. Chesnaye NC, Schaefer F, Groothoff JW, Caskey FJ, Heaf JG, Kushnirenko S, Lewis M, Mauel R, Maurer E, Merenmies J, Shtiza D, Topaloglu R, Zaicova N, Zampetoglou A, Jager KJ, van Stralen KJ. Disparities in treatment rates of paediatric end-stage renal disease across Europe: insights from the ESPN/ERA-EDTA registry. Nephrol Dial Transplant. 2015;30(8):1377–85.
9. Patzer RE, Sayed BA, Kutner N, McClellan WM, Amaral S. Racial and ethnic differences in pediatric access to preemptive kidney transplantation in the United States. Am J Transplant. 2013;13(7):1769–81.
10. Tjaden LA, Noordzij M, van Stralen KJ, Kuehni CE, Raes A, Cornelissen EA, O'Brien C, Papachristou F, Schaefer F, Groothoff JW, Jager KJ, ESPN/ERA-EDTA Registry Study Group. Racial disparities in access to and outcomes of kidney transplantation in children, adolescents, and young adults: results from the ESPN/ERA-EDTA (European Society of Pediatric Nephrology/European Renal Association-European Dialysis and Transplant Association) Registry. Am J Kidney Dis. 2016;67(2):293–301.
11. Harambat J, van Stralen KJ, Schaefer F, Grenda R, Jankauskiene A, Kostic M, Macher MA, Maxwell H, Puretic Z, Raes A, Rubik J, Sørensen SS, Toots U, Topaloglu R, Tönshoff B, Verrina E, Jager KJ. Disparities in policies, practices and rates of pediatric kidney transplantation in Europe. Am J Transplant. 2013;13(8):2066–74.
12. Hogan J, Ranchin B, Fila M, Harambat J, Krid S, Vrillon I, Roussey G, Fischbach M, Couchoud C. Effect of center practices on the choice of the first dialysis modality for children and young adults. Pediatr Nephrol. 2017;32(4):659–67.
13. UK Renal Registry 2020. UK Renal Registry 22nd Annual Report—data to 31/12/2019. Chapter 7: Children and young people on renal replacement therapy (RRT) for end-stage kidney disease (ESKD) in the UK in 2018. Bristol, UK, 2020.
14. Sinha A, Bagga A. Maintenance dialysis in developing countries. Pediatr Nephrol. 2015;30(2):211–9.
15. Ashuntantang G, Osafo C, Olowu WA, Arogundade F, Niang A, Porter J, Naicker S, Luyckx VA. Outcomes in adults and children with end-stage kidney disease requiring dialysis in sub-Saharan Africa: a systematic review. Lancet Glob Health. 2017;5(4):e408–17.
16. Hothi DK, Stronach L, Sinnott K. Home hemodialysis in children. Hemodial Int. 2016;20(3):349–57.

17. McDonald SP, Craig JC, Australian and New Zealand Paediatric Nephrology Association. Long-term survival of children with end-stage renal disease. N Engl J Med. 2004;350(26):2654–62.

18. Gillen DL, Stehman-Breen CO, Smith JM, McDonald RA, Warady BA, Brandt JR, Wong CS. Survival advantage of pediatric recipients of a first kidney transplant among children awaiting kidney transplantation. Am J Transplant. 2008;8(12):2600–6.

19. Amaral S, Sayed BA, Kutner N, Patzer RE. Preemptive kidney transplantation is associated with survival benefits among pediatric patients with end-stage renal disease. Kidney Int. 2016;90(5):1100–8.

20. Chesnaye NC, Schaefer F, Bonthuis M, Holman R, Baiko S, Baskın E, Bjerre A, Cloarec S, Cornelissen EAM, Espinosa L, Heaf J, Stone R, Shtiza D, Zagozdzon I, Harambat J, Jager KJ, Groothoff JW, van Stralen KJ, ESPN/ERA-EDTA Registry Committee. Mortality risk disparities in children receiving chronic renal replacement therapy for the treatment of end-stage renal disease across Europe: an ESPN-ERA/EDTA registry analysis. Lancet. 2017;389(10084):2128–37.

21. Chesnaye NC, van Stralen KJ, Bonthuis M, Harambat J, Groothoff JW, Jager KJ. Survival in children requiring chronic renal replacement therapy. Pediatr Nephrol. 2018;33(4):585–94.

22. ERA-EDTA Registry: ERA-EDTA Registry Annual Report 2018. Section D: Paediatric data reference tables. Amsterdam UMC, location AMC, Department of Medical Informatics, Amsterdam, the Netherlands, 2020.

23. Korevaar JC, Feith GW, Dekker FW, van Manen JG, Boeschoten EW, Bossuyt PM, Krediet RT. NECOSAD Study Group. Effect of starting with hemodialysis compared with peritoneal dialysis in patients new on dialysis treatment: a randomized controlled trial. Kidney Int. 2003;64(6):2222–8.

24. Mitsnefes MM, Laskin BL, Dahhou M, Zhang X, Foster BJ. Mortality risk among children initially treated with dialysis for end-stage kidney disease, 1990–2010. JAMA. 2013;309(18):1921–9.

25. Chesnaye NC, Schaefer F, Groothoff JW, Bonthuis M, Reusz G, Heaf JG, Lewis M, Maurer E, Paripović D, Zagozdzon I, van Stralen KJ, Jager KJ. Mortality risk in European children with end-stage renal disease on dialysis. Kidney Int. 2016;89(6):1355–62.

26. Vidal E, van Stralen KJ, Chesnaye NC, Bonthuis M, Holmberg C, Zurowska A, Trivelli A, Da Silva JEE, Herthelius M, Adams B, Bjerre A, Jankauskiene A, Miteva P, Emirova K, Bayazit AK, Mache CJ, Sánchez-Moreno A, Harambat J, Groothoff JW, Jager KJ, Schaefer F, Verrina E, ESPN/ERA-EDTA Registry. Infants requiring maintenance dialysis: outcomes of hemodialysis and peritoneal dialysis. Am J Kidney Dis. 2017;69(5):617–25.

27. van Stralen KJ, Borzych-Dużalka D, Hataya H, Kennedy SE, Jager KJ, Verrina E, Inward C, Rönnholm K, Vondrak K, Warady BA, Zurowska AM, Schaefer F, Cochat P, ESPN/ERA-EDTA registry, IPPN registry, ANZDATA registry, Japanese RRT registry. Survival and clinical outcomes of children starting renal replacement therapy in the neonatal period. Kidney Int. 2014;86(1):168–74.

28. Tong A, Wong G, McTaggart S, Henning P, Mackie F, Carroll RP, Howard K, Craig JC. Quality of life of young adults and adolescents with chronic kidney disease. J Pediatr. 2013;163(4):1179–85.e5.

29. Tjaden LA, Grootenhuis MA, Noordzij M, Groothoff JW. Health-related quality of life in patients with pediatric onset of end-stage renal disease: state of the art and recommendations for clinical practice. Pediatr Nephrol. 2016;31(10):1579–91.

30. Rees L, Schaefer F, Schmitt CP, Shroff R, Warady BA. Chronic dialysis in children and adolescents: challenges and outcomes. Lancet Child Adolesc Health. 2017;1(1):68–77.

31. Prezelin-Reydit M, Madden I, Macher MA, Salomon R, Sellier-Leclerc AL, Roussey G, Lahoche A, Garaix F, Decramer S, Ulinski T, Fila M, Dunand O, Merieau E, Pongas M, Zaloszyc A, Baudouin V, Bérard E, Couchoud C, Leffondré K, Harambat J. Preemptive kidney transplantation is associated with transplantation outcomes in children: results from the french kidney replacement therapy registry. Transplantation. 2022;106(2):401–11.

32. Marlais M, Martin K, Marks SD. Improved renal allograft survival for pre-emptive paediatric renal transplant recipients in the UK. Arch Dis Child. 2021;106(12):1191–194.

33. Butani L, Perez RV. Effect of pretransplant dialysis modality and duration on long-term outcomes of children receiving renal transplants. Transplantation. 2011;91(4):447–51.

34. Splinter A, Tjaden LA, Haverman L, Adams B, Collard L, Cransberg K, van Dyck M, Van Hoeck KJ, Hoppe B, Koster-Kamphuis L, Lilien MR, Raes A, Taylan C, Grootenhuis MA, Groothoff JW. Children on dialysis as well as renal transplanted children report severely impaired health-related quality of life. Qual Life Res. 2018;27(6):1445–54.

35. Warady BA, Schaefer F, Bagga A, Cano F, McCulloch M, Yap HK, Shroff R. Prescribing peritoneal dialysis for high-quality care in children. Perit Dial Int. 2020;40(3):333–40.

36. Hemodialysis Adequacy 2006 Work Group. Clinical practice guidelines for hemodialysis adequacy, update 2006. Am J Kidney Dis. 2006 Jul;48(Suppl 1):S2–90.

37. National Kidney Foundation. KDOQI Clinical Practice Guideline for Hemodialysis Adequacy: 2015 update. Am J Kidney Dis. 2015;66(5):884–930.

38. Chan CT, Blankestijn PJ, Dember LM, Gallieni M, Harris DCH, Lok CE, Mehrotra R, Stevens PE, Wang AY, Cheung M, Wheeler DC, Winkelmayer WC, Pollock CA. Conference Participants. Dialysis initiation, modality choice, access, and prescription: con-

clusions from a Kidney Disease: Improving Global Outcomes (KDIGO) Controversies Conference. Kidney Int. 2019;96(1):37–47.

39. Abramowicz D, Hazzan M, Maggiore U, Peruzzi L, Cochat P, Oberbauer R, Haller MC, Van Biesen W, Descartes Working Group and the European Renal Best Practice (ERBP) Advisory Board. Does pre-emptive transplantation versus post start of dialysis transplantation with a kidney from a living donor improve outcomes after transplantation? A systematic literature review and position statement by the Descartes Working Group and ERBP. Nephrol Dial Transplant. 2016;31(5):691–7.

40. Grams ME, Massie AB, Coresh J, Segev DL. Trends in the timing of pre-emptive kidney transplantation. J Am Soc Nephrol. 2011;22(9):1615–20.

41. Chadban SJ, Ahn C, Axelrod DA, Foster BJ, Kasiske BL, Kher V, Kumar D, Oberbauer R, Pascual J, Pilmore HL, Rodrigue JR, Segev DL, Sheerin NS, Tinckam KJ, Wong G, Knoll GA. KDIGO clinical practice guideline on the evaluation and management of candidates for kidney transplantation. Transplantation. 2020;104(4S1):S11–S103.

42. Menon S, Valentini RP, Kapur G, Layfield S, Mattoo TK. Effectiveness of a multidisciplinary clinic in managing children with chronic kidney disease. Clin J Am Soc Nephrol. 2009;4(7):1170–5.

43. Filler G, Lipshultz SE. Why multidisciplinary clinics should be the standard for treating chronic kidney disease. Pediatr Nephrol. 2012;27(10):1831–4.

44. Boehm M, Winkelmayer WC, Arbeiter K, Mueller T, Aufricht C. Late referral to paediatric renal failure service impairs access to pre-emptive kidney transplantation in children. Arch Dis Child. 2010;95(8):634–8.

45. Pruthi R, Casula A, Inward C, Roderick P, Sinha MD, British Association for Paediatric Nephrology. Early requirement for RRT in children at presentation in the United Kingdom: association with transplantation and survival. Clin J Am Soc Nephrol. 2016;11(5):795–802.

46. Driollet B, Bayer F, Kwon T, Krid S, Ranchin B, Tsimaratos M, Parmentier C, Novo R, Roussey G, Tellier S, Fila M, Zaloszyc A, Godron-Dubrasquet A, Cloarec S, Vrillon I, Broux F, Bérard E, Taque S, Pietrement C, Nobili F, Guigonis V, Launay L, Couchoud C, Harambat J, Leffondré K. Social deprivation is associated with lower access to pre-emptive kidney transplantation and more urgent-start dialysis in the pediatric population. Kidney Int Rep. 2022;7(4):741–51.

47. Smart NA, Titus TT. Outcomes of early versus late nephrology referral in chronic kidney disease: a systematic review. Am J Med. 2011;124(11):1073–80. e2.

48. Jander A, Nowicki M, Tkaczyk M, Roszkowska-Blaim M, Jarmoliński T, Marczak E, Pałuba E, Pietrzyk JA, Siteń G, Stankiewicz R, Szprynger K, Zajaczkowska M, Zachwieja J, Zoch-Zwierz W, Zwolińska D. Does a late referral to a nephrolo-gist constitute a problem in children starting renal replacement therapy in Poland? A nationwide study. Nephrol Dial Transplant. 2006;21(4):957–61.

49. Preka E, Bonthuis M, Harambat J, Jager KJ, Groothoff JW, Baiko S, Bayazit AK, Boehm M, Cvetkovic M, Edvardsson VO, Fomina S, Heaf JG, Holtta T, Kis E, Kolvek G, Koster-Kamphuis L, Molchanova EA, Muñoz M, Neto G, Novljan G, Printza N, Sahpazova E, Sartz L, Sinha MD, Vidal E, Vondrak K, Vrillon I, Weber LT, Weitz M, Zagozdzon I, Stefanidis CJ, Bakkaloglu SA. Association between timing of dialysis initiation and clinical outcomes in the paediatric population: an ESPN/ERA-EDTA registry study. Nephrol Dial Transplant. 2019;34(11):1932–40.

50. Favel K, Dionne JM. Factors influencing the timing of initiation of renal replacement therapy and choice of modality in children with end-stage kidney disease. Pediatr Nephrol. 2020;35(1):145–51.

51. Ricardo AC, Pereira LN, Betoko A, Goh V, Amarah A, Warady BA, Moxey-Mims M, Furth S, Lash JP, Chronic Kidney Disease in Children (CKiD) Cohort Investigators. Parental health literacy and progression of chronic kidney disease in children. Pediatr Nephrol. 2018;33(10):1759–64.

52. Zhong Y, Muñoz A, Schwartz GJ, Warady BA, Furth SL, Abraham AG. Nonlinear trajectory of GFR in children before RRT. J Am Soc Nephrol. 2014;25(5):913–7.

53. Okuda Y, Soohoo M, Tang Y, Obi Y, Laster M, Rhee CM, Streja E, Kalantar-Zadeh K. Estimated GFR at dialysis initiation and mortality in children and adolescents. Am J Kidney Dis. 2019;73(6):797–805.

54. Winnicki E, Johansen KL, Cabana MD, Warady BA, McCulloch CE, Grimes B, Ku E. Higher eGFR at dialysis initiation is not associated with a survival benefit in children. J Am Soc Nephrol. 2019;30(8):1505–13.

55. Hirano D, Inoue E, Sako M, Ashida A, Honda M, Takahashi S, Iijima K, Hattori M, Japanese Society of Pediatric Nephrology. Clinical characteristics at the renal replacement therapy initiation of Japanese pediatric patients: a nationwide cross-sectional study. Clin Exp Nephrol. 2020;24(1):82–7.

56. Dart AB, Zappitelli M, Sood MM, Alexander RT, Arora S, Erickson RL, Kroeker K, Soo A, Manns BJ, Samuel SM. Variation in estimated glomerular filtration rate at dialysis initiation in children. Pediatr Nephrol. 2017;32(2):331–40.

57. Cooper BA, Branley P, Bulfone L, Collins JF, Craig JC, Fraenkel MB, Harris A, Johnson DW, Kesselhut J, Li JJ, Luxton G, Pilmore A, Tiller DJ, Harris DC, Pollock CA, IDEAL Study. A randomized, controlled trial of early versus late initiation of dialysis. N Engl J Med. 2010;363(7):609–19.

58. Bakkaloğlu SA, Kandur Y, Serdaroğlu E, Noyan A, Bayazıt AK, Sever L, Özlü SG, Özçelik G, Dursun İ, Alparslan C. Effect of the timing of dialysis initiation on left ventricular hypertrophy and ınflammation in pediatric patients. Pediatr Nephrol. 2017;32(9):1595–602.

59. Schaefer F, Benner L, Borzych-Dużałka D, Zaritsky J, Xu H, Rees L, Antonio ZL, Serdaroglu E, Hooman N, Patel H, Sever L, Vondrak K, Flynn J, Rébori A, Wong W, Hölttä T, Yildirim ZY, Ranchin B, Grenda R, Testa S, Drożdz D, Szabo AJ, Eid L, Basu B, Vitkevic R, Wong C, Pottoore SJ, Müller D, Dusunsel R, Celedon CG, Fila M, Sartz L, Sander A, Warady BA, International Pediatric Peritoneal Dialysis Network (IPPN) Registry. Global variation of nutritional status in children undergoing chronic peritoneal dialysis: a longitudinal study of the International Pediatric Peritoneal Dialysis Network. Sci Rep. 2019;9(1):4886.

60. Winnicki E, McCulloch CE, Mitsnefes MM, Furth SL, Warady BA, Ku E. Use of the kidney failure risk equation to determine the risk of progression to end-stage renal disease in children with chronic kidney disease. JAMA Pediatr. 2018;172(2):174–80.

61. Furth SL, Pierce C, Hui WF, White CA, Wong CS, Schaefer F, Wühl E, Abraham AG, Warady BA, Chronic Kidney Disease in Children (CKiD). Effect of strict blood pressure control and ACE inhibition on the progression of CRF in Pediatric Patients (ESCAPE) Study Investigators. Estimating time to ESRD in children with CKD. Am J Kidney Dis. 2018;71(6):783–92.

62. Bonthuis M, Harambat J, Bérard E, Cransberg K, Duzova A, Garneata L, Herthelius M, Lungu AC, Jahnukainen T, Kaltenegger L, Ariceta G, Maurer E, Palsson R, Sinha MD, Testa S, Groothoff JW, Jager KJ, ESPN/ERA-EDTA Registry. Recovery of kidney function in children treated with maintenance dialysis. Clin J Am Soc Nephrol. 2018;13(10):1510–6.

63. Schaefer F, Warady BA. Peritoneal dialysis in children with end-stage renal disease. Nat Rev Nephrol. 2011;7(11):659–68.

64. Craig F, Henderson EM, Patel B, Murtagh FEM, Bluebond-Langner M. Palliative care for children and young people with stage 5 chronic kidney disease. Pediatr Nephrol. 2022;37(1):105–112.

65. Hothi DK, Fenton M. The impact of home hemodialysis in children with severe cardiac failure. Hemodial Int. 2020;24(4):E61–6.

66. Feber J, Schärer K, Schaefer F, Míková M, Janda J. Residual renal function in children on haemodialysis and peritoneal dialysis therapy. Pediatr Nephrol. 1994;8(5):579–83.

67. Ha IS, Yap HK, Munarriz RL, Zambrano PH, Flynn JT, Bilge I, Szczepanska M, Lai WM, Antonio ZL, Gulati A, Hooman N, van Hoeck K, Higuita LM, Verrina E, Klaus G, Fischbach M, Riyami MA, Sahpazova E, Sander A, Warady BA, Schaefer F, International Pediatric Peritoneal Dialysis Network Registry. Risk factors for loss of residual renal function in children treated with chronic peritoneal dialysis. Kidney Int. 2015;88(3):605–13.

68. Watson AR, Hayes WN, Vondrak K, Ariceta G, Schmitt CP, Ekim M, Fischbach M, Edefonti A, Shroff R, Holta T, Zurowska A, Klaus G, Bakkaloglu S, Stefanidis CJ, Van de Walle J, European Paediatric Dialysis Working Group. Factors influencing choice of renal replacement therapy in European paediatric nephrology units. Pediatr Nephrol. 2013;28(12):2361–8.

69. Ng DK, Xu Y, Hogan J, Saland JM, Greenbaum LA, Furth SL, Warady BA, Wong CS. Timing of patient-reported renal replacement therapy planning discussions by disease severity among children and young adults with chronic kidney disease. Pediatr Nephrol. 2020;35(10):1925–33.

70. Gutman T, Hanson CS, Bernays S, Craig JC, Sinha A, Dart A, Eddy AA, Gipson DS, Bockenhauer D, Yap HK, Groothoff J, Zappitelli M, Webb NJA, Alexander SI, Goldstein SL, Furth S, Samuel S, Blydt-Hansen T, Dionne J, Michael M, Wenderfer SE, Winkelmayer WC, Currier H, McTaggart S, Walker A, Ralph AF, Ju A, James LJ, Carter S, Tong A. Child and parental perspectives on communication and decision making in pediatric CKD: A Focus Group Study. Am J Kidney Dis. 2018;72(4):547–59.

71. Saggi SJ, Allon M, Bernardini J, Kalantar-Zadeh K, Shaffer R, Mehrotra R, Dialysis Advisory Group of the American Society of Nephrology. Considerations in the optimal preparation of patients for dialysis. Nat Rev Nephrol. 2012;8(7):381–9.

72. Lacson E Jr, Wang W, DeVries C, Leste K, Hakim RM, Lazarus M, Pulliam J. Effects of a nationwide predialysis educational program on modality choice, vascular access, and patient outcomes. Am J Kidney Dis. 2011;58(2):235–42.

73. Rees L, Shaw V, Qizalbash L, Anderson C, Desloovere A, Greenbaum L, Haffner D, Nelms C, Oosterveld M, Paglialonga F, Polderman N, Renken-Terhaerdt J, Tuokkola J, Warady B, Walle JV, Shroff R, Pediatric Renal Nutrition Taskforce. Delivery of a nutritional prescription by enteral tube feeding in children with chronic kidney disease stages 2-5 and on dialysis-clinical practice recommendations from the Pediatric Renal Nutrition Taskforce. Pediatr Nephrol. 2021;36(1):187–204.

74. White CT, Gowrishankar M, Feber J, Yiu V, Canadian Association of Pediatric Nephrologists (CAPN). Peritoneal Dialysis Working Group. Clinical practice guidelines for pediatric peritoneal dialysis. Pediatr Nephrol. 2006;21(8):1059–66.

75. Warady BA, Bakkaloglu S, Newland J, Cantwell M, Verrina E, Neu A, Chadha V, Yap HK, Schaefer F. Consensus guidelines for the prevention and treatment of catheter-related infections and peritonitis in pediatric patients receiving peritoneal dialysis: 2012 update. Perit Dial Int. 2012;32(Suppl. 2):S32–86.

76. Teitelbaum I, Glickman J, Neu A, Neumann J, Rivara MB, Shen J, Wallace E, Watnick S, Mehrotra

R. KDOQI US Commentary on the 2020 ISPD practice recommendations for prescribing high-quality goal-directed peritoneal dialysis. Am J Kidney Dis. 2021;77(2):157–71.

77. Borzych-Duzalka D, Shroff R, Ariceta G, Yap YC, Paglialonga F, Xu H, Kang HG, Thumfart J, Aysun KB, Stefanidis CJ, Fila M, Sever L, Vondrak K, Szabo AJ, Szczepanska M, Ranchin B, Holtta T, Zaloszyc A, Bilge I, Warady BA, Schaefer F, Schmitt CP. Vascular access choice, complications, and outcomes in children on maintenance hemodialysis: findings from the International Pediatric Hemodialysis Network (IPHN) Registry. Am J Kidney Dis. 2019;74(2):193–202.

78. Boehm M, Bonthuis M, Noordzij M, Harambat J, Groothoff JW, Melgar ÁA, Buturovic J, Dusunsel R, Fila M, Jander A, Koster-Kamphuis L, Novljan G, Ortega PJ, Paglialonga F, Saravo MT, Stefanidis CJ, Aufricht C, Jager KJ, Schaefer F. Hemodialysis vascular access and subsequent transplantation: a report from the ESPN/ERA-EDTA Registry. Pediatr Nephrol. 2019;34(4):713–21.

79. Shroff R, Calder F, Bakkaloğlu S, Nagler EV, Stuart S, Stronach L, Schmitt CP, Heckert KH, Bourquelot P, Wagner AM, Paglialonga F, Mitra S, Stefanidis CJ, European Society for Paediatric Nephrology Dialysis Working Group. Vascular access in children requiring maintenance haemodialysis: a consensus document by the European Society for Paediatric Nephrology Dialysis Working Group. Nephrol Dial Transplant. 2019;34(10):1746–65.

80. Chand DH, Swartz S, Tuchman S, Valentini RP, Somers MJ. Dialysis in children and adolescents: the pediatric nephrology perspective. Am J Kidney Dis. 2017;69(2):278–86.

81. Shroff R, Sterenborg RB, Kuchta A, Arnold A, Thomas N, Stronach L, Padayachee S, Calder F. A dedicated vascular access clinic for children on haemodialysis: two years' experience. Pediatr Nephrol. 2016;31(12):2337–44.

82. Maggiore U, Abramowicz D, Budde K, Crespo M, Mariat C, Oberbauer R, Pascual J, Peruzzi L, Schwartz Sorensen S, Viklicky O, Watschinger B, Oniscu GC, Heemann U, Hilbrands LB, ERA-EDTA DESCARTES Working Group. Standard work-up of the low-risk kidney transplant candidate: a European expert survey of the ERA-EDTA Developing Education Science and Care for Renal Transplantation in European States Working Group. Nephrol Dial Transplant. 2019;34(9):1605–11.

83. Stojanovic J, Adamusiak A, Kessaris N, Chandak P, Ahmed Z, Sebire NJ, Walsh G, Jones HE, Marks SD, Mamode N. Immune desensitization allows pediatric blood group incompatible kidney transplantation. Transplantation. 2017;101(6):1242–6.

84. Rees L, Kim JJ. HLA sensitisation: can it be prevented? Pediatr Nephrol. 2015;30(4):577–87.

85. Hebert SA, Swinford RD, Hall DR, Au JK, Bynon JS. Special considerations in pediatric kidney transplantation. Adv Chronic Kidney Dis. 2017;24(6):398–404.

86. Dharnidharka VR, Fiorina P, Harmon WE. Kidney transplantation in children. N Engl J Med. 2014;371(6):549–58.

87. Fox TG, Nailescu C. Vaccinations in pediatric kidney transplant recipients. Pediatr Nephrol. 2019;34(4):579–91.

88. Brubaker AL, Stoltz DJ, Chaudhuri A, Maestretti L, Grimm PC, Concepcion W, Gallo AE. Superior hypertension management in pediatric kidney transplant patients after native nephrectomy. Transplantation. 2018;102(7):1172–8.

89. Pickles C, Kaur A, Wallace D, Brix C, Lennon R, Plant N, Shenoy M. Bilateral native nephrectomies for severe hypertension in children with stage 5 chronic kidney disease leads to improved BP control following transplantation. Pediatr Nephrol. 2020;35(12):2373–6.

90. Kizilbash SJ, Huynh D, Kirchner V, Lewis J, Verghese PS. Timing of native nephrectomy and kidney transplant outcomes in children. Pediatr Transplant. 2021;25(5):e13952.

91. Chandar J, Chen L, Defreitas M, Ciancio G, Burke G 3rd. Donor considerations in pediatric kidney transplantation. Pediatr Nephrol. 2021;36(2):245–57.

92. Van Arendonk KJ, James NT, Orandi BJ, Garonzik-Wang JM, Smith JM, Colombani PM, Segev DL. Order of donor type in pediatric kidney transplant recipients requiring retransplantation. Transplantation. 2013;96(5):487–93.

93. Van Arendonk KJ, Chow EK, James NT, Orandi BJ, Ellison TA, Smith JM, Colombani PM, Segev AD. Choosing the order of deceased donor and living donor kidney transplantation in pediatric recipients: a Markov decision process model. Transplantation. 2015;99(2):360–6.

94. Oh J, Wunsch R, Turzer M, Bahner M, Raggi P, Querfeld U, Mehls O, Schaefer F. Advanced coronary and carotid arteriopathy in young adults with childhood-onset chronic renal failure. Circulation. 2002;106(1):100–5.

95. Harambat J, Bonthuis M, van Stralen KJ, Ariceta G, Battelino N, Bjerre A, Jahnukainen T, Leroy V, Reusz G, Sandes AR, Sinha MD, Groothoff JW, Combe C, Jager KJ, Verrina E, Schaefer F, ESPN/ERA-EDTA Registry. Adult height in patients with advanced CKD requiring renal replacement therapy during childhood. Clin J Am Soc Nephrol. 2014;9(1):92–9.

96. Hamilton AJ, Clissold RL, Inward CD, Caskey FJ, Ben-Shlomo Y. Sociodemographic, psychologic health, and lifestyle outcomes in young adults on renal replacement therapy. Clin J Am Soc Nephrol. 2017;12(12):1951–61.

97. Vogelzang JL, van Stralen KJ, Jager KJ, Groothoff JW. Trend from cardiovascular to non-cardiovascular late mortality in patients with renal replacement therapy since childhood. Nephrol Dial Transplant. 2013;28(8):2082–9.

98. Groothoff JW, Offringa M, Grootenhuis M, Jager KJ. Long-term consequences of renal insufficiency in children: lessons learned from the Dutch LERIC study. Nephrol Dial Transplant. 2018;33(4):552–60.

99. Modi ZJ, Lu Y, Ji N, Kapke A, Selewski DT, Dietrich X, Abbott K, Nallamothu BK, Schaubel DE, Saran R, Gipson DS. Risk of cardiovascular disease and mortality in young adults with end-stage renal disease: an analysis of the US Renal Data System. JAMA Cardiol. 2019;4(4):353–62.

100. Kramer A, Stel VS, Geskus RB, Tizard EJ, Verrina E, Schaefer F, Heaf JG, Kramar R, Krischock L, Leivestad T, Pálsson R, Ravani P, Jager KJ. The effect of timing of the first kidney transplantation on survival in children initiating renal replacement therapy. Nephrol Dial Transplant. 2012;27(3):1256–64.

101. Vogelzang JL, van Stralen KJ, Noordzij M, Diez JA, Carrero JJ, Couchoud C, Dekker FW, Finne P, Fouque D, Heaf JG, Hoitsma A, Leivestad T, de Meester J, Metcalfe W, Palsson R, Postorino M, Ravani P, Vanholder R, Wallner M, Wanner C, Groothoff JW, Jager KJ. Mortality from infections and malignancies in patients treated with renal replacement therapy: data from the ERA-EDTA registry. Nephrol Dial Transplant. 2015;30(6):1028–37.

Management of Peritoneal Dialysis in Children

65

Alicia M. Neu, Bradley A. Warady,
and Franz Schaefer

Introduction

Peritoneal dialysis (PD) is the most frequently prescribed maintenance dialysis therapy for children with kidney failure worldwide, particularly in infants and very young children [1–3]. Technical advances and increasing efforts to minimize risk for infection and cardiovascular disease, the leading causes of morbidity and mortality, have contributed to improvements in technique and patient survival among children on maintenance PD [4–7]. However, mortality for children on dialysis remains unacceptably high and notably higher than for children who receive a kidney transplant [2, 3, 7]. Ongoing efforts to further improve outcomes in children on maintenance PD must include prescribing, monitoring and adjusting the dialysis treatment to meet the unique needs of the child [8, 9]. This chapter focuses on the principles involved in developing

and monitoring the PD prescription, establishing a functioning access to perform the dialysis procedure and the infectious and non-infectious complications seen in children on maintenance PD. Kidney failure is an incredibly complex condition and therefore comprehensive care of the child on maintenance peritoneal dialysis must not only include tailoring the PD prescription to provide optimal solute and fluid removal, but also maximizing growth and neurocognitive development, managing anemia, minimizing bone and mineral metabolism disorder and cardiovascular disease, and addressing the psychosocial well-being of the child and their family [8, 9]. Each of these important topics is therefore covered in a separate chapter of this book.

The Peritoneal Dialysis Prescription

The directly modifiable components of the PD prescription include the composition and volume of the dialysis fluid and the schedule by which that fluid is instilled and removed from the peritoneal cavity. Although empiric recommendations for prescribing maintenance PD in children are often used when initiating dialysis, optimal care requires that the PD prescription be modified to meet the unique needs of the individual child or adolescent with kidney failure [8–10]. This requires a basic knowledge of the physiology of dialysis which, in turn, relies on an under-

A. M. Neu (✉)
Division of Pediatric Nephrology, The Johns Hopkins University School of Medicine, Baltimore, MD, USA
e-mail: aneu1@jhmi.edu; aneu@jhmi.edu

B. A. Warady
Division of Pediatric Nephrology, Children's Mercy Kansas City, Kansas City, MO, USA
e-mail: bwarady@cmh.edu

F. Schaefer
Division of Pediatric Nephrology, Center for Pediatrics and Adolescent Medicine,
Heidelberg, Germany
e-mail: franz.schaefer@med.uni-heidelberg.de

standing of the peritoneal membrane as the primary barrier to solute and fluid transport. This chapter therefore begins with a brief overview of the structure of the peritoneal membrane, followed by a discussion of the physiology of dialysis, that is, the driving forces for the exchange of solute and fluid across the peritoneal membrane. The application of these principles to guide selection of the modifiable components of the PD prescription is then presented.

The Peritoneal Membrane

The peritoneal membrane is a thin structure lining the inner surface of the abdominal wall and the majority of visceral organs. It is lined by the mesothelium, a continuous layer of flattened epithelial cells covered with numerous microvilli, and includes a dense network of capillaries distributed within a thin interstitium [11–13]. The pathway for the solute and water exchange between the plasma in the peritoneal capillaries and the dialysate in the peritoneal cavity of the child on PD includes the continuous capillary endothelium, the peritoneal interstitial space, and the mesothelium [14]. Of these, the capillary endothelium appears to be the primary determinant of resistance to transport, and microvascular density is therefore a major determinant of transport characteristics [11, 15–18]. The permeability of the endothelium lining the peritoneal capillaries has been functionally described by the three-pore model proposed by Rippe and colleagues [19]. In this model, the major route for small-solute and water movement is represented by the spaces between the endothelial cells, the so-called small pores, which have a radius of 40–50 Å, slightly larger than albumin (36 Å) [12, 19]. Ultrasmall pores, with a radius of approximately 2.5 Å, are the most abundant type of pores and are involved in sodium-free water transport [12, 19]. Several lines of evidence have demonstrated that the water channel aquaporin-1 corresponds to the ultrasmall pore [20, 21]. The third group of pores is the transendothelial 'large pore' pathways, which have a radius of approximately 250 Å, and which

account for only 0.01% of the total population of capillary pores and through which macromolecules are transported [19].

The Physiology of Dialysis

The driving forces for exchange of solute across the peritoneal membrane include diffusion and convective mass transfer through the small pores in the capillary endothelium. The rate of solute movement by diffusion is determined by the concentration gradient of the solute between the dialysate in the peritoneal cavity and the plasma in peritoneal capillaries, the effective surface area of the peritoneal membrane in contact with the dialysate, the so called "wetted membrane," and the permeability of the peritoneal membrane to that solute, which, in turn, is influenced by the molecular weight of the solute [13, 22]. Convective mass transfer occurs as water moves through small pores from capillaries to dialysate, "dragging along" dissolved solutes. The amount of solute removed by convective mass transfer is, therefore, determined by the amount of water removed and by the membrane permeability, or sieving coefficient for that solute. While small molecular weight solutes, like urea, move by both diffusion and convective mass transfer, the movement of larger molecular weight compounds, including the uremic "middle molecules," is driven primarily by convective mass transfer [23].

The bulk movement of water, or ultrafiltration, is driven by Starling forces, i.e. osmotic and hydrostatic pressure [12, 23]. Figure 65.1 depicts the Starling forces (P, hydrostatic pressure; Π, oncotic or osmotic pressure) that operate across each of the pore types in the three-pore model [12]. Movement of water through the ultrasmall pores is driven by the osmotic gradient between the plasma in peritoneal membrane capillaries and the interstitium and, ultimately, the dialysis fluid in the peritoneal cavity. The osmotic pressure in the plasma is generated primarily by albumin, whereas osmotic pressure in the dialysate is typically generated by crystalloid, i.e. glucose, or the glucose polymer icodextrin. This "water only" movement through the ultrasmall pores explains the transient decrease in dialysate sodium concentration during the early phase of a dialysis dwell, which is referred to as sodium

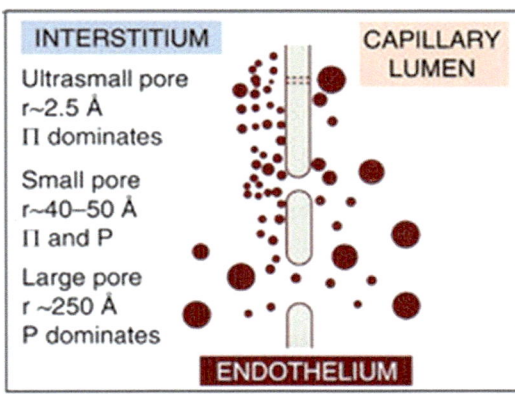

Fig. 65.1 The Starling forces (P, hydrostatic pressure; Π, oncotic pressure) operating across each type of pore in the three-pore model of peritoneal membrane capillary permeability. Å angström, r functional radius. (From [12], with permission)

sieving. Movement of water through small pores is influenced by both hydrostatic and osmotic forces (Fig. 65.1) [12]. In simplest terms, hydrostatic forces in plasma and osmotic forces in the dialysate promote ultrafiltration, while osmotic forces in plasma and hydrostatic pressures in the peritoneal cavity oppose it [24]. Several factors contribute to the generation of these forces; however, the critical component for ultrafiltration during PD is the difference in osmotic pressure between the dialysate and the plasma, which, in turn, is largely dependent on the osmotic agent present in the dialysate [24]. The amount of water removed from the person on PD, or net ultrafiltration, is also influenced by water movement from the peritoneal cavity back to the capillaries in the late stages of a dwell, when the osmotic gradient generated by dialysate glucose may have dissipated, and by uptake of water from the peritoneal cavity into tissue and lymphatics [25, 26]. The contribution of water movement through the relatively rare large pores to net ultrafiltration is felt to be minimal [12].

These principles of solute and fluid movement during PD should be used to guide selection of the various components of the dialysis prescription, including dialysate composition, fill volume and the schedule by which dialysis is instilled and removed from the peritoneal cavity (PD modality/dwell time), to optimize solute and fluid removal.

Determination of Fill Volume

As discussed above, the movement of solutes and water during PD is intrinsically dependent on the amount of peritoneal membrane surface area available for exchange, or the "wetted membrane" [13]. Although the peritoneal membrane has an estimated surface area of 1 m² in adults, computed tomography studies in people on maintenance PD have demonstrated that only 30–60% of this anatomic area is in contact with dialysate [27]. The peritoneal membrane contact area can be influenced by position, increasing in the supine position, and by increasing the volume of the infused dialysate, or fill volume [28]. In children, where body size varies considerably, the concept of scaling the fill volume to body size is intuitive. Fill volume should be based on body surface area (BSA), rather than weight, as the relationship between peritoneal membrane surface area and BSA is constant and age-independent [29]. Body surface area can be calculated from anthropometric data, i.e. height and weight. The most commonly used equation is that of Gehan and George [30]:

$$BSA\ (m^2) = 0.0235 \times (height,\ cm)^{0.42246} \times (weight,\ kg)^{0.51456}$$

As stated above, increasing the fill volume will promote solute and fluid removal by maximizing peritoneal membrane contact area [31]. In addition, increasing fill volume will facilitate movement by diffusion. The impact of fill volume on diffusion rests on the principle of geometry of diffusion, that is, the larger the dialysate volume, the longer the transperitoneal concentration gradient will persist to drive diffusion [32]. However, increasing fill volume also increases intraperitoneal pressure (IPP) which may lead to patient discomfort and other complications including hernia formation, hydrothorax and gastroesophageal reflux (See Non-Infectious Complications) [10, 26, 28, 33]. In addition, elevated IPP may increase lymphatic uptake of fluid, thereby reducing net ultrafiltration [10, 33]. Studies in children on PD revealed that the peritoneal membrane vascular surface area available for exchange increased by a mean of 21% as fill volumes were increased from 800 to 1400 ml/m², with no further improvement as fill volumes increased to 2000 ml/m² [28, 34]. These data support current recommendations that, if required for solute clearance and fluid removal, the fill volume should be gradually increased to an upper limit of 1200–1400 ml/m² in children over age 2 years [10]. Infants may not tolerate such large fill volumes, and an upper limit volume of 800 ml/m² is currently recommended in this age group [10]. The maximal volume for individual children on PD should also be influenced by the child's comfort level and when indicated, an objective measure of IPP [35]. Measurement of IPP can be done at the bedside, using a manometer attached to the PD catheter. The mean IPP is calculated from the pressure measured during inspiration and expiration. Normal ranges of mean IPP for children over age 2 years have been reported to be 7–14 cmH₂O, with an upper tolerated limit of 18 cmH₂O [35, 36].

Choice of PD Fluid

Conventional PD Solutions

PD solutions typically contain an osmotic agent, a buffer and sodium, chloride, calcium and magnesium in varying concentrations, in an effort to provide not only removal of fluid and waste products, but also electrolyte homeostasis, and acid-base and calcium balance. The composition of the most widely used commercially available dialysis solutions attempt to mimic normal plasma, while allowing mass production and storage stability [37]. These constraints led to the selection of glucose in supraphysiologic concentrations as the osmotic agent and lactate alone as the buffer, with a resultant low pH of the dialysis fluid. This allows heat sterilization without caramelization of the glucose, and minimizes precipitation of calcium and magnesium from the solution, which may occur when bicarbonate is used as the buffer [37]. From the description of the Starling forces involved in water movement during PD, it follows that increasing the concentration of glucose in the dialysis fluid increases the osmotic gradient driving ultrafiltration. From a functional standpoint, because glucose is a dif-

fusible solute, it is absorbed from the dialysate to plasma via the small pores, resulting in a time-dependent loss of the crystalloid osmotic gradient. Thus, glucose is unable to provide sustained ultrafiltration during extended exchange dwell times. In addition, absorption of glucose can contribute to anorexia and lead to elevated serum glucose and hyperinsulinemia, even in non-diabetic patients [38]. This increased carbohydrate load can predispose to abnormalities of lipid metabolism and insulin resistance (See Non-Infectious Complications) [37, 39]. In addition to the negative effects associated with glucose absorption, the heat sterilization process used with conventional PD solutions produces high levels of glucose-degradation products (GDP), which are directly toxic to the peritoneal mesothelium and are systemically absorbed [40]. GDPs also enhance production of advanced glycation end products, which along with high concentration of glucose have been implicated in the development of structural changes in the peritoneal membrane including vascular proliferation and progressive fibrosis, both of which contribute to peritoneal membrane failure [31, 37, 41, 42].

Alternate Osmotic Agents

In light of these findings, minimizing the exposure of the peritoneal membrane to hypertonic glucose is a therapeutic aim [43]. Currently, there are two commercially available PD solutions that contain osmotic agents other than glucose; one contains icodextrin and the other amino acids. Icodextrin is a glucose polymer with a molecular weight of approximately 16,000 Daltons, which exerts its osmotic effect through the small pores in the capillary endothelium. Thus, there is little to no salt-free water movement through the ultrasmall pores (sodium sieving) and sodium removal is typically higher than with glucose-based solutions [44]. Because icodextrin does not diffuse through the peritoneal membrane, the osmotic gradient, and therefore ultrafiltration, is typically sustained, and icodextrin solutions are therefore used during dialysis exchanges with a prolonged dwell time [45, 46]. The net ultrafiltration seen in individual people on PD can be variable, probably owing to variability in the peritoneal residual volume, i.e. the amount of non-icodextrin containing fluid remaining in the peritoneal cavity from the previous exchange, which modifies the concentration of icodextrin and, therefore, the osmotic pressure difference between the peritoneal cavity and plasma [47, 48]. Another factor influencing net ultrafiltration is lymphatic absorption of icodextrin, which has been reported to be as much as 45% within 12–14 h in children on PD. [49] Reabsorption may be particularly high in infants on PD, limiting the ultrafiltration achieved with icodextrin in this age group [50]. Finally, a minimum daytime fill volume of 550 ml/m^2 has been suggested to optimize ultrafiltration with icodextrin in children [51]. Icodextrin is metabolized to maltose and a number of oligosaccharides which reach systemic steady state levels within 2 weeks of initiating treatment, and concerns about higher levels of these non-degradable compounds limits the use of icodextrin containing solutions to a single daily exchange [43, 45]. Hypersensitivity reactions have also been reported with icodextrin-containing solutions [45].

Amino acids, in a 1.1% solution, are also used as an osmotic agent in a commercially available, non-glucose PD solution. This solution is as efficient an osmotic agent as a 1.36% glucose-based solution. Amino acid-based solutions initially appeared particularly appealing for children on PD because of the potential nutritional benefit; however, studies revealed conflicting impact on nutrition, as well as increases in blood urea nitrogen and metabolic acidosis [52]. Given these findings, it is not recommended that amino acid solutions be used as a nutritional source in children on PD. [43] The benefits and potential drawbacks of each of the three solutions described here are summarized in Table 65.1 [37].

Biocompatible Solutions

The supraphysiologic concentrations of glucose and the presence of GDPs are not the only contributors to the bio-incompatibility of standard dialysis solutions. Low pH is associated with infusion pain and directly induces neoangiogenesis and mesothelial cell damage [53, 54]. Even at a neutral pH, lactate-based peritoneal dialysis solutions have been associated with impaired mesothelial cell viability and function [55, 56].

Table 65.1 Characteristics of currently available single-chamber peritoneal dialysis solutions, based on osmotic agent. Modified from [37], with permission

Buffer	Potential drawbacks	Potential benefits
Glucose	Low pH High GDP Poor peritoneal membrane biocompatibility Infusion pain Local and systemic glucose exposure	Ease of manufacture Low cost
Icodextrin	Hypersensitivity Low pH Systemic accumulation of oligosaccharides Lactate containing	Sustained ultrafiltration Preservation of RKF Hypertonic glucose replacement Reduced hyperglycemia Desirable effects on metabolic profile and body composition
Amino acid	Low pH Exacerbation of uremic symptoms and acidosis	No GDP Avoid systemic and peritoneal glucose exposure Peritoneal membrane protection Enhanced nutrition in adults

GDP glucose degradation product, *RKF* residual kidney function

The effort to provide truly biocompatible solutions therefore includes not only the use of alternative osmotic agents, but also a solution composition that results in a more neutral pH and reduced exposure to lactate. The development of multi-chamber dialysis solutions has allowed these issues to be addressed at the commercial level. These bags isolate the buffer during storage, thus allowing glucose to be stored at low pH, ensuring stability, and avoiding the creation of GDP during heat sterilization. This also avoids bicarbonate-induced precipitation of calcium and magnesium in the solution [37]. A summary of the benefits and potential drawbacks of the currently available multi-chamber PD solutions is shown in Table 65.2 [37]. All of these solutions provide lower GDP levels than standard glucose-containing solutions. Although numerous in vitro studies have supported the biocompatibility of

Table 65.2 Characteristics of currently available multi-chamber peritoneal dialysis solutions, based on buffer. Modified from [37], with permission

Buffer	Potential drawbacks	Potential benefits
Lactate alone	More physiologic, but not neutral, pH Local and systemic glucose exposure	Lower GDP levels More physiological pH Improved peritoneal membrane biocompatibility Preserved membrane defense
Lactate/bicarbonate	Local and systemic glucose exposure Does not eliminate peritoneal lactate exposure	Lower GDP levels More physiologic pH Improved peritoneal membrane biocompatibility Preserved membrane defense Reduced infusion pain
Bicarbonate alone	Local and systemic glucose exposure	Lower GDP levels More physiologic pH Improved peritoneal membrane biocompatibility Preserved membrane defense Improved correction of acidosis

GDP glucose degradation product

these solutions, a study of peritoneal biopsies in children at the time of PD catheter insertion and then after receiving maintenance PD with neutral pH, low GDP fluids revealed a doubling of peritoneal microvascularization and exchange area within a few months of initiating PD, calling into question the ability of these fluids to preserve membrane function and structure [41]. A subsequent analysis found that the duration of dialysis and dialytic glucose exposure were the primary determinants of the alterations to the peritoneal membrane [57]. Although biocompatible fluids may, in turn, not eliminate the structural changes to the peritoneal membrane, there may be some benefit of using bicarbonate, rather than lactate, as the dialysis solution buffer. A multicenter randomized controlled trial in 37 children on PD compared two multi-chamber, neutral pH, low GDP PD solutions that differed only with regard to the buffer, lactate versus bicarbonate. This study found equivalent correction of metabolic acidosis with the two solutions, but bicarbonate-based solutions were associated with better long-term preservation of peritoneal membrane function as measured by ultrafiltration capacity [58]. In addition, data from the International Pediatric Peritoneal Dialysis Network (IPPN) revealed that young infants exposed to neutral-pH, low-GDP PD solutions exhibited significant catch-up growth, whereas patients using conventional PD fluids showed no improvement in

height standard deviation scores over the same time period. These findings led investigators to speculate that reduction of the inflammatory processes associated with conventional solutions might improve growth in children undergoing maintenance PD [59]. Finally, a Cochrane Review revealed that use of a neutral pH, low GDP PD solution is associated with improved preservation of residual kidney function and urine volume in adults on PD [60]. Given these findings, use of the more biocompatible solutions is encouraged, while recognizing that cost and availability of these solutions may limit widespread use [43]. In fact, data from IPPN reveals significant regional variability in the prescription of neutral pH PD solutions among children on PD enrolled in that registry [61]. When excluding children from the United States, where neutral pH PD solutions are not approved, 8% of children from low-income countries are prescribed these solutions, compared to 68% of children in high-income countries [8, 61].

Determination of PD Modality/Dwell Time

CAPD vs. APD

There are two major PD modalities utilized for maintenance PD, continuous ambulatory peritoneal dialysis (CAPD), in which 3 or 4 exchanges are performed manually during the day with an exchange with a long dwell time conducted overnight, and automated peritoneal dialysis (APD), in which multiple exchanges are provided, typically overnight, by a cycler. The most commonly prescribed APD schedules are continuous cycling PD (CCPD) and nightly or nocturnal intermittent PD (NIPD). Both provide multiple exchanges overnight, but in CCPD, 50–100% of the nightly fill volume is instilled at the end of the APD session for a daytime exchange. For NIPD, no daytime exchange is used, and the person on PD is said to have a dry day with no dialysate being present in the peritoneal cavity. Other modifications can include the addition of a mid-day manual exchange, sometimes referred to as semi-automated PD, and tidal PD, where only a portion of the initially instilled fill volume is drained and replaced with each exchange overnight, with the full volume drained only at the completion of the APD session. Tidal therapy has been found to be particularly beneficial in patients who experience "drain pain."

The selection of PD modality should be individualized for each child based on a number of factors, including age, residual kidney function, nutritional status, tolerance/comfort and the preference of the child and their caregivers [8, 9]. The physiology of PD should be considered so that the modality selected meets the child's solute and fluid removal requirements. Because APD allows more exchanges to be conducted during a 24-h period than CAPD, the peritoneal membrane is exposed to a larger total volume of dialysate in this time period which may enhance clearance of small solutes. In addition, during APD the majority of exchanges occur at night, when the child is in the supine position, which optimizes peritoneal membrane contact area and minimizes increases in IPP [28]. Conversely, CAPD allows increased clearance of middle molecules, which is dependent on the duration of contact between dialysate and the peritoneal membrane [62]. The requirement for fluid removal will also impact modality selection. In CAPD, daytime dwell times are typically 4–6 h long, as more frequent exchanges may be too cumbersome for the child/caregivers to perform. These long dwell times may result in reduced ultrafiltration, due to the loss of glucose-generated osmotic gradient, and necessitate higher glucose-containing solutions

to maintain that gradient. Recall that in the early part of an exchange, sodium-free water movement occurs via the ultrasmall pores. Thus, frequent exchanges with short dwell times characteristic of APD may result in a relatively higher contribution of free water transport to total fluid removal, that is, more water than sodium is removed. Conversely, an exchange with a longer dwell time, as occurs with CAPD, allows more time for convective losses of sodium, but also allows back-diffusion and back-filtration, and may result in net fluid and sodium retention [26].

From a practical standpoint, because a cycler is not required for CAPD, the training and equipment required are less than for APD. However, because APD, is performed at night, this therapy minimizes the restriction on daytime activities, such as school attendance for children and work for adult caregivers, which is a significant benefit associated with the use of this modality [63].

Empiric Dialysis Prescriptions

A typical empiric APD prescription includes 5–10 exchanges over 9–12 h overnight, with an identical fill volume and duration for each exchange. A daytime exchange is usually prescribed, particularly in children who are anuric. More recently the concept of adapted PD, with initial cycles using a relatively small fill volume and short dwell times to maximize ultrafiltration, followed by a larger fill volume with longer dwell times to promote solute clearance, has been suggested as a means of improving dialysis efficiency, and in particular sodium and fluid removal [26, 64]. Not all commercially available PD cyclers are able to provide adapted PD and further prospective crossover studies in children on PD are required for validation. As stated previously, the typical CAPD prescription includes 3–4 exchanges during the day and a long overnight exchange.

Measures of Peritoneal Membrane Function

Because peritoneal membrane transport characteristics may vary considerably between people on PD, and even in a single person over time, it is important to evaluate these characteristics to optimize the PD prescription. Pediatric guidelines recommend evaluating peritoneal membrane function within the first month of initiating PD and then after any event that may impact peritoneal membrane transport capacity, such as peritonitis [65]. The most commonly used test to characterize peritoneal membrane transport capacity is the peritoneal equilibration test or PET, developed by Twardowski [66]. The PET measures the rate at which solutes, specifically urea, creatinine and glucose, equilibrate between the blood and the dialysate. In the PET, dialysate is infused into the peritoneal cavity using a standardized fill volume and glucose concentration. Because the fluid used in the exchange immediately preceding the PET may influence results, the solution used for the PET should also be used for the dialysis session the night prior [67, 68]. Once the dialysis solution is instilled, the concentrations of creatinine and urea in the dialysate and in plasma are measured after 2 and 4 h of dwell time to derive dialysate to plasma ratios (D/P). The concentration of glucose in the dialysate at 2 and 4 h after instillation is compared to the concentration of glucose in the

dialysate at the time of instillation (D/D_0). The D/P and D/D_0 ratios are then compared to standard curves to characterize the child as having high, high average, low average or low peritoneal membrane solute transport capacity [66]. People on PD with low or low average transport capacity may benefit from exchanges with longer dwell times, which will allow maximal diffusion of solutes. Conversely, rapid diffusion of glucose in patients with high peritoneal membrane transport capacity necessitates the use of exchanges with short dwell times to achieve ultrafiltration. The crossing point of the urea and glucose equilibration curves obtained from the standardized PET, referred to as the Accelerated Peritoneal Examination (APEX) time, has been proposed as a means to identify the dwell time to be used to optimize ultrafiltration [69]. The characteristics seen with the various peritoneal membrane transport types, and the percent of children enrolled in the IPPN with each are shown in Fig. 65.2.

Peritoneal Membrane Characteristics

Membrane % Patients	4-Hr Type	Characteristics
20%	High	Very efficient membrane Transports solutes quickly Increased glucose absorption May have difficulty achieving ultrafiltration At risk for low serum albumin
25%	High Average	Efficient membrane Transports solutes fairly well Ultrafilters well
34%	Low Average	Less efficient membrane Transports solutes somewhat slowly Ultrafilters well
21%	Low	Inefficient membrane Transports solutes slowly Difficult to obtain target solute removal when no residual kidney function Ultrafilters very well

Fig. 65.2 Characteristics of the various peritoneal membrane transport types (high, high average, low average and low) and the percentage of children with each of the types enrolled in the registry of the International Pediatric Peritoneal Dialysis Network (personal communication, B Warady)

The PET has been validated in children on PD, using 2.5% dextrose, or 2.3% glucose PD solution and a fill volume of 1100 ml/m² [70, 71]. In infants, the fill volume used for the PET is usually the clinically prescribed fill volume [23]. Figures 65.3 and 65.4 show the standardized D/P creatinine and D/D$_0$ glucose curves, respectively, from which a child's peritoneal membrane transport capacity can be characterized [70]. In a study of 20 children on mainte-nance PD, nearly identical characterization of peritoneal membrane function was found with the D/P creatinine or D/D$_0$ glucose at 2 and 4 h, and it has therefore been suggested that a 2 h or short-PET may be reasonable in children on PD [72]. The sequential PET, in which the standard PET is followed by a "mini-PET," has been proposed as a method for providing more complete characterization of both solute and fluid trans-port [73]. The mini-PET is a modification of the

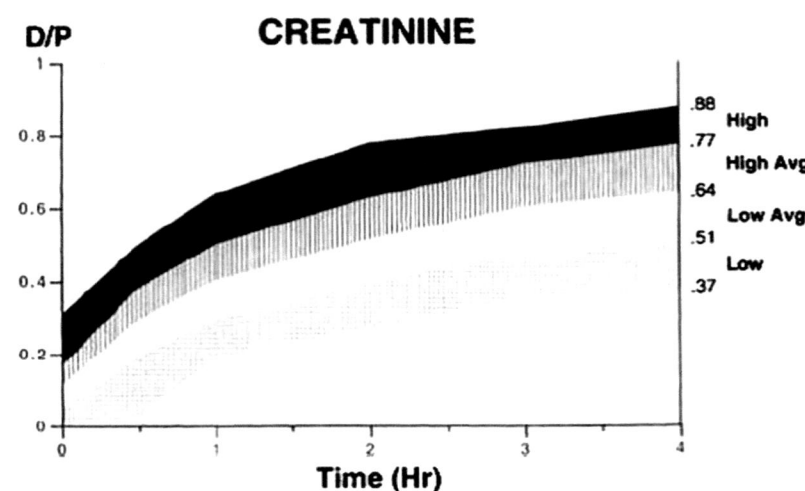

Fig. 65.3 Peritoneal equilibration test results for creatinine. Shaded areas represent high, high average, and low transport rates. The white band represents the low average transport rate. The four categories are bordered by the maximal, mean + 1 SD, mean, mean − 1 SD, and minimal values for the population. D/P, dialysate to plasma ratio. (From [70], with permission)

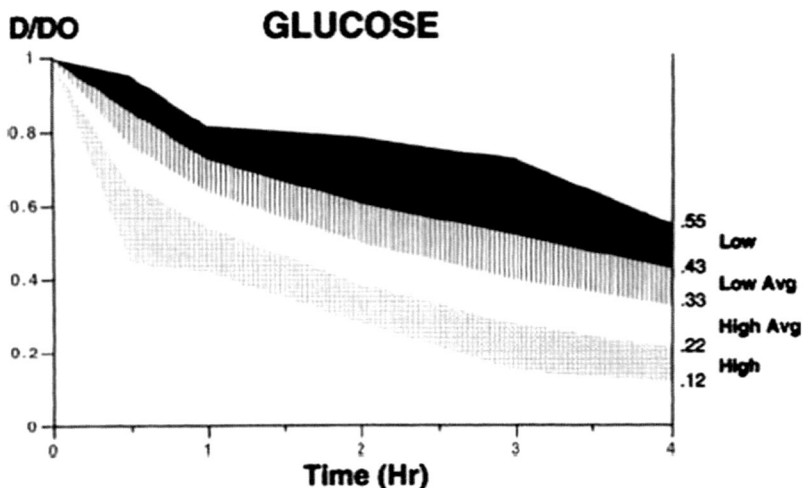

Fig. 65.4 Peritoneal equilibration test results for glu-cose. Shaded areas represent high, low average, and low transport rates. The white band represents the high aver-age transport rate. The four categories are bordered by the maximal, mean + 1 SD, mean, mean − 1 SD, and minimal values for the population. D/D0, dialysate glucose to ini-tial dialysate glucose concentration ratio. (From [70], with permission)

standard PET which uses a 3.86% glucose solution instilled for 1 h. Dialysate sodium concentration is measured just prior to infusion and after 60 min, providing more accurate information about the ultrafiltration capacity and assessment of sodium sieving [74].

Data obtained from the PET can also be used to calculate the mass area transfer coefficient (MTAC) [70, 75, 76]. The MTAC has been variably defined as the area available for solute transport divided by the sum of resistances to peritoneal diffusion. The MTAC represents the maximal clearance of a solute theoretically achievable at a constantly maximal gradient for diffusion, i.e. when the dialysate concentration of the solute remains at zero. Unlike the D/P ratio, MTAC is essentially independent of dialysate glucose or fill volume. Calculation of MTAC requires rigorously performed PD exchanges and complex mathematical equations. However, with the assistance of computer programs, data from a carefully performed PET can be used to derive MTAC. These programs, which have been validated in children on PD, can also be used to predict solute and fluid removal for individualized dialysis prescriptions [77, 78]. It must be recognized that the results predicted by these programs assume optimized conditions and therefore the actual amount of dialysis delivered by any prescription needs to be measured (See Goal-directed Approach to Prescribing PD).

Goal-Directed Approach to Prescribing PD

Solute Clearance

Historically, modification of the empiric PD prescription has been driven by the concept of achieving "dialysis adequacy," i.e. the dose of dialysis delivered is measured and adjustments are made to exceed a minimum dose below which patient outcomes are unacceptable. For decades, adequacy targets focused on the delivered dialysis dose in terms of small solute clearance. Peritoneal dialysis adequacy guidelines recommended the use of urea removal, scaled for the urea volume of distribution, Kt/V_{urea}, to monitor solute clearance and

guidelines published in 2006 in the United States and internationally suggested a minimum target of a total weekly (residual kidney and dialysate) Kt/V_{urea} of 1.8 or 1.7 for adults on PD, respectively [65, 79]. These targets were largely based on studies in adults on PD which suggested improved survival with increasing small solute clearance [80, 81]. However, a reanalysis of data from a large prospective study in Canada and the United States (CANUSA) found the association between small solute clearance and mortality to be completely explained by the clearance contributed by residual kidney function, with no association between increasing dialysate small solute clearance and survival [82]. Similarly, two large prospective randomized trials did not demonstrate an association between increasing small solute clearance and mortality in adults on PD [83, 84]. A retrospective analysis of administrative data in the United States did reveal an increased risk for mortality with a $Kt/V_{urea} < 1.7$ in anuric adults on PD [85].

Although a prospective study of 171 children on PD demonstrated a positive correlation between dialytic creatinine clearance and change in height standard deviation score, and cross-sectional and retrospective studies have suggested improved growth and cardiac function with increasing small solute clearance, there are no large-scale, prospective, randomized studies of the influence of small solute clearance on outcomes in children on PD to more definitely define adequacy targets [86–88]. In light of this, the 2006 guidelines recommended that the total weekly Kt/V_{urea} in children should meet or exceed the adult standard [65].

Measurement of total weekly Kt/V_{urea} should incorporate both dialysate and residual kidney clearance [65]. This is accomplished by collecting the volume of urine from a 24-h period, as well as the peritoneal dialysis effluent from the PD exchanges during those 24 h. The volume is recorded and urea measured on each sample. Blood urea nitrogen concentration is also measured.

The total dialysate Kt/V_{urea} is then calculated by:

(24 h Dialysate/Plasma urea×24 h drained volume × 7) / Volume of distribution of urea

The residual kidney urea clearance is calculated by:

(Volume of 24 h urine in mL×urine urea nitrogen concentration)/(1440 min/day × blood urea nitrogen concentration)

From this, the residual kidney Kt/V_{urea} can be calculated as:

(Kidney urea clearance (ml/min) × 1440 min/day × 7 days)/1000 mL × Volume of distribution of urea.

The total weekly Kt/V_{urea} is the sum of the weekly dialysis and residual kidney Kt/V_{urea} [65].

The volume of distribution of urea, V, is assumed to be equal to total body water. Therefore, accurate estimates of total body water are important to accurately determine Kt/V_{urea}. The gold standard method for determining total body water, the heavy water dilution technique, is rarely applied in the clinical setting. Equations using anthropometric information (height and weight) are more commonly used to estimate total body water, and sex-specific nomograms developed in children on PD are available [89].

Guidelines for children on PD recommend that total weekly Kt/V_{urea} be measured within the first month after initiating dialysis and then at least twice yearly, and following any change in the child's clinical status that could influence solute clearance or ultrafiltration capacity [10, 90]. Given these recommendations, measurement of small solute clearance is standardly performed, and achievement of the minimal target for Kt/V_{urea} in adults and children on PD is used as a measure of the quality of care by dialysis organizations around the globe and regulatory and payment agencies in the United States. However, the data linking small solute clearance to outcomes in people on PD remains relatively weak, with no prospective intervention trials since publication of the 2006 KDOQI guidelines, and prospective cohort and retrospective studies in adults on PD only confirming that patient outcomes are more closely linked with residual kidney function than clearance of solute

by dialysis [91–98]. In addition, it has been increasingly acknowledged that optimal care requires that all aspects of management, including the PD prescription, be driven by the unique needs of the person with kidney failure, and not solely by small solute clearance [8, 91]. In 2018, a Kidney Disease: Improving Global Outcomes (KDIGO) Controversies Conference focused on dialysis proposed a change in terminology from "adequate" to "goal-directed" dialysis, where shared decision-making between the person on PD and the care team is utilized to establish realistic care goals that allow the person on PD to meet their life goals and allow the care team to provide individualized, high quality dialysis care [99]. In this framework, solute removal targets are interpreted and implemented in the context of the overall goals and clinical status of the person on PD [99]. In alignment with this statement, the International Society for Peritoneal Dialysis (ISPD) published new practice points for prescribing high-quality, goal-directed PD in 2020, including specific practice points for children on PD [8, 9, 91]. These documents suggest that modifications to the PD prescription should be based on regular assessment of clinical well-being, volume status (see below) and other laboratory parameters, in addition to Kt/V_{urea}, with a minimum target total weekly Kt/V_{urea} of 1.7 [9]. The guidance document specifically states that children on PD with $Kt/V_{urea} < 1.7$ should not have their PD prescription modified for the sole purpose of achieving the target, if close and repeated assessment of clinical and laboratory parameters suggest that the child is otherwise doing well [9].

The 2020 ISPD guidance document for children on PD also suggests that the PD prescription be adjusted with the goal of achieving a normal serum phosphate level [9]. Because phosphate clearance is related to contact time between dialysate and the peritoneal membrane, optimizing the long daytime exchange is suggested to enhance phosphate removal [100]. It is recognized, however, that phosphate control cannot be achieved with dialytic clearance alone and dietary restriction and phosphate binders are required in most children on peritoneal dialysis [9].

Fluid Removal

Cardiovascular disease, as manifested by hypertension and left ventricular hypertrophy, is unfortunately quite common in children on dialysis, and fluid overload is a major contributor to both [4, 5, 61, 87, 101–104]. PD guidelines have therefore consistently emphasized the importance of adjusting the dialysis prescription to provide adequate salt and water removal [9, 79, 105].

Routine assessments of fluid status should be included in the care of children on PD. Casual blood pressure should be monitored, both in the clinic and at home, and ambulatory blood pressure monitoring may be performed to more accurately assess blood pressure and detect masked hypertension [106]. Central to the evaluation of fluid status is assessing the "dry" body weight of the child on PD, which should be performed routinely. However, determination of fluid overload may be inaccurate when based on clinical assessment alone and is further complicated by the expected weight gain in the growing child. Bioimpedance, if available, may be used as a component of the assessment of fluid status, and a recent study demonstrated that multifrequency whole-body bioimpedance spectroscopy successfully quantified total body water and acute changes of extracellular and intracellular water in children with chronic kidney failure, including those on dialysis [9, 107–109]. Data from the IPPN found that anemia tended to be associated with characteristics of the patient with fluid overload, including low urine output, high ultrafiltration requirements, high transport status on PET, hypertension, and left ventricular hypertrophy [101]. In addition, serum albumin and hemoglobin levels were closely associated, suggesting that fluid overload could result in dilution of both markers [101]. These findings led the authors to speculate that ESA-resistant anemia and hypoalbuminemia may be indicators of "occult" fluid overload in children on PD.

Adjustment to the dialysis prescription should, in turn, be made to achieve "dry weight" and blood pressure control. Efforts to optimize ultrafiltration while avoiding exposure to high glucose containing solutions include the use of icodextrin-containing dialysate for an extended daytime exchange, modifying dwell time using the APEX time, and potentially the use of adapted PD, as discussed previously [9, 26, 69, 110].

The amount of sodium removal required will depend on salt intake. Infants have very low sodium intake from formula or breast milk, and may have significant urinary losses of sodium associated with underlying congenital anomalies of the kidney and urinary tract. As a result, additional sodium losses from dialysis may result in hyponatremia, hypovolemia and hypotension. Therefore, infants on PD often require sodium supplementation [111]. On the other hand, older children and adolescents on PD are typically salt overloaded. In these children, the sodium gap, defined as the difference between the calculated theoretical sodium removal (plasma sodium concentration multiplied by ultrafiltration volume) and the amount actually removed (dialysate sodium concentration multiplied by ultrafiltration volume), is positive, reflecting inadequate sodium removal [112]. Most commercially available PD solutions have a sodium concentration of 132–134 mmol/L, just slightly lower than the concentration in normal serum. Studies of PD solutions containing 115–126 mmol/L sodium in adults on PD have shown increased sodium removal and a lower sodium gap, with associated improvements in blood pressure and fluid status [112–114]. However, very low sodium solutions require slightly higher glucose concentrations to maintain osmolarity and therefore may increase overall glucose exposure [112]. There are currently no studies of the impact of lower sodium-containing dialysis solutions on sodium and fluid balance in children or adolescents on PD.

Peritoneal Dialysis Access

Catheter Configuration

Successful PD requires a catheter that provides reliable, rapid dialysate flow rates without leaks or infections. The first description of placement of an indwelling catheter for maintenance PDs was in 1968 by Tenckhoff, and the Tenckhoff catheter continues to be the most commonly used

PD access in children [3, 115, 116]. Despite significant improvements in catheter design, however, the catheter has continued to be a significant barrier to successful PD because of catheter-related complications. A recent analysis of 824 incident PD catheters in the IPPN revealed that more than 20% required revision and 83% of those revisions occurred in the first year after placement [116]. Need for access revision increased the risk of peritoneal dialysis technique failure or death [116]. This section will review the currently available catheter configurations and placement techniques. Associations between the various configurations and risk for catheter-associated infectious and non-infectious complications, including catheter malfunction, are discussed later in this chapter.

The most commonly used catheters for maintenance PD are constructed of soft material, such as silicone rubber or polyurethane. There are a wide variety of catheter configurations available, which differ in their intraperitoneal configurations (curled or straight), the number of Dacron cuffs (one or two) and the subcutaneous tunnel configuration (straight or "swan-neck"). Figure 65.5 shows the most common combinations of these configurations [117]. Table 65.3 reveals the percentage of catheters with the various configurations in children on PD from large national and international collaborative projects: IPPN, the North American Pediatric Renal Trials and Collaborative Studies (NAPRTCS), and the Standardizing Care to Improve Outcomes in Pediatric End stage kidney disease (SCOPE) collaborative [3, 115, 116]. These data demonstrate that a curled intraperitoneal configuration is most commonly used in children on PD [3, 115, 116].

The next catheter characteristic to consider is the number of Dacron cuffs on the catheter. If a single cuff catheter is used, it is generally recommended that the cuff be positioned between the rectus sheaths in the rectus muscle, and not be located in a superficial position. The addition of a second cuff was prompted by the potential to better secure the catheter and reduce migration of bacteria into the peritoneal cavity. Early data in children on PD demonstrated a lower incidence of infection with catheters having two cuffs,

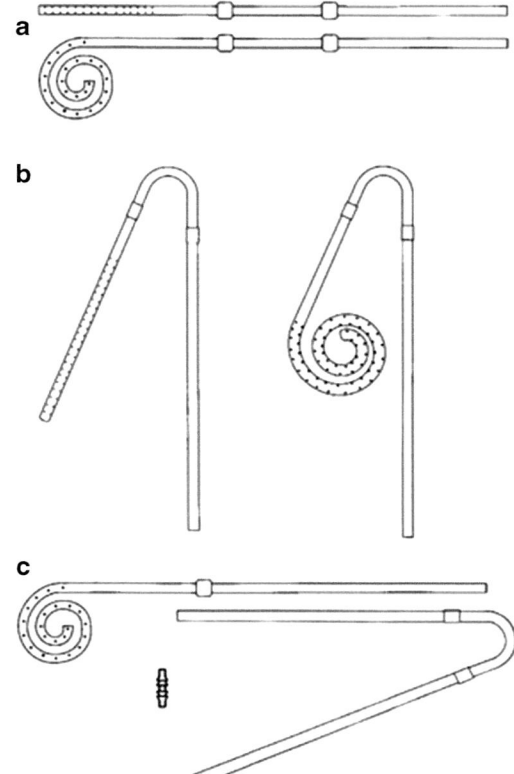

Fig. 65.5 Commonly used peritoneal catheters. (**a**) Catheter with straight tunnel segment, 2 cuffs, and straight or coiled intraperitoneal segment. (**b**) Catheter with preformed arc tunnel segment ("swan neck"), 2 cuffs, and straight or coiled intraperitoneal segment. (**c**) Extended catheter with 1-cuff, coiled-tip abdominal catheter, 2-cuff extension catheter with swan neck. Catheters with a straight tunnel segment are also available with a single cuff. (From [117], with permission)

rather than one [3]. Based on these data, current guidelines recommend use of a 2-cuff PD catheter in children, except possibly in the very small infant in whom it may not be technically feasible [118]. Accordingly, the percentage of children on PD with 2-cuff catheters has increased, from roughly half of children in the NAPRTCS report from 2011, to more than 70% and 80% in recent reports from SCOPE and IPPN, respectively (Table 65.3) [3, 115, 116]. If two cuffs are used, the second cuff should be located at least 2.0 cm from the exit site to reduce the risk for cuff extrusion [117, 119]. If cuff extrusion occurs, prompt

Table 65.3 Catheter configurations from national and international collaborative registries and projects in children on maintenance peritoneal dialysis

Catheter configuration	NAPRTCS [3]	SCOPE [115]	IPPN [116]
	N (%)[a]	N (%)[a]	N (%)[a]
Number of catheters	4687 (100%)	1201 (100%)	2453 (100%)
Intraperitoneal segment			
Tenckhoff Curled	2909 (62.1%)	1070 (89.1%)	1681 (68.5%)
Tenckhoff Straight	1213 (25.9%)	66 (5.5%)	673 (27.4%)
Cuffs			
One	2375 (50.7%)	264 (22.0%)	346 (13.7%)
Two	2124 (45.3%)	873 (72.7%)	2117 (86.3%)
Tunnel			
Swan neck	1590 (33.9%)	793 (66.0%)	1542 (62.9%)
Straight	2895 (61.8%)	313 (26.1%)	911 (37.1%)
Exit-site orientation			
Up	564 (12.0%)	52 (4.3%)	346 (14.1%)
Down	1537 (32.8%)	613 (51.0%)	1299 (53.0%)
Lateral	1816 (16.4%)	459 (38.2%)	808 (32.9%)

NAPRTCS North American Pediatric Renal Trials and Collaborative Studies, *SCOPE* Standardizing Care to Improve Outcomes in Pediatric End Stage Kidney Disease, *IPPN* International Pediatric Peritoneal Dialysis Network
[a] Percentages may not add to 100% due to missing/other

shaving of the cuff off the catheter has been advocated to reduce infection risk [120, 121].

The shape of the extraperitoneal portion, or tunnel, of the catheter can be straight or have a preformed angle ("swan neck"), in which there is an inverted U-shape arc (170–180°) between the deep and the superficial cuffs (Fig. 65.5). The purpose of the catheter arc is to allow the catheter to exit the skin in a downward pointing direction, which may be associated with a decreased likelihood for the accumulation of dirt and debris within the catheter tunnel which, in turn, may reduce the development of a tunnel infection/peritonitis (see Infectious Complications) [3, 122]. In addition, the swan neck configuration allows the distal end of the catheter to enter the peritoneal cavity in an unstressed condition (i.e. without too much torque because of the synthetic material's memory), thereby decreasing the chance for its migration out of the pelvis, and the associated risk for impaired drainage [123, 124]. Since its introduction, the use of swan neck catheters has been increasing in children on PD and is now placed in the majority (Table 65.3) [3, 115, 116].

A modification of the swan neck catheter is the swan neck presternal catheter, which has a very long subcutaneous portion (Fig. 65.5). This catheter has been utilized when it is necessary to make the exit-site remote from the abdomen, such as in infants and children with incontinence, intestinal stomas, and suprapubic catheters, and the catheter exit-site is typically located in the anterior chest wall [125–127]. However, infants with complex congenital anomalies often have minimal subcutaneous tissue over the chest, which makes cuff erosion more likely in that location. One suggested approach to this problem is to place the two cuffs below the costal margin and then have the catheter exit high on the chest wall [126]. Conversely, a single cuff catheter may be used.

Preoperative Evaluation and Preparation

Careful preoperative evaluation is required for all children and adolescents prior to PD catheter placement. The preoperative evaluation should include screening and treatment of constipation, which is common in children with kidney failure and has consistently been associated with an increased risk for post placement PD catheter migration and malfunction [128]. The preoperative physical examination should include evaluation for the presence of hernias. The incidence of hernias is inversely proportional to age, with an overall frequency of 8.0–57.0% [129–132]. The highest frequency of inguinal hernias occurs in the first year of life; they are often bilateral and all require surgical correction. Umbilical hernias can worsen in a child on PD as a result of the increase in intra-abdominal pressure generated by instillation of dialysis solution (see Non-infectious complications). As a result, some have advocated peritoneography or laparoscopic inspection for hernias at the time of catheter placement [130]. If detected, the hernias can then be fixed at the same time the PD catheter is inserted [133, 134].

A critical portion of the pre-catheter assessment is deciding upon the most appropriate location of the exit-site. In infants, the exit-site of the catheter needs to be outside of the diaper area to help prevent contamination. In older children, it should be either above or below the beltline. The presence of a vesicostomy, ureterostomy, colostomy or gastrostomy will also influence the preferred exit-site location. The exit-site must be planned so that it is either on the opposite side of the abdomen from any stoma site or, as stated previously, the exit-site may be placed on the chest to increase the distance from any stoma.

Catheter Placement Technique

Since Moncrief and Popovich first reported on the use of CAPD, there have been a number of modifications of the technique for the implantation of the PD catheter [135]. The two most common PD catheter insertion techniques are open and laparoscopic. Although there are no randomized trials in children comparing outcomes in PD catheters placed using these two approaches, several case series report excellent outcomes with the laparoscopic approach, including excellent revision free survival and a lower incidence of catheter flow problems [117, 136–138]. SCOPE data reveals that more than 65% of catheters in the collaborative were placed using a laparoscopic procedure, with no statistically significant difference in placement technique (open versus laparoscopic) between children with and without peritonitis in the first 60 day after catheter placement [115].

Infectious Complications

PD-associated infections include PD catheter-related infections, i.e. infection at the catheter exit-site and/or the subcutaneous tunnel, and peritonitis. Infectious complications remain the most significant cause of morbidity and PD technique failure in children on maintenance PD [2, 3, 139–141]. In addition, infection is a leading cause of death in children on PD [2, 3, 141]. Analyses of data from large pediatric dialysis registries have revealed associations between many factors and the risk for PD-related infections in children on PD. Recognition of these risk factors is important, as they may prompt modification of care practices, which, in turn, may lower infection rates as well as the rates of patient morbidity and mortality.

Risk Factors and Prevention

Patient Age

Data from collaborative registries have consistently identified young age at dialysis initiation, and specifically age less than 2 years, as a risk factor for peritonitis [3, 122, 142–144]. It seems intuitive that the relatively close proximity of the PD catheter to the diaper region or urinary or gastrointestinal ostomy sites in a small infant would increase the risk for bacterial contamination and subsequent infection. As stated previously, efforts to maximize the distance between the catheter exit-site and the diaper area and stomas are important to decrease the risk for infection [125, 145].

PD Catheter Design, Insertion and Post-operative Exit-Site Care

As discussed previously, early studies of data from children on PD suggested a higher incidence of infection and a higher risk for relapsing peritonitis with a one cuff rather than a two cuff catheter, and current guidelines recommend a catheter with two cuffs in children on maintenance PD [3, 118, 146]. However, more recently the SCOPE collaborative has failed to show any relationship between the number of catheter cuffs and the development of either exit-site/tunnel infections or peritonitis [122, 147]. Data in adults on PD suggest that benefit of a second cuff for infection prevention may have been reduced by widespread adoption of application of antibiotics at the catheter exit-site [117, 148].

While some studies in adults have found the use of the swan neck catheter to be associated with less frequent exit-site/tunnel infections, other studies have been unable to confirm these results [149–151]. As stated previously, one advantage of the swan neck catheter is that it allows a downward, rather than upward, pointing exit-site. Data from NAPRTCS has consistently identified an upward facing exit-site as a risk factor for peritonitis, a finding confirmed by a recent analysis of SCOPE data [3, 122]. Accordingly, current guidelines for children on PD recommend that the exit-site orientation be in the downward or lateral position [118].

Efforts to minimize the risk for peritonitis at the time of catheter placement include the provision of antibiotics prior to surgical incision [118, 152, 153]. Although vancomycin may be slightly more effective than a first-generation cephalosporin in the prevention of post-operative peritonitis, use of the latter is recommended because of concern for the generation of vancomycin resistance [118, 153–155]. The ultimate choice of antibiotic for perioperative prophylaxis should be influenced by the PD unit's antibiotic susceptibility patterns [118, 154]. Current guidelines also recommend that while securing the newly inserted catheter and minimizing movement at the exit site is important, sutures should not be placed at the catheter exit-site at the time of surgical placement, as they may increase risk of bacterial colonization and subsequent infection [118].

In the immediate post-operative period, PD catheter and exit-site care are aimed at optimizing healing and minimizing bacterial colonization [156]. Current guidelines suggest that the sterile dressing placed in the operating room following PD catheter placement remain in place for at least 7 days, and subsequent dressing changes should be performed by trained staff, using aseptic technique, no more frequently than weekly until the exit-site is healed [118, 157]. More frequent dressing changes should be performed only if the dressing becomes loose, damp, or soiled [118]. The catheter should be immobilized to optimize healing and minimize trauma [118, 158]. It is generally recommended that initiation of dialysis be delayed for at least 2 weeks following catheter placement to minimize the risk of leak at the peritoneal insertion site, although exit-site healing may take as long as 6 weeks [156–158]. In support of this, an analysis of SCOPE data demonstrated an association between use of the PD catheter for dialysis within 14 days of placement and an increased risk for early peritonitis, defined as peritonitis occurring within the first 60 days following catheter insertion [115].

Training

Because PD is a home dialysis therapy, appropriate training of the child with kidney failure and caregivers is essential to minimize the risk for infection. Unfortunately, there are no randomized controlled trials to evaluate the relationship between various training elements or the training process itself and outcomes [159–161]. Several observational studies have shown associations between shorter training time (<15 h), training in the 10 days after catheter insertion and small center size with an increased risk for peritonitis [159–164]. Current guidelines for children on PD suggest that training should include the use of a formalized teaching program that has clear objectives and criteria, with incorporation of adult learning principles [118, 159]. The training should be performed by an experienced PD nurse with pediatric training and should include core topics, including those related to infection prevention such as hand hygiene, aseptic technique, exit-site care and appropriate treatment for contamination [118, 159]. It is suggested that PD training should include no more than one child/family simultaneously [118, 159]. A syllabus for teaching PD to patients and caregivers has been published by the ISPD, and includes a checklist for PD assessment and another for PD training [165]. It remains to be determined if widespread use of this syllabus and the associated tools leads to a decrease in infection rates.

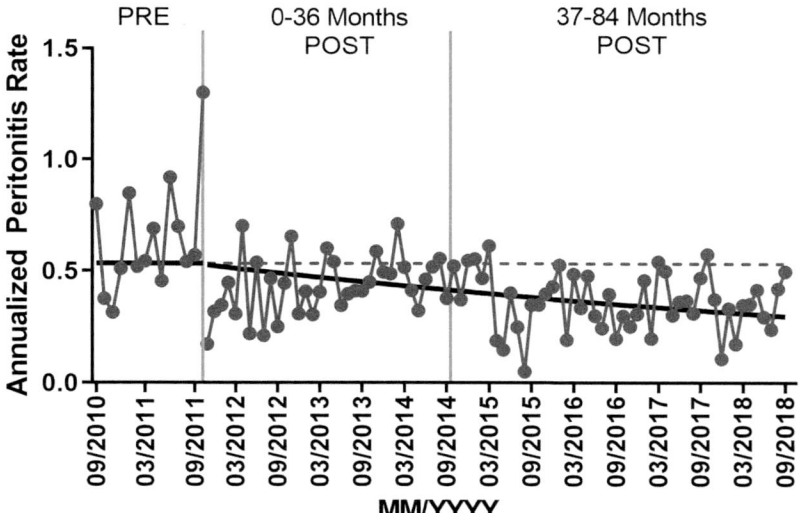

Fig. 65.6 Average monthly peritonitis rates, expressed as annualized rates, among 19 pediatric dialysis centers in the United States participating in the Standardizing Care to Improve Outcomes in Pediatric End Stage Kidney Disease (SCOPE) Collaborative from collaborative launch on October 1, 2011 through September 30, 2018. Differences between peritonitis rates in the 13 months prior to launch (pre-launch period) and the post-launch period were modeled using Generalized Linear Mixed Models techniques and revealed that the decrease in infection rate observed in the first 36 months persisted and there was a significant reduction in the average monthly peritonitis rates from 0.53 (95% CI 0.37, 0.70,) pre-launch to 0.30 infections per patient year (95% CI 0.23, 0.43) at 84 months post launch, p < 0.001. From [170], with permission)

Current guidelines suggest periodic retraining of the persons performing PD in the home, particularly after a peritonitis episode [118, 159]. The Trial on Education and Clinical outcomes for Home PD patients (TEACH), compared PD-related infections in adults on PD randomized to receive home visits for retraining every 1–3 months over a 24-month period compared to no re-training [166]. The study failed to demonstrate a significant difference in peritonitis rates between the two groups, although a sub-analysis demonstrated a significantly lower risk for first peritonitis episodes in patients >60 years of age who received frequent home visits [166]. The SCOPE collaborative includes a "follow up" care bundle, which requires a review of key aspects of hand hygiene, exit-site care, and aseptic technique at each monthly follow up visit in the clinic, redemonstration of competency with these procedures every 6 months, regular scoring of the PD catheter exit-site and treatment of touch contaminations according to ISPD guidelines [118, 167, 168]. SCOPE centers demonstrated a significant increase in compliance with this care bundle over the first 3 years of the collaborative, accompanied by a significant reduction in peritonitis rates [169]. A more recent analysis demonstrated that centers participating in the collaborative for 7 years were able to achieve and then maintain high level compliance with the follow up bundle and had continued reduction in center peritonitis rates over the collaborative's entire post-launch period (Fig. 65.6) [170]. An analysis of SCOPE data at the patient level also demonstrated that compliance with the follow up care bundle was significantly associated with a lower rate of peritonitis [122]. These data suggest that in addition to comprehensive training at the initiation of dialysis, ongoing review with regular testing of competency of PD catheter care and the dialysis procedure may minimize the risk for peritonitis.

Chronic Exit-Site Care

Once the catheter exit-site has healed, regular exit-site care is vital to minimize the risk for PD catheter-related infection. Current guidelines recommend regular cleansing of the exit-site with a sterile antiseptic solution and sterile gauze [118, 171]. Several cleansing agents are available and none has been shown to be superior in the prevention of catheter-related infection [118, 171]. In addition, there is no clear guidance for the optimal frequency of exit-site care, e.g. daily, every other day, or weekly [118, 171]. Not surprisingly, data from the International Pediatric Peritonitis Registry (IPPR) revealed significant variability in exit-site practices around the globe, including the frequency of exit-site care as well as the type of antiseptic agent used [172]. IPPR data also revealed that peritonitis due to *Pseudomonas* species was significantly more common at centers where exit-site care was performed more than twice weekly and where nonsterile cleansing agents (e.g. saline, soap) were used [172]. Among SCOPE participants, compliance with the specific recommendation to review exit-site care at each visit was associated with lower exit-site infection rates [147].

In addition to regular exit-site cleaning, current guidelines suggest application of a topical antibiotic during routine care, in an effort to minimize colonization of the exit-site with *Pseudomonas aeruginosa* (*P. aeruginosa*) and *Staphylococcus aureus* (*S. aureus*), both of which are widely accepted as risk factors for exit-site infection and subsequent peritonitis [118, 171, 173–176]. A number of observational studies, randomized controlled trials and meta-analyses have demonstrated that mupirocin applied to the skin around the exit-site reduces the risk for exit-site infections [118, 153, 171, 177–181]. However, there is concern that routine use of mupirocin may be associated with an increased risk for gram-negative infections and the emergence of mupirocin resistant *Staphylococcus* species [172, 182, 183]. Topical gentamicin is an alternative therapy, and a randomized trial in adults showed that daily application of gentamicin cream to the exit-site was not only effective in reducing exit-site infections caused by *Pseudomonas* species, but it was as effective as topical mupirocin in reducing *S. aureus* infections [180]. There are concerns, however, about the possible development of gentamicin-resistant organisms and an increased risk of fungal infections with this therapy.

Touch Contamination

Accidental contamination of the sterile portions of the PD catheter transfer set or dialysis tubing, or touch contamination, is a leading cause of peritonitis [122, 184, 185]. Current guidelines recommend that contamination prior to the infusion of dialysis fluid into the peritoneal cavity be treated with a sterile transfer set change alone, without antibiotics [118]. If the contaminating event occurs after dialysate has been infused into the peritoneal cavity, both a sterile transfer set change and antibiotic prophylaxis is recommended [118, 163]. Intraperitoneal administration of a first-generation cephalosporin for 1–3 days is typically recommended, unless the patient has a history of methicillin-resistant *S. aureus* (MRSA), in which case a glycopeptide (vancomycin or teicoplanin) should be used [118, 163]. Gram-negative coverage may be appropriate if the contamination may have included enteric organisms, e.g. from stool in a diapered infant [118]. An effluent sample should be obtained for cell count, differential and culture prior to delivery of antibiotics, if possible, and culture results and susceptibility testing used to guide any subsequent antibiotic usage [118].

Ostomies

As stated previously, ostomy sites, including gastrostomy, ureterostomy, nephrostomy and colostomy, may increase the risk of bacterial contamination of an adjacent PD catheter. In fact, data from the IPPN demonstrated an increased risk for peritonitis in the presence of any ostomy [186]. Data in children on PD have not revealed a consistent association between presence of a gastrostomy tube (GT) and risk for infection, including fungal infection; however, among infants on PD enrolled in SCOPE, placement of a GT after PD catheter placement was associated with increased risk for bacterial peritonitis [122, 144, 185, 187–190]. Although data on the subject is limited, current guidelines suggest that an open procedure should be used to place a GT in patients who are already receiving PD, while either open or laparoscopic placement may be used if the gastrostomy is placed prior to initiating PD. [118, 191]. Prophylactic antibiotics, typically a first-generation cephalosporin, and antifungal therapy should be provided during gastrostomy tube placement in a patient with a PD catheter [118].

While an analysis of SCOPE data did not find an association between the presence of a colostomy and the risk for peritonitis in multivariable analysis, a recent study from IPPN revealed a significantly higher rate of peritonitis among patients with a colostomy [122, 192]. The number of children on PD with colostomies in these analyses was relatively small at 14 and 20, respectively [122, 192].

Antibiotic and Antifungal Prophylaxis

Although fungal peritonitis is relatively uncommon in children on PD, it is associated with an increased risk for significant morbidity and mortality [190, 193–195]. Observational data suggests that risk factors for fungal peritonitis include prior treatment with antibiotics, recurrent peritonitis, and immunosuppression [189, 190, 195–199]. Antifungal prophylaxis with either oral nystatin or fluconazole is currently recommended whenever antibiotics are administered to children on PD, although data from SCOPE reveal that this practice is not uniformly implemented, particularly when antibiotics are prescribed for infections other than bacterial peritonitis [118, 190, 200–204].

Prophylactic antibiotic and antifungal therapy should also be provided when children on PD undergo certain procedures, including gastrostomy tube placement, as previously discussed, as well as invasive dental, gastrointestinal or genitourinary procedures [118, 205, 206].

Other Factors

The risk factors listed in this section were largely derived from data collected by observational registries and quality improvement collaboratives that identified associations between various factors and risk for infection among a cohort of children on PD. There are clearly many other factors that may impact the risk for infection in individual children. The dialysis unit should perform a formal review, or apparent cause analysis, of each infection in search of causation [118, 162, 163]. This review should include nurses and physicians

at a minimum. Inclusion of the child on PD and their caregivers/family, social worker, infection preventionist and infectious disease specialist is encouraged. Identification of causation will allow appropriate intervention for the individual, and potentially other children on PD in the unit.

Catheter-Related Infections

Infections of the PD catheter include exit-site and tunnel infections. PD catheter-related infections are associated with an increased risk for peritonitis. However, even without subsequent peritonitis, exit-site and tunnel infections require exposure to antibiotics with the subsequent risk for fungal infection and drug resistant organisms, both of which may require catheter removal [147, 207–209]. Catheter-related infections also carry a high risk of recurrence. In a Japanese multicenter study, 15% of all infections and 40% of MRSA infections relapsed [210].

Routine use of an objective scoring system is recommended to monitor the status of the catheter exit site and to optimize the diagnostic accuracy of exit-site infections. The pediatric Exit Site Score (ESS) considers pericatheter swelling, crust, redness, tenderness and secretion with a score range from 0 to 10 (Table 65.4) [118, 168]. An exit site infection is diagnosed by an ESS >1 in the presence of a pathogenic organism, or >3 irrespective of culture results. A tunnel infection is defined by an ESS >5 [118]. Sonographic examination may help to evaluate the extent of infection along the catheter [211, 212]. Data from SCOPE, which requires scoring of the exit-site at every monthly visit, revealed that an ESS of anything more than

Table 65.4 Catheter exit-site scoring system. From [118], with permission [168]

	0 Points	1 Point	2 Points
Swelling	No	Exit only (<0.5 cm)	Including part of or entire tunnel
Crust	No	<0.5 cm	>0.5 cm
Redness	No	<0.5 cm	>0.5 cm
Pain on pressure	No	Slight	Severe
Secretion	No	Serous	Purulent

zero is associated with an increased risk for an exit-site infection in the following month [147]. However, significant variability in exit-site scoring using this tool has been noted at SCOPE centers, and the collaborative is currently modifying the tool in an effort to promote more consistent scoring and, therefore, greater uniformity in the diagnosis of exit-site infections.

Uncomplicated catheter exit-site infections can be treated with oral antibiotics according to culture results and susceptibilities [118]. Empiric therapy for tunnel infections may be via the oral route; however, intraperitoneal or intravenous antibiotics are often indicated, particularly if signs of severe infection and/or a history of *S. aureus* or *P. aeruginosa* are present. Infections with gram-positive bacteria should be treated with a first-generation cephalosporin or a penicillinase-resistant penicillin. Intraperitoneal or intravenous glycopeptide therapy should be reserved for cases with proven MRSA infection [118]. The use of oral ciprofloxacin for infections due to *P. aeruginosa* had previously been recommended, with the addition of a second antibiotic such as cefepime, piperacillin, or a carbapenem, if resolution of the infection is slow, or there is recurrence [118]. However, recent reports from observational studies have suggested an increased risk for aortic aneurysm or dissection associated with fluoroquinolone use, particularly in the setting of other risk factors such as hypertension, which led the United States' Food and Drug Administration to issue a safety announcement (https://www.fda.gov/Drugs/DrugSafety/ucm628753.htm) [213–216].

Adjunctive therapy for exit-site/tunnel infections should include daily or twice daily dressing changes, and cautious removal of exuberant granulomatous tissue ("proud flesh") with silver nitrate.

Antibiotic treatment should be administered for a minimum of 2 weeks and for at least 7 days beyond complete resolution of the infection. Treatment for at least 3 weeks is recommended for infections caused by *S. aureus* or *P. aeruginosa*. Extension of antibiotic therapy beyond 4 weeks should be avoided. In case of persistence of symptoms or recurrence after discontinuation of antibiotic treatment, the catheter should be removed and replaced [118]. Surgical shaving of the external cuff may be an alternative to catheter removal for

treatment of a persistent exit-site infection if the inner cuff is not involved [121, 217].

Peritonitis

The diagnosis of peritonitis should be considered in any child on PD with abdominal pain and/or cloudy PD effluent, with an effluent white blood cell count of greater than 100/mm^3 and at least 50% polymorphonuclear neutrophils (PMN) confirming the diagnosis [118]. For children on automated PD, the effluent white blood cell count should be obtained from an exchange with the dialysis solution instilled for at least 1–2 h [118]. In this setting, the presence of 50% or more PMN is highly suggestive of peritonitis when the clinical features of peritonitis are present, even if the total white blood cell count is below 100/mm^3. Bacterial growth in the effluent confirms the diagnosis, whereas a negative culture does not rule out a bacterial etiology. The efficiency of microbiological diagnostics can be maximized by incubating the effluent in 3–4 blood culture bottles, and by centrifuging large effluent volumes. A culture-negative rate of less than 10% should be aimed for according to consensus guidelines [218]. However, international surveys have shown that this target is far from being achieved by pediatric PD centers around the globe [172]. Data from the SCOPE collaborative revealed an overall culture negative rate of 26.6% and significant variability in the culture negative rate and culture techniques among centers, although no associations between practices and culture negative rate could be elucidated [219]. In response to these data, the SCOPE collaborative has implemented a standardized PD effluent culture bundle and has already demonstrated a decrease in the both the culture negative rate and the percentage of cultures that are negative per month (unpublished finding). Among culture-positive cases, IPPN discovered wide regional variability in causative organisms, but in general gram-positive organisms predominate, with coagulase-negative *Staphylococci* and *S. aureus* most frequently cultured [122, 172].

Empiric intraperitoneal antibiotic treatment should be initiated as soon as the diagnosis of peritonitis is considered, and include coverage for both gram-positive and gram-negative organisms

[118]. Monotherapy with cefepime may be considered for empiric therapy, while a first-generation cephalosporin or a glycopeptide combined with ceftazidime or an aminoglycoside may be used if cefepime is not available [118]. However, global peritonitis data from children on PD reveals not only significant variability in the causative organisms, but also associated antibiotic susceptibilities, prompting the additional recom-mendation that empiric coverage be guided by the center-specific antibiotic susceptibility pattern [172]. Specifically, the empiric use of glycopep-tides should be restricted to centers where the rate of MRSA exceeds 10%. Antibiotic therapy should be modified based on culture and antibiotic sus-ceptibility results. Dosing recommendations are given in Table 65.5 [118]. If cultures remain ster-ile and signs and symptoms of peritonitis are

Table 65.5 Dosing recommendations for anti-infective agents in children with peritoneal dialysis catheter-related peritonitis. Administration should be via intraperitoneal route unless specified otherwise. Intermittent doses should be applied once daily unless specified otherwise. From [118] with permission

| | Continuous therapy[a] | | |
	Loading dose	Maintenance dose	Intermittent therapy
Aminoglycosides[b]			
Gentamicin	8 mg/L	4 mg/L	
Netilmicin	8 mg/L	4 mg/L	Anuric: 0.6 mg/kg Non-anuric: 0.75 mg/kg
Tobramycin	8 mg/L	4 mg/L	
Amikacin	25 mg/L	12 mg/L	
Cephalosporins			
Cefazolin	500 mg/L	125 mg/L	20 mg/kg
Cefepime	500 mg/L	125 mg/L	15 mg/kg
Cefotaxime	500 mg/L	250 mg/L	30 mg/kg
Ceftazidime	500 mg/L	125 mg/L	20 mg/kg
Glycopeptides[c]			
Vancomycin	1000 mg/L	25 mg/L	30 mg/kg; Repeat dosing 15 mg/kg q 3–5 days
Teicoplanin	400 mg/L	20 mg/L	15 mg/kg q 5–7 days
Penicillins[b]			
Ampicillin	—	125 mg/L	—
Quinolones			
Ciprofloxacin	50 mg/L	25 mg/L	—
Others			
Aztreonam	1000 mg/L	250 mg/L	—
Clindamycin	300 mg/L	150 mg/L	—
Imipenem/Cilastin	250 mg/L	50 mg/L	—
Oral			
Linezolid	<5 years.: 30 mg/kg/day divided TID; 5–11 years: 20 mg/kg/day divided BID; ≥12 years 600 mg/dose BID		
Metronidazole	30 mg/kg/day divided TID (max daily dose 1.2 g)		
Rifampin	10–20 mg/kg/day divided BID (max daily dose 600 mg)		
Antifungals			
Fluconazole	6–12 mg/kg IP, IV or PO q 24–48 h (max daily dose 400 mg)		
Caspofungin	IV only: initial dose 70 mg/m^2 on day 1 (max daily dose 70 mg); Subsequent dosing 50 mg/m^2 daily (max daily dose 50 mg)		

[a] For continuous therapy, the exchange with the loading dose of antibiotics should dwell for 3–6 h, followed by the use of the maintenance dose for all subsequent exchanges

[b] Aminoglycosides and penicillins should not be mixed in dialysis fluid because of the potential for inactivation

[c] Accelerated glycopeptide elimination may occur in patients with residual renal function. If intermittent therapy is used in this setting, the second dose of antibiotic should be time-based on a blood level obtained 2–4 days after the initial dose. Redosing should occur when the blood level is <15 mg/L for vancomycin, or 8 mg/L for teicoplanin. Intermittent therapy is not recommended for patients with residual renal function unless serum drug levels can be monitored in a timely manner

improved, empiric antibiotic therapy should be continued for 2 weeks with the exception of aminoglycosides, which should be discontinued after 72 h in culture-negative peritonitis [118].

General adjunctive measures include the reduction of the peritoneal fill volume during the initial 24–48 h of therapy in children with significant abdominal discomfort, and intraperitoneal administration of 500–1000 IU/L heparin until complete resolution of dialysate cloudiness [118].

Most children with PD-associated peritonitis achieve clinical improvement within two to three days following the initiation of antibiotic treatment [168, 185]. The initial treatment response is predictive of the functional recovery of PD and the risk of peritonitis relapse [142, 146]. Prolonged attempts to treat refractory peritonitis and to "save the catheter" should be avoided to minimize permanent injury to the peritoneal membrane [220]. In children who fail to respond clinically within 72 h of initiation of appropriate antibiotic therapy, repeat effluent cell count, differential and culture should be performed and potential sources of persistent infection should be sought. Treatment failure in peritonitis with *S. aureus* or *P. aeruginosa* points to a concomitant tunnel infection and requires catheter removal [118]. Treatment-resistant peritonitis with anaerobic bacteria or multiple gram-negative organisms is suspicious of intraperitoneal pathology (*e.g.*, ruptured appendix). Catheter removal is also recommended for any bacterial or culture-negative peritonitis that fails to resolve within 5 days of appropriate antibiotic treatment [118, 221, 222].

Ten to twenty percent of peritonitis episodes recur within 4 weeks of completion of antibiotic treatment with the same bacterial strain as indicated by identical antibiotic susceptibilities ('relapsing peritonitis') [146, 168, 185]. Repeated bouts of peritonitis are a risk factor for incomplete functional recovery and PD technique failure [146]. In relapsing peritonitis, empiric therapy should be reinitiated using an antibiotic combination covering the susceptibilities of the previous causative organism. Slime-forming bacteria can survive antibiotic therapy in a biofilm matrix or fibrinous adhesions on catheter surfaces. Accordingly, intraluminal fibrinolytic therapy may expose sequestered bacteria and render them susceptible to antibiotic activity. Local instillation of fibrinolytic agents (urokinase or recombinant tissue plasminogen activator), followed by instillation of high-dose antibiotics, has been shown to be efficacious in preventing further peritonitis relapses [223–225]. Hence, intraluminal fibrinolytic therapy should be considered in patients with a first peritonitis relapse which is not explained by extraluminal pathology such as a tunnel infection or an intraabdominal abscess. If a second relapse occurs, the catheter should be removed as soon as peritonitis is controlled by antibiotic therapy [118].

Fungal peritonitis is an infrequent but potentially serious complication of PD fraught with a high risk of PD technique failure and sometimes life-threatening, systemic infection [189, 190, 195]. Fungal infections represent 1–4% of all peritonitis episodes, although roughly 8% of peritonitis episodes reported to the SCOPE collaborative have been due to fungi [122, 185, 189, 190]. Treatment of fungal peritonitis consists of prompt catheter removal and appropriate antimycotic therapy [193, 226]. Fungi avidly grow on PD catheter surfaces, and resolution of infection is usually not possible as long as the catheter is in place. Fluconazole is the treatment of choice for most *Candida* species due to its excellent bioavailability and peritoneal penetration [227]. Alternative agents are echinocandins (e.g. caspofungin) for non-responding, non-albicans candida, and posaconazole or voriconazole for filamentous fungi such as Aspergillus [227]. Following catheter removal, effective antimycotic therapy should be administered for at least 2 weeks beyond complete resolution of clinical symptoms [118]. Reinitiation of PD following the treatment of fungal peritonitis in children has been successful [189].

Non-Infectious Complications

Non-infectious complications can result in significant morbidity, including the need to terminate PD [116, 228]. Non-infectious PD complications can be divided into catheter-related complications, and complications related to the dialysis procedure itself (Table 65.6) [229–231].

Table 65.6 Non-infectious complications of peritoneal dialysis [229–231]

Catheter related complications
  Obstruction/reduced inflow or outflow
    Migration of catheter out of pelvis
    Catheter kinking
    Catheter blockage
      Fibrin
      Blood clot
      Omentum
    Catheter compression
      Stool/Constipation
      Tumor or other intraabdominal mass
    Peri-Catheter leak
    Catheter cuff extrusion
Complications associated with the dialysis procedure
  Related to increased intraperitoneal pressure
    Subcutaneous leak
    Gastroesophageal reflux and delayed gastric emptying
    Abdominal and back pain
    Hernia
    Hydrothorax
  Related to transfer of solutes during dialysis (electrolyte and metabolic derangements)
    Hypokalemia
    Hypo/hypermagnesemia
    Hyperglycemia
    Hyperinsulinemia
    Hypertriglyceridemia
  Related to exposure of peritoneal membrane to dialysis fluid
    Membrane failure
    Pancreatitis
    Encapsulating peritoneal sclerosis

Catheter-Related Complications

Catheter-related complications include catheter malfunction, i.e. poor inflow and/or outflow, and leaks at the catheter exit-site. A recent analysis of data from the IPPN revealed a catheter revision rate of 1 per 83.2 patient-months, and the leading indication for revision was catheter malfunction, particularly in the first year after placement (Fig. 65.7) [116]. In that study, the need for access revision increased the risk of PD technique failure or death, and access dysfunction due to mechanical causes doubled the risk of technique failure compared with infectious causes [116]. The risk of access revision was associated with younger age, diagnosis of congenital anomalies of the kidney and urinary tract, coexisting ostomies, presence of a swan neck tunnel with curled intraperitoneal portion, and a high gross national income [116].

Catheter malfunction may be caused by obstruction from the omentum, kinking or migration of the catheter out of the pelvis, or blockage by fibrin or clots. Omentectomy at the time of catheter placement may reduce the risk of obstruction, and is practiced in most centers [133, 232, 233]. In practical terms, the omentectomy does not have to be complete. The remnant amount needs to be such that it cannot reach the distal catheter once it is positioned in the pelvis. However, one group of investigators, despite reporting a 20% decrease in the incidence of catheter blockage with omentectomy, calculated that eleven omentectomies would be required to prevent two omental PD catheter blockages. Therefore, the authors felt that nine patients would undergo an unnecessary omentectomy. In their hands, a secondary omentectomy was not difficult, resulting in their conclusion that omentectomies should only be carried out after a blockage occurs [232].

Migration of the catheter out of the pelvis can lead to poor dialysate inflow or outflow, as well as increased pain with dialysis. As mentioned previously, constipation is a risk factor for migration and should be monitored for and treated aggressively. Once migration has occurred, interventional radiology (IR) techniques may be used to reposition the catheter, with laparoscopic repositioning if IR repositioning fails [234]. For catheters that are occluded by fibrin or blood clot, installation of fibrinolytic agents can be very effective in restoring catheter flow [235–237].

Leaking of fluid from the peritoneal cavity through the PD catheter tunnel is a significant risk for the development of peritonitis. As previously discussed, delaying use of the PD catheter for routine dialysis for at least 14 days is advised to minimize the risk for leaks, and subsequent infection [115, 118]. The use of fibrin glue in the PD catheter tunnel has been reported to be both effective in treating established leaks and, when used at the time of catheter implantation, may help prevent the development of peritoneal leaks around catheters that are used soon after being placed [238, 239].

Fig. 65.7 Characterization of 452 access revisions by indication and time on peritoneal dialysis (PD) among children enrolled in the International Pediatric Peritoneal Dialysis Network (IPPN) Registry. ESI, exit site infection; tunnel inf, tunnel infection. (From [116], with permission)

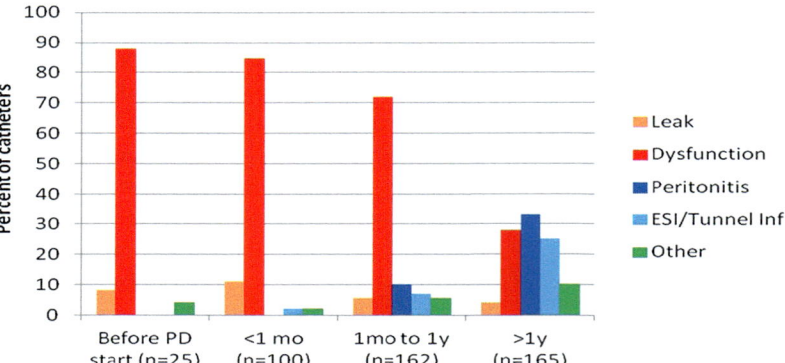

Hemoperitoneum, or blood in the dialysate effluent, is common immediately after PD catheter placement and typically clears with dialysis exchanges. Heparin may be added to the dialysate to reduce the risk of clotting within the PD catheter. Strictly speaking, most cases of hemoperitoneum beyond the post-implantation period are not a complication of PD *per se*, but rather diagnosed because of the ability to visualize peritoneal fluid during the dialysis procedure. A common benign cause of hemoperitoneum in female adolescents and young adult women is menstruation. Blood may appear a few days prior to menstruation and arise from shedding of intraperitoneal endometrial tissue if endometriosis is present, or from the uterus in a retrograde fashion through the fallopian tubes [230, 231]. Hemoperitoneum can also be seen at the time of ovulation. Other causes of hemoperitoneum include trauma, bleeding disorders, anticoagulation therapy, and rupture of a hepatic, ovarian or renal cyst. Finally, bleeding into the peritoneal cavity may be associated with intraperitoneal calcifications, which may occur as a consequence of chronic kidney disease bone and mineral metabolism disorder, or in the setting of encapsulating sclerosing peritonitis (see below) [231].

Complications Related to the Dialysis Procedure

Complications related to the dialysis procedure can be divided into those due to the increased intraperitoneal pressure that arises with instillation of dialysis fluid into the peritoneal cavity, those occurring as a consequence of the transfer of solute between plasma and dialysate during the dialysis exchange (i.e. metabolic or electrolyte derangements), and those that are either directly related to or exacerbated by exposure of the peritoneum and other intra-abdominal organs to dialysis fluid (Table 65.6) [230, 231].

Complications Related to Increased Intraperitoneal Pressure

Since the efficacy of the dialysis procedure is dependent on the area of the peritoneal membrane in contact with the dialysis fluid, increasing this contact area by increasing the fill volume is a therapeutic aim. However, an increase in the fill volume is associated with an increase in the intraperitoneal pressure (IPP) [35]. Elevated IPP can lead not only to patient discomfort and intolerance of the dialysis procedure, but may also increase the risk of dialysis leaks, gastroesophageal reflux, hernia formation and hydrothorax [10, 33, 34]. While leaks at the catheter exit-site occur most frequently around the time of catheter placement, more subtle leaks may occur well after the catheter exit-site has healed [240]. These leaks typically present with accumulation of fluid in the subcutaneous tissue, weight gain, and peripheral and/or genital edema, and often resolve with reduction in fill volume, avoiding a daytime fill, or temporary cessation of PD. Complaints of back or abdominal pain and gastroesophageal reflux may be eased by efforts to lower the IPP, including a reduction of the fill volume, particularly during the day.

As stated previously, hernias are common in children and their frequency is inversely related to age. Ideally, hernias are identified and repaired at the time of PD catheter placement [133, 134, 241]. Hernias may develop after PD is initiated at the sites of surgical incisions or areas of anatomic weakness such as the umbilicus or the linea alba. Small hernias may be followed with careful monitoring for incarceration, with efforts to reduce IPP as described above. However, many hernias in children ultimately require surgical repair.

Hydrothorax in the patient on PD occurs when an elevated IPP causes fluid to enter the pleural space by way of a pleuroperitoneal leak, presumably at the site of a diaphragmatic defect [242]. This defect is almost always on the right side; the presence of the heart and pericardium may limit leak of fluid across the left hemidiaphragm. Hydrothorax usually presents with shortness of breath and chest discomfort and must be differentiated from congestive heart failure. In addition, other causes of transudative pleural effusion, including volume overload, should be ruled out. Diagnosis is typically made by measuring glucose in the fluid obtained by way of thoracocentesis, with an elevated pleural fluid glucose relative to serum glucose verifying the peritoneal dialysate origin of the fluid [231, 242]. Confirmatory tests can include CT peritoneography or a technetium scan, followed by serial imaging [243]. First line treatment of hydrothorax is transient cessation of PD, which may allow closure of the diaphragmatic defect [244]. If conservative therapy fails, chemical pleurodesis with tetracycline, talc or autologous blood may be successful [244, 245]. Other therapeutic options include thoracoscopic pleurodesis, and thoracoscopic or open diaphragmatic repair [231, 244].

Complications Related to Transfer of Solutes During the Dialysis Procedure

The bidirectional transfer of solutes between the plasma in peritoneal capillaries and the dialysate in the peritoneal cavity is the therapeutic goal of the PD procedure. However, the transfer of solutes cannot be precisely controlled and so certain electrolyte and metabolic derangements should be anticipated. The most common of these is hypokalemia, the result of potassium losses into the potassium-free dialysis solution. Liberalization of dietary intake will typically restore normal potassium, but enteral supplementation may be required, particularly in infants or young children on low potassium formulas. The possible association between hypokalemia and the risk for peritonitis should prompt attention to and correction of this issue.

Hypermagnesemia is relatively common in children with kidney failure secondary to reduced kidney clearance of magnesium. Magnesium concentrations in commercially available dialysis solutions range from 0.25–0.75 mmol/L. Elevated serum magnesium levels are typically seen with use of solutions containing 0.75 mmol/L magnesium and high magnesium levels may contribute to adynamic bone disease [246–248]. On the other hand, use of solutions containing both 0.5 mmol/L and 0.25 mmol/L magnesium has been associated with hypomagnesemia in adults on PD [246]. Given the lack of data available on magnesium homeostasis in children on PD, current recommendations suggest choosing a solution that allows maintenance of a high normal serum magnesium, i.e. 0.9–1.0 mmol/L, in this population [43].

Hyperglycemia, hyperinsulinemia and dyslipidemia are present even in the early stages of kidney failure in children [249, 250]. These conditions persist or worsen on dialysis [251–253]. The pathophysiologic mechanisms contributing to disturbances in glucose and lipid metabolism seen in children with kidney failure are quite complex, and beyond the scope of this chapter. It is important to recognize, however, that in people on PD, exposure to glucose-containing dialysis solutions provides a substantial glucose load, which induces insulin resistance and an atherogenic lipid profile [38, 229, 254]. Thus, PD may contribute to the development of disturbances of glucose and lipid metabolism, or exacerbate them if already present. These findings reinforce recommendations to minimize exposure to glucose by using the lowest dialysate glucose concentration possible, with the addition of icodextrin if required to maintain euvolemia [9, 43]. The primary therapeutic approach for dyslipidemia is lifestyle modifications, including nutrition and dietary counseling to address obesity if present. Although several pharmacologic therapies for dyslipidemia are available, given the lack of data on safety and efficacy of these agents in children, KDIGO guidelines suggest that statins or statin/ezetimibe combinations not be initiated in children less than 18 years of age with kidney failure, including those on maintenance dialysis [255].

Complications Related to Exposure of Peritoneal Membrane to Dialysis Fluid

Peritoneal membrane failure, or the inability of the membrane to provide adequate removal of fluid and/or solutes, is an important complication of PD as it typically necessitates conversion to hemodialysis. International and national registry data suggest that 4.2–8% of the children on PD in these large cohorts required transfer to HD due to membrane failure, and the percentage is as high as 27% in smaller series [3, 116, 256]. Severe, persistent or recurrent peritonitis is a significant contributor to membrane failure, but as previously discussed, an increasing body of experimental evidence suggests that exposure of the peritoneal membrane to PD solutions, and high concentrations of glucose in particular, is a predominant contributor to progressive fibrosis [41, 57, 257].

Pancreatitis in people on PD may be caused by the same precipitating factors as in people who are not on PD, such as infection, medications, hypercalcemia and hyperlipidemia. However, irritation from the peritoneal dialysis fluid and/or PD catheter has also been reported as a cause of pancreatitis in people on PD [258]. The presenting symptoms of abdominal pain, emesis and cloudy dialysis effluent may mimic peritonitis, and thus the diagnosis can be missed. The diagnosis should be considered in people on PD with sterile peritonitis, particularly if their symptoms do not improve. Most episodes may be treated conservatively, although recurrence with reintroduction of dialysate into the abdomen may prompt at least the temporary cessation of PD [231].

Encapsulating peritoneal sclerosis (EPS) is a rare, but extremely serious complication of PD defined by the ISPD as 'a clinical syndrome continuously, intermittently or repeatedly presenting with symptoms of intestinal obstruction due to adhesions of a diffusely thickened peritoneum' [259]. EPS has been reported in 0.7–3.3% of adult cohorts, with a mortality rate of 35–69% [259–262]. A 10-year survey of 1472 children on PD revealed a similar prevalence of EPS at 1.5% or 8.7 cases per 1000 patient-years on PD, but a lower mortality rate with 3 deaths among 22 cases after a median follow-up of 4.8 years [263]. Non-PD related risk factors for the development of EPS include previous intra-abdominal surgery, beta-blockers, and cirrhosis with ascites [259]. Among people on PD, the cause of EPS is likely multifactorial, but recurrent infection and long term exposure to dialysate are thought to be the major contributors [259, 261, 264]. As in adults, data from children on PD reveal that increasing time on PD is associated with an increased risk for EPS [263, 265, 266]. Efforts to prevent EPS, therefore, have included pre-emptive transfer to hemodialysis in people who remain on PD for more than 8 years. Ongoing treatment with PD beyond this time period can be considered if the person on PD has a stable dialysate/plasma creatinine (D/P Cr) ratio based on PET, no evidence of high peritoneal transport capacity, no requirement for frequent use of hypertonic dialysis solution, normal or only intermittently elevated serum C-reactive protein level, absence of recurrent peritonitis and clinical stability defined as "good appetite and no signs of fluid overload." [265, 267].

People on PD with EPS typical present with symptoms of bowel obstruction, including abdominal pain, emesis, anorexia, abdominal mass, weight loss, ascites and hemoperitoneum, and EPS is almost universally associated with progressive loss of ultrafiltration [259]. The diagnosis is usually confirmed radiographically, with either ultrasound or CT demonstrating loculated/septated ascites, adherent bowel loops, peritoneal thickening, and peritoneal calcification. Treatment typically consists of transfer to HD and bowel rest with provision of parenteral nutrition [261, 264]. Treatment with several immunosuppressive agents, including prednisolone, sirolimus, mycophenolate mofetil, and tamoxifen, has been reported with variable success [259, 260, 268–271]. EPS can develop in patients on immunosuppression following kidney transplantation, calling into question the role of immunosuppression in this condition [264]. In adults with EPS, surgical intervention at specialized centers has shown improvement in symptoms and survival [272, 273]. Ongoing prospective efforts to monitor peritoneal membrane function and ultrastructural changes in people on PD should provide valuable information about the risk factors for developing EPS and ultimately strategies to minimize the risk for its development [71, 274].

References

1. Harambat J, van Stralen KJ, Kim JJ, Tizard EJ. Epidemiology of chronic kidney disease in children. Pediatr Nephrol (Berlin, Germany). 2012;27(3):363–73.
2. System USRD. 2018 USRDS Annual Data Report: Epidemiology of kidney disease in the United States. Bethesda, MD: National Institutes of Health, National Institute of Diabetes and Digestive and Kidney Diseases; 2018.
3. NAPRTCS 2011 Annual Dialysis Report 2011. https://naprtcs.org.
4. Mitsnefes MM, Laskin BL, Dahhou M, Zhang X, Foster BJ. Mortality risk among children initially treated with dialysis for end-stage kidney disease, 1990-2010. JAMA. 2013;309(18):1921–9.
5. Weaver DJ Jr, Somers MJG, Martz K, Mitsnefes MM. Clinical outcomes and survival in pediatric patients initiating chronic dialysis: a report of the NAPRTCS registry. Pediatr Nephrol (Berlin, Germany). 2017;32(12):2319–30.
6. Chesnaye NC, van Stralen KJ, Bonthuis M, Harambat J, Groothoff JW, Jager KJ. Survival in children requiring chronic renal replacement therapy. Pediatr Nephrol (Berlin, Germany). 2018;33(4):585–94.
7. Ku E, McCulloch CE, Ahearn P, Grimes BA, Mitsnefes MM. Trends in Cardiovascular Mortality Among a Cohort of Children and Young Adults Starting Dialysis in 1995 to 2015. JAMA Netw Open. 2020;3(9):e2016197.
8. Brown EA, Blake PG, Boudville N, Davies S, de Arteaga J, Dong J, et al. International Society for Peritoneal Dialysis practice recommendations: prescribing high-quality goal-directed peritoneal dialysis. Perit Dial Int. 2020;40(3):244–53.
9. Warady BA, Schaefer F, Bagga A, Cano F, McCulloch M, Yap HK, et al. Prescribing peritoneal dialysis for high-quality care in children. Perit Dial Int. 2020;40(3):333–40.
10. Fischbach M, Stefanidis CJ, Watson AR. Guidelines by an ad hoc European committee on adequacy of the paediatric peritoneal dialysis prescription. Nephrol Dial Transplant. 2002;17(3):380–5.
11. Rippe B. Peritoneal physiology. In: Gokal RC, editor. The textbook of peritoneal dialysis. Dordrecht: Kluwer Academic; 1994. p. 68–132.
12. Devuyst O, Rippe B. Water transport across the peritoneal membrane. Kidney Int. 2014;85(4):750–8.
13. Fischbach M, Haraldsson B, Helms P, Danner S, Laugel V, Terzic J. The peritoneal membrane: a dynamic dialysis membrane in children. Ad Perit Dial. 2003;19:265–8.
14. Davies SJ. Peritoneal solute transport--we know it is important, but what is it? Nephrol Dial Transplant. 2000;15(8):1120–3.
15. Schaefer B, Bartosova M, Macher-Goeppinger S, Ujszaszi A, Wallwiener M, Nyarangi-Dix J, et al. Quantitative Histomorphometry of the Healthy Peritoneum. Sci Rep. 2016;6:21344.
16. Rippe B, Rosengren BI, Venturoli D. The peritoneal microcirculation in peritoneal dialysis. Microcirculation (New York, NY : 1994). 2001;8(5):303–20.
17. Rippe B, Venturoli D. Simulations of osmotic ultrafiltration failure in CAPD using a serial three-pore membrane/fiber matrix model. Am J Physiol Renal Physiol. 2007;292(3):F1035–43.
18. Flessner MF. Peritoneal transport physiology: insights from basic research. J Am Soc Nephrol. 1991;2(2):122–35.
19. Rippe B. A three-pore model of peritoneal transport. Perit Dial Int. 1993;13(Suppl 2):S35–8.
20. Carlsson O, Nielsen S, el Zakaria R, Rippe B. In vivo inhibition of transcellular water channels (aquaporin-1) during acute peritoneal dialysis in rats. Am J Phys. 1996;271(6 Pt 2):H2254–62.
21. Ni J, Verbavatz JM, Rippe A, Boisdé I, Moulin P, Rippe B, et al. Aquaporin-1 plays an essential role in water permeability and ultrafiltration during peritoneal dialysis. Kidney Int. 2006;69(9):1518–25.
22. Ronco C, Brendolan A, La Greca G. The peritoneal dialysis system. Nephrol Dial Transplant. 1998;13(Suppl 6):94–9.
23. Fischbach M, Warady BA. Peritoneal dialysis prescription in children: bedside principles for optimal practice. Pediatr Nephrol (Berlin, Germany). 2009;24(9):1633–42; quiz 40, 42
24. Ronco C, Feriani M, Chiaramonte S, Brendolan A, Bragantini L, Conz P, et al. Pathophysiology of ultrafiltration in peritoneal dialysis. Perit Dial Int. 1990;10(2):119–26.
25. Asghar RB, Davies SJ. Pathways of fluid transport and reabsorption across the peritoneal membrane. Kidney Int. 2008;73(9):1048–53.

26. Fischbach M, Zaloszyc A, Schaefer B, Schmitt CP. Optimizing peritoneal dialysis prescription for volume control: the importance of varying dwell time and dwell volume. Pediatr Nephrol (Berlin, Germany). 2014;29(8):1321–7.

27. Chagnac A, Herskovitz P, Weinstein T, Elyashiv S, Hirsh J, Hammel I, et al. The peritoneal membrane in peritoneal dialysis patients: estimation of its functional surface area by applying stereologic methods to computerized tomography scans. J Am Soc Nephrol. 1999;10(2):342–6.

28. Fischbach M, Haraldsson B. Dynamic changes of the total pore area available for peritoneal exchange in children. J Am Soc Nephrol. 2001;12(7):1524–9.

29. Kohaut EC, Waldo FB, Benfield MR. The effect of changes in dialysate volume on glucose and urea equilibration. Perit Dial Int. 1994;14(3):236–9.

30. Gehan EA, George SL. Estimation of human body surface area from height and weight. Cancer Chemother Rep. 1970;54(4):225–35.

31. Fischbach M, Dheu C, Seugé-Dargnies L, Delobbe JF. Adequacy of peritoneal dialysis in children: consider the membrane for optimal prescription. Perit Dial Int. 2007;27(Suppl 2):S167–70.

32. Morgenstern BZ. Peritoneal equilibration in children. Perit Dial Int. 1996;16(Suppl 1):S532–9.

33. Durand PY, Balteau P, Chanliau J, Kessler M. Optimization of fill volumes in automated peritoneal dialysis. Perit Dial Int. 2000;20(Suppl 2):S83–8.

34. Fischbach M, Terzic J, Menouer S, Haraldsson B. Optimal volume prescription for children on peritoneal dialysis. Perit Dial Int. 2000;20(6):603–6.

35. Fischbach M, Terzic J, Laugel V, Escande B, Dangelser C, Helmstetter A. Measurement of hydrostatic intraperitoneal pressure: a useful tool for the improvement of dialysis dose prescription. Pediatr Nephrol (Berlin, Germany). 2003;18(10):976–80.

36. Fischbach M, Terzic J, Menouer S, Bergere V, Ferjani L, Haraldsson B. Impact of fill volume changes on peritoneal dialysis tolerance and effectiveness in children. Adv Perit Dial. 2000;16:321–3.

37. McIntyre CW. Update on peritoneal dialysis solutions. Kidney Int. 2007;71(6):486–90.

38. Delarue J, Maingourd C. Acute metabolic effects of dialysis fluids during CAPD. Am J Kidney Dis. 2001;37(1 Suppl 2):S103–7.

39. Bredie SJ, Bosch FH, Demacker PN, Stalenhoef AF, van Leusen R. Effects of peritoneal dialysis with an overnight icodextrin dwell on parameters of glucose and lipid metabolism. Perit Dial Int. 2001;21(3):275–81.

40. Witowski J, Jörres A, Korybalska K, Ksiazek K, Wisniewska-Elnur J, Bender TO, et al. Glucose degradation products in peritoneal dialysis fluids: do they harm? Kidney Int Suppl. 2003;84:S148–51.

41. Schaefer B, Bartosova M, Macher-Goeppinger S, Sallay P, Voros P, Ranchin B, et al. Neutral pH and low-glucose degradation product dialysis fluids induce major early alterations of the peritoneal membrane in children on peritoneal dialysis. Kidney Int. 2018;94(2):419–29.

42. Nakayama M, Kawaguchi Y, Yamada K, Hasegawa T, Takazoe K, Katoh N, et al. Immunohistochemical detection of advanced glycosylation end-products in the peritoneum and its possible pathophysiological role in CAPD. Kidney Int. 1997;51(1):182–6.

43. Schmitt CP, Bakkaloglu SA, Klaus G, Schroder C, Fischbach M. Solutions for peritoneal dialysis in children: recommendations by the European Pediatric Dialysis Working Group. Pediatr Nephrol (Berlin, Germany). 2011;26(7):1137–47.

44. Rusthoven E, Krediet RT, Willems HL, Monnens LA, Schröder CH. Sodium sieving in children. Perit Dial Int. 2005;25(Suppl 3):S141–2.

45. de Boer AW, Schroder CH, van Vliet R, Willems JL, Monnens LA. Clinical experience with icodextrin in children: ultrafiltration profiles and metabolism. Pediatr Nephrol (Berlin, Germany). 2000;15(1–2):21–4.

46. Michallat AC, Dheu C, Loichot C, Danner S, Fischbach M. Long daytime exchange in children on continuous cycling peritoneal dialysis: preservation of drained volume because of icodextrin use. Adv Perit Dial. 2005;21:195–9.

47. Venturoli D, Jeloka TK, Ersoy FF, Rippe B, Oreopoulos DG. The variability in ultrafiltration achieved with icodextrin, possibly explained. Perit Dial Int. 2009;29(4):415–21.

48. Akonur A, Holmes CJ, Leypoldt JK. Peritoneal residual volume induces variability of ultrafiltration with icodextrin. Perit Dial Int. 2014;34(1):95–9.

49. Canepa A, Verrina E, Perfumo F. Use of new peritoneal dialysis solutions in children. Kidney Int Suppl. 2008;108:S137–44.

50. Dart A, Feber J, Wong H, Filler G. Icodextrin reabsorption varies with age in children on automated peritoneal dialysis. Pediatr Nephrol (Berlin, Germany). 2005;20(5):683–5.

51. Rousso S, Banh TM, Ackerman S, Piva E, Licht C, Harvey EA. Impact of fill volume on ultrafiltration with icodextrin in children on chronic peritoneal dialysis. Pediatr Nephrol (Berlin, Germany). 2016;31(10):1673–9.

52. Canepa A, Perfumo F, Carrea A, Giallongo F, Verrina E, Cantaluppi A, et al. Long-term effect of amino-acid dialysis solution in children on continuous ambulatory peritoneal dialysis. Pediatr Nephrol (Berlin, Germany). 1991;5(2):215–9.

53. Hoff CM. In vitro biocompatibility performance of Physioneal. Kidney Int Suppl. 2003;88:S57–74.

54. Mactier RA, Sprosen TS, Gokal R, Williams PF, Lindbergh M, Naik RB, et al. Bicarbonate and bicarbonate/lactate peritoneal dialysis solutions for the treatment of infusion pain. Kidney Int. 1998;53(4):1061–7.

55. Plum J, Razeghi P, Lordnejad RM, Perniok A, Fleisch M, Fusshöller A, et al. Peritoneal dialysis fluids with a physiologic pH based on either lactate

or bicarbonate buffer-effects on human mesothelial cells. Am J Kidney Dis. 2001;38(4):867–75.

56. Ogata S, Naito T, Yorioka N, Kiribayashi K, Kuratsune M, Kohno N. Effect of lactate and bicarbonate on human peritoneal mesothelial cells, fibroblasts and vascular endothelial cells, and the role of basic fibroblast growth factor. Nephrol Dial Transplant. 2004;19(11):2831–7.

57. Bartosova M, Schaefer B, Vondrak K, Sallay P, Taylan C, Cerkauskiene R, et al. Peritoneal dialysis vintage and glucose exposure but not peritonitis episodes drive peritoneal membrane transformation during the first years of PD. Front Physiol. 2019;10:356.

58. Schmitt CP, Nau B, Gemulla G, Bonzel KE, Holtta T, Testa S, et al. Effect of the dialysis fluid buffer on peritoneal membrane function in children. Clin J Am Soc Nephrol. 2013;8(1):108–15.

59. Rees L, Azocar M, Borzych D, Watson AR, Buscher A, Edefonti A, et al. Growth in very young children undergoing chronic peritoneal dialysis. J Am Soc Nephrol. 2011;22(12):2303–12.

60. Htay H, Johnson DW, Wiggins KJ, Badve SV, Craig JC, Strippoli GF, et al. Biocompatible dialysis fluids for peritoneal dialysis. Cochrane Database of Syst Rev. 2018;10(10):Cd007554.

61. Borzych-Dużałka D, Schaefer F, Warady BA. Targeting optimal PD management in children: what have we learned from the IPPN registry? Pediatr Nephrol (Berlin, Germany). 2021;36(5):1053–63.

62. Kim DJ, Do JH, Huh W, Kim YG, Oh HY. Dissociation between clearances of small and middle molecules in incremental peritoneal dialysis. Perit Dial Int. 2001;21(5):462–6.

63. Chiu MC, Ng CF, Lee LP, Lai WM, Lau SC. Automated peritoneal dialysis in children and adolescents--benefits: a survey of patients and parents on health-related quality of life. Perit Dial Int. 2007;27(Suppl 2):S138–42.

64. Fischbach M, Schmitt CP, Shroff R, Zaloszyc A, Warady BA. Increasing sodium removal on peritoneal dialysis: applying dialysis mechanics to the peritoneal dialysis prescription. Kidney Int. 2016;89(4):761–6.

65. Clinical practice guidelines for peritoneal dialysis adequacy. Am J Kidney Dis. 2006;48:S98–S129.

66. Twardowski ZJ, Nolph KD, Khanna R, Prowant BF, Ryan LP, Moore HL, et al. Peritoneal equilibration test. Perit Dial Bull. 1987;7(3):138–47.

67. Twardowski ZJ, Prowant BF, Moore HL, Lou LC, White E, Farris K. Short peritoneal equilibration test: impact of preceding dwell time. Adv Perit Dial. 2003;19:53–8.

68. Smit W. Estimates of peritoneal membrane function--new insights. Nephrol Dial Transpl. 2006;21(Suppl 2):ii16–9.

69. Fischbach M, Lahlou A, Eyer D, Desprez P, Geisert J. Determination of individual ultrafiltration time (APEX) and purification phosphate time by peritoneal equilibration test: application to individual peritoneal dialysis modality prescription in children. Perit Dial Int. 1996;16(Suppl 1):S557–60.

70. Warady BA, Alexander SR, Hossli S, Vonesh E, Geary D, Watkins S, et al. Peritoneal membrane transport function in children receiving long-term dialysis. J Am Soc Nephrol. 1996;7(11):2385–91.

71. Schaefer F, Langenbeck D, Heckert KH, Schärer K, Mehls O. Evaluation of peritoneal solute transfer by the peritoneal equilibration test in children. Adv Perit Dial. 1992;8:410–5.

72. Warady BA, Jennings J. The short PET in pediatrics. Perit Dial Int. 2007;27(4):441–5.

73. Galach M, Antosiewicz S, Baczynski D, Wankowicz Z, Waniewski J. Sequential peritoneal equilibration test: a new method for assessment and modelling of peritoneal transport. Nephrol Dial Transplant. 2013;28(2):447–54.

74. La Milia V, Di Filippo S, Crepaldi M, Del Vecchio L, Dell'Oro C, Andrulli S, et al. Mini-peritoneal equilibration test: a simple and fast method to assess free water and small solute transport across the peritoneal membrane. Kidney Int. 2005;68(2):840–6.

75. Gruskin AB, Rosenblum H, Baluarte HJ, Morgenstern BZ, Polinsky MS, Perlman SA. Transperitoneal solute movement in children. Kidney Int Suppl. 1983;15:S95–100.

76. Geary DF, Harvey EA, Balfe JW. Mass transfer area coefficients in children. Perit Dial Int. 1994;14(1):30–3.

77. Verrina E, Amici G, Perfumo F, Trivelli A, Canepa A, Gusmano R. The use of the PD Adequest mathematical model in pediatric patients on chronic peritoneal dialysis. Perit Dial Int. 1998;18(3):322–8.

78. Warady BA, Watkins SL, Fivush BA, Andreoli SP, Salusky I, Kohaut EC, et al. Validation of PD Adequest 2.0 for pediatric dialysis patients. Pediatr Nephrol (Berlin, Germany). 2001;16(3):205–211.

79. Lo WK, Bargman JM, Burkart J, Krediet RT, Pollock C, Kawanishi H, et al. Guideline on targets for solute and fluid removal in adult patients on chronic peritoneal dialysis. Perit Dial Int. 2006;26(5):520–2.

80. Adequacy of dialysis and nutrition in continuous peritoneal dialysis: association with clinical outcomes. Canada-USA (CANUSA) Peritoneal Dialysis Study Group. J Am Soc Nephrol. 1996;7(2):198–207.

81. Maiorca R, Brunori G, Zubani R, Cancarini GC, Manili L, Camerini C, et al. Predictive value of dialysis adequacy and nutritional indices for mortality and morbidity in CAPD and HD patients. A longitudinal study. Nephrol Dial Transplant. 1995;10(12):2295–305.

82. Bargman JM, Thorpe KE, Churchill DN. Relative contribution of residual renal function and peritoneal clearance to adequacy of dialysis: a reanalysis of the CANUSA study. J Am Soc Nephrol. 2001;12(10):2158–62.

83. Paniagua R, Amato D, Vonesh E, Guo A, Mujais S. Health-related quality of life predicts outcomes but is not affected by peritoneal clearance: the ADEMEX trial. Kidney Int. 2005;67(3):1093–104.

84. Lo WK, Ho YW, Li CS, Wong KS, Chan TM, Yu AW, et al. Effect of Kt/V on survival and clinical outcome in CAPD patients in a randomized prospective study. Kidney Int. 2003;64(2):649–56.

85. Fried L, Hebah N, Finkelstein F, Piraino B. Association of Kt/V and creatinine clearance with outcomes in anuric peritoneal dialysis patients. Am J Kidney Dis. 2008;52(6):1122–30.

86. Schaefer F, Klaus G, Mehls O. Peritoneal transport properties and dialysis dose affect growth and nutritional status in children on chronic peritoneal dialysis. Mid-European Pediatric Peritoneal Dialysis Study Group. J Am Soc Nephrol. 1999;10(8):1786–92.

87. Bakkaloglu SA, Borzych D, Soo Ha I, Serdaroglu E, Büscher R, Salas P, et al. Cardiac geometry in children receiving chronic peritoneal dialysis: findings from the International Pediatric Peritoneal Dialysis Network (IPPN) registry. Clin J Am Soc Nephrol. 2011;6(8):1926–33.

88. Chadha V, Blowey DL, Warady BA. Is growth a valid outcome measure of dialysis clearance in children undergoing peritoneal dialysis? Perit Dial Int. 2001;21(Suppl 3):S179–84.

89. Morgenstern BZ, Mahoney DW, Warady BA. Estimating total body water in children on the basis of height and weight: a reevaluation of the formulas of Mellits and Cheek. J Am Soc Nephrol. 2002;13(7):1884–8.

90. Clinical Practice Guidelines for Peritoneal Adequacy, Update 2006. Am J Kidney Dis. 2006;48:S91–S7.

91. Boudville N, de Moraes TP. 2005 Guidelines on targets for solute and fluid removal in adults being treated with chronic peritoneal dialysis: 2019 Update of the literature and revision of recommendations. Perit Dial Int. 2020;40(3):254–60.

92. Chang TI, Kang EW, Lee YK, Shin SK. Higher peritoneal protein clearance as a risk factor for cardiovascular disease in peritoneal dialysis patient. PLoS One. 2013;8(2):e56223.

93. Guan JC, Bian W, Zhang XH, Shou ZF, Chen JH. Influence of peritoneal transport characteristics on nutritional status and clinical outcome in Chinese diabetic nephropathy patients on peritoneal dialysis. Chin Med J. 2015;128(7):859–64.

94. Lu YH, Hwang JC, Jiang MY, Wang CT. Comparison of the impact of "fast decline" in residual renal function and "initial anuria" on long-term outcomes in CAPD patients. Perit Dial Int. 2015;35(2):172–9.

95. Hu SL, Joshi P, Kaplan M, Lefkovitz J, Poenariu A, Dworkin LD, et al. Rapid change in residual renal function decline is associated with lower survival and worse residual renal function preservation in peritoneal dialysis patients. Perit Dial Int. 2017;37(4):477–81.

96. Pérez Fontán M, Remón Rodríguez C, da Cunha NM, Borràs Sans M, Rodríguez Suárez C, Quirós Ganga P, et al. Baseline residual kidney function and its ensuing rate of decline interact to predict mortality of peritoneal dialysis patients. PLoS One. 2016;11(7):e0158696.

97. Rumpsfeld M, McDonald SP, Johnson DW. Peritoneal small solute clearance is nonlinearly related to patient survival in the Australian and New Zealand peritoneal dialysis patient populations. Perit Dial Int. 2009;29(6):637–46.

98. Liao CT, Chen YM, Shiao CC, Hu FC, Huang JW, Kao TW, et al. Rate of decline of residual renal function is associated with all-cause mortality and technique failure in patients on long-term peritoneal dialysis. Nephrol Dial Transplant. 2009;24(9):2909–14.

99. Chan CT, Blankestijn PJ, Dember LM, Gallieni M, Harris DCH, Lok CE, et al. Dialysis initiation, modality choice, access, and prescription: conclusions from a Kidney Disease: Improving Global Outcomes (KDIGO) Controversies Conference. Kidney Int. 2019;96(1):37–47.

100. Schmitt CP, Borzych D, Nau B, Wühl E, Zurowska A, Schaefer F. Dialytic phosphate removal: a modifiable measure of dialysis efficacy in automated peritoneal dialysis. Perit Dial Int. 2009;29(4):465–71.

101. Borzych-Duzalka D, Bilginer Y, Ha IS, Bak M, Rees L, Cano F, et al. Management of anemia in children receiving chronic peritoneal dialysis. J Am Soc Nephrol. 2013;24(4):665–76.

102. Kramer AM, van Stralen KJ, Jager KJ, Schaefer F, Verrina E, Seeman T, et al. Demographics of blood pressure and hypertension in children on renal replacement therapy in Europe. Kidney Int. 2011;80(10):1092–8.

103. Mitsnefes MM, Daniels SR, Schwartz SM, Meyer RA, Khoury P, Strife CF. Severe left ventricular hypertrophy in pediatric dialysis: prevalence and predictors. Pediatr Nephrol (Berlin, Germany). 2000;14(10–11):898–902.

104. Mitsnefes M, Stablein D. Hypertension in pediatric patients on long-term dialysis: a report of the North American Pediatric Renal Transplant Cooperative Study (NAPRTCS). Am J Kidney Dis. 2005;45(2):309–15.

105. Clinical Practice Recommendations For Peritoneal Dialysis Adequacy. Am J Kidney Dis. 2006;48:S130–S58.

106. Chaudhuri A, Sutherland SM, Begin B, Salsbery K, McCabe L, Potter D, et al. Role of twenty-four-hour ambulatory blood pressure monitoring in children on dialysis. Clin J Am Soc Nephrol. 2011;6(4):870–6.

107. Frey SM, Vogt B, Simonetti GD, Büscher R, Habbig S, Schaefer F. Differential assessment of fluid compartments by bioimpedance in pediatric patients with kidney diseases. Pediatr Nephrol (Berlin, Germany). 2021;36(7):1843–50.

108. Wühl E, Fusch C, Schärer K, Mehls O, Schaefer F. Assessment of total body water in paediatric patients on dialysis. Nephrol Dial Transplant. 1996;11(1):75–80.

109. Edefonti A, Mastrangelo A, Paglialonga F. Assessment and monitoring of nutrition status in

pediatric peritoneal dialysis patients. Perit Dial Int. 2009;29(Suppl 2):S176–9.

110. Fischbach M, Issad B, Dubois V, Taamma R. The beneficial influence on the effectiveness of automated peritoneal dialysis of varying the dwell time (short/long) and fill volume (small/large): a randomized controlled trial. Perit Dial Int. 2011;31(4):450–8.

111. Fischbach M. Peritoneal dialysis prescription for neonates. Perit Dial Int. 1996;16(Suppl 1):S512–4.

112. Nakayama M, Kasai K, Imai H, Group TRMS. Novel low Na peritoneal dialysis solutions designed to optimize Na gap of effluent: kinetics of Na and water removal. Perit Dial Int. 2009;29(5):528–35.

113. Davies S, Carlsson O, Simonsen O, Johansson AC, Venturoli D, Ledebo I, et al. The effects of low-sodium peritoneal dialysis fluids on blood pressure, thirst and volume status. Nephrol Dial Transplant. 2009;24(5):1609–17.

114. Rutkowski B, Tam P, van der Sande FM, Vychytil A, Schwenger V, Himmele R, et al. Low-sodium versus standard-sodium peritoneal dialysis solution in hypertensive patients: a randomized controlled trial. Am J Kidney Dis. 2016;67(5):753–61.

115. Keswani M, Redpath Mahon AC, Richardson T, Rodean J, Couloures O, Martin A, et al. Risk factors for early onset peritonitis: the SCOPE collaborative. Pediatr Nephrol (Berlin, Germany). 2019;34(8):1387–94.

116. Borzych-Duzalka D, Aki TF, Azocar M, White C, Harvey E, Mir S, et al. Peritoneal dialysis access revision in children: causes, interventions, and outcomes. Clin J Am Soc Nephrol. 2017;12(1):105–12.

117. Crabtree JH, Shrestha BM, Chow KM, Figueiredo AE, Povlsen JV, Wilkie M, et al. Creating and maintaining optimal peritoneal dialysis access in the adult patient: 2019 update. Perit Dial Int. 2019;39(5):414–36.

118. Warady BA, Bakkaloglu S, Newland J, Cantwell M, Verrina E, Neu A, et al. Consensus guidelines for the prevention and treatment of catheter-related infections and peritonitis in pediatric patients receiving peritoneal dialysis: 2012 update. Peritoneal dialysis international: journal of the International Society for Peritoneal Dialysis. 2012;32 Suppl 2:S32–86.

119. Gokal R, Alexander S, Ash S, Chen TW, Danielson A, Holmes C, et al. Peritoneal catheters and exit-site practices toward optimum peritoneal access: 1998 update. (Official report from the International Society for Peritoneal Dialysis). Perit Dial Int. 1998;18(1):11–33.

120. Scalamogna A, De Vecchi A, Maccario M, Castelnovo C, Ponticelli C. Cuff-shaving procedure. A rescue treatment for exit-site infection unresponsive to medical therapy. Nephrol Dial Transplant. 1995;10(12):2325–7.

121. Yoshino A, Honda M, Ikeda M, Tsuchida S, Hataya H, Sakazume S, et al. Merit of the cuff-shaving procedure in children with chronic infection. Pediatr Nephrol (Berlin, Germany). 2004;19(11):1267–72.

122. Sethna CB, Bryant K, Munshi R, Warady BA, Richardson T, Lawlor J, et al. Risk factors for and outcomes of catheter-associated peritonitis in children: the SCOPE collaborative. Clin J Am Soc Nephrol. 2016;11(9):1590–6.

123. Gadallah MF, Mignone J, Torres C, Ramdeen G, Pervez A. The role of peritoneal dialysis catheter configuration in preventing catheter tip migration. Adv Perit Dial. 2000;16:47–50.

124. Lye WC, Kour NW, van der Straaten JC, Leong SO, Lee EJ. A prospective randomized comparison of the Swan neck, coiled, and straight Tenckhoff catheters in patients on CAPD. Perit Dial Int. 1996;16(Suppl 1):S333–5.

125. Chadha V, Jones LL, Ramirez ZD, Warady BA. Chest wall peritoneal dialysis catheter placement in infants with a colostomy. Adv Perit Dial. 2000;16:318–20.

126. Ta A, Saxena S, Badru F, Lee ASE, Fitzpatrick CM, Villalona GA. Laparoscopic peritoneal dialysis catheter placement with chest wall exit site for neonate with stoma. Perit Dial Int. 2019;39(5):405–8.

127. Warchol S, Ziolkowska H, Roszkowska-Blaim M. Exit-site infection in children on peritoneal dialysis: comparison of two types of peritoneal catheters. Perit Dial Int. 2003;23(2):169–73.

128. Flanigan M, Gokal R. Peritoneal catheters and exit-site practices toward optimum peritoneal access: a review of current developments. Perit Dial Int. 2005;25(2):132–9.

129. Hooman N, Esfahani ST, Mohkam M, Derakhshan A, Gheissari A, Vazirian S, et al. The outcome of Iranian children on continuous ambulatory peritoneal dialysis: the first report of Iranian National Registry. Arch Iran Med. 2009;12(1):24–8.

130. Stringel G, McBride W, Weiss R. Laparoscopic placement of peritoneal dialysis catheters in children. J Pediatr Surg. 2008;43(5):857–60.

131. Laakkonen H, Holtta T, Lonnqvist T, Holmberg C, Ronnholm K. Peritoneal dialysis in children under two years of age. Nephrol Dial Transplant. 2008;23(5):1747–53.

132. Lessin MS, Luks FI, Brem AS, Wesselhoeft CW Jr. Primary laparoscopic placement of peritoneal dialysis catheters in children and young adults. Surg Endosc. 1999;13(11):1165–7.

133. Conlin MJ, Tank ES. Minimizing surgical problems of peritoneal dialysis in children. J Urol. 1995;154(2 Pt 2):917–9.

134. Imani PD, Carpenter JL, Bell CS, Brandt ML, Braun MC, Swartz SJ. Peritoneal dialysis catheter outcomes in infants initiating peritoneal dialysis for end-stage renal disease. BMC Nephrol. 2018;19(1):231.

135. Popovich RP, Moncrief JW, Nolph KD. Continuous ambulatory peritoneal dialysis. Artif Organs. 1978;2(1):84–6.

136. Crabtree JH, Burchette RJ. Effective use of laparoscopy for long-term peritoneal dialysis access. Am J Surg. 2009;198(1):135–41.

137. Copeland DR, Blaszak RT, Tolleson JS, Saad DF, Jackson RJ, Smith SD, et al. Laparoscopic

Tenckhoff catheter placement in children using a securing suture in the pelvis: comparison to the open approach. J Pediatr Surg. 2008;43(12):2256–9.

138. Maio R, Figueiredo N, Costa P. Laparoscopic placement of Tenckhoff catheters for peritoneal dialysis: a safe, effective, and reproducible procedure. Perit Dial Int. 2008;28(2):170–3.

139. Chesnaye N, Bonthuis M, Schaefer F, Groothoff JW, Verrina E, Heaf JG, et al. Demographics of paediatric renal replacement therapy in Europe: a report of the ESPN/ERA-EDTA registry. Pediatr Nephrol (Berlin, Germany). 2014;29(12):2403–10.

140. Schaefer F, Borzych-Duzalka D, Azocar M, Munarriz RL, Sever L, Aksu N, et al. Impact of global economic disparities on practices and outcomes of chronic peritoneal dialysis in children: insights from the International Pediatric Peritoneal Dialysis Network Registry. Perit Dial Int. 2012;32(4):399–409.

141. Chesnaye NC, Schaefer F, Groothoff JW, Bonthuis M, Reusz G, Heaf JG, et al. Mortality risk in European children with end-stage renal disease on dialysis. Kidney Int. 2016;89(6):1355–62.

142. Zurowska A, Feneberg R, Warady BA, Zimmering M, Monteverde M, Testa S, et al. Gram-negative peritonitis in children undergoing long-term peritoneal dialysis. Am J Kidney Dis. 2008;51(3):455–62.

143. Sutherland SM, Alexander SR, Feneberg R, Schaefer F, Warady BA. For the International Pediatric Peritonitis R. Enterococcal peritonitis in children receiving chronic peritoneal dialysis. Nephrol Dial Transpl. 2010;25(12):4048–54.

144. Zaritsky JJ, Hanevold C, Quigley R, Richardson T, Wong C, Ehrlich J, et al. Epidemiology of peritonitis following maintenance peritoneal dialysis catheter placement during infancy: a report of the SCOPE collaborative. Pediatr Nephrol (Berlin, Germany). 2018;33(4):713–22.

145. Warchol S, Roszkowska-Blaim M, Sieniawska M. Swan neck presternal peritoneal dialysis catheter: five-year experience in children. Perit Dial Int. 1998;18(2):183–7.

146. Lane JC, Warady BA, Feneberg R, Majkowski NL, Watson AR, Fischbach M, et al. Relapsing peritonitis in children who undergo chronic peritoneal dialysis: a prospective study of the international pediatric peritonitis registry. Clini J Am Soc Nephrol. 2010;5(6):1041–6.

147. Swartz SJ, Neu A, Skversky Mason A, Richardson T, Rodean J, Lawlor J, et al. Exit site and tunnel infections in children on chronic peritoneal dialysis: findings from the standardizing care to improve outcomes in pediatric end stage renal disease (SCOPE) collaborative. Pediatr Nephrol (Berlin, Germany). 2018;33(6):1029–35.

148. Nessim SJ, Bargman JM, Jassal SV. Relationship between double-cuff versus single-cuff peritoneal dialysis catheters and risk of peritonitis. Nephrol Dial Transplant. 2010;25(7):2310–4.

149. Eklund BH, Honkanen EO, Kala AR, Kyllönen LE. Peritoneal dialysis access: prospective randomized comparison of the Swan neck and Tenckhoff catheters. Perit Dial Int. 1995;15(8):353–6.

150. Lo WK, Lui SL, Li FK, Choy BY, Lam MF, Tse KC, et al. A prospective randomized study on three different peritoneal dialysis catheters. Perit Dial Int. 2003;23(Suppl 2):S127–31.

151. Hagen SM, Lafranca JA, IJzermans JN, Dor FJ. A systematic review and meta-analysis of the influence of peritoneal dialysis catheter type on complication rate and catheter survival. Kidney Int. 2014;85(4):920–32.

152. Sardegna KM, Beck AM, Strife CF. Evaluation of perioperative antibiotics at the time of dialysis catheter placement. Pediatr Nephrol (Berlin, Germany). 1998;12(2):149–52.

153. Strippoli GF, Tong A, Johnson D, Schena FP, Craig JC. Antimicrobial agents to prevent peritonitis in peritoneal dialysis: a systematic review of randomized controlled trials. Am J Kidney Dis. 2004;44(4):591–603.

154. Li PK, Szeto CC, Piraino B, de Arteaga J, Fan S, Figueiredo AE, et al. ISPD peritonitis recommendations: 2016 update on prevention and treatment. Perit Dial Int. 2016;36(5):481–508.

155. Berns JS. Infection with antimicrobial-resistant microorganisms in dialysis patients. Semin Dial. 2003;16(1):30–7.

156. Prowant BF, Twardowski ZJ. Recommendations for exit care. Perit Dial Int. 1996;16(Suppl 3):S94–s9.

157. Prowant BF, Warady BA, Nolph KD. Peritoneal dialysis catheter exit-site care: results of an international survey. Perit Dial Int. 1993;13(2):149–54.

158. Twardowski ZJ, Prowant BF. Exit-site healing post catheter implantation. Perit Dial Int. 1996;16(Suppl 3):S51–s70.

159. Bernardini J, Price V, Figueiredo A. Peritoneal dialysis patient training, 2006. Perit Dial Int. 2006;26(6):625–32.

160. Bernardini J, Price V, Figueiredo A, Riemann A, Leung D. International survey of peritoneal dialysis training programs. Perit Dial Int. 2006;26(6):658–63.

161. Campbell DJ, Johnson DW, Mudge DW, Gallagher MP, Craig JC. Prevention of peritoneal dialysis-related infections. Nephrol Dial Transplant. 2015;30(9):1461–72.

162. Holloway M, Mujais S, Kandert M, Warady BA. Pediatric peritoneal dialysis training: characteristics and impact on peritonitis rates. Perit Dial Int. 2001;21(4):401–4.

163. Bender FH, Bernardini J, Piraino B. Prevention of infectious complications in peritoneal dialysis: best demonstrated practices. Kidney Int Suppl. 2006;103:S44–54.

164. Figueiredo AE, Moraes TP, Bernardini J, Poli-de-Figueiredo CE, Barretti P, Olandoski M, et al. Impact of patient training patterns on peritonitis rates in a large national cohort study. Nephrol Dial Transplant. 2015;30(1):137–42.

165. Figueiredo AE, Bernardini J, Bowes E, Hiramatsu M, Price V, Su C, et al. A syllabus for teaching peritoneal dialysis to patients and caregivers. Perit Dial Int. 2016;36(6):592–605.

166. Chang JH, Oh J, Park SK, Lee J, Kim SG, Kim SJ, et al. Frequent patient retraining at home reduces the risks of peritoneal dialysis-related infections: a randomised study. Sci Rep. 2018;8(1):12919.

167. Neu AM, Miller MR, Stuart J, Lawlor J, Richardson T, Martz K, et al. Design of the standardizing care to improve outcomes in pediatric end stage renal disease collaborative. Pediatr Nephrol (Berlin, Germany). 2014;29(9):1477–84.

168. Schaefer F, Klaus G, Muller-Wiefel DE, Mehls O. Intermittent versus continuous intraperitoneal glycopeptide/ceftazidime treatment in children with peritoneal dialysis-associated peritonitis. The Mid-European Pediatric Peritoneal Dialysis Study Group (MEPPS). J Am Soc Nephrol. 1999;10(1):136–45.

169. Neu AM, Richardson T, Lawlor J, Stuart J, Newland J, McAfee N, et al. Implementation of standardized follow-up care significantly reduces peritonitis in children on chronic peritoneal dialysis. Kidney Int. 2016;89(6):1346–54.

170. Neu AM, Richardson T, De Souza HG, Mahon AR, Keswani M, Zaritsky J, et al. Continued reduction in peritonitis rates in pediatric dialysis centers: results of the standardizing care to improve outcomes in pediatric end stage renal disease (SCOPE) collaborative. Pediatr Nephrol. 2021;36(8):2383–91.

171. Szeto CC, Li PK, Johnson DW, Bernardini J, Dong J, Figueiredo AE, et al. ISPD catheter-related infection recommendations: 2017 update. Perit Dial Int. 2017;37(2):141–54.

172. Schaefer F, Feneberg R, Aksu N, Donmez O, Sadikoglu B, Alexander SR, et al. Worldwide variation of dialysis-associated peritonitis in children. Kidney Int. 2007;72(11):1374–9.

173. Piraino B. Staphylococcus aureus infections in dialysis patients: focus on prevention. ASAIO J (American Society for Artificial Internal Organs : 1992). 2000;46(6):S13–7.

174. Blowey DL, Warady BA, McFarland KS. The treatment of Staphylococcus aureus nasal carriage in pediatric peritoneal dialysis patients. Adv Perit Dial. 1994;10:297–9.

175. Kingwatanakul P, Warady BA. Staphylococcus aureus nasal carriage in children receiving long-term peritoneal dialysis. Adv Perit Dial. 1997;13:281–4.

176. Gupta B, Bernardini J, Piraino B. Peritonitis associated with exit site and tunnel infections. Am J Kidney Dis. 1996;28(3):415–9.

177. Strippoli GF, Tong A, Johnson D, Schena FP, Craig JC. Catheter-related interventions to prevent peritonitis in peritoneal dialysis: a systematic review of randomized, controlled trials. J Am Soc Nephrol. 2004;15(10):2735–46.

178. Tacconelli E, Carmeli Y, Aizer A, Ferreira G, Foreman MG, D'Agata EM. Mupirocin prophylaxis to prevent Staphylococcus aureus infection in patients undergoing dialysis: a meta-analysis. Clin Infect Dis. 2003;37(12):1629–38.

179. Bernardini J, Piraino B, Holley J, Johnston JR, Lutes R. A randomized trial of Staphylococcus aureus prophylaxis in peritoneal dialysis patients: mupirocin calcium ointment 2% applied to the exit site versus cyclic oral rifampin. Am J Kidney Dis. 1996;27(5):695–700.

180. Chu KH, Choy WY, Cheung CC, Fung KS, Tang HL, Lee W, et al. A prospective study of the efficacy of local application of gentamicin versus mupirocin in the prevention of peritoneal dialysis catheter-related infections. Perit Dial Int. 2008;28(5):505–8.

181. Xu G, Tu W, Xu C. Mupirocin for preventing exit-site infection and peritonitis in patients undergoing peritoneal dialysis. Nephrol Dial Transplant. 2010;25(2):587–92.

182. Piraino B, Bernardini J, Florio T, Fried L. Staphylococcus aureus prophylaxis and trends in gram-negative infections in peritoneal dialysis patients. Perit Dial Int. 2003;23(5):456–9.

183. Kavitha E, Srikumar R. High-level mupirocin resistance in staphylococcus spp. among health care workers in a tertiary care hospital. Pharmacology. 2019;103(5–6):320–3.

184. Piraino B, Bernardini J, Brown E, Figueiredo A, Johnson DW, Lye WC, et al. ISPD position statement on reducing the risks of peritoneal dialysis-related infections. Perit Dial Int. 2011;31(6):614–30.

185. Warady BA, Feneberg R, Verrina E, Flynn JT, Muller-Wiefel DE, Besbas N, et al. Peritonitis in children who receive long-term peritoneal dialysis: a prospective evaluation of therapeutic guidelines. J Am Soc Nephrol. 2007;18(7):2172–9.

186. Warady BB-DDSF. World wide experience with peritonitis in children: a report from the international pediatric peritoneal dialysis network (IPPN). Perit Dial Int. 2019;39(Supplement 1):S10–S4.

187. Ramage IJ, Harvey E, Geary DF, Hebert D, Balfe JA, Balfe JW. Complications of gastrostomy feeding in children receiving peritoneal dialysis. Pediatr Nephrol (Berlin, Germany). 1999;13(3):249–52.

188. Murugasu B, Conley SB, Lemire JM, Portman RJ. Fungal peritonitis in children treated with peritoneal dialysis and gastrostomy feeding. Pediatr Nephrol (Berlin, Germany). 1991;5(5):620–1.

189. Warady BA, Bashir M, Donaldson LA. Fungal peritonitis in children receiving peritoneal dialysis: a report of the NAPRTCS. Kidney Int. 2000;58(1):384–9.

190. Munshi R, Sethna CB, Richardson T, Rodean J, Al-Akash S, Gupta S, et al. Fungal peritonitis in the standardizing care to improve outcomes in pediatric end stage renal disease (SCOPE) collaborative. Pediatr Nephrol (Berlin, Germany). 2018;33(5):873–80.

191. Ledermann SE, Spitz L, Moloney J, Rees L, Trompeter RS. Gastrostomy feeding in infants and children on peritoneal dialysis. Pediatr Nephrol (Berlin, Germany). 2002;17(4):246–50.

192. Chan EYH, Borzych-Duzalka D, Alparslan C, Harvey E, Munarriz RL, Runowski D, et al. Colostomy in children on chronic peritoneal dialysis. Pediatr Nephrol (Berlin, Germany). 2020;35(1):119–26.

193. Miles R, Hawley CM, McDonald SP, Brown FG, Rosman JB, Wiggins KJ, et al. Predictors and outcomes of fungal peritonitis in peritoneal dialysis patients. Kidney Int. 2009;76(6):622–8.

194. Wang AY, Yu AW, Li PK, Lam PK, Leung CB, Lai KN, et al. Factors predicting outcome of fungal peritonitis in peritoneal dialysis: analysis of a 9-year experience of fungal peritonitis in a single center. Am J Kidney Dis. 2000;36(6):1183–92.

195. Redpath Mahon AC, Richardson T, Neu AM, Warady BA. Factors associated with high-cost hospitalization for peritonitis in children receiving chronic peritoneal dialysis in the United States. Pediatr Nephrol (Berlin, Germany). 2019;34(6):1049–55.

196. Raaijmakers R, Schroder C, Monnens L, Cornelissen E, Warris A. Fungal peritonitis in children on peritoneal dialysis. Pediatr Nephrol (Berlin, Germany). 2007;22(2):288–93.

197. Michel C, Courdavault L, al Khayat R, Viron B, Roux P, Mignon F. Fungal peritonitis in patients on peritoneal dialysis. Am J Nephrol. 1994;14(2):113–20.

198. Goldie SJ, Kiernan-Tridle L, Torres C, Gorban-Brennan N, Dunne D, Kliger AS, et al. Fungal peritonitis in a large chronic peritoneal dialysis population: a report of 55 episodes. Am J Kidney Dis. 1996;28(1):86–91.

199. Bren A. Fungal peritonitis in patients on continuous ambulatory peritoneal dialysis. Eur J Clin Microbiol Infect Dis. 1998;17(12):839–43.

200. Prasad KN, Prasad N, Gupta A, Sharma RK, Verma AK, Ayyagari A. Fungal peritonitis in patients on continuous ambulatory peritoneal dialysis: a single centre Indian experience. J Infect. 2004;48(1):96–101.

201. Lo WK, Chan CY, Cheng SW, Poon JF, Chan DT, Cheng IK. A prospective randomized control study of oral nystatin prophylaxis for Candida peritonitis complicating continuous ambulatory peritoneal dialysis. Am J Kidney Dis. 1996;28(4):549–52.

202. Wadhwa NK, Suh H, Cabralda T. Antifungal prophylaxis for secondary fungal peritonitis in peritoneal dialysis patients. Adv Perit Dial. 1996;12:189–91.

203. Moreiras-Plaza M, Vello-Roman A, Samprom-Rodriguez M, Feijoo-Pineiro D. Ten years without fungal peritonitis: a single center's experience. Perit Dial Int. 2007;27(4):460–3.

204. Restrepo C, Chacon J, Manjarres G. Fungal peritonitis in peritoneal dialysis patients: successful prophylaxis with fluconazole, as demonstrated by prospective randomized control trial. Perit Dial Int. 2010;30(6):619–25.

205. Dajani AS, Taubert KA, Wilson W, Bolger AF, Bayer A, Ferrieri P, et al. Prevention of bacterial endocarditis: recommendations by the American Heart Association. J Am Dent Assoc (1939). 1997;128(8):1142–51.

206. Wilson W, Taubert KA, Gewitz M, Lockhart PB, Baddour LM, Levison M, et al. Prevention of infective endocarditis: guidelines from the American Heart Association: a guideline from the American Heart Association Rheumatic Fever, Endocarditis, and Kawasaki Disease Committee, Council on Cardiovascular Disease in the Young, and the Council on Clinical Cardiology, Council on Cardiovascular Surgery and Anesthesia, and the Quality of Care and Outcomes Research Interdisciplinary Working Group. Circulation. 2007;116(15):1736–54.

207. van Diepen AT, Tomlinson GA, Jassal SV. The association between exit site infection and subsequent peritonitis among peritoneal dialysis patients. Clin J Am Soc Nephrol. 2012;7(8):1266–71.

208. van Diepen AT, Jassal SV. A qualitative systematic review of the literature supporting a causal relationship between exit-site infection and subsequent peritonitis in patients with end-stage renal disease treated with peritoneal dialysis. Perit Dial Int. 2013;33(6):604–10.

209. Lloyd A, Tangri N, Shafer LA, Rigatto C, Perl J, Komenda P, et al. The risk of peritonitis after an exit site infection: a time-matched, case-control study. Nephrol Dial Transplant. 2013;28(7):1915–21.

210. Hoshii S, Wada N, Honda M. A survey of peritonitis and exit-site and/or tunnel infections in Japanese children on PD. Pediatr Nephrol (Berlin, Germany). 2006;21(6):828–34.

211. Vychytil A, Lorenz M, Schneider B, Hörl WH, Haag-Weber M. New criteria for management of catheter infections in peritoneal dialysis patients using ultrasonography. J Am Soc of Nephrol. 1998;9(2):290–6.

212. Kwan TH, Tong MK, Siu YP, Leung KT, Luk SH, Cheung YK. Ultrasonography in the management of exit site infections in peritoneal dialysis patients. Nephrology (Carlton, Vic). 2004;9(6):348–52.

213. Lee CC, Lee MT, Chen YS, Lee SH, Chen YS, Chen SC, et al. Risk of aortic dissection and aortic aneurysm in patients taking oral fluoroquinolone. JAMA Intern Med. 2015;175(11):1839–47.

214. Pasternak B, Inghammar M, Svanstrom H. Fluoroquinolone use and risk of aortic aneurysm and dissection: nationwide cohort study. BMJ (Clinical Research ed). 2018;360:k678.

215. Daneman N, Lu H, Redelmeier DA. Fluoroquinolones and collagen associated severe adverse events: a longitudinal cohort study. BMJ Open. 2015;5(11):e010077.

216. Lee CC, Lee MG, Hsieh R, Porta L, Lee WC, Lee SH, et al. Oral fluoroquinolone and the risk of aortic dissection. J Am Coll Cardiol. 2018;72(12):1369–78.

217. Macchini F, Testa S, Valadè A, Torricelli M, Leva E, Ardissino G, et al. Conservative surgical management of catheter infections in children on peritoneal dialysis. Pediatr Surg Int. 2009;25(8):703–7.

218. Piraino B, Bailie GR, Bernardini J, Boeschoten E, Gupta A, Holmes C, et al. Peritoneal dialysis-related infections recommendations: 2005 update. Perit Dial Int. 2005;25(2):107–31.

219. Davis TK, Bryant KA, Rodean J, Richardson T, Selvarangan R, Qin X, et al. Variability in culture-negative peritonitis rates in pediatric peritoneal dialysis programs in the United States. Clin J Am Soc Nephrol. 2021;16(2):233–40.

220. Piraino B. Peritoneal dialysis catheter replacement: "save the patient and not the catheter". Semin Dial. 2003;16(1):72–5.

221. Szeto CC, Chow KM, Wong TY, Leung CB, Wang AY, Lui SF, et al. Feasibility of resuming peritoneal dialysis after severe peritonitis and Tenckhoff catheter removal. J Am Soc Nephrol. 2002;13(4):1040–5.

222. Choi P, Nemati E, Banerjee A, Preston E, Levy J, Brown E. Peritoneal dialysis catheter removal for acute peritonitis: a retrospective analysis of factors associated with catheter removal and prolonged postoperative hospitalization. Am J Kidney Dis. 2004;43(1):103–11.

223. Williams AJ, Boletis I, Johnson BF, Raftery AT, Cohen GL, Moorhead PJ, et al. Tenckhoff catheter replacement or intraperitoneal urokinase: a randomised trial in the management of recurrent continuous ambulatory peritoneal dialysis (CAPD) peritonitis. Perit Dial Int. 1989;9(1):65–7.

224. Klaus G, Schafer F, Querfeld U, Soergel M, Wolf S, Mehls O. Treatment of relapsing peritonitis in pediatric patients on peritoneal dialysis. Adv Perit Dial. 1992;8:302–5.

225. Duch JM, Yee J. Successful use of recombinant tissue plasminogen activator in a patient with relapsing peritonitis. Am J Kidney Dis. 2001;37(1):149–53.

226. Robitaille P, Merouani A, Clermont MJ, Hebert E. Successful antifungal prophylaxis in chronic peritoneal dialysis: a pediatric experience. Perit Dial Int. 1995;15(1):77–9.

227. Matuszkiewicz-Rowinska J. Update on fungal peritonitis and its treatment. Perit Dial Int. 2009;29(Suppl 2):S161–5.

228. Rinaldi S, Sera F, Verrina E, Edefonti A, Gianoglio B, Perfumo F, et al. Chronic peritoneal dialysis catheters in children: a fifteen-year experience of the Italian Registry of Pediatric Chronic Peritoneal Dialysis. Perit Dial Int. 2004;24(5):481–6.

229. Bender FH. Avoiding harm in peritoneal dialysis patients. Adv Chronic Kidney Dis. 2012;19(3):171–8.

230. McCormick BB, Bargman JM. Noninfectious complications of peritoneal dialysis: implications for patient and technique survival. J Am Soc Nephrol. 2007;18(12):3023–5.

231. Saha TC, Singh H. Noninfectious complications of peritoneal dialysis. South Med J. 2007;100(1):54–8.

232. Lewis M, Webb N, Smith T, Roberts D. Routine omentectomy is not required in children undergoing chronic peritoneal dialysis. Adv Perit Dial. 1995;11:293–5.

233. Phan J, Stanford S, Zaritsky JJ, DeUgarte DA. Risk factors for morbidity and mortality in pediatric patients with peritoneal dialysis catheters. J Pediatr Surg. 2013;48(1):197–202.

234. Savader SJ, Lund G, Scheel PJ, Prescott C, Feeley N, Singh H, et al. Guide wire directed manipulation of malfunctioning peritoneal dialysis catheters: a critical analysis. J Vasc Intervent Radiol. 1997;8(6):957–63.

235. Shea M, Hmiel SP, Beck AM. Use of tissue plasminogen activator for thrombolysis in occluded peritoneal dialysis catheters in children. Adv Perit Dial. 2001;17:249–52.

236. Sakarcan A, Stallworth JR. Tissue plasminogen activator for occluded peritoneal dialysis catheter. Pediatr Nephrol (Berlin, Germany). 2002;17(3):155–6.

237. Krishnan RG, Moghal NE. Tissue plasminogen activator for blocked peritoneal dialysis catheters. Pediatr Nephrol (Berlin, Germany). 2006;21(2):300.

238. Sojo ET, Grosman MD, Monteverde ML, Bailez MM, Delgado N. Fibrin glue is useful in preventing early dialysate leakage in children on chronic peritoneal dialysis. Perit Dial Int. 2004;24(2):186–90.

239. Rusthoven E, van de Kar NA, Monnens LA, Schröder CH. Fibrin glue used successfully in peritoneal dialysis catheter leakage in children. Perit Dial Int. 2004;24(3):287–9.

240. Rahim KA, Seidel K, McDonald RA. Risk factors for catheter-related complications in pediatric peritoneal dialysis. Pediatr Nephrol (Berlin, Germany). 2004;19(9):1021–8.

241. Washburn KK, Currier H, Salter KJ, Brandt ML. Surgical technique for peritoneal dialysis catheter placement in the pediatric patient: a North American survey. Adv Perit Dial. 2004;20:218–21.

242. Leblanc M, Ouimet D, Pichette V. Dialysate leaks in peritoneal dialysis. Semin Dial. 2001;14(1):50–4.

243. Nishina M, Iwazaki M, Koizumi M, Masuda R, Kakuta T, Endoh M, et al. Case of peritoneal dialysis-related acute hydrothorax, which was successfully treated by thoracoscopic surgery, using collagen fleece. Tokai J Exp Clin Med. 2011;36(4):91–4.

244. Chow KM, Szeto CC, Li PK. Management options for hydrothorax complicating peritoneal dialysis. Semin Dial. 2003;16(5):389–94.

245. Bakkaloglu SA, Ekim M, Tumer N, Gungor A, Yilmaz S. Pleurodesis treatment with tetracycline in peritoneal dialysis-complicated hydrothorax. Pediatr Nephrol (Berlin, Germany). 1999;13(7):637–8.

246. Hutchinson AJ. Serum magnesium and end-stage renal disease. Perit Dial Int. 1997;17(4):327–9.

247. Wei M, Esbaei K, Bargman JM, Oreopoulos DG. Inverse correlation between serum magnesium and parathyroid hormone in peritoneal dialysis patients: a contributing factor to adynamic bone disease? Int Urol Nephrol. 2006;38(2):317–22.

248. Wei M, Esbaei K, Bargman J, Oreopoulos DG. Relationship between serum magnesium, parathyroid hormone, and vascular calcification in

patients on dialysis: a literature review. Perit Dial Int. 2006;26(3):366–73.

249. Saland JM, Pierce CB, Mitsnefes MM, Flynn JT, Goebel J, Kupferman JC, et al. Dyslipidemia in children with chronic kidney disease. Kidney Int. 2010;78(11):1154–63.

250. Wilson AC, Schneider MF, Cox C, Greenbaum LA, Saland J, White CT, et al. Prevalence and correlates of multiple cardiovascular risk factors in children with chronic kidney disease. Clin J Am Soc Nephrol. 2011;6(12):2759–65.

251. Mitsnefes MM. Cardiovascular disease in children with chronic kidney disease. J Am Soc Nephrol. 2012;23(4):578–85.

252. Bakkaloglu SA, Ekim M, Tumer N, Soylu K. The effect of CAPD on the lipid profile of pediatric patients. Perit Dial Int. 2000;20(5):568–71.

253. Bakkaloglu SA, Saygili A, Sever L, Noyan A, Akman S, Ekim M, et al. Assessment of cardiovascular risk in paediatric peritoneal dialysis patients: a Turkish Pediatric Peritoneal Dialysis Study Group (TUPEPD) report. Nephrol Dial Transplant. 2009;24(11):3525–32.

254. Burkart J. Metabolic consequences of peritoneal dialysis. Semin Dial. 2004;17(6):498–504.

255. Kidney Disease: Improving Global Outcomes Lipid Work G. KDIGO Clinical Practice Guideline for Lipid Management in Chronic Kidney Disease. Kidney Int Suppl. 2013;3(3):259–305.

256. Verrina E, Edefonti A, Gianoglio B, Rinaldi S, Sorino P, Zacchello G, et al. A multicenter experience on patient and technique survival in children on chronic dialysis. Pediatr Nephrol (Berlin, Germany). 2004;19(1):82–90.

257. Yoshino A, Honda M, Fukuda M, Araki Y, Hataya H, Sakazume S, et al. Changes in peritoneal equilibration test values during long-term peritoneal dialysis in peritonitis-free children. Perit Dial Int. 2001;21(2):180–5.

258. Flynn CT, Chandra PKG, Shadur CA. Recurrent pancreatitis in a patient on CAPD. Perit Dial Int. 1986;6(2):102.

259. Kawaguchi Y, Kawanishi H, Mujais S, Topley N, Oreopoulos DG. Encapsulating peritoneal sclerosis: definition, etiology, diagnosis, and treatment. International Society for Peritoneal Dialysis Ad Hoc Committee on Ultrafiltration Management in Peritoneal Dialysis. Perit Dial Int. 2000;20(Suppl 4):S43–55.

260. Kawanishi H, Kawaguchi Y, Fukui H, Hara S, Imada A, Kubo H, et al. Encapsulating peritoneal sclerosis in Japan: a prospective, controlled, multicenter study. Am J Kidney Dis. 2004;44(4):729–37.

261. Jagirdar RM, Bozikas A, Zarogiannis SG, Bartosova M, Schmitt CP, Liakopoulos V. Encapsulating peritoneal sclerosis: pathophysiology and current treatment options. Int J Mol Sci. 2019;20(22):5765.

262. Balasubramaniam G, Brown EA, Davenport A, Cairns H, Cooper B, Fan SL, et al. The Pan-Thames EPS study: treatment and outcomes of encapsulating peritoneal sclerosis. Nephrol Dial Transplant. 2009;24(10):3209–15.

263. Shroff R, Stefanidis CJ, Askiti V, Edefonti A, Testa S, Ekim M, et al. Encapsulating peritoneal sclerosis in children on chronic PD: a survey from the European Paediatric Dialysis Working Group. Nephrol Dial Transplant. 2013;28(7):1908–14.

264. Brown EA, Van Biesen W, Finkelstein FO, Hurst H, Johnson DW, Kawanishi H, et al. Length of time on peritoneal dialysis and encapsulating peritoneal sclerosis: position paper for ISPD. Perit Dial Int. 2009;29(6):595–600.

265. Honda M, Warady BA. Long-term peritoneal dialysis and encapsulating peritoneal sclerosis in children. Pediatr Nephrol (Berlin, Germany). 2010;25(1):75–81.

266. Hoshii S, Honda M. High incidence of encapsulating peritoneal sclerosis in pediatric patients on peritoneal dialysis longer than 10 years. Perit Dial Int. 2002;22(6):730–1.

267. Kawaguchi Y, Saito A, Kawanishi H, Nakayama M, Miyazaki M, Nakamoto H, et al. Recommendations on the management of encapsulating peritoneal sclerosis in Japan, 2005: diagnosis, predictive markers, treatment, and preventive measures. Perit Dial Int. 2005;25(Suppl 4):S83–95.

268. Summers AM, Clancy MJ, Syed F, Harwood N, Brenchley PE, Augustine T, et al. Single-center experience of encapsulating peritoneal sclerosis in patients on peritoneal dialysis for end-stage renal failure. Kidney Int. 2005;68(5):2381–8.

269. Kuriyama S, Tomonari H. Corticosteroid therapy in encapsulating peritoneal sclerosis. Nephrol Dial Transplant. 2001;16(6):1304–5.

270. Rajani R, Smyth J, Koffman CG, Abbs I, Goldsmith DJ. Differential Effect of sirolimus vs prednisolone in the treatment of sclerosing encapsulating peritonitis. Nephrol Dial Transplant. 2002;17(12):2278–80.

271. Lafrance JP, Letourneau I, Ouimet D, Bonnardeaux A, Leblanc M, Mathieu N, et al. Successful treatment of encapsulating peritoneal sclerosis with immunosuppressive therapy. Am J Kidney Dis. 2008;51(2):e7–10.

272. Latus J, Ulmer C, Fritz P, Rettenmaier B, Biegger D, Lang T, et al. Encapsulating peritoneal sclerosis: a rare, serious but potentially curable complication of peritoneal dialysis-experience of a referral centre in Germany. Nephrol Dial Transplant. 2013;28(4):1021–30.

273. Kawanishi H, Shintaku S, Moriishi M, Dohi K, Tsuchiya S. Seventeen years' experience of surgical options for encapsulating peritoneal sclerosis. Adv Perit Dial. 2011;27:53–8.

274. Korte MR, Boeschoten EW, Betjes MG, Registry EPS. The Dutch EPS Registry: increasing the knowledge of encapsulating peritoneal sclerosis. Neth J Med. 2009;67(8):359–62.

Management of Hemodialysis in Children

66

Daljit K. Hothi, Rukshana C. Shroff, and Benjamin Laskin

Abbreviations

AAMI	Association for the Advancement of Medical Instrumentation
ACE	Angiotensin converting enzyme
ARB	Angiotensin II receptor antagonists
BMI	Body mass index
BP	Blood pressure
BUN	Blood urea nitrogen
BVM	The Blood Volume Monitor ™
cIMT	Carotid intima-media thickness
CKD	Chronic kidney disease
CRP	C-reactive protein
DDS	Dialysis disequilibrium syndrome
DOPPS	Dialysis Outcomes and Practice Patterns Study
ECV	Extracellular volume
eKt/V	Equilibrated Kt/V
ESA	Erythropoiesis stimulating agent
ESKD	End-stage kidney disease
G	Urea generation rate
HD	hemodialysis
HDF	Hemodiafiltration
IVC	Inferior vena cava
IVC	Intracellular volume
K	Urea clearance
KDOQI	National Kidney Foundation Dialysis Outcomes Quality Initiative
KoA	Mass transfer coefficient of urea
K_{uf}	Ultrafiltration coefficient
LAVI	Left atrial volume indexed to height
L-carnitine	Levocarnitine
LMWH	Low molecular weight heparin
LV	Left ventricular
LVH	Left ventricular hypertrophy
NCDS	National Cooperative Dialysis Study
NIVM	Non-invasive blood volume monitoring
nPCR	Normalized protein catabolic rate
PTH	Parathyroid hormone
RBV	Relative blood volume
spKt/v	Single pool method
TAC-urea	Timed-average-concentration of urea
TBV	Total blood volume
TBW	Total body water
UF	Ultrafilter/ultrafiltration
UFH	Unfractionated heparin
URR	Urea reduction rate
USRDS	United States Renal Data System
V	Volume of distribution unless otherwise specified

D. K. Hothi (✉) · R. C. Shroff
Great Ormond Street Hospital for Children NHS Foundation Trust, London, UK
e-mail: Daljit.Hothi@gosh.nhs.uk; r.shroff@ucl.ac.uk

B. Laskin
Division of Nephrology, The Children's Hospital of Philadelphia, Philadelphia, PA, USA
e-mail: LaskinB@email.chop.edu

© The Author(s), under exclusive license to Springer Nature Switzerland AG 2023
F. Schaefer, L. A. Greenbaum (eds.), *Pediatric Kidney Disease*,
https://doi.org/10.1007/978-3-031-11665-0_66

Introduction

Hemodialysis (HD) was introduced as a treatment for uremia at the end of World War II [1]. A decade later, Mateer et al. reported the first experience using HD to treat five uremic adolescents using 15 meter cellophane tubing and a 32 liter dialysis bath. Each dialysis procedure was 13 h, and although the metabolic and fluid status of their patients improved, there were challenges related to anticoagulation of the circuit and achieving normal plasma calcium and potassium concentrations [2]. Maintenance HD was not practical because vascular access required cannulae placed in the radial artery and saphenous vein prior to each session. This problem was overcome by the development of silastic arteriovenous cannula by Scribner et al [3] which were inserted in the forearm vessels and could be used for repeated blood access. What followed was the report by Fine et al [4] describing the use of HD for maintenance treatment of end-stage kidney disease (ESKD) in five adolescents who were dialyzed three times weekly for 7–8 h per session using a concentrated dialysis solution mixed with tap water. A urea clearance of 45 ml/min resulted in a urea reduction rate (URR) of 48% during each 7–8 h treatment. While maintenance HD was now a realistic option for children with ESKD, technical difficulties persisted in small children and the need for 20 h of treatment per week required long periods of time in the hospital.

In 1971, Kjellstrand et al. reported their experience treating 10 children <15 kg [5]. Applying data from adults receiving dialysis, the authors recommended a urea clearance in children based on body weight, with a goal urea clearance of 2–3 ml/kg/min during each dialysis session. This clearance, multiplied by the number of hours of dialysis, allowed an accurate prediction of the expected fall in urea during a single HD session. This reduced the risk of disequilibrium syndrome from excessive reductions in urea and established a standard formula for dialysis urea clearance in children that is still used today.

Despite the initial success of the Scribner shunt, clotting and infection of the vascular access remained common. Arteriovenous fistulae reduced this problem and remain the gold standard for dialysis access. However, creation of fistulae in small children is technically challenging and requires surgical expertise and a critical mass of patients to maintain skills, which are not available in many pediatric centers [6]. These technical challenges, combined with the desire to avoid repeated needle punctures in small children, led Mahan et al. to use a Hickman central venous catheter for prolonged HD vascular access in children [7]. Central venous catheters have since become the most widely used HD access [8]. While allowing children to obtain puncture-free HD, catheters have a high rate of clotting, infection, and decreased blood flow and therefore should only be used for long-term access when creation of a suitable fistula or access to expert fistula teams is not possible.

Technological improvements over the last 50–60 years have made HD widely available for children with ESKD. While overall and cause-specific mortality have decreased for children initiating maintenance dialysis over the last several decades, children with ESKD continue to experience unacceptably high rates of morbidity and mortality compared to the healthy pediatric population [9]. Improvements in dialysis equipment, medications, and consensus treatment guidelines are likely responsible for better patient outcomes (Fig. 66.1) [9]. Today, children often receive less than half the weekly HD treatment time compared to when the therapy first became widely available, as described above [4]. To dramatically improve outcomes further may require a fundamental change to the "standard" thrice weekly HD prescription. Initial pediatric experiences using short daily or nocturnal HD dialysis and hemodiafiltration (HDF) have been very positive, although widespread application remains futuristic due to logistic and funding barriers in some countries.

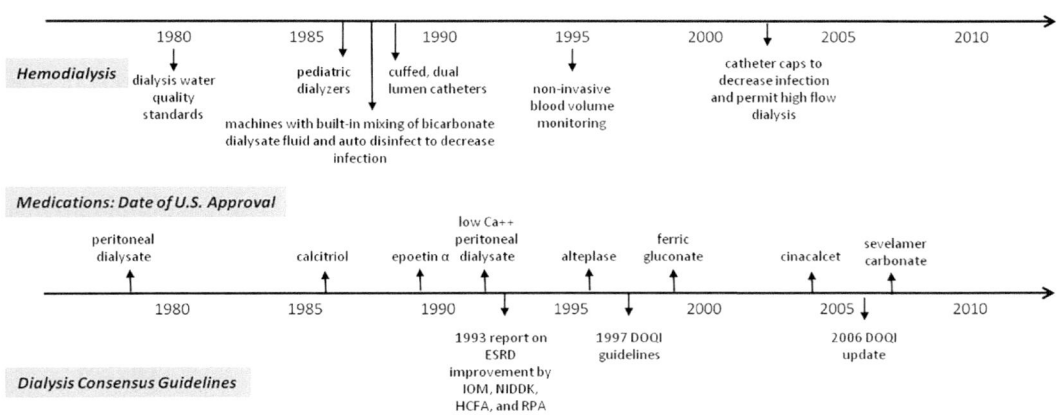

Fig. 66.1 Improvements in hemodialysis from 1980–2010

Prescribing Hemodialysis

Most of the HD literature reports on adults, with less data available in pediatric patients. In theory, the principles learned from adults are universal and applicable to children, but adjustments are required to accommodate the spectrum of age, weight, growth, and physiological development that are specific to children. Ideally, children should receive ESKD treatment at specialized pediatric centers with the necessary technical expertise, staffing, and multidisciplinary resources (physicians, nurses, psychologists, dieticians, social workers, teachers, and child-life specialists) to provide optimal care [10]. The two primary objectives of HD are to clear metabolic waste products and to UF excess fluid. To achieve these goals, the prescriber must calculate adequate clearance and estimate the patient's dry weight. To complete the HD prescription, one must then choose the blood flow rate, dialyzer, extracorporeal tubing, dialysate electrolyte composition and temperature, and anticoagulation.

Adequacy

The publication of the National Cooperative Dialysis Study (NCDS) in 1981 [11, 12] addressed how dialysis might best reduce patient morbidity and mortality by comparing four groups of patients with high or low timed-average-concentration of urea (TAC-urea) and with either long (4.5–5 h) or short (2.5–3.5 h) dialysis sessions. The results showed that the TAC-urea was the most important determinant of patient morbidity and hospitalization. In a subsequent analysis of the NCDS using a single-pool urea kinetic model, Gotch and Sargent argued for the use of Kt/Vurea to measure the adequacy of dialysis [13]. This unitless measure is an estimate of the clearance of urea from the blood during a dialysis session, standardized by total body water (which reflects the urea distribution volume). Kt/Vurea has become the standard measure of the delivered dialysis dose and the adequacy of dialysis.

Various methods for calculating Kt/V have been proposed. The single pool (spKt/V) method assumes urea is removed from a single pool and so a delayed postdialysis sample is not required. However, this method overestimates urea clearance because it ignores urea rebound postdialysis from access recirculation, cardiopulmonary recirculation, and tissue redistribution. Access recirculation becomes insignificant within 15–20 s of the blood flow being reduced to <50–80 ml/min. Cardiopulmonary recirculation only occurs with arteriovenous access and not with central lines. Cardiopulmonary recirculation is a result of blood returning to the dialyzer after circuiting the heart and lungs without passing through the other tissues and ceases 1–2 min after slowing blood flow. Conversely, urea tissue rebound continues over a longer time because there is diminished blood flow to muscle, which has high urea content, during dialysis [14]. Urea rebound is minimized by using either of the following two methods proposed by National Kidney Foundation Dialysis Outcomes Quality Initiative (KDOQI) guidelines [15]. With the slow blood flow method, the dialysate is turned off and the UF is minimized at the end of dialysis. The blood flow is then decreased to <100 ml/min for 15 s and then the urea sample is obtained. Using the stop dialysate method, the same protocol is used, except the blood flow is maintained at a normal rate for 3 min prior to drawing the postdialysis urea sample. Standardization is important, especially because different results for Kt/V have been shown in children depending on which day of the week laboratory studies are performed [16].

The double pool Kt/V recognizes that postdialysis rebound of plasma urea may be substantial. Therefore, a urea sample drawn 60 min postdialysis is required to avoid the overestimation of urea removal. This method is probably the most accurate estimate of Kt/V, but the need for a delayed postdialysis blood sample and lack of validation studies have limited its use.

Calculating Kt/V with urea kinetic modeling requires sophisticated computer algorithms which may not be available in many pediatric dialysis units. However, websites including Hypertension Dialysis and Clinical Nephrology (www.hdcn.com) and www.Kt-v.net provide programs for calculation of single and double pool Kt/V measurements, some of which have been used in pediatric studies [17]. The major advantage of kinetically modeled methods to estimate Kt/V is that they also provide an estimate of the urea generation rate from which the normalized protein catabolic rate (nPCR), an estimate of dietary protein intake, can be calculated. Nevertheless, several potential inaccuracies are intrinsic to the measurement of kinetically derived Kt/V. Urea clearance (K)

for individual dialyzers is derived from the manufacturer's specifications, which do not account for recirculation or reductions in dialyzer efficacy due to clotting of dialysis fibers or interruptions in treatment from kinked lines. Also, determining the urea distribution volume (V) may be imprecise, particularly in children [18].

To overcome these limitations, more simplified equations for calculating Kt/Vurea have been proposed [19]. One such formula [Kt/V = − Log n (R − 0.008 t) + (4–3.5 R) UF/BW] estimates the spKt/V where R is the ratio of the predialysis to postdialysis urea, t is the time of dialysis in hours, UF is the UF volume in liters, and BW is body weight in kg. This formula varies by only 6% from formal urea kinetic modeling in children [17]. To correct for postdialysis urea rebound, additional equations have been developed to calculate the equilibrated Kt/V (eKt/V) in patients with arteriovenous [eKt/V = spKt/V − (0.6 × spKt/V/T) + 0.03] or venovenous [eKt/V = spKt/V − (0.47 × spKt/V/T) + 0.02] access. Standardized (stdKt/V) formulas are available to estimate the Kt/V over a week, which are useful in patients regularly receiving more frequent or intensified dialysis regimens, or for those requiring occasional extra sessions for UF [18, 20].

Finally, the URR measures the percentage decrease in blood urea during a dialysis session. The URR as a marker of dialysis adequacy was evaluated retrospectively in 13,473 patients, and the mortality rate increased by 28% when URR values of <60% were obtained [21]. Despite its validation as a measure of morbidity, URR is not recommended as the primary measure of dialysis adequacy because significant variations of Kt/Vurea may be obtained with each URR value, particularly when URR is greater than 65%. Also, with increasing UF, URR underestimates urea removal. Nonetheless, targeting a URR of <50% for the first several treatments in a patient initiating chronic dialysis is a useful means of preventing dialysis disequilibrium. As no upper limit of Kt/Vurea has been established, care must be taken with aggressive treatment. Even in patients who have been on dialysis for a long time as excessive urea removal can lead to symptoms of dialysis disequilibrium.

KDOQI guidelines published in 2000 recommended that the delivered dose of HD in both adults and children should be measured using formal urea kinetic modeling with a spKt/V urea of at least 1.2. In 2002, the HEMO Study randomized 1846 patients on conventional thrice weekly HD to either a standard or high-dose of dialysis as well as to a low-flux or high-flux dialyzer. In high-dose patients, the URR was 75% and spKt/V 1.71, compared with standard-dose patients whose Kt/V was 1.32 with a URR of 66%. Neither dialysis dose nor dialyser flux affected the relative risk of death. The authors concluded that there was no major benefit from a higher dialysis dose than recommended by KDOQI or from the use of high-flux dialysis membranes [22].

However, dialysis dose may be associated with mortality in association with body mass index (BMI). In patients with lower BMI, a URR of >75% was associated with a lower risk of death compared to patients with a URR of 70–75% [23]. Daugirdas et al. found that by normalizing Kt/V to body surface area (BSA), most children less than 10 years of age would receive less dialysis compared to older patients, despite acceptable eKt/V and stdKt/V values [18]. Theoretically, it is tempting to postulate that there may be a survival advantage in increasing the HD dose in women and patients with a low BMI, such as children.

The Dialysis Outcomes and Practice Patterns Study (DOPPS) review of 22,000 adult HD patients from seven countries found that a higher dialysis dose, as reflected by a higher Kt/V, was important and an independent predictor of lower mortality. Survival was greatest when combining a higher Kt/V with a longer treatment time. For every 30 min longer on HD, the relative risk of mortality was reduced by 7% [24]. Reports from the Australian and New Zealand Dialysis and Transplant Registry and the United States support that longer treatment times, notably those >4–4.5 h, are associated with a lower risk of death, independent of adequate clearance [25, 26]. Such research establishes the basis for intensified dialysis programs (see below), namely a move away from conventional 3–4 h, three-times-per-week dialysis to more frequent and/or more prolonged dialysis sessions.

The KDOQI guidelines for HD adequacy were revised in 2005 to recommend a minimum spKt/V urea of 1.2 per session, with a target spKt/V of 1.4 and URR of 70%. These recommendations were consistent with the minimal Kt/V reported in the HEMO Study and also the European Guidelines for Hemodialysis, which endorsed a spKt/V of 1.4–1.5 [27]. However, no large scale studies have assessed HD adequacy in children. Buur and colleagues compared two urea kinetic models with direct quantification of urea removal and found that although each method produced different results, correlation between the methods was very high [28]. The authors commented that for practical purposes, and to limit blood sampling, one of the direct single-pool methods of urea kinetic modeling should be used. A study of 8 children <18 years of age compared an online urea monitor (UM 1000™, Baxter Healthcare) with single and double-pool formulas and separately with single-needle dialysis [29]. The study reported considerable differences in Kt/V urea between single and double pool formulae and concluded that online urea monitoring was inaccurate during single-needle dialysis.

Despite the limited data in children, expert working groups have developed guidelines for HD in children both in Europe and North America [10] together with European adult guidelines [27]. These are summarized in Table 66.1. We recommend maintaining a spKt/Vurea between 1.4–1.8 in children dialysed for 3–4 h per session. It is imperative that the prescribed dialysis dose for an individual child should be based on more than just an estimate of urea removal. Achieving optimal dialysis must also include a careful clinical assessment including growth, nutrition, cardiovascular health (especially blood pressure (BP)), anemia treatment, and the bone and mineral health of a developing child [30].

Table 66.1 Published guidelines for hemodialysis adequacy

Source	Urea Clearance	Other
KDOQI, adults	Minimum spKt/V $\approx$ 1.2target spKt/V $\approx$ 1.4	URR $\approx$ 65%URR $\approx$ 70%
European, adults	eKt/V > 1.2spKt/V $\approx$ 1.4	Double-pool urea kinetics preferred
KDOQI, children	spKt/V > 1.4	Assess nutrition (nPCR)optimize ultrafiltration
European, children	eKt/V $\geq$ 1.2–1.4	Assess nutrition (nPCR)monitor growth and cardiac function

Estimation of Dry Weight

UF is targeted to an estimated 'dry weight.' Dry weight is most commonly defined as the post-HD weight at which the patient is close to euvolemia without experiencing symptoms. Overestimation of the dry weight places patients at risk of developing volume-dependent hypertension, left ventricular hypertrophy (LVH), and congestive heart failure. An underestimation of the dry weight increases the risk of symptoms from intradialytic volume depletion. In children, growth and changes in lean body mass and body habitus necessitate regular and frequent re-evaluation of the dry weight to detect subtle differences in the ratio of total body water to body mass. This is especially important in infants and young children receiving HD for ESKD as they are growing rapidly, Therefore, tests for evaluating dry weight have to be easily accessible, reproducible, and ideally non-invasive.

The clinical examination is the most widely used test, but at best it only provides a crude assessment of volume status. In children with ESKD, even the most sensitive signs are rendered imprecise. For example, as dialysis patients have fluid removed there are a number of factors that can result in hypotension (cardiac dysfunction, low vascular tone, hypoalbuminemia, medications) and thus changes in orthostatic vital signs are not diagnostic of true hypovolemia. Jugular venous distension, though infrequently assessed in children, is a useful sign in the assessment of central venous pressure, provided heart failure is absent [31].

Biochemical markers including plasma atrial natriuretic peptide and brain natriuretic peptide correlate with increased plasma volume in ESKD [32], but levels can also remain elevated in volume contracted individuals and hence they lack the ability to detect volume depletion. Brain natriuretic peptide appears superior to atrial natriuretic peptide in predicting LVH and dysfunction. However, in the context of defining dry weight, results have been variable [33].

Ultrasound guided supine inferior vena cava (IVC) diameter measurement and its decrease on deep inspiration, better known as the collapse index (CI = end expiratory IVC diameter minus end inspiratory IVC diameter)/end expiratory IVC diameter), have been shown to correlate with right atrial pressure and circulating blood volume [34]. Results are influenced by wide interpatient variability, lack of validated normal values for children, the timing of the measurement in relation to dialysis, and the presence of heart failure or tricuspid regurgitation. As a result of these limitations, although it is a non-invasive test which could conceivably become available at most centers, it cannot reliably predict dry weight in children.

Bioelectrical impedance technology can directly assess extracellular volume (ECV), intracellular volume (ICV) and total body water (TBW) by detecting differences in the degree of resistance (impedance) as electric currents pass through each fluid compartment. At low frequencies, current cannot cross cell membranes and only flows through ECV; at higher frequencies it flows through both the ICV and ECV. Three methods for assessing dry weight using bioimpedance are available: (1) The normovolemia/hypervolemia slope method uses whole body multi-frequency bioimpedance spectroscopy to measure the ECV (Fig. 66.2) [35]; (2) The resistance-reactance graph method uses whole body single-frequency bioimpedance analysis to estimate TBW, but is unable to separate ECV from ICV, and therefore only useful when trying to

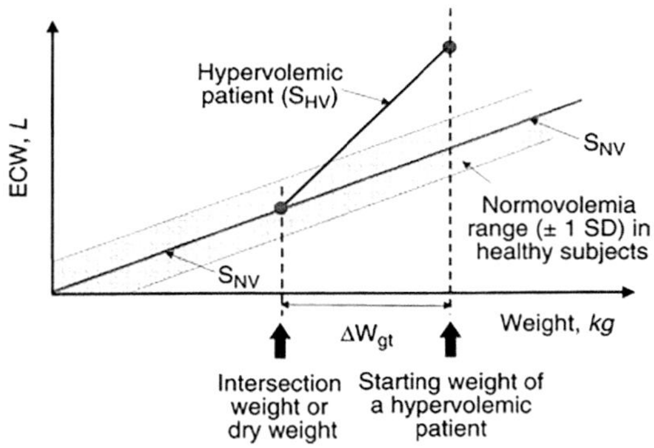

Fig. 66.2 Bioelectrical impedance to estimate dry weight using the normovolemia/hypervolemia slope method with whole body multi-frequency bioimpedance spectroscopy

differentiate between excessive body water and true weight gain [36]; (3) The continuous intradialytic calf bioimpedance method records changes in extracellular resistance in real-time, generating a curve whose slope flattens as excess ECV is removed, dry weight defined as flattening of the curve over a period of 20 minutes [37]. Premature flattening of the curve may occur in the presence of venous thrombosis or lymphatic edema. The value of bioimpedance techniques to estimate dry weight in pediatrics is unknown and limited by incomplete data in children and from patients with ESKD, and the inherent underestimation of TBW with multi-frequency bioimpedance methods. Importantly, changes in electrolyte, red cell, and protein concentrations and patient temperature are all known to influence bioimpedance. Bioimpedance may be used more frequently as increasing evidence from clinical studies validate its assessment of fluid status [38, 39].

Finally, on-line non-invasive blood volume monitoring (NIVM) is commonly used in clinical practice. NIVM provides information on intradialytic blood volume changes and vascular refilling rates. The magnitude of blood volume changes differs between patients and dialysis sessions, but if combined with post-dialytic vascular compartment refilling rates, dry weight can be assessed. Vascular refilling typically occurs in the first 10 min after stopping UF and is characterized by an increase in the relative blood volume (RBV), which can continue for up to 60 min. Steuer et al.

achieved a twofold reduction in intradialytic symptoms using NIVM in 6 hypotension prone adults, without reducing the UF volume or increasing treatment times [40]. Others have shown an increase in the UF potential, lowering of the dry weight, improved patient well-being and reduced hospitalization due to fluid overload.

NIVM is based on the principle of mass conservation: the concentration of measured blood constituents (hemoglobin/haematocrit/plasma protein) confined to the vascular space is proportional to changes in the vascular volume. Individual NIVM devices differ by their intrinsic sensing technique. Optical devices measure the absorbance of monochromatic light via an optoprobe in the arterial line to estimate the hematocrit because the optical density of whole blood is a measure of red blood cell concentration. The Crit-line™ (Fresenius) is a stand alone device, while the Hemoscan™ (Hospal-Dasco, Medolla, Italy) is a component of the dialysis machine. Blood density monitors are dependent on the total protein concentration (plasma protein concentration + mean cellular hemoglobin concentration). The Blood Volume Monitor™ (BVM, Fresenius AG, Bad Homburg, Germany) measures the velocity of sound through blood, as a reflection of blood density, by means of a cell inserted in the pre-pump segment of the arterial line. Schneditz et al. demonstrated a 2% difference in RBV changes between the Crit-line and BVM which developed 1 h into dialysis and persisted thereafter [41].

NIVM is used to divide patients into 4 groups. Group 1: Absence of postdialysis refilling with no symptoms suggestive of intradialytic hypovolemia or post-dialytic fatigue: the patient is likely to be at their dry weight. Group 2: Postdialysis refill, lack of a substantial change in blood volume during HD, and no intradialytic or post dialytic symptoms: indicative of extracellular fluid expansion and the need to lower the patient's dry weight. Group 3: Absence of postdialysis refill, intradialytic and/or post dialytic symptoms: indicative of hypovolemia and the need to increase the dry weight. Group 4: Postdialysis refill but intradialytic symptoms of hypovolaemia: indicative of slow vascular refilling rates, but ECV expansion at the end of dialysis. This suggests that the dry weight needs to be reduced incrementally and slowly following changes to the dialysis prescription to increase the UF potential. Extended duration of dialysis sessions may be necessary.

Information on blood volume status can be particularly helpful in the pediatric HD setting as the prevalence of intra- and interdialytic morbidity may be underestimated because children often do not verbalize early warning symptoms. Jain et al. show reduced dialysis associated morbidity with NIVM, with the greatest impact on children weighing less than 35 kg [42]. Michael observed improved targeting of the dry weight in children, which reduced the requirement for antihypertensive medication [43]. Using a constant dialysate sodium concentration of 140 mmol/L, Jain also defined a safe UF rate as an RBV change of <8% per hour in the first 90 mins and then <4% thereafter, with no more than a 12% net RBV change per dialysis session [42]. Hothi et al. reported in 11 pediatric HD patients that the gradient of the RBV curve in the first hour, as well as changes in heart rate, were the strongest predictors of treatment-related complications [44].

In summary, evaluating a patient's dry weight can be a challenge. The limitations and benefits of the available tests to estimate dry weight are summarized in Table 66.2. As of yet no gold stan-dard has been defined and for the majority, applicability in pediatrics has not been validated. We recommend the use of NIVM combined with clinical assessment. NIVM also offers the advantage of accurate assessment of the patient's hemoglobin, allowing for tracking of responses to changes in erythropoietin stimulating agent and iron administration. This is especially important in young children in whom frequent blood draws for lab testing can exacerbate anemia secondary to ESKD and blood loss from HD.

Blood Flow Rate

The blood flow rate is a major determinant of solute clearance on dialysis. With increased blood flow, more solute is delivered to the dialyzer, resulting in higher dialyser "flow limited clearance." However, clearance is also determined by the membrane's permeability to the solute, which is known as "membrane limited clearance." With poorly permeable solutes, increasing the blood flow will only produce a mild increase in clearance (Fig. 66.3). The dialyser flow clearance is limited and starts leveling off at blood flows of 250–300 ml/min, and therefore some adult dialy-

Table 66.2 Summary of Methods for Assessing Dry Weight [246]

Modality	Pros	Cons
Biochemical markers	-ease of use -noninvasive	-wide variability -poor correlation with volume depletion -not available at most laboratories -inaccurate in patients with congestive heart failure
Inferior vena cava diameter	-correlated with right heart pressure and intravascular volume -noninvasive	-no normative values for children -technician dependent -cost -limited availability -unclear which time after HD to measure
Bioimpedance	-measures ECFV and ICFV, estimating fluid shifts from various compartments -strong correlation with ultrafiltration volume	-limited normative values for children -unclear which time after HD to measure -cost -underestimates volume shifts from trunk
Non-invasive blood volume monitoring	-ease of use -ease of interpretation -decreases risk of intradialytic hypotension -validated use in children	-no standardization across devices -requires active intervention by providers -only measures fluid shifts from intravascular space and refilling rates Cost

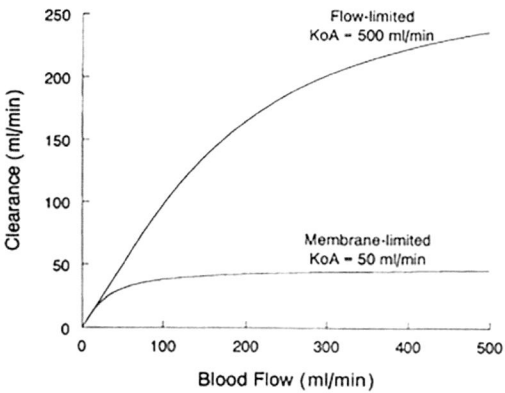

Fig. 66.3 Blood flow-limited and membrane-limited clearance

sis units have set this as their maximum blood flow rate.

The effective blood flow rate is largely determined by the vascular access, especially in pediatrics. For chronic HD we recommend a blood flow rate that is equivalent to 4–6 ml/kg/min urea clearance obtained from dialyser urea clearance estimates provided by the manufacturer. In infants, a minimum blood flow of 20–30 ml/min avoids the risk of clotting the circuit. Effective blood flows are often lower than those prescribed due to partially occlusive pumps, malposition of the vascular access needle, access failure, tubing diameter changes, and shear effects. The efficacy of dialysis is also reduced by recirculation effects, which are more pronounced with higher dialyzer blood flows, vascular access inflows lower than dialyzer blood flow, stenosis at the access outflow, single lumen access particularly with small stroke volumes, increased length of blood lines, and small needle and tubing diameter [45]. This places infants with blood flows determined by small, high resistance double-lumen central venous catheters or single lumen catheters with high recirculation rates at the highest risk of inadequate dialysis with conventional dialysis regimens. This can be improved by increasing the dialysis time, which in our experience is best tolerated by increasing the frequency and not the duration of treatment.

Choice of Dialyser

When selecting a dialyser for maintenance HD, several membrane characteristics need to be taken into consideration [10]. To improve efficacy, dialysers are designed to maximize the surface area available for diffusion. Two designs have predominated, namely hollow fibre and parallel plate dialysers. In the latter, parallel layers of membranes are separated by flat supporting structures. Their greatest disadvantage is their high compliance and thus large filling and priming volumes. Therefore, in children, they have largely been replaced by hollow fibre dialysers, which consist of a bundle of capillaries potted at both ends into a plastic tubular housing unit with sealing material. Hollow fibre dialysers have virtually no compliance and lower priming volumes, but the sealing materials are at risk of releasing solvents or ethylene oxide after gas sterilization, and thus producing anaphylactic reactions. As a general rule, the dialyser membrane surface area (which is readily available on the label of most dialysers) should be approximately equal to the patient's BSA. It is important to regularly assess the choice/size of the dialyser in growing children and those who are receiving inadequate dialysis.

Because the dialysis membrane is in direct contact with the patient's blood, it can initiate leucocyte and complement activation. The extent of the inflammatory response reflects the biocompatibility of the material that makes the dialyser. Three types of membranes are presently available, those made from unmodified cellulose, modified/regenerated cellulose, and synthetic membranes. Unmodified cellulose membranes, such as cuprophan, are relatively inexpensive but also the most bioincompatible. The modified cellulose membranes such as the cellulose acetate or hemophan® have some or all of the hydroxyl groups esterified to make them more biocompatible. However, such modifications may result in increased activation of the coagulation cascade and thus increase the anticoagulation requirement of the HD circuit. Synthetic membranes are made from polysulfone, polycarbonate, polyamide or polyacryl-polyamide acrylate. These membranes are relatively biocompatible, except for the negatively charged AN69 polyacrylonitrile membranes, which are known to cause hypotension, inflammatory hyperemia, oedema and pain secondary to a bradykinin mediated reactions. Dialysis patients most at risk are infants requiring blood to prime their HD circuit [46] and children that are concurrently taking angiotensin converting enzyme (ACE) inhibitors[47] or angiotensin II receptor antagonists (ARB) [48]. Synthetic membranes are generally more hydrophobic than cellulose membranes and therefore have higher adsorption properties [49]. Their increased ability to bind proteins may be partly responsible for their improved biocompatibility, and also makes them the membrane of choice for therapies such as albumin dialysis or in the treatment of acute toxicities where the undesired toxin is highly protein bound.

Membrane solute permeability refers to the clearance of middle molecular weight molecules, and is assessed by measuring the rate of β2-microglobulin clearance. Solute permeability is determined by the number of pores, the size of the pores, and the membrane wall thickness. A highly permeable membrane is one that is thin, with a high pore density and large diameter pores. Efficiency, represented as the KoA or mass transfer coefficient of urea, is a measure of urea clearance, a surrogate marker of small molecule clearance. Traditionally, membranes have been characterized as low-flux or high-flux according to their solute permeability. High-flux membranes are highly permeable membranes that can permit convective solute clearance of molecules weighing between 5000–25,000 Daltons, but urea clearance rates vary. Highly efficient membranes have high urea clearance rates but differ in their hydraulic permeability, and thus may be limited in their ability to clear middle molecules (Table 66.3).

A useful measure of the hydraulic permeability of a membrane is the K_{UF}, the UF coefficient, defined as the volume of UF produced per hour per mmHg transmembranous pressure, which is determined at a blood flow of 200 ml/min. K_{UF} is most directly influenced by the membrane's mean pore size. In turn, the mean pore size influences the solute sieving coefficient and molecular weight cut-off for a membrane. High-flux dialysers with larger mean pore sizes have a higher molecular weight cut-off and are most efficient in clearing larger uremic compounds. The UF rate and the dialyzer membrane's sieving coefficient are the most important determinants of convective solute removal [50]. Therefore, in consideration of predominantly convective therapies such as hemofiltration or HDF, high-flux dialysers are required.

Analyzing the United States Renal Data System (USRDS) database, Bloembergen et al. demonstrated a 20% decrease in the relative risk of death for modified cellulose and synthetic membranes compared with cellulose membranes [51]. In a retrospective analysis of 715 patients, Woods et al [52] compared mortality in a group treated exclusively with low-flux polysulfone dialysers with another treated for at least 3 months with high-flux polysulfone dialysers. The high-flux group had a significant 65% reduction in the risk of death compared with the low-flux group. A Kaplan-Meier analysis suggested a higher 5-year survival in the high-flux group, but a statistically significant difference was only seen after 4 years of dialysis.

In conclusion, epidemiological studies suggest improved morbidity and mortality in dialysis patients treated with modified cellulose or synthetic membranes but few have been able to demonstrate whether the effects were due to differences in flux, biocompatibility or middle

Table 66.3 Dialyser classification [247]

Class	Surface area	K_{UF} (ml/h/mmHg)	Urea clearance	β2 microglobulin clearance
Conventional	< 1.5 m²	< 12	Moderate	Negligible
High efficiency	> 1.5 m²	> 12	High (KoA > 600 ml/min)	Negligible
Mid-flux	Variable	12–30	Variable	Moderate
High-flux	Variable	> 30	Variable	High (>20 ml/min)

molecule clearance. Few, if any, paediatric centers practice dialyzer reuse. Reuse is associated with a reduction in the incidence of "first use" reactions, but may be associated with allergic reactions to residual sterilizing agents, such as formaldehyde. Inadequate sterilization of dialyzers may cause pyrogen reactions or frank infection, manifest by fever, chills and rigors [53].

Extracoporeal Circuit

Multiple dialysis machines are on the market, each with different sizes, weights, capabilities for home therapy, and interfaces with providers (reviewed in [54]). Regarding the extracorporeal circuit, during pediatric dialysis, if the total blood volume of the circuit is greater than 10% of the estimated total blood volume (TBV) a circuit prime with 5% albumin or blood is recommended. Even though traditionally blood has been preferred, these recommendations come from an era when severe anaemia was the rule for children with ESKD. However, minimizing exposure to blood products may decrease the risk of human leukocyte antigen sensitization in young children awaiting transplantation. The TBV is approximately equal to 100 ml/kg body weight in neonates and 80 ml/kg for infants and children. As a general rule, we use blood primes if the patient is anaemic. To avoid the risk of clotting the circuit, priming can be achieved with packed red blood cells diluted with normal saline or 5% albumin to achieve a final haemtocrit of 30–35%. Alternatively, the circuit can be primed with undiluted packed red blood cells from the blood bank when manipulation of the product is not permitted. The potassium load to the patient can be minimized by using fresh blood, and once priming is completed, recirculating the blood through the dialyser for 10 min, without connecting to the patient. At the end of dialysis, we do not recommend retransfusing the blood back into the infant, and if a blood transfusion is required, to give this during the dialysis session infused through a peripheral line or via a Y-connection at the venous return site to reduce the possibility of clotting the circuit.

Dialysate Water

Dialysate contaminants can be both chemical and biological, and can cause significant morbidity. It is therefore imperative that each dialysis unit ensures that disinfection practices are in place to achieve these standards, combined with regular surveillance to ensure that they are sustained. Dialysate quality is known to be an important component of the biocompatibility of the HD procedure and therefore also contributes to the chronic inflammation of dialysis [55]. In vitro studies have shown that bacterial products can cross both high-flux and low-flux dialysis membranes and stimulate synthesis of inflammatory mediators such as cytokines within the blood compartment [56]. The degree of cytokine stimulation is related to the concentration of endotoxin and other 'cytokine-inducing substances' in the dialysate compartment [57, 58] and the permeability of the dialysis membranes to these substances. In general, polysulfone and polyamide based membranes are effective barriers to endotoxins because of their high adsorptive properties [59] whereas high-flux membranes and low-flux cellulose based membranes are less protective [60, 61]. With an increasing use of high-flux membranes, especially with HDF therapy, a very high degree of water purity is essential (see section on 'backfiltration' below).

Water Purification Systems

A standard water treatment device consists of a water softener, an activated carbon filter, a sediment filter, and a reverse osmosis system [62]. Water softeners contain a resin that exchanges sodium cations for calcium, magnesium, and other polyvalent cations. Water softening not only prevents hard water, but also protects the reverse osmosis membrane used in the final step of water treatment from the build-up of scale and subsequent failure. The resin is regenerated periodically with concentrated sodium chloride solution, which also reduces bacterial growth in the resin bed. Activated carbon filters remove chloramines and organic solvents, but tend to release carbon particles and therefore require a sediment filter placed downstream. The final purification step is performed by reverse osmosis where the water is forced through a semipermeable polyamide or poly-sulfone membrane at 14–28 bar. This step removes 90–99% of inorganic and organic substances, pyrogens, bacteria, and particulate matter. The purified water is pumped from the reverse osmosis module to the individual treatment stations in a recirculating ring loop which delivers the water produced in excess back to the reverse osmosis module, avoiding wastage of high-quality water. The ring loops themselves require regular disinfection, and this is performed either by heat or chemical disinfection.

Testing Water Quality

The International Organization for Standardization (ISO) has published a series of standards addressing fluids for extracorporeal therapies. Specifically, ISO 11663:2009, Quality of dialysis fluid for hemodialysis and related therapies, requires that replacement fluid used for HDF be sterile and pyrogen-free; the currently accepted norms for ultrapure dialysate are defined as containing <0.1 colony-forming unit/ml and <0.03 endotoxin unit/ml. In addition, the chemical composition of water must be tested at least once per year [63].

Dialysate Composition

The composition of the dialysate fluid will influence the exchange of electrolytes during the dialysis treatment and thus ultimately creates an opportunity to modify adverse events during dialysis and the net transfer of electrolytes to or from the patient.

Sodium

Following a sodium load, even in the presence of renal failure, the mechanisms responsible for preserving plasma tonicity will maintain plasma sodium within narrow limits by changing the plasma volume. During HD, dialysate sodium generates a crystalloid osmotic pressure and thus influences fluid shift between the different body compartments, but it also permeates the dialysis membrane and thus has the potential for becoming a sodium load.

Diffusive sodium transport is proportional to the difference in sodium activity between blood and dialysate compartments. Dialysate sodium activity is approximately 97% of the measured sodium concentration, but varies with changes in dialysate temperature, pH, and the presence of additional ions. The proportion of plasma water free sodium ions that are unbound to protein and other anions can be measured by direct ionemetry. Plasma sodium activity is influenced by the Donnan effect: negatively charged proteins (mainly albumin) produce a small electrical potential difference across the membrane (negative on the plasma side) that prevents movement of the positively charged sodium ions. In the absence of UF, the concentration of dialysate sodium needed to achieve isotonic dialysis can be approximated by correcting the blood sodium measured by direct ionometry for a Donnan factor of 0.967.

Hyponatremic dialysis causes osmotic fluid shift from the extracellular to intracellular compartment, contributing to dialysis disequilibrium and intradialytic hypotension. Hypernatremic dialysis transfers sodium to the patient, causing interstitial edema, interdialytic thirst, increased interdialytic weight gain and worsening hypertension. A therapeutic advantage can be gained by manipulating the dialysate sodium concentration throughout dialysis, known as sodium profiling, and typically utilizes a sodium concentration that falls in a step, linear, or exponential fashion (Fig. 66.4). The higher dialysate sodium at the start allows a diffusive sodium influx to counterbalance the rapid decline in plasma osmolarity due to clearance of urea and other small molecular weight solutes. Low dialysate sodium at the end aids diffusive clearance of the sodium load and minimizes hypertonicity. Compared with a constant dialysate sodium bath, profiling has been shown to increase stability of intradialytic blood volume and reduce both intradialytic cramps and interdialytic fatigue in children and adults [64,

Fig. 66.4 Sodium profiling options

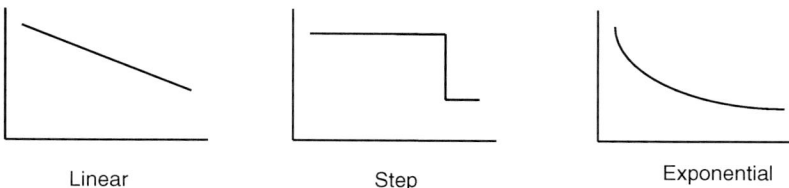

Linear   Step   Exponential

65]. Compared with exponential profiles, step profiles are most effective at attenuating postdialytic hypotension and early intradialytic hypotension, while linear profiles best reduce cramps and late intradialytic hypotension. Sodium profiling is also indicated in the prevention of dialysis dysequilibrium.

The difficulty with sodium profiling is finding the concentration gradient that offers the benefits of cardiovascular stability without exposing the patient to a small but repeated sodium load. A net sodium gain of 1 mmol/L will result in a 1.3% expansion of the extracellular space. Based on concerns of inducing hypervolemia, neutral sodium balance profiles may be preferred. Protocols of isonatremic dialysate are similar, with time averaged dialysate sodium 2–3 mmol/L lower (Donnan effect) than the predialysis sodium [66]. Results indicate benefits similar to those described with sodium profiling, but with a significant decrease in the interdialytic weight gain and thirst score [67, 68]. The difference is likely to be due to an improvement in sodium balance, but as neutral balance is unlikely even with the 'isonatraemic' protocols we recommend monitoring for changes in interdialytic weight gain and BP.

Potassium

One of the key objectives of HD is to maintain the plasma potassium levels within a narrow normal range, both during the intradialytic and interdialytic periods. The risk of arrhythmia, QT dispersion [69] and ventricular ectopic beats is increased with hypokalemia and also if the rate of decline is rapid early in dialysis, even if the actual plasma potassium levels are normal. This is one of the postulated mechanisms for the phenomenon of sudden cardiac death in HD patients. Conversely, failure to normalize serum potassium levels is also arrhythmogenic [70].

The challenge is that HD can only remove potassium from the extracellular compartment and that comprises 2% of total body potassium. In addition net potassium removed is influenced by a number of dialysis related factors. During HD, approximately 85% of potassium is removed by diffusion and this is influenced by the serum:dialysate potassium gradient. The rate of potassium removal is highest in the first hour of dialysis and then declines as the serum:dialysate potassium gradient falls. Therefore the greatest fall in plasma potassium levels are in the first hour, with a more gradual reduction in the subsequent 2 h, and almost no change in the plasma potassium level in the fourth and fifth hours as the serum:dialysate concentrations reach equilibrium. Postdialysis the plasma potassium rebounds and again the serum:dialysate gradient appears to influence the magnitude of this rebound, with a rapid postdialysis rebound of potassium levels with higher gradients compared with smaller gradients [71]. Convective clearance of potassium by UF accounts for approximately 6% of the total potassium mass removed. The glucose content of dialysate solutions is important with high glucose–containing dialysate solutions resulting in higher potassium removal as a result of osmotic shifts of intracellular potassium to the extracellular space [72]. The other major factor is the dialysate bicarbonate. Higher dialysate bicarbonate concentrations result in a rise in serum bicarbonate levels during HD, enhancing Na^+/K^+-ATPase activity with a larger shift of potassium into the intracellular space and a lowering of serum potassium levels, but total body potassium removal is not improved [73].

Optimizing the management of potassium removal in patients on HD involves reducing large intradialytic potassium shifts as well as providing adequate potassium removal to minimize hyperkalemia. However, there is no consensus on how best to achieve this. As a general rule, we would recommend dialyzing children against a potassium bath of 2 mmol/L. If patients are hyperkalemic and asymptomatic, use a 1 mmol/L potassium bath for the first 1–2 h of dialysis, and then switch to 2 mmol/L for the second half of dialysis. We discourage the use of zero potassium dialysate solutions unless the patient is severely hyperkalemic and symptomatic. If predialysis serum potassium levels are low or low normal, a potassium bath of 3–4 mmol/L may be required.

Bicarbonate

Acetate was originally used as the buffer in dialysate as it was inexpensive, offered equimolar conversion to bicarbonate, and was bacteriostatic. However, 10% of patients, especially women, are poor metabolizers of acetate. The high plasma acetate levels led to impaired lipid and ketone bodies metabolism, vasodilatation, depressed left ventricular function, intradialytic hypotension, and hypoxaemia, particularly in the first hour [74]. Consequently, most centers switched to sodium bicarbonate.

The preparation of bicarbonate based dialysate requires a second proportioning pump that mixes solution or dry powder bicarbonate to water, and an 'acid' compartment containing a small amount of acetate or lactate, sodium, potassium, calcium, magnesium, chloride and glucose. During the mixing procedure, the acid in the acid concentrate reacts with an equimolar amount of bicarbonate to generate carbonic acid and carbon dioxide. The generation of carbon dioxide causes the final solution pH to fall to approximately 7–7.4. It is this lower pH, combined with the lower concentrations of calcium and magnesium that prevents precipitation from occurring in the final solution. Cartridge systems containing pure,

dry sodium bicarbonate powder are often preferred as they are less conducive to bacterial growth, and liquid bicarbonate has to be used within 8 h of opening the container to avoid significant bicarbonate loss.

Dialysis aims to correct the metabolic acidosis of ESKD by the removal of organic anions and restoration of the bicarbonate deficit. Plasma bicarbonate levels rise by 4–5 mmol/L and then fall to predialysis levels by 48 h. The adjusted survival of HD patients decreases with predialysis serum bicarbonate levels <18 mmol/L and >24 mmol/L [11], suggesting a "U" shaped correlation with mortality. The severity of metabolic acidosis also correlates with bone disease [75], muscle wasting [76], and ß2-microglobulin levels [77]. With standard dialysate bicarbonate concentrations of 35 mmol/L, the HEMO study showed that 25% of patients had predialysis levels below 19 mmol/L. [78] Increasing the dialysate bicarbonate concentration to 39–40 mmol/L will improve the predialysis bicarbonate levels but in some will result in a transient alkalosis. This has a hypothetical risk of facilitating calcific uremic arteriolopathy, reducing phosphate removal because of shift of phosphate into cells, and intradialytic vascular instability by causing a sudden drop in the plasma potassium and calcium levels.

Alkalosis has been shown to rapidly reduce dangerously high serum potassium levels, albeit with a potentially increased postdialysis rebound effect [79]. Finally on a more experimental level, the use of citric acid in place of acetic acid in the dialysate acid concentrate was shown to improve both acidosis and delivered dose of dialysis [80]. The role for citrate is expanding in the dialysis community; however, caution is advised as it increases aluminum absorption and therefore plasma aluminum levels must be monitored.

Calcium

Owing to fear of inducing extra-skeletal calcium deposition, KDOQI guidelines suggest maintaining plasma calcium levels in the low normal range. Using a dialysate calcium concentration of 1.25 mmol/L permits higher doses of vitamin D and calcium based phosphate binders in the management of hyperparathyroidism. In a proportion of patients this can lead to hypocalcaemia and worsening hyperparathyroidism [81]. Hypocalcaemia also depresses myocardial contractility and reduced vascular reactivity [82] and thus increases the risk of intradialytic hypotension. This forms the basis for the short-term use of a higher calcium bath. In our experience, the only situation requiring routine use of 1.5 mmol/L calcium baths are in patients receiving nocturnal HD, who have a reduced need for calcium containing phosphate binders and increased calcium clearance [83].

Phosphate

Phosphate is the major anion in the intracellular compartment and the steep gradient between the intracellular and extracellular compartments is maintained by active transport systems. The factors that limit the removal of excessive phosphate are dialysis clearance and the kinetics of phosphate distribution within the body. During dialysis, plasma phosphate levels initially fall, but thereafter plateau or increase, with a postdialysis rebound effect persisting for up to 4 h [84]. The implication is slow mobilization of phosphate from the intracellular stores and bone and phosphate generation from reserves triggered by falling extracellular [85] or intracellular levels [86]. The point at which phosphate generation is initiated appears to correlate with predialysis phosphate levels. There is also evidence for a "switching on" effect to protect against critically low intracellular phosphate levels.

Phosphate supplementation to dialysate may occasionally be required in severely hypophosphatemic patients with tubulopathies, severely malnourished children who develop hypophosphataemia secondary to refeeding syndrome, and those receiving more frequent, daily, or nocturnal HD.

Magnesium

Typically the concentration of magnesium in dialysate is 0.5–1 mmol/L. If magnesium containing phosphate binders are used, a lower concentration may be required to avoid hypermagnesemia. Conversely low magnesium levels can result in cramping and arrhythmias and therefore higher magnesium baths may help to improve cardiovascular stability and reduce intradialytic symptoms.

Glucose

Glucose concentration of dialysate usually approximates 100–200 mg/dL (6–11 mmol/L). This level of glucose should ensure patients remain normoglycemic unless hyperglycemic or hypoglycemic at the start. If hyperglycemic, a dialysate glucose in the recommended range will remove glucose, and if hypoglycemic the dialysate will provide supplemental glucose. There is a theoretical risk of inducing hypertriglyceridemia by addition of glucose to dialysate but this should not be significant with dialysate values of 100–200 mg/dL. If the patient is hyperkalemic, less potassium might be removed when dialysate glucose is elevated, causing hyperinsulinemia, which pushes potassium into cells. However, this should not be a problem with the dialysate glucose levels recommended above.

Dialysis Flow Rate

Typically, dialysate flow rates of 300–500 ml/min are employed. During infant dialysis, the practice within our unit is to start with a dialysate flow rate of 300 ml/min. If clearance is inadequate, increasing the dialysate flow rate can produce improvements, but eventually plateaus. The HEMO Study provided in vivo confirmation of increased hemodialyzer mass transfer-area coefficients for urea at high dialysate flow rates [87]. A subsequent study showed that the relative gains in spKt/V for increasing the dialysate flow rate from 300 to 500 ml/min and 500 to 800 ml/min were 11.7% ± 8.7% and 9.9% ± 5.1%, respectively [88].

Dialysate Temperature

By modifying skin blood flow, we can control heat exchange between the body and the environment. This is mediated by two sympathetic nervous system effects, an adrenergic vasoconstrictor and a lesser understood sympathetic vasodilator. During times of increased body core temperature, tonic sympathetic vasoconstriction is relaxed and active vasodilatation is initiated [89] and the skin blood flow rate can increase from a baseline of 5–10% of the total body cardiac output to approximately 60% [90, 91].

Traditionally, dialysate temperatures have been set at ≥37 °C, based to match physiological normal values and to compensate for losses of heat in the extracorporeal circuit. Both of these assumptions have in fact been found to be untrue. In a study of adult HD patients, 62.5% of 128 patients had predialysis body temp below 36.5, with marked inter- and intra-individual differences [92]. There is growing evidence in both adults and children of a net gain rather than loss of heat during dialysis. This is the result of higher resting energy expenditure in HD patients compared to the normal population, especially in those with residual renal function [93]. Secondly, UF activates sympathetic vasoconstriction, reducing skin blood flow and therefore heat exchange, with a direct correlation between UF volume and net heat gain [94]. If the accumulation of heat causes an increase in the body core temperature, UF induced vasoconstriction is overridden by active vasodilatation. Blood is redistributed to the skin [95], and the peripheral vascular resistance falls, resulting in decreased cardiac refilling and hypotension [51]. Fine and Penner [92] showed that dialysis patients with subnormal body temperature (below 36 °C) dialyzed against a 37 °C dialysate had a 15.9% incidence of symptomatic hypotensive episodes, which fell to 3.4% with 35 °C dialysate.

The hemodynamic advantage of "cool" HD has been documented, but may be uncomfortable for patients and reduce urea clearance as a result of compartmental dysequilibrium. Application of thermoneutral (no gain or removal of thermal energy from the extracorporeal circuit) and isothermic (patient temperature is kept constant) dialysis is technically possible, but the dialysis circuit has to be adapted to accommodate a feedback control circuit. A more practical option is to individualize the dialysate temperature based on the patient's predialysis temperature. Even then, efforts may be hampered by the current standards of the Association for the Advancement of Medical Instrumentation (AAMI) that requires the dialysate temperature at the dialyser to be maintained within ±1.5 °C of its set point.

Infants have an increased susceptibility to hypothermia. As a result, infants have traditionally been dialysed against higher dialysate temperatures of 37.5 °C to 38 °C. Alternatively, one may consider more physiological dialysate temperatures with the use of external warming methods to maintain normothermia. The impact of either strategy on thermal balance and cardiovascular stability has not been studied.

Anticoagulation

Anticoagulation of the extracorporeal circuit is usual but not mandatory and should be determined by estimating the risk of bleeding against that of clotting the circuit, which results in blood loss and reduced dialysis efficacy. In children, unfractionated heparin (UFH) remains the agent of choice for systemic anticoagulation, but low molecular weight heparin (LMWH) and citrate have been used.

UFH is a mixture of polyanionic branched glycosaminoglycans that bind with high affinity to antithrombin causing a structural change, converting it from a slow to a very rapidly (1000 times) acting inhibitor of thrombin. It interacts with other components of the coagulation cascade, producing a combined effect of inhibiting fibrin formation and thrombin-induced platelet activation and increasing vessel wall permeability. The polyanionic nature of heparin allows non-selective binding to other proteins and cell membranes. This mediates the adverse effects associated with UFH use such as activation of lipoprotein lipase causing increased generation of free fatty acids, which can induce platelet aggregation, and loss of bone mass resulting in osteoporosis [96, 97].

UFH has to be administered intravenously as intestinal absorption from oral therapy is poor. Following a bolus injection, the non-specific interactions reduce bioavailability to approximately 30%. Consequently, an initial bolus is usually recommended to saturate these non-specific binding sites as the dose-response relationship becomes almost linear thereafter. UFH is metabolized by the liver, and the kidney clears desulfated fragments. Owing to a marked inter-individual sensitivity to heparin and the possibility of heparin inactivation in the extracorporeal circuit, it is essential to individualize heparin requirements during dialysis and review dosing needs with time (Fig. 66.5).

The consensus on the desired degree of anticoagulation varies amongst different dialysis units, ranging between 25 to 300% above baseline. In our experience, for the majority of patients, adequate anticoagulation is achieved with activated clotting time 50% above the baseline. Standard regimens consist of a bolus dose of 15–20 units/kg of heparin at the start of dialysis followed by a continuous infusion of 15–20 units/kg/h, stopping the heparin infusion over the last 30 min of dialysis. In children weighing less than 10 kg, the likelihood of clotting is increased. Nonetheless, safe, effective anticoagulation with lower activated clotting time target ranges is possible with tight heparin regimens [98].

In high-risk groups, there is a 10–30% risk of bleeding with unfractionated heparin. Alternative options include regional anticoagulation with citrate, use of prostacyclin infusion, high flow rate HD, calcium free dialysate with calcium infusion back to the patient in a closely monitored setting, or modification of the standard heparin regimen. Low dose heparin or

Fig. 66.5 Tight heparin regimen

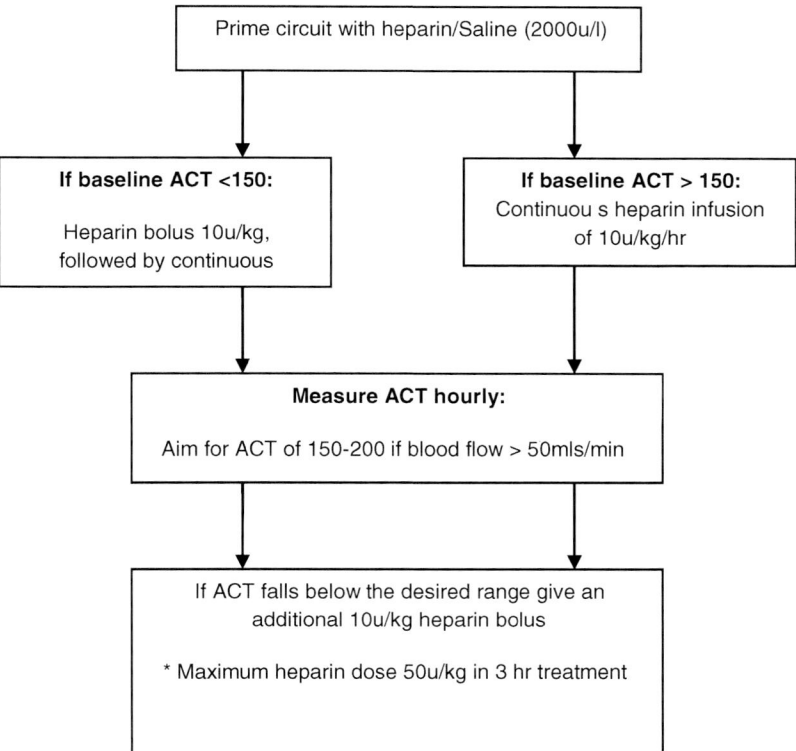

heparin free dialysis combined with regular intermittent saline flushes is possible without compromising dialysis dose or causing unwanted bleeding complications in children at increased of bleeding [98].

LMWH is composed of smaller molecules prepared from UFH through enzymatic or chemical depolymerization. They act predominantly by inhibiting factor Xa, but also cause a variable degree of thrombin inactivation. Following a single subcutaneous injection, bioavailability reaches 100%, but with differences in interindividual sensitivity, fixed dosing is inappropriate. LMWHs are principally cleared by the kidney, and therefore in ESKD the drug's pharmacokinetics are unpredictable.

Due to the prolonged half-life in kidney failure and lack of a commercially available antidote, there has been a reluctance to use LMWH. However, several adult trials show that sustained intradialytic anticoagulation can be achieved following a single bolus dose at the start of dialysis, making it a very convenient option. The negative charge of the LMWH complexes makes them impermeable across dialysis membranes and therefore, in spite of their low molecular weight, there is no relevant elimination either through HD or hemofiltration [99, 100]. One meta-analysis comparing the safety and efficacy of LMWH compared with UFH showed no difference in preventing extracorporeal thrombosis and demonstrated comparable bleeding risks [101].

The use of LMHH was first described in children on HD by Bianchetti et al. who successfully hemodialyzed 7 children for an average time of 4 h, using enoxaparin 24–36 mg/M^2 [102]. More recently, Davenport has reviewed the issue of anticoagulation for children on HD and has proposed doses for LMWH in children receiving HD [103].

It has become our routine practice to use LMWH in our home HD population in London. All patients are commenced on 50 units/kg of dalteparin as a single intravenous dose at the start of dialysis. The dose is then adjusted in 20% increments according to percentage of visible clot formation in the dialyser at the end of dialy-

sis, predialysis anti-Xa levels and, in those with fistulae, the presence of prolonged bleeding times after removing fistulae needles. All patients with fistulae are also placed on low dose aspirin. No patient has lost a circuit from excessive clotting. The final dose of dalteparin ranges from 21 to 58 units/kg, with a trend for infants and young children to be on higher doses of dalteparin (52–58 units/kg) compared with teenagers (21–41 units/kg). Those switching from an evening dialysis schedule to nocturnal schedule require on average a 50% increase in their dalteparin dose. The anti-Xa level 1 h after dosing ranged from 0.13–0.6 and predialysis anti-Xa levels suggests no bioaccumulation of dalteparin.

Citrate is a small molecule and is dialyzable, with an extraction coefficient similar to that of urea, and any citrate that escapes into the systemic circulation is rapidly cleared by the tricarboxylic acid pathway, primarily in the liver and skeletal muscle. Citrate exerts its anticoagulant effect by chelating ionized calcium ions, preventing activation of calcium-dependent procoagulants. Regional anticoagulation of the extra-corporeal circuit without systemic effects is achieved by infusing citrate solution through the arterial limb of the circuit, removal of citrate through dialysis and then neutralizing its anticoagulant effect by infusion of calcium into the venous limb of the circuit, making it a very attractive option for patients with a bleeding risk despite a lack of supportive data in children on maintenance dialysis.

Each method of anticoagulation is associated with specific side-effects. Heparin-induced thrombocytopenia is mediated by heparin-dependent IgG antibodies that bind to platelets, causing platelet activation and subsequent risk of thromboembolic events, characterized by markedly increased thrombin levels. Several alternatives to heparin are commercially available, but only danaparoid sodium use has been documented in pediatric HD, reporting stabilization of both thrombocytopenia and thromboembolic risk [104]. However, it has 30% cross-reactivity with platelet-heparin antibodies [105]. The direct thrombin inhibitor, hirudin, is efficacious but its half-life is prolonged in renal failure and it is associated with anaphylactic reactions [106, 107]. Argatroban, a synthetic direct thrombin inhibitor shows the greatest promise owing to its rapid onset of action, a half-life ranging from 39–51 min, hepatic metabolism, and the fact that it can be used in dialysis patients with no dose adjustment as only a 20% systemic clearance is seen even with high-flux dialyzers. Complications reported with citrate dialysis include hypocalcemia resulting in arrhythmias and paresthesias, hypernatremia, volume expansion, and metabolic alkalosis (one molecule of trisodium citrate is metabolized to 3 molecules of bicarbonate). Citrate toxicity with metabolic acidosis can occur from citrate accumulation due to ineffective dialysis clearance or poor metabolism secondary to impaired synthetic liver function. It is diagnosed biochemically by an increased anion gap acidosis and high total plasma calcium combined with low or normal plasma ionized calcium (so-called citrate lock).

Additionally, evidence suggests a role of citrate in attenuating the chronic inflammatory response to HD, which is linked to atherosclerosis, arteriosclerosis and malnutrition [108]. The use of citrate in pediatrics is growing through its application in plasmapharesis and continuous renal replacement therapy and because its actions are easily neutralized with calcium. These factors make it an attractive option, but until protocols are simplified and validated in children, it cannot presently be recommended as an alternative to heparin for routine dialysis therapy.

Commonly Encountered Hemodialysis Complications Dialysis Disequilibrium Syndrome (DDS)

Dialysis disequilibrium occurs as a result of changes in osmolarity inducing water shifts from the extracellular to the intracellular compartment across the highly permeable blood brain membrane. It manifests during or immediately after HD as a self-limiting entity, but recovery can take several days. Symptoms typically include nausea, vomiting, headache, blurred vision, muscular twitching, disorientation, hypertension, tremors, seizures and coma, but others such as muscular cramps, anorexia, restlessness, and dizziness have been reported. The diagnosis is often one of exclusion.

The exact pathophysiology of disequilibrium remains unknown, although two mechanisms have been proposed. Both mechanisms support that rapid changes in brain volume disrupt the blood brain barrier and cerebral autoregulation. The reverse urea effect postulates that urea is cleared from plasma more rapidly than from brain tissue, resulting in a transient osmotic gradient and cerebral oedema. The second theory is based on the observation of a paradoxical acidaemia of the cerebral spinal fluid and cerebral cortical grey matter in patients and animals treated with rapid HD. This is accompanied by increased brain osmole activity due to displacement of sodium and potassium ions and enhanced organic acid production. The increased intracellular osmolarity induces fluid shifts with subsequent cytotoxic oedema.

The dialysis prescription can be adjusted to reduce the rate of plasma urea clearance by using a smaller dialyser, decreasing the blood or dialysate flow rate, or switching to more frequent, shorter, treatments. Intradialytic osmotic shifts can be minimized with the use of sodium profiles or higher dialysate sodium concentrations, the substitution of bicarbonate for acetate in the dialysate, or if the patient is grossly fluid overloaded, sequential HD in which an initial period of UF alone is followed by conventional dialysis. Mannitol is an osmotically active solute that artificially increases plasma osmolarity at the time of rapid urea clearance. It rapidly lowers intracranial pressure within minutes of administration and has a peak effect at 20–40 min. A maximal intradialytic dose of 1 g/kg is recommended once a week in high risk patients. If more frequent dosing is required, a smaller dose of 0.5 g/kg is advised, as mannitol accumulates in renal failure (half-life: 36 h) and can cause a rebound rise in the intracranial pressure, especially in the face of acidosis. Other adverse effects include nausea, vomiting, lower limb oedema, thrombophlebitis, headache and chest pain. An alternative to mannitol is infusion of 3–5% sodium chloride or the use of higher dialysate sodium baths. Concurrent antiepileptic therapy is required with both therapies if the patient is seizing.

Intradialytic Hypotension

The major barrier to achieving optimal UF is the development of hemodynamic instability, manifesting as intradialytic hypotension. Hypotension occurs in about 20–30% of treatments, can result in underdialysis because of treatment interruptions, and may leave the patient volume overloaded. Frequent hypotensive episodes may accelerate a decline in residual renal function and potentially lead to serious vascular complications such as cerebral, cardiac, and mesenteric ischaemia. In children, the UF goal is often higher because of nutritional supplements or poor adherence to fluid restrictions.

As fluid is removed, plasma refilling, passive venoconstriction and active increases in heart rate, heart contractility and arterial tone are working simultaneously to preserve the effective plasma volume. As a result, even with a UF volume equal to the entire plasma volume, the measured blood volume only changes by 10–20%. Impaired compensatory responses cause hypotension in the face of total body water expansion. Most of the plasma volume resides in the veins, with a marked difference in the venous capacitance between organs. During fluid removal, the ability to mobilize blood from the splanchnic venous pool is vital for preserving the central blood volume. Venous tone is affected by vasoactive hormones, the sympathetic nervous system, and upstream filling pressures. The De-Jager Krogh phenomenon refers to the transmission of upstream arterial pressure through the capillaries to the veins causing venous distension and altered venous capacitance. During arteriolar constriction the distending pressure to the vein is reduced and blood is extruded centrally towards the heart to maintain cardiac refilling. Conversely, factors that cause arterial dilatation, such as antihypertensive medications, increase venous capacitance, reduce cardiac filling pressures and,

through transmission of increased hydrostatic pressure to the capillary bed, inhibit vascular refilling. Adenosine is thought to augment splanchnic blood pooling through an inhibitory effect on norepinephrine release and by causing regional vasodilatation. It is hypothesized that during a sudden, but not gradual intradialytic hypotensive episode, ischaemia leads to increased metabolism of adenosine triphosphate and generation of adenosine [109].

The sympathetic nervous system is the principal control mechanism of arteriolar tone and therefore of central BP. Patients with ESKD show increased basal level of peripheral sympathetic activity [110]. In HD patients prone to hypotension, a paradoxical decrease in sympathetic activity is seen at the time of a hypotensive episode [110], which results in a rapid decline in the peripheral vascular resistance and increased vascular bed capacitance. Problems with sympathetic end-organ responsiveness and the efferent parasympathetic baroreceptor pathway have also been reported, but the underlying mechanism remains unexplained. Some believe this may be a heightened manifestation of the Bezold-Jarisch reflex, a cardiodepressor reflex resulting in a sudden loss of sympathetic tone causing abrupt severe hypotension accompanied by bradycardia. It is postulated that conditions associated with reduced cardiac refilling pressures such as LVH, diastolic dysfunction, or structural heart defects stimulate cardiac stretch receptors and thus is a maladaptive variant of the Bezold-Jarisch reflex resulting in hypotension.

The final and interconnecting component relating to intradialytic hypotension is plasma refilling, the movement of fluid from the extravascular to the vascular compartment under the influences of hydraulic, osmotic, and oncotic pressure gradients at the capillary wall. If UF rates exceed refilling rates the intravascular volume will fall. Arterial vasoconstriction decreases hydrostatic pressures in the capillary bed, facilitating vascular refilling. The oncotic pressure, which is effectively the plasma protein concentration, promotes refilling. Plasma sodium and glucose mobilizes fluid from the intracellular space as a result of increased plasma tonicity

[111]. Finally, refilling is facilitated by greater tissue hydration and occurs at a faster rate when the interstitial space is overloaded. Hypovolaemia within the uremic milieu can augment ineffective venoconstriction, inadequate cardiac refilling, reduced plasma refilling and activation of the Bezold-Jarish reflex leading to sudden hypotension.

Haemodynamic stability during dialysis is improved by withholding antihypertensive medications on dialysis days, avoiding food during dialysis, cooling dialysate, using bicarbonate buffers, high sodium dialysate, and treating intradialytic hypocalcaemia. In some patients, the intradialytic BP can be artificially maintained by pharmacological measures. One study demonstrated that prophylactic caffeine administration, an adenosine antagonist, reduced the occurrence of sudden intradialytic hypotensive episodes [112]. A more widely used alternative is midodrine, a prodrug of a specific α-1 adrenergic receptor agonist, desglymidodrine. It maintains intradialytic BP by mediating constriction of both arterial and venous capacitance vessels and preventing venous pooling while increasing the central BP. Administered orally route, it achieves peak levels at 1 h, and has a half-life of 3 h. We have used it in children successfully, starting with doses of 2.5 mg, incrementally increased to 10 mg. A systematic review of 9 trials, using midodrine doses of 2.5–10 mg given 15–30 min before dialysis, reported a benefit in 6 trials with attenuation of the drop in BP during dialysis, and a decrease in number of hypovolaemia related symptoms. No serious adverse events were described, but minor reactions such as scalp paraesthesia, heartburn, flushing, headache, weakness and neck soreness were reported [113].

Modifying the UF rate throughout dialysis to allow adequate vascular refilling may optimize fluid removal. This is the rationale behind UF profiles. The plasma refilling capacity increases proportionately with interstitial volume expansion. Decreasing stepwise or linear profiles start with high UF rates at the time of maximal tissue hydration, progressively reducing the rate in line with decreasing interstitial hydration in the hope of maintaining the crucial balance between fluid

removal and vascular refilling. Intermittent profiles aim to provide periods of active mobilization of interstitial fluid into the vascular space when UF rates are low, making it amenable to removal during periods of high UF rates (Fig. 66.6).

Donauer et al. reported less symptomatic hypotension with the decreasing profiles, but the intermittent profile was associated with an increased incidence of symptomatic hypotension and postdialysis fatigue [114]. The incidence of intradialytic hypotension was highest with UF rates greater than 1.5 times the average. Ronco et al. observed hypotension at a rate of 6.7/100 treatments when the UF rate was 0.3 ml/min/kg, increasing to 15.8 at an UF rate of 0.4 ml/min/kg, 25.6 at a rate of 0.5 ml/min/kg, and 67.4 at a rate of 0.6 ml/min/kg [115]. In children, application of these figures would suggest that hypotension

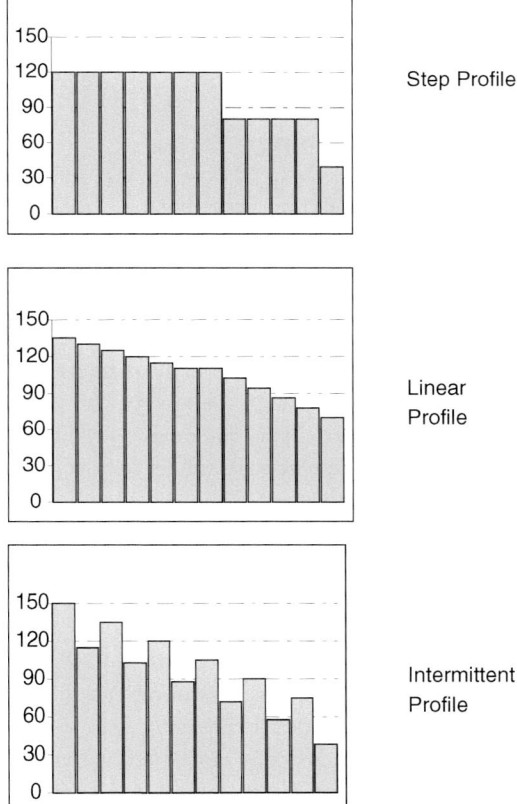

Fig. 66.6 Ultrafiltration profiles

may occur in 25.6 of 100 treatments if a UF rate of 30 ml/kg/h (300 ml/h in a 10 kg child) is exceeded. This data has not been validated in children, but in our experience increasing the UF rate increases the likelihood of intradialytic morbidity. UF profiles will inevitably result in higher UF rate for part of the treatment; the maximal UF rate has to be factored in when considering the most appropriate profile for a patient.

Combining UF profiles with sodium profiles can induce plasma hypertonicity through utilization of a high UF rate during a high-sodium period, and thus provide a greater driving force for plasma refilling. It has been shown to be superior to either sodium or UF profiles alone in attenuating intradialytic symptoms and cardiovascular instability. Finally, the supportive measures for managing hemodynamic instability in high risk patients have a ceiling effect and in resistant cases patients may need to be switched to alternative dialysis programs. HDF, short daily HD, and home nocturnal HD can all potentially be of benefit in these situations.

Myocardial Stunning

Acutely, intradialytic hypotension requires immediate action to stop or reduce the severity of symptoms that may precede or follow the drop in BP. These include a temporary suspension of UF, a 5 ml/kg fluid bolus, and in resistant cases, premature discontinuation of the dialysis treatment. Such measures, although necessary, have an adverse impact on dialysis outcomes by reducing UF goals and adequacy of solute removal. Of greater concern, however, is the evidence linking repeated episodes of intradialytic hypotension with a more severe effect on morbidity and mortality. Several observational studies in adult patients with essential hypertension have described a "J" shaped curve between BP and mortality [116]. The same trend has been described in adult dialysis patients, with a suggestion that hypertension is associated with morbidity, but mortality is more closely associated with hypotension [117]. Zager et al. reported a fourfold increase in the relative risk of cardiac-

related death in adults patients with predialysis systolic BP less than 110 mmHg compared with a systolic BP between 140 to 149 mmHg, and a 2.8-fold increase in relative risk for a cardiac-related death with postdialysis systolic BP less than 110 mm Hg compared with systolic BP 140 to 149 mmHg [118].

Frequent intradialytic hypotensive episodes have been implicated in accelerating the decline in residual renal function and precipitating serious vascular complications. There is growing evidence from isotopic, electrocardiographic, biochemical and echocardiographic studies implicating HD as a source of recurrent ischemic injury. Silent intradialytic ST depression [119, 120] associated with acute changes in serum cardiac troponin levels both in adults [121, 122] and children [123] have been demonstrated. Using single photon emission computed tomography, McIntyre et al. demonstrated an acute reduction in global and segmental myocardial blood flow in adults during dialysis with matched reductions in segmental contractile function, even in patients without angiographically proven epicardial coronary artery disease [124]. A direct correlation was seen between the degree of myocardial dysfunction and intradialytic BP changes and UF volume [125]. Such transient myocardial ischemia with resultant reversible regional left ventricular dysfunction is known as myocardial stunning [126]. In the model of coronary heart disease, repeated stunning is progressive and leads to myocardial hibernation, defined as ischaemic, and non-infarcted myocardium that exists in a state of contractile dysfunction [127]. In dialysis patients, myocardial stunning also appears to be progressive. In a 12 month follow-up of adult HD patients, the presence of acute HD induced regional myocardial dysfunction negatively influenced survival, increased the likelihood of cardiac arrhythmias [128], and resulted in regional fixed systolic dysfunction and a reduction in global systolic function [125, 129] with resultant congestive heart failure. Records from the USRDS have shown that HD associated de novo and recurrent congestive heart failure is highly relevant as it is associated with a 2-year mortality as high as 51% [130]. The left atrial volume is commonly driven by intravascular volume overload and progressive diastolic dysfunction. In a single observational study, the strongest predictor of left atrial volume indexed to height (LAVI) was the presence of stunning. LAVI was a better predictor of mortality than left ventricular (LV) mass index, but both factors became statistically insignificant during a multi-confounder analysis with the addition of myocardial stunning [131].

Of greater concern, perhaps, has been the demonstration of dialysis induced acute regional myocardial dysfunction in 15 children aged 2–17 years. This was associated with varying degrees of compensatory hyperkinesis in unaffected segments and thus the global LV function was maintained throughout HD. In children, intradialytic systolic BP reduction was significantly associated with segmental left ventricular dysfunction, but no correlation was seen with actual intradialytic systolic BP or dialysis vintage [132, 133]. Interestingly, patients on peritoneal dialysis do not appear to have an increased risk of myocardial stunning, despite changes in systemic hemodynamics [134].

We know HD poses a significant hemodynamic challenge. It is conceivable that other vulnerable vascular beds with defective vasoregulation may also be susceptible to significant episodic dialysis-related ischemia. The gut for example is also a high-flow vascular bed. Translocation of endotoxin across the gut wall causes endotoxinaemia and becomes a profoundly pro-inflammatory stimulus. In both children and adults with chronic kidney disease (CKD), circulating endotoxin levels were 1000 times greater than in patients without CKD and almost quadrupled from predialysis levels after initiating HD [135]. Serum endotoxin levels correlated with intradialytic instability, systemic inflammation and dialysis-induced myocardial stunning [135]. One group have even postulated that postdialysis fatigue is a clinical manifestation of cardiac ischemia and cardiac fatigue [136]. The acute cardiac injury that occurs as a direct effect of the HD procedure may be attenuated by altering the dialysis prescription. Cooling, biofeedback and frequent dialysis have all been demonstrated in adults to lower the risk of myocardial stunning [137–139].

Intradialytic or Paradoxical Hypertension

Hypertension is endemic in HD patients and is most often due to salt and volume overload, which responds to UF. The prevalence of hypertension in children receiving HD is reported at 65–69% in studies conducted in Europe and the United States [140, 141]. Intradialytic or paradoxical hypertension is less well-characterized but nonetheless important. Estimates of its frequency are hampered by the lack of a standardized definition. Suggested definitions include an increase in mean arterial pressure of more than 15 mmHg during or immediately after dialysis or an increase in BP that is resistant to fluid removal. Estimates of the incidence in adults range from 5–15%, with no pediatric data available [142].

The pathogenesis of intradialytic hypertension is complex and poorly understood. There may be an iatrogenic aetiology with mobilization of extracellular fluid or in response to osmotic agents such as sodium, mannitol, or concentrated albumin solutions or dialysis induced hypokalemia. Dolson et al. demonstrated significant rebound hypertension at 1 h postdialysis in patients dialyzed against lower potassium baths [143]. In these instances, the hypertension is frequently transient and improves with UF.

Sustained hypertension is commonly due to failure to achieve an appropriate dry weight [144]. However, some patients manifest refractory intradialytic hypertension despite appropriate UF. It is speculated that overzealous UF activates the renin-angiotensin system with resultant vasoconstriction. In support of this theory is the lower incidence of hypertension in anephric HD patients.

Sympathetic nervous system overactivity is well documented in CKD secondary to a number of mediators, including angiotensin II, afferent renal nerve stimulation, impaired brain nitric oxide synthesis and increased production of catecholamines [145–149]. Studies have shown enhanced endothelin I production during dialysis in hypertensive patients, especially those exhibiting paradoxical hypertension [150–152]. This raises the possibility that paradoxical hypertension is secondary to an imbalance of nitric oxide and endothelin I production [153]. Pearl et al. suggested a role for a new pressor protein a 30-kD extra-renal enzyme related to the coagulation factor β-FXIIa that exhibits cardiotonic and pressor activity in rats. The serum of three anephric children produced characteristic pressor responses, suggesting in vivo activation of this protein as a contributory factor in their hypertension [154].

Finally, a number of antihypertensive drugs are removed by dialysis and this conceivably may result in paradoxical hypertension. As a general rule, the beta blockers (atenolol, nadolol, metoprolol), angiotensin converting enzyme (ACE) inhibitors (captopril, enalapril, lisinopril, ramipril) and vasodilators such as minoxidil, nitroprusside and diazoxide are removed, by a variable degree, during dialysis. Calcium channel blockers such as amlodipine and angiotensin receptor blockers (ARBs), such as losartan, are generally not cleared during HD. No data exists for α-blockers such as doxazosin. The management of intradialytic hypertension should start with an assessment of the dry weight and salt and fluid intake. Treatment options include further salt and water restrictions, and where feasible, augmentation of urine output with loop diuretics. The dialysate composition should be examined for the sodium, potassium and calcium content to ensure that the dialysis procedure does not result in acute hypokalemia or a net transfer of sodium and calcium load. Consideration should be given to replacing conventional HD prescriptions with intensive HD or HDF. If hypertension persists despite appropriate salt and water control, blockade of the renin-angiotensin system with ACE inhibitors or ARBs have been shown to improve BP control and reduce sympathetic tone in HD patients. If this produces insufficient BP control, the addition of α-blockers, β-blockers or centrally acting antihypertensive such as methyldopa is physiologically logical. Attention should be paid to the timing of BP medications to ensure they do not contribute to intradialytic hypotension. Similarly, if drug removal by HD is contributing to suboptimal BP control, consideration should be given to switching to an agent that is not significantly removed by dialysis such as calcium channel blockers. Finally, the incidence of hypertension in dialysis patients appears to have increased in the post-erythropoiesis stimulating agent (ESA) era. This may relate to increased viscosity, increased peripheral vascular resistance or a direct effect of ESAs on the vascular endothelium. While there are no published studies showing a direct relationship between hemoglobin and hypertension, effort should be made to avoid excessive hemoglobin values in patients with intradialytic hypertension.

Left Ventricular Hypertrophy

LVH is common in dialysis patients. At the initiation of dialysis, 69–82% of children show evidence of LVH [155] and during maintenance dialysis 40–75% of children have LVH [156]. Several factors increase the risk of developing cardiac hypertrophy, including chronic hypervolemia, a hyperdynamic circulation secondary to arteriovenous fistulae or anemia, increasing arterial stiffness and elevated parathyroid hormone (PTH) levels [157]. There is emerging evidence from established animal models of CKD implicating a klotho-independent, causal role for FGF23 in the pathogenesis of LVH. This raises the possibility of FGF23 being directly involved in the high rates of LVH and mortality in HD patients [158]. Somewhat surprisingly, both adult data and now pediatric data from the ESCAPE trial have failed to demonstrate any relationship between office BP or ambulatory BP and left ventricular mass [159].

Cardiac hypertrophy in combination with continued mechanical stress triggers pathways that result in myocardial remodeling characterized by decreased capillary density and reduced coronary flow reserve predisposing the heart and other organs to ischemic injury. Fortunately, cardiac hypertrophy in HD patients is amenable to treatment, with evidence of resolution in patients on intensified dialysis programmes and HDF.

Endothelial Dysfunction

Endothelial dysfunction is thought to be the initiating step in atherosclerosis and arteriosclerosis. It starts early in renal failure, progressing in dialysis as a number of pathophysiological pathways contribute. HD is pro-inflammatory as a consequence of an immune mediated response to bio-incompatible membranes, blood contact with non-sterile dialysate solution and "back-leaking" of dialysate across the membrane. UF changes endothelial cell dynamics through its effects on blood viscosity and laminar shear stress [160]. Intradialytic hypotension and resultant ischemia causes apoptosis of the vascular endothelium. Finally, reduced clearance of asymmetric dimethylarginine, decreased bioavailability of endothelial nitric oxide, activation of angiotensin II, hyperhomocystinemia and hyperlipidemia are postulated mechanisms for endothelial dysfunction. Compounding these effects, uremia is also associated with reduced hematopoiesis and capacity for repair. In adults, endothelial progenitor cells are reduced, with pronounced functional impairment [161, 162], and HD depletes this source further. In contrast, the pool of smooth muscle cell progenitor cells are preserved and with it the potential for adverse remodeling [163]. Little is known about circulating endothelial progenitor cells in children, but there is clinical evidence of endothelial dysfunction with loss of flow-mediated dilatation and increased aortic pulse wave velocity in children on dialysis [164, 165]. Encouragingly, the degree of endothelial injury is attenuated by switching adults HD patients to either HDF or home nocturnal HD [166, 167].

Sudden Cardiac Death

Sudden cardiac death is a common phenomenon in dialysis patients that appears to be temporally related to the HD procedure. In adults, the risk of sudden death is 1.7 times higher in the 12 h period starting with the dialysis procedure and 3 times higher in the 12 h before HD at the end of the weekend interval [168]. Cardiac arrests are 50% higher for HD patients 3 months after dialysis initiation. The risk remains higher in HD compared with peritoneal dialysis for up to 2 years on maintenance dialysis, but then the trend reverses at 3 years of maintenance dialysis. The most vulnerable patients are infants aged 0–4 years, with

a five- to ten-fold increase risk of cardiac arrest compared to other age groups [169].

The precise aetiology of sudden cardiac death remains elusive but a number of dialysis specific and uremic factors have been implicated. Myocardial interstitial fibrosis, LVH, endothelial dysfunction, cardiac and vascular calcification, microvascular disease with decreased perfusion reserve and diminished ischemia tolerance are all prevalent in dialysis patients and increase the vulnerability of the heart. This, in combination with dialysis related acute fluid shifts, acid-base disturbances, rapid electrolyte shifts and autonomic imbalance with abnormal sympathetic activity, places patients at risk of sudden cardiac death.

Clinically the only modifiable risk factor for fatal cardiac events is manipulation of the dialysate potassium. Patients who suffered a cardiac arrest at the time of dialysis were twice as likely to be dialyzed against a 0 or 1.0 mEq/L potassium dialysate compared to controls, despite no difference in predialysis potassium levels [170]. Kovesdy et al. found that serum potassium between 4.6 and 5.3 mEq/L was associated with the best survival, but levels below 4.0 mEq/L or higher than 5.6 mEq/L were associated with increased mortality [171]. As a result, there is a growing consensus of nephrologists advising against zero potassium dialysate baths.

Atherosclerosis, Arteriosclerosis, and Calcification

Calcification of the cardiovascular system is accelerated in dialysis patients. Studies of young adults who developed ESKD during childhood found a high prevalence of abnormal carotid intima-media thickness (cIMT), diminished arterial wall compliance and coronary artery calcification [172, 173]. Such vascular and cardiac aberrations were also demonstrated in children on dialysis [174]. The vascular abnormalities positively correlated with serum phosphorus levels, while cIMT and cardiac calcification scores also correlated with intact PTH levels and dosage of vitamin D. Patients with mean intact PTH levels greater than twice the upper limit of normal demonstrated stiffer vessels and increased cIMT and cardiac calcification scores. In contrast, 1,25-dihydroxy vitamin D levels showed a U-shaped distribution, with a significantly greater cIMT and calcification score in patients with low and high 1,25-dihydroxy vitamin D levels compared with patients with normal levels. Calcification was most frequently observed in patients with the lowest 1,25-dihydroxy vitamin D and the highest high-sensitivity C-reactive protein (CRP) [175]. Litwin et al. reported vascular abnormalities in children with CKD, but again found the most marked changes in the dialysis patients. The degree of arteriopathy correlated with conventional cardiovascular disease risk factors such as hypertension and dyslipidemia in predialysis CKD and with hyperphosphatemia, hyperparathyroidism and treatment with calcium-containing phosphate binders in dialysis patients [176]. In contrast, in a study examining the effects of dialysate calcium concentrations on changes in arterial stiffness, increased pulse wave velocity was seen even in the group dialysing using the lowest dialysate calcium [177]. Therefore, it is highly probably that factors other than simple net calcium influx and efflux during dialysis are involved in the pathogenesis of accelerated vascular calcification in HD patients.

Inflammation

Inflammation predicts mortality in dialysis patients and may contribute to cardiovascular risk. CRP, an acute phase protein, is a recognized marker of inflammation, but is also reported to be predictive of mortality, structural heart changes such as LVH, and higher coronary calcification scores. Data has also implicated CRP in the pathogenesis of vascular inflammation and atherosclerosis [178]. Plasma CRP levels increase with declining kidney function and then continue to rise after initiation of HD, with levels correlating with the length of the dialysis session [179]. It has been postulated that an interaction of circulating monocytes with bio-incompatible membranes, blood contact with non-sterile dialysate solution and "back-leaking" of dialysate across the membrane results in a chronic inflammatory state. However because there is a high incidence of pre-dialytic inflammation [180], the dialysis procedure is unlikely to be the only factor associated with inflammation [181]. Changes in CRP may also represent an acute inflammatory stimulus [182]. Additionally, vitamin D deficiency has been correlated with inflammatory cytokine levels (IL-10 and SIL-2R) in children receiving HD [183].

The dialysis prescription can be modified to become less inflammatory by using ultrapure dialysate and synthetic biocompatible membranes. Both ACE inhibitors and statins, more commonly recognized for their respective roles in treating hypertension and hypercholesterolemia, have been reported to have anti-inflammatory actions [184, 185]. Finally, lifestyle and dietary changes may be associated with decreasing inflammation and uremic toxins (p-cresyl sulfate and indoxyl sulfate), although data is limited in children [186].

Malnutrition

Protein malnutrition and growth delay commonly occurs in underdialyzed patients and may be associated with mortality in children [187, 188]. Measurement of the nPCR has become an indirect measure of daily protein intake in stable dialysis patients. Measurement of nPCR has traditionally relied on the availability of formal urea kinetic modeling and is included with the web-based programs (www.hdcn.com, and www.Kt-v.net) alluded to above. Goldstein, however, has demonstrated strong agreement between nPCR calculated from urea kinetic modeling and the formula [$nPCR = 5.43 \times G/V + 0.17$] [187]. This calculation requires a blood urea nitrogen (BUN) level 30 s after a mid-week dialysis session, documentation of the time until the next dialysis session, and a BUN value prior to the second dialysis session. In this formula the urea generation rate (G) is calculated as G (mg/min) = (predialysis $BUN_2 \times$ predialysis V) $-$ (postdialysis $BUN_1 \times$ postdialysis V)/T, where V is total body water estimated from $0.58 \times$ body weight, and T is time in minutes from the end of the mid-week dialysis treatment to the beginning of the next dialysis treatment. Validation of this formula has eliminated the need for complicated computer modeling in order to measure nPCR and estimate daily protein intake. A subsequent report, which compared the values of nPCR calculated as above with a simplified formula using only pre- and postdialysis BUN specimens from the same mid-week session has found there is a significant and variable difference between the two methods and invalidates the simplified formula [189].

Although nPCR values are a useful guide to protein intake, because nPCR values may be influenced by factors other than nutrient intake, these values should be interpreted in combination with a review of weight gain and the dietary history. Goldstein et al [190] demonstrated a substantial increase in nPCR associated with improvement in nutritional status of three adolescents treated with intradialytic total parenteral nutrition. However, Van Hoek et al. in a comparison of protein intake from dietary records kept by children, with an estimate of nPCR calculated using an on-line urea monitor, showed significant variation, and PCR significantly underestimated the prescribed and recorded protein intake [33]. These authors concluded that use of their online urea kinetic monitor is therefore not recommended for estimation of nPCR. Also, as reported by Grupe et al. [191], nPCR may be significantly affected by factors other than nutrient intake in as many as 25% of patients.

The safety of enteral intake during dialysis should be assessed on a patient-by-patient basis as blood is diverted to the splanchnic circulation, potentially increasing the risk of intradialytic hypotension. In patients able to tolerate enteral intake during dialysis, it offers an opportunity to provide nutritional supplements. Intradialytic parenteral nutrition is an alternative method of providing calories and protein to undernourished patients during HD. While this increases the amount of fluid needed to remove, utilizing a constant UF to parallel the infusion can minimize excessive UF rates. Use of recombinant growth hormone is another important means of maximizing growth in children on

HD, assuming their nutritional status has first been optimized [192].

Dialysis-Related Carnitine Disorder

Levocarnitine (L-carnitine) facilitates the transport of fatty acids across the inner mitochondrial membrane and is thus a critical co-factor for normal energy production in cardiac and skeletal muscle. There is evidence of reduced plasma free carnitine levels in HD patients, with an inverse relationship between muscle carnitine and duration on dialysis [193]. Within a single dialysis session, clearance is 30 times greater than would be expected in a healthy individual [194] and HD results in an abnormal acylcarnitine:free carnitine ratio (normal <0.25).

Low carnitine may be associated with anaemia that is hyporesponsive to ESAs, intradialytic hypotension, cardiac dysfunction, fatigue, muscle cramping, and reduced exercise tolerance [195]. The National Kidney Foundation Interdisciplinary Consensus Panel recommends L-carnitine [196] supplementation for those patients with these clinical findings even in the absence of a low plasma carnitine levels. As measuring skeletal muscle L-carnitine concentrations is not feasible, some advocate a trial of therapy with discontinuation at 9–12 months if no benefits are observed [196]. Repeated doses of 20 mg/kg given intravenously at the end of dialysis appear to be the most beneficial, as oral carnitine is not recommended in ESKD due to the toxicity of metabolites which accumulate in kidney failure.

Hyperhomocysteinaemia

Homocysteine is a non-protein forming amino acid that results from methionine metabolism. Only 1–2% of total homocysteine circulates freely in the blood in a reduced form, 70–90% is protein bound, and the rest exists in oxidized forms. Studies have shown that plasma homocysteine concentrations start rising in CKD and are inversely related to glomerular filtration rate.

ESKD results in hyperhomocysteinaemia from altered metabolism and impaired clearance. There is conflicting evidence on the impact of hyperhomocysteinemia on outcomes. A meta-analysis reported a positive association between hyperhomocysteinemia and atherosclerosis, ischemic heart disease, stroke, and thrombosis [197]. Conversely, others have found no significant or even an inverse association between plasma homocysteine levels, cardiovascular events, and mortality in ESKD patients [198]. In addition to being a potential marker of inflammation, homocysteine, like β2-microglobulin, can also be a marker of middle molecule clearance in patients receiving more frequent, longer duration, or convective treatment modalities (detailed below).

Treatment options for hyperhomocystinaemia have included folate and vitamin B12 supplementation to achieve supranormal plasma levels and intravenous N-acetylcysteine [199]. An alternative therapeutic strategy involves using high-flux dialysers to achieve greater clearance, but this has not impacted predialysis plasma concentrations [200]. With these therapeutic options, plasma homocysteine levels improve, but normalization is uncommon.

Future Directions

Hemodiafiltration

Conventional HD is based on diffusive transport of solutes across a semipermeable membrane and is effective in removing small uremic retention solutes, such as urea, and correcting electrolyte and fluid imbalances. However, as clearance is inversely proportional to the molecular weight of the toxin (and also depends on its protein binding and tissue distribution), conventional HD does not clear large or protein-bound toxins effectively, and fails to adequately correct the uremic milieu [201, 202]. In HDF, solute clearance involves a combination of diffusion and convection. HDF optimizes the removal of middle (up to 300–500 Dalton (Da) molecular weight) and larger molecules (greater than 15–50 kilo Da).

Definition of HDF Therapy

The European Dialysis Working Group (EUDIAL) has defined HDF as a blood purification therapy that combines diffusive and convective solute removal by UF of 20% or more of the blood volume processed through a high-flux dialyzer and maintenance of fluid balance by sterile replacement fluid infused directly into the patient's blood [202, 203]. Sterile replacement fluid is obtained in large amounts by on-line filtration of standard dialysate through a series of bacteria- and endotoxin-retaining filters [203]. A high-flux membrane is defined as one that has an UF coefficient greater than 20 mL/h/mmHg transmembrane pressure/m^2 and a sieving coefficient for β2-microglobulin of greater than 0.612.

Importance of Convective Volume

A high convective volume is a fundamental requirement for HDF [202, 204]. The convective volume is the sum of the net UF volume (i.e., the amount of fluid removed during a dialysis session based on the interdialytic weight gain) and the amount of substitution fluid (i.e., the sterile replacement fluid given as replenishment for the removal of extra fluid during HDF).

The effectiveness of a membrane to UF fluid is described by the UF coefficient (KUF):

$$KUF = QUF/\Delta P$$
(volume of UF per unit time, divided by the pressure gradient across the membrane, also called the transmembrane pressure gradient [TMP])

Theoretically, the convective volume should be prescribed as a proportion of plasma water volume processed rather than blood volume processed, but blood volume processed is displayed on the machine control panel, and hence this term is commonly used. An UF volume equivalent to 20% of the total blood volume processed for the treatment was chosen by the EUDIAL group because randomized controlled trials in adults [205–207] and a pooled individual participant data analysis [208] suggest that any improved survival associated with HDF occurs when the convective volume exceeds 20 L/session.

Depending on where the replacement volume is infused in the dialysis circuit, there are different modalities of HDF: pre-, post-, mid- or mixed-dilution HDF. Post-dilution, where the replacement fluid is infused downstream of the dialyser, usually into the venous bubble-trap, is the most commonly performed.

The phenomenon of 'backfiltration,' which commonly occurs during high-flux HD [209] (but not in low-flux HD), can achieve some convective clearance, but this is low and unreliable, and called the 'poor man's HDF'! Backfiltration occurs because the hydrostatic pressure of both blood and dialysis fluid decrease as they pass through the dialysis filter. Since blood and dialysis fluid pass through the filter in counter-current directions, the resulting TMP may become negative at the venous side, especially when the venous blood pressure is low. In adults it has been shown that the convective volume achieved by back-filtration is no more than 1–10 L per session depending on the dialyser type, and can vary throughout the dialysis session depending on TMP. Importantly, given the phenomenon of backfiltration, it has been suggested that dialysis fluid used for high-flux HD should also be sterile and pyrogen-free.

Essential Requirements for Performing HDF

High Flux Membranes

Only highly permeable membranes, defined as membranes characterized by an UF coefficient (KUF) greater than 20 mL/h/mmHg transmembrane pressure/m^2 and a sieving coefficient (S) for β2-microglobulin of greater than 0.6 [202, 203, 210], are suitable for HDF. A high-flux membrane allows a larger and pre-defined convective flow as required for HDF. In practice, the KUF should be high enough to allow 50 mL/m/m^2 BSA (equivalent to 2 mL/min/kg body weight) convective flow in post-dilution HDF. The albumin loss through a high-flux

membrane should be <0.5 g in a 4-h HD session [210–212].

As with conventional HD, the dialyser surface area must be equal to (or slightly higher) than the BSA for maintenance dialysis, so that the internal volume of the dialyser and blood lines is less than the safe extracorporeal blood volume permissible (i.e. less than 10 ml/kg body weight). For HDF a biocompatible dialyzer must be selected; biocompatibility is assessed by complement activation, thrombogenicity, contact activation and cytokine generation [63, 211]. European recommendations state that ultrapure dialysate must be used with synthetic high-flux membranes [63].

Ultrapure Water for HDF

Sterile, non-pyrogenic fluid that is used to maintain fluid balance is called replacement fluid or substitution fluid. This can be provided as a sterilized, packaged solution (like intravenous fluid) or as an on-line prepared solution. In all modern HDF machines, the replacement fluid is generated on-line by filtering dialysis fluid through bacteria- and endotoxin-retentive filters to prepare a sterile and pyrogen-free solution that is immediately infused into the patient. Strict safety standards and regulatory oversight are required as large volumes of fluid are removed from, and added to, blood during on-line therapies. Water purification systems are discussed separately in this chapter. Bacteria- and endotoxin-retentive filters installed on the inlet dialysis fluid circuit are the key components of the on-line HDF safety system. Those filters are disinfected after each dialysis treatment according to manufacturer's recommendations and replaced periodically to ensure proper operation of the cold sterilization process.

Dialysis Machines with Accurate Ultrafiltration Control

Today almost all new dialysis machines allow for both HD and HDF. These machines are suitable for children from 10–17 kg body weight, and require a pediatric circuit with low extracorporeal volumes. These systems can be used in a pressure-control mode (fixed TMP and variable substitution flow rate) or a volume-control mode (the target substitution volume or the substitution flow rate are set). Some machines offer an automatic substitution mode, in which the substitution rate is automatically regulated in response to variations in patient- and treatment-related parameters throughout the session.

Writing a HDF Prescription

The following points need to be considered when writing an HDF prescription:

1. A high-flux membrane with surface area equal to the child's BSA is used.
2. Double needle circuits—HDF is rarely ever performed with single-needle circuits given the high convective volume goals.
3. The total extracorporeal circuit should be less than 10 ml/kg body weight. Pediatric blood lines (36–105 ml volume) with or without the possibility to do on-line HDF and to monitor blood volume variation are available.
4. Blood flow: HDF requires an optimal arterial blood flow of 5–8 mL/min/kg body weight or 150 to 250 mL/m² BSA per minute. An optimal blood flow can be achieved through either a fistula or a central venous line, although in most cases a fistula allows a higher blood flow rate. Both the diffusive clearance of molecules with a high K0A and the substitution volume in post-dilution HDF depend on the blood flow rate.
5. Dialysate flow of twice the blood flow is sufficient to optimize the diffusive blood purification process using highly permeable membranes for HDF.
6. Replacement fluid that is generated on-line from the dialysate must be ultrapure (<0.1 CFU/ml and <0.03 endotoxin unit/ml, as per European guideline Dialysate purity 2002, European Pharmacopoeia 2009) [63] as

discussed earlier. The microbiologic purity (bacterial count and endotoxin level) should be determined at intervals of 1–3 months.

7. Convective flow is equal to total UF flow, that is, the sum of the desired UF volume and the replacement fluid. The convective flow needs to be maximal, but is limited by the risk of the filter clotting. Modern dialysis machines automatically adjust the convective volume throughout the session in order to optimize this convective flow without increasing the coagulation risk. In pre-dilution HDF, the convective flow is set at 100% of blood flow. The actual substitution volume obtained per session has to be monitored regularly in order to ensure that the goal of 23 L/1.73 m² per session in post-dilution and 75–100% of blood volume treated in pre-dilution is achieved.
8. The dialysate and substitution fluid are produced 'on-line' by the dialysis machine by dilution of acid concentrate and bicarbonate powder with dialysis water produced by the water treatment system. Dialysate composition is similar to that used in HD, but careful attention to dialysate sodium concentration is important in order to maintain sodium balance and for hemodynamic tolerance of the session [63]. To avoid the risk of positive sodium balance, the dialysate sodium concentration required is lower than in conventional HD, particularly when high convective volumes are infused, as with pre-dilution HDF. Sodium is predominantly drained in ultrafiltered water by convection [213]. A low dialysate sodium enables additional sodium removal by diffusion, but it may be associated with a risk of intradialytic hypotension and disequilibrium syndrome. Conversely, a high dialysate sodium increases hemodynamic tolerance, but causes sodium and water overload that leads to hypertension and increased thirst post-session.
9. Anticoagulation to prevent filter clotting can be achieved with a single dose of LMWH that is effective for a 4-h session. Alternatively, a continuous heparin infusion may be used.

To attain a high convective volume, one needs a high blood flow rate because filtration fraction depends on blood flow and cannot be higher than 35%; optimization of substitution volume by automated programs in new dialysis machines; and careful monitoring of the dialysis prescription and blood results to ensure that all dialysis related parameters are achieved [214–216]. In the HDF, Hearts and Height (3H) study (described in detail below), median convection volumes of 13.4 L/m^2 were achieved in children [217], which is comparable to the 23 L per 1.73 m^2 per session that proved beneficial in the pooled adult studies [208]. Importantly, the convection volume was independent of patient related factors such as age, gender, access type or dialyser used, but strongly correlated with the blood flow rate [217], implying that convection volume is a modifiable factor that can be manipulated and optimized by the dialysis team.

Potential Advantages of HDF Over Conventional HD

HDF is thought to be superior to conventional HD in the following key areas:

1. Clearance of toxins across a wide molecular weight range: HDF has been shown to clear 70–80% of β2-microglobulin compared to HD [218], and increase removal of inflammatory cytokines, with reduction in inflammation and oxidative stress [219].
2. Improved hemodynamic stability: HDF increases UF and improves intradialytic hemodynamic stability [220], leading to less intradialytic hypotension [221], reduced incidence of strokes [221] and faster recovery time postdialysis, even in children [222].
3. Biocompatibility and reduced inflammation: The use of ultrapure dialysate and increased removal of inflammatory cytokines reduces inflammation and oxidative stress [219].

Clinical Studies

A Cochrane review suggests that there is no clear benefit of HDF over HD, but these meta-analyses combine outcomes of both hemofiltration as well as HDF studies as 'convective therapies' and do not interpret outcomes based on convective volumes [223]. The Estudio de Supervivencia de Hemodiafiltración On-line (ESHOL) randomized controlled trial (RCT) comparing HDF vs. high-flux HD in adults, and achieving convective volumes of 23 L/session, has shown that patients on high volume HDF have a survival benefit compared to those on high-flux HD [206]. Pooled data [208] from the three RCTs (including the Turkish [207] and CONTRAST [205] studies) has indicated a critical dose-response relationship between the magnitude of the convective volume and survival, with a goal of at least 23 L per session.

In children, Fischbach et al. showed improved growth, with children achieving a normal height at or above their target mid-parental height [224, 225], reduced inflammation [225], regression of LVH [226, 227], improved anaemia control [214] and reduced postdialysis recovery time [222, 224] in a small number of children undergoing daily HDF. However, this study utilised 6 days per week HDF in the pre-dilution mode, making it difficult to ascertain the benefits of HDF vs. longer dialysis therapy times. A small single-centre study also suggests that switching children from nocturnal in-centre HD to nocturnal in-centre HDF may significantly improve BP, phosphate and PTH control [228]. Further single-centre studies have shown improvements in left ventricular function within a short period of HDF therapy [229]. Studies have shown that when HD patients are switched to HDF, keeping all other dialysis related parameters constant, a significant improvement in inflammation, antioxidant capacity and endothelial risk profile is achieved within 3 months [219], suggesting that even in children who have a short anticipated time on dialysis, HDF is superior to conventional HD. A report from the Italian Registry suggests that HDF use in Italy has been limited to approximately a quarter of patients on extracorporeal dialysis, in particular to those with high dialysis vintage, younger age or a long expected waiting time to renal transplantation [230].

The International Paediatric Hemodialysis Network (IPHN) has performed a multicenter observational study to test the hypothesis that HDF improves the cardiovascular risk profile, growth, nutritional status and health-related quality of life in children compared to conventional HD—the HDF, Hearts and Height (3H) study [217, 222]. The 3H study suggests that HDF halts the progression of increasing carotid intima-media thickness, is associated with an increase in height standard deviation score and improves patient-related outcomes compared to HD [222]. Children on HDF had improved blood pressure and hemodynamic stability, reduced inflammatory markers and lower $\beta2$-microglobulin compared to children on HD [222]. The annualised change in vascular measures correlated with improved BP control and clearances on HDF. In a post-hoc analysis of the 3H data, it was shown that children on HD had a significant and sustained increase in BP over 1 year compared to a stable BP in those on HDF, despite an equivalent dialysis dose.Improved fluid removal as well as clearance of middle molecular weight uraemic toxins by HDF were strongly correlated with improved vascular outcomes in HDF [231]. Although mechanisms of improved growth in HDF are not clear, the 3H study showed an inverse correlation between height SDS increase and serum $\beta2$-microglobulin, suggesting that clearance of middle-molecular weight compounds may partly alleviate growth hormone resistance in dialysis patients. In the HDF cohort, patient related outcome measures that are primarily associated with fluid status, such as the postdialysis recovery time, headaches, dizziness and cramps, were less frequent and severe compared to HD patients, leading to an improvement in school attendance as well as physical activity [222]. Importantly, HDF is a safe treatment, with no reduction in serum albumin levels, and no difference in the rate of change of residual renal function [222] compared to conventional HD.

Intensified Hemodialysis Options

Our current standard of three times weekly hemodialysis evolved during the 1960s from one 24 h treatment per week, to twice weekly treatments of 16–24 h each, and finally three weekly sessions of 8–10 h performed at home. By the time United States Medicare program adopted its ESKD program in 1973, the three times per weekly schedule offered the optimal balance between patient outcome, quality of life, and cost. Remarkably, the first patient treated with these prolonged sessions lived for more than a decade. More than 50 years later, similar outcomes have become difficult to achieve [232].

To improve the health of patients receiving three times weekly in-center hemodialysis, researchers have trialed alternative, intensified dialysis regimens. These methods include short daily hemodialysis, nocturnal home hemodialysis, and in-center nocturnal hemodialysis. In 2010, the Frequent Hemodialysis Network, sponsored by the National Institutes of Health, published their findings in 245 adults randomized to three times versus six times per week in-center hemodialysis. After 1 year of treatment, those in the more frequent group averaged about 5 sessions per week and demonstrated improvements in mortality, LVH, reported physical health, hypertension, and hyperphosphatemia. However, they were also more likely to receive vascular access interventions compared to the three times per week treatment group [11]. A treatment benefit was not observed among adults randomized to 6 times per week home nocturnal hemodialysis [233].

Smaller, uncontrolled studies in children have also supported the potential benefits of intensified dialysis regimens. As mentioned above, Fischbach et al. reported their experience treating 12 children (median age 7 years) in France with 5–6 times per week in center HDF. After a median follow-up of 11 months, dietary restrictions could be lifted and BP and phosphate control improved [234]. Observations by the same group have also noted decreased LVH and postdialysis fatigue with six times per week treatments [225]. In children, weekly treatment times of 15–18 h have been associated with improved growth [224, 227, 235, 236].

The success noted by the investigators in France has prompted others to trial alternative dialysis regimens in children. Four children treated at The Hospital for Sick Children had improved dietary intake, BP control, and school attendance with home nocturnal hemodialysis [237]. Calcium and phosphate metabolism improved, even requiring dialysate phosphate supplementation during therapy [83]. These experiences have been expanded to a larger group of children in Europe, resulting in no postdialysis recovery time and improved energy and quality of life. Patient selection criteria for home therapy have included weight >20 kg, adequate family support and supervision, and the necessary technology to operate the dialysis equipment [237, 238]. While the therapy may represent a 30% cost savings compared with in-center treatment, the requirements for staffing and family resources are high [237]. Future technology may allow home HD to be performed in infants.

In the United States, a published report of four children treated with 6 times per week, in-center or home hemodialysis used the NxStage™, which provides sterile dialysis fluid without the requirement for home modifications for a reverse osmosis water treatment system [239, 240]. After a 16 week pilot study, these children no longer needed antihypertensive therapy and had improved BP control as measured by 24 h ambulatory monitoring, without reporting treatment-related complications [240].In London, we have dialysed 15 children aged from 3 to 17 years on the NxStage™ system. We are currently using 3 circuits: the standard CAR172 circuit, CAR124 for those developing intradialytic thrombocytopenia and CAR125 for children weighing less than 18 kg. Routinely children start on 5 h of dialysis 4 evenings/week (except infants) [241]. From 2 months onwards, we discuss the possibility of switching to nocturnal HD where appropriate. All children report reduced or no postdialysis recovery times, greater energy and improved quality of life scores and vastly improved school attendance, social and family lives. All the children on 20 h or more of dialysis/week are free of diet and fluid restrictions; appetites have improved with better growth. Cardiac echocardiograms were normal at baseline in 6/11, in the 5 remaining signs of LVH and/or fluid overload had regressed within 6 months. PTH levels were successfully maintained within twice upper limit of normal in all except 2 teenagers who became calcium deficient on 1.5 mmol/l calcium dialysate baths [241]. In our experience, one advantage that intensified home HD holds over all other dialysis treatment is in the management of patients with ESKD and cardiac failure, where intensified dialysis prescriptions have resulted in the complete resolution of the cardiac failure [242].

Combining the benefits of more frequent treatments, the quality of life advantages offered by nocturnal therapy, and the safety and convenience of monitoring available in the clinic, investigators in Germany have reported their experience in 16 children and adolescents treated with in-center, nocturnal hemodialysis. Children were prospectively enrolled over an almost 5 year period and there were over 2000 treatments provided. Participants were treated 8 h per session for 3 days per week and each treatment was monitored by a pediatric nephrologist and 2 dialysis nurses. During the study, quality of life improved and children missed fewer days of school. Nutrition indices improved, phosphate levels decreased, and the number of antihypertensive medications decreased compared to matched control patients [243].

While pediatric studies have been mostly uncontrolled and have included a small number of subjects, most demonstrate that intensified hemodialysis is associated with improved quality of life, biochemical markers (especially phosphate clearance), growth, nutrition, and BP control [244]. Nevertheless, significant barriers exist, precluding the more wide-spread adoption of these potentially beneficial options for children with ESKD. These include financial hurdles related to treatment costs, transportation, missed work for parents, and equipment and supplies for those choosing home therapy [244]. Missed time from school and other social activities is a concern for children treated with non-nocturnal, more frequent in-center hemodialysis. We must also be mindful of patient, caregiver, and provider burnout in a patient population already struggling with the management of a very significant chronic disease [237, 239, 241, 243].

It is clear that change is needed to improve the health and survival of children with ESKD. Health-related quality of life remains poor in children with CKD, especially in those receiving HD, in whom daily life activities are greatly limited [245]. While the data suggest that the current treatment is not optimal and more intensified treatment may offer benefit, we must also not minimize the subjective input of our patients. To this end, a 16 year old female, after being switched to three times per week long nocturnal hemodialysis, noted, "regular dialysis was hell and I never want to go back to it again." [243]

Acknowledgements We thank Taylor Moatz and Denis Geary for their assistance with the prior versions of this chapter.

References

1. Kolff WJ BH. Artificial kidney: dialyzer with great area. Acta Medica Scandinav1944.
2. Mateer FMGL, Danowski TS. Hemodialysis of the uremic child. AMA Am J Dis Child. 1995;89(6):645–55.
3. Scribner BH, Buri R, Caner JE, Hegstrom R, Burnell JM. The treatment of chronic uremia by means of intermittent hemodialysis: a preliminary report. Trans Am Soc Artif Intern Organs. 1960;10-11(6):114–22.
4. Fine RNDPJ, Lieberman E, Donnell GN, Gordon A, Maxwell MH. Hemodialysis in children with chronic renal failure. Pediatrics. 1985;73(5):705–13.
5. Kjellstrand CM, Shideman JR, Santiago EA, Mauer M, Simmons RL, Buselmeier TJ. Technical advances in hemodialysis of very small pediatric patients. Proc Clin Dial Transplant Forum. 1971;1:124–32.
6. Sousa CN, Gama M, Andrade M, Faria MS, Pereira E. Haemodialysis for children under the age of two years. J Ren Care. 2008;34(1):9–13.
7. Mahan JDMM, Nevins TE. The Hickman catheter: a new hemodialysis access device for infants and small children. Kidney Int. 1983;24(5):694–7.
8. Fadrowski JJ, Hwang W, Neu AM, Fivush BA, Furth SL. Patterns of use of vascular catheters for hemodialysis in children in the United States. Am J Kidney Dis. 2009;53(1):91–8.
9. Mitsnefes MM, Laskin BL, Dahhou M, Zhang X, Foster BJ. Mortality risk among children initially treated with dialysis for end-stage kidney disease, 1990–2010. JAMA. 2013;309(18):1921.
10. Fischbach M, Edefonti A, Schroder C, Watson A. European pediatric dialysis working G. hemodialysis in children: general practical guidelines. Pediatr Nephrol. 2005;20(8):1054–66.
11. Lowrie EG, Lew NL. Commonly measured laboratory variables in hemodialysis patients: relationships among them and to death risk. Semin Nephrol. 1992;12(3):276–83.
12. Lowrie EG, Laird NM, Parker TF, Sargent JA. Effect of the hemodialysis prescription of patient morbidity: report from the National Cooperative Dialysis Study. N Engl J Med. 1981;305(20):1176–81.
13. Gotch FA, Sargent JA. A mechanistic analysis of the National Cooperative Dialysis Study (NCDS). Kidney Int. 1985;28(3):526–34.
14. Daugirdas JT. Simplified equations for monitoring kt/V, PCRn, eKt/V, and ePCRn. Adv Ren Replace Ther. 1995;2(4):295–304.
15. Geddes CC, Traynor J, Walbaum D, Fox JG, Mactier RA. A new method of post-dialysis blood urea sampling: the 'stop dialysate flow' method. Nephrol Dial Transplant. 2000;15(4):517–23.
16. Nguyen C, Bednarz D, Brier ME, Imam A, Chand DH. A comparison of laboratory values in pediatric hemodialysis patients: does day of the week matter? Nephrol Dial Transplant. 2012;27(2):816–9.
17. Goldstein SL, Sorof JM, Brewer ED. Natural logarithmic estimates of kt/V in the pediatric hemodialysis population. Am J Kidney Dis. 1999;33(3):518–22.
18. Daugirdas JT, Hanna MG, Becker-Cohen R, Langman CB. Dose of dialysis based on body surface area is markedly less in younger children than in older adolescents. Clin J Am Soc Nephrol. 2010;5(5):821–7.
19. Daugirdas JT. Second generation logarithmic estimates of single-pool variable volume Kt/V: an analysis of error. J Am Soc Nephrol. 1993;4(5):1205–13.
20. Leypoldt JK. Urea standard kt/V(urea) for assessing dialysis treatment adequacy. Hemodial Int. 2004;8(2):193–7.
21. Owen WF Jr, Lew NL, Liu Y, Lowrie EG, Lazarus JM. The urea reduction ratio and serum albumin concentration as predictors of mortality in patients undergoing hemodialysis. N Engl J Med. 1993;329(14):1001–6.
22. Eknoyan G, Beck GJ, Cheung AK, Daugirdas JT, Greene T, Kusek JW, et al. Effect of dialysis dose and membrane flux in maintenance hemodialysis. N Engl J Med. 2002;347(25):2010–9.
23. Port FK, Ashby VB, Dhingra RK, Roys EC, Wolfe RA. Dialysis dose and body mass index are strongly associated with survival in hemodialysis patients. J Am Soc Nephrol. 2002;13(4):1061–6.
24. Saran R, Bragg-Gresham JL, Levin NW, Twardowski ZJ, Wizemann V, Saito A, et al. Longer

treatment time and slower ultrafiltration in hemodialysis: associations with reduced mortality in the DOPPS. Kidney Int. 2006;69(7):1222–8.

25. Flythe JE, Curhan GC, Brunelli SM. Disentangling the ultrafiltration rate-mortality association: the respective roles of session length and weight gain. Clin J Am Soc Nephrol. 2013;8(7):1151–61.

26. Marshall MR, Byrne BG, Kerr PG, McDonald SP. Associations of hemodialysis dose and session length with mortality risk in Australian and New Zealand patients. Kidney Int. 2006;69(7): 1229–36.

27. European best practices guidelines for hemodialysis [part I]. Nephrol Dial Transplant. 2002;17(suppl7):17–20.

28. Buur T, Bradbury MG, Smye SW, Brocklebank JT. Reliability of haemodialysis urea kinetic modelling in children. Pediatr Nephrol. 1994;8(5):574–8.

29. Van Hoeck KJ, Lilien MR, Brinkman DC, Schroeder CH. Comparing a urea kinetic monitor with Daugirdas formula and dietary records in children. Pediatr Nephrol. 2000;14(4):280–3.

30. Goldstein SL. Adequacy of dialysis in children: does small solute clearance really matter? Pediatr Nephrol. 2004;19(1):1–5.

31. Ishibe SPA. Methods of assessment of volume status and intercompartmental fluid shifts in hemodialysis patients: implications in clinical practice. Semin Dial. 2004;17(1):37–43.

32. Kouw PMKJ, Cheriex EC, Olthof CG, de Vries PM, Leunissen KM. Assessment of postdialysis dry weight: a comparison of techniques. J Am Soc Nephrol. 1993;4:98–104.

33. Nishikimi TFY, Tamano K, Takahashi M, Suzuki T, Minami J, et al. Plasma brain natriuretic peptide levels in chronic hemodialysis patients: influence of coronary artery disease. Am J Kidney Dis. 2001;37:1201–8.

34. Krause I, Birk E, Davidovits M, Cleper R, Blieden L, Pinhas L, et al. Inferior vena cava diameter: a useful method for estimation of fluid status in children on haemodialysis. Nephrol Dial Transplant. 2001;16(6):1203–6.

35. Chamney PWKM, Rode C, Kleinekofort W, Wizemann V. A new technique for establishing dry weight in hemodialysis patients via whole body bioimpedance. Kidney Int. 2002;61(6):2250–8.

36. Piccoli ARB, Pillon L, Bucciante G. New method for montoring body fluid variation by bioimpedance analysis: the RXc graph. Kidney Int. 1994;46(2):534–9.

37. Zhu FKM, Sarkar S, Kaitwatcharachai C, Khilnani R, Leonard EF, et al. Adjustment of dry weight in hemodialysis patients using intradialytic continuous multifrequency bioimpedance of the calf. Int J Artif Organs. 2004;27(2):104–9.

38. Moissl U, Arias-Guillen M, Wabel P, Fontsere N, Carrera M, Campistol JM, et al. Bioimpedance-guided fluid management in hemodialysis patients. Clin J Am Soc Nephrol. 2013;8(9):1575–82.

39. Marsenic O, Booker K, Studnicka K, Wilson D, Beck A, Swanson T, et al. Use of ionic dialysance to calculate kt/V in pediatric hemodialysis. Hemodial Int. 2011;15(Suppl 1):S2–8.

40. Steuer RR, Leypoldt JK, Cheung AK, Harris DH, Conis JM. Hematocrit as an indicator of blood volume and a predictor of intradialytic morbid events. ASAIO J. 1994;40(3):M691–6.

41. Schneditz D, Roob JM, Vaclavik M, Holzer H, Kenner T. Noninvasive measurement of blood volume in hemodialysis patients. J Am Soc Nephrol. 1996;7(8):1241–4.

42. Jain SR, Smith L, Brewer ED, Goldstein SL. Noninvasive intravascular monitoring in the pediatric hemodialysis population. Pediatr Nephrol. 2001;16(1):15–8.

43. Michael MBE, Goldstein SL. Blood volume monitoring to achieve target weight in pediatric hemodialysis patients. Pediatr Nephrol. 2004;19(4):432–7.

44. Hothi DK, Harvey E, Goia CM, Geary D. Blood-volume monitoring in paediatric haemodialysis. Pediatr Nephrol. 2008;23(5):813–20.

45. Vanholder RCRS. Adequacy of dialysis: a critical analysis. Kidney Int. 1997;42(3):540–58.

46. Lacour F, Maheut H. AN 69 membrane and conversion enzyme inhibitors: prevention of anaphylactic shock by alkaline rinsing? Nephrologie. 1992;13(3):135–6.

47. Kammerl MC, Schaefer RM, Schweda F, Schreiber M, Riegger GA, Kramer BK. Extracorporal therapy with AN69 membranes in combination with ACE inhibition causing severe anaphylactoid reactions: still a current problem? Clin Nephrol. 2000;53(6):486–8.

48. John B, Anijeet HK, Ahmad R. Anaphylactic reaction during haemodialysis on AN69 membrane in a patient receiving angiotensin II receptor antagonist. Nephrol Dial Transplant. 2001;16(9):1955–6.

49. Clark WR, Macias WL, Molitoris BA, Wang NH. Plasma protein adsorption to highly permeable hemodialysis membranes. Kidney Int. 1995;48(2):481–8.

50. Henderson L. Biophysics of ultrafiltration and hemofiltration. Replacement of renal function by dialysis. 4th ed. Dordrecht: Kluwer Academic Publishers; 1996. p. 114–45.

51. Bloembergen WE, Hakim RM, Stannard DC, Held PJ, Wolfe RA, Agodoa LY, et al. Relationship of dialysis membrane and cause-specific mortality. Am J Kidney Dis. 1999;33(1):1–10.

52. Woods HF, Nandakumar M. Improved outcome for haemodialysis patients treated with high-flux membranes. Nephrol Dial Transplant. 2000;15(Suppl 1):36–42.

53. Coppo R, Amore A, Cirina P, Scelfo B, Giacchino F, Comune L, et al. Bradykinin and nitric oxide generation by dialysis membranes can be blunted by alkaline rinsing solutions. Kidney Int. 2000;58(2):881–8.

54. Polaschegg HD. Hemodialysis machine technology: a global overview. Expert Rev Med Devices. 2010;7(6):793–810.

55. Ward RA. Ultrapure dialysate. Semin Dial. 2004;17(6):489–97.

56. Laude-Sharp M, Caroff M, Simard L, Pusineri C, Kazatchkine MD, Haeffner-Cavaillon N. Induction of IL-1 during hemodialysis: transmembrane passage of intact endotoxins (LPS). Kidney Int. 1990;38(6):1089–94.

57. Urena P, Herbelin A, Zingraff J, Lair M, Man NK, Descamps-Latscha B, et al. Permeability of cellulosic and non-cellulosic membranes to endotoxin subunits and cytokine production during in-vitro haemodialysis. Nephrol Dial Transplant. 1992;7(1):16–28.

58. Lonnemann G, Sereni L, Lemke HD, Tetta C. Pyrogen retention by highly permeable synthetic membranes during in vitro dialysis. Artif Organs. 2001;25(12):951–60.

59. Jaber BL, Gonski JA, Cendoroglo M, Balakrishnan VS, Razeghi P, Dinarello CA, et al. New polyether sulfone dialyzers attenuate passage of cytokine-inducing substances from pseudomonas aeruginosa contaminated dialysate. Blood Purif. 1998;16(4):210–9.

60. Lonnemann G, Behme TC, Lenzner B, Floege J, Schulze M, Colton CK, et al. Permeability of dialyzer membranes to TNF alpha-inducing substances derived from water bacteria. Kidney Int. 1992;42(1):61–8.

61. Schindler R, Krautzig S, Lufft V, Lonnemann G, Mahiout A, Marra MN, et al. Induction of interleukin-1 and interleukin-1 receptor antagonist during contaminated in-vitro dialysis with whole blood. Nephrol Dial Transplant. 1996;11(1):101–8.

62. Boccato C, Evans D, Lucena R, Vienken J. Good Dialysis Practice., vol. 8. Lengerich: Pabst Science Publishers; 2015.

63. European Directorate for the Quality of Medicines. Purified water. In: European Pharmacopoeia 9.4; 2018: 5665-5667. https://www.edqm.eu/sites/default/files/institutional-brochure-edqm.pdf. Accessed 7 July 2019

64. Moret K, Aalten J, van den Wall BW, Gerlag P, Beerenhout C, van der Sande F, et al. The effect of sodium profiling and feedback technologies on plasma conductivity and ionic mass balance: a study in hypotension-prone dialysis patients. Nephrol Dial Transplant. 2006;21(1):138–44.

65. Sadowski RH, Allred EN, Jabs K. Sodium modeling ameliorates intradialytic and interdialytic symptoms in young hemodialysis patients. J Am Soc Nephrol. 1993;4(5):1192–8.

66. Song JH, Lee SW, Suh CK, Kim MJ. Time-averaged concentration of dialysate sodium relates with sodium load and interdialytic weight gain during sodium-profiling hemodialysis. Am J Kidney Dis. 2002;40(2):291–301.

67. de Paula FM, Peixoto AJ, Pinto LV, Dorigo D, Patricio PJ, Santos SF. Clinical consequences of an individualized dialysate sodium prescription in hemodialysis patients. Kidney Int. 2004;66(3):1232–8.

68. Song JH, Park GH, Lee SY, Lee SW, Lee SW, Kim MJ. Effect of sodium balance and the combination of ultrafiltration profile during sodium profiling hemodialysis on the maintenance of the quality of dialysis and sodium and fluid balances. J Am Soc Nephrol. 2005;16(1):237–46.

69. Covic A, Diaconita M, Gusbeth-Tatomir P, Covic M, Botezan A, Ungureanu G, et al. Haemodialysis increases QT(c) interval but not QT(c) dispersion in ESKD patients without manifest cardiac disease. Nephrol Dial Transplant. 2002;17(12):2170–7.

70. Ichikawa H, Nagake Y, Makino H. Signal averaged electrocardiography (SAECG) in patients on hemodialysis. J Med. 1997;28(3–4):229–43.

71. Blumberg A, Roser HW, Zehnder C, Müller-Brand J. Plasma potassium in patients with terminal renal failure during and after haemodialysis; relationship with dialytic potassium removal and total body potassium. Nephrol Dial Transplant. 1997;12:1629–34.

72. Zehnder C, Gutzwiller JP, Huber A, Schindler C, Schneditz D. Low-potassium and glucose free dialysis maintains urea but enhances potassium removal. Nephrol Dial Transplant. 2001;16:78–84.

73. Basile C, Libutti P, Lisi P, Teutonico A, Vernaglione L, Casucci F, Lomonte C. Ranking of factors determining potassium mass balance in bicarbonate haemodialysis. Nephrol Dial Transplant. 2015;30:505–13.

74. Dolan MJ, Whipp BJ, Davidson WD, Weitzman RE, Wasserman K. Hypopnea associated with acetate hemodialysis: carbon dioxide-flow-dependent ventilation. N Engl J Med. 1981;305(2):72–5.

75. Kraut JA. Disturbances of acid-base balance and bone disease in end-stage renal disease. Semin Dial. 2000;13(4):261–6.

76. Mehrotra R, Kopple JD, Wolfson M. Metabolic acidosis in maintenance dialysis patients: clinical considerations. Kidney Int Suppl. 2003;88:S13–25.

77. Sonikian M, Gogusev J, Zingraff J, Loric S, Quednau B, Bessou G, et al. Potential effect of metabolic acidosis on beta 2-microglobulin generation: in vivo and in vitro studies. J Am Soc Nephrol. 1996;7(2):350–6.

78. Uribarri J, Levin NW, Delmez J, Depner TA, Ornt D, Owen W, et al. Association of acidosis and nutritional parameters in hemodialysis patients. Am J Kidney Dis. 1999;34(3):493–9.

79. Heguilen RM, Sciurano C, Bellusci AD, Fried P, Mittelman G, Rosa Diez G, et al. The faster potassium-lowering effect of high dialysate bicarbonate concentrations in chronic haemodialysis patients. Nephrol Dial Transplant. 2005;20(3):591–7.

80. Ahmad S, Callan R, Cole JJ, Blagg CR. Dialysate made from dry chemicals using citric acid increases dialysis dose. Am J Kidney Dis. 2000;35(3):493–9.

81. Fernandez E, Borras M, Pais B, Montoliu J. Low-calcium dialysate stimulates parathormone secretion and its long-term use worsens secondary hyperparathyroidism. J Am Soc Nephrol. 1995;6(1):132–5.

82. Fellner SK, Lang RM, Neumann A, Spencer KT, Bushinsky DA, Borow KM. Physiological mechanisms for calcium-induced changes in systemic arterial pressure in stable dialysis patients. Hypertension. 1989;13(3):213–8.

83. Hothi DK, Harvey E, Piva E, Keating L, Secker D, Geary DF. Calcium and phosphate balance in adolescents on home nocturnal haemodialysis. Pediatr Nephrol. 2006;21(6):835–41.

84. Fischbach M, Boudailliez B, Foulard M. Phosphate end dialysis value: a misleading parameter of hemodialysis efficiency. French Society for Pediatric Nephrology. Pediatr Nephrol. 1997;11(2):193–5.

85. Pogglitsch H, Estelberger W, Petek W, Zitta S, Ziak E. Relationship between generation and plasma concentration of anorganic phosphorus. In vivo studies on dialysis patients and in vitro studies on erythrocytes. Int J Artif Organs. 1989;12(8):524–32.

86. Spalding EM, Chamney PW, Farrington K. Phosphate kinetics during hemodialysis: evidence for biphasic regulation. Kidney Int. 2002;61(2):655–67.

87. Leypoldt JK, Cheung AK, Agodoa LY, Daugirdas JT, Greene T, Keshaviah PR. Hemodialyzer mass transfer-area coefficients for urea increase at high dialysate flow rates. The hemodialysis (HEMO) study. Kidney Int. 1997;51(6):2013–7.

88. Schneditz D, Kaufman AM, Polaschegg HD, Levin NW, Daugirdas JT. Cardiopulmonary recirculation during hemodialysis. Kidney Int. 1992;42(6):1450–6.

89. Van Someren EJ, Raymann RJ, Scherder EJ, Daanen HA, Swaab DF. Circadian and age-related modulation of thermoreception and temperature regulation: mechanisms and functional implications. Ageing Res Rev. 2002;1(4):721–78.

90. Bennett LA, Johnson JM, Stephens DP, Saad AR, Kellogg DL Jr. Evidence for a role for vasoactive intestinal peptide in active vasodilatation in the cutaneous vasculature of humans. J Physiol. 2003;552(Pt 1):223–32.

91. Johnson JMPD. Section 4: environmental physiology. In: Fregly MJ, Blatteis CM, editors. Handbook of physiology. New York: Oxford University Press; 1996. p. 215–43.

92. Fine A, Penner B. The protective effect of cool dialysate is dependent on patients' predialysis temperature. Am J Kidney Dis. 1996;28(2):262–5.

93. Ikizler TA, Wingard RL, Sun M, Harvell J, Parker RA, Hakim RM. Increased energy expenditure in hemodialysis patients. J Am Soc Nephrol. 1996;7(12):2646–53.

94. Rosales LM, Schneditz D, Chmielnicki H, Shaw K, Levin NW. Exercise and extracorporeal blood cooling during hemodialysis. ASAIO J. 1998;44(5):M574–8.

95. Maggiore Q, Dattolo P, Piacenti M, Morales MA, Pelosi G, Pizzarelli F, et al. Thermal balance and dialysis hypotension. Int J Artif Organs. 1995;18(9):518–25.

96. Nelson-Piercy C. Hazards of heparin: allergy, heparin-induced thrombocytopenia and osteoporosis. Baillieres Clin Obstet Gynaecol. 1997;11(3):489–509.

97. Greer IA. Exploring the role of low-molecular-weight heparins in pregnancy. Semin Thromb Hemost. 2002;28(Suppl 3):25–31.

98. Geary DF, Gajaria M, Fryer-Keene S, Willumsen J. Low-dose and heparin-free hemodialysis in children. Pediatr Nephrol. 1991;5(2):220–4.

99. Bohler J, Schollmeyer P, Dressel B, Dobos G, Horl WH. Reduction of granulocyte activation during hemodialysis with regional citrate anticoagulation: dissociation of complement activation and neutropenia from neutrophil degranulation. J Am Soc Nephrol. 1996;7(2):234–41.

100. Ljungberg B, Jacobson SH, Lins LE, Pejler G. Effective anticoagulation by a low molecular weight heparin (Fragmin) in hemodialysis with a highly permeable polysulfone membrane. Clin Nephrol. 1992;38(2):97–100.

101. Klingel R, Schwarting A, Lotz J, Eckert M, Hohmann V, Hafner G. Safety and efficacy of single bolus anticoagulation with enoxaparin for chronic hemodialysis. Results of an open-label post-certification study. Kidney Blood Press Res. 2004;27(4):211–7.

102. Bianchetti MG, Speck S, Muller R, Oetliker OH. Simple coagulation prophylaxis using low-molecular heparin enoxaparin in pediatric hemodialysis. Schweiz Rundsch Med Prax. 1990;79(23):730–1.

103. Davenport A. Alternatives to standard unfractionated heparin for pediatric hemodialysis treatments. Pediatr Nephrol. 2012;27(10):1869–79.

104. Evenepoel P, Maes B, Vanwalleghem J, Kuypers D, Messiaen T, Vanrenterghem Y. Regional citrate anticoagulation for hemodialysis using a conventional calcium-containing dialysate. Am J Kidney Dis. 2002;39(2):315–23.

105. Koster A, Meyer O, Hausmann H, Kuppe H, Hetzer R, Mertzlufft F. In vitro cross-reactivity of danaparoid sodium in patients with heparin-induced thrombocytopenia type II undergoing cardiovascular surgery. J Clin Anesth. 2000;12(4):324–7.

106. Fischer KG. Hirudin in renal insufficiency. Semin Thromb Hemost. 2002;28(5):467–82.

107. Greinacher A, Lubenow N, Eichler P. Anaphylactic and anaphylactoid reactions associated with lepirudin in patients with heparin-induced thrombocytopenia. Circulation. 2003;108(17):2062–5.

108. Lim W, Cook DJ, Crowther MA. Safety and efficacy of low molecular weight heparins for hemodialysis in patients with end-stage renal failure: a meta-analysis of randomized trials. J Am Soc Nephrol. 2004;15(12):3192–206.

109. Woolliscroft JO, Fox IH. Increased body fluid purine levels during hypotensive events. Evidence for ATP degradation. Am J Med. 1986;81(3):472–8.

110. Converse RL Jr, Jacobsen TN, Jost CM, Toto RD, Grayburn PA, Obregon TM, et al. Paradoxical

withdrawal of reflex vasoconstriction as a cause of hemodialysis-induced hypotension. J Clin Invest. 1992;90(5):1657–65.

111. Ligtenberg G, Barnas MG, Koomans HA. Intradialytic hypotension: new insights into the mechanism of vasovagal syncope. Nephrol Dial Transplant. 1998;13(11):2745–7.

112. Shinzato T, Miwa M, Nakai S, Morita H, Odani H, Inoue I, et al. Role of adenosine in dialysis-induced hypotension. J Am Soc Nephrol. 1994;4(12):1987–94.

113. Prakash S, Garg AX, Heidenheim AP, House AA. Midodrine appears to be safe and effective for dialysis-induced hypotension: a systematic review. Nephrol Dial Transplant. 2004;19(10):2553–8.

114. Donauer J, Kolblin D, Bek M, Krause A, Bohler J. Ultrafiltration profiling and measurement of relative blood volume as strategies to reduce hemodialysis-related side effects. Am J Kidney Dis. 2000;36(1):115–23.

115. Ronco C, Feriani M, Chiaramonte S, Conz P, Brendolan A, Bragantini L, et al. Impact of high blood flows on vascular stability in haemodialysis. Nephrol Dial Transplant. 1990;5(Suppl 1):109–14.

116. Port S, Garfinkel A, Boyle N. There is a non-linear relationship between mortality and blood pressure. Eur Heart J. 2000;21(20):1635–8.

117. Foley RN, Parfrey PS, Harnett JD, Kent GM, Murray DC, Barre PE. Impact of hypertension on cardiomyopathy, morbidity and mortality in end-stage renal disease. Kidney Int. 1996;49(5):1379–85.

118. Zager PG, Nikolic J, Brown RH, Campbell MA, Hunt WC, Peterson D, et al. "U" curve association of blood pressure and mortality in hemodialysis patients. Medical directors of dialysis clinic. Inc Kidney Int. 1998;54(2):561–9.

119. Conlon PJ, Krucoff MW, Minda S, Schumm D, Schwab SJ. Incidence and long-term significance of transient ST segment deviation in hemodialysis patients. Clin Nephrol. 1998;49(4):236–9.

120. Foley RN, Parfrey PS, Kent GM, Harnett JD, Murray DC, Barre PE. Serial change in echocardiographic parameters and cardiac failure in end-stage renal disease. J Am Soc Nephrol. 2000;11(5):912–6.

121. Tarakcioglu M, Erbagci A, Cekmen M, Usalan C, Cicek H, Ozaslan J, et al. Acute effect of haemodialysis on serum markers of myocardial damage. Int J Clin Pract. 2002;56(5):328–32.

122. Wayand D, Baum H, Schatzle G, Scharf J, Neumeier D. Cardiac troponin T and I in end-stage renal failure. Clin Chem. 2000;46(9):1345–50.

123. Lipshultz SE, Somers MJ, Lipsitz SR, Colan SD, Jabs K, Rifai N. Serum cardiac troponin and subclinical cardiac status in pediatric chronic renal failure. Pediatrics. 2003;112(1 Pt 1):79–86.

124. McIntyre CW, Burton JO, Selby NM, Leccisotti L, Korsheed S, Baker CS, et al. Hemodialysis-induced cardiac dysfunction is associated with an acute reduction in global and segmental myocardial blood flow. Clin J Am Soc Nephrol. 2008;3(1):19–26.

125. Burton JO, Jefferies HJ, Selby NM, McIntyre CW. Hemodialysis-induced cardiac injury: determinants and associated outcomes. Clin J Am Soc Nephrol. 2009;4(5):914–20.

126. Braunwald E, Kloner RA. The stunned myocardium: prolonged, postischemic ventricular dysfunction. Circulation. 1982;66(6):1146–9.

127. Wijns W, Vatner SF, Camici PG. Hibernating myocardium. N Engl J Med. 1998;339(3):173–81.

128. Burton JO, Korsheed S, Grundy BJ, McIntyre CW. Hemodialysis-induced left ventricular dysfunction is associated with an increase in ventricular arrhythmias. Ren Fail. 2008;30(7):701–9.

129. Burton JO, Jefferies HJ, Selby NM, McIntyre CW. Hemodialysis-induced repetitive myocardial injury results in global and segmental reduction in systolic cardiac function. Clin J Am Soc Nephrol. 2009;4(12):1925–31.

130. U.S. Renal Data System. USRDS 2007 Annual Data Report: Atlas of Chronic Kidney Disease and End-Stage Renal Disease in the United States. Bethesda, MD: National Institutes of Health, National Institute of Diabetes and Digestive and Kidney Diseases. p. 2007.

131. Haq IJH, Burton JO, Mcintyre RCW. Left atrial volume is associated with hemodialysis-induced ischaemic cardiac injury (myocardial stunning) and reduced survival. Am Soc Nephrol. 2009:F-PO1431.

132. Hothi DK, Rees L, McIntyre CW, Marek J. Hemodialysis-induced acute myocardial dyssynchronous impairment in children. Nephron Clin Pract. 2013;123(1–2):83–92.

133. Hothi DK, Rees L, Marek J, Burton J, McIntyre CW. Pediatric myocardial stunning underscores the cardiac toxicity of conventional hemodialysis treatments. Clin J Am Soc Nephrol. 2009;4(4):790–7.

134. Selby NM, McIntyre CW. Peritoneal dialysis is not associated with myocardial stunning. Perit Dial Int. 2011;31(1):27–33.

135. McIntyre CW, Harrison LE, Eldehni MT, Jefferies HJ, Szeto CC, John SG, et al. Circulating endotoxemia: a novel factor in systemic inflammation and cardiovascular disease in chronic kidney disease. Clin J Am Soc Nephrol. 2011;6(1):133–41.

136. Dubin RF, Teerlink JR, Schiller NB, Alokozai D, Peralta CA, Johansen KL. Association of segmental wall motion abnormalities occurring during hemodialysis with post-dialysis fatigue. Nephrol Dial Transplant. 2013;28(10):2580–5.

137. Jefferies HJ, Burton JO, McIntyre CW. Individualised dialysate temperature improves intradialytic haemodynamics and abrogates haemodialysis-induced myocardial stunning, without compromising tolerability. Blood Purif. 2011;32(1):63–8.

138. Jefferies HJ, Virk B, Schiller B, Moran J, McIntyre CW. Frequent hemodialysis schedules are associated with reduced levels of dialysis-induced cardiac injury (myocardial stunning). Clin J Am Soc Nephrol. 2011;6(6):1326–32.

139. Selby NM, Lambie SH, Camici PG, Baker CS, McIntyre CW. Occurrence of regional left ventricular dysfunction in patients undergoing standard and biofeedback dialysis. Am J Kidney Dis. 2006;47(5):830–41.

140. Kramer AM, van Stralen KJ, Jager KJ, Schaefer F, Verrina E, Seeman T, et al. Demographics of blood pressure and hypertension in children on renal replacement therapy in Europe. Kidney Int. 2011;80(10):1092–8.

141. Lin JJ, Mitsnefes MM, Smoyer WE, Valentini RP. Antihypertensive prescription in pediatric dialysis: a practitioner survey by the Midwest pediatric nephrology consortium study. Hemodial Int. 2009;13(3):307–15.

142. Chen J, Gul A, Sarnak MJ. Management of intradialytic hypertension: the ongoing challenge. Semin Dial. 2006;19(2):141–5.

143. Dolson GM, Ellis KJ, Bernardo MV, Prakash R, Adrogue HJ. Acute decreases in serum potassium augment blood pressure. Am J Kidney Dis. 1995;26(2):321–6.

144. Cirit M, Akcicek F, Terzioglu E, Soydas C, Ok E, Ozbasli CF, et al. 'Paradoxical' rise in blood pressure during ultrafiltration in dialysis patients. Nephrol Dial Transplant. 1995;10(8):1417–20.

145. Klein IH, Ligtenberg G, Oey PL, Koomans HA, Blankestijn PJ. Enalapril and losartan reduce sympathetic hyperactivity in patients with chronic renal failure. J Am Soc Nephrol. 2003;14(2):425–30.

146. Blankestijn PJ. Sympathetic hyperactivity in chronic kidney disease. Nephrol Dial Transplant. 2004;19(6):1354–7.

147. Hansen J, Victor RG. Direct measurement of sympathetic activity: new insights into disordered blood pressure regulation in chronic renal failure. Curr Opin Nephrol Hypertens. 1994;3(6):636–43.

148. Koomans HA, Blankestijn PJ, Joles JA. Sympathetic hyperactivity in chronic renal failure: a wake-up call. J Am Soc Nephrol. 2004;15(3):524–37.

149. Neumann J, Ligtenberg G, Klein II, Koomans HA, Blankestijn PJ. Sympathetic hyperactivity in chronic kidney disease: pathogenesis, clinical relevance, and treatment. Kidney Int. 2004;65(5):1568–76.

150. El-Shafey EM, El-Nagar GF, Selim MF, El-Sorogy HA, Sabry AA. Is there a role for endothelin-1 in the hemodynamic changes during hemodialysis? Clin Exp Nephrol. 2008;12(5):370–5.

151. Raj DS, Vincent B, Simpson K, Sato E, Jones KL, Welbourne TC, et al. Hemodynamic changes during hemodialysis: role of nitric oxide and endothelin. Kidney Int. 2002;61(2):697–704.

152. Surdacki A, Sulowicz W, Wieczorek-Surdacka E, Herman ZS. Effect of a hemodialysis session on plasma levels of endothelin-1 in hypertensive and normotensive subjects with end-stage renal failure. Nephron. 1999;81(1):31–6.

153. Chou KJ, Lee PT, Chen CL, Chiou CW, Hsu CY, Chung HM, et al. Physiological changes during hemodialysis in patients with intradialysis hypertension. Kidney Int. 2006;69(10):1833–8.

154. Pearl RJ, Papageorgiou PC, Goldman M, Amfilochiadis AA, Boomsma F, Rojkjaer R, et al. Possible role of new pressor protein in hypertensive anephric hemodialysis patients. Pediatr Nephrol. 2003;18(10):1025–31.

155. Mitsnefes MM, Daniels SR, Schwartz SM, Khoury P, Strife CF. Changes in left ventricular mass in children and adolescents during chronic dialysis. Pediatr Nephrol. 2001;16(4):318–23.

156. Ulinski T, Genty J, Viau C, Tillous-Borde I, Deschenes G. Reduction of left ventricular hypertrophy in children undergoing hemodialysis. Pediatr Nephrol. 2006;21(8):1171–8.

157. Mitsnefes MM, Kimball TR, Kartal J, Witt SA, Glascock BJ, Khoury PR, et al. Progression of left ventricular hypertrophy in children with early chronic kidney disease: 2-year follow-up study. J Pediatr. 2006;149(5):671–5.

158. Faul C, Amaral AP, Oskouei B, Hu MC, Sloan A, Isakova T, et al. FGF23 induces left ventricular hypertrophy. J Clin Invest. 2011;121(11):4393–408.

159. Colan SD, Sanders SP, Ingelfinger JR, Harmon W. Left ventricular mechanics and contractile state in children and young adults with end-stage renal disease: effect of dialysis and renal transplantation. J Am Coll Cardiol. 1987;10(5):1085–94.

160. Boulanger CM, Amabile N, Guerin AP, Pannier B, Leroyer AS, Mallat CN, et al. In vivo shear stress determines circulating levels of endothelial microparticles in end-stage renal disease. Hypertension. 2007;49(4):902–8.

161. Choi JH, Kim KL, Huh W, Kim B, Byun J, Suh W, et al. Decreased number and impaired angiogenic function of endothelial progenitor cells in patients with chronic renal failure. Arterioscler Thromb Vasc Biol. 2004;24(7):1246–52.

162. Herbrig K, Pistrosch F, Oelschlaegel U, Wichmann G, Wagner A, Foerster S, et al. Increased total number but impaired migratory activity and adhesion of endothelial progenitor cells in patients on long-term hemodialysis. Am J Kidney Dis. 2004;44(5):840–9.

163. Westerweel PE, Hoefer IE, Blankestijn PJ, de Bree P, Groeneveld D, van Oostrom O, et al. End-stage renal disease causes an imbalance between endothelial and smooth muscle progenitor cells. Am J Physiol Renal Physiol. 2007;292(4):F1132–40.

164. Kari JA, Donald AE, Vallance DT, Bruckdorfer KR, Leone A, Mullen MJ, et al. Physiology and biochemistry of endothelial function in children with chronic renal failure. Kidney Int. 1997;52(2):468–72.

165. Lilien MR, Koomans HA, Schroder CH. Hemodialysis acutely impairs endothelial function in children. Pediatr Nephrol. 2005;20(2):200–4.

166. Chan CT, Li SH, Verma S. Nocturnal hemodialysis is associated with restoration of impaired endothelial progenitor cell biology in end-stage renal disease. Am J Physiol Renal Physiol. 2005;289(4):F679–84.

167. Ramirez R, Carracedo J, Merino A, Nogueras S, Alvarez-Lara MA, Rodriguez M, et al. Microinflammation induces endothelial damage in hemodialysis patients: the role of convective transport. Kidney Int. 2007;72(1):108–13.

168. Bleyer AJ, Hartman J, Brannon PC, Reeves-Daniel A, Satko SG, Russell G. Characteristics of sudden death in hemodialysis patients. Kidney Int. 2006;69(12):2268–73.

169. Herzog CA, Mangrum JM, Passman R. Sudden cardiac death and dialysis patients. Semin Dial. 2008;21(4):300–7.

170. Karnik JA, Young BS, Lew NL, Herget M, Dubinsky C, Lazarus JM, et al. Cardiac arrest and sudden death in dialysis units. Kidney Int. 2001;60(1):350–7.

171. Kovesdy CP, Regidor DL, Mehrotra R, Jing J, McAllister CJ, Greenland S, et al. Serum and dialysate potassium concentrations and survival in hemodialysis patients. Clin J Am Soc Nephrol. 2007;2(5):999–1007.

172. Ganesh SK, Stack AG, Levin NW, Hulbert-Shearon T, Port FK. Association of elevated serum PO(4), ca × PO(4) product, and parathyroid hormone with cardiac mortality risk in chronic hemodialysis patients. J Am Soc Nephrol. 2001;12(10):2131–8.

173. Oh J, Wunsch R, Turzer M, Bahner M, Raggi P, Querfeld U, et al. Advanced coronary and carotid arteriopathy in young adults with childhood-onset chronic renal failure. Circulation. 2002;106(1):100–5.

174. Shroff RC, Donald AE, Hiorns MP, Watson A, Feather S, Milford D, et al. Mineral metabolism and vascular damage in children on dialysis. J Am Soc Nephrol. 2007;18(11):2996–3003.

175. Shroff R, Egerton M, Bridel M, Shah V, Donald AE, Cole TJ, et al. A bimodal association of vitamin D levels and vascular disease in children on dialysis. J Am Soc Nephrol. 2008;19(6):1239–46.

176. Litwin M, Wuhl E, Jourdan C, Trelewicz J, Niemirska A, Fahr K, et al. Altered morphological properties of large arteries in children with chronic renal failure and after renal transplantation. J Am Soc Nephrol. 2005;16(5):1494–500.

177. Charitaki E, Davenport A. Do higher dialysate calcium concentrations increase vascular stiffness in haemodialysis patients as measured by aortic pulse wave velocity? BMC Nephrol. 2013;14(1):189.

178. Calabro P, Willerson JT, Yeh ET. Inflammatory cytokines stimulated C-reactive protein production by human coronary artery smooth muscle cells. Circulation. 2003;108(16):1930–2.

179. Docci D, Bilancioni R, Buscaroli A, Baldrati L, Capponcini C, Mengozzi S, et al. Elevated serum levels of C-reactive protein in hemodialysis patients. Nephron. 1990;56(4):364–7.

180. Panichi V, Migliori M, De Pietro S, Taccola D, Bianchi AM, Giovannini L, et al. C-reactive protein and interleukin-6 levels are related to renal function in predialytic chronic renal failure. Nephron. 2002;91(4):594–600.

181. McIntyre C, Harper I, Macdougall IC, Raine AE, Williams A, Baker LR. Serum C-reactive protein as a marker for infection and inflammation in regular dialysis patients. Clin Nephrol. 1997;48(6):371–4.

182. Sezer S, Kulah E, Ozdemir FN, Tutal E, Arat Z, Haberal M. Clinical consequences of intermittent elevation of C-reactive protein levels in hemodialysis patients. Transplant Proc. 2004;36(1):38–40.

183. Youssef DM, Elshal AS, Abo Elazem AA. Assessment of immune status in relation to vitamin D levels in children on regular hemodialysis. Saudi J Kidney Dis Transpl. 2012;23(2):267–73.

184. Chang JW, Yang WS, Min WK, Lee SK, Park JS, Kim SB. Effects of simvastatin on high-sensitivity C-reactive protein and serum albumin in hemodialysis patients. Am J Kidney Dis. 2002;39(6):1213–7.

185. Vernaglione L, Cristofano C, Muscogiuri P, Chimienti S. Does atorvastatin influence serum C-reactive protein levels in patients on long-term hemodialysis? Am J Kidney Dis. 2004;43(3):471–8.

186. Hyun HS, Paik KH, Cho HY. P-Cresyl sulfate and indoxyl sulfate in pediatric patients on chronic dialysis. Korean J Pediatr. 2013;56(4):159–64.

187. Srivaths PR, Wong C, Goldstein SL. Nutrition aspects in children receiving maintenance hemodialysis: impact on outcome. Pediatr Nephrol. 2009;24(5):951–7.

188. Franke D, Winkel S, Gellermann J, Querfeld U, Pape L, Ehrich JH, et al. Growth and maturation improvement in children on renal replacement therapy over the past 20 years. Pediatr Nephrol. 2013;28(10):2043–51.

189. Srivaths PR, Sutherland S, Alexander S, Goldstein SL. Two-point normalized protein catabolic rate overestimates nPCR in pediatric hemodialysis patients. Pediatr Nephrol. 2013;28(5):797–801.

190. Goldstein SL, Baronette S, Gambrell TV, Currier H, Brewer ED. nPCR assessment and IDPN treatment of malnutrition in pediatric hemodialysis patients. Pediatr Nephrol. 2002;17(7):531–4.

191. Grupe WE, Harmon WE, Spinozzi NS. Protein and energy requirements in children receiving chronic hemodialysis. Kidney Int Suppl. 1983;15:S6–10.

192. Youssef DM. Results of recombinant growth hormone treatment in children with end-stage renal disease on regular hemodialysis. Saudi J Kidney Dis Transpl. 2012;23(4):755–64.

193. Evans AM, Faull RJ, Nation RL, Prasad S, Elias T, Reuter SE, et al. Impact of hemodialysis on endogenous plasma and muscle carnitine levels in patients with end-stage renal disease. Kidney Int. 2004;66(4):1527–34.

194. Evans A. Dialysis-related carnitine disorder and levocarnitine pharmacology. Am J Kidney Dis. 2003;41(4 Suppl 4):S13–26.

195. Miller B, Ahmad S. A review of the impact of L-carnitine therapy on patient functionality in main-

tenance hemodialysis. Am J Kidney Dis. 2003;41(4 Suppl 4):S44–8.

196. Eknoyan G, Latos DL, Lindberg J. National Kidney Foundation carnitine consensus C. practice recommendations for the use of L-carnitine in dialysis-related carnitine disorder. National Kidney Foundation carnitine consensus conference. Am J Kidney Dis. 2003;41(4):868–76.

197. Wald DS, Law M, Morris JK. Homocysteine and cardiovascular disease: evidence on causality from a meta-analysis. BMJ. 2002;325(7374):1202.

198. van Guldener C. Why is homocysteine elevated in renal failure and what can be expected from homocysteine-lowering? Nephrol Dial Transplant. 2006;21(5):1161–6.

199. Scholze A, Rinder C, Beige J, Riezler R, Zidek W, Tepel M. Acetylcysteine reduces plasma homocysteine concentration and improves pulse pressure and endothelial function in patients with end-stage renal failure. Circulation. 2004;109(3):369–74.

200. House AA, Wells GA, Donnelly JG, Nadler SP, Hebert PC. Randomized trial of high-flux vs low-flux haemodialysis: effects on homocysteine and lipids. Nephrol Dial Transplant. 2000;15(7):1029–34.

201. Henderson LW, Colton CK, Ford CA. Kinetics of hemodiafiltration. II. Clinical characterization of a new blood cleansing modality. J Lab Clin Med. 1975;85:372–91.

202. Blankestijn PJ, Ledebo I, Canaud B. Hemodiafiltration: clinical evidence and remaining questions. Kidney Int. 2010;77:581–7.

203. Tattersall JE, Ward RA. Online haemodiafiltration: definition, dose quantification and safety revisited. Nephrol Dial Transplant. 2013;28:542–50.

204. Eknoyan G, Beck GJ, Cheung AK, Daugirdas JT, Greene T, Kusek JW, Allon M, Bailey J, Delmez JA, Depner TA, Dwyer JT, Levey AS, Levin NW, Milford E, Ornt DB, Rocco MV, Schulman G, Schwab SJ, Teehan BP, Toto R. Effect of dialysis dose and membrane flux in maintenance hemodialysis. N Engl J Med. 2002;347:2010–9.

205. Grooteman MP, van den Dorpel MA, Bots ML, Penne EL, van der Weerd NC, Mazairac AH, den Hoedt CH, van der Tweel I, Levesque R, Nube MJ, Ter Wee PM, Blankestijn PJ. Effect of online hemodiafiltration on all-cause mortality and cardiovascular outcomes. J Am Soc Nephrol. 2012;23:1087–96.

206. Maduell F, Moreso F, Pons M, Ramos R, Mora-Macia J, Carreras J, Soler J, Torres F, Campistol JM, Martinez-Castelao A. High-efficiency postdilution online hemodiafiltration reduces all-cause mortality in hemodialysis patients. J Am Soc Nephrol. 2013;24:487–97.

207. Ok E, Asci G, Toz H, Ok ES, Kircelli F, Yilmaz M, Hur E, Demirci MS, Demirci C, Duman S, Basci A, Adam SM, Isik IO, Zengin M, Suleymanlar G, Yilmaz ME, Ozkahya M. Mortality and cardiovascular events in online haemodiafiltration (OL-HDF) compared with high-flux dialysis: results from the Turkish OL-HDF study. Nephrol Dial Transplant. 2013;28:192–202.

208. Peters SA, Bots ML, Canaud B, Davenport A, Grooteman MP, Kircelli F, Locatelli F, Maduell F, Morena M, Nube MJ, Ok E, Torres F, Woodward M, Blankestijn PJ. Haemodiafiltration and mortality in end-stage kidney disease patients: a pooled individual participant data analysis from four randomized controlled trials. Nephrol Dial Transplant. 2016;31:978–84.

209. Ronco C. Backfiltration: a controversial issue in modern dialysis. Int J Artif Organs. 1988;11:69–74.

210. Ward RA, Beck W, Bernardo AA, Alves FC, Stenvinkel P, Lindholm B. Hypoalbuminemia: a price worth paying for improved dialytic removal of middle-molecular-weight uremic toxins? Nephrol Dial Transplant. 2019;34(6):901–7.

211. Boure T, Vanholder R. Which dialyser membrane to choose? Nephrol Dial Transplant. 2004;19:293–6.

212. Ronco C, Clark WR. Haemodialysis membranes. Nat Rev Nephrol. 2018;14:394–410.

213. Canaud B, Kooman J, Selby NM, Taal M, Francis S, Kopperschmidt P, Maierhofer A, Kotanko P, Titze J. Sodium and water handling during hemodialysis: new pathophysiologic insights and management approaches for improving outcomes in end-stage kidney disease. Kidney Int. 2019;95:296–309.

214. Chapdelaine I, de Roij van Zuijdewijn CL, Mostovaya IM, Levesque R, Davenport A, Blankestijn PJ, Wanner C, Nube MJ, Grooteman MP, Blankestijn PJ, Davenport A, Basile C, Locatelli F, Maduell F, Mitra S, Ronco C, Shroff R, Tattersall J, Wanner C. Optimization of the convection volume in online post-dilution haemodiafiltration: practical and technical issues. Clin Kidney J. 2015;8:191–8.

215. Mostovaya IM, Grooteman MP, Basile C, Davenport A, de Roij van Zuijdewijn CL, Wanner C, Nube MJ, Blankestijn PJ. High convection volume in online post-dilution haemodiafiltration: relevance, safety and costs. Clin Kidney J. 2015;8:368–73.

216. Penne EL, van Berkel T, van der Weerd NC, Grooteman MP, Blankestijn PJ. Optimizing haemodiafiltration: tools, strategy and remaining questions. Nephrol Dial Transplant. 2009;24:3579–81.

217. Shroff R, Bayazit A, Stefanidis CJ, Askiti V, Azukaitis K, Canpolat N, Agbas A, Anarat A, Aoun B, Bakkaloglu S, Bhowruth D, Borzych-Duzalka D, Bulut IK, Buscher R, Dempster C, Duzova A, Habbig S, Hayes W, Hegde S, Krid S, Licht C, Litwin M, Mayes M, Mir S, Nemec R, Obrycki L, Paglialonga F, Picca S, Ranchin B, Samaille C, Shenoy M, Sinha M, Smith C, Spasojevic B, Vidal E, Vondrak K, Yilmaz A, Zaloszyc A, Fischbach M, Schaefer F, Schmitt CP. Effect of haemodiafiltration vs conventional haemodialysis on growth and cardiovascular outcomes in children - the HDF, heart and height (3H) study. BMC Nephrol. 2018;19:199.

218. Cheung AK, Rocco MV, Yan G, Leypoldt JK, Levin NW, Greene T, Agodoa L, Bailey J, Beck GJ, Clark W, Levey AS, Ornt DB, Schulman G, Schwab S, Teehan B, Eknoyan G. Serum beta-2 microglobulin levels predict mortality in dialysis patients: results of the HEMO study. J Am Soc Nephrol. 2006;17:546–55.

219. Agbas A, Canpolat N, Caliskan S, Yilmaz A, Ekmekci H, Mayes M, Aitkenhead H, Schaefer F, Sever L, Shroff R. Hemodiafiltration is associated with reduced inflammation, oxidative stress and improved endothelial risk profile compared to high-flux hemodialysis in children. PLoS One. 2018;13:e0198320.

220. Locatelli F, Altieri P, Andrulli S, Bolasco P, Sau G, Pedrini LA, Basile C, David S, Feriani M, Montagna G, Di Iorio BR, Memoli B, Cravero R, Battaglia G, Zoccali C. Hemofiltration and hemodiafiltration reduce intradialytic hypotension in ESRD. J Am Soc Nephrol. 2010;21:1798–807.

221. Morena M, Jaussent A, Chalabi L, Leray-Moragues H, Chenine L, Debure A, Thibaudin D, Azzouz L, Patrier L, Maurice F, Nicoud P, Durand C, Seigneuric B, Dupuy AM, Picot MC, Cristol JP, Canaud B. Treatment tolerance and patient-reported outcomes favor online hemodiafiltration compared to high-flux hemodialysis in the elderly. Kidney Int. 2017;91:1495–509.

222. Shroff R, Smith C, Ranchin B, Bayazit AK, Stefanidis CJ, Askiti V, Azukaitis K, Canpolat N, Agbas A, Aitkenhead H, Anarat A, Aoun B, Aofolaju D, Bakkaloglu SA, Bhowruth D, Borzych-Duzalka D, Bulut IK, Buscher R, Deanfield J, Dempster C, Duzova A, Habbig S, Hayes W, Hegde S, Krid S, Licht C, Litwin M, Mayes M, Mir S, Nemec R, Obrycki L, Paglialonga F, Picca S, Samaille C, Shenoy M, Sinha MD, Spasojevic B, Stronach L, Vidal E, Vondrak K, Yilmaz A, Zaloszyc A, Fischbach M, Schmitt CP, Schaefer F. Effects of hemodiafiltration versus conventional hemodialysis in children with ESKD: the HDF, heart and height study. J Am Soc Nephrol. 2019;30:678–91.

223. Nistor I, Palmer SC, Craig JC, Saglimbene V, Vecchio M, Covic A, Strippoli GF. Haemodiafiltration, haemofiltration and haemodialysis for end-stage kidney disease. Cochrane Database Syst Rev. 2015:CD006258.

224. Fischbach M, Terzic J, Menouer S, Dheu C, Seuge L, Zalosczic A. Daily on line haemodiafiltration promotes catch-up growth in children on chronic dialysis. Nephrol Dial Transplant. 2010;25:867–73.

225. Fischbach M, Fothergill H, Seuge L, Zaloszyc A. Dialysis strategies to improve growth in children with chronic kidney disease. J Ren Nutr. 2011;21:43–6.

226. Fischbach M, Attal Y, Geisert J. Hemodiafiltration versus hemodialysis in children. Int J Pediatr Nephrol. 1984;5:151–4.

227. Fischbach M, Terzic J, Menouer S, Dheu C, Soskin S, Helmstetter A, Burger MC. Intensified and daily hemodialysis in children might improve statural growth. Pediatr Nephrol. 2006;21:1746–52.

228. Bacchetta J, Sellier-Leclerc AL, Bertholet-Thomas A, Carlier MC, Cartier R, Cochat P, Ranchin B. Calcium balance in pediatric online hemodiafiltration: beware of sodium and bicarbonate in the dialysate. Nephrol Ther. 2015;11:483–6.

229. Fadel FI, Makar SH, Zekri H, Ahmed DH, Aon AH. The effect of on-line hemodiafiltration on improving the cardiovascular function parameters in children on regular dialysis. Saudi J Kidney Dis Transpl. 2015;26:39–46.

230. Paglialonga F, Vidal E, Pecoraro C, Guzzo I, Giordano M, Gianoglio B, Corrado C, Roperto R, Ratsch I, Luzio S, Murer L, Consolo S, Pieri G, Montini G, Edefonti A, Verrina E. Haemodiafiltration use in children: data from the Italian pediatric dialysis registry. Pediatr Nephrol. 2019;34:1057–63.

231. De Zan F, Smith C, Duzova A, Bayazit A, Stefanidis CJ, Askiti V, Azukaitis K, Canpolat N, Agbas A, Anarat A, Aoun B, Bakkaloglu SA, Borzych-Dużałka D, Bulut IK, Habbig S, Krid S, Licht C, Litwin M, Obrycki L, Paglialonga F, Ranchin B, Samaille C, Shenoy M, Sinha MD, Spasojevic B, Yilmaz A, Fischbach M, Schmitt CP, Schaefer F, Vidal E, Shroff R. Hemodiafiltration maintains a sustained improvement in blood pressure compared to conventional hemodialysis in children-the HDF, heart and height (3H) study. Pediatr Nephrol. 2021. Epub ahead of print. PMID: 33629141

232. Scribner BH, Cole JJ, Ahmad S, Blagg CR. Why thrice weekly dialysis? Hemodial Int. 2004;8(2):188–92.

233. Rocco MV, Lockridge RS Jr, Beck GJ, Eggers PW, Gassman JJ, Greene T, et al. The effects of frequent nocturnal home hemodialysis: the frequent hemodialysis network nocturnal trial. Kidney Int. 2011;80(10):1080–91.

234. Fischbach M, Dheu C, Seuge L, Menouer S, Terzic J. In-center daily on-line hemodiafiltration: a 4-year experience in children. Clin Nephrol. 2008;69(4):279–84.

235. Fischbach M, Terzic J, Laugel V, Dheu C, Menouer S, Helms P, et al. Daily on-line haemodiafiltration: a pilot trial in children. Nephrol Dial Transplant. 2004;19(9):2360–7.

236. Tom A, McCauley L, Bell L, Rodd C, Espinosa P, Yu G, et al. Growth during maintenance hemodialysis: impact of enhanced nutrition and clearance. J Pediatr. 1999;134(4):464–71.

237. Geary DF, Piva E, Tyrrell J, Gajaria MJ, Picone G, Keating LE, et al. Home nocturnal hemodialysis in children. J Pediatr. 2005;147(3):383–7.

238. Geary DF, Piva E, Gajaria M, Tyrrel J, Picone G, Harvey E. Development of a nocturnal home hemodialysis (NHHD) program for children. Semin Dial. 2004;17(2):115–7.

239. Warady BA, Fischbach M, Geary D, Goldstein SL. Frequent hemodialysis in children. Adv Chronic Kidney Dis. 2007;14(3):297–303.

240. Goldstein SL, Silverstein DM, Leung JC, Feig DI, Soletsky B, Knight C, et al. Frequent hemodialysis with NxStage system in pediatric patients receiving maintenance hemodialysis. Pediatr Nephrol. 2008;23(1):129–35.

241. Hothi DK, Stronach L, Harvey E. Home haemodialysis. Pediatr Nephrol. 2013;28(5):721–30.

242. Hothi DK, Fenton M. The impact of home hemodialysis in children with severe cardiac failure. Hemodial Int. 2020;24(4):E61–6.

243. Hoppe A, von Puttkamer C, Linke U, Kahler C, Booss M, Braunauer-Kolberg R, et al. A hospital-based intermittent nocturnal hemodialysis program for children and adolescents. J Pediatr. 2011;158(1):95–9, 9 e1

244. Muller D, Zimmering M, Chan CT, McFarlane PA, Pierratos A, Querfeld U. Intensified hemodialysis regimens: neglected treatment options for children and adolescents. Pediatr Nephrol. 2008;23(10):1729–36.

245. Kilis-Pstrusinska K, Medynska A, Chmielewska IB, Grenda R, Kluska-Jozwiak A, Leszczynska B, et al. Perception of health-related quality of life in children with chronic kidney disease by the patients and their caregivers: multicentre national study results. Qual Life Res. 2013;22(10):2889–97.

246. Ishibe S, Peixoto AJ. Methods of assessment of volume status and intercompartmental fluid shifts in hemodialysis patients: implications in clinical practice. Semin Dial. 2004;17(1):37–43.

247. Clark WR, Ronco C. Determinants of haemodialyser performance and the potential effect on clinical outcome. Nephrol Dial Transplant. 2001;16(Suppl 5):56–60.

Immunosuppression in Pediatric Kidney Transplantation

67

Burkhard Tönshoff, Anette Melk,
and Britta Höcker

Introduction

Ideally, a recipient (host) would accept a kidney transplant without induction of an antigen-specific response. However, it is not currently possible to induce specific immunologic tolerance, and transplantation requires immunosuppressive therapies. The goal is to use immunosuppressive agents that are not only potent and selective, but allow reversibility of their action, can be reliably delivered and display long-term safety. Most therapies alter immune response mechanisms but are not immunologically specific, and a careful balance is required to find the dose that prevents rejection of the graft, while minimizing the risks of over-immunosuppression leading to infection and cancer.

Current immunosuppressive agents reduce acute rejection, but do not induce tolerance. A few patients with organ transplants can successfully withdraw their immunosuppressive therapy without rejecting their grafts for long periods of time. However, these are rare exceptions, and such patients may eventually reject, even after years as this operational state of prope tolerance is unstable and poorly understood. The hunt for biomarkers to harness this "operational" tolerance state has remained elusive [1]. Even though antigen-specific T cells with reactivity to the foreign antigen persist in the host indefinitely, some graft and host adaptation must occur, since the level of immunosuppression required long-term is very low compared to the levels required within the first weeks post-transplant. This adaptation makes long-term immunosuppression possible; however, the long-term risk of cancer in the immunosuppressed patient remains increased. Thus, the distinction between immunosuppression and tolerance induction is partly artificial: any immunosuppression involves some apparent antigen-specific adaptation, i.e. down-regulation of the host response to the graft; and many tolerance protocols involve some non-specific immunosuppressive therapies.

The goal of immunosuppressive therapy is to prevent acute rejection while minimizing drug side effects. In children who undergo renal transplantation, immunosuppression is divided into 3 categories: (i) Induction therapy, i.e. intense immunosuppression administered during the perioperative period to prevent acute rejection, (ii) maintenance therapy, i.e. immunosuppressive treatment to prevent acute rejection after the peri-

B. Tönshoff (✉) · B. Höcker
Department of Pediatrics I, University Children's
Hospital Heidelberg, Heidelberg, Germany
e-mail: Burkhard.toenshoff@med.uni-heidelberg.de;
britta.hoecker@med.uni-heidelberg.de

A. Melk
Department of Pediatric Kidney, Liver and Metabolic
Diseases, Children's Hospital, Hannover Medical
School, Hannover, Germany
e-mail: melk.anette@mh-hannover.de

© The Author(s), under exclusive license to Springer Nature Switzerland AG 2023
F. Schaefer, L. A. Greenbaum (eds.), *Pediatric Kidney Disease*,
https://doi.org/10.1007/978-3-031-11665-0_67

operative period, and (iii) immunosuppressive therapy to treat graft rejection. In general, immunosuppression should be most intense during the first 3 months after transplantation when the risk of acute rejection and allograft loss is greatest. Immunosuppression is tapered slowly to a maintenance level by 6–12 months post-transplant. The goal remains to find the best combination of immunosuppressive agents that optimizes allograft survival by preventing rejection episodes while limiting drug toxicities. Although data from adult renal transplantation trials are used to help guide management decisions in pediatric patients, immunosuppression must often be modified because of the unique clinical effects of some of these agents in children, including their impact on longitudinal growth and development.

Allograft survival rates vary among the various immunosuppressive agents due to patient-specific clinical characteristics, such as age, ethnicity, obesity, hyperlipidemia, hypertension, proteinuria, delayed allograft function and some donor-related factors such as living-related versus deceased kidney donation. Immunosuppressive agents should therefore be chosen in part based on patient characteristics. Other issues to be considered are related to the immunologic history of the patient, such as ABO compatibility and the degree of HLA matching, pre-sensitization, re-transplantation, history of acute rejection episodes and the risk of recurrent disease.

The common immunosuppressive agents used in pediatric renal transplantation include glucocorticoids (steroids), azathioprine (AZA), mycophenolate mofetil (MMF), the calcineurin inhibitors tacrolimus (TAC) and ciclosporin (CSA), the mammalian target of rapamycin (mTOR) inhibitors sirolimus (SRL) and everolimus (EVR), antibodies to cell surface antigens on lymphocytes, including anti-thymocyte globulin (ATG), anti-CD25 antibodies (anti-interleukin-2 [IL-2] receptor antibodies), alemtuzumab (a humanized anti-CD52 pan-lymphocytic monoclonal antibody) and belatacept, a co-stimulation blocker of T cells. The structures of some immunosuppressives are shown in Fig. 67.1 [2]. Our discussion will focus on these agents and how they inhibit the immune response.

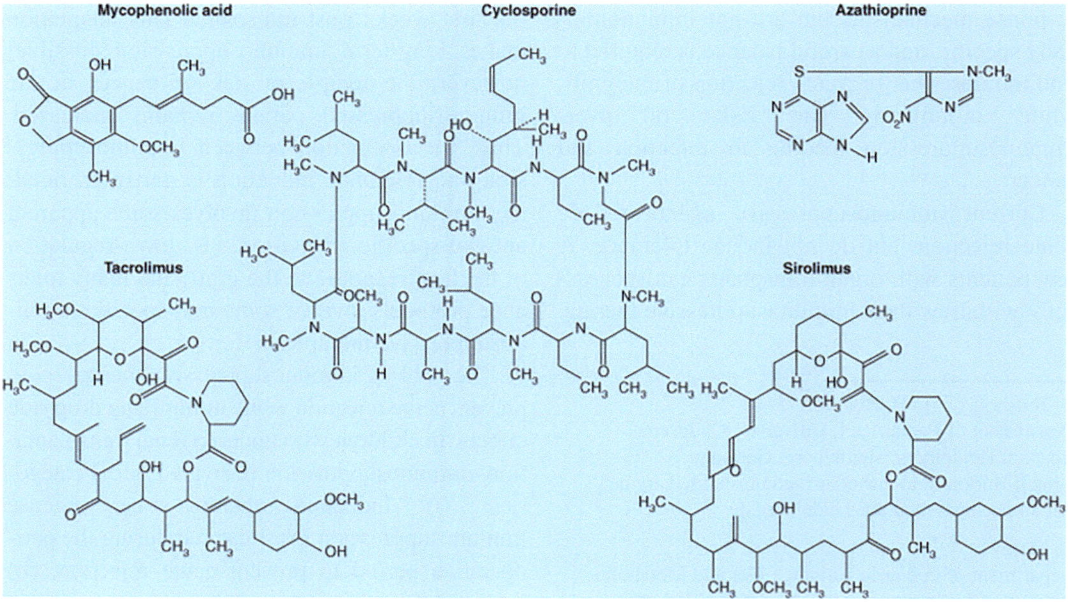

Fig. 67.1 Structure of mycophenolic acid, ciclosporin, azathioprine, tacrolimus, and sirolimus. These are all small molecules with molecular weights of 320, 1203, 277, 804, and 914, respectively. (Used with permission from Johnson RJ, Feehally J (eds): Comprehensive Clinical Nephrology, 2nd ed. Philadelphia: Elsevier; 2003) [2]

The Immune Response

By the time transplant surgery is completed, the graft has undergone acute injury leading to an increased expression of major histocompatibility complex (MHC) molecules by cells within the graft that are either constitutively expressed (class I, HLA-A and HLA-B) or inducible (class II, HLA-DR) antigens. Injury recruits lymphocytes and antigen-presenting cells (APCs), typically monocytes, macrophages, and dendritic cells from the host. These injury-related events may influence the probability of rejection and thereby contribute to the superior outcome in transplants from live donors (with less injury) vs. those from deceased donors.

Allorecognition of donor MHC molecules may occur either by the direct route (host T cells recognize donor MHC on donor cells) or indirectly (host T cells recognize donor MHC as peptides in the MHC groove of host APCs). T cell receptors (TCR) engaging MHC–peptide complexes provide signal 1. Co-stimulatory signals from the APC engaging receptors on the T cells provide signal 2 (Fig. 67.2) [3]. The major co-stimulatory molecules of the APC are B7–1/B7–2, which bind

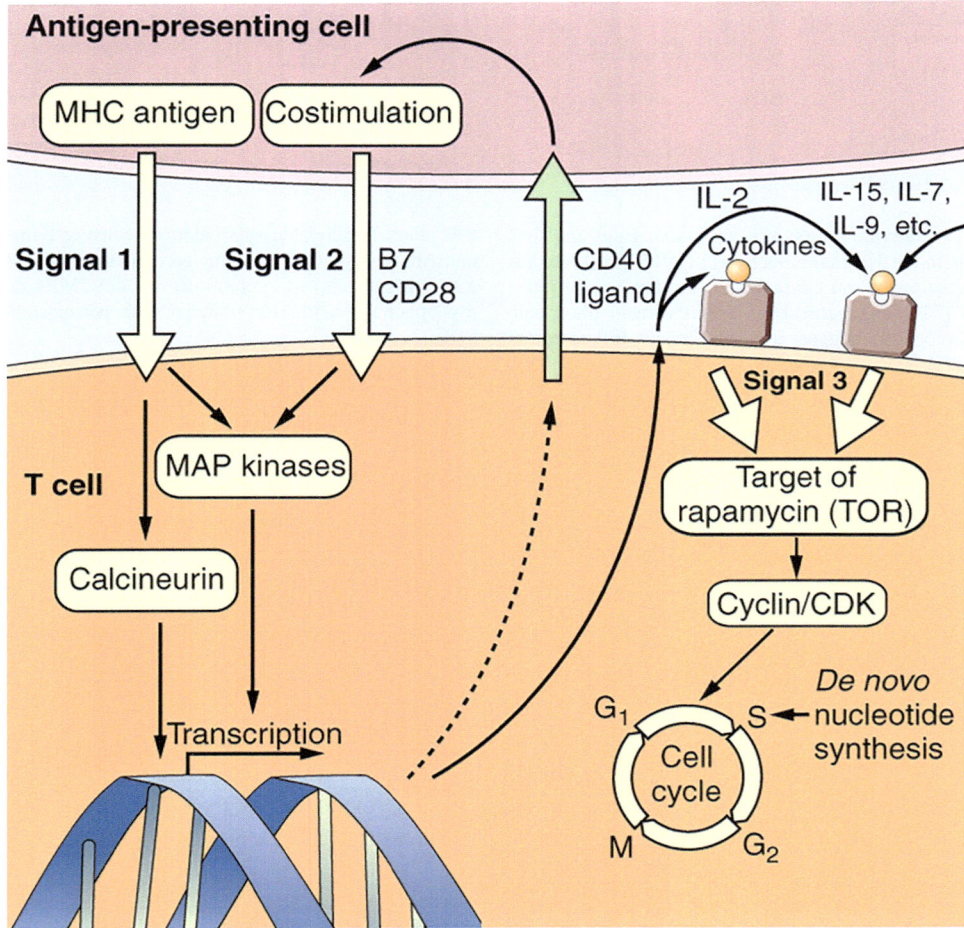

Fig. 67.2 The 3 events in T cell activation. Engagement of the T cell receptor with the antigenic peptide in the context of self–MHC class II molecule leads to the activation of the calcineurin pathway and results in the induction of cytokine genes (e.g., IL–2) (signal 1). Signal 2, the co-stimulatory signal, involves the engagement of CD28 with members of the B7 family. This synergizes with signal 1 to induce cytokine production. Interaction between cytokine production and its corresponding receptor leads to induction of cell division, probably through the target of rapamycin (TOR) pathway. This constitutes signal 3. (Used with permission from Feehally J, Floege J, Johnson RJ (eds.): Comprehensive Clinical Nephrology, 3rd ed. Philadelphia: Mosby, 2007) [3]

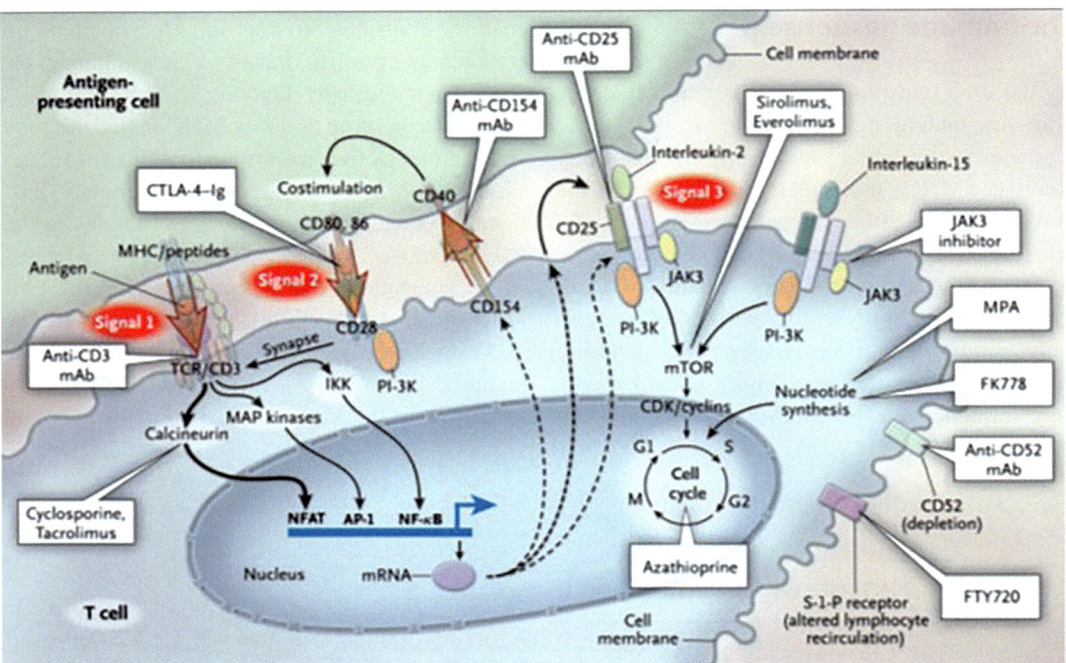

Fig. 67.3 Individual immunosuppressive drugs and sites of action in the 3-signal model. Anti-CD154 antibody has been withdrawn from clinical trials but remains of interest. FTY720 engagement of sphingosine-1-phosphate (S-1-P) receptors triggers and internalizes the receptors and alters lymphocyte recirculation, causing lymphopenia. Antagonists of chemokine receptors (not shown) are also being developed in preclinical models. MPA denotes mycophenolic acid. (Reproduced with permission from [4])

CD28 on the T cells. Activated T cells express CD40L that can activate the APC by engaging CD40 on the APC, and Fas ligand (FasL), which binds Fas on other lymphocytes or other cells to induce apoptosis in the Fas-bearing cell. Activation of signals 1 and 2 is followed by T cell activation with production of many cytokines. Cytokines, such as IL–2, engage specific receptors on the T cells to provide signal 3, the signal for cell division and clonal expansion. The engagement of CD40 by CD40L and the cytokines and growth factors from T cells regulate the T cell response, recruit and activate inflammatory cells, and alter adhesion molecules to cause mononuclear cells to accumulate in the graft. Depending on the type and degree of signaling, full activation of the T cell may occur, or T cells may undergo partial activation, apoptosis, anergy, or neglect (ignoring the antigen). T cells also bind *via* CD40L to CD40 on B cells, thereby directing the switch from IgM to IgG production by B cells and promoting the maturation of IgG-producing B cells.

Chemotactic factors (chemokines) and expression of adhesion proteins and foreign (MHC) antigens mediate localization (homing) of CD4 and CD8 T cells to the graft endothelium. Lymphocyte recirculation depends on the ability to enter and leave lymphoid tissue. CD8 T cells that recognize peptide in the groove of class I MHC become cytotoxic T cells (CTL). Graft rejection is associated with infiltration by cytotoxic CD8 lymphocytes. Delayed type hypersensitivity may also be involved in T cell-mediated damage. Antibody-mediated injury may also occur and causes damage to endothelium. A summary of the effects of immunosuppressive drugs is presented in Fig. 67.3 [3].

Classification of Immunosuppressive Agents

Immunosuppressive and immunomodulatory drugs can be pharmacologically categorized on the basis of their mechanism of action. The 3-signal model of T cell activation and proliferation is helpful in understanding the molecular mechanisms and site of action of various immunosuppressive drugs. Figure 67.3 depicts a schematic representation of the 3-signal model along with the site of action of common immunosuppressive drugs [4]. Signal 1 features APCs (macrophages and dendritic cells) presenting the foreign antigen to the T lymphocyte, activating the TCR, which further relays the signal through the transduction apparatus known as the CD3 complex. Signal 2 is a non-antigen-specific co-stimulatory signal which occurs as a result of binding of the B7 molecule on the APC to CD28 on the T cell. Both signal 1 and signal 2 activate signal transduction pathways: the calcium–calcineurin pathway, mitogen-activated protein (MAP) pathway, and the nuclear factor-κB (NF-κB) pathway. This in turn leads to increased expression of IL-2, which through its receptor (IL-2R) activates the cell cycle (signal 3). Signal 3 activation requires the enzyme mTOR for translation of mRNA and cell proliferation. Thus, various drugs act on different cellular signals and achieve immunosuppression by a number of mechanisms: depleting lymphocytes, diverting lymphocyte traffic, or blocking lymphocyte response pathways.

Induction Immunosuppressive Therapy

Induction refers to the administration of an intensive immunosuppressive regimen during the perioperative period. The rationale behind this approach is that the risk of acute rejection is greatest in the first weeks and months after transplantation. Induction therapies often involve the use of polyclonal or monoclonal antibodies to achieve rapid and profound early immunosuppression. Polyclonal antibodies used for this purpose include those against thymocytes (e.g., commercially available rabbit or equine preparations); monoclonal antibodies include basiliximab (a chimeric human–murine anti-CD25 or anti–IL-2R antibody) and alemtuzumab (an anti-CD52 antibody targeting both B and T cells), which is not always readily available.

A number of trials have been and are being conducted in adult and pediatric renal transplant recipients to look into the effects of prophylactic antibody induction therapies. Evaluation of any induction protocol requires consideration of the following factors: (i) Incidence and severity of delayed allograft function or primary non-function, including post-transplant dialysis requirements; (ii) incidence of acute rejection; (iii) incidence, type, and severity of associated infections; (iv) long-term allograft survival and function; (v) mortality and morbidity, including length of hospitalization, (vi) cost, and (vii) incidence and type of malignancy during long-term follow-up. Several studies from single centers and registries, as well as meta-analyses, have found that induction with antibodies may be superior to non-antibody-based regimens, especially in high-risk groups [5]. Unfortunately, most if not all published studies have addressed only some of the above issues. As a result, although each protocol may have specific advantages and disadvantages in a particular patient population, none is yet proven to be superior when all the above factors are considered. The optimal prophylactic induction immunosuppressive therapy to prevent renal transplant rejection remains therefore controversial. Figure 67.4 presents the induction antibody use from 2007–2018, as reported in the Scientific Registry of Renal Transplant Recipients (SRTR) 2018 annual report, indicating that administration of ATG has increased while that of anti-IL-2R and no induction have decreased over time. This is in contrast to reports from the Cooperative European Paediatric Renal Transplant Initiative (CERTAIN) Registry showing that 60% of pediatric kidney transplant recipients in Europe do not receive any induction therapy, 35% receive basiliximab and 5% ATG [6]. Hence, the frequency and type of the chosen immunosuppressive anti-lymphocyte regimens for induction therapy vary markedly between North America and Europe and probably reflect differences in patient characteristics and estimated immunological risk, but is unfortunately not based on comprehensive clinical trials.

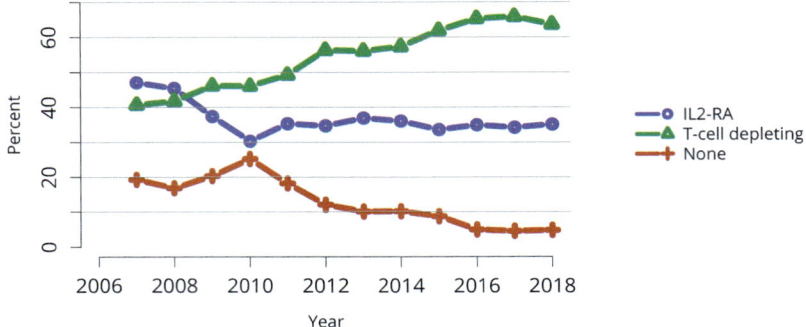

Fig. 67.4 Induction agent use in pediatric kidney transplant recipients in the United States of America. Immunosuppression at transplant reported to the Organ Procurement and Transplantation Network (OPTN) (https://pubmed.ncbi.nlm.nih.gov/31898417). IL2-RA, interleukin-2 receptor antagonist

In fact, induction therapy produces the greatest benefits in groups at high risk of allograft rejection. These high-risk groups include African-Americans, recipients of kidneys with prolonged cold ischemia time, and those at high immunologic risk, particularly individuals who are presensitized. The sequential induction regimen of thymoglobulin followed by a combination of TAC and MMF with or without steroids is recommended in these high-risk groups.

Lymphocyte Depleting Antibodies

Polyclonal Antibodies

Because of the redundancy of the immune system, polyclonal antibodies, which have a broad specificity, should theoretically be more effective in induction therapy than monoclonal anti-lymphocyte agents. Anti-thymocyte globulin (ATGAM) is a purified gamma globulin solution obtained by immunization of horses with human thymocytes. It contains antibodies to a wide variety of human T cell surface antigens, including the major MHC antigens. Thymoglobulin is a rabbit-derived polyclonal antibody preparation approved for the treatment of rejection and induction therapy by the US Federal Drug Administration (FDA). As for ATGAM, thymoglobulin contains antibodies to a wide variety of T cell antigens and MHC antigens.

Polyclonal antibodies act in 3 ways: by activating or altering the function of lymphocytes, by lysing lymphoid cells, and by altering the traffic of lymphoid cells and sequestering them. These antibodies are potently immunosuppressive, but often produce side effects. By triggering T cells, they generate significant first-dose effects, with the release of tumor necrosis factor alpha (TNFα), interferon γ (IFN-γ), and other cytokines, causing a first-dose reaction (flu-like syndrome, fever, and chills).

Dosage of Thymoglobulin

Thymoglobulin induction is usually dosed from 1 to 6 mg/kg per dose, and the duration may range from 1 to 10 days, although a more typical regimen is 1.5 mg/kg per dose for 3–5 days [7–10]. In animal models, higher initial doses of shorter duration approximating a human-equivalent dose of 6 mg/kg were associated with more peripheral and central lymphocyte depletion and better allograft survival [11]. Based on these models, the optimal induction dose is felt to total 6 mg/kg [9, 12]. Total doses of 5.7 mg/kg, on average given as 1.5 mg/kg per day, have been shown to produce similar outcomes as higher doses in high-risk recipients who received an average of 10.3 mg/kg [10]. Higher doses and prolonged duration of induction agents are thought to be associated with an increased risk of infection and the potential development of lymphoma, whereas cumulative doses of less than 3 mg/kg may not effectively prevent acute rejection [13].

Efficacy and Safety

Few studies have compared the relative efficacy of thymoglobulin and ATGAM for induction therapy. In one study in adult renal transplant recipients, 72 patients were randomly assigned in a double-blind 2:1 fashion to receive intravenous doses of thymoglobulin at 1.5 mg/kg or ATGAM at 15 mg/kg intra-operatively, then daily for at least 6 days [14]. The delayed graft function rate was only 1 percent for both groups. At 1 year, the thymoglobulin group had a significantly lower acute rejection rate (4% vs. 25%, respectively) and higher allograft survival (98% vs. 83%). The lower rejection rate was thought to be due in part to a more sustained lymphopenia with thymoglobulin, while the exceptionally low delayed graft function rate seen in both groups may have been due to the intra-operative use of the ATGs. Both antibodies have the ability to block a number of adhesion molecules, cytokines, chemokines, and their receptors, which may contribute to ischemia reperfusion injury and delayed graft function. At 5 years, allograft survival was significantly better in the thymoglobulin arm (77% vs. 57%, respectively) [15]. Two cases of post-transplant lymphoproliferative disorder (PTLD) developed with ATGAM, while none were observed with thymoglobulin. The mean 5-year serum creatinine concentration was similar in both groups.

In pediatric renal transplant recipients, a historical cohort study compared the rates of survival, rejection, and infection in patients who received induction therapy with ATGAM (n = 127) or thymoglobulin (n = 71) [16]. Maintenance immunosuppression included CSA, AZA or MMF, and prednisone. Mean follow-up was 90 ± 25 months for ATGAM recipients and 32 ± 15 months for thymoglobulin recipients.

Overall, the incidence of acute rejection was lower in thymoglobulin recipients vs. ATGAM recipients (33% vs. 50%, P = 0.02). Epstein-Barr virus (EBV) infection was higher in thymoglobulin recipients versus ATGAM recipients (8% vs. 3%, P = 0.002). But the two groups did not significantly differ in patient and graft survival rates, incidence of chronic rejection, EBV lymphoma, or other infections. The authors concluded that thymoglobulin induction was associated with a reduced incidence of acute rejection and an increased incidence of EBV infection in pediatric renal transplant recipients.

IL-2 Receptor Antibodies

Full T cell activation leads to the calcineurin-mediated stimulation of the transcription, translation, and secretion of IL-2, a key autocrine growth factor that induces T cell proliferation. Thus, an attractive therapeutic option is abrogation of IL-2 activity via the administration of anti-IL-2R antibodies. Currently, only basiliximab, a chimeric monoclonal antibody, is commercially available and has been approved by the FDA for use in renal transplantation in adults and pediatric patients (Fig. 67.5). The IL-2R consists of 3 transmembrane protein chains: CD25, CD122, and CD132. CD25 is present on nearly all activated T cells, but not on resting T cells. IL-2 induces clonal expansion of activated T cells. Although CD25 does not transduce the signal, it is responsible for the association of IL-2 with the β- and γ-chains, which triggers the activated T cell to undergo rapid proliferation. This antibody binds to activated T cells and render them resistant to IL-2 by blocking, shedding or internalizing the receptor; it may also deplete and sequester some activated T cells. However, IL-2R functions are partially redundant because other cytokine receptors have overlapping functions, e.g., IL-15R. Therefore, saturating IL-2R produces stable, but relatively mild immunosuppression, and is only effective in combination with other immunosuppressants.

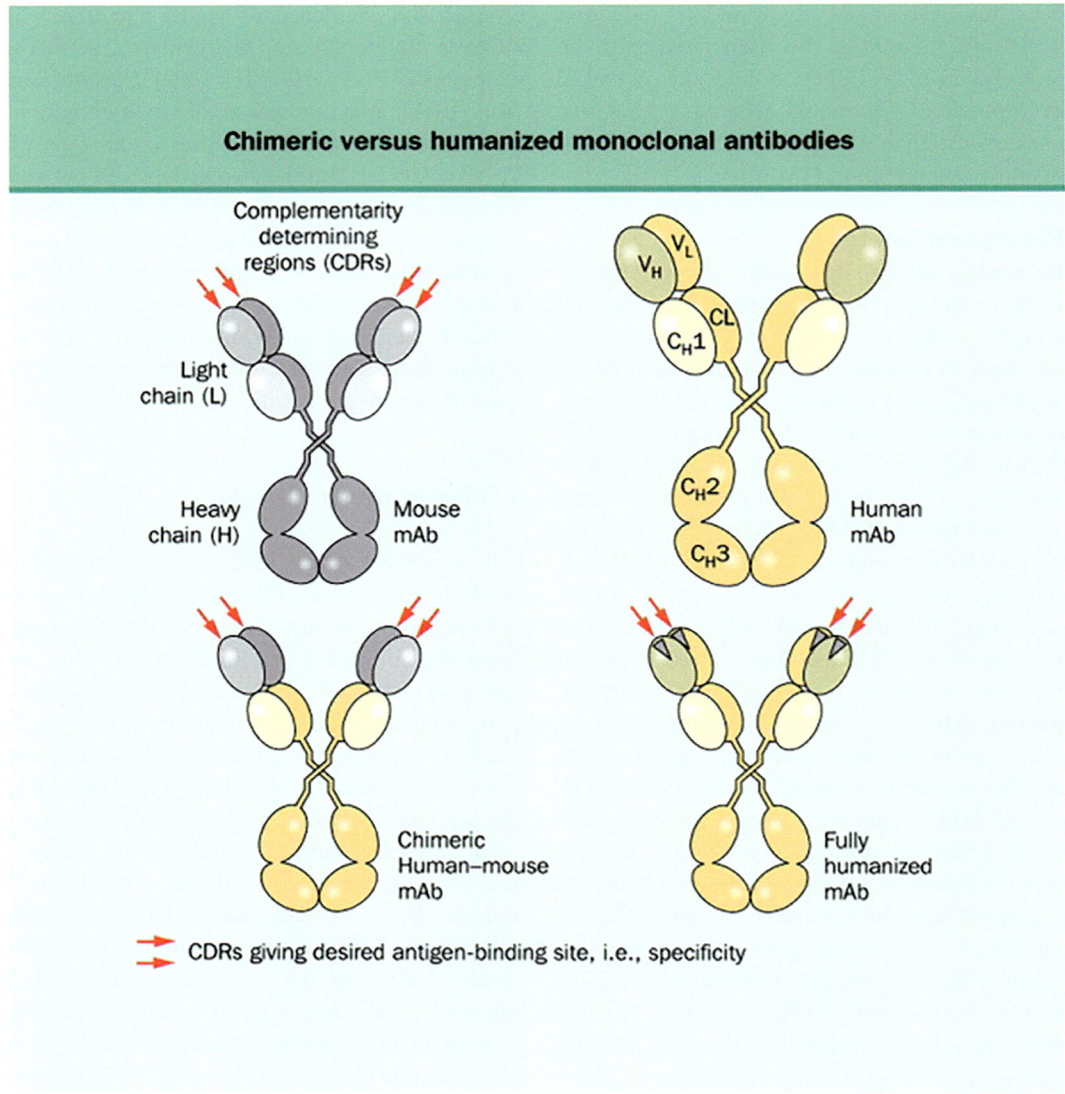

Fig. 67.5 Chimeric vs. humanized monoclonal antibodies. (Used with permission from Feehally J, Floege J, Johnson RJ (eds.): Comprehensive Clinical Nephrology, 3rd ed. Philadelphia: Mosby, 2007) [3]

Dosage of Basiliximab

The dosing schedule for basiliximab is the following: intravenous administration of two 10 mg doses to children <35 kg in weight and two 20 mg doses to children ≥35 kg in weight, with the first dose given within 2 h prior to surgery, and the second on post-transplant day 4. In the 14 patients who were evaluated for the pharmacokinetics and pharmacodynamics of basiliximab and received concomitant immunosuppression with CSA and AZA, the mean duration of IL-2R saturation was 42 ± 16 days [17]. In a larger study of 82 patients who received basiliximab in combination with MMF, MMF reduced basiliximab clearance and thereby prolonged CD25 saturation from 5 to 10 weeks [18].

Efficacy and Safety

The effectiveness of IL-2R antibody therapy was best reported in a meta-analysis involving 38 trials that enrolled nearly 5000 patients that assessed the impact of therapy on allograft loss and rejection [19]. Data were derived from published trials and abstracts of completed and ongoing trials. From these 38 trials, 14 trials enrolling 2410 patients compared IL-2R antagonists with placebo for at least one outcome. Compared with placebo, IL-2R antagonists reduced acute rejection rates at 6 months (relative risk [RR 0.66], CI 0.59–0.74) and 1 year (RR 0.67, CI 0.60–0.75), but the incidence of graft loss was the same.

In pediatric renal transplant recipients, two large prospective randomized controlled trials showed that induction therapy with basiliximab in patients with low to medium immunological risk on maintenance therapy (TAC in conjunction with AZA, or CSA in conjunction with MMF) did not lead to a statistically significant reduction in the incidence of acute rejection episodes [20, 21]. As a result, there is presently no consensus amongst pediatric renal transplantation centers regarding the use of and regimen for immunosuppressive induction therapy. Considerations in choosing the appropriate agent include the efficacy in the patient population (e.g., recipients with high or low risk of graft loss), the side effect profile, and the concomitant immunosuppressive therapy (steroid avoidance, early steroid withdrawal, or conventional steroid therapy).

Comparison of Basiliximab with Thymoglobulin

Few studies have compared the use of different induction immunosuppressive regimens. In adult patients at increased risk of acute rejection, thymoglobulin is more effective than basiliximab in preventing rejection [22–25]. A multicenter, international, randomized, prospective study of 278 first deceased-donor kidney transplant recipients compared the safety and efficacy of a 5-day course of thymoglobulin (n = 141) or 2 doses of basiliximab (n = 137) [26]. Recipients and donors were chosen based upon characteristics that would predict an increased risk of rejection or delayed graft function. Patients in both arms were administered CSA, MMF, and prednisone for maintenance immunosuppression, and received antiviral prophylaxis with ganciclovir. The primary endpoint

was a composite of acute rejection, delayed allograft function, transplant loss, and death. At 1 year, there was no difference between thymoglobulin and basiliximab in the incidence of the composite endpoint. However, thymoglobulin was associated with a significantly lower acute rejection rate (16% vs. 26%), and incidence of acute rejection that required antibody treatment (1.4% vs. 8%). Although overall adverse event and serious adverse event rates were similar, thymoglobulin was associated with a higher incidence of infection (86% vs. 75%), but lower incidence of cytomegalovirus (CMV) disease (8% vs. 18%).

At 5-year follow-up, the incidence of acute rejection and need for antibody treatment of acute rejection remained lower among those treated with thymoglobulin, compared with basiliximab (16% vs. 30% and 3% vs. 12%, respectively) [22]. Patients treated with thymoglobulin also had a significantly lower composite endpoint of acute rejection, graft loss, and death at 5 years (39% vs. 52%) and incidence of treated CMV infection (7% vs. 17%); however, the incidence of malignancy did not differ. Hence, the relative benefits of thymoglobulin were sustained over a 5-year period.

Alemtuzumab

Alemtuzumab (Campath-1H, MabCampath) is a humanized IgG1 monoclonal antibody directed against CD52, a glycoprotein expressed on mononuclear cells, including T and B lymphocytes, monocytes, and natural killer cells [23]. Its efficacy for induction and maintenance immunosuppression with low-dose calcineurin inhibitors (CNIs) was first introduced by Calne et al. [24] and later supported by the Pittsburgh group [25] in adults and children. Alemtuzumab induction has been associated with lower rates of acute rejection than basiliximab and daclizumab in low immunological risk patients and was associated with similar efficacy as compared with rabbit anti-thymocyte globulin in high-risk patients [26]. Although most of these studies have involved adult kidney transplant recipients, there is also pediatric experience that supports this efficacy claim, especially in highly sensitized, high-risk children [27, 28]. A significant reduction of white blood cell and absolute lymphocyte counts, up to 1 year post-transplant, has been observed in children receiving alemtuzumab treatment [29].There is no currently recommended dose for children, but 0.3 mg/kg per dose has been most frequently used in pediatric studies [30]. The most common number of doses administered was 2 doses, with a range from 1 to 4 doses during the first week post-transplant. Due to infusion-related reactions, pre-medication with methylprednisolone, acetaminophen, and diphenhydramine is recommended in addition to administration of anti-emetics to avoid nausea and vomiting. The major side effect that limits the use of alemtuzumab is profound lymphopenia, which may contribute to significant adverse events, including infections, autoimmune complications, and malignancies [30]. The Cooperative Clinical Trials in Pediatric Transplantation program of the National Institute of Allergy and Infectious Disease has completed a multicenter pilot trial of alemtuzumab induction in pediatric kidney transplant recipients with initial maintenance immunosuppression of TAC and MMF, but the results have yet to be published.

Recommendations

There is currently no consensus for immunosuppressive induction therapy following kidney transplantation in children. At the present time, no consistent evidence exists that induction therapy is beneficial or cost-effective in low-risk patients on triple therapy with CNIs in conventional doses, MMF and steroids. According to 2 prospective, randomized, controlled trials, induction therapy with basiliximab in pediatric patients with low or normal immunological risk on maintenance therapy with either TAC in conjunction with AZA or CSA in combination with MMF did not lead to a statistically significant reduction in the incidence of acute rejection episodes [20, 21]. In contrast, the Kidney Disease: Improving Global Outcomes clinical practice guidelines recommend induction therapy for all adult patients, with an IL-2R blocker as first line for those not at high immunological risk [31]. There is some evidence favoring the use of IL-2R blockers over no induction in adult renal

transplantation [32]. However, it has been pointed out in the more recent literature that these studies mainly used outdated maintenance regimens [33]. No large randomized trial has examined the effect of IL-2R antibodies or rabbit ATG induction vs. no induction in patients receiving TAC, mycophenolic acid (MPA) and steroids. With this triple maintenance therapy, the addition of induction may achieve an absolute risk reduction for acute rejection of only 1–4% in standard-risk patients without improving renal allograft or patient survival. In contrast, rabbit ATG induction lowers the relative risk of acute rejection by almost 50% vs. IL-2R antibodies in patients with high immunological risk. These recent data raise questions about the need for IL-2R antibodies in kidney transplantation, as it may no longer be beneficial in standard-risk transplantation. Although augmentation of immunosuppression by IL-2R antibody induction may allow steroid minimization, it may be inferior to rabbit ATG in high-risk situations. Updated evidence-based guidelines are necessary to support clinicians deciding whether and what induction therapy is required for their transplant patients today [33]. Studies in the US and Europe have investigated the potential of IL-2R antibodies or thymoglobulin in replacement of steroids with promising results (see section in this chapter on "Steroid Withdrawal or Avoidance"). Another potential application is delayed graft function when the use of CNIs should be avoided.

Maintenance Immunosuppressive Therapy

Maintenance immunosuppressive therapy is administered to kidney transplant recipients for prevention of acute rejection. Although an adequate level of immunosuppression is required to dampen the immune response to the allograft, the level of chronic immunosuppression is slowly decreased over time to help lower the overall risk of infection and malignancy. The type of immunosuppression may also be modified to decrease the risk of developing chronic antibody-mediated rejection, the most common underlying long-term cause of allograft loss.

Conventional maintenance regimens consist of a combination of immunosuppressive agents that differ in their mechanism of action. This strategy minimizes morbidity and mortality associated with each class of agent while maximizing overall effectiveness. Such regimens vary by transplant center and geographic area. There are a number of important issues to consider when deciding upon the immunosuppressive protocol to administer in a particular patient. First, the risk of acute rejection and allograft loss is highest in the first 3 months post-transplant. As a result, immunosuppression should be at its highest during this period (see section in this chapter on "Induction Immunosuppressive Therapy"). Second, the occurrence of the most serious side effects of immunosuppressive therapy, infections and malignancy, correlate with the total amount of immunosuppression. It is therefore essential that immunosuppression is gradually tapered to a maintenance level by 6–12 months post-transplant.

Allograft survival rates vary among the various immunosuppressive agents due to patient-specific clinical characteristics and co-morbidities, such as age, ethnicity, obesity, hyperlipidemia, hypertension, proteinuria, and/or delayed allograft function. The choice of immunosuppression should consider these factors, but also take into account the "immunologic" history of the patient. Transplant physicians must reflect the following questions: Is the patient sensitized? Is this the first kidney transplant or a re-transplant? How many acute rejection episodes has the patient had? What is the degree of HLA matching?

The optimal maintenance immunosuppressive therapy in pediatric kidney transplantation is not established. The major immunosuppressive agents currently used in various combination regimens are TAC, CSA (in standard form or microemulsion), MMF, EVR, SRL, AZA and steroids (primarily oral prednisone or methylprednisolone). We and most transplant centers currently utilize a maintenance regimen consisting of triple immunosuppression therapy with a CNI (TAC or CSA), an anti-metabolite (MMF or AZA), and methylprednisolone. EVR or SRL are also used by some transplant centers in triple therapy regimens, often in place of the CNI or the antimetabolite. Within the North American Pediatric Renal Trials and Collaborative Studies (NAPRTCS) registry, marked changes in the type of maintenance immunosuppression and dosing strategies have been observed over time [34]. These are substantially caused by the introduction of newer drugs such as MMF and TAC. In the transplant era 2008–2017, the most popular immunosuppressive regimen at post-transplant day 30, utilized in 48.9% of patients, was triple therapy with TAC, MMF and prednisone (Table 67.1).

Table 67.1 Observed drug utilization rates in North American pediatric renal transplant recipients among transplanted grafts with ≥30 days function that have occurred since 1996. (Data are from [34])

	Transplant era 1996–2001				Transplant era 2002–2007				Transplant era 2008–2017			
	30 days	1 year	3 years	5 years	30 days	1 year	3 years	5 years	30 days	1 year	3 years	5 years
Prednisone/CSA/MMF	35.4	38.1	30.6	22.4	9.7	8.6	7.9	7.5	1.7	1.9	0.5	0.7
Prednisone/CSA/AZA	23.1	17.7	14.2	8.9	0.8	0.8	0.6	0.7	0.1	0.2	0.3	0.4
Prednisone/CSA	10.7	4.4	3.8	3.5	1.5	0.8	0.3	0.8	0.4	0.3	0.2	0.0
Prednisone/TAC/MMF	14.3	19.6	24.4	30.1	51.3	49.6	44.2	42.1	48.9	41.7	38.6	33.1
Prednisone/TAC/AZA	2.3	4.9	6.5	6.9	1.7	2.4	2.7	3.9	2.0	2.3	4.3	6.7
Prednisone/TAC	4.2	5.0	6.7	6.9	4.1	5.8	6.7	6.2	2.9	8.2	8.0	6.7
TAC/MMF	0.4	1.1	1.7	2.5	10.7	9.4	11.5	13.1	33.8	27.3	26.5	27.5
Other combination	9.5	9.2	12.0	17.3	20.1	22.7	26.0	25.8	10.1	18.1	21.6	25.3

Glucocorticoids

Glucocorticoids, developed in the early 1950s, represent one of the principal agents used for both maintenance immunosuppression and treatment of acute rejection.

Mechanism of Action

Steroids have both anti-inflammatory and immunosuppressive actions [35]. Lymphopenia and monocytopenia occur with the inhibition of lymphocyte proliferation, survival, activation, homing, and effector functions. Steroids suppress production of MHC molecules and numerous cytokines and vasoactive substances, including IL-1, TNFα, IL-2, chemokines, prostaglandins (*via* inhibition of phospholipase A2), and proteases. Steroids also cause neutrophilia (often with a left shift), but neutrophil chemotaxis and adhesion are inhibited. They also affect non-hematopoietic cells.

Steroids exert their effect by binding to glucocorticoid receptors (GR), which belong to a family of ligand-regulated transcription factors called nuclear receptors. GR are normally present in the cytoplasm in an inactive complex with heat shock proteins (hsp90, hsp70, and hsp56). The binding of steroids to the GR dissociates hsp from the GR and forms the active steroid–GR complex, which migrates to the nucleus and dimerizes on palindromic DNA sequences, called the glucocorticoid response element (GRE), in many genes. The binding of GR in the promoter region of the target genes can lead to either induction or suppression of gene transcription (e.g., of cytokines). GR also exert effects by interacting directly with other transcription factors independent of DNA binding. One principal effect of steroids on immune and inflammatory responses may be attributable to their ability to affect gene transcription by regulating key transcription factors involved in immune regulation: activator protein-1 (AP-1) and NF-κB. The regulation of NF-κB by steroids may be via induction of IkB, the inhibitor of NF-κB. Other effects of steroids are mediated through the release of a regulatory protein, lipocortin, which inhibits phospholipase A2, thereby inhibiting the production of leukotrienes

and prostaglandins. The total immunosuppressive effect of steroids is complex, reflecting effects on cytokines, adhesion molecules, apoptosis, and activation of inflammatory cells.

Pharmacokinetics and Drug Interactions

The major steroids used are prednisone or prednisolone (given orally with comparable efficacy) and methylprednisolone (given orally or intravenously with 25% more potency). These agents are rapidly absorbed and have short plasma half-lives (60–180 min), but long biological half-lives (18–36 h). The effect of prednisone (dose per body weight) is greater in the setting of renal failure or hypalbuminemia, in women, and in the elderly, but less prednisone effect is observed in children. Certain drugs can decrease steroid efficacy by increasing metabolism: rifampicin, phenytoin, phenobarbital, and carbamazepine. In contrast, increased steroid effects may be observed in patients receiving oral contraceptives, estrogens, ketoconazole, and erythromycin.

Administration

In many transplant centers, the initial dose of steroids is usually administered during surgery as intravenous methylprednisolone, at doses between 2 and 10 mg/kg body weight. The oral dose of steroids used for maintenance therapy varies between 15 and 60 mg/m² per day (0.5–2 mg/kg body weight per day), which is gradually tapered over time to approximately 3–5 mg prednisone per m² body surface area, usually taken as a single morning dose. Alternate-day dosing is often administered 6–12 months post-transplant to minimize the effect of steroids on growth.

Side Effects

Steroids have multiple side effects in children, including growth impairment, susceptibility to infections, cushingoid appearance, body disfigurement, acne, cardiovascular complications, hypertension, hyperglycemia, aseptic bone necrosis, osteopenia, cataracts, poor wound healing, and psychological effects (Table 67.2). The

Table 67.2 Semi-quantitative comparison of safety profiles of current primary immunosuppressive compounds

	Tacrolimus	Ciclosporin	Mycophenolate mofetil	Sirolimus/ everolimus	Glucocorticoids
Nephrotoxicity[a]	++(+)	+++	–	+	–
Hyperlipidemia	+(+)	++	–	+++	++
Hypertension	++	+++	–	–	+
Neurotoxicity	+++	+++	–	–	+
Post-transplant diabetes mellitus	+++	++	–	–	++
Bone marrow suppression	–	–	++	++	–
Gastrointestinal adverse effects[b]	+	+	+++	+	–
Hepatotoxicity	+	+	–	+	–
Esthetical changes	+	++	–	–	++
Wound healing problems[c]	–	–	+	++	+
Pulmonary toxicity	–	–	–	+	–
Fetal toxicity	+	+	++	NA	–
Osteoporosis	+	+	–	?	++
Inhibition of longitudinal growth	–	–	–	+	+++

– indicates the drug has no effect on this adverse effect, + indicates mild, ++ indicates moderate, +++ indicates severe, ? indicates clinical data available but insufficient to provide conclusions, *NA* no information available
[a] Sirolimus without calcineurin inhibitor
[b] Gastrointestinal disorders: diarrhoea, abdominal pain, nausea and vomiting, ileus, rectal disorders, mucosal ulcerations
[c] Wound healing problems including lymphocele formation

negative impact that steroids have on appearance may play a role for poor adherence, especially in the body image conscious adolescent. The risk for infection is excessive if high-dose pulse therapy is prolonged (typically >3 g per 1.73 m²). Steroids dosage should therefore be decreased gradually during rejection treatment even if serum creatinine fails to improve. Interestingly, steroids are not associated with an increased risk of malignancy. One of the most important reasons for stopping steroids or switching to alternate-day therapy is statural growth impairment, which is frequently observed in those on continuous treatment.

Steroid Withdrawal or Avoidance

Because of the multiple adverse effects of maintenance steroid therapy, attempts have been made to withdraw or minimize steroid therapy in children with a renal allograft [36–40]. There are two major strategies in steroid minimization in pediatric kidney transplantation: (i) *Late steroid withdrawal* (>1 year post-transplantation) and (ii) either *complete steroid avoidance* or *early steroid withdrawal* (<7 days post-transplantation). In the *late steroid withdrawal* approach, the patients suitable for minimization are identified by a stable post-transplant clinical course and renal function. In *late steroid withdrawal*, there is no need for an antibody induction in the perioperative period [41]. In *early withdrawal or complete avoidance* protocols, the criteria of suitability are predefined before transplantation (e.g., low immunological risk), and antibody induction is used in all patients [42–47]. There is also an *intermediate* approach, combining elements from *early and late withdrawal* protocols, in which antibody induction is used; however, the decision of *steroid withdrawal* is delayed until 6–9 months post-transplant, when stable renal graft function (sometimes combined with a normal protocol biopsy) allows identification of suitable candidates (as in the late withdrawal approach) [48]. *Steroid withdrawal* has the advantage over *steroid avoidance* that immunologically high-risk patients and those with unstable graft function can easily be identified beforehand and be excluded from steroid-free immunosuppression.

Late steroid withdrawal without induction therapy was investigated in a trial of 42 patients with low immunologic risk who were maintained on CSA, MMF, and steroids. At 1 year post-transplant, patients were randomly assigned to either steroid continuation or withdrawal over a 3-month period [40]. At 1 year follow-up, the steroid withdrawal group had increased catch-up growth, lower arterial blood pressure, and a better carbohydrate and lipid profile than those on continuous steroid therapy. In a subsequent follow-up report, longitudinal growth in the steroid withdrawal group continued to be superior to

controls; catch-up growth was especially pronounced in pre-pubertal patients off steroids (Fig. 67.6) [41]. Although the relative height gain after steroid withdrawal was less pronounced in pubertal patients, they still benefited from cessation of steroid treatment. Also, the prevalence of the metabolic syndrome declined in the withdrawal group from 39% at baseline to 6% 2 years after discontinuing steroid therapy [41]. Allograft function remained stable in the withdrawal group compared with controls, and the incidence of acute rejections was similar in the steroid withdrawal and control groups (4% vs. 11%, respectively). An earlier retrospective case–control study had reported a beneficial effect of *late ste-*

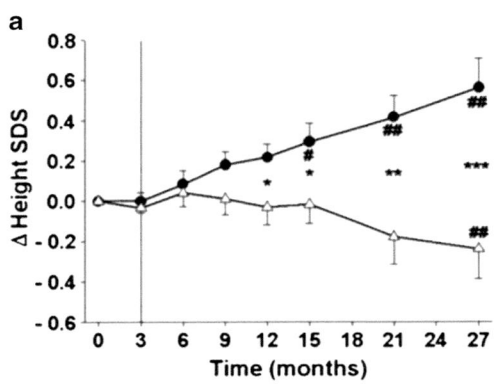

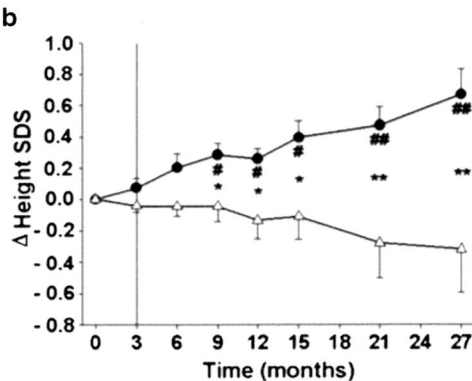

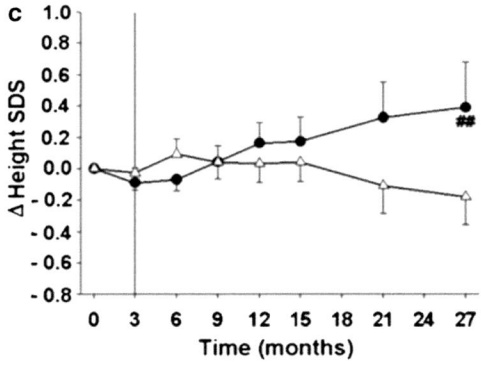

Fig. 67.6 Randomized controlled trial on late steroid withdrawal: Change of height SDS (mean ± SEM) in the steroid withdrawal group (filled circles) and the control group (open triangles) during the 27-month study period. Panel A, all patients; panel B, pre-pubertal patients; panel C, pubertal patients. *$P < 0.05$ vs. control; **$P < 0.01$ vs. control; ***$P < 0.001$ vs. control; #$P < 0.05$ vs. baseline;

##$P < 0.01$ vs. baseline. (Used with permission of Oxford University Press from Höcker B, Weber L, Feneberg R, Drube J, John U, Fehrenbach H, et al. Improved growth and cardiovascular risk after late steroid withdrawal: 2-year results of a prospective, randomized trial in paediatric renal transplantation. Nephrol Dial Transplant 2010; 25:617–624) [41]

roid withdrawal (mean time 1.5 ± 1.3 years post-transplant) on growth in similarly treated (pre-pubertal) children. The patients in this study who had steroids withdrawn also had better blood pressure control with a lower requirement for antihypertensive therapy [49].

More recently, a single-center study has reported on efficacy and safety of a different regimen combining the *intermediate withdrawal of steroids* (>6 months and <1 year) with minimization of exposure to CSA. The protocol initially included a 2-dose basiliximab induction, standard exposure to CSA (C$_0$ 150–200 µg/L) and prednisolone. This was followed by adding EVR at 2 weeks (C$_0$ 4–6 µg/L), reducing CSA exposure by half (C$_0$ 75–100 µg/L), and then steroid withdrawal at 9 months in patients with a normal protocol biopsy. Results of the open-label uncontrolled trial have been promising, without acute rejection and a 100% 3-year graft survival [48, 50–52], while another study on *intermediate steroid withdrawal* (2 doses of basiliximab and sequential replacement of tapered steroids with MMF at 6 months post-transplant under protocol biopsy) reported an acute rejection rate of 13% [53]. Another *intermediate steroid withdrawal* protocol was used in a US multicenter trial, during which patients received 2 doses of basiliximab, combined with SRL, TAC or CSA, and steroids. After 6 months and a protocol biopsy without signs of rejection, patients were randomized to withdraw or maintain steroids [37]. It should be noted that during the first phase of the trial (prior to randomization) 6.9% of the patients developed PTLD. This was mainly seen in young EBV-naïve children, receiving an EBV-seropositive renal allograft; however, this complication should not be regarded as directly related to steroid minimization but rather to initial over-immunosuppression [53].

Early steroid withdrawal or *steroid avoidance* may eventually be found to provide the best overall risk-to-benefit ratio with maintenance immunosuppressive therapy in renal transplantation. *Early steroid withdrawal* or *steroid avoidance* protocols have been used successfully and have undergone extensive evaluation both in the US and in Europe. However, many of these protocols have chosen low-risk individuals and utilized intensive induction therapy with extended daclizumab induction therapy or thymoglobulin, TAC, and MMF [42]. A randomized, controlled study in 196 pediatric kidney transplant recipients investigated the efficacy and safety of *early steroid withdrawal*. Two doses of daclizumab in patients treated with a regimen of TAC and MMF allowed *early steroid withdrawal* on day 5 post-transplant [45]. There was a comparable rate of biopsy-proven acute rejection after 6 months in patients off steroids compared with controls (10.2% vs. 7.1%). In addition, pre-pubertal patients with *early steroid withdrawal* showed better growth and lipid and glucose metabolism profiles compared to controls, without increases in graft loss. These favorable effects were confirmed in a follow-up study over a 2-year observation period [54]. The *steroid avoidance* strategy was examined in a North American, randomized, controlled, multicenter study [55]. One hundred thirty children receiving primary kidney transplants were randomized to steroid-free or steroid-based immunosuppression, with concomitant TAC, MMF and standard dose daclizumab (steroid-based group) or extended dose daclizumab (steroid-free group). Follow-up was 3 years post-transplant. Recipients under 5 years of age showed improved linear growth under a steroid-free regimen compared to controls on steroids. No differences in the rates of biopsy-proven acute rejection were observed at 3 years post-transplant (16.7% in steroid-free vs. 17.1% in steroid-based; P = 0.94). Patient survival was 100% in both arms; graft survival was 95% in the steroid-free and 90% in the steroid-based arms (P = 0.30) at 3 years follow-up. Over the 3-year follow-up period, the steroid-free group had lower systolic blood pressure (P = 0.017) and cholesterol levels (P = 0.034) (Fig. 67.7). The authors concluded that *complete steroid avoidance* is safe and effective in unsensitized children receiving primary kidney transplants [55].

Despite these encouraging results, *steroid withdrawal* or *avoidance* following kidney transplantation remains a controversial issue. Although the benefits of using steroid-free protocols in pediatric patients are obvious, they may increase

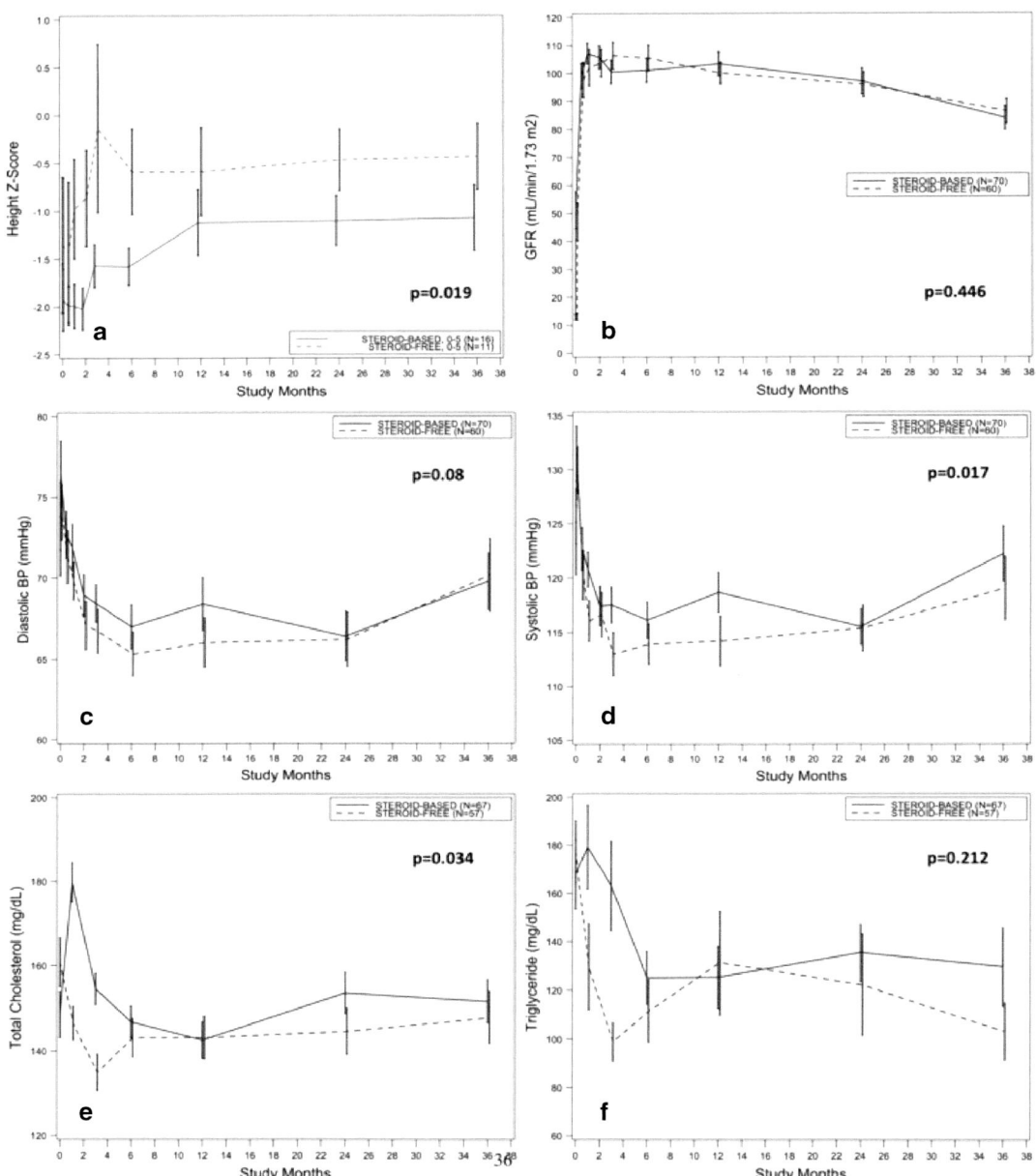

Fig. 67.7 North American randomized controlled multi-center study on steroid avoidance: Estimated group mean standardized change in growth (Z-score) among infants and young children (**a**), mean eGFR level (by Schwartz method) (**b**), mean diastolic (**c**) and systolic (**d**) blood pressure levels and serum cholesterol (**e**) and triglyceride (**f**) levels from transplantation up to 3 years. (Used with permission of John Wiley and Sons from Sarwal MM, Ettenger RB, Dharnidharka V, Benfield M, Mathias R, Portale A, et al. Complete corticosteroid avoidance is effective and safe in children with renal transplants: a multicentre randomized trial with three years follow-up. Am J Transpl 2012; 12: 2719–29) [55]

risk in patients with certain immunological constellations. Further studies need to identify new monitoring tools to assess the immunologic

safety to allow successful and safe conversion of patients to steroid-free immunosuppression at later times after transplantation, even after having initially started on a steroid-based maintenance immunosuppression protocol.

Recurrent Kidney Disease

Because recurrent disease is the fourth most common cause of graft loss in children undergoing kidney transplantation, there have been concerns that steroid withdrawal may be associated with an increased risk of graft loss. Although information is limited, a study demonstrated no difference in graft survival due to recurrent disease in children (4–18 years of age) treated with a rapid prednisone discontinuation protocol compared with historical controls who received steroid therapy [56]. However, more data are needed to ensure there is not an untoward increased risk of recurrent disease, for example lupus erythematosus-associated nephritis, following steroid withdrawal.

Calcineurin Inhibitors

CSA, a lipophilic cyclic peptide of 11 amino acid residues, and TAC, a macrolide antibiotic, are drugs with similar mechanisms of action that have become major maintenance immunosuppressive agents used in transplantation.

Mechanism of Action

CSA and TAC act by inhibiting the calcium-dependent serine phosphatase calcineurin, which normally is rate-limiting in T cell activation (Fig. 67.8). Calcineurin is activated by the engagement of the T cell receptor, followed by activation of tyrosine kinases and phospholipase C-γ1, release of inositol triphosphate, release of calcium stored in the endoplasmic reticulum, and opening of membrane calcium channels. Calcineurin provides an essential step for transducing signal 1 to permit cytokine and CD40L

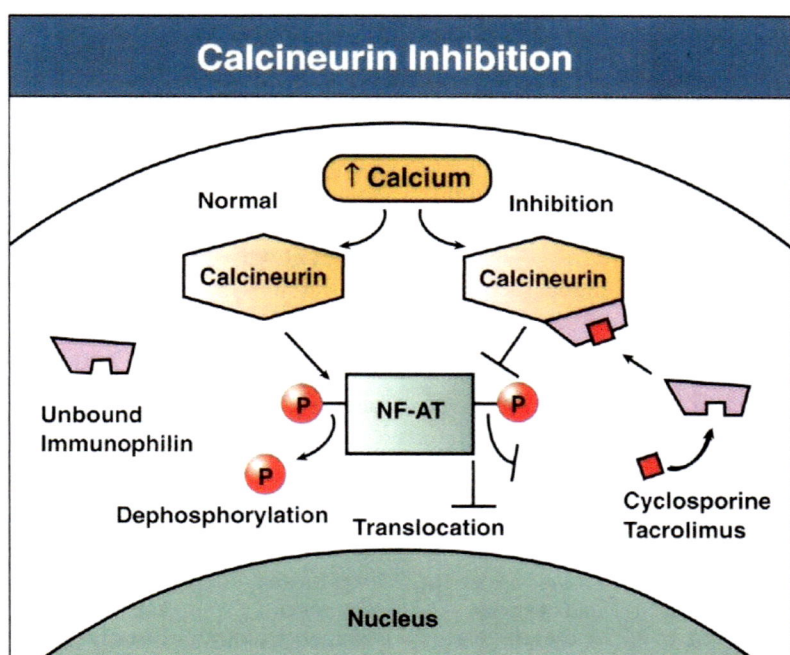

Fig. 67.8 Calcineurin inhibition. During normal T cell activation, calcium release activates calcineurin's phosphatase activity, causing dephosphorylation of the transcription factor nuclear factor of activated T cells (NF-AT) and subsequent translocation to the nucleus. Ciclosporin and tacrolimus form a complex with immunophilins (cyclophilin or FK-binding protein 12, respectively), which bind calcineurin and sterically inhibit the phosphatase activity, preventing dephosphorylation and nuclear translocation of NF-AT. (Used with permission from Floege J, Johnson RJ, Feehally J, (eds.): Comprehensive Clinical Nephrology, 4th ed. St. Louis: Elsevier, 2010)

transcription. A high cytoplasmic calcium concentration activates calcineurin, which then dephosphorylates regulatory sites in key transcription factors, the 'nuclear factors of activated T lymphocytes' (NFAT$_p$ and NFAT$_c$). This causes the NFAT proteins to translocate (with calcineurin) into the nucleus and bind to their DNA target sequences in the promoters of cytokine genes. Calcineurin has been implicated in the dephosphorylation of transcription factor Elk-1, and indirectly in the activation of Jun/AP-1 and NF-κB.

CSA and TAC cross cell membranes freely and bind to immunophilins (cyclophilin and FK-binding protein 12 [FKBP12], respectively), which are ubiquitous and abundant intracellular proteins with isomerase activity. The active complex then binds to a site on calcineurin and blocks its interactions with key substrates. The inactivation of calcineurin bound to CSA–cyclophilin or TAC–FKBP12 is the key to the immunosuppressive effect and some of the toxic effects of these drugs. While inhibition of calcineurin has many effects on the T cell, the best studied is the blocking of the translocation of the NFAT proteins from the cytoplasm into the nucleus.

CSA and TAC partially inhibit the calcineurin pathway at therapeutic blood levels (e.g., trough levels of 200 μg/L CSA or 5–20 μg/L TAC) [57]. However, even partial inhibition of calcineurin reduces the transcription of many genes associated with T cell activation (e.g., IL-2, IFN-γ, granulocyte–macrophage colony-stimulating factor (GM-CSF), TNF-α, IL-4, CD40L). Therefore, the functional consequence of partial calcineurin inhibition is probably a quantitative limitation in cytokine production, CD40L expression, and lymphocyte proliferation. The effect of CSA and TAC on calcineurin *in vivo* is rapidly reversible, emphasizing the importance of patient compliance, drug monitoring, and reliable formulations for delivery. The effects on non-T cells could also be clinically significant.

Pharmacokinetics and Drug Interactions

CSA and TAC are both variably absorbed and are metabolized extensively by the liver via the cyto-chrome P450 system. CSA is excreted primarily by the biliary system. The absorption of some CSA preparations may be bile-dependent, and therefore may be reduced in the presence of cholestatic liver disease. The absorption of the microemulsion formulations of CSA or TAC is bile-independent. Neither CSA nor TAC pharmacokinetics are affected by alterations in renal function. Both CSA and TAC bind to cells and to plasma components (primarily lipoproteins for CSA and albumin for TAC) in the blood; consequently, they must be assayed in whole-blood. Many drugs and agents can affect CSA and TAC levels through effects on their absorption or metabolism (see Table 67.3).

Since the absorption of CSA is decreased and its metabolism increased in children compared to adults, relatively higher dosages are required in pediatric patients. CSA is usually administered initially as 8–15 mg/kg daily in divided doses (or intravenously using one third the oral dose over a 24-h period) during the induction phase, with target trough blood levels of 150–300 μg/L for the first 3–6 months post-transplant. Doses are reduced after 3–6 months (typically 4–6 mg/kg daily); long-term target trough blood levels of 75–125 μg/L appear to provide comparable patient and graft survival as higher blood levels, but with less risk of malignancy [58]. A microemulsion form of CSA (Neoral™, Novartis, East Hanover, NJ) gives more reliable and slightly higher absorption, and may allow a slightly lower dose. Generic forms of CSA are available, but oral formulations of CSA may not be equivalent and readily interchangeable. Knowledge of the characteristics of the oral formulations is necessary before switching between them.

TAC is 20- to 30-fold more potent than CSA, and is therefore administered at a 20-fold lower dose. Initial dosing is usually 0.2–0.3 mg/kg daily in two divided doses orally (or 0.05–0.1 mg/kg daily intravenously over 24 h), and target trough levels are 5–15 μg/L. Since TAC is more water-soluble than CSA, it is not as dependent upon bile salts for absorption. However, food intake can reduce the absorption of TAC by up to 40 percent; thus, it is recommended that this agent be taken on an empty

Table 67.3 Examples of common drug interactions of immunosuppressants used in solid-organ transplantation: ciclosporin, tacrolimus, sirolimus, and everolimus

Common types of drug interactions	Examples of interacting drugs
Co-administration of drugs that inhibit CYP3A metabolism and/or P-gp efflux can increase immunosuppressant whole blood concentrations, leading to significant toxicities	Amiodarone ART-boosting agents (e.g., ritonavir, cobicistat) Azole antifungals (e.g., fluconazole, posaconazole, voriconazole) HIV protease inhibitors (e.g., atazanavir, nelfinavir, saquinavir) Macrolide antibiotics (except azithromycin) Non-dihydropyridine calcium-channel blockers Ombitasvir-paritaprevir-ritonavir with or without dasabuvir (an HCV, direct-acting antiviral regimen) Grapefruit juice
Co-administration of drugs that induce CYP3A metabolism and/or P-gp efflux pumping can decrease immunosuppressant whole blood concentrations, increasing the risk of organ rejection	CYP3A-inducing anti-seizure drugs (e.g., carbamazepine, fosphenytoin, oxcarbazepine, phenobarbital, phenytoin, primidone) Enzalutamide Nafcillin Rifamycins (e.g., rifabutin, rifampin, rifapentine) St. John's wort
Co-administration of nephrotoxic drugs with cyclosporine or tacrolimus can cause additive or synergistic kidney injury	Aminoglycosides Amphotericin B Colchicine Nonsteroidal anti-inflammatory drugs (NSAIDs)
Co-administration of drugs that increase serum potassium with cyclosporine or tacrolimus may cause severe hyperkalemia	ACE inhibitors/ARBs Amiloride Spironolactone Triamterene Trimethoprim, trimethoprim-sulfamethoxazole (cotrimoxazole)
Co-administration of statin drugs with cyclosporine can increase statin levels and risk of myotoxicity	Atorvastatin Lovastatin Pitavastatin Rosuvastatin Simvastatin

CYP cytochrome P450 metabolism, *P-gp* P-glycoprotein drug efflux pump, *ART* HIV antiretroviral therapy, *HIV* human immunodeficiency virus, *HCV* hepatitis C virus, *ACE* angiotensin-converting enzyme, *ARB* angiotensin II receptor blocker

stomach [59]. In addition, TAC is best absorbed in the morning. There is also an extended release formulation of TAC available that is designed to be given once per day with similar efficacy and safety.

Genetic polymorphisms in genes encoding TAC-metabolizing enzymes partly explain the inter-patient variability in TAC pharmacokinetics [60]. The key enzymes involved in the metabolism of TAC are CYP3A4 and CYP3A5 [61]. Individuals are considered expressers of CYP3A5 if they carry at least one CYP3A5*1 allele, whereas individuals homozygous for the CYP3A5*3 allele are classified as CYP3A5

non-expressers. In addition to CYP3A5*3, the CYP3A5*6 and CYP3A5*7 variant alleles can also lead to non-functional CYP3A5 protein [62]. There are ethnic distribution differences of CYP3A5 variant alleles, with expressers (carriers of the CYP3A5*1 variant allele) being more frequently found among non-Caucasian populations. Approximately 10–40% of Caucasians are CYP3A5 expressers, 33% of Asians and 55% of African-Americans [63]. CYP3A5 expressers require a TAC dose that is approximately 1.5–2-fold higher than non-expressers to reach the same exposure [64, 65]. This implies that, following a standard, bodyweight-based TAC dose,

CYP3A5 expressers are prone to have sub-therapeutic TAC concentrations whereas non-expressers are expected to have supra-therapeutic TAC concentrations [66].

Efficacy: Comparison of Ciclosporin and Tacrolimus

To help assess the relative efficacy of TAC and CSA, a 2005 meta-analysis and meta-regression was performed based upon 30 trials consisting of 4102 adult patients [67]. Despite a certain variability between studies, the overall conclusion from data in adults is that TAC-based immunosuppression is associated with decreased acute rejection rates, superior long-term renal function and more favorable cardiovascular risk profile than CSA-based immunosuppression, which translates into improved long-term renal allograft survival. This statement is supported by the results of the SYMPHONY trial, which compared standard immunosuppression vs. 3 regimens with low-dose or no CNI in *de novo* single-organ renal transplant patients over 1 year [68]. In this prospective, randomized, open-label study with 4 parallel arms, 1645 adult patients in 15 countries were randomized to standard immunosuppression with normal-dose CSA (target trough level 150-300 µg/L for 3 months, 100-200 µg/L thereafter), MMF (1 g bid) and steroids, or to one of three regimens consisting of daclizumab induction, MMF (1 g bid) and steroids potentiated by a low-dose of either CSA (50–100 µg/L), TAC (3-7 µg/L) or SRL (4-8 µg/L). The low-dose TAC group was significantly superior to all other groups with respect to glomerular filtration rate (GFR) and biopsy-proven acute rejection (p < 0.01) and to normal-dose CSA and low-dose SRL for graft survival (pair-wise p < 0.05). The authors concluded that immunosuppression consisting of daclizumab induction, MMF, low-dose TAC and corticosteroids provides the most optimal balance between efficacy (control of acute rejection) and toxicity (preserving graft function and graft survival) [68].

In pediatric patients, the efficacy and safety of TAC and CSA were compared in one multicenter trial in 196 patients, who were randomly assigned to receive either TAC or CSA microemulsion administered concomitantly with AZA and steroids [69]. TAC therapy resulted in a significantly lower incidence of acute rejection (36.9% vs. 5.91% with CSA therapy (59.1%); P = 0.003) and of steroid-resistant rejection (7.8% vs. 25.8%, P = 0.001) compared with the CSA group. The difference was also significant for biopsy-confirmed acute rejection (16.5% vs. 39.8%, P < 0.001). At 1 year post-transplant, patient survival was similar (96.1% vs. 96.6%); ten grafts were lost in the TAC group compared with 17 in the CSA group (P = 0.06). The TAC group had a significantly better eGFR. A follow-up study at 4 years showed that patient survival was similar (94% vs. 92%, P = 0.86), but graft survival significantly favored TAC (86% vs. 69%; P = 0.025) [70]. The mean eGFR was superior in TAC-treated patients vs. those on CSA (Fig. 67.9). Cholesterol remained significantly higher with CSA throughout follow-up. Three patients in each arm developed PTLD. Incidence of insulin-dependent diabetes mellitus did not differ. From these studies, the authors concluded that TAC was significantly more effective than CSA in preventing acute rejection and preserving renal function in pediatric renal recipients.

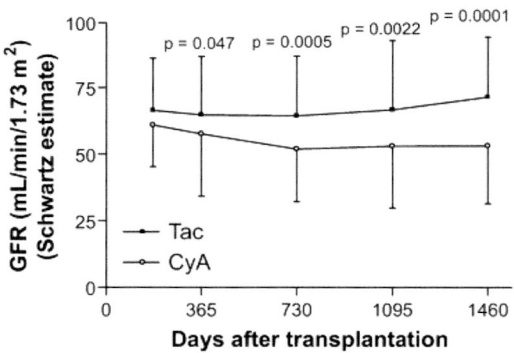

Fig. 67.9 Mean glomerular filtration rate (±1 SD) over 4 years post-transplant. Multicenter trial in 196 pediatric patients, who were randomly assigned to receive either tacrolimus or ciclosporin administered concomitantly with azathioprine and corticosteroids. (Used with permission of John Wiley and Sons from Filler G, Webb NJ, Milford DV, Watson AR, Gellermann J, Tyden G, et al. Four-year data after pediatric renal transplantation: a randomized trial of tacrolimus vs. cyclosporin microemulsion. Pediatr Transplant. 2005; 9:498–503) [70]

A retrospective study of the NAPRTCS database of 986 pediatric renal transplant recipients who were treated either with CSA, MMF and steroids (n = 766) or TAC, MMF and steroids (n = 220) revealed that TAC and CSA, in combination with MMF and steroids, produce similar rejection rates and graft survival in pediatric renal transplant recipients [71]. However, TAC was associated with improved graft function at 1 and 2 years post-transplant (Fig. 67.10). There was no difference in time to first rejection, as well as in risk of rejection or graft failure at 1 or 2 years post-transplant. TAC-treated patients were significantly less likely to require antihypertensive medication at 1 and 2 years post-transplant. TAC-treated patients had a higher mean eGFR at both 1 year (99 vs. 78 mL/min/1.73 m^2, P = 0.0003) and 2 years post-transplant (97 vs. 73 mL/min/1.73 m^2, P < 0.0001). Hence, there is evidence that TAC is superior to CSA (conventional or microemulsion form) in preventing acute rejection after kidney transplantation in adult and pediatric populations. It also seems more effective in improving long-term graft survival in adults.

Side Effects

CSA and TAC have similarities and differences in their toxicity profiles (Table 67.2). Both can cause nephrotoxicity, hyperkalemia, hyperuricemia with occasional gouty attacks, hypomagnesemia secondary to urinary loss, hypertension, diabetes mellitus, and neurotoxicity, especially tremor. In the European pediatric study, the incidence of hypomagnesaemia was significantly higher in the TAC-treated group (34%) compared with the CSA-treated group (12.9%) [69]. Similarly, diarrhea was more frequent in TAC-treated patients (13.6% vs. 3.2%). Hypertrichosis, gum hyperplasia and flu syndrome were reported only in CSA-treated patients, and tremor was reported only in TAC-treated patients [69]. These results are similar to that found in adults, where tremor is consistently more common with TAC, and hirsutism and gum disease more common with CSA [72]. Also, hypertension and hyperlipidemia are more commonly observed with CSA. Interestingly, higher CSA doses are more likely to induce higher blood pressure in older

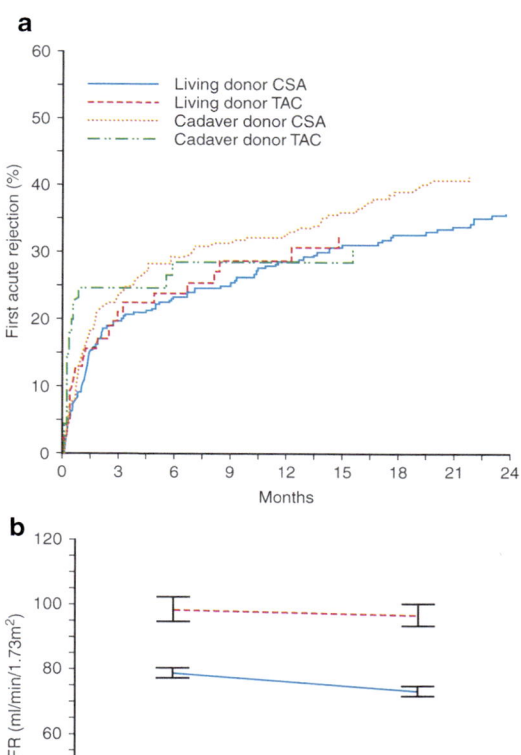

Fig. 67.10 (a) Kaplan–Meier estimates of the percentage of patients experiencing a first acute rejection in the first 2 years post-transplant, by treatment group: tacrolimus (TAC), mycophenolate mofetil (MMF) and steroids vs. ciclosporin (CSA), MMF and steroids and donor source. Patients were included in this analysis if they were transplanted between 1997 and 1999 and had a 2-year follow-up in the database. (b) Mean eGFR as calculated by the Schwartz formula at 1 and 2 year post-transplant in patients treated with TAC, MMF and steroids or CSA, MMF and prednisone. (Used with permission of John Wiley and Sons from Neu AM, Ho PL, Fine RN, Furth SL, Fivush BA. Tacrolimus vs. cyclosporine A as primary immunosuppression in pediatric renal transplantation: a NAPRTCS Study. Pediatr Transplant. 2003; 7:217–22) [71]

girls compared to boys [73]. In the NAPRTCS study, during which CNIs were used in combination with MMF and steroids, TAC-treated patients were significantly less likely to require antihypertensive medications at 1 and 2 years post-transplant [71]. This is similar to adults, where a lower systemic blood pressure was reported in TAC-treated patients in several studies [72]. In the European pediatric study, the mean total cholesterol levels were reported to decline in the TAC group and increase in the CSA group at the end of 6 months [69]. In the multicenter analysis from the European CERTAIN Registry, the prevalence of dyslipidemia was 95% before transplantation, and 88% at 1 year post-transplant [74]; the use of TAC and MMF was associated with significantly lower concentrations of all lipid parameters compared to regimens containing CSA and mTOR inhibitors. Regimens consisting of CSA, MPA, and corticosteroids as well as of CSA, mTOR inhibitors, and steroids were associated with a 3- and 25-fold increased risk of having more than one pathologic lipid parameter as compared to the use of TAC, MMF, and steroids [74]. Similarly, several studies in adults have shown remarkably lower lipid levels in TAC-treated patients than in those receiving CSA [72]. The improved lipid profiles on TAC may contribute to a better long-term outcome with less cardiovascular morbidity in adult patients.

On the other hand, tremor and glucose intolerance are more common with TAC. In the pediatric multicenter European study, there was no difference in the incidence of new onset insulin-dependent diabetes mellitus between TAC- (3%) and CSA-treated patients (2.2%) [69, 70]. Although in early clinical trials of TAC, a significantly higher incidence of diabetes mellitus was reported in TAC-treated adult patients than in recipients on CSA, the incidence of diabetes mellitus under TAC immunosuppression has become less frequent in recent randomized trials comparing these two CNIs [75]. Post-transplant diabetes regresses after dose reduction in some but not all patients. Both the reduction of steroid dosage and low target trough TAC concentrations contribute to this marked reduction of the incidence of diabetes mellitus under TAC immunosuppression in both adults and children [69, 72]. CSA may also be associated with coarsening of facial features, especially in children. Bone pain that is responsive to calcium-channel blockers may also occur with CSA use and sometimes may require changing to TAC.

The most common serious problem with CNIs is nephrotoxicity, with both a reversible vasomotor component and an irreversible component. Both CSA and TAC can cause acute elevations in serum creatinine that reverse with reduction of the dose, apparently caused by renal vasoconstriction, which may be mediated by calcineurin inhibition. Chronically, CSA and TAC can induce interstitial fibrosis and tubular atrophy with characteristic hyalinosis of the afferent arteriole [76]. This lesion appears to result from long-standing renal vasoconstriction, perhaps mediated in part by an increase in local vasoconstrictor tone (increased angiotensin II, endothelin-1, thromboxane, and sympathetic nerve transmitters) and an inadequate vasodilatory response (impaired nitric oxide formation). The importance of this lesion is apparent from studies in cardiac and liver transplant recipients, in whom CSA or TAC use is associated with chronic kidney disease progressing to end-stage kidney disease (ESKD) in a significant fraction of patients [77]. This problem was more relevant at a time when higher doses of CSA were administered for longer periods. Fortunately, currently, CSA and TAC toxicity is associated with only mild to moderate declines in renal function. However, as the number of patients with long-standing non-renal transplants rises, there is increasing concern about future ESKD in this population. In these cases, it is important to establish the diagnosis of CNI toxicity by renal biopsy and reduce or stop calcineurin inhibition whenever possible [75, 78, 79]. Experimentally, CSA nephropathy is exacerbated in the presence of salt restriction/volume depletion and is lessened by treatment with angiotensin-converting enzyme (ACE) inhibitors, calcium-channel blockers, vasodilators (hydralazine), and steroids.

CSA and TAC treatment can cause hemolytic uremic syndrome, probably through endothelial dysfunction. This complication, which is usually associated with elevated drug levels, may respond to temporary withdrawal of CSA or TAC, plasma exchange, switching to another CNI, or conversion to another immunosuppressive drug class.

There is no difference in the incidence of PTLD between TAC- and CSA-treated recipients when used in combination with AZA/steroids [1% (1/103) vs. 2.1% (2/93)] [69] or when given in conjunction with MMF/steroids (1.4% vs. 2%) [71]. This is similar to adults, in whom recent large, randomized studies showed no differences in the incidence of malignancy between patients treated with TAC or CSA [72].

Therapeutic Drug Monitoring

CSA is a drug with a narrow therapeutic index and broad intra-individual and inter-individual pharmacokinetic variability. Serious clinical consequences may occur because of underdosing or overdosing. Hence, individualization of CSA dosage by therapeutic drug monitoring is required. The traditional monitoring strategy for CSA is based on pre-dose trough level measurements (C_0). However, C_0 shows a relatively poor correlation with CSA exposure (area under the concentration-time curve [AUC]) and with clinical outcome [80]. Studies on the pharmacokinetic and pharmacodynamic relationship of CSA have shown that CSA induces a partial inhibition of calcineurin activity, the rate-limiting step in the activation of primary human T lymphocytes and the target of the CSA/cyclophilin complex [81]. The greatest calcineurin inhibition and the maximum inhibition of IL-2 production occur in the first 1–2 h after dosing. Calcineurin is only partially inhibited in patients, which can result in rejection even when CSA blood concentrations are in the putative therapeutic range. From these observations, it was hypothesized that the CSA AUC_{0-4} (absorption profile) or the C_2 concentration (sample 2 h after oral intake) may be a better predictor of immunosuppressive efficacy than the CSA AUC_{0-12}. However, a prospective, randomized study in adult renal transplant recipients did not show any advantage of C_2 monitoring strategy in the early post-transplant period compared to a C_0 monitoring strategy, but led to significantly higher CSA doses and blood levels than C_0 monitoring [82]. In a large study in pediatric renal transplant recipients, CSA absorption profiles predicted the risk of acute rejection, while the single pharmacokinetic parameters C_0 or C_2 did not [83]. A disadvantage of C_2 monitoring is the fact that it requires a timed blood sample within a narrow time window (±15 min) that necessitates further organizational requirements for physicians and nursing staff, which may be judged differently between transplant centers. In our center, we routinely monitor CSA therapy by 12-h pre-dose trough concentrations. We aim for the following trough levels in combination with MMF therapy and prednisone: 120–200 μg/L during months 0–3 post-transplant and 80–160 μg/L thereafter. We feel that a monitoring strategy based on CSA C_2 concentrations in the stable period post-transplant is an additional tool in preventing chronic CSA-induced nephrotoxicity. In patients with low or normal immunological risk, who are on additional maintenance therapy with MMF, we aim for CSA C_2 concentrations between 300–600 μg/L beyond the first year post-transplant; C_2 concentrations are monitored every 3–6 months.

When TAC is utilized, a monitoring strategy based on trough levels is in general sufficient because trough levels are good indicators of systemic exposure. In most transplant centers, doses are adjusted to attain target whole-blood trough concentrations of 8–12 μg/L during the first 3 months post-transplant, between 5 and 10 μg/L during months 4–12, and 4–8 μg/L thereafter [84]. It must be emphasized that these target ranges are dependent on the concomitant immunosuppressive therapy. In the SYMPHONY trial, for example, low tacrolimus exposure (trough levels between 3 and 7 μg/L) in the first year post-transplant, in conjunction with MMF, prednisone and daclizumab induction, was associated with excellent efficacy and little TAC-associated toxicity [68]. However, although TAC trough level goals in the low-dose TAC group of the Symphony study were protocol specified at 3–7 μg/L, the achieved levels were 6.4 and 6.5 μg/L at 12 and 36 months post-transplant, respectively. Hence, a more appropriate interpretation of the SYMPHONY trial is that, in combination with MMF, TAC trough level goals of 5–8 μg/L

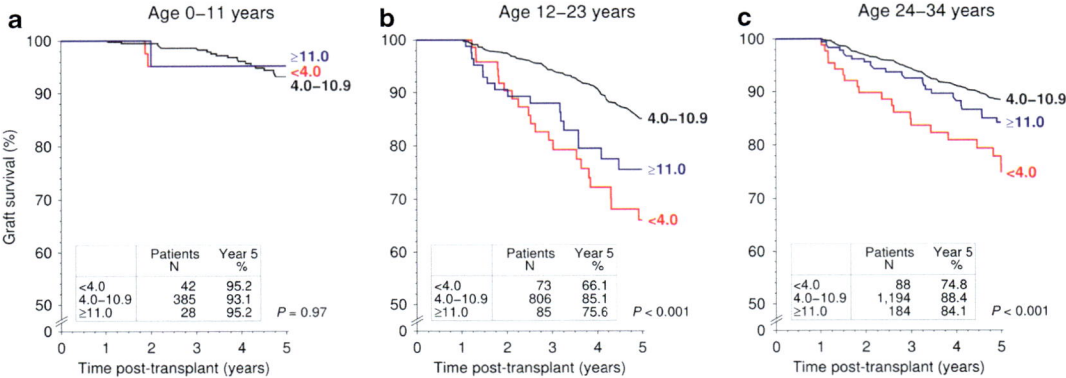

Fig. 67.11 Association of 1-year tacrolimus trough level (ng/mL) with graft survival during post-transplant years 2–5 for the age groups (**a**) 0–11, (**b**) 12–23, and (**c**) 24–34 years at the time of transplantation. Log rank P values of Kaplan–Meier analysis are shown. (Reproduced from [86], with permission)

should be considered as standard of care in adult patients. In addition, recent studies in adult kidney allograft recipients lend support to maintain TAC trough levels above 5 μg/L in order to reduce the risk of *de novo* donor-specific antibodies [85].

Recent registry data indicate that that a more consistent and less variable exposure to the main immunosuppressant TAC later than 1 year post-transplant is associated with a better 5-year graft survival, especially in adolescents and young adults (Fig. 67.11) [86]. In adolescent and young adult patients, the risk of premature graft loss associated with a low 1-year TAC trough level <4.0 ng/mL was 2.38-fold higher compared to a trough level of 4.0–10.9 ng/mL, whereas the risk was not significantly increased in recipients aged 0–11 years. In 24–34-year-old adult patients, the risk of premature graft loss due to a low 1-year TAC trough level <4.0 ng/mL was 1.94-fold increased, but still lower than in adolescent and young adult patients. Importantly, trough levels in the range of 4.0–10.9 ng/mL resulted in a good 5-year graft survival of 85% in the group of 12–23-year-old recipients, comparable to the 88% survival rate observed in 24–34-year-old adult patients (Fig. 67.11). Hence, it appears that optimal TAC exposure can at least partially counteract the enhanced immunoreactivity in this high-risk age group.

Antimetabolic Agents: Azathioprine

AZA, developed by Nobel Prize laureates Elion and Hitchings in the1950s, has been widely used in renal transplantation for 4 decades. AZA is a purine analog derived from 6-mercaptopurine (6-MP).

Mechanism of Action

AZA is metabolized in the liver to 6-MP and further converted to the active metabolite thioinosinic acid (TIMP) by the enzyme hypoxanthine–guanine phosphoribosyltransferase. Some but not all of the immunosuppressive activity of AZA is attributable to 6-MP. AZA acts mainly as an antiproliferative agent by interfering with normal purine pathways, by inhibiting DNA synthesis, and by being incorporated into DNA, thereby affecting the synthesis of DNA and RNA [64]. By inhibiting the synthesis of DNA and RNA, AZA suppresses the proliferation of activated B and T lymphocytes. In addition, AZA has been shown to reduce the number of circulating monocytes by arresting the cell cycle of promyelocytes in the bone marrow. The anti-proliferative action of AZA probably explains much of its observed effects on the immune system and its toxicity. AZA shows some selectivity in its effects with certain cell types and different kinds of immune reactions [87]. For instance, it has been shown that primary immune responses are more susceptible to AZA than secondary responses despite the fact that there is a more rapid proliferation of lymphocytes during a secondary response.

Pharmacokinetics and Drug Interactions

AZA is administered orally at 1.5 mg/kg per day in conjunction with CNIs and 2.5 mg/kg per day when used without CNIs. Higher initial doses (5 mg/kg per day) combined with monitoring of 6-thioguanine nucleotide levels in red blood cells are associated with an approximately 20 percent reduction in the acute rejection rate as compared to lower doses [88]. It is metabolized in the liver to 6-MP and further converted to the active metabolite TIMP. Because 6-MP is degraded by xanthine oxidase, allopurinol, a xanthine oxidase inhibitor, will increase the levels of TIMP. Severe leukopenia can occur if allopurinol, used for the treatment of hyperuricemia and gout, is given with AZA. Thus, allopurinol should generally be avoided in patients treated with AZA. If, however, the patient has severe gout and allopurinol must be used, AZA doses must be reduced by about two-thirds, and the white blood cell count must be carefully monitored. AZA eventually has to be discontinued in many such patients. A possible alternative is switching from AZA to MMF, which does not interact with allopurinol.

Side Effects

The major side effect of AZA is bone marrow suppression. All 3 hematopoietic cell lines can be affected, leading to leukopenia, thrombocytopenia, and anemia. The hematologic side effects are dose-related and can occur late in the course of therapy. They are usually reversible upon dose reduction or temporary discontinuation of the drug. AZA should be temporarily withheld if the white cell count falls below 3000/mm^3 or if the count drops by 50 percent between blood draws. Recovery usually occurs within 1–2 weeks. The drug can then be restarted at a lower dose and increased gradually to the usual maintenance dose while monitoring the white cell count. Occasionally, AZA has to be discontinued because of recurrent or persistent leukopenia. The mean cell volume is commonly increased in patients on full-dose AZA, and red cell

aplasia can eventually result. Interactions between AZA and ACE inhibitors have been reported, causing anemia and leukopenia.

Another potentially serious side effect of AZA, which requires decreasing the dose or even stopping the drug, is hepatotoxicity. This complication is manifested by abnormal liver function tests, usually showing a cholestatic picture. The diagnosis of AZA-induced liver disease is one of exclusion, and the patient should be evaluated for other more serious causes of hepatic dysfunction. AZA has also been linked to the development of skin cancer, the most common malignancy in renal transplant patients. As a result, patients taking AZA for a prolonged period should be instructed to avoid direct exposure to sunlight or to use heavy sun screens when exposed. Other side effects include increased susceptibility to infection and hair loss.

Antimetabolic Agents: Mycophenolate Mofetil

MMF impairs lymphocyte function by blocking purine biosynthesis via inhibition of the enzyme inosine monophosphate dehydrogenase (IMPDH). MMF was developed as a replacement for AZA for maintenance immunosuppression. It is not nephrotoxic and has less bone marrow toxicity than AZA. However, gastrointestinal toxicity can occur, usually manifested by gastritis and diarrhea. MMF is currently available in intravenous, capsule, and liquid formulations.

Mechanism of Action

MPA, the active ingredient of the prodrug MMF, acts by blocking *de novo* purine synthesis in lymphocytes. Purines can be generated either by *de novo* synthesis or by recycling (salvage pathway). Lymphocytes preferentially use *de novo* purine synthesis, whereas other tissues such as brain use the salvage pathway. MPA uncompetitively inhibits IMPDH, which is the rate-limiting enzyme in the *de novo* synthesis of guanosine monophosphate (GMP) (Fig. 67.12). Inhibition of IMPDH creates a relative deficiency of GMP and a relative excess of adenosine monophosphate (AMP). GMP and AMP levels act as a con-

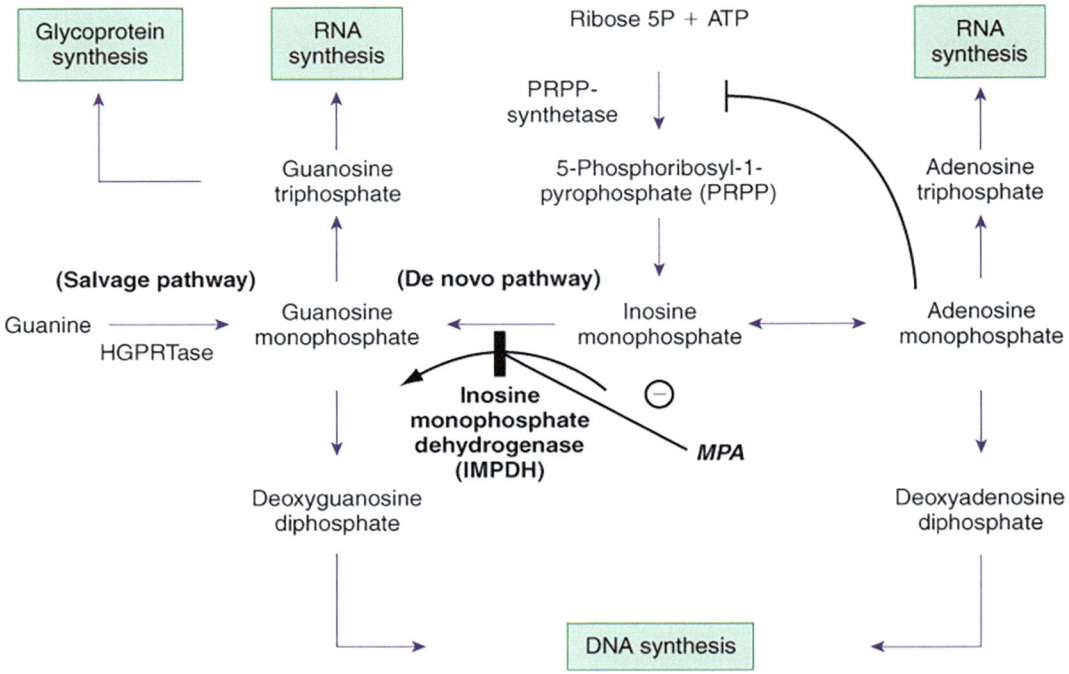

Fig. 67.12 Immunosuppressive mechanism of mycophenolic acid. By inhibiting inosine monophosphate dehydrogenase (IMPDH), mycophenolic acid (MPA) antagonizes the *de novo* pathway of purine synthesis on which lymphocytes particularly depend. Accumulation of adenosine monophosphate inhibits 5-phosphoribosyl-1- pyrophosphate (PRPP) activity thereby diminishing the substrate of IMPDH. Depletion of guanosine phosphates inhibits DNA and RNA synthesis. Lymphocytes lack the salvage pathway of purine synthesis, which depends on the activity of the enzyme hypoxanthine guanosine phosphoribosyl transferase (HGPRTase)

trol on *de novo* purine biosynthesis, which is essential for T and B lymphocyte proliferation, but not for division in other cells. Therefore, MMF, by blocking IMPDH, creates a block in *de novo* purine synthesis that selectively interferes with proliferative responses of T and B lymphocytes, inhibiting clonal expansion, and thus inhibiting antibody production, the generation of cytotoxic T cells, and the development of delayed type hypersensitivity. Furthermore, MPA impairs the ability of dendritic cells to present antigen, suppresses the recruitment of monocyte lineage cells, suppresses the glycosylation of adhesion molecules, inhibits vascular smooth muscle proliferation, improves endothelial function, and inhibits mononuclear cell recruitment into allografts and nephritic kidneys [89]. MPA also decreases cytokine-induced nitric oxide synthesis and prevents the formation of reactive species

such as peroxynitrite. Furthermore, MPA exhibits antioxidant effects in experimental nephropathies. These properties of MPA likely augment its immunosuppressive properties by limiting fibrosis and vascular sclerosis after immunological injury [90].

Dosage and Pharmacokinetics

MMF, a semi-synthetic ethyl ester of MPA, is rapidly and completely absorbed and hydrolyzed by esterases to yield the active drug MPA. The recommended dose in pediatric patients in conjunction with CSA is 1200 mg/m^2 per day in two divided doses, the recommended MMF dose in conjunction with TAC is 800 mg/m^2 per day in two divided doses. However, recent data from a large, prospective, randomized study in both pediatric and adult renal transplant recipients on fixed dose MMF vs. a concentration-controlled regimen, the FDCC study, indicate that a higher initial MMF dose, for example 1800 mg MMF/ m^2 per day in conjunction with CSA and 1200 mg MMF/m^2 per day in conjunction with TAC for the first 2–4 weeks post-transplant, is required to achieve adequate MPA exposure in the majority of patients [91, 92]. The MMF dose should be reduced with active CMV infection. When MMF is associated with diarrhea (a side effect of MMF, see below), dividing the daily dosing to 3–4 doses per day may be effective in controlling the diarrhea.

The difference in MMF dosing depending on the concomitant CNI is explained by a pharmacokinetic interaction of CSA with the main MPA metabolite 7-O-MPA glucuronide (7-O-MPAG). CSA inhibits the multidrug resistance protein 2-mediated transport of 7-O-MPAG into the bile. MPAG is subject to enzymatic and non-enzymatic hydrolysis in bile and more importantly in the intestine, thereby liberating the unconjugated drug MPA, which is then reabsorbed into the systemic circulation. This enterohepatic circulation is responsible for a secondary MPA peak occurring 6–12 h after administration. The impact of the enterohepatic cycle on the MPA plasma concentration varies within and between individuals due to factors such as meal times or co-medication of drugs that interrupt the enterohepatic circulation (e.g., bile acid sequestrants, antibiotics). These factors should be considered when evaluating MPA concentrations (particularly pre-dose concentrations) in clinical practice. Furthermore, genetic differences and disease can affect enterohepatic cycling and thus the bioavailability of MPA [93]. If CSA doses are tapered, the pre-dose concentrations of MPA significantly increase, and after complete discontinuation of CSA they can reach about twice the values seen in patients still on CSA co-therapy. When using MMF in combination with TAC or SRL, lower MMF doses can be used to achieve comparable MPA exposure, guided by therapeutic drug monitoring, to that seen with CSA [93]. However, an uncritical approach used by some centers to reduce the MMF dose generally by 50% when co-administered with TAC or SRL is not advisable.

Table 67.4 Drug-Drug-Interactions between mycophenolate mofetil and frequently used co-medications

Drug	Effect	Site of interaction
Antacids	MPA AUC ↓	Absorption
Cholestyramine	MPA AUC ↓ MPAG AUC ↓	Absorption
Corticosteroids	MPA trough ↓ MPA AUC ↓ MPAG ↑	Glucuronidation
Ciclosporin	MPA trough ↓ MPA AUC ↓	Enterohepatic cycling
Metronidazole	MPA AUC ↓ MPAG AUC ↓	Enterohepatic cycling, suppression of anaerobic bacterial glucuronidase
Norfloxacin	MPA AUC ↓ MPAG AUC ↓	Enterohepatic cycling, suppression of anaerobic bacterial glucuronidase
Phosphate binder	MPA AUC ↓ Cmax ↓	Absorption

AUC area under the concentration time-curve, *Cmax* maximal (peak) plasma concentration, *MPA* mycophenolic acid, *MPAG* mycophenolic acid-glucuronide

The metabolism of MPA due to glucuronidation can also be affected by drug induction. Steroids are known inducers of UDP-glucuronosyltransferases *in vitro*, and there is evidence that this may hold true *in vivo*. In one study, for example, the effect of steroid withdrawal on MPA bioavailability was studied in 26 kidney transplant recipients [94]. When steroids were completely withdrawn 12 months post-transplant, a 33% increase in the mean dose-normalized MPA pre-dose concentrations and MPA-AUCs was observed compared with concentrations at 6 months, when the patients were still receiving maintenance doses of steroids. The relevant drug-drug interactions are summarized in Table 67.4.

An important pharmacokinetic property of MPA is its extensive and tight protein binding particularly to serum albumin. The free MPA fraction in individuals with conserved renal function ranges from 1% to 3%. Based on *in vitro* studies, the free MPA fraction is responsible for the pharmacological activity of the drug. Furthermore, it is an important determinant of the

MPA clearance. Of the factors evaluated for their effect on MPA protein binding, serum albumin was the most important. In patients with delayed graft function or renal impairment, there are many factors which can affect MPA protein binding. These may lead to substantially elevated free MPA concentrations despite total MPA levels similar to those found in patients with relatively preserved renal function [95, 96].

Efficacy

Following the success of the early MMF studies in adults, MMF was investigated in pediatric renal transplant recipients in open-label studies with historical controls, since randomized, controlled trials were quite difficult to carry out due to the relatively small numbers of pediatric kidney transplants performed each year. Since studies in adult renal transplant recipients had previously established the superiority of MMF over AZA or placebo in reducing the risk of acute rejection, it was important for the pediatric transplant community to have prompt access to open-label studies. Data from 3 large multicenter studies [97–101] and one smaller study [102] provided support for the safety and efficacy of MMF in the pediatric renal transplant population when used with CSA and prednisone. Induction therapy was optional in one study [97] and not used in the other two studies [99, 102]. The incidence of acute rejection within the first 6 months to 1 year for patients receiving MMF in these studies ranged from 28% to 37% [97, 99, 101]. Those studies comparing MMF patient groups to historical controls reported significant reductions in the incidence of acute rejection with MMF vs. AZA [99, 101]. There was also a significant improvement in the incidence of acute rejection between patients receiving MMF and those receiving AZA at 3 years in a follow-up report to one study [100]. In one large study [97], no differences in the incidence of acute rejection were observed when results were stratified by age. Long-term (3-year) graft and patient survival were excellent, with a 30% incidence of acute rejection [98]. MMF has a role in the prevention and/or treatment of chronic rejection. Among

children with chronic rejection, some evidence suggests that substituting MMF for AZA may improve renal function [103, 104].

Side Effects

The major toxicity of MMF is gastrointestinal, mainly diarrhea, possibly as a result of the high concentrations of acyl-MPAG in the gut. MMF is devoid of intrinsic renal, cardiovascular or metabolic toxicities, but can increase the risk for CMV infections, leukopenia, and perhaps, mild anemia (Table 67.2). MPA has been associated with protection from *Pneumocystis jirovecii* pneumonia (PJP) and may actually have some anti-PJP activity because *Pneumocystis jirovecii* has IMPDH activity. MMF should not be used in pregnant transplant patients since its safety in pregnancy has not yet been established.

In the MMF suspension trial in pediatric renal transplant recipients, MMF safety was evaluated based on the occurrence of adverse events, including the development of opportunistic infections and malignancies. The most frequently noted adverse events were hematological problems such as leukopenia and gastrointestinal disorders like diarrhea, which occurred in 25% and 16% of all patients, respectively, and were observed more often in the youngest age group. In general, the risk of developing side effects declined with increasing age.

Therapeutic Drug Monitoring

Patients on standard-dose MMF therapy show considerable between-patient variability in pharmacokinetic parameters. This variability is attributable to factors that influence exposure to MMF, such as renal function, serum albumin levels, concomitant medications such as CSA that inhibit enterohepatic recirculation of the active metabolite of MMF, MPA, (Table 67.4) and genetic polymorphisms of MPA-metabolizing enzymes. This variability is clinically relevant, as higher plasma concentrations of MPA are correlated with reduced risk of acute rejection after kidney transplantation [96, 105]. These findings have suggested that individualizing the dose regimen of MMF may further improve clinical outcomes compared with a standard-dose regimen.

There has been considerable debate regarding the utility of measuring MPA levels. Advocation for MPA monitoring is based on the premise that monitoring will result in avoiding both underdosing, which prevents rejection, and overdosing, which increases the risk of adverse reactions [105]. One study in adults, for example, showed significantly fewer treatment failures and acute rejection episodes in the monitoring arm compared with the fixed dose arm with no significant difference in side effects [106]. Within this study, MPA exposure and MMF dosing were higher in the monitoring arm based on 3 levels measured over the first 3 h post-dose. Awareness of the potential for a more personalized dosing has led to development of methods to estimate MPA AUC based on the measurement of drug concentrations in only a few samples. This approach is feasible clinically, and has proven successful in terms of correlation with outcome [107]. An MPA-AUC > 40 mg x L/12 h has been recommended for sufficient MPA exposure for the prevention of acute rejection episodes [92]. In general, monitoring of MPA exposure by MPA pre-dose plasma levels is more popular in clinical practice than monitoring of the MPA-AUC by a limited sampling strategy, but less precise. Therefore, some transplant centers monitor MPA pre-dose and target levels between 1.5 and 4 mg/L. In addition, they use levels as a measure of adherence.

Target of Rapamycin (TOR) Inhibitors

SRL (sirolimus, rapamycin) is a macrocyclic triene antibiotic that is produced by the actinomycete *Streptomyces hygroscopicus.* SRL was approved in September 1999 by the US FDA and in December 2000 by the European Medicines Agency for use in adult renal transplant recipients. EVR is an analog of SRL that has similar effectiveness and side effect profile.

Mechanism of Action

SRL displays a novel mechanism of immunosuppressive action. Interaction with at least two intracellular proteins is required to elicit its anti-proliferative activity. SRL first binds to the cytosolic immunophilin FK-binding protein 12 (FKBP12). In contrast to the TAC-FKBP12 complex, the complex of SRL with FKBP12 does not inhibit calcineurin activity. Instead, this complex binds to and inhibits the activation of mTOR, a key regulatory kinase. This inhibition suppresses cytokine-mediated T-cell proliferation, inhibiting the progression from the G1 to the S-phase of the cell cycle. Thus, SRL acts at a later stage in the cell cycle than do the CNIs CSA and TAC. SRL can, therefore, be used in combination with the CNIs to produce a synergistic effect [108].

Dosage and Pharmacokinetics

EVR is available as tablets and dispersible tablets for administration in water. The current evidence from pediatric renal transplantation suggests that EVR should be administered at an initial dose of 0.8 mg/m² body surface area twice daily when given in combination with CSA therapy, adjusted to target a trough concentration of 3–8 µg/L [109, 110]. There is a well-documented drug-drug interaction between mTOR inhibitors and CSA [111], arising from a shared metabolic pathway via the cytochrome P450 CYP3A4 isoenzyme system, and the fact that both are substrates for the drug transporter P-glycoprotein. EVR exposure is increased by up to three-fold in patients receiving concomitant CSA [112, 113], while TAC exerts only a minimal effect [113, 114]. In patients receiving EVR with concomitant TAC, a dose of 2 mg/m² body surface area twice daily is therefore appropriate [112]. Similarly, SRL bioavailability is higher in the presence of CSA than TAC [115, 116].

SRL is available as tablets form and an oral solution. Data on target doses and blood concentrations for SRL in pediatric transplant recipients are more limited than for EVR. The half-life of SRL increases with age in children [117]. Twice-daily dosing and daily dosing is therefore recommended in young children and older recipients, respectively. However, there is no clear guidance regarding the age or body weight when the switch should be considered. One trial used 13 years of age as a cutoff point [118]. In a pharmacokinetic study of 13 children receiving SRL in a CNI-free regimen, with a median age of 15.5 years, the authors concluded that twice-daily dosing was required in this setting due to more rapid metabolism of SRL in the absence of concomitant CNI therapy [119]. High SRL trough concentrations (>10 µg/L) either with or without concomitant CNI appear inadvisable in children in view of the high risk of toxicity and discontinuation. One small prospective study (n = 19) converted pediatric kidney transplant patients to a CNI-free regimen of SRL with MMF using a single SRL loading dose of 5–7 mg/m^2 body surface area, then a daily dose of 2–4 mg/m^2 body surface area adjusted to target a SRL trough concentration of 5–10 µg/L, and achieved a low rate of rejection with a good renal response [118].

EVR and SRL are both macrolide derivatives and share many pharmacokinetic features, including a close correlation between total exposure and trough concentration, low absorption that varies between and within patients, and differences in absorption between adults and children [111, 120]. However, EVR is the 40-O-(2-hydroxyethyl) derivative of SRL, a modification that results in some important pharmacokinetic differences between the two drugs. EVR is more hydrophilic than SRL and is absorbed more rapidly from the gut with more systemic clearance than SRL [121]. As a result, the elimination half-life of EVR is shorter than for SRL (mean 28 h vs. 62 h) [122, 123]. The clinical effect is that no loading dose is required for EVR whereas a loading dose of 3 times the maintenance dose has been recommended for starting SRL in adults to accelerate achievement of steady-state concentration [124]. EVR is administered twice a day in pediatric and adult patients whereas once daily dosing is appropriate for SRL in older children and adult patients (see above for considerations regarding SRL dosing in younger children).

Efficacy

The most frequent reason to include an mTOR inhibitor in the immunosuppressive regimen is to facilitate a reduction in CNI exposure, or to eliminate CNI therapy entirely. The current evidence suggests that *de novo* administration of EVR with low-exposure CNI therapy in children undergoing renal transplantation is efficacious and safe.

The recently published 36-month, multicenter, open-label randomized study investigated EVR with reduced-dose TAC and steroid elimination from month 5 post-transplant compared with a standard-dose TAC regimen with MMF and steroids (control) [125]. The incidence of composite efficacy failure (biopsy-proven acute rejection [BPAR], renal allograft loss, or death) at month 36 was 9.8% vs. 9.6% for EVR with reduced-dose TAC and MMF with standard-dose TAC, respectively, which was driven by BPARs. Kidney allograft loss was low (2.1% vs. 3.8%) with no deaths. Mean eGFR rate at 3 years post-transplant was comparable between groups. Growth in pre-pubertal patients on EVR with reduced-dose TAC without steroids was better (P = 0.05) vs. MMF with standard-dose TAC and steroids. The overall incidence of adverse events and serious adverse events was comparable between groups. Rejection was the leading adverse event for study drug discontinuation in the EVR with reduced-dose TAC group. The authors concluded that, although adverse events-related study drug discontinuation was higher, an EVR with reduced-dose TAC regimen represents an alternative treatment option that enables steroid withdrawal as well as CNI reduction in pediatric kidney transplant recipients [125].

Use of *de novo* EVR with complete CNI avoidance has not been explored in large trials in pediatric transplant recipients, but is unlikely to be preferable to concomitant reduced-exposure CNI. Primarily mTOR-based, CNI-free immunosuppression is associated with a significantly increased risk of the development of DSA [126]. Switching maintenance patients to an mTOR inhibitor to facilitate CNI minimization can improve renal allograft function or avoid further functional deterioration, particularly when undertaken before irreversible damage has developed. Late switch below an eGFR of 40 mL/min/1.73 m^2, however, may be associated with an increase in pre-existing proteinuria, favoring early conversion. It remains unresolved whether CNI therapy should be reduced or, indeed, eliminated in maintenance patients regardless of whether renal dysfunction is believed to be due to CNI-related nephrotoxicity. Currently, many transplant centers use mTOR inhibitors as part of a maintenance immunosuppressive regimen only in the following patient subsets in which this drug class may have particular utility: (i) Patients, who have histologically proven CNI nephrotoxicity despite low levels and doses of the CNI; (ii) patients with malignancy (e.g., skin cancers and Kaposi sarcoma), either in remission or being actively treated; (iii) patients after treatment of B cell PTLD; (iv) patients with recurrent CMV viremia, because EVR has anti-CMV activity *in vitro* and is associated with less CMV replication and disease *in vivo* compared to MMF [127, 128]. Notably, the incidence of EBV or BK polyomavirus infection is not lower in EVR- compared to MMF-treated patients [125].

Side Effects

Clinically relevant adverse effects of SRL and EVR that require a specific therapeutic response or can potentially influence short- and long-term patient morbidity and mortality as well as graft survival include hypercholesterolemia, hypertriglyceridemia, infectious and non-infectious pneumonia, anemia, lymphocele formation and impaired wound healing (Table 67.2). These drug-related adverse effects are important determinants in the choice of a tailor-made immunosuppressive drug regimen that matches the individual patient risk profile. Equally important in the latter decision is the lack of severe intrinsic nephrotoxicity associated with SRL and EVR and its advantageous effects on hypertension, post-transplantation diabetes mellitus and esthetic changes induced by CNIs. Mild and transient thrombocytopenia, leukopenia, gastrointestinal adverse effects and mucosal ulcerations are all minor complications of SRL and EVR therapy that have less impact on the decision for choosing this drug as the basis for tailor-made immunosuppressive therapy.

An additional side effect in the setting of CNI withdrawal and mTOR inhibitor introduction is aggravation of proteinuria in patients with pre-existing proteinuria by a still incompletely defined mechanism. Available data are consistent with the hypothesis that the increase of proteinuria is causally related to CNI withdrawal and not

because of initiation of an mTOR inhibitor [129]. On the other hand, it cannot be excluded that SRL and EVR might also affect glomerular permeability in some patients. The potential complication of increased proteinuria, which is an independent risk factor for decreased long-term kidney allograft function, should therefore be considered when converting from a CNI-based to an mTOR-containing maintenance therapy. Preliminary results show that mTOR inhibitor treatment may impair gonadal function after kidney transplantation, but the clinical significance of these effects is unknown [129, 130].

Generic Immunosuppressive Drugs

The number of immunosuppressive drugs prescribed to prevent rejection is relatively small. Not more than 10 different compounds have been used over a period of 50 years. For most of these drugs, the patents have expired (AZA, CSA, TAC, MMF, SRL), or will expire within the next few years (EVR, mycophenolate sodium) [131]. Policy makers consider generic drugs an attractive option to enable savings on medication cost, allowing the savings to be used for funding high-cost medicines. Generic immunosuppressive drugs are available in Europe, Canada, and the US. Between countries, there are large differences in the market penetration of generic drugs in general, and for immunosuppressive drugs in particular. To allow for safe substitution, a number of criteria need to be fulfilled. Generic substitution should not be taken out of the hands of the treating physicians. Generic substitution can only be done safely if initiated by the prescriber, and in well-informed and prepared patients. Payers should refrain from forcing pharmacists to dispense generic drugs in patients on maintenance treatment with brand drugs. Instead, together with transplant societies, they should design guidelines on how to implement generic immunosuppressive drugs into clinical practice. Substitutions must be followed by control visits to check if the patient is taking the medication correctly and if drug exposure remains stable. Inadvertent, uncontrolled

12. Stevens RB, Mercer DF, Grant WJ, Freifeld AG, Lane JT, Groggel GC, et al. Randomized trial of single-dose versus divided-dose rabbit anti-thymocyte globulin induction in renal transplantation: an interim report. Transplantation. 2008;85:1391–9.

13. Goggins WC, Pascual MA, Powelson JA, Magee C, Tolkoff-Rubin N, Farrell ML, et al. A prospective, randomized, clinical trial of intraoperative versus postoperative thymoglobulin in adult cadaveric renal transplant recipients. Transplantation. 2003;76:798–802.

14. Brennan DC, Flavin K, Lowell JA, Howard TK, Shenoy S, Burgess S, et al. A randomized, double-blinded comparison of thymoglobulin versus ATGAM for induction immunosuppressive therapy in adult renal transplant recipients. Transplantation. 1999;67:1011–8.

15. Hardinger KL, Schnitzler MA, Miller B, Lowell JA, Shenoy S, Koch MJ, et al. Five-year follow up of thymoglobulin versus ATGAM induction in adult renal transplantation. Transplantation. 2004;78:136–41.

16. Khositseth S, Matas A, Cook ME, Gillingham KJ, Chavers BM. Thymoglobulin versus ATGAM induction therapy in pediatric kidney transplant recipients: a single-center report. Transplantation. 2005;79:958–63.

17. Sterkers G, Baudouin V, Ansart-Pirenne H, Maisin A, Niaudet P, Cochat P, et al. Duration of action of a chimeric interleukin-2 receptor monoclonal antibody, basiliximab, in pediatric kidney transplant recipients. Transplant Proc. 2000;32:2757–9.

18. Höcker B, Kovarik JM, Daniel V, Opelz G, Fehrenbach H, Holder M, et al. Pharmacokinetics and immunodynamics of basiliximab in pediatric renal transplant recipients on mycophenolate mofetil comedication. Transplantation. 2008;86:1234–40.

19. Webster AC, Playford EG, Higgins G, Chapman JR, Craig JC. Interleukin 2 receptor antagonists for renal transplant recipients: a meta-analysis of randomized trials. Transplantation. 2004;77:166–76.

20. Grenda R, Watson A, Vondrak K, Webb NJ, Beattie J, Fitzpatrick M, et al. A prospective, randomized, multicenter trial of tacrolimus-based therapy with or without basiliximab in pediatric renal transplantation. Am J Transplant. 2006;6:1666–72.

21. Offner G, Toenshoff B, Höcker B, Krauss M, Bulla M, Cochat P, et al. Efficacy and safety of basiliximab in pediatric renal transplant patients receiving cyclosporine, mycophenolate mofetil, and steroids. Transplantation. 2008;86:1241–8.

22. Brennan DC, Schnitzler MA. Long-term results of rabbit antithymocyte globulin and basiliximab induction. N Engl J Med. 2008;359:1736–8.

23. Ratzinger G, Reagan JL, Heller G, et al. Differential CD52 expression by distinct myeloid dendritic cell subsets: implications for alemtuzumab activity at the level of antigen presentation in allogeneic graft-host interactions in transplantation. Blood. 2003;101:1422–9.

24. Calne R, Friend P, Moffatt S, et al. Prope tolerance, perioperative campath 1H, and low-dose cyclosporin monotherapy in renal allograft recipients. Lancet. 1998;351:1701–2.

25. Tan HP, Donaldson J, Basu A, et al. Two hundred living donor kidney transplantations under alemtuzumab induction and tacrolimus monotherapy: 3-year follow-up. Am J Transplant. 2009;9:355–66.

26. Calne R, Watson CJ. Some observations on prope tolerance. Curr Opin Organ Transplant. 2011;16:353–8.

27. Shapiro R, Ellis D, Tan HP, et al. Antilymphoid antibody preconditioning and tacrolimus monotherapy for pediatric kidney transplantation. J Pediatr. 2006;148:813–8.

28. Tan HP, Donaldson J, Ellis D, et al. Pediatric living donor kidney transplantation under alemtuzumab pretreatment and tacrolimus monotherapy: 4-year experience. Transplantation. 2008;86:1725–31.

29. Kim IK, Choi J, Vo AA, et al. Safety and efficacy of alemtuzumab induction in highly sensitized pediatric renal transplant recipients. Transplantation. 2017;101:883–9.

30. Ona ET, Danguilan RA, Africa J, et al. Use of alemtuzumab (Campath-1H) as induction therapy in pediatric kidney transplantation. Transplant Proc. 2008;40:2226.

31. Kidney Disease: Improving Global Outcomes (KDIGO) Transplant Work Group. KDIGO clinical practice guideline for the care of kidney transplant recipients. Am J Transplant. 2009;9(Suppl 3):S1–155.

32. Webster AC, Ruster LP, McGee R, et al. Interleukin 2 receptor antagonists for kidney transplant recipients. Cochrane Database Syst Rev. 2010;20:CD003897.

33. Hellemans R, Bosmans JL, Abramowicz D. Induction therapy for kidney transplant recipients: do we still need anti-IL2 receptor monoclonal antibodies? Am J Transplant. 2017;17:22–7.

34. Chua A, Cramer C, Moudgil A, et al. Kidney transplant practice patterns and outcome benchmarks over 30 years: the 2018 report of the NAPRTCS. Pediatr Transplant. 2019;23:e13597.

35. Franchimont D. Overview of the actions of glucocorticoids on the immune response: a good model to characterize new pathways of immunosuppression for new treatment strategies. Ann N Y Acad Sci. 2004;1024:124–37.

36. Ingulli E, Tejani A. Steroid withdrawal after renal transplantation. In: Tejani AH, Fine RM, editors. Pediatric renal transplantation. New York: Wiley-Liss; 1994. p. 221–38.

37. Benfield MR, Bartosh S, Ikle D, Warshaw B, Bridges N, Morrison Y, et al. A randomized double-blind, placebo controlled trial of steroid withdrawal after pediatric renal transplantation. Am J Transplant. 2010;10:81–8.

38. Sutherland S, Li L, Concepcion W, Salvatierra O, Sarwal MM. Steroid-free immunosuppression in pediatric renal transplantation: rationale for and

[corrected] outcomes following conversion to steroid based therapy. Transplantation. 2009;87:1744–8.

39. Barletta GM, Kirk E, Gardner JJ, Rodriguez JF, Bursach SM, Bunchman TE. Rapid discontinuation of corticosteroids in pediatric renal transplantation. Pediatr Transplant. 2009;13:571–8.

40. Höcker B, Weber LT, Feneberg R, Drube J, John U, Fehrenbach H, et al. Prospective, randomized trial on late steroid withdrawal in pediatric renal transplant recipients under cyclosporine microemulsion and mycophenolate mofetil. Transplantation. 2009;87:934–41.

41. Höcker B, Weber L, Feneberg R, Drube J, John U, Fehrenbach H, et al. Improved growth and cardiovascular risk after late steroid withdrawal: 2-year results of a prospective, randomized trial in paediatric renal transplantation. Nephrol Dial Transplant. 2010;25:617–24.

42. Sarwal MM, Vidhun JR, Alexander SR, Satterwhite T, Millan M, Salvatierra O Jr. Continued superior outcomes with modification and lengthened follow-up of a steroid-avoidance pilot with extended daclizumab induction in pediatric renal transplantation. Transplantation. 2003;76(9):1331–9.

43. Shapiro R, Ellis D, Tan HP, Moritz ML, Basu A, Vats AN, et al. Antilymphoid antibody preconditioning and tacrolimus monotherapy for pediatric kidney transplantation. J Pediatr. 2006;148(6):813–8.

44. Chavers BM, Chang C, Gillingham KJ, Matas A. Pediatric kidney transplantation using a novel protocol of rapid (6-day) discontinuation of prednisolone: 2-year results. Transplantation. 2009;88(2):237–41.

45. Grenda R, Watson A, Trompeter R, Tönshoff B, Jaray J, Fitzpatrick M, et al. A randomized trial to assess the impact of early steroid withdrawal on growth in pediatric renal transplantation: the TWIST study. Am J Transplant. 2010;10:828–36.

46. Delucchi A, Valenzuela M, Lillo A, Guerrero JL, Cano F, Azocar M, et al. Early steroid withdrawal in pediatric renal transplant: five years of follow-up. Pediatr Nephrol. 2011;26(12):2235–44.

47. Grenda R, Webb NJA. Steroid minimization in pediatric renal transplantation: early withdrawal or avoidance? Pediatr Transplant. 2011;14:961–7.

48. Pape L, Offner G, Kreuzer M, Froede K, Drube J, Kanzelmeyer N, et al. De novo therapy with everolimus, low-dose cyclosporine A, basiliximab and steroid elimination in pediatric kidney transplantation. Am J Transplant. 2010;10(10):2349–54.

49. Höcker B, John U, Plank C, Wühl E, Weber LT, Misselwitz J, et al. Successful withdrawal of steroids in pediatric renal transplant recipients receiving cyclosporine A and mycophenolate mofetil treatment: results after four years. Transplantation. 2004;78:228–34.

50. Pape L, Lehner F, Blume C, Ahlenstiel T. Pediatric kidney transplantation by de novo therapy with everolimus, low-dose cyclosporine a and ste-

roid elimination: 3-year data. Transplantation. 2011;92(6):658–62.

51. Cibrik D, Silva HT Jr, Vathsala A, Lackova E, Cornu-Artis C, Walker RG, et al. Randomized trial of everolimus-facilitated calcineurin inhibitor minimization over 24 months in renal transplantation. Transplantation. 2013;95(7):933–4.

52. Ferraresso M, Belingheri M, Ginevri F, Murer L, DelloStrologo L, Cardillo M, et al. Three-year safety and efficacy of everolimus and low-dose cyclosporine in de novo pediatric kidney transplant patients. Pediatr Transplant. 2014 Jun;18(4):350–6.

53. McDonald RA, Smith JM, Ho M, Lindblad R, Ikle D, Grimm P, et al. Incidence of PTLD in pediatric renal transplant recipients receiving basiliximab, calcineurin inhibitor, sirolimus and steroids. Am J Transplant. 2008;8:984–9.

54. Webb N, Douglas S, Rajai A, Roberts SA, Grenda R, Marks SD, et al. Corticosteroid-free kidney transplantation improves growth: two-year follow-up of the TWIST randomised controlled trial. Transplantation. 2015 Jun;99(6):1178–85.

55. Sarwal MM, Ettenger RB, Dharnidharka V, Benfield M, Mathias R, Portale A, et al. Complete corticosteroid avoidance is effective and safe in children with renal transplants: a multicentre randomized trial with three year follow-up. Am J Transpl. 2012;12:2719–29.

56. Chavers BM, Rheault MN, Gillingham KJ, Matas AJ. Graft loss due to recurrent disease in pediatric kidney transplant recipients on a rapid prednisone discontinuation protocol. Pediatr Transplant. 2012;16:704.

57. Batiuk TD, Kung L, Halloran PF. Evidence that calcineurin is rate-limiting for primary human lymphocyte activation. J Clin Invest. 1997;100:1894–901.

58. Dantal J, Hourmant M, Cantarovich D, Giral M, Blancho G, Dreno B, et al. Effect of long-term immunosuppression in kidney-graft recipients on cancer incidence: randomised comparison of two cyclosporin regimens. Lancet. 1998;351:623–8.

59. Venkataramanan R, Jain A, Warty VW, Abu-Elmagd K, Furakawa H, Imventarza O, et al. Pharmacokinetics of FK 506 following oral administration: a comparison of FK 506 and cyclosporine. Transplant Proc. 1991;23:931–3.

60. Andrews LM, Li Y, De Winter BCM, et al. Pharmacokinetic considerations related to therapeutic drug monitoring of tacrolimus in kidney transplant patients. Expert Opin Drug Metab Toxicol. 2017;13:1225–36.

61. De Jonge H, De Loor H, Verbeke K, et al. In vivo CYP3A4 activity, CYP3A5 genotype, and hematocrit predict tacrolimus dose requirements and clearance in renal transplant patients. Clin Pharmacol Ther. 2012;92:366–75.

62. Tang JT, Andrews LM, Van Gelder T, et al. Pharmacogenetic aspects of the use of tacrolimus in renal transplantation: recent developments and

ethnic considerations. Expert Opin Drug Metab Toxicol. 2016;12:555–65.

63. Kuehl P, Zhang J, Lin Y, et al. Sequence diversity in CYP3A promoters and characterization of the genetic basis of polymorphic CYP3A5 expression. Nat Genet. 2001;27:383–91.

64. Picard N, Bergan S, Marquet P, et al. Pharmacogenetic biomarkers predictive of the pharmacokinetics and pharmacodynamics of immunosuppressive drugs. Ther Drug Monit. 2016;38(Suppl 1):S57–69.

65. Billing H, Höcker B, Fichtner A, et al. Single-nucleotide polymorphism of CYP3A5 impacts the exposure to Tacrolimus in pediatric renal transplant recipients: a Pharmacogenetic substudy of the TWIST trial. Ther Drug Monit. 2017;39:21–8.

66. Andrews LM, De Winter BC, Tang JT, et al. Overweight kidney transplant recipients are at risk of being overdosed following standard bodyweight-based tacrolimus starting dose. Transplant Direct. 2017;3:e129.

67. Webster AC, Woodroffe RC, Taylor RS, Chapman JR, Craig JC. Tacrolimus versus ciclosporin as primary immunosuppression for kidney transplant recipients: meta-analysis and meta-regression of randomised trial data. BMJ. 2005;331:810.

68. Ekberg H, Tedesco-Silva H, Demirbas A, Vítko S, Nashan B, Gürkan A, et al. ELITE-Symphony study. Reduced exposure to calcineurin inhibitors in renal transplantation. N Engl J Med. 2007;357(25):2562–75.

69. Trompeter R, Filler G, Webb NJ, Watson AR, Milford DV, Tyden G, et al. Randomized trial of tacrolimus versus cyclosporin microemulsion in renal transplantation. Pediatr Nephrol. 2002;7:141–9.

70. Filler G, Webb NJ, Milford DV, Watson AR, Gellermann J, Tyden G, et al. Four-year data after pediatric renal transplantation: a randomized trial of tacrolimus vs. cyclosporin microemulsion. Pediatr Transplant. 2005;9:498–503.

71. Neu AM, Ho PL, Fine RN, Furth SL, Fivush BA. Tacrolimus vs. cyclosporine as primary immunosuppression in pediatric renal transplantation: a NAPRTCS study. Pediatr Transplant. 2003;7:217–22.

72. Tanabe K. Calcineurin inhibitors in renal transplantation: what is the best option? Drugs. 2003;3:1535–48.

73. Sugianto RI, Schmidt BMW, Memaran N, Duzova A, Topaloglu R, Seeman T, König S, Dello Strologo L, Murer L, Özçakar ZB, Bald M, Shenoy M, Buescher A, Hoyer PF, Pohl M, Billing H, Oh J, Staude H, Pohl M, Genc G, Klaus G, Alparslan C, Grenda R, Rubik J, Krupka K, Tönshoff B, Wühl E, Melk A. Sex and age as determinants for high blood pressure in pediatric renal transplant recipients: a longitudinal analysis of the CERTAIN registry. Pediatr Nephrol. 2020;35(3):415–26.

74. Habbig S, Volland R, Krupka K, Querfeld U, DelloStrologo L, Noyan A, Yalcinkaya F, Topaloglu R, Webb NJ, Kemper MJ, Pape L, Bald M, Kranz B, Taylan C, Höcker B, Tönshoff B, Weber LT. Dyslipidemia after pediatric renal transplantation-the impact of immunosuppressive regimens. Pediatr Transplant. 2017;21(3)

75. Toenshoff B, Hoecker B. Treatment strategies in pediatric solid organ transplant recipients with calcineurin inhibitor-induced nephrotoxicity. Pediatr Transplant. 2006;10:721–9.

76. Nankivell BJ, Borrows RJ, Fung CL, O'Connell PJT, Allen RD, Chapman JR, et al. The natural history of chronic allograft nephropathy. N Engl J Med. 2003;349:2326–33.

77. Ojo AO, Held PJ, Port FK, Wolfe RA, Leichtman AB, Young EW, et al. Chronic renal failure after transplantation of a nonrenal organ. N Engl J Med. 2003;349:931–40.

78. Höcker B, Tönshoff B. Treatment strategies to minimize or prevent chronic allograft dysfunction in pediatric renal transplant recipients: an overview. Paediatr Drugs. 2009;11:381–96.

79. Höcker B, Tönshoff B. Calcineurin inhibitor-free immunosuppression in pediatric renal transplantation: a viable option? Paediatr Drugs. 2011;13:49–69.

80. Oellerich M, Armstrong VW. Two-hour cyclosporine concentration determination: an appropriate tool to monitor neoral therapy? Ther Drug Monit. 2002;24:40–6.

81. Halloran PF, Helms LM, Kung L, Noujaim J, et al. The temporal profile of calcineurin inhibition by cyclosporine in vivo. Transplantation. 1999;68:1356–61.

82. Kyllonen LE, Salmela KT. Early cyclosporine C0 and C2 monitoring in de novo kidney transplant patients: a prospective randomized single-center pilot study. Transplantation. 2006;81:1010–5.

83. Weber LT, Armstrong VW, Shipkova M, Feneberg R, Wiesel M, Mehls O, et al. Members of the German study group on pediatric renal Transplantion. Cyclosporin a absorption profiles in pediatric renal transplant recipients predict the risk of acute rejection. Ther Drug Monit. 2004;26:415–24.

84. Gaston RS. Maintenance immunosuppression in the renal transplant recipient: an overview. Am J Kidney Dis. 2001;38:25–35.

85. Wojciechowski D, Wiseman A. Long-term immunosuppression management: opportunities and uncertainties. Clin J Am Soc Nephrol. 2021;16:1264–71.

86. Gold A, Tönshoff B, Döhler B, Süsal C. Association of graft survival with tacrolimus exposure and late intra-patient tacrolimus variability in pediatric and young adult renal transplant recipients-an international CTS registry analysis. Transpl Int. 2020;33:1681–92.

87. Elion GB. The pharmacology of azathioprine. Ann N Y Acad Sci. 1993;685:400–7.

88. Bergan S, Rugstad HE, Bentdal O, Sodal G, Hartmann A, Leivestad T, et al. Monitored high-dose azathioprine treatment reduces acute rejection epi-

sodes after renal transplantation. Transplantation. 1998;66:334–9.

89. Allison AC, Eugui EM. Mechanisms of action of mycophenolate mofetil in preventing acute and chronic allograft rejection. Transplantation. 2005;80:181–90.

90. van Leuven SI, Kastelein JJ, Allison AC, Hayden MR, Stroes ES. Mycophenolate mofetil (MMF): firing at the atherosclerotic plaque from different angles? Cardiovasc Res. 2006;69:341–7.

91. van Gelder T, Silva HT, de Fijter JW, Budde K, Kuypers D, Tyden G, et al. Comparing mycophenolate mofetil regimens for de novo renal transplant recipients: the fixed-dose concentration-controlled trial. Transplantation. 2008;86(8):1043–51.

92. Tönshoff B, David-Neto E, Ettenger R, Filler G, van Gelder T, Goebel J, et al. Pediatric aspects of therapeutic drug monitoring of mycophenolic acid in renal transplantation. Transplant Rev (Orlando). 2011;25:78–89.

93. Shipkova M, Armstrong VW, Oellerich M, Wieland E. Mycophenolate mofetil in organ transplantation: focus on metabolism, safety and tolerability. Expert Opin Drug Metab Toxicol. 2005;1:505–26.

94. Cattaneo D, Perico N, Gaspari F, Gotti E, Remuzzi G. Glucocorticoids interfere with mycophenolate mofetil bioavailability in kidney transplantation. Kidney Int. 2002;62:1060–7.

95. Weber LT, Shipkova M, Lamersdorf T, Niedmann PT, Wiesel M, Mandelbaum A, et al. Pharmacokinetics of mycophenolic acid (MPA) and determinants of MPA free fraction in pediatric and adult renal transplant recipients. German Study group on Mycophenolate Mofetil Therapy in Pediatric Renal Transplant Recipients. J Am Soc Nephrol. 1998;9:1511–20.

96. Weber LT, Shipkova M, Armstrong VW, Wagner N, Schütz E, Mehls O, et al. The pharmacokinetic-pharmacodynamic relationship for total and free mycophenolic acid in pediatric renal transplant recipients: a report of the German study group on mycophenolate mofetil therapy. J Am Soc Nephrol. 2002;13:759–68.

97. Bunchman T, Navarro M, Broyer M, Sherbotie J, Chavers B, Tönshoff B, et al. The use of mycophenolate mofetil suspension in pediatric renal allograft recipients. Pediatr Nephrol. 2001;16:978–84.

98. Hoecker B, Weber LT, Bunchman T, Rashford M, Toenshoff B. Tricontinental MMF suspension study group. Mycophenolate mofetil suspension in pediatric renal transplantation: three-year data from the tricontinental trial. Pediatr Transplant. 2005;9:504–11.

99. Staskewitz A, Kirste G, Tönshoff B, Weber LT, Böswald M, Burghard R, et al. Mycophenolate mofetil in pediatric renal transplantation without induction therapy: results after 12 months of treatment. German Pediatric Renal Transplantation Study Group. Transplantation. 2001;71:638–44.

100. Jungraithmayr T, Staskewitz A, Kirste G, Böswald M, Bulla M, Burghard R, et al. Pediatric renal trans-plantation with mycophenolate mofetil-based immunosuppression without induction: results after three years. Transplantation. 2003;75:454–61.

101. Cransberg K, Marlies Cornelissen EA, Davin JC, Van Hoeck KJ, Lilien MR, Stijnen T, et al. Improved outcome of pediatric kidney transplantations in the Netherlands–effect of the introduction of mycophenolate mofetil? Pediatr Transplant. 2005;9:1004–11.

102. Ferraris JR, Ghezzi LF, Vallejo G, Piantanida JJ, Araujo JL, Sojo ET, et al. Improved long-term allograft function in pediatric renal transplantation with mycophenolate mofetil. Pediatr Transplant. 2005;9:178–82.

103. Ferraris JR, Tambutti ML, Redal MA, Bustos D, Ramirez JA, Prigoshin N, et al. Conversion from azathioprine to mycophenolate mofetil in pediatric renal transplant recipients with chronic rejection. Transplantation. 2000;70:297–301.

104. Henne T, Latta K, Strehlau J, Pape L, Ehrich JH, Offner G. Mycophenolate mofetil-induced reversal of glomerular filtration loss in children with chronic allograft nephropathy. Transplantation. 2003;76:1326–30.

105. Van Gelder T, Meur YL, Shaw LM, Oellerich M, DeNofrio D, Holt C, et al. Therapeutic drug monitoring of mycophenolate mofetil in transplantation. Ther Drug Monit. 2006;28:145–54.

106. Le Meur Y, Büchler M, Thierry A, Caillard S, Villemain F, Lavaud S, et al. Individualized mycophenolate mofetil dosing based on drug exposure significantly improves patient outcomes after renal transplantation. Am J Transplant. 2007;7:2496–503.

107. Bergan S, Brunet M, Hesselink DA, et al. Personalized therapy for mycophenolate: consensus report by the International Association of Therapeutic Drug Monitoring and Clinical Toxicology. Ther Drug Monit. 2021;43:150–200.

108. Kahan BD, Camardo JS. Rapamycin: clinical results and future opportunities. Transplantation. 2001;72:1181–93.

109. Ettenger R, Hoyer PF, Grimm P, et al. Multicenter trial of everolimus in pediatric renal transplant recipients: results at three year. Pediatr Transplant. 2008;12:456–63.

110. Pape L, Ahlenstiel T, Ehrich JH, et al. Reversal of loss of glomerular filtration rate in children with transplant nephropathy after switch to everolimus and low-dose cyclosporine a. Pediatr Transplant. 2007;11:291–5.

111. Kirchner GI, Meier-Wiedenbach I, Manns MP. Clinical pharmacokinetics of everolimus. Clin Pharmacokinet. 2004;43:83–95.

112. Kovarik JM, Curtis JJ, Hricik DE, et al. Differential pharmacokinetic interaction of tacrolimus and cyclosporine on everolimus. Transplant Proc. 2006;38:3456–8.

113. Kovarik JM, Kalbag J, Figuerredo J, et al. Differential influence of two cyclosporine formu-

lations on everolimus pharmacokinetics: a clinically relevant pharmacokinetic interaction. J Clin Pharmacol. 2002;42:95–9.

114. Brandhorst G, Tenderich G, Zittermann A, et al. Everolimus exposure in cardiac transplant recipients is influenced by concomitant calcineurin inhibitor. Ther Drug Monit. 2008;30:113–6.

115. Ciancio G, Burke GW, Gaynor JJ, Mattiazzi A, Roth D, Kupin W, et al. A randomized longterm trial of tacrolimus and sirolimus versus tacrolimus and mycophenolate mofetil versus cyclosporine (Neoral) and sirolimus in renal transplantation. I. Drug interactions and rejection at one year. Transplantation. 2004;77:244–51.

116. Wu FL, Tsai MK, Chen RR, Sun SW, Huang JD, Hu RH, et al. Effects of calcineurin inhibitors on sirolimus pharmacokinetics during staggered administration in renal transplant recipients. Pharmacotherapy. 2005;25:646–53.

117. Ettenger R, Hoyer PF, Grimm P, Webb N, Loirat C, Mahan JD, et al. Multicenter trial of everolimus in pediatric renal transplant recipients: results at three year. Pediatr Transplant. 2008;12:456–63.

118. Höcker B, Feneberg R, Köpf S, Weber LT, Waldherr R, Wühl E, et al. SRL-based immunosuppression vs. CNI minimization in pediatric renal transplant recipients with chronic CNI nephrotoxicity. Pediatr Transplant. 2006;10:593–601.

119. Schachter AD, Meyers KE, Spaneas LD, Palmer JA, Salmanullah M, Baluarte J, et al. Short sirolimus half-life in pediatric renal transplant recipients on a calcineurin inhibitor-free protocol. Pediatr Transplant. 2004;8:171–7.

120. Mahalati K, Kahan BD. Clinical pharmacokinetics of sirolimus. Clin Pharmacokinet. 2001;40:573–85.

121. Crowe A, Bruelisauer A, Duerr L, Guntz P, Lemaire M. Absorption and intestinal metabolism of SDZ-RAD and rapamycin in rats. Drug Metab Dispos. 1999;27:627–32.

122. Rapamune. Summary of product characteristics. New York: Pfizer; 2011.

123. Certican. Basic prescribing information. Basel: Novartis Pharma AG; 2012.

124. Zimmermann J, Kahan BD. Pharmacokinetics of sirolimus in stable renal transplant patients after multiple oral dose administration. J Clin Pharmacol. 1997;37:405–15.

125. Tönshoff B, Tedesco-Silva H, Ettenger R, et al. Three-year outcomes from the CRADLE study in de novo pediatric kidney transplant recipients receiving everolimus with reduced tacrolimus and early steroid withdrawal. Am J Transplant. 2021;21:123–37.

126. Grimbert P, Thaunat O. mTOR inhibitors and risk of chronic antibody-mediated rejection after kidney transplantation: where are we now? Transpl Int. 2017;30:647–57.

127. Tedesco-Silva H, Felipe C, Ferreira A, et al. Reduced incidence of cytomegalovirus infection in kidney transplant recipients receiving everolimus and reduced tacrolimus doses. Am J Transplant. 2015;15:2655–64.

128. Höcker B, Zencke S, Pape L, et al. Impact of everolimus and low-dose cyclosporin on cytomegalovirus replication and disease in pediatric renal transplantation. Am J Transplant. 2016;16:921–9.

129. Ganschow R, Pape L, Sturm E, Bauer J, Melter M, Gerner P, et al. Growing experience with mTOR inhibitors in pediatric solid organ transplantation. Pediatr Transplant. 2013;17:694–706.

130. Tönshoff B. The use of everolimus in pediatric kidney transplantation. Pediatr Transplant. 2014;18:323–4.

131. van Gelder T. What is the future of generics in transplantation? Transplantation. 2015;99:2269–73.

132. Dharnidharka VR, Lamb KE, Zheng J, et al. Across all solid organs, adolescent age recipients have worse transplant organ survival than younger age children: a US national registry analysis. Pediatr Transplant. 2015;19:471–6.

133. Shaw RJ, Palmer L, Blasey C, Sarwal M. A typology of non-adherence in pediatric renal transplant recipients. Pediatr Transplant. 2003;7:489–93.

134. Rubik J, Debray D, Iserin F, et al. Comparative pharmacokinetics of tacrolimus in stable pediatric allograft recipients converted from immediate-release tacrolimus to prolonged-release tacrolimus formulation. Pediatr Transplant. 2019;23:e13391.

135. Rubik J, Debray D, Kelly D, et al. Efficacy and safety of prolonged-release tacrolimus in stable pediatric allograft recipients converted from immediate-release tacrolimus - a phase 2, open-label, single-arm, one-way crossover study. Transpl Int. 2019;32:1182–93.

136. Noble J, Jouve T, Janbon B, et al. Belatacept in kidney transplantation and its limitations. Expert Rev Clin Immunol. 2019;15:359–67.

137. Moudgil A, Dharnidharka VR, Feig DI, Warshaw BL, Perera V, Murthy B, et al. Phase I study of single-dose pharmacokinetics and pharmacodynamics of belatacept in adolescent kidney transplant recipients. Am J Transplant. 2019;19:1218–23.

138. Chambers ET. Role of low-dose calcineurin inhibitor regimens in pediatric kidney transplantation. Am J Transplant. 2021;21:11–2.

Non-Infectious Post-Transplant Complications: Disease Recurrence and Rejection

68

Lyndsay A. Harshman, Sharon M. Bartosh, and Stephen D. Marks

Introduction

With improved screening for immunological sensitization and newer immunosuppressants, the early renal allograft survival rates have increased considerably over the past three decades. However, the risk of renal allograft loss due to non-infectious complications—such as rejection or recurrence of primary disease—remains a worrisome and stark reality for some pediatric kidney transplant recipients (pKTR). This chapter will discuss the causes of allograft dysfunction, including recurrence of primary kidney disease, rejection, and acute post-operative complications. The investigations and management of these conditions will be considered with particular emphasis on the diagnosis and treatment of graft dysfunction.

Recurrence of Primary Kidney Disease in the Allograft

Overall, recurrence of disease accounts for 7–8% of graft losses in pKTR and is the fourth most common cause of allograft loss after chronic rejection, acute rejection, and death with a functioning graft [1]. Recurrent diseases leading to allograft loss are most commonly glomerulonephritis (70–80%) and inherited metabolic diseases (Table 68.1) [1].

Disease recurrence may render the graft unsalvageable and lead to years of patient and graft life lost [2]. General features of disease recurrence may include renal allograft dysfunction with elevated serum creatinine, hypertension, oligoanuria, hematuria, and/or proteinuria. Recurrence may occur at variable time points post-transplant, with some diseases, such as C3 glomerulopathy (C3G) and focal and segmental glomerulosclerosis (FSGS), having the potential to recur within hours to days after transplant.

In a competing risk analysis of 1955 European children transplanted before age 20 years, the highest rates of allograft failure were seen in

L. A. Harshman
Division of Pediatric Nephrology, Dialysis, and Transplantation, University of Iowa Stead Family Department of Pediatrics, Iowa City, IA, USA
e-mail: lyndsay-harshman@uiowa.edu

S. M. Bartosh
Division of Pediatric Nephrology and Pediatric Kidney Transplantation, Department of Pediatrics, University of Wisconsin, Madison, WI, USA
e-mail: smbartosh@wisc.edu

S. D. Marks (✉)
Paediatric Nephrology and Transplantation, Department of Paediatric Nephrology, Great Ormond Street Hospital for Children NHS Foundation Trust, London, UK

NIHR Great Ormond Street Hospital Biomedical Research Centre, University College London Great Ormond Street Institute of Child Health, London, UK
e-mail: Stephen.Marks@gosh.nhs.uk

Table 68.1 Estimated rates of disease recurrence following transplantation. (Reproduced with permission from Cochat et al., [1])

Primary disease	Recurrence rate	Graft loss to recurrence
FSGS	14–50%	40–60%
Atypical HUS	20–80%	10–83%
Typical HUS	0–1%	0–1%
MPGN type 1	30–77%	17–50%
MPGN type 2	66–100%	25–61%
SLE nephritis	0–30%	0–5%
IgA nephritis (Berger disease)	35–60%	7–10%
Henoch–Schönlein nephritis	31–100%	8–22%
Primary hyperoxaluria type 1	90–100%	80–100%

those children with immune-mediated kidney disease compared to children with end-stage kidney disease (ESKD) secondary to congenital anomalies of the kidney and urinary tract (CAKUT) [3]. Statistically significant differences in 5-year allograft losses were seen for children with FSGS (25.7%) and membranoproliferative glomerulonephritis (MPGN) (32.4%) compared to transplant recipients with CAKUT (14.4%) as the cause of their ESKD [3].

Focal and Segmental Glomerulosclerosis

Nature and Frequency of Primary Disease

FSGS is the third most common primary diagnosis in children and adolescents, accounting for 10–13.2% of cases in children older than 12 years of age, with nearly 50% of affected patients progressing to ESKD [4]. The percentage of children listed as having either FSGS or other glomerular disease as the cause of their ESKD has been decreasing over the past decade, perhaps related to improved therapeutics and success in treating glomerulonephritis in children. Despite improvements in treatment, glomerulonephritis (non FSGS) is the identified cause of ESKD in 6.5% of children undergoing kidney transplantation in the USA [5].

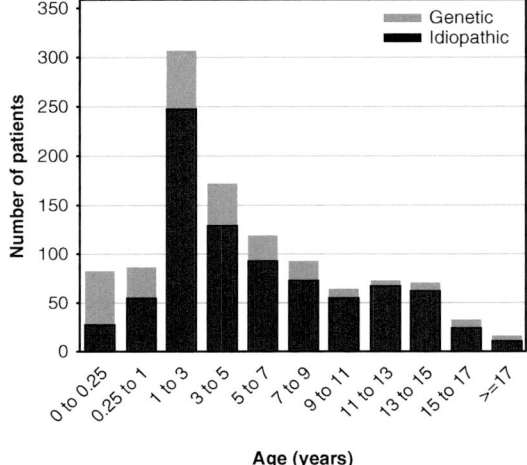

Fig. 68.1 Age at first disease manifestation in children with and without an identified genetic cause of steroid-resistant nephrotic syndrome [13]

Although most cases of FSGS are sporadic (idiopathic), familial forms have been linked to mutations in genes encoding slit diaphragm in addition to other proteins, including nephrin, podocin, WT1, alph-actin-4, CD2AP and TRPC6 [6–12]. The percentage of children having an identified gene mutation is variable depending on the age of the child [13]. In children presenting with NS in the first 3 months of life, 85% have pathogenic mutations. The percentage of children with identifiable mutations decreases with age (for example, 50% in those 4–12 months and approximately 10% in teenagers; Fig. 68.1).

Investigations into podocyte biology and circulating permeability factors have shed light on the pathogenesis of FSGS. A candidate circulating factor, soluble urokinase-type plasminogen activator receptor (suPAR) has been identified to potentially explain the pathophysiology of FSGS at least in some cases of primary, non-familial FSGS [14–16]. The prognostic value of suPAR in the prediction of disease recurrence post-transplant, however, remains unclear [2, 17–20].

Considerations for Transplant Planning: Predicting Risk for Recurrence

In children with ESKD secondary to FSGS, considerations for transplant planning and donor selection are related to the risk of disease recurrence [13]. Much of the early literature relating to recurrence risk did not differentiate between idiopathic cases of FSGS and genetic causes of FSGS. Since genetic FSGS is presumably due to structural alterations in podocyte proteins of the native kidneys, one would not predict recurrence of disease for these patients. Screening for genetic mutations has become a routine part of pre-transplantation evaluation in patients who develop ESKD due to FSGS to allow for appropriate counseling of families and to anticipate the risk of recurrence [6, 21, 22]. Unfortunately, the genotype-phenotype relationship for recurrence risk is not always clear, especially when identified variants are of unknown pathogenic significance.

The clinical course of FSGS prior to ESKD can provide important insight to risk for recurrence. For example, initial steroid responsiveness that evolves to secondary steroid resistance appears to have a higher risk of recurrent disease. In contrast, patients with initial steroid resistance were more likely to have a genetic cause of FSGS and a significantly lower likelihood of developing recurrence post-transplant [23]. Additional clinical risk factors for recurrence include: an aggressive clinical course of primary FSGS with rapid progression to ESKD within 3 years of diagnosis and younger age at onset of nephrotic

syndrome [24–26]. The role of race in predicting recurrence of FSGS has been evaluated by several groups. Although African American children tend to have a more aggressive course of initial disease, they do not appear to be at higher risk of recurrence and may be at a lower risk compared to white children [27–29].

Donor type, induction immunosuppression regimen, and timing of corticosteroid withdrawal have all been evaluated using large international registry studies to describe risk for FSGS recurrence after kidney transplant. The TANGO (post-transplant glomerular disease) study evaluated a cohort of 176 patients who presented with nephrotic syndrome and had biopsy proven idiopathic FSGS [30, 31]. FSGS recurrence rate was 32%, with a median time to recurrence of 1.5 months. Among those who had FSGS recurrence, 39% lost their allograft over a median of 5 years. There was a higher risk of recurrence with older age at primary FSGS onset, white race, lower BMI at transplant, and native nephrectomies. No differences were seen for donor type (living or deceased), human leucocyte antigen (HLA) mismatch, induction immunosuppression regimen, pre-transplantation plasmapheresis (PE), or time to ESKD from disease occurrence.

The impact of FSGS on renal allograft survival in children is greatest in transplants after living donation, resulting in loss of the expected living donor allograft survival advantage [28, 32–34]. This effect is particularly evident in adolescents [32]. For this reason, the rationale for use of living donors in children with ESKD secondary to FSGS should be based on factors other than better outcomes typically associated with living donor transplantation [21]. Since the risk of recurrence of FSGS in a second allograft has, in some series, been reported to be as high as 100% [35], further attempts to transplant after allograft loss due to recurrence should be carefully considered [1].

While practices regarding pre-transplant native nephrectomies vary and some experts have supported bilateral native nephrectomy prior to transplantation [36, 37], others have not confirmed this recommendation [38, 39]. While there may be reasons to perform native nephrectomy prior to kidney transplantation, such as persistence of nephrosis and abnormal coagulation increasing the risk of thrombosis, there is not convincing evidence that native nephrectomies affect FSGS recurrence risk in the pediatric population.

There are no clear data to support a single induction immunosuppression regimen to minimize risk for post-transplant FSGS recurrence. Raafat et al., [40] evaluated retrospective data for 35 pKTR between 1968–1997 at a single center. They found a potentially higher risk of FSGS recurrence associated with use of anti-lymphocyte globulin, with seven of eight patients receiving anti-thymocyte globulin (ATG) experiencing a recurrence. Hubsch et al. [41] compared the incidence of recurrence following induction with ATG and the IL-2 receptor blocker daclizumab. In contrast to data from Rafaat et al., Hubsch found a significantly higher risk of recurrence with daclizumab as induction therapy. More recent multicenter, retrospective data from the North American Pediatric Renal Trials Collaborative Study (NAPRTCS) evaluated patients transplanted between 2002 and 2016, comparing patients with FSGS to other glomerular diseases [34]. Among the cohort of 2010 patients, there was no association between induction agent(s) and allograft survival. Lastly, there are no data supporting use of rituximab as a primary transplant induction agent for prevention of recurrence of FSGS.

As with the data for induction immunosuppression, published literature is mixed as to the impact of corticosteroid avoidance and early corticosteroid withdrawal on potential for FSGS recurrence. Clinical practice regarding use of corticosteroids following transplant is variable. A descriptive survey was performed by the European Society for Pediatric Nephrology to evaluate current practices for recurrence of FSGS after pediatric kidney transplantation [42]. Within this professional cohort, corticosteroids were prescribed for different durations following transplant: (a) life-long (37%); (b) for 3–12 months (17%); (c) 1–2 years (15%); and (4) other or unknown (31%).

Kukla et al., [43] studied the effect of rapid corticosteroid discontinuation on disease recurrence among adult transplant recipients with a history of glomerulonephritis, including recipients with FSGS. They found that corticosteroid avoidance was associated with a higher rate of recurrent glomerulonephritis, but no apparent increase in risk of allograft loss. The 1-, 5-, and 7-year recurrence rate in the glomerulonephritis group completing a rapid corticosteroid discontinuation protocol was 6.7%, 13.7%, and 19.2% and in historic glomerulonephritis recipients maintained on corticosteroids it was 2.4%, 3.8%, and 5.3%, respectively ($P < 0.0001$). Within this sample, rapid corticosteroid discontinuation was also associated with a higher adjusted risk of recurrent disease for all glomerulonephritis types (hazard ratio 4.86; 95% confidence interval 2.34–10.07; $P < 0.0001$). The results of early corticosteroid withdrawal in adult FSGS recipients compared to a historic control group of FSGS patients who received a kidney transplant in parallel with corticosteroid-based immunosuppression was reported by Boardman et al., [44]. There was no significant difference in recurrent FSGS, time to recurrence, or allograft loss.

Given the mixed and limited results across available literature, the use of long-term corticosteroids should be weighed in the context of duration and risk-benefit ratio considering the increased risk for development of new onset diabetes mellitus after transplantation, hyperlipidemia and poor growth.

Treatment of FSGS Recurrence

When FSGS is the cause of ESKD, recurrence is one of the major risk factors for premature allograft loss and has been reported to occur in 14–60% of first transplants and up to 80% of subsequent transplants [1, 25, 27–29, 35, 45–47]. In the NAPRTCS report, 6.6% of index graft failures were due to recurrent disease, with 48% secondary to recurrence of FSGS [48]. There are many approaches for the treatment of recurrent FSGS, and conclusions are limited by small sample sizes and heterogeneity in treatment. The CERTAIN study group recommended initial treatment with early PE or immunoadsorption—

possibly combined with intravenous rituximab—and an angiotensin-converting enzyme inhibitor or angiotensin receptor blocker [21]. If there is inadequate response or patients are dependent on apheresis modalities, then the use of high dose cyclosporin, rituximab, or LDL apheresis should be considered.

Rarely, recurrence may occur intraoperatively at the time of transplant, and approximately 30% of patients with FSGS recurrence have histological evidence of recurrence within the first few days after transplant, with allograft loss in half of these cases [49, 50]. Recurrent disease should be suspected if there is significant proteinuria, which is often accompanied by hypoalbuminemia and other features of nephrotic syndrome. The diagnosis is confirmed histologically with the demonstration of podocyte foot process effacement and without the classical segmental sclerosis of glomeruli [51].

Optimal management of recurrent FSGS remains controversial due to the paucity of well-designed randomized trials and lack of control groups and is often approached in a multimodal manner using various combinations of high dose cyclosporin, cyclophosphamide, intravenous rituximab, PE, immunoadsorption (IA) and LDL-apheresis. To date, no controlled clinical trials comparing different treatment strategies have been performed, and current management recommendations have been adapted from anecdotal reports and small case series.

High dose cyclosporin, with doses of 13–35 mg/kg/day or intravenously at 3 mg/kg/day for up to 3 weeks, has been used for treatment of post-transplant recurrence of FSGS and has been found in retrospective series to achieve remission in approximately 75% of pKTR [52–54]. The reported studies are confounded by the inclusion of patients who had also received plasma exchange in addition to high dose cyclosporin, although the best outcomes were observed when combination therapy was utilized [55]. The CERTAIN study group recommended initial treatment with early PE or immunoadsorption—possibly combined with intravenous rituximab—and an angiotensin-converting enzyme inhibitor or angiotensin receptor blocker [21]. If there is inadequate response or patients are dependent on apheresis modalities, then the use of high dose cyclosporin, rituximab, or LDL apheresis should be considered.

Pre-emptive rituximab monotherapy has not been shown to prevent recurrence of nephrotic syndrome post-transplantation [56]. The addition of rituximab to PE may be considered, with 44–50% of patients treated with rituximab achieving complete remission and 20–25% achieving partial remission, and the reported number of doses given varying from 1 to 6 [57–61]. The optimal timing of rituximab administration and the required number of doses remain unclear. Likewise, a correlation between CD19/CD20 B-cell depletion and clinical efficacy has not been demonstrated. Side effects of rituximab include hypogammaglobulinemia and increased risk for infection.

Due to the successful treatment of children with steroid-dependent or frequently relapsing nephrotic syndrome with oral cyclophosphamide, this treatment has also been used to treat FSGS recurrence. Experience with oral cyclophosphamide in this setting is quite limited but has been reported to be well tolerated and to lead to long-term remission in some patients [35, 45, 62]. In one series of pediatric subjects, a cumulative dosage of 115–121 mg/kg of cyclophosphamide was used over a 3-month period to induce remission following disease recurrence [63].

Clinical and experimental evidence supports the existence of a circulating factor responsible for FSGS, with several candidate factors proposed including galactose, cardiotrophin-like cytokine-1 and soluble urokinase receptor (suPAR) [64]. Due to the possibility of a circulating permeability factor causing progressive podocyte injury leading to FSGS (primary or recurrent), the use of extracorporeal systems aimed at removal of this factor such as PE, IA, and low-density lipoprotein-apheresis (LDL-A) have been introduced. Several groups have reported the favorable effects of PE on remission of recurrent FSGS and on overall allograft survival although these retrospective case series differed in numbers of patients treated, underlying immunosuppression regimens, definition of recurrence, and ethnicity of the patients [1, 25, 50, 54, 65–68]. Different PE protocols have been reported, with colloid replacement including 4.5–5% albumin, intravenous gamma globulin and fresh frozen plasma. In most reports, PE was started early, within 7 days of developing proteinuria. The outcome of PE in recurrent FSGS may be linked to the number of sessions performed, typically ranging from 5 to 13 treatments. After initiation of PE, the time to remission is also highly variable, ranging from 5 to 27 days in the reported literature. Immediately post-transplant, the exclusive use of 5% albumin should be avoided due to the increased risk of post-operative bleeding. Some centers recommend prophylactic use of PE even before nephrotic syndrome develops [67], although others have not found that pre-emptive therapy is effective [65, 69]. It is important to note that in reported cases, PE is almost universally used in conjunction with immunosuppressive therapy, including corticosteroids, cyclophosphamide and calcineurin inhibitors (CNIs).

Another therapy for recurrent FSGS which could potentially remove inciting circulating factors is IA [66, 70, 71]. A comprehensive review of the extracorporeal therapies, particularly with respect to the technical aspects, has recently been published [72]. Case series data suggests that IA seems to have comparable efficacy to PE although there are no head-to-head comparisons; thus, the exact mechanism of IA remains unclear. In a multicenter French study of recurrent FSGS in children, 10 of 12 treated with IA responded (eight with complete remission and two with partial remission) [68]. A decrease in proteinuria occurred within the first 10 sessions. Within 3 months of IA, eight pKTR were IA dependent, with two patients able to maintain remission without IA.

Apoproteins play a role in lipid transport and possibly in maintaining the integrity of the glomerular filtration barrier. Loss of these factors may play a role in the pathogenesis of recurrent FSGS [73]. There are many proposed mechanisms through which hyperlipidemia, hypercholesterolemia, and abnormal lipoproteins ultimately lead to progressive renal disease involving oxidative stress, vasoactive substances, and inflammatory factors [74]. LDL-A is a primary selective extracorporeal system that has been studied in FSGS [72]. In addition to inducing remission, LDL-A is purported to improve response rate to corticosteroid and immunosuppressive therapy. Currently, LDL-A is commonly performed using the Liposorber LA-15 system, which was approved by the FDA in the USA for a Humanitarian Device Exemption in 2013 for use in the treatment of pediatric patients with drug-refractory FSGS as well as post-transplant FSGS.

Lastly, renin-angiotensin-aldosterone blockade may be considered in post-transplant recurrence of FSGS, particularly to help diminish protein excretion and to address the suggested role of angiotensin in the role in the pathogenesis of recurrent FSGS [24, 75].

Atypical Hemolytic Uremic Syndrome

Nature and Frequency of Primary Disease

The prevalence of atypical hemolytic uremic syndrome (aHUS) in patients less than 20 years of age is estimated at 2.21–9.4 per million people [76] with the highest disease prevalence occurring in children between 0–4 years of age [77]. Uncontrolled overactivation of the alternative complement pathway (ACP) at the level of the endothelium is a primary immunological feature of aHUS [78]. There are known genetic abnormalities within the ACP which predispose to aHUS, including complement factor H (CFH), complement factor I (CFI), complement component C (C3), complement factor B (CFB), and membrane cofactor protein (MCP). In addition, some patients have aHUS secondary to autoantibodies to CFH. The clinical hallmark of aHUS is a thrombotic microangiopathy (TMA) with a microangiopathic hemolytic anemia, thrombocytopenia and renal dysfunction. Direct kidney injury is largely driven by damage to the glomerular endothelium from the complement-associated membrane attack complex (MAC) composed of complement components (C) C5b-9 [79]. Kidney damage results in acute kidney injury, difficult to control hypertension, microscopic hematuria, and proteinuria.

Considerations for Transplant Planning

Kidney transplantation should be delayed at least 6 months after starting rescue therapy with eculizumab (a recombinant, humanized monoclonal antibody against the complement protein C5 [80]) as there may be limited recovery of kidney function that occurs within the first several months of eculizumab initiation [81–83]. Furthermore, aHUS-associated hematological features and extra-renal manifestations should be resolved prior to transplantation [81].

The risk for aHUS recurrence post-transplant is strongly linked with several pathogenic complement-based mutations. CFH, CFI, and C3 mutations have the highest risk for aHUS recurrence (68–90%, 70–80%, and 40–50%, respectively) [84]. It is important to note that approximately 30–50% of patients with aHUS have no identifiable genetic mutation or CFH autoantibody using currently available testing platforms [85, 86]. Pediatric patients and families should meet with a genetic counselor having expertise in complement-mediated genetic abnormalities. When counseling families of children and young people affected with aHUS without identification of a genetic mutation or autoantibody, it should be emphasized that there still may be an underlying genetic contribution to aHUS that could confer recurrence risk post-kidney transplant.

The diagnosis of aHUS has implications for evaluation of potential living donors. For example, kidney donation from a living-related donor has historically not been advised given the potential for the related donor to have the same genetic susceptibility factor(s) as the recipient [87]. As noted, if there is no identifiable complement genetic mutation in the patient, then living-related donation is contraindicated given the risk for an unidentified, underlying genetic mutation

which could adversely impact the donor [88]. Conversely, if a pathogenic gene variant is identified in the recipient and not present in a potential living-related donor (and the donor has no other evidence of abnormal complement activation), then living-related donation may be feasible [87]. Living donation may, in fact, confer a decreased risk for complement activation secondary to ischemia-reperfusion injury typically encountered with deceased donation [89].

Risk Factors for Recurrence and Treatment of Recurrence

Most aHUS recurrences occur within the first year following kidney transplant. The strongest risk factor for aHUS recurrence is the presence of genetic complement abnormalities [86, 87, 90]. Feitz et al. [84] provide an excellent review of the estimated risk for aHUS recurrence based on complement gene mutation. The development and availability of eculizumab has drastically changed how transplant nephrologists approach prevention of aHUS recurrence. For patients with a known genetic mutation conferring risk for recurrence, intravenous eculizumab should be initiated within 24 h prior to transplantation, with an additional dose on the first post-operative day [87].

Current guidelines from the Kidney Disease Improving Global Outcomes (KDIGO) consensus report provide expert opinion regarding prophylaxis strategies against aHUS recurrence post-transplant based on a risk-assessment strategy (Table 68.2). For example, patients with persistently negative factor H autoantibody and/or isolated MCP mutations can potentially be transplanted without prophylactic eculizumab [81, 91]. In this situation, the child should be followed closely post-transplant for disease recurrence, with a low threshold to initiate intravenous eculizumab therapy. Markers of disease recurrence might include dropping C3, anemia, thrombocytopenia, low haptoglobin, elevated lactate dehydrogenase, new onset hypertension, microscopic hematuria, and/or proteinuria.

There are no data to support that nephrectomy prior to or coincident with transplant decreases

Table 68.2 Expert opinion regarding prophylaxis strategies against aHUS recurrence post-transplant based on a risk-assessment strategy. (Reproduced with permission from Loirat et al., [91])

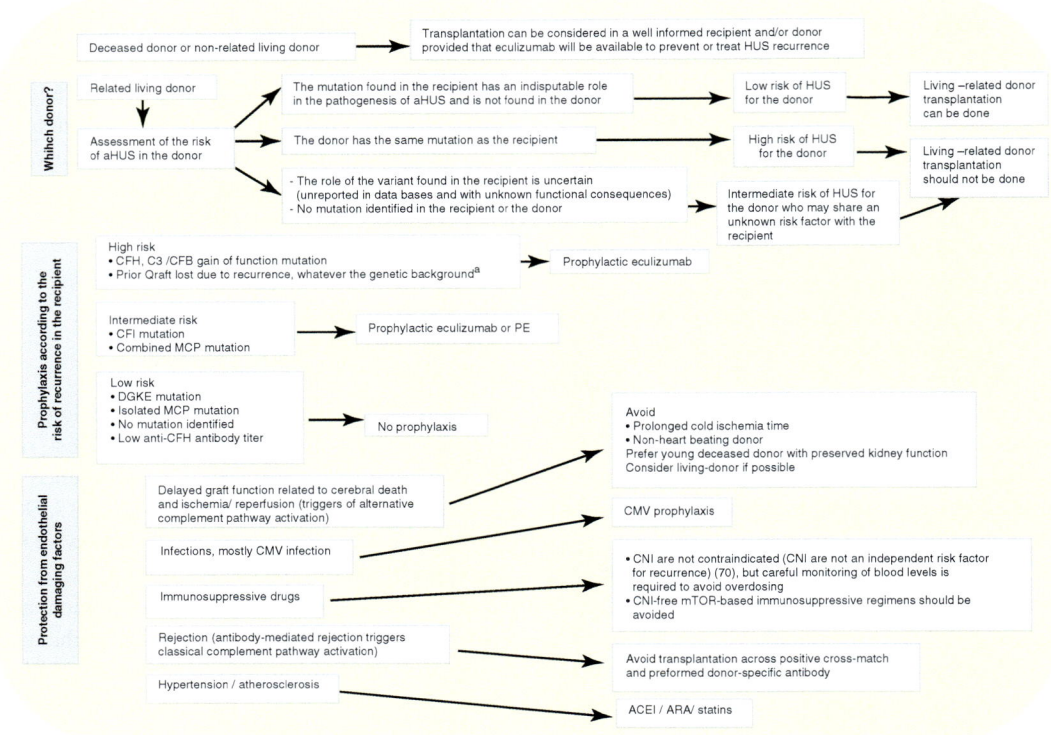

risk for recurrence. Available, limited data suggest that targeted transplant protocols attempting to minimize endothelial damage may decrease risk for aHUS recurrence in patients not receiving prophylactic eculizumab. For example, induction therapy with basiliximab (interleukin-2 receptor blocker) may be preferable to use of lymphocyte depleting agents [92] in addition to decreasing the target trough CNI levels [93]. A case series [94] demonstrated excellent patient and allograft outcomes using an induction regimen with intravenous basiliximab, reduced-dose tacrolimus, and high-dose mycophenolate mofetil (MMF) in conjunction with early, strict blood pressure control, statin therapy, and angiotensin-converting enzyme inhibition to diminish the risk for endothelial injury that might up-regulate complement activation within the allograft. Acute rejection is an additional risk factor for aHUS recurrence; thus, intensified monitoring for aHUS recurrence may be required during rejection episodes [95].

Risk of Disease Recurrence in the Era of Eculizumab

Prior to the widespread use of eculizumab, kidney transplantation was not a viable option for many aHUS patients given the substantial morbidity and mortality associated with disease recurrence. Without eculizumab, the risk of recurrent disease after kidney transplantation was estimated to be 50–80%, with an overall 5-year graft survival of $36 \pm 7\%$ in patients with a recurrence compared with $70 \pm 8\%$ in patients without a recurrence [96, 97]. In the absence of effective anti-complement treatment, nearly 30% of the pediatric patients and half of adult patients with aHUS who survived in the acute phase of disease recurrence required long-term dialysis [85, 96]. The 2016 KDIGO consensus report on aHUS suggests that withdrawal of eculizumab should not be considered in patients treated for post-transplant recurrence until there are data demonstrating the safety of this approach [91]. Limited case-series data suggest that cessation of eculizumab after the first year post-transplant may be a viable, safe option [98]; however, there is currently limited consensus to support this approach.

Additional Post-Transplant Considerations

Due to the risk for sepsis from encapsulated organisms, recipients receiving eculizumab should receive meningococcal and pneumococcal vaccinations prior to transplantation with additional booster vaccinations as necessary following transplantation [99]. The recipient additionally requires prophylactic antimicrobial coverage with ciprofloxacin or penicillin-V for the duration of eculizumab use [99]. The use of eculizumab, MMF, and CNI constitutes triple immunosuppression; thus, terminal CNI levels can potentially be targeted at the lowest end of the clinician's goal

range to avoid overimmunosuppression and infectious complications. For example, this may correlate with targeting tacrolimus levels to 3–5 ng/mL after the first 12 months post transplantation in the absence of rejection (expert opinion).

C3 Glomerulopathy

Nature and Frequency of C3G

C3 glomerulopathy (C3G) is an umbrella term that encompasses both C3 glomerulonephritis (C3GN) and dense deposit disease (DDD). C3G is caused by overactivation of the alternative complement pathway. Abnormal complement activation typically may result from loss of function of one of the complement regulatory proteins (factor H or factor I) or from gain-of-function mutations in C3 that lead to resistance to regulation by factor H [100] (see Fig. 68.2). Overactivation of the complement pathway can

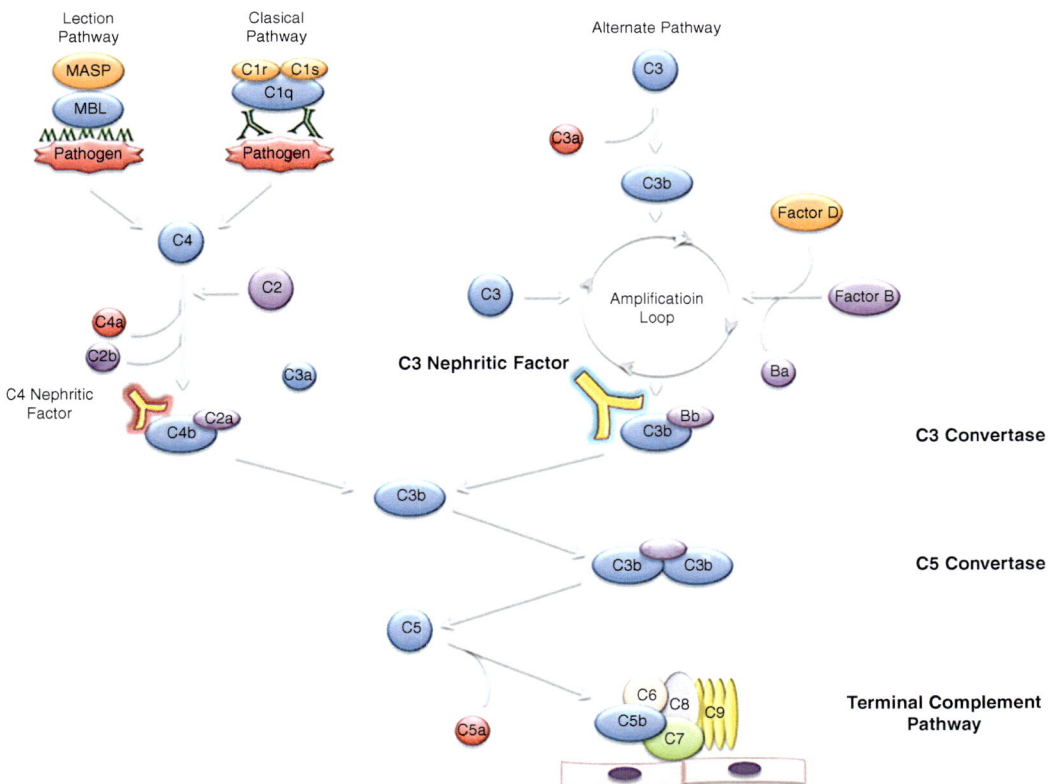

Fig. 68.2   Complement Inhibition in C3G. (Figure used with permission from Nester et al., [100])

also be secondary to generation of a C3 convertase-stabilizing autoantibody, C3 nephritic factor (C3NeF), or production of an autoantibody to factor H. Ultimately, these abnormalities result in overactivity of the C3 convertase and consumption of complement. Thus, low C3 level is a feature of C3G in approximately 75% of cases [78, 101].

C3GN and DDD have an overlapping spectrum of pathological and clinical features. Clinical features are consistent with active glomerulonephritis: nephrotic range proteinuria, microscopic hematuria, hypertension, and renal dysfunction with elevated serum creatinine. The diagnosis of C3G requires a percutaneous renal biopsy demonstrating significant C3 deposition within the kidney, specifically the glomerulus. C3 deposition occurs in the *absence* of immunoglobulin deposition on pathological examination (e.g., negative/ near absent immunoglobulin G, immunoglobulin A, and immunoglobulin M) [102, 103]. Electron microscopy findings of electron-dense, "sausage-shaped" deposits within the glomerular basement membrane are pathognomonic of DDD whereas in C3G the deposits are less dense and primarily located within the mesangium.

C3G is an ultra-rare disease with an incidence of around 0.2–1 per 1,000,000 [104, 105]. C3G i has a 10-year kidney survival of 50%, leading to eventual need for kidney replacement therapy [78].

Considerations for Transplant Planning

As with aHUS, planning for transplant in the setting of C3G should include an evaluation with a team experienced in the genetics of complement-mediated kidney disease. This evaluation should include genetic testing of complement genes, measurement/assessment of complement function, and screening for complement autoantibodies. Mutation screening of complement regulatory genes (e.g., CFH, CFI), activation protein genes (C3, CFB), autoantibodies (C3NeF and antibodies to CFH), and assessment of copy number variation across the CFH-CFH-related (CFHR) locus should be done on a case-by-case basis given the need for expert interpretation and clinical validation [81, 102]. Genetic and functional studies may provide insight regarding utility and efficacy of targeted anti-complement therapy (e.g., eculizumab or novel anti-complement therapies in development) should C3G recur following transplant.

Living-related donor kidney transplantation should be approached with caution for both the presumed healthy donor and recipient with C3G. Current international recommendations are that all potential *recipients* of a living-related kidney be screened for genetic abnormalities within the complement system [81]. If a genetic abnormality is found, the donor should subsequently be tested. The presence of an identical genetic abnormality may not constitute an absolute contraindication to donation; however, the individual case be evaluated in conjunction with expert teams in complement genetics and C3G. Furthermore, for donors with identified complement genetic abnormalities, the donor team must disclose the theoretical risks that donation may trigger new disease onset.

There are no published data supporting a specific induction agent; thus, selection is based on center preference. There are no data to support pre- or peri-transplant nephrectomy to prevent disease recurrence. The presence of active disease, specifically heavy proteinuria, is a relative contraindication to transplantation; transplantation should be delayed until there is resolution of nephrotic-range proteinuria, which may require nephrectomies in some patients [81].

Risk Factors for Recurrence and Treatment of C3G Recurrence

C3G recurs at a high rate, with allograft loss due to C3G in approximately 50% of those patients [81]. Patients and families should be counseled on the high risk for disease recurrence. The reported recurrence rate of C3GN is estimated as greater than 50% [106, 107]. The recurrence rate of DDD is much higher and approaches 80–100% [108, 109].

Pediatric patients have lower long-term graft survival. It has been hypothesized that this may be due to more significant complement disruption and aggressive disease in children compared to adults. In one case series, 10-year graft survival was 11% and 21% in pediatric and adult allograft recipients, respectively [110].

Pre-transplantation C3 levels may also predict allograft outcomes. In one small case series, low C3 levels were present pre-transplantation in more than 50% of patients with recurrence; C3 levels were normal pre-transplantation in all patients without recurrence [111]. Other factors associated with an increased risk of C3G recurrence include high levels of circulating autoantibodies (C3NeF and FH autoantibody), rapid progression to ESKD in the native kidneys (crescentic disease) and living-related kidney transplantation [112].

Diagnosis of C3G recurrence requires pathological features of the disease and should be supported by clinical history. Following transplant, patients with history of C3G should be closely followed for signs of recurrence, including proteinuria, hematuria, reducing complement C3 levels and elevated serum creatinine. Up to 90% of C3G allograft recipients will show histological C3 deposition [109, 113]. Data support that protocol biopsies from C3G transplant recipients can show deposition of C3 as early as the first month post-transplant in the absence of clinical disease [113, 114]. Furthermore, glomerular C3 deposition in the absence of other clinicopathological findings is independently associated with a higher risk of allograft failure [114].

Unfortunately, even when recurrence is diagnosed early therapeutic options in the setting of recurrence are very limited. The decision to utilize any therapy for C3G recurrence should be done in parallel with clinical and pathological data as well as comprehensive complement biomarker assessment. There are insufficient data to recommend routine use of plasma exchange for C3G recurrence unless there is an identified complement factor deficiency, such as CFH [81, 102]. Insufficient data exist to support routine use of eculizumab for C3G recurrence [81, 102]. One study [115, 116] suggests that the lowest incidence of allograft loss (33%) among patients with recurrent C3G are those treated with eculizumab. Among those who received no treatment for C3G due to stable allograft function, there is a high incidence of allograft loss of 32% in C3GN and 53% in DDD [115]. Consideration to plasma exchange and/or eculizumab should incorporate assessment of patient complement biomarkers [115]. For example, soluble membrane attack complex levels may help to select good responders to eculizumab.

Due to the mechanistic complexity of C3G, there may not be a single therapeutic option, such as eculizumab for aHUS, that provides comprehensive treatment of C3G recurrence. More promising, perhaps, is the development of complement inhibitors (e.g., inhibition of C3 or complement factor B) which could provide targeted therapy for recurrence of C3G following transplant. Early clinical trial (phase II) data for the novel complement factor B agent, LNP023, demonstrate resolution of proteinuria and stability of kidney function in native kidneys [117]. Data from allograft recipients with C3G recurrence have not been published. With the current lack of treatment options for C3G recurrence post-transplant, loss of a prior allograft due to recurrent C3G indicates a high risk of recurrence upon subsequent transplantation and this should be a major consideration in determining candidacy for re-transplant [112].

IgA-Mediated Kidney Disease

IgA vasculitis (IgAV; previously Henoch-Schönlein purpura) and IgA nephropathy (IgAN) are thought to be related diseases with nearly identical pathology. IgA dominant mesangial deposits are characteristic of both IgAV and IgAN. IgAV is classically described in children, whereas, IgAN occurs more often in early adulthood. IgAV, unlike IgAN, has extrarenal manifestations, including a purpuric lower extremity rash. IgA vasculitis and IgAN are comparatively rare causes of ESKD in pediatric patients.

IgA Vasculitis

Based on limited data, the recurrence rate of IgAV) after transplantation is similar to that of IgAN. A matched retrospective cohort study patients with IgAV in the Organ Procurement and Transplantation Network/United Network for Organ Sharing (OPTN/UNOS) database reported allograft failure from recurrent disease in 13.6%, but no difference in 10-year allograft survival compared to the matched cohort [118].

In a study from six European transplant centers [119], overall allograft survival rates were 84%, 66%, and 56% at 5, 10 and 15 years, respectively. Histologic recurrence occurred in 33% on for-cause biopsies. Clinical recurrence occurred in five patients at a median time of 96 months post-transplant. Allograft loss occurred in three patients resulting in an actuarial risk of allograft loss from recurrence in a first graft of 7.5% at 10 years post-transplant. Severity of disease at presentation and type of immunosuppression post-transplant did not affect recurrence. Although not reaching significance, 60% of those with clinically significant recurrence had living donors compared to 16% of living donors in the cohort who did not experience.

IgA Nephropathy

Nature and Frequency of IgA Nephropathy

IgAN is characterized by a highly variable course ranging from a benign condition to rapidly progressive renal failure and affecting 10–20% of all persons undergoing kidney biopsy, rendering IgAN the most prevalent primary chronic glomerular disease worldwide [120]. Prevalence of IgAN differs among populations of different ancestries, being most frequent among persons of Asian descent, rare in those of African descent, and with an intermediate prevalence among those with European descent.

IgAN is thought to occur due to a primary, inherited defect leading to preferential production of IgA with galactose-deficient O-glycans in the hinge-region. IgA deficient in galactose elicits the production of anti-glycan autoantibodies that lead to the formation and subsequent glomerular deposition of immune complexes. IgA-based activation of alternative complement pathway plays a critical role in the pathogenesis of IgAN. For example, C3 is frequently involved in the formation of circulating immune deposits inducing mesangial stress, podocyte damage and progressive deterioration of kidney function. On this basis, IgAN can be classified as an autoimmune glomerular disease. While the pathogenesis of the disease resulting in IgA1 subclass deficient in galactose is not completely clarified, genome-wide association studies have identified multiple susceptibility loci for IgAN implicating independent defects in adaptive and innate immunity, and alternative complement pathways that potentially influence the different pathogenetic steps towards development of disease [121].

IgAN generally has an indolent course, with a 10-year native kidney survival rate of 90% in adults and children with normal renal function at diagnosis; however, 71% of patients will demonstrate worsened hematuria and/or proteinuria in upwards of 20 years follow-up [122]. Clinical risk factors for progression to ESKD include heavy proteinuria, decreased estimated glomerular filtration rate (eGFR) at diagnosis and uncontrolled hypertension, although the ability to accurately predict individual patient-level risk remains limited [123].

Risk Factors for Recurrence

The reported frequency of histologic or clinically significant recurrence of IgAN post-transplantation varies in the literature. An excellent review of recurrence rates cis available [124]. The recurrence rate in a study from the Australia and New Zealand Dialysis and Transplantation Registry (ANZDATA) was 5.4% and 10.8% at 5 and 10 years, respectively, with a median time to recurrence of 4.6 years [125]. Analysis of data from the ANZDATA showed no increased risk of recurrence in a second allograft after loss of a first allograft to recurrence despite prior reports of increased risk.

Recurrence of IgAN can be "histologic only" when diagnosed on protocol biopsies in asymptomatic patients or "clinical" when associated with urinary abnormalities and/or graft dysfunction. Histologic recurrence in protocol biopsies in adults, with or without evidence of clinical disease, is common, with IgA mesangial deposition being found in up to 32–58% of grafts [126, 127]. In children with IgAN, the recurrence of IgA deposits in the allograft following transplantation is very common, but clinically relevant recurrent disease has been reported to be infrequent [128]. Hematuria, the hallmark of IgAN in the native kidney, is not a reliable manifestation of recurrence, being absent in 52% of cases diagnosed by protocol biopsy [126]. Given the lack of a prospective study involving allograft protocol biopsies in pKTR, the true risk of significant allograft dysfunction and allograft loss from recurrent disease in the pediatric population remains unclear.

No single parameter, including age, gender, race, donor source, HLA typing, pre-transplantation course or biochemical characteristics of serum IgA, has been shown to reliably predict recurrence. Risk factors for recurrence in IgAN have been suggested to be younger age at transplant, male gender, and rapidly progressive course of original disease, but there is not consensus. Furthermore, one study of native kidney biopsies in adults with IgAN showed that younger age at onset of IgAN and greater burden of crescents predicted recurrence after transplant [129]. Longer time following transplantation may also be a risk factor for disease recurrence and supports the suggestion that recurrence may be a time-dependent event [127]. The relationship between donor type and recurrence of disease is discussed below.

Considerations for Transplant Planning

The relationship between the risk of recurrence and the donor type remains controversial, with conflicting reports in the literature [130–135]. There have been no large, prospective studies defining the risk of recurrence in patients with

IgAN who receive either living donor or deceased donor renal allograft although there are large registry reports. An analysis of ANZDATA found recurrence was significantly more frequent in the zero HLA-mismatched living donors at 17% vs 7% in the cohort overall. In this report, allograft survival was the same for recipients of zero HLA-mismatched donors and those with one or more HLA mismatches (and no recurrence), suggesting loss of the survival advantage expected with zero HLA-mismatched transplants [136]. The authors concluded that despite increased recurrence risk, since allograft survivals were similar, there is no reason to avoid living donor-recipient pairs with zero HLA-mismatches in IgAN. In the same study, there were no differences seen in recurrence rates in those with HLA B12, B35 or DR4. A more recent report from the same registry, showed a 10-year recurrence rate of 16.7% in living donors, 7.1% in living-unrelated donors and 9.2% with deceased donors, with a significant HR of 1.7 for living-related vs deceased donors [137].

Genome wide association studies have identified abnormalities in the cCFH and CFHR genes in patients with IgAN [121, 138, 139]. Although it is unclear whether these variants increase the risk of recurrence following transplant, familial IgAN should be rigorously excluded in potential living-related donors since familial IgAN is associated with a high risk of ESKD [140].

The effect of immunosuppression regimen on IgA recurrence risk is unclear. Despite initial enthusiasm, newer immunosuppressants seem ineffective in preventing recurrence [141]. Retrospective data suggest that induction with ATG or anti-lymphocyte globulin is associated with a lower risk of recurrence compared to interleukin receptor-2 blockade [142–144].

Corticosteroid avoidance has become a major goal in pediatric kidney transplantation and has been successful in select transplant recipients [145, 146]. There are conflicting reports on the effect of rapid corticosteroid withdrawal or corticosteroid avoidance on IgAN recurrence risk and allograft survival. In a retrospective analysis of adults in the OPTN/UNOS database with IgAN receiving a first kidney transplant, early corticosteroid withdrawal was associated with increased risk of recurrence compared to patients in the corticosteroid continuation group. Patient survival and death-censored allograft survival were not different [147]. Similarly, in an analysis of the ANZDATA of adult recipients of a primary transplant for IgAN, corticosteroid use was strongly associated with a reduced risk of recurrence, after adjusting for age, sex, HLA mismatch, dialysis duration and transplant era [148]. In this report, 12.6% of graft loss was attributed to recurrence. Conversely, a study of pediatric patients within the OPTN database reported that receiving a corticosteroid avoidance regimen in patients with a pre-transplantation diagnosis of glomerular kidney disease was not associated with an increased risk of allograft failure, although this study was unable to examine recurrence rates [149].

Treatment of IgAN Recurrence

Just as with native kidney IgAN, no therapy for recurrent IgAN has been shown to be effective. In the setting of disease recurrence, KDIGO guidelines recommend treatment strategies to reduce proteinuria, optimize blood pressure, and reduce inflammation [150].

Use of corticosteroids as well as intravenous rituximab to treat recurrence in small numbers of patients has been described [151–153]. Data from Japan have reported favorable outcomes after tonsillectomy in patients with recurrent IgAN, but these results have not been confirmed in other populations [154–156]. The effect of fish oil on recurrent IgAN has not been systematically examined for risk reduction or treatment of IgAN. One study reported a reduction in proteinuria and stabilization of kidney function after budesonide administration in native kidney IgAN patients, possibly by targeting the intestinal mucosa directly, suggesting a possible role in patients with recurrence post-transplant [157].

Impact of IgAN on Graft Function and Survival

Recurrent disease was thought to have little impact on allograft outcomes; however, recent studies with longer duration of follow-up suggest that recurrent disease may contribute substantially to allograft injury. The rate of allograft loss due to recurrence of IgAN varies based on time from transplant, with less early allograft loss attributed to IgAN and significantly more at 10 years post-transplant [52, 54]. True estimates of allograft loss purely attributable to disease recurrence are difficult given the interplay with acute or chronic rejection and calcineurin toxicity, particularly if histology close to the time of graft loss is not available [127, 158, 159].

Lupus Nephritis

Nature and Frequency of Disease

Systemic lupus erythematosus (SLE) is an autoimmune inflammatory disease that is characterized by antibodies directed against self-antigens, resulting in multiorgan damage. SLE in children is more severe than in adults, and there is a higher incidence of lupus nephritis (LN) [160, 161]. Risk factors for development of ESKD due to LN include International Society of Nephrology and the Renal Pathology Society class IV LN, male gender, black race, hypertension, nephrotic syndrome, anti-phospholipid antibodies, high glomerular staining for monocyte chemoattractant protein-1, chronicity on biopsy, poor response to induction therapy, and occurrence of nephritic kidney flare [162, 163]. Lupus nephritis is responsible for approximately 3% of ESKD leading to transplantation in North America [48].

Risk for Disease Recurrence

The reported risk for recurrent lupus nephritis (RLN) after renal transplantation has been quite variable, ranging from <5% [112] to between 30–50% [164] in studies implementing protocol biopsies to evaluate serially for recurrence. The variability in reported recurrence rates has been attributed to varying indications for renal allograft biopsy across transplant centers; single-center versus registry-based study design; follow-up duration; and varying races and ethnicities in study samples [165].

Large-scale data derived from UNOS between 1987 and 2006 estimated period prevalence as well as predictors of RLN and assessed the effects of RLN on both allograft failure and recipient survival [166]. The period prevalence of RLN within the cohort was 2.44%. Non-Hispanic black race, female gender, and age < 33 years were independent risk factors for RLN. In another study, pre-transplantation antiphospholipid auto-antibodies confer a higher risk for RLN [167].

Considerations for Transplant Planning

Data are mixed regarding the impact of donor type on RLN. Data from over 30 years ago suggest that grafts from deceased donors are a better option for patients with lupus nephritis than grafts from living-related donors based on lower 1-year graft survival, presumably due to possible familial inheritance through the HLA system [168, 169]. In contrast, more recent data show no difference in allograft loss between the two types of donors [170].

Pre-transplantation clinical condition and immunosuppressive history are important considerations in transplant planning. KDIGO guidelines recommend that lupus should be clinically quiescent and that the patient is receiving minimal (no) immunosuppression prior to transplantation [112]. Delay of transplantation may be necessary for those patients who have received high levels of pre-transplantation immunosuppression or long-term glucocorticoid therapy to minimize the cumulative risk of prior therapy on top of the need for potent induction immunosuppression at the time of transplant [171]. As noted previously, the presence of antiphospholipid autoantibodies should be carefully considered in transplant planning due to the risk of vascular thrombosis and early allograft failure [172, 173]. Anticoagulation in the peri- and post-transplant period should be considered in patients with antiphospholipid autoantibodies to reduce the risk of vascular thrombosis [112, 174]; however, this risk should be balanced by the potential for bleeding in the immediate post-transplant period [173].

The post-transplant immunosuppression for LN patients does not differ from that normally used. The OPTN/UNOS database was utilized to compare rates of allograft loss due to disease recurrence between transplant patients receiving cyclosporin plus azathioprine (CSA + AZA) compared to those receiving cyclosporin plus MMF (CSA + MMF) [175]. There was no difference in the rates of allograft loss due to RLN among recipients receiving either CSA + AZA or CSA + MMF maintenance immunosuppressive therapy at 10-year follow-up. In patients with LN recurrence, an intensification of immunosuppression should be reserved for the exceptional cases showing a severe (life threatening) lupus flare due to the potential risks of serious or lethal infection post-transplant [165].

Impact of RLN on Graft Function and Survival

Retrospective multicenter data from the North American Pediatric Renal Transplant Cooperative Study (NAPRTCS) database demonstrated that kidney transplant outcomes in young patients with LN were comparable to those seen in an age-, ancestry-, and gender-matched control group, in spite of an unexplained increase in recurrent rejections in the living donor LN patients [176].

In an analysis of UNOS data, allograft failure occurred in 93% of those with RLN, 86% of those with rejection, and 19% of control subjects without rejection [166]. Although recipients with RLN had a fourfold greater risk for allograft failure compared with control subjects without rejection, only 7% of allograft failure episodes were attributable to RLN compared with 43% due to rejection. Mortality was similar (11–18%) between those with RLN, rejection, and controls.

Acute Graft Dysfunction in the Early Post-Operative Period

Graft Thrombosis

One cause of acute graft dysfunction in the early post-operative period is graft thrombosis. Around

2–3% of all renal grafts in the pediatric population thrombose and not surprisingly this is seen more frequently in the early post-transplant period [177, 178]. Thrombosis is encountered more commonly in younger children, particularly those less than 2 years of age at the time of transplant and in those receiving a deceased donor graft [177–180]. The size of the native vessels is undoubtedly a contributing factor, and the frequent discrepancy between donor and recipient vessels increases the surgical difficulty of the anastomosis. Previously, high rates of thrombosis were seen when very young donors were used and this is one of the reasons why children under the age of 5–6 years are now usually excluded from being donors [35, 181]. Thrombosis is now the third most common cause of graft loss, accounting for 9.8% of losses overall and for 7% of index graft losses since January 2000 [182].

Thrombosis is reported to occur more commonly in grafts from deceased donors, in those with prolonged cold ischemic time beyond 24 h and in retransplants [177, 180, 181]. Furthermore, there are data to suggest that pr—transplantation peritoneal dialysis increases the risk of thrombosis [181, 183]. Interestingly, the most recent NAPRTCS data suggest that the previously reported risk factors may not be significant and that the use of IL-2 receptor blockers more than halves the risk of graft thrombosis [178]. Further studies are required to establish the true risk factors for this often devastating complication.

There is an apparent higher incidence of thrombophilic risk factors in the ESKD population. In one study of pediatric pre-transplantation patients, 27% were found to have an increased risk of thrombophilia, whereas another group found that almost 90% of children screened pre-transplantation had at least one thrombotic risk factor [182]. There was a higher risk in the "non-anatomical" etiological group of patients where lupus anticoagulant was commonly detected [48]. The routine use of prophylactic anticoagulation remains controversial and the evidence for its use is limited. Currently, there are many different protocols, ranging from no anticoagulation, tailored anticoagulation according to risk and the use of one or more anticoagulants routinely. One study has compared the use of routine unfractionated heparin with historical controls given no anticoagulation and found no reduction in the rate of allograft thrombosis [177]. Others have reported reduced thrombosis rates with the use of low-molecular-weight heparin [184, 185]. Several units where patients are routinely screened for thrombophilic risk factors have shown good outcomes using anticoagulation protocols stratified for risk, but the numbers of patients included have been small and it is difficult to extrapolate the data to the general pediatric ESKD population [150, 185]. Until there is a large, randomized, controlled trial, the benefit of anticoagulation remains undetermined.

Obstruction

Obstruction to the flow of urine from the allograft can occur at any time but is most common in the early post-operative period. Complete obstruction will result in no urine output, but partial obstruction may only be detected on ultrasound. The scan may show dilatation of the renal pelvis with or without urine in the bladder depending on the level of the obstruction. The major concerns with obstruction are the increased pressure on the ureteric anastomosis with the risk of rupture and the long-term effects of increased pressure on the renal parenchyma. There are many reasons for the early increased risk of obstruction, including intravesical clots, stenosis of the ureter, particularly at the anastomosis site, and external compression or kinking of the ureter due to hematomas and other fluid collections. There is inevitable bleeding at the time of transplant, and it is not unusual for clots to form. The majority of patients post-transplant will have either a urethral or suprapubic catheter to drain the bladder, or rarely a urinary diversion, and this should facilitate the passage of clots, though it is possible for clots to block the catheter and flushing of the catheter is often required in the first few days after the transplant. Inadequate drainage of urine can also be the result of dislodgement of the catheter. Many centers also routinely place a stent into the ureter of the allograft at the time of transplantation and this generally remains in situ for 2–6 weeks to minimize the risk of stenosis or effects of external compression. External compression of the ureter may be caused by a hematoma, a urinoma, a lymphocele, stool, or any other mass in the vicinity of the graft. Ultrasound will usually be able to follow the length of the ureter and will detect any mass compressing it. Transplant ureters are also at risk of kinking, especially if a large adult donor has been used without appropriate trimming of the ureter. Rarely, further surgical intervention is necessary.

Beyond the early post-operative period, obstruction is more frequently encountered in patients with known bladder problems and in those with incomplete bladder emptying. Double voiding regimes, clean intermittent catheterization or indwelling catheter drainage may be necessary to relieve the obstruction.

Urine Leak

This potentially devastating complication is fortunately rare, and the incidence appears to be decreasing. Leakage is usually due to ureteral necrosis around the anastomosis site, and urine then collects in the abdomen. If an abdominal drain has been placed at the time of surgery, the drain fluid can easily be tested for the creatinine concentration, which would be comparable to that of the urine rather than the blood. If there is no drain, then fine needle aspiration of the fluid and measurement of the creatinine concentration will aid in the diagnosis. Occasionally, nuclear medicine imaging studies may also be considered. The adult literature has demonstrated poorer wound healing in patients treated with sirolimus and subsequent increased urine leak [186].

Investigation of Delayed Graft Function and Peri-Operative Allograft Dysfunction

If no urine is obtained post-operatively, then a systematic approach should identify the cause. Assessment of the patient, ensuring that there is adequate volume replacement to maintain a good blood pressure and central venous pressure is critical. The position of the urinary catheter should be assessed, and it should be checked for any blockage. A Doppler ultrasound will demonstrate the degree and pattern of renal perfusion. If the kidney looks well-perfused and the patient is well-hydrated, then the most likely cause of the delayed graft function (DGF) is acute tubular necrosis, although most would advocate an early biopsy to rule out hyperacute rejection.

If good urine volumes were present but then decrease, factors such as inadequate fluid replacement or a blocked catheter should be considered initially. These problems are common and are easily resolved. If the patient is assessed to be normo- or hypervolemic, then a trial of a loop diuretic may be appropriate. If there is still no response, then more serious complications such as urinary leak, graft thrombosis and hyperacute rejection need to be investigated. A Doppler ultrasound, with or without a mercaptoacetyltriglycine or diethylenetriamine pentaacetic acid scan, will assess the perfusion of the kidney. Ultrasound will also detect obstruction to the kidney, fluid collections around the kidney suggestive of a urine leak or lymphocele, and clots in the bladder. A renal biopsy is required to rule out rejection. In exceptional cases, surgical re-exploration is required to assess the viability of the kidney.

Treatment of Delayed Graft Function

By the most used definition of DGF, dialysis will be required. Data from the OPTN show that 50% recover adequate function by the tenth post-transplant day. The use of CNIs is often minimized or delayed until good graft function is obtained. These patients are often treated with ATG, until graft function improves, or for a maximum of 10 days, as an alternative to CNIs, as there is evidence to suggest less DGF with ATG [187].

Acute Rejection and Chronic Allograft Dysfunction

Acute rejection and chronic allograft dysfunction require clinical, immunological, and histopathological input to understand and appropriately treat. With the advent of new techniques for detecting anti-HLA antibodies and a better understanding of histological changes, it is becoming easier to define the causes of acute rejection and chronic allograft dysfunction, although it is important to remember that more than one factor may be operating in any individual patient. Interstitial fibrosis and tubular atrophy (IFTA) are the final common pathway of chronic allograft dysfunction; however, early investigation may pinpoint the underlying mechanism involved and allow intervention prior to irreversible allograft fibrosis.

International data from single center reports and registries have shown improved long-term patient and renal allograft survival rates for children and young people after kidney transplantation, including the NAPRTCS [48]. Most studies have shown improvement inpatient and renal allograft survival rates over the last three decades, which may be due to changes in immunosuppressive drug regimens, improvements in HLA matching, and a reduction in cold ischemia times. Pre-emptive and living donor renal transplantation are preferred given improved outcomes for living donation as compared to deceased donation with donation after brain death (DBD) and donation after circulatory death (DCD). A national study from the United Kingdom showed 1-year DBD renal allograft survival for those transplanted from 2012 to 2016 was 98%, compared with 72% for those transplanted from 1987 to 1991 [188]. Within this cohort, renal allograft survival for first kidney only transplants at 1, 5, 10, 20 and 25 years were 89%, 79%, 65%, 42% and 33%, respectively. Superior survival with living donation was maintained throughout the study period with 25-year renal allograft survival at 33% compared with 31% from deceased donation (p < 0.0001). These are similar to long-term data published from the Dutch LERIC study; 20-year allograft survival was 49% and 29% for LD and DD, respectively [189]. The 20-year allograft survival in Norway of allografts children since 1970 was 45%; 52% of these allografts were pre-emptive and 84% were from LD [190].

Predictors of Pediatric Renal Allograft Survival

Renal allograft function is calculated using eGFR, which requires the plasma creatinine and height according to modified Schwartz or other formulae, although other serum markers such as cystatin C have been proposed as providing increased accuracy [191].

Living donation confers a distinct advantage over deceased donation as the process of brain death and longer cold ischemia may predispose to acute tubular injury and DGF. DGF, prior transplantation, primary renal disease, and degree of HLA matching appear to influence long-term allograft outcome [192]. Recipient age is a predictor for graft survival, with older children having better early allograft survival but worse 5-year allograft survival [193]. Pre-transplantation dialysis and early acute rejection adversely affect allograft survival [194]. Additionally, some studies have found a deceased donor age over 40 years and prolonged cold ischemia time to be predictive of reduced allograft survival [195].

Proteinuria is common after pediatric renal transplantation, occurring in up to 80% of patients and can be glomerular or tubular in origin. Proteinuria can be both a contributor to and sign of chronic allograft damage [196]. A reduction in nephron mass results in increased intra-glomerular pressure in the remaining nephrons, causing proteinuria, which is injurious to the kidney via glomerular and interstitial inflammation, resulting in interstitial fibrosis and glomerulosclerosis [192]. Proteins entering the interstitium are processed by dendritic cells [197]. It has even been postulated that activated dendritic cells may then predispose to the development of rejection [194]. Transplant glomerulopathy is associated with proteinuria, presumably linked to damage to the glomerular basement membrane following antibody mediated rejection [198]. The use of mammalian target of rapamycin inhibitors has also been associated with the development of proteinuria [199].

Chronic Allograft Dysfunction

Allograft lifespan can be influenced by a variety of factors including peri-implantation injuries, history of allograft rejection, cardiovascular disease, and (recurrent) infection—all of which may influence the rate of decline of renal allograft function. However, the contribution of each of these factors will vary in individual patients. Post-transplant factors can be divided into early or implantation stresses and later injuries to the allograft. It is likely that multiple factors operate in individual patients. Over the last decade, there has been an appreciation that repeated episodes of stress damage the allograft resulting in nephron loss. This cumulative burden of injury eventually results in allograft failure [200].

Pre-Implantation Injury

Long-term outcome data clearly demonstrate that LD transplantation confers a survival advantage compared with deceased donation. This is observed in living-related and unrelated donors, suggesting that reduction in cold ischemia time and avoidance of brain death are important factors. The process of brain death, through hemodynamic and neuro-hormonal changes, reduces the viability of DD kidneys, although optimal management of brain-dead donors and their kidneys can improve outcome [201–203].

Advanced donor age for living and deceased donors is associated with a worse long-term outcome in adult recipients, which may represent reduced functional renal mass, although other factors such as donor hypertension or arteriosclerosis may be important [204]. However, older donor age is associated with a greater risk of renal allograft failure for pediatric recipients. Donor organ quality is also important; more functioning nephrons lead to better outcomes. The presence of interstitial fibrosis on implantation biopsies (reflecting nephron loss) is predictive of late outcome as is glomerular size, which is an inversely related surrogate for renal mass [205–207]. Extended criteria donors are rarely used in pediatric practice, and include donors older than 60 years, or 50–59 years with two out of three of the following: hypertension, cerebro-

vascular cause of death or plasma creatinine >130 µmol/l (1.5 mg/dL), as they have a 70% increased risk of long-term allograft failure compared with standard criteria donors [208].

Implantation Injury

Cold ischemia, preservation injury and ischemia/reperfusion injury, with or without the effects of brain death, cause allograft injury and DGF, which may result in nephron loss if there is incomplete recovery. There is increased expression of cytokines, adhesion molecules and HLA molecules with ischemia, and DGF can be associated with acute rejection episodes and worse outcomes.

Post Implantation Injury

There are further stresses on the transplanted kidney, including acute or chronic rejection, recurrent disease, hypertension, hyperlipidemia, nephrotoxic medications, and bacterial and viral infections. These insults may cause further loss of nephrons with increasing IFTA. Rejection, as the major cause of chronic allograft dysfunction, is discussed in detail below.

The significant contribution of the immune system to chronic allograft dysfunction is supported by reduced allograft survival in the setting of previous acute rejection episodes, in highly sensitized patients, where there is de novo production of anti-donor HLA antibodies, and where there is evidence of under-immunosuppression.

Acute Allograft Dysfunction and Rejection

Acute allograft dysfunction or transplant acute kidney injury may result from pre-renal, renal, and post-renal conditions. The commonest pre-renal conditions include hypovolemia caused by dehydration (including viral gastroenteritis), hypotension and renal arterial or venous thrombosis, although thrombosis is rare after the immediate post-operative period. Intrinsic renal disease is more common with acute rejection, nephrotoxicity (including CNI nephrotoxicity) and infection (including bacterial infections, such as transplant pyelonephritis, and viral infections) and recurrent and de novo glomerulonephritis (see above). Post-renal causes are detailed below and include transplant ureteric stent obstruction and dislodgement, ureteropelvic and ureterovesical junction obstructions, bladder dysfunction and rarely perirenal hematoma or fluid. Percutaneous renal transplant biopsies may be required to make the correct diagnosis; these are called indication biopsies as opposed to protocol or surveillance biopsies, which are routinely performed at a specific time point post-transplant.

Allograft Rejection

The Banff Classification was originally devised in 1991 and was introduced to standardize reporting of acute and chronic rejection (Table 68.3) [209]. The Banff criteria have subsequently been updated on a regular basis to reflect increased understanding of antibody-mediated rejection and place more emphasis on the type rather than the degree of rejection [210–212]. Four main types of acute rejection are defined: T cell medi-

ated rejection (TCMR) with or without vasculitis and AMR with or without vasculitis [213]. Antibody mediated vascular rejection (AMR with vasculitis) is associated with a poor outcome. A better understanding of the underlying mechanisms of rejection will allow more appropriate treatment and hopefully better outcomes. There is improved long-term survival with aggressive treatment of early TCMR, as early TCMR can rapidly lead to renal allograft loss if left untreated. However, it may result in a degree of nephron loss and IFTA, which will still be evident in later percutaneous renal biopsies but will not have progressed.

Chronic Allograft (Late) Rejection

Chronic allograft dysfunction has been intensively studied over the last decade, resulting in increased understanding of late acute and chronic rejection. Rejection episodes occurring 3–6 months after transplantation are labeled acute or chronic depending on the speed of development, severity of allograft dysfunction and the

Table 68.3 Acute allograft rejection according to the Banff 2017 classification. (Table used with permission from Haas et al., 2018 [256])

Acute T cell–mediated rejection (TCMR)
- Ia >25% interstitial inflammation with moderate tubulitis (t2)
- Ib >25% interstitial inflammation with severe tubulitis (t3)
- IIa mild-to-moderate intimal arteritis (v1)
- IIb severe intimal arteritis (v2)
- III transmural arteritis and/or fibrinoid necrosis (v3)

Acute antibody-mediated rejection (ABMR): Should have all three criteria below
Histologic evidence of tissue injury:
- Acute tubular injury
- Microvascular inflammation (g > 0 and/or ptc > 0)
- Arteritis (v > 0)
- Thrombotic microangiopathy without apparent cause
Evidence of current/recent antibody interaction with endothelium:
- Positive C4d staining of peritubular capillaries
- Moderate microvascular inflammation (g + ptc ≥ 2)
- Increased expression of gene transcripts in biopsy tissue strongly associated with ABMR
Serologic evidence of donor-specific antibodies (DSA):
- Positive C4d staining/presence of ABMR-associated gene transcripts may substitute for DSA

Key: i0—No inflammation or in <10% of unscarred cortical parenchyma. i1—Inflammation in 10–25% of unscarred cortical parenchyma. i2—Inflammation in 26–50% of unscarred cortical parenchyma. i3—Inflammation in more than 50% of unscarred cortical parenchyma

t0—No mononuclear cells in tubules or single focus of tubulitis only, t1—Foci with 1–4 mononuclear cells/tubular cross section (or 10 tubular cells), t2— 5–10 mononuclear cells and t3—Foci with >10 mononuclear cells/tubular cross section or the presence of ≥2 areas of tubular basement membrane destruction accompanied by i2/i3 inflammation and t2 elsewhere. G: glomerulitis, none (g0), segmental or global glomerulitis in 75% of glomeruli (g3), PTC: peritubular capillaries- at least 1 leukocyte in ≥10% of cortical PTC but 10 leukocytes in most severely involved PTC (ptc3)

biopsy findings. Late acute rejection is associated with a worse outcome [214]. The timing of a biopsy for allograft dysfunction is predictive; indication biopsies (performed for allograft dysfunction) in adult recipients after 12 months are associated with worse outcome than a biopsy performed during the first post-transplant year [215]. Dorje et al. report similar findings with AMR; allograft survival at 4 years was 75% in those with early AMR in the first 3 months post-transplant, compared with 40% in those with AMR diagnosed after 3 months [216]. Non-adherence or suboptimal immunosuppression were more common in the group with later AMR.

There is increasing research on the link between late allograft dysfunction and subsequent allograft loss. Previously, used causes of allograft loss have often been imprecise diagnoses such as chronic allograft nephropathy (CAN) or IFTA [209, 217]. These terms describe the final common pathway of several different processes and have been shown to be unhelpful in determining the underlying cause of allograft failure. Recruitment to a large multicenter study of factors that affect long-term kidney transplant function was commenced in 2005 [218]. Biopsies performed for allograft dysfunction were frequently reported by local pathologists as showing CAN or CNI toxicity. However, further follow-up showed no difference in outcome for patients with or without a diagnosis of CAN. This study demonstrated that late allograft dysfunction in a previously stable allograft was associated with a high risk of renal allograft loss. Further reports showed that a diagnosis of CNI toxicity was associated with a reduced rather than increased risk of allograft failure, and, unexpectedly, a high incidence of antibody-mediated rejection was found on biopsies for late allograft dysfunction [219, 220].

A precise diagnosis of allograft failure was made in a detailed prospective study of adult kidney transplant recipients of whom 19% had allograft loss, which was correlated with findings on earlier indication biopsies, clinical and serological data [221]. The causes of allograft failure were rejection in 64% of cases, glomerulonephritis in 18%, polyoma virus in 7% and intercurrent events in 11%. The most common cause of allograft failure was AMR, with all allografts that failed from rejection having some degree of AMR, whereas no losses were attributable to TCMR alone. A substantial proportion of AMR losses were associated with non-adherence. Neither a diagnosis of IFTA alone without evidence of inflammation nor CNI toxicity were common causes of allograft failure in this study. Antibody mediated rejection is the most common cause of late allograft loss, and it is important to differentiate late acute rejection into TCMR or AMR to allow appropriate treatment.

Antibody Mediated Rejection

Endothelial inflammation and injury in the microvasculature of the kidney allograft is the underlying pathology in AMR [222]. This can be due to donor specific anti-HLA antibodies (DSA) causing direct toxicity to antigen expressing endothelial cells through activation of the classical complement cascade or through cell-mediated toxicity after binding to the Fc receptors of mononuclear cells [223, 224]. The spectrum of histological lesions range from mild changes with acute tubular necrosis to severe changes with vascular fibrinoid necrosis [225]. There is swelling of the injured endothelia in the glomeruli and peritubular capillaries, which are infiltrated with mononuclear cells. The Banff criteria for AMR include signs of microcirculatory inflammation and the presence of complement split product C4d staining, which reflects activation of the classical complement pathway [226]. The Banff criteria require both of these markers to be present for the diagnosis of AMR, with or without the presence of DSA, although it is now appreciated that C4d staining is not always present in AMR [227].

Chronic injury in AMR is characterized by remodeling of the microvasculature and larger arteries. There is multilayering of the basement membrane in the peritubular capillaries, often with associated secondary IFTA, with or without C4d staining. The changes on electron microscopy may be present before there are obvious changes on light microscopy. The glomeruli are enlarged, and the capillary walls are thickened with duplication of the glomerular basement membrane causing double contours with interposition of mesangial matrix, usually with an increase in mesangial matrix. There may be subendothelial accumulation of deposits on electron microscopy. These chronic changes are referred to as transplant glomerulopathy (TG), which is associated with a poor outcome despite treatment [228]. There is now better understanding of the role of the endothelium and microcirculatory inflammation and repair in AMR [229].

The presence of C4d staining of peritubular capillaries has been associated with a worse outcome than C4d negative AMR, but the category of C4d negative AMR is now established and is well-recognized as a cause of allograft loss [230]. Deposition of C4d has been shown to have a high specificity but a poor sensitivity for AMR [231]. Fifty percent of AMR is missed if reliance is placed on the presence of C4d to make a diagnosis. Signs of microcirculatory injury, including glomerulitis, are a better predictor of late allograft loss than the presence of C4d.

Deposition of C4d on biopsy is associated with basement membrane multilayering, TG and the accumulation of mononuclear cells within the peritubular capillaries. Deposition of C4d in biopsies from low immunological risk patients which show normal glomerular morphology is associated with the development of TG on later biopsies. C4d deposits in the absence of other signs of AMR can be seen in ABO incompatible transplantation and may be a sign of accommodation [212, 232]. Molecular studies have shown that the presence of inflammatory cells in areas of fibrosis contribute to rejection and are predictive of outcome. It is therefore recommended that fibrotic areas should be included when calculating the degree of inflammatory infiltrate on a percutaneous renal biopsy [233]. Gene expression analysis has also proved useful in discriminating biopsies classified histologically as showing borderline histological changes of rejection into those patients with and without rejection [234]. However, there is the hope for point of care testing of biomarkers in pediatric renal transplantation to predict rejection in the future. Studies linking findings on indication biopsies with later allograft loss have used a broader diagnosis of AMR than traditional Banff criteria with the requirement for microcirculatory inflammation, DSA or C4d.

Donor Specific Antibody

The consequences of developing de novo DSA on allograft outcome has been known for some time [235]. In both adults and children, the natural history of de novo DSA in pKTR is well-documented, with evidence of complement activation leading to renal allograft injury [134, 236]. The development of sensitive solid-phase assays has helped to detect the presence of DSA and establish its role as a major cause of late allograft dysfunction and failure. The sensitivity of the assay and the cut-off median fluorescent intensity (MFI) used will affect the ability to distinguish de novo DSA from antibody present prior to transplantation. Using rigorous methods to exclude antibody already present in the recipient at the time of transplantation, no de novo DSA was detected prior to 6 months, 2% had developed DSA by 1 year and the median time to develop DSA was 4.6 years in adult kidney transplant recipients, although other adult studies have found that de novo antibodies can develop earlier [237, 238]. The prevalence of de novo DSA in pediatric renal transplant populations has been reported to be between 14 and 34% and can be associated with allograft loss [239].

HLA molecules are expressed on peritubular capillaries and can be upregulated during infectious or inflammatory processes by interferon gamma. This may result in cellular rejection or allow the expansion of B cells producing DSA. Early cellular rejection has been shown to be a risk factor for DSA development [240]. More intense peritubular capillaritis during cellular rejection is associated with the development of DSA. The degree of immunosuppression is important; reduction in immunosuppression or the use of less potent immunosuppressants is associated with the development of DSA. DSA occur more frequently with the use of cyclosporin than with tacrolimus, with everolimus compared to cyclosporin and with azathioprine compared to MMF [241]. HLA mismatching is a predictor of the development of DSA, especially HLA class II mismatch. In addition younger age predicts development of DSA, which may reflect a more robust immune system in the young or non-adherence [242]. De novo DSA precedes the onset of allograft dysfunction by months or years. Most DSA is directed against class II HLA, including DQ and DP, which are not included in most matching algorithms. There are other non-DSA anti-HLA and non-HLA antibodies. Anti-HLA antibodies that are not donor specific have been reported to be pathogenic in some studies, whereas in other studies there has been no association with outcome [243]. The development of de novo DSA post-transplant has been associated with 10-year allograft survival that is almost 40% lower than those without DSA [244].

Ginevri has published a detailed study in pediatric renal transplant recipients [245]. Thirty-seven of 82 consecutive recipients of first allografts developed de novo anti-HLA antibodies; 19 had DSA (6 also had non-DSA) and 18 had non-DSA only. Two patients who had only HLA Class I mismatches developed only HLA Class I DSA. The other 17 had mismatches at both HLA Class I and class II; 11 developed HLA Class II antibody and 6 developed both HLA Class I and II. HLA Class II DSA were almost exclusively directed against DQ. In the non-DSA group, 15 developed mostly HLA Class I with or without HLA Class II antibodies that recognized cross-reactive epitope group specificities related to the donor mismatch. The MFI of the non-DSA were significantly lower than the MFI of the DSA. DSA appeared at a median time of 2 years post-transplant with a range of 3–60 months. DSA were more likely to remain detectable compared with non-DSA and were more common in patients receiving cyclosporin compared with tacrolimus. Renal allograft function decreased significantly in the DSA group during 4.3 years of follow-up. Five allografts were lost in the DSA groups; four were due to AMR. Seventeen (89%) DSA patients needed an indication biopsy compared to 44% in the non-DSA group and 11% in those with no antibody (p < 0.0001). Eleven of the biopsies showed AMR, and 8 were C4d positive. One recipient in the non-DSA group had evidence of microcirculatory inflammation in keeping with probable AMR. These data suggest that it is prudent to monitor DSA post transplantation.

Prevention and Treatment of Rejection

Prevention of chronic allograft dysfunction confers significant health and economic benefits and is likely to be a more successful strategy than treatment. Many preventative strategies have been touched on already, including the use of living donors, which carries an allograft survival benefit, as does the appropriate selection of deceased donors. Optimal management of the deceased donor can attenuate the effects of ischemia reperfusion injury [246]. Prevention and treatment of rejection is an important part of post-transplant management. In our opinion, the most effective way to prevent allograft rejection is through regular adherence counseling, increasing parent-patient engagement in post-transplant care, and close laboratory and clinical follow-up after transplant.

Early acute rejection is most likely to be TCMR and this is usually responsive to corticosteroid treatment and indeed recent improvements in early allograft survival have been attributed in part to newer, more potent immunosuppressants which have significantly reduced early acute rejection rates. Accurate diagnosis of early rejection episodes into either T or B cell-mediated with or without a vascular component is important in determining outcome.

The treatment of late AMR remains a challenge. The outcome after late AMR is worse than for early AMR, where good results have been obtained using PE or intravenous immunoglobulin (IVIG) and rituximab [247–250]. There are no RCT data available regarding the treatment of late AMR but a number of different agents have been tried. High-dose corticosteroids, IVIG, PE, IA, rituximab and bortezomib have been used [251]. Baseline immunosuppression is commonly augmented to include MMF and tacrolimus [252]. Varying results have been reported, which are likely to be influenced by the baseline function of the allograft and the degree of injury that has already occurred by the time of AMR diagnosis [253]. Rituximab, used in combination with other therapies, and bortezomib both appear less effective for late AMR than early AMR [254]. Many reports describe reduced immunosuppression or non-adherence prior to the development of AMR; prevention of late AMR is likely to be a more effective strategy than treatment. Late TCMR seems more amenable to treatment and in studies of late allograft dysfunction does not appear to be a cause of allograft loss.

Adequate Immunosuppression

Late allograft dysfunction is often due to AMR with non-adherence or under-immunosuppression as the underlying mechanisms. Non-adherence and under-immunosuppression with lower doses of tacrolimus, cyclosporin and MMF may in part be related to a concern that calcineurin nephrotoxicity contributes to chronic allograft dysfunction. Calcineurin nephrotoxicity is a concern clinically, but not a frequent cause of allograft loss. The Mycophenolic Renal Transplant Registry of the de novo use of MMF showed that reductions in dose during the first-year posttransplant were associated with increased rejection, and if tacrolimus levels were also low, with increased allograft failure [255]. An observational analysis of over 25,000 low-risk, adult recipients showed that withdrawing maintenance cyclosporin, tacrolimus or MMF, or reducing the dose below certain thresholds after the first posttransplant year, was associated with a significant risk of allograft failure. These data indicate the importance of adequate immunosuppression for allograft survival.

Conclusion

Transplant planning and care require a thorough understanding of the underlying cause of ESKD and close monitoring for non-infectious complications in the post-operative period. In most instances, transplantation confers significantly reduced morbidity and mortality and improve-

ments in quality of life. Rejection remains a lifelong concern for kidney transplants, as does the risk for disease recurrence in certain populations. For most, the risk of disease recurrence is low; however, exceptions are notable in the case of complement-mediated kidney disease where risk for disease recurrence may be greater than 50%. Most patients with recurrent disease due to glomerulonephritis still have generally equivalent patient and allograft survival compared to those with non-recurrent etiologies, such as CAKUT.

Despite scientific advances, the management of disease recurrence and allograft rejection in pediatric kidney transplant recipients remains challenging; however, emerging therapies for high-risk diseases, such as aHUS and C3G, provide hope for improved allograft survival amongst these pediatric kidney diseases at highest risk for recurrence. Our understanding of optimal treatment for both allograft rejection and recurrent disease is limited by the lack of systematic, randomized studies, particularly in pediatric patients. Systematic use of international registries and prospective multicenter collaborative studies is necessary to allow improvement in pretransplantation risk evaluation and facilitate data-driven yet individualized post-transplantation management.

References

1. Cochat P, et al. Disease recurrence in paediatric renal transplantation. Pediatr Nephrol. 2009;24(11):2297–108.
2. Cravedi P, Kopp JB, Remuzzi G. Recent progress in the pathophysiology and treatment of FSGS recurrence. Am J Transplant. 2013;13(2):266–74.
3. Van Stralen KJ, et al. Impact of graft loss among kidney diseases with a high risk of post-transplant recurrence in the paediatric population. Nephrol Dial Transpl. 2013;28(4):1031–8.
4. Kiffel J, Rahimzada Y, Trachtman H. Focal segmental glomerulosclerosis and chronic kidney disease in pediatric patients. Adv Chronic Kidney Dis. 2011;18(5):332–8.
5. Hart A, et al. OPTN/SRTR 2018 annual data report: kidney. Am J Transplant. 2020;20(Suppl s1):20–130.
6. Weber S, Tonshoff B. Recurrence of focal-segmental glomerulosclerosis in children after renal transplantation: clinical and genetic aspects. Transplantation. 2005;80(1 Suppl):S128–34.

7. Preston R, Stuart HM, Lennon R. Genetic testing in steroid-resistant nephrotic syndrome: why, who, when and how? Pediatr Nephrol. 2019;34(2):195–210.

8. Winn MP. Approach to the evaluation of heritable diseases and update on familial focal segmental glomerulosclerosis. Nephrol Dial Transplant. 2003;18(Suppl 6):vi14–20.

9. Pollak MR. The genetic basis of FSGS and steroid-resistant nephrosis. Semin Nephrol. 2003;23(2):141–6.

10. Winn MP, et al. A mutation in the TRPC6 cation channel causes familial focal segmental glomerulosclerosis. Science. 2005;308(5729):1801–4.

11. Billing H, et al. NPHS2 mutation associated with recurrence of proteinuria after transplantation. Pediatr Nephrol. 2004;19(5):561–4.

12. Bertelli R, et al. Recurrence of focal segmental glomerulosclerosis after renal transplantation in patients with mutations of podocin. Am J Kidney Dis. 2003;41(6):1314–21.

13. Trautmann A, et al. Spectrum of steroid-resistant and congenital nephrotic syndrome in children: the PodoNet registry cohort. Clin J Am Soc Nephrol. 2015;10(4):592–600.

14. Wei C, et al. Circulating urokinase receptor as a cause of focal segmental glomerulosclerosis. Nat Med. 2011;17(8):952–60.

15. Wei C, et al. Circulating suPAR in two cohorts of primary FSGS. J Am Soc Nephrol. 2012;23(12):2051–9.

16. Shuai T, et al. Serum soluble urokinase type plasminogen activated receptor and focal segmental glomerulosclerosis: a systematic review and meta-analysis. BMJ Open. 2019;9(10):e031812.

17. Winnicki W, et al. Diagnostic and prognostic value of soluble urokinase-type plasminogen activator receptor (suPAR) in focal segmental glomerulosclerosis and impact of detection method. Sci Rep. 2019;9(1):13783.

18. Reiser J, Wei C, Tumlin J. Soluble urokinase receptor and focal segmental glomerulosclerosis. Curr Opin Nephrol Hypertens. 2012;21(4):428–32.

19. Harel E, et al. Further evidence that the soluble urokinase plasminogen activator receptor does not directly injure mice or human podocytes. Transplantation. 2020;104(1):54–60.

20. Franco Palacios CR, et al. Urine but not serum soluble urokinase receptor (suPAR) may identify cases of recurrent FSGS in kidney transplant candidates. Transplantation. 2013;96(4):394–9.

21. Weber LT, et al. Clinical practice recommendations for recurrence of focal and segmental glomerulosclerosis/steroid-resistant nephrotic syndrome. Pediatr Transplant. 2021;25(3):e13955.

22. Sadowski CE, et al. A single-gene cause in 29.5% of cases of steroid-resistant nephrotic syndrome. J Am Soc Nephrol. 2015;26(6):1279–89.

23. Ding WY, et al. Initial steroid sensitivity in children with steroid-resistant nephrotic syndrome predicts post-transplant recurrence. J Am Soc Nephrol. 2014;25(6):1342–8.

24. Newstead CG. Recurrent disease in renal transplants. Nephrol Dial Transplant. 2003;18(Suppl 6):vi68–74.

25. Seikaly MG. Recurrence of primary disease in children after renal transplantation: an evidence-based update. Pediatr Transplant. 2004;8(2):113–9.

26. Ponticelli C. Recurrence of focal segmental glomerular sclerosis (FSGS) after renal transplantation. Nephrol Dial Transplant. 2010;25(1):25–31.

27. Tejani A, Stablein DH. Recurrence of focal segmental glomerulosclerosis posttransplantation: a special report of the north American pediatric renal transplant cooperative study. J Am Soc Nephrol. 1992;2(12 Suppl):S258–63.

28. Nehus EJ, et al. Focal segmental glomerulosclerosis in children: multivariate analysis indicates that donor type does not alter recurrence risk. Transplantation. 2013;96(6):550–4.

29. Huang K, et al. The differential effect of race among pediatric kidney transplant recipients with focal segmental glomerulosclerosis. Am J Kidney Dis. 2004;43(6):1082–90.

30. Uffing A, et al. A large, international study on post-transplant glomerular diseases: the TANGO project. BMC Nephrol. 2018;19(1):229.

31. Uffing A, et al. Recurrence of FSGS after kidney transplantation in adults. Clin J Am Soc Nephrol. 2020;15(2):247–56.

32. Baum MA, et al. Outcome of renal transplantation in adolescents with focal segmental glomerulosclerosis. Pediatr Transplant. 2002;6(6):488–92.

33. Baum MA, et al. Loss of living donor renal allograft survival advantage in children with focal segmental glomerulosclerosis. Kidney Int. 2001;59(1):328–33.

34. Koh LJ, et al. Risk factors associated with allograft failure in pediatric kidney transplant recipients with focal segmental glomerulosclerosis. Pediatr Transplant. 2019;23(5):e13469.

35. Dall'Amico R, et al. Prediction and treatment of recurrent focal segmental glomerulosclerosis after renal transplantation in children. Am J Kidney Dis. 1999;34(6):1048–55.

36. Fujisawa M, et al. Long-term outcome of focal segmental glomerulosclerosis after Japanese pediatric renal transplantation. Pediatr Nephrol. 2002;17(3):165–8.

37. Odorico JS, et al. The influence of native nephrectomy on the incidence of recurrent disease following renal transplantation for primary glomerulonephritis. Transplantation. 1996;61(2):228–34.

38. Fuentes GM, et al. Long-term outcome of focal segmental glomerulosclerosis after pediatric renal transplantation. Pediatr Nephrol. 2010;25(3):529–34.

39. Sener A, et al. Living-donor renal transplantation of grafts with incidental renal masses after ex-vivo partial nephrectomy. BJU Int. 2009;104(11):1655–60.

40. Raafat R, et al. Role of transplant induction therapy on recurrence rate of focal segmental glomerulosclerosis. Pediatr Nephrol. 2000;14(3):189–94.

41. Hubsch H, et al. Recurrent focal glomerulosclerosis in pediatric renal allografts: the Miami experience. Pediatr Nephrol. 2005;20(2):210–6.

42. Bouts A, et al. European Society of Pediatric Nephrology survey on current practice regarding recurrent focal segmental glomerulosclerosis after pediatric kidney transplantation. Pediatr Transplant. 2019;23(3):e13385.

43. Kukla A, et al. Recurrent glomerulonephritis under rapid discontinuation of steroids. Transplantation. 2011;91(12):1386–91.

44. Boardman R, et al. Early steroid withdrawal does not increase risk for recurrent focal segmental glomerulosclerosis. Transplant Proc. 2005;37(2):817–8.

45. Cheong HI, et al. Early recurrent nephrotic syndrome after renal transplantation in children with focal segmental glomerulosclerosis. Nephrol Dial Transplant. 2000;15(1):78–81.

46. First MR. Living-related donor transplants should be performed with caution in patients with focal segmental glomerulosclerosis. Pediatr Nephrol. 1995;9(Suppl):S40–2.

47. Hwang JH, et al. Outcome of kidney allograft in patients with adulthood-onset focal segmental glomerulosclerosis: comparison with childhood-onset FSGS. Nephrol Dial Transplant. 2012;27(6):2559–65.

48. North American Pediatric Renal Transplant Cooperative Study Annual Report. 2014.

49. D'Agati VD, Kaskel FJ, Falk RJ. Focal segmental glomerulosclerosis. N Engl J Med. 2011;365(25):2398–411.

50. Straatmann C, et al. Success with plasmapheresis treatment for recurrent focal segmental glomerulosclerosis in pediatric renal transplant recipients. Pediatr Transplant. 2014;18(1):29–34.

51. Kowalewska J. Pathology of recurrent diseases in kidney allografts: membranous nephropathy and focal segmental glomerulosclerosis. Curr Opin Organ Transplant. 2013;18(3):313–8.

52. Shishido S, et al. Combination of pulse methylprednisolone infusions with cyclosporine-based immunosuppression is safe and effective to treat recurrent focal segmental glomerulosclerosis after pediatric kidney transplantation. Clin Transpl. 2013;27(2):E143–50.

53. Raafat RH, et al. High-dose oral cyclosporin therapy for recurrent focal segmental glomerulosclerosis in children. Am J Kidney Dis. 2004;44(1):50–6.

54. Ingulli E, Tejani A. Incidence, treatment, and outcome of recurrent focal segmental glomerulosclerosis posttransplantation in 42 allografts in children—a single-center experience. Transplantation. 1991;51(2):401–5.

55. Mowry J, et al. Treatment of recurrent focal segmental glomerulosclerosis with high-dose cyclosporine a and plasmapheresis. Transplant Proc. 1993;25(1 Pt 2):1345–6.

56. Aunon P, et al. Pre-emptive rituximab in focal and segmental glomerulosclerosis patients at risk of recurrence after kidney transplantation. Clin Kidney J. 2021;14(1):139–48.

57. Grenda R, et al. Long-term effect of rituximab in maintaining remission of recurrent and plasmapheresis-dependent nephrotic syndrome post-renal transplantation - case report. Pediatr Transplant. 2011;15(6):E121–5.

58. Grenda R, et al. Rituximab is not a "magic drug" in post-transplant recurrence of nephrotic syndrome. Eur J Pediatr. 2016;175(9):1133–7.

59. Dello Strologo L, et al. Use of rituximab in focal glomerulosclerosis relapses after renal transplantation. Transplantation. 2009;88(3):417–20.

60. Garrouste C, et al. Rituximab for recurrence of primary focal segmental glomerulosclerosis after kidney transplantation: clinical outcomes. Transplantation. 2017;101(3):649–56.

61. Araya CE, Dharnidharka VR. The factors that may predict response to rituximab therapy in recurrent focal segmental glomerulosclerosis: a systematic review. J Transp Secur. 2011;2011:374213.

62. Kershaw DB, et al. Recurrent focal segmental glomerulosclerosis in pediatric renal transplant recipients: successful treatment with oral cyclophosphamide. Clin Transpl. 1994;8(6):546–9.

63. Nathanson S, et al. Recurrence of nephrotic syndrome after renal transplantation: influence of increased immunosuppression. Pediatr Nephrol. 2005;20(12):1801–4.

64. Konigshausen E, Sellin L. Circulating permeability factors in primary focal segmental glomerulosclerosis: a review of proposed candidates. Biomed Res Int. 2016;2016:3765608.

65. Gonzalez E, et al. Preemptive plasmapheresis and recurrence of focal segmental glomerulosclerosis in pediatric renal transplantation. Pediatr Transplant. 2011;15(5):495–501.

66. Belson A, et al. Long-term plasmapheresis and protein a column treatment of recurrent FSGS. Pediatr Nephrol. 2001;16(12):985–9.

67. Ohta T, et al. Effect of pre-and postoperative plasmapheresis on posttransplant recurrence of focal segmental glomerulosclerosis in children. Transplantation. 2001;71(5):628–33.

68. Allard L, et al. Treatment by immunoadsorption for recurrent focal segmental glomerulosclerosis after paediatric kidney transplantation: a multicentre French cohort. Nephrol Dial Transplant. 2018;33(6):954–63.

69. Verghese PS, et al. The effect of peri-transplant plasmapheresis in the prevention of recurrent FSGS. Pediatr Transplant. 2018;22(3):e13154.

70. Dantal J, et al. Effect of plasma protein adsorption on protein excretion in kidney-transplant recipients with recurrent nephrotic syndrome. N Engl J Med. 1994;330(1):7–14.

71. Fencl F, et al. Recurrence of nephrotic proteinuria in children with focal segmental glomerulosclerosis: early treatment with plasmapheresis and immunoadsorption should be associated with better prognosis. Minerva Pediatr. 2016;68(5):348–54.

72. Raina R, et al. Extracorporeal therapies in the treatment of focal segmental glomerulosclerosis. Blood Purif. 2020;49(5):513–23.
73. Candiano G, et al. Apolipoproteins prevent glomerular albumin permeability induced in vitro by serum from patients with focal segmental glomerulosclerosis. J Am Soc Nephrol. 2001;12(1):143–50.
74. Raina R, Krishnappa V. An update on LDL apheresis for nephrotic syndrome. Pediatr Nephrol. 2019;34(10):1655–69.
75. Mizuiri S, et al. Post-transplant early recurrent proteinuria in patients with focal glomerulosclerosis—angiotensin II immunostaining and treatment outcome. Clin Transpl. 2005;19(Suppl 14):12–9.
76. Yan K, et al. Epidemiology of atypical hemolytic uremic syndrome: a systematic literature review. Clin Epidemiol. 2020;12:295–305.
77. Jenssen GR, et al. Incidence and etiology of hemolytic-uremic syndrome in children in Norway, 1999-2008—a retrospective study of hospital records to assess the sensitivity of surveillance. BMC Infect Dis. 2014;14:265.
78. Servais A, et al. Acquired and genetic complement abnormalities play a critical role in dense deposit disease and other C3 glomerulopathies. Kidney Int. 2012;82(4):454–64.
79. Thurman JM, Nester CM. All things complement. Clin J Am Soc Nephrol. 2016;11(10):1856–66.
80. Rother RP, et al. Discovery and development of the complement inhibitor eculizumab for the treatment of paroxysmal nocturnal hemoglobinuria. Nat Biotechnol. 2007;25(11):1256–64.
81. Goodship TH, et al. Atypical hemolytic uremic syndrome and C3 glomerulopathy: conclusions from a "kidney disease: improving global outcomes" (KDIGO) controversies conference. Kidney Int. 2017;91(3):539–51.
82. Povey H, et al. Renal recovery with eculizumab in atypical hemolytic uremic syndrome following prolonged dialysis. Clin Nephrol. 2014;82(5):326–31.
83. Licht C, et al. Efficacy and safety of eculizumab in atypical hemolytic uremic syndrome from 2-year extensions of phase 2 studies. Kidney Int. 2015;87(5):1061–73.
84. Feitz WJC, et al. The genetics of atypical hemolytic uremic syndrome. Med Genet. 2018;30(4):400–9.
85. Fremeaux-Bacchi V, et al. Genetics and outcome of atypical hemolytic uremic syndrome: a nationwide French series comparing children and adults. Clin J Am Soc Nephrol. 2013;8(4):554–62.
86. Noris M, et al. Relative role of genetic complement abnormalities in sporadic and familial aHUS and their impact on clinical phenotype. Clin J Am Soc Nephrol. 2010;5(10):1844–59.
87. Zuber J, et al. Use of eculizumab for atypical haemolytic uraemic syndrome and C3 glomerulopathies. Nat Rev Nephrol. 2012;8(11):643–57.
88. Loirat C, Fremeaux-Bacchi V. Hemolytic uremic syndrome recurrence after renal transplantation. Pediatr Transplant. 2008;12(6):619–29.
89. Noris M, Ruggenenti P, Remuzzi G. Kidney transplantation in patients with atypical hemolytic uremic syndrome: a therapeutic dilemma (or not)? Am J Kidney Dis. 2017;70(6):754–7.
90. Zuber J, et al. New insights into postrenal transplant hemolytic uremic syndrome. Nat Rev Nephrol. 2011;7(1):23–35.
91. Loirat C, et al. An international consensus approach to the management of atypical hemolytic uremic syndrome in children. Pediatr Nephrol. 2016;31(1):15–39.
92. Noris M, Remuzzi G. Managing and preventing atypical hemolytic uremic syndrome recurrence after kidney transplantation. Curr Opin Nephrol Hypertens. 2013;22(6):704–12.
93. Renner B, et al. Cyclosporine induces endothelial cell release of complement-activating microparticles. J Am Soc Nephrol. 2013;24(11):1849–62.
94. Duineveld C, et al. Living donor kidney transplantation in atypical hemolytic uremic syndrome: a case series. Am J Kidney Dis. 2017;70(6):770–7.
95. Artz MA, et al. Renal transplantation in patients with hemolytic uremic syndrome: high rate of recurrence and increased incidence of acute rejections. Transplantation. 2003;76(5):821–6.
96. Verhave JC, Wetzels JF, van de Kar NC. Novel aspects of atypical haemolytic uraemic syndrome and the role of eculizumab. Nephrol Dial Transplant. 2014;29(Suppl 4):iv131–41.
97. Noris M, Remuzzi G. Atypical hemolytic-uremic syndrome. N Engl J Med. 2009;361(17):1676–87.
98. Wijnsma KL, et al. Eculizumab in atypical hemolytic uremic syndrome: strategies toward restrictive use. Pediatr Nephrol. 2019;34(11):2261–77.
99. Benamu E, Montoya JG. Infections associated with the use of eculizumab: recommendations for prevention and prophylaxis. Curr Opin Infect Dis. 2016;29(4):319–29.
100. Nester CM, Smith RJ. Complement inhibition in C3 glomerulopathy. Semin Immunol. 2016;28(3):241–9.
101. Sethi S, et al. C3 glomerulonephritis: clinicopathological findings, complement abnormalities, glomerular proteomic profile, treatment, and follow-up. Kidney Int. 2012;82(4):465–73.
102. Pickering MC, et al. C3 glomerulopathy: consensus report. Kidney Int. 2013;84(6):1079–89.
103. Hou J, et al. Toward a working definition of C3 glomerulopathy by immunofluorescence. Kidney Int. 2014;85(2):450–6.
104. Smith RJ, et al. New approaches to the treatment of dense deposit disease. J Am Soc Nephrol. 2007;18(9):2447–56.
105. Smith RJH, et al. C3 glomerulopathy - understanding a rare complement-driven renal disease. Nat Rev Nephrol. 2019;15(3):129–43.
106. Denton MD, Singh AK. Recurrent and de novo glomerulonephritis in the renal allograft. Semin Nephrol. 2000;20(2):164–75.

107. Floege J. Recurrent glomerulonephritis following renal transplantation: an update. Nephrol Dial Transplant. 2003;18(7):1260–5.

108. Braun MC, et al. Recurrence of membranoproliferative glomerulonephritis type II in renal allografts: the north American pediatric renal transplant cooperative study experience. J Am Soc Nephrol. 2005;16(7):2225–33.

109. Zand L, et al. Clinical findings, pathology, and outcomes of C3GN after kidney transplantation. J Am Soc Nephrol. 2014;25(5):1110–7.

110. Angelo JR, Bell CS, Braun MC. Allograft failure in kidney transplant recipients with membranoproliferative glomerulonephritis. Am J Kidney Dis. 2011;57(2):291–9.

111. Alasfar S, et al. Membranoproliferative glomerulonephritis recurrence after kidney transplantation: using the new classification. BMC Nephrol. 2016;17:7.

112. Chadban SJ, et al. KDIGO clinical practice guideline on the evaluation and management of candidates for kidney transplantation. Transplantation. 2020;104(4S1 Suppl 1):S11–S103.

113. Lu DF, et al. Clinical features and outcomes of 98 children and adults with dense deposit disease. Pediatr Nephrol. 2012;27(5):773–81.

114. Panzer SE, et al. Glomerular C3 deposition is an independent risk factor for allograft failure in kidney transplant recipients with transplant glomerulopathy. Kidney Int Rep. 2019;4(4):582–93.

115. Gonzalez Suarez ML, et al. Treatment of C3 glomerulopathy in adult kidney transplant recipients: a systematic review. Med Sci (Basel). 2020;8(4):44.

116. Gonzalez Suarez ML, et al. Outcomes of kidney transplant patients with atypical hemolytic uremic syndrome treated with eculizumab: a systematic review and meta-analysis. J Clin Med. 2019;8(7):919.

117. Wong EK, et al. LNP023: a novel oral complement alternative pathway factor B inhibitor safely and effectively reduces proteinuria in C3 glomerulopathy. American Society of Nephrology. 2020: Virtual.

118. Samuel JP, et al. Long-term outcome of renal transplantation patients with Henoch-Schonlein purpura. Clin J Am Soc Nephrol. 2011;6(8):2034–40.

119. Kanaan N, et al. Recurrence and graft loss after kidney transplantation for henoch-schonlein purpura nephritis: a multicenter analysis. Clin J Am Soc Nephrol. 2011;6(7):1768–72.

120. Donadio JV, Grande JP. IgA nephropathy. N Engl J Med. 2002;347(10):738–48.

121. Gharavi AG, et al. Genome-wide association study identifies susceptibility loci for IgA nephropathy. Nat Genet. 2011;43(4):321–U68.

122. Ronkainen J, et al. Long-term outcome 19 years after childhood IgA nephritis: a retrospective cohort study. Pediatr Nephrol. 2006;21(9):1266–73.

123. Barbour SJ, Reich HN. Risk stratification of patients with IgA nephropathy. Am J Kidney Dis. 2012;59(6):865–73.

124. Moroni G, et al. Immunoglobulin a nephropathy. Recurrence after renal transplantation. Front Immunol. 2019:10.

125. Jiang SH, Kennard AL, Walters GD. Recurrent glomerulonephritis following renal transplantation and impact on graft survival. BMC Nephrol. 2018;19(1):344.

126. Ortiz F, et al. IgA nephropathy recurs early in the graft when assessed by protocol biopsy. Nephrol Dial Transpl. 2012;27(6):2553–8.

127. Odum J, et al. Recurrent mesangial Iga nephritis following renal-transplantation. Nephrol Dial Transpl. 1994;9(3):309–12.

128. Habib R, et al. Glomerular-lesions in the transplanted kidney in children. Am J Kidney Dis. 1987;10(3):198–207.

129. Avasare RS, et al. Predicting post-transplant recurrence of IgA nephropathy: the importance of crescents. Am J Nephrol. 2017;45(2):99–106.

130. Andresdottir MB, et al. Exclusive characteristics of graft survival and risk factors in recipients with immunoglobulin a nephropathy: a retrospective analysis of registry data. Transplantation. 2005;80(8):1012–8.

131. Wang AY, et al. Recurrent IgA nephropathy in renal transplant allografts. Am J Kidney Dis. 2001;38(3):588–96.

132. Freese P, et al. Clinical risk factors for recurrence of IgA nephropathy. Clin Transpl. 1999;13(4):313–7.

133. Han SS, et al. Impact of recurrent disease and chronic allograft nephropathy on the long-term allograft outcome in patients with IgA nephropathy. Transpl Int. 2010;23(2):169–75.

134. Kim YS, et al. Live donor renal allograft in end-stage renal failure patients from immunoglobulin a nephropathy. Transplantation. 2001;71(2):233–8.

135. Ponticelli C, et al. Kidney transplantation in patients with IgA mesangial glomerulonephritis. Kidney Int. 2001;60(5):1948–54.

136. McDonald SP, Russ GR. Recurrence of IgA nephropathy among renal allograft recipients from living donors is greater among those with zero HLA mismatches. Transplantation. 2006;82(6):759–62.

137. Kennard AL, Jiang SH, Walters GD. Increased glomerulonephritis recurrence after living related donation. BMC Nephrol. 2017;18(1):25.

138. Kiryluk K, et al. Discovery of new risk loci for IgA nephropathy implicates genes involved in immunity against intestinal pathogens. Nat Genet. 2014;46(11):1187–96.

139. Zhai YL, et al. Rare variants in the complement factor H-related protein 5 gene contribute to genetic susceptibility to IgA nephropathy. J Am Soc Nephrol. 2016;27(9):2894–905.

140. Schena FP, et al. Increased risk of end-stage renal disease in familial IgA nephropathy. J Am Soc Nephrol. 2002;13(2):453–60.

141. Chandrakantan A, et al. Recurrent IgA nephropathy after renal transplantation despite immunosuppressive regimens with mycophenolate mofetil. Nephrol Dial Transplant. 2005;20(6):1214–21.

142. Berthoux F, et al. Antithymocyte globulin (ATG) induction therapy and disease recurrence in renal transplant recipients with primary IgA nephropathy. Transplantation. 2008;85(10):1505–7.

143. Berthoux F, et al. Prognostic value of serum biomarkers of autoimmunity for recurrence of IgA nephropathy after kidney transplantation. J Am Soc Nephrol. 2017;28(6):1943–50.

144. Pascual J, et al. Alemtuzumab induction and recurrence of glomerular disease after kidney transplantation. Transplantation. 2007;83(11):1429–34.

145. Nehus E, Goebel J, Abraham E. Outcomes of steroid-avoidance protocols in pediatric kidney transplant recipients. Am J Transplant. 2012;12(12):3441–8.

146. Zhang H, et al. Steroid avoidance or withdrawal regimens in paediatric kidney transplantation: a meta-analysis of randomised controlled trials. PLoS One. 2016;11(3):e0146523.

147. Leeaphorn N, et al. Recurrence of IgA nephropathy after kidney transplantation in steroid continuation versus early steroid-withdrawal regimens: a retrospective analysis of the UNOS/OPTN database. Transpl Int. 2018;31(2):175–86.

148. Clayton P, McDonald S, Chadban S. Steroids and recurrent IgA nephropathy after kidney transplantation. Am J Transplant. 2011;11(8):1645–9.

149. Nehus EJ, et al. Graft survival of pediatric kidney transplant recipients selected for de novo steroid avoidance-a propensity score-matched study. Nephrol Dial Transplant. 2017;32(8):1424–31.

150. Kasiske BL, et al. KDIGO clinical practice guideline for the care of kidney transplant recipients: a summary. Kidney Int. 2010;77(4):299–311.

151. Messina M, et al. Treatment protocol with pulse and oral steroids for IgA nephropathy after kidney transplantation. J Nephrol. 2016;29(4):575–83.

152. Matsukuma Y, et al. Effect of steroid pulse therapy on post-transplant immunoglobulin a nephropathy. Nephrology (Carlton). 2018;23(Suppl 2):10–6.

153. Chancharoenthana W, et al. Rituximab for recurrent IgA nephropathy in kidney transplantation: a report of three cases and proposed mechanisms. Nephrology (Carlton). 2017;22(1):65–71.

154. Kennoki T, et al. Proteinuria-reducing effects of tonsillectomy alone in IgA nephropathy recurring after kidney transplantation. Transplantation. 2009;88(7):935–41.

155. Hotta K, et al. Tonsillectomy ameliorates histological damage of recurrent immunoglobulin a nephropathy after kidney transplantation. Nephrology (Carlton). 2013;18(12):808–12.

156. Ushigome H, et al. Efficacy of tonsillectomy for patients with recurrence of IgA nephropathy after kidney transplantation. Clin Transpl. 2009;23(Suppl 20):17–22.

157. Fellstrom BC, et al. Targeted-release budesonide versus placebo in patients with IgA nephropathy (NEFIGAN): a double-blind, randomised, placebo-controlled phase 2b trial. Lancet. 2017;389(10084):2117–27.

158. Briganti EM, et al. Recurrent glomerulonephritis and risk of renal allograft loss. N Engl J Med. 2002;347(19):1531–2.

159. Andresdottir MB, et al. Favorable outcome of renal transplantation in patients with IgA nephropathy. Clin Nephrol. 2001;56(4):279–88.

160. Amaral B, et al. A comparison of the outcome of adolescent and adult-onset systemic lupus erythematosus. Rheumatology (Oxford). 2014;53(6):1130–5.

161. Feng X, et al. Associations of clinical features and prognosis with age at disease onset in patients with systemic lupus erythematosus. Lupus. 2014;23(3):327–34.

162. Marks SD, et al. Clinicopathological correlations of paediatric lupus nephritis. Pediatr Nephrol. 2007;22(1):77–83.

163. Lee BS, et al. Clinical outcomes of childhood lupus nephritis: a single center's experience. Pediatr Nephrol. 2007;22(2):222–31.

164. Norby GE, et al. Recurrent lupus nephritis after kidney transplantation: a surveillance biopsy study. Ann Rheum Dis. 2010;69(8):1484–7.

165. Ponticelli C, Moroni G, Glassock RJ. Recurrence of secondary glomerular disease after renal transplantation. Clin J Am Soc Nephrol. 2011;6(5):1214–21.

166. Contreras G, et al. Recurrence of lupus nephritis after kidney transplantation. J Am Soc Nephrol. 2010;21(7):1200–7.

167. Moroni G, et al. The long-term prognosis of renal transplantation in patients with lupus nephritis. Am J Kidney Dis. 2005;45(5):903–11.

168. Winchester RJ, Nunez-Roldan A. Some genetic aspects of systemic lupus erythematosus. Arthritis Rheum. 1982;25(7):833–7.

169. Cats S, et al. Increased vulnerability of the donor organ in related kidney transplants for certain diseases. Transplantation. 1984;37(6):575–9.

170. Albuquerque BC, et al. Outcome and prognosis of patients with lupus nephritis submitted to renal transplantation. Sci Rep. 2019;9(1):11611.

171. Ponticelli C, Moroni G. Renal transplantation in lupus nephritis. Lupus. 2005;14(1):95–8.

172. Wagenknecht DR, et al. Risk of early renal allograft failure is increased for patients with antiphospholipid antibodies. Transpl Int. 2000;13(Suppl 1):S78–81.

173. Vaidya S, Gugliuzza K, Daller JA. Efficacy of anticoagulation therapy in end-stage renal disease patients with antiphospholipid antibody syndrome. Transplantation. 2004;77(7):1046–9.

174. McIntyre JA, Wagenknecht DR. Antiphospholipid antibodies and renal transplantation: a risk assessment. Lupus. 2003;12(7):555–9.

175. Pham PT, Pham PC. The impact of mycophenolate mofetil versus azathioprine as adjunctive therapy to cyclosporine on the rates of renal allograft loss due to glomerular disease recurrence. Nephrol Dial Transplant. 2012;27(7):2965–71.

176. Bartosh SM, Fine RN, Sullivan EK. Outcome after transplantation of young patients with systemic lupus erythematosus: a report of the north American

pediatric renal transplant cooperative study. Transplantation. 2001;72(5):973–8.

177. Al Midani A, et al. Low-dose aspirin reduces the rate of renal allograft thrombosis in pediatric renal transplant recipients. Exp Clin Transplant. 2020;18(2):157–63.

178. Smith JM, et al. Decreased risk of renal allograft thrombosis associated with interleukin-2 receptor antagonists: a report of the NAPRTCS. Am J Transplant. 2006;6(3):585–8.

179. Kari JA, et al. Renal transplantation in children under 5 years of age. Pediatr Nephrol. 1999;13(9):730–6.

180. Singh A, Stablein D, Tejani A. Risk factors for vascular thrombosis in pediatric renal transplantation: a special report of the north American pediatric renal transplant cooperative study. Transplantation. 1997;63(9):1263–7.

181. McDonald RA, et al. Pretransplant peritoneal dialysis and graft thrombosis following pediatric kidney transplantation: a NAPRTCS report. Pediatr Transplant. 2003;7(3):204–8.

182. Kranz B, et al. Outcome after kidney transplantation in children with thrombotic risk factors. Pediatr Transplant. 2006;10(7):788–93.

183. Vats AN, et al. Pretransplant dialysis status and outcome of renal transplantation in north American children: a NAPRTCS study. North American pediatric renal transplant cooperative study. Transplantation. 2000;69(7):1414–9.

184. Broyer M, et al. Preventive treatment of vascular thrombosis after kidney transplantation in children with low molecular weight heparin. Transplant Proc. 1991;23(1 Pt 2):1384–5.

185. Alkhunaizi AM, et al. Efficacy and safety of low molecular weight heparin in renal transplantation. Transplantation. 1998;66(4):533–4.

186. Valente JF, et al. Comparison of sirolimus vs. mycophenolate mofetil on surgical complications and wound healing in adult kidney transplantation. Am J Transplant. 2003;3(9):1128–34.

187. Goggins WC, et al. A prospective, randomized, clinical trial of intraoperative versus postoperative thymoglobulin in adult cadaveric renal transplant recipients. Transplantation. 2003;76(5):798–802.

188. Mumford L, et al. The impact of changing practice on improved outcomes of paediatric renal transplantation in the United Kingdom: a 25 years review. Transpl Int. 2019;32(7):751–61.

189. Groothoff JW. Long-term outcomes of children with end-stage renal disease. Pediatr Nephrol. 2005;20(7):849–53.

190. Tangeraas T, et al. Long-term outcome of pediatric renal transplantation: the Norwegian experience in three eras 1970-2006. Pediatr Transplant. 2008;12(7):762–8.

191. Tsampalieros A, Lepage N, Feber J. Intraindividual variability of the modified Schwartz and novel CKiD GFR equations in pediatric renal transplant patients. Pediatr Transplant. 2011;15(7):760–5.

192. Anderson S, et al. Control of glomerular hypertension limits glomerular injury in rats with reduced renal mass. J Clin Invest. 1985;76(2):612–9.

193. Ishitani M, et al. Predictors of graft survival in pediatric living-related kidney transplant recipients. Transplantation. 2000;70(2):288–92.

194. Hochheiser K, et al. Kidney dendritic cells become pathogenic during crescentic glomerulonephritis with proteinuria. J Am Soc Nephrol. 2011;22(2):306–16.

195. Johnson RW, et al. Outcome of pediatric cadaveric renal transplantation: a 10 year study. Kidney Int Suppl. 1996;53:S72–6.

196. Bateman RM, et al. 36th international symposium on intensive care and emergency medicine : Brussels, Belgium. 15–18 march 2016. Crit Care. 2016;20(Suppl 2):94.

197. Teteris SA, Hochheiser K, Kurts C. Isolation of functional dendritic cells from murine kidneys for immunological characterization. Nephrology (Carlton). 2012;17(4):364–71.

198. Amer H, et al. Proteinuria after kidney transplantation, relationship to allograft histology and survival. Am J Transplant. 2007;7(12):2748–56.

199. Butani L. Investigation of pediatric renal transplant recipients with heavy proteinuria after sirolimus rescue. Transplantation. 2004;78(9):1362–6.

200. Halloran PF, et al. An integrated view of molecular changes, histopathology and outcomes in kidney transplants. Am J Transplant. 2010;10(10):2223–30.

201. Gasser M, et al. The influence of donor brain death on short and long-term outcome of solid organ allografts. Ann Transplant. 2000;5(4):61–7.

202. Rosendale JD, et al. Aggressive pharmacologic donor management results in more transplanted organs. Transplantation. 2003;75(4):482–7.

203. Treckmann J, et al. Machine perfusion versus cold storage for preservation of kidneys from expanded criteria donors after brain death. Transpl Int. 2011;24(6):548–54.

204. Noppakun K, et al. Living donor age and kidney transplant outcomes. Am J Transplant. 2011;11(6):1279–86.

205. Mueller TF, Solez K, Mas V. Assessment of kidney organ quality and prediction of outcome at time of transplantation. Semin Immunopathol. 2011;33(2):185–99.

206. Randhawa PS, et al. Biopsy of marginal donor kidneys: correlation of histologic findings with graft dysfunction. Transplantation. 2000;69(7):1352–7.

207. Azevedo F, et al. Glomerular size in early protocol biopsies is associated with graft outcome. Am J Transplant. 2005;5(12):2877–82.

208. Rao PS, Ojo A. The alphabet soup of kidney transplantation: SCD, DCD, ECD—fundamentals for the practicing nephrologist. Clin J Am Soc Nephrol. 2009;4(11):1827–31.

209. Solez K, et al. International standardization of criteria for the histologic diagnosis of renal allograft rejection: the Banff working classifica-

tion of kidney transplant pathology. Kidney Int. 1993;44(2):411–22.

210. Racusen LC, et al. Antibody-mediated rejection criteria - an addition to the Banff 97 classification of renal allograft rejection. Am J Transplant. 2003;3(6):708–14.

211. Sis B, et al. Banff '09 meeting report: antibody mediated graft deterioration and implementation of Banff working groups. Am J Transplant. 2010;10(3):464–71.

212. Haas M, et al. C4d and C3d staining in biopsies of ABO- and HLA-incompatible renal allografts: correlation with histologic findings. Am J Transplant. 2006;6(8):1829–40.

213. Lefaucheur C, et al. Antibody-mediated vascular rejection of kidney allografts: a population-based study. Lancet. 2013;381(9863):313–9.

214. Smith JM, Ho PL, McDonald RA. Renal transplant outcomes in adolescents: a report of the north American pediatric renal transplant cooperative study. Pediatr Transplant. 2002;6(6):493–9.

215. Einecke G, et al. Antibody-mediated microcirculation injury is the major cause of late kidney transplant failure. Am J Transplant. 2009;9(11):2520–31.

216. Dörje C, et al. Early versus late acute antibody-mediated rejection in renal transplant recipients. Transplantation. 2013;96(1):79–84.

217. Nankivell BJ, et al. The natural history of chronic allograft nephropathy. N Engl J Med. 2003;349(24):2326–33.

218. Gourishankar S, et al. Pathological and clinical characterization of the 'troubled transplant': data from the DeKAF study. Am J Transplant. 2010;10(2):324–30.

219. Gaston RS, et al. Evidence for antibody-mediated injury as a major determinant of late kidney allograft failure. Transplantation. 2010;90(1):68–74.

220. El-Zoghby ZM, et al. Identifying specific causes of kidney allograft loss. Am J Transplant. 2009;9(3):527–35.

221. Sellarés J, et al. Understanding the causes of kidney transplant failure: the dominant role of antibody-mediated rejection and nonadherence. Am J Transplant. 2012;12(2):388–99.

222. Colvin RB, Smith RN. Antibody-mediated organ-allograft rejection. Nat Rev Immunol. 2005;5(10):807–17.

223. Cornell LD, Smith RN, Colvin RB. Kidney transplantation: mechanisms of rejection and acceptance. Annu Rev Pathol. 2008;3:189–220.

224. Akiyoshi T, et al. Role of complement and NK cells in antibody mediated rejection. Hum Immunol. 2012;73(12):1226–32.

225. Racusen LC, et al. The Banff 97 working classification of renal allograft pathology. Kidney Int. 1999;55(2):713–23.

226. Regele H, et al. Capillary deposition of complement split product C4d in renal allografts is associated with basement membrane injury in peritubular and glomerular capillaries: a contribution of humoral immunity to chronic allograft rejection. J Am Soc Nephrol. 2002;13(9):2371–80.

227. Solez K, Racusen LC. The Banff classification revisited. Kidney Int. 2013;83(2):201–6.

228. de Kort H, et al. Microcirculation inflammation associates with outcome in renal transplant patients with de novo donor-specific antibodies. Am J Transplant. 2013;13(2):485–92.

229. Drachenberg CB, Papadimitriou JC. Endothelial injury in renal antibody-mediated allograft rejection: a schematic view based on pathogenesis. Transplantation. 2013;95(9):1073–83.

230. Sis B, et al. Endothelial gene expression in kidney transplants with alloantibody indicates antibody-mediated damage despite lack of C4d staining. Am J Transplant. 2009;9(10):2312–23.

231. Sis B, et al. A new diagnostic algorithm for antibody-mediated microcirculation inflammation in kidney transplants. Am J Transplant. 2012;12(5):1168–79.

232. Couzi L, et al. Incidence and outcome of C4d staining with tubulointerstitial inflammation in blood group-incompatible kidney transplantation. Transplantation. 2015;99(7):1487–94.

233. Mengel M, et al. Scoring total inflammation is superior to the current Banff inflammation score in predicting outcome and the degree of molecular disturbance in renal allografts. Am J Transplant. 2009;9(8):1859–67.

234. de Freitas DG, et al. The nature of biopsies with "borderline rejection" and prospects for eliminating this category. Am J Transplant. 2012;12(1):191–201.

235. Martin S, et al. Posttransplant antidonor lymphocytotoxic antibody production in relation to graft outcome. Transplantation. 1987;44(1):50–3.

236. Kim JJ, et al. The clinical spectrum of de novo donor-specific antibodies in pediatric renal transplant recipients. Am J Transplant. 2014;14(10):2350–8.

237. Wiebe C, et al. Evolution and clinical pathologic correlations of de novo donor-specific HLA antibody post kidney transplant. Am J Transplant. 2012;12(5):1157–67.

238. Willicombe M, et al. De novo DQ donor-specific antibodies are associated with a significant risk of antibody-mediated rejection and transplant glomerulopathy. Transplantation. 2012;94(2):172–7.

239. Miettinen J, et al. Donor-specific HLA antibodies and graft function in children after renal transplantation. Pediatr Nephrol. 2012;27(6):1011–9.

240. Liefeldt L, et al. Donor-specific HLA antibodies in a cohort comparing everolimus with cyclosporine after kidney transplantation. Am J Transplant. 2012;12(5):1192–8.

241. Piazza A, et al. Post-transplant donor-specific antibody production and graft outcome in kidney transplantation: results of sixteen-year monitoring by flow cytometry. Clin Transpl. 2006;323–36.

242. Everly MJ, et al. Reducing de novo donor-specific antibody levels during acute rejection diminishes renal allograft loss. Am J Transplant. 2009;9(5):1063–71.

243. Nickerson PW, Rush DN. Antibodies beyond HLA. Am J Transplant. 2013;13(4):831–2.

244. Hidalgo LG, et al. De novo donor-specific antibody at the time of kidney transplant biopsy associates with microvascular pathology and late graft failure. Am J Transplant. 2009;9(11):2532–41.

245. Ginevri F, et al. Posttransplant de novo donor-specific hla antibodies identify pediatric kidney recipients at risk for late antibody-mediated rejection. Am J Transplant. 2012;12(12):3355–62.

246. Schnuelle P, et al. Effects of donor pretreatment with dopamine on graft function after kidney transplantation: a randomized controlled trial. JAMA. 2009;302(10):1067–75.

247. Sun Q, et al. Late and early C4d-positive acute rejection: different clinico-histopathological subentities in renal transplantation. Kidney Int. 2006;70(2):377–83.

248. Péfaur J, et al. Early and late humoral rejection: a clinicopathologic entity in two times. Transplant Proc. 2008;40(9):3229–36.

249. Lefaucheur C, et al. Comparison of combination plasmapheresis/IVIg/anti-CD20 versus high-dose IVIg in the treatment of antibody-mediated rejection. Am J Transplant. 2009;9(5):1099–107.

250. Montgomery RA, et al. Humoral immunity and antibody-mediated rejection in solid organ transplantation. Semin Immunol. 2011;23(4):224–34.

251. Marks SD. Treatment strategies to treat antibody-mediated rejection and to reduce donor-specific antibodies. Pediatr Transplant. 2014;18(5):417–9.

252. Gubensek J, et al. Plasma exchange and intravenous immunoglobulin in the treatment of antibody-mediated rejection after kidney transplantation: a single-center historic cohort study. Transplant Proc. 2013;45(4):1524–7.

253. Gupta G, et al. Late antibody-mediated rejection in renal allografts: outcome after conventional and novel therapies. Transplantation. 2014;97(12):1240–6.

254. Walsh RC, et al. Proteasome inhibitor-based primary therapy for antibody-mediated renal allograft rejection. Transplantation. 2010;89(3):277–84.

255. Langone A, et al. Does reduction in mycophenolic acid dose compromise efficacy regardless of tacrolimus exposure level? An analysis of prospective data from the mycophenolic renal transplant (MORE) registry. Clin Transpl. 2013;27(1):15–24.

256. Haas M, et al. The Banff 2017 kidney meeting report: revised diagnostic criteria for chronic active T cell-mediated rejection, antibody-mediated rejection, and prospects for integrative endpoints for next-generation clinical trials. Am J Transplant. 2018;18(2):293–307.

Prevention and Treatment of Infectious Complications in Pediatric Renal Transplant Recipients

Jodi M. Smith, Sarah J. Kizilbash, and Vikas R. Dharnidharka

Introduction

Over the last few decades, significant advances have been made in the outcomes of pediatric kidney transplant recipients, with marked improvement in patient survival and early allograft survival. However, the more potent immunosuppressive therapy that successfully reduced the incidence of acute rejection has resulted in a higher incidence of infectious complications [1]. This increase has manifested as (1) an increase in the total frequency of infection [2]; (2) infection becoming the primary reason for post-transplant hospitalization [3]; and (3) the successive emergence of new viral infections in the past several decades. Specifically, cytomegalovirus (CMV) infections have been common in kidney transplant recipients since the 1980s, followed by Epstein Barr virus (EBV) related post-transplant lymphoproliferative disorder (PTLD) since the 1990s, and BK virus associated allograft nephropathy (BKVAN) in the last 15 years. Infections are not only a significant source of morbidity and hospitalization, but they also can lead to graft loss and patient death. Even when adjusting for death, infections represent an additional risk factor for worse graft survival [4–6], thus in part accounting for the less significant improvement in longer-term allograft survival [7]. Excessive PTLD resulted in the early termi-

J. M. Smith (✉)
Department of Pediatrics, University of Washington School of Medicine, Seattle, WA, USA
e-mail: jodi.smith@seattlechildrens.org

S. J. Kizilbash
Department of Pediatrics, University of Minnesota, Minneapolis, MN, USA
e-mail: kizil010@umn.edu

V. R. Dharnidharka
Department of Pediatrics, Washington University School of Medicine, St. Louis, MO, USA
e-mail: vikasD@wustl.edu

© The Author(s), under exclusive license to Springer Nature Switzerland AG 2023
F. Schaefer, L. A. Greenbaum (eds.), *Pediatric Kidney Disease*,
https://doi.org/10.1007/978-3-031-11665-0_69

nation of a large multi-center immunosuppression trial in pediatric kidney transplantation in the US [8]. Hospitalizations due to infection occurred in 47% of children within the first 3 years after kidney transplant, higher than in adults with a kidney transplant or in children on dialysis [2]. Unlike adults, the total incidence of infections did not drop in children in more recent years. From 2019 onwards, the global SARS-COV-2 (COVID19) pandemic greatly affected organ transplant recipients.

Special Considerations in Pediatric Transplantation

Organ transplant recipients are at greater risk for infection than immunocompetent individuals. The immunosuppressive medications currently in use are non-selective in nature, suppressing immune responses to alloantigens, as well as to infectious organisms. An organ transplant is a major surgical procedure with the infection risks of any major surgery. Chronic kidney failure itself suppresses the immune system to some extent. Cytopenias are common post-transplant due to medication side-effects, and can raise the infection risk.

Further, children are exposed to some unique infection risks. Many of the main viral infections that occur post–transplant are associated with higher morbidity when they are primary infections. A primary viral infection is defined as infection in a recipient who is seronegative at the time of transplant, with no prior immunity. Reactivation infection occurs in the setting of a patient who is seropositive and has some prior immunity. Pediatric patients are at higher risk for primary infection due to higher rates of recipient seronegativity at the time of transplant. Recent US data demonstrated that approximately 50% of pediatric kidney transplant recipients were EBV seronegative and 65% were CMV seronegative at the time of transplant compared to 10% EBV and 40% CMV seronegativity among adults [9]. The grafts to children come most often from adult (therefore most likely seropositive) donors, thereby introducing the virus at transplant.

Viral Infections

Cytomegalovirus

CMV, now called human herpesvirus 5 (HHV5), a double-stranded DNA virus of the herpes virus family, is perhaps the single most important pathogen in solid organ transplantation [10]. CMV not only causes significant morbidity by direct infection, but its immuno-modulatory effects also predispose to other infectious complications [10]. CMV infection and CMV disease are different from each other. CMV infection is defined as evidence of CMV replication regardless of symptoms (differs from latent CMV). CMV disease is defined as evidence of CMV infection with attributable symptoms. Three patterns of CMV infection may be seen post-transplantation: Primary infection, reactivation infection, and superinfection. Primary infection occurs in transplant patients who were CMV seronegative prior to transplant, most commonly via transmission from a graft from a seropositive donor [10–12]. Without preventative therapy, the incidence of CMV disease in such recipients is 50–65% [10]. Reactivation infection is due to activation of latent virus in seropositive recipients, while superinfection is activation of virus from a seropositive donor in a seropositive recipient. Infection with CMV usually presents in the first few months post-transplant and can manifest as CMV syndrome, characterized by fever, myalgias, malaise, leukopenia and thrombocytopenia, or CMV disease, in which there is clinical evidence of organ involvement by the infection [10, 13]. The transplanted kidney is at higher risk for CMV infection than are the native organs, but pulmonary, liver and gastrointestinal tract infection are common, regardless of the organ transplanted [14–16]. As stated above, in addition to causing direct infection, CMV has significant indirect effects, including an increase in the overall state of immunosuppression leading to increased risk for opportunistic infection [10]. CMV infection has been demonstrated to increase the risk of EBV-associated PTLD [10, 16]. In addition, CMV and acute rejection are interrelated. CMV infection is a risk factor for acute rejection, while rejection leads to release of tumor necrosis factor, triggering the process that ultimately leads to CMV replication [17].

Prevention of CMV infection can be accomplished with either (1) universal prophylaxis: the administration of anti-CMV therapy to all patients except seronegative recipients of a seronegative organ; or (2) preemptive therapy: viral monitoring and initiation of the treatment dose of anti-viral medication when a certain positive threshold is reached. There is some controversy as to the optimal strategy, as both methods have advantages and disadvantages. Consensus guidelines from the American Society of Transplantation (AST), Kidney Disease: Improving Global Outcomes (KDIGO), and The Transplantation Society International CMV Consensus Group recommend universal prophylaxis for high risk patients (seronegative recipients of seropositive organs or seropositive recipients of seropositive organs in the setting of anti-T-cell antibody immunosuppression), based on the available data suggesting better graft survival and clinical outcomes [11, 12]. Preemptive therapy has not been well studied in pediatrics. Although several agents are available for prophylaxis, valganciclovir has revolutionized both CMV prevention and treatment [18]. It is a prodrug of ganciclovir and is approximately 60% bioavailable, which is tenfold more than ganciclovir [19]. While the dosing of valganciclovir is well established in adults, the dosing in pediatric patients is somewhat more complex due to the dependence on metabolic activation, renal clearance and variable absorption. Since 2009, the manufacturer recommends normalization of the adult dose for BSA and creatinine clearance. Other centers have employed a weight based approach. Due to the

challenges, particularly in infants and young children, ganciclovir levels may be helpful to guide therapy. Leukopenia is a common side effect of valganciclovir therapy. The duration of prophylaxis is an area of debate. Consensus recommendations guide the duration of therapy based on the serostatus of the donor and recipient [11, 12] (Table 69.1). For CMV Donor (D)+/Recipient (R)- patients, 3–6 months of prophylaxis with oral ganciclovir or valganciclovir is recommended. For CMV R+ patients, 3 months is recommended but 6 months should be considered if anti-lymphocyte induction is used. No prophylaxis is recommended in the CMV D−/R- patient. In addition, treatment of rejection with antilymphocyte antibodies in at risk recipients (D+/R-) should prompt re-initiation of prophylaxis or preemptive therapy for 1–3 months [11, 12, 22]. For treatment of CMV disease in pediatric patients, IV ganciclovir is recommended [12]. Therapy should continue until the CMV is no longer detectable. Reduction of immunosuppression in life-threatening CMV disease is indicated in cases of persistent disease despite treatment.

Late onset CMV disease is defined as disease occurring after prophylaxis has been discontinued and has been reported in 25–40% of patients on universal prophylaxis [20, 23]. Late onset CMV is associated with significant morbidity and high mortality, underscoring the ability of anti-viral prophylaxis to delay but not prevent

Table 69.1 Recommendations for duration of CMV prophylaxis [20, 21]

CMV D+/R-	• 3–6 months of prophylaxis with oral ganciclovir or valganciclovir is recommended. • In addition, treatment of rejection with antilymphocyte antibodies in at risk recipients (D+/R-) should prompt re-initiation of prophylaxis or preemptive therapy for 1–3 months.
CMV D+/ R+ CMV D−/R+	• 3 months is recommended but 6 months should be considered if anti-lymphocyte induction is used.
CMV D−/R-	• No prophylaxis is recommended.

Table 69.2 Expert recommendations regarding BK virus screening

	2003 Polyoma-virus associated nephropathy interdisciplinary group [24]	2009 AST infectious diseases group [25]	2009 KDIGO transplant work group [12]
Screening	Urine screening, various techniques, every 3 months till month 24 (grade A-II) and annually thereafter till fifth year post-transplant (grade B-III) or with allograft dysfunction Biopsy if urine BK DNA > 1 × 10^7, VP1 mRNA >6.5 × 10^5 or plasma DNA > 1 × 10^4	Urine screening every 3 months in first 2 years then annually until fifth year post-transplant (grade II-B). If plasma screening performed, then at monthly intervals Biopsy if urine BK DNA > 1 × 10^7, VP1 mRNA > 6.5 × 10^5 or plasma DNA > 1 × 10^4	Plasma BK nucleic acid testing monthly for first 3–6 months, then every 3 months till month 12, or if elevated serum creatinine or after treatment for acute rejection
Intervention	Various approaches discussed, none specifically endorsed	Reduce immunosuppression for presumptive BKVN (plasma BKV loads >1 × 10^4 for >3 weeks)	Reduce immunosuppression if plasma nucleic acid load persistently >1 × 10^4

Adapted from [139]

CMV. Thus, careful clinical follow-up and virologic monitoring is recommended after completion of prophylaxis.

Antiviral drug resistance should be suspected and tested for in the setting of a patient who has had cumulative ganciclovir exposure of more than 6 weeks and there are rising viral loads or progressive disease after 2 weeks at full dose [11]. Risk factors include prolonged antiviral drug exposure (median 5–6 months), ongoing active viral replication, lack of prior CMV immunity (D+/R-), and inadequate drug delivery. Currently, genotype testing includes the UL97 kinase and UL54 DNA polymerase, with the UL97 mutation appearing in 90% of cases.

The timing and frequency of screening for CMV is largely center-specific and influenced by donor and recipient CMV serostatus, as well as whether universal or preemptive therapy is employed. Published guidelines recommend regular monitoring using a quantitative viral load assay for the first year post-transplant; however, the duration and frequency may vary depending on the type of CMV prevention strategy [11, 12]. Table 69.2 summarizes the characteristics of many commonly used assays for the different viral infections. The recent development of an international standard for CMV is promising as it will permit determination of appropriate standardized trigger points for intervention and allow comparison among sites.

Epstein-Barr Virus

EBV is another herpes virus that causes significant morbidity post-transplantation. Distinctions are made between EBV infection and disease. Active, asymptomatic EBV infection is defined by the presence of a detectable EBV viral load as measured by a nucleic acid amplification assay. Uncommonly, asymptomatic infection may also be identified in lymphoid rich histopathologic specimens. EBV disease is defined by the presence of active EBV infection with symptoms or signs attributable to the virus. The spectrum of clinical manifestations of EBV in transplant recipients includes nonspecific viral syndrome, mononucleosis, lymphoproliferative disorders and malignant lymphomas.

Like CMV, EBV commonly infects immunocompetent people sometime in childhood and establishes a prolonged latency in reticuloendothelial cells. Thus, the patterns of infection are identical to CMV: primary infection (often from the graft of a seropositive donor), reactivation or superinfection. Again, like CMV, the primary infection in an immunosuppressed transplant recipient is more virulent. Unlike CMV, EBV infection does not seem to have many indirect effects except for the development of PTLD. PTLD is a major complication and is covered in detail in the next chapter. This section deals with EBV infection only.

Prospective viral surveillance studies revealed that subclinical EBV infection occurs in 35–40% of pediatric renal transplant recipients [6, 26]. In a recent cohort study of adult kidney transplant recipients, 40% had subclinical viremia [27]. EBV viremia often precedes the development of EBV disease and PTLD by 4–16 weeks [28, 29]. Thus, early identification of EBV viremia may allow for intervention that could prevent progression to EBV disease and PTLD. KDIGO recommends the following post-transplant EBV screening schedule for high risk D+/R- patients: once in the first week after transplant; at least monthly for the first 3–6 months; then at least every 3 months until the end of the first year with re-initiation of monitoring after treatment for acute rejection. While D−/R− patients might be at decreased risk of developing EBV disease compared to D+/R−, they are still at increased risk relative to R+ patients and therefore warrant close monitoring. Some centers may choose to measure EBV loads more frequently. Beyond the first year, selective monitoring, such as in those with persistently high viral loads or in those with higher than normal immunosuppression, may be performed based on center preferences. Some centers recommend continued monitoring for an indefinite period for all patients. For seropositive individuals, selective monitoring may be considered in the setting of increased immunosuppression or clinical concern.

The reader should note that PCR techniques to detect EBV DNA amplification vary greatly based on the type of sample and laboratory standards. Thus, PCR values from peripheral blood leukocytes and whole blood generally correlate with each other but not with PCR values from plasma [30, 31]. To date, there is no defined standard sample site for EBV. In practice, the most important strategy is to follow the viral load in the same lab using the same type of sample consistently over time and to be careful to not compare viral loads from one lab to another.

There is no universally accepted treatment for subclinical EBV infection post-transplant. Options include reduction of immunosuppression, antiviral therapy, intravenous immunoglobulin (IVIG), and monoclonal antibody therapy directed toward infected B lymphocytes

[21, 29, 32–34]. Currently, the only consensus recommendation is for a reduction of immunosuppression in EBV seronegative patients with an increasing EBV viral load. The utility of antiviral therapy to prevent PTLD is controversial, with little evidence to support the role of acyclovir or ganciclovir in response to an elevated or rising EBV viral load without a concomitant reduction of immunosuppression. These agents seem to delay the onset of infection rather than reducing its incidence. Two studies suggest that anti-viral prophylaxis has an additional benefit of preventing the progression from EBV disease to PTLD [19, 35]. IVIG does not appear to be of added benefit [36]. Preemptive use of rituximab in response to subclinical EBV infection began in the hematopoietic stem cell population and has recently been reported in the adult kidney transplant population [37, 38]. It is important to remember, however, that children, in particular, can develop a chronic high load carrier state without ever progressing to PTLD [39–44]. Nevertheless, the majority of reports indicate that higher EBV PCR values are associated with a greater risk for subsequent PTLD [45–47]. An EBV vaccine, directed against an EBV-glycoprotein, was tested in the United Kingdom but failed [48]. Unlike with CMV, we are not aware of any cost-benefit analysis of EBV monitoring or preventative treatment strategies.

BK Virus and BKVAN

BK virus (BKV) was first isolated from the urine of a kidney transplant recipient in the 1970s [49], but it was not until the late 1990s that this virus emerged as a significant problem in kidney transplantation [50, 51]. BKV is a part of the polyoma group of viruses. Though this virus is not from the herpesvirus group, it shares the characteristics of herpesviruses of infecting most immunocompetent people during childhood and establishing a prolonged latency. Unlike the herpesviruses, the virus does not establish latency in reticuloendothelial cells but in the uroepithelium. This propensity for the uroepithelium is responsible for the clinical manifestations: hemorrhagic cystitis in bone marrow transplant recipients and allograft nephropathy in kidney transplant recipients. The incidence of BKVAN in pediatric kidney transplantation appears to be the same as in adult kidney transplants at 3–8% [52–56]. Risk factors include the intensity of immunosuppression, recent treatment for acute rejection, and placement of a ureteral stent, though the data implicating specific immunosuppressive agents is conflicting [54, 57–59].

BKVAN and BKV infection are two separate entities. BKVAN is defined as the presence of virus in the renal parenchyma, with accompanying evidence of either tubulointerstitial nephritis or elevated serum creatinine, as defined by a working group of the AST [2]. BKVAN is more prevalent in the medulla of the kidney, so at least one core should be deep enough to include medulla. A negative biopsy result does not rule out BKVAN due to the possibility of sampling error and the focal nature of the infection, so sensitivity is not 100%. In cases where the biopsy is negative, but there is high clinical suspicion for BKVAN, a repeat biopsy may be indicated. The histologic patterns of BKVAN have been divided into three types, as reviewed by Liptak et al. and the AST Transplant Infectious Diseases Group [25, 60]: Type A has intranuclear viral inclusions only, Type B has additional acute inflammation but very little chronic fibrosis, and Type C has significant chronic fibrosis and atrophy. The value of this classification lies in its prognostic value of clinical outcomes: the incidence of progression to end-stage kidney disease (ESKD) was only 13% with Type A, 55% with Type B and 100% with Type C [61]. BKVAN represents a diagnostic challenge because the condition may resemble acute rejection. Symptoms are often minimal or absent. Serum creatinine elevations are found on clinical lab monitoring. Since the treatment of acute rejection (intensifying immunosuppression) is the opposite of the treatment of BKVAN (reduction in immunosuppression), making the correct diagnosis is critical.

Early identification of BKV infection (detectable viral load in blood or urine) may permit intervention that may prevent BKVAN. Data suggest that the BK viremia precedes BKVAN by a median of 8 weeks [24]. BKV viral load >10,000 copies/L has a high positive predictive value for BKVAN [59]. Indications for biopsy vary among centers but many include viral load >10,000 copies/L with or without an elevated creatinine.

Routine screening is the most important tool used to identify patients at risk for BKVAN. Various schedules of surveillance are shown in Table 69.3. Intervention options include reduction of immunosuppression and use of other agents such as cidofovir, leflunomide, or IVIG. Stepwise immunosuppression reduction is recommended for kidney transplant recipients with plasma BKV-DNAemia of >1000 copies/ml sustained for 3 weeks or increasing to >10,000 copies/ml, reflecting probable and presumptive BKVAN, respectively [64]. The approach to immunosuppression reduction varies among centers, with varying levels of supporting evidence, and includes the following: (1) switching from tacrolimus to cyclosporine (CSA) or sirolimus; (2) mycophenolate mofetil (MMF) to azathioprine or sirolimus or leflunomide; (3) decreasing tacrolimus (trough levels <6 ng/ml), MMF (dosing ≤1 g/day), and CSA (trough levels 100–150 ng/ml); or (4) decreasing tacrolimus or MMF (maintain or switch to dual therapy with calcineurin inhibitor (CNI) and prednisone, sirolimus/prednisone, MMF/prednisone) [12]. While the reduction of immunosuppression raises concerns about the unintended consequence of rejection, several studies have reported successful preemptive intervention with no increase in rejection [65, 66].

There are virtually no randomized controlled trials to test any of these strategies head to head for any of the viral infections. Anti-viral therapy against BKV is more complicated than for CMV or EBV, since acyclovir, ganciclovir or their analogues are not active against BKV. Cidofovir is one anti-viral drug that has been tried with some success [67, 68]. Higher doses of cidofovir can be very nephrotoxic. Probenecid in combination with the higher dose cidofovir or intermediate dose cidofovir prevents the nephrotoxicity [69]. Fluoroquinolones are not recommended for either prophylaxis or treatment [64].

Table 69.3 Recommended vaccinations for pediatric transplant candidates and recipients [62, 63]

Vaccine	Inactivated/live attenuated (I/LA)	Recommended before transplant[a]/ strength of recommendation	Recommended after transplant/ strength of recommendation	Monitor vaccine titers?	Quality of evidence
Influenza, injected	I	Yes/A	Yes/A	No	II
Hepatitis B	I	Yes/A	Yes[b]/B	Yes[b]	II
Hepatitis A	I	Yes/A	Yes/A	Yes	II
Pertussis	I	Yes/A	Yes/A	No	III
Diphtheria	I	Yes/A	Yes/A	No	II
Tetanus	I	Yes/A	Yes/A	No	II
Polio, inactivated	I	Yes/A	Yes/A	No	III
Hemophilus influenzae	I	Yes/A	Yes/A	Yes[c]	II
Streptococcus pneumoniae[d] (conjugated/ polysaccharide)	I/I	Yes/A	Yes/A	Yes[c]	III
Neisseria meningitidis[e]	I	Yes/A	Yes/A	No	III
Rabies[f]	I	Yes/A	Yes/B	No	III
Varicella	LA	Yes/A	No/D	Yes	II
Measles	LA	Yes/A	No/D	Yes	II
Mumps	LA	Yes/A	No/D	Yes	III
Rubella	LA	Yes/A	No/D	Yes	II
Bacille Calmette-Guérin [g]	LA	Yes/B	No/D	No	III
Smallpox[h]	LA	No/C	No/D	No	III
Anthrax	I	No/C	No/C	No	III

Adapted from (a) Advisory Committee for Immunization Practices 2013; (b) The American Society of Transplantation (AST) Handbook of Transplant Infections, 2011

[a]Whenever possible, the complete complement of vaccines should be administered before transplantation. Vaccines noted to be safe for administration after transplantation may not be sufficiently immunogenic after transplantation. Some vaccines, such as Pneumovax, should be repeated regularly (every 3–5 years) after transplantation

[b]Routine vaccine schedule recommended prior to transplant and as early in the course of disease as possible; vaccine poorly immunogenic after transplantation, and accelerated schedules may be less immunogenic. Serial hepatitis B surface antibody titers should be assessed both before and after transplantation to assess ongoing immunity

[c]Serologic assessment recommended if available

[d]Children older than 5 years should receive 23-valent pneumococcal polysaccharide vaccine. Children less than 2 years should receive conjugated pneumococcal vaccine. Those 2 years–5 years of age should receive vaccination based on age and number of previous immunizations with conjugated pneumococcal vaccine

[e]Vaccination with conjugated meningococcal vaccine recommended in United States for all children aged 11–12 years of age and adolescents at high school entry or 15 years of age, whichever comes first

[f]Not routinely administered. Recommended for exposures, or potential exposures due to vocation or avocation

[g]The indications for Bacille Calmette-Guérin administration in the United States are limited to instances in which exposure to tuberculosis is unavoidable and where the measures to prevent its spread have failed or are not possible

[h]Transplant recipients who are face-to-face contacts of a patient with smallpox should be vaccinated; vaccinia immune globulin may be administered concurrently if available. Those who are less intimate contacts should not be vaccinated

Varicella

Varicella-zoster virus (VZV) is the most infectious of the human herpesviruses. Primary infection with VZV results in chickenpox. Following primary infection, the virus remains in the body in a latent state from which it may be reactivated, resulting in cutaneous herpes zoster, or shingles. Most adult kidney transplant recipients have experienced primary infection in childhood and, therefore, are at risk for reactivation and the development of herpes zoster with the introduction of immunosuppressive medication post-transplant [70]. Historically many children were VZV naive at the time of transplantation and primary infection was a significant cause of morbidity and mortality [71, 72]. With the development of a safe and effective VZV vaccine, routine immunization of pediatric kidney transplant candidates has been documented to reduce the incidence of primary VZV infection post-transplantation [73]. Given these findings, it is recommended that all transplant candidates over 9–12 months of age receive immunization with the VZV vaccine [74]. Studies in children with chronic kidney disease and on dialysis suggest that two doses, rather than one, may be necessary to elicit protective antibody levels, so it is recommended that antibody levels be obtained at least 4 weeks following immunization, and a second dose given if necessary [74–76]. Although some studies have evaluated the use of this vaccine in post-transplant patients, both the American Academy of Pediatrics Committee on Infectious Diseases and the Centers for Disease Control and Prevention's Advisory Committee on Immunization Practices (ACIP) advise against the use of this live viral vaccine in immunocompromised patients [77, 78]. Thus, it is imperative that immunization be provided and protective antibody levels documented prior to transplant whenever possible.

Patients who are varicella-naive at the time of transplant, i.e. no history of chicken pox or VZV immunization, or fail to develop protective antibody after immunization, and who are exposed to varicella should receive prophylactic therapy. Previous recommendations included the delivery of varicella zoster immune globulin (VZIG); however, this product is no longer being manufactured [79]. In North America, an investigational VZIG product, VariZIG (Cangene Corporation, Winnipeg, Canada) has become available under an investigational new drug application and the ACIP recommends that use of this product be requested if an immunocompromised patient is exposed to varicella infection [79]. If this product is not available, IVIG, which contains some anti-varicella antibody, may be given. Any prophylactic therapy should be given as soon as possible, up to 96 hours after exposure. Patients who develop infection, either primary or secondary, should receive treatment with intravenous or oral acyclovir, with consideration of reduction of immunosuppression [12, 80, 81].

COVID-19

The coronavirus disease 2019 (COVID-19), characterized by significant respiratory and multiorgan disease, is caused by the novel severe acute respiratory syndrome coronavirus 2 (SARS–COV–2). This virus first emerged in December 2019 in Wuhan, China [82]. Droplets expelled during talking, coughing, sneezing, or eating are the most common mode of transmission. Transmission may also occur through aerosol; however, it is unclear if this is a significant mode of transmission outside of laboratory settings. Common symptoms of COVID-19 infection include fever, dry cough, shortness of breath, fatigue, myalgias, nausea and vomiting, diarrhea, headaches, weakness and rhinorrhea. Common complications include pneumonia, acute respiratory distress syndrome, liver injury characterized by elevation of liver enzymes, cardiac injury marked by troponin elevation, acute heart failure, myocarditis, prothrombotic coagulopathy, acute kidney injury, and acute cerebral vascular disease. Rare complications include cytokine storm and macrophage activating syndrome. Patients become contagious about 2–3 days prior to the onset of symptoms until about 8 days after symptom onset [82]. Nearly 80% of patients with COVID-19 have mild manifestations, 15% develop severe illness and 5% become critical.

Data are emerging on the impact of COVID-19 on kidney transplant recipients. The incidence of COVID-19 in solid organ transplant (SOT) recipients is 10- to 15-fold higher than in the general immunocompetent population and adult SOT patients with COVID-19 appear to be at higher risk of poor outcomes on the basis of their chronically immunosuppressed state and underlying medical comorbidities [67, 68]. Initial reports in pediatric kidney transplant recipients demonstrate a decreased risk for infection and less severe disease when compared to adult kidney transplant recipients [83, 84].

Transplant Candidate Considerations

Vaccination is recommended to occur prior to transplantation, ideally completing the vaccine series a minimum of 2 weeks prior to transplant. Living donor candidates should self-quarantine or follow strict social distancing for a 14 day period prior to the transplant. All candidates should also have a negative nucleic acid amplification test (NAT) documented prior to surgery.

Post-Transplant Vaccination

The AST recommends vaccination against SARS CoV-2 using the locally approved vaccines for pediatric kidney transplant recipients [85]. Information about COVID-19 vaccine responses in transplantation is rapidly evolving. However, antibody responses to COVID-19 vaccines in transplant recipients are diminished compared with the general population [86–97]. Data suggest that providing a third dose of mRNA vaccine to SOT recipients that have previously received two doses of mRNA vaccine can increase antibody titers to SARS-CoV-2 [98–100]. In a recent, double-blind, randomized placebo-controlled trial, a third dose mRNA vaccine provided 2 months after the second dose significantly increased antibody titers, neutralizing antibody, and cellular immune response to SARS-CoV-2 compared to a third dose placebo [94]. Based on

this, a third dose of mRNA vaccine is recommended for SOT recipients who have previously completed a 2-dose mRNA vaccine series. The use of a third dose should, until further evidence is available, be based on individual patient's unique situation and must depend on local availability of vaccines and local regulations. In addition, vaccination is recommended for all eligible household and close contacts. Routine antibody testing following vaccination is not recommended by the FDA.

COVID-19 and Donor Considerations

The AST published guidelines for organ donor screening for COVID-19. All deceased donors should be tested for SARS-CoV-2 infection using RT-PCR from the upper respiratory tract within 72 hours, but ideally as close to organ recovery as possible. For donors previously known to have had COVID-19, organ acceptance can be considered if the following circumstances are met: negative SARS-CoV-2 RT-PCR testing from the respiratory tract, symptoms of COVID-19 have resolved, AND at least 21 days have transpired since the date of disease onset. Data regarding the safety of organ donation from donors with previous COVID-19 are limited at this time and consultation with transplant infectious disease experts is recommended. Living donors should be advised to follow universal masking precautions and strict social distancing for 14 days prior to donation. All living donors should undergo respiratory tract SARS-CoV-2 RT- PCR testing within 3 days of donation. Donors should be encouraged to self-quarantine after the preoperative COVID-19 test [101].

Bacterial Infections

Urinary Tract Infection

Urinary tract infection (UTI) is the most common bacterial infection in kidney transplant recipients, in both adults [102, 103] and children [104].

UTIs develop in 20–60% in the first year post-transplant and 40–80% by 3 years post-transplant [2, 102–105]. UTI is not only a cause of morbidity but is also associated with higher rates of graft loss and patient death [106, 107]. Early UTI (within 6 months of transplant) elevated the risk for graft loss in children, while late UTI did not [108]. The urogenital tract is the most common entry point for systemic sepsis [109]. Numerous risk factors have been identified for UTIs post-transplant. Urologic anomalies such as neurogenic bladder, urinary tract obstruction, vesicoureteral reflux, bladder augmentation, ureteral stents and intermittent catheterization have all been associated with an increased risk of UTI post-transplant [105, 110–112]. UTI risk is highest in the first 3–6 months post-transplant but some risk remains at later time points. While the organisms implicated are usually the same as in immunocompetent individuals, such as Enterobacter species (e.g., *Escherichia coli* and *Klebsiella*), a higher percentage of UTIs in transplant patients are due to unusual organisms such as *Pseudomonas* species [113]. Clinical symptoms may include fever, dysuria, graft tenderness and foul-smelling or cloudy urine. In some patients, symptoms may be masked due to immunosuppression. A rise in serum creatinine may occur and can mimic acute rejection. UTIs can also precipitate acute rejection.

The diagnosis of UTI is usually made by urine culture, though patients on trimethoprim-sulfamethoxazole prophylaxis for *Pneumocystis jiroveci* may not demonstrate positive cultures. Treatment is with antimicrobial therapy. Initially, the antimicrobial prescribed should cover the common gram negative organisms, such as the beta-lactams or the quinolones [114]. Once the organism is known, the most specific and cost-effective antimicrobial can be prescribed. Treatment route and total duration are determined by the severity of infection, recipient age, and other risk factors. Kidney allograft pyelonephritis can be associated with bacteremia and significant morbidity. If allograft pyelonephritis is suspected, hospitalization and treatment with intravenous antibiotics for up to 14 days is recommended [12]. Shorter 5–7 day oral courses,

as are used in immunocompetent individuals, can be used for milder cystitis episodes in older children [92]. KDIGO suggests that all kidney transplant recipients receive UTI prophylaxis with daily trimethoprim-sulfamethoxazole for at least 6 months post-transplant based on data showing a decrease in the frequency of UTIs [115]. For patients who are allergic to trimethoprim-sulfamethoxazole, the recommended alternative is nitrofurantoin. Currently, the available evidence does not support routine treatment of asymptomatic bacteriuria [114].

Other Bacterial Infections

Other bacterial infections, such as wound infections, line sepsis and pneumonia are seen with significant frequency in kidney transplant recipients. Wound infections and line sepsis are commonly due to gram-positive *staphylococcus* and *streptococcus*.

Pneumonia can be due to multiple etiologies (bacterial, viral or fungal), but bacterial pathogens are responsible for approximately 44% of cases [116]. In adult transplant recipients, cellulitis and bacterial abscesses are frequent problems, largely due to co-morbid diabetes mellitus. In general, these complications are less common in the pediatric population. The treatment of these infections is generally no different than standard treatment in immunocompetent hosts, though duration of therapy may be longer.

Bartonella henselae infection (also known as cat-scratch disease) has been reported in pediatric organ transplant recipients, including kidney transplants [117]. This infection typically presents as fever and lymphadenopathy, and thus must be included in the differential diagnosis for PTLD. However, unlike PTLD, this infection is treated with antimicrobial therapy.

The incidence of *Mycobacterium tuberculosis* infection in kidney transplant recipients varies geographically, occurring in less than 2% of kidney transplant recipients in North America and Europe, but 5–15% in Asia and Africa [118–120]. This infection may present at any time post-transplant, but is most common in the first post-transplant year [119]. *M. tuberculosis* infection presents with a myriad of symptoms, including weight loss, cough, fever and lymphadenopathy, again mimicking PTLD. The diagnosis of tuberculosis in the transplant recipient is similar to that in other populations, although the tuberculin skin test may be positive in only a third of kidney transplant recipients with tuberculosis [120]. Early diagnosis is best achieved by staining for acid-fast bacilli or using PCR from sputum, bronchoalveolar lavage or gastric aspirates. Interferon-gamma release assays such as QuantiFERON and T-SPOT.TB are alternative methods used to detect latent infection. Management of tuberculosis is complex and evolving and has long been directed by recommendations developed, updated and disseminated by expert panels [12, 120–122]. A four-drug regimen, similar to the regimen recommended in the general population, should be used in case of active tuberculosis after transplantation [123]. Rifampin is associated with numerous drug interactions through its activation of the CYP3A4 pathway which can impact levels of CNIs and mTOR inhibitors, sometimes necessitating higher CNI doses. Alternatively, rifabutin could be used instead of rifampicin given its milder interactions [123].

Other Infections

Pneumocystis Jiroveci Pneumonia

Pneumocystis jiroveci was previously known as *Pneumocystis carinii* and classified as a protozoal disease. The classification has evolved based on DNA sequence analysis such that *P. jirovecii* is now classified as a fungus. Human pneumocystis is now called jirovecii as *Pneumocystis carinii* only infects rats. *P. jirovecii* pneumonia (PJP) is an important opportunistic infection that has fortunately decreased in frequency due to the widespread use of sulfamethoxazole/trimethoprim prophylaxis in the immediate post-transplant period. Patients typically present with fever, dyspnea and nonproductive cough, interstitial infiltrate on chest x-ray and hypoxemia. Elevated lactate dehydrogenase and hypercalcemia are characteristic biochemical findings supporting the diagnosis. The diagnosis is established by demonstration of pneumocystis in lung secretions obtained from bronchoalveolar lavage or in tissue from lung [124]. Gomori stain or toluidine blue staining will demonstrate the cysts and Giemsa staining will identify the sporozoites. CMV infection is the major differential diagnosis. Many children may have dual infection, in which CMV infection predisposed to superinfection with *P. jirovecii*. Treatment recommendations include high dose intravenous trimethoprim-sulfamethoxazole, corticosteroids and a reduction in immunosuppression. Chemoprophylaxis with three times a week oral sulfamethoxazole/trimethoprim (5 mg/kg trimethoprim component/dose) has reduced the incidence of PJP from 3.7% to 0% [125]. Daily dosing may be easier for patient adherence and is recommended by KDIGO [12]. Prophylaxis is recommended in all transplant recipients for 3–6 months post-transplant. Some also advocate its use after anti-rejection therapy, particularly with anti-T cell antibodies.

Parasitic Infections

Although several parasitic infections have been reported in pediatric recipients of solid organ or bone marrow transplantation, there are few reports of such infections in pediatric kidney recipients. Several parasitic infections deserve mention, however, as they have been reported as transmitted by the transplanted graft in adult kidney transplant recipients. *Strongyloides stercoralis* is an intestinal nematode that infects tens of millions of people worldwide. It is endemic in tropical and sub-tropical regions. The highest rate of infection in the US is in the Southeast [126]. *S. stercoralis* may remain in the human intestinal tract without symptoms for decades, and then cause disseminated infection with the introduction of immunosuppressive medication post-transplant [126]. In addition, there are case reports of transmission of strongyloidiasis by kidney transplantation in an adult recipient [127]. Interestingly, CSA but not tacrolimus has effects against *S. stercoralis* and may reduce the risk for disseminated strongyloidiasis [128, 129]. Active infection typically presents with cutaneous, gastrointestinal and pulmonary symptoms as well as eosinophilia [130]. With disseminated disease, fever, hypotension, and central nervous system symptoms may be present [130]. In uncomplicated infections, diagnosis is made by detection of larvae in stool, although 25% of infected patients may have negative stool examinations [131]. In disseminated disease, larvae may be found in stool, sputum, bronchoalveolar lavage fluid, and peritoneal and pleural fluid [126, 132]. Serologic testing using ELISA may also be of value, but may be falsely negative in immunocompromised hosts [132, 133]. Thiabendazole, previously the treatment of choice for *S. stercoralis,* has been replaced by ivermectin, with albendazole as an alternative [134].

Other parasitic infections reported in kidney transplant recipients as transmitted by the transplanted graft include Chagas' disease and malaria [126, 135, 136]. Chagas' disease is caused by *Trypanosoma cruzi* and is found only in the southern US, Mexico and Central and South America. The manifestations of Chagas' disease classically include megaesophagus, megacolon, and cardiac disease, although CNS involvement has been reported in kidney transplant recipients [135]. The diagnosis is routinely made serologically and treatment typically consists of benznidazole or nifurtimox. Post-transplant malaria, transmitted from donors living in high-risk areas, is a frequent occurrence [136]. The discussion of these infections is meant to illustrate the potential problem of parasitic infections post-transplant. Policies to screen potential recipients and donors for these and other parasitic infections should be based on the presence of risk factors, including residence in or travel to an endemic area.

Fungal Infections

In general, serious invasive fungal infections such as aspergillosis are less common in pediatric kidney transplant recipients than thoracic organ recipients. Candida is the most common organism affecting kidney transplant recipients, either as oral and esophageal thrush, vaginitis, nail infection or UTI. The diagnosis of thrush is by clinical examination or demonstration of hyphae on a smear. Candidal UTI is diagnosed by urine culture. Treatment for topical candida is by topical nystatin or clotrimazole. Prophylactic measures include oral clotrimazole lozenges, nystatin, or fluconazole for 1–3 months post-transplant and for 1 month after treatment with an anti-lymphocyte antibody [12]. Treatment of invasive disease typically requires amphotericin. Fluconazole may be used for treatment of less severe disease, or for infections that have stabilized after initial therapy with amphotericin. Dose adjustment and close monitoring of the levels of CNIs are necessary when fluconazole is used due to the drug-drug interactions. In addition, there are potential drug-drug interactions between CNIs and clotrimazole [137].

Immunizations

One of the cornerstones of preventative care in pediatrics is the delivery of routine childhood immunizations. Unfortunately, the complicated medical care required by many children with chronic kidney disease may result in only sporadic delivery of routine well-child care, including immunizations. Complete immunization is especially important in children with ESKD as they approach transplantation given the increased risk for vaccine preventable disease post-transplant. In general, children with chronic kidney disease should receive immunizations according to the recommendations for healthy children in the region. Because they may also be more susceptible to or at risk for more serious infection from pathogens that are not typically problematic in healthy children, candidates for or recipients of kidney transplantation may also benefit from supplemental or additional vaccinations [76]. Table 69.3 provides a list of vaccinations recommended specifically for pediatric transplant candidates and recipients. Because children with chronic kidney disease and on dialysis may have sub-optimal response to many immunizations, or lose immunity prior to transplantation, it is important not only to ensure timely delivery of routine childhood immunizations, but also to monitor antibody titers or levels and revaccinate when indicated [138]. This is especially true of the live viral vaccines, including measles, mumps, rubella and varicella zoster vaccine, which are contraindicated in the immunosuppressed patient post-transplant.

In the post-transplant period, immunizations may be given after immunosuppressive medications have reached a baseline level, typically 6 to 12 months post-transplant. Again, live viral vaccines are generally contraindicated in the post-transplant period. Because the presence of immunosuppressive medications may impair response to vaccines, maximal protection requires universal immunization of health care workers, family members and household contacts [74]. In particular, annual immunization with injectable influenza vaccine is required [74].

References

1. Husain S, Singh N. The impact of novel immunosuppressive agents on infections in organ transplant recipients and the interactions of these agents with antimicrobials. Clin Infect Dis. 2002;35(1):53–61.
2. Dharnidharka VR, Caillard S, Agodoa LY, Abbott KC. Infection frequency and profile in different age groups of kidney transplant recipients. Transplantation. 2006;81(12):1662–7.
3. Dharnidharka VR, Stablein DM, Harmon WE. Post-transplant infections now exceed acute rejection as cause for hospitalization: a report of the NAPRTCS. Am J Transplant. 2004;4(3):384–9.
4. U.S.R.D.S. USRDS 2003 Annual Data Report: Atlas of End-Stage Renal Disease in the United States. Bethesda, MD: National Institutes of Health, National Institute of Diabetes and Digestive and Kidney Diseases. p. 2003.
5. Dharnidharka VR, Martz KL, Stablein DM, Benfield MR. Improved survival with recent post-transplant lymphoproliferative disorder (PTLD) in children with kidney transplants. Am J Transplant Off J Am Soc Transplant Am Soc Transplant Surg. 2011;11(4):751–8.
6. Smith JM, Corey L, Bittner R, Finn LS, Healey PJ, Davis CL, et al. Subclinical viremia increases risk for chronic allograft injury in pediatric renal transplantation. J Am Soc Nephrol. 2010;21(9):1579–86.
7. Dharnidharka VR, Lamb KE, Zheng J, Schechtman KB, Meier-Kriesche HU. Lack of significant improvements in long-term allograft survival in pediatric solid organ transplantation: a US national registry analysis. Pediatr Transplant. 2015;19(5):477–83.
8. McDonald RA, Smith JM, Ho M, Lindblad R, Ikle D, Grimm P, et al. Incidence of PTLD in pediatric renal transplant recipients receiving basiliximab, calcineurin inhibitor, sirolimus and steroids. Am J Transplant. 2008;8(5):984–9.
9. Matas AJ, Smith JM, Skeans MA, Lamb KE, Gustafson SK, Samana CJ, et al. OPTN/SRTR 2011 annual data report: kidney. Am J Transplant. 2013;13(Suppl 1):11–46.
10. Pereyra F, Rubin RH. Prevention and treatment of cytomegalovirus infection in solid organ transplant recipients. Curr Opin Infect Dis. 2004;17(4):357–61.
11. Kotton CN, Kumar D, Caliendo AM, Asberg A, Chou S, Danziger-Isakov L, et al. Updated international consensus guidelines on the management of cytomegalovirus in solid-organ transplantation. Transplantation. 2013;96(4):333–60.
12. Chapman JR. The KDIGO clinical practice guidelines for the care of kidney transplant recipients. Transplantation. 2010;89(6):644–5.
13. Keough WL, Michaels MG. Infectious complications in pediatric solid organ transplantation. Pediatr Clin N Am. 2003;50(6):1451–69. x
14. Dummer JS, Hardy A, Poorsattar A, Ho M. Early infections in kidney, heart, and liver transplant recipients on cyclosporine. Transplantation. 1983;36(3):259–67.
15. Smyth RL, Scott JP, Borysiewicz LK, Sharples LD, Stewart S, Wreghitt TG, et al. Cytomegalovirus infection in heart-lung transplant recipients: risk factors, clinical associations, and response to treatment. J Infect Dis. 1991;164(6):1045–50.
16. Fishman JA, Rubin RH. Infection in organ-transplant recipients. N Engl J Med. 1998;338(24):1741–51.
17. Tolkoff-Rubin NE, Fishman JA, Rubin RH. The bidirectional relationship between cytomegalovirus and allograft injury. Transplant Proc. 2001;33(1–2):1773–5.
18. Paya C, Humar A, Dominguez E, Washburn K, Blumberg E, Alexander B, et al. Efficacy and safety of valganciclovir vs. oral ganciclovir for prevention of cytomegalovirus disease in solid organ transplant recipients. Am J Transplant. 2004;4(4):611–20.
19. Marks WH, Ilsley JN, Dharnidharka VR. Posttransplantation lymphoproliferative disorder in kidney and heart transplant recipients receiving thymoglobulin: a systematic review. Transplant Proc. 2011;43(5):1395–404.
20. Helantera I, Kyllonen L, Lautenschlager I, Salmela K, Koskinen P. Primary CMV infections are common in kidney transplant recipients after 6 months valganciclovir prophylaxis. Am J Transplant. 2010;10(9):2026–32.
21. McDiarmid SV, Jordan S, Kim GS, Toyoda M, Goss JA, Vargas JH, et al. Prevention and preemp-

tive therapy of postransplant lymphoproliferative disease in pediatric liver recipients. Transplantation. 1998;66(12):1604–11.

22. Akalin E, Bromberg JS, Sehgal V, Ames S, Murphy B. Decreased incidence of cytomegalovirus infection in thymoglobulin-treated transplant patients with 6 months of valganciclovir prophylaxis. Am J Transplant. 2004;4(1):148–9.

23. Arthurs SK, Eid AJ, Pedersen RA, Kremers WK, Cosio FG, Patel R, et al. Delayed-onset primary cytomegalovirus disease and the risk of allograft failure and mortality after kidney transplantation. Clin Infect Dis. 2008;46(6):840–6.

24. Hirsch HH, Brennan DC, Drachenberg CB, Ginevri F, Gordon J, Limaye AP, et al. Polyomavirus-associated nephropathy in renal transplantation: interdisciplinary analyses and recommendations. Transplantation. 2005;79(10):1277–86.

25. Hirsch HH, Randhawa P. BK virus in solid organ transplant recipients. Am J Transplant. 2009;9(Suppl 4):S136–46.

26. Li L, Chaudhuri A, Weintraub LA, Hsieh F, Shah S, Alexander S, et al. Subclinical cytomegalovirus and Epstein-Barr virus viremia are associated with adverse outcomes in pediatric renal transplantation. Pediatr Transplant. 2007;11(2):187–95.

27. Bamoulid J, Courivaud C, Coaquette A, Chalopin JM, Gaiffe E, Saas P, et al. Subclinical Epstein-Barr virus viremia among adult renal transplant recipients: incidence and consequences. Am J Transplant Off J Am Soc Transplant Am Soc Transplant Surg. 2013;13(3):656–62.

28. Rowe DT, Qu L, Reyes J, Jabbour N, Yunis E, Putnam P, et al. Use of quantitative competitive PCR to measure Epstein-Barr virus genome load in the peripheral blood of pediatric transplant patients with lymphoproliferative disorders. J Clin Microbiol. 1997;35(6):1612–5.

29. Paya CV, Fung JJ, Nalesnik MA, Kieff E, Green M, Gores G, et al. Epstein-Barr virus-induced posttransplant lymphoproliferative disorders. ASTS/ASTP EBV-PTLD task force and the mayo clinic organized international consensus development meeting. Transplantation. 1999;68(10):1517–25.

30. Wadowsky RM, Laus S, Green M, Webber SA, Rowe D. Measurement of Epstein-Barr virus DNA loads in whole blood and plasma by TaqMan PCR and in peripheral blood lymphocytes by competitive PCR. J Clin Microbiol. 2003;41(11):5245–9.

31. Hill CE, Harris SB, Culler EE, Zimring JC, Nolte FS, Caliendo AM. Performance characteristics of two real-time PCR assays for the quantification of Epstein-Barr virus DNA. Am J Clin Pathol. 2006;125(5):665–71.

32. Humar A, Michaels M. American Society of Transplantation recommendations for screening, monitoring and reporting of infectious complications in immunosuppression trials in recipients of organ transplantation. Am J Transplant. 2006;6(2):262–74.

33. Roychowdhury S, Peng R, Baiocchi RA, Bhatt D, Vourganti S, Grecula J, et al. Experimental treatment of Epstein-Barr virus-associated primary central nervous system lymphoma. Cancer Res. 2003;63(5):965–71.

34. Lee TC, Savoldo B, Rooney CM, Heslop HE, Gee AP, Caldwell Y, et al. Quantitative EBV viral loads and immunosuppression alterations can decrease PTLD incidence in pediatric liver transplant recipients. Am J Transplant. 2005;5(9):2222–8.

35. Funch DP, Walker AM, Schneider G, Ziyadeh NJ, Pescovitz MD. Ganciclovir and acyclovir reduce the risk of post-transplant lymphoproliferative disorder in renal transplant recipients. Am J Transplant. 2005;5(12):2894–900.

36. Hadou T, Andre JL, Bourquard R, Krier-Coudert MJ, Venard V, Le Faou A. Long-term follow-up of Epstein-Barr virus viremia in pediatric recipients of renal transplants. Pediatr Nephrol. 2005;20(1):76–80.

37. van Esser JW, Niesters HG, van der Holt B, Meijer E, Osterhaus AD, Gratama JW, et al. Prevention of Epstein-Barr virus-lymphoproliferative disease by molecular monitoring and preemptive rituximab in high-risk patients after allogeneic stem cell transplantation. Blood. 2002;99(12):4364–9.

38. Martin SI, Dodson B, Wheeler C, Davis J, Pesavento T, Bumgardner GL. Monitoring infection with Epstein-Barr virus among seromismatch adult renal transplant recipients. Am J Transplant. 2011;11(5):1058–63.

39. D'Antiga L, Del Rizzo M, Mengoli C, Cillo U, Guariso G, Zancan L. Sustained Epstein-Barr virus detection in paediatric liver transplantation. Insights into the occurrence of late PTLD. Liver Transpl. 2007;13(3):343–8.

40. Bingler MA, Feingold B, Miller SA, Quivers E, Michaels MG, Green M, et al. Chronic high Epstein-Barr viral load state and risk for late-onset posttransplant lymphoproliferative disease/lymphoma in children. Am J Transplant. 2008;8(2):442–5.

41. Green M, Soltys K, Rowe DT, Webber SA, Mazareigos G. Chronic high Epstein-Barr viral load carriage in pediatric liver transplant recipients. Pediatr Transplant. 2009;13(3):319–23.

42. Nasimuzzaman M, Kuroda M, Dohno S, Yamamoto T, Iwatsuki K, Matsuzaki S, et al. Eradication of Epstein-Barr virus episome and associated inhibition of infected tumor cell growth by adenovirus vector-mediated transduction of dominant-negative EBNA1. Mol Ther. 2005;11(4):578–90.

43. Moudgil AMK, Moore T, Harmon WE, Dharnidharka VR. Significance of persistent asymptomatic EBV viral load in pediatric renal transplant (TX) recipients. Am J Transplant. 2012;12(S3):445A.

44. Tanaka E, Sato T, Ishihara M, Tsutsumi Y, Hisano M, Chikamoto H, et al. Asymptomatic high Epstein-Barr viral load carriage in pediatric renal transplant recipients. Pediatr Transplant. 2011;15(3):306–13.

45. Kenagy DN, Schlesinger Y, Weck K, Ritter JH, Gaudreault-Keener MM, Storch GA. Epstein-Barr virus DNA in peripheral blood leukocytes of patients with posttransplant lymphoproliferative disease. Transplantation. 1995;60(6):547–54.

46. Savoie A, Perpete C, Carpentier L, Joncas J, Alfieri C. Direct correlation between the load of Epstein-Barr virus-infected lymphocytes in the peripheral blood of pediatric transplant patients and risk of lymphoproliferative disease. Blood. 1994;83(9):2715–22.

47. Allen UD, Farkas G, Hebert D, Weitzman S, Stephens D, Petric M, et al. Risk factors for post-transplant lymphoproliferative disorder in pediatric patients: a case-control study. Pediatr Transplant. 2005;9(4):450–5.

48. Rees L, Tizard EJ, Morgan AJ, Cubitt WD, Finerty S, Oyewole-Eletu TA, et al. A phase I trial of epstein-barr virus gp350 vaccine for children with chronic kidney disease awaiting transplantation. Transplantation. 2009;88(8):1025–9.

49. Gardner SD, Field AM, Coleman DV, Hulme B. New human papovavirus (B.K.) isolated from urine after renal transplantation. Lancet. 1971;1(7712):1253–7.

50. Ramos E, Drachenberg CB, Papadimitriou JC, Hamze O, Fink JC, Klassen DK, et al. Clinical course of polyoma virus nephropathy in 67 renal transplant patients. J Am Soc Nephrol. 2002;13(8):2145–51.

51. Hirsch HH, Steiger J. Polyomavirus BK. Lancet Infect Dis. 2003;3(10):611–23.

52. Smith JM, Dharnidharka VR, Talley L, Martz K, McDonald RA. BK virus nephropathy in pediatric renal transplant recipients: an analysis of the north American pediatric renal trials and collaborative studies (NAPRTCS) registry. Clin J Am Soc Nephrol. 2007;2(5):1037–42.

53. Vats A. BK virus-associated transplant nephropathy: need for increased awareness in children. Pediatr Transplant. 2004;8(5):421–5.

54. Ginevri F, De Santis R, Comoli P, Pastorino N, Rossi C, Botti G, et al. Polyomavirus BK infection in pediatric kidney-allograft recipients: a single-center analysis of incidence, risk factors, and novel therapeutic approaches. Transplantation. 2003;75(8):1266–70.

55. Haysom L, Rosenberg AR, Kainer G, Waliuzzaman ZM, Roberts J, Rawlinson WD, et al. BK viral infection in an Australian pediatric renal transplant population. Pediatr Transplant. 2004;8(5):480–4.

56. Alexander RT, Langlois V, Tellier R, Robinson L, Hebert D. The prevalence of BK viremia and urinary viral shedding in a pediatric renal transplant population: a single-center retrospective analysis. Pediatr Transplant. 2006;10(5):586–92.

57. Mengel M, Marwedel M, Radermacher J, Eden G, Schwarz A, Haller H, et al. Incidence of polyomavirus-nephropathy in renal allografts: influence of modern immunosuppressive drugs. Nephrol Dial Transplant. 2003;18(6):1190–6.

58. Nickeleit V, Singh HK, Mihatsch MJ. Polyomavirus nephropathy: morphology, pathophysiology, and clinical management. Curr Opin Nephrol Hypertens. 2003;12(6):599–605.

59. Brennan DC, Agha I, Bohl DL, Schnitzler MA, Hardinger KL, Lockwood M, et al. Incidence of BK with tacrolimus versus cyclosporine and impact of preemptive immunosuppression reduction. Am J Transplant. 2005;5(3):582–94.

60. Liptak P, Kemeny E, Ivanyi B. Primer: histopathology of polyomavirus-associated nephropathy in renal allografts. Nat Clin Pract Nephrol. 2006;2(11):631–6.

61. Drachenberg CB, Papadimitriou JC, Hirsch HH, Wali R, Crowder C, Nogueira J, et al. Histological patterns of polyomavirus nephropathy: correlation with graft outcome and viral load. Am J Transplant. 2004;4(12):2082–92.

62. Bridges CB, Woods L, Coyne-Beasley T. Advisory Committee on Immunization Practices (ACIP) recommended immunization schedule for adults aged 19 years and older—United States, 2013. MMWR Surveill Summ. 2013;62(Suppl 1):9–19.

63. Sharma TLL, editor. Immunizations after pediatric solid organ transplant and hematopoietic stem cell transplant: Wiley-Blackwell; 2011.

64. Hirsch HH, Randhawa PS, Practice ASTIDCo. BK polyomavirus in solid organ transplantation-guidelines from the American Society of Transplantation infectious diseases Community of Practice. Clin Transpl. 2019;33(9):e13528.

65. Hardinger KL, Koch MJ, Bohl DJ, Storch GA, Brennan DC. BK-virus and the impact of preemptive immunosuppression reduction: 5-year results. Am J Transplant. 2010;10(2):407–15.

66. Weiss AS, Gralla J, Chan L, Klem P, Wiseman AC. Aggressive immunosuppression minimization reduces graft loss following diagnosis of BK virus-associated nephropathy: a comparison of two reduction strategies. Clin J Am Soc Nephrol. 2008;3(6):1812–9.

67. Akalin E, Azzi Y, Bartash R, et al. Covid-19 and kidney transplantation. N Engl J Med. 2020;382:2475–7.

68. Yi SG, Rogers AW, Saharia A, et al. Early experience with COVID-19 and solid organ transplantation at a US high-volume transplant center. Transplantation. 2020;104(11):2208–14.

69. Araya CE, Lew JF, Fennell RS 3rd, Neiberger RE, Dharnidharka VR. Intermediate-dose cidofovir without probenecid in the treatment of BK virus allograft nephropathy. Pediatr Transplant. 2006;10(1):32–7.

70. Gourishankar S, McDermid JC, Jhangri GS, Preiksaitis JK. Herpes zoster infection following solid organ transplantation: incidence, risk factors and outcomes in the current immunosuppressive era. Am J Transplant. 2004;4(1):108–15.

71. Lynfield R, Herrin JT, Rubin RH. Varicella in pediatric renal transplant recipients. Pediatrics. 1992;90(2 Pt 1):216–20.

72. Kashtan CE, Cook M, Chavers BM, Mauer SM, Nevins TE. Outcome of chickenpox in 66

pediatric renal transplant recipients. J Pediatr. 1997;131(6):874–7.

73. Broyer M, Tete MJ, Guest G, Gagnadoux MF, Rouzioux C. Varicella and zoster in children after kidney transplantation: long-term results of vaccination. Pediatrics. 1997;99(1):35–9.

74. Guidelines for vaccination of solid organ transplant candidates and recipients. Am J Transplant. 2004;4(Suppl 10):160–3.

75. Furth SL, Hogg RJ, Tarver J, Moulton LH, Chan C, Fivush BA. Varicella vaccination in children with chronic renal failure. A report of the southwest pediatric nephrology study group. Pediatr Nephrol. 2003;18(1):33–8.

76. Neu AM, Fivush BA. Immunization of children with renal disease. In: Kaplan BS, Meyers KEC, editors. Pediatric nephrology and urology: the requisites in pedicatrics. 54. Philadelphia, PA. Elsevier Mosby; 2004. p. 33–40.

77. Recommendations of the Advisory Committee on Immunization Practices: Programmatic strategies to increase vaccination rates—assessment and feedback of provider-based vaccination coverage information. MMWR Morb Mortal Wkly Rep. 1996;45(10):219–20.

78. Recommendations for the use of live attenuated varicella vaccine. American Academy of Pediatrics Committee on infectious diseases. Pediatrics. 1995;95(5):791–6.

79. A new product (VariZIG) for postexposure prophylaxis of varicella available under an investigational new drug application expanded access protocol. MMWR Morb Mortal Wkly Rep. 2006;55(8):209–10.

80. Nyerges G, Meszner Z, Gyarmati E, Kerpel-Fronius S. Acyclovir prevents dissemination of varicella in immunocompromised children. J Infect Dis. 1988;157(2):309–13.

81. Prober CG, Kirk LE, Keeney RE. Acyclovir therapy of chickenpox in immunosuppressed children—a collaborative study. J Pediatr. 1982;101(4):622–5.

82. Wiersinga WJ, Rhodes A, Cheng AC, Peacock SJ, Prescott HC. Pathophysiology, transmission, diagnosis, and treatment of coronavirus disease 2019 (COVID-19): a review. JAMA. 2020;324:782–93.

83. Varnell C Jr, Harshman LA, Smith L, et al. COVID-19 in pediatric kidney transplantation: the improving renal outcomes collaborative. Am J Transplant. 2021;21(8):2740–8.

84. Bansal N, Ovchinsky N, Foca M, Lamour JM, Kogan-Liberman D, Hsu DT, Beddows K, Abraham L, Coburn M, Cunningham R, Nguyen T, Hayde N. COVID-19 infection in pediatric solid organ transplant patients. Pediatr Transplant. 2021;11:e14156. https://doi.org/10.1111/petr.14156. Online ahead of print. PMID: 34633125

85. AST Statement about Vaccine Efficacy in Organ Transplant Recipients. Accessed 27 Oct 2021 at ast ishlt guidance vaccine 08132021FINAL DRAFT2. pdf (myast.org).

86. Boyarsky BJ, Werbel WA, Avery RA, Tobian AAR, Massie AB, Segev DL, Garonzik-Wang JM. Antibody response to 2-dose SARS-CoV-2 mRNA vaccine series in solid organ transplant recipients. JAMA. 2021;325(21):2204–6.

87. Benotmane I, Gautier-Vargas G, Cognard N, Olagne J, Heibel F, Braun-Parvez L, et al. Weak anti-SARS-CoV-2 antibody response after the first injection of an mRNA COVID-19 vaccine in kidney transplant recipients. Kidney Int. 2021;99(6):1487–9.

88. Sattler ASE, Weber U, Potekhin A, Bachmann F, Budde K, Storz E, Proß V, Bergmann Y, Thole L, Tizian C, Hölsken O, Diefenbach A, Schrezenmeier H, Jahrsdörfer B, Zemojtel T, Jechow K, Conrad C, Lukassen S, Stauch D, Lachmann N, Choi M, Halleck F, Kotsch K. Impaired humoral and cellular immunity after SARS-CoV2 BNT162b2 (Tozinameran) prime-boost vaccination in kidney transplant recipients. MedRxv. 2021; https://doi.org/10.1101/2021.04.06.21254963.

89. Yi SG, Knight RJ, Graviss EA, Nguyen DT, Ghobrial RM, Gaber AO, et al. Kidney transplant recipients rarely show an early antibody response following the first COVID-19 vaccine administration. Transplantation. 2021;105(7):e72–3.

90. Havlin JSM, Dvorackova E, et al. Immunogenicity of BNT162b2 mRNA COVID19 vaccine and SARS-CoV-2 infection in lung transplant recipients. J Heart Lung Transplant. 2021;40(8):754–8.

91. Miele M, Busa R, Russelli G, Sorrentino MC, Di Bella M, Timoneri F, et al. Impaired anti-SARS CoV-2 humoral and cellular immune response induced by Pfizer-BioNTech BNT162b2 mRNA vaccine in solid organ transplanted patients. Am J Transplant. 2021;21(8):2919–21.

92. Cucchiari D, Egri N, Bodro M, Herrera S, Del Risco-Zevallos J, Casals-Urquiza J, et al. Cellular and humoral response after mRNA-1273 SARS-CoV-2 vaccine in kidney transplant recipients. Am J Transplant. 2021;21(8):2919–21.

93. Rozen-Zvi B, Yahav D, Agur T, Zingerman B, Ben-Zvi H, Atamna A, et al. Antibody response to SARS-CoV-2 mRNA vaccine among kidney transplant recipients: a prospective cohort study. Clin Microbiol Infect. 2021;27(8):1173.e1–4.

94. Hall VG, Ferreira VH, Ierullo M, et al. Humoral and cellular immune response and safety of two-dose SARS-CoV-2 mRNA-1273 vaccine in solid organ transplant recipients. Am J Transplant. 2021;21(12):3980–9. https://doi.org/10.1111/ajt.16766.

95. Grupper A, Rabinowich L, Schwartz D, Schwartz IF, Ben-Yehoyada M, Shashar M, et al. Reduced humoral response to mRNA SARS-Cov-2 BNT162b2 vaccine in kidney transplant recipients without prior exposure to the virus. Am J Transplant. 2021;21(8):2719–26.

96. Khoury DS, Cromer D, Reynaldi A, Schlub TE, Wheatley AK, Juno JA, Subbarao K, Kent SJ, Triccas JA, Davenport MP. Neutralizing antibody

levels are highly predictive of immune protection from symptomatic SARS-CoV-2 infection. Nat Med. 2021;27(7):1205–11. https://doi.org/10.1038/s41591-021-01377-8.

97. Herrera S, Colmenero J, Pascal M, Escobedo M, Castel MA, Sole-González E, Palou E, Egri N, Ruiz P, Mosquera M, Moreno A, Juan M, Vilella A, Soriano A, Farrero M, Bodro M. Cellular and humoral immune response after mRNA-1273 SARS-CoV-2 vaccine in liver and heart transplant recipients. Am J Transplant. 2021;21(12):3971–9. https://doi.org/10.1111/ajt.16768. Epub ahead of print

98. Kamar N, Abravanel F, Marion O, Couat C, Izopet J, Del Bello A. Three doses of an mRNA Covid-19 vaccine in solid-organ transplant recipients. N Engl J Med. 2021;385(7):661–2. https://doi.org/10.1056/nejmc2108861.

99. Werbel WA, Boyarsky BJ, Ou MT, Massie AB, Tobian AAR, Garonzik-Wang JM, Segev DL. Safety and immunogenicity of a third dose of SARS-CoV-2 vaccine in solid organ transplant recipients: a case series. Ann Intern Med. 2021;174(9):1330–2. https://doi.org/10.7326/l21-0282.

100. Stumpf J, Tonnus W, Paliege A, Rettig R, Steglich A, Gembardt F, Kessel F, Krooger H, Arndt P, Sradnick J, Frank K, Tonn T, Hugo C. Cellular and humoral immune responses after three doses of BNT162b2 mRNA SARS-Cov-2 vaccine in kidney transplant. Transplantation. 2021;105(11):e267–9.

101. SARS-CoV-2 (Coronavirus, 2019-nCoV): Recommendations and Guidance for Organ Donor Testing. 2021. https://www.myast.org/sites/default/files/Donor%20Testing_07.07.21.pdf. Accessed 30 Nov 2021

102. Maraha B, Bonten H, van Hooff H, Fiolet H, Buiting AG, Stobberingh EE. Infectious complications and antibiotic use in renal transplant recipients during a 1-year follow-up. Clin Microbiol Infect. 2001;7(11):619–25.

103. Martinez-Marcos F, Cisneros J, Gentil M, Algarra G, Pereira P, Aznar J, et al. Prospective study of renal transplant infections in 50 consecutive patients. Eur J Clin Microbiol Infect Dis. 1994;13(12):1023–8.

104. Chavers BM, Gillingham KJ, Matas AJ. Complications by age in primary pediatric renal transplant recipients. Pediatr Nephrol. 1997;11(4):399–403.

105. Silva A, Rodig N, Passerotti CP, Recabal P, Borer JG, Retik AB, et al. Risk factors for urinary tract infection after renal transplantation and its impact on graft function in children and young adults. J Urol. 2010;184(4):1462–7.

106. Abbott KC, Swanson SJ, Richter ER, Bohen EM, Agodoa LY, Peters TG, et al. Late urinary tract infection after renal transplantation in the United States. Am J Kidney Dis. 2004;44(2):353–62.

107. Muller V, Becker G, Delfs M, Albrecht KH, Philipp T, Heemann U. Do urinary tract infections trigger chronic kidney transplant rejection in man? J Urol. 1998;159(6):1826–9.

108. Dharnidharka VR, Agodoa LY, Abbott KC. Effects of urinary tract infection on outcomes after renal transplantation in children. Clin J Am Soc Nephrol. 2007;2(1):100–6.

109. Wagener MM, Yu VL. Bacteremia in transplant recipients: a prospective study of demographics, etiologic agents, risk factors, and outcomes. Am J Infect Control. 1992;20(5):239–47.

110. Chuang P, Parikh CR, Langone A. Urinary tract infections after renal transplantation: a retrospective review at two US transplant centers. Clin Transpl. 2005;19(2):230–5.

111. Takai K, Tollemar J, Wilczek HE, Groth CG. Urinary tract infections following renal transplantation. Clin Transpl. 1998;12(1):19–23.

112. Kamath NS, John GT, Neelakantan N, Kirubakaran MG, Jacob CK. Acute graft pyelonephritis following renal transplantation. Transpl Infect Dis. 2006;8(3):140–7.

113. So S, Simmons R. Infections following kidney transplantation in children. In: Patrick CC, editor. Infections in immunocompromised infants and children. New York: Churchill Livingstone; 1992. p. 215–30.

114. Goldman JD, Julian K. Urinary tract infections in solid organ transplant recipients: Guidelines from the American Society of Transplantation Infectious Diseases Community of Practice. Clin Transpl. 2019;33(9):e13507.

115. Fox BC, Sollinger HW, Belzer FO, Maki DG. A prospective, randomized, double-blind study of trimethoprim-sulfamethoxazole for prophylaxis of infection in renal transplantation: clinical efficacy, absorption of trimethoprim-sulfamethoxazole, effects on the microflora, and the cost-benefit of prophylaxis. Am J Med. 1990;89(3):255–74.

116. Chang GC, Wu CL, Pan SH, Yang TY, Chin CS, Yang YC, et al. The diagnosis of pneumonia in renal transplant recipients using invasive and noninvasive procedures. Chest. 2004;125(2):541–7.

117. Dharnidharka VR, Richard GA, Neiberger RE, Fennell RS 3rd. Cat scratch disease and acute rejection after pediatric renal transplantation. Pediatr Transplant. 2002;6(4):327–31.

118. Jha V, Chugh KS. Posttransplant infections in the tropical countries. Artif Organs. 2002;26(9):770–7.

119. Singh N, Paterson DL. Mycobacterium tuberculosis infection in solid-organ transplant recipients: impact and implications for management. Clin Infect Dis. 1998;27(5):1266–77.

120. Sakhuja V, Jha V, Varma PP, Joshi K, Chugh KS. The high incidence of tuberculosis among renal transplant recipients in India. Transplantation. 1996;61(2):211–5.

121. API TB Consensus Guidelines 2006. Management of pulmonary tuberculosis, extra-pulmonary tuberculosis and tuberculosis in special situations. J Assoc Physicians India. 2006(54):219–34.

122. Taylor Z, Nolan CM, Blumberg HM. Controlling tuberculosis in the United States. Recommendations

from the American Thoracic Society, CDC, and the Infectious Diseases Society of America. MMWR Recomm Rep. 2005;54(RR-12):1–81.

123. Subramanian AK, Theodoropoulos NM. Infectious Diseases Community of Practice of the American Society of T. Mycobacterium tuberculosis infections in solid organ transplantation: Guidelines from the infectious diseases community of practice of the American Society of Transplantation. Clin Transpl. 2019;33(9):e13513.

124. Djamin RS, Drent M, Schreurs AJ, Groen EA, Wagenaar SS. Diagnosis of Pneumocystis carinii pneumonia in HIV-positive patients. Bronchoalveolar lavage vs. bronchial brushing. Acta Cytol. 1998;42(4):933–8.

125. Elinder CG, Andersson J, Bolinder G, Tyden G. Effectiveness of low-dose cotrimoxazole prophylaxis against Pneumocystis carinii pneumonia after renal and/or pancreas transplantation. Transpl Int. 1992;5(2):81–4.

126. Patel R. Infections in recipients of kidney transplants. Infect Dis Clin N Am. 2001;15(3):901–52, xi

127. Hoy WE, Roberts NJ Jr, Bryson MF, Bowles C, Lee JC, Rivero AJ, et al. Transmission of strongyloidiasis by kidney transplant? Disseminated strongyloidiasis in both recipients of kidney allografts from a single cadaver donor. JAMA. 1981;246(17):1937–9.

128. Nolan TJ, Schad GA. Tacrolimus allows autoinfective development of the parasitic nematode Strongyloides stercoralis. Transplantation. 1996;62(7):1038.

129. Schad GA. Cyclosporine may eliminate the threat of overwhelming strongyloidiasis in immunosuppressed patients. J Infect Dis. 1986;153(1):178.

130. DeVault GA Jr, King JW, Rohr MS, Landreneau MD, Brown ST 3rd, McDonald JC. Opportunistic infections with Strongyloides stercoralis in renal transplantation. Rev Infect Dis. 1990;12(4):653–71.

131. Sato Y, Kobayashi J, Toma H, Shiroma Y. Efficacy of stool examination for detection of Strongyloides infection. Am J Trop Med Hyg. 1995;53(3):248–50.

132. Harris RA Jr, Musher DM, Fainstein V, Young EJ, Clarridge J. Disseminated strongyloidiasis. Diagnosis made by sputum examination. JAMA. 1980;244(1):65–6.

133. Abdalla J, Saad M, Myers JW, Moorman JP. An elderly man with immunosuppression, shortness of breath, and eosinophilia. Clin Infect Dis. 2005;40(10):1464, 535–6

134. Drugs for Parasitic Infections. The Medical Letter [Internet]. 2004; 46:66.

135. Ferraz AS, Figueiredo JF. Transmission of Chagas' disease through transplanted kidney: occurrence of the acute form of the disease in two recipients from the same donor. Rev Inst Med Trop Sao Paulo. 1993;35(5):461–3.

136. Turkmen A, Sever MS, Ecder T, Yildiz A, Aydin AE, Erkoc R, et al. Posttransplant malaria. Transplantation. 1996;62(10):1521–3.

137. Vasquez E, Pollak R, Benedetti E. Clotrimazole increases tacrolimus blood levels: a drug interaction in kidney transplant patients. Clin Transpl. 2001;15(2):95–9.

138. Soni R, Horowitz B, Unruh M. Immunization in end-stage renal disease: opportunity to improve outcomes. Semin Dial. 2013;26(4):416–26.

139. Dharnidharka VR, Abdulnour HA, Araya CE. The BK virus in renal transplant recipients-review of pathogenesis, diagnosis, and treatment. Pediatr Nephrol. 2011;26(10):1763–74.

Long-Term Outcome of Kidney Failure in Children

Jaap W. Groothoff

Introduction

…The patient remained unconscious during dialysis, showing cramps from time to time …suddenly he vomited, showing massive gingival bleeding…13 h the patient started shaking after a piece of wood had been placed in the device against the spatter of dialysate…an example of a smooth dialysis session….

These thrilling notes are from Willem Kolffs' thesis in which he describes the first dialysis sessions ever performed in humans. The experiments took place during World War II in Kampen, a small town in the Netherlands [1]. Only one of the 12 patients, notably a sympathizing Nazi, survived the treatment. After the war Kolff emigrated to the United States where he developed the first production artificial kidney, the Kolff Brigham Artificial Kidney, which laid the foundation for modern hemodialysis treatment.

Yet, it would take until the end of the 1960s before chronic kidney replacement therapy (KRT) became available on a routine basis for children with end-stage kidney disease (ESKD). Initially, many physicians were reluctant to start such invasive therapy in children. Among those who refused to start dialysis in children were some very distinguished pediatric nephrologists. As both the dialysis technique and supportive therapy improved during the 70s and 80s chronic renal replacement therapy in children became gradually more accepted. In particular, better nutrition, the introduction of bicarbonate-buffer replacing acetate in hemodialysis, the introduction of continuous cycling peritoneal dialysis, the use of recombinant human erythropoietin and growth hormone therapy, and the introduction of cyclosporine after transplantation contributed to a marked decrease in morbidity and mortality and increase of children taken into therapy.

Despite all these improvements in therapy, RRT in children remained controversial at least until the early nineties of the last century. Even today, many physicians feel uncomfortable in offering chronic RRT to young children and question whether it should be offered to all children, especially in case of multiple comorbidities [2]. The fear for acute casualties has been replaced by concerns about the long-term prospects for children on RRT. One of the first questions parents ask when confronted with the necessity of chronic dialysis or transplantation for their child is what his or her future will be like. Will he or she ever be able to participate in society as an independent individual and have an acceptable life?

Unfortunately, even to date few extensive data exist on long-term outcome. This chapter reviews the very few late outcome studies performed to

J. W. Groothoff (✉)
Emma Children's Hospital, Amsterdam UMC/
Location University of Amsterdam,
Amsterdam, The Netherlands
e-mail: j.w.groothoff@amsterdamumc.nl;
j.w.groothoff@amc.uva.nl

date. By definition, these data are based on out-comes of patients who started RRT in the early experimental years of dialysis and transplantation in children. Extrapolation of outcomes to the current generation of children on RRT is therefore hazardous as both the treatment quality and policies have importantly changed over time. Most western registry data show, for instance, a significant and continuous rise in pre-emptive transplantation rates in children over time [3–5]. Yet, despite all improvements, the most important problems of dialysis and transplantation have not been solved to date. Therefore, the situation of the first generation of now middle-aged patients with pediatric chronic renal replacement therapy may indeed give at least an impression of the potential threats for the current generation of children with ESKD.

Chronic Pediatric Renal Replacement Therapy in Developing Countries

A shortcoming of this review is that the reported data apply to patients from highly developed countries. Few data exist on the situation in resource limiting settings, but from the few existing reports it is obvious that the situation there is incomparable with that in developed countries. In some countries, chronic renal replacement therapy in children does not even exist at all. In an IPNA survey in 2017 among all countries with more than 300,000 inhabitants and a response rate of 80%, chronic RRT for children was reported to be absent in 10 out of 94 countries [6]. However, this is most likely an underreport, as nearly all not-responding countries were low-income countries. Also, the existence of a program for pediatric renal replacement therapy does not automatically imply access to RRT for all children. In China and India, for instance, the world's largest countries with 32% of the global childhood population, the estimated prevalence of pediatric RRT was in 2017 less than 10% of that observed in Western countries [6]. A recent report from Nigeria described outcomes of peritoneal dialysis in children aged 3–11 years for

acute kidney injury after 18 months of follow up and reported 27.6% mortality [7]. A report from India mentioned 72% one-year survival, falling to 30% after 106 months of 66 children median aged 12.3 years on PD [8]. Another recent paper on country disparity within Europe showed that children on RRT from low-income countries have less access to transplantation but equal graft survival of those who received a kidney graft. Access to transplantation should also therefore be also the main aim for countries with limited financial means [9].

Course of Treatment Over Time

"A child with end-stage renal disease should receive a kidney transplant as soon as possible; a child that cannot be transplanted should not be started on chronic renal replacement therapy at all."

This paradigm has been a guideline for most pediatric nephrologists. Unfortunately, there are several circumstances in which dialysis is the only—temporary—option for children with ESRD. Moreover, as renal grafts may fail over time, the longer a patient is on RRT the higher is the chance that a patient will have a sequence of periods of living with a functioning graft alternating with periods on dialysis.

Most outcome studies have followed patients either on dialysis or after transplantation, ignoring the fact that most patients living with RRT for decades spend variable periods on both treatment modalities. The interpretation of such studies is troublesome, as it is the cumulative time spent on dialysis vs. the time with a functioning renal graft that predominantly affects the overall outcome.

In a long-term study of all 249 Dutch patients born before 1979 who started RRT before age 15 years between 1972 and 1992 with follow-up to 2010 (the LERIC study), patients spent on average 25.5 years on RRT. Of this cumulative time, 19.7 (0.03–39.6) years (77%) were spent with a functioning graft and 5.8 (0–36.5) years on dialysis. Among the 231 (93%) transplant recipients, 71 (31%) lived with a single transplant -not necessarily their first- for more than 20 consecutive years, up to 37.2 years. Transplantation was performed twice in 84 patients (36.4%), three times in 43 (18.6%), four times in 8 (3.5%), five times in 1 (0.4%) and six times in 3 patients (1.3%). Patients changed treatment modality between 1 and 11 times during the study period. Only 2 of the 249 patients (0.8%) lived with a functioning graft during the entire follow-up (median survival 25.3 years) while 18 patients (7.2%) only received dialysis (median survival 3.7 years) [10].

In an equally long follow-up study using data of the Australian and New Zealand database (ANZDATA) concerning 1634 patients with RRT onset <19 years between 1963 and 2002, patients received RRT for on average for 11.3 years, of which 3.5 years were spent on dialysis and 7.8 years (69%) with a functioning graft [11]. The difference towards a longer time on dialysis in the latter study is probably explained by the 10 years earlier observation period [11].

Possibly, the average lifetime on dialysis may further decrease in the future as the last decade has shown a trend towards more pre-emptive transplantations in children, at least in the Western countries. All registry data show rises in rates of pre-emptive transplantation, varying from 26% in 1997–2001 to 32.9% in 2007–2011 in the United Kingdom (p < 0.05), from 10% to 25% between 1992 and 2007 in Canada and from 9.6% in 1985–1989 to 18.4% in 2000–2004 in the countries connected to the ERA-EDTA database [3–5]. According to the ANZDATA base, the proportion of children who underwent transplantation as the initial RRT modality had remained stable over time, being about 19–20% of all children starting RRT. On the other hand, the incidence of pre-emptive transplantation in children increased from 0.58 transplantations per million age related population (pmarp) in 1967–1971 to 1.65 transplants pmarp in 2002–2006 [12].

A recent report from the ESPN/ERA-EDTA database showed a 2% increase from 26.4 per million age-related population (pmarp) in 2007 to 32.1 pmarp between 2007 and 2016 of the prevalence of pediatric transplant recipients aged <15 years, with an unchanged incidence (5.5–6.6 pmarp), reflecting a better graft survival and promising a prolonged time on transplantation over time [13]. These shifts will certainly impact on the course of RRT as well as the impact on adult life in the current population of children with ESRD.

Impact of RRT Modality Over Time: Transplantation vs. Dialysis

All late outcome studies favor early transplantation in children with ESKD, which appears to have a beneficial effect on overall mortality, morbidity and psychosocial development. In the LERIC study, the cumulative duration of dialysis in relation to years with a renal graft was the strongest factor associated with nearly all adverse outcomes, especially with cardiovascular death, but also with impaired cognitive performance, loco motor disorders and social independency [10, 14–18]. The impact of dialysis on physical condition is also reflected by the sharp difference in physical health perception of dialysis and transplanted patients. On the other hand, the ANZDATA data showed that a short period of dialysis (up to 2 years) did not affect overall mortality, a finding that was confirmed by ERA-EDTA data on mortality in young adults with pediatric-onset ESKD [11]. None of the studies showed significant differences in outcome of peritoneal dialysis and hemodialysis.

Although dialysis is the most unfavorable mode of RRT, transplantation is associated with considerable late morbidity. Disabling co-morbidity was reported by 40% of all transplant recipients in the LERIC study of whom most patients were transplanted at time of investigation [19]. Apart from clinical bone disease, the most frequently reported disabling problems were severe daily headaches, tremors and severe itching, most of them appearing in transplanted patients. Malignancies, infection, hypertension related LVH and arterial wall stiffening are the most life-threatening problems after transplantation. Although current insight shows a much lower mortality in transplant recipients with childhood ESKD than in patients who remain on dialysis, with the passage of time the 'dark side of Camelot' may become more lucid. The longer the period of transplantation, the more patients become at risk for life-threatening infections and malignancies at relatively young age [20]. The current trend towards the use of more potent, and hence potentially more carcinogenic, immunosuppressive therapy may bear significant future consequences.

Mortality

According to long-term outcome studies, the overall mortality of patients with pediatric onset of chronic renal replacement therapy is about 30 times as high as among people of the same age without the need for RRT [10, 20–23]. Mortality rates per 100 patients decreased in most long-term outcome studies from 4.4 (ANZDATA) and 3.6 (LERIC) in 1972–1983 to 1.2–1.8 years after 1983 (ANZDATA, LERIC, Canadian Registry) [4, 10, 11, 20]. After on average 30 years of cRRT, the Dutch cohort study showed a U-shaped course of mortality risk over time: the added mortality risk, expressed as Mortality Rate Ratio, was extremely high during the first years of RRT in 72–'89, then decreased from 53 to 19.7 in the following period '90–'99, but increased again to 26.8 in the period '00–'10 [20]. After on average 30 years of RRT, mortality risk in the Dutch cohort study showed a U-shaped course over time: the added mortality risk, expressed as Mortality Rate Ratio, was extremely high in the 1970s and 1980s, decreased from 53 to 19.7 in the 1990s, but increased again to 26.8 in the first decade of this century [20]. This suggests that the added mortality risk may increase with ageing.

To some extent, these figures may overestimate the mortality risk for children currently on RRT as the dialysis technique certainly has improved over time and more children are transplanted pre-emptively. All studies on patients with ESKD indeed show a substantial decrease in mortality over the last 40 years, especially in the very young age groups. Yet, at the same time, this trend toward improvement of survival of ESKD has also slowed dramatically during the last 25 years [10, 11]. In fact, the survival trends are quite disappointing,

considered the experimental nature of renal replacement therapy among children during the early years. Both McDonald's study on the ANZDATA and the Dutch cohort showed no increase in survival after 1983 [10, 11]. These outcomes are in line with other registry data. A Canadian registry study on survival rates of pediatric dialysis and transplantation since 1992 showed no improvement over time [4]. The USRDS data show a slightly different picture; here the mortality hazard ratio among transplanted patients decreased from to 0.83 in 1988–1994, dropped further to 0.77 in 1995–1997, stabilized between 1998–2001 and further dropped to 0.69 in 2002–2006. Yet, the latest figure might be biased by the maximum time to follow up as the authors also showed an increase of mortality with increasing time, becoming significant after 10 years of transplantation. Ageing and, more importantly, return to dialysis seem to explain this effect. Taken this into account, one can conclude that the actual mortality risk has not changed since the mid 90ies.

The lack of improvement might have been due at least partly to a shift towards acceptance of more severely disabled and younger children for chronic renal replacement therapy over the last two decades. Unfortunately, data on the referral and selection of children for chronic RRT do not exist, yet from oral communication this tendency over time towards accepting sicker children for chronic RRT accounts for most Western countries. Nevertheless, it is beyond discussion that the stable mortality rate over the last 20 years is unacceptably high.

Low-income countries that do offer chronic RRT to children show fewer favorite outcomes with respect to survival compared to high income countries. A recent report from the ESPN/ERA-EDTA database showed important disparities between European low- and high-income countries. A high-income country like France had a mortality rate (9.2) of more than 3 SDs better, in contrast to relatively low-income countries like Russia (35.2), Poland (39.9), Romania (47.4), and Bulgaria (68.6) had mortality rates more than 3 SDs worse than the European average. At the same time, the number of children on RRT was significantly lower in low income compared to high income countries. Public health expenditure was inversely associated with mortality risk (per SD increase, aHR 0.69, 95% CI 0.52–0.91) and explained 67% of the variation in renal replacement therapy mortality rates between countries. Child mortality rates showed a significant association with renal replacement therapy mortality, albeit mediated by macroeconomics (e.g., neonatal mortality reduced from 1.31 [95% CI 1.13–1.53], p = 0.0005, to 1.21 [0.97–1.51], p = 0.10). After accounting for country distributions of patient age, the variation in renal replacement therapy mortality rates between countries increased by 21% [24].

Factors Associated with Mortality

Age of onset of RRT before 6 years, a long-time burden of hypertension, onset of RRT before 1982 and most significantly, the cumulative duration of dialysis during RRT were associated with

premature death in the LERIC study. The risk ratios with respect to overall mortality of a relatively long period of dialysis and relatively long-standing hypertension were 7.2 and 3.1, respectively. Patients who started RRT between 1972 and 1982 had a 1.7-fold chance of premature death compared to those who started between 1982 and 1992, and patients aged below 6 years a 2.2-fold risk compared to older patients [10].

These outcomes are in line with those of the larger ANZDATA study and the Canadian Registry. In the ANZDATA study, the hazard ratio for death among those who started RRT before 12 months of age was 3.7 as compared to those who started at 15–19 years, and of those who started RRT between 1963 and 1972 the risk ratio was 4.2 compared to 1993–2002. In the Canadian study, the hazard ratio of patients aged younger than 1 year at onset of RRT and of those aged 2–10 were 7.8 and 1.5, respectively, compared to patients aged 10–18 years [4] (Fig. 70.1).

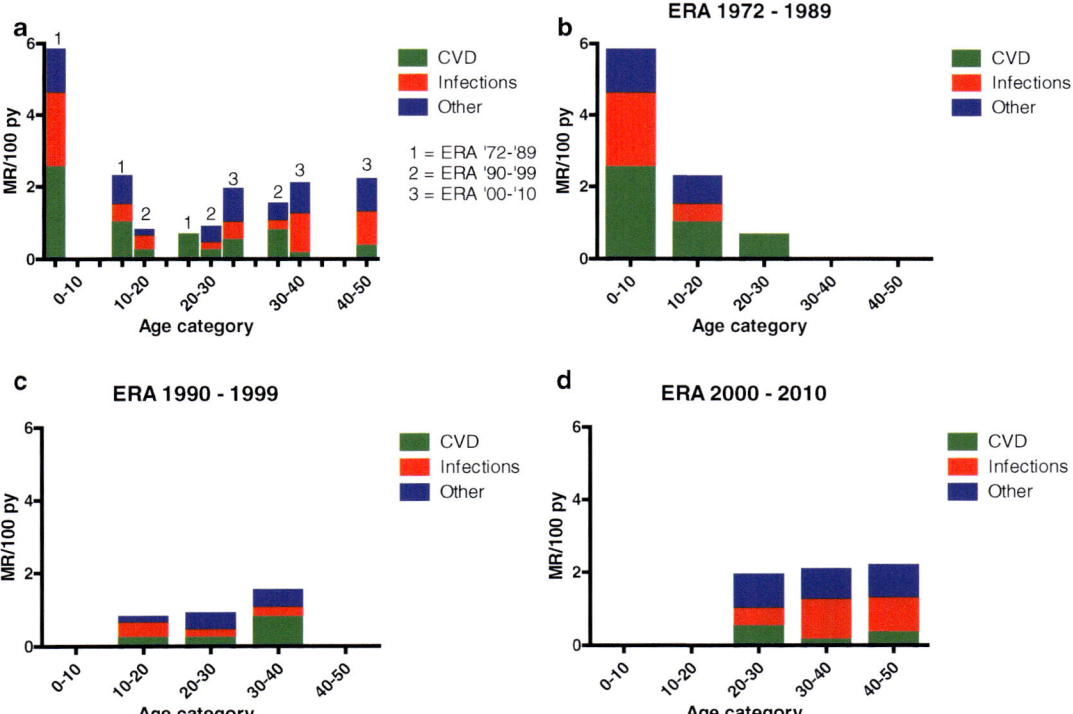

Fig. 70.1 CVD, infections and other causes related mortality rates per 100 persons in the LERIC Cohort (all Dutch patients with ESKD at age <15 years in 1972–1992 with follow-up to 2010) per age category per ERA (**a**), in the ERA 1972–1989 per age category (**b**) in the ERA 1990–1999 per age category (**c**) and in the ERA 2000–2010 per age category (**d**). (From Ref. [20]: Vogelzang JL et al, Nephrol Dial Transplant. 2013;28:2082–2089)

Rates of survival also varied with the type of renal replacement therapy. Overall mortality rates were 4.8 per 100 patient-years among patients receiving hemodialysis, 5.9 among those receiving peritoneal dialysis, and 1.1 among those with a functioning renal transplant. The Canadian Registry study showed that graft failure with return to dialysis was strongly associated with greater mortality risk in an adjusted model compared with a functioning graft (HR 7.2) [4]. According to both the ANZDATA and the ERA-EDTA registry study a short period of dialysis did not influence mortality; patients with pre-emptive transplantation had equal mortality to those with a maximum period of 2 years dialysis vintage [11, 13] (Fig. 70.2).

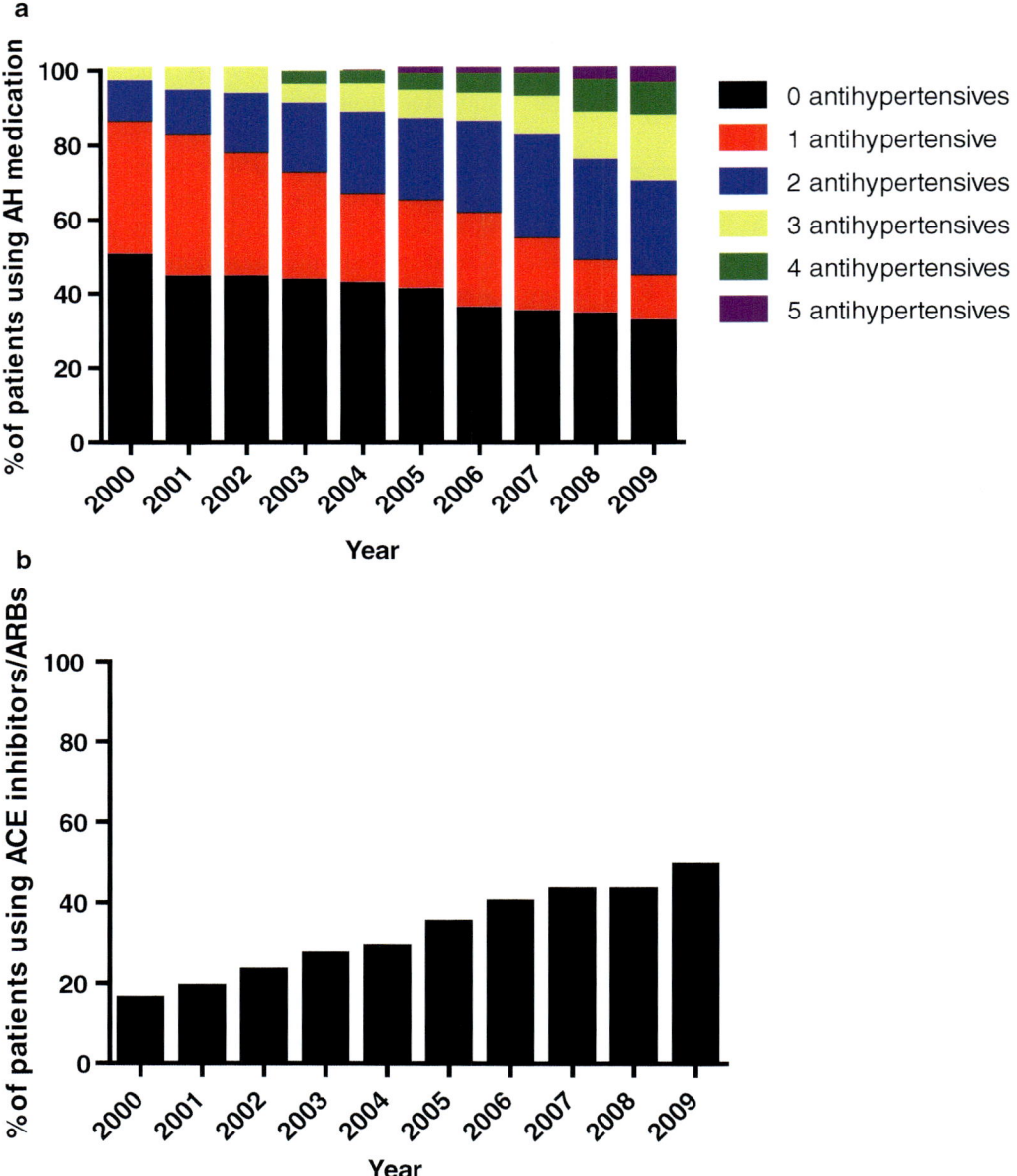

Fig. 70.2 Number of antihypertensive used per patient in each calendar years (**a**) and ACE-inhibitor (**b**) prescriptions in the LERIC Cohort (all Dutch patients with ESKD at age <15 years in 1972–1992 with follow-up to 2010) over time. (From Ref. [42]: Vogelzang JL et al, Nephrol Dial Transplant. 2013;28:2545–2552)

Causes of Death

Cardiovascular disease accounts for most casualties in pediatric RRT, followed by infection and malignancies, at least according to most outcome studies. Between 35 and 50% of all deaths are attributed to cardiovascular disease [10, 11, 20, 22, 25–27] Although one has to be cautious in interpreting "cardiac death" as a genuine cause of death, these figures reflect the excess risk of cardiovascular disease in children with ESRD. Prolonged hypertension has been shown to be independently associated with increased morality [10]. Other recent studies show that left ventricular hypertrophy (LVH) occurs early in children with ESRD and that it is strongly associated with hypertension [28–30]. Mitsnefes et al. found that 69% of all children already had LVH at the onset of dialysis therapy which persisted for 2 years after transplantation in 56% and that regression of the LVH could be induced by controlling systolic blood pressure [28–30]. These data emphasize the pivotal role of blood pressure in both dialyzed and transplanted children. Both the ESPN registry and NAPTRCS have shown that uncontrolled hypertension occurs in 40–65% of patients [28, 31].

Despite the high prevalence of hypertension in transplanted patients, the overall cardiovascular profile of conventional dialysis is by far more adverse than that of kidney transplantation. In line with this notion, late outcome studies have identified extended time spent on dialysis as the strongest predictor for premature death from cardiovascular disease. Patients on dialysis who do not receive a transplant have a four times higher risk of death than transplant recipients; in patients who have spent more time on dialysis than with a renal graft, mortality rates are seven times higher [10, 11]. A long-term outcome report on pediatric transplant data of the USRDS showed that after the first post-transplant year, each additional year with a functioning graft was associated with a 16% decrease of cardiovascular mortality [32]. The same study showed a significant 6% increase in mortality risk for each year on dialysis prior to transplantation, whereas the ANZDATA and the ERA-EDTA data only found an increase in mor-

tality risk of patients with a pre-transplant dialysis period of more than 2 years [11, 31, 32]. Nevertheless, the beneficial effect of transplantation on survival is beyond discussion.

In adults, increasing the intensity of hemodialysis, especially nocturnal hemodialysis, has shown to be effective in reducing cardiovascular disease, improve overall condition and quality of life and prolong survival [33]. Frequent hemodialysis ideally preformed as nocturnal home hemodialysis should be considered in children who cannot be transplanted and are long-time bound to dialysis treatment.

A younger age at onset of RRT was consistently identified as a considerable mortality risk factor across all studies [10, 11, 26, 32]. However, it is encouraging to notice that the survival of very young patients has improved over time. Considering the fact that more infants have been accepted for chronic RRT during the last 20 years, it seems that we indeed have overcome a great deal of the specific technical problems concerning delivering RRT to very young children, at least in terms of survival.

Trends Over Time in Causes of Death: From Cardiovascular Disease to Infections?

Up to the late 1990s, few physicians, internists as well as pediatric nephrologists were fully aware of the extreme cardiovascular burden that threatened their patients. Growing awareness and adjustment of therapy accordingly might be the basis of a remarkable trend in change of outcome according to some very recent data. In an extension of the Dutch LERIC study, a significant shift from cardiovascular disease to infections as main cause of death was found [20]. In this study following up to 2010 all Dutch patients with RRT onset before 15 years of age between 1972 and 1992, the overall mortality rate as well as the added risk to the overall population, the Mortality Rate Ratio (MRR), stabilized over time. At the same time, the MRR for cardiovascular death decreased from 660 in 1972–1989 to 70 in 1990–1999 and further to 20 in 2000–2010. Conversely,

Fig. 70.3 Infection-non infection for Hospital Admission Rate Ratio according to decade and Renal Replacement Therapy modality in the LERIC Cohort. *p < 0.001 vs. decade 2000–2010. Whiskers represent 95% CI> *HD* hemodialysis, *PD* peritoneal dialysis, *Tx* transplantation (From Ref. [46]: Lofaro D et al, Pediatr Neph. 2016)

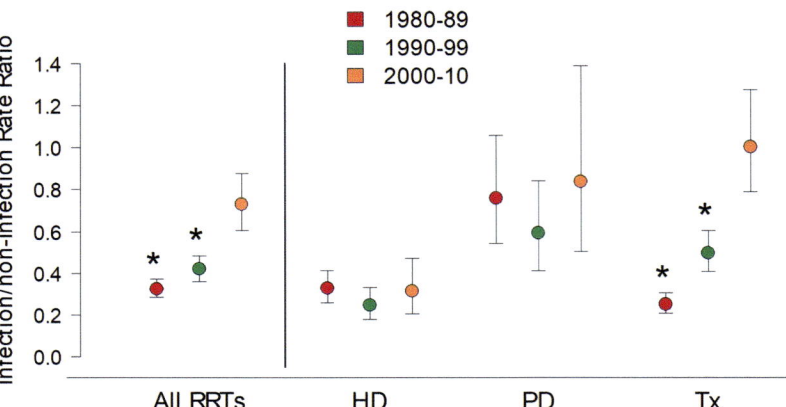

the MRR for infectious death showed a U-shaped curve; it decreased from 503 in 1972–1989 to 102 in 1990–1999 and increased again to 350 in 2000–2010. In the period 2000–2010, infections became the most prevalent cause of death (44%). In 2000–2010 cardiovascular mortality had decreased by 91% since 1972–1989 (p = 0.003) whereas infectious mortality had doubled over time, although not significantly (adjusted HR 2.12, p = 0.09) [20] (Fig. 70.3).

More recent data confirm this trend of infections gradually replacing cardiovascular disease as the most important cause of death. Recent USRDS data show a declining burden of cardiovascular mortality among the dialysis patients of all ages over the last years (MR 120 in 2001 to MR 83 in 2008 per 1000 patient years without changes in other causes of death over time (MR 100 per 1000 patient years in 1998, 2001 and 2008) [34]. This trend was similar in patients aged 20–44 years, with the cardiovascular MR declining from 40.5 per 1000 patient years in 2001 to 31.3 in 2008 [34]. Also ANZDATA showed decreasing cardiovascular mortality rates for all dialysis patients (MR 9.0 in 1992 to 6.4 in 2005 per 1000 patient years), but not among the younger patients aged 35–54 years [35].

Co-morbidity

Many studies have shown that end-stage renal disease affects many organs, especially the cardiovascular system and the loco motor system,

and that it has an important impact on the overall physical condition of patients. Yet, very little data exist on the exact physical burden of pediatric ESKD later in life. In the LERIC study, 40% of survivors aged between 20 and 40 years. 75% being carriers of a functioning renal graft at time of investigation, indicated an important co-morbidity that significantly affected their activities of daily life, ranging from chronic fatigue to symptoms of cardiovascular disease or disabilities due to loco motor disorders [19].

Cardiovascular Disease

Asymptomatic cardiovascular disease, to an extent that it might induce sudden death, has been reported to be highly prevalent in transplanted as well as in dialysis patients with pediatric ESKD [10, 14, 18, 22, 30, 36, 37]. Yet, for transplanted patients, previous dialysis vintage is the strongest factor for developing cardiac and vascular abnormalities [10]. In a German single center late outcome study of 283 patients that had been transplanted between 1970 and 1997 and of whom 42 patients had died, in 50% of cardiovascular disease, CT scans were performed in 39 survivors, aged between 19 and 39 years [22]. Coronary artery calcifications were present in 92% of patients; calcium scores exceeded the 95th age- and sex-specific percentiles tenfold on average. Carotid IMT was significantly increased compared with matched control subjects. Both coronary calcium scores and IMT were associated with cumulative dialysis and ESKD time and the cumulative serum calcium-phosphate product [22]. In the Dutch LERIC study, nearly 50% of all living male and 40% of all female patients aged between 20 and 42 years were found to have moderate to severe left ventricular hypertrophy (LVH), 75% being transplanted at the time of investigation in 2000 [18]. Like LVH, cardiac valve calcification and arterial wall stiffening caused by media proliferation and secondary calcification are highly prevalent in young adults with childhood ESRD, both in dialysis and transplant recipients [14, 22]. All these abnormalities are associated with an increased risk of death. Coronary ischemia and cardiac conduction defects due to myocardial calcification are the most probable links between aortic valve calcification and mortality. Aortic valve calcification may occur early in ESKRD patients and reflects a more generalized artery disease with calcification of the coronary arteries and the myocardium [38]. Vascular calcification appears to already start at a young age. Eifinger et al. described coronary calcifications in 16-year-old dialysis patients [38]. Chronic hypertension, a high calcium phosphate product and a chronic state of inflammation are among the most important potential determinants of cardiovascular disease in ESKD [36, 39–41].

Yet, as previously discussed, increased awareness among physicians of the impact of pediatric ESKD on the cardiovascular system might profoundly change outcomes in the near future. To our surprise, we found in the extension of the LERIC study in 2010 that between 2000 and 2010, most people had died of infections and only 1 due to CVD [20]. Among the survivors, the prevalence of cardiovascular risk factors decreased from 41.3% in 2000 to 18.8% in 2010. The odds ratios in 2010 relative to 2000 for left ventricular hypertrophy, hypertension and hypercholesterolemia were 0.26, 0.22 and 0.04, respectively. The rate of non-fatal cardiovascular events dropped, although not significantly, from 1.75 in 1972–2000 to 0.95 in 2000–2010 per 100 patient years. RAS antagonists and cholesterol lowering medication were significantly more often prescribed in the period 2000–2010 (OR 7.4 and 11.5) [42]. Trends were similar among those who survived and those who did not survive the last decade. Although a causal relationship between the two cannot be inferred from this study, our data strongly suggest that strict blood pressure control, with preferential use of RAS antagonists, and reduction of dyslipidemia may be effective in reducing cardiac threat in patients with end-stage renal disease even after a long-lasting burden of cardiovascular disease (Fig. 70.4).

Fig. 70.4 Histogram of occurrence of PTLD against time since transplantation (Data from the Australian and New Zealand Transplant Registry. (Used with permission from Ref. [60]: Faul RJ et al, Transplantation. 2005:80:193–197)

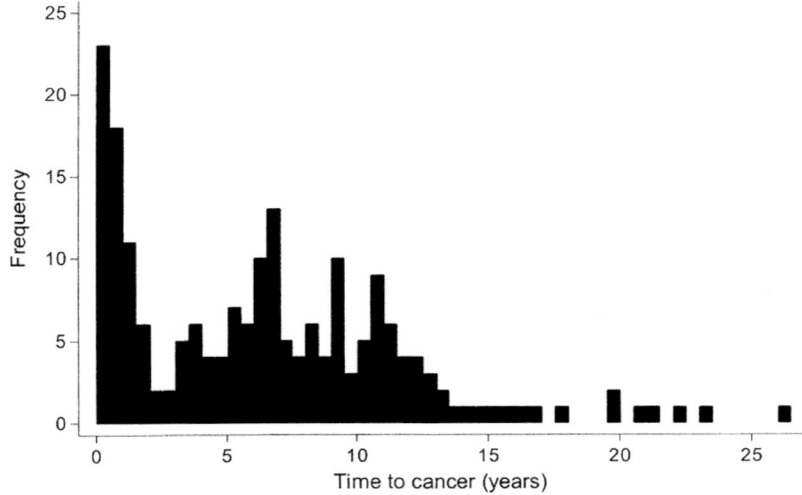

Infections

In adults, infections are the leading cause of death in the first year after kidney transplantation [43]. In a single center study, only 7 out of 129 consecutively transplanted patients did not have an infection for which medical intervention was necessary [44]. Urinary tract infections (69.8%) and CMV infection/reactivation were most prevalent. Yet, USRDS data show that infections, especially urinary tract infections are also highly prevalent much later after transplantation. In a retrospective cohort study on 28,942 Medicare renal transplant recipients the cumulative incidence of urinary tract infections was 60% for women and 47% for men at 3 years after transplantation. Late urinary tract infection was significantly associated with an increased risk of subsequent death (adjusted hazard ratio-AHR 2.93) and graft loss (AHR 1.85). The association of urinary tract infection with death persisted after adjusting for cardiac and other infectious complications, and regardless of whether urinary tract infection was assessed as a composite of outpatient/inpatient claims, primary hospitalized infections, or solely outpatient infections [44]. This contrasts somewhat with findings in children; according to USRDS data the risk for graft loss was increased for early but not late urinary tract infection. This finding might, however, be biased by a relatively short follow-up time [45].

Data on the prevalence of severe infections over a very long time in pediatric ESKD come from the LERIC study. This study shows an increasing importance of infections over time. Between 2000 and 2010, 34 out of 186 patients died; 44% of these died of infections in contrast to only 12% of cardiovascular disease. There was a 60% reduction of the number of hospitalizations over time, from 1202 in the period 1980–1989 to 484 in 2000–2010. This was entirely due to a reduction in non-infection-related hospitalizations by 74%, whereas infection-related hospitalizations in allograft recipients did not change at all. Consequently, the hospital admission incidence rate ratio of infections and other causes increased from 0.25 to 1.0 over time in transplanted patients [46]. Urinary tract infections (UTI) became more prevalent over time in transplanted patients; the UTI/non-UTI infections hazard rate ratio in transplanted patients for which hospitalization was required increased from 0.42 in 1980–1999 to 0.72 in 2000–2010 [46].

Most of the transplanted patients in LERIC have a relatively mild immunosuppression as compared to currently used strategies. In adult studies, there is some evidence suggesting that the incidence of infection is associated with the intensity of the immunosuppressive regime. Most studies show that the dose rather than the type of immunosuppression is responsible for the increased risk of infections. The ELITE (Efficacy Limiting Toxicity Elimination)-Symphony study compared outcome of either low-dose of ciclosporin, tacrolimus or sirolimus with standard dose ciclosporin and with equal MMF dose in both groups. Opportunistic infections were more common in the standard-dose ciclosporin group [47]. Infections were also more common if patients use a standard dose of ciclosporin as compared to low-dose ciclosporin combined with everolimus [48]. The TERRA (Tacrolimus Evaluation in Renal Transplantation with Rapamycin) study compared 0.5 mg with 2.0 mg sirolimus and equal dose tacrolimus in both groups; more infections were found in the 2 mg sirolimus group [49].

In conclusion, ageing in pediatric RRT goes with a high risk for premature death by infections. Urinary tract infections are probably the most prevalent late life-threatening infections. Lowering of the immunosuppressive load, especially in patients with a prolonged rejection-free period after transplantation, might help reducing the number of fatal infections in these patients.

Malignancies

Incidence

In young adults with pediatric ESKD, the cumulative incidence of cancer varies between 0.8 and 17%. Malignancy is believed to occur about ten times more frequently than expected for age [50–54]. The most prevalent forms of malignancies seen are non-Hodgkin lymphomas and above all, skin cancer at older age. Cancer was found in 24 cases of all 536 transplanted children in Sweden since 1970 with a mean follow-up of 12.5 (0.04–34) years [52]. In a French single center study with 20 years follow-up, 16 malignancies were found in 219 kidney transplant recipients at a median age of 20.8 (4.1–36.5) years [53]. A large German long-term follow-up study of transplanted children with a mean follow-up of 13 years showed a relatively low percentage of malignancies of 2.6% [25]. In a long-term follow-up study on 187 renal transplant recipients who had reached adulthood at time of assessment, Bartosh et al. found 12% malignancies [50].

The NAPRTCS reported recently on the prevalence among "more than 10,000" pediatric transplant recipients since 1987 and found 35 cases of malignancy, including 5 cases of renal cell carcinoma [54]. The estimated prevalence of 72.1 cases per 100,000 person-years reflects a 6.7-fold increased risk compared with the general population [54].

Yet most studies suffer from a relatively short follow-up period and the distribution over time after onset of RRT suggests that most casualties might come at a later age. In the 10 years extension of the Dutch LERIC study, 54 (21%) of the originally 249 patients had developed 105 *de novo* malignancies after an average RRT time of 23 years (age survivors 30–50 years) [55]. In this study, the Cancer-free survival after 10, 20, 30 and 35 years of follow-up was 97%, 87%, 68% and 58% respectively. The mean age at malignancy diagnosis was 36.9 (range 11.1–50.4) years. The mean interval from first transplantation to diagnosis of cancer was 23.7 (range 0.1–36.2) years. Death was attributed to the malignancy in 13 out of the 54 (24%) patients who developed cancer at time of assessment [55].

Type of Cancer

Post-Transplant Lymphoproliferative Disease (PTLD)

The term Post-transplantation lymphoproliferative disorder (PTLD) stands for different types of lymphoid neoplasms that may develop after kidney organ transplantation. The World Health Organization (WHO) distinguishes four subtypes of PTLD: an early, a polymorphic, a monomorphic and a classical Hodgkin-lymphoma-like type, each with its different therapeutic approach. The risk of PTLD is biphasic in time. The highest incidence is within the first year after transplantation. These so-called early onset PTLD types are for 95% associated with Epstein-Barr virus (EBV) and have a relatively good prognosis. A second peak occurs after 5–10 years [56]. Late onset PTLD is related to the impact of relative high burden of immunosuppressive therapy most often independent from EBV and has a worse prognosis than the early onset form [56, 57]. PTLD occurs in about 0.8–2.8% in kidney transplant recipients [58–60].

Pathophysiology of EBV Associated PTLD

EBV-related PTLD occurs because of a de novo EBV infection or reactivation from latent B-cells driven by immunosuppressive therapy. An EBV-seronegative recipient who gets an allograft from an EBV-seropositive donor (D+/R-) may undergo a primary EBV infection, a situation which is the most important risk factor for PTLD. This explains why PTLD occurs 2–8 times more often in pediatric than adult transplant recipients [56, 61]. EBV is a lymphotropic virus which enters the B-lymphocytes during the initial infection and remains in the host nucleus in a state of latency for that individual's lifetime. This latent state is associated with EB nuclear antigen production and Latent Membrane Proteins which protect the B-cell from apoptosis and stimulate ongoing viral application which is controlled by a cytotoxic T cell driven EB specific surveillance. Impairment of this cytotoxic T-cell protection is believed to be essential for developing PTLD [62]. Lack of T-cell protection leads to uncontrolled viral replication and an increase of virus-carrying B-cells in the circulation [62]. Cytokine responses, induced by immunosuppression, may lead to uncontrolled B-cell proliferation and ultimately neoplastic PTLD.

Risk Factors for PTLD

Epstein-Barr Virus (EBV)

EBV seronegativity and the use of potent immunosuppressive therapy are the two most important PTLD risk factors. In children, over 70% of PTLD is EBV-associated. The risk of being EBV naïve has been established in various studies. Sero-negativity of EBV is associated with a 4–7 times overall increased risk and a 20 times increased risk with in the first years after transplantation [63–65].

CMV/Hepatitis C

Reports on the role of CMV and hepatitis C are conflicting. Studies from the 1990s have revealed a four-to-six-fold excess risk of PTLD of CMV sero-mismatch (i.e., a negative recipient and a positive donor) after non-renal transplantation [66]. A *de novo* CMV infection was associated with polyclonal B-cell proliferation. The same role has been suggested for hepatitis C [67], but neither the CMV nor the hepatitis C link could be confirmed by large registry reports from the USRDS and ANZDATA [60, 68].

Immunosuppressive Therapy

All longitudinal evaluations of the incidence of PTLD show a trend over time toward increased incidence and earlier onset of PTLD up to 2000–2005. The exact role of immunosuppressive drugs in this trend remains to be elucidated. The concurrent increase in potency of the immunosuppressive therapy and incidence of PTLD is obvious, but links between the use of specific drugs and PTLD are unclear. It is believed that MMF is of less influence than calcineurin inhibitors but that statement is not supported by hard evidence and even contradicted by some case reports [69]. The previously supposed protective effect of mTOR is also contradicted by recent data [70].

Other

Apart from the increased overall risk of children, UNOS data have shown that young male Caucasians were at greatest risk for PTLD [65] A complete HLA-DR mismatch associates with a twofold increased risk, probably as a result of the greater immunosuppressive requirements [71].

Monitoring and early detection. Elevated EBV levels in mononuclear cells or in plasma assessed by PCR is the key to early detection of PTLD. The most important monitor is serial EBV quantitative PCR assessment as a rising level is more predictive than a single positive EBV quantitative PCR. EBV+ PTLD most often occurs in the first 1–2 years post-transplant, so monitoring should be intensified during this period [72]. Unfortunately, there is no standardized assay for EBV quantitation. Thresholds for elevation of the EBV load therefore differ per individual lab [72]. A negative EBV PCR does not exclude PTLD. Unexplained anemia, leukopenia or thrombocytopenia and high uric acid and LDH levels are non-specific abnormalities that are associated with PTLD or another malignant blood or lymph disease. Patients should be checked for tonsil abnormalities; if they do occur, a biopsy is indicated. Radiological monitoring includes MRI, CT and positive positron emission tomography (PET) scanning to evaluate the spread of PTLD. In case of CNS involvement, a lumbar puncture with cerebral spinal fluid (CSF) analysis (EBV PCR in CSF fluid) is indicated. Histopathologic examination of the tumor can only determine the definitive diagnosis.

A new development in monitoring is the detection of a certain viral load as proxy for decrease of immuno-competence [73]. Data of a study in 96 heart and lung transplant recipients suggest that a high anellovirus load may be indicative of over-immunosuppression. In line with this, metagenomic shotgun sequencing of tissues from PTLD patients showed that more than 50% of the specimens contained anellovirus sequences, and the anellovirus levels, but not EBV levels, were associated with death within 5 years in a univariate analysis [74]. This presumes that virome changes, and even specific viruses such as anellovirus, may provide indirect measures of the immune status which can promote the development of EBV+ PTLD.

Therapy/prevention of PTLD. Reduction of immunosuppressive therapy in case of an increase in EBV load in EBV-seronegative recipients and incase of EBV disease in all recipients is the first step in preventing PTLD (KDIGO level 2D and 1C) [75]. Rituximab is the cornerstone of 1e first line therapy of PTLD. In a multicenter trial, 152 transplant recipients with CD20 + PTLD that was unresponsive to immunosuppression reduction, were initially treated with 4 doses of weekly rituximab. In case of complete remission, rituximab treatment was continued with another 4 gifts; other patients received 4 R-CHOP courses. The overall response and CR rates were 88% and 70%, respectively; the most significant prognostic factor respect to overall survival and time to progression was the response to the first 4 courses of rituximab with [76].

Skin Tumors

Skin cancer is the most frequent malignancy after transplantation, also after pediatric transplantation, but hardly occurs in childhood. Most tumors only become manifest 10–15 years after transplantation. According to IPTTRS data, 16 out of 101 skin cancers found in pediatric solid-organ transplant recipients developed during childhood [77], 10 of them being squamous cell carcinomas (predominantly of the lower lip) and 6 melanomas. Death occurred in 8 patients, five from squamous cell carcinoma and three from melanoma [77].

The mean age at onset of skin cancer has been reported to be about 27 years [51, 54, 77–79]. However, recent data of the LERIC study shows that most tumors occur at later age. In the Dutch study, the risk for non-melanoma skin cancer (NMSC) was over 200 times higher than in the age-related population. Of all 249 patients, 63 had died in 2000 and 97 in 2010. At that time, 39 patients had developed 82 non-melanoma skin cancers (78% of all tumors). The mean age at developing a NMSC was 39 (range 22–50) years [55].

UV exposure and human papilloma virus (HPV) in combination with immunosuppression are thought to be the most important causative factors for the development of post-transplant skin tumors. UV radiation is probably one of the most important factors [78] This explains the

extremely high incidence in Australia, a country with a majority of genetically ill-protected Caucasian people and a very high sun exposure, with a 93% proportion of skin cancer among all post-transplant malignancies [80]. Sun protection is therefore of utmost importance, in combination with Vitamin D supplementation to avoid Vitamin D deficiency.

Skin cancer may appear in the absence of any pre-existing skin lesion, but is often preceded by actinic keratosis, which suggests the involvement of HPV in its pathogenesis. Additional evidence for the role of HPV comes from a study on post-transplant squamous cell carcinomas (SCC) that occurred in a cohort of 500 allograft recipients; HPV DNA could be detected in nearly 50% of all SCC [81, 82].

Calcineurin inhibitors have been regarded as most important immunosuppressive drugs that may increase the risk of skin cancer [83]. CNIs may express their oncogenic effect by interference with the p53 pathway and nucleotide excision repair and by promotion of malignant cell differentiation [84, 85]. In contrast, mTOR inhibitors have anti-tumor properties. Indeed, several studies have showed that diversion to mTOR in transplanted patients with NMSC could prevent the occurrence of new tumors [86, 87]. A recent study showed that the combination of low dose CNI and sirolimus could also be effective as prevention against new tumors [88].

Squamous cell carcinoma and basal cell carcinoma (non-melanoma skin cancers, NMSC). Squamous cell carcinoma (SCC) accounts for more than 50% of all skin cancers after transplantation. The ratio of basal cell carcinoma (BCC) to SCC is reversed in transplant patients compared with the general population in which basal cell carcinoma is the most common one. SCC was 81 times more prevalent in a cohort of Danish renal allograft recipients than in the general population [82]. The predominance of SCC over basal cell carcinoma (BCC) is more pronounced in pediatric than in adult transplant recipients (SCC: BCC 2.8:1 vs. 1.7:1) [77]. SCC is for the most part found in parts of the body exposed to daylight [80]. In pediatric transplant recipients, lip cancers account for 23% of all skin cancers [77].

Skin cancers may develop rapidly, and recurrences are common. In the LERIC study NMSC was most common to recur and/or metastasize of all malignancies. Including metastases, 114 NMSC (78 SCC and 36 BCC) occurred in 39 patients at a mean age of 39 (21.8–50.4) years [55]. The Incidence Rate and Incidence Rate Ratio's for SCC were 1.5 and 744, respectively. The IRR was 992 in the 25–30 and 2610 in the 45–50 year age group. Two patients died of SCC; far more patients had important morbidity because of SCC metastases.

Melanoma

Melanoma seems to be more prevalent in pediatric than in adult transplant recipients (12 vs. 5%) [77]. The Dutch cohort study counted 5 melanomas on 105 malignancies, occurring at a mean age of 29 years [55]. Data of the IPTTRS and the Dutch cohort study suggest an earlier onset of melanoma compared to NMSC. The IPTTRS noted 25% of deaths were due to melanoma [55, 77].

Melanocytic nevi, a risk factor for melanoma, may develop in excess after transplantation [89]. In transplantation, melanoma can be transmitted by the donor. Any person with a history of melanoma should be excluded from donation [90]. It has been speculated that growth hormone use might increase the growth rate of melanocytic nevi, but to date no association between GH therapy and the occurrence of melanomas has been found [91]. Sun protection and removal of suspect nevi are the most important protective measures.

Kaposi's Sarcoma

Kaposi's sarcoma is caused by HHV8 virus infection. The Norwegian study found 3 times more Kaposi Sarcoma's in kidney transplant recipients than in the general population [92]. The IPTTRS reported 2% Kaposi sarcoma's, nearly all of which occurred during childhood [78]. Only one child presented with skin cancer. All had various visceral localizations. The age of occurrence ranged from 5 to 17 years, the onset was typically within a few months after trans-plantation. Six of the eight reported patients had a fatal outcome.

Other Tumors

There are very few data on other solid tumors after pediatric renal transplant recipients. The NAPRTCS transplant registry found a rate of non-lymphoproliferative solid tumors of 72.1 per 100,000 person-years which implies a 6.7-fold increased risk compared with the general pediatric population (10.7 cases per 100,000 person-years). Non-LPD malignancy was diagnosed in 35 subjects at a median of 726 days post-transplant. The most common type of malignancy was renal cell carcinoma. No specific type of immunosuppression was identified as a risk factor [54]. In the LERIC study, 9 solid non-skin/non lymphoproliferative tumors were found, consistent with 158 per 100,000 patient years, at a mean age of 41.7 years [55]. All 9 tumors were from different origin.

Other Somatic Co-morbidities

Bone disease and motor disabilities. Whereas cardiovascular disease and infections have proven to be the most life-threatening co-morbidities, chronic fatigue in dialysis patients and motor disabilities as a result of metabolic bone disease are the most frequently reported daily problems of young adults with childhood ESRD [16, 19, 50]. As expected, in a cohort of patients that has grown up in the pre-growth hormone era, more than two-thirds of the LERIC patients were severely growth retarded [16]. A more surprising and more worrisome finding was the extent and severity of clinically manifest metabolic bone disease that we found in the LERIC patients. More than one-third had daily complaints or disabilities related to metabolic bone disease. About 18% were disabled as a result of bone disease [16]. Very few data exist on this evidently under-exposed problem. Although conclusive evidence is lacking, most of these problems seem to be related to chronic inactivity, inadequately managed CKD-MBD, a high burden of corticosteroids and an increased total duration of renal replacement therapy [93]. Bone mineral densities (BMD) are lower than −2.5 SDS in over 50% of adult patients with childhood ESRD [16]. However, in a 10-year extension of the LERIC study, no association of low BMD with clinical bone disease, such as fractures, daily pain or motor disabilities, could be found (unpublished data).

Itching is a frequently mentioned complaint of both dialysis and transplanted patients [94].

Psychosocial Consequences

Cognitive Functioning

Neurocognitive dysfunction is a well-recognized complication of pediatric CKD. Many studies have found evidence of several neuropsychological deficits, including IQ, academic achievement, memory, and executive functioning [95–99]. This deficit is reflected by cognitive dysfunction at adult age. Cognitive and learning impairment is also more prevalent in middle-aged adult patients with childhood ESKD than in the age-matched population [15, 100]. In the LERIC study mean IQ scores of adults aged 20–40 years with childhood ESKD were on average ten points lower than in the aged matched Dutch population, which is in line with the results of IQ studies performed in children [15, 101, 102]. Impaired schooling and cognition appear to be induced by a long period of dialysis during youth. The LERIC study found no difference in intellectual performance between patients who were on dialysis and those who were transplanted by the time of investigation. In theory, chronic aluminum intoxication as a result of chronic use of aluminum-containing phosphate binders could have influenced the cognitive development of our patients. Yet, no evidence was found for this [15]. On the contrary, the compatible results of recent IQ studies in ESRD children indicate that abandoning aluminum-containing phosphate binders has not shown beneficial effects on intellectual development [15, 103]. Most deficits are found in tasks requiring concentration, memory and most of all general knowledge. Consequently, early

educational intervention in young patients on dialysis might prevent most of these impairments. In spite of improvements in identification and treatment, CKD causes both direct and indirect insults to a variety of organ systems. In contrast with the Dutch study, the educational attainment of pediatric transplanted patients with a median age of 25.7 years in a Swedish study was in line with the general population. The problem of this study is that 40% of the cohort did not participate and no information about the characteristics of these non-participants was provided [104].

Previous studies of children with CKD suggest that toddlers and children with CKD are at increased risk for delays in neuro-cognitive development [105]. In a large North American study (CKiD) on 386 children with CKD 2–4 (mean GFR 41), the overall neuro-cognitive functioning was within the average range for the entire group, but 21% to 40% of participants scored at least one SD below the mean on measures of intelligence quotient (IQ), academic achievement, attention regulation, or executive functioning. A higher GFR was associated with lesser risk for poor performance on measures of executive function. Significant proteinuria was associated with lower verbal IQ, full-scale IQ, and attention scores [106].

In an accompanying analysis, CKiD cohort participants with hypertension scored lower on visual-spatial organization, planning, constructive abilities, and nonverbal reasoning [107]. Results from these studies highlight the importance of recognizing neurocognitive dysfunction in children with CKD early on because of the significant impact it may have on school performance and the opportunity it presents for prompt intervention [108].

Quality of Life

Transplant Patients
According to most studies, adult patients with a functioning renal graft achieve normal scores on self-assessment of mental and physical health for most domains. In the LERIC study, data on quality

of life were assessed in 2000 in 131 of 186 surviving patients aged 20–40 years with mean onset of RRT at age 11 years. In transplanted patients, only scores on social functioning and general health perception were slightly lower than in the age related general Dutch population. All other scores were within the normal range [17]. Equally good outcomes were found in an Italian follow up study on transplanted patients at aged 18–34 years who were transplanted a median age of 15 years [109]. In contrast, a study from Japan noted lower mean scores, especially of those related to the mental quality of life, in kidney allograft recipients of the same age [110]. Remarkably, in this study, nearly all scores of hemodialysis patients awaiting transplantation appeared to be similar to those of transplanted patients. In contrast, dialysis patients not awaiting transplantation (i.e. not on a transplant waiting list for medical or personal reason) had much lower scores [110]. Most available studies emphasize the improvement of the quality of life after renal transplantation [111–113]. However, for some young adults, transplantation not always had the wellness and health that they hoped it would have, as was shown in a more recent review on adult perspectives of living with kidney failure. Young adults with pediatric ESRD most often have a driving desire to *be* "normal," whereas those diagnosed later in early adulthood often feel an "unbearable loss" and hope *to return* to their previous state of "normal" [114].

Dialysis Patients

Not unexpectedly, in the LERIC study patients aged 20–40 years with pediatric onset of ESRD who were on dialysis at time of assessment indicated more often an impaired quality of life than the general population in all physical domains: activities that require good physical condition (Physical Functioning), social activities that require a good physical condition = Role Limitations due to physical health (Role Physical), social functioning (SF), general health perception (GH) and the so-called physical component summary (PCS). Yet the same patients reported an impaired quality of life for the mental domains equally or even less often than aged-matched Dutch citizens [17].

These results sharply contrast with data derived from dialysis patients with onset of ESRD in adulthood [115–117]. Patients with adult onset of disease appear to have a substantially poorer quality of life, particularly in Physical domains and General Health perceptions, but also in domains related to the mental quality of life.

In the LERIC study, outcomes of patients on dialysis were compared with age-matched dialysis patients with adult-onset ESRD from the NECOSAD-2 study. The latter concerned Dutch patients who were only on RRT since 1 year. In all domains except one, scores of NECOSAD patients were significantly lower than those found in the general population, whereas the LERIC dialysis patients had normal mental scores [17].

The high scores on mental health in LERIC are on the other hand consistent with findings in other studies of adolescents and adults with chronic illness since childhood, including sickle cell patients, cystic fibrosis and asthma [118–120]. Different expectations of life and different coping strategies by children and adults may explain the difference in mental status of patients with pediatric and those with adult onset of disease. Carr et al. have reasoned that health-related quality of life is to a large extent based on the difference between health expectations and health experiences [121].

Effect of Age at Assessment

Quality of Life (QoL) scores seem to be age dependent to some extent. At both late adolescent and very old age, patients score on average lower than at middle age [111, 122–124]. Using another scoring system, a Finnish group assessed QoL at young adult age years in 21 patients transplanted at very young age (mean 2.4 years) and found significantly lower scores than in age-matched controls, contrary to the Dutch and Italian late outcome studies. Significantly lower scores were found regarding mobility, usual activities, mental functioning and vitality [123]. There was a clear tracking effect, as scores per patient were comparable to those measured 10 years before. These outcomes mimic more the QoL scores found in children with ESRD [125].

Trend Over Time

Most favorable outcomes in transplanted patients are reported after at most 10–20 years of follow up. The QoL assessment in the Dutch LERIC study was repeated in 2010 after a mean duration of about 30 years of RRT in surviving patients aged by then 30–50 years. The scores in physical domains were significantly lower in 2010 than in 2000. These concern limitations of daily activities and social participation by physical impairment or pain ('Physical Functioning,' 'Role Physical' and 'Bodily Pain') as well as General Health perception. The decrease of physical QoL over time also accounted for transplanted patients [126]. The deterioration of physical QoL is partly explained by a normal effect of ageing in line with the trend in the general population as older age is an important negative predictor of perceived physical health status [124].Nevertheless, the ongoing decay superposed on lower scores on some domains could become a significant problem for these patients in the near future, adversely influencing their social functioning. In the LERIC study, one transplanted woman aged 32 years illustrated this by questionnaire comments: "Much more often than 10 years ago, even when I was on dialysis, I feel very tired nowadays, reason why I recently have decided to stop working for a while."

According to the same study, all domains relating to psychosocial functioning had remained stable over the last 10 years.

Co-morbidity was associated with an increased risk of impaired QoL in the domains 'Physical Functioning,' 'Role Physical' and 'Bodily Pain.' Having disabilities was associated with an increased risk of impaired QoL regarding Physical Functioning, Vitality and Bodily Pain. Notably, the current RRT modality at time of investigation was not correlated with impaired QoL in any domain. However in case lifetime on dialysis exceeded lifetime on renal transplant, there was an increased risk of impaired participation in social activities by physical strain.

Regarding the socio-demographic variables, being employed appeared to be associated with a lower risk of impaired QoL in the domains of Physical Functioning, Vitality and General

Health perception. Having offspring was associated with a lower risk of impaired QoL regarding Social Functioning and an income equal to or above the national average of €2500 (about $ 3200) gross per month was associated with a lower risk of RP [126].

Although in line with positive outcomes on mental health perception for other chronic diseases of childhood with shorter follow-up time, the universally high scores on mental health after 30 years of RRT with a concurrent decline in physical health and subsequently physical QoL are striking. Nearly 80% of patients stated that their disease had brought them something positive in life. The perceived benefits of having ESRD included more satisfaction with (small things in) life, having developed a sense of perseverance and positive responses from friends and relatives [126].

Social Outcome

Employment

A review from a social work perspective of data on late social consequences of pediatric kidney transplantation showed a significant impact on many aspects of social development including education, peer/intimate relationships, employment and overall well-being. Young adults, kidney transplanted at childhood, are more likely to live with their parents and less likely to have a partner. Social isolation, fear to disclose their disease status to peers and difficulties to establish intimate relationships are more prevalent than in the general population [127].

Social outcome was assessed in the LERIC study in 2000 and in 2010. In 2000, 67.4% was employed, about 85% for more than 50% time equivalent [128]. Involuntary unemployment occurred in 19.1% vs. 6.4% in the Dutch population. Most patients (53%) had low skilled and only 10% had high skilled professions, a situation significantly different from the average Dutch population [128]. In 2010, 61.8% were employed of whom 81.8% had at least 50% full time equivalent paid work. However, different from the situation in 2000, there was a very significant difference between patients on dialysis of whom only 31.3% were still employed, and transplanted patients [126]. Apart from dialysis as RRT modality, having motor disabilities was the most important risk factor for becoming unemployed. Patients also mentioned increasing chronic fatigue as an important reason for becoming unemployed. Some patients, however, reported that their employment contract was not renewed as a direct result of the disclosure of their dialysis patient status to the employer. Unemployment was related to patients' low subjective health perception, an apparent failure to adjust to their disease, rather than to their objective physical condition, or to whether they were transplanted or on dialysis [126]. Among 42 transplanted patients aged 20–38 years in a Swedish long-term follow up study 54% were part-time or full time employed, 14% were unemployed (compared to 5.3% in the general population, p = 0.059) and 21% received education [104].

A positive change was a significant trend towards more highly educated occupations. Also the educational level had on average increased over time. Among the patients, 22.1% had completed a high vocational training or scientific degree, compared to 31.2% in the general Dutch population (P > 0.05) [126] 34.8% of the patients had an income equal to or above the national modal income of €2500 (about US$ 3200) gross per month, a significantly smaller proportion compared to the general population (61.1%) [126].

In a very recent French outcome study of 624 patients transplanted in childhood, fewer patients than expected had a high-level degree (Q3-year university level: 14.8 vs. 30.2% general population) and fewer women had a baccalaureate degree (49.2 vs. 76.5%), but these differences were less marked than in the Dutch study [129, 130]. Mean incomes were much lower than in the French population [130]. While the distribution of professional occupations was representative of the French society, more patients were unemployed (18.5% vs. 10.4%; p < 0.01). Independent factors for poor social outcome with respect to professional career were ESRD onset in infancy, the presence of co-morbidity and disabilities, a low educational level of the parents or patient, female gender and being (again) on dialysis at

time of assessment [130]. Interestingly, patients less often had a permanent contract than the average French employee (66.8 vs. 81.8%) [130]. This might reflect the observed reluctance of employers against a long-term professional commitment with renal patients, as also observed in the LERIC study. The relatively good overall outcome of the French study might be slightly biased by the fact that more non-responders than responders had graft failure at time of investigation and that the cumulative duration on dialysis was also higher in the non-responder group [130].

Interestingly, nearly 50% of the French transplanted patients indicated to have suffered from discrimination, either at school (60.8%), from employers (27.8%) or work colleagues (19.9%) and even from friends (19.3%) [130]. In the Dutch cohort, 35.2% of patients lost their job between 2000 and 2010, in 32.3% because they were fired—sometimes as part of a 'reorganization' and in 45.2% for medical reasons. In 12.1%, employers indicated that the disease state of the patient influenced their achievements. About 21% of patients felt that their disease had a significant negative influence on their professional achievements and career [126].

Partnership and Independency

In the first evaluation of the LERIC study in 2000 patients showed to have significant difficulties in finding a partner. Of all 144 patients, 31.9% lived alone, 34% lived with a partner, and 49 (34%) still lived with their parents. The odds ratio of living with parents, as a measure of dependency, vs. living alone or with a partner was 3.3 (95% CI, 2.3–4.7) for LERIC patients compared with age-matched Dutch inhabitants [128]). The odds ratio of living with a partner was 0.3 (95% CI, 0.2–0.4) for LERIC patients compared with age-matched Dutch controls. These figures are in line with those of the French follow-up study of pediatric transplanted patients of the same age as the LERIC study at time of assessment (31.1% partnership, 35.7% living with parents) [130]. In 2010, the situation in the LERIC cohort was completely changed: 67.4% was married or lived with a partner and 28 (31.5%) had offspring compared to respectively 74.4% (P > 0.05) and 64.8%

(P < 0.05) in the general population [126]. This delay in starting a relationship could reflect a genuine delay in sexual maturity or a late 'social maturity' as has been described in patients with a chronic illness [131]. Patients with disabilities and patients from Southern more than from Northern European countries tend to remain living with their parents [25, 101, 126, 129, 130]. In an older study, patients reported on average successful partnerships after pediatric kidney transplantation, but fewer than in the general population had children and 40% reported not to be sexually active [132]. Men appear to have problems finding a life partner more often than women [129, 132].

Conclusions

Although the prospects of end-stage kidney disease in children have improved over the last 30 years, the risk for premature death remains extremely high and adult life comes with considerable physical troubles. Cardiovascular disease has been recognized for more than a decade as most important threat in pediatric ESKD. Recent data indicate that adjusted therapeutic approaches and changes in lifestyle may be very effective in reducing the risk for premature cardiac death in this population. On the other hand, physicians should be aware for a potential increase in life-threatening infections and malignancies as a result of more potent immunosuppressive therapy after transplantation. Co-morbidities, most importantly motor disabilities have an important impact on social life in adulthood, especially with respect to finding a job and a life partner. Despite all physical discomfort, the mental health perception of adult patients with pediatric ESKD is remarkably good. Most patients are highly motivated to fully participate in society and to join the work force, well-adjusted to their situation.

In appreciation of the insights gained from long-term outcome research in patients with childhood-onset ESKD, the following should be the principles of modern pediatric renal replacement therapy in order to optimize late outcomes in these patients: Reduction of RRT time on dialysis to the absolute minimum; propagation of pre-emptive and living-related transplantation; personalization of immunosuppressive therapy; aggressive prevention of CKD bone-mineral disease in order to avoid later motor disabilities; timely start of intensified dialysis regimes (preferably frequent nocturnal home hemodialysis) in patients who are not eligible for transplantation; and finally, active and early stimulation of development towards independency.

A Patient's Story

"I am 41 years old, live with my boyfriend in this beautiful apartment. Currently I am in between 2 jobs, partly because, over the last few years, I often feel quite exhausted, despite the fact that I have a well-functioning renal graft at this moment.

I used to work as a radio reporter at the local radio of Utrecht and as a stand-up comedian. The radio work was very exciting, making documentaries and interviews that was actually my dream as a young girl. My father was photographer. As a Moluccan son of a military servant of the Dutch Indian (former "Dutch India"— currently Indonesia), he moved to Holland in the fifties where he met my mother. She worked as a nursery-class teacher and has Dutch as well as Russian-Jewish blood. Combativeness and urge for moving both run in the family.

I was 3 years old when I turned ill. I remember having a sore throat and getting medicines that didn't work. I felled extremely tired, but our house doctor was not impressed, everybody feels occasionally tired. It took months before they realized that something was wrong. Then, I was hospitalized for 3 months, where I had to stay in bed and live on an awful diet. Later, they transferred me to the Sophia Children's (university) Hospital of Rotterdam where the doctors told me that my kidneys were very sick and would slowly get ruined. Gradually the troubles came. I blew up like a balloon for which I felt awfully ashamed. At school I was abused, children called me a stupid Chinese. Between my third and 11th year, I was more often in the hospital than at home. At a certain time, my mother quit her job to join me at the hospital as she always did, unlike my father.

I do not know why they have waited so long with starting dialysis, because in a way it came as a relief. I had to dialyze 3 times per week for 4–5 h per time. Fortunately, my doctors were wonderful. They gave me much attention and explained everything to me. After 6 months, I got my first transplantation. That kidney lasted 10 years. Once in a while I had to go to the hospital for treatment of a rejection. At age 22, when I had entered university to study Dutch language, I was back on dialysis. I had never noticed that my kidney function was deteriorating, which is a frightening experience. Even today I am still nervous about my creatinine when I have am at the out clinic.

Then I got problems with my shunt. I had to turn to peritoneal dialysis. Not a big deal, but very tiresome to combine with my study. Luckily, I was rid of my dialysis hang-over. I have never understood how people could drive home themselves after a hemo session. I was always exhausted, even though I nicely kept my diet and fluid restriction. I have always experienced the day of dialysis as a totally wasted day. Actually, you only lived 3 days per week. With PD, things were different; I was freer, changed bags on the train, airplane, airfield, whatever. At first, I felled embarrassed to do so, but very rapidly it became quite normal.

The hospital feels like my second home; it is all very familiar, the smell of the ward, the nurses, the smell of antiseptics, the idea that you can drop down and people will help you immediately. I always thought that if I would get a child, I would call her Sophia, after the name of the hospital. I never regretted to go to the hospital. There were always people that I knew very well and who always paid attention to you. That is a very particular thing. Up to your 18th, people always listen to you and treat you as a person and suddenly at the internal department you become a number and you have to do everything by yourself. Behave as a mature person, but not too clever or candid!

Later I have learned to speak freely about my disease but when I entered university, nobody knew about my illness, even not when I was back on dialysis. I dialyzed in the evening, so I always had to find an excuse for not joining my friends at the pub or the movie. At first this was not a big problem. Many people had a job in the evening, but then friends started asking questions about my scars, so I had to disclose my disease, which actually turned out to be a big relief.

During my school time at home, I always felt extremely tired after a hemo session—there was no EPO at that time -, yet my mother always forced me first to clean my room or do a little job, before she allowed me to lie down. Later I have learned to appreciate her behavior. Many parents treat their sick children as princesses, which I think is disastrous. Most of the times, you are spared anyway. I always got attention from everybody. People were always worried about me, always asked about me, even the most distant acquaintances of my parents. That was a big frustration for my sister. So, even although my parents try to avoid it, I got pampered by my environment. The first time, that I realized this was at work, where nobody new about my situation. I could be heavily upset when people did not understand why I was not willing to work over-time or demanded a day off. I always thought, 'man, if you would know my situation ...' Later, I sometimes used by illness when I thought that people were whining.

When I started working at the radio, I told nobody at work about my situation. I just wanted to work for a maximum of 20 h a week and I thought it was of no once business to know why. Unfortunately, I got problems with my knees which was due to bone necrosis caused by long time prednisone use. I had to be operated and to disclose my disease status. My direct colleagues were all shocked and people started to behave differently. You could feel that they thought, that lady will be out for a long time, so we probably have to look for someone else. And with all those medicines, this will of course happen more often. These things were never openly discussed, but suddenly things were taken out of my hands and my contract was not extended. I received a letter in which I was thanked for everything, they wished me good luck and appreciated how I had handled my disease. But I learned my lesson. Never disclose your disease if not absolutely necessary to your employer!

During my time at the university, I first realized how awful it is not to be able to comply with the activities of your friends. They really could feel offended when I turned down their invitations to go out at evening. As in my world, everybody knows that there are good and bad days and that if you feel good, you want to enjoy your day which always means that you have to pay for it the next day.

I think that I am less ambitious than my healthy peers, that I am more realistic and easier pleased with small things. I have no driving license, I am not married, I rent my house, have no children. I have probably consciously avoided all these obligations, yet the thought of never having children is most depressing. Currently my graft function is too bad, my doctor advised against it. I do not see it as a problem to have a child with my disease, even when I would have to start dialysis again.

Getting mad is my biggest fear. When I was 29 years old, I got psychotic. I had visions how my parents must had felt when I got sick and religious delusions. I thought that I had special medical gifts and I was convinced to be pregnant of a twin. I was isolated for 3 weeks in a psychiatric hospital, because I was intruding other patients with my special medical gifts. When I recovered I realized that it was all due to a strange chemical reaction inside my head and not due to some unprocessed emotions. I always thought that to be bull shit. In the seventies, I had to encounter a pediatric psychologist and had to talk about my disease, how I dealt with it. She noticed from my drawings that I drew too many clouds, clearly a sign that I could not express my anger. Me, not able to show anger, that was totally absurd! She showed me that I was observed from a one-way screen by at least 10 people. One of the most terrible things you could do to a child! Every time, I was at the hospital afterwards, I checked the room for one-way screens. Anyway, the point was that I had no anger, I just liked the doctors. I was never sad when I had to go to the hospital. I always stood immediately ready with my suitcase. I was eager to help the doctors and was never afraid of the blood punctures. I always stuck out my arm and told the doctor what I thought would be the best vein to attack with the needle. To some extent, it was nice to return, as it was part of my family, I knew all the nurses and doctors and there were funny things to do on the ward. The worst thing about it was the sadness of my parents.

The psychosis has changed my attitude. I previously thought that I could rationally solve all my problems, now I have learned to be more honest. It has taught me that nothing is certain in life. And then suddenly, I was asked my former employer at the radio if I would be interested to come back. The work at the radio really helped me to overcome my psychosis."

References

1. Kolff WJ. De Kunstmatige Nier (the artificial kidney). Kampen: J.H. Kok; 1946.
2. Wightman AG, Freeman MA. Update on ethical issues in pediatric dialysis: has pediatric dialysis become morally obligatory? Clin J Am Soc Nephrol. 2016;11(8):1456–62.
3. Kramer A, Stel VS, Geskus RB, Tizard EJ, Verrina E, Schaefer F, et al. The effect of timing of the first kidney transplantation on survival in children initiating renal replacement therapy. Nephrol Dial Transplant. 2012;27(3):1256–64.
4. Samuel SM, Tonelli MA, Foster BJ, Alexander RT, Nettel-Aguirre A, Soo A, et al. Survival in pediatric dialysis and transplant patients. Clin J Am Soc Nephrol. 2011;6(5):1094–9.
5. Pruthi R, O'Brien C, Casula A, Braddon F, Lewis M, Maxwell H, et al. UK renal registry 15th annual report: chapter 4 demography of the UK paediatric renal replacement therapy population in 2011. Nephron Clin Pract. 2013;123(Suppl 1):81–92.
6. Ploos van Amstel S, Noordzij M, Warady BA, Cano F, Craig JC, Groothoff JW, et al. Renal replacement therapy for children throughout the world: the need for a global registry. Pediatr Nephrol. 2018;33(5):863–71.
7. Alao MA, Ibrahim OR, Asinobi AO, Akinsola A. Long-term survival of children following acute peritoneal dialysis in a resource-limited setting. Kidney Res Clin Pract. 2020;39(4):469–78.
8. Prasad N, Rangaswamy D, Patel M, Gulati S, Bhadauria D, Kaul A, et al. Long-term outcomes in children on chronic continuous ambulatory peritoneal dialysis: a retrospective cohort study from a developing country. Pediatr Nephrol. 2019;34(11):2389–97.
9. Bonthuis M, Cuperus L, Chesnaye NC, Akman S, Melgar AA, Baiko S, et al. Results in the ESPN/ERA-EDTA registry suggest disparities in access to kidney transplantation but little variation in graft survival of children across Europe. Kidney Int. 2020;98(2):464–75.
10. Groothoff JW, Gruppen MP, Offringa M, Hutten J, Lilien MR, Van De Kar NJ, et al. Mortality and causes of death of end-stage renal disease in children: a Dutch cohort study. Kidney Int. 2002;61(2):621–9.
11. McDonald SP, Craig JC. Long-term survival of children with end-stage renal disease. N Engl J Med. 2004;350(26):2654–62.
12. Orr NI, McDonald SP, McTaggart S, Henning P, Craig JC. Frequency, etiology and treatment of childhood end-stage kidney disease in Australia and New Zealand. Pediatr Nephrol. 2009;24(9):1719–26.
13. Bonthuis M, Vidal E, Bjerre A, Aydog O, Baiko S, Garneata L, et al. Ten-year trends in epidemiology and outcomes of pediatric kidney replacement therapy in Europe: data from the ESPN/ERA-EDTA registry. Pediatr Nephrol. 2021;36(8):2337–48.
14. Groothoff JW, Gruppen MP, Offringa M, de Groot E, Stok W, Bos WJ, et al. Increased arterial stiffness in young adults with end-stage renal disease since childhood. J Am Soc Nephrol. 2002;13(12):2953–61.
15. Groothoff JW, Grootenhuis M, Dommerholt A, Gruppen MP, Offringa M, Heymans HS. Impaired cognition and schooling in adults with end stage renal disease since childhood. Arch Dis Child. 2002;87(5):380–5.
16. Groothoff JW, Offringa M, Van Eck-Smit BL, Gruppen MP, Van De Kar NJ, Wolff ED, et al. Severe bone disease and low bone mineral density after juvenile renal failure. Kidney Int. 2003;63(1):266–75.
17. Groothoff JW, Grootenhuis MA, Offringa M, Gruppen MP, Korevaar JC, Heymans HS. Quality of life in adults with end-stage renal disease since childhood is only partially impaired. Nephrol Dial Transplant. 2003;18(2):310–7.
18. Gruppen MP, Groothoff JW, Prins M, van der Wouw P, Offringa M, Bos WJ, et al. Cardiac disease in young adult patients with end-stage renal disease since childhood: a Dutch cohort study. Kidney Int. 2003;63(3):1058–65.
19. Groothoff JW. Late somatic and psycho-social consequences of renal insufficiency in children. EDTNA ERCA J. 2004;30(4):222–5.
20. Vogelzang JL, van Stralen KJ, Jager KJ, Groothoff JW. Trend from cardiovascular to non-cardiovascular late mortality in patients with renal replacement therapy since childhood. Nephrol Dial Transplant. 2013;28(8):2082–9.
21. McDonald SP, Craig JC. Australian, New Zealand paediatric nephrology A. Long-term survival of children with end-stage renal disease. N Engl J Med. 2004;350(26):2654–62.
22. Oh J, Wunsch R, Turzer M, Bahner M, Raggi P, Querfeld U, et al. Advanced coronary and carotid arteriopathy in young adults with childhood-onset chronic renal failure. Circulation. 2002;106(1):100–5.
23. Alexander RT, Foster BJ, Tonelli MA, Soo A, Nettel-Aguirre A, Hemmelgarn BR, et al. Survival and transplantation outcomes of children less than 2 years of age with end-stage renal disease. Pediatr Nephrol. 2012;27(10):1975–83.
24. Chesnaye NC, Schaefer F, Bonthuis M, Holman R, Baiko S, Baskin E, et al. Mortality risk disparities in children receiving chronic renal replacement therapy for the treatment of end-stage renal disease across Europe: an ESPN-ERA/EDTA registry analysis. Lancet. 2017;389(10084):2128–37.
25. Offner G, Latta K, Hoyer PF, Baum HJ, Ehrich JH, Pichlmayr R, et al. Kidney transplanted children come of age. Kidney Int. 1999;55(4):1509–17.
26. van der Heijden BJ, van Dijk PC, Verrier-Jones K, Jager KJ, Briggs JD. Renal replacement therapy in children: data from 12 registries in Europe. Pediatr Nephrol. 2004;19(2):213–21.
27. Adamczuk D, Roszkowska-Blaim M. Long-term outcomes in children with chronic kidney disease stage 5 over the last 40 years. Arch Med Sci. 2017;13(3):635–44.

28. Mitsnefes M, Stablein D. Hypertension in pediatric patients on long-term dialysis: a report of the North American pediatric renal transplant cooperative study (NAPRTCS). Am J Kidney Dis. 2005;45(2):309–15.

29. Mitsnefes MM, Kimball TR, Witt SA, Glascock BJ, Khoury PR, Daniels SR. Left ventricular mass and systolic performance in pediatric patients with chronic renal failure. Circulation. 2003;107(6):864–8.

30. Mitsnefes MM, Khoury PR, McEnery PT. Early posttransplantation hypertension and poor long-term renal allograft survival in pediatric patients. J Pediatr. 2003;143(1):98–103.

31. Kramer AM, van Stralen KJ, Jager KJ, Schaefer F, Verrina E, Seeman T, et al. Demographics of blood pressure and hypertension in children on renal replacement therapy in Europe. Kidney Int. 2011;80(10):1092–8.

32. Foster BJ, Dahhou M, Zhang X, Platt RW, Hanley JA. Change in mortality risk over time in young kidney transplant recipients. Am J Transplant. 2011;11(11):2432–42.

33. Rocha S, Fonseca I, Silva N, Martins LS, Dias L, Henriques AC, et al. Impact of pediatric kidney transplantation on long-term professional and social outcomes. Transplant Proc. 2011;43(1):120–4.

34. Chavers BMMJSG. Trends in mortality in pediatric dialysis; 2015. www.usrds.org.

35. Roberts MA, Polkinghorne KR, McDonald SP, Ierino FL. Secular trends in cardiovascular mortality rates of patients receiving dialysis compared with the general population. Am J Kidney Dis. 2011;58(1):64–72.

36. Mitsnefes MM, Laskin BL, Dahhou M, Zhang X, Foster BJ. Mortality risk among children initially treated with dialysis for end-stage kidney disease, 1990-2010. JAMA. 2013;309(18):1921–9.

37. Mitsnefes MM. Cardiovascular disease in children with chronic kidney disease. J Am Soc Nephrol. 2012;23(4):578–85.

38. Eifinger F, Wahn F, Querfeld U, Pollok M, Gevargez A, Kriener P, et al. Coronary artery calcifications in children and young adults treated with renal replacement therapy. Nephrol Dial Transplant. 2000;15(11):1892–4.

39. Mitsnefes MM, Daniels SR, Schwartz SM, Khoury P, Strife CF. Changes in left ventricular mass in children and adolescents during chronic dialysis. Pediatr Nephrol. 2001;16(4):318–23.

40. Shroff R, Long DA, Shanahan C. Mechanistic insights into vascular calcification in CKD. J Am Soc Nephrol. 2013;24(2):179–89.

41. Shroff R, Degi A, Kerti A, Kis E, Cseprekal O, Tory K, et al. Cardiovascular risk assessment in children with chronic kidney disease. Pediatr Nephrol. 2013;28(6):875–84.

42. Vogelzang JL, Heestermans LW, van Stralen KJ, Jager KJ, Groothoff JW. Simultaneous reversal of risk factors for cardiac death and intensified ther-

apy in long-term survivors of paediatric end-stage renal disease over the last 10 years. Nephrol Dial Transplant. 2013;28(10):2545–52.

43. Galindo Sacristan P, Perez Marfil A, Osorio Moratalla JM, de Gracia GC, Ruiz Fuentes C, Castilla Barbosa YA, et al. Predictive factors of infection in the first year after kidney transplantation. Transplant Proc. 2013;45(10):3620–3.

44. Abbott KC, Swanson SJ, Richter ER, Bohen EM, Agodoa LY, Peters TG, et al. Late urinary tract infection after renal transplantation in the United States. Am J Kidney Dis. 2004;44(2):353–62.

45. Dharnidharka VR, Agodoa LY, Abbott KC. Effects of urinary tract infection on outcomes after renal transplantation in children. Clin J Am Soc Nephrol. 2007;2(1):100–6.

46. Lofaro D, Vogelzang JL, van Stralen KJ, Jager KJ, Groothoff JW. Infection-related hospitalizations over 30 years of follow-up in patients starting renal replacement therapy at pediatric age. Pediatr Nephrol. 2016;31(2):315–23.

47. Ekberg H, Tedesco-Silva H, Demirbas A, Vitko S, Nashan B, Gurkan A, et al. Reduced exposure to calcineurin inhibitors in renal transplantation. N Engl J Med. 2007;357(25):2562–75.

48. Nashan B, Curtis J, Ponticelli C, Mourad G, Jaffe J, Haas T, et al. Everolimus and reduced-exposure cyclosporine in de novo renal-transplant recipients: a three-year phase II, randomized, multicenter, open-label study. Transplantation. 2004;78(9):1332–40.

49. Vitko S, Wlodarczyk Z, Kyllonen L, Czajkowski Z, Margreiter R, Backman L, et al. Tacrolimus combined with two different dosages of sirolimus in kidney transplantation: results of a multicenter study. Am J Transplant. 2006;6(3):531–8.

50. Bartosh SM, Leverson G, Robillard D, Sollinger HW. Long-term outcomes in pediatric renal transplant recipients who survive into adulthood. Transplantation. 2003;76(8):1195–200.

51. Coutinho HM, Groothoff JW, Offringa M, Gruppen MP, Heymans HS. De novo malignancy after paediatric renal replacement therapy. Arch Dis Child. 2001;85(6):478–83.

52. Simard JF, Baecklund E, Kinch A, Brattstrom C, Ingvar A, Molin D, et al. Pediatric organ transplantation and risk of premalignant and malignant tumors in Sweden. Am J Transplant. 2011;11(1):146–51.

53. Koukourgianni F, Harambat J, Ranchin B, Euvrard S, Bouvier R, Liutkus A, et al. Malignancy incidence after renal transplantation in children: a 20-year single-centre experience. Nephrol Dial Transplant. 2010;25(2):611–6.

54. Smith JM, Martz K, McDonald RA, Harmon WE. Solid tumors following kidney transplantation in children. Pediatr Transplant. 2013;17(8):726–30.

55. Ploos van Amstel S, Vogelzang JL, Starink MV, Jager KJ, Groothoff JW. Long-term risk of cancer in survivors of pediatric ESRD. Clin J Am Soc Nephrol. 2015;10(12):2198–204.

56. Shapiro R, Nalesnik M, McCauley J, Fedorek S, Jordan ML, Scantlebury VP, et al. Posttransplant lymphoproliferative disorders in adult and pediatric renal transplant patients receiving tacrolimus-based immunosuppression. Transplantation. 1999;68(12):1851–4.

57. Engels EA, Jennings LW, Everly MJ, Landgren O, Murata K, Yanik EL, et al. Donor-specific antibodies, immunoglobulin-free light chains, and BAFF levels in relation to risk of late-onset PTLD in liver recipients. Transplant Direct. 2018;4(6):e353.

58. Robinson CH, Coughlin CC, Chanchlani R, Dharnidharka VR. Post-transplant malignancies in pediatric organ transplant recipients. Pediatr Transplant. 2020;25:e13884.

59. Dharnidharka VR, Webster AC, Martinez OM, Preiksaitis JK, Leblond V, Choquet S. Post-transplant lymphoproliferative disorders. Nat Rev Dis Primers. 2016;2:15088.

60. Faull RJ, Hollett P, McDonald SP. Lymphoproliferative disease after renal transplantation in Australia and New Zealand. Transplantation. 2005;80(2):193–7.

61. Samant H, Vaitla P, Kothadia JP. Post transplant lymphoproliferative disorders. Island, FL: StatPearls Treasure; 2020.

62. Tanner JE, Alfieri C. The Epstein-Barr virus and post-transplant lymphoproliferative disease: interplay of immunosuppression, EBV, and the immune system in disease pathogenesis. Transpl Infect Dis. 2001;3(2):60–9.

63. Babcock GJ, Decker LL, Freeman RB, Thorley-Lawson DA. Epstein-barr virus-infected resting memory B cells, not proliferating lymphoblasts, accumulate in the peripheral blood of immunosuppressed patients. J Exp Med. 1999;190(4):567–76.

64. Dharnidharka VR, Sullivan EK, Stablein DM, Tejani AH, Harmon WE. North American Pediatric Renal Transplant Cooperative S. Risk factors for post-transplant lymphoproliferative disorder (PTLD) in pediatric kidney transplantation: a report of the North American Pediatric Renal Transplant Cooperative Study (NAPRTCS). Transplantation. 2001;71(8):1065–8.

65. Knight JS, Tsodikov A, Cibrik DM, Ross CW, Kaminski MS, Blayney DW. Lymphoma after solid organ transplantation: risk, response to therapy, and survival at a transplantation center. J Clin Oncol. 2009;27(20):3354–62.

66. Manez R, Breinig MC, Linden P, Wilson J, Torre-Cisneros J, Kusne S, et al. Posttransplant lymphoproliferative disease in primary Epstein-Barr virus infection after liver transplantation: the role of cytomegalovirus disease. J Infect Dis. 1997;176(6):1462–7.

67. Buda A, Caforio A, Calabrese F, Fagiuoli S, Pevere S, Livi U, et al. Lymphoproliferative disorders in heart transplant recipients: role of hepatitis C virus (HCV) and Epstein-Barr virus (EBV) infection. Transpl Int. 2000;13(Suppl 1):S402–5.

68. Caillard S, Dharnidharka V, Agodoa L, Bohen E, Abbott K. Posttransplant lymphoproliferative disorders after renal transplantation in the United States in era of modern immunosuppression. Transplantation. 2005;80(9):1233–43.

69. O'Neill BP, Vernino S, Dogan A, Giannini C. EBV-associated lymphoproliferative disorder of CNS associated with the use of mycophenolate mofetil. Neuro-Oncology. 2007;9(3):364–9.

70. Sampaio MS, Cho YW, Shah T, Bunnapradist S, Hutchinson IV. Association of immunosuppressive maintenance regimens with posttransplant lymphoproliferative disorder in kidney transplant recipients. Transplantation. 2012;93(1):73–81.

71. Opelz G, Dohler B. Pediatric kidney transplantation: analysis of donor age, HLA match, and posttransplant non-Hodgkin lymphoma: a collaborative transplant study report. Transplantation. 2010;90(3):292–7.

72. Martinez OM, Krams SM. The immune response to Epstein Barr virus and implications for post-transplant LYMPHOPROLIFERATIVE disorder. Transplantation. 2017;101(9):2009–16.

73. De Vlaminck I, Khush KK, Strehl C, Kohli B, Luikart H, Neff NF, et al. Temporal response of the human virome to immunosuppression and antiviral therapy. Cell. 2013;155(5):1178–87.

74. Dharnidharka VR, Ruzinova MB, Chen CC, Parameswaran P, O'Gorman H, Goss CW, et al. Metagenomic analysis of DNA viruses from post-transplant lymphoproliferative disorders. Cancer Med. 2019;8(3):1013–23.

75. KDIGO Clinical Practice Guideline for the Care of Kidney Transplant Recipients; 2009. https://kdigo.org/wp-content/uploads/2017/02/KDIGO-2009-Transplant-Recipient-Guideline-English.pdf.

76. Trappe RU, Dierickx D, Zimmermann H, Morschhauser F, Mollee P, Zaucha JM, et al. Response to rituximab induction is a predictive marker in B-cell post-transplant Lymphoproliferative disorder and allows successful stratification into rituximab or R-CHOP consolidation in an international, prospective, multicenter phase II trial. J Clin Oncol. 2017;35(5):536–43.

77. De PI. Novo malignances in pediatric organ transplant recipients. Pediatr Transplant. 1998;2(1):56–63.

78. Bouwes Bavinck JN. Epidemiological aspects of immunosuppression: role of exposure to sunlight and human papillomavirus on the development of skin cancer. Hum Exp Toxicol. 1995;14(1):98.

79. Euvrard S, Kanitakis J, Cochat P, Claudy A. Skin cancers following pediatric organ transplantation. Dermatol Surg. 2004;30(4 Pt 2):616–21.

80. Hardie IR, Strong RW, Hartley LC, Woodruff PW, Clunie GJ. Skin cancer in Caucasian renal allograft recipients living in a subtropical climate. Surgery. 1980;87(2):177–83.

81. Euvrard S, Chardonnet Y, Pouteil-Noble C, Kanitakis J, Chignol MC, Thivolet J, et al. Association of skin malignancies with various and multiple car-

cinogenic and noncarcinogenic human papillomaviruses in renal transplant recipients. Cancer. 1993;72(7):2198–206.

82. Jensen AO, Svaerke C, Farkas D, Pedersen L, Kragballe K, Sorensen HT. Skin cancer risk among solid organ recipients: a nationwide cohort study in Denmark. Acta Derm Venereol. 2010;90(5):474–9.

83. Kaufmann RA, Oberholzer PA, Cazzaniga S, Hunger RE. Epithelial skin cancers after kidney transplantation: a retrospective single-Centre study of 376 recipients. Eur J Dermatol. 2016;26(3):265–70.

84. Hojo M, Morimoto T, Maluccio M, Asano T, Morimoto K, Lagman M, et al. Cyclosporine induces cancer progression by a cell-autonomous mechanism. Nature. 1999;397(6719):530–4.

85. Wheless L, Jacks S, Mooneyham Potter KA, Leach BC, Cook J. Skin cancer in organ transplant recipients: more than the immune system. J Am Acad Dermatol. 2014;71(2):359–65.

86. Geissler EK, Schlitt HJ. The potential benefits of rapamycin on renal function, tolerance, fibrosis, and malignancy following transplantation. Kidney Int. 2010;78(11):1075–9.

87. Salgo R, Gossmann J, Schofer H, Kachel HG, Kuck J, Geiger H, et al. Switch to a sirolimus-based immunosuppression in long-term renal transplant recipients: reduced rate of (pre-)malignancies and nonmelanoma skin cancer in a prospective, randomized, assessor-blinded, controlled clinical trial. Am J Transplant. 2010;10(6):1385–93.

88. Preterre J, Visentin J, Saint Cricq M, Kaminski H, Del Bello A, Prezelin-Reydit M, et al. Comparison of two strategies based on mammalian target of rapamycin inhibitors in secondary prevention of non-melanoma skin cancer after kidney transplantation, a pilot study. Clin Transpl. 2021;35(3):e14207.

89. Smith CH, McGregor JM, Barker JN, Morris RW, Rigden SP, MacDonald DM. Excess melanocytic nevi in children with renal allografts. J Am Acad Dermatol. 1993;28(1):51–5.

90. Dreno B. Skin cancers after transplantation. Nephrol Dial Transplant. 2003;18(6):1052–8.

91. Zvulunov A, Wyatt DT, Laud PW, Esterly NB. Lack of effect of growth hormone therapy on the count and density of melanocytic naevi in children. Br J Dermatol. 1997;137(4):545–8.

92. Jensen P, Hansen S, Moller B, Leivestad T, Pfeffer P, Geiran O, et al. Skin cancer in kidney and heart transplant recipients and different long-term immunosuppressive therapy regimens. J Am Acad Dermatol. 1999;40(2 Pt 1):177–86.

93. Bonthuis M, Busutti M, van Stralen KJ, Jager KJ, Baiko S, Bakkaloglu S, et al. Mineral metabolism in European children living with a renal transplant: a European society for paediatric nephrology/european renal association-European dialysis and transplant association registry study. Clin J Am Soc Nephrol. 2015;10(5):767–75.

94. Krajewski PK, Krajewska M, Szepietowski JC. Pruritus in renal transplant recipients: current state of knowledge. Adv Clin Exp Med. 2020;29(6):769–72.

95. Brouhard BH, Donaldson LA, Lawry KW, McGowan KR, Drotar D, Davis I, et al. Cognitive functioning in children on dialysis and post-transplantation. Pediatr Transplant. 2000;4(4):261–7.

96. Harshman LA, Johnson RJ, Matheson MB, Kogon AJ, Shinnar S, Gerson AC, et al. Academic achievement in children with chronic kidney disease: a report from the CKiD cohort. Pediatr Nephrol. 2019;34(4):689–96.

97. Chen K, Didsbury M, van Zwieten A, Howell M, Kim S, Tong A, et al. Neurocognitive and educational outcomes in children and adolescents with CKD: a systematic review and meta-analysis. Clin J Am Soc Nephrol. 2018;13(3):387–97.

98. Matsuda-Abedini M, Fitzpatrick K, Harrell WR, Gipson DS, Hooper SR, Belger A, et al. Brain abnormalities in children and adolescents with chronic kidney disease. Pediatr Res. 2018;84(3):387–92.

99. Gipson DS, Hooper SR, Duquette PJ, Wetherington CE, Stellwagen KK, Jenkins TL, et al. Memory and executive functions in pediatric chronic kidney disease. Child Neuropsychol. 2006;12(6):391–405.

100. Qvist E, Pihko H, Fagerudd P, Valanne L, Lamminranta S, Karikoski J, et al. Neurodevelopmental outcome in high-risk patients after renal transplantation in early childhood. Pediatr Transplant. 2002;6(1):53–62.

101. Broyer M, Le Bihan C, Charbit M, Guest G, Tete MJ, Gagnadoux MF, et al. Long-term social outcome of children after kidney transplantation. Transplantation. 2004;77(7):1033–7.

102. Bawden HN, Acott P, Carter J, Lirenman D, MacDonald GW, McAllister M, et al. Neuropsychological functioning in end-stage renal disease. Arch Dis Child. 2004;89(7):644–7.

103. Gipson DS, Duquette PJ, Icard PF, Hooper SR. The central nervous system in childhood chronic kidney disease. Pediatr Nephrol. 2007;22(10):1703–10.

104. Karrfelt HM, Berg UB. Long-term psychosocial outcome after renal transplantation during childhood. Pediatr Transplant. 2008;12(5):557–62.

105. Johnson RJ, Warady BA. Long-term neurocognitive outcomes of patients with end-stage renal disease during infancy. Pediatr Nephrol. 2013;28(8):1283–91.

106. Hooper SR, Gerson AC, Butler RW, Gipson DS, Mendley SR, Lande MB, et al. Neurocognitive functioning of children and adolescents with mild-to-moderate chronic kidney disease. Clin J Am Soc Nephrol. 2011;6(8):1824–30.

107. Lande MB, Gerson AC, Hooper SR, Cox C, Matheson M, Mendley SR, et al. Casual blood pressure and neurocognitive function in children with chronic kidney disease: a report of the children with chronic kidney disease cohort study. Clin J Am Soc Nephrol. 2011;6(8):1831–7.

108. Wong CJ, Moxey-Mims M, Jerry-Fluker J, Warady BA, Furth SL. CKiD (CKD in children) prospective cohort study: a review of current findings. Am J Kidney Dis. 2012;60(6):1002–11.

109. Tozzi AE, Mazzotti E, Di Ciommo VM, Dello Strologo L, Cuttini M. Quality of life in a cohort of patients diagnosed with renal failure in childhood and who received renal transplant. Pediatr Transplant. 2012;16(8):840–5.

110. Fujisawa M, Ichikawa Y, Yoshiya K, Isotani S, Higuchi A, Nagano S, et al. Assessment of health-related quality of life in renal transplant and hemodialysis patients using the SF-36 health survey. Urology. 2000;56(2):201–6.

111. Jofre R, Lopez-Gomez JM, Moreno F, Sanz-Guajardo D, Valderrabano F. Changes in quality of life after renal transplantation. Am J Kidney Dis. 1998;32(1):93–100.

112. Rebollo P, Ortega F, Baltar JM, Alvarez-Ude F, Alvarez Navascues R, Alvarez-Grande J. Is the loss of health-related quality of life during renal replacement therapy lower in elderly patients than in younger patients? Nephrol Dial Transplant. 2001;16(8):1675–80.

113. Manu MA, Radulescu S, Harza M, Manu R, Capsa D, Sinescu I. Quality of life assessed by SF-36 health survey in renal transplant patients. Transplant Proc. 2001;33(1–2):1927–8.

114. Bailey PK, Hamilton AJ, Clissold RL, Inward CD, Caskey FJ, Ben-Shlomo Y, et al. Young adults' perspectives on living with kidney failure: a systematic review and thematic synthesis of qualitative studies. BMJ Open. 2018;8(1):e019926.

115. Merkus MP, Jager KJ, Dekker FW, Boeschoten EW, Stevens P, Krediet RT. Quality of life in patients on chronic dialysis: self-assessment 3 months after the start of treatment. The Necosad study group. Am J Kidney Dis. 1997;29(4):584–92.

116. Merkus MP, Jager KJ, Dekker FW, De Haan RJ, Boeschoten EW, Krediet RT. Quality of life over time in dialysis: the Netherlands cooperative study on the adequacy of dialysis. NECOSAD Study Group. Kidney Int. 1999;56(2):720–8.

117. Neto JF, Ferraz MB, Cendoroglo M, Draibe S, Yu L, Sesso R. Quality of life at the initiation of maintenance dialysis treatment—a comparison between the SF-36 and the KDQ questionnaires. Qual Life Res. 2000;9(1):101–7.

118. Gee L, Abbott J, Conway SP, Etherington C, Webb AK. Validation of the SF-36 for the assessment of quality of life in adolescents and adults with cystic fibrosis. J Cyst Fibros. 2002;1(3):137–45.

119. McClish DK, Penberthy LT, Bovbjerg VE, Roberts JD, Aisiku IP, Levenson JL, et al. Health related quality of life in sickle cell patients: the PiSCES project. Health Qual Life Outcomes. 2005;3:50.

120. Lee TA, Hollingworth W, Sullivan SD. Comparison of directly elicited preferences to preferences derived from the SF-36 in adults with asthma. Med Decis Mak. 2003;23(4):323–34.

121. Carr AJ, Gibson B, Robinson PG. Measuring quality of life: is quality of life determined by expectations or experience? BMJ. 2001;322(7296):1240–3.

122. Haavisto A, Korkman M, Sintonen H, Holmberg C, Jalanko H, Lipsanen J, et al. Risk factors for impaired quality of life and psychosocial adjustment after pediatric heart, kidney, and liver transplantation. Pediatr Transplant. 2013;17(3):256–65.

123. Haavisto A, Jalanko H, Sintonen H, Holmberg C, Qvist E. Quality of life in adult survivors of pediatric kidney transplantation. Transplantation. 2011;92(12):1322–6.

124. Hathaway DK, Winsett RP, Johnson C, Tolley EA, Hartwig M, Milstead J, et al. Post kidney transplant quality of life prediction models. Clin Transpl. 1998;12(3):168–74.

125. Splinter A, Tjaden LA, Haverman L, Adams B, Collard L, Cransberg K, et al. Children on dialysis as well as renal transplanted children report severely impaired health-related quality of life. Qual Life Res. 2018;27(6):1445–54.

126. Tjaden LA, Vogelzang J, Jager KJ, van Stralen KJ, Maurice-Stam H, Grootenhuis MA, et al. Long-term quality of life and social outcome of childhood end-stage renal disease. J Pediatr. 2014;165(2):336–42 e1.

127. Puma L, Doyle M. Long-term psychosocial outcomes of adults transplanted in childhood: a social work perspective. Pediatr Transplant. 2021;25(1):e13859.

128. Groothoff JW, Grootenhuis MA, Offringa M, Stronks K, Hutten GJ, Heymans HS. Social consequences in adult life of end-stage renal disease in childhood. J Pediatr. 2005;146(4):512–7.

129. Tjaden LA, Maurice-Stam H, Grootenhuis MA, Jager KJ, Groothoff JW. Impact of renal replacement therapy in childhood on long-term socioprofessional outcomes: a 30-year follow-up study. J Pediatr. 2016;171(189–95):e1–2.

130. Mellerio H, Alberti C, Labeguerie M, Andriss B, Savoye E, Lassalle M, et al. Adult social and professional outcomes of pediatric renal transplant recipients. Transplantation. 2014;97(2):196–205.

131. Rees L, Shroff R, Hutchinson C, Fernando ON, Trompeter RS. Long-term outcome of paediatric renal transplantation: follow-up of 300 children from 1973 to 2000. Nephron Clin Pract. 2007;105(2):c68–76.

132. Morel P, Almond PS, Matas AJ, Gillingham KJ, Chau C, Brown A, et al. Long-term quality of life after kidney transplantation in childhood. Transplantation. 1991;52(1):47–53.

Part XIV

Drugs and Toxins

Drug Use, Dosing, and Toxicity in Kidney Disease

71

Matthias Schwab, Simon U. Jaeger, and Guido Filler

Abbreviations

ABC	ATP binding cassette
AIN	Acute interstitial nephritis
ATN	Acute tubular necrosis
BSA	Body surface area
CL	Clearance
GFR	Glomerular filtration rate
LSS	Limited sampling strategy
MATE1	Multidrug and toxin extrusion protein 1
MDR	Multidrug resistance
MRP	Multidrug resistance-associated proteins
OAT1	Organic anion transporter 1
OAT3	Organic anion transporter 3
OATs	Organic anion transporters and organic cation transporters
OCTs	Organic cation transporters
PAH	Paraminohippuric
SCr	Serum creatinine
SLC	Solute carrier

M. Schwab (✉) · S. U. Jaeger
Dr. Margarete Fischer-Bosch Institute of Clinical Pharmacology, Stuttgart, Germany

Division of Clinical Pharmacology, University Hospital Tuebingen, Tuebingen, Germany
e-mail: matthias.schwab@ikp-stuttgart.de;
simon.jaeger@ikp-stuttgart.de;
simon.jaeger@med.uni-tuebingen.de

G. Filler
Departments of Pediatrics, Medicine, and Pathology and Laboratory Medicine, University of Western Ontario, London, ON, Canada
e-mail: guido.filler@lhsc.on.ca

Introduction

The interplay between xenobiotics (including most drugs) and the living organism (in this context the patient) is traditionally viewed from two perspectives, and this chapter is organized along them:

- How does the organism (patient) affect the drug? *Pharmacokinetics* or *drug disposition* are the terms used to describe the body's handling of drugs. This topic includes drug dosing in kidney disease and it will be discussed in the section "Drug Handling by the Kidneys: Principles of Pharmacokinetics/Drug Disposition."
- How does the drug affect the organism (patient)? *Pharmacodynamics* describe the drug's effects, i.e., both desired (therapeutic) and unwanted (adverse) effects. This topic includes most aspects of nephrotoxicity, and it will be discussed in the section "Drug Injury to the Kidney: Nephrotoxicity."

© The Author(s), under exclusive license to Springer Nature Switzerland AG 2023
F. Schaefer, L. A. Greenbaum (eds.), *Pediatric Kidney Disease*,
https://doi.org/10.1007/978-3-031-11665-0_71

Drug Handling by the Kidneys: Principles of Pharmacokinetics/ Drug Disposition

Generally, the effects of drugs depend on the concentration at the site of action. The concentration is a result of the way and speed at which the body deals with the drug.

Obviously, drug handling by the organism is time-dependent and quantitative. This is why numbers are useful to describe a drug's pharmacokinetic features and why equations provide the most appropriate tools to describe the underlying processes [1].

Drug handling by the organism includes processes that are usually encompassed by the LADME acronym—*l*iberation, *a*bsorption, *d*istribution, *m*etabolism, and *e*xcretion. While liberation, absorption and distribution are rarely critical for individual variation of pharmacokinetics, elimination is the central process that, with repeated administration of drugs at steady state, determines the relationship between dose (D) and concentration (C$_{ss}$).

Clearance is the best parameter to describe the body's overall capacity of eliminating a specific xenobiotic. Clearance is defined as the volume (usually plasma) that is cleared of the compound within a particular period of time. The usual units of expression are liter per hour (L/h) or milliliter per minute (ml/min).

$$\frac{D \cdot F}{\tau} = C^{ss} \cdot Cl \qquad (71.1)$$

- D = dose
- F = bioavailability
- τ = dose interval

- C$_{ss}$ = concentration at steady state
- Cl = clearance

Clearance determines the maintenance dose rate required to achieve a target plasma concentration of a drug, and therefore its effect, at steady state.

As a consequence, dose reduction is required to avoid toxic concentrations (C^{ss}) in individuals and situations with impaired clearance (Eq. 71.1). For the selection of the dose that is appropriate for a specific patient, it is important to consider by which route the drug leaves the body and whether or not that particular organ works properly.

The bile and the urine provide aqueous environments for xenobiotics to leave the body from systemic circulation. Xenobiotics need to be water-soluble to take these routes. It is the biological purpose of metabolism, predominantly in the liver, by chemical alteration to facilitate water solubility of xenobiotics. While the majority of drugs first undergo hepatic metabolism, some other drugs, which are water-soluble by themselves, skip metabolism and are excreted unchanged via the bile or urine. Xenobiotics with a molecular weight of less than 400 to 500 g/mol undergo excretion via the kidneys [2–4]. Larger molecules prefer the biliary route for excretion.

While the liver is important for both metabolism and biliary excretion, the kidneys are essential for excretion and thus have a predominant role in disposing xenobiotics. Most drugs, before leaving the body by the kidney route, undergo metabolism. In fact, some drugs (e.g., allopurinol, morphine, meperidine) have active metabolites which are cleared by the kidney.

Kidney drug clearance is the net result of three processes, i.e., glomerular filtration, tubular secretion, and tubular reabsorption (Eq. 71.2).

$$\text{Renal clearance} = \text{glomerular filtration} + \text{tubular secretion} - \text{tubular reabsorption} \qquad (71.2)$$

Glomerular Filtration of Drugs

The extent of a drug's glomerular filtration depends heavily on its binding to plasma proteins. The proteins that are relevant for drug binding, i.e., albumin and α1-glycoprotein, do not cross the glomerular membrane unless the patient is nephrotic. Thus, the protein-bound component cannot be filtered, and only the free fraction (f_u, fraction unbound) undergoes glomerular filtration. Beyond this, functional integrity of the glomeruli, the drug's molecular size, and kidney plasma flow (which is a marker of nephron endowment) determine glomerular filtration.

Glomerular filtration rate (GFR) and Cl are equal for drugs that are not bound to proteins and do not undergo secretion and reabsorption (Eq. 71.2). Inulin is an example of an exogenous substance without plasma protein binding; assessment of its clearance is the gold standard of measuring GFR [5].

For drugs and drug metabolites primarily eliminated by glomerular filtration, drug elimination declines as kidney function decreases and drug will accumulate if the dosing regimen is not adjusted. There are not many drugs that are subject to exclusive glomerular filtration; most drugs are actually excreted through active tubular transport.

Tubular Secretion of Drugs

As outlined above, most drugs excreted by the kidneys are eliminated by active tubular transport. Organic anion transporters (OATs) and organic cation transporters (OCTs) have an important role in the excretion of drugs. They are members of the solute carrier (SLC) transporter family. The energy required for the transport is provided by a gradient of the drug to be transported or by a co-transported ion (e.g., sodium).

In addition to OATs and OCTs, ATP binding cassette (ABC) transporters are important. Hydrolysis of ATP provides the energy. ABC transporters that are important for the renal elimination of drugs are some multidrug resistance (MDR) proteins, i.e., MDR1 (ABC1), multidrug resistance-associated proteins (MRP), i.e., MRP2 (ABCC2), MRP4 (ABCC4) and MRP5 (ABCC5), and BCRP (ABCG2). Figure 71.1 gives an overview of the localization of SLC transporters in human proximal tubule epithelial cells.

The active kidney tubular secretion of drugs and drug metabolites by relatively nonspecific anionic and cationic transport systems in the proximal tubule contribute substantially to the amount of drug eliminated by the kidney. The tubular secretion of basic and acidic drug molecules involves three steps:

1. *Drug uptake from blood by transporters in the basolateral membrane*

   At least two systems perform the basolateral uptake of organic acids into the tubular cell, a Na^+-dependent (linked to Na^+/α-ketoglutarate co-transport and subsequent exchange of α-ketoglutarate with organic anions by OAT1) and a Na^+-independent anion transporter. The basolateral uptake of organic cations with primary, secondary, tertiary, or quaternary amine structure is mediated by OCTs and depends on membrane potential. OCT2 is responsible for the uptake of numerous drugs such as cimetidine, famotidine, ranitidine, metformin, and cisplatin.

2. *Drug diffusion through the cytosol*

3. *Drug transport into the lumen by transporters in the brush-border membrane*

   The efflux of organic acids is performed by OATs such as OAT4. Two organic cation antiporters, OCTN1/2 (organic cation transporter novel), organize the efflux of organic cations. OCTN2 physiologically mediates the reabsorption of L-carnitine and thus organizes the homeostasis of the kidney carnitine pool. MDR1, localized in the luminal membrane of the proximal tubule, is involved in the secretion of lipophilic basic and neutral drugs (e.g., anthracyclines, vinca alkaloids, taxanes, quinidine, and digoxin). Other ABC transporters, such as MRP2 and MRP4, transport glucuronides. Interactions by competition may occur with the simultaneous administration of drugs which are substrates of these transporters.

Fig. 71.1 Localization of solute carrier transporters in human proximal tubular epithelial cells implicated in drug-related nephrotoxicity. Representative immunofluorescence pictures show localization of organic cation transporter 2 in the basolateral membrane and *MATE1* in the luminal membrane of proximal tubule epithelial cells in cryosections from human kidney. *Cl* – chloride, *MATE1* multidrug and toxin extrusion proteins 1, *OA* – organic anion, *OC* + organic cation, *UC* uncharged compound, *ZI* zwitterion, *α-KG2* α-ketoglutarate. (Modified from Fisel et al. [6])

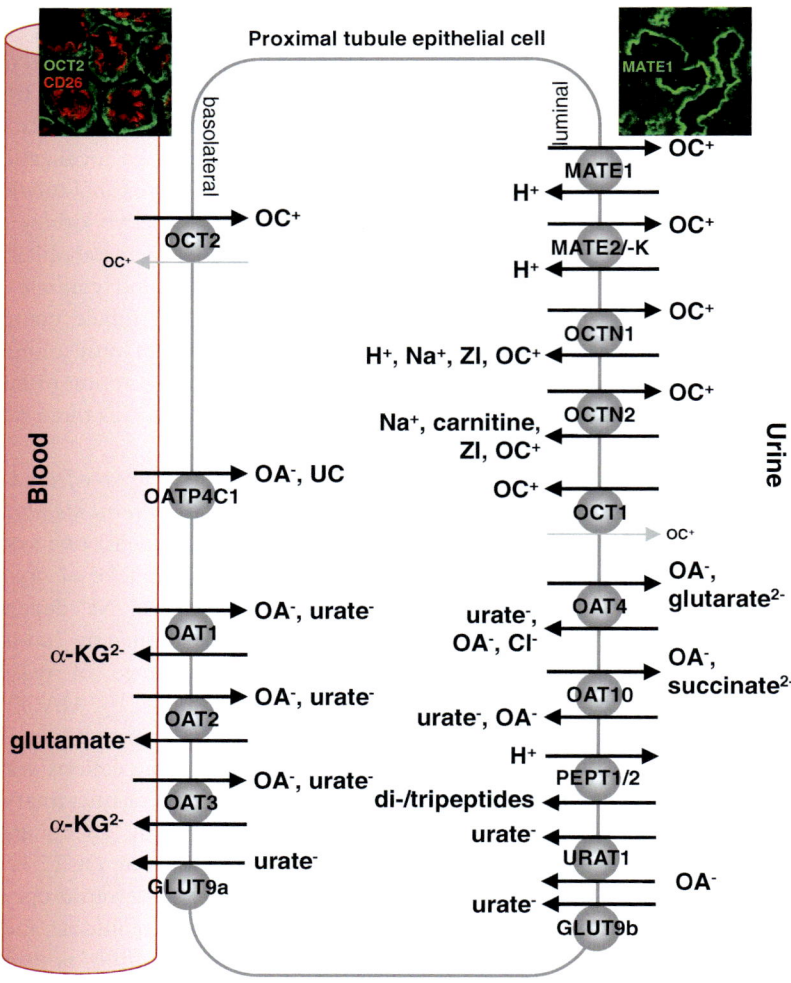

Thus, cimetidine, by inhibiting the OCT2-mediated uptake of cisplatin into tubular cells, reduces its nephrotoxicity. This transport system is an elimination pathway for many drugs such as penicillins. For instance, probenecid competitively inhibits the tubular secretion of organic anions such as penicillins. In consequence, plasma levels of weak organic acids such as penicillins will increase.

Tubular Reabsorption of Drugs

As the filtered urine becomes increasingly concentrated in the proximal tubule, a concentration gradient towards the intercellular space and vas-cular lumen develops. As a result, lipophilic compounds are reabsorbed to a larger degree.

Reabsorption is the passive diffusion of non-ionized (non-charged) drug from the filtrate into the kidney tubular cell. Reabsorption of acids and bases depends on their pK_a and urinary pH. Basic urine (e.g., urine pH > 7.5) favors the ionized form of acidic drugs and limits their reabsorption, whereas reabsorption of basic drugs is enhanced in basic urine because the nonionized form of the drug is favored. Alteration of urinary pH thus affects the renal clearance of acidic and basic drugs because predominance of ionized drug reduces their tubular reabsorption. This intervention, together with increasing urinary flow ("forced diuresis"), has been used in the past to treat intoxications. With hemodialysis and hemofiltration, safer and more effective methods of elimination are available now.

Kidney Failure Induced Alterations in Drug Disposition

Kidney dysfunction affects the disposition of renally cleared drugs. The clinical significance of decreased kidney function on a drug dosing regimen is a function of:

- the therapeutic index (TI), i.e. the amount of a therapeutic agent that causes the therapeutic effect relative to the amount that causes toxicity. The TI varies widely among drugs. Drugs with a high TI such as penicillins have a wide therapeutic window, have less side effects and are considered to be less toxic. Drugs with a low therapeutic index such as aminoglycosides or vancomycin require therapeutic drug monitoring to achieve plasma concentrations in the therapeutic window and limit toxicity and adverse effects of the drug.
- the percentage of total drug elimination that is due to renal clearance. E.g., the angiotensin converting enzyme inhibitor fosinopril is subject to both kidney and liver clearance and will not accumulate in kidney failure, whereas Enalapril is exclusively cleared by the kidneys and will accumulate with worsening kidney function [7].
- the degree of kidney failure.

The most difficult task is obtaining an accurate assessment of kidney function, e.g., GFR [5]. The GFR is estimated by measuring the rate at which the kidney removes a substance from the blood (e.g., kidney clearance). Endogenous compounds (e.g., creatinine, cystatin C) [5, 8], exogenous compounds that are specifically administered to measure the GFR (e.g., inulin), or compounds primarily eliminated by glomerular filtration that are administered as part of clinical care (e.g., gentamicin or vancomycin) are used for measurement.

Age-Related Development of Kidney Function

The developmental increase in GFR involves active nephrogenesis, a process that begins at 9 weeks and is complete by 36 weeks of gestation, followed by postnatal changes in blood flow, both to the kidney and inside the kidney [9, 10] (Fig. 71.2). In the postnatal period, the mean arterial pressure increases, consequently altering the glomerular hydraulic pressure and increasing the GFR. When GFR is indexed to body surface area, GFR increases rapidly after birth in term neonates from 10 to 15 ml/min/1.73 m^2 in the first days of life to values of 90–110 ml/min/1.73 m^2 at the age of 12–18 months [2, 3]. In preterm infants GFR rises more slowly and reaches adult values only by 2 years of age [11, 12].

Similarly, to the above-mentioned factors, tubular secretory pathways are immature at birth and gain full capacity during the first year of life [14]. In preterm neonates sodium excretion for example is inversely correlated to gestational age, mostly due to tubular immaturity [15]. Also, loss of bicarbonate and glucose may necessitate supplementation in preterm neonates. Other tubular functions are impaired such as organic cation transporters (OAT); these have been reported to mature functionally over the first weeks of life and reach adult levels around 7–8 months post-partum. For example, para-amino hippurate (PAH), a substrate of OAT1, is used as a marker for blood flow as the tubular secretion is approximately 100% at first pass through the nephron. PAH is therefore used to test for drug-induced inhibition of OAT1 that would lead to a reduced uptake of PAH. The expression of the luminal drug transporter P-glycoprotein changes significantly during maturation, as illustrated by the threefold difference in digoxin dosing between children and adults. Of note, the inter-individual variation in tubular maturation seems to be much greater than the variations seen in GFR maturation. As these tubular transport mechanisms play an important role in drug excretion, preterm birth can be expected to have an impact on kidney drug handling, although different mechanisms are impor-

Fig. 71.2 Summary of the effect of postnatal development on the processes of active tubular secretion— represented by the clearance of para-aminohippuric acid and the glomerular filtration rate, both of which approximate adult activity by 6–12 months of age. (From Kearns et al. [13])

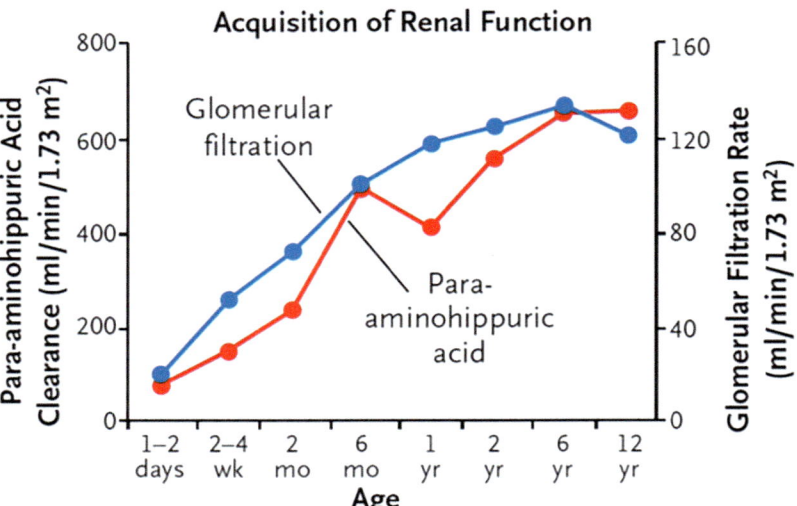

Dialysis

The impact of dialysis on drug disposition is determined largely by the extent of drug removal by the dialysis procedure. During dialysis, drug clearance is a composite of ongoing drug removal by kidney, hepatic, and other intrinsic clearance pathways and the additional clearance provided by dialysis.

The physicochemical properties of a drug such as molecular size, protein binding, and volume of distribution largely determine its dialyzability [16, 17]. Additional factors specific to the dialysis prescription such as the type of dialyzer and blood/dialysate flow rates can also impact drug removal.

In general, drug removal is considered clinically significant when >25% of the administered dose is removed by dialysis. Only a drug present within the systemic circulation in the unbound form is available for removal by dialysis. Uremic solutes that accumulate in CKD are known to increase the free fraction of some drugs, making them more easily dialyzable.

High-flux dialyzers can remove drugs with molecular weights of up to 40,000 Da. Failure to recognize the extent of dialytic drug removal and provide supplemental dosing is needed can result in underdosing and therapeutic compromise. For instance, vancomycin (~1450 Da) is cleared minimally with conventional low-flux dialysis but is extensively removed by high-flux dialyzers (dialytic clearance between 45–131 ml/min with high-flux polysulfone dialysis membranes) [18, 19]. Other drugs that exhibit the same characteristic include carbamazepine, cisplatin, daptomycin, fluorouracil, ranitidine, and valproic acid.

Drugs cannot be directly removed from tissue stores but must be redistributed from the tissue sites into the vascular space to be available for elimination by any dialysis procedure. Drugs that have a small V_d (e.g. <0.7 L/kg) are generally restricted to the blood compartment and therefore more accessible for removal during dialysis. In contrast, drugs with a large V_d are distributed into the tissues and are generally minimally impacted by dialysis. Although drug usually moves from the blood compartment to dialysis fluid, drug can also be absorbed from the dialysis fluid into the blood compartment when the dialysis fluid drug concentration exceeds the serum concentration. The bidirectional movement of drugs is exploited for the antibiotic treatment of peritonitis in patients on peritoneal dialysis where therapeutic blood concentrations can be achieved by intra-peritoneal administration.

Drugs with a large V_d are also more susceptible to the rebound effect following dialysis.

Examples of drugs with a substantial rebound effect include gentamicin and vancomycin. Gentamicin concentrations rebound by up to 25% several hours following the completion of a dialysis session [20]. Vancomycin exhibits a similar rebound as plasma concentrations decrease by 38% immediately following dialysis but are only 16% lower than the pre-dialysis concentration 5 h post-dialysis [21].

The efficiency of drug removal is greatest for hemodialysis, followed by continuous kidney replacement therapies (CKRTs), and least by peritoneal dialysis. Although drug removal by CKRT and peritoneal dialysis is less efficient than hemodialysis, the total drug removal may be equivalent because CKRT and peritoneal dialysis are performed for a longer period of time.

Guidelines for Drug Dosing in Children with Kidney Failure

The optimal drug prescription for a child with kidney failure considers the multiple factors impacting drug disposition and response and is best achieved by using an individualized approach. Although drug lists and dosing tables can be helpful to identify those drugs that require attention in children with kidney failure (Table 71.1), such guidelines fall short when it comes to providing dosing recommendations because optimal therapy must be individualized according to the degree of kidney failure, concurrent medications, and developmental factors—all

of which can impact the disposition of a drug. Table 71.1 should be interpreted with caution since systematic clinical data from trials in children of different age groups and across wide GFR ranges are still limited.

Thus, the provision of safe and effective therapy in children with kidney failure is best accomplished using an individualized systematic approach (Fig. 71.3). The design of a successful therapeutic regimen begins with an estimate of the child's residual kidney function and an estimate of the relative contribution of kidney elimination to the total drug elimination obtained from the literature. Reference books such as the *Pediatric Drug Handbook*, *Physicians' Desk Reference*, and *Micromedex* are excellent sources for information on drug disposition—and most references are available as electronic documents that can be used on hand-held devices for point-of-care therapeutic decisions.

Although children receiving dialysis by definition have very poor kidney function, it is inappropriate to assume that there is no kidney elimination because many children maintain a significant amount of residual kidney function. Failure to account for the continued kidney elimination of drug may result in insufficient drug dosing and therapeutic failure. If one assumes that drug protein binding, distribution, and metabolism are not altered to a clinically significant degree in kidney failure (an assumption likely true for most drugs), a dosing adjustment factor Q can be estimated using the following equation (Eq. 71.3):

$$Q = 1 - \left[\text{fraction renal elimination} \cdot \left(1 - \frac{\text{child's Cl}_{cr}}{\text{normal Cl}_{cr}} \right) \right] \qquad (71.3)$$

- Cl_{cr} = creatinine clearance [ml/min/1.73 m^2]

The appropriate dose amount or dosing interval for a child with reduced kidney function is generated by applying the dosing adjustment factor Q to either the normal dose amount (Q × normal dose = adjusted dose) or normal dosing interval (normal dosing interval ÷ Q = adjusted dosing

interval). The dosage adjustment factor estimates the change that occurs in elimination associated with kidney failure but does not account for any additional clearance by dialysis. If appropriate, supplemental doses may be required to replace the dialysis-related drug losses.

Whether a change is made in the dose amount or dosing interval depends on the therapeutic goal

Table 71.1 Drug dosing guidelines for common therapeutic agents according to Filler et al. [22]

Drugs	Normal DOSE/day Not to exceed adult dose	Dose at GFR 50–30	Dose at GFR 30–10	Dose at GFR < 10	MW	Plasma protein binding	%eliminated by kidney	Elimination t½ with normal GFR
Aminoglycosides								
Amikacin	15–22.5 mg/kg div Q8 h	Q12–18 h	Q18–24 h	Q48–72 h	585.6	<11%	>95	2–3 h
Gentamicin	6–7.5 mg/kg div Q8 h	Q12–18 h	Q18–24 h	Q48–72 h	477.6	<30%	>95	5–>100 h
Tobramycin	6–7.5 mg/kg div Q8 h	Q12–18 h	Q18–24 h	Q48–72 h	467.5	<30%	>95	2–3 h
Carbapenems								
Imipenem + cilastin	60–100 mg/kg div Q6 h	7–13 mg/kg/dose Q8 h	7.5–12.5 mg/kg/dose Q12 h	7.5–12.5 mg/kg/dose Q24 h	Imipenem: 299.3	Imipenem 13–21% cilastin 40%	70	1 h
Meropenem	30–100 mg/kg div Q8 h	20–40 mg/kg/dose Q12 h	10–20 mg/kg/dose Q12 h	10–20 mg/kg/dose Q24 h	383.5	2%	70	1 h
Cephalosporins								
Cefaclor	20–40 mg/kg div Q8–12 h	Normal	Normal	50% dose	367.8	25%	80	40 min
Cephalexin	25–100 mg/kg div Q6–8 h	Normal	Q8–12 h	Q12–24 h	347.4	10.60%	~100	1–1.5 h
Cefazolin	50–150 mg/kg div Q8 h	60%, Q12 h	25%, Q12 h	10%, Q24 h	454.5	74–86%	80–100	2 h
Cefixime	8 mg/kg div Q12–24 h	75%	75%	50%	453.4	76–91%	20–35	3–4 h
Cefotaxime	100–200 mg/kg div Q6–8 h	35–70 mg/kg, Q8–12 h	35–70 mg/kg, Q12 h	35–70 mg/kg, Q24 h	619.6	31–50%	80	1.4–1.9 h
Cefotiam	50–100 mg/kg	50 mg/kg Q12 h	50 mg/kg Q24 h	50 mg/kg Q48 h	525.6	76–91%	80	0.9–1.2 h
Ceftazidime	100–150 mg/kg div Q8 h				546.6	17%	80–90	1.8–2.2 h
Ceftriaxone	50–100 mg/kg Q24 h	Normal	Normal	Normal	554.6	85–95%	67	6–9 h
Cefuroxime	75–150 mg/kg div Q8 h	Normal	Normal dose Q8–12 h	Normal, Q24 h	424.4	33–50%	95	1–1.5 h

Drugs	Normal DOSE/day Not to exceed adult dose	Dose at GFR 50–30	Dose at GFR 30–10	Dose at GFR < 10	MW	Plasma protein binding	%eliminated by kidney	Elimination t½ with normal GFR
Cefuroxime axetil	20–30 mg/kg div Q12 h	Normal	Normal dose Q24 h	Normal Q48 h	510.5	33–50%	95	1–1.5 h
Glycopeptides								
Teicoplanin	10 mg/kg/dose Q12 h × 3 then 3–10 mg/kg Q24 h	50% ?	Avoid ?	Avoid ?	1893.7	71.9–80.5%, higher in older children	42–58	21–58 h
Vancomycin	40–60 mg/kg div Q6 h	10 mg/kg Q12 h	Q18–24 h	Single dose of 10 mg/kg, then follow levels	1449.3	55%	80–90	4–11 h
Ciprofloxacin	20–30 mg/kg div Q12 h	Normal	Q18 h	Q24 h	331.3	16–43%	30–50	3–5 h
Macrolides								
Azithromycin	10 mg/kg × 1 day, then 5 mg/kg Q24 h × 4 days	Normal	Normal	Normal	749	7–51%	6	54.5 h
Clarithromycin	15 mg/kg div Q12 h	Normal	8 mg/kg Q12 h	4 mg/kg Q24 h	748	42–70%	20–40	3–7 h
Erythromycin	30–50 mg/kg PO div Q6–8 h	Normal	Normal	50–75% Q6–8 h	734	73–81%	2–5	1.5–2 h
Nitroimidazoles								
Metronidazole	30 mg/kg div Q6–8 h	Normal	Normal	4 mg/kg/dose Q8 h	171.2	<20%	60–80	6–14
Penicillins								
Amoxicillin	20–50 mg/kg div Q8 h	Normal	8–20 mg/kg/dose Q12 h	8–20 mg/kg/dose Q24 h	365.4	17–20%	60	1–2 h
Amoxicillin + clavulanic acid (dosed by amoxicillin component)	Variable, dependent on formulation 25–50 mg/kg div Q8 h	Normal	8–20 mg/kg/ dose Q12 h	8–20 mg/kg/dose Q24 h	602.7	Amoxicillin 17–20% Clavulanate 25%	Amoxicillin 50–70 Clavulanate 25–40	1–1.5 h
Ampicillin	50–400 mg/kg div Q6 h	Normal	Q8–12 h	Q12–24 h	349.4	10–18%	90	1–1.8 h

(continued)

Table 71.1 (continued)

Drugs	Normal DOSE/day Not to exceed adult dose	Dose at GFR 50–30	Dose at GFR 30–10	Dose at GFR < 10	MW	Plasma protein binding	% eliminated by kidney	Elimination t½ with normal GFR
Other antibiotics								
Clindamycin	PO 20–40 mg/kg div Q6–8 h	Normal	Normal	Normal	425	60–95%	10	2–3 h
Doxycycline	2–4 mg/kg div Q12–24 h	Normal	Normal	Normal	444.4	80–85%	23	12–15 h
Trimethoprim/ sulfamethoxazole TMP/SMZ Dosed by TMP component	Variable PO 6–12 mg/kg div Q12 h	Normal	GFR15–30 50% dose	GFR < 15 avoid	543.6	TMP 44% SMX 70%	TMP IV 17–42.4 TMP PO 66.8 SMX IV 7–12.7 SMX PO 30	TMP 4–8 h/ SMX 9–12 h
Nitrofurantoin	5–7 mg/kg div Q6 h	Avoid	Contrain-dicated	Contrain-dicated	238.2	~40–60%	40	0.3–1 h
Antifungal agents								
Amphotericin B	0.25–1.5 mg/kg Q24 h	Normal	Normal	Q24–36 h	924.1	90%	2–5	12–40 h
Fluconazole	3–12 mg/kg Q24 h	50%	50%	50%	306.3	11–12%	80	15–25 h
Itraconazole	5–10 mg/kg div Q12–24 h	Normal	Normal	50%	705.6	99%	0	Parent: 36/ metabolite: 18
Antituberculosis agents								
Ethambutol	PO 15–25 mg/kg Q24 h	Normal	Q24–36 h	Q48 h	204.3	20–30%	50	2.5–3.6 h
Isoniazid	10–15 mg/kg Q24 h	Normal	Normal (use with caution)	Normal (use with caution)	137.1	10–15%	75–95	2.3–4.9 h
Pyrazinamide	15–30 mg/kg Q24 h	Normal	Normal	50–100%	123.1	50%	4	6.7 h
Rifampin	10–20 mg/kg div Q12–24 h	Normal	Normal	Normal	822.9	80%	Up to 30%	3–5 h
Antivirals								
Acyclovir	30–60 mg/kg div Q8 h	Normal dose Q12 h	Normal dose Q24 h	50% dose Q24 h	225.2	9–33	60–90	2–3 h

Drugs	Normal DOSE/day Not to exceed adult dose	Dose at GFR 50–30	Dose at GFR 30–10	Dose at GFR < 10	MW	Plasma protein binding	%eliminated by kidney	Elimination t½ with normal GFR
Ganciclovir	IV 5–10 mg/kg div Q12–24 h	50% dose Q24 h	25% dose Q24 h	25% dose 3 times week post-hemodialysis	255.2	1–2%	80–99	2.5–6.5 h
Indinavir	1050–1500 mg/m² div Q8 h	Not studied	Not studied	Not studied	613.8	60%	<20%	1.4–2.2 h
Lamivudine	8 mg/kg div BID	Normal Q24 h	50% dose Q24 h	25% dose Q24 h	229.3	<36%	70	0.5–4 h
Valacyclovir	60 mg/kg div Q8 h	Normal Q12 h	Normal Q24 h	50% dose Q24 h	324.3	13.5–17.9%	88%	1.3–2.5
Valganciclovir	Once daily using formula	Formula	Formula	Formula	354.4	1–2%	80–90%	2–7 h
Zidovudine	Varied	Normal	Normal	50% dose Q8 h	267.2	25–38%	63–95	1–2 h
Anticonvulsants								
Carbamazepine	10–30 mg/kg	Normal	Normal	75%	236.3	75–90%	1–3%	Single dose 40 h/ maintenance 36 h
Clonazepam	0.05–0.5 mg/kg	Normal	Normal	Normal	315.7	85%	Majority	23–36 h
Ethosuximide	15–40 mg/kg div Q12 h	50–75% (use with caution)	50–75% (use with caution)	No data (use with caution)	141.2	<10%	10–20	30 h
Phenobarbital	4–8 mg/kg div Q12–24 h	No data	No data	No data	232.2	35–50%	≤ 75	
Phenytoin	5 mg/kg	Normal	66%	50%	252.3	90–95%		
Sodium valproate	10–100 mg/kg (plasma levels 5–100 mg/L)	Normal	Reduce or avoid	Avoid	166.2	80–90%	~100	13–17
Antihypertensive drugs								
ACE-inhibitors								
Captopril	0.3–3.15 mg/kg	50%—Normal	25–50%	25–50%	217.3	25–30%	~65	4–5 h
Enalapril	0.1–0.3 mg/kg	25–50%	12.5–25%	6.25–12.5%	376.4	50–60%	61	35 h

(continued)

Table 71.1 (continued)

Drugs	Normal DOSE/day Not to exceed adult dose	Dose at GFR 50–30	Dose at GFR 30–10	Dose at GFR < 10	MW	Plasma protein binding	%eliminated by kidney	Elimination t½ with normal GFR
Ramipril	0.1–0.2 mg/kg Q24 h	>40 ml/min = no adjustment; <40 ml/min = 25% dose	25%	25%	416.5	73%	60	>50 h
ARB-inhibitors								
Irbesartan	75–300 mg	Normal	Normal	Normal	428.5	90%	~20	11–15 h
Losartan	0.7–1.4 mg/kg	Normal	Normal	Normal	422.9	>98%	~35	1.5–2.5 h
B-blockers								
Atenolol	0.5–2 mg/kg	Normal	50%	25%	266.3	6–16%	100	6–10 h
Bisoprolol	0.2 mg/kg	Normal	50%	Normal	325.4	30%	50	10–12 h
Carvedilol	Low-dose: 0.2–12.5 mg/kg High-dose: 0.4–25 mg/kg	Normal	Normal	Normal	406.5	>98%	~35	7 h
Metoprolol	1–6 mg/kg	No data	No data	No data	267.4	12%	~95	3–4 h(though 2–9,5 reported)
Propanolol	1–4 mg/kg div Q8–12 h	Normal	Normal	Normal	259.3	93%	<1	4–6 h
Ca-antagonists								
Amlodipine	0.1–0.5 mg/kg	Normal	Avoid	Avoid	408.9	93%	~95	10–36 (with repetitive dosing, 45)
Nifedipine	0.5–2 mg/kg	Normal	Normal	Normal	346.3	92–98%	70–80	4 h

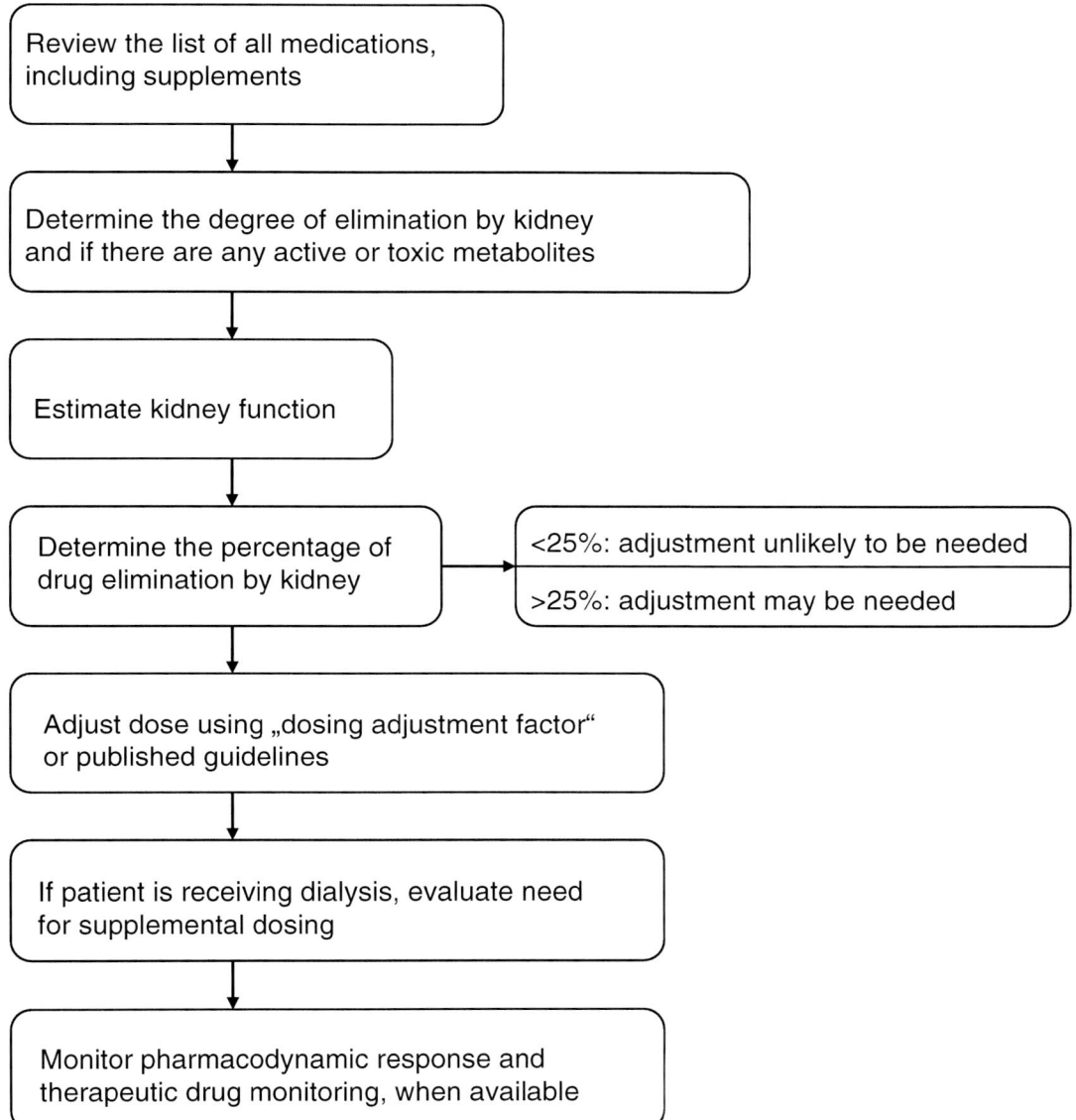

Fig. 71.3 Guidelines for drug dosing in children with kidney failure

and relationships between drug concentrations and clinical response and toxicity. In general, increasing the dosing interval will increase the variation between peak and trough blood concentration and would be most appropriate for drugs whose effects are based on achieving a certain peak drug level (e.g., aminoglycosides). In contrast, a decrease in variations between peak and trough blood concentration will be observed when a normal dosing interval is maintained but

the dose amount is decreased. This dosing adjustment would be most appropriate for drugs that should be maintained at a relatively stable blood concentration, such as cephalosporins or blood pressure medications.

Once the prescribed drug dosing schedule has been adjusted for kidney failure, a supplemental dose or dosing adjustment may be required for children receiving dialysis when >25% of a drug is removed during the dialysis procedure.

Supplemental dosing is given to replace the amount of drug removed by dialysis and may be achieved as a partial or full dose administered after hemodialysis, or an increase in the dosing amount or frequency in children receiving peritoneal dialysis or CRRT. When possible, routine maintenance drugs should be provided after hemodialysis. Guidelines for drug dosing during dialysis are available in selected references [16].

The determinants of drug disposition and action in children with kidney failure and on dialysis are frequently altered such that changes in the dosing regimens are necessary to avoid toxicity or inadequate treatment. In view of the many factors capable of altering both the disposition and action of a given drug, it is important to individualize drug therapy for the known alterations associated with age, kidney failure, and dialysis.

Therapeutic Drug Monitoring

Humans are not equal, and it is increasingly appreciated that this inequality pertains to pharmacokinetics also. Much of what carries the label "personalized medicine" is related to pharmacokinetics.

Target concentration strategy is a concept where pharmacokinetics plays a critical role. This strategy is useful as an adjunct in initiating and monitoring drug therapy when certain criteria are met. Most important is a close concentration-response relationship, which means the plasma concentration of a drug must correlate quantitatively with the intensity or probability of therapeutic or toxic effects across the patient population. The strategy becomes particularly attractive when a therapeutic endpoint is difficult to quantify, i.e., with the non-occurrence of epileptic seizures. The strategy is ideal when the aim is to maintain a therapeutic effect for which a systemic exposure within a given range is necessary. Drug administration in a constant-rate input or multiple-dose regimens is possible when the potential for organ toxicity or rejection may be predicted from the trough or peak concentration.

Multiple dosing regimens are usually based on the total body clearance such that the dosing rate is taken as the product of the clearance and the desired steady-state plasma concentration of the drug. For drugs eliminated by the kidneys, it is widely accepted that the kidney clearance is proportional to GFR [23].

For drugs with a narrow therapeutic index and poor correlations of trough levels with efficacy and adverse effects, limited sampling strategy (LSS) models have been developed to estimate the area under the concentration time curve. Ting et al. published different LSS approaches [24]. Many LSS studies utilize blood sampling within the first 4 h (C2 and C4) or the first 8 h (C1, C4, and C8) postdose with multiple regression analysis.

Drug Injury to the Kidney: Nephrotoxicity

Kidney dysfunction and toxicity secondary to medications are common, but the real incidence of drug-induced nephrotoxicity is difficult to determine. Approximately 18% of acute tubular necrosis (ATN) or acute interstitial nephritis (AIN) cases can be attributed to nephrotoxic medication. The incidence of nephrotoxic injury due to antibiotics such as aminoglycosides is even higher, up to 36% [25].

Fortunately, most episodes of drug-induced kidney injury, if diagnosed and treated early, are reversible, with *a restitution ad integrum* after cessation of the causing medication. Chronic kidney damage may occur with prolonged exposure to drugs such as analgesics and calcineurin inhibitors and will lead to chronic tubulointerstitial inflammation, papillary necrosis or prolonged proteinuria. A close follow-up is necessary to avoid kidney failure [26].

Nephrotoxic drugs require therapeutic drug monitoring (TDM) to maintain a balance between efficacy and toxicity. This is particularly important if a drug has a narrow target range, significant pharmacokinetic variability, a reasonable relationship between plasma concentration and clinical effects, an established therapeutic window, and availability of a cost-effective assay. Most places offer TDM for aminoglycosides (acute tubular necrosis), vancomycin (acute interstitial nephritis), calcineurin inhibitors (cyclosporine: acute tubular necrosis, chronic interstitial nephritis, thrombotic microangiopathy; tacrolimus: acute tubular necrosis), antifungal drugs (amphotericine: acute tubular necrosis, distal tubular renal acidosis), antiepileptic drugs (mostly not nephrotoxic), lithium (chronic interstitial nephritis, glomerulonephritis, rhabdomyolysis), and digoxin (not nephrotoxic) [27]. For some drugs like acyclovir (acute interstitial nephritis, crystal nephropathy) [28] or ganciclovir (crystal nephropathy), which should have TDM, this is not widely available. It is important not note that toxicity may be more related to the area under the time concentration curve (AUC) than the pre-dose trough level. For instance, switching from BID dosing of cyclosporine to TID dosing may substantially reduce the AUC [29]. Some other drugs may not be increasing the active drug, but rather metabolites, which then account for toxicity. An example is mycophenolic assay, where the main metabolite mycophenolic acid glucuronide (MPAG) accumulates with decreased kidney function, rendering it intolerable with low eGFR [30].

An increasing number of observational studies report on early drug-related nephrotoxicity in humans. The investigations concern nephrotoxicity from antibiotics (particularly aminoglycosides), angiotensin-converting enzyme (ACE) inhibitors, non-steroidal anti-inflammatory drugs and antifungal agents [31]. Also, there is growing interest in the long-term effects of drugs on the neonatal kidney. A recent up-to-date summary of nephrotoxic drugs with particular impact on children highlighted additional underlying pathophysiological mechanisms [32]. Figure 71.4 summarises the clinically relevant information. In the following paragraph we describe selected mechanisms of drug nephrotoxiciy and include some examples of nephrotoxic drugs.

Regarding toxic effects on nephrogenesis drugs administered to pregnant women and to neonates born preterm may influence kidney development. Nephrogenesis ceases at approximately 36 weeks gestation in humans so that most toxic effects on nephrogenesis may be expected in treatment with drugs during pregnancy. In premature-born neonates nephrogenesis has not completed at time of birth. Many of them will be treated with drugs in the vulnerable phase of kidney development. An adequately functioning RAS is essential for kidney development. The use of angiotensin converting enzyme inhibitors (ACEIs) in pregnancy can therefore negatively influence nephrogenesis and lead to neonatal kidney failure (ACEI fetopathy). Mutations in genes coding for renin, ACE and AT1 cause autosomal recessive kidney tubular dysgenesis and fetal hypotension [33]. Both inherited and acquired defects of the RAS can alter kidney hemodynamics with deleterious effects on kidney development.

Aminoglycosides are well-known for their nephrotoxic effect on the developing fetal kidney. These drugs will result in tubular alterations and low nephron number. Offsprings of pregnant rats treated with aminoglycoside are born with lower nephron numbers and subsequently develop glomerulosclerosis with aging. Unfortunately these drugs are still commonly used as first-line treatment of infections in premature neonates although alternative treatment options with less adverse effects on nephrogenesis are available, such as cephalosporins and carbapenems [34, 35].

Pathophysiologic Mechanisms of Drug Nephrotoxicity

Direct Tubular Cell Toxicity

This damage is at least in part dose-dependent, is generally of surreptitious onset (with symptoms often undetected in the early stages), and is characterized by acute tubular necrosis (with loss of a proportion of kidney proximal tubular cells). This mode of toxicity is typical for the aminoglycosides, where it has been reported in 20–35% of exposed children [25], and for antivirals such as aciclovir, foscarnet, cidofovir, adenovir and tenofovir [36]. Cisplatin induced nephrotoxicity is

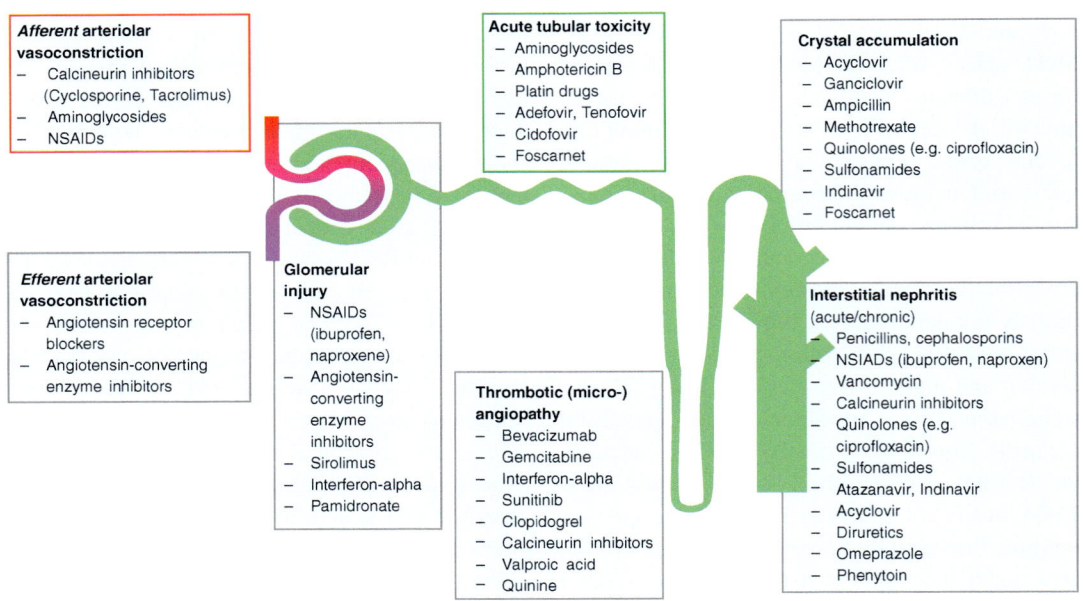

Fig. 71.4 Nephrotoxic drugs in children with related pathophysiological mechanisms. Modified from Tjon and Teoh [32]

frequent (up to 80%) [37] and linked to the accumulation of toxic metabolites with subsequent inflammation and cellular damage. The cyclophosphamide analogon ifosfamide causes proximal tubular dysfunction (Fanconi syndrome) in up to 30% of exposed children and the toxic damage is conferred by the metabolite chloroacetaldehyde. Other drugs associated with this type of damage are amphotericin B, calcineurin inhibitors, methotrexate, pamidronate, pentamidine, and cocaine.

Generally, transient enzymuria and a Fanconi-like syndrome are early signs of proximal tubular damage. These often remain undetected but may be followed by urine sediment disorders (granular, hyaline, and cellular casts) and kidney failure.

Acute Interstitial Nephritis and Immunologically Mediated Kidney Toxicity

Immunologic kidney toxicity is mediated by inflammation of the interstitium and tubules. It occurs on an allergic basis in an idiosyncratic,

dose-independent manner with a predominance of lymphocytes, monocytes, eosinophils and plasma cells within the interstitium, and active urinary sediment [38]. Clinical and laboratory signs such as fever, rash and eosinophiluria are rare (<10%) and therefore, if indicated, the diagnosis can be confirmed with certainty only by kidney biopsy. Interstitial nephrotoxicity is typical of antibiotics such as beta-lactams, quinolones, rifampin, macrolides, sulfonamides, vancomycin, most NSAIDs, diuretics (thiazides, loop diuretics, and triamterene), anticonvulsants (phenytoin), cimetidine and ranitidine, allopurinol, and antivirals (acyclovir, indinavir, atazanavir), etc.

If acute interstitial nephritis is diagnosed, potential nephrotoxic drugs should be discontinued immediately.

Chronic interstitial nephritis is more complex and associated with drugs such as calcineurin inhibitors (cyclosporin A, tacrolimus) and carmustine. In contrast to acute interstitial nephritis, the prognosis of chronic interstitial nephritis is rather poor. Data from post-transplant patients treated with cyclosporine indicate a high frequency of cyclosporine-induced interstitial nephrotoxicity resulting in chronic rejection [39].

Arteriolar Vasoconstriction

Decreased kidney blood flow and GFR due to dose-dependent reversible vasoconstriction affecting primarily the afferent but also the efferent arterioles (prerenal dysfunction with intact tubular function) is the main pathophysiogical mechanism of acute kidney toxicity typical for calcineurin inhibitors, NSAIDs, angiotensin-converting enzyme (ACE) inhibitors, and angiotensin receptor blockers. The synthesis of strong vasoconstrictors such as angotensin II, leukotrienes and endothelin is stimulated and endothelial nitric oxide concentrations are reduced.

Prostaglandins contribute to the regulation of kidney perfusion and GFR—with their vasodilating properties opposing the action of vasoconstrictive substances. Thus, subjects suffering from conditions associated with high levels of vasoconstrictive substances (such as hypovolemia, cardiac failure, sepsis, and hypertension) may develop kidney damage when treated with NSAIDs which induce a reduction of prostaglandin synthesis.

Kidney dysfunction associated with antihypertensive therapy is a result of excessive lowering of blood pressure. Since kidney blood flow and kidney perfusion are maintained during treatment with ACE inhibitors despite the adverse effects on glomerular function, kidney function readily returns to pretreatment levels when the drug is discontinued.

Crystal Accumulation

The pH-dependent precipitation of insoluble crystals in the distal tubular lumen is a nephrotoxic mechanism occurring mostly with antiviral drugs (e.g. acyclovir, ganciclovir), sulphonamides, methotrexate, indinavir, etc. Crystalluria after fluoroquinolone administration is rare, and may occur in the condition of dehydration. Among the factors that increase the likelihood of kidney crystal deposition, severe volume contraction is the most important. Uric acid and calcium phosphate crystals contribute to tumor lysis associated nephrotoxicity after chemotherapy for malignancies.

Proteinuric Glomerular Dysfunction

Some drugs can cause nephrotic range proteinuria due to podocyte toxicity. These include NSAIDs, captopril, interferon-alpha, pamidronate, MTOR inhibitors (sirolimus, everolimus), tiopronin, etc. Discontinuation of the drug usually leads to resolution of proteinuria, although irreversible lesions have also been reported.

Vascular Injury/Thrombotic Microangiopathy

Thrombotic microangiopathy has been associated with a wide range of drugs, including cyclosporin A, tacrolimus, gemcitabine, clopidogrel, sunitib, valproic acid, bevacizumab, etc. The main pathologic finding is presence of hyaline thrombi in the microvessels of many organs, including glomerular thrombosis. The manifestations can include fever, hemolytic anemia, thrombocytopenic purpura, kidney dysfunction, central nervous system involvement (thrombotic thrombocytopenic purpura, TTP), and predominance of kidney failure with anemia and thrombocytopenia (hemolytic uremic syndrome).

Alterations of Fluids and Electrolytes

Examples of alteration of fluids and electrolytes are excess of sodium and water removal; metabolic alkalosis and hypokalemia induced by excessive use of diuretics; and hyperkalemia and metabolic acidosis secondary to pharmacologic hyporeninemic hypoaldosteronism as induced by NSAID and tacrolimus.

Other Mechanisms

Additional specific mechanisms of drug nephrotoxicity include osmotic nephrosis (related mainly to mannitol and immunoglobulins) and rhabdomyolysis (e.g. codein, corticosteroids). Osmotic nephrosis is characterized by vacuolization and swelling of renal proximal tubular cells as consequence of glucose and sucrose reabsorption by pinocytosis. Thrombolytic agents often disrupt or dissolve protective thrombi covering ulcerated plaques, thereby releasing cholesterol plaques into the circulation leading to occlusion of small-diameter arteries of the kidney (i.e., arcuate and interlobular arteries, terminal arterioles and glomerular capillaries). Cholesterol embolization with anticoagulants, such as warfarin and heparin, or thrombolytic agents (streptokinase and tissue-plasminogen activator) is sometimes observed weeks or months after initiation of therapy.

Ten Rules for Prevention of Drug-Induced Kidney Damage

- **Rule 1**: **Alternatives**. *Do not use nephrotoxic drugs if alternatives are available.*

- The simplest way to prevent drug-induced nephrotoxicity is to avoid the use of these drugs. Knowledge of drug safety is a useful element for preventing iatrogenic dysfunction. Lack of nephrotoxicity is one of the parameters to be considered in the choice of drug therapy. Before prescribing a potentially nephrotoxic drug, the risk-to-benefit ratio and the availability of alternative drugs should be considered.

- Nephrotoxic drugs should be avoided whenever possible, especially in high-risk situations. Critically ill children are not ideal candidates for potentially nephrotoxic drug treatment, although pediatricians may not always have valid alternative choices. E.g., aminoglycosides have two unique pharmacodynamic properties: their postantibiotic effect and concentration-dependent killing. However, aztreonam is a reasonable alternative to aminoglycoside therapy in children and low-birth-weight infants with gram-negative infections at risk of nephrotoxicity.
- **Rule 2: High-Risk Patients**. *Do not use nephrotoxic drugs in high-risk patients.*

- Chronic kidney failure and a preexisting kidney injury are major risk factors for most nephrotoxins. Diabetes mellitus increases vulnerability to aminoglycosides, nonsteroidal anti-inflammatory drugs (NSAIDs), and ACE inhibitors. Sepsis itself is a major risk for nephrotoxicity. Significant volume depletion is a risk factor for NSAID-induced nephrotoxicity.
- Volume management is essential for prevention. Generally, pretreatment hydration can reduce the nephrotoxic potential of many drugs, including amphotericin B, aminoglycosides, NSAIDs, cisplatin, and indinavir. A "diuretic holiday" (a period off diuretics) is suggested before starting an ACE inhibitor. Modifiable risk factors should be corrected. In many cases, patients are routinely prehydrated before the administration of a nephrotoxic drug. In such cases, it is mandatory to accurately monitor urine output and avoid intravascular volume overload.
- Novel biomarkers such as kidney injury molecule-1 (KIM-1) may be helpful to early identify children with aminoglycoside-induced tubular toxicity (see Chap. 51) [25].
- **Rule 3: Choice of Compound**. *Choose the least nephrotoxic compound.*
- For the kidney, netilmicin is better than gentamicin, teicoplanin is better than vancomycin, and lipid formulations of amphotericin B are better than conventional formulations. Ceftazidime seems the safest cephalosporin for the kidney. Analgesics other than NSAIDs are preferred in children with compromised hemodynamic status or volume depletion.
- **Rule 4: Dosage and Monitoring**. *Use correct dosage and therapeutic drug monitoring, if required.*
- The correct drug dosage should be prescribed. For many years, it has been debated whether TDM of aminoglycosides and vancomycin will decrease toxicity—especially at the kidney level. Probably it depends on the patient population, with high-risk patients benefiting more. However, a tailored TDM is generally associated with lower nephrotoxicity.
- **Rule 5**: **Concomitance**. *Do not use concomitant nephrotoxic drugs.*

- Specific combinations of drugs (such as cephalosporins and aminoglycosides, cephalosporins and acyclovir, and vancomycin and aminoglycosides) may result in synergistic nephrotoxicity. The combination aminoglycoside-vancomycin is believed to increase the nephrotoxic risk up to sevenfold.
- **Rule 6**: **Duration**. *Limit the duration of treatment.*
- Prolonged duration of treatment has been associated with increased aminoglycoside and amphotericin B nephrotoxicity. In adult studies, aminoglycoside-related nephrotoxicity may reach approximately 55% of cases according to the duration of the treatment (high risk with duration >10 days). Moreover, repeated courses of aminoglycoside therapy a few months apart can enhance nephrotoxicity.
- **Rule 7**: **Diagnosis**: *Seek to diagnose kidney damage early.*
- Kidney function (and particularly the GFR) should be frequently monitored during the administration of a potentially nephrotoxic drug. Cystatin C, a marker of glomerular function in the "creatinine blind range" (GFR 60 to 90 ml/min/1,73m^2), and urinary biomarkers of nephrotoxicity (microglobulins, enzymes, and growth factors) can be used for early noninvasive identification of kidney damage occurring in the course of drug therapy. Moreover, they are helpful in establishing its extent and monitoring its time course.
- **Rule 8**: **Damage**. *Stop drug administration if damage occurs.*
- In many cases, the most important first step in treating drug-induced nephropathy is to stop the offending drug. This is true in many cases, such as for acute interstitial nephritis, nephritic syndrome, drugs associated with TTP-HUS, and obstructive nephropathy.
- **Rule 9**: **Pediatric Drugs**. *Use caution when using new drugs in pediatrics.*
- It is important to be cautious in administering drugs to children outside the terms indicated in the product license (off-label use as regards the dose, age group, route of administration, different indication) or in an unlicensed manner (formulations modified, extemporaneous preparations, imported medicines, chemicals used as drugs).
- The lack of approval for pediatric use does not imply a drug is contraindicated or disapproved. It simply means that insufficient data are available to grant approval status and the risks/benefits balance (including nephrotoxicity) cannot be evaluated.
- This suggestion should be extended to obstetricians because increasing reports of kidney damage in newborns are related to drugs administered to the mother.
- **Rule 10**: **Kidney Failure Dosing**. *Modify dose and/or interval dosing in kidney failure.*

- Normal kidney function is important for the excretion and metabolism of many drugs. Kidney failure alters drug clearance and requires modification in dosage regimens to optimize therapeutic outcome and minimize the risk of toxicity. This is a key point for prevention and is recommended as an essential component of any computer-based prescription system to minimize medical errors and adverse drug events, including drug-induced nephrotoxicity.

Acknowledgement For this current chapter, parts of two chapters from the edition 2014 (Chap. 64 on Drug Use and Dosage in Kidney Failure by Dr. Douglas L. Blowey and Chap. 65 on Causes and Manifestation of Nephrotoxicity by Dr. Vassilios Fanos and Dr. Laura Cuzzolin) have been used.

References

1. Birkett DJ. Pharmacokinetics made easy, Rev., 2. ed., reprint. Australian prescriber. Sydney: McGraw-Hill; 2006.
2. Yang X, Han L. Roles of renal drug transporter in drug disposition and renal toxicity. Adv Exp Med Biol. 2019;1141:341–60.
3. Parvez HRC. Molecular responses to xenobiotics. Amsterdam: Elsevier; 2001.
4. König J, Müller F, Fromm MF. Transporters and drug-drug interactions: important determinants of drug disposition and effects. Pharmacol Rev. 2013;65(3):944–66.
5. Filler G, Yasin A, Medeiros M. Methods of assessing renal function. Pediatr Nephrol. 2014;29(2):183–92.

6. Fisel P, Renner O, Nies AT, Schwab M, Schaeffeler E. Solute carrier transporter and drug-related nephrotoxicity: the impact of proximal tubule cell models for preclinical research. Expert Opin Drug Metab Toxicol. 2014;10(3):395–408.

7. Regulski M, Regulska K, Stanisz BJ, Murias M, Gieremek P, Wzgarda A, Niznik B. Chemistry and pharmacology of angiotensin-converting enzyme inhibitors. Curr Pharm Des. 2015;21(13):1764–75.

8. Filler G, Bökenkamp A, Hofmann W, Le Bricon T, Martínez-Brú C, Grubb A. Cystatin C as a marker of GFR--history, indications, and future research. Clin Biochem. 2005;38(1):1–8.

9. van den Anker JN, Schwab M, Kearns GL. Developmental pharmacokinetics. Handb Exp Pharmacol. 2011;205:51–75.

10. Arant BS. Developmental patterns of renal functional maturation compared in the human neonate. J Pediatr. 1978;92(5):705–12.

11. Guignard JP, Torrado A, Da CO, Gautier E. Glomerular filtration rate in the first three weeks of life. J Pediatr. 1975;87(2)

12. Aperia A, Broberger O, Elinder G, Herin P, Zetterström R. Postnatal development of renal function in pre-term and full-term infants. Acta Paediatr Scand. 1981;70(2):183–7.

13. Kearns GL, Abdel-Rahman SM, Alander SW, Blowey DL, Leeder JS, Kauffman RE. Developmental pharmacology—drug disposition, action, and therapy in infants and children. N Engl J Med. 2003;349(12):1157–67.

14. Hayton WL. Maturation and growth of renal function: dosing renally cleared drugs in children. AAPS PharmSci. 2000;2(1):E3.

15. Siegel SR, Oh W. Renal function as a marker of human fetal maturation. Acta Paediatr Scand. 1976;65(4):481–5.

16. Veltri MA, Neu AM, Fivush BA, Parekh RS, Furth SL. Drug dosing during intermittent hemodialysis and continuous renal replacement therapy: special considerations in pediatric patients. Paediatr Drugs. 2004;6(1):45–65.

17. Blowey BL, Leeder JS, Blowey DL. Drug administration and pharmacogenomics in children receiving acute or chronic renal replacement therapy. In: Warady BA, Alexander SR, Schaefer F, editors. Pediatric dialysis. Cham: Springer; 2021. p. 683–707.

18. DeSoi CA, Sahm DF, Umans JG. Vancomycin elimination during high-flux hemodialysis: kinetic model and comparison of four membranes. Am J Kidney Dis. 1992;20(4):354–60.

19. Pallotta KE, Manley HJ. Vancomycin use in patients requiring hemodialysis: a literature review. Semin Dial. 2008;21(1):63–70.

20. Ernest D, Cutler DJ. Gentamicin clearance during continuous arteriovenous hemodiafiltration. Crit Care Med. 1992;20(5):586–9.

21. Blowey DL, Warady BA, Abdel-Rahman S, Frye RF, Manley HJ. Vancomycin disposition following intra-peritoneal administration in children receiving peritoneal dialysis. Perit Dial Int. 2007;27(1):79–85.

22. Filler G, Kirpalani A, Urquhart BL. Handling of drugs in children with abnormal renal function. In: Avner E, Harmon W, Niaudet P, Yoshikawa N, Emma F, Goldstein S, editors. Pediatric nephrology. Berlin, Heidelberg: Springer; 2016.

23. Rowland M, Tozer TN. Clinical pharmacokinetics and pharmacodynamics: concepts and applications. 4th ed. Philadelphia, PA: Wolters Kluwer Health/Lippincott William & Wilkins; 2011.

24. Ting LSL, Villeneuve E, Ensom MHH. Beyond cyclosporine: a systematic review of limited sampling strategies for other immunosuppressants. Ther Drug Monit. 2006;28(3):419–30.

25. McWilliam SJ, Antoine DJ, Smyth RL, Pirmohamed M. Aminoglycoside-induced nephrotoxicity in children. Pediatr Nephrol. 2017;32(11):2015–25.

26. Choudhury D, Ahmed Z. Drug-associated renal dysfunction and injury. Nat Clin Pract Nephrol. 2006;2(2):80–91.

27. Medeiros MFG. Drug dosing in abnormal kidney function in children. In: Emma F, Goldstein S, Bagga A, Bates CM, Shroff R, editors. Pediatric nephrology. Berlin, Heidelberg: Springer; 2021.

28. Vomiero G, Carpenter B, Robb I, Filler G. Combination of ceftriaxone and acyclovir - an underestimated nephrotoxic potential? Pediatr Nephrol. 2002;17(8):633–7.

29. Filler G, de Barros VR, Jagger JE, Christians U. Cyclosporin twice or three times daily dosing in pediatric transplant patients - it is not the same! Pediatr Transplant. 2006;10(8):953–6.

30. Filler G, Alvarez-Elías AC, McIntyre C, Medeiros M. The compelling case for therapeutic drug monitoring of mycophenolate mofetil therapy. Pediatr Nephrol. 2017;32(1):21–9.

31. Zaffanello M, Bassareo PP, Cataldi L, Antonucci R, Biban P, Fanos V. Long-term effects of neonatal drugs on the kidney. J Matern Fetal Neonatal Med. 2010;23(Suppl 3):87–9.

32. Tjon J, Teoh CW. Medication-induced nephrotoxicity in children. Curr Pediatr Rep. 2020;8(3):122–33.

33. Lacoste M, Cai Y, Guicharnaud L, Mounier F, Dumez Y, Bouvier R, Dijoud F, Gonzales M, Chatten J, Delezoide A-L, Daniel L, Joubert M, Laurent N, Aziza J, Sellami T, Amar HB, Jarnet C, Frances AM, Daïkha-Dahmane F, Coulomb A, Neuhaus TJ, Foliguet B, Chenal P, Marcorelles P, Gasc JM, Corvol P, Gubler MC. Renal tubular dysgenesis, a not uncommon autosomal recessive disorder leading to oligohydramnios: role of the renin-angiotensin system. J Am Soc Nephrol. 2006;17(8):2253–63.

34. Schreuder MF, Bueters RR, Huigen MC, Russel FGM, Masereeuw R, van den Heuvel LP. Effect of drugs on renal development. Clin J Am Soc Nephrol. 2011;6(1):212–7.

35. Schreuder MF, Bueters RRG, Allegaert K. The interplay between drugs and the kidney in premature neonates. Pediatr Nephrol. 2014;29(11):2083–91.

36. Rao S, Abzug MJ, Carosone-Link P, Peterson T, Child J, Siparksy G, Soranno D, Cadnapaphornchai MA, Simões EAF. Intravenous acyclovir and renal dysfunction in children: a matched case control study. J Pediatr. 2015;166(6):1462–8.e1–4.

37. Ruggiero A, Ferrara P, Attinà G, Rizzo D, Riccardi R. Renal toxicity and chemotherapy in children with cancer. Br J Clin Pharmacol. 2017;83(12):2605–14.

38. Joyce E, Glasner P, Ranganathan S, Swiatecka-Urban A. Tubulointerstitial nephritis: diagnosis, treatment, and monitoring. Pediatr Nephrol. 2017;32(4):577–87.

39. Nankivell BJ, Borrows RJ, Fung CL-S, O'Connell PJ, Allen RDM, Chapman JR. The natural history of chronic allograft nephropathy. N Engl J Med. 2003;349(24):2326–33.

Complementary Therapies for Renal Diseases

72

Cecilia Bukutu and Sunita Vohra

Abbreviations

b.i.d.	Bis in die (twice a day)
BUN	Blood urea nitrogen
CAM	Complementary and alternative medicine
cfu	Colony-forming unit
CI	Confidence interval
CKD	Chronic kidney disease
CKD	Chronic kidney disease
Cr	Creatinine
CrCl	Creatinine clearance
dl	Decilitre
ESKD	End stage kidney disease
ESWL	Extracorporeal Shockwave lithotripsy
FDA	Food and Drug Administration
g	Grams
GFR	Glomerular filtration rate
GTP	Guanosine triphosphate
Hz	Hertz
IgA	Immunoglobulin A
IgAN	Immunoglobulin A nephropathy
IU	International unit
kg	Kilogram
MD	Mean difference
mg	Milligram
ml	Millilitres
Mol/L	Moles per liter
n-3 LCPUFA	n-3 Long-chain polyunsaturated fatty acid
NHP	Natural health product
O3FA	Omega-3 fatty acids
PAC	Proanthocyanidin
RCT	Randomized Control Trial
RR	Relative risk
SD	Standard deviation
TCM	Traditional Chinese medicine
TEAS	Transcutaneous electrical acupoint stimulation
TENS	Transcutaneous electrical nerve stimulation
TNF-α	Tumor necrosis factor-alfa
TwHF	Tripterygium wilfordii Hook F
US	United States
UTI	Urinary tract infection
VAS	Visual analog scale
µg	Microgram

C. Bukutu
Faculty of Science, Dept of Public Health, Concordia University of Edmonton (CUE), Edmonton, AB, Canada
e-mail: cecilia.bukutu@concordia.ab.ca

S. Vohra (✉)
Faculty of Medicine and Dentistry (FoMD), Depts of Pediatrics and Psychiatry, University of Alberta, Edmonton, AB, Canada
e-mail: svohra@ualberta.ca

© The Author(s), under exclusive license to Springer Nature Switzerland AG 2023
F. Schaefer, L. A. Greenbaum (eds.), *Pediatric Kidney Disease*,
https://doi.org/10.1007/978-3-031-11665-0_72

Introduction

Complementary therapies have been described as "health care approaches that are not typically part of conventional medical care or that may have origins outside of usual Western practice" [1]. Thus complementary therapies are a term that includes a diverse range of products and practices (e.g., natural health products [NHPs], massage therapy, acupuncture, etc.) used in the prevention or treatment of illness or the promotion of health and well-being.

The distinction between conventional medicine and complementary therapies is not always well defined or fixed [1]. As complementary therapies do not have a well-demarcated border, the inclusion or exclusion of dietary modifications, vitamins, and prayer/spirituality as complementary therapies remains unresolved [2]. This chapter focuses on evidence regarding NHPs, traditional Chinese medicine (TCM), and massage therapy. First, we review core relevant concepts, including definitions, epidemiology of complementary therapy use (including reasons for use and lack of disclosure), NHP quality and regulation, and legal and ethical issues related to the use of complementary therapies.

Natural Health Products, TCM, and Massage Therapy

In Canada, NHPs are defined in the *Natural Health Products Regulations* as vitamins and minerals, herbal medicines, homeopathic remedies, traditional medicines such as TCMs, probiotics, and other products like amino acids and essential fatty acids [3]. In the United States (US), these products are more commonly referred to as "dietary supplements" [4].

TCM is an ancient medical system that includes acupressure, acupuncture, breathing exercises, NHPs, moxibustion, oriental massage, qi gong, and tai chi [5]. An important concept in TCM is qi, a life energy with various mental, physical, and spiritual manifestations. This energy is said to flow throughout the body, along the meridian system, allowing for the integration of internal organs and

other body structures. If one's qi is flowing in an orderly fashion, the person is healthy. Disorderly flow causes disease. One of TCM's aims is to restore the orderly flow of qi (Table 72.1) [9].

Yin-yang is another important concept in TCM, in which yin and yang represent opposing but complementary qualities [10]. The philosophical and physiologic implications of yin-yang imbalance in TCM theory are complicated and beyond the scope of this chapter. It can be confusing; for example, the term *kidney* in TCM has a very different meaning than it does in conventional Western medicine. In TCM theory, it does not imply the physical organ; instead, in TCM theory, the kidney's main function is to store energy that governs conception, growth, development, sexual maturation, reproduction, and pregnancy [10].

Table 72.1 Principles of selected Traditional Chinese Medicine (TCM) therapies

Therapy	General principles
Acupressure	Pressing and/or massaging various acupuncture points (acupoints) using fingers, palms, elbow, feet or special devices on the body's meridians [6].
Acupuncture	The Chinese art of stimulating the pathways of energy (14 main meridians plus branches) by puncturing, pressing, heating, using electrical current, or using herbal medicines [7].
Moxibustion	Moxibustion is the process where dried moxa herb (a mugwort) is burned usually just above but sometimes directly on the skin over acupuncture points. The herb may be in the form of incense sticks or wool [8].
Oriental massage	A wide range of therapeutic techniques involving the manipulation of muscles and soft tissues, including kneading, rubbing, tapping, friction, vigorous or relaxing, deep or superficial [7].
Qigong	Exercises aimed at bringing about harmony, as well as improving health and longevity. Healing methods involve breathing, movement, the mind, and the eyes [7].
Tai chi	Balanced gentle movements, incorporating a combination of meditation and breathing, are designed to dissolve physical and karmic layers of tension in both the physical body and the energy body, and to open up the spiritual space inside [7].

In massage therapy, pressure is used to manipulate the body's soft tissues to impact the circulatory, lymphatic, musculoskeletal, and nervous systems, and in so doing enhance the body's self-healing ability [11]. Aromatherapy generally refers to the use of massage therapy in conjunction with aromatic plant extracts, also known as essential oils [12].

Epidemiology of Complementary Therapy Use

There is widespread use of complementary therapies worldwide [13] with varying prevalence rates: 10–40% in different European countries; 40–60% in the USA [14]; 49% in Australia; 75% in Africa, and between 21.6–90% in Saudi Arabia [15, 16]. A US survey of complementary therapies use in the past 12 months found that 4 in 10 adults and 1 in 9 children and youth had used complementary products or therapies [17]. In a Canadian 2011 survey (n = 2001), 71% of respondents reported using one or more NHPs [18], while in a 2016 survey 56% of Canadians reported having used at least one complementary therapy in in the last 12 months [19]. The prevalence of complementary use tends to be higher among individuals with conditions that are chronic, serious, or recurrent [20–22]. A systematic review reported that prevalence rates for complementary therapy use among children/adolescents range from 10.9% to 87.6% for lifetime use and from 8% to 48.5% for current use [23]. The review also found variance in lifetime prevalence by type of complementary therapy: homeopathy 0.8–39% (highest in Germany, United Kingdom, and Canada) and herbal medicine use 0.8–85.5% (highest in Germany, Turkey, and Brazil) [23].

There is a high prevalence of complementary therapy consumption among adult renal patients. The use of complementary therapies in the previous 6 months among patients (N = 278) at a nephrology outpatient clinic in India was 66.3% [24]. A Saudi cross-sectional study (N = 315) reported that 54.9% of chronic kidney disease (CKD) patients were current complementary therapy users [15]. An earlier survey in Egypt reported a similar complementary therapy prevalence rate (52%) among outpatient nephrology clinic attendees (N = 1005) [25]. In a German survey, regular complementary therapy use was reported by 57% of dialysis patients (n = 119) and 49% of kidney transplant patients (n = 45) [26]. In a Thai survey of 421 adults with CKD, 45% had used NHPs in the past year, and a 2004 US survey found 29% of CKD patients used NHPs (n = 250) [27]. A Canadian study reported that 45% of patients (n = 100) with CKD had used NHPs [28], and 25.2% of 206 CKD patients in a Turkish study reported having used complementary therapies at least once following their renal diagnosis [29].

Parents who use complementary therapies are likely to offer these to their children. Although no complementary therapies prevalence studies among pediatric kidney patients were identified, studies show the main predictors of complementary therapy use to be higher parental income and education, older children [23], female children and the existence of comorbid medical condition [30]. The prevalence of complementary therapy use increases to over 50% in children who have chronic [31, 32] recurrent or incurable conditions [22]. For adults and children, complementary therapy use often occurs in combination with conventional care [32].

Reasons for complementary therapy use may include a desire to improve and cure the disease [31]; having an expectation of benefits of complementary therapies; and dissatisfaction with conventional medicine due to lack of cure, side effects, or higher costs [27, 33, 34]. Some adults mention long wait times and insufficient time spent with their physician as reasons for using complementary therapies. Many complementary therapy users value the long appointments that complementary therapy practitioners provide and feel their concerns can therefore be addressed more thoroughly [34, 35]. Other commonly cited reasons for complementary therapy use include increased personal control regarding treatment, and the perception of complementary therapies as more natural, and therefore safer, than Western medical treatments [27, 33].

Despite common use, many physicians remain unaware about their patients' complementary therapies use. Only 20% to 65% of families discuss their complementary therapies use with their physician [22]. A US complementary therapies user study (N = 7493) found that 42.3% (n = 3094) did not discuss complementary therapies use with their primary care physicians [36]. Among adults with kidney disease, non-disclosure of complementary therapy use can be as high as 72% [37]. Lack of disclosure usually occurs because patients may not think it is relevant, healthcare providers do not ask, concerns about the healthcare provider's knowledge regarding complementary therapies or patients feel their healthcare provider would disapprove of their complementary therapies use [36, 38, 39].

Regulation of complementary therapy practices varies significantly within and among countries [13, 40]. For example, the regulation of complementary therapy practices within the US is inconsistent (some complementary therapy practices are regulated in some states, and not others). Different states can have different requirements for practitioners or different regulations regarding scope of practice [41]. In the United Kingdom, with the exception of osteopaths and chiropractors, most complementary therapy providers are largely unregulated [41, 42]; conversely, in Canada, regulation of chiropractors, naturopaths, homeopaths, osteopaths, TCM practitioners, acupuncturists, and massage therapists often varies by province [41]. In Canada, various provincial professional medical bodies have produced guidelines that address how physicians should deal with complementary therapies and practitioners [43, 44].

Natural Health Product Quality and Regulation

NHPs have complex product quality issues. Heterogeneity in product quality is common for various reasons. For example, for any given herbal product (e.g., *Echinacea*) there may be several plant species (*Echinacea purpurea, Echinacea pallida, Echinacea angustifolia)* with different phytochemical constituents and different physiologic effects [9]. Moreover differences in growing conditions, time of harvesting, parts used (e.g., aerial vs. root), and extraction methods used to prepare the herbal product may vary, compounding differences within and among manufacturers [45]. Some manufacturers have tried to reconcile this problem by standardizing some herbal products to a marker compound specific to that particular plant [46].

NHP product quality suffers from issues related to species misidentification, adulteration, and contamination. Various techniques, including microscopy, mass spectrometry and, more recently, DNA barcoding have been used to identify NHP quality issues [47]. Using DNA barcoding techniques, Newmaster and colleagues [46] found that 59% of herbal products sold on the North American herbal market were contaminated, and McCutcheon's [48] examination of Chinese herbal medicines found that 7% to 23.7% were adulterated [48]. Other reports of NHP quality concerns include a case of neonatal androgenization reported in Toronto where a pregnant mother consumed what she believed to be Siberian ginseng, but was actually Chinese silk vine [48].; herbal products being contaminated with bacteria, fungi, herbicides, and heavy metals; and cases of adulteration of NHPs with pharmaceutical agents [49]. Some herbal products have been found to be mislabeled, a problem that is often associated with the absence of regulation [48]. A 2003 US study found that 10% (6 of 59) of products marketed as *Echinacea* actually contained no *Echinacea* [50, 51].

Different regulatory approaches have been adopted internationally with regard to NHPs, In the US, the 1994 Dietary Supplements and Health Education Act reclassified NHPs as dietary supplements (i.e., neither food nor drug), and thereby exempted them from the usual safety and regulatory rules set by the Food and Drug Administration (FDA).[41, 52] As such, dietary supplements can be marketed without proven safety or efficacy, and it is the responsibility of the FDA to demonstrate that a supplement is unsafe, which can be challenging. In Canada, Health Canada's Natural and Non-prescription Health Products Directorate regulates NHPs under the NHPs Regulations. Although Health Canada has not attempted to standardize NHPs, its regulations demand that manufacturers meet label claims and eliminate contamination and adulteration from products sold in the Canadian marketplace [3]. In order to help consumers to select and safely use NHPs, Health Canada has proposed regulation amendments to make NHP labels easier to read and understand [3]

Legal and Ethical Considerations

A number of legal and ethical considerations surround the use of complementary therapies. While many patients report that complementary therapy use helps them feel better, use of complementary therapies may delay the use of known effective treatment. Physicians should always inquire about complementary therapy use, monitoring high-risk patients such as those on dialysis, and consider the possibility of NHP-drug interactions as many patient mix NHPs with prescription medications. Clinicians may be hesitant to encourage the use of complementary therapies, as it is unfamiliar [53]. A survey of clinicians (N = 195) in Quebec found that 86.7% believed it was their role to advise patients on complementary therapies, but only 33.1% reporting being able to do so [54] Studies show that most medical students believe that integrative medicine information and education is important to their future practice and improves patient care [55].

Medical school curriculum is evolving to include more information about complementary therapies. For example, a Thai survey found that 50% of medical schools had integrated traditional, complementary, and alternative medicine training in their curriculum [56]. In the US over 50% of medical schools now include some complementary therapies education in their curriculum, with the majority of courses offered as electives [57–59]. At the same time, the number of US hospitals that offer complementary and integrative medicine as an ancillary clinical service has increased, with different hospitals addressing issues related to scope of practice, licensure and malpractice liability differently in their models of integrative health care [57]. There are over 12 residency programs that offer board-certified fellowships (by the American Board of Integrative Medicine or the Academic Consortium for Integrative Medicine and Health) in Integrative Medicine, with opportunities for elective residency experiences in the US [60]. Across North American, there has also been an increase in academic pediatric integrative medicine programs that develop and promote evidence-based integrative approach within Children's hospitals [22]. In Canadian medical programs, few formal courses on complementary therapies are offered as part of medical training [55]. Established in 2008, the Academic Consortium for Integrative Medicine and Health is a group of more than 70 universities, many of which offer educational courses for students and continuing education courses for practicing providers [55].

If a patient expresses interest in using complementary therapies for his or her illness, the physician should review the literature and advise accordingly. If there are sufficient safety and efficacy data, physicians may choose to recommend complementary therapies or refer their patient to a licensed complementary therapy provider [21] (see Fig. 72.1). If efficacy is uncertain, but the therapy is likely to be safe, patients may choose to try the therapy while their clinician continues to monitor them. If a therapy is felt to be unsafe, the patient should be advised to discontinue its use [9].

This chapter reviews the best available evidence with regard to NHPs, TCM and massage therapy. When pediatric evidence is unavailable, evidence from studies conducted among adults is discussed. Because limiting research by language can promote bias, our searches were conducted without language restriction.

It is important to highlight that the methodological quality of randomized controlled trials (RCTs) examining complementary therapies have been assessed and found equivalent to that

b *Evidence supports safety, but evidence regarding efficacy is inconclusive.*	a *Evidence supports both safety and efficacy.*
Therapeutic posture: Tolerate, provide caution, and closely monitor effectiveness.	**Therapeutic posture:** Recommend and continue to monitor.
Clinical examples: Acupuncture for chronic pain; homeopathy for seasonal rhinitis; dietary fat reduction for certain types of cancer; mind-body techniques for metastatic cancer; massage therapy for low-back pain; self- hypnosis for pain from metastatic cancer.	**Clinical examples:** Chiropractic care for acute low-back pain; acupuncture for chemotherapy-induced nausea and dental pain; mind-body techniques for chronic pain and insomnia.
Potential liability risk: Conceivably liable but probably acceptable.	**Potential liability risk:** Probably not liable.

— Efficacy ——————————————————————————————▶

d *Evidence indicates serious risk or inefficacy.*	c *Evidence supports efficacy, but evidence regarding safety is inconclusive.*
Therapeutic posture: Avoid and actively discourage.	**Therapeutic posture:** Consider tolerating, provide caution, and closely monitor safety.
Clinical examples: Injections of unapproved substances; use of toxic herbs or substances; dangerous delay or replacement of curative conventional treatments; inattention to known herb-drug interactions (for example, St. John's wort and indinavir or cyclosporine)	**Clinical examples:** St. John's wort for depression; saw palmetto for benign prostatic hyperplasia; chondroitin sulfate for osteoarthritis; *Ginkgo biloba* for cognitive function in dementia; acupuncture for breech presentation.
Potential liability risk: Probably liable.	**Potential liability risk:** Conceivably liable but more than likely acceptable.

(left vertical axis labeled **S a f e t y**)

Fig. 72.1 Potential malpractice liability risk associated with complementary and integrative medical therapies [61]. (Used with permission from Cohen MH, Eisenberg DM. Potential physician malpractice liability associated with complementary and integrative medical therapies. Ann Intern Med. 2002;136(8):596–60)

of conventional interventions, while complementary therapies' systematic reviews have tended to be of better quality than those of conventional therapies [62, 63]. While this is reassuring regarding the overall quality of complementary therapies evidence, there have been calls for improvement in specific areas, such as Chinese TCM studies [64].

Nephrotic Syndrome

Various studies have examined complementary therapy treatments in children with nephrotic syndrome, including TCM and dietary modification. We identified several RCTs and systematic reviews of Chinese herbal medicines in the treatment of children with nephrotic syndrome.

TCM

Deng and colleagues [65] have published a systematic review that investigates the effect of Chinese medicine prescription on nephrotic syndrome.

Feng and associates [66] performed a Cochrane review that examined the benefits and harms of administering Huangqi or Huangqi formulations alone (oral solution or intravenous injection) or in addition to other drug therapies in treating nephrotic syndrome [66]. Haungqi is a traditional Chinese herbal medicine and is a root of *Huangqi membranaceus* (Fisch) Bge. var. *mongholicus* (Bge) Hsiao or *Huangqi membranaceus* (Fisch) Bge. or *Hedysarum polybotrys* Hand. –Mazz (fam. *Leguminoseae)* [66]. Haungqi and its formulations have been used commonly for nephrotic syndrome in China [66]. In the review, nine Chinese studies (n = 461 participants) were included; five included children only, one study was of adults only and three studies included both adults and children. Compared to control interventions, Huangqi and Huangqi formulations were found to have positive effects in treating nephrotic syndrome by increasing plasma albumin and reducing urine albumin excretion, blood cholesterol, triglycerides. At 3 months, more patients who had taken Huangqi showed improvement (relative risk (RR) 0.41, 95% confidence interval (CI) 0.20 to 0.84). However, due to small sample sizes and other methodological concerns including lack of blinding and unclear randomization, the evidence was insufficient to support the use of Huangqi formulations for the treatment of nephrotic syndrome. No adverse effects of Huangqi formulations were reported.

A previous systematic review [67] examined various interventions for preventing infections in children with nephrotic syndrome. Twelve studies (n = 762), all carried out in China, were included. Nine studies assessed prophylactic pharmacotherapy (e.g., intravenous immune globuli, Bacillus Calmette-Guerin) compared to placebo, no or other treatment. Three studies investigated the efficacy of the Chinese medicinal herbs tiaojining (one study) and Huangqi (astragalus) granules (2 studies). Tiaojining is a compound of six primary Chinese medicinal herbs (Shengdi, Zhimu, Zexie, Shanyurou, Xianlinpi, and Baihuasheshecao) associated with immunomodulation effects. *Huangqi astragalus* granules contain astragalus polysaccharides, astragaloside, amino acids and various microelements associated with improved immune function. The authors noted that the trials included in the review were of very poor methodological quality because most studies did not describe the methods used for randomization, blinding or withdrawals.

We describe here the three RCTs included in the Wu et al. [67] review that investigated the efficacy of Chinese medicinal herbs for nephrotic syndrome, one about tiaojining and two about Huangpi (astragalus) granules. The first study evaluated the efficacy of tiaojining for reducing the risk of infection among children with nephrotic syndrome (n = 60; aged 1–13 years) [68]. Children in the treatment group received 8 weeks of prednisone combined with various doses of tiaojining 3 times/day based on their age. Children in the control group received prednisone for the same duration. At the end of treatment tiaojining was effective in preventing infection, with a relative risk (RR) of 0.59 (95% CI 0.43 to 0.81, p = 0.001). No adverse events or safety data were presented.

The second study was a parallel group RCT in which 92 children (aged 2–13.7 years) were assigned to either prednisone in combination with Huangpi granules (dose between 7.5 and 15 g b.i.d. based on age) or control (prednisone) for 3 months [69]. The third study was a smaller parallel RCT, which allocated 38 children (aged 1.5–7 years) to either prednisone with 15 g of Huangqi granules for 3–6 months or control (prednisone only) [70]. When both studies were combined, Huangqi granules showed a significant beneficial effect (RR 0.62, 95% CI 0.47 to 0.83) in reducing the risk of infection in children with nephrotic syndrome. Both studies reported that no adverse events were observed. Although these findings seem promising, these studies had methodological limitations and no recommendations for use can be made without larger and better designed studies.

Tripterygium wilfordii Hook F (TwHF) is a traditional herbal medicine that has been used as an immunosuppressive agent to decrease proteinuria and preserve kidney function [71]. A systematic review published in 2013 evaluated the benefits of taking two standardized types of TwHF (ethanol-ethyl acetate extract and chloroform methanol extract only) alone or in combination with other drug therapies in primary nephrotic syndrome patients. The review included 10 Chinese RCTs (9 involving adults only and one involving both adults and children) with 630 patients. The main outcomes measured were complete or partial remission. Treatment with TwHF was administered for 4 to 8 weeks at dosages ranging from 0.5 mg/kg/day to 2.0 mg/kg/day, while the follow-up period ranged from 3 to 18 months. In 4 trials (n = 293) comparing TwHF to control, TwHF significantly increased complete or partial remission. The evidence was not statistically significant when comparing TwHF to prednisone or cyclophosphamide. No serious adverse events of TwHF were observed. The authors concluded that TwHF may have an add-on effect on remission in patients with primary nephrotic syndrome. The authors had major concerns regarding the poor quality of the included studies and called for better studies with larger sample size and adequate follow-up.

Standardised TwHF preparations are purported to be less toxic and have fewer serious adverse effects than non-standardised preparations [72]. Some common adverse events associated with standardised TwHF include gastrointestinal tract disturbances, leukopenia, thrombocytopenia, rash, skin pigmentation, and malfunction of the reproductive system [73]. These adverse effects reportedly resolve after adjusting the dose or discontinuing TwHF treatment [66, 74]. In Chinese clinical practice, many physicians are unwilling to use TwHF in children due to potential reproductive system complications [75]. Serious adverse events associated with use of non-standardized TwHF include severe liver dysfunction, aplastic anaemia, and death [72]. More evidence is needed regarding long-term use and safety of TwHF in children with

nephrotic syndrome before recommendations can be made for its clinical use.

An earlier RCT carried out by Wang et al. (2005) [76] compared the effects of Tripterygium glycosides with that of cyclophosphamide in 80 children (aged 1–13 years) with relapsing primary nephrotic syndrome. Children in the experimental group (n = 39) received 1 mg/kg of tripterygium glycosides orally 2 or 3 times each day for 3 months. The control group (n = 41) received 10 mg/kg/day of cyclophosphamide by intravenous pulse over 3–6 months. All children also received tapering doses of prednisone over a period of 12–18 months. After follow-up for 3–7 years, no significant differences in the relapse rates in the two groups were observed (p > 0.05). The researchers concluded that treatment with tripterygium glucosides and prednisone was as effective as cyclophosphamide and prednisone, although this study was not designed as an equivalence trial. More side effects were reported in the control (n = 21) than the experimental group (n = 2), but in both groups symptoms resolved after treatment was discontinued. The control group side effects included one case of rising guanosine triphosphate (GTP) levels, 3 cases of transient leukocytopenia, 11 cases of alopecia, and 6 cases of gastrointestinal disturbance. The experimental group had a case of transient leukocytopenia and another of rising GTP. Safety information regarding tripterygium glycosides beyond this trial are unknown; therefore, more studies are needed.

The efficacy of Chai-Ling-Tang (Sairei-to), a preparation of 10 Chinese medicinal plants, was evaluated in 69 children (aged 5–12 years) with steroid-dependent nephrotic syndrome [77]. Over 3 weeks, children in the experimental group (n = 37) received tapering doses of prednisone until they had protein-free urine and consistent doses of Chai-Ling-Tang for 1.5 years. The control group (n = 32) received tapering doses of prednisone plus 2.5 mg/kg/day of cyclophosphamide for 8 weeks. All study participants were monitored for at least 2 years. No significant differences were reported between the experimental and control group in terms of outcomes measured, including relapse time, time to absence of proteinuria, amount of prednisone intake, and side effects. Chai-Ling-Tang was therefore equivalent to cyclophosphamide in treating steroid-dependent nephrotic syndrome. The authors suggested that Chai-Ling-Tang could be used as an alternative where patients are either non-responsive or have severe side effects from cyclophosphamide. Beyond this RCT, the safety of Chi-Ling-Tang is not known. More research is needed before any considerations for its routine clinical use in pediatric patients with nephrotic syndrome.

Immunoglobulin A (IgA) Nephropathy

There has been a substantial amount of research conducted on the effectiveness of omega-3 fatty acids (O3FA) as a therapy for individuals with IgA nephropathy (IgAN). Most of the research comes from studies involving adult patients, with a few that included children. There are also RCTs that assessed the usefulness of TCM and Vitamin E in IgAN patients.

Omega-3 Fatty Acids

A 2017 meta-analysis [78] of 9 RCTs (N = 444) evaluated the effects of O3FA on renal function and subsequent end-stage kidney disease (ESKD) events in patients with IgAN (7 RCTs) and CKD (2 RCTs). Two trials were in the US, 2 in Japan, 3 in Europe and 2 in Australia. Participants ranged from 23 to 106 patients, and follow-up ranged from 2 to 76.8 months. O3FA supplementation was significantly associated with both a lower risk of proteinuria (SMD: -0.31; 95% CI: -0.53 to -0.10; p = 0.004) and ESKD (RR: 0.49; 95% CI: 0.24 to 0.99; p = 0.047). There was no evidence to suggest that O3FA has an effect on creatinine clearance (CrCl) and estimated glomerular filtration rate (eGFR). There was no mention of adverse effects in this meta-analysis. The limitations of the meta-analysis included pooled data (due to unavailability of data), and not having sufficient relevant trials to conduct subgroup analyses for ESKD or examine for publication bias [78].

Chou et al. (2012) [79] conducted a meta-analysis to evaluate the effects of O3FA on GFR and proteinuria in IgAN. The review included 5 RCTs reported between 1989 and 2009 and included 233 adults. One hundred and sixteen patients received O3FA and 117 patients received no treatment (3 studies) or placebo (2 studies). Patients received therapy for 6–48 months. There was no significant difference in renal function between O3FA and control groups. No significant differences in renal function or proteinuria were observed when analysis was based on comparing patients who received high (> 3 g/day) and low ($\leq$ 3 g/day) O3FA doses. In addition, no dose-effect relationships between O3FA and renal function or proteinuria were observed. This meta-analysis included a small number of RCTs with study design limitations that included small sample size, short duration and variable stages of renal disease. The authors concluded that there was no evidence to suggest that O3FA has significant effects on renal function compared to controls.

An earlier meta-analysis published in 2009 [80] combined evidence from 17 RCTs to determine the effectiveness of n-3 long-chain polyunsaturated fatty acid (n-3 LCPUFA; also known as OSFA) supplementation on change in urine protein excretion and GFR in 626 adults with various chronic kidney conditions [80]. The underlying conditions in the patients were IgA nephropathy (5 trials), diabetes (7 trials), lupus (1), and kidney disease of mixed etiology (3). One trial included in the review did not report the underlying kidney disease of the study participants. Four of the IgAN trials included in this review were the same studies included in the 2012 meta-analysis [58]. The dose of n-3 LCPUFAs administered ranged from 0.7 to 5.1 g/day and follow-up was 6 weeks to 48 months. Supplementation with n-3 LCPUFA significantly reduced urine protein excretion compared to control, but there was no effect on GFR. Side effects were reported in 5 of the 17 trials and included; gastrointestinal side effects including nausea, fish aftertaste, and smell/taste of fish on eructation [80].

In a US based double blind RCT, Hogg et al. [81] compared the efficacy of prednisone or O3FA to placebo in 96 children and young adults with IgAN. A total of 23 patients were randomly assigned to receive O3FA 4 g/day (1.88 g/day of eicosapentaenoic acid, 1.48 g/day docosahexaenoic acid) for 2 years. Another 33 patients received alternate day prednisone at 60 mg/m^2 for 3 months, then 40 mg/m^2 for 9 months and 30 mg/m2 for 12 months. The last group of 31 patients received placebo. The main outcome measure was time to failure, defined as an eGFR ≤60% of baseline. The investigators found no differences with respect to time to failure between the three groups. Significantly more patients in the prednisone group compared to the placebo group experienced heartburn (48 vs. 16%; p = 0.018), and increased appetite (73 vs. 32%; p = 0.001). Other adverse events such as weight gain and anxiety were not statistically different between the two groups.

The current body of evidence assessing the efficacy of fish oils for the treatment of IgAN is from relatively small trials. More evidence from large, randomized, double-blind, placebo-controlled studies is required. Fish oils are considered extremely safe for adults when taken in recommended doses. Common adverse effects of fish oil supplements include fishy after-taste and gastrointestinal complaints such as nausea and dyspepsia [82]. Fish oil ingestion above 3 g/day may result in an increased risk of bleeding, especially in patients taking warfarin [82]. Based on this safety information, the inclusion of fish oils at recommended dosages in the treatment of adult IgA patients may be considered. The potential use of fish oils in children warrants further examination.

TCM

An RCT conducted in pediatric patients (n = 62) found that treatment with both TCM and Western medicine improved symptoms in pediatric patients with renal biopsy diagnosed IgAN [83]. Children (aged 5–14 years) were randomized to receive TCM and Western medicine (n = 34) or Western medicine only (n = 28) for 6 months. The Western medicine group took dipyridamole, captopril, common threewingnut, prednisone or cyclophosphamide according to their illness condition. Based on the clinical features, a range of TCM preparations such as Huang Qi (RadixAstragali seu Hedysari), Jian Qu (Massa Medicata Fermentata Fujianensis), fresh Mao Gen (Radix Rubi Parvifolii) and Lu Gen (Rhizoma Phragmitis) were prescribed, leading to considerable variability in TCM preparations and dosing used between patients. Eight children dropped out from the study; 2 from the TCM group and 6 from Western medicine group. After 6 months of treatment, there was no significant difference in efficacy between the two groups. The cure plus marked effect rate in the group treated with both TCM and Western medicine was higher compared to the group treated with Western medicine alone. One adverse event occurred in a patient who received TCM and Western medicine: the patient had increased alanine aminotransferase, which returned to normal after 1 week of "liver-protecting treatment" (not specified).

Safety information regarding TCM beyond the adverse effect described in the study is unknown. More studies and safety information are required before TCM herbals can be recommended for routine clinical use.

Vitamin E

A pilot double-blind, placebo-controlled trial found reduced protein/creatinine ratios in 55 children with early or mild IgAN (biopsy-proven) who were given vitamin E as antioxidant therapy [84]. Children were randomized to receive placebo (n = 28) or vitamin E capsules (n = 27). The dose of vitamin E amount was 400 IU/day if they weighed less than 30 kg and 800 IU/day if they weighed more than 30 kg. Thirty-eight patients completed 1 year of the follow-up, with no side effects reported in either the vitamin E or the placebo group. At study conclusion, there was no significant difference in GFR or in hematuria. The urine protein to creatinine ratio was significantly better in the vitamin E group (0.61; 1.37 mg/mg) vs. the placebo group (0.24; 0.38 mg/mg; p = 0.013). This small pilot study supports the use of vitamin E in pediatric patients with mild IgAN. However, larger studies investigating the long-term treatment effects of taking vitamin E in patients with mild to severe IgAN are needed.

Vitamin E is generally considered to be a safe, inexpensive product, with no clinically relevant side effects [84] when taken at recommended dosages for short periods of time.

Urolithiasis

A number of studies have assessed complementary therapies for urolithiasis and renal colic. The research has mainly focused on adults and the efficacy of acupuncture, with one study each investigating the efficacy of massage and probiotics in treating urolithiasis.

Acupuncture

Acupuncture involves the insertion of fine sterile needles into specific acupuncture points on various parts of the body.

A systematic review investigated the role of complementary therapies (including acupuncture) in decreasing analgesia requirement and alleviating anxiety during extracorporeal shockwave lithotripsy (ESWL) [85]. The systematic review included only studies published in English; they had sample sizes from 35 to 100 patients. In the five studies (4 RCTs and 1 prospective design without a control), 235 adult kidney stone disease (KSD) patients received different types of acupuncture: electro-acupuncture (2 studies), sham acupuncture and electro-acupuncture (2 studies), sham acupuncture, electro-acupuncture and auricular acupuncture (2 studies), and unspecified acupuncture (one study) d. The primary outcome measures across the studies were visual analogue scale (VAS) for pain and the State-Trait Anxiety Inventory (STAI) for anxiety. Four studies reported a statistically significant lowered pain and/or anxiety score. Two studies also reported a decrease in analgesia or opiate use. No major or minor side effects were noted with the use of acupuncture. The reviewers concluded that acupuncture reduced pain as well as anxiety and should be considered for use in outpatient urological procedures [85].

An RCT [86] in Turkey compared the efficacy of diclofenac, acetaminophen and acupuncture in treating urolithiasis-driven renal colic. Adult patients (N = 121) were divided into 3 groups: Group A (n = 40) was treated with 1 g of intravenous acetaminophen over 15 min, Group B (n = 41) was treated with acupuncture applied to the urinary bladder meridian points the side with acute renal colic pain (UB-21 to 24, UB-45 to 48), and Group C (n = 40) was treated with a 75-mg intramuscular injection of diclofenac sodium. VAS and verbal rating scale (VRS) were used to assess drop in pain intensity after 10, 30, 60, and 120 min. After 10 min, the largest decrease in VAS and VRS scores was observed in patients who received acupuncture ($p < 0.05$). At subsequent intervals (30, 60, and 120 min) either diclofenac or acetaminophen had higher decreases in VAS and VRS scores compared to acupuncture. Adverse effects were reported in individuals who received acetaminophen (one patient had an allergic reaction and another reported dizziness and vomiting) and diclofenac (one patient had rash, and 2 patients had abdominal burning/pain). No adverse effects were reported in the patients that received acupuncture treatment. The authors concluded that acupuncture is a viable alternative treatment modality for renal colic.

A RCT conducted in Tunisia [87] randomized 115 renal colic patients into two groups. The first group (n = 61) received 0.1 mg/kg intravenous morphine every 5 min until the pain score as measured using the VAS dropped by at least 50% of its baseline value. The second group (n = 54) received a 30-min acupuncture session where needles were inserted to urinary bladder meridian points on the side of the pain (UB21–24, UB26, UB45–49). VAS was used to assess pain intensity at baseline and at 10, 20, 30, 45, and 60 min after treatment. From the tenth minute until the end of the intervention, acupuncture was associated with a faster and higher analgesic effect compared to morphine ($P < 0.05$). Forty-two side effects (namely, dizziness, nausea and vomiting and drowsiness) were reported in the morphine group compared to 3 (1 needle blockage and 2 reports of itching/rash/bleeding at needle insertion point) in the acupuncture group ($P < 0.001$). The investigators suggested that acupuncture represents an effective alternative treatment for patients with high risk of adverse events due to morphine and its use be further assessed [87].

A Chinese RCT evaluated the clinical effects of body and auricular acupuncture compared to medication in treating renal colic in 60 participants (aged 16–45 years) [88]. Renal colic patients in the intervention group received body acupuncture (acupoints: bilateral Zusanli (ST36), Yanglingquan (GB 34), and Ashi points on the affected side) and auricular acupuncture (ear points: Shenmen (TF 4), Kidney (CO 10), and Bladder (CO 9) for 30 min). Patients in the medication group received an intramuscular injection with pethidine 50 mg and atropine 1 mg. Pain relief and analgesic effects were measured using a patient numeric rating scale. Patients in both groups reported reduced pain. The total effective rate was higher in the acupuncture group (89.7%) than in the medication group (77.4%); (p < 0.05). The researchers concluded that acupuncture could be used as an alternative to pethidine and atropine in treating renal colic.

Hodzic et al. (2007) [89] investigated whether acupuncture could lower or replace the need for analgesics in ESWL of kidney stones in adult patients (aged 17–85 years) in Germany. The control group (n = 78) received 50 mg pethidine plus 10 mg diazepam. Patients randomized into the treatment group (n = 86) received acupuncture at various acupoints. The main outcome was self-rated pain scores. Pain sensation was rated prior to ESWL and for every minute until 21 min after the therapy started, and for 10 min after therapy stopped. All patients who reported a pain sensation higher than 5, received analgesics delivered intravenously. Twenty percent of recruited patients refused acupuncture treatment and were excluded from the study. There was no mention of adverse events. The mean pain score throughout the treatment was significantly less for the treatment group (2.6) vs. the control group (3.2) (p < 0.0001). Acupuncture was reported to provide significantly more effective analgesia than pethidine and diazepam. It is important to note that 23% (n = 20) of patients in the acupuncture group needed additional pain medication [89].

Another RCT assessed the clinical effectiveness of electro-acupuncture compared to a combination of tramadol and midazolam in relieving pain during outpatient ESWL [90]. Thirty-five adults with kidney stones were allocated to undergo lithotripsy with a third generation lithotriptor following treatment with either electro-acupuncture (treatment group; n = 17) or tramadol/midazolam (control group; n = 18) for sedation and analgesia. For patients in the treatment group, the same licensed acupuncturist administered 20-min electro-acupuncture stimulation with 2–4 Hz frequency for 30 min prior to ESWL. Patients in the control group received treatment with tramadol (1.5 mg/kg) 30 min before the start of lithotripsy and midazolam (0.06 mg/kg) 5 min before ESWL. The main outcome, pain intensity, was measured using a VAS. Although the electro-acupuncture group was found to have lower VAS compared to the medication group, this finding was not statistically significant. Similarly, there was no significant difference in stone-free rates between the two groups. There were no adverse effects in the electro-acupuncture group. Participants in the control group experienced moderate adverse events such as orthostatic hypotension and dizziness, which did not warrant their removal from the study. The authors concluded that electro-acupuncture is an effective alternate pain relieving method without any demonstrable side effects.

In an earlier RCT, Lee and colleagues [91] investigated the effect of acupuncture compared to a conventional analgesic (Avafortan, which has since been discontinued) in the treatment of 38 adult males with renal colic from urolithiasis [91]. Patients were randomized to either receive acupuncture treatment (n = 22), or an intramuscular injection of Avafortan (n = 16). Renal colic pain scores were evaluated before treatment and 30 min following treatment. There was no significant difference in the reduction in mean pain score between the two groups, but acupuncture had a significantly faster analgesic onset than Avafortan (p < 0.05). Nearly half (n = 7) of the Avafortan group experienced side effects; 3 cases of skin rash, 2 cases of tachycardia and one case of facial flushing and drowsiness. Patients in the acupuncture group did not experience any adverse effects. The authors contended that acupuncture could be a good alternative for the treatment of renal colic.

Serious adverse events associated with acupuncture are rare. In a prospective survey of 229,230 patients (mean age 46 years) 8.6% patients reported experiencing at least one adverse event [92]. Bleeding (6.1% of patients) and pain (1.7% of patients) were the most common adverse events reported. A systematic review evaluating the safety of pediatric needle acupuncture calculated a mild adverse event incidence per patient of 168 in 1422 patients (11.8%; 95% CI: 10.1% −13.5%). In the review, adverse events included bleeding, pain, bruising and worsening of symptoms. Although rare, serious adverse events associated with acupuncture in children have occurred such as infections, thumb deformations, cardiac rapture (a fatal consequence of myocardial infarction) and hospitalization [64]. Some of the acupuncture related serious adverse events may have been avoidable as they were likely caused by substandard practice. The evidence suggests pediatric acupuncture is safe where it is performed by appropriately trained acupuncture practitioners [64, 93].

Massage

A retrospective RCT assessed the use of vibration massage therapy after ESWL in 103 adults with lower caliceal stones [94]. Patients in the experimental group (n = 51) received ESWL and 20- to 25-min sessions of vibration massage therapy (applied at a speed of 3800 rpm) in 2-day intervals for 2 weeks. The control group (n = 52) received ESWL alone. The stone-free rates in the experimental and control groups were 80% and 60%, respectively (p = 0.003). The rate of stone recurrence was significantly higher in the control group than in the experimental group (p = 0.0006). However, there were more reports of renal colic in the experimental group (p = 0.03) than in the control group. No trials investigating the use of vibration massage therapy in children were identified.

While therapeutic massage generally carries a low risk of complications, information pertaining to the safety of vibration massage is unknown.

Probiotics

Probiotics have been described as live microorganisms which can provide a health benefit to the host when ingested in adequate amounts [95].

A small pilot study investigated whether a mixture of freeze-dried lactic acid bacteria could reduce oxaluria in 6 adults with idiopathic calcium oxalate urolithiasis and hyperoxaluria [96]. During a 4-week period, all patients received 8×10^{11} freeze-dried lactic acid bacteria (*L. acidophilus, L. plantarum, L. brevis, S. thermophilus, B. infantis*) and did not eat foods rich in oxalate (e.g. spinach, chocolate, peanuts, cocoa and rhubarb). There was a significant decrease in 24-h oxalate excretion compared to baseline (p < 0.05). The treatment was associated with a mean reduction in oxaluria of approximately 30 mg/day [96]. The reduced levels were sustained for at least 1 month after the end of treatment.

Probiotics are generally safe in healthy individuals, and some probiotics (*L. acidophilus*, *Lactobacillus* GG, *Saccharomyces* sp.) have been found safe for use in children, when administered in appropriate doses [97]. Case reports of serious infections including bacteremia, fungemia, endocarditis, liver abscess, septicemia and meningitis have been associated with probiotics [95, 98]. The risk of adverse effects associated with probiotics is high in patients that are immunocompromised, including those with indwelling medical devices [95, 98].

Urinary Tract Infections

Various NHPs have been used as a prophylaxis for urinary tract infections (UTIs) including cranberry, probiotics and vitamin A. The evidence evaluating the efficacy of cranberry juice in pediatrics is increasing, while the number of pediatric trials evaluating probiotics and vitamin A remains limited. Studies often have small sample sizes and other methodological limitations.

Cranberry

In vitro evidence suggests that proanthocyanidins (tannins) and fructose found in cranberries have antibacterial activity [98] via preventing bacteria from adhering to the walls of the bladder and thus decrease the development of UTIs [99].

In 1998 Jepson and colleagues [100] published a systematic review of cranberry trials for the prevention of UTIs which they updated in 2004, 2008 and in 2012 [101]. The 2012 update included 24 studies which compared the effectiveness of cranberry in different forms and combinations (concentrate juice, tablets, liquid concentrate syrup and capsules/tablets) to placebo, no treatment, water, methenamine hippurate, antibiotics or lactobacillus. Due to design and data shortcomings, 11 studies were excluded, leaving 13 studies (2462 participants) for the meta-analyses. Studies were analysed together and separately by participant subgroups (e.g., children with first or subsequent UTI, participants with a history of recurrent lower UTI, and pregnant women). Cranberry products did not significantly reduce the risk of repeat UTI across the combined 13 studies (overall RR 0.86, 95% CI 0.71 to 1.04) or any subgroup populations analysed. Although not significant, the pediatric subgroup analysis, which compared cranberry juice to placebo/control, suggested the greatest effect (RR 0.48, 95% CI 0.19 to 1.22). Many of the studies reported low compliance and a high number of withdrawal/dropout due to problems with the palatability/acceptability of the cranberry product, mainly the cranberry juice. The authors concluded that cranberry products compared to placebo was not effective in most population groups, and that any benefit in sub-groups is likely very small.

The three pediatric RCTs included in the review are described. The largest pediatric RCT investigating the efficacy of cranberry juice in preventing UTI recurrences was performed in Finland and involved 263 children (1–16 years) with a verified UTI in the previous 2 months [102]. Children were randomized to receive 1 or 2 daily doses of up to 300 ml per day of cranberry juice containing 41 grams cranberry concentrate (n = 129) or placebo (n = 134) for 6 months and

monitored for UTI recurrences over 12 months. Nearly 45% of participants in this study were toddlers, the mean age being 3.8 years (standard deviation (SD) 2.5) in the cranberry group and 4.5 years (SD 2.9) in the placebo. Eight children were excluded from the study due to protocol violations leaving 255 children included in the analysis. There were no significant differences observed in the proportion of children that had at least one UTI after entering the study; 20 vs. 28 children in the intervention and controls, respectively. The UTI incidence per person-year at risk was 0.16 episodes lower in the cranberry group (95% CI, 2.31 to −.01; p = 0.035) [102]. Twenty-seven children dropped out: 16 from the cranberry group and 11 from the placebo group. The authors only cited the main reason for withdrawal, which was reluctance to drink the juice (7 from the intervention and 6 from the placebo groups).

The second RCT [103] compared the effectiveness of cranberry juice vs. *Lactobacillus* in preventing the recurrence of UTIs in 84 girls (aged 3–14 year; mean age 7.5) in Italy. The girls were randomized to receive, for a 6-month period, either: a daily 50 ml dose of cranberry juice containing 7.5 g of cranberry concentrate and 1.7 g of lingonberry concentrate juice in 50 ml of water, without sugar additives (n = 28); 100 ml of *Lactobacillus* drink containing 4×10^7 cfu of *Lactobacillus* GG/100 ml on 5 days a month (n = 27); or control (n = 29). Four children dropped out due to poor compliance to the protocol, two from the control group and one from each of the other groups. During the 6 months of observation, reduction in UTIs was significant (p < 0.05) for the cranberry group compared to the other groups: UTI occurrence was 5/27 (18.5%) in the cranberry group; 11/26 (42.3%) in the *Lactobacillus* group; and 18/27 (48.1%) in the control group.

The third RCT [104] recruited children (aged 1 month to 13 years) with more than two UTIs in the last 6 months. Children (n = 192) in the treatment group received a nocturnal dose of 0.2 ml/kg of cranberry syrup (5 ml of the syrup contained 36 mg of highly bioactive proanthocyanidin (PACs); n = 75). Children in the control group ingested 0.2 ml/kg of a color-masked suspension of trimethoprim at a concentration of 8 mg/ml just before the evening meal (n = 117) for a year. The incidence of UTIs was 18.9% (n = 18) in the trimethoprim group (95% CI:11%–26.3%) and 8.4% (n = 8) (95% CI: 2.8%–13.9%) in the cranberry group. However, there was no significant difference between the two groups. Adverse reports included: gastrointestinal intolerance (5 in the trimethoprim group and 2 in the cranberry group) and a case of rash in each group. The authors concluded that cranberry syrup was non-inferior to trimethoprim in preventing recurrent UTIs.

In 2015 Durham and colleagues evaluated the use of cranberry products for the prevention of UTIs in pediatric patients in a literature review. Of the eight trials reviewed: 3 were in healthy children [102, 103, 105] and 5 in children with underlying urogenital abnormalities [104, 106–109]. The literature review concluded that cranberry products may be an effective option for preventing recurrent UTIs in healthy children, while in children with anatomical abnormalities the findings were inconclusive. In two trials that compared the effectiveness of cranberry juice to antibiotics in children with underlying urogenital abnormalities, cranberry juice was found to have comparable efficacy to antibiotics [104, 108]. This finding is important as cranberry juice could be an alternative to the use of antibiotics at a time when overuse of antimicrobial agents and antibiotic resistance is on the rise [110].

A Taiwanese RCT [111] not included in the previously described reviews evaluated the effects of highly concentrated cranberry juice in preventing repeat UTI's in boys aged 6–18 years (55 uncircumcised and 12 circumcised). Over a 6-month period, uncircumcised boys in group A (n = 28) drank 120 mL of cranberry juice daily and in group B (control) drank placebo. A third control group C of circumcised boys also drank a placebo juice. The main outcome was a confirmed urine culture of symptomatic UTI. The results showed that recurrent UTI's was 25%, 37% and 33.3% in groups A (cranberry), B and C, respectively. No adverse effects were observed in the study. The findings support the use of con-

centrated cranberry juice to reduce the number of repeated episodes of UTI in uncircumcised boys compared to placebo (in circumcised and uncircumcised boys).

Cranberry products (mostly as juice) have been observed to decrease the risk of UTIs in healthy children, and in children with urogenital abnormalities cranberries appear to be just as effective as antibiotic prophylaxis. The primary adverse effects reported by children following cranberry juice intake are mild: sour taste and a lingering aftertaste [99]. No serious adverse effects have been reported from cranberry fruit; however, large intake of cranberry products should be used with caution to prevent the potential for gastrointestinal distress and diarrhea. The use of sweetened cranberry products should be used with caution in diabetic and overweight individuals as it unnecessarily exposes them to carbohydrates and calories [110].

It is safe to use cranberry in clinical practice; however, it is important to note that information regarding the amount and concentration of pro-anthocyanidins (PACs) in commercially available cranberry juice products may not be known. In addition, PACs are degradable molecules, which means the manufacturing data and storage practices are crucial factors in determining the bioavailability of PACs.

Probiotics

A RCT compared the effect of probiotic and placebo in preventing UTIs in children (4 months to 5 years) with uncomplicated UTI [112]. Children (N = 181) were randomized to receive a probiotic mixture of Lactobacillus acidophilus, Lactobacillus rhamnosus, Bifidobacterium bifidum, and Bifidobacterium lactis (n = 91) or placebo (n = 90) for a total of 18 months of therapy. The primary outcome measure was being UTI free (composite cure) during the study period. At 18 months, compared to children who received placebo, the composite cure was significantly (p = 0.02) higher in children treated with probiotics (96.7% vs 83.3%, respectively). The researchers reported that there were no specific adverse events among the participants who received the probiotic mixture during the course of therapy.

The findings by Sadeghi-Bojd (2020) [112] are consistent with those reported in an RCT [113] that compared probiotic to antibiotic prophylaxis for the prevention of UTIs in 129 children with persistent primary vesicoureteral reflux (VUR) for 1 year prior to the study [113]. Children were randomized to receive probiotics twice daily (*Lactobacillus acidophilus* 10^8 colony forming units (cfu) twice a day, n = 60) or once a day antibiotic (trimethoprim/sulfamethoxazole 2/10 mg/kg, n = 60) at bedtime. The incidence of UTIs was 18.3% in the probiotic group and 21.6% in the antibiotic group, but the difference was not statistically significant. Two children from the probiotic group and one from the antibiotic group dropped out due to noncompliance. The authors concluded that probiotics prophylaxis was as effective as antibiotic prophylaxis in preventing UTIs in children with persistent primary VUR [113].

An earlier double blind RCT assessed whether probiotics could prevent UTIs in 585 preterm infants (birth weight < 1500 g or gestational age < 33 weeks) [114]. Newborns were randomized to receive standard milk enriched with 6×10^9 cfu of *Lactobacillus* GG (n = 295) or standard milk with placebo (n = 290) once a day beginning with the first feed and continued until they were discharged (mean 48 days). The occurrence of UTIs in the babies receiving probiotic-enriched milk was less compared to that observed in the control group (3.4% vs. 5.8%). This difference was, however, not statistically significant.

Unlike the above studies a meta-analysis that included 10 studies (N = 2865; 61.5% boys) found no beneficial effect of probiotics in preventing UTIs (RR = 0.94; 95% CI 0.85–1.03; p = 0.19) and recurrence (RR = 0.93; 95% CI 0.85–1.02; p = 0.14) in children and adolescents [115]. When probiotics were used as adjuvant therapy to antibiotics, the incidence of UTI was reduced (RR = 0.92; 95% CI 0.85–0.99; p = 0.02). The studies in the meta-analysis included children with the following characteristics: admitted into intensive care (4 studies, n = 1681); with vesicoureteral reflux (3 studies, n = 333); first-time UTI (1 study, n = 80), preterm (1 study, n = 585) and preterm with acute pyelonephritis (1 study, n = 186). The outcomes measured were incidence of UTI (5 studies), recurrence of UTI (4 studies), and both were evaluated in one study. The meta-analysis had several limitations (7 studies were of poor quality) that prevent generalizing the findings. Moreover, most studies were conducted in preterm infants or children that were admitted into intensive care.

An earlier 2015 [116] systematic review (N = 725) that included 9 trials (4 included children) comparing the effectiveness of probiotic use to no treatment, placebo or antibiotics in children and adults with complicated UTI also reported no significant benefit for probiotics. Adverse effects reported in the studies included diarrhoea, nausea, vomiting, constipation, and vaginal symptoms. The reviewers noted that most studies had small sample sizes and poor methodological reporting limiting rigorous evaluation [116].

Current evidence on the efficacy of probiotics in preventing or reducing the recurrence of UTI in children is inconclusive. Additional research with larger sample sizes is needed to provide more conclusive evidence and to answer many unresolved questions such as what is the most effective probiotic strain, the ideal combination of strains, effective doses, and the safety of long-term use.

Vitamin A

Vitamin A has anti-inflammatory properties, which in animal studies have been demonstrated to reduce the damage to kidneys after glomerulonephritis [117].

An Iranian RCT evaluated the efficacy of vitamin A supplementation in combination with antibiotics for improving UTI symptoms and preventing renal scarring in girls (N = 90, aged 2–12 years) with acute pyelonephritis (APN) [118]. Children were randomized to receive 10 days of oral vitamin A (n = 36) or placebo (n = 38) in addition to antibiotics during the acute phase of infection. Sixteen girls were lost to follow-up. The main outcomes were duration of UTI symptoms during trial treatment period and renal scarring as measured by 99 mTc-DMSA scan. The duration of fever (vitamin A: 1.8 days, placebo: 3.1, p = 0.0026), urinary frequency (1.3 vs. 2.8, p = 0.003) and poor feeding (2.3 vs. 4.2, p = 0.005) were significantly less in the vitamin A group than in the placebo group. The vitamin A group showed renal lesion improvement on DMSA scan compared to the placebo group: 63.8% (23 patients) vs. 21% (8 patients), respectively (P < 0.0001) [118] No vitamin A intolerance or adverse effects were observed in the study. The researchers concluded that vitamin supplementation was effective in improving UTI clinical symptoms and reducing scarring following APN, but called for larger studies with longer follow-up.

A meta-analysis [119] of four studies assessed the efficacy of vitamin A administration in addition to antibiotic therapy on renal damage in children aged 1–144 months (N = 248) after APN (120 in the experimental group and 128 in the control group). Three studies were performed in Iran and one was performed in China. The doses and duration of vitamin A were slightly different across studies. Vitamin A was inversely associated with renal damage (relative risk 0.53, 95% confidence interval 0.43–0.67) when compared with placebo after an average follow-up of 5 months. Although vitamin A may have a preventive effect on renal damage in children with APN, these findings need to be further investigated because the few studies in the meta-analysis were of low methodological quality (risk of selection and attrition bias) [119].

A small Turkish RCT not included in the meta-analysis [119] examined the effectiveness of a high dose of vitamin A in preventing UTIs in 24 children (mean age 6.3 ± 1.09 years) with non-complicated lower recurrent UTI [120]. All children received 10 days of antimicrobial therapy and were also randomly assigned to vitamin A (n = 12) or placebo (n = 12). After eradication of infection, children in both groups received antimicrobial prophylaxis and were followed for 1 year. Among children who received vitamin A supplementation, the recurrence rate of UTIs was

reduced from 3.58 to 0.75 (p = 0.002) in the first 6 months. During the same period, UTI recurrence rate in the placebo also decreased, but was not statistically significant. There was no mention of adverse events. The authors concluded that vitamin A may have a beneficial role as an adjuvant for treatment of recurrent UTI [120].

Vitamin A is safe at usual doses; however, when taken at more than 25,000 IU, toxicity may include elevated intracranial pressure, severe liver injury (cirrhosis), bone and cartilage damage, and diarrhea [121]. Because vitamin A is fat soluble, it can be stored in the human body and released long after it is taken. There have been two reports of vitamin A toxicity in two hemodialysis patients who had consumed large quantities of vitamin A. The two patients had serum vitamin A levels of 220 ug/dl and 380 ug/dl respectively (normal vitamin A is between 30–95 ug/dl) [122].

Larger and adequately designed studies are needed to confirm whether vitamin A is an effective prophylaxis that alleviates renal scarring (damage) and to determine what dosage is safe for long-term use in the prevention of UTIs in children.

Vitamin D

Vitamin D is known to have an effect on bone and mineral homeostasis in the human body. What is not yet known is its immunoregulatory role in enhancing the body's defenses against bacterial and viral infections [123].

A 2014 small RCT [124] in Iran investigated the effect of Vitamin D supplementation on prevention of recurrent UTI in 68 children and adolescents. Study participants either received Vitamin D (1000 IU/daily) (n = 33) or placebo (n = 32) for 6 months. The differences in the frequency of UTIs was not significantly different between the two groups studied (P = 0.72). There was no mention of adverse effects. The author concluded that vitamin D at the dose levels taken in this study had no significant effect on preventing recurrent UTI, and suggested that more research is required with higher doses of vitamin D and longer follow-up [124].

Chronic Kidney Disease

Complementary therapies that have been used to treat symptoms associated with CKD include NHPs such as folic acid, L-arginine, rhubarb, and various TCM herbal medicines. More conventional approaches have included evaluations of a low-protein diet.

Folic Acid

One of the leading causes of death among CKD patients is cardiovascular disease. Some research has been conducted to evaluate the effects of folic acid supplementation on endothelial function and homocysteine levels. Bennett-Richards et al. [125] performed a crossover RCT involving 25 children (aged 7–17 years) with CKD, who over an 8-week period received 5 mg/m² of folic acid per day, followed by an 8-week washout period, and 8 weeks of placebo [125]. Twenty-three children completed the study. During the folic acid phase, homocysteine levels decreased (10.3 mol/L to 8.6 mol/L, p = 0.03), while no decrease in levels was observed during the placebo period. In addition, during the folic acid phase, endothelial-dependent flow-mediated dilatation improved significantly from 7.21 (2.8%) to 8.47 (3.01%) (p = 0.036). The authors speculated that, although folic acid supplementation in adults with CKD have largely been negative, the positive finding in children may be linked to the timing of treatment because atherosclerosis in children is at an earlier stage of its natural history. Folic acid is safe when taken at recommended dosages. More studies in pediatric populations are needed with relevant clinical outcomes before folic acid supplementation can be recommended in pediatric CKD.

Oral L-Arginine

In a crossover RCT, Bennett-Richards et al. [126] examined the effect of dietary supplementation with oral L-arginine on the response of the endothelium to shear stress in 21 children (aged 7–17 years) with CKD and documented endothelial dysfunction. During the treatment phase, each child received 2.5 g/m² or 5 g/m² of oral L-arginine three times a day for a 4-week period.

This was followed by a rest period of 4 weeks and then 4 weeks of placebo. Twenty-one children completed the study as 4 children withdrew (2 due to L-arginine taste complaints, one due to L-arginine related nausea and another received a renal transplant). After the treatment phase, a significant rise in levels of plasma L-arginine was observed; however, there was no significant change in endothelial-dependent dilation. Hence, dietary supplementation with L-arginine was not useful in the treatment of children with CKD. L-arginine at the dosage used resulted in some children experiencing metabolic side effects, namely increased urea and extracellular acidosis [126]. The authors suggested that this could have also contributed to the negative results observed in the study.

Rhubarb

A systematic review that included 18 randomized and quasi-randomized trials (n = 1322) assessed the use of rhubarb in adult patients with CKD [127]. The included trials compared different forms of rhubarb, including tablets and decoctions, to conventional medicine (e.g. captopril) and TCM herbs. The doses and parts of the plant used were not specified. Rhubarb was found to be significantly more effective in treating CKD than conventional medicine alone. However, there was no significant difference in effectiveness between rhubarb and other TCM herbs for treating CKD. Although rhubarb was effective in reducing the symptoms of CKD, it was not possible to determine whether it could slow or stop long-term progression due to the small number of patients. Half the included trials reported adverse events, but these were not described.

Rhubarb is possibly safe for most people when used for short periods (i.e., less than 8 days) and in low doses [128]. Rhubarb has been associated with side effects such as abdominal pain and diarrhea [128]. Long-term use of rhubarb can result in several adverse effects, including electrolyte depletion, edema, colic, atonic colon, and hyperaldosteronism. Rhubarb leaves contain oxalic acid and are considered toxic if ingested [128]. Patients with renal disorders should be cautious and monitored closely when using rhubarb as potential electrolyte disturbances may occur [128]. Individuals with renal stones are not advised to consume rhubarb because of its high oxalate content [129]. Rhubarb safety and dosing information for children is limited and not conclusive.

TCM Herbs

The effectiveness of TCM herbs as a supplement treatment to conventional drugs in the treatment of CKD was assessed in an RCT including 248 adults [130]. For a year, the TCM group (n = 120) received conventional drugs (including prednisone and furosemide) in combination with 5 different herbal decoctions which were individualized in terms of type used and dosage. The TCM herbs were selected to supplement the kidney (as described by TCM theory) and invigorate blood flow. Details related to the composition of the TCM herb decoctions can be found in the original article. The control group (n = 128) received conventional medicine for a year. Significant differences between the two groups were found in improved symptoms (92.5% for TCM vs. 49.2% for control group, p < 0.01) and in improved CRCL (56 ml/min for TCM vs. 37 ml/min for control group, p < 0.01). There was no mention of side effects in the study, and safety information regarding the various TCM herbs used is unknown. Further research is required to determine if the results can be replicated in children.

Protein Restriction

A Cochrane review [131] assessed the effectiveness of a protein-restricted diet in delaying the start of maintenance dialysis and maintaining nutrition in children with CKD. The review included 2 studies (250 children) which compared outcomes for 124 children receiving a protein restricted diet to 126 children on a control diet. The protein-restricted diet given to children was equivalent to the lowest safe protein intake recommended by the World Health Organization (0.8 to 1.1 g/kg/day). The reviewers found no significant differences in the number of renal deaths (RR 1.12, 95% CI 0.54 to 2.33), progression of kidney disease as measured by CRCL at 2 years (mean difference 1.47, 95% CI −1.19 to 4.14) or

growth. Thus, the authors concluded that reducing protein intake does not appear to have a significant impact in delaying the progression to ESKD in children. A major limitation for this review was that only two studies were identified. Of these, one had a small sample size (n = 24) and the larger study (n = 226) had significant loss to follow-up [131].

The larger study included in the above systematic review was a multicenter randomized trial involving 226 children (aged 2 to 18) with CKD from 25 pediatric nephrology centers across Europe [132]. After a 6 month run in period, children were first stratified into one of two groups (progressive or non-progressive disease). They were then further stratified into 3 renal disease groups. Children were then randomly assigned into either a diet or control group. Over a 2-year period, the intervention group received a low protein, 0.8 to 1.1 g/kg of protein a day, with adjustments made for age, while the control group had no protein intake restrictions. After 2 years in the study, 112 participants agreed to continue for an additional year. GFR was estimated every 2 months by CRCL. No statistically significant differences in the decline of CRCL were found, suggesting little value in protein restriction in pediatric CKD. There was significant loss of follow-up. No adverse effects were reported, including growth impairment due to the protein-restricted diet.

The smaller study included in the protein diet restriction systematic review was a multicenter RCT which evaluated the effect of a low-protein intake in a group of 24 infants (aged 8 months) with CKD [133]. Infants were randomized to receive a low protein (1.4 ± 0.3 g/kg/day, (protein: energy ratio 5.6%) or control protein (2.4 ± 0.4 g/kg/day, protein: energy ratio 10.4%) formula for 10 months. During the 2-month run-in period prior to randomization, all infants were fed formula with intermediate protein (protein: energy ratio of 8%). An assessment of GFR over time could not be conducted due to the short follow-up period and lack of progression to ESKD in patients. At 18 months, the low protein group had significantly lower standard deviation scores for length compared to the control group (−2.6+ 1.2 vs. −1.7 + 1.4),raising safety concerns of a low protein diet in this young population. It is recommended that extra caution be employed when considering any protein restrictions until larger prospective RCTs provide more data on efficacy and safety in children. Although there were no dropouts due to adverse events, 2 infants from each group had possible protein deficiency (based on poor weight gain) or excess protein (defined as blood urea nitrogen (BUN) greater than 80 mg/dl or BUN/serum creatinine ratio greater than 60). These infants were given their individual group formula combined (50:50) with the intermediate (8%) protein: energy ratio formula until the end of the study.

Rheum Officinale

Rheum officinale (Da Huang, a medicinal herb) is a type of rhubarb from the family *Polygonaceae*, and has been used by TCM practitioners for its strong cathartic action, and more recently, to delay progression of CKD [134].

A systematic review [134] which examined the effectiveness of *Rheum officinale* (Da Huang) in treating or preventing the progression of CKD found no evidence to recommend its use. The systematic review included 682 patients from 9 studies. Seven of the trials compared *Rheum officinale* with no treatment and 2 compared it to captopril. The main outcome was changes in two blood markers that indicate progression of CKD: serum creatinine (Cr) and BUN. Compared with no treatment, *Rheum officinale* had a positive effect on Cr (MD −87.49 µmol/L, 95% CI −139.25 to −35.72) and BUN (MD −10.61 mmol/L, 95% CI −19.45 to −2.21). The studies had various methodological shortcomings that included lack of reporting on group allocation or blinding (all studies) and small or relatively small sample size (all studies). Only one small trial (n = 30) reported on adverse effects: two-thirds of the study participants experienced diarrhea when taking more than 3 g/day of *Rheum officinale*. Despite the seemingly positive results, the authors highlighted that there was no high quality evidence to indicate that treatment with *Rheum officinale* can improve CKD or delay its

progression. Well-designed RCTs are needed to better assess if there are benefits from *Rheum officinale* for CKD patients. More safety information about *Rheum officinale* is also needed.

Topical Herbal Medicine

Zhang H et al. [135] evaluated if the topical application of herbal medicine delays the progress of renal disease and improves its complications in CKD patients. The review included 23 trials, all published in Chinese, that compared external use of herbal medicine (e.g. herbal paste, herbal body/foot bathing or fuming) with no treatment, placebo, or conventional treatment. Commonly prescribed ingredients in the herbal paste and bathing formulas were Radix et Rhizoma Rhei (Da huang), Radix Salviae Miltiorrhiza (Dan shen), Rhizoma Chuanxiong (Chuan xiong), Radix Angelicae Sinensis (Dang gui), and Radix Astragali (Huang qi). The authors suggested that herbal paste and bathing or fuming treatment may be effective in delaying renal disease progression, improving kidney function, and improving some kidney complications in CKD patients. However, because of the low quality and poor reporting practices of the included trials, the authors were unable to reach a more definitive conclusion. Instead, they expressed a need for the current findings to be confirmed through larger, well-designed clinical trials with longer follow-up (greater than the 2 weeks to 2 months employed in the majority of studies included in the review) and appropriate primary outcome measures (GFR, ESKD, and all-cause mortality).

Bicarbonate

An open label RCT found that supplementation with bicarbonate was effective in slowing progression of CKD and in improving the nutritional status of 134 adults attending a predialysis clinic in the United Kingdom [136]. Patients were randomized to receive 1.82 ± 0.80 g/day oral supplementation with sodium bicarbonate (n = 67) or usual care (n = 67) for 2 years. The main primary and secondary outcomes were change in CrCl and dietary protein intake, respectively. Side effects were similar between the two groups, and included worsening of hypertension and edema. A small proportion (6.5%) of patients in the supplementation group did not like the taste of bicarbonate. Compared with the control group, decline in CrCl was significantly slower in patients who received bicarbonate supplementation (5.93 vs. 1.88 ml/min 1.73 m^2; p < 0.0001). Fewer patients supplemented with bicarbonate developed ESKD (6.5 vs. 33%; relative risk 0.13; 95% confidence interval 0.04 to 0.40; p < 0.001). Compared to the control group, nutritional status, as measured by dietary protein intake, also improved significantly in the bicarbonate supplementation group (p < 0.007). The observed benefits and tolerability of bicarbonate supplementation, inexpensive and simple strategy, warrants further investigation of efficacy and safety through multi-centre double-blind RCTs in adults and children.

Traditional Chinese Medicine (TCM)

A meta-analysis of 39 Chinese RCTs investigated the efficacy and safety of TCM alone or in combination with Western medicine in reducing the risk of kidney damage in children (N = 3643) with Henoch-Schönlein Purpura (HSP) [137]. The RCT had a follow-up period between 2 weeks and 1 year and interventions included TCM self-preparation, TCM differentiation, Xijiao Dihuang Decoction, and Chinese patent medicines. In 7 RCTs (n = 582), adverse effects were significantly (p < 0.05) higher in children in the control 7.6% (20 cases of 263 patients) than treatment group 3.5% (12 of 319 patients). TCM significantly (P < 0.01) improved the treatment effect (OR: 4.31, 95% CI [3.34, 5.57], reduced the risk of kidney damage (RR: 0.36; 95% CI [0.21, 0.61], and rate of HSP recurrence (RR: 0.43, 95% CI [0.34, 0.54]. Although this study showed that TCM is an effective treatment for HSP, the RCTs included had several limitations, including small sample size, inconsistent follow-up, and poor to moderate quality of some of the studies. Large multi-centre trials are required to confirm these results.

A prospective, controlled, open-label study [138] of 150 children (aged 5–16 years) with HSP and proteinuria examined the efficacy and effectiveness taking a Traditional Chinese herbal

decoction Qingre-Lishi-Yishen Formula (QLYF). All (N = 150) children received oral glucocorticoid and cyclophosphamide intravenous pulse regimen (Western medicine), and 100 of the 150 also received QLYF (integrated therapy). Children were followed up for 2 years. The main outcome measures were: adverse events and short- and long-term clinical effects. Compared to children that received the Western medicine only, children who received the integrated therapy had lower adverse event rates of respiratory infection, urinary infection, hepatoxicity, poor appetite, cardiotoxicity, and neutropenia(p < 0.05). The integrated therapy group also had lower levels of 24-h urine protein, urine blood cell count, occurrence of secondary TCM syndrome, and recurrence rate (p < 0.05).

Zhang et al. [139] and Ding et al. [140] published a protocols for a large multi-centre prospective studies to investigate the effectiveness and safety of Chinese Herbal Medicine (CHM) for the treatment of HSP in children [139, 140]. These findings are not yet available for inclusion in this review.

Uremic Pruritus

Although no pediatric studies were identified, various complementary therapies, such as acupuncture, acupressure, thermal therapy, homeopathy and aromatherapy, have been evaluated in the treatment of uremic pruritus in adults undergoing dialysis.

Acupuncture

Kim and associates [141] examined the effectiveness of acupuncture for uremic pruritus in patients with ESKD. Their review included three parallel RCTs, a controlled clinical trial, and two uncontrolled observational studies (case series). Needle acupuncture was assessed in four studies and electro-acupuncture in 2 studies. All studies used standardized acupuncture protocols, and primary endpoints such as the pruritus score and symptom relief were measured. Although all the included trials reported beneficial effects of acupuncture, the majority of studies had high risk of bias as measured by the Cochrane criteria. The authors also cited publication bias as a potential limitation to the review and considered the evidence insufficient and inconclusive to support the usefulness of acupuncture as effective treatment for uremic pruritus in patients with ESKD.

Evidence from the three RCTs included in the above systematic review will be described, starting with the most recent study which investigated the efficacy of applying acupuncture at a single acupoint in treating refractory uremic pruritus in 40 hemodialysis patients (mean age of 62 years) in China [142]. Patients allocated to receive intervention had a 1-inch 34-gauge acupuncture needle inserted at Quchi (LI11) for an hour three times a week for a month. Patients in the control group had a 1-inch 34-gauge needle inserted 2 cm lateral to the Quchi (LI11) acupoint, for the same time period. The main outcomes captured through a pruritus score questionnaire included severity, distribution and frequency of uremic pruritus and related sleep disturbance. Outcomes were measured before and after 1 month and 3 months of treatment. Within the acupuncture group compared to baseline (38.3 ± 4.3), pruritus scores significantly decreased after acupuncture at 1 month (17.3 ± 5.5) and 3 months (16.5 ± 4.9; p = 0.001). Pruritus scores were not significantly different in the control group at 38.3 ± 4.3, 37.5 ± 3.2 and 37.1 ± 5, respectively. Two patients from the acupuncture group and one in the control group experienced elbow soreness which resolved after 1 day, and three patients in the acupuncture group had minimal bleeding. The authors concluded that acupuncture at the Quchi (LI11) acupoint was an easy, safe and effective means of relieving uremic pruritus.

An earlier study compared the effects of needle acupuncture to oral antihistamine for uremic pruritus in 68 adult hemodialysis patients (mean age 43.6) [143]. Patients in the intervention group (n = 34) received 30-min acupuncture sessions twice a week for 4 weeks. The control group (n = 34) received 4 mg of chlorpheniramine and a topical dermatitis ointment (no ingredient details were provided) three times daily for 2 weeks. Patients were then observed for the alleviation of pruritus. A significantly higher effective rate of 95% was observed in the acupuncture group, compared to an effective rate of 70.6% in the control group (p < 0.01). In the acupuncture group, this improvement was maintained in 16 patients for 3 months and 18 patients for 1 month. Once treatment administration stopped, uremic pruritus recurred in all patients in the control group.

The largest study included in the systematic review compared the efficacy of acupuncture to oral calcitriol in treating uremic pruritus in 150 hemodialysis adult patients [144]. Patients in the intervention group (n = 80) received acupuncture for 20 min, twice or three times per week for a total of 16 weeks. During the same period, the control group received oral calcitriol. Within group changes in the acupuncture and control group were similar, with an 88% response rate. No adverse events occurred in this study.

Adult efficacy and safety data for acupuncture are promising and some clinicians may want to consider including acupuncture for patients with uremic pruritus.

Acupressure

Acupressure is part of TCM and involves pressing and/or massaging various acupuncture points on the body [145].

A non-randomized control trial published in 2013 investigated the effect of acupressure on uremic pruritus in 78 adult patients receiving hemodialysis [146]. Using a transcutaneous electrical nerve stimulation (TENS), acupressure apparatus patients in the intervention group (n = 38) received acupressure at the SP6, ST36, SP10, and LI11 points three times/week for 6 weeks and a total of 18 sessions. Patients in the control group received no acupressure. Outcome points were captured using a VAS and a pruritus score. The presence or absence of adverse effects was not reported. Mean VAS and pruritus scores significantly decreased at week 6 (p < 0.001) in the acupuncture group compared to the control group. This decrease showed a stable trend in weeks 12 and 18 (p > 0.05). Throughout the study, patients in the acupuncture group were also observed to use less medication than the control (p < 0.001). Acupressure was concluded to be effective in reducing pruritus in hemodialysis patients.

An earlier RCT also showed that acupressure decreases pruritic symptoms in 60 adult dialysis patients [145]. Patients in the treatment group (n = 30) received 15–20 min sessions of acupressure three times a week for 5 weeks, either immediately before or after dialysis. The control group (n = 30) received no other treatment. Between the acupuncture and control groups, significant differences in mean pruritus scores at 6, 12 and 18 weeks after baseline were found, with the acupressure group having lower scores (p < 0.0001).

Acupressure is believed to be quite safe as it is a non-invasive procedure that does not involve needle insertion. Some clinicians may choose to consider it in treatment in their patients with uremic pruritus.

Thermal Therapy

A RCT that employed convenience sampling [147] compared the effectiveness of thermal therapy to non-thermal therapy on uremic pruritus and biochemical parameters in 49 hemodialysis patients. For various reasons, 8 patients (thermal group = 3, non-thermal group = 5) dropped out of the study, leaving 41 patients. The intervention group (n = 21) was treated with 40 °C thermal therapy with far infrared rays, a type of electromagnetic wave with a wavelength of 4 ~ 1000 µm [147], at the Sanyinjiao (SP6) acupoint once a day for 15 min on 2 days a week for a total of 18 sessions. The control group (n = 20) had a plain adhesive patch placed on the same acupoint plus routine care. Uremic pruritus improved in both groups, with a larger decrease in pruritus scores in the thermal group (p < 0.001) as compared with the non-thermal group. There was, however, no difference in pruritus scores between the two groups. No side effects related to the intervention were observed. The effectiveness of thermal therapy for uremic pruritus treatment warrants further investigation.

Homeopathy

Homeopathy is the use of substances that cause a particular symptom (e.g., rash) in healthy individuals to treat unwell patients with the same symptom (e.g., "like cures like"), with the belief that progressive dilution of the substance strengthens the remedy. Cavalcanti et al [148] performed an RCT to evaluate the effect of individualized homeopathic treatment on uremic pruritus in 20 adults from 5 dialysis centres. The experimental group (n = 11) received a homeopathic treatment and the control group (n = 9) were given placebo. All patients were assessed individually by a homeopath that was free to change the prescription based on reassessments of the patients after treatment had begun. During the study, 40 homeopathic medications were prescribed and each patient in the homeopathic group received more than one type of homeopathic remedy. At each point of observation, that is after 15, 30, 45, and 60 days of follow-up, pruritus scores were found to have decreased significantly (p < 0.05) in the treatment group. However, at the end of the study, post-treatment pruritus scores between the two groups were not significantly different. The authors concluded that homeopathy may be a valuable option in relieving uremic pruritus.

Side effects associated with homeopathy are generally rare and not severe. Some side-effects reported include allergic reactions and symptom aggravation [149].

Aromatherapy

A pre and post-clinical study [150] using convenience sampling assessed the effect of aromatherapy on pruritus relief in 24 adult patients receiving hemodialysis. Over a 2-week period, participants received 6 sessions of 7 min of hand massage in the non-fistulated hand with 3–5 ml of lavender, mint, and tea tree oils at 5% concentration. Four patients withdrew from the study; two objected to the oil odor, one had incontinence linked to the greasy oil sensation, and one patient was lost to follow-up. In the twenty patients that completed the study, the average pruritus score decreased significantly from 7.40 (1.18) at pre-intervention to 5.85 (1.69) at post-intervention (t = 5.43, p < 0.001), suggesting that aromatherapy can significantly relieve pruritus in hemodialysis patients.

A previous study also showed positive results when using aromatherapy and massage for the treatment of uremic pruritus in 29 adult dialysis patients [151]. Patients in the experimental group (n = 13) received aromatherapy (lavender or tea tree oil) using massage 3 times a week for 4 weeks. The control group (n = 16) received no treatment. In the experimental group, the mean pruritus score decreased significantly from 5.69 (SD = 1.25) before treatment to 2.69 (SD = 1.03) after treatment (p $^<$ 0.001). Pruritus scores were significantly lower in the experimental group vs. the control group (t = 6.60, p = 0.001) after the treatment period. The investigators suggested that the massage component of the aromatherapy may have confounded the findings and recommended future studies also provide massage to the control group.

Some aromatherapy oils have been linked to adverse effects such headache, nausea, and allergic reactions [12]. Although aromatherapy was found to be useful in the studies discussed with mild adverse effects, generalization and application of this therapy for uremic pruritus still requires further investigation using better designed studies with larger sample sizes and longer follow-up periods.

Chinese Herbal Bath Therapy

A meta-analysis [152] of 17 RCTs (N = 970; study sample size ranged from 24 to 156 adult patients) assessed the efficacy of Chinese herbal bath therapy (CHBT) in the treatment of uremic pruritus in adult hemodialysis (HD) patients. In CHBT, decoction or extract of Chinese medicine is poured into warm water and then patients bathe in it [152]. Patients in the treatment group bathed in baths that included 11 Chinese herbs for a period ranging between 2 weeks and 3 months (mean = 4.7 weeks). During the same time period, the control group used standard medical treatment alone or in combination with sham CHBT, clean hot water bath, or calamine lotion. At the end of the treatment period, the outcomes measures were pruritus level (measured using the VAS or the symptom score scale) and the total effective rate. None of the RCTs mentioned adverse events. CHBT plus basic treatment sig-

nificantly (p < 0.00001) reduce the VAS score (MD = − 2.38; 95% confidence intervals [CI], − 3.02 to − 1.74) and the symptom score (MD = − 8.42; 95% confidence intervals [CI], − 12.47 to − 4.36) and had a higher total effectiveness rate (risk ratio [RR] = 1.46; 95% CI, 1.31 to 1.63). The authors noted that the quality of RCTs was poor to moderate. The majority of studies suffered from unclear randomization and concealment, lack of blinding and selective reporting [152].

Although findings suggest CHBT improves pruritic symptoms in individuals with uremic pruritus further investigation, with better designed (large sample size, randomization) studies is warranted to determine efficacy and safety.

End Stage-Renal Disease (ESKD)

Studies have investigated the efficacy of complementary therapies such as O3FA, acupuncture and acupressure, in reducing fatigue and depression and improving the quality of sleep and life among adult patients with ESKD. The findings from these studies suggest some positive effects and warrant further examination in pediatric populations.

O3FA

A multi-center clinical trial conducted in Iran investigated the efficacy of O3FA on inflammatory markers, namely C-reactive protein and tumor necrosis factor-alfa (TNF-α), in 45 patients with ESKD (aged 15–63 years) [82]. For 2 months, study participants received 3 g of O3FA per day (1 g omega-3 Pearl 3 times a day). Nine patients withdrew from the study: 5 for personal reasons; 2 underwent kidney transplantation and one died. After 2 months, TNF-α serum levels decreased significantly from 6.91 ± 15.25 to 2.35 ± 8.02, p = 0.038 among the 37 patients who completed the study. Adverse effects associated with O3FA included nausea, diarrhea and an unfavorable smell. The authors concluded that O3FA has a positive effect in reducing inflammatory markers in ESKD patients, but acknowledged that a larger study with a longer duration of treatment was needed. Future studies would benefit from the addition of a control group, randomization, and blinding.

Acupressure

A recent double blind RCT conducted in two hospitals in Iran found that acupressure in conjunction with routine care improves the sleep quality of ESKD adult patients [153]. Over 4 weeks, patients in the intervention group (n = 22) received routine care and acupressure on the Shenmen (He7) and He Gu (Li4) points in the hands and Sanyingjao (sp6) point in the feet, while the control group (n = 22) received routine care only. After the intervention, significant differences between the acupressure group and the control group were recorded for the global Pittsburgh Sleep Quality Index score (p < 0.001) and all sleep quality indices: subjective sleep quality (p < 0.001), sleep latency (p < 0.001), sleep duration (p < 0.001), sleep efficiency (p = 0.006), sleep disturbance (p < 0.001), the use of sleeping medication (p = 0.028), and daytime dysfunction (p < 0.001). Although these preliminary findings support the effectiveness of acupressure in improving sleep quality in ESKD adult patients, the study was small and would benefit from replication.

Kim et al. [154] conducted a systematic review of the evidence from 7 RCTs of acupressure in the management of symptoms in patients with ESKD. In the studies, acupressure was used to alleviate sleep disorder, muscle cramps, uremic pruritus, fatigue, and depression experienced by ESKD patients. Acupressure treatment was compared to usual care (n = 3), sham acupressure (n = 2), transcutaneous electrical stimulation (n = 1), sleep medication (n = 1) or an undefined control (n = 1). Across 6 RCTs the follow-up period ranged between 4–18 weeks from baseline, while in one study only the immediate effects of acupressure were reported. Although in 5 trials there were some suggested benefits of acupressure compared to usual care (n = 3), sleep medication (n = 1), and undefined control intervention (n = 1), the authors could not draw any definitive conclusions regarding the efficacy of

acupuncture until larger trials with clearer methodology and better reporting were conducted. None of the studies included in the review reported any adverse events. Six of the 7 trials included in the systematic review will be briefly described. One trial which evaluated acupressure for uremic pruritus was described in an earlier section of this chapter.

Dai and associates [155] investigated the therapeutic effect of lower extremity point massage for improving quality of sleep in 82 ESKD patients with sleep disorders. Patients in the treatment group (n = 42) received 20 to 30 min lower extremity point massage, once a day, for 4 weeks. During the same time period, patients in the control group (n = 40) took 1 mg of estazolam tablets orally half an hour before sleep. Patients who received acupressure reported significantly better sleep quality and lower rates of sleep disturbance-related disorders than patients in the control group.

A double-blind RCT by Tsay et al. [156] allocated 105 adult ESKD patients experiencing sleep disturbances to either receive manual acupressure (n = 35), placebo (n = 32), or control (n = 31). The acupressure group received 14 min of acupoint massage during hemodialysis three times a week for 4 weeks. The placebo group received sham acupressure, which involved massage on non-acupoints 1 cm from the meridian, at the same frequency and duration as the acupressure group. The control group received only standard care. Sleep quality and quality of life scores as measured by the Pittsburgh Sleep Quality Index in the acupressure group were significantly improved compared to the usual care (control) group, but not when compared to the placebo (sham acupressure) group.

Tsay et al. [157] conducted another RCT, this time to examine the effect of acupressure, transcutaneous electrical acupoint stimulation (TEAS) and routine care on sleep quality, depression and fatigue in 108 adult patients with ESKD. Over 4 weeks, patients in the acupressure (n = 36) and TEAS group (n = 36) received manual acupressure for 20 min 3 times weekly plus usual care for a total of 12 sessions. The control group received usual care only. Sleep quality, fatigue and depression were significantly improved in the acupressure and TEAS group compared to the control group. No differences were observed between the acupressure and the TEAS group.

In yet another study, Tsay [158] compared the effect of acupressure, placebo and control on fatigue in 106 ESKD patients. Patients in the acupressure group (n = 35) received acupressure massage 3 times a week for 4 weeks, and the placebo group (n = 35) received a massage at locations with no acupoints at the same frequency as the acupressure group. The control group (n = 36) received no intervention. Patients in the acupressure group had significantly lower scores of fatigue than patients in the control group, but no difference was observed between the acupressure and placebo group. The authors concluded that acupressure provided an alternative method for health care providers to use to manage ESKD patients with fatigue.

A smaller study also found positive effects of acupressure on fatigue and depression in 58 hemodialysis patients [159]. Over a 4-week period, patients either received 12 min of acupressure (n = 28) plus 3 min of lower limb massage three times a week or routine care (n = 30; control group). After the 4-week study period, fatigue (p = 0.04) and depression (p = 0.045) were significantly improved among patients that received acupressure compared to patients who received routine care (control). The authors noted that the lack of a sham acupressure group meant that a placebo effect could not be ruled out.

Another study included in the review was a small RCT which examined the effects of acupressure plus routine care (n = 23) or routine care alone (control; n = 21) on pain associated with muscle leg cramps in 44 hemodialysis patients [160]. Routine care included stopping ultrafiltration and providing hypertonic solution. Patients in the acupressure group received acupressure at acupoints for 1 to 2 min. The rate of treatment response (pain resolving time ≤ 8 min) was significantly (p < 0.01) greater among the acupressure group compared to the control group.

Summary

A substantive body of evidence regarding the use, efficacy and safety of complementary therapies exists and is growing. This chapter examined current research evidence on interventions used to prevent or treat symptoms associated with kidney conditions with a specific focus on pediatric patients. The information provided allows for better informed discussions between medical/health care providers and patients or families with an interest in using complementary therapies for their children. The information provided can be used as a guide or resource by pediatric health care providers as they treat patients with kidney disease and consider seeking and referring patients to relevant local qualified complementary therapists.

References

1. National Center for Complementary and Integrative Health (NCCIH). Are You Considering a Complementary Health Approach? [Internet]. 2021 [cited 2021 March 2] https://www.nccih.nih.gov/health/are-you-considering-a-complementary-health-approach

2. Surette S, Vanderjagt L, Vohra S. Surveys of complementary and alternative medicine usage: a scoping study of the paediatric literature. Complement Ther Med. 2013;21(Suppl 1):S48–53.

3. Government of Canada. Natural Health Products. [Internet]. 2021 [cited 2021 Mar 2]; https://www.canada.ca/en/health-canada/services/drugs-health-products/natural-non-prescription.html

4. Office of Dietary Supplements. National Institutes of Health. Dietary Supplement Health and Education Act of 1994. Public Law 103–417. 103rd Congress. [cited 2021 March 2] https://ods.od.nih.gov/About/DSHEA_Wording.aspx.

5. National Center for Complementary and Integrative Health (NCCIH). Traditional Chinese Medicine: What You Need To Know? [Internet]. 2021 [cited 2021 March 2] https://www.nccih.nih.gov/health/traditional-chinese-medicine-what-you-need-to-know

6. WebMed. Acupressure points and massage treatment. [Internet]. 2021 [cited 2021 March 2]; https://www.webmd.com/balance/guide/acupressure-points-and-massage-treatment

7. Institute of Medicine (US) Committee on the Use of Complementary and Alternative Medicine by the American Public. Complementary and Alternative

Medicine in the United States. Washington, DC: National Academies Press (US); 2005. APPENDIX A, CAM Therapies, Practices, and Systems. https://www.ncbi.nlm.nih.gov/books/NBK83796/

8. Merck Manual Consumer Version. Moxibustion [Internet] 2021 [cited 2021 March 2]; https://www.merckmanuals.com/home/special-subjects/integrative-complementary-and-alternative-medicine/moxibustion.

9. Sandhu GK, Vohra S. Complementary and alternative treatments for renal diseases. In: Geary D, Schaefer F, editors. Comprehensive pediatric nephrology. Philadelphia, PA: Elsevier; 2007. p. 1017–26.

10. Maciocia G. Diagnosis in Chinese medicine. Edinburgh, Toronto: Churchill Livingstone; 2004.

11. Freeman L, Lawlis GF. Mosby's complementary and alternative medicine: a research-based approach. Orlando, FL: Mosby Inc.; 2001.

12. Cooke B, Ernst E. Aromatherapy: a systematic review. Br J Gen Pract. 2000;50(455):493–6.

13. World Health Organization. WHO Global Report on Traditional and Complementary Medicine 2019. World Health Organization; 2019. [Google Scholar].

14. Clarke TC, Black LI, Stussman BJ, Barnes PM, Nahin RL. Trends in the use of complementary health approaches among adults: United States, 2002–2012. Natl Health Stat Report. 2015;79:1–16.

15. AlAnizy L, AlMatham K, Al Basheer A, AlFayyad I. Complementary and alternative medicine practice among Saudi patients with chronic kidney disease: a cross-sectional study. Int J Nephrol Renovasc Dis. 2020;13:11–8.

16. Sait KH, Anfinan NM, Eldeek B, et al. Perception of patients with cancer towards support management services and use of complementary alternative medicine-a single institution hospital-based study in Saudi Arabia. Asian Pac J Cancer Prev. 2014;15:2547–54.

17. Barnes PM, Bloom B, Nahin RL. Complementary and alternative medicine use among adults and children: United States, 2007. Natl Health Stat Report. 2008;12:1–23.

18. Ipsos Reid. Natural Health Product Tracking Survey - 2010 Final Report. 2011;Report No.: POR 135–09, HCPOR-09-25.

19. Esmail N. Complementary and alternative medicine: use and public attitudes 1997, 2006, and 2016. Vancouver: Fraser Institute; 2017. https://www.fraserinstitute.org/sites/default/files/complementary-and-alternative-medicine-2017.pdf

20. Gardiner P, Phillips R, Shaughnessy AF. Herbal and dietary supplement—drug interactions in patients with chronic illnesses. Am Fam Physician. 2008;77(1):73–8.

21. Cohen MH, Hrbek A, Davis RB, Schachter SC, Eisenberg DM. Emerging credentialing practices, malpractice liability policies, and guidelines governing complementary and alternative medical practices and dietary supplement recommendations: a descriptive study of 19 integrative health care centers in the United States. Arch Intern Med. 2005;165(3):289.

22. Vohra S, Surette S, Mittra D, Rosen LD, Gardiner P, Kemper KJ. Pediatric integrative medicine: pediatrics' newest subspecialty? BMC Pediatr. 2012;12:123.

23. Italia S, Wolfenstetter SB, Teuner CM. Patterns of complementary and alternative medicine (CAM) use in children: a systematic review. Eur J Pediatr. 2014;173:1413–28.

24. Castelino LR, Nayak-Rao S, Shenoy MP. Prevalence of use of complementary and alternative medicine in chronic kidney disease: a cross-sectional single-center study from South India. Saudi J Kidney Dis Transpl. 2019;30(1):185–93. PMID: 30804280

25. Osman NA, Hassanein SM, Leil MM, NasrAllah MM. Complementary and alternative medicine use among patients with chronic kidney disease and kidney transplant recipients. J Ren Nutr. 2015;25(6):466–71. https://doi.org/10.1053/j.jrn.2015.04.009. Epub 2015 Jun 17

26. Nowack R, Balle C, Birnkammer F, Koch W, Sessler R, Birck R. Complementary and alternative medications consumed by renal patients in southern Germany. J Ren Nutr. 2009;19(3):211–9.

27. Tangkiatkumjai M, Boardman H, Walker DM. Potential factors that influence usage of complementary and alternative medicine worldwide: a systematic review. BMC Complement Med Ther. 2020;20(1):363. https://doi.org/10.1186/s12906-020-03157-2.

28. Spanner ED, Duncan AM. Prevalence of dietary supplement use in adults with chronic renal insufficiency. J Ren Nutr. 2005;15(2):204–10.

29. Gottschling S, Gronwald B, Schmitt S, Schmitt C, Langler A, Leidig E, et al. Use of complementary and alternative medicine in healthy children and children with chronic medical conditions in Germany. Complement Ther Med. 2013;21(Suppl 1):S61–9.

30. Wang C, Preisser J, Chung Y, Li K. Complementary and alternative medicine use among children with mental health issues: results from the National Health Interview Survey. BMC Complement Altern Med. 2018;18(1):241. https://doi.org/10.1186/s12906-018-2307-5.

31. Machado LCB, Alves C. Complementary and alternative medicine in Brazilian children and adolescents with type 1 diabetes mellitus. Pediatr Endocrinol Diabetes Metab. 2017;23(2):64–9. https://doi.org/10.18544/PEDM-23.02.0075.

32. Dannemann K, Hecker W, Haberland H, Herbst A, Galler A, Schafer T, et al. Use of complementary and alternative medicine in children with type 1 diabetes mellitus - prevalence, patterns of use, and costs. Pediatr Diabetes. 2008;9(3 Pt 1):228–35.

33. Sirois FM. Motivations for consulting complementary and alternative medicine practitioners: a comparison of consumers from 1997-8 and 2005. BMC Complement Altern Med. 2008;29(8):16.

34. Qureshi W, Shah S, Singh NP. Prevalence of complementary and alternative medicine in patients with chronic kidney disease in India. Am J Kidney Dis. 2013;61(4):B66.

35. Ernst E. Prevalence of complementary/alternative medicine for children: a systematic review. Eur J Pediatr. 1999;158(1):7–11.

36. Jou J, Johnson PJ. Nondisclosure of complementary and alternative medicine use to primary care physicians: findings from the 2012 National Health Interview Survey. JAMA Intern Med. 2016;176(4):545–6. https://doi.org/10.1001/jamainternmed.2015.8593.

37. Tangkiatkumjai M, Boardman H, Praditpornsilpa K, Walker DM. Prevalence of herbal and dietary supplement usage in Thai outpatients with chronic kidney disease: a cross-sectional survey. BMC Complement Altern Med. 2013;13:153.

38. Chang HY, Chang HL, Siren B. Exploring the decision to disclose the use of natural products among outpatients: a mixed-method study. BMC Complement Altern Med. 2013;13(1):319.

39. Robinson A, McGrail MR. Disclosure of CAM use to medical practitioners: a review of qualitative and quantitative studies. Complement Ther Med. 2004;12(2–3):90–8.

40. Thakkar E, Anklam A, Xu F, Ulberth J, Li B, Li M, Hugas N, Sarma S, Crerar S, Swift T, Hakamatsuka V, Curtui W, Yan X, Geng W, Slikker WT. Regulatory landscape of dietary supplements and herbal medicines from a global perspective. J Regul Toxicol Pharmacol. 2020;114:104647.

41. Trebilcock MJ, Ghimire KM. Regulating alternative medicines: disorder in the Borderlands. CD Howe Institute Commentary; 2019. p. 541.

42. National Health Service. NHS Careers. Complementary and alternative Medicine (CAM) [Internet]. 2018 [cited 2021 Feb 14]; https://www.nhs.uk/conditions/complementary-and-alternative-medicine/

43. Canadian Medical Protective Association. Alternative medicine - what are the medico-legal concerns? [Internet] 2012 [cited 2021 Mar 2]; https://www.cmpa-acpm.ca/en/advice-publications/browse-articles/2012/alternative-medicine-what-are-the-medico-legal-concerns

44. Boon H. Regulation of complementary/alternative medicine: a Canadian perspective. Complement Ther Med. 2002;10(1):14–9.

45. Zhang J, Wider B, Shang H, Li X, Ernst E. Quality of herbal medicines: challenges and solutions. Complement Ther Med. 2012;20(1–2):100–6.

46. Newmaster SG, Grguric M, Shanmughanandhan D, Ramalingam S, Ragupathy S. DNA barcoding detects contamination and substitution in North American herbal products. BMC Med. 2013;11:222.

47. Srirama R, Santhosh Kumar JU, Seethapathy GS, Newmaster SG, Ragupathy S, Ganeshaiah KN, Uma Shaanker R, Ravikanth G. Species adulteration in the herbal trade: causes, consequences and mitigation. Drug Saf. 2017;40(8):651–61. https://doi.org/10.1007/s40264-017-0527-0.

48. McCutcheon AR, Beatty D. Herb quality. In: Chandler F, editor. Herbs: everyday reference for health professionals. Ottawa: Canadian Pharmacists Association; 2000. p. 25–33.

49. Marcus DM, Grollman AP. The consequences of ineffective regulation of dietary supplements. Arch Intern Med. 2012;172(13):1035–6.

50. Gilroy CM, Steiner JF, Byers T, Shapiro H, Georgian W. Echinacea and truth in labeling. Arch Intern Med. 2003;163(6):699–704.

51. Posadzki P, Watson L, Ernst E. Contamination and adulteration of herbal medicinal products (HMPs): an overview of systematic reviews. Eur J Clin Pharmacol. 2013;69(3):295–307.

52. National Institutes of Health. Dietary Supplement Health and Education Act of 1994. Public Law 103–417 [Internet]. 1994 [cited 2021 Mar 2]; http://ods.od.nih.gov/About/DSHEA_Wording.aspx.

53. Cohen MH. Legal issues in caring for patients with kidney disease by selectively integrating complementary therapies. Adv Chronic Kidney Dis. 2005;12(3):300–11.

54. Gaboury I, Johnson N, Robin C, Luc M, O'Connor D, Patenaude J, Pélissier-Simard L, Xhignesse M. Complementary and alternative medicine: do physicians believe they can meet the requirements of the Collège des médecins du Québec? Can Fam Physician. 2016;62(12):e772–5. PMID: 27965354; PMCID: PMC5154669

55. Cutshall SM, Khalsa TK, Chon TY, Vitek SM, Clark SD, Blomberg DL, Mustafa R, Bhagra A. Curricular development and implementation of a longitudinal integrative medicine education experience for trainees and health-care professionals at an Academic Medical Center. Glob Adv Health Med. 2019;8:2164956119837489. https://doi.org/10.1177/2164956119837489.

56. Peltzer K, Pengpid S. A survey of the training of traditional, complementary, and alternative medicine in universities in Thailand. J Multidiscip Healthc. 2019;12:119–24. https://doi.org/10.2147/JMDH.S189644.

57. Cowen VS, Cyr V. Complementary and alternative medicine in US medical schools. Adv Med Educ Pract. 2015;6:113–7. https://doi.org/10.2147/AMEP.S69761.

58. Karpa K. Development and implementation of an herbal and natural product elective in undergraduate medical education. BMC Complement Altern Med. 2012;12:57.

59. Frenkel M, Frye A, Heliker D, Finkle T, Yzaguirre D, Bulik R, et al. Lessons learned from complementary and integrative medicine curriculum change in a medical school. Med Educ. 2007;41(2):205–13.

60. American Board of Physician Specialties. Integrative Medicine Fellowships. 2021. https://www.abpsus.org/integrative-medicine-fellowships/. Accessed 14 Feb 2021.

61. Cohen MH, Eisenberg DM. Potential physician malpractice liability associated with complementary and integrative medical therapies. Ann Intern Med. 2002;136(8):596–60.

62. Klassen TP, Pham B, Lawson ML, Moher D. For randomized controlled trials, the quality of reports of complementary and alternative medicine was as good as reports of conventional medicine. J Clin Epidemiol. 2005;58(8):763–8.

63. Lawson ML, Pham B, Klassen TP, Moher D. Systematic reviews involving complementary and alternative medicine interventions had higher quality of reporting than conventional medicine reviews. J Clin Epidemiol. 2005;58(8):777–84.

64. Adams D, Wu T, Yasui Y, Aung S, Vohra S. Systematic reviews of TCM trials: how does inclusion of Chinese trials affect outcome? J Evid Based Med. 2012;5(2):89–97.

65. Deng Y, Zhang L, Wen A, Xu D, Wang W, Hou Y, Liu Z, Yang L, Shen T, Luo Q, Wu W, Ou Y. Effect of Chinese medicine prescription on nephrotic syndrome. Medicine. 2020;99(23):e20622.

66. Feng M, Yuan W, Zhang R, Fu P, Wu T. Chinese herbal medicine Huangqi type formulations for nephrotic syndrome. Cochrane Database Syst Rev. 2013;6:CD006335.

67. Wu HM, Tang JL, Cao L, Sha ZH, Li Y. Interventions for preventing infection in nephrotic syndrome. Cochrane Database Syst Rev. 2012;4:003964.

68. Li RH, Peng ZP, Wei YL, Liu CH. Clinical observation on Chinese medicinal herbs combined with prednisolone for reducing the risk of infection in children with nephrotic syndrome. Inf J Chin Med. 2000;7(10):60–1.

69. Chen J, Chen SQ. Preventive effects of Huangqi on infection in children with nephrotic syndrome. Zhongguo Zhong Xi Yi Jie He Za Zhi. 2008;28(5):467–9.

70. Kang GG. Preventive effects of Huangqi on secondary infection in children with simple nephrotic syndrome. Chin J Integr Tradit West Nephrol. 2005;6(12):718.

71. Chen Y, Gong Z, Chen X, Tang L, Zhao X, Yuan Q, et al. Tripterygium Wilfordii Hook F (a traditional Chinese medicine) for primary nephrotic syndrome. Cochrane Database Syst Rev. 2013;8:CD008568.

72. Wen ZH, Xu WH, Lai SL. Causal relationship of adverse reactions with tripterygium in 38 patients. Zhongyao Xinyao Yu Linchuang Yaoli. 1999;10(1):50–3.

73. Bao J, Dai SM. A Chinese herb Tripterygium Wilfordii Hook F in the treatment of rheumatoid arthritis: mechanism, efficacy, and safety. Rheumatol Int. 2011;31(9):1123–9.

74. Goldbach-Mansky R, Wilson M, Fleischmann R, Olsen N, Silverfield J, Kempf P, et al. Comparison of Tripterygium wilfordii Hook F versus sulfasalazine in the treatment of rheumatoid arthritis: a randomized trial. Ann Intern Med. 2009;151(4):229–40, W49–51

75. Chen YZ, Zhao XZ, Yuan Q. Tripterygium wilfordii Hook F (a traditional Chinese medicine) for primary nephrotic syndrome (protocol). Cochrane Database Syst Rev. 2010;7:CD008568.

76. Wang YP, Liu AM, Dai YW, Yang C, Tang HF. The treatment of relapsing primary nephrotic syndrome in children. J Zhejiang Univ Sci B. 2005;6(7):682–5.

77. Liu XY. Therapeutic effect of chai-ling-tang (saireito) on the steroid-dependent nephrotic syndrome in children. Am J Chin Med. 1995;23(3–4):255–60.

78. Hu J, Liu Z, Zhang H. Omega-3 fatty acid supplementation as an adjunctive therapy in the treatment of chronic kidney disease: a meta-analysis. Clinics (Sao Paulo). 2017;72(1):58–64. https://doi.org/10.6061/clinics/2017(01)10.

79. Chou HH, Chiou YY, Hung PH, Chiang PC, Wang ST. Omega–3 fatty acids ameliorate proteinuria but not renal function in IgA nephropathy: a meta-analysis of randomized controlled trials. Nephron Clin Pract. 2012;121(1–2):c30–5.

80. Miller ER, Juraschek SP, Appel LJ, Madala M, Anderson CA, Bleys J, et al. The effect of n–3 long-chain polyunsaturated fatty acid supplementation on urine protein excretion and kidney function: meta-analysis of clinical trials. Am J Clin Nutr. 2009;89(6):1937–45.

81. Hogg RJ, Lee J, Nardelli N, Julian BA, Cattran D, Waldo B, et al. Clinical trial to evaluate omega-3 fatty acids and alternate day prednisone in patients with IgA nephropathy: report from the southwest pediatric nephrology study group. Clin J Am Soc Nephrol. 2006;1(3):467–74.

82. Tayyebi-Khosroshahi H, Houshyar J, Dehgan-Hesari R, Alikhah H, Vatankhah AM, Safaeian AR, et al. Effect of treatment with omega-3 fatty acids on C-reactive protein and tumor necrosis factor-alfa in hemodialysis patients. Saudi J Kidney Dis Transpl. 2012;23(3):500–6.

83. Zhou N, Shi X, Shen Y. The short-term therapeutic effects of TCM for IgA nephropathy in children. J Tradit Chin Med. 2011;31(2):115–9.

84. Chan JC, Mahan JD, Trachtman H, Scheinman J, Flynn JT, Alon US, et al. Vitamin E therapy in IgA nephropathy: a double-blind, placebo-controlled study. Pediatr Nephrol. 2003;18(10):1015–9.

85. Saraogi M, et al. Role of complementary medicine (music, acupuncture, acupressure, TENS and audio-visual distraction) in shockwave lithotripsy (SWL): a systematic review from EAU sections of urolithiasis (EULIS) and uro-technology (ESUT). Urology. 2020;145:38–51.

86. Kaynar M, et al. Comparison of the efficacy of diclofenac, acupuncture, and acetaminophen in the treatment of renal colic. Am J Emerg Med. 2015;33(6):749–53.

87. Beltaief K, Grissa MH, Msolli MA, Bzeouich N, Fredj N, Sakma A, Boubaker H, Bouida W, Boukef R, Nouira S. Acupuncture versus titrated morphine in acute renal colic: a randomized controlled trial. J

Pain Res. 2018;11:335–41. https://doi.org/10.2147/JPR.S136299.

88. Huang L, Li J. Clinical study on the treatment of renal colic by body and auricular acupuncture. J Acupunct Tuina Sci. 2011;9(2):104–6.

89. Hodzic J, Golka K, Selinski S, Pourvali H, Sommerfeld HJ. Analgesia with acupuncture in extracorporeal shock wave lithotripsy of kidney stones—first results. Urologe A. 2007;46(7):740. 742-4, 746-7

90. Resim S, Gumusalan Y, Ekerbicer HC, Sahin MA, Sahinkanat T. Effectiveness of electro-acupuncture compared to sedo-analgesics in relieving pain during shockwave lithotripsy. Urol Res. 2005;33(4):285–90.

91. Lee YH, Lee WC, Chen MT, Huang JK, Chung C, Chang LS. Acupuncture in the treatment of renal colic. J Urol. 1992;147(1):16–8.

92. Witt CM, Pach D, Brinkhaus B, Wruck K, Tag B, Mank S, et al. Safety of acupuncture: results of a prospective observational study with 229,230 patients and introduction of a medical information and consent form. Forsch Komplementmed. 2009;16(2):91–7.

93. White A. A cumulative review of the range and incidence of significant adverse events associated with acupuncture. Acupunct Med. 2004;22(3):122–33.

94. Kosar A, Ozturk A, Serel TA, Akkus S, Unal OS. Effect of vibration massage therapy after extracorporeal shockwave lithotripsy in patients with lower caliceal stones. J Endourol. 1999;13(10):705–7.

95. Didari T, Solki S, Mozaffari S, Nikfar S, Abdollahi M. A systematic review of the safety of probiotics. Expert Opin Drug Saf. 2014;13(2):227–39.

96. Campieri C, Campieri M, Bertuzzi V, Swennen E, Matteuzzi D, Stefoni S, et al. Reduction of oxaluria after an oral course of lactic acid bacteria at high concentration. Kidney Int. 2001;60(3):1097–105.

97. Charrois TL, Sandhu G, Vohra S. Probiotics. Pediatr Rev. 2006;27(4):137–9.

98. Thomas DW, Greer FR. American Academy of Pediatrics Committee on Nutrition, American Academy of Pediatrics Section on Gastroenterology, Hepatology, and Nutrition. Probiotics and prebiotics in pediatrics. Pediatrics. 2010;126(6):1217–31.

99. Shamseer L, Vohra S. American Academy of Pediatrics provisional section on complementary, holistic, and integrative medicine. Complementary, holistic, and integrative medicine: cranberry. Pediatr Rev. 2007;28(8):e43–5.

100. Jepson R, Mihaljevic L, Craig J. Cranberries for treating urinary tract infections. Cochrane Database Syst Rev. 1998;4:CD001322.

101. Jepson RG, Williams G, Craig JC. Cranberries for preventing urinary tract infections. Cochrane Database Syst Rev. 2012;10:CD001321.

102. Salo J, Uhari M, Helminen M, Korppi M, Nieminen T, Pokka T, et al. Cranberry juice for the prevention of recurrences of urinary tract infections in children: a randomized placebo-controlled trial. Clin Infect Dis. 2012;54(3):340–6.

103. Ferrara P, Romaniello L, Vitelli O, Gatto A, Serva M, Cataldi L. Cranberry juice for the prevention of recurrent urinary tract infections: a randomized controlled trial in children. Scand J Urol Nephrol. 2009;43(5):369–72.

104. Uberos J, Nogueras Ocana M, Fernández Puentes V, Rodríguez Belmonte R, Narbona López E, Molina Carballo A, et al. Cranberry syrup vs trimethoprim in the prophylaxis of recurrent urinary tract infections among children: a controlled trial. Open Access J Clin Trials. 2012;4:31–8.

105. Afshar K, Stothers L, Scott H, MacNeily AE. Cranberry juice for the prevention of pediatric urinary tract infection: a randomized controlled trial. J Urol. 2012;188(4 Suppl):1584–7.

106. Foda MM, Middlebrook PF, Gatfield CT, Potvin G, Wells G, Schillinger JF. Efficacy of cranberry in prevention of urinary tract infection in a susceptible pediatric population. Can J Urol. 1995;2:98–102

107. Schlager TA, Anderson S, Trudell J, Hendley JO. Effect of cranberry juice on bacteriuria in children with neurogenic bladder receiving intermittent catheterization. J Pediatr. 1999;135:698–702.

108. Nishizaki N, Someya T, Hirano D, et al. Can cranberry juice be a substitute for cefaclor prophylaxis in children with vesicoureteral reflux? Pediatr Int. 2009;51:433–4.

109. Mutlu H, Ekinci Z. Urinary tract infection prophylaxis in children with neurogenic bladder with cranberry capsules: randomized controlled trial. ISRN Pediatr. 2012;2012:317280.

110. Durham SH, Stamm PL, Eiland LS. Cranberry products for the prophylaxis of urinary tract infections in pediatric patients. Ann Pharmacother. 2015;49(12):1349–56.

111. Wan K-S, et al. Cranberries for preventing recurrent urinary tract infections in uncircumcised boys. Altern Ther Health Med. 2016;22:6.

112. Sadeghi-Bojd S, et al. Efficacy of probiotic prophylaxis after the first febrile urinary tract infection in children with normal urinary tracts. J Pediatr Infect Dis Soc. 2020;9(3):305–10.

113. Lee SJ, Shim YH, Cho SJ, Lee JW. Probiotics prophylaxis in children with persistent primary vesicoureteral reflux. Pediatr Nephrol. 2007;22(9):1315–20.

114. Dani C, Biadaioli R, Bertini G, Martelli E, Rubaltelli FF. Probiotics feeding in prevention of urinary tract infection, bacterial sepsis and necrotizing enterocolitis in preterm infants. A prospective double-blind study. Biol Neonate. 2002;82(2):103–8.

115. Hosseini M, Yousefifard M, Ataei N, Oraii A, Mirzay Razaz J, Izadi A. The efficacy of probiotics in prevention of urinary tract infection in children: a systematic review and meta-analysis. J Pediatr Urol. 2017;13(6):581–91. https://doi.org/10.1016/j.jpurol.2017.08.018. Epub 2017 Oct 9

116. Schwenger EM, Tejani AM, Loewen PS. Probiotics for preventing urinary tract infections in adults and children. Cochrane Database Syst Rev. 2015;12:CD008772.

117. Schaier M, Lehrke I, Schade K, Morath C, Shimizu F, Kawachi H, et al. Isotretinoin alleviates renal damage in rat chronic glomerulonephritis. Kidney Int. 2001;60(6):2222–34.

118. Kahbazi M, Sharafkhah M, Yousefichaijan P, Taherahmadi H, Rafiei M, Kaviani P, Abaszadeh S, Massoudifar A, Mohammadbeigi A. Vitamin a supplementation is effective for improving the clinical symptoms of urinary tract infections and reducing renal scarring in girls with acute pyelonephritis: a randomized, double-blind placebo-controlled, clinical trial study. Complement Ther Med. 2019;42:429–37. https://doi.org/10.1016/j.ctim.2018.12.007. Epub 2018 Dec 12

119. Zhang GQ, Chen JL, Zhao Y. The effect of vitamin A on renal damage following acute pyelonephritis in children: a meta-analysis of randomized controlled trials. Pediatr Nephrol. 2016;31:373–9. https://doi.org/10.1007/s00467-015-3098-2.

120. Yilmaz A, Bahat E, Yilmaz GG, Hasanoglu A, Akman S, Guven AG. Adjuvant effect of vitamin a on recurrent lower urinary tract infections. Pediatr Int. 2007;49(3):310–3.

121. Burrowes JD, Van Houten G. Use of alternative medicine by patients with stage 5 chronic kidney disease. Adv Chronic Kidney Dis. 2005;12(3):312–25.

122. Fishbane S, Frei GL, Finger M, Dressler R, Silbiger S. Hypervitaminosis A in two hemodialysis patients. Am J Kidney Dis. 1995;25(2):346–9.

123. Walker VP, Modlin RL. The Vitamin D connection to pediatric infections and immune function. Pediatr Res. 2009;65:106R–13R.

124. Merrikhi A, Ziaei E, Shahsanai A, Kelishadi R, Maghami-Mehr A. Is Vitamin D supplementation effective in prevention of recurrent urinary tract infections in the pediatrics? A randomized triple-masked controlled trial. Adv Biomed Res [Serial Online]. 2018. [cited 2021 Feb 13];7:150.

125. Bennett-Richards K, Kattenhorn M, Donald A, Oakley G, Varghese Z, Rees L, et al. Does oral folic acid lower total homocysteine levels and improve endothelial function in children with chronic renal failure? Circulation. 2002;105(15):1810–5.

126. Bennett-Richards KJ, Kattenhorn M, Donald AE, Oakley GR, Varghese Z, Bruckdorfer KR, et al. Oral L-arginine does not improve endothelial dysfunction in children with chronic renal failure. Kidney Int. 2002;62(4):1372–8.

127. Li Z, Qing P, Ji L, Su B, He L, Fan J. Systematic review of rhubarb for chronic renal failure. Chin J Evid Based Med. 2004;4:468–73.

128. WebMed. Rhubarb [Internet]. 2021 [cited 2021 March 2]; https://www.webmd.com/vitamins/ai/ingredientmono-214/rhubarb#:~:text=Rhubarb%20 can%20cause%20some%20side,loss%2C%20 and%20irregular%20heart%20rhythm.

129. Huang Q, Lu G, Shen HM, Chung M, Ong CN. Anticancer properties of anthraquinones from rhubarb. Med Res Rev. 2007;27(5):609–30.

130. Zhang M, Zhang D, Zhang W, Liu S, Zhang M. Treatment of chronic renal failure by supplementing the kidney and invigorating blood flow. J Tradit Chin Med. 2004;24(4):247–51.

131. Chaturvedi S, Jones C. Protein restriction for children with chronic kidney disease. Cochrane Database Syst Rev. 2007;4:CD006863.

132. Wingen AM, Fabian-Bach C, Schaefer F, Mehls O. Randomised multicentre study of a low-protein diet on the progression of chronic renal failure in children. Lancet. 1997;349(9059):1117–23.

133. Uauy RD, Hogg RJ, Brewer ED, Reisch JS, Cunningham C, Holliday MA. Dietary protein and growth in infants with chronic renal insufficiency: a report from the southwest pediatric nephrology study group and the University of California, San Francisco. Pediatr Nephrol. 1994;8(1):45–50.

134. Wang H, Song H, Yue J, Li J, Hou YB, Deng JL. Rheum officinale (a traditional Chinese medicine) for chronic kidney disease. Cochrane Database Syst Rev. 2012;7:CD008000.

135. Zhang H, Ho YF, Che C, Lin Z, Leung C, Chan LS. Topical herbal application as an adjuvant treatment for chronic kidney disease–a systematic review of randomized controlled clinical trials. J Adv Nurs. 2012;68(8):1679–91.

136. de Brito-Ashurst I, Varagunam M, Raftery MJ, Yaqoob MM. Bicarbonate supplementation slows progression of CKD and improves nutritional status. J Am Soc Nephrol. 2009;20(9):2075–84.

137. Bing L, Yang M, He G-L, Gao X-G, Li L, Zhai W-S. Efficacy and safety of Chinese herbs for the prevention of the risk of renal damage in Henoch-Schonlein purpura in children: meta-analysis of randomized controlled trials and GRADE evaluation. Evidence Based Complement Alternat Med. 2019;2019:4089184. https://doi.org/10.1155/2019/4089184.

138. Fan L, Yan H, Zhen X, Wu X, Hao J, Hou L, Han L. Safety and efficacy evaluation of traditional Chinese medicine (Qingre-Lishi-Yishen Formula) based on treatment of regular glucocorticoid combined with cyclophosphamide pulse in children suffered from moderately severe Henoch-Schonlein purpura nephritis with nephrotic proteinuria. Evid Based Complement Alternat Med. 2020;2020:3920735. https://doi.org/10.1155/2020/3920735.

139. Zhang J, Lv J, Pang S, et al. Chinese herbal medicine for the treatment of Henoch-Schönlein purpura nephritis in children: a prospective cohort study protocol. Medicine (Baltimore). 2018;97(24):e11064. https://doi.org/10.1097/MD.0000000000011064.

140. Ding Y, Zhang X, Ren X, et al. Traditional Chinese medicine versus regular therapy in Henoch-Schönlein purpura nephritis in children: study protocol for a randomized controlled trial. Trials. 2019;20:538. https://doi.org/10.1186/s13063-019-3484-3.

141. Kim KH, Lee MS, Choi SM. Acupuncture for treating uremic pruritus in patients with end-stage renal disease: a systematic review. J Pain Symptom Manag. 2010;40(1):117–25.

142. Che-yi C, Wen CY, Min-Tsung K, Chiu-Ching H. Acupuncture in haemodialysis patients at the Quchi (LI11) acupoint for refractory uraemic pruritus. Nephrol Dial Transplant. 2005;20(9):1912–5.

143. Gao H, Zhang W, Wang Y. Acupuncture treatment for 34 cases of uremic cutaneous pruritus. J Tradit Chin Med. 2002;22(1):29–30.

144. Rui H, Lin W, Sha J. Observation on therapeutic effect of 80 cases of uremic cutaneous pruritus treated with acupuncture. Zhongguo Zhen Jiu. 2002;22:235–6.

145. Jedras M, Bataa O, Gellert R, Ostrowski G, Wojtaszek E, Lange J, et al. Acupressure in the treatment of uremic pruritus. Dial Trans Plant. 2003;32(1):8–10.

146. Kilic AN, Tasci S, Karatas N. Effect of acupressure on patients in Turkey receiving hemodialysis treatment for uremic pruritus. Altern Ther Health Med. 2013;19(5):12–8.

147. Hsu MC, Chen HW, Hwu YJ, Chanc CM, Liu CF. Effects of thermal therapy on uremic pruritus and biochemical parameters in patients having haemodialysis. J Adv Nurs. 2009;65(11):2397–408.

148. Cavalcanti AM, Rocha LM, Carillo R Jr, Lima LU, Lugon JR. Effects of homeopathic treatment on pruritus of haemodialysis patients: a randomised placebo-controlled double-blind trial. Homeopathy. 2003;92(4):177–81.

149. Endrizzi C, Rossi E, Crudeli L, Garibaldi D. Harm in homeopathy: aggravations, adverse drug events or medication errors? Homeopathy. 2005;94(4):233–40.

150. Shahgholian N, Dehghan M, Mortazavi M, Gholami F, Valiani M. Effect of aromatherapy on pruri-

tus relief in hemodialysis patients. Iran J Nurs Midwifery Res. 2010;15(4):240.

151. Ro YJ, Ha HC, Kim CG, Yeom HA. The effects of aromatherapy on pruritus in patients undergoing hemodialysis. Dermatol Nurs. 2002;14(4):231–4, 237-8, 256; quiz 239

152. Xue W, Zhao Y, Yuan M, Zhao Z. Chinese herbal bath therapy for the treatment of uremic pruritus: meta-analysis of randomized controlled trials. BMC Complement Altern Med. 2019;19(1):103. https://doi.org/10.1186/s12906-019-2513-9.

153. Shariati A, Jahani S, Hooshmand M, Khalili N. The effect of acupressure on sleep quality in hemodialysis patients. Complement Ther Med. 2012;20(6):417–23.

154. Kim KH, Lee MS, Won Kang K, Choi S. Role of acupressure in symptom management in patients with end-stage renal disease: a systematic review. J Palliat Med. 2010;13(7):885–92.

155. Dai X, Xing X, Shi Y, Jiang W, Zhou M. Lower extremity point massage for improving quality of sleep in patients with end-stage renal disease: a clinical study of 42 cases. J Tradit Chin Med. 2007;48:44–6.

156. Tsay S, Chen M. Acupressure and quality of sleep in patients with end-stage renal disease— a randomized controlled trial. Int J Nurs Stud. 2003;40(1):1–7.

157. Tsay S, Cho Y, Chen M. Acupressure and transcutaneous electrical acupoint stimulation in improving fatigue, sleep quality and depression in hemodialysis patients. Am J Chin Med. 2004;32(03):407–16.

158. Tsay S. Acupressure and fatigue in patients with end-stage renal disease–a randomized controlled trial. Int J Nurs Stud. 2004;41(1):99–106.

159. Cho YC, Tsay SL. The effect of acupressure with massage on fatigue and depression in patients with end-stage renal disease. J Nurs Res. 2004;12(1):51–4.

160. Zhu L, Pan X, Zhou C, Huang K. Effects of adjunctive acupressure for muscle cramps of lower extremities in patients undergoing hemodialysis. Mod J Integr Tradit Chin West Med. 2006;17:2347–8.

Environmental Nephrotoxins

Jie Ding and Ruth A. Etzel

There are a large number of environmental chemicals that are potentially toxic to the kidneys [1]. Children may be exposed to these chemicals in toys, consumer products, household pesticides, and as contaminants of food and drink. This chapter will provide information about some of the chemicals that the pediatrician should consider when a child presents with renal injury of unknown etiology. In order to determine the possibility of exposure to nephrotoxic chemicals, a careful environmental history should be performed as part of the complete history and physical examination [2, 3]. Table 73.1 lists agents that should be considered in the environmental history. Table 73.2 shows the most likely site of renal injury for selected toxicants [4].

J. Ding (✉)
Pediatric Department, Peking University First
Hospital, Beijing, China

R. A. Etzel
The George Washington University,
Washington, DC, USA

© The Author(s), under exclusive license to Springer Nature Switzerland AG 2023
F. Schaefer, L. A. Greenbaum (eds.), *Pediatric Kidney Disease*,
https://doi.org/10.1007/978-3-031-11665-0_73

Table 73.1 Environmental toxicants and renal dysfunction

Ammonia	Acute nephrotoxicity, oliguria, hematuria
Arsenic	Cortical necrosis, hematuria, leukocyturia, glucosuria
Barium	Renal insufficiency, hemoglobinuria, degeneration of kidney, acute renal failure
Cadmium	Acute renal failure, necrosis of tubular cells, Fanconi syndrome
Carbon tetrachloride	Acute renal failure, aminoaciduria, oliguria
Chloromethane	Albuminuria, proteinuria, anuria, increased serum creatinine and serum BUN
Chromate and chromium (VI)	Necrosis of tubular cells
Copper sulfate	Necrosis of tubular cells
Fluoride	Interstitial nephritis
Lead	Chronic nephropathy, Fanconi syndrome, renal insufficiency
Methyl parathion	Acute nephrotoxicity
Mercury	Glomerular dysfunction, acute nephritic syndrome
Naphthalene	Tubular necrosis, oliguria, anuria, proteinuria, hemoglobinuria, increased serum creatinine and serum BUN
Pentachlorophenol	Renal tubular degeneration, metabolic imbalance
Thallium	Proteinuria, decreased creatinine clearance, increased blood urea
Uranium	Chronic nephritis, renal sclerosis
1,2 dibromomethane	Acute nephrotoxicity
1,2 dichloromethane	Acute nephrotoxicity
1,2 dichloropropane	Acute nephrotoxicity

Source: Adapted from: Agency for Toxic Substances and Disease Registry, Priority Health Conditions: An Integrated Strategy to Evaluate the Relationship between Illness and Exposure to Hazardous Substances. Atlanta, Georgia: U.S. Department of Health and Human Services, Public Health Service, Agency for Toxic Substances and Disease Registry, 1993, page 98

Table 73.2

Site affected/mechanism	Short-term toxicity	Long-term toxicity
Prerenal failure/hemodynamic alteration	Cocaine; animals	
Kidney failure	Ethylene glycol; potassium bichromate; animals Mushrooms; melamine; creatine; licorice	*Cortinarius* intoxication
Glomerular damage/ proteinuria	Mercury; animals	Mercury; gold; bismuth Glycol ether solvents
Hemolytic uremic syndrome/ thrombotic Microangiopathy	Animals	
Proximal tubular injury (Fanconi syndrome)	Lead, cadmium, mercuric chloride; aristolochic acid Ecstasy; *l*-lysine	Heavy metals; *l*-lysine
Interstitial nephritis	Traditional herbal medicines, cat's claw, creatine	Aristolochic acid; lead, *l*-lysine
Tubular necrosis (acute) or degeneration (chronic)	Heavy metals (mercury); potassium bichromate; animals; fish gallbladders; traditional herbal medicines; chromium; yellow oleander	Germanium; pennyroyal
Crystalliation/nephrolithiasis	Ethylene glycol; melamine; silica-containing milk Thickener; star fruit	Cranberry; ephedra; vitamin C
Immune vasculitis/lupus		Silica; yohimbe

Reprinted from: Bacchetta J, Dubourg L, Juillard L, Cochat P. Non-drug-induced nephrotoxicity. Pediatr Nephrol. 2009;24 (12):2291–2300. (table on page 2297)

Cadmium

Cadmium is nephrotoxic [5]. Cadmium has a biological half-life of 10–30 years in humans. At birth, cadmium is present only at very low levels, but the whole-body cadmium burden can reach 20–30 mg by the age of 50 years and in people with occupational exposure it can reach 200–300 mg. Cadmium concentrates in the kidneys. Increased proteinuria is the earliest sign of cadmium nephropathy. A study of children 6–17 years of age living near a previous zinc smelter in Pennsylvania showed that urine concentrations of N-acetyl-β-D-glucosaminidase, alanine aminopeptidase and albumin were positively associated with the children's urine cadmium concentrations, but the findings did not remain statistically significant after adjusting for urinary creatinine and other potential confounders [6]. Food is the major source of cadmium for children. A study in France showed that a high proportion of children exceeded the tolerable weekly intake of cadmium in the diet during the first 3 years of childhood [7]. A study in Mexico documented an association between early-life dietary cadmium exposure and kidney function in 9-year-old children [8]. Cadmium is estimated to contribute, along with other metals, to the global burden of foodborne disease [9]. Children may also be exposed to cadmium by drinking water, inhalation of cadmium-containing particles from ambient air or cigarette smoke, ingestion of contaminated soil and dust, or use of inexpensive metal jewelry containing cadmium [10, 11].

The primary route of excretion is through the urine. The rate of excretion is low, in part because cadmium binds tightly to metallothionein, a transport and storage protein synthesized in response to cadmium and zinc exposure, preventing excretion into the tubules. In addition, the majority of filtered cadmium is reabsorbed in the renal tubules.

Clinical Effects

Acute and Short-Term Effects
Large oral exposure can produce renal toxicity. A tragic episode of industrial dumping of cad-

mium into the environment occurred in the Jinzu and Kakehashi river basins in Japan, leading to contamination of locally grown rice. This event produced widespread human exposure and a syndrome of renal disease coupled with brittle bones referred to as "Itai-itai" (ouch-ouch) disease. The disease was particularly common among women [12, 13], perhaps because of their higher prevalence of iron deficiency and, therefore, greater cadmium absorption.

Chronic Toxicity
Cadmium is well recognized as a toxicant in occupational exposures. Chronic occupational exposures most commonly produce renal toxicity; microproteinuria is one of the earliest signs.

Epidemiological studies among people living in cadmium-polluted areas of Japan have documented that ß2-microglobulinuria regularly occurs following a lifetime accumulation of 2000 mg cadmium or more [14]. Cui et al. reported early renal effects from cadmium exposure in children and adults living in the tungsten-molybdenum mining areas of South China [15]. Kidney damage also may occur at lower levels of cadmium; a study by Wang et al. in China suggested that adverse tubular renal effects (increased levels of N-acetyl-β-D-glucosaminidase and β2-microglobulin) occur in children even at the current low cadmium levels in the Chinese general population [16].

Diagnosis
While the cadmium concentration in blood reflects recent exposure, urinary cadmium concentration more closely reflects total body burden because cadmium accumulates in the kidney and is considered the gold standard measure of cumulative exposure. Twenty-four–hour urine collections are standard, but spot urine measures in conjunction with urinary creatinine to adjust for urine volume can also be used to assess exposure. However, the kidney is also a prime target of cadmium toxicity, and if renal damage from cadmium exposure occurs, the excretion rate may increase sharply and urinary

cadmium concentrations will no longer reflect body burden.

In adults, 24-h urinary cadmium excretion should be <10 µg/g of creatinine. There is no child-specific standard. On the basis of data from the National Health and Nutrition Examination Survey, the geometric mean urinary cadmium concentration in children 6–11 years of age is 0.075 µg/L per gram of creatinine. From occupational monitoring studies, the first signs of renal abnormalities in adults typically occur at 2 µg/g of creatinine and include microproteinuria—in particular, β_2-microglobulin and α_1-microglobulin are spilled. At urinary cadmium concentrations of 4 µg/g of creatinine, enzymes such as N-acetyl-B-glucosaminidase (NAG) are found in urine; signs of more significant glomerular damage (such as albumin in the urine and decreases in glomerular filtration rate) are seen. In the final stages of cadmium nephropathy, glycosuria, wasting of calcium and phosphate, and altered calcium metabolism are seen [17].

Prevention of Exposure

There is no effective treatment for cadmium toxicity or exposure, thus prevention of exposure is important. Chelation therapy has been shown to mobilize tissue cadmium and increase renal cadmium concentrations, increasing renal toxicity. Children younger than 6 years should not be given or allowed to play with inexpensive metal jewelry. Cadmium should also not be used in consumer products unless absolutely necessary, particularly not in products designed to be used by or with children. Reducing children's exposure to secondhand smoke has obvious health benefits beyond reducing cadmium exposure. Consumption of liver and kidney from exposed animals are potential sources of high dietary cadmium. Exposure to environmental cadmium can be prevented by reducing environmental levels in soil, in water used to irrigate food crops, and by reducing drinking water levels of cadmium. Cadmium concentrations in drinking water supplies are typically less than 1 µg/L (1 part per billion).

Lead

Exposure to high levels of lead causes kidney damage. Children may be exposed to lead in a variety of ways in and near their homes [18]. Studies of adolescents working in auto shops in low and middle income countries and children living near lead smelters have documented significant increases in urinary biomarkers of kidney tubular dysfunction such as N-acetyl-β-D-glucosaminidase, retinol binding protein, and α-1-microglobulin [19–23].

Chronic exposures to low levels of lead also cause proximal tubular injury characterized by proximal tubule nuclear inclusion bodies that progresses to tubulo-interstitial disease and fibrosis. Lead accumulation eventually results in decreased renal clearance, tubular reabsorption and glomerular filtration rate [24]. The association between blood lead and lower estimated GFRs has been documented in a representative sample of US adolescents who participated in the third National Health and Nutrition Examination Survey (1988–1994). More than 99% of the adolescents had blood lead levels below 10 µg/dL. Adolescents with lead in the highest quartile (>3 µg/dL) had 6.6 mL/min/1.73 m^2 lower estimated GFR compared to those in the first quartile (<1 µg/dL) [25].

Diagnosis

The exposure history is essential to making a diagnosis of lead poisoning. When taking the history of exposure, it is important to document the occupation and hobbies of the parents and all home occupants, age of the home, and use of ceramic dishes and fold medicines. Essential questions in the environmental history are shown in Table 73.3. The physical examination should include careful evaluation and documentation of hearing, language, and other developmental milestones. It is rare to see a purplish line on the gums (lead line), but if present it usually indicates severe and prolonged lead poison-

Table 73.3 The Environmental History—focus on lead

When obtaining the environmental history of a child with suspected lead poisoning, the following questions and actions should be included:

- What is the age and general condition of the residence or other structure (school) in which the child spends time?
- Is there evidence of chewed or peeling paint on woodwork, furniture or toys?
- How long has the family lived in that residence?
- Have there been recent renovations or repairs to the house or building?
- Are the windows new?
- Are there other sites at which the child spends significant amounts of time?
- What is the condition or composition of indoor play areas?
- Do outdoor play areas contain bare soil that may be contaminated?
- How does the family attempt to control dust and dirt?
- Does smoke or dust come from external sources close to the building?
- Are there any point sources near the home, such as smelters, metallurgic industries, battery recycling activity (even inactive) or open burning of waste?
- What was the previous use of the land before the building was constructed?
- To what degree does the child exhibit hand-to-mouth activity?
- Does the child exhibit pica?
- Are the child's hands washed before meals and snacks?
- Has anyone in the household ever had lead poisoning?
- What are the occupations of adult household members?
- Are the clothes and shoes used for working activities brought into the house or washed with the home laundry?
- Is the family or any member of the family involved in scavenger activities?
- Is there any work done with lead—For example, car battery recycling, radiator repairs or recuperation of metals—In or around the home?
- What are the hobbies of household members? For example, do they include fishing and preparing weights, working with ceramics or stained glass, hunting and preparing shots for guns, or handicraft activities that use tin or lead solders?
- Are painted materials or waste materials burned in household fireplaces or used as combustibles?
- Are there any local idiosyncratic sources or uses of lead?
- Does the child receive or have access to imported food, food of unsecure origin, cosmetics or folk remedies?
- Is food prepared or stored in glazed pottery or metal vessels?
- Does the family use foods stored in soldered cans?

ing [26]. The best index of exposure is a measurement of blood lead concentration [26]. Suggested laboratory tests to evaluate lead poisoning include a blood lead concentration, CBC with peripheral smear, BUN and creatinine level, and urinanalysis (looking for proteinuria, glucosuria, and aminoaciduria, seen in acute poisoning). In 2012 the US Centers for Disease Control and Prevention defined a reference level of 5 µg/dL to identify children with exposure to lead [27].

Management

Management of lead poisoning includes finding and eliminating the source of the lead, instructing the parents in proper hygienic measures (personal and household), and following up closely. Assessing the nutritional status of the child is important because iron and calcium deficiencies enhance the absorption of lead and aggravate pica [26]. Because most children in the United States with higher blood lead concentrations live in or frequently visit a home with lead paint, successful therapy depends on eliminating the child's exposure. Management that does not control environmental exposure to lead is inadequate. A thorough investigation of the child's environment and family lifestyle for sources of lead should be undertaken.

Deteriorated lead paint is the most common source of exposure in the United States. Other sources that should be considered include tableware, cosmetics such as surma and kohl, home remedies, dietary supplements of calcium, tap water, and parental occupation. Some children have elevated blood lead levels without access to lead paint. Blood lead levels should fall after the child reaches 2 years of age, and a stable or increasing blood lead level after that age is likely to be due to ongoing exposure. Specific attention should be paid to treating iron deficiency and ensuring adequate calcium and zinc intake.

Chelation therapy for children with blood lead levels of 20–44 µg/dL may reduce blood lead concentrations but has not been documented to reverse or diminish cognitive impairment or other behavioral or neuropsychological effects of lead [28]. If the blood lead level is greater than 45 µg/dL and the exposure has been controlled, treatment should begin. A pediatrician experienced in managing children with lead poisoning should be consulted [29].

Mercury

Mercuric salts are usually colorless or white crystals or intensely colored yellow or red powders; they include mercuric oxide (antiseptic and disinfecctant), mercuric cyanide and mercuric oxide (topical antiseptics), and mercuric nitrate (used in working with felt). Mercurous salts are typically colorless, white or light yellow powders; they include mercurous acetate (antibacterial agent), mercurous chloride or calomel (cathartic, diuretic, antiseptic, and antisyphilitic agent), mercurous nitrate (used to blacken brass) and mercurous oxide (used to make electrical batteries) [30].

Children may be exposed to mercury through uses of mercury compounds at home or in school, or in working environments such as small scale artisanal gold mining [31]. Residents in the gold mining communities and downstream of the gold mining communities consume fish that may be heavily contaminated with methylmercury, and it impacts their kidney function [32]. Mercury is used in skin-lightening creams, Chinese traditional

medicine (especially for rheumatoid arthritis), and hair-dyeing agents. In a study of 509 infants exposed to phenylmercury fungicide on cloth diapers [33] urinary excretion of gamma-glutamyl-transpeptidase increased in a dose-dependent manner when urinary mercury exceeded approximately 220 µg/L. This effect was completely reversible and was no longer detectable when the children were re-examined 2 years later.

Acute mercury poisoning presents with acute tubular necrosis, especially with involvement of the proximmal tubules. Chronic low-dose exposure to mercuric salts or elemental mercury vapor can present with edema, proteinuria and normal renal function. Chronic mercury exposure can induce an immunological form of glomerular disease. This form of mercury injury to the kidney is a common form of mercury-induced nephropathy [34–36]. Findings of this membranous nephropathy may include thickened glomerular basement membrane and mildly proliferative mesangial cells and deposits of IgG1 subclasses along the glomerular capillary loops [37].

Diagnosis

The exposure history is essential to making a diagnosis of mercury poisoning. When taking the history of exposure, it is important to document the occupation and hobbies of all home occupants, use of medicines, folk remedies and antiseptics. Essential questions in the environmental history are shown in Table 73.4. A 24 h urine specimen collected in an acid-washed plastic container is appropriate for patients who have been chronically exposed to elemental mercury or mercury salts. A first morning void can provide a close approximation of a 24-h collection, particularly if it is adjusted for the concentration of the urine (using the amount of creatinine present).

A urine mercury concentration of less than 8 µg/L in adults is considered background [37]. Urinary mercury concentrations from 12 to 100 µg/L are associated with subtle changes on some tests, even before overt symptoms occur. Background or toxic urinary mercury concentrations have not been determined for children [30].

Table 73.4 The Environmental History—focus on mercury

When obtaining the environmental history of a child with suspected mercury exposure, the following questions and actions should be included:
- What are the occupations and hobbies of adult household members?
- Has there been recent application of mercury-containing caulks, latex paints, and other materials in constructing or renovating homes and other buildings?
- Has there been recent use of folk medicines? (these may contain mercury compounds.)
- Has there been a recent move? (previous tenants may have spilled mercury.)
- Has there been recent use of cosmetics containing mercury? (mercury is contained in some mascaras and wave fixatives and some skin lighteners sold outside the US.)
- Has there been use of over-the-counter preparations such as nasal sprays, contact lens solutions, and topical antiseptics?
- Has there been use of elemental mercury in a school laboratory?
- Has the child been playing with mercury? (children are attracted to elemental mercury because of its unique properties.)

Management

Proper management includes finding and eliminating the source of the mercury. When a patient has ingested mercury salts, the goals of therapy are to remove mercury from the body and to prevent dehydration and shock. Inorganic mercury can be removed from the gastrointestinal tract by emesis, catharsis or lavage. It is imperative that adequate intravenous fluids be administered to prevent dehydration and to reduce the concentration of mercury in the kidneys. BAL or another appropriate chelating agent should be administered immediately; its usefulness depends on rapid administration [30].

Prognosis

If mercury exposure ceases, complete remission is expected [37].

Uranium

Exposure to uranium can damage the proximal tubules of the kidney [38]. A case series described a family in Connecticut, who discovered that their private well was contaminated with naturally occurring uranium. Twenty four hour measurements of urine uranium were obtained on all 7 family members, but only the youngest child (age 3) had an elevated β-2-microglobulin excretion rate [39]. They had lived in the house for the previous 5 years, and the 3-year-old had derived a major portion of her nutritional intake from infant formula that was prepared by mixing powdered formulas with contaminated well water. Soil and water can also become contaminated from depleted uranium in areas where armed conflict has occurred.

Diagnosis

The exposure history is essential to making a diagnosis of uranium poisoning. When taking the history of exposure, it is important to document the source of the family's water. If the child lives in an area where armed conflict has occurred, the physician should inquire if children play in areas where depleted uranium penetrators have impacted, if children have ingested heavily contaminated soil, and if a buried penetrator feeds uranium directly into a well. Environmental movement of depleted uranium from buried penetrators into local water supplies is likely to be very slow. Over decades levels of uranium could increase in local water supplies [40].

Urine analysis for uranium is the best test to determine whether a patient has been exposed to large amounts of uranium.

Management

Because well water used for drinking or to reconstitute infant formula may be contaminated with uranium, families who use well water should consider having the water tested. Most large municipal water supplies maintain uranium levels less than the U.S. EPA maximum contaminant level of 30 µg/L.

Table 73.5 Characteristic renal manifestations of exposure to selected pesticides

Manifestation	Characteristic of these poisonings	Occurs with these agents
Proteinuria	Inorganic arsenicals	Cadmium compounds
Hematuria	Copper compounds	Phosphorous
Sometimes leading	Sodium fluoride	Phosphides
To oliguria	Naphthalene	Phosphine
Acute renal failure	Borate	Chlorophenoxy compounds
With azotemia	Nitrophenols	Creosote
	Pentachlorophenol	Organotin compounds
	Sodium chlorate	
	Sulfuryl fluoride	
	Paraquat	
	Diquat	
	Arsine	
	Ethylene dibromide	
Dysuria, hematuria, pyuria	Chlordimeform	
Polyuria	Cholecalciferol	Fluoride
Hemoglobinuria	Naphthalene	
	Sodium chlorate	
	Arsine	
Wine-red urine (porphyrinuria)	Hexachlorobenzene	
Smoky urine	Creosote	
Glycosuria		Organotin compounds
Ketonuria		Borate

Source: Environmental Protection Agency. Recognition and Management of Pesticide Poisonings. 6th edition, 2013. Washington, DC: US Environmental Protection Agency, Office of Pesticide Programs

Pesticides

Many pesticides are toxic to the kidney; pesticides such as paraquat and diquat are particularly toxic [41]. Paraquat and diquat are bipyridyl herbicides that are widely used, primarily in agriculture and by government agencies and industries for control of weeds [42].

When humans are exposed to these herbicides the proximal convoluted tubules show vacuolation and cell necroses [43, 44]. Proteinuria, hematuria, glucosuria or all of the features of the Fanconi syndrome may occur. Severely poisoned patients develop acute oliguric renal failure. Characteristic manifestations of poisoning with other pesticides are shown in Table 73.5.

Diagnosis

Pesticide poisonings may go unrecognized because of the failure to take a proper exposure history. The exposure history is essential to making a diagnosis. When taking the history of exposure, it is important to document the location of the family's home and the occupation

Table 73.6 Environmental History—focus on pesticides

When obtaining the environmental history of a child with suspected exposure to pesticides, the following questions and actions should be included:

- Are pesticides (e.g., bug or weed killers, flea and tick sprays, collars, powders, or shampoos) used in your home or garden or on your pet?
- Has anyone in the family worked with pesticides that they might have brought home?
- Does parent or any household member have a hobby with exposure to pesticides?
- Has the patient ever lived near a facility which could have contaminated the surrounding area (plant, dump site)?
- Does the patient's drinking water come from a private well, city water supply and/or grocery store?
- If pesticides are used:
  - Is a licensed pesticide applicator used?
  - Are children allowed to play in areas recently treated with pesticides?
  - Where are the pesticides stored?
  - Is food handled properly (e.g., washing of raw fruits and vegetables)?

and hobbies of all home occupants. Essential questions in the environmental history are shown in Table 73.6.

Management

If poisoning with paraquat or diquat is suspected based on the environmental history, a simple colorimetric test can be used to identify paraquat and diquat in the urine, and to give a rough indication of the magnitude of absorbed dose [42]. To one volume of urine add 0.5 volume of freshly prepared 1% sodium dithionate (sodium hydrosulfite) in 1-normal sodium hydroxide (1.0 N NaOH). Observe color at the end of 1 min. A blue color indicates the presence of paraquat in excess of 0.5 mg/L. Both positive and negative controls should be run to ensure that the dithionate has not undergone oxidation in storage [42]. Diquat in urine yields a green color with the dithionate test. Both paraquat and diquat can also be measured in blood and urine [42]. Treatment should be managed in conjunction with a pediatric toxicologist, and includes immediate gastrointestinal decontamination with an adsorbent such as activated charcoal, Bentonite, or Fuller's Earth (2 gm/kg for children under 12 years.)

Arsenic

Arsenic has been classified as a known human carcinogen [10]. Children's most common exposure to arsenic is from contaminated drinking water. Other major sources of children's exposure are foods including rice, organic rice syrup, other grains, fruits, and juices [45].

Chronic exposure to arsenic is associated, in a dose-related fashion, with an increased risk of bladder cancer [10, 46–53]. Arsenic also has been associated with an excess risk of cancers of the kidney [10, 54–56]. The chronic consumption of water contaminated with arsenic in a concentration of 500 parts per million is associated with an estimated risk of 1 in 10 people developing bladder cancer. At a concentration of 50 parts per billion (ppb), cancer mortality is estimated to be in the range of 0.6 to 1.5 per 100, or approximately 1 in 100. At 10 ppb, the US Environmental Protection Agency drinking water standard since 2006, the risk of bladder cancer is 1–3 per 1000 [57].

Infancy and childhood appear to be susceptible periods during which exposure to arsenic can have lasting effects [58]. Exposure to arsenic during pregnancy and childhood is associated with a greater risk of increased occurrence of kidney cancer than exposure during adulthood [59].

Diagnosis

The exposure history is essential to making a diagnosis of arsenic poisoning. When taking the history of exposure, it is important to document the source of the family's water.

Management

Because well water used for drinking or to reconstitute infant formula may be contaminated with arsenic, families who use well water should consider having the water tested. Most large municipal water supplies maintain arsenic levels less than the EPA standard of 0.010 mg/L.

Ochratoxin A

Exposures to certain ochratoxins can cause kidney damage. Ochratoxins are natural toxins produced by fungi including *Aspergillus ochraceus*, *Aspergillus ostianus*, and *Penicillium verrucosum* that grow on cereal grains (barley, oats, rye, corn and wheat) and contaminate foods and drinks such as milk powder, coffee, wine and beer [60]. Ochratoxin A is a potent nephrotoxin [61]. Outbreaks of **Balkan nephropathy**, a fatal, chronic renal disease occurring in limited areas of Bulgaria, the former Yugoslavia, and Romania, have been linked with exposure to ochratoxin A [62–65]. Levels of ochratoxin A are elevated in the blood of patients with Balkan nephropathy [66].

In the United States, ochratoxin exposure is highest in infants and young children who consume large amounts of oat-based cereals [67]. Infants may also be exposed through breast milk if the mother has consumed foods contaminated with ochratoxin [68, 69].

Although the primary route of children's exposure to ochratoxin has previously been assumed to be through ingestion, there is growing evidence that inhalation can be an important route of exposure [70]. A case report linked exposure to ochratoxin A to focal segmental glomerulosclerosis in a 5-year-old girl who was diagnosed after presenting with enuresis. The child had a significantly elevated urine concentration of ochratoxin A (9.1 parts per billion (limit of detection 2.0 parts per billion). She probably had been exposed to ochratoxin from a home environment that was water damaged and moldy [71].

Apart from its nephrotoxicity, chronic exposure to ochratoxin A is associated with tumors of the upper urinary tract in adults. In view of substantial evidence from animal experiments supporting the carcinogenicity of ochratoxin A, the substance is categorized as possibly carcinogenic to humans (Group 2B) [66].

Diagnosis

The exposure history is essential to making a diagnosis of kidney damage from ochratoxin. When taking the history of exposure, it is important to collect a dietary history and to carefully document the condition of the home environment, with special attention to a history of the child's exposure to water damaged and moldy indoor areas.

Management

Investigations are ongoing to study the use of aspartame, a structural analogue of ochratoxin A and phenylalanine, in preventing the toxic effects of ochratoxin A exposure on the kidneys [72]. Aspartame competitively prevents the binding of ochratoxin to serum albumin. Investigations are also being conducted to study ways to reduce the genotoxic effects of ochratoxin. The quantity of DNA adducts that are induced by ochratoxin A in animals can be reduced dramatically by pretreatment of the animals with aspirin and indomethacin, which inhibit prostaglandin H synthase [73].

Aristolochic Acid

Aristolochic acids belong to the *Aristolochia* genus of plants which are often used as herbal medicines [74]. The kidney injury caused by aris-

tolochic acids was identified from a group of women who used the herbal weight-loss regimen *Guang Fang Ji*, which contains aristolochic acid [75]. The kidney disease caused by exposure to aristolochic acids is now formally termed **aristolochic acid nephropathy**. Cases of aristolochic acid nephropathy have been reported in Europe [76–81], the United States [82] Australia [83], Japan [84], Korea [85], China [86, 87], Taiwan [86], and Hong Kong [88]. In addition, some cases of Balkan endemic nephropathy have documented exposure to aristolochic acid [89]. In the area close to tributaries of the Danube River in Bosnia, Bulgaria, Croatia, Romania, and Serbia there is a weed, *A. Clematitis*. Seeds of this weed contain aristolochic acid. The contamination of wheat flour with the seed has been associated with some cases of Balkan endemic nephropathy. Many studies show an association between the exposure with high- dose and/or long-lasting aristolochic acid exposure and kidney disease as well as urothelial cancer. The mechanism for aristolochic acid nephropathy might be apoptosis in tubular cells, whereas the urothelial cancer might be caused by DNA adducts [90].

Diagnosis

There is no specific diagnostic feature for aristolochic acid nephropathy. However, a clinical inquiry for the possible use of herbal medicines containing aristolochic acid should be taken in patients with unexplained progressive decline in glomerular filtration rate.

Patients with aristolochic acid nephropathy usually have proximal tubular dysfunction, such as glycosuria and low molecular weight proteinuria. Urinalysis reveals few erythrocytes and leukocytes, and mild proteinuria. Anemia often is unusually prominent relative to the degree of GFR impairment.

Ultrasonography usually demonstrates contracted kidneys. Unfortunately, there are no defined biomarkers for diagnosing aristolochic acid nephropathy.

Kidney biopsy reveals extensive interstitial fibrosis associated with tubular atrophy and low numbers of chronic inflammatory cells. The most specific pathologic feature is that injury decreases from the outer to the inner cortex [91–93].

Although no strict criteria for diagnosing aristolochic acid nephropathy are available, a set of criteria allowing the definite, probable and possible diagnosis of aristolochic acid nephropathy has been proposed [94]. A definite diagnosis can be made in the patient with impaired renal function and any 2 of 3 additional findings: renal pathology demonstrating hypocellular fibrosis decreasing from the outer to the inner renal cortex, phytochemical analysis proving the intake of products containing aristolochic acid, or the detection of AA–DNA adducts in renal or urinary tract tissue. If only one of the additional findings is present in patients with impaired renal function together with urothelial cancer at the time of presentation, a probable diagnosis can be made. A possible diagnosis can be made in patients with unexplained renal dysfunction and a history of taking herbal medicines likely containing aristolochic acid.

Management

There are no randomized clinical trials supporting an evidence-based therapeutic strategy. The discontinuation of ingestion of products containing aristolochic acid is certainly essential. A study on steroid treatment for aristolochic acid nephropathy showed significant slowing of progressive renal failure in 12 patients [95].

Melamine

The Chinese Epidemic

In 2008, an epidemic of melamine contamination from formula milk was associated with urinary tract stones in young children in China. Nearly 230,000 children were diagnosed with urinary stones revealed through a targeted screening program. Melamine contamination was detected in 22 commercial brands of formula. The level of melamine in contaminated formula was 2.5 mg/kg in many brands of milk powder, exceeding the estimated tolerable daily intake level (0.063 mg/kg body weight) multifold [96]. It appeared that melamine was added to milk powder to boost the protein content, because melamine is 66% nitrogen by mass.

Non-epidemic Exposures

Melamine is prevalent in the environment and the effects of low-level exposures to children have not been clarified. A study in the US found concentrations of melamine and cyanuric acid in children's urine to be higher than levels reported in children from other countries [97]. Cyanuric acid was associated with increased KIM-1 concentrations, suggesting kidney injury.

Pathogenesis of Renal Injury Induced By Melamine-Related Urinary Stones

Almost all the available data on the toxicology and toxicokinetics was obtained by animal experiments that included dogs, cats, rats and mice. Melamine and cyanuric acid are not metabolized and are eliminated from the kidneys unchanged [98–100]. Crystals form mostly in the distal tubules from melamine and cyanuric acid [101–103].

Kidney injury is thought to be induced by the crystals or via obstruction of urine flow [101–104]. In a study of rats administered a diet containing melamine, stone formation was associated with injury to renal tubular epithelial cells, apoptosis and inflammation [105]. Gut microbiota can convert melamine to cyanuric acid *in vitro*, implicating a role of intestinal microbiota in the pathogenesis of melamine-related renal injury [106].

Clinical Manifestations

Three quarters of the children with urinary stones caused by melamine-contaminated formula in the Chinese epidemic were asymptomatic [107]. A few patients presented with dysuria, hematuria, and unexplained crying when urinating; these patients usually had obstruction caused by urinary stones. A small portion of patients (about 5%) with acute obstructive renal failure caused by melamine-induced urinary stones presented with nausea, vomiting, edema and anuria [108].

Infants were the major victims because of their high exposure to milk powder formula. However, the age at diagnosis of melamine-associated urinary stones ranged from 1.5 months to 10 years [108]. The incidence of melamine-associated urinary stones was 3.1 times higher in male than in female subjects; the excess risk of males was most marked in boys younger than 1 year of age [109, 110].

Diagnosis

The exposure history is essential to making a diagnosis of melamine-associated urinary stones. When taking the history of exposure, it is important to document the feeding mode, formula brand, duration and amount of daily feeding.

Ultrasonography of the kidneys along with the ureters and the bladder is the first choice to detect stones, hydronephrosis and obstruction caused by melamine-associated calculi [111–113]. The location and number of stones should be reported. Abdominal X-ray and CT urography can be performed if the stone or hydronephrosis cannot be confirmed by ultrasonography [114].

Management

The management of melamine-related urinary stones in the Chinese epidemic included a conservative treatment approach, extracorporeal shock wave lithotripsy and surgical intervention. The decision regarding the approach usually was made by taking into account symptoms, stone size, stone numbers and location, etc. In children with non-obstructive melamin-related stones smaller than 4 mm without serious clinical symptoms, only oral fluid prescription was increased [113]. In case of stones larger than 4 mm, management included infusion of fluids, forced diuresis and urinary alkalization aiming for urine pH between 6.0 and 6.5. A follow-up study after 4 years showed that among 45 children treated conservatively melamine-related urinary stones had disappeared in 34 children, partially discharged in six, were unchanged in four and had grown in size in one child [115]. Hence, the vast majority of children with melamine-related stones without serious clinical symptoms, recovered with time.

Many medical teams opted for extracorporeal shock wave lithotripsy (ESWL) for children with

a single melamine-related urinary stone who failed conservative treatment. In a cohort of 189 young children ESWL was performed on stones 3.8–25 mm in size located in the renal pelvis (n = 141), proximal ureter (n = 17), mid ureter (n = 5), or distal ureter (n = 26). Most children (95%) required only one lithotripsy session. During 28 months of follow-up there was not a single case with a severe complication of lithotripsy [116].

Few children (5.6% according to a meta-analysis of 2164 cases) underwent surgical intervention because of failure of conservative treatment or obstructive kidney failure [108]. Surgery included minimally invasive percutaneous nephrolithotomy using ureteroscope and pneumatic intracorporeal lithotripsy, and lithotripsy with cystoscopy or ureteroscopy.

Per- and Polyfluoroalkylated Substances

Per- and polyfluoroalkylated substances (PFAS) are synthetic chemicals that repel both water and fat and are highly heat resistant. These substances are used in many consumer products including stain-repellant fabrics and carpets, food packaging, floor care and cleaning products and personal care products. Their half-life in humans is several years. PFAS are eliminated via the kidneys by tubular excretion. PFAS are suspected to cause cellular and tubular histological changes in the kidneys via oxidative stress, enhanced endothelial permeability and other molecular pathways [117].

Few studies addressed the relationship of PFAS exposure with children's kidney function. A study of children found an eGFR decrease of 0.75 mL/min/1.73 m² decrease per quartile increase in per-fluorooctanoic acid (PFOA) concentration [118]. Two pediatric studies linked serum PFA concentrations to high uric acid levels [119, 120]. A study among adolescents and young adults in Taiwan who had abnormal urinalysis found that children with CKD had higher serum PFUA concentrations [121]. Given their renal mode of elimina-

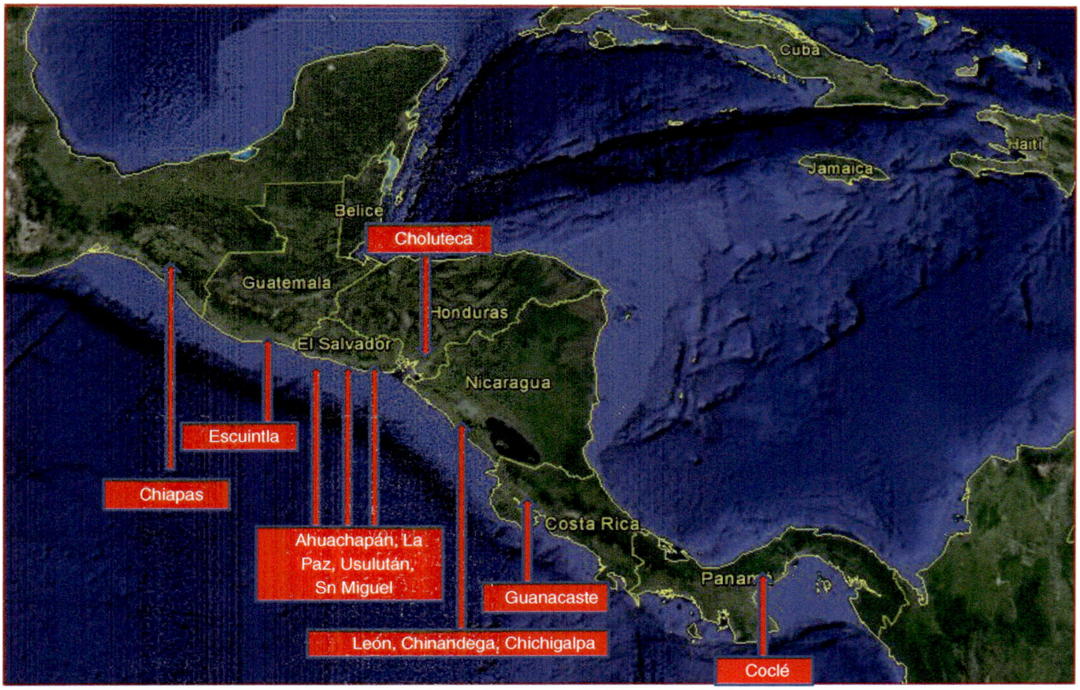

Fig. 73.1 Locations of studies of chronic kidney disease of unknown etiology in Central America. (Courtesy of Dr. Juan Jose Amador of Boston University)

tion, it is still controversial whether CKD may be the cause rather than the consequence of PFAS accumulation. However, in a recent long-term follow-up study in pre-diabetic adults, baseline PFAS concentrations were inversely correlated with long-term eGFR, with a reduction by 2.3 mL/min/1.73 m² per PFAS concentration quartile [122].

Chronic Kidney Disease of Unknown Etiology

Among young adults (primarily men) in Central American countries, an epidemic of non-proteinuric chronic kidney disease of unknown etiology has been occurring for at least the past 25 years on the Pacific coast (see Fig. 73.1). Young men working in the sugar-cane fields appear to be most severely affected [123–126]. There is some evidence that the initial damage may be occurring at an early age [127]). A urine dipstick study conducted in the

city of León among 423 pre-school children documented some level of proteinuria in 51% of the children in the study and hematuria in 20% [128].

Similar epidemics have been reported in Sri Lanka, India, and Egypt [129–131]. Investigators have evaluated the potential role of a variety of medicines, agrochemicals, arsenic, leptospirosis, and heat and strenuous labor combining to cause volume depletion, but a definitive etiology has not yet been identified [132–141].

Diagnosis
This is a diagnosis of exclusion. A thorough occupational and exposure history are essential if considering a diagnosis of chronic kidney disease of unknown etiology. When taking the history of exposure, the clinician should document the parents' occupation, and whether the child accompanies the parents to work. Adolescent work history should be obtained. Inquiries should be made about the source of the family's water.

References

1. Zheng LY, Sanders AP, Saland JM, Wright RO, Arora M. Environmental exposures and pediatric kidney function and disease: a systematic review. Environ Res. 2017;158:625–48.

2. American Academy of Pediatrics Council on Environmental Health. Taking an environmental history and giving anticipatory guidance. In: Etzel RA, editor. Pediatric environmental health. 4th ed. Itasca, IL: American Academy of Pediatrics; 2019. p. 47–67.

3. Paulson JA, Gordon L. The environmental history and examination: the key to diagnosis of environmental diseases. In: Landrigan PJ, Etzel RA, editors. Textbook of children's environmental health. New York, NY: Oxford University Press; 2014. p. 475–81.

4. Bacchetta J, Dubourg L, Juillard L, Cochat P. Non-drug-induced nephrotoxicity. Pediatr Nephrol. 2009;24(12):2291–300.

5. Weidemann DK, Weaver VM, Fadrowski JJ. Toxic environmental exposures and kidney health in children. Pediatr Nephrol (Berlin, Germany). 2016;31(11):2043–54.

6. Noonan CW, Sarasua SM, Campagna D, Kathman SJ, Lybarger JA, Mueller PW. Effects of exposure to low levels of environmental cadmium on renal biomarkers. Environ Health Perspect. 2002;110(2):151–5.

7. Jean J, Sirot V, Hulin M, Le Calvez E, Zinck J, Noël L, et al. Dietary exposure to cadmium and health risk assessment in children – results of the French infant total diet study. Food Chem Toxicol. 2018;115:358–64.

8. Rodríguez-López E, Tamayo-Ortiz M, Ariza AC, Ortiz-Panozo E, Deierlein AL, Pantic I, et al. Early-life dietary cadmium exposure and kidney function in 9-year-old children from the PROGRESS cohort. Toxics. 2020;8(4):83.

9. Gibb HJ, Barchowsky A, Bellinger D, Bolger PM, Carrington C, Havelaar AH, et al. Estimates of the 2015 global and regional disease burden from four foodborne metals – arsenic, cadmium, lead and methylmercury. Environ Res. 2019;174:188–94.

10. National Toxicology Program. 12th Report on Carcinogenics. Research Triangle Park, NC: National Toxicology Program; 2011. http://ntp.niehs.nih.gov/?objectid=03C9AF75-E1BF-FF40-DBA9EC0928DF8B15. Accessed 30 May 2014.

11. New York State Department of Health. Cadmium in Children's Jewelry. http://www.health.state.ny.us/environmental/chemicals/cadmium/cadmium_jewelry.html.

12. Horiguchi H, Oguma E, Sasaki S, Miyamoto K, Ikeda Y, Machida M, et al. Comprehensive study of the effects of age, iron deficiency, diabetes mellitus, and cadmium burden on dietary cadmium absorption in cadmium-exposed female Japanese farmers. Toxicol Appl Pharmacol. 2004;196(1):114–23.

13. Kobayashi E, Suwazono Y, Uetani M, Inaba T, Oishi M, Kido T, et al. Estimation of benchmark dose as the threshold levels of urinary cadmium, based on excretion of total protein, beta 2-microglobulin, and N-acetyl-β-d-glucosaminidase in cadmium nonpolluted regions in Japan. Environ Res. 2006;101(3):401–6.

14. Nogawa K, Honda R, Kido T, Tsuritani I, Yamada Y, Ishizaki M, et al. A dose-response analysis of cadmium in the general environment with special reference to total cadmium intake limit. Environ Res. 1989;48(1):7–16.

15. Cui X, Cheng H, Liu X, Giubilato E, Critto A, Sun H, et al. Cadmium exposure and early renal effects in the children and adults living in a tungsten-molybdenum mining areas of South China. Environ Sci Pollut Res. 2018;25(15):15089–101.

16. Wang D, Sun H, Wu Y, Zhou Z, Ding Z, Chen X, et al. Tubular and glomerular kidney effects in the Chinese general population with low environmental cadmium exposure. Chemosphere. 2016;147:3–8.

17. Roels HA, Hoet P, Lison D. Usefulness of biomarkers of exposure to inorganic mercury, Lead, or cadmium in controlling occupational and environmental risks of nephrotoxicity. Ren Fail. 1999;21(3–4):251–62.

18. Organization WH. Childhood lead poisoning. Geneva: WHO; 2010. http://www.who.int/ceh/publications/childhoodpoisoning/en/index.html

19. Oktem F, Arslan MK, Dundar B, Delibas NK, Gultepe M, Ergurhan Ilhan I. Renal effects and erythrocyte oxidative stress in long-term low-level lead-exposed adolescent workers in auto repair workshops. Arch Toxicol. 2004;78(12):681–7.

20. Sönmez F, Dönmez O, Sönmez HM, Keskinoğlu A, Kabasakal C, Mir S. Lead exposure and urinary N-acetyl beta D glucosaminidase activity in adolescent workers in auto repair workshops. J Adolesc Health. 2002;30(3):213–6.

21. Fels L. Adverse effects of chronic low level lead exposure on kidney function-a risk group study in children. Nephrol Dial Transpl. 1998;13(9):2248–56.

22. Verberk MM, Willems TEP, Verplanke AJW, Wolff FAD. Environmental Lead and renal effects in children. Archiv Environ Health. 1996;51(1):83–7.

23. Bernard AM, Vyskocil A, Roels H, Kriz J, Kodl M, Lauwerys R. Renal effects in children living in the vicinity of a Lead smelter. Environ Res. 1995;68(2):91–5.

24. Gonick H. Nephrotoxicity of cadmium & lead. Indian J Med Res. 2008;128(4):335–52.

25. Fadrowski JJ, Navas-Acien A, Tellez-Plaza M, Guallar E, Weaver VM, Furth SL. Blood lead level and kidney function in US adolescents: the third National Health and Nutrition Examination Survey. Arch Intern Med. 2010;170(1):75–82.

26. Agency for Toxic Substances and Disease Registry. Case studies in environmental medicine: lead toxicity. 2010. http://www.atsdr.cdc.gov/csem/lead/docs/lead.pdf.

27. Advisory Committee on Childhood Lead Poisoning Prevention to the Centers for Disease Control and Prevention. Low Level Lead Exposure Harms Children: A Renewed Call for Primary Prevention. 2012. http://www.cdc.gov/nceh/lead/acclpp/final_document_030712.pdf.

28. Dietrich KN. Effect of chelation therapy on the neuropsychological and behavioral development of Lead-exposed children after school entry. Pediatrics. 2004;114(1):19–26.

29. American Academy of Pediatrics Council on Environmental Health. Lead. In: Etzel RA, editor. Pediatric environmental health. 4th ed. Itasca, IL: American Academy of Pediatrics; 2019. p. 557–84.

30. Agency for Toxic Substances and Disease Registry. Case studies in environmental medicine: pediatric environmental health. 2002. http://www.atsdr.cdc.gov/HEC/CSEM/pediatric/docs/pediatric.pdf.

31. World Health Organization. Children's exposure to mercury compounds. Geneva: WHO; 2010. http://www.who.int/ceh/publications/children_exposure/en/index.html

32. Gibb H, O'Leary KG. Mercury exposure and health impacts among individuals in the artisanal and small-scale gold mining community: a comprehensive review. Environ Health Perspect. 2014;122(7):667–72.

33. Gotelli C, Astolfi E, Cox C, Cernichiari E, Clarkson T. Early biochemical effects of an organic mercury fungicide on infants: "dose makes the poison". Science. 1985;227(4687):638–40.

34. Tubbs RR, Gephardt GN, McMahon JT, Pohl MC, Vidt DG, Barenberg SA, et al. Membranous glomerulonephritis associated with industrial mercury exposure:study of pathogenetic mechanisms. Am J Clin Pathol. 1982;77(4):409–13.

35. Agner E, Jans H. Mercury poisoning and nephrotic syndrome in two young siblings. Lancet. 1978;312(8096):951.

36. Onwuzuligbo O, Hendricks AR, Hassler J, Domanski K, Goto C, Wolf MTF. Mercury intoxication as a rare cause of membranous nephropathy in a child. Am J Kidney Dis. 2018;72(4):601–5.

37. Li S-J, Zhang S-H, Chen H-P, Zeng C-H, Zheng C-X, Li L-S, et al. Mercury-induced membranous nephropathy: clinical and pathological features. Clin J Am Soc Nephrol. 2010;5(3):439–44.

38. Arzuaga X, Rieth SH, Bathija A, Cooper GS. Renal effects of exposure to natural and depleted uranium: a review of the epidemiologic and experimental data. J Toxicol Environ Health Part B. 2010;13(7–8):527–45.

39. Magdo HS, Forman J, Graber N, Newman B, Klein K, Satlin L, et al. Grand rounds: nephrotoxicity in a young child exposed to uranium from contaminated well water. Environ Health Perspect. 2007;115(8):1237–41.

40. https://royalsociety.org/-/media/Royal_Society_Content/policy/publications/2002/9954-Summary.pdf.

41. International Programme on Chemical Safety. Environmental Health Criteria 119. Principles and methods for the assessment of nephrotoxicity associated with exposure to chemicals. http://www.inchem.org/documents/ehc/ehc/ehc119.htm.

42. Environmental Protection Agency. Recognition and management of pesticide poisonings. 6th edition. 2013. http://www2.epa.gov/pesticide-worker-safety.

43. Lock E. The effect of paraquat and diquat on renal function in the rat. Toxicol Appl Pharmacol. 1979;48(2):327–36.

44. Lock EA, Ishmael J. The acute toxic effects of paraquat and diquat on the rat kidney. Toxicol Appl Pharmacol. 1979;50(1):67–76.

45. Food and Drug Administration. Arsenic in rice and rice products; 2013. http://www.fda.gov/food/foodborneillnesscontaminants/metals/ucm319870.htm.

46. Bates MN, Smith AH, Cantor KP. Case-control study of bladder cancer and arsenic in drinking water. Am J Epidemiol. 1995;141(6):523–30.

47. Kurttio P, Pukkala E, Kahelin H, Auvinen A, Pekkanen J. Arsenic concentrations in well water and risk of bladder and kidney cancer in Finland. Environ Health Perspect. 1999;107(9):705–10.

48. Tsuda T, Babazono A, Yamamoto E, Kurumatani N, Mino Y, Ogawa T, et al. Ingested arsenic and internal cancer: a historical cohort study followed for 33 years. Am J Epidemiol. 1995;141(3):198–209.

49. Smith AH, Goycolea M, Haque R, Biggs ML. Marked increase in bladder and lung cancer mortality in a region of Northern Chile due to arsenic in drinking water. Am J Epidemiol. 1998;147(7):660–9.

50. Hopenhayn-Rich C. Lung and kidney cancer mortality associated with arsenic in drinking water in Cordoba, Argentina. Int J Epidemiol. 1998;27(4):561–9.

51. Wu M-M, Kuo T-L, Hwang Y-H, Chen C-J. Dose-response relation between arsenic concentration in well water and mortality from cancers and vascular diseases. Am J Epidemiol. 1989;130(6):1123–32.

52. Chiou H-Y, Chiou S-T, Hsu Y-H, Chou Y-L, Tseng C-H, Wei M-L, et al. Incidence of transitional cell carcinoma and arsenic in drinking water: a follow-up study of 8,102 residents in an Arseniasis-endemic area in Northeastern Taiwan. Am J Epidemiol. 2001;153(5):411–8.

53. Meliker JR, Slotnick MJ, AvRuskin GA, Schottenfeld D, Jacquez GM, Wilson ML, et al. Lifetime exposure to arsenic in drinking water and bladder cancer: a population-based case-control study in Michigan, USA. Cancer Causes Control. 2010;21(5):745–57.

54. Ferreccio C, Smith AH, Durán V, Barlaro T, Benítez H, Valdés R, et al. Case-control study of arsenic in drinking water and kidney cancer in uniquely exposed Northern Chile. Am J Epidemiol. 2013;178(5):813–8.

55. Steinmaus C, Ferreccio C, Acevedo J, Yuan Y, Liaw J, Durán V, et al. Increased lung and bladder cancer incidence in adults after in utero and early-life arsenic exposure. Cancer Epidemiol Biomark Prev. 2014;23(8):1529–38.

56. Steinmaus CM, Ferreccio C, Romo JA, Yuan Y, Cortes S, Marshall G, et al. Drinking water arsenic in northern Chile: high cancer risks 40 years after exposure cessation. Cancer Epidemiol Biomark Prev. 2013;22(4):623–30.

57. National Research Council. Arsenic in Drinking Water: 2001 Update. Washington, DC: National Academies Press; 2001. http://www.nap.edu/books/0309076293/html/.

58. Naujokas MF, Anderson B, Ahsan H, Aposhian HV, Graziano JH, Thompson C, et al. The broad scope of health effects from chronic arsenic exposure: update on a worldwide public health problem. Environ Health Perspect. 2013;121(3):295–302.

59. Yuan Y, Marshall G, Ferreccio C, Steinmaus C, Liaw J, Bates M, et al. Kidney cancer mortality: fifty-year latency patterns related to arsenic exposure. Epidemiology. 2010:103–8.

60. Etzel RA. Mycotoxins and human disease. In: Proft T, editor. Microbial toxins: molecular and cellular biology. Norfolk: Horizon Bioscience; 2005. p. 449–72.

61. Agriopoulou S, Stamatelopoulou E, Varzakas T. Advances in occurrence, importance, and mycotoxin control strategies: prevention and detoxification in foods. Foods. 2020;9(2):137.

62. Petkova-Bocharova T, Castegnaro M. Ochratoxin A contamination of cereals in an area of high incidence of Balkan endemic nephropathy in Bulgaria. Food Addit Contam. 1985;2(4):267–70.

63. Maaroufi K, Achour A, Zakhama A, Ellouz F, El May M, Creppy EE, et al. Human nephropathy related to ochratoxin A in Tunisia. J Toxicol. 1996;15(3):223–37.

64. Pfohl-Leszkowicz A, Manderville RA. Ochratoxin A: an overview on toxicity and carcinogenicity in animals and humans. Mol Nutr Food Res. 2007;51(1):61–99.

65. Bui-Klimke TR, Wu F. Ochratoxin a and human health risk: a review of the evidence. Crit Rev Food Sci Nutr. 2015;55(13):1860–9.

66. International Agency for Research on Cancer (IARC). IARC summary and evaluation, ochratoxin A. Volume 56, 1993. http://www.inchem.org/documents/iarc/vol56/13-ochra.html.

67. Mitchell NJ, Chen C, Palumbo JD, Bianchini A, Cappozzo J, Stratton J, et al. A risk assessment of dietary Ochratoxin a in the United States. Food Chem Toxicol. 2017;100:265–73.

68. Muñoz K, Blaszkewicz M, Campos V, Vega M, Degen GH. Exposure of infants to ochratoxin A with breast milk. Arch Toxicol. 2014;88(3):837–46.

69. Hassan AM, Sheashaa HA, Fattah MFA, Ibrahim AZ, Gaber OA, Sobh MA. Study of ochratoxin A as an environmental risk that causes renal injury in breast-fed Egyptian infants. Pediatr Nephrol. 2005;21(1):102–5.

70. Iavicoli I, Brera C, Carelli G, Caputi R, Marinaccio A, Miraglia M. External and internal dose in subjects occupationally exposed to ochratoxin a. Int Arch Occup Environ Health. 2002;75(6):381–6.

71. Hope JH, Hope BE. A review of the diagnosis and treatment of Ochratoxin A inhalational exposure associated with human illness and kidney disease including focal segmental glomerulosclerosis. J Environ Public Health. 2012;2012:835059.

72. Baudrimont I, Sostaric B, Yenot C, Betbeder A-M, Dano-Djedje S, Sanni A, et al. Aspartame prevents the karyomegaly induced by ochratoxin A in rat kidney. Arch Toxicol. 2001;75(3):176–83.

73. Obrecht-Pflumio S, Grosse Y, Pfohl-Leszkowicz A, Dirheimer G. Protection by indomethacin and aspirin against genotoxicity of ochratoxin A, particularly in the urinary bladder and kidney. Arch Toxicol. 1996;70(3–4):244–8.

74. Heinrich M, Chan J, Wanke S, Neinhuis C, Simmonds MSJ. Local uses of Aristolochia species and content of nephrotoxic aristolochic acid 1 and 2—A global assessment based on bibliographic sources. J Ethnopharmacol. 2009;125(1):108–44.

75. Vanherweghem JL, Tielemans C, Abramowicz D, Depierreux M, Vanhaelen-Fastre R, Vanhaelen M, et al. Rapidly progressive interstitial renal fibrosis in young women: association with slimming regimen including Chinese herbs. Lancet. 1993;341(8842):387–91.

76. Pourrat J, Montastruc J, Lacombe J, Cisterne J, Rascol O, Dumazer P. Nephropathy associated with Chinese herbal drugs. 2 cases. Presse Med (Paris, France: 1983). 1994;23(36):1669.

77. Pena JM, Borras M, Ramos J, Montoliu J. Rapidly progressive interstitial renal fibrosis due to a chronic intake of a herb (Aristolochia pistolochia) infusion. Nephrol Dial Transpl. 1996;11(7):1359–60.

78. Stengel B, Jones E. End-stage renal insufficiency associated with Chinese herbal consumption in France. Nephrologie. 1998;19(1):15–20.

79. Lord GM, Tagore R, Cook T, Gower P, Pusey CD. Nephropathy caused by Chinese herbs in the UK. Lancet. 1999;354(9177):481–2.

80. Krumme B, Endmeir R, Vanhaelen M, Walb D. Reversible Fanconi syndrome after ingestion of a Chinese herbal 'remedy' containing aristolochic acid. Nephrol Dial Transpl. 2001;16(2):400–2.

81. Laing C, Hamour S, Sheaff M, Miller R, Woolfson R. Chinese herbal uropathy and nephropathy. Lancet. 2006;368(9532):338.

82. Meyer MM, Chen T-P, Bennett WM, editors. Chinese herb nephropathy. Baylor University Medical Center Proceedings. Taylor & Francis; 2000.

83. Chau W, Ross R, Li JYZ, Yong TY, Klebe S, Barbara JA. Nephropathy associated with use of a Chinese herbal product containing aristolochic acid. Med J Aust. 2011;194(7):367–8.

84. Tanaka A, Nishida R, Maeda KA, Sugawara A, Kuwahara T. Chinese herb nephropathy in Japan presents adult-onset Fanconi syndrome: could different components of aristolochic acids cause a

different type of Chinese herb nephropathy? Clin Nephrol. 2000;53(4):301–6.

85. Lee S, Lee T, Lee B, Choi H, Yang M, Ihm C-G, et al. Fanconi's syndrome and subsequent progressive renal failure caused by a Chinese herb containing aristolochic acid. Nephrology. 2004;9(3):126–9.

86. Yang C-S, Lin C-H, Chang S-H, Hsu H-C. Rapidly progressive fibrosing interstitial nephritis associated with Chinese herbal drugs. Am J Kidney Dis. 2000;35(2):313–8.

87. Yang L, Su T, Li XM, Wang X, Cai SQ, Meng LQ, et al. Aristolochic acid nephropathy: variation in presentation and prognosis. Nephrol Dial Transpl. 2011;27(1):292–8.

88. Poon W-T, Lai C-K, Chan AY-W. Aristolochic acid nephropathy: the Hong Kong perspective. Hong Kong J Nephrol. 2007;9(1):7–14.

89. Ivic M. Etiology of endemic nephropathy. Lijec Vjesn. 1969;91(12):1273–81.

90. Jha V. Herbal medicines and chronic kidney disease. Nephrology. 2010;15:10–7.

91. Cosyns J-P, Jadoul M, Squifflet J-P, De Plaen J-F, Ferluga D, de Strihou CVY. Chinese herbs nephropathy: a clue to Balkan endemic nephropathy? Kidney Int. 1994;45(6):1680–8.

92. Depierreux M, Van Damme B, Houte KV, Vanherweghem JL. Pathologic aspects of a newly described nephropathy related to the prolonged use of Chinese herbs. Am J Kidney Dis. 1994;24(2):172–80.

93. Edwards KL, Wang JY, Snappin K, Sonicki Z, Miletic-Medved M, Grollman AP, et al. Abstract 1837: exposure to aristolochic acid is associated with endemic (Balkan) nephropathy. Cancer Res. 2010;70(8_Supplement):1837.

94. Gökmen MR, Cosyns J-P, Arlt VM, Stiborová M, Phillips DH, Schmeiser HH, et al. The epidemiology, diagnosis, and management of aristolochic acid nephropathy. Ann Intern Med. 2013;158(6):469.

95. Vanherweghem J-L, Abramowicz D, Tielemans C, Depierreux M. Effects of steroids on the progression of renal failure in chronic interstitial renal fibrosis: a pilot study in Chinese herbs nephropathy. Am J Kidney Dis. 1996;27(2):209–15.

96. Guan N, Fan Q, Ding J, Zhao Y, Lu J, Ai Y, et al. Melamine-contaminated powdered formula and urolithiasis in young children. N Engl J Med. 2009;360(11):1067–74.

97. Sathyanarayana S, Flynn JT, Messito MJ, Gross R, Whitlock KB, Kannan K, et al. Melamine and cyanuric acid exposure and kidney injury in US children. Environ Res. 2019;171:18–23.

98. Allen LM, Briggle TV, Pfaffenberger CD. Absorption and excretion of cyanuric acid in long-distance swimmers. Drug Metab Rev. 1982;13(3):499–516.

99. Mast RW, Jeffcoat AR, Sadler BM, Kraska RC, Friedman MA. Metabolism, disposition and excretion of [14C]melamine in male Fischer 344 rats. Food Chem Toxicol. 1983;21(6):807–10.

100. Baynes RE, Smith G, Mason SE, Barrett E, Barlow BM, Riviere JE. Pharmacokinetics of melamine in pigs following intravenous administration. Food Chem Toxicol. 2008;46(3):1196–200.

101. Puschner B, Poppenga RH, Lowenstine LJ, Filigenzi MS, Pesavento PA. Assessment of melamine and cyanuric acid toxicity in cats. J Vet Diagn Investig. 2007;19(6):616–24.

102. Dobson RLM, Motlagh S, Quijano M, Cambron RT, Baker TR, Pullen AM, et al. Identification and characterization of toxicity of contaminants in pet food leading to an outbreak of renal toxicity in cats and dogs. Toxicol Sci. 2008;106(1):251–62.

103. Kobayashi T, Okada A, Fujii Y, Niimi K, Hamamoto S, Yasui T, et al. The mechanism of renal stone formation and renal failure induced by administration of melamine and cyanuric acid. Urol Res. 2010;38(2):117–25.

104. Cianciolo RE, Bischoff K, Ebel JG, Van Winkle TJ, Goldstein RE, Serfilippi LM. Clinicopathologic, histologic, and toxicologic findings in 70 cats inadvertently exposed to pet food contaminated with melamine and cyanuric acid. J Am Vet Med Assoc. 2008;233(5):729–37.

105. Lu X, Gao B, Wang Y, Liu Z, Yasui T, Liu P, et al. Renal tubular epithelial cell injury, apoptosis and inflammation are involved in melamine-related kidney stone formation. Urol Res. 2012;40(6):717–23.

106. Zheng X, Zhao A, Xie G, Chi Y, Zhao L, Li H, et al. Melamine-induced renal toxicity is mediated by the gut microbiota. Sci Transl Med. 2013;5(172):172ra22.

107. Hopenhayn-Rich C, Biggs ML, Smith AH. Lung and kidney cancer mortality associated with arsenic in drinking water in Cordoba, Argentina. Int J Epidemiol. 1998;27(4):561–9.

108. Wang P-X, Li H-T, Zhang L, Liu J-M. The clinical profile and prognosis of Chinese children with melamine-induced kidney disease: a systematic review and meta-analysis. Biomed Res Int. 2013;2013:868202.

109. Guan N, Yao C, Huang S, Hu B, Zhang D, Fang Q, et al. Risk factors of melamine-contaminated milk powder related urolithiasis: a multicenter nested case-control study. Beijing Da Xue Xue Bao Yi Xue Ban. 2010;42(6):690–6.

110. J-m L, Ren A, Yang L, Gao J, Pei L, Ye R, et al. Urinary tract abnormalities in Chinese rural children who consumed melamine-contaminated dairy products: a population-based screening and follow-up study. CMAJ. 2010;182(5):439–43.

111. Melamine-contamination event [Internet]. 2008 [updated 2009 February 16]. http://www.who.int/foodsafety/fs_management/infosan_events/en/index.html. Accessed 30 May 2014

112. He Y, Jiang G-P, Zhao L, Qian J-J, Yang X-Z, Li X-Y, et al. Ultrasonographic characteristics of urolithiasis in children exposed to melamine-tainted powdered formula. World J Pediatr. 2009;5(2):118–21.

113. Proposed therapy for infants affected by melamine-contaminated milk powder [Internet]. 2008 [updated 2008 September 12;cited 2008 October 20]. www.moh.gov.cn/publicfiles/business/htmlfiles/mohyzs/s3586/200809/37772.htm.

114. Li X, Shen Y, Sun N. Analysis 2 cases of Melamine-induced stones in the upper urinary tract accompanied with acute renal failure. Chin J Emerg Med. 2008;17(12):1247–9.

115. Yang L, Wen JG, Wen JJ, Su ZQ, Zhu W, Huang CX, et al. Four years follow-up of 101 children with melamine-related urinary stones. Urolithiasis. 2013;41(3):265–6.

116. Jia J, Shen X, Wang L, Zhang T, Xu M, Fang X, et al. Extracorporeal shock wave lithotripsy is effective in treating single melamine induced urolithiasis in infants and young children. J Urol. 2013;189(4):1498–502.

117. Stanifer JW, Stapleton HM, Souma T, Wittmer A, Zhao X, Boulware LE. Perfluorinated chemicals as emerging environmental threats to kidney health. A scoping review. Clin J Am Soc Nephrol. 2018;13(10):1479–92.

118. Watkins DJ, Josson J, Elston B, Bartell SM, Shin H-M, Vieira VM, et al. Exposure to perfluoroalkyl acids and markers of kidney function among children and adolescents living near a chemical plant. Environ Health Perspect. 2013;121(5):625–30.

119. Kataria A, Trachtman H, Malaga-Dieguez L, Trasande L. Association between perfluoroalkyl acids and kidney function in a cross-sectional study of adolescents. Environ Health. 2015;14(1):1–13.

120. Qin X-D, Qian Z, Vaughn MG, Huang J, Ward P, Zeng X-W, et al. Positive associations of serum perfluoroalkyl substances with uric acid and hyperuricemia in children from Taiwan. Environ Pollut. 2016;212:519–24.

121. Lin C-Y, Wen L-L, Lin L-Y, Wen T-W, Lien G-W, Hsu SH, et al. The associations between serum perfluorinated chemicals and thyroid function in adolescents and young adults. J Hazard Mater. 2013;244:637–44.

122. Lin PD, Cardenas A, Hauser R, Gold DR, Kleinman KP, Hivert MF, et al. Per- and polyfluoroalkyl substances and kidney function: follow-up results from the diabetes prevention program trial. Environ Int. 2021;148:106375.

123. Wesseling C, Crowe J, Hogstedt C, Jakobsson K, Lucas R, Wegman DH. The epidemic of chronic kidney disease of unknown etiology in Mesoamerica: a call for interdisciplinary research and action. Am J Public Health. 2013;103(11):1927–30.

124. Torres C, Aragón A, González M, López I, Jakobsson K, Elinder C-G, et al. Decreased kidney function of unknown cause in Nicaragua: a community-based survey. Am J Kidney Dis. 2010;55(3):485–96.

125. Peraza S, Wesseling C, Aragon A, Leiva R, García-Trabanino RA, Torres C, et al. Decreased kidney function among agricultural workers in El Salvador. Am J Kidney Dis. 2012;59(4):531–40.

126. Wijkström J, Leiva R, Elinder C-G, Leiva S, Trujillo Z, Trujillo L, et al. Clinical and pathological characterization of Mesoamerican nephropathy: a new kidney disease in Central America. Am J Kidney Dis. 2013;62(5):908–18.

127. Ramirez-Rubio O, McClean MD, Amador JJ, Brooks DR. An epidemic of chronic kidney disease in Central America: an overview. J Epidemiol Community Health. 2012;67(1):1–3.

128. Pastora Coca IV, Palma Villanueva YA, Salinas Centeno MJ. Prevalence of hematuria and/or proteinuria and its relationship with some risk factors in pre-school population of the city of Leon, April–August 1998.

129. Athuraliya NTC, Abeysekera TDJ, Amerasinghe PH, Kumarasiri R, Bandara P, Karunaratne U, et al. Uncertain etiologies of proteinuric-chronic kidney disease in rural Sri Lanka. Kidney Int. 2011;80(11):1212–21.

130. Machiraju R, Yaradi K, Gowrishankar S, Edwards K, Attaluri S, Miller F, et al. Epidemiology of Udhanam endemic nephropathy. J Am Soc Nephrol. 2009;20:643A.

131. Wang IJ, Wu YN, Wu WC, Leonardi G, Sung YJ, Lin TJ, et al. The association of clinical findings and exposure profiles with melamine associated nephrolithiasis. Arch Dis Child. 2009;94(11):883–7.

132. Cohen J. Mesoamerica's mystery killer. Science. 2014;344:143–7.

133. Weaver VM, Fadrowski JJ, Jaar BG. Global dimensions of chronic kidney disease of unknown etiology (CKDu): a modern era environmental and/or occupational nephropathy? BMC Nephrol. 2015;16:145.

134. Correa-Rotter R, García-Trabanino R. Mesoamerican nephropathy. Semin Nephrol. 2019;39(3):263–71.

135. Lunyera J, Mohottige D, Von Isenburg M, Jeuland M, Patel UD, Stanifer JW. CKD of uncertain etiology: a systematic review. Clin J Am Soc Nephrol. 2016;11(3):379–85.

136. Stalin P, Purty AJ, Abraham G. Distribution and determinants of chronic kidney disease of unknown etiology: a brief overview. Indian J Nephrol. 2020;30(4):241.

137. Ordunez P, Nieto FJ, Martinez R, Soliz P, Giraldo GP, Mott SA, et al. Chronic kidney disease mortality trends in selected Central America countries, 1997–2013: clues to an epidemic of chronic interstitial nephritis of agricultural communities. J Epidemiol Community Health. 2018;72(4):280–6.

138. O'Callaghan-Gordo C, Shivashankar R, Anand S, Ghosh S, Glaser J, Gupta R, et al. Prevalence of and

risk factors for chronic kidney disease of unknown aetiology in India: secondary data analysis of three population-based cross-sectional studies. BMJ Open. 2019;9(3):e023353.

139. Global South Contributions to Universal Health: The Case of Cuba. Epidemic of Chronic Kidney Disease of Nontraditional Etiology in El Salvador: Integrated Health Sector Action and South–South Cooperation. MEDICC Rev. 2019;21(4):46–52.

140. Wanigasuriya KP, Peiris H, Ileperuma N, Peiris-John RJ, Wickremasinghe R. Could ochratoxin A in food commodities be the cause of chronic kidney disease in Sri Lanka? Trans R Soc Trop Med Hyg. 2008;102(7):726–8.

141. Ordunez P, Saenz C, Martinez R, Chapman E, Reveiz L, Becerra F. The epidemic of chronic kidney disease in Central America. Lancet Glob Health. 2014;2(8):e440–e1.

Index

© The Editor(s) (if applicable) and The Author(s), under exclusive license to Springer Nature
Switzerland AG 2023
F. Schaefer, L. A. Greenbaum (eds.), *Pediatric Kidney Disease*,
https://doi.org/10.1007/978-3-031-11665-0